Psycho-oncology

Psycho-oncology

Edited by

JIMMIE C. HOLLAND

Chair, Department of Psychiatry and Behavioral Sciences
Memorial Sloan-Kettering Cancer Center
New York, New York

Associate Editors

William Breitbart
Paul B. Jacobsen
Marguerite S. Lederberg
Matthew Loscalzo
Mary Jane Massie
Ruth McCorkle

New York   Oxford
OXFORD UNIVERSITY PRESS
1998

Oxford University Press

Oxford   New York
Athens   Auckland   Bangkok   Bogota
Bombay   Buenos Aires   Calcutta   Cape Town
Dar es Salaam   Delhi   Florence   Hong Kong   Istanbul
Karachi   Kuala Lumpur   Madras   Madrid
Melbourne   Mexico City   Nairobi   Paris
Singapore   Taipei   Tokyo   Toronto   Warsaw

and associated companies in
Berlin   Ibadan

Library of Congress Cataloging-in-Publication Data
Psycho-oncology/edited by Jimmie C. Holland
associate editors, William Breitbart ... [et al.].
p.   cm.   Includes bibliographical references and index.
ISBN 0-19-510614-8
1. Cancer—Psychological aspects.   2. Cancer—Patients—Mental health.
I. Holland, Jimmie C.   II. Breitbart, William, 1951–   .
[DNLM: 1. Neoplasms—psychology.   2. Neoplasms—complications.
3. Neoplasms—therapy.
QZ 200 P9743 1998]   RC262.P7825   1998
616.99 ′4′ 0019—dc21, DNLM/DLC,
for Library of Congress   97-26914

1 3 5 7 9 8 6 4 2

Printed in the United States of America
on acid-free paper

Preface

Nearly a decade ago, Julia Rowland, psychologist, and I edited the *Handbook of Psychooncology*. Written in the late eighties, its seven hundred forty-nine pages easily covered the available information about the psychological issues in the care of patients with cancer. The rationale for the edited volume was to provide a single resource in which the widely scattered information could be found; the corollary was that the book be written in non-jargon language that would make it readable and useful to all disciplines working in oncology, from the classical clinical disciplines to the mental health professionals who were increasingly being invited to join cancer centers and participate in multidisciplinary research teams. At that time, it was feasible to develop the Handbook by asking only individuals from our own cancer center to participate. They based their reviews on the sparse but growing empirical research and their experiences with patients. The Preface noted that the authors had learned from the "true experts," our patients with cancer and their families, whose courage in the face of illness taught us many lessons about living and dying. While we proudly touted the presence of a new subspecialty on the scene, psycho-oncology, it was in fact in its infancy. Almost ten years later, it is reassuring to look back and see that the field did continue to grow and that it has made and continues to make significant contributions to both patient care and research.

Lewis Thomas, in the Foreword to that Handbook, observed that the time was right for such a volume. He noted:

The clinical oncologists of all stripes have, for too long, overlooked or ignored the psychological factors that may, for all we know at present, play a surprisingly large role in individual susceptibility to neoplasia. They are certainly influential in affecting the course of treatment, the adaptation to the illness, and hence, in some ways, not all of which are yet understood, affect the outcome of treatment.

He felt that intensive cancer treatment had

come to be an extremely technical undertaking, . . . involving the strenuous efforts of highly specialized professionals, each taking his or her responsibility for a share of the patient's problem, but sometimes working at a rather impersonal distance from the patient as an individual. To many patients, stunned by the diagnosis, suffering numerous losses and discomforts, moved from place to place for one procedure after another, the experience is bewildering and frightening; at worst, it is like being trapped in the workings of a huge piece of complicated machinery. . . .

Within less than a decade, the term psycho-oncology, viewed at first with deep suspicion by most oncologists, has at last emerged as a respectable field for both application and research. In my own view, having passed through both stages as a skeptical clinician and administrator, the appearance on the scene of psychiatrists and experimental psychologists has so vastly improved the lot of cancer patients as to make these new professionals indispensable.

This present volume describes the many ways in which mental health professionals have indeed contributed to improving the lot of the cancer patient. The parts of the book reveal the whole new areas that have come under psycho-oncology's purview. First, there is a large section of the book devoted to the present understanding of psychological, social, and behavioral factors that contribute to cancer risk and survival. Changing habits and behaviors to reduce the toll of preventable cancer deaths has come very much into the domain of behavioral psycho-oncology. Smoking cessation is reviewed by Gritz and colleagues; sun exposure by Berwick. Research showing the impact of social class and socioeconomic factors in altering risk is also reviewed, by Balfour and Kaplan. Social ties, coping, treatment adherence, are all critiqued by experts as to their role in risk and survival. Fox provides a critical review of such research, fulfilling his long-respected role of monitor of the quality of the science in this area. Two chapters explore the brain—

endocrine–immune connections and how they may contribute to risk and survival.

Advances in cancer treatment bring new psychological issues. Several parts of the book are devoted to the vastly extended "worried well" population emerging from the cancer information today—people who are physically healthy but who bear the knowledge of a positive tumor marker (without clinical signs of disease) or those who have a strong family history of a particular cancer and who must deal with whether to pursue gene testing or not. These individuals vary in their responses—from denial leading to refusal to follow surveillance guidelines to anxiety levels causing almost constant self-monitoring and almost immobilizing anxiety. The psychological issues raised are clinically very important to assure appropriate screening behaviors. Counseling with genetic testing, and attention to its psychological, social, and ethical consequences, is a critical part of the national agenda for dealing with this new issue.

Ten years has led to a widely expanded discussion of interventions. Many controlled trials have shown efficacy for psychosocial interventions which represent a far wider array of ways to improve patients' quality of life, using psychological, psychoeducational, and behavioral methods. The management of psychiatric disorders complicating cancer is greatly enhanced by the array of psychopharmacological agents available to relieve distressing psychological symptoms, and many of these agents have been found useful in the control of the pain, nausea and vomiting, and fatigue that often accompany cancer. Group therapies have become familiar in most settings. Nontraditional therapies, such as art, meditation, and alternative and complementary therapies, have come into greater use in traditional medical settings. Greater appreciation of spiritual and religious beliefs and the importance of including spiritual care in total patient care has occurred, with greater collaboration and dialogue with members of the clergy.

The ethical issues of cancer care have received far more attention. First, this related to clinical trials and the ethics of informed consent, as outlined by Dubler and Post. The more recent agenda, coming out of the public debate about physician-assisted suicide, has been devoted to end-of-life and palliative care; Emanuel provides a critique of this area. Psycho-oncology is particularly attuned to the complexity of issues that are intertwined with psychology and ethics, as outlined by Lederberg. Special issues in care of the

family of the cancer patient, the psychological care of children with cancer, and patients with special needs, such as the elderly and underserved populations, are presented and discussed.

Last, the research agenda for psycho-oncology has become more central to oncology in general as the outcome measures for treatments have come to include not only length of survival but quality of life as well. The valid measurement of quality of life, a multidimensional construct that involves subjective evaluation of the domains of living that are important to people, has become a major research endeavor. Methods are being developed and refined to relate scores to clinical situations and treatment decisions. Cella provides a useful overview of the status of this research area. Ingham and Portenoy outline research methods in evaluation of pain and symptoms common in palliative care, providing a basis for clinical trials of interventions.

In 1997, it is encouraging that far greater attention is being given to patients' own reports of their symptoms and their quality of life. Dr. Thomas, who died in 1995, would be pleased that psycho-oncology has indeed achieved a "respectable place in application and research" in cancer. Care is more patient-centered, less fragmented, and the treatment teams more commonly include a mental health professional. Almost all cancer centers have an identified psycho-oncology unit, although often small, with a staff responsible for identifying and treating patients having trouble coping with illness and treatment. The larger units are engaged in training and in conducting psychosocial and behavioral research as well. In the late nineties, an exciting new agenda for psycho-oncology is being developed, based on advances in oncology that have themselves led to new forms of psychological and social problems. Fortunately, the field itself has generated a body of solid research that has defined clinical problems more clearly, has provided empirical data on interventions and their efficacy, and has devised research methods that include quality of life as a bona fide treatment goal.

I thank the co-editors who have joined me in this endeavor, Drs. Breitbart, Jacobsen, Lederberg, Loscalzo, Massie, and McCorkle. Each has done excellent editorial work. They represent the major disciplines working in psycho-oncology today. The authors of the chapters have been outstanding in their willingness to write, and sometimes revise, their contributions to fit them into the whole. Jeff House at Oxford University Press has provided the guidance to assure that the effort came to fruition. And last, and most important, my co-editors join me in giving much thanks to Ivelisse Belardo and Wanda Cintron, who truly made it possible to compile the chapters and collate the large amount of information. We are saddened by the untimely death of Ms. Cintron in November 1996. It is a source of great sadness that she is not here to share in the pleasure of the publication of the book. This Preface is dedicated to her memory, with great appreciation for her contributions to this volume and to our lives and our work.

April 1997   J.C.H
New York, N.Y.

Contents

PART I   INTRODUCTION

1. Societal Views of Cancer and the Emergence of Psycho-oncology   **3**
   Jimmie C. Holland

2. Biology of Cancer for the Psycho-oncologist   **16**
   James F. Holland

PART II   PSYCHOLOGICAL AND BEHAVIORAL FACTORS IN CANCER RISK

PAUL B. JACOBSEN, EDITOR

3. Smoking Cessation and Cancer Prevention   **27**
   Paul M. Cinciripini, Ellen R. Gritz, Janice Y. Tsoh, and Karyn L. Skaar

4. Alcohol and Cancer   **45**
   Jeremy C. Lundberg and Steven D. Passik

5. Diet and Cancer   **49**
   Barbara L. Winters

6. Sun Exposure and Cancer Risk   **58**
   Marianne Berwick

7. Compliance with Cancer Treatment   **67**
   Jean L. Richardson and Kathleen Sanchez

8. Social Class/Socioeconomic Factors   **78**
   Jennifer L. Balfour and George A. Kaplan

9. Personality and Coping   **91**
   Maggie Watson and Steven Greer

10. Social Ties and Cancer   **99**
    Vicki S. Helgeson, Sheldon Cohen, and Heidi L. Fritz

11. Psychosocial Factors in Cancer Incidence and Prognosis   **110**
    Bernard H. Fox

12. Psychoneuroimmunology: Implications for Psycho-oncology   **125**
    Dana H. Bovbjerg and Heiddis B. Valdimarsdottir

13. Psychoneuroendocrinology and Cancer   **135**
    Dominique L. Musselman, J. Steven McDaniel, Maryfrances R. Porter, and Charles B. Nemeroff

PART III   PSYCHOLOGICAL ISSUES IN CANCER SCREENING

PAUL B. JACOBSEN, EDITOR

14. Psychological Responses to Tumor Markers   **147**
    Debra L. Fertig and Daniel F. Hayes

15. Psychosocial Issues in Cancer Screening   **161**
    Joanne DiPlacido, Ann Zauber, and William H. Redd

PART IV   HIGH GENETIC RISK OF CANCER

JIMMIE C. HOLLAND, EDITOR

16. Genetics for the Psycho-oncologist   **175**
    Alexander Kamb and Mark H. Skolnick

17. Genetic Counseling for the Oncology Patient   **186**
    Elizabeth Gettig, Joan H. Marks, and John J. Mulvihill

18. Psychological, Social, and Ethical Issues in Gene Testing   **196**
    Kathryn M. Kash and Caryn Lerman

PART V   PSYCHOLOGICAL ADAPTATION TO CANCER

RUTH McCORKLE, EDITOR

19. Psychological and Social Factors in Adaptation   **211**
    Stacie M. Spencer, Charles S. Carver, and Alicia A. Price

20. Psychosocial Adaptation of Cancer Survivors   **223**
    Alice B. Kornblith

PART VI   PSYCHOLOGICAL RESPONSES TO TREATMENT

RUTH McCORKLE, EDITOR

21. Surgery   **257**
    Paul B. Jacobsen, Andrew J. Roth, and Jimmie C. Holland

22. Radiotherapy   **269**
    Donna B. Greenberg

23. Chemotherapy, Hormonal Therapy, and Immunotherapy   **277**
    M. Tish Knobf, Jeannie V. Pasacreta, Alan Valentine, and Ruth McCorkle

24. Bone Marrow Transplantation   **289**
    Michael A. Andrykowski and Richard P. McQuellon

PART VII   PSYCHOLOGICAL ISSUES RELATED TO SITE OF CANCER

RUTH McCORKLE, EDITOR

25. Central Nervous System Tumors   **303**
    Steven D. Passik and Patricia L. Ricketts

26. Head and Neck Cancer   **314**
    Alyson B. Moadel, Jamie S. Ostroff, and Stimson P. Schantz

27. Gastrointestinal Cancer   **324**
    Jürg Bernhard and Christoph Hürny

28. Lung Cancer   **340**
    Linda Sarna

29. Genitourinary Malignancies   **349**
    Andrew J. Roth and Howard I. Scher

30. Gynecologic Cancer   **359**
    Sarah S. Auchincloss and Cheryl F. McCartney

31. Skin Neoplasms and Malignant Melanoma   **371**
    Fawzy I. Fawzy and Nancy W. Fawzy

32. Breast Cancer   **380**
    Julia H. Rowland and Mary Jane Massie

33. Sarcoma   **402**
    David K. Payne and Jeremy C. Lundberg

34. Hematopoietic Dyscrasias   **406**
    Lynna M. Lesko

35. HIV Infection and AIDS-Associated Neoplasms   **417**
    Barry Rosenfeld

36 Tumors of Unknown Primary Site   **427**
    Leonard B. Saltz, Steven D. Passik, and Jeremy C. Lundberg

PART VIII   MANAGEMENT OF SPECIFIC SYMPTOMS

WILLIAM BREITBART, EDITOR

37. Palliative and Terminal Care   **437**
    William Breitbart, Juan R. Jaramillo, and Harvey M. Chochinov

38. Pain   **450**
    William Breitbart and David K. Payne

39. Cancer Cachexia   **468**
    Stewart B. Fleishman

40. Nausea and Vomiting   **476**
    Gary R. Morrow, Joseph A. Roscoe, and Jane T. Hickok

41. Fatigue   **485**
    Donna B. Greenberg

42. Sexual Dysfunction   **494**
    Leslie R. Schover

43. Neuropsychological Impact of Cancer and Cancer Treatments   **500**
    Susan E. Walch, Tim A. Ahles, and Andrew J. Saykin

PART IX   PSYCHIATRIC DISORDERS
MARY JANE MASSIE, EDITOR

44. Adjustment Disorders   **509**
    James J. Strain

45. Depressive Disorders   **518**
    Mary Jane Massie and Michael K. Popkin

46. Suicide   **541**
    William Breitbart and Suzanne Krivo

47. Anxiety Disorders   **548**
    Russell Noyes Jr., Craig S. Holt, and Mary Jane Massie

48. Delirium   **564**
    William Breitbart and Kenneth R. Cohen

49. Substance Abuse Disorders   **576**
    Steven D. Passik and Russell K. Portenoy

50. Alcoholism and Cancer   **587**
    Jeremy C. Lundberg and Steven D. Passik

51. Posttraumatic Stress Disorder   **595**
    Steven D. Passik and Kathy L. Grummon

52. Somatoform and Factitious Disorders and Cancer   **608**
    Charles V. Ford

53. Schizophrenia   **614**
    John L. Shuster

54. Personality Disorders   **619**
    Philip R. Muskin

55. Chemotherapeutic Agents and Neuropsychiatric Side Effects   **630**
    Stewart B. Fleishman and Glenn R. Kalash

56. Metabolic Disorders and Neuropsychiatric Symptoms   **639**
    William Breitbart and Simon E. Wein

PART X   INTERVENTIONS
MATTHEW LOSCALZO, EDITOR

57. Screening Procedures for Psychosocial Distress   **653**
    James R. Zabora

58. Brief Crisis Counseling   **662**
    Matthew Loscalzo and Karlynn BrintzenhofeSzoc

59. Psychoeducational Interventions   **676**
    Fawzy I. Fawzy and Nancy W. Fawzy

60. Psychotherapeutic Issues   **694**
    Barbara M. Sourkes, Mary Jane Massie, and Jimmie C. Holland

61. Group Therapies   **701**
    James L. Spira

62. Cognitive-Behavioral Interventions   **717**
    Paul B. Jacobsen and Danette M. Hann

63. Studies of Life-Extending Psychosocial Interventions   **730**
    Catherine Classen, Sandra E. Sephton, Susan Diamond, and David Spiegel

64. Art Psychotherapy   **743**
    Paola Luzzatto and Bonnie Gabriel

65. Telephone Counseling   **758**
    Julia A. Bucher, Peter S. Houts, Myra Glajchen, and Diane Blum

66. Meditation   **767**
    Jon Kabat-Zinn, Ann Ohm Massion, James R. Hebert, and Elana Rosenbaum

67. Religion and Spiritual Beliefs   **780**
    Marc A. Musick, Harold G. Koenig, David B. Larson, and Dale Matthews

68. Spiritual Assessment, Screening, and Intervention   **790**
    George Fitchett and George Handzo

69. Bedside Interventions   **809**
    Jeannie V. Pasacreta and Ruth McCorkle

70. Alternative and Complementary Therapies   **817**
    Brian D. Doan

71. Rehabilitation   **828**
    Richard Tunkel and Steven D. Passik

PART XI   PERSONS WITH SPECIAL NEEDS

RUTH McCORKLE, EDITOR

72. The Older Patient   **839**
    Betty R. Ferrell and Bruce Ferrell

73. Underserved Patients   **845**
    R Eric Weston, Bruce D. Rapkin, Randolph G. Potts, and Meredith Y. Smith

74. The Patient from a Different Culture   **857**
    Maria Die-Trill

75. Psychosocial Sequelae of Perceived Environmental Exposures   **867**
    Karolynn Siegel

PART XII   THE CHILD WITH CANCER

JIMMIE C. HOLLAND, EDITOR

76. Biology of Childhood Cancers   **881**
    Peter G. Steinherz and Joseph Simone

77. Psychological Problems of Curative Cancer Treatment   **897**
    Maria Die-Trill and Margaret L. Stuber

78. Pediatric Palliative Care and Pain Management   **907**
    Gerri Frager and Barbara Shapiro

79. Long-Term Adaptation, Psychiatric Sequelae, and PTSD   **923**
    James M. Hill and Margaret L. Stuber

80. Psychosexual Sequelae   **930**
    Karolyn Woolverton and Jamie Ostroff

81. Cognitive Sequelae of Treatment in Children   **940**
    Susan E. Walch, Tim A. Ahles, and Andrew J. Saykin

82. Psychotherapy   **946**
    Barbara M. Sourkes

83. Pediatric Psychopharmacology   **954**
    Ladd Spiegel

84. Behavioral Interventions in Pediatric Oncology   **962**
    Katherine N. DuHamel, Suzanne M. Johnson Vickberg, and William H. Redd

PART XIII   PSYCHOLOGICAL ISSUES FOR THE FAMILY

MATTHEW LOSCALZO, EDITOR

85. The Family of the Cancer Patient   **981**
    Marguerite S. Lederberg

86. Family Therapy: A Systems Approach to Cancer Care   **994**
    Jane Jacobs, Jamie Ostroff, and Peter Steinglass

87. Palliative Home Care—Impact on Families   **1004**
    Sherry R. Schachter and Nessa Coyle

88. Bereavement: A Special Issue in Oncology   **1016**
    Harvey M. Chochinov, Jimmie C. Holland, and Laurence Y. Katz

PART XIV   STAFF SUPPORT AND TRAINING IN PSYCHO-ONCOLOGY

MARGUERITE S. LEDERBERG, MARY JANE MASSIE, EDITORS

89. Oncology Staff Stress and Related Interventions   **1035**
    Marguerite S. Lederberg

90. Establishing a Psycho-oncology Unit in a Cancer Center   **1049**
    Jimmie C. Holland

91. Training Psychiatrists and Psychologists in Psycho-oncology   **1055**
    Steven D. Passik, Charles V. Ford, and Mary Jane Massie

92. Principles of Training Social Workers in Oncology   **1061**
    Elizabeth D. Smith, Katherine Walsh-Burke, and Chris Crusan

93. Education of Nurses in Psycho-oncology   **1069**
    Ruth McCorkle, Marilyn Frank-Stromborg, and Jeannie V. Pasacreta

94. Principles of Training Medical Staff in Psychosocial and Communication Skills   **1074**
Debra Roter and Lesley Fallowfield

PART XV   ETHICAL ISSUES IN ONCOLOGY: A PSYCHOLOGICAL FRAMEWORK

MARGUERITE S. LEDERBERG, EDITOR

95. Truth Telling and Informed Consent   **1085**
Nancy Neveloff Dubler and Linda Farber Post

96. Ethics of Treatment: Palliative and Terminal Care   **1096**
Ezekiel J. Emanuel

97. Global Issues of Resource Allocation in Health Care   **1112**
Charles L. M. Olweny

98. Understanding the Interface Between Psychiatry and Ethics   **1123**
Marguerite S. Lederberg

PART XVI   RESEARCH METHODS IN PSYCHO-ONCOLOGY

WILLIAM BREITBART, EDITOR

99. Quality of Life   **1135**
David Cella

100. Pain and Physical Symptom Assessments   **1147**
Jane Ingham and Russell K. Portenoy

PART XVII   INTERNATIONAL ASPECTS

JIMMIE C. HOLLAND, ANTHONY MARCHINI, EDITORS

101. International Psycho-oncology   **1165**
Jimmie C. Holland and Anthony Marchini

PART XVIII   POLICY ISSUES

JIMMIE C. HOLLAND, EDITOR

102. Bridging the Gap Between Research, Clinical Practice, and Policy   **1173**
Jessie C. Gruman and Rena Convissor

Index   **1177**

Contributors

TIM A. AHLES, Ph.D.
Center for Psyscho-oncology Research
Dartmouth Medical School
Lebanon, New Hampshire

MICHAEL A. ANDRYKOWSKI, Ph.D.
Department of Behavioral Science
University of Kentucky College of Medicine
Lexington, Kentucky

SARAH S. AUCHINCLOSS, M.D.
Department of Psychiatry and Behavioral Sciences
Memorial Sloan-Kettering Cancer Centre
New York, New York

JENNIFER L. BALFOUR, M.P.H.
Human Population Laboratory
California Department of Health Services
Berkeley, California

JÜRG BERNHARD, Ph.D.
Quality of Life Office
Swiss Institute for Applied Cancer Research (SIAK)
Berne, Switzerland

MARIANNE BERWICK, Ph.D., M.P.H.
Department of Epidemiology and Biostatistics
Memorial Sloan-Kettering Cancer Center
New York, New York

DIANE BLUM, A.C.S.W.
Cancer Care, Inc.
New York, New York

DANA H. BOVBJERG, Ph.D.
Department of Psychiatry and Behavioral Sciences
Memorial Sloan-Kettering Cancer Center
New York, New York

WILLIAM BREITBART, M.D. (*Editor*)
Department of Psychiatry and Behavioral Sciences
Memorial Sloan-Kettering Cancer Center
New York, New York

KARLYNN BRINTZENHOFESZOC, D.S.W.
Psychosocial Research
Johns Hopkins Oncology Center
Baltimore, Maryland

JULIA A. BUCHER, R.N., Ph.D.
Department of Behavioral Science
Pennsylvania State University
Hershey, Pennsylvania

CHARLES S. CARVER, Ph.D.
Department of Psychology
University of Miami
Coral Gables, Florida

DAVID CELLA, Ph.D.
Centre on Outcomes, Research, and Education
Evanston Northwestern Health Care
Evanston, Illinois

HARVEY M. CHOCHINOV, M.D.
Winnipeg Health Sciences Centre
Winnipeg, Manitoba
Canada

PAUL M. CINCIRIPINI, Ph.D.
Department of Behavioral Science
University of Texas M.D. Anderson Cancer Center
Houston, Texas

CATHERINE CLASSEN, Ph.D.
Department of Psychiatry and Behavioral Sciences
Stanford University School of Medicine
Stanford, California

KENNETH R. COHEN, M.D.
Department of Psychiatry and Behavioral Sciences
Memorial Sloan-Kettering Cancer Center
New York, New York

SHELDON COHEN, Ph.D.
Department of Psychology
Carnegie Mellon University
Pittsburgh, Pennsylvania

RENA CONVISSOR, M.P.H.
Center for Advancement of Health
Washington, DC

NESSA COYLE, R.N.
Pain and Palliative Care Service
Memorial Sloan-Kettering Cancer Center
New York, New York

CHRIS CRUSAN, M.S.W.
Johns Hopkins Oncology Center
Johns Hopkins School of Medicine
Baltimore, Maryland

SUSAN DIAMOND, M.S.W.
Department of Psychiatry and Behavioral Sciences
Stanford University School of Medicine
Stanford, California

MARIA DIE-TRILL, Ph.D.
Hospital Universitario
Madrid, Spain

JOANNE DIPLACIDO, Ph.D.
Department of Psychology
Central Connecticut State University
New Britain, Connecticut

BRIAN D. DOAN, M.D.
Psychology Service
Toronto-Sunnybrook Regional Cancer Centre
North York, Ontario
Canada

NANCY NEVELOFF DUBLER, LL.B.
Division of Bioethics
Montefiore Hospital and Medical Center
Bronx, New York

KATHERINE N. DUHAMEL, Ph.D.
Donald H. Ruttenberg Cancer Centre
Mount Sinai School of Medicine
New York, New York

EZEKIEL J. EMANUEL, M.D., Ph.D.
Department of Clinical Bioethics
Warren G. Magnuson Clinical Center
National Institutes of Health
Bethesda, Maryland

LESLEY FALLOWFIELD, Ph.D.
Department of Oncology
CRC Communication and Counselling Research Centre
London, England

FAWZY I. FAWZY, M.D.
Department of Psychiatry and Behavioral Sciences
UCLA School of Medicine
Los Angeles, California

NANCY W. FAWZY, R.N., D.N.Sc.
John Wayne Cancer Center
St. John's Hospital
Santa Monica, California

BETTY R. FERRELL, Ph.D., F.A.A.N.
Department of Nursing Research and Education
City of Hope National Medical Center
Duarte, California

BRUCE FERRELL, M.D.
Geriatric Medicine
Veterans Adminstration Hospital
Sepulveda, California

DEBRA L. FERTIG, M.D.
Dana Farber Partners Cancer Care
Harvard Medical School
Boston, Massachusetts

REV. GEORGE FITCHETT
St. Lukes Medical Centre
Rush-Presbyterian
Chicago, Illinois

STEWART B. FLEISHMAN, M.D.
Division of Hematology/Oncology
Long Island Jewish Medical Center
New Hyde Park, New York

CHARLES V. FORD, M.D.
Neuropsychiatric Clinic
University of Alabama School of Medicine
Birmingham, Alabama

BERNARD H. FOX, Ph.D.
Department of Psychiatry
Boston University School of Medicine
Boston, Massachusetts

GERRI FRAGER, M.D.
Pediatric Palliative Care
Children's Hospital
Halifax, Nova Scotia
Canada

MARILYN FRANK-STROMBORG, Ed.D., F.A.A.N.
Oncology Clinical Specialist Program
School of Nursing
Northern Illinois University
DeKalb, Illinois

HEIDI L. FRITZ, M.S.
Department of Psychology
Carnegie Mellon University
Pittsburgh, Pennsylvania

BONNIE GABRIEL, M.P.S.-A.T.
Department of Psychiatry and Behavioral Sciences
Memorial Sloan-Kettering Cancer Center
New York, New York

ELIZABETH GETTIG, M.S.
Department of Human Genetics
University of Pittsburgh
Pittsburgh, Pennsylvania

MYRA GLAJCHEN, D.S.W.
Department of Pain Medicine and Palliative Care
Beth Israel Medical Center
New York, New York

DONNA B. GREENBERG, M.D.
Department of Psychiatry
Massachusetts General Hospital
Boston, Massachusetts

STEVEN GREER, M.D., F.R.C.Psych.
Institute of Cancer Research
University of London
London, England

ELLEN R. GRITZ, Ph.D.
Department of Behavioral Science
University of Texas M.D. Anderson Cancer Center
Houston, Texas

JESSIE C. GRUMAN, Ph.D.
Center for Advancement of Health
Washington, DC

KATHY L. GRUMMON, Ph.D.
Department of Psychiatry
Beth Israel Medical Center
New York, New York

REV. GEORGE HANDZO
Department of Chaplaincy
Memorial Sloan-Kettering Cancer Center
New York, New York

DANETTE M. HANN, Ph.D.
Psychosocial Oncology Program
H. Lee Moffitt Cancer Center and Research Institute
Tampa, Florida

DANIEL F. HAYES, M.D.
Lombardi Cancer Center
Georgetown University School of Medicine
Washington, DC

JAMES R. HEBERT, M.S.P.H., Sc.D.
University of Massachusetts at Worcester
Worcester, Massachusetts

VICKI S. HELGESON, Ph.D.
Department of Psychology
Carnegie Mellon University
Pittsburgh, Pennsylvania

JANE T. HICKOK, M.D., M.P.H.
University of Rochester Cancer Center
University of Rochester School of Medicine
Rochester, New York

JAMES M. HILL, Ph.D.
Department of Psychiatry
New Jersey Medical School
University of Medicine and Dentistry of New Jersey
Newark, New Jersey

JAMES F. HOLLAND, M.D.
Department of Neoplastic Diseases
Mount Sinai School of Medicine
New York, New York

JIMMIE C. HOLLAND, M.D. (*Editor*)
Chair, Department of Psychiatry and Behavioral Sciences
Memorial Sloan-Kettering Cancer Center
New York, New York

CRAIG S. HOLT, Ph.D.
Department of Psychiatry
University of Iowa College of Medicine
Iowa City, Iowa

PETER S. HOUTS, Ph.D.
Department of Behavioral Science
Pennsylvania State University
Hershey, Pennsylvania

CHRISTOPH HÜRNY, M.D.
Burgerspital
St. Gallen, Switzerland

JANE INGHAM, M.B.B.S., F.R.A.C.P.
Georgetown University School of Medicine
Washington, DC

JANE JACOBS, Ed.D.
Ackerman Family Institute
New York, New York

PAUL B. JACOBSEN, Ph.D. (*Editor*)
Psychosocial Oncology Program
H. Lee Moffitt Cancer Center and Research Institute
Tampa, Florida

JUAN R. JARAMILLO, M.D.
Department of Psychiatry
Albert Einstein School of Medicine
Bronx, New York

JON KABAT-ZINN, Ph.D.
University of Massachusetts at Worcester
Worcester, Massachusetts

GLENN R. KALASH, D.O.
Department of Psychiatry
Jamaica Hospital Medical Center
Jamaica, New York

ALEXANDER KAMB, Ph.D.
Ventana Genetics, Inc.
Salt Lake City, Utah

GEORGE A. KAPLAN, Ph.D.
Department of Epidemiology
University of Michigan School of Public Health
Ann Arbor, Michigan

KATHRYN M. KASH, Ph.D.
Strang Cancer Prevention Center
New York, New York

LAURENCE Y. KATZ, M.D.
Winnipeg Health Sciences Centre
Winnipeg, Manitoba
Canada

M. TISH KNOBF, R.N., M.S.N., F.A.A.N.
Yale University School of Nursing
New Haven, Connecticut

HAROLD G. KOENIG, M.D., M.H.Sc.
Program on Religion, Aging, and Health
Duke University Medical Center
Durham, North Carolina

ALICE B. KORNBLITH, Ph.D.
Department of Psychiatry and Behavioral Sciences
Memorial Sloan-Kettering Cancer Center
New York, New York

SUZANNE KRIVO, B.S.
Cornell University Medical College
New York, New York

DAVID B. LARSON, M.D., M.P.H.
National Institute for Healthcare Research
Rockville, Maryland

MARGUERITE S. LEDERBERG, M.D. (*Editor*)
Department of Psychiatry and Behavioral Sciences
Memorial Sloan-Kettering Cancer Center
New York, New York

CARYN LERMAN, Ph.D.
Lombardi Cancer Center
Georgetown University School of Medicine
Washington, DC

LYNNA M. LESKO, M.D., Ph.D.
International Clinical Research
Boehringer-Ingelheim Pharmaceuticals Inc.
Ridgefield, Connecticut

MATTHEW LOSCALZO, M.S.W. (*Editor*)
Oncology Social Work
Johns Hopkins Oncology Center
Johns Hopkins Scool of Medicine
Baltimore, Maryland

JEREMY C. LUNDBERG, B.S.
Department of Psychiatry and Behavioral Sciences
Memorial Sloan-Kettering Cancer Center
New York, New York

PAOLA LUZZATTO, Ph.D., A.T.R.-B.C.
Department of Psychiatry and Behavioral Sciences
Memorial Sloan-Kettering Cancer Center
New York, New York

ANTHONY MARCHINI, M.S.
Department of Psychiatry and Behavioral Sciences
Memorial Sloan-Kettering Cancer Center
New York, New York

JOAN H. MARKS, M.S.
Human Genetics and Health Advocacy Program
Sarah Lawrence College
Bronxville, New York

MARY JANE MASSIE, M.D. (*Editor*)
Department of Psychiatry and Behavioral Sciences
Memorial Sloan-Kettering Cancer Center
New York, New York

ANN OHM MASSION, M.D.
University of Massachusetts at Worcester
Worcester, Massachusetts

DALE MATTHEWS, M.D.
Georgetown University School of Medicine
Washington, DC

CHERYL F. MCCARTNEY, M.D.
University of North Carolina School of Medicine
Chapel Hill, North Carolina

RUTH MCCORKLE, Ph.D. (*Editor*)
School of Nursing
University of Pennsylvania
Philadelphia, Pennsylvania

J. STEVEN MCDANIEL, M.D.
Department of Psychiatry and Behaviorial Sciences
Emory University School of Medicine
Atlanta, Georgia

RICHARD P. MCQUELLON, Ph.D.
Comprehensive Cancer Center
Wake Forest University School of Medicine
Winston-Salem, North Carolina

ALYSON B. MOADEL, Ph.D.
Department of Epidemiology and Social Medicine
Albert Einstein College of Medicine
Bronx, New York

GARY R. MORROW, M.S., Ph.D.
University of Rochester Cancer Center
University of Rochester School of Medicine
Rochester, New York

JOHN J. MULVIHILL, M.D.
Department of Human Genetics
University of Pittsburgh
Pittsburgh, Pennyslvania

MARC A. MUSICK, M.A.
Department of Sociology
Duke University
Durham, North Carolina

PHILIP R. MUSKIN, M.D.
Department of Psychiatry
Columbia-Presbyterian Medical Center
New York, New York

DOMINIQUE L. MUSSELMAN, M.D.
Department of Psychiatry and Behavioral Sciences
Emory University School of Medicine
Atlanta, Georgia

CHARLES B. NEMEROFF, M.D., Ph.D.
Department of Psychiatry and Behavioral Sciences
Emory University School of Medicine
Atlanta, Georgia

RUSSELL NOYES, Jr., M.D.
Department of Psychiatry
University of Iowa College of Medicine
Iowa City, Iowa

CHARLES L. M. OLWENY, M.D.
WHO Centre for Quality of Life Research
St. Boniface General Hospital
Winnipeg, Manitoba
Canada

JAMIE S. OSTROFF, Ph.D.
Department of Psychiatry and Behavioral Sciences
Memorial Sloan-Kettering Cancer Center
New York, New York

JEANNIE V. PASACRETA, Ph.D., R.N., C.S.
Yale University School of Nursing
New Haven, Connecticut

STEVEN D. PASSIK, Ph.D.
Department of Psychiatry (Psychology)
Indiana University School of Medicine
Indianapolis, Indiana

DAVID K. PAYNE, Ph.D.
Department of Psychiatry and Behavioral Sciences
Memorial Sloan-Kettering Cancer Center
New York, New York

MICHAEL K. POPKIN, M.D.
Department of Psychiatry
Hennepin County Medical Center
Minneapolis, Minnesota

RUSSELL K. PORTENOY, M.D.
Department of Pain Medicine and Palliative Care
Beth Israel Medical Center
New York, New York

MARYFRANCES R. PORTER, B.A.
Department of Psychology
University of Denver
Denver, Colorado

LINDA FARBER POST, B.S.N., M.A., J.D.
Division of Bioethics
Montefiore Hospital and Medical Center
Bronx, New York

RANDOLPH G. POTTS, Ph.D.
University of Hartford
Hartford, Connecticut

ALICIA A. PRICE, Ph.D.
Department of Psychology
University of Miami
Coral Gables, Florida

BRUCE D. RAPKIN, Ph.D.
Department of Psychiatry and Behavioral Sciences
Memorial Sloan-Kettering Cancer Center
New York, New York

WILLIAM H. REDD, Ph.D.
Donald H. Ruttenberg Cancer Center
Mount Sinai School of Medicine
New York, New York

JEAN L. RICHARDSON, Dr.P.H.
Department of Preventive Medicine
USC/Norris Comprehensive Cancer Center
University of Southern California
Los Angeles, California

PATRICIA L. RICKETTS, B.A.
Department of Psychology
Long Island University
Brooklyn, New York

JOSEPH A. ROSCOE, M.A
University of Rochester Cancer Center
University of Rochester School of Medicine
Rochester, New York

ELANA ROSENBAUM, M.S.W.
University of Massachusetts at Worcester
Worcester, Massachusetts

BARRY ROSENFELD, Ph.D.
Department of Psychology
Long Island University
Brooklyn, New York

DEBRA ROTER, Dr.P.H.
School of Public Health
Johns Hopkins University
Baltimore, Maryland

ANDREW J. ROTH, M.D.
Department of Psychiatry and Behavioral Sciences
Memorial Sloan-Kettering Cancer Center
New York, New York

JULIA H. ROWLAND, Ph.D.
Department of Psychiatry
Georgetown University School of Medicine
Washington, DC

LEONARD B. SALTZ, M.D.
Department of Medicine
Memorial Sloan-Kettering Cancer Center
New York, New York

KATHLEEN SANCHEZ, M.P.H.
Department of Preventive Medicine
USC/Norris Comprehensive Cancer Center
University of Southern California
Los Angeles, California

LINDA SARNA, D.N.Sc., R.N., F.A.A.N.
School of Nursing
University of California at Los Angeles
Los Angeles, California

ANDREW J. SAYKIN, Psy.D.
Department of Psychiatry
Dartmouth Medical School
Lebanon, New Hampshire

SHERRY R. SCHACHTER, R.N.
Department of Psychiatry and Behavioral Sciences
Memorial Sloan-Kettering Cancer Center
New York, New York

STIMSON P. SCHANTZ, M.D.
Department of Surgery
Memorial Sloan-Kettering Cancer Center
New York, New York

HOWARD I. SCHER, M.D.
Department of Medicine
Memorial Sloan-Kettering Cancer Center
New York, New York

LESLIE R. SCHOVER, Ph.D.
The Cleveland Clinic Cancer Center
The Cleveland Clinic Foundation
Cleveland, Ohio

SANDRA E. SEPHTON, Ph.D.
Department of Psychiatry and Behavioral Sciences
Stanford University School of Medicine
Stanford, California

BARBARA SHAPIRO, M.D.
Department of Pediatrics
University of Pennsylvania School of Medicine
Philadelphia, Pennsylvania

JOHN L. SHUSTER, M.D.
Department of Psychiatry and Behavioral Neurobiology
University of Alabama School of Medicine
Birmingham, Alabama

KAROLYNN SIEGEL, Ph.D.
Columbia University School of Public Health
New York, New York

JOSEPH SIMONE, M.D.
Huntsman Comprehensive Cancer Center
Salt Lake City, Utah

KARYN L. SKAAR, Ph.D.
Department of Behavioral Science
University of Texas M.D. Anderson Cancer Center
Houston, Texas

MARK H. SKOLNICK, Ph.D.
Myriad Genetics, Inc.
Salt Lake City, Utah

ELIZABETH D. SMITH, D.S.W.
National Catholic School of Social Work
The Catholic University of America
Washington, DC

MEREDITH Y. SMITH, Ph.D.
Department of Psychiatry and Behavioral Sciences
Memorial Sloan-Kettering Cancer Center
New York, New York

BARBARA M. SOURKES, Ph.D.
Montreal Children's Hospital
McGill University School of Medicine
Montreal, Quebec
Canada

STACIE M. SPENCER, Ph.D.
Department of Psychology
University of Pittsburgh
Pittsburgh, Pennsylvania

DAVID SPIEGEL, M.D.
Department of Psychology and Behavioral Sciences
Stanford University School of Medicine
Stanford, California

LADD SPIEGEL, M.D.
Department of Psychiatry and Behavioral Sciences
Memorial Sloan-Kettering Cancer Center
New York, New York

JAMES L. SPIRA, Ph.D., M.P.H.
Division of Health Psychology
Naval Medical Center
San Diego, California

PETER STEINGLASS, M.D.
Ackerman Family Institute
New York, New York

PETER G. STEINHERZ, M.D.
Department of Pediatrics
Memorial Sloan-Kettering Cancer Center
New York, New York

JAMES J. STRAIN, M.D.
Department of Psychiatry
Mount Sinai School of Medicine
New York, New York

MARGARET L. STUBER, M.D.
Department of Psychiatry
University of California at Los Angeles
Los Angeles, California

JANICE Y. TSOH, Ph.D.
Department of Behavioral Science
University of Texas M.D. Anderson Cancer Center
Houston, Texas

RICHARD TUNKEL, M.D.
Rehabilitation Service
Memorial Sloan-Kettering Cancer Center
New York, New York

HEIDDIS B. VALDIMARSDOTTIR, Ph.D.
Department of Psychiatry and Behavioral Sciences
Memorial Sloan-Kettering Cancer Center
New York, New York

ALAN VALENTINE, M.D.
Department of Neuro-Oncology
University of Texas M.D. Anderson Cancer Center
Houston, Texas

SUZANNE M. JOHNSON VICKBERG, B.A.
Department of Psychology
City University of New York
New York, New York

SUSAN E. WALCH, Ph.D.
Center for Psycho-Oncology Research
Dartmouth Medical School
Lebanon, New Hampshire

KATHERINE WALSH-BURKE, D.S.W.
Department of Social Work
Springfield College
Springfield, Massachusetts

MAGGIE WATSON, Ph.D.
Psychological Medicine
Royal Marsden Hospital and Institute of Cancer Research
Sutton, Surrey
England

SIMON E. WEIN, M.D.
Sharrett Institute of Oncology
Hadassah Medical Center
Jerusalem, Israel

R. ERIC WESTON, Ph.D.
Department of Psychiatry and Behavioral Sciences
Memorial Sloan-Kettering Cancer Center
New York, New York

BARBARA L. WINTERS, Ph.D., M.Ed., R.D.
American Health Foundation
New York, New York

KAROLYN WOOLVERTON, Ph.D.
Department of Psychiatry and Behavioral Sciences
Memorial Sloan-Kettering Cancer Center
New York, New York

JAMES R. ZABORA, M.S.W.
Patient and Family Services
Johns Hopkins Oncology Center
Johns Hopkins School of Medicine
Baltimore, Maryland

ANN ZAUBER, Ph.D.
Department of Epidemiology and Biostatistics
Memorial Sloan-Kettering Cancer Center
New York, New York

Psycho-oncology

1

INTRODUCTION

1

Societal Views of Cancer and the Emergence of Psycho-oncology

JIMMIE C. HOLLAND

Psychological and social issues related to cancer were not actively studied until the last two decades. As they have come under study by small groups of clinicians and investigators around the world, the subspecialty of psycho-oncology (also called psychosocial or behavioral oncology) has emerged within the broader field of oncology. It addresses the psychological, social, and behavioral dimensions of cancer from two perspectives: the psychological responses of patients at all stages of disease and their families (psychosocial); and the psychological, social, and behavioral issues that influence morbidity and mortality (psychobiological). This book seeks to explain these two dimensions in depth to provide the reader with a base from which to understand and treat patients and to understand and to counsel healthy people, especially those at enhanced risk of cancer because of their behaviors, habits, or life-styles (1).

This important but neglected area has been slow in development for several reasons: the stigma associated with psychological and emotional issues in medical illness; the limited funds that have been available for research and training; the small number of psychosocial clinicians and investigators in cancer centers worldwide, often lacking the critical mass to develop research and training programs; the necessity to develop valid instruments to quantitate data in these domains, long viewed as "soft science" by the scientific community; the focus of the field of oncology on cure with, consequently, less attention to symptom control, quality of life, and the well-being of the patient. This aspect is particularly poignant when one recognizes that each advance made by oncologists in treatment methods over the years has created side effects and problems with which patients had to cope (e.g., hair loss and vomiting associated with chemotherapy).

The dynamic relationship continues between advances in treatment and diagnosis and the creation of new psychological and social problems which require study as evidenced by DNA testing of healthy individuals for cancer risk and biomarkers (See Chapters 14 and 15). New challenges in psycho-oncology are posed by each advance in oncologic diagnostics and therapeutics, and we seek to assist patients in meeting them.

Psycho-oncology has brought attention to these areas through several avenues: training in counseling and communication skills; developing behavioral and psychosocial interventions; measurement of subjective symptoms and states (pain, nausea, dyspnea, anxiety, depression, delirium); and quantitative measurement of quality of life as an outcome variable in clinical trials research. On the side of reducing cancer risk and mortality, the contributions of psycho-oncology have also been significant: understanding behavioral factors in cancer control and prevention; developing smoking cessation methods based on psychological principles; studying ways of changing risk behaviors; and creating a cadre of investigators with expertise in behavioral change of life-style and habits as well as clinical investigators in quality of life research (2).

Equally important, however, is how society views these advances and the social climate that results from attitudes and knowledge of the public about cancer and its treatment. Thus, the experience of an individual who has cancer is greatly influenced by the historical epoch in which it occurs, and the nature of cancer treatment and the societal views at that given time. Table 1.1 outlines the three factors that primarily influence psychological adaptation: those that are society-derived (attitudes and knowledge); those that are patient-derived (the personal attributes of the individuals (coping skills, philosophy); their social envir-

TABLE 1.1. *Factors which Determine Psychological Adjustment to Cancer*

SOCIETY-DERIVED
Open discussion of diagnosis vs. unrevealed secret
Knowledge of treatment options, prognosis, and participation as partner
Popular beliefs (stress causes cancer)
PATIENT-DERIVED
Intrapersonal
Coping ability; emotional maturity at time of cancer; philosophic, spiritual, or religious beliefs which influence coping
Developmental stage at time of cancer and meaning of curtailed goals (e.g., marriage, children)
Interpersonal
Spouse, family, friends (social support)
CANCER-DERIVED
Site, stage, symptoms (especially pain) and prognosis
Treatment required (surgery, radiation, chemotherapy) and sequelae (immediate and delayed)
Altered body structure of function; rehabilitation/restoration available
Psychological management by the treating staff

onment (social supports and tangible resources); and those that are disease-derived (the medical facts of stage at diagnosis, site and treatment).

No disease has sustained as strong a negative stigma through the centuries as has cancer. Old attitudes and myths about it have persisted despite new information that invalidated them. They remain strong even today. For these reasons, one who attempts to understand the attitudes and beliefs about cancer today, or attempts to understand a particular patient's response, must be aware of these powerful social forces derived from the past. The intertwining of these issues is reflected in this chapter which traces the changes in the treatment of cancer and the concurrent attitudes (Table 1.2). Table 1.2 also shows the parallel views toward medicine and death. The role of psychiatrists, and later health psychologists, is documented. This information provides the historical base for understanding patients' responses today.

This chapter outlines psychological issues in cancer and the early interface of knowledge of cancer and treatment with social attitudes, the growth and development of oncology as a specialty in medicine, the emergence of psycho-oncology in the late 1970s, and finally the maturing relationship between oncology and the social sciences in recent years, and the development of a subspecialty of psycho-oncology.

EARLY ATTITUDES OF SOCIETY TOWARD CANCER

In the 1800s, a definitive diagnosis of cancer was unusual and no treatment was available. Surgical extirpation became possible only after general anesthesia came into use after mid-century. Even then, cure was rare; death was the expected outcome for most cancer patients. Adequate methods to control the pain and distressing symptoms associated with advanced disease were also few. Little was known about the causes of cancer and, thus, an aura of fear and dread surrounded cancer.

By the early part of the twentieth century, three major diseases predominated in the Western world: heart disease, tuberculosis, and cancer. Heart disease never aroused the same abhorrence and fear as tuberculosis and cancer. A diagnosis of either was a death sentence and caused the person to be stigmatized, isolated, and humiliated, a fate similar to that of persons with leprosy and syphilis. Most people feared that cancer was contagious also.

There were other special problems associated with cancer: uncontrolled pain, nonhealing, fungating, foul-smelling tumors, debilitation, and loss of attractiveness and self-esteem. All contributed to the special revulsion associated with the diagnosis of a malignant tumor. The visibility of cancer of the breast and genital organs, and the resemblance of these inoperable lesions to the gummas of syphilis, frequently led to the erroneous assumption of sexual transmission, adding further to the patient's shame, stigma, and guilt. The information that someone had cancer was whispered among family members and was often withheld from children in the family. The diagnosis was rarely publicly stated. Obituaries never gave cancer as a cause of death; instead a euphemism such as " a lingering illness"—which was known to mean cancer—was employed.

TABLE 1.2. *Events Altering Perceptions of Cancer*

Decade	Advances in Medicine and Cancer	Attitudes Toward Cancer	Attitudes Toward Death	Psychiatry and Psychology
1800s	Mortality high from infectious diseases; tuberculosis common Effective cancer treatment unknown Introduction of anesthesia and antisepsis, opening way for surgical excision of cancer (1847)	Cancer equals death; diagnosis not revealed Stigma, shame, guilt associated with having cancer; fears of transmission	Patient is "in God's hands"; physician's role seen to comfort; *"death is part of life"*; person died at home	Concern only with major, mental illness; psychiatrists called "alienists" Psychiatric hospitals largely removed from general hospitals; by 1850s, efforts to bring psychiatry into medicine
1900–1920s	Successful surgical removal of some early cancers Radiation used for palliation American Cancer Society (ACS) started (1913)	In 1890s, efforts in Europe & U.S. to inform public of warning signs of cancer Era of home remedies and quack cures for cancer	Doctors assumed authoritarian and paternalistic role, did not reveal diagnosis or medications; "trust me and don't worry" philosophy	First psychiatric unit in a general hospital, Albany, N.Y. (1902) Psychobiological approach of Adolf Meyer Psychophysiologic approach to disease by Cannon
1930s	National Cancer Institute and International Union against Cancer formed (1937)	ACS visitor–volunteer programs for cancer patients with functional deficits (colostomy, laryngectomy)	Deaths in hospitals; embalming, elaborate funerals; person "only sleeping" as euphemism for death	Beginning psychiatric consultation and psychiatric units in general hospitals Psychosomatic movement begun; strong psychoanalytic orientation
1940s	Nitrogen mustards, developed in World War II, found to have antitumor action First remission of acute leukemia by use of drug	Pervasive pessimism of public and doctors about outcome of cancer treatment	Expression of grief encouraged; concern for handling of death Funeral "industry"	Search for cancer personality and life events as cause of cancer First scientific study of acute grief Role for social workers defined in U.S.
1950s	Beginning of cancer chemotherapy; first cure of choriocarcinoma by drugs alone (1951)	Debates about the practice of not revealing cancer diagnosis reach the public, who are better informed about issues in medicine	Post World War II concerns about informed consent and patient autonomy	First papers on psychological reactions to cancer (1951–1952); psychiatrists favor revealing cancer diagnosis First psychiatric unit established at Memorial Sloan-Kettering Cancer Center (MSKCC) (1950) under Sutherland
1960s	Combined modalities lead to first survivors of childhood leukemia and Hodgkin's disease Hospice movement started Tobacco related to lung cancer	More optimism Survivors concerns are heard Public concern grows for prevention research in cancer	U.S. federal guidelines for patient participation in research	Kubler-Ross's influence important in U.S. Thanatology begun and interest in "death with dignity" Behavioral studies of life style and habits which increase cancer risk
1970s	National Cancer Plan, 1972, with rehabilitation and cancer control, psychosocial included Informed consent for treatment protocols; increased patient autonomy Two cooperative groups,* CALGB & EORTC, established committees to study quality of life (QOL) and psychosocial issues	Diagnosis usually revealed in U.S. and several others countries Guidelines for protection of patients' rights	Prognosis more likely not revealed First hospice in U.S. (1974) Guidelines for care of hopelessly ill — do not resuscitate (DNR) (1976)	First support for psychosocial studies First National Conference on psychosocial research (1975) Psychosocial Collaborative Oncology Group (PSYCOG) began Project Omega (1977–84) Study of children with cancer Psychiatry Service at MSKCC established (1977)

(continued)

TABLE 1.2. *Events Altering Perceptions of Cancer — Continued*

Decade	Advances in Medicine and Cancer	Attitudes Toward Cancer	Attitudes Toward Death	Psychiatry and Psychology
1980s	ACS assisted in development of psycho-oncology; four conferences on research methods ACS-Peer Review Committee established for psychosocial research (1989) Better analgesics and antiemetics developed Federal Drug Administration in U.S. mandates quality of life in cancer trials of new anticancer agents (1985)	More cancer survivors Formation of national (U.S.) coalition of cancer survivors U.S. consumer and women's movement Concern for quality of life and symptom control increases Pain initiatives for public and professional education	Impact of U.S. President's Commission for study of ethical problems in medicine Health proxy assignment encouraged in U.S. U.S. physicians required to discuss wishes about resuscitation (DNR)	International Psycho-oncology Society (1984) National and regional psycho-oncology societies formed in U.S. Health psychologists contribute to clinical care and research in cancer Development of psychobiological research (psychoneuroimmunology)
1990s	First overall reduction in cancer mortality reported in U.S. Increased global interest in palliative medicine; chairs established in U.K., Canada, and Australia Cooperative trials groups include QOL (quality of life) in outcome measures	Increased public concern about cigarettes and cancer Social and legal pressure on tobacco companies in U.S. Active smoking cessation research	Public and professional debate about physician-assisted suicide New educational and research interest in care at the end of life (Project on Death in America)	Increasing support for nursing and social work research Third World Congress of Psycho-Oncology (Beaune, 1992) Kobe, 1995, New York, 1996 Behavioral, psychosocial, and psychopharmacologic intervention trials

*CALGB, Cancer and Leukemia Group B; EORTC, European Organization for Research in the Treatment of Cancer

The word cancer carried such dread that the doctor revealed the diagnosis only to the family and never to the patient. The Death of Ivan Ilyich by Tolstoy provided a literary example of the isolation that a patient in the nineteenth century felt when his physician and family refused to acknowledge that he was dying of cancer. He recognized his serious condition, yet all those around him maintained a pretense that he was scarcely ill. His servant alone acknowledged his condition (3).

Early in the twentieth century, surgery began to offer a possible cure for cancer when the tumor could be removed before it had spread, but success depended on "getting it all out." For the first time, educating the public about the possibility of cure became important. Educational programs encouraging people to seek consultation for suspicious symptoms began, representing the first attempt to alter the negative attitudes toward cancer. The first pioneering effort in public cancer education began in Europe in the 1890s when Winter, a gynecologist in East Prussia, urged women to become better informed about the danger signals of cancer. A newspaper campaign in East and West Prussia in 1903 publicized the early warning signs of cancer. Childe began a similar campaign in England to educate the public that cancer,

when diagnosed early, was not a death warrant; early cancer could be cured by surgery. Childe also advocated the establishment of cancer control societies worldwide to create a more informed public (4).

The American Society for Control of Cancer was formed in 1913. The mandate of this organization, later renamed the American Cancer Society (ACS), was to "disseminate knowledge concerning the symptoms, treatment and prevention of cancer" (5). To counter the ignorance, fatalism and fears, warning signals of cancer were publicized; emphasis was placed on information as a way to combat fear by such slogans as "Fight cancer with knowledge." Figures 1–1 and 1–2 show the nature of the early education efforts. Physicians equally needed education to counter their pessimism about the treatment of cancer. Despite the greater public information, however, many people neglected the danger signals and appeared only after delaying for months in seeking consultation, which led to a fatal outcome.

As part of the American Cancer Society's efforts, a special Women's Field Army was developed to teach women about the early symptoms of breast and uterine cancer and to reduce their embarrassment and reluctance to consult a male physician for gynecological problems. In this regard, the first consumer awareness article to appear in the popular press was published in 1912 in the *Ladies Home Journal*. It said in part:

Be careful of persistent sores and irritations, external and internal. Be watchful of yourself, without undue worry. At the first suspicious symptoms, go to a good physician and demand the truth . . . The risk is not in surgery, but in delayed surgery.—(5).

Early surgical efforts were directed toward developing increasingly radical procedures and wider excisions in an attempt to attain eradication of the tumor. Although the efforts offered cure to a few, the prognosis continued to be dire for tumors that were not surgically resectable. In cases not curable by surgery, the doctor's role was one of offering comfort and "laying on of hands."

In fact, at the time the general physicians had little medical education and the public distrusted their care. People tried to "be their own doctors" and home remedies abounded for all diseases, but particularly for incurable diseases such as cancer. Patterson in his excellent history of social attitudes about cancer noted that Oliver Wendell Holmes said, "if the whole of matera medica, as used now, could be sunk to the bottom of the sea, it would be better for mankind—and worse for the fishes" (4). Quack cures abounded. A common belief, early in the twentieth century, was that disease was the result of cold and could be treated with heat. Patients were encased in hot bricks and given hot baths, along with emetics to cleanse their bodies of harmful waste, a treatment known as Thompsonism. Homeopathy ("like cures like") was popular, as well as chiropractic. Both persist today and the use of alternative therapies has become more common in traditional medicine (see Chapter 70). By the 1930s, reflecting newer medical use of radiation, alternatives treatments consisted of electric and cosmic "energy" cures. As immune defenses became better understood, alternatives took on a more "natural" and less harsh approach, represented later by treatments such as laetrile and Krebiozen.

In the nineteenth century, psychiatrists were known as alienists, whose major role was to remove the mentally ill from society, by placing them in mental hospitals. By 1850, however, there was keen interest in teaching psychological medicine to medical students and physicians who cared for medical patients in general hospitals (6). In 1902, a psychiatric ward was placed in a general hospital in Albany, New York, representing the first effort to bring psychiatry into the general medical care setting. The psychobiological concepts of Adolph Meyer had an impact on psychiatric thought, which was felt in the first quarter of the

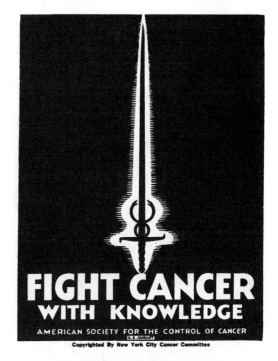

FIG. 1–1. Reprinted with permission from Patterson JT. *The Dread Disease: Cancer and Modern American Culture.* Cambridge, MA: Harvard University Press; 1987.

century. The psychophysiological experiments of Walter Cannon furthered interest in what later became psychosomatic medicine. Typically, however, psychiatrists had no role in the understanding or care of cancer patients until they began to participate in debates about revealing the diagnosis of cancer in the 1960s.

CANCER TREATMENT ADVANCES AND EARLY PSYCHOSOCIAL EFFORTS

In the 1920s, radium was added as a treatment for cancer; however, it mainly offered only palliation after surgical failure (7). The patient and family knew it meant incurable disease. The search for new treatments became a major focus of biomedical research.

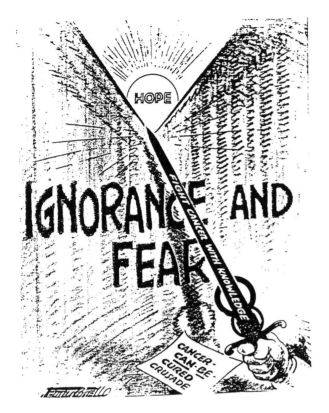

FIG. 1–2. Reprinted with permission from Patterson JT. *The Dread Disease: Cancer and Modern American Culture.* Cambridge, MA: Harvard University Press; 1987.

The International Union Against Cancer, composed of national cancer societies, and the U.S. National Cancer Institute (NCI) were both established in 1937. The NCI model has been highly successful as a governmental agency for biomedical research and has been emulated throughout the world.

Consonant with the greater research effort in the 1940s, new support for cancer patients was initiated through the American Cancer Society's field and service "visitor" programs. Trained volunteers provided information and counseling for patients with specific cancers whose treatment resulted in major functional loss; concrete services such as transportation and providing bandages for nonhealing skin lesions were important. It soon became apparent that the best providers of information were other patients and their families. Surgeons began to ask patients who had had a laryngectomy or colostomy to speak with patients anticipating similar surgery. This was often a critical intervention in encouraging a person to consent to a radical procedure leading to loss of voice or normal bowel function. Laryngectomy and ostomy clubs

developed as the first cancer self-help groups. In the 1950s, the ACS took over Reach-to-Recovery, which has led to its worldwide expansion as the most successful self-help program.

Despite widespread endorsement by patients, these organizations had an uphill battle to gain acceptance in the medical community. Except in special situations, physicians were slow to acknowledge that there was a unique and useful role for patients to support and encourage others with the same diagnosis and treatment. Such efforts were viewed by many as an intrusion into the doctor–patient relationship, even though few adverse effects were reported. The strong bias against encouraging patients to talk to one another continued to the last quarter of this century.

The development in the late 1940s of the first anti-cancer agent initiated the use of chemotherapy in cancer treatment. Chemotherapy became the third modality, along with surgery and radiation. The first responses of acute leukemia to nitrogen mustard, a drug that was developed in World War II research on war gases, were seen in the early 1950s. The first cure of a cancer, choriocarcinoma, by a single chemotherapeutic agent, methotrexate, was also achieved in the early 1950s. Use of chemotherapy led to the creation of the subspecialty of medical oncology, with its own professional standards and certification within the field of internal medicine. The rapid increase in the number of medical oncologists quickly provided a group of physicians who were trained in administering chemotherapy and who could provide care throughout the course of the illness, reducing the fragmentation of care.

The introduction of chemotherapy to the treatment armamentarium dramatically altered the prognosis for several previously fatal tumors of children and young adults, notably acute childhood leukemia and Hodgkin's disease. These cures of previously fatal cancers in the 1960s did much to reduce the pessimism about treatment of cancer.

The psychosocial issues in cancer changed dramatically as treatments became more successful. Initially, when childhood tumors and many adult cancers were uniformly fatal, efforts were directed toward assisting the patient and family to adapt to the inevitable outcome. It was considered more humane to shield the patient from the frightening word equated with death. Doctors, who saw their role as protectors, chose to withhold the news as long as possible. The primary psychological issue was dealing with death, by avoiding discussion of it. The survivors were few and they chose not to reveal it because of the stigma.

A GROWING INTERFACE BETWEEN PSYCHIATRY, PSYCHOLOGY, AND ONCOLOGY

Between the 1930s and 1950s, increasing numbers of psychiatric consultation services and psychiatric units in general hospitals resulted in rising concern about the psychological care of medically ill patients. The first two studies of psychological adaptation to cancer came from the psychiatric group at the Massachusetts General Hospital. They reported the patterns of change in communication as patients reached advanced stages of illness. Communication became more limited and discussion of actual diagnosis and prognosis did not occur, perhaps reflecting that patients sensed the expectation of others to remain silent. Guilt was also a prominent psychological response related to the stigma (8,9). Ruth Abrams, a social worker, was an important contributor to these early observations of the psychosocial aspects of care.

Early papers about psychological adaptation dealt also with how patients responded to radical surgery. Since the assumption was that the widest possible resection offered the best chance for cure, extensive procedures developed for gynecologic and breast cancer, in particular. Major physical and functional deficits were the cost of possible cure. In 1950, Arthur Sutherland, a psychiatrist, established the first psychiatric unit in a cancer hospital at the Memorial Sloan-Kettering Cancer Center. It was devoted to the study of the psychosocial consequences of cancer and surgical treatment. The group carried out several seminal studies describing responses to colostomy and radical mastectomy (10,11). Important insights into the psychological issues confronting the patient facing death were also provided by Eissler and Norton, who described patients who were in analysis and developed cancer (12,13).

At about the same time that Sutherland's group was exploring the impact of radical surgery and psychiatrists were studying psychosomatic diseases, the first debates began to arise about the wisdom of never revealing the diagnosis of cancer. A group of oncologists and psychiatrists suggested to the "never tellers," who constituted more than 90% of physicians polled in a survey by Oken in 1961, that more harm was being done by telling a lie which led to loss of trust in the physician (14). Doctors working with cancer began to change their practice in this regard and found that both they and the patient were more comfortable when false pretenses were dropped. Over the next 25 years, the public's sophistication about diseases, the development of informed consent guidelines, and the increasingly successful treatment of cancer contributed

to the far more open discussion of cancer diagnosis, treatment, and prognosis. The same questions asked in a survey in 1977 showed that 97% of the doctors studied generally told patients their cancer diagnosis (15). However, the candor of American doctors in revealing cancer was not matched in most other countries. The custom of "not telling" continues in many. (See Chapter 101 on International Psycho-oncology.) However, the general trend is moving gradually toward fuller disclosure by both physicians and patients. The factors which contributed to this change and greater emphasis on psychological aspects of care are outlined in Table 1.3.

The wide publicity given to the work of Elizabeth Kubler Ross sharply focused medical and public attention on the psychological dimension of patients dying with cancer. Kubler-Ross's seminal work on open communication with the dying cancer patient heralded the beginning of the thanatology movement in this country and brought American attitudes toward death under scrutiny (16). Her work underscored the tendency of doctors and staff to avoid the discussion of death as they had avoided revealing the diagnosis of cancer. She observed that death was a taboo subject that was spurned by the healthy as well. The thanatology movement encouraged exploration of social attitudes about death, and better communication with cancer patients during terminal stages of disease, and it contributed to the hospice and palliative care movement in the United States.

Because Kubler-Ross's work focused on cancer patients' reactions to the anticipation of death, it had a profound impact on professionals, especially on nurses who were the primary persons speaking with patients about these feelings. Dr. Kubler-Ross spoke at all major cancer centers and recounted her experiences with dying patients, with a remarkably charismatic delivery. For some years, attention was directed toward her "stages of dying," assuming that the course of cancer was a predictable and inexorable

TABLE 1.3. *Factors Contributing to Greater Emphasis on Psychological and Social Issues in Cancer*

Societal attitudes shifting away from fatalism about cancer

Trend toward revealing diagnosis in many countries

Patient participation in treatment decisions (autonomy, informed consent)

Increased doctor–patient dialogue

Development of valid instruments for measuring subjective symptoms and quality of life (QOL)

Recognition that effective cancer prevention and screening is dependent on changing behaviors downhill path from diagnosis to death, with equally predictable psychological stages. While all the emotions are seen, they vary widely and do not occur in stages. Nevertheless, the impact on public and professionals was quite profound. Her book was widely read.

These changes toward more open disclosure were enhanced further in the 1970s by the consumer and women's movements in the United States, and by the greater concern for patient autonomy and patients' rights. The patient–doctor dialogue changed. (See Chapters 95–98 on ethical issues.) Federal guidelines were promulgated in relation to patient participation in experimental research, with institutional boards of oversight required in any institution carrying out research in humans.

The growth of the liaison–consultation division of psychiatry beginning in the early 1970s had an impact on cancer patient care by providing consultation to staff on management of difficult cases, often patients with anxiety, depression, or delirium. Nurses and social workers had previously carried the burden of support, irrespective of the level of patients' distress. Multidisciplinary teaching rounds and support groups began to focus on psychological and behavioral problems, ethical dilemmas, conflicts between patient, and stress on staff (17). Psychological and social issues have increasingly attracted health psychologists to the field, both as clinicians and as investigators. They have been major contributors to research, particularly bringing cognitive and behavioral interventions to the bedside. Psychological and behavioral issues related to prevention, early detection, and compliance with cancer treatment came under study, especially behaviors enhancing cancer risk, such as cigarette smoking. (See Chapter 3.) Nurse clinicians and investigators, social workers, and sociologists have also made major contributions to psycho-oncologic knowledge and skills.

Very little support for psychosocial research in cancer existed before 1970. However, with the advent of the National Cancer Plan in 1972 and the establishment of the Division of Cancer Control and Rehabilitation, demonstration projects (but not research studies) to improve rehabilitation were funded (18). The first conference that brought together the handful of psychosocial researchers was held in San Antonio in 1975 (19). The American Cancer Society became concerned that psychosocial and behavioral issues received little attention. They sponsored several workshops that reviewed the status of the research methods, and the goals and directions in education and training (20,21). The result was the development of a national advisory committee and a peer review committee to evaluate behavioral and psychosocial research proposals.

In 1967, Cicely Saunders opened St. Christopher's Hospice in London, a hospice that focused on improving symptom control and palliative care of terminally ill patients, composed largely of patients with cancer. In addition, it became a center for training professionals in supportive care and for research studies in symptom control, especially pain. Three years later in 1970, Feigenberg, a Swedish psychiatrist at the Radiumhemmet, Karolinska Institute in Stockholm, established the Psychosomatic Unit to which he brought a new psychoanalytic perspective to patients' care (22). In 1971, the Faith Courtauld Unit was formed at King's College in London under Greer and Pettingale and focused on psychological research in cancer. The group under Greer moved to the Royal Marsden Hospital in the 1980s as the Psychosocial Research Unit.

Also in the 1970s, several organizations contributed significantly to collaborative research and education. The International Working Group on Dying, Death, and Bereavement began in 1974 as a cross-cultural group interested in education in psychosocial aspects of advanced and terminal illness. It has provided a continuing forum at a global level for discussion of these issues. In the late 1970s, two cancer collaborative clinical trials groups became multimodality in scope and added committees to conduct psychosocial and quality of life research. The Cancer and Leukemia Group B (CALGB) established the Psychiatry Committee in 1976, chaired by Holland, as part of its initial multimodality effort mandated by the NCI. At about the same time, the National Cancer Institute funded the multicenter Psychosocial Collaborative Oncology Group (PSYCOG) under Schmale's leadership, which conducted research until the mid 1980s, developing research tools and addressing prevalence of psychosocial problems.

The European Organization for Research in the Treatment of Cancer (EORTC) added a committee on Quality of Life, chaired initially by van Dam. This has been a potent force in developing psychometric assessment and research in quality of life. Under Aaronson, these efforts culminated in the establishment of a World Health Organization Collaborating Center in Quality of Life Measurement. A second WHO Center for Study of Quality of Life Measurement in Developing Countries was begun by Olweny in Winnipeg, Manitoba, Canada.

For a decade, beginning in 1978, Weisman headed Project Omega at the Massachusetts General Hospital.

With Worden, they contributed to conceptual approaches, research methods, and information about patients' responses to cancer at all stages in cancer.

CURRENT STATUS

The status of psycho-oncology as a subspecialty of oncology is confirmed by its activities in four broad areas: inclusion of psycho-oncology in services for patients; growth of educational and training programs; research addressing psychosocial issues; and publications of research and scholarly papers. Significant challenges, however, exist in each area for continued growth of the field (see Table 1.4 for outline of the major issues).

Clinical Programs
Most cancer centers and divisions have an identified staff member or members responsible for providing psychological and social support. The units vary from a single individual who requests the consultative participation of other professionals, to a fully developed multidisciplinary team providing a broad array of services designed to assist patients with significant distress or overt psychiatric disorders, and to provide support for their families and for the staff. (See Chapter 90 on setting up a psycho-oncology unit.) There are currently only a few centers in the world, however, that have psycho-oncologic programs which are large enough to incorporate research and training.

The composition of the staff of these programs varies. The staffing is usually multidisciplinary and may include a psychologist, social worker, psychiatrist, nurse, or clergy, with consultation available from the unrepresented disciplines. Some programs depend heavily on volunteers, who give important psychological and practical support to patients, especially in North America.

Education and Training
Several organizations in Europe and North America have contributed to the early professional development of psycho-oncologists. The European International Psychosomatic Study Group and, in France, Psychology and Cancer each provided early networks studying cancer from different, but important perspectives. The German Psychosocial Postcare Unit and Training Center was an early proponent of training. The British Psychosocial Oncology Group has been a significant force since 1983, holding regular meetings and publishing monographs that have represented pioneering efforts in the field. A psycho-

TABLE 1.4. *Challenges to Psycho-oncology*

CLINICAL CARE
Impact of health care policy to support adequate psychosocial care
TRAINING
Set standards for training and curriculum
Develop training centers for clinical and research training
Obtain support for training of young investigators and clinicians
RESEARCH
Continue development of quality of life measurement which can be used by clinicians in treatment decisions
Controlled trials of interventions
Psychobiological studies
Behavioral research in prevention and detection

social society has developed in Italy as well as an active organization of psychologists interested in studying these issues of cancer in Europe. Growing out of the efforts within the EORTC network of psychosocial clinicians and researchers, the European Society of Psychosocial Oncology (ESPO) was formed in 1986 under Zittoun.

The International Psycho-oncology Society (IPOS) was formed in 1984 as a recognition of the need for communication among the small, scattered groups with interests in psycho-oncology. It has served as a source of international exchange through a newsletter and as a research tool for identifying training opportunities for psychosocial researchers to study in different countries and to learn new clinical and research skills. In 1988, the board of directors requested that the society develop guidelines for a psycho-oncology curriculum, which was published in 1995 (23). With encouragement from IPOS, the Mexican and Japanese psycho-oncology societies were formed: by Romero in Mexico in 1984 and by Kawano in Japan in 1985. Argentina and Brazil have led the way toward a South American group, and an Australian society is being planned. The Belgian society is well established. In 1988, the American Society of Psychiatric-Oncology/AIDS was formed. There are now over 20 national societies. Regional societies are the European Society of Psychosocial Oncology, the Pan African Psycho-Oncology Society, and the Nordic Society. The International Psycho-Oncology Society serves as an umbrella organization. (See Chapter 101 on International Psycho-Oncology.)

Several events occurred in 1989. The European School of Oncology conducted the first course on psychosocial issues in cancer in Venice (24). Initial meetings were held in Brazil and India. The first joint British and European Psychosocial Oncology Society meeting was also held. The WHO Expert Committee on Pain Relief/Supportive Care, in Geneva, utilized experts to develop a psychosocial component.

The first joint European Society of Psychosocial Oncology and International Psycho-oncology Society meeting took place in 1990 in Hamburg. In 1991, the two organizations and the Psychiatry Service, Memorial Sloan-Kettering Cancer Center, presented the fourth Update on Psycho-oncology New York City. In 1992, the first Psychosocial World Congress was held in Beaune, France; the second was held in Kobe, Japan, in 1995. The Third World Congress of Psycho-Oncology was held in New York in 1996 with almost one thousand health professionals attending. The international educational activities have grown exponentially over the last decade.

Research

As assessment methods improved, and as more and better psychometric tools were developed or adapted for use with cancer patients, the quality of scientific investigation improved. In addition, more studies have undertaken to collect concurrent quantitative psychological and biological data, especially psycho-neuroimmune. There is also increasing consideration being given to cross-cultural research topics. Research efforts fall into several major areas: adaptation to illness and interventions; quality of life measurement; behavioral interventions in cancer prevention; and psychobiological research with immunologic and neuroendocrine variables. A research model can now be presented which identifies the issues (Fig. 1–3).

The problem of securing adequate funding for psycho-oncologic research and research training is fundamental to the further recognition and development of psycho-oncology as a legitimate subspecialty. The most hopeful signs are those arising from patients and families who increasingly demand greater concern for their quality of life related to cancer treatment and outcome. Their pressure, exerted in part by cancer survivors themselves and by those committed to psycho-oncology, is the driving force which is influencing publicly elected officials to alter their health care policy to recognize and support these needs. This should, in turn, encourage funding for this dimension of health care. Despite the fact that patients have repeatedly stated that they want this included in care, it has consistently been neglected.

Publications

Another measure of the development of a field is the presence of publications, journals, and texts which reflect the body of knowledge constituting the field. Major textbooks of both oncology and psychiatry in the United States have included chapters on psychosocial issues in cancer since the early 1980s. The British Psychosocial Oncology Group has encouraged publication of several books developed from their annual meetings. The *Handbook of Psychooncology* provided a comprehensive review of the current practices and references in all major areas in 1989 (1). The European School of Oncology published a monograph in 1990, *Psychosocial Aspects of Oncology*, bringing together a largely European faculty (24). The *Journal of Psychosocial-Oncology* has been published since 1982 and is devoted to these issues; *Psycho-Oncology: Journal of the Psychological, Social, and Behavioral Dimensions of Cancer* started in 1992 and has published papers from investigators representing all continents.

RESEARCH IN PSYCHO-ONCOLOGY

A central research area is quality of life assessment and its integration into clinical trials and patient care. This area today is directed toward obtaining patients' view of their function in the key areas of their lives: physical, psychological, social, work, and sexual. Scales which measure each domain and global dimensions have been developed. Aaronson, for the EORTC, and Cella in the United States have led in multilingual instrument development, using a modular approach with a generic core of questions for all patients and a cancer site-specific module for patients with specific neoplasms. (See Chapter 99 by Cella on measurements.) Patient-centered data are now being gathered far more routinely in clinical trials, which helps in making decisions and in studying the psychosocial predictors of adaptation and survival.

Research and controlled trials of psychosocial interventions will need to expand in patients receiving both curative and palliative care. The positive impact of interventions on psychological symptoms and well-being is outlined by Fawzy and Fawzy in Chapter 59. The data show a positive outcome on quality of life and reduction of troubling symptoms. However, controlled trials are needed to compare the different approaches and to test psychotropic agents for specific symptoms.

There are two new categories of patients being seen by psycho-oncologists that present new psychological problems. The healthy person, who has an elevated

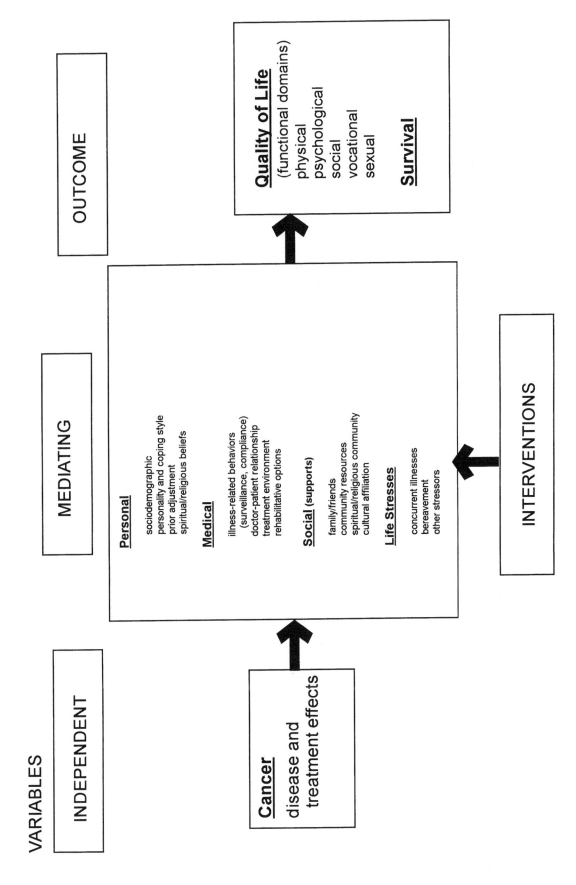

FIG. 1–3. Model of research in psycho-oncology.

tumor marker for a specific tumor (e.g., PSA for prostate or CA125 for ovarian cancer), but who has no evidence of disease on physical examination. High levels of anxiety are seen in these patients, which impact upon their ability to adhere to surveillance procedures. The other new group of "worried well" are those at high genetic risk of cancer. Some deny their risk and refuse close follow-up, creating a problem in early detection. The availability of DNA testing for several genetic mutations adds anxiety as these individuals are offered the opportunity to be tested to find out their actual risk status. Those who choose to be tested must deal with the potential for possible adverse psychological and social consequences, such as employers and insurance companies learning about their results. The ethics, policy, and psychological issues are in need of study. (See Chapter 18 by Kash and Lerman.) The major challenges to the field are: enhancing clinical care; implementing current knowledge by developing a curriculum with support for training; in research, by expanding quality of life assessment, developing controlled trials of interventions, and conducting studies that examine psychological and biological variables.

SUMMARY

In summary, the psychological domain of cancer has begun to be actively explored in the past twenty years by small groups in cancer centers around the world. Psychotherapy and a range of psychotherapeutic, psychosocial, behavioral and psychoeducational interventions are effective for patients who are identified and treated. Clearly, psycho-oncology has begun to fill a need in overall cancer care. Much will depend on the future development of a cohort of individuals who are skilled in this area, and who can lead psycho-oncology units in cancer centers, interact with other disciplines, and develop research studies that address the major issues, many of which arise out of new oncologic discoveries or treatments. There will need to be a continuing and growing effort to ensure patient-centered care that incorporates concern for quality of life, especially in supportive and palliative care. As noted by Greer in 1994, "The most immediately important task of psycho-oncology is to close the yawning gap between current knowledge and actual clinical care of patients" (25).

REFERENCES

1. Holland JC. Historical overview. In: Holland JC, Rowland JH, eds. *Handbook of Psychooncology: Psychological Care of the Patient with Cancer*. New York: Oxford University Press; 1989: 3–12.
2. Holland JC. Psycho-oncology: Overview, obstacles and opportunities. *Psycho-Oncology*. 1992; 1:1–13.
3. Tolstoy L. The Death of Ivan Ilyich (original work in Russian). In: *Great Short Works of Leo Tolstoy*. New York: Harper & Row; 1967: 247–302.
4. Patterson JJ. *The Dread Disease: Cancer and Modern American Culture*. Cambridge, MA: Harvard University Press; 1987.
5. American Cancer Society. *Fact Book for the Medical and Related Professional*. New York: American Cancer Society; 1980.
6. Lipowski ZJ. Holistic-medical foundations of American psychiatry: a bicentennial. *Am J Psychiatry*. 1981; 138:888–895.
7. Shimkin M. *Contrary to Nature*. Washington DC: US Department of Health and Human Services. Public Health Service; 1977; National Institutes of Health Publ. No. 76-7291977.
8. Shands HC, Finesinger JE, Cobb S, Abrams RD. Psychological mechanisms in patients with cancer. *Cancer*. 1951; 4:1159–1170.
9. Abrams RD, Finesinger JE. Guilt reactions in patients with cancer. *Cancer*. 1953; 6:474–482.
10. Sutherland AM, Orbach CE, Dyk RB, Bard M. The psychological impact of cancer and cancer surgery: I. Adaptation to the dry colostomy: Preliminary report and summary of findings. *Cancer*. 1952; 5:857–872.
11. Bard M, Sutherland AM. Psychological impact of cancer and its treatment. IV. Adaptation to radical mastectomy. *Cancer*. 1955; 8:656–672.
12. Eissler KR. *The Psychiatrist and the Dying Patient*. New York: International Universities Press; 1955.
13. Norton J. Treatment of a dying patient. *Psychoanal Stud Child*. 1963; 18:541–560.
14. Oken D. What to tell cancer patients: A study of medical attitudes. *J Am Med Assoc*. 1961; 175:1120–1128.
15. Novack DH, Plumer R, Smith RL, Ochitill H, Morrow GR, Bennet JM. Changes in physicians' attitudes toward telling the cancer patient. *J Am Med Assoc*. 1979; 241:897–900.
16. Kubler-Ross E. *On Death and Dying*. New York: Macmillan; 1969.
17. Artiss LK, Levine AS. Doctor-patient relation in severe illness: A seminar for oncology Fellows. *N Engl J Med*. 1973; 288:1210–1214.
18. Burke LD. A national planning program for cancer rehabilitation. In: Burchenal J, Oettgen HF, eds. *Cancer: Achievements, Challenges and Prospects for the 1980s*. New York: Grune & Stratton, 1981; 2:771–791.
19. Cullen JW, Fox BH, Ison RN, eds. *Cancer: The Behavioral Dimensions*. Washington, D.C.: National Cancer Institute; 1976; DHEW Publ. No. (NIH) 76-1074.
20. American Cancer Society Working Conference. The psychological, social, and behavioral medicine aspects of cancer: Research and professional education needs and directions for the 1980s. *Cancer*. 1982; 50:1919–1978.
21. American Cancer Society Workshop Conference. Methodology in behavioral and psychosocial cancer research. *Cancer*. 1984; 53:2217–2384.

22. Feinberg L. *Terminal Care: Friendship Contracts with Dying Cancer Patients*. New York: Brunner & Mazel; 1980.

23. Die Trill M, Holland JC. A model curriculum for training in psycho-oncology. *Psycho-Oncology*. 1995; 4:169–183.

24. Holland JC, Zittoun R, eds. *Psychosocial Aspects of Oncology*. Berlin: Springer-Verlag; 1990; European School of Oncology Monograph.

25. Greer S. Psycho-oncology: its aims, achievements and future tasks. *Psycho-Oncology*. 1994; 3:87–103.

2

Biology of Cancer for the Psycho-oncologist

JAMES F. HOLLAND

CELL BIOLOGY

Normal cells are exquisite structures organized to carry on the business of life. During embryonic development cell programming unfolds to limit the functions of cells as they join tissues to become component members of organ systems. There the cells exercise specific limited functions throughout life. The cellular stem cells in the bone marrow retain the capacity to differentiate into erythroid, myeloid, or lymphoid precursors dependent on environmental stimuli. Similarly, glandular epithelium may, upon environmental stimuli, transform to squamous epithelium (metaplasia) even in adult life. Thus cells have limited plasticity to adapt.

As the embryo ages, certain cells must be replaced by developing organ structures. Through intrinsic messages not yet elucidated, or because of cellular secretions that influence nearby cellular survival, these cells undergo programmed cell death. The program, distinct from necrosis, initiates a cascade of genetic events leading to enzymatic hydrolysis of DNA and consequent cellular death. This process is known as *apoptosis*, the term adopted from the Greek for falling leaves. The analogy derives from the shedding of only part of the tree with survival of the main organism. A potential apoptotic pathway exists in nearly every cancer cell. This pathway is under active investigation because it is such a desirable therapeutic target (1).

The environmental stimuli that a cell encounters can be totally exogenous, as from the diet or the atmosphere, or can be secreted by a remote cell and transmitted through the circulation (endocrine effect), secreted by a nearby cell and transmitted through the interstitial fluid (paracrine effect), or secreted by the cell itself, providing molecules to the cell surface (autocrine effect). At the cell surface such stimulatory molecules can interact with receptor molecules. Receptor molecules characteristically have a portion outside the cell, a transmembrane domain, and a domain within the cytoplasm. External domains have unique molecular architectures that react only with an extremely narrow range of ligands. The ligands that bind are growth-promoting or regulatory molecules, or drugs of similar conformation that mimic or block the normal reactions. After the ligand binds to the receptor, a configurational change due to electrostatic forces may occur, informing the intracytoplasmic domain that the receptor is occupied. This initiates an intracellular reaction, often a catalytic phosphorylation of an amino acid constituent of the intracellular domain: tyrosine, threonine, or serine, the three amino acids with hydroxyl groups available to accept a phosphate group. The signal is most often transmitted farther by additional intracellular pathways, some of which involve compounds moving through the cytoplasm to or through the nuclear membrane. There they may interact directly with DNA, or with nuclear proteins that then interact with DNA. This entire process is called *signal transduction* (2).

MOLECULAR BIOLOGY

Physical exposure of a specific gene allows the complementary ribonucleotides to assemble along it, uridylate for deoxyadenylate, cytidylate for deoxyguanylate, adenylate for thymidylate and guanylate for deoxycytidylate. All DNA components are deoxyribonucleotides, and RNA components are ribonucleotides. The ribonucleotides get assembled by DNA-directed RNA polymerases into a faithful RNA copy of the gene. Because there are unused sequences in the gene called introns, the RNA portions to be used, coded by the exons, must be enzymatically excised and ligated to make messenger RNA while the unused RNA in the introns is hydrolyzed and reprocessed.

Messenger RNA is transported out of the nucleus to ribosomes. There, each triplet nucleotide in the message, a codon, specifies a particular amino acid. Transport RNAs, by unique alignment of their nucleotides on the messenger RNA codon, sequentially deliver the particular amino acids that form the specific protein. This protein may be a structural or enzymatic component of the organism. A newly synthesized enzyme may catalyze a specific cellular process which constitutes the response of the cell to the stimulus. This entire sequential reaction from stimulus to response may transpire in an extraordinarily short time, often minutes.

Cancer cell behavior differs from the normal cell in reproduction and survival. Because of mutation, the gene product of a tumor suppressor gene may be unable to carry out its normal functions of limiting cell growth, or inaugurating a cell into apoptosis, the pathway for programmed death of the cell. Such tumor suppressor genes as *P53* (for a protein weighing 53,000 daltons, 53 kDa), *RB* (for retinoblastoma) or *WT1* (for Wilms' tumor) may have single nucleotide substitutions that change a codon, leading to change in a single amino acid in the protein. Such a mutation can affect electrostatic charge or protein folding and thus biochemical behavior. For example, normal P53 protein has so short a half-life it is not found by immunoperoxidase staining in cells. Mutant P53, often due to a single point mutation, has a much longer intracellular half-life, but lacks the ability to inhibit cell growth. Thus, a cell positive for P53 by immunoperoxidase staining is, paradoxically, one that lacks normal P53 activity. High proportions of different cancers, approximating 50% overall, lack normal tumor suppressor activity. Tumor suppressor proteins interact, at least in part, with enzymes that are crucial for mechanistically advancing the cell through the different phases of the cell cycle.

G_0 represents cells not in cycle; G_1, the first gap, a resting and preparatory phase; S the phase in which DNA is synthesized, G_2 a second gap during which preparation for mitosis occurs; and M mitosis, which completes cell division. In the absence of tumor suppressor gene function, the cell can pass continuously through the cell cycle, missing the gap periods during which repair of biochemical mistakes occurs by multiple enzymes that survey, edit, and correct DNA structure. Tumor suppressor proteins can also be inactivated by complexing with proteins of viral origin, thereby allowing uninhibited cell growth. This complexing of viral proteins with growth regulatory proteins appears to be a defensive mechanism evolved to prevent unlimited viral growth that would kill the cell. This complexing mechanism appears to operate, for example, in the case of human papilloma viruses 16 and 18, which are associated with cancer of the cervix.

Oncogenes are genes that ordinarily are no longer expressed in adult cells, but which by mutation or dis-

regulation are amplified in number or in transcriptional activity to produce gene products that favor growth. Such gene products may be secreted cytokines which stimulate the producing cell itself (autocrine) or nearby cells (paracrine secretion). An oncogene may also code for mutated receptor molecules that are abnormal in their external domains; they can behave as if permanently switched on, thereby stimulating intracellular growth pathways.

Thus, there is no final common pathway to cancer. A series of mechanisms exists by which genetic alteration in a cell can produce not only excess stimulation but decreased inhibition of growth. Multiple lesions acquired sequentially are usually necessary before a normal cell becomes a cancer cell. There are some 50 known oncogenes and 10 or more tumor suppressor genes so far discovered.

Loss of heterozygosity (LOH) occurs when a chromosome or a chromosomal segment is missing, leaving a single allele on the remaining chromosome. This condition, hypothesized by Knudson to account for the early onset and bilaterality of familial retinoblastoma means that only a single mutation must occur in the cell on the remaining allele. In an ordinary cell with two alleles, each must usually be affected before a mutation leads to cancer. It has been estimated that more than 1 billion free radicals per cell can be produced every hour, some of which can react with DNA, which speaks to the extraordinary reparative capacity of the cell (3). Defects in repair enzymes (from mutations in the DNA that coded for them) are also potentially oncogenic.

METASTASIS

Cancer cells do not abide by the ordinary complex regulation that governs normal tissues. Cancers are not restricted to an anatomical locus, nor do they reach a specified size and stop growing as do normal tissues. Cancer cells invade through the basement membrane (the distinction between carcinoma in situ and invasive cancer) and destroy nearby cells and structures by proteolytic mechanisms. They secrete angiogenic factors which stimulate the ingrowth of blood vessels, providing a much richer source of nutrition than can be attained through diffusion of intercellular fluids. Cancer cells can invade these new (and old) blood vessels and nearby lymphatics and be mechanically transferred to distant parts of the body. There, dependent upon surface adhesion molecules of the tumor cell and of the endothelium in the target organ, cancer cells may attach. If not killed by white blood cells, they can migrate out of the vessel there and can grow to small size. Dependent upon the balance of angiogenic and angiostatic factors, the cells can inaugurate a neocirculation and become a growing metastatic focus of tumor (4).

The lymph node, liver, lung, skeleton, and brain are tissues most frequently involved with metastatic disease. The cancers of tissues drained by the portal vein often involve the liver first, whereas tissues outside the portal circulation often involve the lung first. Tumor metastases to regional draining lymph nodes are indicative of the possibility that systemic spread has occurred with much higher frequency than in patients who do not have nodal involvement. The absence of lymph node involvement does not guarantee an absence of distant metastases, however.

SYMPTOMATOLOGY

Cancers create symptoms by impinging on nerves in the region, by obstructing hollow visceral conduits, by ulceration onto a mucosal surface, and by occupancy of visceral substance with resultant lack of function. Skeletal pain from stretching of the periosteum or vertebral collapse, visceral pain from invasion or stretching of the liver capsule, and sciatic pain from invasion of retroperitoneal tissues are representative. Compromise of the sigmoid or rectal lumen can be manifest by constipation or by bypass diarrhea, culminating in complete obstruction. Partial esophageal obstruction leads to dysphagia and partial gastric obstruction to anorexia, early satiety, and eventual vomiting. Obstruction of the biliary outflow tract produces jaundice. Urinary tract obstruction may be asymptomatic if a single ureter is involved, may lead to uremia if bilateral, or may be acutely symptomatic if bladder or urethral obstruction occurs. Ulceration on a mucosal surface leads to bleeding, irritation, and infection, serving as a portal of entry for bacteria. Carcinoma of the bronchus can lead to all three symptom complexes. Brain dysfunction, liver dysfunction, and marrow dysfunction relate to space occupancy of the organ mass by cancer cells. More often, brain dysfunction is associated with edema surrounding the neoplasm, and liver dysfunction with impingement on intrahepatic bile ducts. It is remarkable how much reserve there is in brain, liver, marrow, and lung, when only nodular metastases are present as distinct from permeating cells.

Neoplasms also serve as internal parasitic twins, so altering metabolism as to cause anorexia, fever, weight loss, cachexia, and, perhaps the most common symptom of all, fatigue. Although these symptoms are attributed to futile metabolic cycles that waste energy and to cytokines, the exact pathogenesis is not established.

Since many other benign conditions can cause pain, dysfunction, fatigue, and nearly all the symptoms referred to above, it is the obligation of a physician, particularly an oncologist, to prove that the patient does not have cancer as an explanation for symptoms. Regrettably, many physicians do not include cancer in the differential diagnosis of mild organ dysfunctional states. Many doctors empirically treat constipation, anorexia, abdominal pain, cough, intermenstrual bleeding, and even palpable lumps as though they were unquestionably benign diseases, with reassurance, symptomatic treatments, and absence or long delay of diagnostic inquiry. There are very few symptoms of any kind that last two weeks or more that do not deserve explanation rather than symptomatic treatment. Cancer should enter the differential diagnosis of nearly every symptom complex of obscure nature. Unfortunately, the patient himself or herself often makes the diagnosis of cancer by experiencing a symptom too bothersome to overlook. It is the role of the physician and oncologist to detect such neoplasms before they become sufficiently obvious for a layman to make the diagnosis.

DIAGNOSIS

Every cancer must be histologically or cytologically confirmed. Even in the most frail patient, sonographically guided or computerized tomographically guided needle aspiration can be performed. A surgical specimen (sometimes with a cutting needle instead of a knife) is far more valuable in allowing characterization of the tissue behavior. Important information above and beyond the simple proposition of malignancy or benignity can be more readily derived from a tissue section.

Every patient on presentation should be assessed for potential curability. It is convenient to codify this using the clinical TNM system, which classifies tumors by size and invasion, classifies nodes as palpable or not, and describes metastases as present or not. Pathologic staging is more valuable, allowing better assessment of tumor size and invasiveness, pathological proof of node involvement, and rigorous determination of the presence or absence of metastases (Table 2.1).

SURGERY

Every patient on presentation should be approached with the concept of potential curability. Not a few tumors can be cured surgically, despite the presence

TABLE 2.1. *TNM Classification of Breast Cancer**

T_0	No evidence of primary tumor
T_{IS}	In situ cancer
T_2	Tumor 2 cm or less in greatest dimension
T_1	Tumor more than 2 cm but not more than 5 cm in greatest dimension
T_3	Tumor more than 5 cm in greatest dimension
T_4	Tumor of any size with direct extension to chest wall or skin
N_0	Homolateral axillary nodes not considered to contain tumor
N_1	Movable homolateral axillary nodes considered to contain tumor
N_2	Homolateral axillary nodes containing tumor and fixed to one another or to other structures
N_3	Homolateral supraclavicular or infraclavicular nodes containing tumor, or edema of arm
M_0	No evidence of distant metastases
M_1	Distant metastasis present, including skin involvement beyond the breast area

Stage I	T_1	N_0	M_0
Stage II	T_{0-2}	N_1	M_0
Stage IIIA	T_3	N_{0-1}	M_0
	T_{0-3}	N_2	M_0
Stage IIIB	T_4	N_{0-2}	M_0
	T_{0-4}	N_3	M_0
Stage IV	T_{0-4}	N_{0-3}	M_1

*The prefix p as in pT_1 indicates the stage is based on pathologic rather than clinical data.

TABLE 2.2. *Some Types of Cancer Surgery*

BIOPSY

Needle aspirate for cytology (often guided by ultrasound or CT scan)

Needle, cutting, for tissue (e.g. breast, prostate)

Incisional

Excisional

LAPAROSCOPY; THORACOSCOPY; MEDIASTINOSCOPY

Biopsy

Staging

Resection

RESECTION

Local

Elective node dissection

Radical with en bloc removal of lymphatics

Amputation

Metastatectomy (e.g. lung, liver, skin)

RECONSTRUCTION

Internal fixation for fractures

Limb-sparing endoprosthesis for bone tumors

Gastrointestinal

    Esophageal reconstruction

Genitourinary

    Artificial bladder

Breast reconstruction

    With prosthesis

    With autologous tissue

Maxillofacial

    With free grafts and microvascular anastomoses

PALLIATION AND SUPPORT

Diversions

    Tracheostomy

    Gastroenterostomy

    Colostomy

    Biliary (stenting; bypass)

    Ureteral (stenting; percutaneous nephrostomy)

Aspiration

    Seroma drainage

    Paracentesis

    Thoracentesis; pleurodesis

Vascular Access

Neurosurgical

    Laminectomy

    Vertebrectomy

    Epidural catheter for narcotics

    Cordotomy

    Myelotomy

    Ventricular access

    Ventricular shunt

of lymph node metastases and even single hepatic or pulmonary metastasis. Surgery also plays a role during the course of continuing cancer illness to relieve or bypass obstructions; to excise recurrences when they are painful and regionally confined and in selected cases to resect other metastases; to provide venous access; and occasionally to provide neurosurgical control of intractable pain. Orthopedic surgical approaches to appendicular pathologic fractures are mandatory (Table 2.2).

RADIOTHERAPY

Radiation therapy is indispensable to the practice of oncology. X-rays result from electrons hitting a metallic target; when X-rays enter tissue, they impart their energy by displacing orbital electrons, predominantly resulting in ionization of water. The free radicals formed interact with DNA and other critical molecules, leading to point mutations and single-strand and double-strand breaks in DNA. If unrepaired, they may lead to apoptosis, or to cells that produce such mutant forms that at the next division they are nonviable. Radiotherapy affects normal tissues as well as the neoplasm, and thus meticulous attention to proper geometric planning is a critical part of radiation oncology. This assures that the tumor receives the selected dose; that there is not a geographic miss of a margin of the tumor, and that the dose is distributed to normal tissues in such a way that none sustains a highly toxic insult. It is necessary, for example, to protect the spinal cord, the larynx, the lungs, the liver, the kidneys, and the small intestine from excessive dose (5), since these tissue are particularly sensitive to radiation. Fractionation of radiation treatments allows better recovery of normal tissues than of tumor tissues, which accounts for protraction of radiation therapy over several weeks when curative intent is the goal (Table 2.3).

The advantages of radiotherapy are that it can be delivered to tissues that cannot be resected, or tissues that could be resected but with great disadvantage because of the consequences of surgery. Thus, lumpectomy with radiation to the breast is indistinguishable from modified radical mastectomy in outcome, except for the preservation of the breast. This example provides evidence, too, that surgery and radiotherapy can combine with advantage, since radiation is more effective in killing small cell volumes which are well oxygenated rather than large tumors with hypoxic centers.

It has been shown in recent years that radiation has a significant additional role to play after resection of carcinoma of the rectum, many extensive head and neck cancers, and soft-tissue sarcomas. Radiotherapy and chemotherapy have displaced surgery in carcinoma of the anus, in advanced carcinoma of the cervix, and in some carcinomas of the esophagus and head and neck cancer. Ocular tumors less commonly require enucleation than earlier because of radiation treatments of ocular melanoma and of retinoblastoma. Lymphomas in their localized form are still potential indications for radiotherapy, and in their disseminated form may be optimally treated in some instances by chemotherapy and radiotherapy.

Radiotherapy is of extreme usefulness in palliating cancer pain in an isolated area. This is particularly true for skeletal metastases, where pain can be the dominant aspect of metastatic cancer. Disseminated pain in many body regions simultaneously is not well treated by radiation, however, since treatment of the most troublesome site often relieves that dominant symptom to be replaced by another which, previously muted, now seems equally bad.

CHEMOTHERAPY

The effectiveness of chemotherapy in metastatic disease, particularly in childhood tumors, led to major implementation of chemotherapy immediately after surgery as adjuvant treatment. Intuitively it seemed easier to eradicate presumptive micrometastatic deposits than gross disease, and this was experimentally proved in murine tumors. The success of adjuvant postoperative therapy has supported the use of chemotherapy prior to operative treatment (neoadjuvant chemotherapy) as a means of eliminating micrometastatic disease and of making the primary tumor more readily resectable. Among the tumors in which adjuvant and neoadjuvant chemotherapy have substantial benefit are osteosarcomas, other childhood sarcomas, breast cancer, ovarian cancer, colonic cancer, rectal cancer, testicular cancer, and some stages of lung cancer.

Favorable adjuvant results have been reported in a few studies of gastric cancer, head and neck cancer, esophageal cancer, and bladder cancer. Chemotherapy is the primary modality in leukemias, metastatic testicular cancer, and in disseminated lymphomas. For metastatic cancer, hormonal therapies and chemotherapy are the main approaches, keeping in mind that there are several hormones and tens of chemotherapeutic compounds, each of which has relatively specialized indications (Table 2.4). The major consideration in chemotherapy is selective toxicity to tumor rather than normal tissues, which determines the risk–benefit ratio. Many patients who are not cured can be palliated for months to years by chemotherapeutic regimens that shrink their tumors and provide improved performance. Combinations of drugs are important to this end (Table 2.5).

TABLE 2.3. *Some Types of Radiation Therapy*

TELETHERAPY
X-rays—Linear Accelerators, 4–24 MV
Gamma rays
Electrons
Neutrons
Protons
STEREOTACTIC RADIOSURGERY

BRACHYTHERAPY
^{137}Cesium
^{198}Iridium
^{125}Iodine
MONOCLONAL ANTIBODY RADIOIMMUNOTHERAPY

TABLE 2.4. *Common Oncologic Drugs and Some of their Indications*

Oncologic Drug	Indication
ALKYLATING AGENTS	
Nitrogen mustard, mechlorethamine, HN_2, Mustargen®	Hodgkin's disease
Cyclophosphamide, Cytoxan®, Endoxan®	Lymphomas, breast cancer, BMT [a]
Phenylalanine mustard, PAM, Alkeran®	Myeloma
Chlorambucil, Leukeran®	Chronic lymphocytic leukemia
Busulfan, Myleran®	Chronic myeloid leukemia
Thiotepa, Thioplex®	Breast, BMT, intravesical bladder
Ifosfamide, Ifex®	Sarcomas
Cisplatin, platinum, DDP, Platinol®	Squamous carcinomas, lung, testis, ovary, bladder, sarcomas, BMT
Carboplatin, Paraplatin®	Squamous carcinoma, lung, ovary, BMT
Carmustine, BCNU, BiCNU®	Lymphomas, melanoma, BMT
Lomustine, CCNU, CeeNU®	Lymphomas, melanoma, BMT
Procarbazine, Matulane®	Hodgkin's disease
Dacarbazine, DTIC, DTIC-Dome ®	Sarcomas, Hodgkin's disease
ANTIBIOTICS	
Doxorubicin, Adriamycin®	Lymphomas, breast, ovary, bladder, sarcomas
Daunorubicin, Cerubidine®	Acute leukemia
Idarubicin, Idamycin®	Acute leukemia
Mitomycin C, Mutamycin®	Colon, breast
Dactinomycin, actinomycin D, Cosmegen®	Sarcomas
Mitoxantrone, Novantrone®	Lymphomas, breast
ANTIMETABOLITES	
Methotrexate, Mtx	Breast, lymphomas, leukemias, sarcomas
Fluorouracil, 5-FU	Breast, colon, squamous carcinomas
Floxuridine, fluorodeoxyuridine, FudR	Intraarterial for liver metastases
Cytarabine, Cytosine arabinoside, ara C, Cytosar®	Acute leukemia
Mercaptopurine, 6-MP, Purinethol®	Acute leukemia
Gemcitabine, Gemzar®	Pancreas
Fludarabine phosphate, Fludara®	Lymphomas, CLL [b]
Cladribine, 2-chlorodeoxyadenosine, CDA, Leustatin®	Lymphomas, CLL
Azacytidine	Myelodysplastic syndromes
Hydroxyurea, Hydrea®	Chronic myeloid leukemia, radiosensitization
BOTANICALS	
Paclitaxel, Taxol®	Breast, lung, ovary, bladder, squamous carcinoma
Docetaxel, Taxotere®	Breast, lung, ovary, bladder, squamous carcinoma
Vincristine, VCR, Oncovin®	Lymphomas, leukemia, breast
Vinblastine, VLB, Velban®	Lymphomas, breast
Vinorelbine, VRB, Navelbine®	Lymphomas, breast
Etoposide, VP16, Vepesid®	Lung, lymphomas, testis
Irinotecan, CPT11, Camptosar®	Colon
Topotecan, Hycamtin®	Ovary, lung
HORMONES AND THEIR ANALOGS	
Prednisone	Lymphomas, leukemias, breast
Dexamethasone, Decadron®	Lymphomas, leukemias, breast, myeloma
Diethylstilbestrol, DES	Breast, prostate
Tamoxifen, Nolvadex®	Breast
Aminoglutethide, Cytadren®	Breast
GNRH [c] agonists	
Leuprolide—Lupron®	Prostate, breast
Goserelin—Zoladex®	Prostate, breast

(continued)

TABLE 2.4. *Common Oncologic Drugs and Some of their Indications — Continued*

Oncologic Drug	Indication
Flutamide, Eulexin®	Prostate
Bicalutamide, Casodex®	Prostate
IMMUNOMODULATORS	
Interferon-α	Lymphomas, chronic myeloid leukemia
Interleukin-2	Kidney, melanoma, post chemotherapy
HOST SUPPORT	
Filgrastim, GCSF[d], Neupogen®	Granulocytopenia
Sargramostin, GMCSF[e], Leukine®	Granulocytopenia
Epoetin, Erythropoietin, Epogen®	Anemia
Antibiotics	Infection
Analgesics	Pain
Narcotics	Pain

[a]BMT = bone marrow transplantation
[b]CLL = chronic lymphocytic leukemia
[c]GNRH = gonadotropin releasing hormone
[d]GCSF = granulocyte colony stimulating factor
[e]GMCSF = granulocyte macrophage colony stimulating factor

Because of the discovery of qualitatively different targets in cancer cells compared to normal cells, such as oncogenes and mutated tumor suppressor genes, there is new promise of more specific therapies. New agents may target a particular metabolic pathway. Tumor-specific antibodies may serve as blockers of particular receptors, or as vehicles for toxins or radio-isotopes.

TABLE 2.5. *Common Combination Chemotherapy Regimens for Selected Cancers*

BREAST CANCER		
CMF	Cytoxan, methotrexate, fluorouracil	
CMFVP	CMF, vincristine and prednisone	
CAF	Cytoxan, adriamycin, fluorouracil	
AC	Adriamycin, cytoxan	
ATC	Adriamycin, taxol, cytoxan (sequentially)	
LYMPHOMA		
MOPP	Mustard, vincristine (oncovin), prednisone, procarbazine	Hodgkin's disease
ABVD	Adriamycin, bleomycin, vinblastine, dacarbazine	Hodgkin's disease
COP	Cytoxan, vincristine (oncovin), prednisone	Non-Hodgkin's lymphomas
CHOP	Cytoxan, doxorubicin (hydroxydaunorubicin), vincristine, prednisone	Non-Hodgkin's lymphomas
OTHER CANCERS		
AP	Adriamycin, cisplatin	Ovary, osteosarcoma
FU-LV	Fluorouracil and leukovorin	Colon
FU-LV-P	Fluorouracil, leukovorin, cisplatin	Head and neck squamous cell
TP	Taxol, cisplatin	Ovary
TCb	Taxol, carboplatin	Lung
MVAC	Methotrexate, vinblastine, adriamycin, cisplatin	Bladder
AraC and DNR	Cytarabine and daunorubicin	Acute myeloid leukemia
C, P, BCNU	Cytoxan, cisplatin, BCNU	Bone marrow transplantion
C, Cb, ThioTEPA	Cytoxan, carboplatin, thiotepa	Bone marrow transplantion

No cancer is treated so well that we could not do better. We can confidently expect continuing advances at an accelerated rate. Herein lies the hope for patient and doctor alike. Part of the oncologist's task is to show that brighter horizon to the patient, which makes holding the course easier to justify. The horizon that will come into view as the world turns is brighter still.

REFERENCES

1. Bresnick E. Biochemistry of cancer. In: Holland JF, Frei E III, Bast RC Jr., Kufe DW, Morton DL, Weichselbaum RR, eds. *Cancer Medicine*, 4th ed. Baltimore: Williams & Wilkins; 1997: 143–164.
2. Hannun Y. Signal transduction. In: Holland JF, Frei E III, Bast RC Jr., Kufe DW, Morton DL, Weichselbaum RR, eds. *Cancer Medicine*, 4th ed. Baltimore: Williams & Wilkins; 1997: 65–84.
3. Reid TM, Loeb LA. Mutagenic specificity of oxygen radicals produced by human leukemia cells. *Cancer Res.* 1992; 52:1082–1086.
4. Folkman, J. Tumor angiogenesis. In: Holland JF, Frei E III, Bast RC Jr., Kufe DW, Morton DL, Weichselbaum RR, eds. *Cancer Medicine*, 4th ed. Baltimore: Williams & Wilkins; 1997: 181–206.
5. Weichselbaum RR, Chen G, Hallahan DE. Biological and physical basis of radiation oncology. In: Holland JF, Frei E III, Bast RC Jr., Kufe DW, Morton DL, Weichselbaum RR, eds. *Cancer Medicine*, 4th ed. Baltimore: Williams & Wilkins; 1997: 697–726.

II

PSYCHOLOGICAL AND BEHAVIORAL FACTORS IN CANCER RISK

EDITOR: PAUL B. JACOBSEN

3

Smoking Cessation and Cancer Prevention

PAUL M. CINCIRIPINI, ELLEN R. GRITZ, JANICE Y. TSOH, AND
KARYN L. SKAAR

SCOPE OF THE PROBLEM

Tobacco use has been implicated in one of every six deaths in the United States and has been described as the single most important preventable cause of premature death and disability in our country (1). Accounting for approximately 434,000 deaths annually (2), cigarette smoking has been related to 21% of all deaths due to coronary heart disease; 30% of total cancer mortality; 87% of all lung cancer deaths; and 82% of deaths from chronic obstructive pulmonary disease (1,3).

The percentage of total deaths attributable to all types of cancer has risen from 16.3% in 1965, to 23.7% in 1991, with much of the increase due to the effects of smoking, particularly for lung cancer incidence and mortality (4). As shown in Table 3.1, data from the American Cancer Society's prospective studies on cancer prevention (CPS-I and CPS-II) (5) document a substantial rise in smoking-attributable mortality for cancer of the lung, oral cavity, pharynx, larynx, and esophagus (1,6). Compared with nonsmokers, smokers exhibit a dose-dependent increase in the risk of dying from lung (1), pancreatic (7), head and neck, and renal cancer (8); as well as a twofold increase in risk for developing bladder cancer (9) and leukemia (10), and a threefold risk increase for myeloma (10). Environmental tobacco exposure may also account for a small but important increase in the risk of lung cancer in healthy nonsmokers and a significant increase in respiratory problems in young children and infants (11).

Particular concern has been expressed for the rising cancer risk experienced by women and minorities. Between 1960 and 1987, age-adjusted cancer mortality rates for African American males were significantly higher than that of their Caucasian counterparts (269.2 vs. 213.4 per 100,000) (12), which was due in part to the differences in the lung cancer mortality rates observed between the two populations (88.5 vs. 73.2) (13). Although African American men reportedly smoke fewer cigarettes per day than Caucasian males (14), the decline in smoking behavior that has characterized large segments of the U.S. population has been less pronounced in this group of smokers (15). Moreover, in contrast to previous years, lung cancer deaths since 1987 no longer appear to be rising among males, while those for women have continued to increase, except for the very young (13,14,16). It is most significant that lung cancer has now surpassed breast cancer as the leading cause of cancer-related death among women (17).

SMOKING CESSATION AND CANCER RISK

It is clear that former smokers live longer than continuing smokers and that the benefits of quitting extend into the later age groups. In comparison to continuing smokers, people who quit smoking before age 50 show a 50% reduction in risk for all causes of death in the subsequent 16 years, and by age 64, their risk of mortality is similar to that of never smokers of the same age. As shown in Table 3.2, factors such as health status and age at cessation, duration of abstinence, and level of tobacco exposure will determine the magnitude of risk reduction achieved. In the case of cancer mortality, changes may also vary by site. For example, a 30%–50% reduction in lung cancer mortality risk has been noted for both genders and all histologic types after 10 years of nonsmoking, while for cancer of the bladder or kidney the risk to former smokers may be reduced 50% within a few years following smoking cessation. A 50% reduction in risk for cancer of the oral cavity and esophagus has been observed as soon as 5 years after cessation, with further reductions becoming apparent over longer periods of time (17).

TABLE 3.1. *Risk of Cancer Mortality in Smokers Relative to Nonsmokers (≥35 Years Old)*

Cause of Death (cancer type)	Smoking Attributable Mortality[a]			
	Males		Females	
	CPS-I[a]	CPS-II[a]	CPS-I	CPS-II
Lung and bronchus	11.9	23.2*	2.70	12.80*
Urinary bladder	2.90	2.86	2.87	2.58
Kidney, renal pelvis	1.84	2.95	1.43	1.41
Oral and pharyngeal	6.33	27.48*	1.96	5.59*
Pancreas	2.34	2.14	1.39	2.33
Larynx	10.0	10.48	3.81	17.78*
Esophagus	3.62	7.60*	1.94	10.25*

Sources: Refs 5 and 1.

[a]CPS-I and CPS-II samples consisted 1.02 and 1.5 million, predominantly older, educated, middle class Caucasians (93%–97%), who were assessed from 1959 to 1965 and 1982 to 1986, respectively. Lung cancer data is provided through 1988, from Ref. (5).

In a 26-year follow-up of over 200,000 U.S. veterans, 23% of excess cancer deaths were attributed to the earlier smoking of those who had quit in the year prior to assessment. Relative to nonsmokers, the estimated risk for the development of cancer for current vs. former smokers was: 11.6 vs 3.6 for lung carcinoma; 13.7 vs 5.0 for cancer of the larynx; 3.4 vs 1.5 for oral cancer, and 2.2 vs 1.3 for cancer of the bladder.

A major weakness of this study, however, was the reliance on a single assessment of smoking behavior made 26 years before the determination of the cancer diagnosis (8).

The longer time frame required for a reduction in risk of lung cancer is also supported in a recent study of female lung cancer patients; even after 15 years of abstinence, lung cancer mortality remained substan-

TABLE 3.2. *Overall Mortality Ratios Among Current and Former Smokers, Relative to Never Smokers, by Sex and Duration of Abstinence and Cigarette Intake*

Consumption (cigarettes/day)	Current smokers	Duration of abstinence (years)					
		< 1	1–2	3–5	6–10	11–15	≥ 16
FORMER SMOKERS							
Males							
1–20	2.22	2.49	2.38	2.03	1.63	1.38	1.06
≥21	2.43	2.77	2.64	2.25	2.04	1.77	1.27
Females							
1–19	1.60	1.58	1.96	1.41	1.14	1.10	1.01
≥20	2.10	3.39	2.58	2.03	1.60	1.38	1.15
FORMER SMOKERS EXCLUDING THOSE WITH ILLNESS*							
Males							
1–20	2.34	2.06	2.05	1.89	1.48	1.29	1.01
≥21	2.73	1.85	2.15	1.90	1.77	1.65	1.19
Females							
1–19	1.82	0.76	1.26	1.42	1.01	1.09	1.00
≥20	2.46	3.33	2.15	1.44	1.46	1.18	0.95

Source: Data from ACS CPS-II appearing in the 1989 Surgeon Generals Report (1).

*Former smokers with heart disease, cancer, stroke or other serious illness at time of enrollment into the study were excluded.

tially higher for former smokers than for women who had never smoked (population attributable risk = 59%) (18). This is noteworthy, in light of the fact that women may have more difficulty quitting than men (19). a fact which could further compromise the expected reduction in their cancer risk due to smoking cessation.

Risk of head and neck cancer is dually influenced by both smoking and alcohol intake. After adjusting for level of consumption of both substances (20). a 30% reduction in the risk of oral cancer among smokers who quit 1–9 years earlier, and a 50% reduction for those who stopped more than 10 years ago was observed. Relative to current smokers, Kabat (21) also showed a significant reduction in risk of oral cancer for both males (3.5 vs. 1.11) and females (4.34 vs. 1.39) who had quit smoking 1–9 years earlier, but no further risk reduction was evident after 10 or more years of abstinence. For pancreatic cancer, a progressive reduction in risk was associated with cumulative years of cessation in a Chinese sample, but a full 10 years were required before the risk of former smokers equaled that of nonsmokers (22).

Biomarkers of Carcinogenesis

Smoking cessation can also have a direct and positive effect on reducing the levels of PAH–DNA and 4-ABP–Hb adducts (see below). DNA adducts are thought to reflect a crucial step in cancer induction, and are formed as chemical carcinogens are absorbed by the body, bioactivated by drug-metabolizing enzymes (e.g., cytochrome P450s) and bonded with cellular macromolecules. Polycyclic aromatic hydrocarbons (PAHs) are potent respiratory carcinogens found in cigarette smoke. The PAH benzo[a]pyrene forms DNA adducts in the lung that correspond to the mutations found in the K-*ras* oncogene in lung cancer tissue and in the *p53* tumor-suppressor gene, associated with cancer of the lung, head and neck, and urinary bladder. The arylamine 4-aminobiphenyl (4-ABP) is a potent human bladder carcinogen also present in tobacco smoke, which forms adducts with hemoglobin (Hb). It is thought to be a principal component in smoking-related bladder carcinogenesis (for review see Ref. (23)).

Substantial reduction (50%–75%) in PAH–DNA and 4-ABP–Hb adducts have been observed after 10 weeks of nonsmoking. The estimated half-life of these compounds, after adjusting for background environmental tobacco exposure, was 9–13 and 7–9 weeks, respectively (24). Variability in the rate of PAH–DNA and 4-ABP–Hb decline may reflect genetic differences in metabolic detoxification (i.e., *N*-acetylation polymorphism (*NAT2*)), which may be slower among

smokers (25). Such findings may have relevance to cancer prevention strategies, since changes in these biomarkers may function as an intermediate indicator of the reduction in cytogenetic damage attributable to smoking cessation.

BENEFITS OF CESSATION TO CANCER PATIENTS

Relative 5-year survival rate for all cancers now stands at 56% (26) and a growing body of sound epidemiological, clinical, and biological evidence, supports the inclusion of smoking cessation treatment within the spectrum of the cancer care continuum. Smoking cessation may have a favorable impact on cancer treatment efficacy, complications, the development of further disease, and overall cancer and noncancer mortality. While such benefits may be particularly important among those with early stage disease and smoking-related tumors, the impact of smoking cessation on a wide array of cancer treatment modalities and outcomes, including surgical recovery, radiotherapy, chemotherapy, and prevention of second malignant tumors, is only beginning to be studied (27).

Surgical Recovery

The absence of chronic sympathetic stimulation produced by nicotine (e.g., increased heart rate, blood pressure, and platelet aggregation), and the improved oxygen-carrying capacity of the blood owing to reduced levels of carboxyhemoglobin, may decrease the risk of deep venous thrombosis, pulmonary embolism, and impaired wound healing following surgery (28–30). While it is recommended that patients stop smoking at least two months prior to surgery (31) to achieve maximal risk reduction, surgeons typically have only two weeks between diagnosis and treatment in which to insist upon cessation. Even this brief period of abstinence can result in a beneficial diminution of bronchial secretion, reducing postoperative complications and improving pulmonary rehabilitation (28) and surgical approaches to speech rehabilitation in head and neck cancer patients (32).

Radiotherapy

The outcome and side effects of radiation therapy for tumors of the aerodigestive tract can also be affected by smoking cessation in several ways. Head and neck cancer patients who smoke during radiotherapy experience lower response rates, poorer survival (33), and exacerbated side effects, including oral mucositis, loss of taste, and xerostomia. Long-term complications include soft-tissue and bone necrosis (34–36), and greater difficulty regaining satisfactory voice quality following treatment for laryngeal cancer (37). Interestingly, relative to surgically treated patients, head and neck cancer patients treated with primary radiotherapy may also be among the most difficult to treat behaviorally for smoking cessation, given the lesser level of physical impairment imposed by their cancer treatment (38). Smoking may also interfere with the radiation-induced early inflammatory connective-tissue reaction of the lung, and suppress the therapeutic ionizing radiation-induced tissue response among patients treated with radiation to the thorax, following breast conservation surgery (39). Finally, an elevated risk for lung cancer has been noted among smokers irradiated for Hodgkin's disease (40) or a primary breast cancer (41).

Chemotherapy

Long-term pulmonary toxicity (reduced capacity to expire carbon monoxide) has been reported for smokers treated with high-dose vs. low-dose combination chemotherapy for testicular cancer (42,43). In addition, the suppression of immune function which results from malignancy itself, or from treatment with corticosteroids, cytotoxic chemotherapy, or irradiation, may be exacerbated in smokers who, due to smoking alone, may be at greater risk for decreased natural killer cell activity and increased lymphocyte chromosomal abnormalities (44–46). Interestingly, suppression of immune function has also been related to symptoms of psychological depression (47), a factor which may add to the cessation difficulty of this group. Smokers with a history of depression (48) are more likely to be nicotine dependent, and those who experience relatively high levels of negative affect during cessation (dysphoria, tension, anxiety) may be least likely to quit (49,50).

Second Malignant Tumors (SMT) and Survival

It has been suggested that continued smoking following cancer diagnosis may increase a patient's risk of developing second malignant or primary tumors (SMT) or a recurrence of the disease. The connection between smoking and the development of further disease is plausible given the "field cancerization" concept (51), which posits that extensive cytologic changes (e.g., *p53* mutations) brought about by chronic tobacco exposure can lead to the development of multiple independent tumors (52–55). Studies supporting this hypothesis have shown that failure to quit after initial diagnosis of lung or head and neck cancer is associated with a higher risk of SMTs and a shorter survival time (56–62). Although such findings have not

been uniform (63–65), additional support for this concept is provided by the observation of dose-dependent relationships between smoking, SMTs, and survival. For example, male smokers diagnosed with laryngeal cancer showed relative risks for SMTs of the oral cavity and pharynx (24.5), esophagus (6.1), and lung (2.3) that were significantly elevated over those of the general population and proportional to their level of tobacco exposure (e.g., heavy smokers had higher risk than light smokers) (66). Among females, age-adjusted survival time following lung cancer diagnosis was significantly lower for those who have ever smoked (18 months) vs. nonsmokers (33 months) and inversely related to total cigarettes smoked per day and duration of smoking (67). Lower survival rates for smokers vs. nonsmokers at cancer diagnosis have also been reported for prostate (68), breast (69), and invasive cervical cancer (70). For breast cancer, survival decreases as a function of dose (cigarettes/day) and smoking duration (years) (69).

Thus, smoking cessation could substantially decrease the risk of SMTs and lengthen the duration of survival. For example, a fourfold increase in risk of developing second aerodigestive tract tumors was noted in current vs. former smokers diagnosed with an oral cancer. However, the risk of SMTs decreased after 5 years of smoking cessation (71). Further prospective studies of the effects of smoking cessation are needed for all the smoking-related cancers. Studies that evaluate both physical and psychosocial outcomes, as well as focusing on high-risk patient groups (e.g., those with premalignant lesions, known genetic vulnerabilities, or occupational exposures), would be particularly valuable.

SMOKING CESSATION TREATMENT EFFICACY

Smoking and Self-Quitting in the General Population

Adult smoking prevalence has decreased dramatically over the past 25 years, ranging from 42.4% in 1965 to approximately 25.0% in 1993, or about 48 million current smokers (58,72). Although about half the population of those who have ever smoked (90 million people) have already stopped smoking (72), the decline in smoking prevalence appears to have plateaued in recent years. As shown in Figure 3–1, the difficulty of smoking cessation is highlighted by the fact that 70% of current smokers report wanting to stop smoking completely, with 34% making a serious annual attempt at cessation (stop for at least one day). However, only 2.5% of all smokers actually succeed in being abstinent for a year (73).

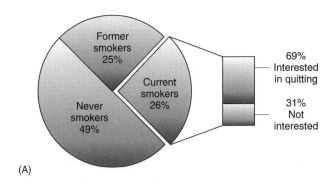

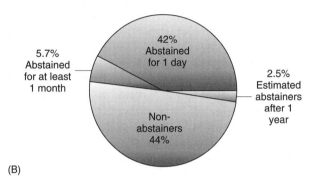

FIG. 3–1. (A) Percent never, current, and former smokers in the U.S. (1994) (adapted from the 1994 Supplement to the NHIS (NHIS-2000) (72)). (B) Levels of abstinence among U.S. smokers (1990–91) in the previous year (adapted from NHIS-HPDP (73)). Note in 1994, 46.4% of current everyday smokers reported abstaining for one day (72). The comparable figure for 1990 is 42.1% and is depicted in the lower figure.

Interestingly, the majority of former smokers (85%) report a preference for quitting on their own (74), using "cold turkey" (85%), gradual reduction (13%), or some other self-help approach to cessation. Only 15% report using assisted or more intensive treatments (e.g., physician's advice, counseling, nicotine replacement, etc.) to quit. These findings are consistent with the suggestion that most smokers are reluctant to take advantage of assisted forms of treatment (75).

However, the high prevalence of self-quitting among former smokers should not be interpreted as an endorsement for the effectiveness of a single unassisted cessation attempt. Such statistics most likely reflect the cumulative effect of multiple cessation attempts carried out over a period of several years (76). Preference for self-cessation methods is more likely attributable to their low cost (minimal to free) and ready access (e.g., widespread availability of self-help/public health materials), combined with the presence of psychosocial (e.g., poor recognition of difficulty of cessation and reluctance to ask for assistance) and economic (poor third-party reimbursement) barriers to assisted forms of treatment. Indeed, in a prospective evaluation of over 5000 self-quitters, continuous abstinence of only 4.3% was reported at the 1-year follow-up (77). Similarly, one-year continuous abstinence estimates of 1%–5% have also been reported in controlled studies of self-help materials (78–80).

It will be interesting to document the characteristics of smokers as the prevalence of smoking declines in the total population. It is possible that fewer smokers will succeed at self-quitting and that many of those who continue to smoke may comprise a difficult-to-treat constituency. For example, a high proportion of these smokers may have a history of major depression and/or problems with managing negative moods while quitting (i.e., dysphoria, depression, sadness, tension) (48). Such factors are inversely related to success of cessation (81–84). Indeed, the co-morbidity between smoking and depression (and other psychiatric disorders) has been observed as early as age 16 in national samples, suggesting that emotional impairment may be an influential factor in the cessation difficulty of future generations of smokers (85). Other factors which adversely influence cessation success in the clinic population, such as nicotine dependence (86,87), insufficient psychosocial support for quitting (88,89), and impaired coping skills and poor self-efficacy for cessation (90), could also become more widespread in the general population of smokers, as those with more psychological resources successfully quit on their own.

Thus, cessation approaches which fail to take these factors into account may be less effective than those that do. Traditional self-help interventions, while cheap and popular, are insufficient for managing such complex psychological and pharmacological treatment issues. Although more difficult to implement, assisted methods of intervention (i.e., counseling) target many of these constructs and typically result in higher abstinence rates on any one cessation attempt (50). If our hypotheses about the increased cessation difficulty experienced by present smokers are correct, then the next generation of population-based treatments may need to incorporate the more intensive cessation strategies previously reserved for the clinic if they are to meet the challenge posed by smokers who have fewer psychological resources. For example, this may involve greater use of nicotine replacement therapy and/or cognitive behavioral interventions.

CURRENT TREATMENT RECOMMENDATIONS

Synopsis of the AHCPR Smoking Cessation Guidelines

In 1996, the Agency for Health Care Policy and Research (AHCPR) and the Centers for Disease Control (CDC) convened a private panel to review the existing literature on smoking cessation and develop a set of guidelines for practicing clinicians, smoking cessation specialists, and health care administrators/insurers, to deliver and support effective smoking cessation interventions (91). Approximately 3000 smoking studies were reviewed, from which over 300 were selected for inclusion in the guidelines database and metaanalysis. Selected studies met the following inclusion criteria: randomized controlled trials of a smoking cessation interventions; follow-up cessation rates at least 5 months past the quit date; and publication between 1975 and 1994 in a peer-reviewed English-language journal. Using this database, the guideline panel reviewed the efficacy of various types and components of smoking cessation interventions, including provider screening for tobacco use and cessation advice; self-help, individual or group counseling methods; minimal, brief, and intensive behavioral intervention; intervention content; treatment duration, number of sessions; and provision of nicotine replacement therapy.

A brief overview of the panel's recommendations is presented below, and a summary of selected and salient comparisons from the AHCPR report are provided in Table 3.3.[1] The major recommendations of the guidelines, to all health care providers can be summarized as follows.

1. Effective smoking cessation treatments are available and every patient who smokes should be offered one or more of these treatments.
2. It is essential that clinicians determine and document the tobacco use status of every patient treated in a health care setting.
3. Brief cessation treatments are effective and at least a minimal intervention should be provided to every patient who uses tobacco.
4. A dose–response relationship exists between the intensity and duration of treatment and its effectiveness. In general, the more intense the intervention, the more effective it is in producing long-term abstinence from tobacco.

---

1. It should be noted that the panel's analysis was limited to those comparisons and recommendations for which sufficient and reliable data were available. Our summary highlights only those recommendations most relevant to cancer prevention and control.

5. Three treatment elements, in particular, are effective, and one or more of these elements should be included in smoking cessation treatment:
   (a) Nicotine replacement therapy (nicotine patches or gum).
   (b) Social support (clinician provided encouragement and assistance)
   (c) Skills training/problem solving (techniques on achieving and maintaining abstinence).
6. Effective reduction of tobacco use requires that health care systems make institutional changes that result in systematic identification of, and intervention with, all tobacco users at every visit.

The AHCPR guidelines have particular relevance to medical oncologists, surgeons, psychologists, nurses, dentists, health educators, social workers, etc. whose direct treatment of cancer patients as well as work in cancer prevention offers unique opportunities to intervene on the smoking behavior of their patients. The recommendations may serve as a starting point from which to implement smoking cessation programs and conduct future intervention research in cancer prevention.

Cessation Screening Advice and Providers

The AHCPR panel recommended that providers in primary care settings, which would include cancer screening and detection clinics, implement a systematic assessment to identify *all* smokers. Expanding the "vital signs" to include documentation of smoking status, for every patient at every visit, has been suggested for this purpose. The "four As" model of smoking cessation (Ask, Advise, Assist, Arrange) was recommended as a strategy to be used by primary care clinicians (92). The model includes strong personalized messages to encourage/motivate a quitting attempt; advice/information on preparing to quit and coping with withdrawal, making a commitment to abstinence; and arranging social support and follow-up. Referrals to other specialty providers are encouraged if desired by the smoker. Implementation of a smoking status screening system alone increases provider behavior (assessment of smoking status), but, as shown in Table 3.3 the direct involvement of physicians and other providers in smoking cessation intervention significantly enhances long-term abstinence. Indeed, the largest increment in success was observed after smokers were exposed to providers from multiple disciplines, (e.g., medicine, psychology, nursing).

TABLE 3.3. *Efficacy of Smoking Cessation Treatment Interventions and Components**

Intervention/Component	Reference Group	Estimated odds ratio (95% C.I.)†	Estimated cessation rate (95% C.I.)
SCREENING, ADVICE AND PROVIDERS			
System in place to identify smokers	No system	2.0 (0.8–4.8)	6.4 (1.3-11.6)
Physician advice to quit	No advice	1.3 (1.1–1.6)	10.2 (8.5–12.0)
Multiple Providers across disciplines	No provider	3.8 (2.6–5.6)	25.5 (18.1–32.7)
INTERVENTION FORMAT			
Self-help	No Contact	1.2 (0.97–1.6)	9.3 (7.3–11.4)
Individual Counseling	No Contact	2.2 (1.9–2.4)	15.1 (13.6–16.5)
Group Counseling	No Contact	2.2 (1.6–3.0)	15.3 (11.4–19.2)
INTENSITY LEVEL			
Minimal contact (≤3 min)	No contact/self-help	1.2 (1.0–1.5)	10.7 (8.9–12.5)
Brief Counseling (≥3 to10 min)	No contact/self-help	1.4 (1.2–1.7)	12.1 (10.0–14.3)
Counseling (> 10 min)	No contact/self-help	2.4 (2.1–2.7)	18.7 (16.8–20.6)
TREATMENT DURATION			
2 to < 4 weeks	< 2 weeks	1.6 (1.3–2.0)	5.6 (12.9–18.3)
4 to 8 weeks	< 2 weeks	1.6 (1.2–2.1)	16.1 (12.4–19.7)
> 8 weeks	< 2 weeks	2.7 (2.2–3.2)	23.8 (20.6–27.1)
TREATMENT FREQUENCY			
2–3 sessions	< 1 session	2.0 (1.6–2.4)	18.8 (15.8–21.9)
4–7 sessions	< 1 session	2.5 (2.2–2.9)	22.6 (19.9–25.3)
> 7 sessions	< 1 session	1.7 (1.2–2.5)	16.7 (11.4–22.0)
TREATMENT CONTENT			
Intratreatment social support	No contact	1.8 (1.4–2.5)	15.2 (11.3–19.1)
Problem solving/skills training	No contact	1.6 (1.4–2.5)	13.7 (10.3–17.1)
NICOTINE REPLACEMENT (see text)		OR range:	See text
Transdermal nicotine patch: 4 metaanalyses	Placebo	2.2–2.6	
Nicotine gum: 3 metaanalyses	Placebo/no gum	1.4–1.6 (1.4–1.8)	

*This table was adapted from the AHCPR Clinical Practice Guideline for Smoking Cessation (88).

†Only odds ratios with a 95% confidence interval that does not include 1.0 (reference) are significant at the 0.05 level.

INTERVENTION FORMAT

Self-Help, Individual, and Group Interventions

The panel noted that cessation rates attributed to different self-help modalities (e.g., books, manuals, audiotapes, community referral lists, pamphlets, etc.) did not appreciably differ from each other or from controls receiving no self-help material controls. A slight increase in cessation rates was noted for three studies providing telephone hotline support for *smoker*-initiated calls (odds ratio (OR) = 1.4 (1.1,1.8)), and in one study (OR = 1.9 (1.2, 2.9)) which combined several types of self-help materials. The panel recommended that phone call-in support be considered, if feasible, when establishing a self-help intervention program.

On the other hand, interventions that offer person-to-person contact (i.e., group or individual counseling) provide a substantial treatment advantage over self-help materials alone. As shown in Table 3.3, either individual or group counseling may be expected to double the cessation rates relative to no-contact controls. However, the analyses found no significant difference between the two counseling formats.

Patient–Provider Interaction Intensity, Duration, and Frequency

One of the most robust findings in the AHCPR review was the presence of a dose–response relationship between treatment efficacy, intensity, and duration of person–person (provider to patient) contact. As shown in Table 3.3, in comparison to self-help interventions, the more time providers spend (Intensity Level) with smokers in a treatment session, the higher the likelihood of cessation. The highest cessation rates were observed for provider counseling sessions lasting longer than 10 minutes,[2] but brief contact lasting 3–10 minutes, and even minimal contact lasting less than 3 minutes, progressively improved a smoker's chance of success over that of controls. In addition, both the duration of treatment in weeks and the number of treatment sessions improved the odds of cessation even after controlling for treatment intensity[3] (length of session). As shown in Table 3.3, significant improvements in cessation probability were observed for interventions involving 4–7 sessions carried out over an 8-week period or more.

Treatment Content

The panel also examined the efficacy of various treatment components. This analysis included 39 studies whose primary treatment content involved one or more of the following elements: aversive (rapid) smoking; setting a quit day; counseling for diet or motivation or exercise; contingency contracting; relaxation; cigarette (brand) fading; intra- or extra-treatment social support, and problem solving/skills training. The results indicated that cessation counseling, involving general problem solving/skills training (relapse prevention, stress management, etc.), and/or supportive care provided by the clinician within the treatment session, significantly raised cessation rates over no-contact controls (see Table 3.3).

Although analysis of the individual components was problematic (e.g., some strategies were not well isolated and conceptually similar treatments varied in implementation by investigator), two broad treatment approaches—problem solving/skills training and social support—emerged as the most efficacious among those reviewed. The problem solving/treatment skills component consisted of such counseling elements as the recognition of high-risk situations (e.g., being around other smokers, alcohol consumption); enhancement of coping skills designed to alter or ameliorate risk of relapse (e.g., use of distraction, avoidance and planning for unanticipated events); countering negative mood with stress reduction and reinforcement enhancement strategies; and basic information about smoking and successful quitting (e.g., nature and course of withdrawal, the addictive aspects of smoking,

etc.). The social support treatment component referred to provider behavior that encouraged the patient to quit, by communicating belief in the patient's ability, providing basic information about withdrawal, showing concern and a willingness to help the patient, and providing opportunities to discuss cessation difficulties (such as feelings of ambivalence, or fears of quitting) and accomplishments (such as successful urge resistance).

In conclusion, the AHCPR guidelines provide substantial evidence that dividends in cessation success may be expected with interventions which last relatively longer, involve more clinical contact, and provide increasing levels of problem solving/skills training and social support. The benefits of increased counseling time are apparent even at the lower levels of treatment contact (3–10 min) and are suggestive for brief contact (< 3 minutes) as well, but are markedly greater at the upper level of treatment intensity (> 10 minutes). It is recommended that counseling focus on problem solving skills and social support and last as many weeks as feasible given available resources (the longer the better), but clinicians should strive to meet with quitting smokers on at least four occasions (presumably per quit attempt).

Nicotine Replacement Therapy (NRT)

The AHCPR panel also reviewed the results of five metaanalyses on the efficacy of the transdermal nicotine patch, and three analyses focusing on nicotine gum. It was concluded that all smokers should be encouraged to use the nicotine patch or gum for smoking cessation, except in the presence of special circumstances (i.e., need for abstinence from all sources of nicotine).

Transdermal nicotine (TN) has been shown to be an effective form of treatment that significantly improves cessation rates across diverse settings and populations. Use of TN approximately doubles 6- to 12-month cessation rates over that of a comparable placebo regardless of the intensity of the associated psychosocial intervention; that is, *relative* treatment differences between patch and placebo are unaffected by the intensity of the psychological intervention with which it is paired. This is true even when the patch is provided alone or paired with a low-intensity behavioral intervention. However, *absolute* cessation rates observed with the active patch are enhanced when it is used in conjunction with more vs. less intense psychological interventions. For example, mean cessation rates reported for the active patch plus high vs. low intensity psychological interventions (93) were 41.5% (37.6%–45.4%) vs. 22.8% (21%–24.7%) at the end of treat-

---

2. Studies in this group also included ones with sessions lasting 20–30 minutes.

3. These factors are often interrelated, i.e., more intense interventions are given more often and over longer periods of time.

ment (EOT); and 26.5% (26.5%–30.6%) vs. 19.5% (17.2%–22.1%) at 6 months after the quit date.

The metaanalyses for the nicotine gum studies produced similar results. The gum appears to improve 12-month cessation rates by 40%–60% compared with control interventions. However, the effect sizes for gum vs. placebo or no-gum conditions were higher when administered with more vs. less intensive psychological therapy. One analysis showed no difference in 1-year abstinence rates for gum vs. control conditions when each were combined with a brief behavioral intervention (94). Thus, unlike the patch, the gum may be less effective when only minimal forms of psychological intervention are used but, similarly to the patch, cessation rates are likely to improve with increasing intensity of adjuvant therapy.

Studies using the 2 mg and 4 mg forms of the nicotine gum were also reviewed. It was noted that the 4 mg gum was more effective with heavier smokers (>20/day), while the 2 mg gum seemed efficacious with lighter smokers. For either dose, noncompliance with chewing frequency and use duration reduced the effectiveness of the gum. Although compliance improves with concurrent psychological therapy, the nicotine patch may still be preferred to the gum, given its ease of use and consistent nicotine dosing.

Nicotine Replacement Update

Studies of NRT published since work on the AHCPR guidelines concluded have addressed several additional treatment issues. These include TN use in the general population; its dose effects, and interactions with other treatment variables; repeated use of TN following relapse; long-term use of nicotine gum; efficacy of new forms of NRT, such as nicotine nasal spray and inhalers; and results of clinical trials combining patch and gum use. Results of these studies are summarized below.

Nicotine Replacement in the General Population

While the efficacy of the nicotine patch seems well established in clinical trials, there has been limited experience with its use in the general population of smokers. The FDA has approved transdermal nicotine replacement for over-the-counter (OTC) distribution in late 1996, and studies which focus on its use outside of the clinical setting are most important. For example, the 1993 California Tobacco Survey (95) was conducted in the first year after the patch became available by prescription and has provided initial information on patch effectiveness for a large sample of current and former smokers (who had quit within the previous year). The results showed that 11% of those who made a cessation attempt in the previous year had tried the patch. Among patch users, a 15.8% abstinence rate was observed 1 year after their cessation attempt, which was significantly higher than the 7.1% rate observed for patch nonusers. The majority (91.2%) of patch users who relapsed used the patch for less than 2 months and relapsed either before (35.4%) or simultaneous (42.7%) with discontinuation of the patch. Only 12.6% of the relapsers sustained abstinence 1 month after stopping transdermal nicotine. Univariate logistic regression showed that patch users were significantly more likely to be female, Caucasian, older (45–64 years) and better-educated smokers, who smoked heavily and were motivated to quit. Among smokers who received other forms of assistance in their cessation attempt—physician advice, self-help materials, counseling, etc.—the addition of TN significantly enhanced treatment outcome. One-year abstinence rates of 18% were noted for those receiving the patch vs. 10.9% for those who did not. However, patch use did not improve cessation rates among smokers receiving no additional assistance: 15.4% vs. 14% 6-month abstinence rates were observed with and without the patch, respectively.

These figures must be interpreted with caution, however, given the bias created by patient self-selection into patch vs. no-patch treatments and the lack of comparability between use of the term "assistance" as defined in the 1993 survey and in the clinical trial literature. In the survey, assistance included self-help materials, advice, or counseling. In clinical studies, these categories refer to three distinct areas of behavioral intervention. In addition, the survey reflected patch use in only one area of the country and was conducted in just the first year following the commercial availability of the patch. Observations of TN use made a year later show higher rates of smoker use (19%) (96) and higher rates of long-term abstinence (23.4%–29%) (89,94). TN use will undoubtably increase with the OTC availability of the patch.

Even with these caveats in mind, the increase in the cessation rates attributable to the patch plus assistance found in the 1993 survey is in clear agreement with the AHCPR findings described above. However, the absence of a patch effect when no assistance is provided is at variance with the AHCPR review, since a modest increase in cessation rates is expected with the patch even when no concomitant therapy is provided. It would be important to clarify this finding in future population studies, since many smokers may try the patch once it becomes available OTC, but they may be less inclined to avail themselves of additional treatment.

Dose Effects, Interactions, and the Cessation Process Using TN

The TN studies reviewed in the AHCPR guideline provided a maximum dose of 22 mg/day (mean levels about 9–17 ng/ml), which yields an average 54%–69% replacement of baseline nicotine (97). Recently, the efficacy of a higher dose patch preparation (44 mg/day) was compared to the 22 mg and 11 mg patches in a physician/nurse counseling smoking cessation program (98). The 44 mg nicotine patch produced a higher percentage of cotinine replacement (99% of baseline for subjects smoking 40 cigarettes/day) and more withdrawal symptom relief, and was found to be safe for heavy smokers (> 30 cigarettes/day). However, no differences were found in 6–12-month abstinence rates across the three doses.

Recently, both the dose of the patch and the intensity of behavioral counseling (99) were varied in a randomized trial of 504 smokers assigned to receive either the 44 mg (high) or 22 mg (low) patches, and either a self-help, physician/nurse individual intervention, or behavioral group counseling condition. One month after the quit date, high-dose patch users were abstinent significantly more often than low-dose users (67% vs. 60%) though they experienced significantly more side effects. Physician/nurse (66%) and group counseling methods (68%) were associated with higher abstinence rates than the self-help intervention (56%), although the self-help treatment was more effective with the high-dose (68%) vs. low-dose (44%) patch. None of these treatment differences were maintained at the 6-month follow-up. Abstinence for all conditions ranged from 25% to 34%. Although these figures are within the range of abstinence expected for the patch plus counseling (> three visits) conditions, the lack of an effect due to counseling intensity is at variance with earlier findings (100). This could be due to in part to problems in the implementation of the intervention, and/or to artificially high abstinence rates in the (control) condition.

There also appears to be a beneficial effect of combining transdermal nicotine replacement and intensive psychological treatment on the mediating behaviors targeted by the behavioral intervention to increase smoking cessation. For example, in a study comparing smokers treated with the nicotine patch plus behavioral group counseling (BTP) to those receiving the behavioral counseling alone (BT), as expected abstinence rates were significantly higher in the BTP vs. BT group at the EOT (79% vs. 63%) and 3-month follow-up (p < 0.01), though effects weakened 6 months after cessation (39% vs. 22%) (101). However, in addition to an anticipated reduction in nicotine withdrawal symptoms due to use of the patch, less emotional distress was observed among the BTP group, along with an increased level of coping behavior and attenuating concomitant rise in self-efficacy. Thus, TN seemed to enhance the effectiveness of counseling, by reducing symptoms of negative affect and improving the effectiveness of coping behavior.

Dose Effects of Nicotine Gum and Self-Help Intervention

Both the 2 mg and 4 mg gum preparations are now available OTC and, as suggested by the guideline review and subsequent study, the 4 mg may be more effective than the 2 mg gum for highly dependent smokers (91,102). Manipulation of dose by instructing patients to chew more of the 2 mg gum does not seem to enhance treatment efficacy (103), while instructions to chew the gum on a fixed schedule (1 per hour) improves abstinence over ad lib administration (104). Interestingly, a similar advantage for smoking cigarettes on a fixed schedule, prior to cessation, has also been noted. This finding is discussed in more detail later in this chapter.

While it appears from the clinical data reviewed by the AHCPR panel that the effectiveness of nicotine gum may be dependent on at least brief behavioral support, a recent study combining self-help materials and nicotine gum suggests that in highly motivated smokers the gum may be effective even when no other behavioral support is provided. Significant differences in 6-month abstinence rates were noted for gum vs. no gum conditions (21% vs. 16%), but self-help materials added little to the effects of the gum alone (105). These findings are at odds with previous reviews (94), but seem readily attributable to high abstinence in the control condition (20%). This study was unusual in the sense that strong financial incentives were provided for cessation ($100 at 6 months) and only smokers who could achieve 24 hours of abstinence were entered into the trial. Such measures are not typical in the clinical trials literature.

Treatment Recycling and Long-term Use of NRT

The studies of NRT reviewed by the AHCPR have typically followed patients 6–12 months after treatment, with no information being provided regarding the future cessation success of those who failed in their initial quit attempt. However, in one study conducted subsequent to the review, relapsers from an earlier clinical trial of TN and behavioral counseling were provided with a second round of TN treatment, similar to the earlier intervention (106). The results showed that the active patch outperformed the placebo, but cessation rates at the 6-month follow-up were minimal (6.3% active vs. 2.5% placebo). The repeated treatment occurred 6–12 months after the initial failure, and it was unclear whether higher abstinence rates might have been obtained had the second attempt been made shortly after relapse.

Another strategy for sustaining abstinence has been the extended use of nicotine replacement, within a single cessation attempt. Although this has not been studied systematically for the patch, most studies report that smokers use the patch for less than the 8–12 weeks recommended by the manufacturers. In the case of the gum, however, up to 20% of successful abstainers report continued use for a year or more after their quit date (107). Concerns about terminating gum use among successful abstainers after 6 months of use were addressed in a recent study, and revealed that gum use could be abruptly stopped or tapered/without promoting relapse (98).

Summary. Studies that vary the dose of NRT suggest that in the case of TN abstinence is unlikely to improve with a higher patch dose (44 vs. 22 mg), though side effects may increase substantially. However, the 4 mg dose of nicotine gum may be more effective than 2 mg, especially for heavier smokers, with little increase in adverse reactions observed. The dose–effect does not seem attainable simply by chewing more of the 2 mg gum, though some advantage may be observed when the gum is used on a fixed schedule of time. Studies examining the effects of NRT and behavioral intervention have also generally shown little or no improvement in efficacy when the gum is administered without a minimal level of behavioral treatment, while the patch appears effective even with brief behavioral support. Absolute differences in abstinence have been noted when gum or patch is paired with increasing levels of counseling intensity, although the results of two recent studies have run counter to these expectations. Studies on the long-term use of gum by abstainers and repeated exposure to TN among relapsers show no effects on relapse due to stopping the gum after 6 months of use and significant, albeit small, increases in abstinence have been observed after a second trial of TN within 6–12 months of relapse from a previous cessation attempt. Finally, treatment with the nicotine patch may also produce a favorable influence on negative affect and coping

behavior above that which can be expected from the behavioral treatment alone.

Combined Patch and Gum Use

Recent studies by Kornitzer (108) and Puska (109) have evaluated the combined use of transdermal nicotine and nicotine gum, and suggested that use of both types of NRT may be more effective than either alone, but only within 12–24 weeks of combined therapy. Kornitzer compared continuous abstinence rates associated with patch plus gum (P + G), patch plus placebo gum (P + PG) and placebo patch + placebo gum (PP + PG), in 374 smokers receiving a 24-week step-down dose regimen of transdermal nicotine (15/10/5 mg/day) plus ad libitum nicotine gum. Odds ratios in favor of the P + G vs. P + PG treatment, were significant at week 24 (27.5% vs. 15.3%) but not at week 52 (18.1% vs. 12.7%) six months after the treatment concluded. No significant differences were observed in the PP + PG vs. P + PG comparison, producing the unusual finding of no active vs. placebo patch difference (15.7% vs. 14.7% at week 24) among those receiving concurrent placebo gum. Although the authors report no significant differences in gum and patch use between the groups, only about half the subjects used the patch on a daily basis and considerable variability was also observed for daily use of the gum (0–16 pieces per day). The lack of a patch effect among placebo gum users is inconsistent with the doubling of abstinence rates reported earlier for the patch (91). The most likely explanation is the unusually high abstinence rate (13.3%) observed for the patch/gum placebo condition at week 52, which may be attributed to the systematic, yet poorly documented, effects of provider intervention (i.e., the study was conducted in multiple worksites by occupational physicians and nurses who met with subjects individually and contacted them by phone).

The study by Puska compared the effectiveness of brief cessation advice by public health nurses, plus either the patch plus ad lib gum (P + G) or placebo patch plus gum (PP + G), in 10 health centers in North Karelia. Step-down patch dosing and ad lib gum use regimens were implemented for 18 weeks, similar to the Kornitzer study. Significant differences in abstinence were observed in favor of the combined treatments through the twelfth week of treatment (39.3% vs. 28%) but not at the 1-year follow-up (24% vs. 17%).

Nicotine Nasal Spray and Inhaler

Schneider (110) studied the effects of a new type of NRT, the nicotine nasal spray (NNS), on 225 smokers randomized to active or placebo treatment. Patients were instructed to administer one spray per nostril (1 ng nicotine total), in response to smoking urges and were provided with a self-help booklet for smoking cessation. Continuous, "no-slip" abstinence rates for the NNS and placebo groups, respectively, were 43% vs. 20% at week 6; and 18% vs. 8% at 1 year. Attrition and side effects were very high: drop-out by day 2 of this study averaged 25% and 40% for the NSS and placebo groups, respectively, and the vast majority of participants experienced throat, nose, and eye irritation resulting from either active or placebo nasal spray.

The nicotine inhaler is another new nicotine replacement device, which delivers 13 ng nicotine per puff, although it takes about 80 puffs to achieve the full dose of nicotine available in most cigarettes. One-year abstinence rates of 15.2% vs. 5.0% have been reported (111) for active vs. placebo inhalers in one controlled trial, which also used brief behavioral support. Coughing and throat irritation were the most common side effects of the inhaler device.

Summary. It is too early to tell what the proper place of NNS and the inhaler will be in the NRT armamentarium. Presently, the NNS is an FDA-approved device but the inhaler is not. Overall abstinence rates relative to placebo are significantly different for both devices and are comparable to the lower range of abstinence expected with either the patch or gum, plus minimal or no behavioral intervention. However, side effects and attrition are considerably greater. It has been suggested that acute administration of nicotine via spray or inhaler could help prevent relapse or promote recovery from a slip, but data on such events are lacking. Smoker-controlled (contingent) administration of nicotine, that is, gradually reducing cigarettes while trying to quit, seems to attenuate the development of effective coping strategies (112), whereas, noncontingent use (i.e., smoking on a fixed schedule prior to quitting) does not. It is unclear whether such drawbacks would arise from the contingent use of NNS or the inhaler (i.e., when used on demand), but it seems plausible for NNS, since it produces a blood nicotine profile, and CNS effects, similar to that of smoking a cigarette (113).

Self-Selection of NRT

In an interesting study of patient treatment selection, smokers were randomly assigned to either gum, patch, nasal spray, inhaler or nicotine lozenges conditions, or to a condition in which they were free to select their own form of nicotine replacement through a process of

trial and error (114). This study is quite unusual because all subjects were medically ill but indicated an unwillingness to quit smoking completely. Thus, smokers were instructed to use as much NRT as they wished yet to smoke as much as needed to "feel comfortable." No change in abstinence was reported. However, cigarette intake decreased significantly in the free-choice group only, and 93% of the these smokers reported an increased motivation to quit. Perhaps self-directed exposure to NRT may enhance cessation motivation; however, such results are meaningful only if future cessation behavior is affected.

In conclusion, there seems to be little reason to vary from the AHCPR recommendation for use of the nicotine patch or gum as the preferred methods of nicotine replacement, for combining these approaches with as much problem solving/coping skills training and provider initiated emotional support as feasible. New studies suggest that combined patch and gum use may have promise, particularly in the control of early withdrawal symptoms. This may be an especially important focus in future interventions, since forestalling any experimentation with smoking in the early days of abstinence may enhance the smokers' chances of achieving long-term abstinence (115). Studies on the effectiveness of other forms of NRT, such as the NNS and the inhaler, have recently begun, but their place in the NRT approach to cessation is unclear. Problems with side effects, attrition, and the possibility that contingent use of a smoking-like burst of self-administered nicotine may reduce behavioral coping efficacy, require further study. Interestingly, exposing unmotivated smokers to all forms NRT seems to improve their cessation motivation, but the effects on future cessation behavior remain unrealized.

SELF-HELP AND BEHAVIORAL TREATMENT UPDATE

Self-Help

As discussed in the AHCPR review section, the effects of traditional self-help interventions for smoking cessation—pamphlets, manuals, etc.—have been quite limited. Recently, however, favorable cessation effects have been noted with a new type of self-help intervention, described as personalized or tailored feedback. This method incorporates information provided by the subject on certain aspects of their smoking behavior, (readiness to quit, barriers to cessations etc.) into specific written or counselor-delivered suggestions for behavior change. For example, in a study of family practice patients, volunteer smokers were provided with either computer-generated and tailored letters focused on motivational and behavioral strategies for cessation, nontailored general health education letters, or no-letters at all. Relative to the education and no letter control conditions (7.3%), the effects of tailoring on 6-month abstinence rates (19.1%–30.7%) were significant, but only among moderate to light smokers (116). In a similar study, nonvolunteer smokers within a health maintenance organization (HMO) were provided with either a traditional self-help manual; a self-help manual plus letters tailored to their motivation to quit, self-efficacy, and stage of change; or both the manual and the letters plus *provider*-initiated telephone counseling. The 3-month outcome for this largely unmotivated group of smokers showed that only the combination of all three procedures resulted in higher quit rates than self-help alone, and that these effects were significant only for precontemplators (9% vs. 3%) (117). However, in a study of community volunteers, who were presumably more motivated to quit, abstinence rates were highest for both tailored letters alone and those who received tailored letters plus telephone counseling, in comparison to those who were provided with only a self-help manual (118).

In addition to its use with tailored approaches to cessation, the use of telephone counseling alone has generated substantial interest in the treatment community. Phone intervention may have several advantages over traditional treatment modalities, including its relatively low cost, personalized nature, and ease of access for most smokers. A recent study compared the efficacy of self-help materials alone either to a single telephone counseling session, or to multiple counseling sessions scheduled early in the cessation process (119). Results indicated that both single (7.5%) and multiple (9.9%) phone counseling conditions produced significantly higher abstinence rates at the 12-month follow-up, in contrast to the self-help (5.4%) intervention alone. A dose–response relationship was observed between the number of counseling sessions and 12-month continuous abstinence rates, suggesting that an increment in abstinence might be expected as additional phone sessions are provided. Multisession telephone counseling was effective in reducing relapse rates, and the delivery of the intervention during the first week after quitting was found to be essential.

The results of these studies suggest that personalized feedback may be a promising addition to self-help smoking cessation aids. However, for some smokers, especially the less motivated ones, the personal contact of telephone counseling may be required to sufficiently make use of the tailored information. Provider-initiated phone counseling, applied early in the cessation process and on multiple occasions, appears to provide significant reduction in the risk of relapse among those who actually make a cessation attempt and to enhance long-term abstinence rates, albeit such differences are small. Future configurations of telephone counseling intervention may enhance the AHCRP-recommended focus on problem solving/skills and social support, and incorporate other proactive treatments in the early days of cessation, e.g., NRT.

Other Behavioral Interventions—Scheduled Smoking

As discussed above, gradual reduction and abrupt (cold turkey) cessation methods are used by the vast majority of self-quitters in their cessation attempts (74). Alhough they are popular, little direct research has been done to evaluate these common approaches to cessation. Some of our most popular self-help manuals (79,80,120,121) advise people to "gradually cut down on their own" and most studies require abrupt cessation prior to initiation of NRT. However, we recently examined the efficacy of these approaches by instructing smokers to smoke for three weeks prior to a target date using one of the following schedules: a fixed time schedule and progressively longer intercigarette intervals; a fixed schedule with no increase in the intercigarete cigarette intervals; smoker-controlled gradual reduction in total daily frequency; or no controlled variation in frequency or intercigarete interval (cold turkey). Abstinence rates at 1 year posttreatment were 44%, 32%, 18%, and 22% for the four groups, respectively, indicating that both types of scheduled smoking (with and without reductions in intercigarette interval) outperformed traditional methods of a gradual reduction and cold turkey cessation. Significant reduction in symptoms of negative affect, nicotine withdrawal, and urges to smoke were also observed with scheduled smoking, with related improvements in coping behavior. This suggests that progressively longer but tolerable delays in smoking may facilitate coping and reduce the reinforcing properties of cigarette smoking (112).

Cessation with Cancer Patients

Although we have limited experience with smoking cessation interventions in cancer patients or a high-risk population, the smoking cessation studies described thus far have provided a wealth of data examining treatment efficacy, vulnerability to relapse, psychopharmacological issues, and important subject characteristics of successful and unsuccessful abstainers. It seems reasonable to assume that many factors related to the smoking behavior of noncancer patients will apply equally to cancer patients or to smokers at high risk for cancer (genetically susceptible/environmentally exposed). The content of the intervention and the specific motivational or supportive aspects of treatment may vary, however, in order to account for specific factors unique to the patient's disease or circumstance.

For example, high self-quit rates have been reported in retrospective analysis of lung cancer survivors (52%) (122), while somewhat lower rates (40%) have been reported in prospective studies when patients receive no formal intervention (123). Among head and neck cancer patients treated with surgical intervention, self-quit rates of 65% were reported 3–15 months after surgery (124). Interestingly, those who continued smoking were less likely to have received postoperative radiotherapy; to have had less extensive disease; to have had disease of the oral cavity; and to be better educated. This last point is at variance with population studies in which lower education is related to smoking prevalence (1).

These studies point to the opportunity both to achieve high quit rates in a cancer patient population and to better understand the specific factors of treatment related to either sustained abstinence or relapse. Many smoking cessation programs designed for the general population have focused on specific techniques for preventing relapse, but application of these principles to a cancer patient population has begun only recently. For example, one prospective randomized clinical trial of a smoking cessation program tailored to head and neck patients evaluated limited vs. extensive physician intervention (27). It showed that, unlike the general population of these, many smokers were highly dependent, long-time users who seemed motivated to quit and expressed high levels of self-efficacy. Overall, 1-year continuous abstinence rates for smokers completing this trial were high (64.6%) (38). Although both levels of physician intervention were equally effective, those treated with primary radiotherapy showed 12-month continuous abstinence rates of 36%, while those experiencing total laryngectomy or other surgical procedures evidenced abstinence rates of 87% and 68.8%, respectively. Presumably, the surgical patients experienced a period of rigidly enforced abstinence prior to and during their hospitalization and were limited in relapse potential by the physical barriers imposed by their surgery. Primary radiation, on the other hand provided less extensive barriers to continued smoking. Interestingly, as indicated above, surgery followed by radiotherapy has also been associated with a decreased probability of relapse (124).

For patients with early stage disease or genetically susceptible to cancer, techniques adapted from the clinical trials literature may also be used, for example, motivational interviewing, NRT, personalized feedback, affect management, or scheduled smoking. Surprisingly, there is little clinical research with these groups. At present, however, it may be important to focus on risk information and motivational enhancement with this population, as well as on providing extensive smoking cessation intervention. For example, personalized risk information involving the CYP2D6 genotype (a biomarker related to lung cancer susceptibility) has been associated with increased ratings of fear, perceived vulnerability to lung cancer, perceived health benefits of quitting smoking, and advanced stage of readiness to quit. However, the feedback alone seems insufficient for producing cessation (125). Although we may apply specific motivational/psychological strategies to meet the needs of a cancer patient population, we must also make use of reliable cessation methods and not rely exclusively on the motivational enhancements provided by the cancer treatment setting.

ACKNOWLEDGMENTS

Special thanks go to Ms. Deborah K. Watkins for technical support on the manuscript.

REFERENCES

1. *Reducing the Health Consequences of Smoking: 25 Years of Progress.* A Report of the Surgeon General. U.S. Washington, D.C.: Department of Health and Human Services, Public Health Service, Centers for Disease Control, Centers for Chronic Disease Prevention and Health Promotion, Office on Smoking and Health; 1989.
2. *Centers for Disease Control. Smoking-attributable Mortality and Years of Potential Life Lost—United States, 1988.* Centers for Disease Control; 1991.
3. U.S. Department of Health and Human Services. *The Health Consequences of Smoking: Cancer.* A Report of the Surgeon General. U.S. Washington, D.C.: Department of Health and Human Services, Public Health Service, Centers for Disease Control, Centers for Chronic Disease Prevention and Health Promotion, Office on Smoking and Health; 1982.
4. Garfinkel L. Probability of Developing or Dying of Cancer, United States, 1991. *Stat* 1995:31–37.
5. Thun MJ, Day-Lally C, Myers DG. Trends in tobacco smoking and mortality from cigarette use in cancer prevention studies I (1959–1965) and II (1982–1988). *Am J Public Health.* 1995;85:1223–1229. (Changes in Cigarette-Related Disease Risks and Their Implication for Prevention and Control. Washington, D.C.: National Institutes of Health.)
6. Thun MJ, Day-Lally CA, Calle EE, Flanders WD, Heath CW. Excess mortality among cigarette smokers:

Changes in a 20-year interval. *Am J Public Health.* 1995;85:1223–1230.

7. Howe GR, Jain M, Burch JD, Miller AB. Cigarette smoking and cancer of the pancreas: evidence from a population-based case-control study in Toronto, Canada. *Int J Cancer.* 1991;47:323–328.

8. McLaughlin JK, Hrubec Z, Heineman EF, Blot WJ, Fraumeni JF. Smoking and cancer mortality among U.S. veterans: A 26-year follow-up. *Int J Cancer.* 1990;105:190–193.

9. Whitmore WF Jr. The treatment of invasive cancers of the bladder. *J Urol.* 1988;94:337–343.

10. Mills PK, Newell GR, Beeson WL, Fraser GE, Phillips RL. History of cigarette smoking and risk of leukemia and myeloma: results from the Adventist health study. *J Natl Cancer Inst.* 1990;82:1832–1836.

11. National Institutes of Health NCI. *Respiratory health effects of passive smoking: Lung cancer and other disorders, smoking and tobacco control.* Monograph 4; 1993.

12. Boring CC, Squires TS, Tong T. Cancer statistics. *CA Cancer J Clin.* 1993;43:7–26.

13. U.S. Department of Health and Human Services. *Strategies to Control Tobacco Use in the United States.* A Report of the Surgeon General. Washington D.C.: U.S. Department of Health and Human Services, Public Health Service, Centers for Disease Control, Centers for Chronic Disease Prevention and Health Promotion, Office on Smoking and Health; 1991.

14. U.S. Department of Health and Human Services. *Preventing Tobacco Use Among Young People.* A Report of the Surgeon General. Washington D.C.: U.S. Department of Health and Human Services, Public Health Service, Centers for Disease Control, Centers for Chronic Disease Prevention and Health Promotion, Office on Smoking and Health; 1994.

15. Fiore MC, Novotny TE, Pierce JP, Hatziandren EJ, Patel KM, Davis RM. Trends in cigarette smoking in the United States. The changing influence of gender and race. *J Am Med Assoc.* 1989;261:49–55.

16. Devesa SS, Bolt WJ, Fraumeni JF Jr. Declining lung cancer rates among young men and women in the United States. A cohort analysis. *J Nat Cancer Inst.* 1989;81:1568–1571.

17. U.S. Department of Health and Human Services. *The Health Benefits of Smoking Cessation.* A Report of The Surgeon General. Washington, D.C.: U.S. Department of Health and Human Services, Public Health Service, Centers for Disease Control, Centers for Chronic Disease Prevention and Health Promotion, Office on Smoking and Health; 1990.

18. Alavanja MCR, Brownson RC, Benichou J, Swanson C, Boice JD. Attributable risk of lung cancer in lifetime nonsmokers and long-term ex-smokers (Missouri, United States). *Cancer Causes Control.* 1995;6:209–216.

19. Gritz ER, Nielsen IR, Brooks LA. Smoking cessation and gender: the influence of physiological, psychological, and behavioral factors. *J Am Med Women's Assoc.* 1996;51:35–42.

20. Macfarlane GJ, Zheng T, Marshall JR, et al. Alcohol, tobacco, diet and the risk of oral cancer—a pooled analysis of three case-control studies. *Eur J Cancer Part B, Oral Oncol.* 1995;31B:181–187.

21. Kabat GC, Chee JC, Wynder EL. The role of tobacco, alcohol use, and body mass index in oral and pharyngeal cancer. *Int J Epidemiol.* 1994;23:1137–1144.

22. Ji BT, Chow WH, Mclaughlin DQ, et al. Cigarette smoking and alcohol consumption and the risk of pancreatic cancer —a case-control study in Shanghai, China. *Cancer Causes Control.* 1995;6:369–376.

23. Vineis P, Bartsch H, Caporaso N, et al. Genetically based *N*-acetyltransferase metabolic polymorphism and low-level environmental exposure to carcinogens. *Nature.* 1994;369:154–156.

24. Mooney LA, Santella LC, Jeffrey AM, et al. Decline of DNA damage and other biomarkers in peripheral blood following smoking cessation. *Cancer Epidemiol Biomarkers Prev.* 1995;4:627–634.

25. Vineis P. The use of biomarkers in epidemiology: the example of bladder cancer. *Toxicol. Lett.* 1992;64/65:463–467.

26. American Cancer Society. *Cancer Facts and Figures.* Atlanta: American Cancer Society; 1996.

27. Gritz ER, Carr CR, Rapkin DA, Chang C, Beumer J, Ward PH. A smoking cessation intervention for head and neck cancer patients: trial design, patient accrual, and characteristics. *Cancer Epidemiol Biomarkers Prev.* 1991;1:67–73.

28. Benowitz NL. Pharmacologic aspects of cigarette smoking and nicotine addiction. *N Engl J Med.* 1988;319:1318–1330.

29. Dresler CM, Roper C, Patterson GA, Cooper JD. Effect of physician advice on smoking cessation in patients undergoing thoracotomy. *ABS Chest.* 1993;104:18S.

30. U.S. Department of Health and Human Services. *The Health Consequences of Smoking: Nicotine Addiction,* A Report of the Surgeon General. Washington, D.C.: U.S. Department of Health and Human Services, Public Health Service, Centers for Disease Control, Centers for Chronic Disease Prevention and Health Promotion, Office on Smoking and Health; 1988.

31. Warner MA, Kenneth PO, Warner ME, Lennon RL, Conover A, Jansson-Schumacher U. Role of preoperative cessation of smoking and other factors in postoperative pulmonary complication: a blinded prospective study of coronary artery bypass patients. *Mayo Clin Proc.* 1989;64:609–619.

32. Ariyan S (ed.). *Cancer of the Head and Neck.* St. Louis: C.V. Mosby; 1987.

33. Browman GP, Wong G, Hodson I, et al. Influence of cigarette smoking on the efficacy of radiation therapy in head and neck cancer. *N Engl J Med.* 1993;328:159–163.

34. Million RR, Cassisi NJ. *Management of Head and Neck Cancer: A Multidisciplinary Approach.* Philadelphia: J.B. Lippincott; 1984.

35. Wang CC. *Radiation Therapy for Head and Neck Neoplasms: Indications, Techniques, and Results.* Chicago: Year Book Medical Publishers; 1990.

36. Whittet HB, Lund JV, Brockbank M, Feyerbend C. Serum cotinine as an objective marker for smoking habit in head and neck malignancy. *J Laryngol Otol.* 1991;105:1036–1039.

37. Karim AB, Snow GB, Siek HT, Njo KH. The quality of voice in patients irradiated for laryngeal carcinoma. *Cancer.* 1983;51:47–49.

38. Gritz ER, Carr CR, Rapkin D, et al. Predictors of long-term smoking cessation in head and neck cancer patients. *Cancer Epidemiol Biomarkers Prev.* 1993;2:261–270.

39. Bjermer L, Franzen L, Littbrand B, Nilsson K, Angstrom T, Henriksson R. Effects of smoking and irradiated volume on inflammatory response in the lung of irradiated breast cancer patients evaluated with bronchoalveolar lavage. *Cancer Res.* 1991;50:2027–2030.

40. Tucker MA, Coleman CN, Cox RS, Varghese A, Rosenberg SA. Risk of second cancers after treatment for Hodgkin's disease. *N Engl J Med.* 1988;318:76–80.

41. Neugut AI, Murray T, Santos J, et al. Increased risk of lung cancer after breast cancer radiation therapy in cigarette smokers. *Cancer.* 1994;73:1615–1620.

42. Hansen SW, Groth S, Sorensen PG, Rossing N, Rorth M. Enhanced pulmonary toxicity in smokers with germ-cell cancer treated with cis-platinum, vinblastine and bleomycin: a long-term follow-up. *Eur J Cancer Clin Oncol.* 1989;25:733–736.

43. Lehne G, Johansen B, Fossa SD. Long-term follow-up of pulmonary function in patients cured from testicular cancer with combination chemotherapy including bleomycin. *Br J Cancer.* 1993;68:555–558.

44. Ghosh R, Ghosh PK. The effect of tobacco on the frequency of sister chromatid exchanges in human lymphocyte chromosomes. *Cancer Genet Cytogenet.* 1987;27:15–19.

45. Tollerud DJ, Clark JW, Bronn LM, et al. Association of cigarette smoking with decreased numbers of circulating natural killer cells. *Am Rev Respir Dis.* 1989;139:194–198.

46. Tucker JD, Ashworth LK, Johnston GR, Allen NA, Carrano AV. Variation in the human lymphocyte sister chromatid exchange frequency: results of a long-term longitudinal study. *Mutat Res.* 1988;204:435–444.

47. Kaplan HI, Sadock BJ. *The Brain and Behavior. Synopsis of Psychiatry Behavioral Sciences Clinical Psychiatry*, 6th ed. Baltimore: Williams & Wilkins.

48. Breslau N, Kilbey MM, Andreski P. Nicotine dependence and major depression. *Arch Gen Psychiatry.* 1993;50:31–35.

49. Perkins KA. Sex differences in nicotine versus non nicotine reinforcement at determinants of tobacco smoking. *Exp Clin Psychopharmacol.* 1996;4:1–12.

50. Cinciripini PM. Current trends in smoking cessation research: psychological therapy, nicotine replacement, and changes in smoking behavior. *Cancer Bull.* 1995;47:259–263.

51. Slaughter DP, Southwick HW, Smejkal W. "Field cancerizations" in oral stratified squamous epithelium: clinical implications of multicentric origin. *Cancer.* 1953;5:963–968.

52. Hong WK, Lippman SM, Wolf GT. Recent advances in head and neck cancer-larynx preservation and cancer chemoprevention. *Cancer Res.* 1993;53:5113–5120.

53. Brennan JA, Jay OB, Koch WM, et al. Association between cigarette smoking and mutation of the p53 gene in squamous-cell carcinoma of the head and neck. *New Engl J Med.* 1995;332:712–717.

54. Boyle JO, Hakim J, Koch W. The incidence of p53 mutations increasers with progression of head and neck cancer. *Cancer Res.* 1993;53:4477–4480.

55. Sidransky D, Mikkelsen T, Schwechheimer K, Rosenblum ML, Cavanee W, Vogelstein B. Clonal expansion of p53 mutant cells is associated with brain tumor progression. *Nature.* 1992;355:846–847.

56. Johnson BE, Ihde DC, Matthews MJ, et al. Non-small-cell lung cancer survival. *J Am Med Assoc.* 1986;80:1103–1110.

57. Johnston WD, Ballantyne AJ. Prognostic effect of tobacco and alcohol use in patients with oral tongue cancer. *Am J Surg.* 1977;134:444–447.

58. Johnston-Early A, Cohen MH, Minna JD, et al. Smoking abstinence and small cell lung cancer survival. *J Am Med Assoc.* 1980;244:2175–2179.

59. Moore C. Cigarette smoking and cancer of the mouth, pharynx and larynx. *J Am Med Assoc.* 1971;218:553–558.

60. Silverman S, Gorsky M, Greenspan D. Tobacco usage in patients with head and neck carcinomas: a follow-up study on habit changes and second primary oral/oro-phayngeal cancers. *J Am Dent Assoc.* 1983;106:33–35.

61. Stevens MH, Gardner JW, Parkin JL, Johnson LP. Head and neck cancer survival and lifestyle change. *Arch Otolaryngol.* 1983;109:746–749.

62. Wynder EL, Dodo H, Bloch DA, Gantt RC, Moore DS. Epidemiologic investigation of multiple primary cancer of the upper alimentary and respiratory tracts I: a retrospective study. *Cancer.* 1969;24:730–739.

63. Bergman S, Sorenson S. Smoking and effect of chemotherapy in small cell lung cancer. *Eur Respir J.* 1988;1:932–937.

64. Castigliano SG. Influence of continued smoking on the incidence of second primary cancers involving mouth, pharynx, and larynx. *J Am Dent.* 1968;77:580–585.

65. Schottenfeld D, Gantt RC, Wynder EL. The role of alcohol and tobacco in multiple primary cancers of the upper digestive system, larynx and lung: a prospective study. *Prev Med.* 1974;3:277–293.

66. Hiyama T, Sato T, Yoshino K, Tsukuma H, Hanai A, Fujimoto I. Second primary cancer following laryngeal cancer with special reference to smoking habits. *Jap J Cancer Res.* 1992;83:334–339.

67. Goodman MT, Kolonel LN, Wilkens LR, Yoshizawa CN, Marchand LL. Smoking history and survival among lung cancer patients. *Cancer Causes Control.* 1990;1:155–163.

68. Bako G, Dewar R, Hanson J, Hill G. Factors influencing the survival of patients with cancer of the prostate. *J Can Dent Assoc.* 1982;127:727–729.

69. Calle EE, Miracle-McMahill HL, Thun MJ, Heath J. Cigarette smoking and risk of fatal breast cancer. *Am J Epidemiol.* 1994;139:1001–1007.

70. Kucera H, Enzelsberger H, Eppel W, Weghaupt K. The influence of nicotine abuse and diabetes mellitus on the results of primary irradiation in the treatment of carcinoma of the cervix. *Cancer.* 1987;60:1–4.

71. Day GL, Blot WJ, Shore RE, et al. Second cancers following oral and pharyngeal cancers: role of tobacco and alcohol. *J Natl Cancer Inst.* 1994;86:131–137.

72. CDC. Cigarette smoking among adults - United States, 1994. *Morbid Mortal Weekly Rep.* 1996;45:588–590.

73. CDC. Smoking cessation during previous year among adults—United States 1990 &1991. *Morbid Mortal Weekly Rep.* 1993;42:504–507.

74. Fiore MC, Novotny TE, Pierce JP, et al. Methods used to quit smoking in the United States. *J Am Med Assoc.* 1990;263:2760–2765.

75. Hollis JF, Lichtenstein E, Vogt TM. Nurse-assisted counseling for smokers in primary care. *Ann Intern Med.* 1993;118:521–525.

76. DeClemente CC, Velicer WF, Hughes SL. An empirical typology of subjects within stage of change. *Addict Behav.* 1995;20:299–320.

77. Cohen S, Lichtenstein E, Prochaska JO. Debunking myths about self-quitting. Evidence from ten prospective studies of persons quitting smoking by themselves. *Am Psychol.* 1989;44:1955–1965.

78. Schwartz J. Methods for smoking cessation. *Clin Chest Med.* 1991;12:737–753.

79. Orleans CT, Schoenbach VJ, Quade D, Salmon MA, Porter CQ, Kaplan BH. Self-help quit smoking interventions: effects of self-help materials, social support instructions, and telephone counseling. *J Consult Clin Psychol.* 1991;59:439–448.

80. Curry SJ, Wagner EH, Grothaus LC. Evaluation of intrinsic and extrinsic motivation interventions with a self-help smoking cessation program. *J Consult Clin Psychol.* 1991;59:318–324.

81. Glassman AH. Cigarette smoking: Implications for psychiatric illness. *Am J Psychiatry.* 1993;150:546–553.

82. Brandon TH, Copeland AL, Saper ZL. Programmed therapeutic messages as a smoking treatment adjunct: reducing the impact of negative affect. *Health Psychol.* 1995;14:41–47.

83. Brown RA, Lewinsohn PM, Wagner EF. Comorbidity of cigarette smoking and psychiatric disorders in adolescents. Presented at The Second Annual Meeting of the Society for Research on Nicotine and Tobacco. Washington, D.C.; 1996.

84. Cinciripini PM, Lapitsky LG, Wallfisch A, Haque H, Van Vunakis H. Smoking cessation and depressed mood: Does transdermal nicotine replacement enhance success? Presented at the Society for Behavioral Medicine Annual Meeting. San Diego, CA; 1995.

85. Brown RA, Lewinsohn PM, Wagner EF. Comorbidity of cigarette smoking and psychiatric disorders in adolescents. Presented at The Society for Research on Nicotine and Tobacco (SRNT) 2nd annual scientific conference. Washington, D.C.; 1996.

86. Killen JD, Fortmann SP, Kraemer HC. Who will relapse? symptoms of nicotine dependence predict long-term relapse after smoking cessation. *J Consult Clin Psychol.* 1992;60:797–801.

87. Rosales TA. DSM-III-R nicotine dependence in the national commorbidity survey (NCS). Presented at The Society for Research on Nicotine and Tobacco (SRNT) 2d annual scientific conference. Washington, D.C.; 1996.

88. Digiusto E, Bird KD. Matching smokers to treatment: self-control versus social support. *J Consult Clin Psychol.* 1995;63:290–295.

89. Orleans CT, Resch N, Noll E, Keintz MK, Rimer BK. Use of transdermal nicotine in a state-level prescription plan for the elderly. *J Am Med Assoc.* 1994;271:601–607.

90. Marlatt GA, Gordon JR. *Relapse Prevention Maintenance Strategies in the Treatment of Addictive Behaviors*, 2d ed. New York: The Guilford Press; 1985.

91. Fiore MC, Bailey WC, Cohen SJ, et al. *Smoking Cessation Guideline Panel.* Washington, D.C.: U.S. Department of Health and Human Services, Public Health Service, Centers for Disease Control, Centers for Chronic Disease Prevention and Health Promotion, Office on Smoking and Health 1996;18:1–125.

92. Fiore MC, Jorenby DE, Schensky AE, Smith SS, Bauer RR, Baker TB. Smoking status as the new vital sign: Effect on assessment and intervention in patients who smoke. *Mayo Clin Proc.* 1995;70:209–213.

93. Fiore MC, Epps RP, Manley MW. Missed opportunity: teaching medical students about tobacco cessation and prevention. *J Am Med Assoc.* 1994;271:624–626.

94. Cepeda-Benito. A meta-analytic review of the efficacy of nicotine chewing gum in smoking treatment programs. *J Consult Clin Psychol.* 1993;61:822–830.

95. Pierce JP, Gilpin E, Farkas AJ. Nicotine patch use in the general population: results from the 1993 California tobacco survey. *J Natl Cancer Inst.* 1995;87:87–93.

96. Willey C, Laforge R, Prochaska J, Levesque D. Transdermal nicotine usage in a randomly selected population based sample of smokers. Presented at The Society of Behavioral Medicine. San Diego; 1995.

97. Hurt RD, Dale LC, Fredrickson PA, et al. Nicotine patch therapy for smoking cessation combined with physician advice and nurse follow-up. *J Am Med Assoc.* 1994;271:595–600.

98. Hurt RD, Offord KP, Lauger GG, et al. Cessation of long-term nicotine gum use: a prospective, randomized trial. *Soc Study Addict Alcohol.* 1995;90:407–413.

99. Jorenby DE, Stevens SS, Fiore MC, et al. Varying nicotine patch dose and type of smoking cessation counseling. *J Am Med Assoc.* 1995;274:1347–1352.

100. Fiore MC, Smith SS, Jorenby DE, Baker TB. The effectiveness of nicotine patch for smoking cessation. *J Am Med Assoc.* 1994;271:1940–1947.

101. Cinciripini PM, Cinciripini LG, Wallfisch A, Haque W. Behavior therapy and the transdermal nicotine patch: effects on cessation outcome, affect, and coping. *J Consult Clin Psychol.* 1996;64:314–323.

102. Garvey AJ, Kinnunen T, Doherty K, Vokonas PS. Effects of nicotine gum on smokers differing in level of dependence. Paper presented at The Society for Research on Nicotine and Tobacco. Washington, D.C.; 1996.

103. Gross J, Johnson J, Sigler L, Stitzer ML. Dose Effects of Nicotine Gum. *Addict Behav.* 1995;20:371–381.

104. Killen JD, Fortmann SP, Newman B, Varady A. Evaluation of a treatment approach combining nicotine gum with self fluted behavioral treatments for smoking relapse prevention. *J Consult Clin Psychol.* 1990;58:85–92.

105. Fortmann SP, Killen JD. Nicotine gum and self-help behavioral treatment for smoking relapse prevention: Results from a trial using population-based recruitment. *J Consult Clin Psychol.* 1995;63:460–468.

106. Gourlay SG, Forbes A, Marriner T, Pethica D, McNeil JJ. Double blind trial of repeated treatment with trans-

dermal nicotine for relapsed smokers. *Br Med J.* 1995;311:363–366.

107. Hughes JR, Gust SW, Keenan R, Fenwick JW, Skoog K, Higgins ST. Long-term use of nicotine vs. placebo gum. *Arch Intern Med.* 1991;151.

108. Kornitzer M, Boutsen M, Draxaix M, Thijs J, Gustavsson G. Combined use of nicotine patch and gum in smoking cessation: a placebo-controlled clinical trial. *Prev Med.* 1995;24:41–47.

109. Puska P, Korhonen J, Vartiainen E, Urjanheimo E-L, Gustavsson G, Westin A. Combined use of nicotine patch and gum compared with gum alone in smoking cessation: a clinical trial in North Karelia. *Tobacco Control.* 1995;4:231-235.

110. Schneider NG, Olmstead R, Mody FV, et al. Efficacy of a nicotine nasal spray in smoking cessation: a placebo-controlled, double-blind trial. *Addiction.* 1995;90:1671–1682.

111. Tonnesen PFV, Hansen M. Effect of nicotine chewing gum in combination with group counseling on the cessation of smoking. *N Engl J Med.* 1988;318:15–18.

112. Cinciripini PM, Lapitsky LG, Seay S, Wallfisch A, Kitchens K, Van Vunakis H. The effects of smoking schedules on cessation outcome: Can we improve on common methods of gradual and abrupt nicotine withdrawal? *J Consult Clin Psychol.* 1995;63:388–399.

113. Henningfield JE. Nicotine medications for smoking cessation. *N Engl J Med.* 1995;333:1196–1203.

114. Fagerstrom KO, Westin A, Lunell E, Tejding LR. Aiding reduction of smoking with nicotine replacement medications. A strategy for the hopeless? Presented at The Society for Research on Nicotine and Tobacco. Washington, D.C.; 1996.

115. Kenford SL, Fiore MC, Jorenby DE, Smith SS, Wetter D, Baker TB. Predicting smoking cessation—who will quit with and without the nicotine patch. *J Am Med Assoc.* 1994;271:589–594.

116. Strecher VJ, Kreuter M, Boer D, Hospers KS, Skinner CS. The effects of computer-tailored smoking cessation messages in family practice settings. *J Fam.* 1994;39:262–270.

117. Curry SJ, McBride C, Grothaus LC, Louie D, Wagner EH. Self-help with non volunteer smokers: a randomized trial of self-help materials, personalized feedback and telephone counseling with non volunteer smokers. *J Consult Clin Psychol.* 1995;63:1005–1014.

118. Prochaska JO, DiClementee CC, Velicer WF, Rossi JS. Standardized, individualized, interactive, and personalized self-help programs for smoking cessation. *Health Psychol.* 1993;12:399–405.

119. Zhu SH, Stretch V, Balabanis M, Rosbrook B, Sadler G, Pierce JP. Telephone counseling for smoking cessation: effects of single-session and multiple-session interventions. *J Consult Clin Psychol.* 1996;64:202–211.

120. American Lung Association. *A Lifetime of Freedom from Smoking.* American Lung Association; 1986.

121. U.S. Department of Health and Human Services. *Clearing the Air: How to Quit Smoking and Quit for Keeps.* Washington, D.C.: U.S. Department of Health and Human Services, Public Health Service, Centers for Disease Control, Centers for Chronic Disease Prevention and Health Promotion, Office on Smoking and Health; 1987.

122. Davison G, Duffy M. Smoking habits of long-term survivors of surgery for lung cancer. *Thorax.* 1982;37:331–333.

123. Gritz ER, Nisenbaum R, Elashoff R, Holmes EC. Smoking behavior following diagnosis in patients with Stage I non-small cell lung cancer. *Cancer Causes Control.* 1991;2:105–112.

124. Ostroff JS, Jacobsen PB, Moadel AB, et al. Prevalence and predictors of continued tobacco use after treatment of patients with head and neck cancer. *Cancer.* 1995;75:569–576.

125. Lerman C, Gold K, Audrain J, et al. Incorporating biomarkers of exposure and genetic susceptibility into smoking cessation treatment: effects on smoking-related cognitions, emotions, and behavior change. *Health Psychol.* 1997;16:87–99.

4

Alcohol and Cancer

JEREMY C. LUNDBERG AND STEVEN D. PASSIK

ALCOHOL CONSUMPTION AND ITS LINK TO CANCER

Inadequate public attention has been given to the link between alcohol consumption and the development of cancer. The lay public may be confused about health problems related to alcohol because of the reported health benefits of moderate alcohol consumption, such as in preventing coronary artery disease (1). Although alcohol has never been shown to be a carcinogen, research suggests that alcohol has a definite role in the development of certain types of cancers (2). The American Cancer Society estimates that 18,000 cancer deaths will be related to excessive alcohol use, frequently in combination with tobacco use, and recommends that decreased alcohol consumption may decrease an individual's risk for neoplasms of the head, neck and liver (3). Cancers of the oral cavity, pharynx, larynx, esophagus have been shown to be directly related to alcohol use; while studies examining the role of alcohol use in the development of colo-rectal, stomach, breast, pancreatic, and liver cancers have resulted in conflicting data and have become the focal point of controversy (4). In addition, the exact biophysiological mechanisms affected by alcohol that result in cancer are unclear at this time. The following section will summarize recent hypotheses about the theoretical role of alcohol in the development of site-specific neoplasms.

Head and Neck Neoplasms

An estimated 75% of all oral and pharyngeal cancers in the United States are caused by smoking and alcohol use (5). Similarly, approximately 80% of patients diagnosed with squamous-cell neoplasms in the head and neck have a prior history of excessive alcohol and tobacco use (6). Given that alcoholic individuals tend also to smoke tobacco heavily, research suggests that the heavy consumption of both alcohol and tobacco may have a co-carcinogenic effect in the esophagus, mouth, pharynx, and larynx. Although it is difficult to obtain a sample of nonsmoking alcohol drinkers, high rates of head and neck neoplasm have also been reported in nonsmokers. A study by Blot found that heavy drinking in the absence of smoking resulted in a 5.8-fold increased risk for the development of head and neck neoplasms, thus suggesting that alcohol alone is sufficient to induce oral tumors (5). Researchers have suggested that the ingestion of ethanol increases mucosal permeability allowing carcinogens to penetrate tissue (6). However, a critical review of the literature by Garro and Lieber concluded that there was a lack of convincing evidence to support this theory (7). In contrast, researchers have found the risk of oral cancers to increase in users of mouthwashes that have a high alcohol content. Winn and colleagues found that mouthwashes high in alcohol (greater than 25%) presented the highest relative risk (8). This hypothesis is supported by a Canadian study in which it was found that alcohol produced a greater effect on neoplasms of the extrinsic larynx than on the intrinsic larynx (9). Because individuals do not typically ingest mouthwash, the evidence suggests that role of alcohol in oral carcinogenesis may be topical and not systemic in nature (4).

Poor nutrition and diet, frequently present in alcoholic individuals, is also strongly associated with head and neck cancers. A study by Zeigler of female smokers in North Carolina found that the highest risk for oral and pharyngeal cancer was found in heavy drinkers who consumed low amounts of fruits and vegetables (10). Blot concluded that drinking enhances the deleterious effect of poor nutrition (4).

Liver Carcinoma

The development of primary carcinoma of the liver is practically nonexistent in developed countries, except in the presence of preexisting cirrhosis (11). In 1987, cirrhosis of the liver was the ninth leading cause of death in the United States, claiming 26,351 lives (12). Although not all cases of cirrhosis are directly related to alcohol abuse, the National Institute on Alcohol Abuse and Alcoholism considers the rate of cirrhosis an indicator of current trends of alcohol-related mortality (13). Reports of cirrhosis in patients with liver carcinoma (hepatoma) range from 60% to 90%. Liver cancer may result from the induction of cirrhosis and other liver damage as consequence of the ingestion of alcohol, that may predispose individuals to hepatic tumor development (4,14–16).

The precise biological mechanisms in the liver that are affected by alcohol are unclear. Studies have provided support for a number of hypotheses. The first hypothesis focuses on the depletion of vitamin A stored in the liver. Vitamin A, which is responsible for the maintenance and repair of cell membranes and layers found inside tubular and hollow organs such as the mouth and throat, is severely depressed following alcohol consumption. In animal models, ethanol-consuming rats deficient in vitamin A developed an increased risk of upper respiratory and digestive tract cancers (7). A second hypothesis contends that enzymes necessary for metabolizing and deactivating carcinogens are impaired by the intake of alcohol. A final hypothesis is based upon research that has found acetaldehyde, the product of ethanol metabolism, to represent a possible carcinogen (17). Although research has demonstrated a number of preliminary hypotheses, further investigation is needed on the relationship of alcohol and the development of carcinoma of the liver.

Breast Cancer

The American Cancer Society estimated that approximately 182,000 women and 1400 men in the United States were diagnosed breast cancer in 1995 (3). Since the late 1970s, researchers have debated whether alcohol consumption increases the risk for the development of breast cancer (18). As with other sites, the exact biological mechanisms affected by alcohol in relation to breast cancer are unclear at this time. It is possible that the effect of alcohol on breast tissue is topical. Researchers have found that alcohol is distributed evenly, via the bloodstream, throughout the body, including breast tissue (19). For example, a study by Mennella and Beauchamp found alcohol in the breast milk of lactating women following ingestion (20).

Other hypotheses involve the systemic effects of alcohol on cancer risk factors that have produced mixed results. For example, researchers have found that alcohol may lead to early menopause—a protective factor against breast cancer—and increased levels of estrogen and other hormone levels that may be potential risk factors (21). A more recent study by Longnecker and colleagues found that, regardless of age, alcohol consumption was clearly associated with breast cancer risk even at moderate levels of alcohol consumption (22).

Colorectal and Pancreatic Carcinoma

The consumption of alcohol has been thought to be associated with the development of neoplasms in colorectal sites and the pancreas. In 1990, Stemmermann and colleagues reported a link between heavy alcohol consumption and the development of rectal carcinoma (23). Researchers have theorized that alcohol competes for detoxification by the liver, thus allowing other carcinogens to escape to the colorectal region in toxic form (24). A meta-analysis of the available data on the relationship between alcohol consumption and colorectal carcinoma concluded that the evidence is not strong enough to establish a causal relationship between the two variables, providing only a modest association in heavy drinkers (17,25). The authors point out that beer tends to be more strongly associated with colorectal cancer, suggesting that it is not alcohol itself but some other component of beer that may be responsible for the increased risk. Although the findings are speculative, carcinogens, such as nitrosamine and asbestos fibers, have been found in a range of beers and other types of alcoholic beverages (26–28).

Tumors of the pancreas and their relationship to the consumption of alcohol have been studied extensively. A pooled analysis by Bouchardy and others of three case-controlled studies in Italy, France, and Switzerland found no evidence for an association between alcohol consumption and pancreatic cancer (29). These findings were supported by Farrow and Davis in the United States (30).

ALCOHOL AND CANCER: POSSIBLE BIOCHEMICAL PATHWAYS

Although alcohol has never been shown to be a carcinogen, evidence suggests that the active metabolizing of alcohol may influence the initiation and promotion of carcinogenesis, the first two stages of carcinogenesis, followed by progression. The following summary will examine ways in which alcohol affects each of the three stages (4,7,31).

During the initiation stage, carcinogens are metabolized—chemically altered—within cells, which damages genetic material by attaching to specific sites (forming adducts) on DNA molecules. The genetic damage is converted into a defect (mutation) that can be inherited during cell reproduction. The initiation process is irreversible. However, the process will not continue unless the mutated genes are expressed, thus allowing for abnormal cell growth and the ability to divide unchecked. Mutations can induce the expression of genes involved in tumor formation (oncogenes), while inhibiting the expression of genes responsible for tumor suppression. Alcohol metabolites can affect initiation. In rats, acetaldehyde, the result of metabolized ethanol, has been shown to cause mutations and induce nasal tumors when inhaled in vapor form (32,33). Acetaldehyde has also been found to inhibit the activation of DNA repair enzymes that would return the DNA to its normal state (34).

Promotion is the second stage of carcinogenesis. Promoters act through their ability to induce gene expression and cell division (31). Gene expression, vitamin A metabolism, immunoresponse suppression, and enhanced cell division have all been shown to be affected by alcohol. Vitamin A levels have been shown to decrease in the liver following consumption of alcohol. The suppression of the body's immune system has been studied in drinkers of alcohol. Studies indicate that the numbers of helper T cells and suppresser T cells are reduced in alcoholic individuals. This effect is reversible, at least partially, given abstinence. More importantly, alcohol has been shown to inhibit the effectiveness of natural killer (NK) cells, thought to be important in the destruction of virus-infected and cancerous cells (35,36). It is important to note that NK cell activity may be enhanced following the ingestion of very low doses of alcohol (37). The exact nature alcohol plays in inhibiting the response of the immune system is unclear and requires further investigation.

Progression is the last stage of carcinogenesis and signifies the transition from benign to fully malignant cells. Although the process is not fully understood, cells undergo further genetic changes that lead to increased unrestricted growth and the ability to metastasize. Whether or not alcohol contributes to the progression of cancer is unclear at this time.

Further investigation is necessary to examine the exact biological mechanisms that are affected by alcohol consumption. Theories that examine the role of nutritional deficiencies and hormonal disruptions have also been reported, but are beyond the scope of this chapter.

SUMMARY

Alcohol, either alone or in combination with tobacco, is a significant risk factor related to lifestyle for cancers of the mouth, esophagus, pharynx, larynx, and primary liver carcinoma. It may increase risk of breast cancer, but does not appear related to colorectal (though beer consumption is) or pancreatic neoplasms. Public education, especially about the role of excessive alcohol consumption in cancers of head and neck and liver lags far behind the campaign for reducing cigarette smoking. The problem may lie in the fact that cigarette smoking should not be continued in moderate amounts, where as moderate alcohol consumption is a part of this society's lifestyle in general. Separating "moderate" from "excessive" may be a harder differentiation than an out and out recommendation of total abstinence, as can be made for tobacco use.

REFERENCES

1. Kannel WB, Wilson PW. An update on coronary risk factors. *Med Clin N Am.* 1995; 79:951–971.
2. Garro AJ, Espina N, Lieber CS. Alcohol and cancer. *Alcohol Health Res World.* 1992; 16(1):81–86.
3. American Cancer Society. *Cancer Facts and Figures—1995.* Atlanta: American Cancer Society; 1995.
4. Blot WJ. Alcohol and cancer. *Cancer Res (Suppl).* 1992; 52:2119–2123.
5. Blot WJ, McLaughlin JK, Winn DM, et al. Smoking and drinking in relation to oral and pharyngeal cancer. *Cancer Res.* 1988; 48:3282–3287.
6. Rothman K, Keller A. The effect of joint exposure to alcohol and tobacco on risk of cancer of the mouth and pharynx. *J Chronic Dis.* 1972; 25:711–716.
7. Garro AJ, Lieber CS. Alcohol and Cancer. *Ann Rev Pharmacol Toxicol.* 1990; 30:219–249.
8. Winn DM, Blot WJ, McLaughlin JK, et al. Mouthwash use and oral conditions in the risk of oral and pharyngeal cancer. *Cancer Res.* 1991; 51:3044–3047.
9. Elwood JM, Pearson JC, Skippen DH, Jackson SM. Alcohol, smoking, social and occupational factors in the aetiology of cancer of the oral cavity, pharynx, and larynx. *Int J Cancer.* 1984; 34:603–612.
10. Zeigler RG. Alcohol-nutrient interactions in cancer etiology. *Cancer.* 1986; 58:1942–1948
11. Holland JC. Behavioral and psychosocial risk factors in cancer: human studies. In: Holland JC and Rowland JH eds. *Handbook of Psychooncology: Psychological Care of the Patient with Cancer.* New York: Oxford University Press, 1990:291–299.
12. Grant B, Zoebeck T, Pickering R. Surveillance Report No. 15: Liver cirrhosis mortality in the United States, 1973–87. Washington, D.C. National Institute on Alcohol Abuse and Alcoholism, 1990.
13. Stinson FS, DeBakey SF. Alcohol-related mortality in the United States. *Br J Addict.* 1992; 87:777–783.
14. Lieber CS, Seitz HK, Garro AJ, Worner TM. Alcohol-related diseases and carcinogenesis. *Cancer Res.* 1979; 39:2863–2886.

15. Tuyns AJ. Alcohol and Cancer. *Alcohol Health Res World*. 1978; 2:20–31.

16. Tuyns AJ. Cancer risks derived from alcohol. *Med Oncol*. 1987; 4:241–244.

17. Longnecker MP. Alcohol consumption in relation to risk of cancers of the breast and large bowel. *Alcohol Health Res World*. 1992; 16(3):223–229.

18. Williams RR. Breast and thyroid cancer and malignant melanoma promoted by alcohol-induced pituitary secretion of prolactin, T.S.H., and M.S.H. *Lancet*. 1976; 7967:996–999.

19. Frezza M, Di Padova C, Pozzato G, Terpin M, Baraona E, Lieber CS. High blood alcohol levels in women: the role of decreased gastric alcohol dehydrogenase activity and first-pass metabolism. *N Engl J Med*. 1990; 322(2):95–99.

20. Mennella JA, Beauchamp GK. The transfer of alcohol to human milk. Effects on flavor and the infant's response. *N Engl J Med*. 1991; 325(14):981–985.

21. Gavaler JS, VanThiel DH. Reproductive consequences of alcohol abuse: males and females compared and contrasted. *Mutat Res*. 1987; 186:269–277.

22. Longnecker MP, Newcomb PA, Mittendorf PA, et al. Risk of breast cancer in relation to lifetime alcohol consumption. *J Nat Cancer Inst*. 1995; 87(12):923–929.

23. Stemmermann GN, Nomura AMY, Chyou PH, Yoshizawa C. Prospective study of alcohol intake and large bowel cancer. *Dig Dis Sci*. 1990; 35(11):1414–1420.

24. Seitz HK, Simanowski UA. Ethanol and colorectal carcinogenesis. In: Sietz HK, Simanowski UA, Wright NA, eds. *Colorectal Cancer: From Pathogenesis to Prevention*. Heildelberg: Springer-Verlag, 1989:177–189.

25. Longnecker MP, Orza MJ, Adams ME, Vioque J, Chalmers TC. A meta-analysis of alcoholic beverage consumption in relation to risk of colorectal cancer. *Cancer Causes Control*. 1990; 1(1):59–68.

26. Walker EA, Castegnaro M, Garren L, Touissaint G, Kowalski B. Intake of volatile nitrosamines from consumption of alcohols. *J Natl Cancer Center*. 1979; 63:947–951.

27. Biles B, Emerson TR. Examination of fibers in beer. *Nature*. 1979; 219:93–94.

28. Cunningham HM, Pontefract R. Asbestos fibers in beverages and drinking water. *Nature*. 1971; 232:332–333.

29. Bouchardy C, Clavel F, La Vecchia C, Raymond L, Boyle P. Alcohol, beer and cancer of the pancreas. *Int J Cancer*. 1990; 45:842–846.

30. Farrow DC, Davis S. Risk of pancreatic cancer in relation to medical history and the use of tobacco, alcohol and coffee. *Int J Cancer*. 1990; 45:816–820.

31. Garro AJ, Espina N, Lieber CS. Alcohol and cancer. *Alcohol Health Res World*. 1992; 16(1):81–86.

32. Dellarco VL. A mutagenicity assessment of acetaldehyde. *Mut Res*. 1988; 195:1–20.

33. Woutersen RA, Appelman LM, Feron VJ, Van Der Heijden CA. Inhalation toxicity of acetaldehyde in rats. II. Carcinogenicity study: Interm results after 15 months. *Toxicology*. 1984; 31:123–133.

33. Espina N, Lieber CS, Garro AJ. In vitro and in vivo inhibitory effect of ethanol and acetaldehyde on O6-methylguanine transferase. *Carcinogenesis*. 1988; 9(5):761–766.

35. Roselle GA, Mendenhall CL, Grossman CJ, Weesner RE. Lymphocyte subset alterations in patients with alcoholic hepatitis. *J Clin Lab Immunol*. 1988; 26:169–173.

36. Roselle GA. Alcohol and the immune system. *Alcohol Health Res World*. 1992; 16(1):16–22.

37. Saxena Q, Saxena R, Adler W. Regulation of natural killer activity in vivo. Part IV. High natural activity in alcohol-drinking mice. *Indian J Exp Biol*. 1981; 19(1):1001–1006.

5

Diet and Cancer

BARBARA L. WINTERS

The findings from comprehensive reviews (1–3) of cancer-related risks clearly buttress the argument that certain dietary patterns can modify the risk for cancer. However, dietary data do not demonstrate that dietary risk reduction lifestyles are practiced. Evidence on current dietary intakes and disease risks suggests that the dietary patterns of a considerable portion of our population leave much to be desired (4–6). This includes the diets of age groups ranging from children to the elderly, and of socioeconomic groups ranging from the poor and disadvantaged to the affluent.

Ideally, a cancer risk-reduction diet should be implemented at the start of life. If dietary habits in adulthood are less than optimal, it is pivotal to provide adults with the essential knowledge, environment, and behaviors to help maximize the nutritional quality of life by diminishing high-risk dietary behaviors. This chapter will review fundamental data and provide scientific support relative to dietary factors as they may impact cancer prevention lifestyles. Included is a review of the inadequacies and excesses in dietary intakes and general public health recommendations on optimal dietary choices. Lifestyle guidelines to reduce cancer risk through nutritional modifications are also provided

DIET AND CANCER—INADEQUACIES AND EXCESSES

Although reality dictates that people eat diets, not single foods or nutrients, the connection between diet and cancer is often related to specific nutrient intakes. A widely used definition of a nutrient is "a substance obtained from food and used in the body to promote growth, maintenance, and/or repair" (7). The generally recognized classes of nutrients are carbohydrates, proteins, fats, vitamins, minerals, and water. Nonnutrient food components such as phytochemicals include, but are by no means limited to, such elements as allyl sul-

fides, phytates, isoflavones, lignans, isothiocyanates, indoles, and ellagic acid (8). These phytochemicals are linked with various metabolic pathways associated with the development of cancer (9).

Dietary elements including naturally occurring nutrients, synthetic components and nonnutritional factors, can either inhibit or facilitate the carcinogenic process (10–11). Imbalances, that is, excesses or inadequacies in defined nutrients and/or nonnutrients, are one means by which diet contributes to cancer etiology.

Dietary Inadequacies

A significant inadequacy in the Western diet is the low intake of fruits and vegetables (12). This inadequacy has been linked epidemiologically to increased risk of several cancers (9,12–14). In 82% of 156 reviewed studies, it was found that fruit and vegetable consumption provided significant protection against cancer (9). People who eat greater amounts of fruits and vegetables have approximately one-half the risk and, if diagnosed, lower mortality rates from cancer (12–15). The risks associated with a diet low in fruits and vegetables are derived in part from inadequate levels of antioxidants such as vitamin C (ascorbic acid), vitamin A, and beta-carotene (16). Other carotenoids such as lycopene, a superior antioxidant, also could be deficient. In addition, consuming a diet rich in fruits and vegetables provides a milieu of phytochemicals that appear to possess health-protective qualities (17).

Fiber

The increased cancer risks associated with low intakes of fruits and vegetables also relate to fiber intake. This is because many fruits and vegetables are excellent sources of fiber, as are cereals and grains. Inadequate intake of fiber has been significantly linked to the increased incidence of colon (18–22), breast (23,24), and prostate cancer (25). The anticarcinogenic action of fiber relative to colorectal cancer has been attributed to its ability to reduce exposure to carcinogens through dilution of the gut contents. Fiber also increases stool transit time and so decreases the length of time that carcinogens are in contact with the colon (26). Data also support a protective role for dietary fiber with hormone-related cancers, perhaps due to fiber's ability to reduce intestinal reabsorption of androgens and estrogens (23).

Although there is substantial support for the anticarcinogenic effect of fiber in the diet, some studies have reported a lack of effect (27–29). The inconsistencies in the reports have been attributed to disagreements by experts on the best way to measure levels of different fibers in epidemiological studies (27). The inconsistencies have also been related to the fact that both the physical forms and the chemical compositions of fiber are probably biologically important. Epidemiological studies need more detailed dietary intake data to address this point.

Inadequate Levels of Micronutrients

Specific micronutrient deficiencies have been linked to increases in several cancers (30). For example, under certain circumstances, deficiencies of riboflavin and iron are associated with an increase in esophageal cancer (31). The geographic differences in thyroid cancer occurrence have been attributed to imbalances in iodine intake (32). Low intake of calcium has been associated with increased risk of intestinal cancer (33), and selenium intake below recommended dietary levels has been associated with increased risk for human prostate, lung, and colon cancers (34).

It is important to point out that our knowledge of the risks and benefits associated with micronutrient intake and of the cancer prevention properties of many micronutrients is still evolving. It may be that synergistic effects of micronutrients is important or that an excess intake of one micronutrient increases risk. Until more data are obtained and clinical trials are conducted, changes in total dietary patterns are preferable for the general public over modifications in specific micronutrients.

Inadequate Levels of Nonnutrient Food Components

Experimental evidence demonstrates that a number of nonnutrient food components have anticarcinogenic properties (35). Epidemiological studies of the risk reduction properties of fruits and vegetables suggest that their beneficial effects (24) may relate to their roles as dietary sources of nonnutritive factors. For instance, certain diphenoic lignans and isoflavanoid phytoestrogens appear to be antiestrogenic and anti-

carcinogenic (36). The intake of soy (37), a major source of isoflavonoid phytoestrogens, is associated with lower risk of cancers such as breast cancer. Similarly, the lower incidence of aggressive prostate cancer in Asian countries relative to Western populations has been linked to the intake of soy (38) in those countries. Typically, Western diets are quite low in isoflavones; perhaps constituting a deficiency. Research is ongoing in this regard as well as into numerous other nonnutritive factors (24).

Dietary Excesses: Fat and Calories

Evidence is considerable that excessive consumption of total calories or specific food components can create a condition of metabolic overload (39). The key concern with metabolic overload is excessive fat intake. Population studies have shown that fat intake greater than 20% of total calories is strongly associated with an increased incidence of colon (26), breast (40), prostate (41), and possibly pancreatic cancer (42). Animal studies also reveal that dietary fat influences cancer development in the breast (43), colon (44), pancreas (45), and prostate (46), although specific exceptions have been observed.

In general, the fat hypothesis has been supported by intercountry comparisons that involve correlation studies examining the effect of fat over wide ranges of intake (47). Conversely, there have been inconsistent findings in cohort and case-control studies that examine fat in smaller ranges (48–51). Insufficient variation in fat intake in countries like the United States may make it impossible to establish potential differences even if they do exist. Within a defined population such as exists in this country, virtually everyone may be "overexposed" in terms of calorie and especially fat (52) intake. Another difficulty with these studies is that the research populations may be underreporting fat intake because of a "social desirability" bias (53).

The overexposed control group phenomenon appears to be responsible, in part, for the results noted in case-control studies (54) and cohort studies in which no significant change in breast cancer risk were found relative to fat intake. Before any conclusions are drawn from these studies alone, the composite of research on the relationship of fat intake to breast cancer must be weighed. The extensive evidence from animal (55–58) and ecological studies (59) demonstrates the strength of association between fat intake and breast cancer. Furthermore, this relationship is supported by a substantial amount of data on the plausible biological effects of fat on breast tissue biomechanisms such as hormone metabolism (60–63), oxidative damage (64), and immune function (65).

Cancer Risk and Specific Fatty Acids and Oils. While all fats provide identical caloric loads, there are distinctive effects of different fats on carcinogenesis. In rodent models, omega-6 polyunsaturated fats (e.g., corn, sunflower, and safflower oil) are strong cancer promoters, particularly the omega-6 fatty acid, linoleic acid. In contrast, the omega-9 monounsaturated oils (e.g., olive, peanut, and canola oil) appear neutral. Data also suggests that omega-3 polyunsaturated fats (marine based/fish oils) are protective (66,67). The relationship between specific fats and cancer also holds true for the metastatic process. The growth and metastasis of transplantable human breast tumors is suppressed by high levels of omega-3 fatty acids, but enhanced by omega-6 fatty acids (68).

Human studies substantiate the effect of different fats on carcinogenesis. Recent dietary studies support the observation that consumption of omega-9-rich, monounsaturated fat does not increase the risk of breast cancer. Women in southern Europe who consume more monounsaturated fat (olive oil) than their northern neighbors have a lower incidence of breast cancer (69,70). In contrast, several studies suggest that the high consumption of animal fat from red meat rich in saturated fat increases the incidence of cancer. Meat and whole milk intake, which contribute approximately 40% and 20%, respectively, of fat in the adult American diet, are positively associated with prostate cancer (71–73). In two prospective studies, men who consumed higher amounts of red meat and animal fat had approximately twice the risk of prostate cancer as men who consumed low amounts (41,73). Red meat is not only an important source of saturated fat in the diet, it is also a major contributor to dietary cholesterol, thus having negative effects on both carcinogenesis and cardiovascular incidence. Overall data suggests that red meat consumption may be excessive in Western cultures (27).

Excess Calories. Some experiments have been interpreted as suggesting that the effect of a high-fat diet is entirely attributable to increased caloric intake. Analysis of the collective literature, however, reveals a specific enhancing effect of dietary fat, with a separate enhancing effect of calories (74). Nonetheless, as distinct from fat, excess caloric intake may be of importance in humans, especially where overnutrition leads to obesity. Interestingly, in animal models, the only modulation of diet that consistently maintains maximal longevity is caloric restriction (75). In part, this relates to the effect on cell cycling, itself a key factor in carcinogenesis and longevity.

Health Benefits: Reducing Excess Intakes of Carcinogens

Excessive pickling, salting, and smoking of foods has been associated with increased carcinogenesis (10,76,77). During the cooking process of primarily meats and fish, a variety of heterocyclic amines are formed in the browning reaction, producing potent multiorgan DNA-reactive agents (78). Excess intake of these heterocyclic amines has been postulated as being an initiating agent for breast, colon, and stomach cancers (79). Similarly, nitroamines, formed from common precursors in the diet, are postulated to be initiating agents for cancer (80) and have been linked with the high rates of esophageal cancer in China.

Reducing the formation of, and thus the exposure to these carcinogens illustrates the potential for modification of diet to affect cancer rates. An excellent example is the decline of stomach cancer in the Western world. Stomach cancer rates in the United States have decreased from 38 deaths per 100,000 white males in 1930 to 7 per 100,000 in 1985; and from 29 deaths per 100,000 white females to 4 per 100,000 (81). This reduction is related to the diminished use of salt and nitrates for preserving foods in favor of canning, freezing, and refrigeration.

DIET AND NUTRITIONAL STRATEGIES FOR CANCER RISK REDUCTION

The preceding discussion provides sound evidence that nutritional excesses and inadequacies have a significant impact on cancers. The following material reviews practical public health and childhood targeted approaches to reducing risk of cancer and other diseases (82) through dietary modification.

Public Health Measures

Those working in the public health sector are looked upon to make recommendations to the public as to the type and amount of foods people should consume for optimal health. Tables 5.1 to 5.3 summarize guidelines for the prevention of disease, and include the most recent dietary recommendations of several groups. The recent recommendations of the Committee on Diet and Health of the National Academy of Sciences, the *Dietary Guidelines for Americans* (83,84), and the *Food Guide Pyramid* (85), published by the U.S. Department of Agriculture, are general recommendations for chronic disease reduction. These recommendations focus on decreasing risks of a variety of chronic degenerative diseases and conditions while ensuring sufficient intake of essential nutrients.

The American Cancer Society (86) (ACS) Guidelines for Adults address a total dietary pattern for lowering cancer risk. In most respects, the ACS Guidelines are close to the more general recommendations. However, the ACS Guildelines provide additional detail in some areas. There is also a nationwide campaign to promote increased consumption of fruits and vegetables. The National Cancer Institute sponsored, "5-a-Day for Better Health" program (87) is designed to encourage the consumption of at least five servings of fruits and vegetables per day. Unfortunately, at present, the average American eats only about one and one-half servings of vegetables per day and less than one serving of fruit per day (88).

TABLE 5.1. *Dietary Guidelines for Americans, 1995*

Eat a variety of foods.

Balance the food you eat with physical activity. Maintain or improve your weight.

Choose a diet with plenty of grain products, vegetables, and fruits.

Choose a diet low in fat, saturated fat, and cholesterol.

Choose a diet moderate in sugars.

Choose a diet moderate in salt and sodium.

If you drink alcoholic beverages, do so in moderation.

Source: Ref. 83.

TABLE 5.2. *U.S. Department of Agriculture Food Guide Pyramid, 1992*

FOOD CATEGORIES AND RECOMMENDED SERVINGS PER DAY	
Bread, cereal, rice, and pasta group:	6–11 servings
Fruit group:	2–4 servings
Vegetable group:	3–5 servings
Meat, poultry, fish, dry beans, eggs, and nuts group:	2–3 servings (total amount equal to 5–7 oz cooked lean meat, poultry, or fish per day, with a serving size of 2–3 oz for lean meat poultry or fish, and ½ cup cooked dry beans, 1 egg, or 2 tablespoons peanut butter as 1 oz of meat)
Milk, yogurt, and cheese group:	2–3 servings
Fats, oils, and sweets:	use sparingly

Source: Ref. 85.

TABLE 5.3. *Cancer-specific Guidelines, American Cancer Society, 1991*

Maintain a desirable body weight.

Eat a varied diet.

Include a variety of fruits and vegetables in the daily diet.

Eat more high-fiber foods such as whole-grain cereals, legumes, vegetables, and fruits.

Cut down total fat intakes.

Limit consumption of alcoholic beverages, if you drink at all.

Limit consumption of salt-cured, smoked, or nitrate-preserved foods.

Source: Ref. 86.

Childhood Risk Reduction

Risk Reduction Behaviors and Childhood: The rationale for implementing measures aimed at cancer prevention in childhood is based on the following: (*1*) the high prevalence of the disease, especially among adults; (*2*) the often insidious onset of cancer and its frequently poor prognosis when diagnosed; and (*3*) the knowledge that many of the risk factors are life-style-related and thus preventable (89,90). Dietary practices during childhood may be exceptionally important in cancer incidence and prevention. For example, during developmental maturation in puberty, the breast is especially sensitive to carcinogens. This has led to the suggestion that dietary intervention programs to reduce the incidence of breast cancer should be targeted at early adolescent girls (91). It has been speculated that dietary habits during childhood may affect the incidence of prostate cancer.

Dietary modifications to reduce disease risk at the preschool rather than adult age is preferable because patterns of risk are apparent at this time when lifestyle habits are being formed. In addition, with the development of technology to detect genetic conditions that predispose individuals to cancer, it is critical to institute risk-reduction strategies as early as possible. This is also the time when young parents are often eager for advice on child care and when visits to pediatricians are frequent in those families that have ready access to and funds for health care (89).

Implementation of an effective cancer prevention program for children and adolescents from a public health perspective leads logically to dietary habits learned in families and in the schools. Families can be very influential in determining a child's health-related values, beliefs, and practices (92). Risk-reduction school programs ideally should be an important part of a comprehensive school education program (93). Designed to affect knowledge, attitudes, and health behaviors, risk-reduction school programs should help children adopt lifestyles that promote health and prevent disease (94–99). One such comprehensive health education program is the "Know Your Body" (KYB), program, developed by the American Health Foundation. The KYB program is designed to empower students with the skills and experience needed to adopt proactive health promoting behaviors that include cancer risk reduction (99–100). High-risk programs, such as those practiced in the physician's office, complement the population approach (89) and include counseling and preventive treatment for children at increased future cancer risk.

AN OPTIMAL CANCER RISK REDUCTION DIET AND SPECIFIC DIETARY GUIDELINES

A major focus for cancer prevention must be a simplified approach to ensuring optimal nutrition and balance of dietary components. The optimal diet is defined as one that would lead to a significant reduction in disease and at the same time would feasibly be consumed by the majority of people. As a general guide, the American Health Foundation recommends a 25:25 diet for adults, which comprises 25% or fewer calories from fat and 25 grams of fiber (101) (see Table 5.4).

As cancer is a chronic condition that develops over time, with certain cancers having their inceptions during childhood (102), guidelines are needed for a cancer-preventive lifestyle beginning in childhood. Whereas the current level of fat intake for children is around 35% (103), the dietary recommendation for children after the age of 2 is for no more that 30% of their total calories from fat (104,105). The average dietary fiber intake of children and adolescents is about 12 g per day which, like that of adults, is probably only about half of an optimal intake (106). The optimal fiber intake (in grams) for children is "age plus 5" (89). Therefore the recommended fiber intake for a 3-year-old is 8 g per day (3 + 5), whereas an 11-year-old should consume 16 g per day.

TABLE 5.4. *The 25/25 Plan*

Eat no more than 25% of calories from fat
A typical adult woman eating 1800 calories should eat no more than 50 grams of fat per day
A typical adult man eating 2200 calories should eat no more than 60 grams of fat per day
Adults should eat 25 grams of fiber daily

Specific Diet and Nutritional Guidelines for Risk-Reduction Life-Styles

Public health measures to modify life-style practices are important. As important are specific guidelines aimed at maximizing the nutritional quality of life for primary prevention as well as those aimed at reducing the incidence of recurrence. In addition, nutritional messages for cancer risk-reduction practices must include the larger advocacy of healthy life-style choices and must also provide guidance and means to achieve the recommendations. The following eight guidelines are aimed to maximize the nutritional quality of life.

1. *Place diet in the context of overall risk reduction strategies.* When it comes to health promotion and risk reduction, guidelines cannot focus on diet alone, on a single type of cancer, or even on cancer alone. Dietary recommendations must be in the context of recommendations for appropriate exercise levels, smoking cessation, stress reduction, and moderation in alcohol consumption (107).

2. *Remember that recommendations for cancer risk reduction and cancer treatment often differ.* Dietary recommendations for one purpose are not necessarily correct for another purpose. Nutritional measures for cancer treatment vary depending upon the type, location, and severity of the disease and the age of the individual (108). The best source of information on disease-specific and age-specific recommendations is a nutritionist with an expertise in nutrition and oncology.

3. *Supports and barriers to dietary changes. "Do not assume that dietary change is always easy."* For a variety of reasons, including physical, social, and psychological, an individual may have difficulty achieving dietary modifications. Intentions to change do not automatically lead to the corresponding behavior (109). Likewise, nutrition knowledge does not always translate into healthy behavior. A nutritional regimen that does not fit into the individual's cultural or age-related needs may be ignored or followed inconsistently (93).

4. *Discourage individuals from "blaming the cook" or blaming themselves for cancer.* Individuals with cancer, or those aiming at preventing cancer, often believe that what they eat or what they have eaten is solely responsible for causing disease. People need to be informed that diet is only one of many genetic and environmental factors related to the development and recurrence of cancer (109).

5. *People eat for taste, not primarily for nutritional or health reasons.* When the focus is on nutrition, we must consider the palatability of the food. Chefs, dietitians, food scientists, and other experts can be called upon to establish an interdisciplinary approach to changing what we serve and how we eat (109). For long-term life-style modifications, dietary risk reduction plans should be tailored to fit the individual's favored foods and cultural preferences (93).

6. *Avoid "good food/bad food" terminology for the general public, children and cancer patients of all ages.* In considering individual foods, "good food/bad food" terminology does not encourage healthy food consumption practices (109). There are dietary practices that are "good" or better than others in the sense that some patterns are more likely to foster good health than others. However, nutritionists have been aware for years that distributing lists of bad or "forbidden" foods often promotes a sense of guilt. This can result in individuals using diet as a means to express defiance or anger. Effective strategies for shaping eating behavior and healthy lifelong eating habits recognize that occasional lapses are inevitable and are unlikely to be critical in the long term. Importantly, they emphasize positive choices and the social desirability of eating and drinking in healthy ways.

7. *Keep open and listen when individuals talk about their alternative practices (yet unproven or questionable remedies) related to nutrition.* Individuals and the public should be provided with strategies to deal with questionable remedies. Questionable remedies can decrease the quality of life, cause financial burden, and may be harmful. They may also be harmless and provide psychological benefit to an individual (109). There is also the potential that alternative practices may have beneficial effects that have not yet been proven via the conventional rigors of scientific inquiry. The National Institutes of Health (NIH) has established the Office of Alternative Medicines (OAM) whose charge is to investigate alternative cancer treatments. The OAM and other organizations such as the American Cancer Society and the FDA Office of Consumer Affairs, can provide objective reviews of alternative treatments and help identify situations of outright fraud (110).

8. *Remember that research is ongoing and recommendations change as new data are generated.* There are ongoing trials investigating various nutritive (e.g., vitamin A, ascorbic acid, fiber sources) and nonnutritive substances including lignans, phytoestrogens, and many other compounds that may inhibit or promote carcinogenesis. As results become available, revisions of recommendations may be made. Radical changes in recommendations are unlikely. In contrast, we expect to see more quantitative dietary guidelines emerge from results of ongoing studies.

SUMMARY AND CONCLUSIONS

Because the most common neoplasms in industrial countries remain irremediable for many patients, identifying effective preventive regimens has added urgency. Diet has for some time been considered a reasonable and safe way to try to prevent cancer. All professionals owe their patients an informed and balanced perspective, and should be sensitive to the need to support individuals as they adopt dietary changes.

Clearly, prevention through dietary change is worth "preaching" even at the point when a patient reaches an oncologist (111–113). This is demonstrated by epidemiological and animal studies that support a beneficial role for diet after cancer has occurred (11,43,56). Healthy changes at the time of diagnosis of cancer may make a difference in recurrence and survival (112,113). Human studies supporting the benefit of dietary modifications to prevent disease recurrence are ongoing. For example, the Women's Intervention Nutrition Study (WINS) is looking at the effect of a low-fat diet (15% of calories as fat) on the reduction in recurrence of breast cancer (114). As more cancers are cured, recurrence prevention will become a more frequent goal.

In conclusion, the potential for preventing cancer and other disease by improving nutrition is considerable. A body of research supports the importance of a varied diet, of the protective role of fruits and vegetables and dietary fiber, and of eating a low-fat diet in reducing cancer risk. The data are not conclusive, however, about the cancer-preventing properties of a number of specific micronutrients because the optimal levels of intake of differing micronutrients are yet to be defined (115). Our knowledge of the risks and benefits associated with them is still evolving. Thus it is preferable overall to recommend prevention through modification of total dietary patterns rather than through the administration of individual agents, the exception being the case of very high-risk populations where potent chemopreventive agents are being tested. Childhood targeted strategies may have the greatest potential for reducing overall cancer morbidity and mortality. Relatively small modifications in poor dietary habits, if carried into adulthood, could significantly reduce eventual cancer incidence.

REFERENCES
1. Micozzi MS, Moon TE. *Macronutrients: Investigating Their Role in Cancer*. New York: Marcel Dekker; 1992.

2. Moon TE, Micozzi MS. *Nutrition and Cancer Prevention: Investigating the Role of Micronutrients.* New York: Marcel Dekker; 1989.

3. Rowland IR. *Nutrition, Toxicity, and Cancer.* Boca Raton, FL: CRC Press; 1991.

4. Life Sciences Research Office, Federation of American Societies for Experimental Biology. *Nutrition Monitoring in the United States: An Update Report on Nutrition Monitoring.* Hyattsville, MD: US Department of Agriculture; September 1989. (DHHS publication no. (PHS) 89-1255.)

5. National Center for Health Statistics. *Health, United States, 1990.* Hyattsville, MD: US Department of Health and Human Services; 1991. (DHHS publication no. (PHS) 91-1232.)

6. Anderson SA. Core indicators of nutritional state for difficult to sample populations. *J Nutr.* 1990; 120:917–954.

7. Whitney EN, Hamilton EMN. *Understanding Nutrition,* 2d ed. St. Paul, MN: West Publishing; 1981.

8. Block A, Thomson CA. Position of the American Dietetic Association: phytochemicals and functional foods. *J Am Diet Assoc.* 1995; 95:493–496.

9. Block G, Patterson B, Sunbar A. Fruit, vegetables and cancer prevention: a review of the epidemiological evidence. *Nutr Cancer.* 1992; 18(1):1–29.

10. Williams, GM, Weisburger JH. Chemical carcinogenesis. In: Amdur MO, Doull J, Klaasen CD, eds. *Casarett and Doull's Toxicology. The Basic Sciences of Poisons,* 4th ed. New York: Pergamon Press, 1991; 127.

11. Wattenberg LW. Inhibition of carcinogenesis by minor dietary constituents. *Cancer Res.* 1992; 52:2085s.

12. Zeigler RG. Vegetables, fruits, and carotenoids and the risk of cancer. *Am J Clin Nutr.* 1991; 53(suppl):251S–259S.

13. Trichopoulos D, Ouanos D, Day NE, et al. Diet and cancer of stomach: a case-control study in Greece. *Int J Cancer.* 1985; 36:291.

14. Chyou PH, Nomura AMY, Hankin JH, Stemmerman GN. A case-cohort study of diet and stomach cancer. *Cancer Res.* 1990; 50:7501.

15. Steinmetz K, Potter J. Vegetables, fruit and cancer. I. Epidemiology. *Cancer Causes Control.* 1991; 2(suppl): 325–357.

16. Hwang H, Dwyer J, Russell RM. Diet, Helicobacter pylori: food preservation and gastric cancer risk: are there new roles for preventative factors? *Nutr Rev.* 1994; 52:75.

17. Cargay AB. Cancer-preventative foods and ingredients. *Food Technol.* 1992; 46(4):65–68.

18. Phillips RL, Garfinkel L, Kuzma JW, et al. Mortality among California Seventh-day Adventists for selected cancer sites. *J Natl Cancer Inst.* 1980; 65:1097–1107.

19. Trock B, Lanza E, Greenwald P. Dietary fiber, vegetables, and colon cancer. *J Natl Cancer Inst.* 1990; 82:650–661.

20. Giovannucci E, Stampfer MJ, Colditz GA, et al. Relation of diet to the risk of colorectal adenoma in men. *J Natl Cancer Intst.* 1992; 84:91–98.

21. McKeowen-Eyssen GE. Fiber intake in different populations and colon cancer risk. *Prev Med.* 1987; 16:532.

22. Freudenheim JL, Graham S. Hovarth PJ, Marshall JR, Haughey BP, Wilkinson G. Risk associated with sources of fiber and fiber components in cancer and rectum. *Cancer Res.* 1990; 50:3295.

23. Rose DP, Goldman M, Connolly JM, Strong LE. High-fiber diet reduces serum estrogen concentrations in premenopausal women. *Am J Clin Nutr.* 1991; 54:520–525.

24. Freudenheim JL, Marshall JR, Vena JE, et al. Premenopausal breast cancer risk and intake of vegetables, fruits, and related nutrients. *J Natl Cancer Inst.* 1996; 88:340–348.

25. Howie BJ, Shultz TD. Dietary and hormonal interrelationships among vegetarian and Seventh-Day Adventist and nonvegetarian men. *Am J Clin Nutr.* 1985; 42:127–134.

26. Reddy BS, Cohen LA, eds. *Diet, Nutrition and Cancer: A Critical Evaluation.* CRC Press: Boca Raton, FL; 1986.

27. Willett WC. Diet and Cancer: What Do We Know Now? *Adv Oncol.* 1995; 11:3–8.

28. Willett WC, Hunter DJ, Sampfer MJ. Dietary fat and the risk of breast cancer. *N Engl J Med.* 1987; 316:22–28.

29. Graham S, Zielezny M, Marshall J, et al. Diet in the epidemiology of post menopausal breast cancer in the New York State cohort. *Am J Epidemiol.* 1992; 136:1327–1337.

30. Williams GM, Wynder EL. Diet and cancer: a synopsis of causes and preventive strategies. In: Watson RR, Mufti SI, eds. *Nutrition and Cancer Prevention.* Boca Raton, FL: CRC Press; 1996: 1–12.

31. Wynder EL, Fryer JH. Etiologic considerations of Plummer–Vinson (Paterson–Kelly) syndrome. *Ann Intern Med.* 1958; 49:1106.

32. Franceschi S, Boyle P, Maisonneuve P, et al. The epidemiology of thyroid carcinoma. *Crit Rev Oncogen.* 1993; 4:25.

33. Garland C, Shekelle RB, Barrett-Connor E, Criqui MH, Rossof AH, Ogelsby P. Dietary vitamin D and calcium and risk of colorectal cancer: a 19-year prospective study in men. *Lancet.* 1985; 1:307.

34. Clark LC, Combs GF, Turnbull BW, et al. Effects of selenium supplementation for cancer prevention in patients with carcinoma of the skin. *J Am Med Assoc.* 1996; 276:1957–1963.

35. Smith TJ, Yang CS. Effects of food phytochemicals or xenobiotic metabolism. In: Huang MJ, Osawa T, Ho CT, Rosen RT, eds. *Food Phytochemicals for Cancer Prevention. I. Fruits and Vegetables.* Washington, D.C.: American Chemical Society; 1994; 17–48.

36. Knight DC, Eden JA. Phyoestorgens—a short review. *Maturitas.* 1995; 22:167–175.

37. Messina M, Barnes S. The role of soy products in reducing risk of cancer. *J Natl Cancer Inst.* 1993; 83(8):541–546.

38. Adlercreutz H. Plasma concentrations of phytoestorgens in Japanese men. *Lancet.* 1993; 50(suppl 201):3–23.

39. Wynder RL, Williams GM. Metabolic overload and carcinogenesis form the viewpoint of epidemiology. In: Somogyi A, Appel KE, Katenkamp A, eds. *Chemical Carinogenesis: The Relevance of Mechanistic Understanding of Toxicological Evaluations.* Munchen: MMV Medizin Verlag; 1993: 17.

40. Boyd NF, Martin LJ, Noffel M, Lockwood GA, Trichler DL. A meta-analysis of studies of dietary fat and breast cancer risk. *Br J Cancer*. 1993; 68:627.

41. LeMarchand L, Kolonel LN, Wilken LR. Animal fat consumption and prostate cancer: a prospective study in Hawaii. *Epidemiology*. 1994; 5:276–282.

42. Lyon JL, Slattery ML, Mahoney AW, Robinson LM. Dietary intake as a risk factor for cancer of the exocrine pancreas. *Cancer Epidemiol Biomarkers Prev*. 1993; 2:513.

43. Welsh CW. Relationship between dietary fat and experimental mammary tumorigenesis: a review and critique. *Cancer Res*. 1992; 52(suppl):2040s.

44. Reddy BS, Burill C, Rigotty J. Effect of diets high in omega-3 and omega-6 fatty acids on initiation and post-initiation stages of colon carcinogenesis. *Cancer Res*. 1991; 51:487.

45. Birt DF, Julius AD, White LT, Pour PM. Enhancement of pancreatic carcinogenesis in hamsters fed a high-fat diet ad libitum and at a controlled calorie intake. *Cancer Res*. 1989; 49:5845.

46. Corr JG, Fair WR, Heston WDW. Diet induced alteration of growth in LNCaP prostatic cancer cells. *Proc Am Assoc Cancer Res*. 1993; 34:131.

47. Goodwin PJ, Boyd NF. Critical appraisal of the evidence that dietary fat intake is related to breast cancer risk in humans. *J Natl Cancer Inst*. 1987; 79:473–485.

48. Lubin JH, Burns PE, Blot WJ, et al. Dietary factors and breast cancer risk. *Int J Cancer*. 1981; 28:685–689.

49. Katsouyanni K. Trichopoulos D, Boyle P, Xirouchaki E, Trichopouplou A. Diet and breast cancer: a case control study in Greece. *Int J Cancer*. 1986; 38:815–820.

50. La Vecchia C, Decarli A, Franceschi S, et al. Dietary factors and the risk of breast cancer. *Nutr Cancer*. 1987; 10:205–214.

51. Van't Veer P, Kok FJ, et al. Dietary fat and the risk of breast cancer. *Int J Epidemiol*. 1990; 19:12–18.

52. Wynder EL, Stellman SD. The "over-exposed" control group. *Am J Epidemiol*. 1992; 135:459–461.

53. Herbert JR, Clemow L, Pbert L, Ockene IS, Ockene JK. Social desirability bias in dietary self-report may compromise the validity of dietary intake measures. *Int J Epidemiol*. 1995; 24:389–398.

54. Hunter DJ, Speigelman D, Adami HO, et al. Cohort studies of fat intake and the risk of breast cancer—a pooled analysis. *N Engl J Med*. 1996; 334:356–361.

55. Katz EB, Boylan ES. Stimulatory effect of high polyunsaturated fat diet on lung metastasis from the 13762 mammary adenocarcinoma in female retired breeder rats. *J Natl Cancer Inst*. 1987; 79:351–358.

56. Rose DP, Connolly JM, Menschter CL. Effect of dietary fat on human brest cancer growth and lung metastases in nude mice. *J Natl Cancer Inst*. 1991; 83:1491–1493.

57. Rose DP, Connolly JM, Liu X-H. Effects of linoleic acid on the growth and metastastasis of two human breast cell lines in nude mice, and the invasive capacity of these cell lines in vitro. *Cancer Res*. 1994; 54:6557–6562.

58. Carroll KK, Gammal EB, Plunkett ER. Dietary fat and mammary cancer. *Can Med Assoc J*. 1968; 98:590–594.

59. Prentice RL, Sheppard L. Dietary fat and cancer: consistency of the epidemiologic data, and disease prevention that may follow from a practical reduction in fat consumption. *Cancer Causes Control*. 1990; 1:81–97.

60. Rose DP. Diet, hormones and cancer. *Annu Rev Public Health*. 1993; 14:1–17.

61. Bennett FC, Ingram DM. Diet and female sex hormone concentrations: an intervention study for the type of fat consumed. *Am J Clin Nutr*. 1990; 52:802–812.

62. Key TJA, Chen J, Wang Dym Pike MC, Boreham J. Sex hormones in women in rural China and Britain. *Br J Cancer*. 1990; 62:631–636.

63. Bradlow HL, Michnovicz JJ, Telang NT, Osborne MD, Goldin BR. Diet, oncogenes and tumor viruses as modulators of estrogen metabolism in vivo and in vitro. *Cancer Prev Detect*. 1991; 516:35–42.

64. Thorgeirsson SS. Endogeneous DNA damage and breast cancer. *Cancer*. 1993; 71:2897–2899.

65. Herbert JR, Barone J, Reddy MM, Backlund JY. Natural killer cell activity in a longitudinal dietary fat intervention trial. *Clin Immunol Immunopathol*. 1989; 54:103–107.

66. Carroll KK. Dietary fat and breast cancer. *Lipids*. 1992; 27:793.

67. Cave WT, Jr. Dietary n-3 (omega-3) polyunsaturated fatty acid effects on animal tumorigenesis. *FASEB J*. 1990; 5:2160.

68. Rose DP, Connolly JM, Effects of dietary omega-3 fatty acids on human breast cancer growth and metastases in nude mice. *J Natl Cancer Inst*. 1993; 85:1743.

69. Martin Morno JM, Willet WC, Gogojo L, et al. Dietary fat, olive oil intake and breast cancer risk. *Int J Cancer*. 1994; 54:774–780.

70. Trichopoulous A, Katsouyanni K, Stuver S. Consumption of olive oil and specific food groups in relation to breast cancer risk in Greece. *J Natl Cancer Inst*. 1995; 87:110–116.

71. Mettlin C, Selenskas S, Natarajan N, Huben R. Beta-carotene and animal fats and their relationship to prostate cancer risk. *Cancer*. 1989; 64:605–612.

72. Snowdon DA, Phillips RL, Choi W. Diet, obesity, and risk of fatal prostate cancer. *Am J Epidemiol*. 1984; 120:244–250.

73. Giovannucci E, Rimm EB, Stampfer MJ, et al. Intake of fat, meat, and fiber in relation to risk of colon cancer in men. *Cancer Res*. 1994; 54:2390–2397.

74. Freedman LS, Clifford C, Messina M. Analysis of dietary fat, calories, body weight, and development of mammary tumors in rats and mice: a review. *Cancer Res*. 19909; 50:5710.

75. Masoro EJ. Carolic restriction and aging in rats. In: Ingram DK, Baker GT III, Shock NW, eds. *The Potential for Nutritional Modulation of Aging Processes*. Food & Nutrition Press; 1991; 123.

76. Kneller, RW, Guo WD, Hsing AW, et al. Risk factors for stomach cancer in sixty-five Chinese Counties. *Cancer Epidemiol Biomarkers Prev*. 1992; 1:113–118.

77. Takahashi M, Kokubo T, Furukawa F, Kurokawa Y, Tatematsu M, Hayashi Y. Effect of high salt diet on rat gastric carcinogenesis induced by N-methyl-N'-nitro-N-nitrosoguanidine. *Gann*. 74; 28:1983.

78. Wakabayashi K, Nagao M, Esumi H, Sugimura T. Food-derived mutagens and carcinogens. *Cancer Res*. 1992; 52(suppl):2092s.

79. Weisburger JH, Williams GM. Food: its role in the etiology of cancer. In: Waldron KW, Johsen IT, Genwick GR, eds. *Food and Cancer Prevention: Chemical and Biological Aspects.* Cambridge, UK: The Royal Society of Chemistry; 1993: 3.

80. Craddock VM. Aetiology of esophageal cancer: some operative factors. *Eur J Cancer Prev.* 1992; I:89.

81. American Cancer Society. *Cancer Facts and Figures—1994.* Atlanta, GA: American Cancer Society; 1994.

82. Shils MD, Olson JA, Shike M, eds. *Modern Nutrition in Health and Disease*, 8th ed. Philadelphia: Lea & Febiger; 1994.

83. United States Department of Agriculture, U.S. Department of Health and Human Serices. *Nutrition and Your Health: Dietary Guidelines for Americans.* 4th ed. Washington, D.C.: US Government Printing Office; 1995.

84. Hahn NI. Variety is still the spice of a healthful diet. *J Am Diet Assoc.* 1995; 95:1096–1098.

85. United States Department of Agriculture (USDA). *USDA's Food Guide Pyramid.* Hyattsville, MD: Human Nutrition Information Services; 1992. (Home and garden bulletin no. 249.)

86. Work Study Group on Diet, Nutrition, and Cancer. American Cancer Society guidelines on diet, nutrition, and cancer. *Cancer.* 1991; 41:335–339.

87. Subar AS, Heimendinger J, Krebs-Smith SM, et al. *5-Day For Better Health: A Baseline Study of Americans' Fruit and Vegetable Consumption.* Rockville, MD: National Cancer Institute; 1991: 7.

88. Patterson B, Block G, Rosenberger WF, et al. Fruits and vegetables in the American diet: data from the NHANES II survey. *Am J Pub Health.* 1990; 80: 1443–49.

89. William CL. Nutrition in childhood: a key component of primary cancer prevention. In: Watson RR, Mufti SI, eds. *Nutrition and Cancer Prevention.* Boca Raton, FL: CRC Press; 1996: 25–50.

90. Committee on Diet, Nutrition and Cancer, Assembly of Life Sciences, National Research Council. *Diet, Nutrition and Cancer.* Washington, D.C.: National Academy Press; 1982.

91. Colditz GA, Fazier AL. Models of breast cancer show that risk is set by events of early life: prevention efforts must shift focus. *Cancer Epidemiol Biomarkers Prev.* 1995; 4:567–571.

92. Gritz ER, Bastani R. Cancer prevention—behavior changes: The short and the long of it. *Prev Med.* 1993: 22:676–688.

93. Wynder EL. Primary prevention of cancer: the case of comprehensive school heatlh education. *Cancer.* 1991; 67:1820.

94. D'Onofrio CN. Making the case for cancer prevention in the schools. *J Sch Health.* 1989; 59:225.

95. Anderson DM, Portnoy B. Diffusion of cancer education into schools. *J Sch Health.* 1989; 59:214.

96. Light L, Contento IR. Changing the course a school nutrition and cancer education curriculum developed by the American Cancer Society and the National Cancer Institute. *J Sch Health.* 1989; 59:205.

97. Corcoran RD, Portnoy B. Risk reduction through comprehensive cancer education: the American Cancer Society plan for youth education. *J Sch Health.* 1989; 59:199.

98. Resnikow K, Cross D, Wynder EL. The role of comprehensive school-based interventions: the result of four Know Your Body studies. *Ann NY Acad Sci.* 1993: 623:285.

99. Walter HJ. Primary prevention of chronic disease among children: the school-based "Know Your Body" intervention trials. *Health Educ Q.* 1989; 16:201.

100. Wynder EL, Williams CL, Laakso K. Screening for risk factors for chronic disease in children from fifteen countries. *Prev Med.* 1981; 10:121.

101. Wynder EL, Weisburger JH, Ng SK. Nutrition: the need to define "optimal intake as a basis for public policy decisions. *Am J Public Health.* 1992; 82:34.

102. Williams C, Bolella M, Williams GM. Cancer prevention beginning in childhood. In: De Vita VT, Jr., Hollman S, Rosenberg SA, eds. *Cancer Prevention.* Philadelphia, PA: Lippincott; 1993: 1.

103. Third National Health and Nutrition Examination Survey 1994 Phase 1, 1988–91. *Morbid Mortal Weekly Rep.* 43:116–125.

104. American Academy of Pediatrics, Committee on Nutrition, American Academy of Pediatrics Committee on Nutrition: statement on cholesterol. *Pediatrics.* 1992: 90:469.

105. Kleinman RD, Finberg LF, Kersh WJ, Laver RV. Dietary guidelines for children: U.S. recommendations. *J Nutr.* 1995; 125:10285–10305.

106. Fulgoni VL, Mackey MA. Total dietary fiber in children's diets. *Ann NY Acad Sci.* 1991; 623:368.

107. American Cancer Society, Inc. *Taking Control: Ten Steps to a Healthier Life and Reduced Cancer Risk.* Atlanta: American Cancer Society; 1985.

108. Dwyer JT. Diet and Nutritional Strategies for Cancer Risk Reduction. *Cancer.* 1993; 72(suppl):1024–1031.

109. Snow L. Folk medical beliefs and their implications for care of patients. *Ann Intern Med.* 1974; 81:82–96.

110. Barrett, S. *Health Schemes, Scams, and Frauds.* New York: Consumer Reports Books; 1990.

111. Cohen LA, Rose DP, Wynder EL. A rationale for dietary intervention in post menopausal breast cancer patients: an update. *Nutr Cancer.* 1993; 19:1–10.

112. Wynder EL, Rose DP, Cohen LA. Nutrition and prostrate cancer: a proposal for dietary intervention. *Nutr Cancer.* 1994; 22:1–10.

113. Chlebowski RT, Rose D, Buzzard IM, et al. Adjuvant dietary fat intake reduction in postmenopausal breast cancer patient management. *Breast Cancer Res Treat.* 1991; 20:73–84.

114. Chledowski RT, Blackburn GL, Buzzard IM, et al. Adherence to a dietary fat intake reduction program in postmenopausal women receiving therapy for early breast cancer. *J Clin Oncol.* 1993; 11:2072–2080.

115. Weisburger JH. Nutritional approach to cancer prevention with emphasis on vitamins, antioxidants, and carotenoids. *Am J Clin Nutr.* 1991; 53:226s–237s.

6

Sun Exposure and Cancer Risk

MARIANNE BERWICK

All substances are poisons; there is none which is not a poison. The right dose differentiates a poison and a remedy (1)
—*Paracelsus (1493–1541)*

Sunlight, critical to human health, provides light and warmth, and aids the body in the formation of vitamin D. Yet too much may be lethal. Excessive exposure to the sun invites the most common cancer of all: skin cancer, melanoma and nonmelanoma. In addition to its more commonly known impact on the skin, sunlight is also an important risk factor for cataract formation (2). This chapter will summarize both aspects of sunlight exposure—its protective aspect as well as its risk for cancer—and so help provide an informed basis for evaluating sun exposure.

The association with melanoma, the most deadly form of skin cancer, is complex. Although "too much" sun exposure may cause melanoma, how much is "too much" is highly individual; the characteristics of susceptibility have not been thoroughly defined. Furthermore, some sun exposure may actually exert a protective effect against colon, breast, ovarian, and prostate cancers (3). Sunlight also benefits a variety of disorders: heart conditions (4,5), psoriasis (6), and "SAD" (seasonal affective disorder) (7,8).

ULTRAVIOLET RADIATION (UVR)

The ultraviolet radiation spectrum is generally divided into three components: UVC, UVB, and UVA.

The divisions of the solar spectrum are important because the proportion of UVR from the bands of the solar spectrum changes with time of day, time of year, and latitude. The properties of each band affect cancer risk differently.

1. The UVC band of radiation lies between 265 and 280 nm. UVC is toxic to life but generally does not reach the earth's surface; the atmosphere filters it out. The amount of UVC reaching the earth will probably not be affected by stratospheric ozone depletion (9).

2. UVB radiation lies between 280 and 320 nm of the solar spectrum. In contrast to UVC, UVB radiation at the earth's surface will certainly increase as the stratospheric ozone layer diminishes. However, current measurement techniques are not sensitive enough, UVB radiation has not been measured consistently enough over time to determine whether it has increased. Until recently, most research on the carcinogenic effects of sunlight had focused on UVB. These effects include DNA damage, decrease in immunologic function, and possible modification of endocrine function. However, of late, the role of UVA in carcinogenesis has become increasingly clear.

3. UVA radiation, between 320 and 400 nm of the solar spectrum, can cause cancer, immunologic suppression, endocrinologic changes, and ocular changes, as well as skin aging. UVA at doses too low to cause skin redness (called erythema) can cause connective-tissue damage and cancer. The erythemal action spectrum, that is the wavelength of UV necessary to cause erythema, is somewhat different from the carcinogenic action spectrum, the wavelengths of UV necessary to induce cancer. At this time, the carcinogenic action spectrum for humans is unknown.

UVB Radiation

Indirect evidence indicates that ultraviolet radiation, particularly UVB, is part of the causal chain for melanoma skin cancer. Melanoma rates among Caucasians have a linear and inverse relationship to latitude (10). For example, during 1986 the incidence for melanoma in Tasmania, Australia, at 42°S, was approximately 15 per 100,000 people; the incidence for melanoma in Queensland, Australia, at 28°S, was approximately 43 per 100,000. Similarly, during 1978–

1982 in the United States the incidence for melanoma in males in Hawaii at 19.5°N was approximately 20 per 100,000 men; the incidence for melanoma in males in Connecticut at 42°N was approximately 9 per 100,000 men (11). Studies of Caucasians born in countries with a higher ambient solar radiation, such as Australia and Israel, show that they have a dramatically higher incidence of melanoma than Caucasian migrants to Australia or Israel from areas with lower ambient solar radiation (12,13). This suggests two alternative, but not mutually exclusive, explanations. The effects of UV are cumulative, so the longer the exposure, the greater the cancer risk, and/or sun exposure early in life is more damaging than long-term exposure.

In addition to being carcinogenic, UVB causes immunologic suppression. UVB damage to DNA initiates a cascade of reactions leading from direct DNA damage to antigen-specific immunosuppression (14–17). The major types of DNA damage caused by UVB include pyrimidine dimer formation (18), DNA strand breaks and DNA–protein cross linkages (19). In patients with *Xeroderma pigmentosum* (a genetic disease in which cells are deficient in DNA repair), sun exposure induces melanoma as well as nonmelanoma skin cancer at rates a thousand-fold greater than in normal individuals, although it acts by different mechanisms (20).

Much information exists on the effects of UV light on the immune system in experimental animals (17,21), but relatively little information on its effects in humans (22). Suppression of contact hypersensitivity (ability to respond to an antigen) in humans has been shown after exposure to UVB (23–25). This suppression occurs at a higher level in subjects with nonmelanoma skin cancer and melanoma, and may be one pathway by which sun exposure causes cancer (25).

UVA Radiation

Epidemiologic and laboratory studies of tanning salons which use UVA radiation predominantly as well as studies of sunscreen use with UVB protection suggest that UVA is important in carcinogenesis.

Because UVA was thought not to be associated with carcinogenesis, tanning salons were thought to be safe. However, several recent epidemiologic studies have shown that the use of tanning salons, where sunlamps emit predominantly UVA rays, was independently associated with melanoma formation, which indicated that UVA might induce melanoma skin cancer. Westerdahl and colleagues (26) reported that people who used suntanning beds had a 30% higher risk of melanoma. If they were younger than age 30 years and

used suntanning beds more than ten times a year their risk for melanoma was almost 8 times higher than older subjects who did not use suntanning beds. Other studies have similar findings (27,28).

Hersey and colleagues (29,30) found a reduced immune function in volunteers both immediately after and two weeks after exposure to commercial suntanning beds. Changes included reduced responses to carcinogens, slightly reduced blood lymphocyte numbers, changes in the proportion of lymphocyte subpopulations, changes in suppressor T cell activity and a depression of natural killer (NK) cell activity.

The use of sunscreens that block UVB but not UVA may be associated with an increase in melanoma rates. Also, most people do not apply sunscreen thickly enough (as directed) to afford the protection signified by the SPF (sun protection factor) on the label (31). Garland (32) first suggested that the use of sunscreens may encourage excessive exposure of the skin to UVA (where 90% to 95% of the ultraviolet energy in the solar spectrum occurs). New biological evidence supports this hypothesis (33), and an epidemiologic study in Sweden has reported an increased risk for melanoma with the use of sunscreens (34). Therefore, traditional means of avoiding overexposure to the sun, such as wearing hats and long sleeves and limiting sunbathing may be more appropriate than a heavy reliance on sunscreens.

The role of UVA in carcinogenesis is an important area for future research.

CURRENT RESEARCH ON SUN EXPOSURE AND CANCER RISK

Sun Exposure Behavior

Human behavior determines sun exposure. *Acute*, or intermittent, sun exposure, produces sunburn; *chronic* exposure, such as occupational exposure, where the skin has adapted to the sun, produces thickening of the stratum corneum and may afford protection for many people. Epidemiologic studies have shown (12,35) that people, such as farmers and construction workers, who are outdoors constantly have a lower relative mortality from melanoma than people who work indoors, such as office workers. Intermittent sun exposure is probably more risky; indoor workers have a higher risk of melanoma incidence and mortality. This has not been shown to be associated with fluorescent light exposure, notwithstanding an early suggestion of an association (36). Attempting to measure intermittent sun exposure or recreational sun exposure becomes problematic because measures of past sun exposure necessarily depend on subject recall of exposure, not a reliable measure (37). Epidemiologic studies have invariably shown weak associations between episodes of sunburn and melanoma incidence (38,39) (Table 6.1). Epidemiologic estimates of the effect of intermittent exposure have ranged from a protective effect reported by MacKie (40) of 0.44 (0.21–0.91) to an adverse risk of 8.41 (3.63–19.6) estimated by Grob (41). In contrast to popular notions, most estimates of the effects of sun exposure on melanoma incidence vary widely and are frequently not statistically significant (38).

Cancer Risk Related to Sun Exposure

Individual pigmentary risk factors are critical determinants of skin cancer risk. Subjects with light skin, light hair color, light eye color, a tendency to freckle, a tendency to burn on first exposure to sunlight, and an inability to tan after repeated exposures have a greater risk of developing all forms of skin cancer. Conversely, light pigmentation and sun exposure may decrease risk of colon, breast, prostate, and ovarian cancer at higher latitudes if the hypothesized association between sun exposure and vitamin D_3 in relation to carcinogenesis is correct.

Sun Exposure and Risk of Nonmelanoma Skin Cancer

Sun exposure plays a relatively clear role in causing nonmelanoma skin cancer (basal cell carcinoma and squamous cell carcinoma) and its precursor lesions, such as actinic keratoses (42). Clinicians diagnose approximately 100,000 squamous cell carcinomas (SCC) and 200,000 basal cell carcinomas (BCC) each year in the United States (43). Approximately 2% of SCC will metastasize (44); BCC rarely metastasizes (45). Mortality from nonmelanoma skin cancers is low, but the associated morbidity (illness) places a burden on the health care system (46) and is expected to increase as the population ages.

Nonmelanoma skin cancers occur primarily at sun-exposed body sites such as the head, neck, and arms, in people who are sensitive to the sun, and possibly among those who have a reduced capacity to repair DNA damage (47). Gallagher and colleagues (48) found no association between risk of SCC and cumulative lifetime sun exposure after accounting for pigmentary factors. In the Nurses' Health Study (a longitudinal study of 200,000 nurses begun in the 1970s), however, Grodstein, Speizer, and Hunter (49,50) concluded that sunburns are an important

TABLE 6.1. *Odds Ratios and 95% Confidence Intervals (CI) for Measures of Intermittent and Chronic Sun Exposure in Case-Control Studies**

Author, Year	Measure of Intermittent Sun Exposure	Odds Ratio (95% CI)	Measure of Chronic Sun Exposure	Odds Ratio (95% CI)
Adam, 1981 (89)	Deliberate tanning of the trunk; yes,no	1.58 (1.01–2.49)	Work time spent outdoors	No definite association
Beral, 1982 (36)	Various measures of recreational sun exposure	No consistent effect	Work outdoors; ever, never	0.93 (0.55–1.61)
MacKie, 1982 (40)	Recreational: ≥ 16 vs. 0 h/wk	0.44 (0.21–0.91)	Occupational: 16+ vs. < 16 h/wk	0.52 (0.23–1.16)
Green, 1984–86 (90–92)	Recreation on the beach: 6000+ vs. 0 h/lifetime	1.30 (0.39–4.29)	Cumulative hours of exposure: 50,000+ vs. < 2000 lifetime	1.70 (0.38–7.54)
Elwood, 1985 (93)	Swimming and beach activities 8+ vs 0 h/wk	1.70 (1.08–2.67)	Occupational summer: 16+ vs. < 16 h/wk	0.90 (0.57–1.41)
Graham, 1985 (94)	Vacations in southern regions: yes vs. no	No relation	Average annual hours 3200+ vs. ≤ 1600 h/yr	0.38 (0.19–0.75)
Holman, 1986 (95)	Recreational outdoor exposure proportion (ROEP): > 69% vs. 0–29%	1.57 (0.87–2.82)	Outdoor work in summer	0.41 (0.22–0.77)
Osterlind, 1988 (96)	Sunbathing: at some time vs. never	1.60 (1.08–2.37)	Working outside in summer	0.70 (0.52–0.93)
Walter, 1990 (27)	Use of sunbeds: ever vs. never	1.54 (0.96–2.46)	Not given	Not given
Beitner, 1990 (97)	Number of sunbaths April–September: > 30 vs. < 20/yr	1.80 (1.22–2.67)	Outdoor workers	0.60 (0.38–0.94)
Grob, 1990 (41)	Leisure sun exposure > 60 vs 0 SU†	8.54 (3.63–19.6)	Outdoor occupation: ever vs never	0.83 (0.55–1.25)

*After Nelemans PJ, Rampen FHJ, Ruiter DJ, Verbeek ALM. An addition to the controversy on sunlight exposure and melanoma risk: A meta-analytical approach. *J Clin Epidemiol.* 1995; 58:1331–1342.
†SU, sun exposure unit = days with at least 2 h of direct exposure.

risk factor for the development of SCC (relative risk (RR) = 2.4; 95%CI = 1.5–4.0 for six or more burns); interestingly, current cigarette smokers had a 50% increase in the risk of SCC compared with those who had never smoked. In the same cohort, Hunter and colleagues (50) found a higher risk of BCC in those who regularly spent time outdoors *and used sunscreen* than in those who regularly spent time outdoors *and did not use sunscreen* (RR = 0.60, 95% CI 0.50–0.70). Gallagher's work, which showed no association between mean annual cumulative summer sunlight exposure and risk of BCC, indirectly supports this finding. When Kricker and colleagues (51) examined the association between sun exposure and risk of BCC, they found that the effect of sun on BCC of the head, neck, and limbs decreased with increasing total exposure, whereas the risk of BCC on the trunk, which is generally exposed only intermittently, increased with increasing sun exposure. These features of nonmelanoma skin cancer are consistent with findings in melanoma skin cancer. A more critical appraisal of the similarities between the two seems to show similar patterns of effects from sun exposure.

Sun Exposure and Cutaneous Melanoma

Sun exposure plays a complex role in causing melanoma skin cancer and its precursor lesions. Pathologists estimate that nevi, both normal and atypical, are the precursor lesions for at least 50% of melanomas, and sun exposure at an early age seems to increase their number (52,53). So far, the strongest known risk factor for melanoma is the number of nevi a person has; the increased risk for increasing numbers of nevi ranges from 1.6 to as high as 50 (38,54) (Table 6.2).

Lifetime sun exposure is difficult to measure; most people cannot recall episodes of sunburn or amount of sun exposure reliably (37). Some studies have found that sunburn increases risk for cutaneous malignant melanoma (CMM), as noted by Whiteman and Green (39). Our own work (55) shows no effect of one sunburn, but an increased risk as the number of burns increases. Westerdahl's data are somewhat similar (26); this group found an increased risk of 1.9 for 3 or more sunburns per year when compared with subjects who had never had a sunburn. To add further complexity to the association of sun exposure and melanoma, our research group (56) has shown that pathologically verified solar damage is associated with increased survival for subjects with melanoma.

A paradoxical relationship may exist whereby in melanoma severe sun exposure initiates melanoma but nonburning sun exposure inhibits it (57,58). In

TABLE 6.2. *Major Risk Factors for Melanoma*

Variable	Odds ratio*	95% CI
Light skin color	2.15	(1.69–2.72)
Total sun exposure		
light	1.00	
moderate	1.04	(0.65–1.66)
heavy	1.80	(1.14–2.86)
very heavy	2.11	(1.18–3.15)
Total nevi†		
0	1.00	
10	1.77	(1.18–2.67)
11–30	3.97	(2.56–6.16)
31–50	5.47	(2.93–10.24)
> 50	4.89	(2.47–9.69)
Positive family history of skin cancer	1.88	(1.40–2.53)
Skin type		
Tendency to burn	1.36	(1.08–1.71)
Inability to tan	2.05	(1.57–2.67)
Light eye color	2.12	(1.65–2.74)
Light hair color	2.03	(1.61–2.56)
Tendency to freckle before age 25	1.70	(1.33–2.17)
Ever severely sunburned	1.26	(0.99–1.61)

Source: Berwick et al. (55).
*Adjusted for age and sex.
†As counted on backs and arms of subjects (with adjustment for the proportion of relevant skin surface examined).

fact, this pattern explains Kricker's finding in BCC as well. Each individual has a different "dangerous dose" of sun depending on their genetic predisposition and cutaneous phenotype, or coloring. This explanation may account for the conflicting results from epidemiologic studies. Several studies have found that the effects of sun exposure differ depending on individual susceptibility; for those who tan poorly, sun exposure increases risk (or shows no effect) compared with those who tan well, and sun exposure protects against melanoma for those who tan well (Table 6.3). White and colleagues (59) reported that tanning ability can modify melanoma risk due to sun exposure in childhood. Poor tanners showed no effect of sun exposure at ages 2–10 or ages 11–20 years. In contrast, people who reported a deep or moderate tan in reaction to chronic sun exposure appeared to be protected from melanoma with increasing sun exposure at ages 2–10 and at 11–20 years. Weinstock and colleagues (60) compared sun-sensitive women wearing swimsuits to non-sun-sensitive women and found that the former had a significantly increased risk with increasing sun exposure and that the latter had a significantly decreased risk with increasing sun exposure. Dubin and colleagues (61) found that a history of severe sunburn with blistering was associated with a nearly threefold risk among poor tanners but protected good tanners.

TABLE 6.3. *Studies on the Interaction Between Sun Exposure and Skin Type*

Author, Year	Measure	Odds Ratio (95% CI)	
Dubin, 1990 (61)	Severe sunburn history		
	Poor tanners		
	never	1.00	
	ever	2.93	(1.34–6.88)
	Dark tanners		
	never	1.00	
	ever	0.79	(0.41–1.50)
Weinstock, 1991 (60)	Annual frequency of swimsuit use outdoors ages 15–20 yr		
	Sun sensitive*		
	0–10	1.00	
	11–30	1.20	(0.6–2.6)
	>30	3.50	(1.3–9.3)
	Sun resistant		
	0–10	1.00	
	11–30	0.60	(0.2–1.4)
	>30	0.30	(0.1–0.8)
White, 1994 (59)	Sun exposure index† at ages 11–20 yr		
	Poor tanners		
	low	1.00	
	medium	0.94	(0.42–2.08)
	high	1.55	(0.61–3.99)
	Dark tanners		
	low	1.00	
	medium	0.50	(0.30–0.85)
	high	0.31	(0.16–0.59)

*Sun-resistant women were those with a sun-sensitive score of less than 0.5.
†Adjusted for type of clothing worn during sun-exposed activities.

Sun Exposure and Non-Hodgkin's Lymphoma

Data for a relationship between sun exposure and cancers other than melanoma have been more limited. Several researchers have suggested that sun exposure plays a causal role in the incidence of non-Hodgkin's lymphoma (62,63). This relationship may be due to the immunosuppressive role of sun exposure, or to the mutation of a tumor suppressor gene which may have a similar function in both non-Hodgkin's lymphoma and cutaneous melanoma. Our group and others are actively investigating this area.

A Beneficial Effect of Sun Exposure and Cancer: Cancer of the Colon, Breast, Prostate, Ovary, and Leukemia

Mortality rates for colorectal and other cancers decrease from north to south; this association has led to the hypothesis that sunlight exposure might be important in preventing some cancers by enhancing vitamin D_3 and calcium formation, which are inversely associated with colorectal cancer incidence (64). In a cohort of 25,000 subjects, even moderately elevated concentrations of 25-hydroxyvitamin D were associated with large reductions in the incidence of colorectal cancer (65).

Melanin, the pigment responsible for dark skin, has long been thought to be photoprotective (66). However, racial pigmentation also determines the magnitude of increase in serum vitamin D_3 levels following whole body exposure to UVB irradiation; serum levels of vitamin D_3 were highest in whites and lowest in blacks (67). Some evidence shows that low levels of sun exposure may result in higher cancer incidence, particularly among subsets of individuals, such as older people who would benefit from exposure to sunlight because of problems with micronutrient absorption or darker-skinned people who may have moved to higher latitudes (3). For example, Pakistani women living in Oslo, Norway, traditionally avoid the sun, have a low dietary intake of vitamin D, use few or no supplements, and have lower serum vitamin D levels (68).

Other cancers, such as breast cancer (69,70), prostate cancer (71–73), and ovarian cancer (74) may be inversely associated with sunlight exposure through a lack of vitamin D produced in the skin.

REACTION AND OVERREACTION TO THE HARM OF SUN EXPOSURE

Since sun exposure is so clearly related to skin cancer, many dermatologists warn that "there is no such thing as a healthy tan." As the data are most consistent with the hypothesis that melanoma and nonmelanoma are induced by intense sun exposure on skin which has not adapted to the sun, but inhibited by nonburning sun exposure (57), a more moderate *and* complex public health message would probably be more effective, both in reaching the public and in reducing the incidence of melanoma morbidity and mortality.

Psychological Research

To date, educational messages and research have focused on motivating people to reduce sun exposure and on ways of increasing the appeal of untanned skin. Along the same lines, most psychological research has focused on sunscreen use and attitudes toward tanning.

Some programs that attempt to change behavior achieved these goals. Fear of cancer has been successfully used as motivation to increase early detection of melanoma. Theobald and colleagues (75) reported that a television show about a young man dying from melanoma motivated 56% of viewers to examine their own skin and 36% to examine someone else's skin. Three months after this show, the proportion of tumors removed in the thin, easily cured stage increased 167%. Dukeshire and Fong (76) found that study participants whose risk for developing skin cancer was greatest and who were most frightened about skin cancer changed their sun-protective intentions the most. Australian research has shown a significant reduction in the number of people who sunburned after a health promotion campaign (77) that significantly increased the use of hats and sunscreen.

On the whole, these educational messages may, however, be based on an inaccurate assessment of the causes of skin cancer (78). Although sunscreen use is important in reducing erythema (sunburn), clear evidence that it is associated with a reduction in melanoma skin cancer is lacking, and the public may realize this. Although people say they know about the carcinogenic effects of sun exposure (79), they do not take what some dermatologists deem are appropriate safeguards. Arthey and Clarke (80) indicate that many people consistently display a high level of knowledge about the adverse consequences of excessive sun exposure and the need for sun protection, but do not decrease their sun exposure. That the current approach to sun behavior change is not ideal is supported both by the current understanding of the complex relationship of sun exposure to melanoma skin cancer and also by the research of Grob and colleagues (81), who reported that many adolescents and mothers were reasonably well informed but considered the risk of sun exposure to be exaggerated by the media.

Most research demonstrates that knowledge alone does not encourage sun protection behavior (79,82). Psychologically based interventions which are also grounded in accurate theory as to the etiologic role of sun exposure and cancer are necessary. In an examination of the effectiveness of different appeals, such as health and appearance, on intentions to engage in sun protection behavior, the appearance-based appeal was most effective (83–85). The perception of suntans as attractive is a barrier to skin cancer control campaigns designed to reduce exposure to the sun (86). People who believed they risked developing skin cancer were most likely to engage in protective behaviors (87,81).

PREVENTION OF SKIN CANCER

Skin Self-Examination

Skin self-examination has been reported to potentially reduce mortality from melanoma (55). This epidemiologic study was the first to study the effect of skin self-examination on lethal melanoma and should be replicated before firm pronouncements are made. In the meantime, promotion of skin self-examination is advisable. Skin self-examination should be done on a routine basis—once a month, once a season, or once a year—but not more than once a month. Ideally, one would involve a partner, or a "buddy" in visualizing the hard-to-see places like the scalp and the back. However, if a partner is not available then two mirrors will work. One should go over the entire body in a methodical manner. Start at the top and work down to the bottom: scalp, ears, face, neck, arms, underarms, chest, abdomen, back, buttocks, genital area, thighs, calves, feet, soles, and between the toes. In examining the skin, one should look for the ABCDs—asymmetry of a mark, border irregularity, color variegation, and diameter larger than a pencil eraser. Any mark which has been changing, or which seems unusual, should be referred to a dermatologist for further examination.

Sun Exposure

The role of sun exposure in cancer etiology is complex, and so advice to patients should not be simplistic. Sunshine should be enjoyed in moderation. Sunburn and other damage from excessive exposure should be avoided. Sunscreens give a false sense of security and it is unclear that they protect against melanoma, although fairly certain that they protect against non-melanoma skin cancer. The best advice is to wear hats and long sleeves, to seek shade, and to avoid long exposure in the midday sun (between the hours of 10a.m. and 3p.m.). It is important to realize that melanoma skin cancer develops in a relatively small proportion of the population; the majority will not get it. Scare tactics are therefore to be avoided and common sense is to be encouraged.

SUMMARY AND FUTURE DIRECTIONS

As epidemiologists and laboratory scientists become more accurate in ascertaining the role of sun exposure in the etiology of melanoma and other cancers, public health educators will be able to make use of the research on motivation for safe sun behavior. Perception of risk appears to be a major *sine qua non* for adopting appropriate sun protection. As the scientific community develops the ability to define risk more carefully and accurately, public health research into behavior change and the public health messages will become more appropriate

The most important aid for the recognition of the healing power and avoidance of the destructive effects of natural and artificial ultraviolet radiation . . . remains still the human intelligence. (88)

REFERENCES

1. Pagel W. *Paracelsus: An Introduction to Philosophical Medicine in the Era of the Renaissance.* New York: S. Karger; 1958.
2. Taylor HR, West SK, Rosenthal FS, et al. Effect of ultraviolet radiation on cataract formation. *N Engl J Med.* 1988; 319(22):1429–1433.
3. Studzinski GP, Moore DC. Sunlight—Can it prevent as well as cause cancer? *Cancer Res.* 1995; 55:4014–4022.
4. Shuh A. Climate therapy—more than the "right" climate. Prevention—cardiac rehabilitation. *Fortschr Med.* 1992; 110(28):18.
5. Solimene U, Sirtori PG, Balsamo V, Miani A Jr, Pirola V. Rehabilitative physiotherapy in Soviet medicine. *Clin Ter.* 1991; 139(3-4):75–79.
6. Snellman E, Aromaa A, Jansen CT, et al. Supervised four-week heliotherapy alleviates the long-term course of psoriasis. *Acta Derm Venereol.* 1993; 73(5):388–92.
7. Tietjen GH, Kripke DF. Suicides in California (1968–1977):absence of seasonality in Los Angeles and Sacramento counties. *Psychiatry Res.* 1994; 53(2):161–72.
8. Sakamoto K, Kamo T, Nakadaira S, Tamura A, Takahashi K. A nationwide survey of seasonal affective disorder at 53 outpatient university clinics in Japan. *Acta Psychiatr Scand.* 1993; 87(4):258–265.
9. Roy CR, Gies HP, Elliott G. The ARL solar ultraviolet radication measurement programme. *Trans Menzies Found.* 1989; 15:71–76.
10. Lancaster HO, Nelson J. Sunlight as a cause of melanoma:a clinical survey. *Med J Aust.* 1957; 1:452–456.
11. Grin-Jorgensen CM, Rigel DS, Friedman RJ. The worldwide incidence of melanoma. In: Balch CM, ed. *Cutaneous Melanoma*, 2d ed. Philadelphia: JB Lippincott; 1992: 27–36.
12. Holman CDJ, Armstrong BK. Cutaneous malignant melanoma and indicators of total accumulated exposure to the sun: an analysis separating histogenetic types. *J Natl Cancer Inst.* 1984; 73:75–82.
13. Katz L, Ben-Tuvia S, Steinitz R. Malignant melanoma of the skin in Israel: effect of migration. In: Magnus K, ed. *Trends in Cancer Incidence: Causes and Practical Implications.* New York: Hemisphere Publishers; 1982: 419–426.
14. Noonan FP, Kripke ML, Pedersen GM, Greene MI. Suppression of contact hypersensitivity in mice by ultraviolet irradiation is associated with defective antigen presentation. *Immunology.* 1981; 43:527–536.
15. Kripke ML, Thorn RM, Lill PH, Civin CI, Pazmino NH, Fisher MS. Further characterization of immunological unresponsiveness induced in mice by ultraviolet radiation. Growth and induction of nonultraviolet-induced tumors in ultraviolet-irradiated mice. *Transplantation.* 1979; 28:212–217.
16. Fisher S, Kripke ML. Suppressor T lymphocytes control the development of primary skin cancers in ultraviolet-irradiated mice. *Science.* 1982; 216:1133–1134.
17. Kripke ML. Ultraviolet radiation and immunology: something new under the sun—presidential address. *Cancer Res.* 1994; 54(23):6102–6105.
18. Brash DE, Rudolph JA, Simon JA, et al. A role for sunlight in skin cancer: UV-induced p53 mutations in squamous cell carcinoma. *Proc Natl Acad Sci USA.* 1992; 88:10124–10128.
19. Kricker A, Armstrong BK, Jones ME, Burton RC. *Health, Solar UV Radiation and Environmental Change.* Lyon: International Agency for Research on Cancer, Lyon; 1993. (IARC Technical Report No. 13.)
20. Kraemer KH, Lee MM, Andrews AD, Lambert WC. The role of sunlight and DNA repair in melanoma and nonmelanoma skin cancer. The xeroderma pigmentosum paradigm. *Arch Dermatol.* 1994; 130(8):1018–1021.
21. Noonan FP, De Fabo EC. Immunosuppression by ultraviolet B radiation: initiation by urocanic acid. *Immunol Today.* 1992; 13:250–254.
22. Pamphilon DH, Alnaqdy AA, Wallington TB. Immunomodulation by ultraviolet light: clinical studies and biological effects. *Immunol Today.* 1991; 12:119–123.
23. Sjovall P, Christesen OB. Local and systemic effect of ultraviolet irradiation (UVB and UVA) on human and allergic contact dermatitis. *Acta Dermatol.* 1986; 66:290–294.
24. Yoshikawa J, Rae V, Ruins-Slot W, Van den Berg JW, Taylor JR, Streilein JW. Susceptibility to effects of UVB radiation on induction of contact hypersensitivity as a risk factor for skin cancer in man. *J Invest Dermatol.* 1990; 95:530–536.
25. Streilen JW, Taylor JR, Vincek V, et al. Immune surveillance and sunlight-induced skin cancer. *Immunol Today.* 1994; 15(4):174–179.
26. Westerdahl J, Olsson H, Ingvar C. At what age do sunburn episodes play a crucial role for the development of malignant melanoma? *Eur J Cancer.* 1994; 30A(11):1647–1654.
27. Walter SD, Marrett LD, From L, Hertzman C, Shannon HS, Roy P. The association of cutaneous malignant melanoma with the use of sunbeds and sunlamps. *Am J Epidemiol.* 1990; 131:232–243.
28. Autier P, Dore JF, Lejeune F, et al. Cutaneous malignant melanoma and exposure to sunlamps or sunbeds: an

EORTC multicenter case-control study in Belgium, France and Germany. EORTC Melanoma Cooperative Group. *Int J Cancer*. 1994; 58(6)809–813.

29. Hersey P, Bradley M, Hasic E, Haran G, Edwards A, McCarthy WH. Immunological effects of solarium exposure. *Lancet*. 1983:545–548.
30. Hersey P, MacDonald M, Henderson C, et al. Suppression of natural killer cell activity in humans by radiation from solarium lamps depleted of UVB. *J Invest Dermatol*. 1988; 90:305–310.
31. Bech-Thomsen N, Wulf HC. Sunbathers' application of sunscreen is probably inadequate to obtain the sun protection factor assigned to the preparation. *Photodermatol Photoimmunol Photomed*. 1992–93; 9(6):242–244.
32. Garland CF, Garland FC, Gorham ED. Rising trends in melanoma. An hypothesis concerning sunscreen effectiveness. *Ann Epidemiol*. 1993; 3(1):103–110.
33. Setlow RB, Grist E, Thompson K, Woodhead AD. Wavelengths effective in induction of malignant melanoma. *Proc Natl Acad Sci USA*. 1993; 90:6666–6670.
34. Westerdahl J, Olsson H, Masback A, Ingvar C, Jonsson N. Is the use of sunscreens a risk factor for malignant melanoma? *Melanoma Res*. 1995; 5(1):59–65.
35. Lee JAH, Strickland D. Malignant melanoma:social status and outdoor work. *Br J Cancer*. 1980; 41:757–763.
36. Beral V, Evans S, Shaw H, Milton G. Malignant melanoma and exposure to fluorescent lighting at work. *Lancet*. 1982; 2:290–293.
37. Berwick M, Chen Y-T. Reliability of reporting of sunburn history in a case-control study of cutaneous malignant melanoma. *Am J Epidemiol*. 1995; 141(11):1033–1037.
38. Armstrong BK. Epidemiology of malignant melanoma: intermittent or total accumulated exposure to the sun? *J Dermatol Surg Oncol*. 1988; 14:835–849.
39. Whiteman D, Green A. Melanoma and sunburn. *Cancer Causes Control*. 1994; 5:564–572.
40. MacKie RM, Aitchison T. Severe sunburn and subsequent risk of primary cutaneous malignant melanoma in Scotland. *Br J Cancer*. 1982; 46:955–960.
41. Grob JJ, Gouvernet J, Aymar T, et al. Count of benign melanocytic nevi as a major indicator of risk for nonfamilial nodular and superficial spreading melanoma. *Cancer*. 1990; 66:387–395.
42. Ananthaswamy HN, Pierceall WE. Molecular mechanisms of ultraviolet radiation carcinogenesis. *Photochem Photobiol*. 1990; 52:1119–1136.
43. Preston DS, Stern RS. Nonmelanoma cancers of the skin. *N Engl J Med*. 1992; 327:1649–1662.
44. Nixon RL, Dorevitch AP, Marks R. Squamous cell carcinoma of the skin. *Med J Aust*. 1986; 144:235–239.
45. Miller SJ. Biology of basal cell carcinoma (Part I). *J Am Acad Dermatol*. 1991; 24:1–13.
46. Johnson ML, Johnson KG, Engel A. Prevalence, morbidity and cost of dermatologic diseases. *J Am Acad Dermatol*. 1984; 11(5 Pt2):930–936.
47. Wei Q, Matanoski GM, Farmer ER, Hedayati MA, Grossman L. DNA repair and aging in basal cell carcinoma:a molecular epidemiology study. *Proc Natl Acad Sci USA*. 1993; 90:1614–1618.
48. Gallagher RP, Hill GB, Bajdik CD, et al. Sunlight exposure, pigmentation factors, and risk of nonmelanocytic

skin cancer. II. Squamous cell carcinoma. *Arch Dermatol*. 1995; 131(2):164–169.
49. Grodstein F, Speizer FE, Hunter DJ. A prospective study of incident squamous cell carcinoma of the skin in the Nurses' Health Study. *J Natl Cancer Inst*. 1995; 87:1061–1066.
50. Hunter DJ, Colditz GA, Stampfer MJ, Rosner B, Willett WC, Speizer FE. Risk factors for basal cell carcinoma in a prospective cohort of women. *Ann Epidemiol*. 1990; 1:13–23.
51. Kricker A, Armstrong BK, English DR, Review: Sun exposure and non-melanocytic skin cancer. *Cancer Causes Control*. 1994; 5:367–392.
52. Harrison SL, MacLennan R, Speare R, Wronski I. Sun exposure and melanocytic naevi in young Australian children. *Lancet*. 1994; 344:1529–1532.
53. English DR, Rouse IL, Zhong X, et al. Cutaneous malignant melanoma and fluorescent lighting. *J Natl Cancer Inst*. 1985; 74:1191–1197.
54. Carli P, Biggeri A, Gianotti B. Malignant melanoma in Italy: risks associated with common and clinically atypical melanocytic nevi. *J Am Acad Dermatol*. 1995; 32(5 Pt l):734–739.
55. Berwick M, Begg C, Fine JA, Roush GC, Barnhill RL. Screening for cutaneous melanoma by skin self-examination. *J Natl Cancer Inst*. 1996; 88(1):17–23.
56. Barnhill RL, Fine JA, Roush GC, Berwick M. Predicting mortality in melanoma, a population-based analysis. *Cancer*. 1996; 78:427–432.
57. Ainsleigh HG. Beneficial effects of sun exposure on cancer mortality. *Prev Med*. 1993; 22:132–140.
58. Koh HK, Kligler BE, Lew RA. Yearly Review: Sunlight and cutaneous malignant melanoma:evidence for and against causation. *Photochem Photobiol*. 1990; 51(6):765–779.
59. White E, Kirkpatrick CS, Lee JAH. Case-control study of malignant melanoma in Washington State. I. Constitutional factors and sun exposure. *Am J Epidemiol*. 1994; 139:857–868.
60. Weinstock MA, Colditz GA, Willett WC, et al. Melanoma and the sun:the effect of swimsuits and a "healthy" tan on the risk of nonfamilial malignant melanoma in women. *Am J Epidemiol*. 1991; 134:462–470.
61. Dubin N, Moseson M, Pasternack BS. Sun exposure and malignant melanoma among susceptible individuals. *Environ Health Perspect*. 1989; 81:139–151.
62. Adami J, Frisch M, Yuen J, Glimelius B, Melbye M. Evidence of an association between non-Hodgkin's lymphoma and skin cancer. *Br Med J*. 1995; 310;1491–1495.
63. Zheng T, Mayne Taylor S, Boyle P, Holford TR, Lin WI, Flannery J. Epidemiology of non-Hodgkin lymphoma in Connecticut 1935-1988. *Cancer*. 1992; 70:840–1849.
64. Garland CF, Garland FC. Do sunlight and vitamin D reduce the likelihood of colon cancer? *Int J Epidemiol*. 1980; 9:227–231.
65. Bostick RM, Potter JD, Sellers TA, McKenzie DR, Kushi LH, Folsom AR. Relation of calcium, vitamin D, and dairy food intake to incidence of colon cancer among older women. *Am J Epidemiol*. 1993; 137:1302–1317.
66. Barker D, Dixon K, Medrano EE, et al. Comparison of the responses of human melanocytes with different mel-

anin contents to ultraviolet B irradiation. *Cancer Res.* 1995; 55:4041–4046.

67. Matsuoka LY, Wortsman J, Haddad JG, Kolm P, Hollis BW. Racial pigmentation and the cutaneous synthesis of vitamin D. *Arch Dermatol.* 1991; 127:536–538.

68. Henriksen C, Brunvand L, Stoltenberg C, Trygg K, Haug E, Pedersen JI. Diet and vitamin D status among pregnant Pakistani women in Oslo. *Eur J Clin Nutr.* 1995; 49(3):211–218.

69. Gorham ED, Garland FC, Garland CF. Sunlight and breast cancer incidence in the USSR. *Int J Epidemiol.* 1990; 19:820–924.

70. Furst CJ, Auer G, Nordevang E, Nilsson B, Holm LE. DNA pattern and dietary habits in patients with breast cancer. *Eur J Cancer.* 1993; 29:1285–1288.

71. Schwartz GG, Hulka BS. Is vitamin D deficiency a risk factor for prostate cancer (Hypothesis)? *Anticancer Res.* 1990; 10:1307–1312.

72. Hanchette CL, Schwartz GG. Geographic patterns of prostate cancer mortality. *Cancer (Phila).* 1992; 70:2861–2869.

73. Schwartz GG, Hulka BS, Morris D, Mohler JL. Prostate cancer and vitamin (hormone) D:a case control study. *J Urol (Suppl).* 1992; 147:294A.

74. Lefkowitz ES, Garland CF. Sunlight, vitamin D, and ovarian cancer mortality rates in US women. *Int J Epidemiol.* 1994; 23(6):1133–1136.

75. Theobald T, Marks R, Hill D, Dorevitch A. "Goodbye sunshine": effects of a television program about melanoma on beliefs, behavior and melanoma thickness. *J Am Acad Dermatol.* 1991; 25(4):717–723.

76. Dukeshire SR, Fong GT. Turning up the heat:using fear appeals to change sun-protective behavior. Pres. American Psychological Association, August 11–15, 1995, New York.

77. Hill D, White, V, Marks R, Borland R. Changes in sun-related attitudes and behaviours, and reduced sunburn prevalence in a population at high risk of melanoma. *Eur J Cancer Prev.* 1993; 2(6):447–456.

78. Young AR, Potten GC, Chadwick CA, Murphy GM, Hawk JLM, Cohen AJ. Photoprotection and 5-MOP photochemoprotection under UVR-induced DNA damage in humans: the role of skin type. *J Invest Dermatol.* 1991; 97:942–948.

79. Rossi JS, Blais LM, Redding CA, Weinstock MA. Preventing skin cancer through behavior change. *Dermatal Clin.* 1995; 13:613–622.

80. Arthey S, Clarke VA. Suntanning and sun protection: a review of the psychological literature. *Soc Sci Med.* 1995; 40(2):265–274.

81. Grob JJ, Guglielmina C, Gouvernet J, Zarour H, Noe C, Bonerandi JJ. Study of sunbathing habits in children and adolescents:application to the prevention of melanoma. *Dermatology.* 1993; 186(2):94–98.

82. Berwick M, Fine J, Bolognia JL. Sun exposure and sunscreen use following a community skin cancer screening day. *Prev Med.* 1992; 21(3):302–310.

83. Jones JL, Leary MR. Effects of appearance-based admonitions against sun exposure on tanning intentions in young adults. *Health Psychol.* 1994; 13(1):86–90.

84. Vail-Smith K, Felts WM. Sunbathing: college students' knowledge, attitudes, and perceptions of risks. *J Am Coll Health.* 1993; 42(1):21–26.

85. Broadstock M, Borland R, Gason R. Effects of suntan on judgements of healthiness and attractiveness by adolescents. *J Appl Soc Psychol.* 1992; 22:157–172.

86. Leary MR, Jones JL. The social psychology of tanning and sunscreen use: self-presentational motives as a predictor of health risk. *J Appl Soc Psychol.* 1993; 1390–1406.

87. von Schirnding Y, Strauss N, Mathee A, Robertson P, Blignaut R. Sunscreen use and environmental awareness among beach-goers in Cape Town, South Africa. *Public Health Rev.* 1991–92; 19(1-4):209–217.

88. Breit R. *Roting und Braunnung durch UVA.* Munich: W. Zucherschwert Verlag; 1987.

89. Adam SA, Sheaves JK, Wright NH, Mosser G, Harris RW, Vessey MP. A case-control study of the possible association between oral contraceptives and malignant melanoma. *Br J Cancer.* 1981; 44:45–50.

90. Green A. Sun exposure and the risk of melanoma. *Aust J Dermatol.* 1984; 25:99–102.

91. Green A, Siskind V, Bain C, Alexander J. Sunburn and malignant melanoma. *Br J Cancer.* 1985; 51:393–397.

92. Green A, Bain C, McLennan R, Siskind V. Risk factors for cutaneous melanoma in Queensland. In: Gallagher RP, ed. *Epidemiology of Malignant Melanoma.* Heidelberg: Springer-Verlag; 1986, 76–97.

93. Elwood JM, Gallagher RP, Hill GB, Pearson JCG. Cutaneous melanoma in relation to intermittent and constant sun exposure: The Western Canada Melanoma Study. *Int J Cancer.* 1985; 35:427–433.

94. Graham S, Marshall J, Haughey B. An inquiry into the epidemiology of melanoma. *Am J Epidemiol.* 1985; 122:606–619.

95. Holman CDJ, Armstrong BK, Heenan PJ. Relationship of cutaneous malignant melanoma to individual sunlight-exposure habits. *J Natl Cancer Inst.* 1986; 76:403–414.

96. Osterlind A, Tucker MA, Stone BJ, Jensen OM. The Danish case-control study of cutaneous malignant melanoma. II. Importance of UV-light exposure. *Int J Cancer.* 1988; 42:319–324.

97. Beitner H, Norell SE, Ringborg U, Wennersten G, Mattson B. Malignant melanoma: aetiological importance of individual pigmentation and sun exposure. *Br J Dermatol.* 1990; 122:43–51.

7

Compliance with Cancer Treatment

JEAN L. RICHARDSON AND KATHLEEN SANCHEZ

Reviews of the literature on patient compliance are numerous and are consistent in the conclusion that many more patients than expected do not adhere to their treatment regimens (1–3). Noncompliance with treatment regimens has been shown to be a problem across a wide range of diseases, age groups, and treatments, with serious implications for the prognosis of the patient. Unfortunately, compliance is rarely monitored in the clinical setting; however, when patients fail to respond to a prescribed treatment it is important to determine whether the underlying problem is noncompliance or an ineffective treatment, because the solutions are different.

Compliance is also a major factor affecting the evaluation of new cancer therapies. It is not possible to determine the benefit of a new therapy without knowing how much of the medication was taken. Although clinical trials are generally evaluated in terms of assignment, important information can be gained by assessing the role of adherence in trial results. If an arm of a trial fails owing to ineffective medication, the solution is to modify the medications already prescribed; but when it fails owing to noncompliance, interventions need to be developed to help the patient adhere.

In this chapter we will review the studies that have examined compliance with follow-up recommendations after an abnormal examination, compliance with cancer treatment protocols for children and adults, and compliance challenges for chemoprevention and dietary protocols. These more recently developed chemoprevention strategies involve the topical application or the ingestion of a chemopreventive agent—often a vitamin—for those with a cancer precursor or early disease, while other trials examine more fundamental changes in dietary intake. Finally, we will examine where there are gaps in the research and why those gaps exist.

COMPLIANCE WITH FOLLOW-UP RECOMMENDATIONS AFTER AN ABNORMAL EXAMINATION

Numerous studies have examined population-based cancer screening programs to detect cancer early, but far fewer have examined the issue of compliance with follow-up examinations subsequent to suggestive findings. In this section we do not deal with the issue of individuals who notice symptoms but fail to refer themselves for initial evaluation, nor do we examine literature that assesses delays that are due to the system of health care; both of these are significant problems and have been reviewed elsewhere (4,5). However, in the case of follow-up after an abnormal finding, individuals are already in contact with the health care system, and they can be easily targeted for intervention. The timeliness of the response is influenced by the individual's knowledge of the importance of the symptoms, their own or family's/friend's experience with these illnesses, access to medical care, their sociodemographic characteristics, and numerous other psychological and knowledge factors. This form of delay is important to consider in a discussion of compliance because stage at diagnosis is the most important determinant of survival and because a patient who delays after being advised to return for definitive diagnosis may also be a less compliant patient during treatment.

Several studies have examined follow-up colonoscopies. Meyers and colleagues (6) found that compliance with surveillance colonoscopy one year following treatment for an index lesion was only 54%. Similarly, low levels with one-year surveillance colonoscopy have been reported by others and range from 31% to 39% (7,8).

Other studies have examined follow-up after an abnormal mammogram. In order to improve adherence with follow-up for abnormal mammograms found during surveillance screening, Lerman and co-workers (9) designed materials that used negative or positive framing styles to explain the results and the importance of continued surveillance. The groups that received the intervention were significantly more likely to have a follow-up mammogram (66%) than the control group (53%); however, message framing style did not make a difference. Similarly, Lantz and colleagues (10) assessed the impact of physician reminder letters and telephone calls in increasing follow-up after abnormal mammograms or pap smears. After six months women who received the reminder letters and telephone calls were more likely to comply with the follow-up procedures (67%) than the control group (43%).

Numerous studies have examined compliance with follow-up recommendations among those having abnormal pap smears. Paskett and colleages (11) notified women with abnormal pap smears with a standard clinic letter and an information sheet explaining the abnormal result. The intervention women received the same materials along with a motivational pamphlet describing reasons for compliance with follow-up visits. The follow-up rate was higher among the intervention (64.2%) than the control group (51%).

Marcus and colleagues (12) designed a much more complex study with eight conditions to increase follow-up after abnormal pap smears. The intervention groups were assigned to *(1)* receive a "personalized" physician follow-up letter and educational pamphlet, or *(2)* view a slide-tape program, or *(3)* receive transportation incentives (bus tokens) or any possible combination of these interventions. Nearly 30% of women in the control group failed to return for clinic visits, however, the findings regarding intervention effects were unclear. The combined personalized letter/pamphlet and slide-tape program increased the return rate for follow-up visits significantly over the control group, although none of the single-strategy interventions was effective.

Lerman and colleagues (13) used telephone counseling that focused on potential barriers to appointment keeping to increase adherence to a diagnostic colposcopy. The purpose of the intervention was to reduce barriers that were related to psychological (e.g., anxiety), educational (e.g., lack of understanding), and lifestyle (e.g., child care) issues. The intervention increased compliance (67%) with scheduled colposcopy over the control group (43%).

Manfredi and colleagues (14) noted that delay in obtaining treatment is, in part, related to noncompliance with referrals. His intervention among low-income patients with several conditions, such as

abnormal pap smears and fecal occult blood, included referral information and telephone counseling. The control group received standard referrals. With this limited intervention, follow-up was improved from 68% in the control group to 89% in the intervention group.

The range of compliance with follow-up after an abnormal test result among control groups ranged from 43% to 70%. The tested interventions improved compliance between 10% and 20%. Delay in seeking treatment has been overcome by increasing a patient's knowledge about symptoms, increasing their belief in early detection strategies, and addressing ways to overcome barriers, including psychological barriers, to follow-up. These reminders have been delivered in writing or by telephone, suggesting that relatively inexpensive interventions can significantly improve compliance. However, as many as one-third of patients still fail to respond to these interventions and virtually nothing is known about how to reach these more resistant individuals.

Delay in seeking treatment has been associated with poor patient–provider communication (15), lack of prompt appointments (11), fear of diagnosis (9) and financial concerns (12). Clearly, fear of cancer, anxiety, and perhaps depression will accompany the news of the abnormal results from these screening tests. Paskett and Rimer (5) suggest several steps to improve follow-up compliance, including *(1)* reduction of time until referral appointment, *(2)* provision of clear instructions for follow-up recommendations, *(3)* use of triage/tracking systems for monitoring compliance (i.e., increasing the intensity for apparently noncompliant patients), *(4)* sharing test results with patients to enlist them as part of the team, *(5)* reduction of barriers to compliance within the medical care system and, *(6)* use of reminder systems. Because this behavior is easily tracked and documented, most providers are capable of including some of these compliance-enhancing strategies into their practice.

COMPLIANCE WITH TREATMENT PROTOCOLS

Pediatric and Adolescent

Several studies have examined compliance with oral medications for pediatric and adolescent cancer patients. Most examine medications used for maintenance chemotherapy in childhood acute lymphoblastic leukemia (ALL) including prednisone, 6-mercaptopurine (6MP) and methotrexate (MTX) (16).

One of the earliest studies using biological markers of pediatric/adolescent compliance with cancer chemotherapy was conducted by Smith and co-workers

(17). Compliance with prednisone was measured by identifying metabolites of prednisone, 17 ketogenic steroids, in the urine. On the basis of urine assays of 19 children under 11 years of age, 14 (73.7%) were classified as compliers, 3 (15.8%) were noncompliers, and 2 (10.5%) were intermittent compliers. For those 8 children over 11 years of age, 3 (37.5%) were compliers, and 5 (62.5%) were noncompliers. Overall, 59% of all urine samples from adolescents and 18% of urine samples from pediatric patients fell below the expected level; 33% of all patients were classified as noncompliant.

Lansky and colleagues (18) similarly assessed compliance with oral prednisone for 31 patients with ALL. No patient was found to be 100% compliant on the three urine samples collected. Eighteen (58%) of the children were classified as compliers while 42% were classified as noncompliers. Tebbi and colleagues (19) studied 46 cancer patients, most with hematologic malignancies, between 2.5 and 23 years old. Serum bioassay and self-reports of compliance with prednisone and 6MP were collected. Serious and occasional noncompliance was found in about one-third of children and was especially problematic in adolescents. Compliance decreased over time from 81% at 2 weeks to 61% at 20 weeks. Festa and colleagues (20) similarly used bioassays to evaluate compliance among 21 young patients with ALL or Hodgkin's disease who were prescribed prednisone. Eleven of the 21 (52%) were found to be nonadherent to treatment. Of 29 adolescents with Hodgkin's disease who were prescribed penicillin for postsplenectomy prophylaxis, confirmation of adherence by urine bioassay of growth inhibition of *Micrococcus luteus* indicated that 14 (48%) were nonadherent.

A few studies stand in contrast to these dismal suggestions of childhood cancer patient noncompliance. MacDougall and colleagues (21) studied children aged 3–14 years with ALL in remission who received oral 6MP daily. 6MP was detected in 81% of first morning urine samples from children receiving an evening oral dose. Since false negative results may be obtained in morning urine samples for those who void during the night, even this high level may be conservative. Davies, Lennard and Lilleyman (22) indicated that of 35 children on maintenance 6MP after remission of ALL, 22 (62.9%) appeared to tolerate the treatment without cytopenia. Among these children, 6 (17.1%) were shown to be noncompliant with their medication, although none of these completely abstained from treatment. A further study by Lennard and Lilleyman (23) showed that of 130 children with ALL, who were prescribed 6MP, 10%–20% did not comply with their prescribed therapy.

Few studies among pediatric populations have specifically addressed children of minority groups. Foucar and colleagues (24) examined survival of 28 Native American, 91 Hispanic white, and 77 nonHispanic white children with ALL. Median survival ranged from 8 months for Native American boys to 140 months for nonHispanic white girls. Both Native American boys and girls, respectively, had delays in receiving prescribed treatments and more problems with compliance. Native American boys achieved lower rates of complete remission than patients in other ethnic groups and stopped maintenance treatment (which was planned to last for 36 months), within the first 12 months after diagnosis.

These results indicate that noncompliance ranges between 10% and 59% among childhood cancer patients and is especially high among adolescents. Adolescent patients have been judged by their providers to be significantly less compliant than younger patients, with almost half rated as being "poor" or "very poor" compliers. In fact, poor compliance was judged by their provider to be a threat to the prognosis of over half of the adolescents studied (25). This provider assessment is consistent with the results of Smith et al. (17) and Tebbie et al. (19).

Data on the determinants of compliance are sparse. In one study compliance was not correlated with several expected determinants including family income level, mother's marital status, complexity of the regimen, side effects, satisfaction with information given, understanding of the disease, or belief in efficacy of the medication (19). Yet, adolescents often suffer more severe side effects as a result of their illness and treatment than younger patients. In addition, adolescents may be more sensitive to changes in appearance caused by cancer treatment. Both of these factors may contribute to the lower compliance rate of adolescent cancer patients.

Tamaroff and colleagues (26) found that adolescent cancer patients who complied had higher levels of understanding of the causality of illness and comprehension of issues related to prognosis. Noncompliers were more reassured by the absence of symptoms, were more prone to use denial in the context of illness-related issues, believed that the medications could cause other serious health problems, and believed the side effects could interfere with their normal activities. Yet, in the two studies reported by Festa and co-workers (20), the purpose and the effects of the medications were different. Prednisone is prescribed as a part of the treatment regimen but has definite cosmetic effects. Penicillin, on the other hand is preventive and has few side effects. The low rate of compliance with each regimen suggests that neither the purpose of the regimen nor the adverse effects accounted for noncompliance, or alternatively they separately accounted for an equal decrement. While side effects may have led to noncompliance with the prednisone, the penicillin may have been affected by the generally low level of compliance with preventive treatments.

A few studies have examined parental variables as potential explanations for low compliance among children with cancer. Lansky and colleagues (18) examined the role of parents and of gender in poor compliance. Although they found no gender difference in compliance, predictors of compliance differed between males and females. Parental variables associated with compliance in boys were hostility, anxiety, and obsessive-compulsive behavior, while parental variables were not associated for girls. Parents seemed to worry less about their daughters and to give them more responsibility.

Surprisingly, Lansky and colleagues (18) found that boys from larger families were more likely to take their oral prednisone than those from smaller families while Tebbie and colleagues (19) showed that patients in families with more children were less compliant as were those in families who had less understanding of the instructions. Compliers were also more likely to agree with their parents regarding who was responsible for the administration of the medication, perhaps indicating that, among those who did not agree, the changes in roles of parents and adolescents may not have been clearly negotiated or communicated, resulting in lower levels of compliance. It is important to note that while Tamaroff and colleagues (26) found that parental supervision of medication taking did not differ between compliers and noncompliers, virtually *none* of the patients (12.9–25.6 years old) was supervised by a parent in their medication taking (26). Reasons most often given for noncompliance by patients and parents were forgetfulness, busy schedules, and nonavailability of medication, although parents were more likely to list busy schedules first and patients were more likely to list forgetfulness first (19). Taken as a whole, these studies suggest that the supervisory role of parents in medication adherence of child cancer patients, especially adolescents, is an important determinant of compliance. Unfortunately, the information is sparse concerning parental correlates of child cancer patient compliance. Furthermore, experimentally tested interventions to address noncompliance of children, especially adolescents, are virtually nonexistent.

Adult

Although adult patients with cancer undergoing treatment far outnumber children undergoing treatment, there are not many more studies of adult compliance than of child compliance. In addition, there are not many studies that examine minority patients with cancer, multimodality treatment, covariates of compliance, or that test interventions to improve compliance.

Richardson and colleagues (27) and Levine and colleagues (28) documented a low level of compliance with prescribed chemotherapy and supportive therapy among patients with hematologic malignancy. Although this was an intervention study, the level of compliance among the control group represents prevailing levels of compliance. Using bioassays, prednisone was consistently present in six-monthly blood samples of only 27% of patients, and for allopurinol it was present for only 22.5% of patients. The level for the metabolite of prednisone was slightly lower and the metabolite of allopurinol more than twice as high, suggesting that many more patients may be intermittent compliers with allopurinol. Nevertheless the self report of compliance with allopurinol was only 53.8%, indicating that patients themselves recognize their low level of compliance. Only 66.5% of appointments for intravenous chemotherapy were kept in the control group.

Feld and colleagues (29) conducted a study of stage II and III lung cancer patients assigned to receive adjuvant chemotherapy with cyclophosphamide, doxorubicin, and cisplatin. Eighty percent received the initial dose, 66% received at least two cycles, but only 53% received all four courses and only 57% of these patients received all four cycles on time.

As with pediatric cancer patients, there are a significant number of studies that indicate that noncompliance is not a major problem. Budman and colleagues (30) showed that 30 of 32 patients completed a course of intravenous outpatient cyclophosphamide, adriamycin, and 5-fluoroacil (CAF) in four months. Moul and colleagues (31) assessed treatment among testicular cancer patients and found that only 7 of 244 (2.9%) refused all or a portion of their cancer therapy. Lee and colleagues (32) monitored patients undergoing treatment for Hodgkin's disease or non-Hodgkin's lymphoma for 65 treatment periods of two weeks each. A medication vial with an electronic device in the cap to indicate bottle openings suggested compliance was high, approaching 100%. Lebovits and colleagues (33) followed breast cancer patients treated with oral cytoxan and/or prednisone and assessed patient nonadherence based on repeat self-report over six months. Though 22 patients (43%) were noncompliant, only 8 of these patients underingested the medication while 12 patients overingested cytoxan and/or prednisone or took the drugs on weeks when they were not prescribed, suggesting that poor understanding of the regimen rather than intentional noncompliance was at issue.

Compliance with clinic appointments is especially important because much of the chemotherapy is given intravenously. The ranges reported for compliance with clinic appointments varied from 66.5% (28) to 77% (34) to 98% (35). Ayers and colleagues (36) examined compliance with clinic appointments for intravenously administered chemotherapy for minority and lower socioeconomic women with breast cancer and found that 63% were classified as compliant (kept 85% of clinic appointments), while 37% were not compliant and four were unclassified. Compliance with follow-up appointments may be influenced by the treatment regimen itself. Young and colleagues (37) examined compliance with follow-up visits for nonseminomatous testicular cancer treated with surgery alone or with chemotherapy. For those treated with surgery alone, chemotherapy is given if there is a relapse, therefore follow-up monitoring is especially important. Yet none of those treated by surgery were compliant with all appointments as compared to 57% for the chemotherapy group. Chemotherapy patients saw their disease as more dangerous than surgical patients and saw their disease as widespread, perhaps leading to their higher level of compliance.

Three studies specifically address the issue of compliance with radiation therapy. Smith and colleagues (38) found high compliance (95%) with radiation therapy after a lumpectomy among medically indigent breast cancer patients. On the other hand, Formenti and colleagues (39) assessed compliance with radiation therapy among Latina cervical cancer patients. Those patients who completed therapy in eight weeks were considered compliant. Only 16% (11/69) completed radiation within that time period, while 64% (44/69) completed it in longer than eight weeks; 20% (14/69) elected to discontinue radiation prematurely.

Jacobs and colleagues (40) examined compliance with a treatment protocol for head and neck cancer patients which included surgery followed by three courses of chemotherapy, followed by radiation therapy. Major unacceptable noncompliance with radiation therapy occurred among 15%–19% of patients. For those who completed less than three courses of chemotherapy, noncompliance with radiation therapy was 33%, suggesting that noncompliance cuts across regimen demands.

Two studies (33,31) indicated that lower socioeconomic status was related to lower levels of compliance. Since both Formenti and colleagues (39) and Richardson and colleagues (27) conducted their research among a low socioeconomic status population, this may also explain their low levels of compliance, although others (38,40) did not find socioeconomic status to be an issue. Formenti and colleagues indicated that expressed concerns were about job loss due to absences, transportation, and child care; in addition, confusion about the etiology and nature of the disease and the chances for cure was present in many of the patients. Three studies by Lebovits (33), Lee (32) and Richardson (41) and their colleagues showed that greater regimen complexity also influenced noncompliance and that compliance decreased over time. Ayers and colleagues (36) found that psychological factors that correlated with compliance included high scores on fighting spirit, anxiety, depression, and vigor scales. High scores on guilt and hostility predicted lower levels of compliance. Richardson and colleagues (41) found little relationship between depression and compliance; however, satisfaction with care was related to higher compliance.

Most chemotherapeutic regimens for the treatment of cancer cause at least one side effect. Clearly, toxicities are a major factor in physician decisions about modifying treatment regimens, but little is known about the role of these side effects on patient noncompliance. Some side effects are easily tolerated or treated and some patients take the occurrence of side effects as an indication that the treatment is working. Nevertheless, side effects have been suggested to be a major deterrent to compliance, although the actual research support for this is slim. The occurrence of side effects cannot be denied; for example, Feld and colleagues (29) found that 89% of patients had mild to severe hair loss, 88% had mild to severe nausea and vomiting, and 65% had hematologic toxic effects. Similarly high rates were documented for hematologic malignancy patients: hair loss (58%), nausea (72%), weakness (58%), and loss of appetite (53%) (42). In this study, adverse effects were more common among younger patients, those who had a poorer prognosis, or those who had a complex treatment regimen. Younger patients also reported greater difficulty dealing with these effects than older patients; this was also found by Nerenz and colleagues (43). While no aspect of compliance correlated with self-report of side effects experienced, the difficulty of dealing with a side effect and interference with daily activities correlated inversely with compliance with clinic appointments. This suggests that patients may skip an appointment to avoid the intravenous drugs thought to be associated with side effects especially nausea, loss of appetite, and hair loss.

There are few experimental intervention studies targeted to improve low compliance rates among patients. This lack of interventions targeted to cancer patients may be partly due to the great difficulty of studying compliance in clinical settings and the expectation that patients with such a serious disease would, of course, comply.

Richardson and colleagues (27) examined the effect of three strategies to improve compliance with therapy for patients with hematologic malignancy: *(1)* a nurse education session to increase knowledge and enhance patient participant compliance; *(2)* a home visit to tailor the daily treatment regimen to the patient and family home environment; *(3)* a shaping component while the patient was still in the hospital to improve the patient's knowledge about medication identification and dosage schedule. Greater efforts aimed at providing information on the part of providers was met with greater satisfaction on the part of patients that lead to greater compliance. Although the three groups did not differ on compliance, the intervention groups had higher levels of compliance than the control group for allopurinol and appointment keeping (92% vs. 61%) but not prednisone.

Both the pediatric and the adult literature indicate that there are a wide range of results concerning the actual level of noncompliance with treatment. The variables that may cause such a wide discrepancy are almost too many to enumerate. While the childhood studies have tended to focus more on one disease, ALL, the adult studies have addressed many diseases and treatment modalities. The populations themselves may differ; the exact inclusion and exclusion criteria for patients may have a major effect; the number of measurement time points and the exact measures used (records, self-report, bioassay) are all affected by different sources and levels of error. Furthermore, the lack of information concerning effective strategies to improve compliance among cancer patients is distressing and cuts across both the pediatric and the adult literature.

COMPLIANCE WITH CANCER CONTROL PROTOCOLS

Within recent years, dietary and chemoprevention interventions have been suggested as a means for preventing cancer. These are based on the results of epidemiological studies that have identified patterns of cancer in populations that suggest dietary causation

or inhibitory characteristics of particular agents. Diet studies are those that contain a dietary prescription. Chemoprevention studies are those where a defined chemical (even though a dietary factor such as a vitamin) is prescribed.

Chemoprevention Intervention Trials
In chemoprevention studies, healthy patients are provided with medications, vitamins, dietary regimens, or other medical or lifestyle recommendations to prevent the development of cancer. In most cases the individuals selected are assumed to be at high risk of developing the disease because of family history, age, or the occurrence of a presumed cancer precursor such as intestinal polyps. Chemoprevention trials have focused on skin, oral mucosa, lung, cervix, bladder, and colon cancer. Most cancer chemoprevention programs are in trial phases and are not widely recommended to the general population (44). Individuals who participate in chemopreventive trials for cancer are more likely to be younger, better educated, and have higher incomes, be regular vitamin users, and have a greater belief in the link between diet and cancer (45), and these characteristics may limit the generalizability of the results.

The success of these trials often depends on the recruitment of large numbers of individuals and the compliance of the individuals with the treatment protocol for many years. A chemoprevention study for familial adenomatous polyposis (in which polyps in the colon at a young age progress to colon cancer within ten years) provides a good example of the issues involved (46). Wheat fiber, and antioxidants such as ascorbic acid (vitamin C) and α-tocopherol (vitamin E), may alter the appearance and growth of polyps. Oral administration of these vitamins with and without a wheat fiber supplement (two small cereal-sized boxes each day) was tested. There was a significant decline in compliance with both fiber and vitamins from the first year of treatment to the second year of treatment. After 8 months on study approximately 80% complied with their fiber recommendation, while at 22 months the rate was approximately 55%; for vitamins the compliance rate dropped from 95% to 85%. Fiber compliance was related to distaste for the fiber supplement and to variations in eating practices such as eating breakfast. Psychological factors such as internal control of health and negative affect were also related to compliance.

In a similar supplementation trial to prevent lung cancer among smokers, β-carotene and retinol were provided. Visit adherence over the course of the study was 74% for males and 70% for females; capsule consumption was 85% and 82%, respectively, over the three-year study, however, adherence did decrease over the course of the study (47).

Several prevention trials involving oral medication to prevent or delay a chronic disease endpoint have indicated surprisingly good levels of compliance, as high as 80%–90% (48,49). Individual counseling, nutritional information, cooking demonstrations, newsletters, and educational materials are always included to increase adherence. Several of these studies conclude that though compliance can be very high, it may not be generalizable. Engstrom (50) attributes the high level of success of these programs to planned and purposeful attempts to improve compliance: selecting a population that is interested in the study by virtue of being composed of volunteers, using a run-in period before randomization (noncompliers declare themselves within 3–4 months), preparing a study booklet and newsletter, using a once-a-day dosing regimen, contacting patients regularly throughout the study, and using incentives to increase compliance.

Dietary Interventions for Women with Breast Cancer

This section will review the feasibility of achieving a high level of patient compliance with a low-fat diet as part of the regimen for women with breast cancer. Low-fat diets, in conjunction with other treatment modalities, have been suggested to improve the prognosis of women with resected local breast cancer (51). However, dietary changes have been shown to be among the most difficult of regimens to follow and maintain for long periods of time.

The argument for reducing fat intake during breast cancer treatment is based on *(1)* epidemiologic observation of stage by stage survival advantages for women in countries with low-fat diets (Japan) versus high-fat diets (United States); *(2)* adverse effects of weight gain on breast cancer patient outcomes; *(3)* animal studies indicating an adverse influence of increased dietary fat intake (especially the fatty acid linoleic acid) on growth and metastatic spread of mammary cancer; and *(4)* direct effects of linoleic acid to stimulate human breast cancer cell growth both in vitro and as solid tumors in nude mice (52). Weight gains of approx 2.5 kilograms have been consistently observed during adjuvant chemotherapy regimens such as CMF and CMFP for stage II breast cancer and may have a detrimental effect on clinical outcome for patients with resected breast cancer. Questions have been raised about the conceptual basis and feasibility of such trials. In particular, the difference in cancer survival between Japanese and American women may not be due to

fat intake per se but may be due to lower body fat mass among Asian women. Body fat is a strong determinant of postmenopausal estrogen levels and may influence tumor growth (53). Other data suggest that greater weight at the time of mastectomy effects outcome, suggesting also that body fat and not fat intake may be the important issue. Finally, if linoleic acid has been shown to be the main form of fat important in tumor growth in animals, then an intervention to decrease all fat intake may not be sufficiently focused.

Buzzard and colleagues (54) examined the effect of a pilot study to assess the efficacy of a low-fat diet (15% of calories from fat) during drug therapy for postmenopausal women with stage II breast cancer. After three months of dietary intervention, the mean fat intake dropped from 38% calories from fat to 23%. Total calorie consumption, serum cholesterol, and weight also decreased significantly.

Chlebowski and colleagues (55) reported results for 290 postmenopausal women with stage I to IIIa breast cancer who were receiving systemic therapy and were randomized to a low-fat diet or to a control group. The majority of those in the intervention and control group were receiving tamoxifen alone (61% and 56%, respectively) while 28% and 32%, respectively, were receiving chemotherapy. Fat intake was significantly lower in the intervention (20.3%) as compared with the control group (31.5%) at six months and was maintained for 24 months. This decrease in fat intake was not accompanied by a decrease in serum cholesterol but was accompanied by a decrease in body weight.

Holm and colleagues (56) also examined the effect of a pilot study to reduce fat intake in stage I–II breast cancer patients in Sweden. The intervention group decreased fat intake from 36% to 22% and maintained this change for two years, the control group decreased by 3.6%. However only 52% of the patients in the intervention group were followed two years later while 89% of the control group had a two year follow-up. The fact that the long-term participation rate was lower in the intervention group is perhaps due to selective retention of compliers. Noncompliers who chose not to be followed in the intervention group could significantly alter the results.

It is not yet clear whether low-fat diets during cancer treatment will improve prognosis. Larger trials of low-fat diets for prevention have been conducted and have shown that dietary fat can be reduced to approximately 20% and maintained for 24 months (57–60). Although self-reports of fat consumption were lower for the intervention groups than the control group in these studies, changes in serum cholesterol and weight were not always consistent with these reports, although weight maintenance could occur with dietary substitutions. These studies suggest that a low-fat diet can be adopted as a long-term life-style change, however; the possibility of biased self-reports cannot be discounted. Lower education, feelings of deprivation, as well as costliness of the diet in time and money negatively influenced long-term adherence (61). Concerns about long-term maintenance of dietary interventions have been examined by Henkin and colleagues (62), who found that 89% of subjects followed dietary recommendations successfully for 12 weeks, but only 30% felt that they maintained the diet long-term.

These trials have, for the most part, used counseling by a dietician as the major intervention strategy. Sessions were generally offered on a weekly schedule which tapered to monthly. Identification of high- and low-fat foods, self-monitoring strategies, recipe modification, and individualized eating plans were emphasized.

It appears that the compliance of individuals on these studies has been high, probably owing to a careful selection process, run-in period, education program, and follow-up plan. These high success rates, in the face of low success rates for weight-loss regimens and community intervention programs, are dependent on highly motivated women who were screened prior to study entry and carefully instructed and followed during the trial. It cannot be assumed that the same success rate would be achieved in the general population.

DIFFICULTIES IN DOING COMPLIANCE RESEARCH

Although the need to understand the reasons for noncompliance is great, both to help the patient and to aid in the development and evaluation of new effective therapies, there are many factors that cause the study of compliance and the evaluation of compliance-gaining interventions to be extremely difficult. These issues are described briefly below.

Cross-sectional studies of compliance have suffered from biases because factors correlated with compliance may not necessarily be predictive in the longitudinal model. Achieving change in variables shown to be significant in the cross-sectional studies will not necessarily result in changes in the dependent variable in longitudinal or experimental studies. Cross-sectional studies have also suffered from the biased sample problem, that is to say, the individuals who will be seen in a clinic cross-sectional sample will be survivors, those who like the clinic staff, those who are more likely to be compliers, and those who adhere to clinic appointments. Studies that have used what has been termed an inception cohort—identifying patients at the start of treatment and following them over their treatment course—are rare.

Part of the reason this design is so rare is that cancer therapy often changes over time as new drugs and regimens are developed; thus compliance criteria continually change. Cancer therapy for the individual also changes over time, often because a regimen appears to not be efficacious for an individual and often because the patient is intolerant of the regimen.

The experimental studies designed to evaluate strategies to improved compliance are also rare. It is difficult to develop and have available a new behavioral intervention and to randomize patients to receive or not receive this intervention. Nurses or physicians who have been trained in the new strategy are reluctant to withhold it from any patient, especially if the intervention involves a new skill in patient teaching or counseling. Patients seek out the information they need and the social support they need. Patients within the same institution discuss not just their treatment plan but also the educational programs they have received, and therefore it is very difficult to keep a control group from being contaminated with the intervention group benefits. The alternative is to assign institutions to intervention or control groups; however, this does not address the issue of institutional comparability. Institutions attract individuals with specific characteristics and thus the generalizability of the findings may be limited.

Statistical power is a major problem because the number of patients with a particular type of cancer and related treatment may be less than expected in a set of institutions. While clinical trials run by national groups achieve power by having many physicians recruit only a few patients each, this is not a feasible approach to behavioral interventions.

Research on compliance, and particularly the predictors of compliance, requires great attention to instrumentation. The use of multiple measurement techniques is necessary. Direct measures of the drug or metabolite in the blood or urine are seen as the most unbiased estimate of compliance; however, even these fail to provide information on the pattern of self-medication. If the drug is taken intermittently and the half-life is short, it may never be detected. In addition, patterns of missed doses cannot be determined in this manner. Self-reports typically provide higher estimates of compliance than blood samples; however, these are distorted by self-presentation biases. Even the newer techniques of pill vial caps with computer chips to record opening and closing do not necessarily document the fact that the medication was taken. Record abstracts are useful sources of information about appointment keeping and procedures administered. The need for multiple measures of compliance is obvious but always cumbersome, expensive, and not always possible to achieve. While these issues all make the conduct of descriptive and intervention trials of compliance very difficult, the inclusion of some measures of compliance in national clinical trials would advance dramatically understanding of the magnitude and importance of compliance.

CONCLUSIONS

We have dealt with several experiences that require very different compliance behaviors: follow-up of abnormal test results, compliance with treatment regimens on the part of children and adults, compliance with chemoprevention regimens for those who have a precursor to cancer, and compliance with a low-fat diet for women with breast cancer.

Compliance is to a large extent determined by the patient's perceptions and beliefs about the characteristics of the disease they are confronting and the options they have in dealing with this disease. The costs of complying for the patient include time, inconvenience, and money. The physical costs of complying with surgery, chemotherapy, or radiation include disfigurement, pain, nausea, vomiting, hair loss, and others. Emotional costs are also involved and may include loss of control and loss of peace of mind. Finally, social costs may also include loss of social role. The dynamics surrounding the costs are highly individualized. The balance of beliefs about treatment efficacy and the values associated with them when compared with the costs suggests that it is the patient's personal weighing of these that causes them to comply or not with their treatment.

Noncompliance should not be considered attributable to the patient alone. The health care environment also has an impact on patient behavior. Health care institutions, providers, and payment systems have been shown in repeated studies to have a major impact on patient behavior. Communication with providers and satisfaction with care are major factors of importance. Although patients may self-regulate their own compliance on the basis of their own values, the costs of complying, and their understanding of the disease and its treatment, clear and accurate communication of information is critical. Most individuals when diagnosed with cancer know very little about the disease itself, the treatment options and effects, the probabilities of treatment success, the side effects associated with specific treatments and how these might be con-

trolled. It is important to them and to the provider to improve their understanding of these issues so that they can become cooperative participants in their own treatment. While patients may weigh their decisions in light of the values that are important to them, it is also very likely that individuals cannot weigh these decisions because they lack the information to do so. Patients are dependent on their medical provider to communicate this information to them in a way they can understand and in an emotionally supportive manner. The patient and the provider will often have a series of decisions and difficulties to experience together during treatment. The stronger and more effective the communication lines, the more the patient can truly be an informed participant in their own health care. Understanding one's disease and what is required in complying with one's treatment regimen is very different from actually complying. Supportive interventions in the form of home visits, significant-other training, and behavioral contracting can be useful in strengthening compliance with medication and treatment regimens in cancer patient populations. However, greater effort aimed at providing information on the part of providers is usually met with greater satisfaction on the part of patients, which leads to greater compliance (41).

In some cases the provider needs to provide specific skills training. This is the case in dietary interventions and may well apply to other repeat behaviors as well. For example, cueing of pill taking by behavioral linkage with other tasks such as tooth brushing has been shown to be helpful. Contracting with patients and family members to improve agreements about responsibility may be especially important for adolescents. Such behavioral strategies can be taught in the clinical setting by nurses or other professionals.

The existing data on patient compliance with treatment regimens are limited but suggest a wide range of compliance levels. Although this may be due to different research methods, the many studies evaluated in this chapter suggest that compliance with regimens may differ by age group, by the demands of the regimen, by socioeconomic status, by social-situational aspects of adherence, by the communication skills of the provider, by whether patients are seen as part of a clinical protocol trial, and by a host of other factors. It would appear that compliance with follow-up of abnormal findings, while ranging from 50% to 70%, can be improved by 10%–20% by the use of telephone counseling procedures, yet the behavior of resistant subjects is unstudied. Dietary compliance can be achieved in the short term and extending out to 24 months by careful one-to-one dietary counseling focusing on knowledge and skills training, although the generalizability of these results is unclear. Compliance with treatment regimens suggests a wide range of compliance, with indications that patient understanding of the disease and supportive communication with providers will improve compliance. Noncompliance is not always intentional and is often due to misunderstanding of the demands of the regimen and lack of attentiveness. In some cases it may be due to poor compliance skills. Compliance is a task-specific behavior and is not an unchangeable characteristic of a situation or of a person. This area of research is poorly studied and fraught with difficulties in study design. Improved patient survival depends upon the ability of the medical and research communities to develop effective strategies to address these issues.

ACKNOWLEDGMENTS
This work was supported by grant #SIG20 from the American Cancer Society and by National Cancer Insitute training grant #T32-CA09492.

REFERENCES

1. Sackett DL, Snow JC. The magnitude of compliance and noncompliance. In: Haynes RB, Taylor DW, Sackett DL. *Compliance in Health Care.* Baltimore: Johns Hopkins University Press; 1979: 11–23.
2. Shope JT. Medication compliance. *Pediatr Clin N Am.* 1981; 28:5–21.
3. Morrow GR, Leirer V, Sheikh J. Adherence and medication instructions: review and recommendations. *J Am Geriatr Soc.* 1988; 36:1147–1160.
4. Caplan LS, Helzlsouer KJ. Delay in breast cancer: A review of the literature. *Public Health Rev.* 1992; 93(20):187–214.
5. Paskett ED, Rimer BK. Psychosocial effects of abnormal pap tests and mammograms: a review. *J Women's Health.* 1995; 4(1):73–82.
6. Myers RE, Bralow SP, Goldstein R, Jacobs M, Wolf TA, Engstrom PF. Surveillance for colorectal neoplasia: is patient adherence following treatment a problem? *Cancer Detect Prev.* 1993; 17(6):609–617.
7. Rozen P, Fireman Z, Baratz M, et al. Screening for colorectal tumors: A progress report of the Tel-Aviv Program. In: Rozen P, Winawer SJ, vol. eds. *Frontiers of Gastrointestinal Research: Secondary Prevention of Colorectal Cancer: An International Perspective.* New York: Karger; 1986: 10:164–181.
8. Woolfson I, Eckholdt G, Wetzel C, et al. Usefulness of performing colonoscopy one year after endoscopic polypectomy. *Dis Colon Rectum.* 1990; 33(5):389–393.
9. Lerman C, Ross E, Boyce A, et al. The impact of mailing psychoeducational materials to women with abnormal mammograms. *Am J Public Health.* 1992; 82(5):729–730.
10. Lantz PM, Stencil D, Lippert MT, Beversdorf S, Jaros L, Remington PL. Breast and cervical cancer screening in a low-income managed care sample: the efficacy of physician letters and phone calls. *Am J Public Health.* 1995; 85:834–836.
11. Paskett ED, White E, Carter WB, Chu J. Improving follow-up after an abnormal pap smear: a randomized control trial. *Prev Med.* 1990; 19:630–641.
12. Marcus AC, Crane LA, Kaplan CP, et al. Improving adherence to screening follow-up among women with abnormal pap smears. *Med Care.* 1992; 30(3):216–230.
13. Lerman C, Hanjani P, Caputo C, et al. Telephone counseling improves adherence to colposcopy among lower-income minority women. *J Clin Oncol.* 1992; 10(2):330–333.
14. Manfredi C, Lacey L, Warnecke R. Results of an intervention to improve compliance with referrals for evaluation of suspected malignancies at neighborhood public health centers. *Am J Public Health.* 1990; 80(1):85–87.
15. Lauver D, Rubin M. Message framing, dispositional optimism and follow-up for abnormal papanicolaou tests. *Res Nurs Health.* 1990; 13:199–207.
16. Davies HA, Lilleyman JS. Compliance with oral chemotherapy in childhood lymphoblastic leukaemia. *Cancer Treat Rev.* 1995; 21(2):93–103.
17. Smith SD, Rosen D, Trueworthy RC, Lowman JT. A reliable method for evaluating drug compliance in children with cancer. *Cancer.* 1979; 43:169–173.
18. Lansky SB, Smith SD, Cairns NU, Cairns GF. Psychological correlates of compliance. *Am J Pediatr Hematol Oncol.* 1983; 5:87–92.
19. Tebbi CK, Cummings KM, Zevon MA, Smith L, Richards M, Mauon J. Compliance of pediatric and adolescent cancer patients. *Cancer.* 1986; 58:1179–1184.
20. Festa RS, Tamaroff MH, Chasalow F, Lanzkowsky P. Therapeutic adherence to oral medication regimens by adolescents with cancer I. Laboratory assessment. *J Pediatr.* 1992; 120:807–811.
21. Macdougall LG, McElligott SE, Ross E, Greef MC, Poole JE. Pattern of 6-mercaptopurine urinary excretion in children with acute lymphoblastic leukaemia: urinary assays as a measure of drug compliance. *Therap Drug Monitor.* 1992; 14:371–375.
22. Davies HA, Lennard L, Lilleyman JS. Variable mercaptopurine metabolism in children with leukemia: a problem of non-compliance? *Br Med J.* 1993; 306:1239–1240.
23. Lennard L, Lilleyman JS. Compliance with 6-mercaptopurine metabolism in UKALL trials. *Br J Hematol.* 1993; 84 (suppl):19.
24. Foucar K, Duncan MH, Stidley CA, Wiggins CL, Hunt WC, Key CR. Survival of children and adolescents with acute lymphoid leukemia. A study of American Indians and Hispanic and non-Hispanic whites treated in New Mexico (1969 to 1986). *Cancer.* 1991; 67(8):2125–2130.
25. Dolgin MJ, Katz ER, Doctors SR, Siegel SE. Caregivers' perceptions of medical compliance in adolescents with cancer. *J Adolesc Health Care.* 1986; 7:22–27.
26. Tamaroff MH, Festa RS, Adesman AR, Walco GA. Therapeutic adherence to oral medication regimens by adolescents with cancer—Part II. Clinical and psychologic correlates. *J Pediatr.* 1992; 120:812–817.
27. Richardson JL, Shelton DR, Krailo M, Levine AM. The effect of compliance with treatment in survival among patients with hematologic malignancies. *J Clin Oncol.* 1990; 8(2):356–364.

28. Levine AM, Richardson JL, Marks G, et al. Compliance with oral drug therapy in patients with hematologic malignancy. *J Clin Oncol.* 1987; 5:1469–1476.

29. Feld R, Rubinstein L, Thomas PA, and the Lung Cancer Study Group. Adjuvant chemotherapy with cyclophosphamide, doxorubicin, and cisplatin in patients with completely resected stage I non-small cell lung cancer. *J Natl Cancer Inst.* 1993; 85(4):299–305.

30. Budman DR, Korzun AH, Aisner J, et al. A feasibility study of intensive CAF as outpatient adjuvant therapy for stage II breast cancer in a cooperative group: CALGB 8443. *Cancer Invest.* 1990; 8(6):571–575.

31. Moul JW, Paulson DF, Walther PJ. Refusal of cancer treatment in testicular cancer patients [letter]. *J Natl Cancer Instit.* 1989; 81(20):1587–1588.

32. Lee CR, Nicholson PW, Souhami RL, Deshmukh AA. Patient compliance with oral chemotherapy as assessed by a novel electronic technique. *J Clin Oncol.* 1992; 10(6):1007–1013.

33. Lebovits AH, Strain JJ, Schleifer SJ, Tanaka JS, Bhardwaj S, Messe MR. Patient noncompliance with self administered chemotherapy. *Cancer.* 1990; 65:17–22.

34. Itano JK, Tanabe PH, Lum J, et al. Compliance and noncompliance in cancer patients. *Advances in Cancer Control: Research and Development.* New York: Alan R. Liss; 1983; pp. 483–495.

35. Carey P, Gjerdingen DK. Follow-up of abnormal papanicolaou smears among women of different races. *J Fam Pract.* 1993; 37(6):583–587.

36. Ayres A, Hoon PW, Franzoni JB, Matheny KB, Cotanch PH, Takanyanagi S. Influence of mood and adjustment to cancer on compliance with chemotherapy among breast cancer patients. *J Psychosom Res.* 1994; 38(5):393–402.

37. Young, BJ, Bultz BD, Russell JA, Trew MS. Compliance with follow-up of patients treatment for non-seminomatus testicular cancer. *Br J Cancer.* 1991; 64(3):606–608.

38. Smith RG, Landry JC, Hughes LL, et al. Conservative treatment of early-stage breast cancer in a medically indigent population. *J Nat Med Assoc.* 1995; 87(7):500–504.

39. Formenti SC, Meyerowitz BE, Ell K, et al. Inadequate adherence to radiotherapy in Latina immigrants with carcinoma of the cervix: potential impact of disease-free survival. *Cancer.* 1995; 75(5):1135–1140.

40. Jacobs JR, Casiano RR, Schuller DE, Pajak TF, Laramore GE, Al-Sarraf M. Chemotherapy as a predictor of compliance. *J Surg Oncol.* 1994; 55(3):143–148.

41. Richardson JL, Marks G, Johnson CA, et al. Path model of multidimensional compliance with cancer therapy. *Health Psychol.* 1987; 6(3):183–207.

42. Richardson JL, Marks G, Levine AM. The influence of disease and side effects of treatment compliance with cancer therapy. *J Clin Oncol.* 1988; 6:1746–1752.

43. Nerenz DR, Leventhal H, Love RR. Factors contributing to emotional distress during cancer chemotherapy. *Cancer.* 1982; 50(5):1020–1027.

44. DeWys WD, Malone WF, Butrum RR, Sestilli MA. Clinical trials in cancer prevention. *Cancer.* 1986; 58:1954–1962.

45. Mettlin C, Cummings KM, Walsh D. Risk factor and behavioral correlates of willingness to participate in cancer prevention trials. *Nutr Cancer.* 1985; 7:189–198.

46. Berenson M, Groshen S, Miller H, DeCosse J. Subject-reported compliance in a chemoprevention trial for familial adenomatous polyposis. *J Behav Med.* 1989; 12(3):233–247.

47. Thornquist MD, Patrick DL, Omenn GS. Participation and adherence among older men and women recruited to the beta carotene and retinol efficacy trial (CARET). *Gerontologist.* 1991; 31(5):593–597.

48. Steering Committee of the Physicians Health Study Research Group. Final report on the aspirin component of the ongoing physicians health study. *N Engl J Med.* 1989; 321:129–135.

49. Albanes DK, Virtamo J, Rautalahti M, et al. Pilot Study: The US-Finland lung cancer prevention trial. *J Nutr Growth Cancer.* 1981; 3:207–214.

50. Engstrom PF. Specific compliance issues in an antiestrogen trial of women at risk for breast cancer. *Prev Med.* 1991; 20:125–131.

51. Chlebowski RT, Grosvenor M. The scope of nutrition intervention trials with cancer-related endpoints. *Cancer.* 1994; 74:2734–2738.

52. Chlebowski RT, Rose DP, Buzzard M, et al. Adjuvant dietary fat intake reduction in postmenopausal breast cancer patient management. *Breast Cancer Res Treat.* 1991; 20:73–84.

53. Willett WC. Dietary fat reduction among women with early breast cancer. *J Clin Oncol.* 1993; 11(11):2061–2062.

54. Buzzard IM, Asp EH, Chlebowski RT, et al. Effect of a low-fat diet on intake of other dietary components. *J Am Diet Assoc.* 1990; 90:45–50.

55. Chlebowski RT, Blackburn GI, Buzzard M, et al. Adherence to a dietary fat intake reduction program in post menopausal women receiving therapy for early breast cancer. *J Clin Oncol.* 1993; 11(11):2072–2080.

56. Holm LE, Nordevang E, Ikkala E, Hallström L, Callmer E. Dietary intervention as adjuvant therapy in breast cancer patients—a feasibility study. *Breast Cancer Res Treat.* 1990; 16:103–109.

57. Boyd NF, Cousins M, Lockwood G, Tritchler D. Dietary fat and breast cancer risk: the feasibility of a clinical trial of breast cancer prevention. *Lipids.* 1992; 27(10):821–826.

58. Heber D, Ashley JM, McCarthy WJ, et al. Assessment of adherence to a low-fat diet for breast cancer prevention. *Prev Med.* 1992; 21:218–227.

59. Insull W Jr, Henderson MM, Prentice RL. Results of a randomized feasibility study of a low-fat diet. *Arch Intern Med.* 1990; 150(2):421–427.

60. Henderson MM, Kushi LH, Thompson DJ, et al. Feasibility of a randomized trial of a low fat diet for the prevention of breast cancer: dietary compliance in the Women's Health Trial Vanguard Study. *Prev Med.* 1990; 19(2):115–133.

61. Urban N, White E, Anderson GL, Curry S, Kristal AR. Correlates of maintenance of a low-fat diet among women in the Women's Health Trial. *Prev Med.* 1992; 21(3):279–291.

62. Henkin Y, Garber DW, Osterlund LC, Darnell BE. Saturated fats, cholesterol, and dietary compliance. *Arch Intern Med.* 1992; 152:1167–1174.

8

Social Class/Socioeconomic Factors

JENNIFER L. BALFOUR AND GEORGE A. KAPLAN

Why include a chapter on socioeconomic status (SES) and cancer in a volume on psycho-oncology? It is simply because SES profoundly affects people and populations with cancer at all stages of the disease. Not only do the risks of developing cancer and the risks of dying from cancer vary across levels of SES, but the experience of living with cancer and fighting the disease also changes with socioeconomic status. When poor persons have cancer, they and their families bear a disproportionate burden of increased morbidity, difficulty in affording medical treatment, and ultimately increased risk of death (1,2). Because SES has such a profound affect on all aspects of cancer, and because SES is a complex phenomenon that pervades social, psychological, medical, and physical experiences, the connection between SES and cancer is at the heart of psycho-oncology.

SOCIOECONOMIC STATUS AND HEALTH

The knowledge that increasing SES is associated with increasing health is very old, extending back to the twelfth century (3). An inverse gradient between SES and poor health has been documented for many diseases, across the lifespan, and in many different populations and places. Poorer people have an increased risk for such diverse outcomes as low birth weight pregnancies, diabetes, accidental death, and coronary heart disease (4–7). This inverse gradient is found using many different measures of SES such as income, education, geographic area of residence, and occupational status. Several explanations have been proposed for the association between SES and ill-health. These include *(1)* experience of material deprivation by the poorest populations, *(2)* poorer access to medical prevention, diagnosis, and treatment, *(3)* a higher prevalence of specific risk factors in lower social classes, *(4)* selection of people with poorer health into the lower social classes through illness, and *(5)* a general sus-

ceptibility to disease that increases as SES decreases (7–11). Evidence has shown that it is not just the poorest groups that suffer a higher rate of disease and death, but that SES shows a graded relationship to disease experience. This inverse pattern of SES and disease is difficult to interpret using any simple explanation. For example, differences in levels of material deprivation are not likely to account for the different health experiences of the most well-off compared to those just below them. The consistency of these gradients suggests that it is important to search for the social, behavioral, psychologic, and physical differences which give rise to the pervasive SES gradient in health (7).

The associations of SES with cancer incidence and SES with cancer survival have been the focus of much investigation. SES gradients are used in many studies of cancer to generate etiologic hypotheses. More recently, the persistence of SES as a risk factor in cancer incidence and mortality has commonly led to statistical adjustment for SES, in order to examine other factors independently of the role of SES. Of course, such an approach offers little opportunity for clarifying why and how SES is related to cancer incidence and mortality. In this chapter we will summarize the data indicating a relationship between SES and cancer incidence and mortality for major cancer sites, discuss in more detail the putative pathways for a few sites, and conclude with some comments on the relevance of this material for research and practice.

SOCIOECONOMIC STATUS AND CANCER

Cancer offers an interesting context in which to examine the impact of SES on disease. Unlike many diseases, which show an inverse pattern between SES and health, cancer affords a contrast between incidence and mortality patterns. Depending on the site of the cancer, SES is associated both directly and inversely with cancer incidence. However, the pattern between SES and cancer survival is consistent across site; as SES decreases, so does the rate of survival from cancer.

There are both exogenous and endogenous pathways by which SES might influence these patterns of cancer onset and progression. The exogenous pathways include influences on life-style, health behaviors, and medical care. Life-style and health behavior changes are then the "real" exposures to cancer initiating and cancer-promoting agents. Therefore, other individual risk factors besides SES are more commonly measured and evaluated in epidemiological studies of cancer, often without investigation of how and why SES might pattern exposure to such factors, or whether these factors account for the variation in cancer outcome explained by SES. The second pathway—endogenous—hypothesizes that SES, through stress, resiliency or other systemic changes, has direct physiological effects on the host (12–14). Most recently, endogenous stress research has developed into the field of psychoneuroimmunology, investigating the link between a person's social and physical environment and changes in the endocrine and immune systems. However, to our knowledge, no research has investigated whether SES is a potential source of endogenous changes (15–17).

Cancer Incidence Patterns

Across different populations from North America, Europe, and Asia, many sites of cancer have incidence rates that follow the general pattern between SES and health; rates increase with decreasing SES (18,19). The cancer sites where incidence increases with lower SES include lung, oral and esophageal, stomach , uterine cervix, and pancreas (20–33). We term these cancers, somewhat naively, "cancers of poverty."

While incidence of cancer and SES have an inverse association at many cancer sites, for other sites there is *increased* incidence of cancer with increasing SES (19). Rimpela (34) dubbed these latter sites "cancers of affluence." Cancers sites for which there is typically a direct association with SES include colon, rectum, testis, prostate, breast, uterine corpus, and skin (28–30,32,33,35–37). Example of cancer incidence patterns by SES for both cancers of poverty and cancers of affluence are presented in Figure 8–1. The data are taken from one study using educational level as a measure of SES. Decreasing educational level is associated with protection from colon cancer and increased risk of lung cancer in men, and with protection from cervical cancer and increased risk of breast cancer in women.

The incidence patterns reviewed above reflect the current association between SES and cancer incidence. These patterns may not have remained constant across time. Lung cancer was very rare prior to the mid-

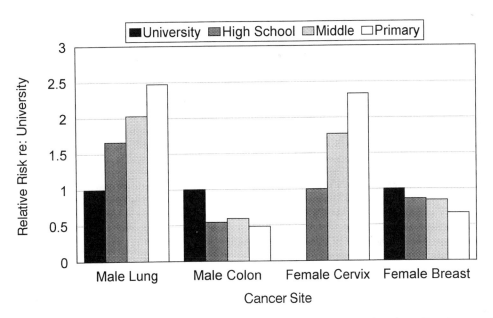

FIG. **8–1.** Cancer incidence by education, site, and SES, Turin, Italy: 1985–87. (Based on data from Faggiano et al. Cancer risk and social inequalities in Italy. *Journal of Epidemiology and Community Health* 1994; 48:447–452.)

twentieth century and was a cancer associated with affluence, whereas now lung cancer in the United States is overwhelmingly a cancer associated with lower SES groups. Despite its very strong inverse association with SES, lung cancer is occasionally found to be a cancer of affluence in some populations. For example, Italian women and residents of Columbia, South America, have lung cancer incidence rates which increase with SES (19,28). Likewise, colon and rectal cancer typically have a direct association with SES, showing higher incidence among white-collar and college-educated men (19,29,35). However, other studies reveal either no gradient or an inverse gradient between SES and colon and rectal cancer (38). One potential explanation is that a change in the association between SES and colon cancer incidence is occurring.

Explaining Cancer Incidence Patterns

Why is cancer incidence associated with SES and why does the relationship vary with cancer site? The most logical explanation is that risk factors for cancer at that site are patterned either directly or indirectly

with SES. Thus, the most pertinent question is "How are the risk factors for cancers of poverty and cancers of affluence associated with SES?"

Table 8.1 presents several of the common cancer sites inversely associated with SES and Table 8.2 presents several of the common cancer sites directly associated with SES, along with the strongest and best-established risk factors for each site. In addition, the direction of the association between the risk factor and SES is presented. Overwhelmingly, the relationship between SES and the major epidemiologic risk factors for cancer incidence have the same direction of association as the relationship between SES and cancer itself. The risk factors are graded by SES, and the cancer incidence follows this same gradient. While there is insufficient space to consider each site in detail, it is instructive to consider three sites which differ in the nature of their risk factor-SES associations.

EXAMPLE 1: LUNG CANCER.   By far the strongest risk factor for lung cancer is tobacco smoking, but other risk factors, such as occupational exposures and air pollution, have also been established (39,40) (see Table 8.1). All

TABLE 8.1. *Cancers of Poverty: Etiologic Factors and Their Relationship with Socioeconomic Status for Selected Cancer Sites*

Cancer Site	Etiologic Factors	Risk Factor Relationship with SES	Citations
Lung	Tobacco	Inverse	(41–44)
	Air Pollution	Inverse	(45–48)
	Occupation	Inverse	
	Nutrition—retinoids	Inverse	
Esophagus	Tobacco	Inverse	(41–44)
	Alcohol	Inverse	
Oral and esophageal	Tobacco	Inverse	(41–44)
	Alcohol	Inverse	
Liver	Alcohol	Inverse	(41–44)
	Viral infection (HBV)	Inverse	(49)
Cervix	Viral infection (HPV)	Inverse	(49)
	Early first marriage	Inverse	(51, 52)
	Multiple sexual partners	Inverse	
	SES of partner	Inverse	
Stomach	Diet		
	High fat	Inverse	(41–44)
	High complex carbohydrates	Inverse	
	Low fruits & vegetables	Inverse	
	Tobacco	Inverse	
	Alcohol	Inverse	

Source: Thomas DB. Cancer. In: Last JM, Wallace RB, eds. *Maxcy-Rosenau-Last Public Health and Preventive Medicine*, 13th ed. Norwalk, CT: Appleton and Lange, 1987. Doll FRS, Peto R. *The Causes of Cancer: Quantitative Estimates of Avoidable Risks of Cancer Today*. New York: Oxford University Press; 1981.

TABLE 8.2. *Cancers of Affluence: Etiologic Factors and Their Relationship with Socioeconomic Status for Selected Cancer Sites*

Cancer Site	Etiologic Factors	Risk Factor Relationship with SES	Citations
Colorectal	White collar work	Direct	(34–35)
	Physical activity	Inverse	(41–44)
	Diet		
	High meat and animal fat	Inverse	
	Low fiber	Inverse	
Breast	Reproductive/Endocrine		
	Nulliparity	Direct	(51, 52)
	Early menarche	Direct	(41–44)
	Older age at menopause	Direct	
	Diet		
	High dietary fat (±)	Inverse	
	Tobacco (±)	Inverse	
	Physical activity (±)	Inverse	
Corpus uteri	Endocrine		
	Nulliparity	Direct	(51, 52)
	Early menarche	Direct	(41–44)
	Older age at menopause	Direct	
	Obesity (±)	Inverse	
Prostate	Nutrition		
	High dietary fat	Inverse	(41–44)
	Occupation	Direct	(36)

Source: Thomas DB. Cancer. In: Last JM, Wallace RB, eds. *Maxcy-Rosenau-Last Public Health and Preventive Medicine*, 13th ed. Norwalk, CT: Appleton and Lange, 1987. Doll FRS, Peto R. *The Causes of Cancer: Quantitative Estimates of Avoidable Risks of Cancer Today*. New York: Oxford University Press; 1981.

of these common risk factors for lung cancer show evidence of an inverse gradient with SES. Thus, a person in a lower SES groups has a greater chance of beginning smoking earlier, smoking for longer period of his or her life, and smoking more cigarettes per day, while having less chance of quitting compared to individuals in higher SES groups (41–44). Lower SES groups may also have higher exposures to occupational hazards and air pollution (45–48). However, some investigators have found that the SES gradient remains even after adjusting for smoking behavior (23), which suggests that levels of tumor inhibiting/promoting factors may vary with SES in some way (see Fig. 8–2). It is also possible that measurement of smoking exposures are too crude to allow its full influence on the SES gradient to be demonstrated.

Further evidence that SES influences cancer incidence through patterns of life-style and behavior is offered by considering trends in the SES-smoking association reported above. For example, in areas where smoking in women is most common among women of higher SES, the association with lung cancer inci-

dence is direct; however, where women with a lower SES level have higher smoking prevalence, as in the United States, smoking patterns have an inverse association with lung cancer incidence. Both the adoption of risk factors at an *individual* level and the pattern of this adoption at a *social* level have profound effects on cancer incidence patterns.

EXAMPLE 2: BREAST CANCER. Epidemiologic analyses indicate that breast cancer incidence is related to a group of reproductive factors: nulliparity, age at first childbirth, earlier menarche, and later menopause. This pattern suggests that endocrine factors play a role in breast cancer, increasing exposure to naturally produced sex hormones such as estrogens (50). Reproductive behavior is profoundly influenced by social factors, SES among them, with poorer women more likely to have children at a younger age and to have more children (51,52). In addition, it is possible for factors such as nutrition to influence the age at menarche and menopause, with good nutrition prolonging the fertile period. Women in higher SES

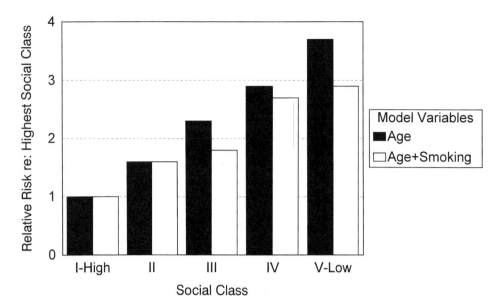

FIG. **8–2.** Age and smoking adjusted incidence of lung cancer in males by SES, The Netherlands. (Based on data from Hein et al. Lung cancer risk and social class. *Danish Medical Bulletin* 1992; 39:173–176.)

groups, because of socially mediated reproductive patterns, experience an increased dose of sex hormones and a higher rate of breast cancer. However, other hypothesized risk factors for breast cancer (for which the evidence is inconclusive) include high dietary fat intake, smoking, and low levels of physical exercise. All of these risk factors are currently inversely associated with SES, and would not account for the pattern of breast cancer incidence.

EXAMPLE 3: COLON CANCER.   Risk of developing colon cancer is directly associated with SES, particularly with SES as measured by occupational grade. The primary risk factors for colon cancer are a diet low in fiber and high in protein and fat and a history of low physical activity (39,40). These risk factors, measured in the 1980s and 1990s, all show an inverse association with SES, whereas the incidence of colon cancer has a direct association (41,42,44,53). Therefore, colon cancer risk behavior does not follow the same pattern with SES as the cancer itself. The inverse association between these risk factors and SES may reflect a changing temporal trend. In the early and middle twentieth century, white-collar jobs were associated with higher rates of sedentary behavior and a diet high in protein and animal fat and low in fiber. Since colon cancer is hypothesized to develop over a very long time, the excess of colon cancer found in white-collar workers as compared to blue-collar workers is a result of behaviors occurring much earlier. In the later part of this century, the dietary and

exercise patterns by SES group have changed. High consumption of meat, dairy, and starch foods and low consumption of fruits and vegetables has become more frequent in the lower SES groups, while the pattern is the opposite in higher SES groups. The same reversal is occurring for physical exercise. While higher SES groups still hold sedentary jobs, as a group they have adopted a higher rate of leisure-time physical activity than have lower social classes. In addition, many low-paying service and manufacturing jobs are now sedentary. If these trends in risk factors continue, a diminishing or reversal in the association of colon cancer incidence and SES might occur. Indeed, such a pattern has been reported in two analyses from the United Kingdom (25).

Patterns of Cancer Mortality

Cancer mortality exhibits a more consistent association with SES. Regardless of the pattern of cancer incidence, SES has an inverse relationships with cancer mortality. The poorer you are, the greater the risk of death and the shorter the survival time (54–59). In one prospective study of SES and cancer mortality, Smith (25) reported that men in the lowest occupational grade had a 50% higher overall mortality from cancer of all sites compared with that of men in the highest; in addition, there was strong evidence of a trend across occupational grade. As well as an overall association with cancer survival, an inverse association between survival from cancer and SES has been documented for the following sites: lung, colon and rectum, breast, uterine cervix, uterine corpus, bladder, lymphomas, prostate, stomach, kidney and brain (23,24,43,58,60–69). Among lower SES groups, cancer recurs more often and at a younger age (55).

While studies find a direct association between SES and cancer mortality, length of survival plays a role in determining the strength of the SES gradient. In general, cancers with poor survival rates exhibit little survival differences by level of SES, while cancers with the highest survival rates tend to have the greatest relative social class differences in survival. Figure 8–3 presents the association between SES and survival for four cancer sites, along with the average 5-year survival rates, which range between 11.2% and 68.8% for each cancer. The figure shows that the risk of death becomes more strongly graded by SES as survival lengthens.

Explaining Patterns of Cancer Mortality

Why do people die sooner from cancer depending on where they are in a social system? While research on cancer incidence focuses primarily on gradients in risk behavior, the consistency of the inverse gradient between SES and survival means that potential pathways for mortality are similar to those used to explain the gradient between SES and health overall. These include material deprivation, especially of access to medical care, and differences in risk factors for cancer progression, such as a reduced ability to fight disease.

An example of the multitude of pathways between SES and cancer mortality is suggested in Figure 8–4 from Dayal (70), which offers a conceptual diagram by which lower SES might lead to lower survival rates.

The fact that cancers with the best survival times exhibit the greatest relative SES gradient, along with the idea these cancers are most amenable to intervention, immediately suggests that medical treatment factors may play a large role in forming the SES differences in survival. The potential differences in medical care can be separated into many aspects of seeking and receiving care: access to regular cancer screening and preventive medicine, symptom recognition, delay in seeking diagnosis, medical treatment offered, medical procedure accepted, and treatment efficacy and adherence. Research on these topic areas, particularly in the United States, has usually focused on racial differences in survival rather than SES differences in survival. The problems of interpreting race as a proxy for SES are addressed later in the chapter. The consequence is that little systematic research on SES differences in medical care for cancer is available, and evidence must be compiled from disparate studies.

Perhaps the most prominent hypothesis for survival differences is diagnosis with later stage tumors or metastases, which then respond less well to cancer treatment. Evidence from several studies suggests that social class plays a role in tumor stage at diagno-

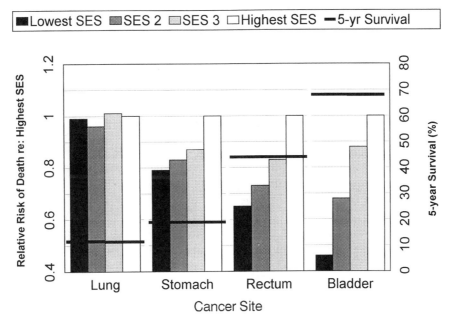

FIG. **8–3.** Association between SES and cancer death at 5 years by cancer site, Finnish men, 1971–1985. (Based on data from: Auvinen et al. Social class and cancer patient survival in Finland. *American Journal of Epidemiology* 1995; 142(10):1089–1102.)

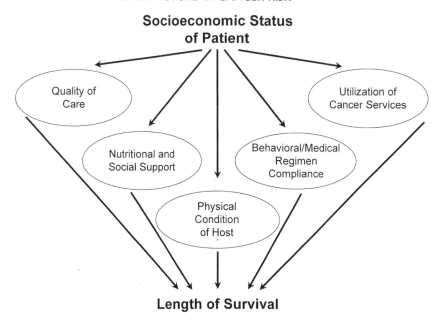

FIG. **8–4.** A plausible pathway through which SES may influence survival for a given stage at diagnosis. (From Dayal HH. Cancer etiology, management and outcome: does it matter who you are? In: *Advances in Cancer Control: The War on Cancer—15 Years of Progress.* New York: Alan R. Liss, 1987:245–253.)

sis. Lower SES groups have the highest rate of diagnosis at the time of autopsy for all sites of cancer in a Finnish population (58). SES is a risk factor for presentation with grade 3 and 4 breast cancer tumors at the time of diagnosis in American women, but the critical measure of SES is different for black (medical insurance type) and white (income) women (71). In contrast, Roberts (72) found that presentation with late stage breast cancer and cervical tumors did not vary by SES in a population with a high proportion of late-stage presenters (30%). In general, while stage of tumor progression at diagnosis does diminish the association between SES and cancer survival, the survival differences remain significant across SES groups (62,66).

It is unknown exactly what causes these differences in time and stage at diagnosis. Hypotheses include differences in symptom recognition, delay in seeking diagnosis, or difficulty accessing treatment. Some support exists for these hypotheses. Roberts (73) found that knowledge of the signs and symptoms of breast cancer differed by social class. A study on black/white differences in breast cancer survival reported that the delay between symptom onset and treatment was longer for those with incomes closer to the poverty line (74). While the mean difference in delay was statistically significant, it was quite small—6 days. However, this same study found that the risk of

ever seeking treatment rose with increasing income. Other studies have found that delay in seeking diagnosis helps explain survival differences by SES for breast and stomach cancer, but that SES differences in colon, rectum, prostate, and lung cancer could not be explained by stage at diagnosis or treatment delay (59,62).

Symptom recognition and delay in seeking treatment are hypotheses in which the responsibility rests on the individual patient; systemic or contextual hypotheses for SES differences in stage at diagnosis include differences in access to medical care, perhaps mediated by insurance status, lack of a personal provider, and feelings of mistrust and fatalism about medical intervention (2). There is good reason to suspect that these factors would be inversely associated with SES, yet they are rarely investigated in relation to SES and cancer survival.

Once cancer has been diagnosed, treatment differences are a potential risk for survival differences across SES groups. There is little evidence on whether treatment is offered or accepted differently by SES category. Treatment differences did not explain survival differences in the Netherlands (59). In contrast, a preliminary report of a recent study in the United States indicates that income is substantially associated with appropriate treatment for lung cancer, and that half of the differences in survival between the lowest and highest income groups studied was attributable to treatment differences (75).

Underlying health differences between SES groups may complicate treatment differences by SES. Since SES is associated inversely with many other health problems, lower SES groups may have serious co-morbid conditions besides the incident cancer, conditions which contraindicate optimum treatment options for cancer (76). In a recent population-based study of cancer patients in Finland, both mortality from all causes and mortality from cancer alone were inversely associated with SES in cancer patients (58). This suggests that unequal survival time in cancer patients is not due to cancer differences alone. Co-morbidity may also be one of several factors which influence progression of tumors through a decrease in host resistance. This possibility is particularly relevant to survival from cancers which have better treatment options and prognosis and thus longer survival times, such as breast and prostate cancer.

Attempts to study the effects of SES on host resistance and cancer survival include research on the endogenous pathways to mortality. In investigating the endogenous pathways, research has focused primarily on psychological adjustment and response to illness with cancer, coping strategies, social support, and presence of stressful life events. Factors such as coping strategies and social support are hypothesized to alter host resistance through a variety of endocrine and immune pathways, and consequently affect cancer survival.

Several early studies on factors influencing host resistance and survival used multiple cancer sites as outcomes. Results from these studies suggest that short-term survivors tend to have high levels of anxiety, be more defensive, be less able to express negative emotions, and be more isolated. Long-term survivors tend to have higher levels of hostility and aggression (77–79). However, these studies have flaws, such as small sample sizes and unclear subject selection, which make it difficult to rely on the results. Much of the current work on host resistance and cancer survival has focused on breast cancer survival in women. Greer and colleagues (80,81) divided women with stage I and II breast cancer into five coping categories. Psychological response to cancer predicted survival at 5-, 10-, and 15-year follow-up, with fighting spirit and denial (positive avoidance) responses protecting against mortality compared with responses characterized as fatalistic, helplessness/hopelessness, and anxious preoccupation. Later research has confirmed these results in women with both early and late stage disease (82–84). Longer survival was associated with

higher levels of hostility, depression, guilt, and total negative affect, and shorter survival was associated with higher anxiety and higher external locus of control. In addition, hopelessness has been shown to be associated with shorter survival in both breast cancer and all cancers (85,86).

Studies examining the association between life events and breast cancer recurrence found that severe life events were associated with significantly increased risk of cancer recurrence, independent of SES (87,88). One study examining the association between life events and breast cancer survival found that both severe life events and lower SES were associated with lower breast cancer survival (89).

Research suggests that amount and quality of social support also influences the length of survival through the endogenous pathway, perhaps through changing social and psychologic coping responses. Social support, measured as support from spouse, family, friends, or medical care providers, is associated with longer survival with cancer in general (90,91) as well as survival with breast, colorectal, and lung cancers (92–95).

While there is good reason to believe that psychosocial factors influence cancer survival, little of the research explores whether these factors help explain the SES gradient in survival. Therefore, the research reviewed above does not explicitly help elucidate the SES differences in cancer survival. While some of the studies adjusted for SES in their analyses, none of them examined how psychological response and coping methods might be graded by SES. Previous research indicates that coping strategies are influenced by SES; as SES decreases, both community and patient samples report increasing avoidant coping (96). Hostility, depression, and social support are all negatively associated with SES in national and community subsamples (97–99). While we might suspect that these SES and psychosocial factors are similarly associated in cancer patients, few studies exist that test these hypotheses.

METHODOLOGIC ISSUES

Our estimation of the magnitude of SES-related differential in cancer mortality and survival, and our understanding of these differentials, are influenced by a number of methodologic challenges. In many studies of cancer incidence and mortality, there is no measurement of SES at all, providing no opportunity to document or understand SES–cancer relationships. Even when SES measures are available, there are still major problems related to the conceptualization of SES and to its measurement.

A wide variety of socioeconomic characteristics have been assessed in relationship to cancer incidence and mortality, among them: being individual income, family income, years of education, occupational grade, and area of residence. The relationship between SES and cancer incidence changes depending on the type of SES measure used. For example, one of the advantages of level of education as a measure of SES is that, for the most common sites of cancer, it is unlikely that the disease itself has influenced the measure of SES, completed many years before most cancers have developed to any clinically significant extent. However, education, in itself is relatively uninformative. We do not know what the more proximal pathways are that link education to cancer risk or survival, or how these differ by site. Other measures of SES may also be importantly associated with the natural history of cancer. For example, income histories, in addition to current income, may provide information about cumulative exposures to health-damaging environments. On the other hand, given the long latency of many cancers, it is questionable whether measures of SES gathered at the time of diagnosis are the most relevant to understanding the contribution of SES. Income itself may be less useful among the elderly, and measures of assets may be a better indicator of the financial reserves and resources which can result in greater access to diagnostic, therapeutic, or rehabilitative services. Occupational histories may provide information about job-related exposures that are not captured by data on "usual" occupation or last occupation.

Another problem with conceptualization and measurement of SES is that many studies use categorizations of race and ethnicity as proxies for SES. This generally results when information on SES has not been collected. However, using race as a proxy for SES can lead to considerable misunderstanding. SES and race/ethnicity constitute different systems of social stratification, with different origins and consequences, and should not be used interchangeably. At the least, interchanging them risks considerable misclassification of SES. While non-Hispanic whites are proportionally overrepresented at higher household incomes, and African-Americans are similarly overrepresented at lower household incomes, inspection of national data indicates that there is considerable overlap in the middle portions of the income distribution. For example, for the United States in 1992, the proportions of white and African-Americans in the second through fourth quintiles of the income distribution differed by less than 10% (100). In such a case, substitution of race/ethnicity information for SES information is inappropriate. Even more importantly, such a substitution will impede understanding of what the pathways are which link SES and cancer. Freeman (101) offers a conceptual figure for the relationship between SES, race, and survival in the United States, suggesting that race is a cultural screen through which aspects of SES are filtered. If this is true, then a dynamic interaction between SES and race should be considered, rather than substitution of one for another or considering the risks from the two variables independently.

Given the limitations of the measures of SES which are used in most epidemiologic studies of cancer incidence and mortality, it is likely that the increased risks associated with variation in SES are underestimated. However, even if we can arrive at better estimates of the associations between SES and cancer outcomes, our understanding will be compromised to the extent that we ignore the temporal structure of cancer. The theory of the biology of cancer separates the process into three rough stages: the first stage, initiation, during which there is an alteration in the cell's genetic structure from a physical, chemical, or genetic agent; the second stage, promotion, characterized by the proliferation of altered, initiated cells; and the third stage, progression, characterized by an increased growth rate of the tumor, increased invasiveness, and metastasis. It is important to note that the promotion stage is believed to be reversible. A period of time lasting from 1.5 to 40 years may elapse between the initial genetic alteration and the clinical presence of disease (102). Given that SES may be related in different ways to tumor initiation, promotion, and progression and at different stages in the natural history of cancer, different aspects of SES may be more or less important at different times during the natural history of disease. Since the development of cancer is so widely varied in time, the temporal measurement of SES becomes crucial. Most of the studies on SES and cancer reviewed in this chapter measured SES at time of diagnosis or not more than three to five years before diagnosis. Examination of secular trends in the association between SES and cancer outcomes could be very informative with respect to intervening pathways.

Substantial variations in patterns and trends between geographic locations exist in the literature reviewed here. Unfortunately, despite the decades of knowledge of the SES-patterning of cancer, we still know very little concerning the question of how SES patterns affect geographic and temporal patterns of cancer.

IMPLICATIONS FOR RESEARCH AND PRACTICE

The strength, consistency, and gradient of association between SES and cancer incidence and mortality provide excellent reasons to believe that these patterns should be of substantial concern to researchers and practitioners in the fields of cancer epidemiology and psycho-oncology. Cancer incidence is graded by SES both inversely and directly, but cancer survival decreases with decreasing social status. However, with the validity of the association established, we must now move beyond examining the overall gradient of SES and cancer incidence or SES and cancer mortality. Furthermore, we must stop assuming that we know what SES signifies in the lives of people, and move beyond simple adjustment on our way to discovering other risk factors. There is much we do not understand or have not explored about SES and its effects on cancer morbidity and mortality.

1. In order to advance in our research, we need to include appropriate measures of SES in all cancer databases. Appropriateness means asking ourselves how we believe SES acts in the population we study, what measure of SES reflects social status most accurately, and at what time in the cancer process might SES be increasing risk. While we know that certain measures of SES are more appropriate at different life stages, data have not been examined to see whether SES has different effects on cancer at different life stages.

2. A second challenge is to determine which part of the course of cancer development is influenced by SES. It is likely that SES may play a different role at different stages of cancer initiation, promotion, and progression. Given our current inability to detect most cancers at the initiation and early progression stages, measuring the effects of SES on cancer initiation or early promotion may be difficult. We know that the length of the promotion stage varies widely. We need to think about timing the measurement of SES to test different hypothetical connections. In the absence of ability to detect cancer biologically, one option is to examine prospective studies where waves of data are available; risk at different times before breast cancer could be investigated.

3. Much of the literature suggests that there is an SES gradient in health because other risk factors are also graded by SES. However, we need to examine the complex association between SES and cancer, and SES and other risk factors for cancer incidence and mortality, more closely. It is unclear whether the more proximal risk factors such as individual behavior or medical care entirely account for the association between SES and cancer. In many studies on cancer incidence and survival, SES remains a significant risk factor after adjustment for these risk factors. It may be possible, with more careful examination of SES, to find other risk factors which also are distributed along a social gradient.

4. Finally, the gradient of individual risk following a gradient of social risk illuminates vital questions that epidemiologic literature is only beginning to examine. Are risk factors only functioning at the individual level? Why do social groups adopt certain patterns that may increase or decrease risk of health and mortality? Why are risk factors clustered and graded by socioeconomic group? These questions suggest that we need to examine, not only whether individual risk factor patterns are graded by SES, but also how SES shapes the social, physical, and psychological environments of populations and how these environments might be associated with risk patterns. For example, cigarette smoking is an individual behavior, but one which changes depending on the cost of tobacco as regulated by sales tax, on the regulations which prohibit or allow smoking, on the availability of cigarettes in stores and vending machines, and on the social expectations of a community. Changing an aspect of the environment has repercussions in the daily lives and health of the people in that environment. If we understand how SES shapes the social, physical, and psychological environments of populations, we may be able to intervene on many risk factors simultaneously.

These questions, if addressed, may lead to a better understanding of how to prevent and treat cancer, and improve quality and duration of life in people with cancer. In the complex terrain covered by psycho-oncology, it may seem to some to be reaching too far to include considerations of SES and cancer. We have tried to argue that SES importantly shapes the natural history of cancer. Further understanding of the role of SES in the origins and consequences of cancer holds promise in our attempts to lower the burden from cancer.

REFERENCES

1. Berkman BJ, Sampson SE. Psychosocial effects of cancer economics on patients and their families. *Cancer.* 1993; 72(9):2846–2849.
2. American Cancer Society. A summary of the American Cancer Society report to the nation: cancer in the poor. *Cancer.* 1989;39:263–265.
3. Antonovsky A. Social class, life expectancy, and overall mortality. *Milbank Memorial Fund Q.* 1967; 45:31–73.
4. Marmot MG, Rose G, Shipley MJ, Hamilton PJS. Employment grade and coronary heart disease in British civil servants. *J Epidemiol Commun Health.* 1978; 32:244–249.

5. Morris JN. Social inequalities undiminished. *Lancet.* 1979; 87–90.

6. Baker SP, O'Neill B, Karpf RS. *The Injury Fact Book.* Lexington, MA: Lexington Books; 1984.

7. Haan MN, Kaplan GA, Syme, SL. Socioeconomic status and health: old observations and new thoughts. In: Bunker JP, Gomby DS, Kehrer BH, eds. *Pathways to Health: The Role of Social Factors.* Menlo Park, CA: Henry J. Kaiser Foundation; 1989:76–135.

8. Syme SL, Berkman LF. Social class, susceptibility and sickness. *Am J Epidemiol.* 1976; 104:1–8.

9. Najman JM. Theories of disease causation and the concept of general susceptibility: a review. *Soc Sci Med.* 1980; 14A(3):231–237.

10. Townsend P, Davidson N, eds. *Inequalities in Health: the Black Report.* Harmondsworth, UK: Penguin Books; 1982.

11. Marmot MG, Shipley MJ, Rose G. Inequalities in death—specific explanations of a general pattern. *Lancet.* 1984; (May 5):1003–1006.

12. Cassel J. The contribution of the social environment to host resistance. *Am J Epidemiol.* 1976; 104(2):107–123.

13. Asterita MF. *The Physiology of Stress.* New York: Human Sciences Press; 1985.

14. Holland JC. Behavioral and psychological risk factors in cancer: human studies. In: Holland JC, Rowland JH, eds. *Handbook of Psycho-oncology.* New York: Oxford University Press; 1989.

15. Fox BH. Current theory of psychogenic effects on cancer incidence and prognosis. *J Psychosoc Oncol.* 1983; 1(1):17–31.

16. Ader R, Felton DL, Cohen N. *Psychoneuroimmunology.* San Diego, CA: Academic Press; 1991.

17. Chrousos GP, Gold PW. The concept of stress system disorders: an overview of physical and behavioral homeostasis. *J Am Med Assoc.* 1992; 276:1244–1252.

18. Williams RR, Horm JW. Association of cancer sites with tobacco and alcohol consumption and socioeconomic status of patients: interview study from the Third National Cancer Survey. *J Natl Cancer Inst.* 1977;58(3):525–547.

19. Faggiano F, Zanetti R, Costa G. Cancer risk and social inequalities in Italy. *J Epidemiol Commun Health.* 1994; 48:447–452.

20. Brown SM, Selvin S, Winkelstein W. The association of economic status with the occurrence of lung cancer. *Cancer.* 1975; 36(5):1903–1911.

21. Hathcock AL, Greenberg RA, Dakan AW. An analysis of lung cancer on a micrographical level. *Soc Sci Med.* 1982; 16(2):1235–1238.

22. Devesa SS, Diamond EL. Socioeconomic and racial differences in lung cancer incidence. *Am J Epidemiol.* 1983; 118(6):818–831.

23. Hein HO, Suadicani P, Gyntelberg F. Lung cancer risk and social class. *Dan Med Bull.* 1992; 39:173–176.

24. van Loon AJM, Goldbohm RA, van den Brandt PA. Lung cancer: is there an association with socioeconomic status in The Netherlands? *J Epidemiol Commun Health.* 1995; 49:65–69.

25. Smith EM. Epidemiology of oral and pharyngeal cancers in the United States: review of recent literature. *J Natl Cancer Inst.* 1979; 63(5):1189–1198.

26. Greenberg RS, Haber MJ, Clark WS, et al. The relation of socioeconomic status to oral and pharyngeal cancer. *Epidemiology.* 1991; 2(3):194–200.

27. Haenszel W, Kurihara M, Locke FB, Shimuzu K, Segi M. Stomach cancer in Japan. *J Natl Cancer Inst.* 1976; 56(2):265–274.

28. Cuello C, Correa P, Haenszel W. Socio-economic class differences in cancer incidence in Cali, Colombia. *Int J Cancer.* 1982; 29(6):637–643.

29. Pukkala E, Teppo L. Socioeconomic status and education as risk determinants of gastrointestinal cancer. *Prev Med.* 1986; 15:127–138.

30. Devesa SS, Diamond EL. Association breast cancer and cervical cancer incidence with income and education among whites and blacks. *J Natl Cancer Inst.* 1980; 65(3):515–528.

31. Fasal E, Simmons ME, Kampert JB. Factors associated with high and low risk of cervical neoplasia. *J Natl Cancer Inst.* 1981; 66(4):631–636.

32. Hakama M, Hakulinen T, Pukkala E, Saxen E, Teppo L. Risk indicators of breast and cervical cancer on ecologic and individual levels. *Am J Epidemiol.* 1982; 116(6):990–1000.

33. Morton WE, Baker HW, Fletcher WS. Geographic pathology of uterine cancers in Oregon: risks of double primaries and effects of socioeconomic status. *Gynecol Oncol.* 1983; 16(1):63–77.

34. Rimpela AH, Pukkala E. Cancers of affluence: positive social class gradient and rising incidence trend in some cancer forms. *Soc Sci Med.* 1987; 24(7):601–606.

35. van Loon AJM, van den Brandt PA, Golbohm RA. Socioeconomic status and colon cancer incidence: a prospective cohort study. *Br J Cancer.* 1995; 71:882–887.

36. Swerdlow AJ, Douglas AJ, Huttly SRA, Smith PG. Cancer of the testis, socioeconomic status, and occupation. *Br J Ind Med.* 1991; 48:670–674.

37. Ewertz M. Risk of breast cancer in relation to social factors in Denmark. *Acta Oncol.* 1988; 27:787–792.

38. Smith GD, Leon D, Shipley MJ, Rose G. Socioeconomic differentials in cancer among men. *Int J Epidemiol.* 1991; 20(2):339–345.

39. Thomas DB. Cancer. In: Last JM, Wallace RB, eds. *Maxcy-Rosenau-Last Public Health and Preventive Medicine*, 13th ed. Norwalk, CT: Appleton and Lange; 1987

40. Doll FRS, Peto R. *The Causes of Cancer: Quantitative Estimates of Avoidable Risks of Cancer Today.* New York: Oxford University Press; 1981.

41. Jeffery RW, French SA, Forster JL, Spry VM. Socioeconomic status differences in health behaviors related to obesity: the Healthy Worker Project. *Int J Obes.* 1991; 15(10):689–696.

42. Hulshol KF, Lowik MR, Kok FJ, et al. Diet and other life-style factors in high and low socio-economic groups. *Eur J Clin Nutr.* 1991; 45(9):441–450.

43. Pugh H, Power C, Goldblatt P, Arber S. Women's lung cancer mortality, socioeconomic status and changing smoking patterns. *Soc Sci Med.* 1991; 32(10):1105–1110.

44. Bennett S. Cardiovascular risk factors in Australia: trends in socioeconomic inequalities. *J Epidemiol Commun Health.* 1995; 49(4):363–372.

45. Winkelstein W, Kantor S, Davis EW, Maneri CS, Mosher WE. The relationship of air pollution and eco-

nomic status to total mortality and selected respiratory system mortality in men. II. Oxides of sulphur. *Arch Environ Health.* 1968; 16(3):410–405.

46. Dayal H, Chiu CY, Sharrar R, et al. Ecologic correlates of cancer mortality patterns in an industrialized urban population. *J Natl Cancer Inst.* 1984; 73(3):565–574.

47. Jacobsen BS. The role of air pollution and other factors in local variations in general mortality and cancer mortality. *Arch Environ Health.* 1984; 39(4):306–313.

48. Kunst AE, Looman CW, Mackenbach JP. Determinants of regional differences in lung cancer mortality in The Netherlands. *Soc Sci Med.* 1993; 37(5):623–631.

49. Morton WE, Horton HB, Baker HW. Effects of socioeconomic status on incidence of three sexually transmitted diseases. *Sex Trans Dis.* 1979; 6(3):206–210.

50. Kelsey JL, Horn-Ross PL. Breast cancer: magnitude of the problem and descriptive epidemiology. *Epidemiol Rev.* 1993; 15(1):7–16.

51. Freidman HL. Changing patterns of adolescent sexual behavior: consequences for health and development. *J Adolesc Health.* 1992; 13(5):345–350.

52. Forrest JD. Timing of reproductive life stages. *Obstet Gynecol.* 1993; 82(1):105–111.

53. Marmot MG, Smith GD, Stansfeld S, et al. Health inequalities among British civil servants: the Whitehall II study. *Lancet.* 1991; 337(8754):1387–1393.

54. Lipworth L, Abelin T, Connelly RR. Socio-economic factors in the prognosis of cancer patients. *J Chron Dis.* 1970; 23(2):105–116.

55. Berg JW, Ross R, Latourette HB. Economic status and survival of cancer patients. *Cancer.* 1977; 39(2):467–477.

56. Jenkins CD. Social environment and cancer mortality in men. *N Engl J Med.* 1983; 308(7):395–398.

57. Schrijvers CTM, Mackenbach JP. Cancer patient survival by socioeconomic status in The Netherlands: a review for six common cancer sites. *J Epidemiol Commun Health.* 1994; 48:441–446.

58. Auvinen A, Karjalainen S, Pukkala E. Social class and cancer patient survival in Finland. *Am J Epidemiol.* 1995; 142(10):1089–1102.

59. Schrijvers CTM, Coebergh JWW, van der Heijden LH, Mackenbach JP. Socioeconomic variation in cancer survival in the southeastern Netherlands, 1980–1989. *Cancer.* 1995; 75(12):2946–2953.

60. Wegner EL, Kolonel LN, Nomura AMY, Lee J. Racial and socioeconomic status differences in survival of colorectal cancer patients in Hawaii. *Cancer.* 1982; 49:2208–2216.

61. Brenner H, Mielck A, Klein R, Ziegler H. The role of socioeconomic factors in the survival of patients with colorectal cancer in Saarland, Germany. *J Clin Epidemiol.* 1991; 44(8):807–815.

62. Auvinen A. Social class and colon cancer survival in Finland. *Cancer.* 1992; 70(2):402–409.

63. Dayal JJ, Power RN, Chiu C. Race and socio-economic status in survival from breast cancer. *J Chron Dis.* 1982; 35:675–683.

64. Steinhorn SC, Myers MH, Hankey BF, Pelham VF. Factors associated with survival differences between black women and white women with cancer of the uterine corpus. *Am J Epidemiol.* 1986; 124(1):85–93.

65. Murphy MFG, Mant DCA, Goldblatt PO. Social class, marital status, and cancer of the uterine cervix in England and Wales, 1950–1983. *J Epidemiol Commun Health.* 1992; 46:378–381.

66. Lamont DW, Symonds RP, Brodie MM, Nwabineli NJ, Gillis CR. Age, socioeconomic status and survival from cancer of cervix in the west of Scotland 1980–87. *Br J Cancer.* 1993; 67:351–357.

67. Dayal HH, Chiu C. Factors associated with racial differences in survival for prostatic carcinoma. *J Chron Dis.* 1982; 3(7)5:553–560.

68. Dayal HH, Polissar L, Dahlberg S. Race, socioeconomic status and other prognostic factors for survival from prostate cancer. *J Natl Cancer Inst.* 1985; 74(5):1001–1006.

69. Chirikos TN, Horner RD. Economic status and survivorship in digestive system cancers. *Cancer.* 1985; 56:210–217.

70. Dayal HH. Cancer etiology, management, and outcome: Does it matter who you are? In: Engstrom PF, Mortenson LE, Anderson PN, eds. *Advances in Cancer Control: The War on Cancer—15 Years of Progress.* New York: Alan R. Liss, 1987: 245–253.

71. Hunter CP, Redmond CK, Chen VW, et al. Breast cancer: factors associated with stage at diagnosis in black and white women. *J Natl Cancer Inst.* 1993; 85(14):1129–1137.

72. Roberts MM, Alexander FE, Elton RA, Rodger A. Breast cancer state, social class and the impact of screening. *Eur J Surg Oncol.* 1990; 16:18–21.

73. Roberts MM, French K, Duffy J. Breast cancer and breast self-examination: what do Scottish women know? *Soc Sci Med.* 1984; 18:791–797.

74. Coates RJ, Bransfield DD, Wesley M, et al. Differences between black and white women with breast cancer in time from symptom recognition to medical consultation. *J Natl Cancer Inst.* 1992; 84:938–950.

75. Holzman D. Better access for the poor may improve lung cancer survival. *J Natl Cancer Inst News.* 1995; 87:1212.

76. Satariano WA, Ragland DR. The effect of comorbidity on 3-year survival of women with primary breast cancer. *Ann Intern Med.* 1994; 120(2):104–110.

77. Blumberg EM, West PM, Ellis FW. A possible relationship between psychologic factors and human cancer. *Psychosom Med.* 1954; 16:277-286.

78. Stavraky KM. Psychological factors in the outcome of human cancer. *J Psychosom Res.* 1968; 12:251–259.

79. Weisman AD, Worden JW. Psychosocial analysis of cancer deaths. *Omega.* 1975; 6(1):61–74.

80. Greer S, Morris T, Pettingale KW. Psychological response to breast cancer: effect on outcome. *Lancet.* 1979; 785–787.

81. Greer S. Psychological response to cancer and survival. *Psychol Med.* 1991; 21:43–49.

82. Derogatis LR, Abeloff MD, Melisaratos N. Psychological coping mechanisms and survival time in metastatic breast cancer. *J Am Med Assoc.* 1979; 242(14):1504–1508.

83. Jamison RN, Burish TG, Wallston KA. Psychogenic factors in predicting survival of breast cancer patients. *J Clin Oncol.* 1987; 5(5):768–772.

84. Dean C, Surtees PG. Do psychological factors predict survival in breast cancer? *J Psychosom Res.* 1989; 33:561–569.

85. Jensen M. Psychobiological factors predicting the course of breast cancer. *J Pers.* 1987; 55:317–342.

86. Stein S, Linn MW, Stein EM. Psychological correlates of survival in nursing home cancer patients. *Gerontologist.* 1989; 29:224–228.

87. Ramirez AJ, Craig TK, Watson JP, et al. Stress and relapse of breast cancer. *Br Med J.* 1989; 298:291–293.

88. Barraclough J, Pinder P, Cruddas M, et al. Life events and breast cancer prognosis. *Br Med J.* 1992; 304:1078–1081.

89. Forsen A. Psychosocial stress as a risk for breast cancer. *Psychother Psychosom.* 1991; 55:176–185.

90. Reynolds P, Kaplan GA. Social connections and risk for cancer: prospective evidence form the Alameda County Study. *Behav Med.*1990; 16(3):101–110.

91. Vogt TM, Mullooly JP, Ernst D, Pope CR, Hollis JF. Social networks as predictors of ischemic heart disease, cancer, stroke and hypertension: incidence, survival and mortality. *J Clin Epidemiol.* 1992; 45(6):659–666.

92. Hilsop TG, Waxler NE, Coldman AJ, Elwood JM, Kan L. The prognostic significance of psychosocial factors in women with breast cancer. *J Chron Dis.* 1987; 40(7):729–735.

93. Spiegel D, Bloom JR, Kraemer HC, Gottheil E. Effect of psychosocial treatment on survival of patients with metastatic breast cancer. *Lancet.* 1989; 2(8668):888–891.

94. Waxler-Morrison N, Hilsop TG, Mears B, Kan L. Effects of social relationships on survival for women with breast cancer: a prospective study. *Soc Sci Med.* 1991; 33(2):177–183.

95. Ell K, Nishimoto R, Mediansky L, Mantell J, Hamovitch M. Social relations, social support and survival among patients with cancer. *J Psychosom Res.* 1992; 36(6):531–541.

96. Holahan CJ, Moos RH. Personal and contextual determinants of coping strategies. *J Pers Soc Psychol.* 1987; 52(5):946–955.

97. Barefoot JC, Peterson BL, Dahlstrom WG, Siegler IC, Anderson NB, Williams RB. Hostility patterns and health implications: correlates of Cook–Medley Hostility scale scores in a national survey. *Health Psychol.* 1991; 10:18–24.

98. Scherwitz L, Perkins L, Chesney M, Hughes G. Cook-Medley Hostility scale and subsets: relationship to demographic and psychological characteristics in young adults in the CARDIA Study. *Psychosom Med.* 1991; 53:36–49.

99. Kaplan GA, Wilson TW, Cohen RC, Kauhanen J, Wu M, Salonen JT. Social functioning and overall mortality: prospective evidence form the Kuopio Ischemic Hearth Disease Risk Factor Study. *Epidemiology.* 1994; 5(5):495–500.

100. *Statistical Abstract of the United States, 1994: The National Data Book on CD-ROM.* Prepared by the Bureau of the Census. Washington, D.C.: Department of Commerce, Bureau of the Census; 1995.

101. Freeman HP. Poverty, race, racism, and survival. *Ann Epidemiol.* 1993; 3:145–149.

102. Pitot HC. *Fundamentals of Oncology,* 3rd ed. New York: Marcel Decker; 1986.

9

Personality and Coping

MAGGIE WATSON AND STEVEN GREER

COPING

Much has been written about the possible effect of stressful life events on the development and course of cancers. But studying the occurrence and nature of stress in isolation is akin to listening for the sound of one hand clapping. At least as important as the stressor are the different ways in which individuals cope with stressful events.

The importance of coping is illustrated in a landmark study by Goodkin and his colleagues (1). They examined the role of stress and coping style in the promotion of cervical intraepithelial neoplasia to invasive squamous cell carcinoma of the cervix. Goodkin found only a weak correlation between stress per se and promotion to carcinoma, but the inclusion of measures of coping made a significant difference: in women with coping styles of pessimism and hopelessness there were strong correlations between stressful events and disease promotion to carcinoma. There is another good reason for measuring coping styles. In most cases, little if anything can be done to prevent stressful experiences; they are, after all, part of life. In order to alleviate the detrimental effects of stressors on the quality of life of the individual and, possibly, on the course of his or her disease, psychotherapeutic intervention must be directed at coping styles. Empirical evidence suggests that coping styles can be altered by therapy (1–4).

Coping has been variously defined. In the present context, it refers to the cognitive and behavioral responses of patients to cancer, comprising: appraisal (i.e., the personal meaning of cancer for the individual) and the ensuing reactions (i.e., what the individual thinks and does to reduce the threat posed by cancer). Although this review examines coping styles, affective responses (i.e., anxiety, depression) have been included. The term *psychologic response* as used here subsumes cognitive, behavioral, and affective responses. Studies of the influence of psychologic response to cancer on disease outcome (5–25) are summarized in Table 9.1 and meet the following minimum criteria: *(1)* the sample contained at least 30 patients, *(2)* the follow-up period was at least one year, *(3)* attempts were made to control for biologic prognostic factors.

In a salient critical review several years ago, Temoshok and Heller (26) likened the difficulty of summarizing reported findings to comparing apples, oranges, and fruit salad. It was an apt description that applies with equal force today. Published studies differ in many respects, including the type, site, and stage of cancer, the measuring instruments used, the kind of psychologic responses that were measured, and duration of follow-up. We need, therefore, to consider methodologic problems inherent in this area of research.

Methodologic Issues

Prospective studies of cancer patients which involve both biologic and psychologic variables are difficult to mount and to carry out. In the first place, such studies are—to put it mildly—not universally looked upon with favor by grant-giving bodies, who still view psycho-oncology with some suspicion. Second, this kind of research requires an unusual ability to overcome territorial boundaries that divide the various disciplines involved in multidisciplinary studies. Last, cooperation from cancer patients may be difficult to obtain, understandably so since they have weightier matters on their minds than completing psychologic questionnaires. For these reasons, it is hardly surprising to find methodologic shortcomings in the literature. Patient samples are, in most cases, based on small numbers as shown in Table 9.1. In some of the cited studies, measures of psychologic responses to cancer were those used for psychiatric patients without standardizing these measures for what is a different population, namely, cancer patients. This problem

TABLE 9.1. *Coping and Disease Outcome*

Study	Cancer	Stage	n	Follow-up	Findings
Weisman and Worden (5)	Breast Colon Hodgkin's Malignant melanoma	Early and advanced	125	18 mo	(i) Long survival *significantly related* to close personal relationships (ii) Brief survival *significantly related* to high emotional distress to which patients responded by passitivity, fatalism, trying to forget
Greer et al. (6) Pettingale et al. (7) Greer et al. (8)	Breast	Mostly I	62	15 yr	(i) Recurrence and death *significantly related* to fatalism, anxious preoccupation, helplessness/hopelessness (ii) Recurrence-free survival *significantly related* to fighting spirit, denial (avoidance)
Derogatis et al. (9)	Breast	Metastatic	35	1 yr	Survival *significantly related* to hostility, guilt, depression
Rogentine et al. (10)	Malignant melanoma	I,II	64	1 yr	Recurrence *significantly related* to low personal adjustment
Temoshok and Fox (11)				3 yr	Recurrence *unrelated* to personal adjustment
Cassileth et al. (12)	(i) Pancreas Stomach Lung Colorectal Glioma	Advanced	204	3–8 yr	(i) Survival *unrelated* to hopelessness
	(ii) Breast Malignant melanoma	II	155	3–8 yr	(ii) Reccurence *unrelated* to hopelessness
Di Clemente and Temoshok (13)	Malignant melanoma	Mostly I	117	26 mo	Recurrence *significantly related* to (a) helplessness/hopelessness in men, (b) fatalism in women
Holland et al. (14)	Breast	II	346	8 yr	Recurrence/survival *unrelated* to psychiatric symptoms (SCL-90)
Hislop et al. (15)	Breast	Mostly I	133	80% for 3 yr	Survival *significantly related* to extroversion, and socially active, "consistent with findings regarding fighting spirit"
Jensen (16)	Breast	Early and metastatic	52	Average 624 days	Recurrence/death *significantly related* to helplessness/hopelessness, repressive personality style
Jamison et al. (17)	Breast	Metastatic	49	Average 45 mo	Survival *unrelated* to anxiety, depression, hostility, self-esteem
Levy et al. (18)	Breast	First recurrence	34	7 yr	Survival *significantly related* to expression of joy, more positive affect
Thomas et al. (19)	Colorectal	Duke's A,B, C_1, C_2	68	3 yr	Recurrence-free survival *significantly related* to fighting spirit in men Recurrence/death *significantly related* to denial in men
Dean and Surtees (20)	Breast	Nonmetastatic	121	6–8 yr	Recurrence-free survival *significantly related* to denial, unrelated to fighting spirit
Buddeberg et al. (21)	Breast	Nonmetastatic	107	3 yr	Recurrence/death *unrelated* to depression, "distraction," "problem tackling"
Morris et al. (22)	Breast	Nonmetastatic	88	5 yr	Recurrence-free survival *significant trend* of worsening prognosis as response varies from fighting spirit to denial through anxious preoccupation to fatalism or helplessness/hopelessness
	Lymphoma	All stages	50		
Fawzy et al. (23)	Malignant melanoma	I, II	68	6 yr	Survival *significantly related* to psychological therapy, higher coping scores indicating "more active-behavioral coping"

(continued)

TABLE 9.1.— *Continued*

Study	Cancer	Stage	*n*	Follow-up	Findings
Andrykowski et al. (24)	Leukemia treated by allogeneic bone marrow transplant	First remission/ chronic phase and later stages	42	Median 714 days	Death *significantly related* to anxious preoccupation
Ratcliffe et al. (25)	(i) Hodgkin's (ii) Non-Hodgkin's lymphoma	92% II, III, IV 46% high-grade disease	63	5yr	Death *significantly related* to high L scores on EPI, depression

has, in fact, been addressed: statistical norms for cancer patients have been reported in respect of the Hospital Anxiety and Depression scale (27), the Profile of Mood States (28) and the Mental Adjustment to Cancer scale (29), which measures specific coping styles.

Another shortcoming is that some authors do not reveal *when* they assessed their patients' psychologic responses. Clearly, results will differ depending on whether such assessments were made immediately after patients were told the diagnosis or after a period of time to allow the acute stress reaction to subside. In the cited studies, psychologic responses were assessed on a single occasion. It would prove informative if such assessments were made more than once during the follow-up period, in order to determine the stability of patients' coping styles. In some studies, the analysis of survival data is open to the following criticisms: duration of survival should be calculated not from the time of psychologic assessment but from the time of diagnosis; and statistical analyses should not be based on comparisons bnetween arbitrarily defined "short-term" and "long-term" survivors; techniques of multivariate analysis using Cox's proportional hazards regression model (30) are preferable (31).

Biologic factors—in particular the site, histology, and stage of the tumor—are unquestionably predominant in determining outcome for all cancers. Consequently, the need to control for these factors is a critical methodologic issue. All the cited studies have controlled for biologic prognostic factors as far as possible. In the longest follow-up study of women with breast cancer (6–8), however, the authors controlled for clinical stage, approximate tumor mass, histologic grade, mammographic appearance, and treatment but were unable to control for lymph node status because, in many cases, axillary node sampling was not carried out. Its importance as a prognostic indicator is well documented, but data on nodal status are not always available because management of the axilla in patients with operable breast cancer remains controversial (32,33). A number of other prognostic indicators for breast cancer have been reported: estrogen receptor (ER) status (33), cathepsin D (34), tumor cyclic AMP binding proteins (35), c-*erb*-2B expression (36), and proliferating cell nuclear antigen score (37). The order of importance of these factors and the independence of each from other prognostic factors is not clear at present. What is required, but so far not available, is a comprehensive prognostic indicator profile. In the meantime, the overriding importance of nodal status makes it essential to control for this factor in studies of the role of psychologic factors in disease outcome of breast cancer.

Provisional Conclusions

We have alluded to some formidable methodologic difficulties which beset this area of enquiry. As a consequence, the evidence currently available does not provide conclusive proof (or disproof) of a relationship between psychological responses to cancer and the course of these diseases. Nonetheless, subject to this important caveat, the following provisional conclusions can be drawn.

Psychiatric Symptoms and Disease Outcome. Seven studies have examined the influence of psychiatric symptoms on disease outcome in patients with breast cancer (5,9,14,17,18,21,22), colorectal cancer (5), malignant melanoma (5), Hodgkin's disease (5,25) and non-Hodgkin's lymphoma (25). The presence of psychiatric symptoms including "emotional distress" was significantly related to good outcome in one study (9) and to poor outcome in three studies (5,18,25); three other studies found psychiatric symptoms and disease outcome to be unrelated (14,17,21). In view of the equivocal results, the relationship between psychiatric symptoms and disease outcome remains an open question.

Coping Styles. In one of the earliest prospective studies of women with early (stages I & II) breast cancer, the authors delineated several broad categories of coping style (6–8,38). Initially based on clinical ratings, these categories have since been validated in patients with various cancers by means of a self-rating questionnaire (38,39). These coping styles were found to be significantly associated with subsequent disease outcome. As mentioned earlier, a drawback of this study was the unavoidable lack of data concerning nodal status. However, in a subsequent study (22) of patients with breast cancer, complete data on nodal status were obtained. In that study, which also included patients with lymphoma, the authors were able to control rigorously for biologic prognostic factors; they reported similar results to those in the earlier study. Three further replication studies have been carried out (13,19,20) and a number of other investigations that used different coping styles have been reported (12,15,16,23,24). The evidence is summarized below.

Fighting spirit—An active coping response in which the patient fully accepts the diagnosis, adopts an optimistic attitude, is determined to fight the disease, and wants to participate in decisions regarding treatment.
> *Significantly related to good disease outcome* (longer survival): Greer et al. (6–8), Morris et al. (22), Hislop et al. (15), Thomas et al. (19) in men only, Fawzy et al. (23)
> *Unrelated to disease outcome*: Dean and Surtees (20)

Avoidance (denial)—The patient either rejects the diagnosis of cancer or, more commonly, minimizes the seriousness, avoids thinking about the illness.
> *Significantly related to good disease outcome*. Greer et al. (6–8), Dean and Surtees (20), Morris et al. (22)
> *Significantly related to poor disease outcome*. Thomas et al. (19) in men only

Fatalism (stoic acceptance)—the patient accepts the diagnosis, has a resigned, fatalistic attitude.
> *Significantly related to poor disease outcome*: Greer et al. (6–8), Di Clemente and Temoshok (13) in women only, Weisman and Worden (5), Morris et al. (22)

Anxious preoccupation—the patient is constantly preoccupied with cancer, fears that any aches and pains indicate spread or recurrence of the disease, seeks frequent reassurance.
> *Significantly related to poor disease outcome*: Greer et al. (6–8), Morris et al. (22), Andrykowski et al. (24)

Helplessness/hopelessness—the patient is engulfed by the diagnosis of cancer, feels like giving up, adopts a totally pessimistic attitude, feels hopeless.

> *Significantly related to poor disease outcome*: Greer et al. (6–8), Di Clemente and Temoshok (13) in men only, Jensen (16), Morris et al. (22).
> *Unrelated to disease outcome*: Cassileth et al. (12).

The evidence summarized here strongly supports the hypothesis that passive coping styles—in particular fatalism, anxious preoccupation and helplessness/hopelessness—are associated with poor subsequent disease outcome. This hypothesis is supported by all the cited studies with a single exception (12). Further support comes from the study by Goodkin et al. (1), which demonstrated a significant association between hopelessness and the promotion of cervical intraepithelial neoplasia to invasive carcinoma of the cervix.

The relationship of passive coping styles to poor disease outcome is not confined to cancer. A recent well-designed study of homosexual men with AIDS reported that "realistic acceptance," which the authors describe as similar to stoic acceptance as above, was a significant predictor of decreased survival time (40). Evidence regarding the effect of fighting spirit and avoidance on disease outcome is a little less convincing. Although the majority of studies that measured these coping styles reported a significant association with good outcome, one study found no relationship between fighting spirit and disease outcome and another study reported denial to be related to poor disease outcome in men. The latter finding may be due to the difficulty of measuring avoidance (denial). This problem appears to have been overcome by the development of a new self-report measure of coping styles among cancer patients (41). On balance, the evidence suggests that fighting spirit is related to a good disease outcome, whereas the role of avoidance remains uncertain.

PERSONALITY

The cancer-prone personality has long been a popular notion, with supporting citations going back as far as Hippocrates and Galen. Despite this there has been a paucity of scientific evidence. However, the recent past has seen the publication of a number of studies that use an acceptable methodology. It is these which form the basis for this review of personality and cancer. Premorbid, psychological characteristics, as risk factors in disease, represent a serious area of study. Psychosomatic medicine is considered quite respectable and it is acknowledged that behavior may contribute to some medical disorders, the most obvious example being smoking, where knowledge of the associated carcinogenic process is well established (although the absence of lung cancer in some smokers is poorly understood). People may adopt life-styles which place them at increased risk of developing specific diseases and quite often it is argued that the way we die reflects the way we live. But where does personality fit into any proposed psychosomatic model of cancer? Drever's *Dictionary of Psychology* (42) describes personality as "the integrated and dynamic organization of the physical, mental, moral, and social qualities of the individual, as that manifests itself to other people . . . ." It is also described as the natural and acquired impulses and complexes and the habits of the person as these are manifested within our social interactions. More often than not, when cancer-prone personality is referred to this usually means a specific personality type. As Drever suggests, these typologies are often stereotypes which include the more extreme characteristics and elements of behavior and, of course, these do not, by definition, represent the normal or average person. In this respect personality typologies are often illustrative of an extreme, and extrapolation is limited when we use such descriptions to try and explain behavior: personality types are not necessarily mutually exclusive categories but rather a continuum of a particular behavior pattern. In this respect the limits of personality theories need to be borne in mind when considering the appropriateness of a model of the cancer-prone personality. Many personality models are also descriptions of temperament, i.e., constitutional processes that determine behavior. We tend to think of temperament as being very strongly determined by genetic factors. The whole notion of a cancer-prone personality is, indeed, deterministic and this is reflected in much of the reported research.

When evaluating the merits of recent research on cancer and personality, the simplest method of scrutiny is in terms of the timing of data collection, i.e., whether psychological assessment is made retrospectively, semiprospectively, or prospectively. A number of studies (43–46) examining personality among those already diagnosed with cancer have provided consistent support for a personality type characterized by unassertiveness, repression of negative emotions (especially anger), with an easy-going and compliant attitude to life. Such results are open to criticism on the basis that it cannot be clearly established that the personality characteristics identified predate onset of the disease. Despite the argument that a personality typology represents a lifelong tendency toward a particular behavior pattern, it is not possible to exclude reactions to recent events (such as the diagnosis of a major life-threatening disease like cancer) as an explanation for current behavior.

Semiprospective studies can, to a certain extent, circumvent this difficulty if people are evaluated regarding personality type before the disease diagnosis is known, either to the investigator or to the person who is the subject of that investigation. For obvious reasons this has been the most commonly used methodology in research on cancer and personality, being relatively easy to implement. One of the earliest studies using this approach was described by Kissen (47). Using a reliable and well-validated method of psychological assessment, comparing those with lung cancer to controls suffering other chest diseases and with the investigator "blind" to the diagnosis, he was able to establish, using this semiprospective design, that those with lung cancer had "a lesser ability to discharge emotion" and this risk factor appeared to be independent of smoking habit. Subsequent work, when summarized, suggests a personality type characterized by abnormal release of emotions (48,49), rationalizing and suppressing feelings (50), less hostility (51), a bottling up of emotions and inability to express anger (52). However, it has become increasingly difficult to conduct acceptable semiprospective studies: the most common argument against their validity is that patients are more knowledgeable now about cancer and have formulated ideas about their diagnosis before this becomes known to them. Scherg (53) has suggested, however, that controlling for knowledge of diagnosis bias appears to strengthen evidence for the personality effect observed, but it is nevertheless an important criticism as many semiprospective studies failed to control for this source of bias and thus are open to the same criticism as those which are retrospective. More commonly, however, it is simply the speed with which a cancer diagnosis is now reached which limits the facility to make prediagnostic psychological assessments. Clearly, the strongest evidence for any psychological risk model will be derived from true prospective studies. However, the number of studies meeting this criterion comes down to less than can be counted on one hand, and few of these actually set out to test the hypothesis that personality type predicts cancer. Most were exploratory epidemiologic studies looking at disease precursors (54–56) with no a priori predictions regarding cancer incidence. Where clear a priori predictions were tested prospectively, the results had not been without controversy. Hagnell (57) found no association between personality and subsequent incidence of cancer, although the data suggested a trend, found only in women, toward a "sub-stable" personality type, which might affect the growth of cancer. Scherg's (58) study of psychological risk factors indicated no evidence of increase in suppression of anger or a "type A" behavior pattern in a large group of women studied. One of the strongest sets of prospective studies was generated by Grossarth-Maticek (59), who reported data from a cohort in Yugoslavia and later, with Eysenck (60), from a German cohort (the Heidelberg studies). Unfortunately, these studies by Grossarth-Maticek, which appeared to provide definitive evidence for a cancer-prone personality, have been unable to withstand close scientific scrutiny (61) and have been largely discredited. Despite the seemingly flimsy evidence for a cancer-prone personality, the notion of a "type C" personality has been received enthusiastically. The idea of a type C personality was promulgated by Morris (62,63) and subsequently elucidated by Temoshok (64). This typology appears to include some of the opposite characteristics of Friedman and Rosenman's (65) type A personality, where the latter is characterized by "intense ambition, competitive drive . . . and a sense of time urgency," which was linked with increased risk of coronary artery disease. The main impact of type A behavior upon increased risk of heart disease was explained by possible life-style factors: long working hours, heavy smoking, and lack of exercise. The type C pattern, which is contrary to type A is characterized by behavior which is appeasing, unassertive, unexpressive of negative emotions (especially anger), and social compliance (65). That this type C behavior pattern has been more frequently observed among those who have developed cancer is an interesting finding. However, the coexistence of a particular behavior pattern with disease is not sufficient in itself to support a notion of causation. Mechanisms for disease promotion need to be identified, and despite the current fashion for a psychoimmunologic model, no clear biologic link between type C behavior, or associated high-risk life-style factors, and cancer, has been found. Furthermore, it is important to remember that personality typologies are stereotypes and only a small proportion of those people evaluated will be "true to type" and show evidence of the focal behavioral characteristics; this is a given in the science of personality types.

PROVISIONAL CONCLUSIONS

In summary, it would appear that it is possible to conceptualize a set of behaviors frequently occurring together which are formulated as a type C personality. That they occur more often in people who have developed cancer is supported by limited evidence. There is no clear evidence, however, from well-designed prospective studies that this, or any other, personality type has a causal role in cancer. Life-style factors are

important precursors (e.g., smoking) but personality per se is not. It would appear that the scientific community is no closer to establishing the validity of the concept of the cancer-prone personality than was Hippocrates some 2000 or more years ago. Despite this, it is clear that the notion of a cancer-prone personality has developed into popular mythology and, as Doan (66) has observed, "we doubt, however, that science alone will ever resolve the controversy over belief in psychological effects on cancer." Such beliefs are apparently perceived (at least in a North American culture) to be "helpful to persons with cancer, even if untrue" (66).

RECOMMENDATIONS

1. In view of the evidence suggesting an association between patients' coping styles and subsequent disease outcome, cancer treatment trials should include measures of coping styles.
2. Comprehensive profiles of biologic prognostic indicators for each of the cancers are required.
3. Large multicentred studies of patients with various cancers are required to define the apparent relationship of coping styles to disease outcome. Such studies should: (1) be based on rigorous experimental design, (2) employ the same standardized measures of coping style, and (3) control for biologic prognostic factors.
4. Psychologic investigations should be initiated to identify the biologic mechanisms mediating possible psychological influences upon the course of cancers.
5. Psychologic therapy that will enable patients with passive and helpless responses to adopt active coping responses should be developed and evaluated in controlled prospective investigations.
6. Large prospective studies setting out a priori predictions regarding cancer and personality are needed.

REFERENCES

1. Goodkin K, Antoni MH, Blaney PH. Stress and hopelessness in the promotion of cervical intraepithelial neoplasia to invasive squamous cell carcinoma of the cervix. *J Psychosom Res.* 1986; 30:67–76.
2. Greer S, Moorey S, Baruch J, et al. Adjuvant psychological therapy for patients with cancer: a prospective randomized trial. *Br Med J.* 1992; 304:675–680.
3. Fawzy FI, Cousins N, Fawzy NW, Kemeny ME, Elashoff R, Morton D. A structured psychiatric intervention for cancer patients. I. *Arch Gen Psychiatry.* 1990; 47:720–725.
4. Burton MV, Parker RW, Farrell A, et al. A randomized controlled trial of preoperative psychological preparation for mastectomy. *Psycho-Oncology.* 1995; 4:1–9.

5. Weisman AD, Worden JW. *Coping and Vulnerability in Cancer Patients*. Boston: Massachusetts General Hospital; 1977.

6. Greer S, Morris T, Pettingale KW. Psychological response to breast cancer; effect on outcome. *Lancet*. 1979; ii:785–787.

7. Pettingale KW, Morris T, Greer S, Haybittle J. Mental attitudes to cancer: an additional prognostic factor. *Lancet*. 1985; 1:750.

8. Greer S, Morris T, Pettingale KW, Haybittle J. Pyschological response to breast cancer and 15 year outcome. *Lancet*. 1990; i:49–50.

9. Derogatis LR, Abeloff MD, Melisaratos N. Psychological coping mechanisms and survival time in metastatic breast cancer. *J Am Med Assoc*. 1979; 242:1504–1508.

10. Rogentine GN, van Kammen DP, Fox BH, et al. Psychological factors in the prognosis of malignant melanoma: a prospective study. *Psychosom Med*. 1979; 41:647–655.

11. Temoshok L, Fox BH. Coping styles and other psychosocial factors related to medical status and to prognosis in patients with cutaneous malignant melanoma as a predictor of follow-up clinical status. In: Fox BH, Newberry BH, eds., *Impact of Psychoendocrine Systems in Cancer and Immunity*. Toronto: Hogrefe; 1984: 258–287.

12. Cassileth BR, Lusk EJ, Miller DS, Brown L, Miller C. Psychological correlates of survival in advanced malignant disease. *N Engl J Med*. 1985; 312:1551–1555.

13. Di Clemente KJ, Temoshok L. Psychological adjustment to having cutaneous malignant melanoma as a predictor of follow-up clinical status. *Psychosom Med*. 1985; 47:81.

14. Holland JC, Korzun AH, Tross S, Cella DF, Norton L, Wood W. Psychosocial factors and disease-free survival in stage II breast carcinoma [abstract]. *Proc Am Soc Clin Oncol*. 1986; 5:237.

15. Hislop GT, Waxler NE, Coldman J, Elwood JM, Kan L. The prognostic significance of psychosocial factors in women with breast cancer. *J Chronic Dis*. 1987; 40:729–735.

16. Jensen MR. Psychobiological factors predicting the course of cancer. *J Pers*. 1987; 55:329–342.

17. Jamison RN, Burish TG, Wallston KA. Psychogenic factors in predicting survival of breast cancer patients. *J Clin Oncol*. 1987; 5:768–772.

18. Levy SM, Lee J, Bagley C, Lippman M. Survival hazards analysis in first recurrent breast cancer patients: seven-year follow-up. *Psychosom Med*. 1988; 50:520–528.

19. Thomas C, Turner P, Madden F. Coping and the outcome of stoma surgery. *J Psychosom Res*. 1988; 32:457–467.

20. Dean C, Surtees PG. Do psychological factors predict survival in breast cancer? *J Psychosom Res*. 1989; 33:561–569.

21. Buddeberg C, Wolf C, Sieber M, et al. Coping strategies and course of disease of breast cancer patients. *Psychother Psychosom*. 1991; 55:151–157.

22. Morris T, Pettingale KW, Haybittle J. Psychological response to cancer diagnosis and disease outcome in patients with breast cancer and lymphoma. *Psycho-Oncology*. 1992; 1:105–114.

23. Fawzy FI, Fawzy NW, Hyn CS, et al. Malignant melanoma: effects of an early structured psychiatric intervention, coping and affective state on recurrence and survival 6 years later. *Arch Gen Psychiatry*. 1993; 50:681–689.

24. Andrykowski MA, Brady MJ, Henslee-Downey PJ. Psychosocial factors predictive of survival after allogenic bone marrow transplantation for leukemia. *Psychosom Med*. 1994; 56:432–439.

25. Ratcliffe MA, Dawson AA, Walker LG. Eysenck Personality Inventory L-scores in patients with Hodgkin's disease and non-Hodgkin's lymphoma. *Psycho-Oncology*. 1995; 4:39–45.

26. Temoshok L, Heller BW. On comparing apples, oranges and fruit salad: a methodological overview of medical outcome studies in psychosocial oncology. In: Cooper CL, ed. *Psychosocial Stress and Cancer*. New York: Wiley, 1984: 231–260.

27. Moorey S, Greer S, Watson M, et al. The factor structure and factor stability of the Hospital Anxiety and Depression scale in patients with cancer. *Br J Psychiatry*. 1990; 158:255–259.

28. Cella DF, Tross S, Orav EJ, Holland JC, Silberfarb PM, Rafla S. Mood states of patients after the diagnosis of cancer. *J Psychosoc Oncol*. 1989; 7:45–54.

29. Watson M, Greer S, Young J, Inayat Q, Burgess C, Robertson C. Development of a questionnaire measure of adjustment to cancer: the MAC scale. *Br J Psychiatry*. 1988; 18:203–209.

30. Cox DR. Regression models and life tables. *J R Stat Soc*. 1972; 34B:187–202.

31. Watson M, Ramirez A. Psychological factors in cancer prognosis. In: CL Coper, M Watson, eds. *Cancer and Stress*. New York: Wiley; 1991:47–71.

32. Morris J, Royle GT, Taylor I. Changes in the surgical management of early breast cancer in England. *J R Soc Med*. 1991; 22:12–14.

33. Sacks NPM, Pitcher ME. Early breast cancer. In: Horwich A, ed. *Oncology*. London: Chapman & Hall; 1995: 513–527.

34. Spyratos F, Maudelonde T, Brouillet J-P. Cathepsin-D: an independent prognosis factor for metastasis of breast cancer. *Lancet*. 1989; 2:1115–1118.

35. Miller WR, Elton RA, Dixon JM, Chetty V, Watson DMA. Cyclic AMP binding proteins and prognosis in breast cancer. *Br J Cancer*. 1990; 61:263–266.

36. Anbazhagan R, Gelber RD, Bettelheim R, Goldhirsch A, Gusterson BA. Association of c-erb-2 expression and S-phase fraction in the prognosis of node positive breast cancer. *Ann Oncol*. 1991; 2:47–53.

37. Tahan SR, Neuberg DS, Dieffenbach A, Yacoub L. Prediction of early relapse and shortened survival in patients with breast cancer by proliferating cell nuclear antigen score. *Cancer*. 1993; 71:3552–3559.

38. Watson M, Greer S, Young J, Inayat Q, Burgess C, Robertson B. Development of a questionnaire measure of adjustment to cancer: the MAC scale. *Psychol Med*. 1988; 18:203–209.

39. Greer S, Morrey S, Watson M. Patients' adjustment to cancer: the Mental Adjustment to Cancer (MAC) scale vs clinical ratings. *J Psychosom Res*. 1989; 33:373–377.

40. Reed GM, Kemeny ME, Taylor SE, Wang H-YJ, Visscher BR. Realistic acceptance as a predictor of decreased survival time in gay men with AIDS. *Health Psychol*. 1994; 13:299–307.

41. Watson M, Law M, dos Santos M, Greer S, Baruch J, Bliss J. The Mini-Mac: further development of the Mental Adjustment to Cancer scale. *J Psychosoc Oncol.* 1994; 12:33–46.

42. Drever, J. *A Dictionary of Psychology.* Harmondsworth, UK: Penguin Books; 1952.

43. Jansen MA, Muenz LR. A retrospective study of personality variables associated with fibrocystic disease and breast cancer. *J Psychosom Res.* 1984; 28:35–42.

44. Watson M, Pettingale KW, Greer S. Emotional control and autonomic arousal in breast cancer patients. *J Psychosom Res.* 1984; 28:467–474.

45. Priestman TJ, Priestman SG, Bradshaw C. Stress and breast cancer. *Br J Cancer.* 1985; 51:493–498.

46. Goldstein DA, Antoni MH. The distribution of repressive coping styles among non-metastatic and metasatic breast cancer patients as compared to non-cancer patients. *Psychol Health.* 1989; 3:245–258.

47. Kissen DM. Personality characteristics in males condusive to lung cancer. *Br J Med Psychol.* 1963; 36:27–36.

48. Greer S, Morris T. Psychological attributes of women who develop breast cancer: a controlled study. *J Psychosom Res.* 1975; 19:147–153.

49. Morris T, Greer S, Pettingale KW, Watson M. Patterns of expression of anger and their psychological correlates in women with breast cancer. *J Psychosom Res.* 1981; 25:111–117.

50. Wirsching M, Hoffmann F, Stierlin H, Weber G, Wirsching B. Prebioptic psychological characteristics of breast cancer patients. *Psychother Psychosom.* 1985; 43:69–76.

51. Grassi L, Molinari S. Pattern of emotional control and psychological reactions to breast cancer: a preliminary report. *Psychol Rep.* 1988; 62:727–732.

52. Cooper CL, Faragher EB. Psychosocial stress and breast cancer: the interrelationship between stress events, coping strategies and personality. *Psychol. Med.* 1993; 23:653–662.

53. Scherg H. Psychosocial factors and disease bias in breast cancer patients. *Psychosom Med.* 1987; 49:302–312.

54. Thomas CB, Duszynski KR, Shaffer JW. Family attitudes reported in youth as potential predictors of cancer. *Psychosom Med.* 1979; 41:287–302.

55. Shekelle RB, Raynor WJ, Ostfeld AM, et al. Psychological depression and seventeen-year risk of death from cancer. *Psychosom Med.* 1981; 43:117–125.

56. Zonderman AB, Costa PT, McCrae RR. Depression as a risk for cancer morbidity and mortality in a nationally representative sample. *J Am Med Assoc.* 1989; 262:1191–1195.

57. Hagnell O. The premorbid personality of persons who develop cancer in a total population investigated in 1947 and 1957. *Ann NY Acad Sci.* 1966; 125:846–855.

58. Scherg H. Psychosocial factors in breast cancer and other cancers in retrospective and prospective view. In: Muthny FA and Haag G, eds. *Onkologie in Psychosozialen Kontext.* Heidelberg: Roland Ansager Verlag; 1993: 27–37.

59. Grossarth-Maticek R. Psychosocial predictors of cancer and internal diseases. *Psychother Psychosom.* 1980; 33:122–128.

60. Grossarth-Maticek R, Eysenck HJ, Vetter H. Personality type, smoking habit and their interaction as predictors of cancer and coronary heart disease. *Pers Individ Differences.* 1988; 9:479–495.

61. *Psychological Inquiry* (1991). Whole issue Vol 2. Number 3. Laurence Erlbaum Associates, Hose and London.

62. Morris T. A 'Type C' for Cancer? Paper presented at the Royal Society of Medicine Clinical Oncology Study Course, London 1977.

63. Morris T. A 'Type C' for Cancer? Low trait anxiety in the pathogenesis of cancer. *Cancer Detect Prev.* 1980; 3:102.

64. Temoshok L. Bio-psychosocial studies on cutaneous malignant melanoma: Psychosocial factors associated with prognostic indicators, progression, psychophysiology and tumour–host response. *Soc Sci Med.* 1985; 20:833–840.

65. Friedman M, Rosenman RH. Association of overt behaviour pattern with blood and cardiovascular findings. *J Am Med Assoc.* 1959; 169:1286–1296.

66. Doan B, Gray RE, Davis CS. Belief in psychological effects on cancer. *Psycho-Oncology.* 1993; 2:139–150.

10

Social Ties and Cancer

VICKI S. HELGESON, SHELDON COHEN, AND HEIDI L. FRITZ

The possible role of the social environment in cancer risk and survival has received considerable attention over the last 15 years. Much of the impetus for this interest derives from increasing evidence that social ties are related to both endocrine and immune responses thought to play a role in the risk for cancer and the progression of disease (1,2). However, evidence for the role of social networks in the onset and progression of cancer has been unclear. Some of the confusion derives from inconsistency in the quality of published studies, from differences in conceptualization of social network variables, and from a failure to consider whether relations with the social network may differ across patient gender, stage of disease, and cancer site. The purpose of this chapter is to evaluate the role of social ties in the onset and progression of cancer. We begin by addressing the plausibility of social environmental influences on the pathogenesis of neoplastic disease. We propose psychologic, behavioral, and biological mechanisms that could link social ties to cancer. Next, we review over 30 studies that have examined the relation of the social environment to cancer. We distinguish between studies of cancer incidence and mortality among healthy people and of length of survival and time to recurrence among those already afflicted with the disease. Finally, we summarize the work we review, discuss its limitations, and propose guidelines for future work.

Social networks can have both positive and negative effects on health and well-being. It is generally believed that positive effects are attributed to strong network ties and to resources that the network can provide when persons are in need (3). Negative effects are primarily attributed to social conflict and social threats to self-esteem and self-concept (4,5). The research linking social networks to cancer has focused on the characteristics of the environment thought to result in beneficial effects on health. For this reason, the term "social support" is often used in describing this literature.

PATHWAYS LINKING THE SOCIAL ENVIRONMENT TO CANCER

How could social networks contribute to the onset and progression of cancer? Figure 10–1 presents a simplified model of the mechanisms by which social ties can influence disease risk and progression. Simply, positive characteristics of the social environment are associated with *cognitive benefits* such as increased access to information, and feelings of control, self-esteem, and optimism, and with *affective benefits* such as the experience of more positive and fewer negative emotions (6). In turn, these psychologic characteristics can influence *behavioral* and *biologic* responses that are thought to play a role in the onset and progression of cancer. For example, greater self-esteem might result in increased motivation to care for oneself. This can be manifest in behaviors associated with decreased risk of cancer incidence and mortality (e.g., quitting smoking, improving diet), early cancer detection (e.g., self-examinations, routine screenings), timely response to symptoms, and improved compliance with medical regimens. Similarly, by preventing negative emotional reactions, social ties can buffer against disturbances of the neuroendocrine and immune systems thought to contribute to disease pathogenesis (see 1,7).

At a more detailed level, the beneficial effects of the social environment are thought to occur as a function of two processes: *(1)* network membership and social interaction directly increase positive cognitions, emotions, and behaviors, and *(2)* social networks help ameliorate the deleterious effects of stressful life events by providing coping resources such as emotional, informational, and instrumental support (3,6). The former is termed the "main (or direct) effect" hypothesis and the latter the "stress-buffering" hypothesis. Either of these hypotheses may explain the relations between social ties and cancer that we report in this review, as studies are not designed to distinguish between the two.

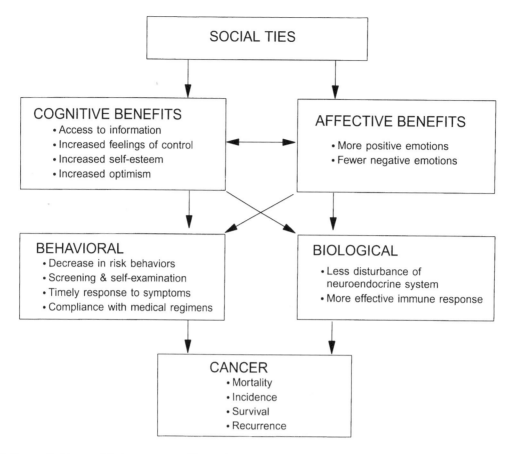

FIG. 10–1. Pathways linking social ties to cancer. The paths identified in the model move in only one direction from social ties to cancer. The absence of alternative paths is not intended to imply that they do not exist.

REVIEW OF THE LITERATURE

We review studies that examine the impact of the social environment on cancer incidence and mortality for healthy persons (Table 10.1), and length of survival and time to recurrence for persons with a prior diagnosis of cancer (see Table 10.2). For the most part, the correlational work we review is limited to prospective studies. By assessing the social environment at study onset and then examining subsequent changes in

TABLE 10.1. *Study of the Relation of the Social Environment to Cancer Incidence and Mortality among Healthy Persons*

Author	Site	n	Sex	Race	Marital	Structure	Function	Outcome
Jenkins (13)	Variety	39 areas			+			Mortality
Krause & Lilienfeld (14)	Variety	not given			+			Mortality
Reynolds & Kaplan (15)	Variety	6,848			0	+ Women, 0 Men	+ women, 0 men	Mortality
Welin et al. (16)	Variety	9,89	100% men		0	+, +		Mortality
Reynolds & Kaplan (15)	Variety	6,848			0	0		Incidence
Zonderman et al. (21)	Variety	9,000+			−			Incidence
Vogt et al. (38)	Healthy	2,603				0		Incidence
Thomas and Duszynski (42)	All sites	20	100% men	100% white			+	Incidence

TABLE 10.2. *Study of the Relation of the Social Environment to Survival and Recurrence among People with Cancer*

Author	Site	n	Sex	Race	Marital	Structure	Function	Intervention	Outcome
Neale et al. (22)	Breast: all stages	1,261	100% women	100% white	+				Survival
Wilkinson et al. (23)	Breast	1,784	100% women		0				Survival
LeMarchand et al. (24)	Breast: all stages	2,956	100% women	Caucasian Japanese Hawaiian Chinese Filipino	0				Survival
Goodwin et al. (25)	Epithelial	27,779		White Hispanic	+				Survival
Waxler-Morrison et al. (26)	Breast: all stages	118	100% women	100% white	−	+,0			Survival
Ell et al. (27)	Breast, lung, colorectal: all stages	294	78% women	83% white	− Breast 0 Lung 0 Colorectal	+	+ Breast		Survival
Dean and Surtees (28)	Breast: local, regional	121	100% women		0				Survival
Funch and Marshall (29)	Breast: local, regional	208	100% women	100% white	0	+,0			Survival
Stavraky et al. (30)	Lung: regional advanced	224	75% men		0		+		Survival
Cassileth et al. (31)	All sites: advanced	204	63% men	76% white	0	0			Survival
Cassileth et al. (32)	All sites: advanced	204	63% men	76% white	−	+			Survival
Reynolds & Caplan (15)	Variety	339	55% women		0	+ men 0 women	0		Survival
Dean and Surtees (28)	Breast: local, regional	121	100% women		0	0			Recurrence
Cassileth et al. (31)	Breast stage 2 skin stages 1,2	149	79% women	78% white	0	0			Recurrence
Cassileth et al. (32)	Breast stage 2 skin stages 1,2	149	79% women	78% white	0	0			Recurrence
Horn et al. (33)	Breast: local, regional	338	100% women		+/−	+,0			2nd cancer
Vogt et al. (38)	Variety	not given				+,0			Survival
Hislop et al. (39)	Breast: all stages	127	100% women	100% white		+			Survival
Richardson et al. (40)	Hematologic	94	63% men	17% white 23% black 55% hispanic		0		+	Survival
Hislop et al. (39)	Breast: all stages	124	100% women	100% white		+			Recurrence
Levy et al. (43)	Breast: stage 1,2	90	100% women				0,+		Recurrence
Spiegel et al. (44)	Breast: metastatic	86	100% women					+	Survival
Fawzy et al. (45)	Melanoma	68	51% women					+	Survival
Fawzy et al. 93	Melanoma	68	51% women					+	Recurrence
Morgenstern et al. (40)	Breast: all stages	136	100% women	100% white				0	Survival
Gellert et al. (47)	Breast: all stages	136	100% women	100% white				0	Survival

health, prospective designs allow us to *exclude* interpretations of the data that suggest that the disease is responsible for changes in social networks and their functions. The better studies also provide control for spurious variables that might be responsible for changes in both social networks and disease status. For example, increased age may be associated with both network shrinkage (i.e., close friends and relatives die) as well as increased risk for cancer. Potential spurious variables that are commonly assessed and statistically controlled include age, socioeconomic status, and (in survival and recurrence studies) stage of disease at diagnosis. This review also includes several provocative, if not as methodologically sophisticated studies, that compare the social characteristics of persons who died of cancer to those of persons in the general population. Finally, we report intervention evaluations that use experimental and quasi-experimental designs and hence provide evidence that is less subject to alternate causal explanations.

The literature includes studies of both structural and functional characteristics of social networks, as well as evaluations of interventions intended to increase available social support. *Structural* measures of the social environment describe the existence of and interconnections between network members. Three types of structural measures have been used in the literature we review: marital status, network size, and social integration. Marital status variables range from a simple married/unmarried dichotomy to more specific categories of married, never married, widowed, divorced, and separated. Network size is assessed by counts of friends and close family members. Number of network members with whom there is regular social contact is intended to provide a marker of social integration. More elaborate measures of social integration assess the range of social roles and social activities in which persons participate. A frequently used measure of social integration is the Social Network Index (SNI) (8)—a composite index that includes marital status, membership in organizations, and frequency and number of social contacts. *Functional* measures of support tap either the perception that resources are available or the receipt of resources from network members through supportive interactions. Typologies of functions typically differentiate emotional, informational, and instrumental support (e.g., 9,10). *Social support interventions* refer to professionally designed attempts to alter patients' social networks and provide one or more support functions. They are generally based on structured or semistructured protocols.

Structural Measures

Marital Status. Being married has been associated with better mental health (11) and with lower all-cause mortality (see Ref. 12 for a review). Typically, the marriage benefit is attributed to the emotional and material resources that can be provided by an intimate relationship. The studies reviewed here are intended as tests of the marriage benefit in relation to cancer.

MORTALITY. Comparisons of cancer mortality rates across geographic areas have provided some support for a health benefit of marriage. Jenkins (13) found more cancer deaths in catchment areas with fewer married couples and more divorced, separated, and widowed people. Kraus and Lilienfeld (14) compared cancer deaths in married and widowed persons to distributions of these two marital status groups in the population and found an increased risk of cancer mortality for widowed persons. It is not clear, however, whether this finding represents a protective effect of marriage or a harmful effect of losing a spouse.

Unfortunately, prospective studies of marital status and mortality do not support a marriage benefit. Reynolds and Kaplan (15) followed 6848 initially healthy adults for 17 years, and Welin and colleagues (16) followed 989 initially healthy men (50–60 years old) for 12 years. Neither of these studies found evidence that marital status as assessed at study onset was associated with subsequent cancer mortality.

INCIDENCE. Many reports have been published examining cancer incidence by comparing the marital status of cancer patients to population data derived from the census. These studies are based on very large samples and hence even very small differences are statistically significant. In general, this literature suggests that: *(1)* marriage has been associated with both lower and higher incidence of cancer, and *(2)* the role of marital status in incidence probably varies by race and gender and possibly by cancer site (see Refs. 17–19). The lack of clear results is further complicated by two methodological problems: misclassification of marital status groups and underenumeration of specific race and marital status groups (20).

Results from prospective population studies fail to support a protective effect of marriage on cancer incidence. In the previously mentioned study conducted by Reynolds and Kaplan (15), there was no relation of marital status to cancer incidence over 17 years for either men or women. Zonderman and colleagues (21) studied over 9000 healthy people and found that married people were *more likely* to be diagnosed with cancer than unmarried people over a 10-year period. The latter study made no mention of whether results applied to both men and women, and neither study explored whether results applied across racial or ethnic groups.

Overall, this literature fails to provide any clear answers in regard to the role of marriage in cancer incidence. It does, however, suggest that the role of marriage in incidence may vary across gender and ethnic groups. It is important to point out that it is unclear whether a marriage benefit would be manifest in increased or decreased cancer incidence. Diagnosis of cancer requires the seeking of care. To the extent that the marriage benefit is derived from spousal help in detection and reduced delay in seeking care, marriage could be associated with a higher incidence of disease.

SURVIVAL. In four archival studies, medical records were abstracted for length of survival and for marital status at the time of cancer diagnosis. Three of the four studies were of women with any stage of breast cancer. A study comparing 10-year survival of married and widowed women found that married women survived longer even when stage of disease at diagnosis, age, socioeconomic status, and delay in seeking treatment were statistically controlled (22). However, studies of 2 to 7-year (23) and 5-year survival (24) comparing married to single and formerly married women found no relation after including appropriate statistical controls. The remaining archival study examined survival from epithelial cancer in 27,779 white and Hispanic men and women (25). Even after including controls for age, gender, stage of disease at diagnosis, and treatment, married patients had a longer survival compared to unmarried patients for all stages of cancer (length of follow-up was variable), but the effect was strongest among patients with localized disease. The overall relative risk of death for being unmarried was 1.23.

In other studies, newly diagnosed patients were recruited and followed for length of survival. These were based on smaller sample sizes than the archival studies reviewed above. Four studies of women with breast cancer showed that marriage is either associated with *poorer* survival or not associated with survival. A study of 118 white women with any stage of disease revealed a lower survival rate for married compared to unmarried people over 1–4 years of follow-up (26). Analyses of data collected from 168 women with breast cancer (length of follow-up not specified) similarly found marriage to be associated with shorter survival (27). The cause of death in that study was not limited to cancer, however. In contrast, two studies of women

with local and regional breast cancer found no relation of marital status to survival ($n = 121$, 6–8 years (28); $n = 208$, 20 years (29)).

Research focusing on other cancer sites or not differentiating sites has generally found little evidence for any relation of marital status to survival. Marital status was not related to 1-year survival among 224 regional and advanced lung cancer patients (30) nor to 5-year survival among 204 white and black men and women with all sites of metastatic cancer (31). Eight-year follow-up of the latter group of patients revealed married people were *more likely* to have died than unmarried people (32), but this finding should be interpreted with caution, as only 6% of patients remained alive at 8-year follow-up. In the study by Ell described earlier (27), there was no association between marital status and survival among people with either lung or colorectal cancer. Finally, in a 17-year prospective study, Reynolds and Kaplan (15) identified 339 people who developed cancer (any site, any stage) during the intervening period, and determined their length of survival. Marital status had no relation to survival from cancer.

In sum, there is no consistent association of marital status with survival from cancer. This inconsistency seems to hold across persons with localized and advanced cancer and across men and women. It is noteworthy that the studies showing protective effects of marriage on survival employed very large samples by extracting data from medical records. It may be that there is a marriage benefit but that the effect size is so small that it is only detectable in studies of this type. In fact, the only study to report an effect size (25) reported a relative risk of only 1.23. A conclusion that sample size provides the answer to the inconsistencies in the literature is insufficient, however, in light of the three smaller prospective studies that found marriage to be associated with *shorter* survival (26,27,32).

RECURRENCE. Two studies examined the relation of marital status to recurrence of cancer and found no association. This included a study of 121 women with local or regional breast cancer that followed patients for 6–8 years after diagnosis (28) and a study of 149 white and black patients with either stage 2 breast cancer or stages 1 and 2 melanoma at either 5-year (31) or 8-year follow-up (32).

One study examined the association of marital status to the development of a *second* primary breast cancer by comparing 338 patients who developed a second cancer with two different control groups of women with an initial diagnosis of breast cancer (33). One control group was randomly selected from the tumor registry ($n = 338$) and the other matched on age and time since diagnosis from the tumor registry ($n = 336$). Marital status interacted with age such that never being married was associated with a decreased risk of second breast cancer among younger women but an increased risk among older women, regardless of which control group served as the comparison. The authors suggest that marital status may reflect reproductive history because their findings parallel reports that not having children reduces risk of breast cancer among women under age 40 and increases risk of breast cancer among women after age 40.

SUMMARY. The literature on marital status is inconsistent. It is possible that more information about the role of marriage in cancer for men and women and for members of different cultural groups may provide more clarity. Although a number of studies have focused exclusively on women by studying breast cancer, few of the studies examined men separately. Research on all-cause mortality shows that marriage is more health protective for men than for women (34,35). There also is reason to believe that marriage may not have the same effect across cultural groups, as different ethnic groups construe marriage differently in terms of support resources. Moreover, it is likely that differences in marital quality may be important, with better relationships providing a marriage benefit and worse relationships conveying the same (or greater) risk as not being married. Such a finding has been documented for other health outcomes (11,36). Finally, it is likely that studies (particularly incidence and mortality studies) that associate marital status to a cancer outcome occurring many years later may include many initially married persons who divorce, remarry, or are widowed by the time the outcome occurs. As a consequence, any beneficial effects of marriage may be diluted by the instability of the measure.

Network Size and Social Integration. A large all-cause mortality literature suggests that although network size does not predict mortality, social integration as indicated by membership in organizations and frequency of social contacts is reliably associated with lower mortality rates (reviews in Refs. 6,37). Here we review the role of these same structural network variables in predicting cancer mortality, incidence, survival, and recurrence.

MORTALITY. As shown in Table 10.1, two studies found some evidence for protective effects of structural measures of support on cancer mortality. A prospective study of 989 men found that more people living in the house and more frequent social activities predicted reduced mortality from cancer (16). These relations did not hold, however, when age, smoking status, and perceived health at the onset of the study were statistically controlled. Reynolds and Kaplan (15) found that greater social integration as assessed by the SNI was associated with reduced mortality, and social isolation (i.e., few close friends and little contact with friends) was associated with increased mortality among women but not among men ($n = 6848$). These relations held even with statistical controls for age, baseline physical health status, income, alcohol use, and smoking status.

INCIDENCE. Neither of the two studies that examined the effects of structural support on cancer incidence found a relation. In a prospective study of 6848 men and women, Reynolds and Kaplan (15) found that the SNI did not predict incidence of cancer for either gender. Similarly, in a study of 2603 men and women, Vogt and colleagues (38) report that none of the network measures assessed at the onset of the study (scope of network, frequency of contact, and size of network) predicted subsequent incidence of cancer over 15 years among either gender.

SURVIVAL. There are seven prospective studies that examine the influence of structural measures of support, aside from marital status, on survival from cancer (see Table 10.2). These studies include a variety of network measures that can be roughly categorized as either markers of social integration or as *counts* of network members. In general, network size does not predict survival, but involvement in a range of social activities is associated with longer survival.

Two studies that measured both network size and markers of social integration support this conclusion. In a 15-year follow-up of 2603 initially healthy men and women, Vogt (38) found that number of domains in which men and women had relationships and frequency of contact with network members were both associated with longer survival from all cancers, but network size was not. These relations held when age, gender, smoking status, socioeconomic status, and baseline health status were statistically controlled. The number of cancer cases was not specified, however. In a study of 208 white women with local and regional breast cancer, active membership in organizations was associated with longer survival over 20 years of follow-up, but number of family and friends was not (29). These findings held when stage of disease at diagnosis, past health status, and socioeconomic status were statistically controlled.

Other studies assessing either a marker of social integration or network size suggest a similar conclusion. Activities involving social interactions were associated with better 1 to 4-year survival rates among 127 women with all stages of breast cancer (39). This relation was upheld after controlling for age, stage of disease at diagnosis, nodal status, and estrogen receptor status. In this same sample of women ($n = 118$), Waxler-Morrison and colleagues (26) found evidence that social contacts with friends were more important than social contacts with relatives. Frequency of contact with friends predicted increased survival, but frequency of contact with relatives did not. Inconsistent with other studies, *number* of friends (but not relatives) also was associated with longer survival. These findings held even with controls for stage of disease at diagnosis and nodal status. In a study of 294 men and women with breast, colorectal, or lung cancer, greater access to distant social ties was associated with increased survival, even when age, stage of disease at diagnosis, and socioeconomic status were statistically controlled (27). In the one study to evaluate network size variables only, neither living alone nor network size was associated with 2 to 5-year survival among 94 patients with hematologic malignancies participating in an intervention (described later (40)).

Three studies using the SNI or a variation of it suggest that greater social integration is associated with longer survival. Recall that the SNI assesses the range of social roles and social activities in which persons participate. The SNI was related to greater likelihood of survival over 1–4 years of follow-up among 118 women with any stage of breast cancer (26) and with longer survival for men but not women in Reynolds and Kaplan's (15) study of 339 initially healthy individuals who developed cancer during the 17 years of their study. Their findings held even when stage of disease and age at diagnosis were statistically controlled. A "social ties" index, composed of the SNI as well as frequency of phone contact and adequacy of number of friends, was administered to 204 patients with all sites of advanced cancer. The index did not predict survival at 5-year follow-up (31), but did predict survival at 8-year follow-up (32). The latter finding must be regarded with caution, however, as only 6% of patients remained alive at 8-year follow-up.

RECURRENCE. Two studies evaluated the associations between social network variables and recurrence. The social ties index developed by Cassileth and colleagues did not predict recurrence among patients with stage 2 breast cancer or stages 1 and 2 melanoma at 5 years

($n = 149$ (31)) or 8 years (32). Hislop's (39) measure of activities involving social interactions, however, was associated with less likelihood of breast cancer recurrence over 1–4 years of follow-up, controlling for age, stage of disease, nodal status, and estrogen receptor status.

SUMMARY. Overall, there is no evidence that structural measures of support predict incidence of new disease. Although there are only a few studies that evaluate whether these measures predict disease mortality or recurrence, the existing evidence is suggestive of a protective effect for persons involved with their social networks. By contrast, there is substantial evidence for relations between social integration and increased survival. Because the majority of studies focus on breast cancer, the generalization of these findings is limited by both gender and site. There is, however, some evidence (e.g., Ref. 15) that social participation may differentially influence men and women. Further gender comparisons may help clarify this issue. Unfortunately, only one study (27) examined whether social integration had a differential impact on localized versus advanced disease, and it found no differential effects.

Functional Measures

Among the different kinds of support, cancer patients report that their need for emotional support is often not met by their social networks, and prospective studies indicate that emotional support is associated with better psychological adjustment to disease (see review in Ref. 41). In this section, we evaluate whether certain resources provided by the social network are similarly associated with disease onset and progression.

MORTALITY. There are no studies that directly examine the influence of functional support on cancer mortality. However, one study of 6848 initially healthy people found that feeling isolated predicted increased mortality from cancer among women but not men (15). Feeling isolated was measured by perceptions of feeling left out and difficulty in getting close to others, which may reflect loneliness rather than perceived lack of support.

INCIDENCE. Cancer incidence was examined in a study of white male medical students who were followed for 9–24 years after graduation (42). The 20 who subsequently developed malignant tumors were compared with a group of healthy individuals matched on age, gender, race, and class in school. Those who developed cancer reported less closeness to their parents at the onset of the study [measured by subjects' attitudes toward their parents (e.g.,. warm, understanding) and perception of parents' attitude toward subject] than people in the matched control group.

SURVIVAL. Two prospective studies indicate effects of emotional support on survival. In a study of lung, colorectal, and breast cancer patients, perceived adequacy of emotional support (which was not defined) predicted survival only among women with localized breast cancer (27). These relations held when age, socioeconomic status, and stage of disease at diagnosis were statistically controlled. In a study of 224 men and women with lung cancer, Stavraky and colleagues (30) evaluated needs for and supplies of different kinds of support (emotional support, network membership, esteem support) as well as the fit between needs and supplies. A high *need* for emotional support (i.e., sympathy, care, and devotion) predicted death at one year, when stage of disease at diagnosis was statistically controlled. The more seriously ill patients may have desired more emotional support, or it may be that the patients who had the least emotional support available expressed the greatest need. Feeling isolated did not predict survival in a follow-up of men and women who developed cancer over a 17-year period (15).

RECURRENCE. Only one study examined the relation of support functions to cancer recurrence. Perceived family support (quality of relationships, availability of help, quality of communication) did not predict recurrence among 81 women with stage I or II breast cancer (43). However, among those whose cancer recurred (*n* = 29), family support predicted longer time to recurrence.

SUMMARY. Given the small number of studies and the diversity of measures across studies, we cannot draw any firm conclusions about the association of functional measures of support and cancer. We note that the majority of the studies focused on the more emotional aspects of support. In addition, the two studies that examined women separately from men found that the protective effects of emotional support are limited to women (15,27).

Support Interventions

Support interventions are limited to those diagnosed with cancer. Four studies have been conducted in which the survival or recurrence rate of people assigned to a support intervention was compared to that of those assigned to a no-treatment control group. The interventions are aimed at two functions of support, emotional support and informational support, although the interventions also may inadvertently increase network size (see Ref. 41).

The three methodologically strong studies show clear benefits of the support intervention on survival. A study in which 86 women with metastatic breast cancer were randomly assigned to an emotional support group (lasting one year) or a no-treatment control group showed an 18-month survival benefit for the intervention group 10 years later (44). The intervention consisted of weekly 90-minute meetings for one year that focused on discussing problems with having a terminal illness and ways to improve relationships. An educational intervention in which 94 men and women were sequentially assigned to experimental or control conditions showed a positive effect on survival three years later (40). The intervention was designed to increase compliance with therapy among patients with hematologic malignancies. A randomized psychosocial intervention that involved group provision of emotional and informational support increased survival and reduced recurrence 5–6 years later among 68 men and women with melanoma (45). Finally, a nonrandomized intervention that involved emotional support, imagery, and counseling for 136 women with breast cancer found effects on survival one year later (46), but the time lag between diagnosis and study participation was longer for intervention participants than nonparticipants, suggesting that the sickest patients may have been selected out of the intervention. The intervention effect was not statistically reliable when the time interval between diagnosis and study participation was controlled in the analysis. In addition, there was no effect of the intervention on survival 10 years later (47).

Summary. The current literature reveals provocative evidence for health benefits of support interventions for people with cancer. However, the studies are few and involve different intervention protocols and different kinds of support. This makes it difficult to draw strong conclusions about the nature of an intervention that would influence survival. We note that the interventions are aimed at two functions of support: emotional support and informational support. None of the studies evaluated whether men or women or people of different races were more likely to derive health benefits from the interventions.

CONCLUSIONS

Only a few studies have evaluated the influence of social networks on cancer mortality and cancer recurrence, but findings suggest health benefits. By contrast, there is substantial evidence that social ties influence cancer survival. Among the social environment variables, there is stronger evidence that social integration and functional support influence cancer than there is for marital status or network size. Support interventions also seem to have health benefits, which can be attributed to increased social network integration or receipt of specific support functions. Thus, it is not the mere existence of a social network but more extensive and meaningful involvement that provides disease-related benefits.

Why would involvement in a social network or receipt of support resources influence neoplastic disease? Earlier, we suggested two proximal pathways: behavioral and biologic. One behavior that may be influenced by social ties is timely response to symptoms—delay in seeking treatment. To the extent that network members reduce delay, an earlier stage and more treatable form of cancer may be diagnosed, which would have beneficial effects on survival and recurrence rates. Two studies found that longer delay periods were associated with diagnosis of a more advanced stage of cancer and reduced survival (22,23), but neither provided evidence for social network influences on delay (only marital status is evaluated (22). Some support for the delay hypothesis, however, is provided by evidence that married people were more likely to be diagnosed with an earlier stage of cancer and more likely to receive treatment for localized and regional disease (25). Another behavioral mechanism that may influence disease progression is compliance with treatment. One of the intervention studies reviewed was aimed at increasing treatment compliance (40). Not only did the intervention influence compliance, but compliance predicted survival. None of the studies we reviewed, however, evaluated whether richer measures of the social environment (i.e., social integration) were associated with behavioral factors, such as delay, treatment adherence, or general health practices, that could have accounted for survival benefits.

A biologic pathway by which the social environment might influence disease progression is immune function. There is increasing evidence that stronger social ties and perceptions of social support are associated with more competent immune responses (at least in vitro; see reviews in Refs. 1,2). This includes two studies in which perceptions of supportive relationships were associated with higher natural killer cell (NK) activity among women with stage I and II breast cancer (48,49). Only one study, however, has evaluated whether immune function mediates the relation between social ties and cancer survival. Fawzy and colleagues (50) found a positive effect of their support intervention on NK activity, but NK activity did not account for the intervention's effect on survival. Thus, it is not yet clear whether the immune system plays a role in linking social networks to cancer.

LIMITATIONS AND FUTURE DIRECTIONS

Much of the literature we have reviewed suffers from methodologic weaknesses and poor reporting. For example, not all studies provide adequate controls for spurious factors such as age, socioeconomic status, or health at study onset. Some studies do not distinguish cancer deaths from deaths due to other causes. Some of the survival studies do not specify the follow-up period, and many studies could provide greater methodologic detail, such as precise sampling techniques and detailed descriptions of the independent variables.

One limitation of the prospective studies reviewed in this chapter is that investigators do not take into consideration that the social environment may change from study onset to termination of data collection (51). For example, in our culture, marital status may vary considerably over the 10- to 15-year follow-ups that are often used in mortality studies. This might account, in part, for why measures of social integration, thought to be stable over long periods of time, are more reliable predictors in this literature (6).

The studies reviewed in this chapter are heavily biased toward women with breast cancer. Other studies typically include people with a variety of cancers with different prognoses. Few studies examine whether findings hold across men and women, across different sites of cancer, and across different stages of disease. Those that do often find differential effects. Some investigations statistically control for variables such as gender, race, age, and stage of disease, but rarely do they stratify the data or otherwise investigate whether they alter the association of social network variables to cancer outcomes.

Most importantly, few studies examine the mechanism by which the social environment could impact on cancer. The two types of mechanisms most proximal to the disease outcome are behavioral and biologic (see Figure 10–1). Future researchers should examine the extent to which the social environment influences behavioral risk factors for incidence or mortality; cancer-specific health behavior (e.g., delay in seeking treatment), which could affect incidence, mortality, survival, and recurrence; or compliance with treatment, which could affect survival and time to recurrence.

Finally, in order to design effective social support interventions, we need a more detailed understanding of how interventions influence the social environment and the various pathways that influence disease outcomes. Interventions may be providing patients with specific support functions (e.g., emotional support) or may be altering the structure of patients' social networks (i.e., increasing network size or social integration). Although the intervention studies reveal provocative effects of support manipulations, generally investigators have failed to examine mechanisms through which support interventions influence disease outcomes. Only by understanding these mechanisms can we develop effective interventions for different populations, cancer sites, and stages of disease.

ACKNOWLEDGMENTS

Preparation of this chapter was supported by a grant from the National Cancer Institute (CA61303) to Vicki Helgeson and a Research Scientist Development Award from the National Institute of Mental Health to Sheldon Cohen (MH00721).

REFERENCES

1. Cohen S, Herbert TB. Health psychology: psychological factors and physical disease from the perspective of human psychoneuroimmunology. *Ann Rev Psychol.* [In press.]
2. Uchino BN, Cacioppo JT, Kiecolt-Glaser JK. The relationship between social support and physiological processes: a review with emphasis on underlying mechanisms and implications for health. *Psychol Bull.* [In press.]
3. Cohen S, Wills TA. Stress, social support and the buffering hypothesis. *Psychol Bull.* 1985; 98:310–357.
4. Wills TA. The helping process in the context of personal relationships. In: Spacapan S, Oskamp S, eds. *Helping and Being Helped: Naturalistic Studies.* Newbury Park, CA: Sage; 1992:17–48.
5. Rook KS, Pietromonaco P. Close relationships: ties that heal or ties that bind? *Adv Pers Relat.* 1987; 1:1–35.
6. Cohen S. Psychosocial models of social support in the etiology of physical disease. *Health Psychol.* 1988; 7:269–297.
7. Herbert TB, Cohen S. Depression and immunity: a meta-analytic review. *Psychol Bull.* 1993; 113:472–486.
8. Berkman LF, Syme SL. Social networks, host resistance, and mortality: A nine-year follow-up study of Alameda County residents. *Am J Epidemiol.* 1979; 109:186–204.
9. House JS, Kahn RL. Measures and concepts of social support. In: Cohen S, Syme SL, eds. *Social Support and Health.* New York: Academic Press; 1985: 83–108.
10. Thoits PA. Social support and psychological well-being: theoretical possibilities. In: Sarason IG, Sarason BR, eds. *Social Support: Theory, Research, and Applications.* Dordrecht, The Netherlands: Martinus Nijhoff; 1985: 51–72.
11. Gove WR, Hughes M, Style CB. Does marriage have positive effects on the psychological well-being of the individual? *J Health Soc Behav.* 1983; 24:122–131.
12. Burman B, Margolin G. Analysis of the association between marital relationships and health problems: an interactional perspective. *Psychol Bull.* 1992; 112:39–63.
13. Jenkins CD. Social environment and cancer mortality in men. *N Engl J Med.* 1983; 308:395–398.
14. Kraus AS, Lilienfeld AM. Some epidemiologic aspects of the high mortality rate in the young widowed group. *J Chron Dis.* 1959; 10:207–217.
15. Reynolds P, Kaplan GA. Social connections and risk for cancer: Prospective evidence from the Alameda County Study. *Behav Med.* 1990; 16:101–110.
16. Welin L, Larsson B, Svardsudd K, Tibblin B, Tibblin G. Social network and activities in relation to mortality from cardiovascular diseases, cancer and other causes: A 12 year follow up of the study of men born in 1913 and 1923. *J Epidemiol Commun Health.* 1992; 46:127–132.
17. Ernster VL, Sacks ST, Selvin S, Petrakis NL. Cancer incidence by marital status: U.S. third national cancer survey. *J Natl Cancer Inst.* 1979; 63:567–585.
18. Newell GR, Pollack ES, Spitz MR, Sider JG, Fueger JJ. Incidence of prostate cancer and marital status. *J Natl Cancer Inst.* 1987; 79:259–262.
19. Swanson GM, Belle SH, Satariano WA. Marital status and cancer incidence: Difference in the black and white populations. *Cancer Res.* 1985; 45:5883–5889.
20. Zhu K, Weiss NS, Schwartz SM, Daling JR. Assessing the relationship between marital status and cancer incidence: Methodological considerations. *Cancer Causes Control.* 1994; 5:83–87.
21. Zonderman AB, Costa PT, McCrae RR. Depression as a risk for cancer morbidity and mortality in a nationally representative sample. *J Am Med Assoc.* 1989; 262:1191–1195.
22. Neale AV, Tilley BC, Vernon SW. Marital status, delay in seeking treatment and survival from breast cancer. *Soc Sci Med.* 1986; 23:305–312.
23. Wilkinson GS, Edgerton F, Wallace HJ, Reese P, Patterson J, Priore R. Delay, stage of disease and survival from breast cancer. *J Chron Dis.* 1979; 32:365–373.
24. LeMarchand L, Kolonel LN, Nomura AMY. The relationship of ethnicity and other prognostic factors to breast cancer survival patterns in Hawaii. *J Natl Cancer Inst.* 1984; 73:1259–1265.
25. Goodwin JS, Hunt WC, Key CR, Samet JM. The effect of marital status on stage, treatment, and survival of cancer patients. *J Am Med Assoc.* 1987; 258:3125–3130.
26. Waxler-Morrison N, Hislop TG, Mears B, Kan L. Effects of social relationships on survival for women with breast cancer: a prospective study. *Soc Sci Med.* 1991; 33:177–183.
27. Ell K, Nishimoto R, Mediansky L, Mantell J, Hamovitch M. Social relations, social support and survival among patients with cancer. *J Psychosom Res.* 1992; 36:531–541.
28. Dean C, Surtees PG. Do psychological factors predict survival in breast cancer? *J Psychosom Res.* 1989; 33:561–569.
29. Funch DP, Marshall J. The role of stress, social support and age in survival from breast cancer. *J Psychosom Res.* 1983; 27:77–83.

30. Stavraky KM, Donner AP, Kincade JE, Stewart MA. The effect of psychosocial factors on lung cancer mortality at one year. *J Clin Epidemiol.* 1988; 41:75–82.

31. Cassileth BR, Lusk EJ, Miller DS, Brown LL, Miller C. Psychosocial correlates of survival in advanced malignant disease? *N Engl J Med.* 1985; 312:1551–1555.

32. Cassileth BR, Walsh WP, Lusk EJ. Psychosocial correlates of cancer survival: A subsequent report 3 to 8 years after cancer diagnosis. *J Clin Oncol.* 1988; 6:1753–1759.

33. Horn PL, Thompson WD, Schwartz SM. Factors associated with the risk of second primary breast cancer: An analysis of data from the Connecticut Tumor Registry. *J Chron Dis.* 1987; 40:1003–1011.

34. Gove WR. Sex, marital status, and mortality. *Am J Sociol.* 1973; 79:45–67.

35. Belle D. Gender differences in the social moderators of stress. In: Barnett RC, Biener L, Baruch GK, eds. *Gender and Stress.* New York: Free Press; 1987: 257–277.

36. Helgeson V. The effects of masculinity and social support on recovery from myocardial infarction. *Psychosom Med.* 1991; 53:621–633.

37. House JS, Landis KR, Umberson, D. Social relationships and health. *Science.* 1988; 241:540–545.

38. Vogt TM, Mullooly JP, Ernst D, Pope CR, Hollis JF. Social networks as predictors of ischemic heart disease, cancer, stroke and hypertension: Incidence, survival and mortality. *J Clin Epidemiol.* 1992; 45:659–666.

39. Hislop TG, Waxler NE, Coldman AJ, Elwood JM, Kan L. The prognostic significance of psychosocial factors in women with breast cancer. *J Chron Dis.* 1987; 40:729–735.

40. Richardson JL, Shelton DR, Krailo M, Levine AM. The effect of compliance with treatment on survival among patients with hematologic malignancies. *J Clin Oncol.* 1990; 8:356–364.

41. Helgeson V, Cohen S. Relation of social support to adjustment to cancer: Reconciling descriptive, correlational, and intervention research. *Health Psychol.* 1996; 15:135–148.

42. Thomas CB, Duszynski KR. Closeness to parents and the family constellation in a prospective study of five disease states: Suicide, mental illness, malignant tumor, hypertension and coronary heart disease. *Johns Hopkins Med J.* 1974; 134:251–270.

43. Levy SM, Herberman RB, Lippman M, D'Angelo T, Lee J. Immunological and psychosocial predictors of disease recurrence in patients with early-stage breast cancer. *Behav Med.* 1991; 17:67–75.

44. Spiegel D, Bloom JR, Kraemer HC, Gottheil E. Effect of psychosocial treatment on survival of patients with metastatic breast cancer. *Lancet.* 1989; 2:888–891.

45. Fawzy FI, Fawzy NW, Hyun CS, et al. Malignant melanoma: effects of an early structured psychiatric intervention, coping, and affective state on recurrence and survival 6 years later. *Arch Gen Psychiatry.* 1993; 50:681–689.

46. Morgenstern H, Gellert GA, Walter SD, Ostfeld AM, Siegel BS. The impact of a psychosocial support program on survival with breast cancer: the importance of selection bias in program evaluation. *J Chron Dis.* 1984; 37:273–282.

47. Gellert GA, Maxwell RM, Siegel BS. Survival of breast cancer patients receiving adjunctive psychosocial support therapy: a 10-year follow-up study. *J Clin Oncol.* 1993; 11:66–69.

48. Levy S, Herberman R, Maluish A, Schlien B, Lippman M. Prognostic risk assessment in primary breast cancer by behavioral and immunological parameters. *Health Psychology.* 1985; 4:99–113.

49. Levy SM, Herberman RB, Whiteside T, Sanzo K, Lee J, Kirkwood J. Perceived social support and tumor estrogen/progesterone receptor status as predictors of natural killer cell activity in breast cancer patients. *Psychosom Med.* 1990; 52:73–85.

50. Fawzy FI, Kemeny ME, Fawzy NW, et al. A structured psychiatric intervention for cancer patients. *Arch Gen Psychiatry.* 1990; 47:729–735.

51. Cohen S, Matthews KA. Social support, type A behavior, and coronary artery disease. *Psychosom Med.* 1987; 49:325–330.

11

Psychosocial Factors in Cancer Incidence and Prognosis

BERNARD H. FOX

The relationship of psychosocial factors to cancer has been a matter of limited interest for centuries, but during the last several decades that interest has grown markedly. The beliefs that various factors cause cancer, identify people who are prone to cancer, and affect the prognosis of cancer are widely held in the lay public, and also by a substantial number of researchers. Earlier in this century many researchers did studies to examine the correctness of observations already reported by physicians about their cancer patients and possibly to discover other such psychosocial attributes (1). Most of these studies were unacceptable scientifically, with too few subjects, lack of control groups, and unstandardized psychosocial measuring instruments. Serious efforts toward more acceptable studies began in the 1950s, and the number of such studies grew rapidly. By the late 1970s enough had been done to warrant several reviews of the overall picture (e.g., Bahnson and Kissen (2), Crisp (3), Fox (4)), and publication of the first book on the behavioral aspects of cancer (5). More recently less extensive reviews have appeared, for example, on both incidence and progression (6) and on cancer progression only (7).

Almost all of the mid-century works were case-control studies, also called retrospective studies. In a case-control study a group of cancer patients is chosen, a group of control subjects, more or less matched to the case group, is selected, and some psychosocial factor is examined in the two groups to see if it can distinguish them. If so, one might conclude that that psychosocial factor is related to the presence of cancer in the case group. Most of the earlier researchers inferred causation in such cases, but that is not necessarily true. A second type of study is known as a cohort, or prospective study. In a cohort study a group of people is examined in respect to one or more selected psychosocial factors before the outcome takes place. After an inter-

val specified by the researcher, the proportion of people in the cohort who were diagnosed with cancer, had a recurrence, or died (depending on the researcher's outcome of interest) during that period is compared with the proportion who did not have the given outcome. If the proportions differ substantially, the researcher concludes that the psychosocial factor is related to the outcome. Again, an inference of causation may be but does not have to be true. The first cohort study on cancer was done by Hagnell (8) in 1966. That work is subject to considerable question, since he ignored some outcomes in his data that contradicted his conclusion (4), and, further, reported very poor reliability in his instrument (9). No further cohort studies appeared until the 1970s.

Case-control studies are more prone to bias than cohort studies. Such biases, whether known or unknown, make it hard to decide which such studies to accept and which to reject. Cohort studies, which are also subject to some biases, but fewer and less damaging ones, are more trustworthy and involve less risk of a false conclusion. A good example of a potential confounding or biasing factor is age difference in the cases and controls. The incidence rate for all cancers during the period 1985–86 in an approximately 10% sample of the U.S. population was 357/100,000 per year among people aged 45–54 (both sexes combined), but was more than double that, 769/100,000, among those 55–64 years old (10).

THE VARIETY OF PSYCHOSOCIAL FACTORS

In the human a great many psychosocial factors (PFs) have been reported to be present in cancer patients. An extensive but incomplete list (59 PFs) appearing in a recently published article (6) is presented in Table 11.1. Another list, referring only to lung cancer patients, presents 32 psychosocial factors (11). In recent years, particular ones have received special attention, some because they were reported in certain high-visibility studies, and some because they were more often reported as having positive connection to a cancer outcome than other factors. This discussion will address the variables noted in Table 11.1 that have received such special attention. They are: stress; bereavement; depressed mood; helplessness and hopelessness; suppression of emotions, especially anger; psychosis, especially schizophrenia; social support; and psychosocial intervention.

STRESS

Stress will be used here to mean the psychological and physiological disequilibrium caused by some event, which will be called a stressor. Stressors can be external to the organism or can arise within the organism.

Animal Stress

A thorough review of studies on animal stress and cancer has been done by Justice (12). He presented a number of variables that have been found to affect the influence of stress on incidence and growth rate of both spontaneous and induced tumors, and on animals' length of survival. Some of these are stress duration, time of stress in relation to tumor implantation, intensity of stressors, site of tumor, source of tumor (viral or nonviral), and exposure to early stress experiences. It is known that animals' responses to stressors include immunosuppression. In almost all virally induced tumors, either spontaneously occurring, as in breast cancer induced by Bittner virus in mice (13), or by transplantation, stress hastens both the appearance of

TABLE 11.1. *A Selected List of Psychosocial Variables That Have Been Associated with Presence of Cancer or its Prognosis*

Stress*	Constricted personality
Animal	Difficulty remembering dreams
Human	Religiosity associated with high risk
Occurrence of events usually deemed stressful, e.g., disasters, divorce, job loss, family illness or death; also the perception that such events were stressful	Strong religiosity associated with spontaneous regression of tumors
Bereavement*	Rigidity
Psychosis, especially schizophrenia*	Conventionality
Depressed mood*	Ego alienation
Suppression of emotions, especially anger*	Poor expression of emotions
Helplessness and hopelessness*	Masochistic character
Social support*	Sexual disorders
Psychotherapeutic intervention*	Extraversion
Hospitalizable depression	Social introversion
High level of neuroticism	Disturbed female identifica-tion (breast cancer)
Low level of neuroticism	Strong, unbalanced nervous system
Severe, long-lasting unresolved emotional conflicts	Weak nervous system
Denial	Submissiveness
Strong repression	Façade of pleasantness
Not excessive repression	Strong expression of emotions
Excessive anxiety, tension and hostility	High verbal IQ and ability to control hostility
Not excessive anxiety	Four validity scales of the MMPI (Minnesota Multiphasic Personality Inventory)
Inhibited sexuality	Nine clinical scales of the MMPI
Parent-child disturbances following bereavement	Warmheartedness, social mindedness
Poor emotional outlet in children	Low score on closeness to parents scale
Low level of psychosomatic symptoms except ulcers	Little need of life adjustment after cancer surgery
Anal personality type	
Early neurosis	

*Starred items have been most intensively studied and will be addressed specifically here.

new tumors and the growth rate of existing tumors. Justice says:

Many researchers in the field of tumor immunology have concluded that the only tumors in animals that are consistently responsive to immune manipulations are those caused by viruses . . . [In regard to nonviral tumors] evidence is offered below that the growth of these tumors is inhibited during exposure to a stressor, so something other than the immune system must be involved. (12)

A famous early study showing stimulation of virally induced tumor growth was done by Riley (13), whose work has been confirmed many times over. A good example of the inhibition of chemically induced tumor growth under stressful stimulation was done by Newberry and Sengbusch (14), whose work has also been confirmed.

It is true that Justice (12) found some exceptions to his generalization. These, however, detract little from the strength of the convincing evidence leading him to that position. They do, however, show that the variables listed above are part of the broad picture, and indicate a complex state of affairs.

If the viral and nonviral view is correct, extrapolation to the human becomes a problem because only about 3–4% of all U.S. human tumors are known or strongly suspected to be virally induced. The most prevalent of these is cervical cancer, thought to be caused and promoted primarily by the papilloma virus, although other viruses, especially herpes 2, and certain bacilli may also be involved (15). If one extrapolated to the human on the basis of these statistics, the logical inference would be that in most cases stress will inhibit tumor development and growth, a very uncertain proposition. For several reasons it is not wise to assume that animal findings in this area are directly duplicated in the human:

1. Humans, guinea pigs, and certain other animals are considerably less sensitive to the effects of glucocorticoid proliferation than the major rodent species used in the laboratory (16) and, indeed, even among the latter, various strains differ in their sensitivity to these corticosteroids.

2. In animals, tumor transplants or heavy doses of carcinogens introduce strong antigens, that is, stimuli to immune recognition and response. Spontaneous human tumors, however, take a long time to develop and probably produce relatively weak or even absent antigen proliferation and hence limited or even absent immune recognition of and response to these antigens.

3. When animals are immunosuppressed, they develop tumors in excess of normal frequency at many sites, each strain being susceptible to concentration of tumors at the site peculiar to that strain—liver, lung, testes, etc. When humans are immunosuppressed they also develop tumors in excess of normal, but most frequently lymphomas. The focus of the immunosuppressive stimulus in man is the immune system itself. In transplant patients, who must be medically immunosuppressed to survive, the relative risk (incidence in the case group compared to the population incidence) of histiocytic lymphoma is on the order of 150, and that of all the non-Hodgkin's lymphomas is about 50. In contrast, the relative risk of other tumors ranges from no elevation to substantial elevation for certain sites, especially skin (not melanoma), but nowhere near the level of lymphomas (17).

In spite of the foregoing, the animal findings are important. They should, however, form the bases for hypotheses about humans, not for conclusions.

Human Stress

Case-Control Studies. This discussion will report on some case-control studies, but will focus on cohort studies. There are several reasons for giving little emphasis to case-control studies when considering psychosocial factors. First, cancer can and does produce physical, psychological and attitudinal changes, mostly negative, that can bias conclusions (18). Second, people with negative affect such as cancer patients are known to increase reports of stressful events when compared to reports of controls (19). Third, with the usual small number of cases in case-control studies, the chance of bias in the patient group is considerably greater than in the usually larger cohort study patient group. In a large cohort study the chances of possibly confounding variables being more or less equally distributed in the later examined positive and negative outcome groups is increased, and, conversely, the chances of a confounder selectively affecting one or the other of these groups is diminished. A limited list of variables that might lead to biased case or control groups in case-control studies, or biased positive or negative outcomes in cohort studies is given in Table 11.2. The possible confounders are divided into demographic, social, or psychological variables, and physical or biological variables. Every one of the listed variables has appeared at least once in a study showing that variable to be related to some outcome measure.

Early case-control studies reported a greater number of stressful events earlier in life in the cancer group than in the controls (21,22). In the 1960s and 1970s few studies addressed that issue, but about as many found no relationship to survival as found a positive

TABLE 11.2. *A Limited List of Variables That Might Confound the Results When the Independent Variable is a Psychosocial Factor**

DEMOGRAPHIC, SOCIAL OR PSYCHOLOGICAL VARIABLES	Degree of patient compliance
Age	Patient's history of malignancies
Race	Delay in diagnosis after symptoms
Social class	Interval between diagnosis and metastasis
Socio-economic status	Immunologic status (several measures)
Marital status	P-53 gene expression
National origin	Tissue histology
Degree of social support (at least 12 different measures)	Family history of malignancy
Geographical environment	Baseline health status
Quality of life scores	Smoking
Differences between hospitals	Habits of alcohol consumption
Adherence to cultural habits and living style	Rise in prolactin level after surgery
An unknown number of the variables listed in Table 11.1	Allogeneic peri-operative blood transfusion
PHYSICAL AND BIOLOGICAL VARIABLES	Pain level
Site of tumor	Duration of followup
Stage	Clark level (melanoma only)
Tumor size	Breslow thickness (melanoma only)
Number of positive nodes	*Besides the above, the following are especially relevant to breast cancer:*
Estrogen receptor status	Uni- or bilateral breast cancer
Degree of cell differentiation	Age at menarche
Degree of angiogenesis or microvascularization	Age at menopause
Karnofsky score (overall and within stage)	Age at first birth
Rate of tumor growth	Oral contraceptive use
Peritumoral lymphatic vessel invasion	Auxometric indicators (20)
Aneuploidy	Menstrual cycle phase in which mastectomy took place
Type of treatment	

*Every one of the variables listed above has appeared in at least one study showing a positive relationship between the variable and some outcome measure.

one (23,24). From the mid 1980s on, a number of studies were done, and we find similar contrary results, with a preponderance of studies showing a positive relationship. A sampling of such studies is: positive relationship found (25–27); no relationship or a reverse one found (28,29). A good example of a study that found an excess of stressful events in the patients' histories is the study of Ramirez and colleagues (27), who looked at frequency of traumatic events between diagnosis of breast cancer and first recurrence among 50 women, comparing it with the frequency during a similar period in 50 patients without recurrence. They found an excess of reported events among those with recurrence. Among the studies finding no excess, a good example is that of Priestman and colleagues (29), who studied 300 women, 100 with malignancy, 100 with benign tumors, and 100 controls. The severity and nature of the stressors did not differ among the groups, but contrary to Ramirez and colleagues (27),

the controls experienced more stressful events than the benign group, and the latter experienced more than those with cancer.

Before taking up cohort studies on stress it is important to examine a bias in case-control studies that was suspected early on (4), but not verified directly until much more recently. It is quite likely that, on the whole, cancer patients tend to recall more stressful events than noncancer controls. A thorough and intensive review of memory as it is influenced by affect has been written by Blaney (30), one of whose conclusions was that people with negative affect report more negative events than people with average or positive affect. Blaney's conclusions are broadly supported in studies specifically relating to recall of stressful events among those with negative affect, e.g., Brett et al. (31) and Cohen et al. (32). Almost all those who have cancer and know it have negative affect to varying degrees. Even if this is true only of a substantial number but not of all cancer patients, their excessive recall of negative events would still be enough to bias the average recall level of the whole.

To my knowledge, however, only one study not subject to the usual case-control biases has been done to examine whether cancer patients' reports exaggerate the frequency or severity of stressful events in the past (33). The Nurses' Health Study of 121,700 nurses aged 30-55 began in 1976. In 1982 a questionnaire was given to the cohort asking about risk factors for melanoma. Those diagnosed with melanoma between 1976 and 1982 were called the prevalent group, $n = 87$. A repeat questionnaire was given to all melanoma patients, and those diagnosed with melanoma between 1982 and 1984 were called incident cases, $n = 34$. A nonmelanoma control group of 234 was also chosen randomly from the cohort and given both questionnaires. Two questions were asked: *(1)* a neutral one, "What was the natural color of your hair at age 21?"; *(2)* a relevant one, "As a child or adolescent, after repeated sun exposures, what kind of tan would you get?" Options were scored from 1 to 4: practically none, light tan, average tan, deep tan (or other). Hair color was dichotomized into red or blond (score = 1) and brown or black (score = 0). The changes in scores from the 1982 questionnaire to the post-1984 one were recorded.

Although this is a nested case-control study, all the possible disease cases were used, and the controls were not selected but randomly determined. When both of these design features are used, a study is no more biased than would be a cohort study. In a comparison of the three groups (Kruskal-Wallis test), none of the groups changed their responses concerning hair color, the respective mean changes being 0.00, 0.00, and 0.02 ($p = 0.84$). As for tanning responses, the prevalent and control groups' means hardly changed (0.03 and 0.06), indicating no recall bias between 1982 and 1984. The incident group's mean score, however, changed by -0.24 ($p = 0.035$), suggesting that the cancer diagnosis affected their perception of the hazardous events earlier in their lives, that is, suggesting recall bias. Whatever recall bias occurred in the the prevalent group in 1982 could not, of course, be determined, but it did not change in the later questionnaire.

Cohort Studies. The earlier cohort studies found no more cancers among stressed than among unstressed members of the cohort. For example, Keehn and colleagues (34) found no greater cancer mortality among 9813 soldiers of World War II discharged for psychoneurosis than among 9942 controls over the period January 1946 to December 1969. Keehn (35) studied cancer mortality among prisoners of war in World War II from 1946 through 1975, and the Korean conflict from 1954 through 1978. No excess cancer mortality was found for either Pacific or European WWII prisoners ($N = 6023$) or for Korean prisoners ($N = 3959$) over their respective controls ($N = 5223$ and $N = 3953$). Lastly, Joffres (36) looked at 4581 Japanese men in Hawaii and found no more stressful events among cancer patients than among controls. While this is a case-control analysis, it should be remarked that if such an analysis is done on all the cases and all the controls in a population, the results are no more biased than those in a cohort study, where all the later cases and later controls are similarly identified. Stronger bias is found in case-control studies where both the controls and cases are samples of a population. In the Joffres study neither were selected beforehand, and it could therefore be judged to be as trustworthy as a parallel cohort study.

There have been relatively few recent cohort studies. An example is that by Barraclough and colleagues, who found no relationship between stressful events and breast cancer survival (37). A widely cited series of studies was done by Grossarth-Maticek and colleagues (38), who found a relationship between stressful events and later cancer. All of his work has been criticized most severely (39), and it will not be further dealt with here.

We are led to a conclusion by these three sets of findings:

1. Case-control studies yield mixed results but are subject to biases.
2. The broadly known cohort studies show no excess of stressful events associated with later cancer incidence, mortality, or survival.
3. It has been shown that both normals and ill people with negative affect report having experienced more stressful events than those with average or positive affect.

The last fact explains much if not all of the case-control findings. It is also the basis for predicting that, in the absence of such bias, there will be no excess of stressful events among the cancer group. The prediction is confirmed by the findings of the cohort studies, where that particular bias cannot exist. The conclusion is that it is quite likely, perhaps even almost certain, that stressful events do not occur more often among those who later get cancer, die of it, or survive a shorter time than controls.

BEREAVEMENT

Among the varieties of stress that have been examined in the literature in regard to later cancer incidence and mortality bereavement is an important category. Holmes and Rahe, in setting up a list of 43 stressful events, gave the ranking of most stressful to loss of spouse (40). Some deaths can produce relief rather than sadness or distress, but the number of such cases is probably relatively small, and an overall measure will average the combination of distressed and relieved. The result will clearly be conservative, since the possible effect of distress in producing cancer will be diminished overall by the lack of reported distress among those experiencing relief.

Some of the earlier case-control studies reported increased cancer incidence among widowed persons. These have been analyzed intensively as have prospective studies up to 1986, and their problems and difficulties have been carefully delineated (41).

In the cohort studies, as before, the bias that may exist in case-control studies has been removed. Bereaved spouses, in almost all the large cohort studies carried out over an extended period, have shown no excess cancer deaths when compared with still-married spouses. In the exceptions the excess lasted six months, a year, or in one study, as long as two years. We know that the development time to diagnosis of most cancers is on the order of years—3, 10, 15—and thus those findings could not have referred to cancer initiation. A 1987 Finnish cohort study on 95,647 persons widowed in 1972 showed no excess deaths during the next four years among 7600 cancer cases (42). In another study, 4032 white persons in Washington County, Maryland, widowed between 1963 and 1974, were followed for approximately 12 years (43), and showed no excess of cancer deaths within any interval of import after bereavement. A third cohort study of a 1% sample of the whole populations of England and Wales from 1971 to 1981, examining the causes of death among widowed persons, reported "No peak of post-bereavement mortality from malignant disease is clearly established in either sex" (41). In a fourth such study on 1782 breast cancer patients, all those diagnosed in Denmark from March 1, 1983 to February 29, 1984, and 1738 controls, Ewertz (44) found no difference in the death rates of married and widowed patients.

In summary, while some studies have reported short-term excess of cancer following bereavement, the large cohort studies have in general not found excess cancer incidence or death over the long term. This conclusion is consistent with the previous one that stress other than bereavement cannot be said to increase later cancer incidence or death.

A few studies have looked at survival among widows, e.g., Neale (45); one or two of these included widowers' survival. Also, one or two studies have looked at disease-free interval. However, the results have been mixed, some finding reduced survival among the widowed, and some not. In either case none of those results can be applied to the current issue, bereavement as a psychosocial factor, since none of the studies on survival even mention the time of bereavement in respect to the cancer.

DEPRESSED MOOD

A considerable number of case-control studies have reported more cancer cases with depressed mood than controls, although a few have not. It is surely curious that the researchers paid little or no attention to the possibility that the knowledge of having cancer might have induced depressed mood (46), or that paraneoplastic syndromes might have produced some cases of depressed mood (47), enough to give an average finding of an excess among cancer cases. That possibility could easily be eliminated in cohort studies.

The first one was done by Shekelle and colleagues (48) on a cohort of 2018 male workers at an electric plant in Chicago. Those workers whose highest scale score among the nine scales of the MMPI was depressed mood showed a cancer death rate 2.3 times the remainder of the cohort over a 17-year period (that is, the relative odds were 2.3). This finding (1981) stood alone for several years, but in 1988 and 1989 a series of further cohort studies appeared. Colleagues of Shekelle's, Persky et al. (49) followed up the same cohort for another 3 years, and observed that while the incidence of cancer among those with depressed mood had fallen to the control rate, the overall mortality risk, though less, was still higher than that of the remainder of the cohort. However, four other cohort studies appeared, all with cohort size greater than that of Shekelle et al. (50–53). None of these showed an excess of cancer deaths among people with depressed mood (Linkins and Comstock (52) later withdrew their exception for smokers). The findings of all of these studies were written about and described in an editorial in the *Journal of American Medical Association* (54). The conclusion was: "Nevertheless, the combined evidence is consistent with a null or weak relationship, the relative risks being distributed around a value of 1.0 or slightly more. It is clearly not consistent with a strong relationship between depressive symptoms and cancer among major segments of the population." Special circumstances in the electric plant where the Shekelle et al. cohort worked could have biased their results: the presence of ubiquitous electric fields in the plant, and widespread distribution of PCB (polychlorinated biphenyl) vapors from condenser and transformer manufacture. Both phenomena have been shown, definitely in animals and probably in humans to yield neurological symptoms and to stimulate cancer incidence (55).

PSYCHOSIS, ESPECIALLY SCHIZOPHRENIA

Many early studies have reported a clear reduction of cancer incidence or mortality among psychotics, especially schizophrenics. These studies have been examined carefully (56,57), and a fundamental error of calculation was discovered. The faulty studies estimated cancer deaths by proportional mortality; that is, they asked what proportion of cancer deaths was due to cancer in a mental patient cohort when compared with the proportion who died of cancer in an age-equivalent normal population. In the properly done studies, however, the question was, what was the absolute cancer death rate in a mental patient cohort when compared with the age-equivalent normal population's absolute cancer death rate? It is quite clear that if the relative proportion of deaths in a hospital sample due to alcoholism, neurologic disease, accidents, suicide, etc. is in excess of the population proportion, which it is in mental hospitals, then the proportion of deaths in the remainder due to other causes, especially cancer, has to be less than that of the population, which it is. Luckily, eight of the studies that were analyzed by the proportionate mortality method reported enough data that absolute mortality rates could also be determined. The newly analyzed data showed either no deficiency of cancer deaths, or even a slight, though nonsignificant, excess among the hospitalized samples (56,57). A later study by Tsuang and colleagues (58), analyzing their data by both methods, verified the reality of the error.

More recent studies tend to support the earlier corrected findings. Gulbinat and colleagues (59) analyzed record linkages for 16,236 schizophrenia patients and cancer in three areas—Århus, Denmark; State of Hawaii; and Nagasaki—over periods of 23, 18, and 18 years, respectively. A total of 895 cancer cases were found. They said, "There is no evidence of any uniform and consistent general reduction, or general increase of cancer risk in schizophrenia." Jørgensen and Mortensen (60) studied causes of death in 21,615 first-admitted patients diagnosed with reactive psychosis over the period 1970–88. The standard mortality ratio (similar to the relative risk) for cancer deaths in men was 1.21, and for women, 1.18, both significant at $p < 0.05$. This finding contradicts the idea of reduced cancer mortality, and gives weak support for the idea of increased cancer mortality among patients with reactive psychosis. Parenthetically, the authors recommend reconsidering reactive psychosis as a separate diagnostic term, since so many of them were later diagnosed as schizophrenic or depressed.

Thus, one can lay to rest the view often repeated even today, view that psychotics, especially schizophrenics, have fewer cancer deaths than normals.

HELPLESSNESS AND HOPELESSNESS, AND FIGHTING SPIRIT

No cohort studies could be found that examined whether helplessness–hopelessness (h-h) or fighting spirit (f-s) could predict incidence of cancer, although in an animal model uncontrollable stress (producing a reaction that seems to resemble humans' loss of hope) made the animals more susceptible to developing cancer (61). Further, it has been suggested that

Hopelessness might in some way be analogous to the kind of behavior shown by [most] animals transferred to other cages, which become the most submissive members of the new animal group . . . The finding of a fighting spirit as being associated with longer survival among breast cancer patients . . . is not inconsistent with the findings of Sklar and Anisman (1981) [62] that mice that fought persistently when placed in a new social environment did not suffer increased tumor load. (63)

Submissive animals did suffer an increased tumor load.

Many researchers believe that a h-h coping reaction in cancer patients affects the immune and hormonal systems severely enough to shorten survival time. Predictive studies of cancer *incidence* involving depressed mood might be considered to address h-h, but instruments devised to measure the two responses have limited commonality, and studies of the two conditions should not be grouped together or dealt with as parallels. Moreover, most locus of control studies have failed to reveal a connection between external locus of control, theoretically the response one might predict in a person with a h-h attitude, and later cancer incidence.

As for f-s, one might conceive that type A personalities have a fighting spirit, and that such people might be less likely to get cancer. No cohort studies addressing the relationship between f-s and cancer incidence could be found other than those involving type A, and there were only two of those. Faragher and Cooper (64) used a modified Bortner scale for type A on a group of 1463 women attending a screening clinic just before breast cancer diagnosis, and 727 normal women. They said,

Although statistically significant, the differences between the four study groups [cancer, cyst, benign, normal] with respect to the individual personality traits are numerically small; most of the mean differences were less than one unit on the Likert scale, so probably of little clinical importance. (64)

The other study (65) was a prospective one, done on the original cohort whose members Friedman and Rosenman interviewed to derive their type A concept. In a 22-year follow-up of those 3154 men, cancer mortality was determined using Cox proportional hazard analyses. The univariate analysis yielded an overall relative hazard (RH, approximating relative risk) of 1.53, confidence interval (CI) = 1.14–2.05, $p < 0.005$. Lung cancer and type A personality were not related (RH = 0.98). Controlling for age and smoking, the CI for the hazard function became 0.94–1.70, $p = 0.12$. Finally, when alcohol-related tumors were taken into account in the equation for non-lung cancers only, the CI for that group was 0.87–1.89, $p = 0.28$.

Many early researchers, observing a h-h reaction in a number of cancer patients, inferred that it caused shorter survival, without considering the possibility that the disease itself, or the realization of having the disease, might have brought about the coping reaction. A number of studies have explored the relationship between coping styles and cancer survival. The first major study ($n = 62$) was carried out by Greer and Morris (66). They reported a greater percentage of 5-year survivals among those breast cancer patients, mostly stage I, a few stage II, who showed either denial (not many) or fighting spirit, and shorter survival among those showing h-h or stoic acceptance. Later these categories were changed somewhat, but the basic h-h and fighting spirit findings were the same. Greer's group confirmed the earlier results in 10- and 15-year follow-ups (67). Buddeberg and colleagues (68) have concluded that, based on their repeated measurements of coping style in women with breast cancer—nine times in three years—patients' approaches to dealing with their disease varied considerably from occasion to occasion. Others have verified that conclusion (69). Several other studies have reported that cancer patients who used the h-h response as a coping mechanism died earlier than those who showed fighting spirit or denial, e.g., Jensen (70), Schmale and Iker (71).

On the other hand, a number of studies have shown no such relationship [e.g., Buddeberg et al. (68)] or only partial relationship [e.g., Cassileth et al. (72)

Dean and Surtees (73)]. An important study appeared recently in which the h-h response was subjected to a careful multivariate analysis (74). The cohort was made up of 243 patients with mixed diagnoses: breast 62, lymphoma 32, lung 30, other 129; and mixed prognoses: good 81, medium 62, poor 110. Several questionnaires were presented, including Beck's Hopelessness Scale. The latter was examined for scalability and some items making the measure unscalable were eliminated, as well as three items for cause, leaving a total of 14 acceptably scaled items. Several variables were felt to be possibly relevant to a feeling of hopelessness, and were measured: sex, age, marital status, education, economic status, personal functioning, and prognosis. Kaplan–Meier survival curves showed a clear survival advantage for those getting low and medium scores on the Beck scale (almost superposed curves) over those getting high scores on the scale. However, following standard procedure, a Cox regression was performed ($N = 216$) with the factors just mentioned entered as covariates. Hopelessness was not significantly related to survival: relative hazard = 1.04, $p = 0.195$, CI = 0.98–1.09. Only prognosis and personal functioning were significantly related to survival, and were the only substantial contributors to the outcome. Obviously there was an interaction among them and hopelessness that led to the latter's reduced relationship to survival. Even if one were to maintain that the nonsignificance of the p value showed a type II error, a relative risk of 1.04 is not very great, and hardly suggests a ponderable role for hopelessness as a predictor of survival. Similarly, Cody and colleagues found no relationship of h-h to survival (75) in a study of 209 newly diagnosed lung cancer patients.

Generally, the evidence, while not overwhelming, weighs heavily toward thinking that h-h is not a strong contributor to survival. It is possible, however, that it can affect survival in a few special cases. The difficulty is that even if that is so, we have no idea as to what kinds of cases.

SUPPRESSION OF EMOTIONS, ESPECIALLY ANGER

Many studies have reported that cancer patients, on average, are not so prone to express emotions, especially anger, as well people. The latter behavior is generally interpreted as anger suppression (76), not unconscious repression, although that view is not universally accepted (77). In any case, not all cancer patients are suppressors of emotion. Temoshok described what she called a type C personality (she actually said opposite in character to the better known type A) (78). They were, she said, "cooperative and appeasing, unassertive, patient, unexpressive of negative emotions (particularly anger), and compliant with external authorities." The term "Type C" was first used by Morris and Greer (79) in 1980 to describe people "emotionally contained," especially when confronted by stress.

A number of studies affirming and denying the existence of the phenomenon, both in foreign-language (1) and English-language publications, were reported early on, e.g., Kissen (80). In 1975 a major work supporting this distinction between cancer patients and controls was done by Greer and Morris (81). Following their study, a flurry of positive and negative studies appeared, continuing to the present. Gross (76) describes and discusses many germane studies.

The majority of those reporting positive results believe this emotional suppression to be a stable personality style; others think it is a state brought on by the disease. The question is not a trifling issue, as will be shown below. The studies can be divided into two types, those discussing whether suppression of emotions can distinguish cancer patients from others, and those discussing whether suppression of emotions can predict either cancer incidence/mortality or duration of survival.

I analyzed the study outcomes of 24 studies, 12 asking whether suppression of emotional expression can distinguish groups of cancer patients from others, and 12 asking whether suppression can predict incidence, mortality or survival. (The list, of which 14 were discussed by Gross (76), can be obtained from the author on request.) Four of the 18 studies examined by Gross were omitted for cause (no statistical work, etc.). Among the studies on distinction of the groups, five decided yes, four decided no, and three had mixed results (e.g., one measure was positive, another negative; or out of three age groups, only one was positive.) Among the predictive studies, three decided yes, six decided no, and three had mixed results (e.g., measures taken at or near mastectomy and those taken 3 months later gave opposite results; or p for mortality was 0.008, but p for recurrence was 0.48).

Two recent papers may clarify the situation in regard to the distinction studies. Kreitler and colleagues (82) examined three groups of women prior to surgery: two for possible breast cancer and one with surgery unrelated to breast cancer. All were tested with measures of anxiety and what Kreitler and colleagues called repression of emotions, the latter being measured with a combination of the Taylor Manifest Anxiety Scale and the Marlowe–Crowne Social Desirability Scale, assessing defensiveness. After sur-

gery, the possible cancer patients were told the results of their biopsies. Before surgery the three groups, cancer patients ($N = 40$), benign patients ($N = 32$), and nonsurgical patients ($N = 26$) did not differ on either of the measures. After surgery the three groups were all less anxious, but the repression scores among the cancer group rose markedly (18.00%), while the other two group scores rose minimally (benign, 3.35%, noncancer, 0.17%). A further analysis using the McNemar χ^2, comparing number of patients in the four categories of possible change, R→N, R→R, N→R, N→N (repression = R, non-repression = N), showed significance only for the cancer group.

In a second paper, Servaes and colleagues (83) gave 43 breast cancer patients and 47 age-matched healthy women four instruments, two investigating their tendencies to express or suppress emotions, and two whether such tendencies were deliberate. Alexithymia scales were included. The results showed no differences in measures of alexithymia, but significantly higher scores on the scales measuring intention to suppress emotional expression. The authors say, "The results thus suggest that lack of emotional expression in cancer patients results from purposeful inhibition of expression and appeasing others rather than from a disturbance of emotional processing (alexithymia)."

Thus, regarding the issue mentioned above of whether suppression is a stable trait or brought on by the realization that one has cancer, the second option finds support in the Kreitler et al. study (82). Moreover, the findings by Servaes and colleagues (83) are consistent with this view. Finally, support for the tendency of cancer patients to misrepresent their true feelings comes from the several studies examining their scores on the lie scales of various instruments (81) and social desirability measures (84). These were uniformly elevated. In the only cohort study found that examined whether lie scale scores could predict survival, high scorers had shorter survival (85). The studies by Kreitler (82) Servaes et al. (83) and Ratcliffe (85) urgently need replication.

In sum, the aggregate evidence on suppression that suggests a distinction between cancer patients and others is strong; however, the phenomenon does not seem to be universal. The evidence is very strong that suppression of emotion does not predict incidence of cancer, and it is likely that suppression does not predict survival. Because there are so many variables that can affect the outcomes in such studies, a yes or no state of affairs is not very probable. I believe that the most influential variables are site of disease, early or late stage of disease, the patient's gender, his or her age, the instruments used, and possible sampling bias.

SOCIAL SUPPORT

The presence of social support is known to be inversely related to overall mortality. However, the major diseases involved in most of these studies showing this are cerebrovascular and cardiovascular, and cancer mortality is only occasionally mentioned in these overall mortality studies. Those specifically aimed at cancer incidence or mortality report inconsistent results, more, perhaps, showing no relationship than a relationship. In survival studies, however, where a significant finding is reported, poor social support tends to accompany shorter survival. The measures of social support differ considerably, which may be one reason for the inconsistent findings. Some of the measures examined are number of social contacts; number of supportive friends; number of support persons; employment status; size of social network; frequency of contact with friends; same for relatives; level of need for social support; difference between level of need and level of received support. Other measures have been studied. Of course, other factors affecting survival ought to be controlled, but various studies control for different possible confounders. This issue merits close attention.

Some major studies should be mentioned. Reynolds and Kaplan (86) studied whether social support was related to cancer incidence over a period of 17 years in an initial cohort of 6848 adults. They measured 11 social support elements: social network index level (four levels, from least connected to most connected); number of contacts; feeling of isolation; marital status; friend/relative contacts; church group membership; other group memberships; and church attendance. Only age at diagnosis and stage at diagnosis were controlled. The degree of men's social support showed no relationship to their subsequent cancer incidence, but among women, those reporting social isolation had a greater cancer incidence than those not isolated. Women who reported not only the fact of isolation but also the feeling of social isolation were at especially high risk of later cancers, particularly hormone-related cancers. They also studied cancer survival among 154 men and 185 women from the cohort, and found that men who were least connected (level 1 of the social network index) survived a significantly shorter time than those at other levels, but that women showed no such relationship. None of the other social support variables were related to survival duration.

Joffres and colleagues (87) studying a cohort of 4581 men of Japanese ancestry in Hawaii, found that "among eight items related to social networks, two were significantly associated with cancer incidence in multivariate analysis, but one of these associations was in the direction opposite to that of the social support hypothesis."

Ell and colleagues (88) studied 294 cancer patients, 168 breast, 76 colorectal, and 50 lung. They analyzed breast and combined lung and colorectal separately, and localized ($n = 138$) and nonlocalized ($N = 156$) separately. Their results differed by site and also by stage, but since no analysis was done by site *and* stage, the results are uncertain. Moreover, results for the only distinguishing measures, emotional support, marital status, stage and role limitation, cannot be taken at face value because sex was not controlled in any of the multivariate analyses, and that would obviously have had a substantial role in the picture. While their caution that results probably differ by stage and by site is reasonable, that conclusion cannot firmly be derived from their own data.

Vogt and colleagues (89) did a more careful cohort study of 2603 health maintenance organization (HMO) members. They analyzed the 15-year risk of incurring five different outcomes, death, ischemic heart disease, hypertension, cancer and stroke, so only a few variables could be controlled. They were age, sex, smoking, socioeconomic status (SES), and baseline health status. The three social predictor measures were network scope (number of domains in which a person had social contacts), network size (summed number of persons comprising the whole network), and network frequency (number of contacts overall). The analysis compared the highest tertile against the lowest. None of the network predictors were associated with cancer incidence, even in a Cox multivariate analysis. Both scope and frequency were associated with improved cancer mortality, and size marginally so. Unfortunately, no site, stage, or duration of survival data were avaliable. Even more unfortunately, they failed to give the numbers of cases for any of the analyzed cancers.

Neale and colleagues (90) examined 10-year survival among 1261 breast cancer patients, after adjusting for age, SES, stage, and delay in seeking treatment for symptoms. Using a Cox regression that took account of the control variables, they found no effect for delay, but reported that widows did not survive as long as married women. Thus, marital status was important in this cohort. Neale and colleagues mention many possible reasons in the literature for this finding, including greater social exclusion than married women.

Goodwin and colleagues (91) confirmed the results of Neale et al. (90) correcting for stage and whether treated or not. They gave further possible reasons for the increased survival of married women. One was that the effect of marital status followed a clear gradient, the younger the patient, the greater the effect of marriage on survival. This does away with much of the contradiction between these findings and those of Cassileth and colleagues (72), most of whose patients were old and in late disease stage.

Waxler-Morrison and colleagues (92) confirmed other studies showing a connection between greater social involvement and longer survival of cancer patients. Her cohort of 133 breast cancer patients, moreover, was controlled for age, stage, nodal status, histologic grade, and estrogen receptor status.

Funch and Marshall (93) studied 208 white female breast cancer patients, measuring social support in an interview at diagnosis that covered the five previous years. After 20 years the survival pattern of the cohort was determined for all patients. Marital status and number of friends were not related to survival; involvement in organizations was. On theoretical grounds, a subanalysis by age group was undertaken. Those in the youngest and oldest groups (premenopausal = 15–45 years and post-menopausal = 61–90 years) survived longer when their social involvement was high than when it was low. Those in the perimenopausal group (46–60 years) showed no difference in survival in regard to social involvement. These findings are not impressive, but show the variability one finds in these studies.

Overall, the general evidence points toward no relationship between social involvement and incidence of cancer. However, in regard to cancer survival, the general evidence does point toward such a relationship, although in most cases the relative risk (where determined) was low, less than 1.5. A few studies found a mixed relationship of social involvement and survival; for example, one age group showed a positive relationship, where others did not (93), and patients with certain tumors did, while others did not (88).

The caution mentioned above can be made more specific after one looks at a number of studies. Many variables influence results in studies such as these, and so far as they can be controlled, an attempt should be made to do so. The list of the variables dealt with in the studies mentioned in this section should surely have included others such as pain, Karnofsky score, and interval from diagnosis to study entry, but only the following were mentioned: age, sex, marital status, stress, baseline health status, cancer history, delay in diagnosis, site, stage, positive nodes, tumor histology, estrogen receptor status, whether in treatment, and type of treatment. Last, duration of follow-up is important because several studies noted stronger effects early in the follow-up period and weaker effects later.

PSYCHOTHERAPEUTIC INTERVENTIONS

Several studies report on the success of psychotherapeutic intervention in extending survival and disease-free interval. Certain ones have been prominently disseminated throughout the scientific community because they seem to have followed good procedure. Yet there are differences in their results which could well have been brought about by procedural differences. The best-known study is that of Spiegel and colleagues (94). They studied 86 patients with metastatic breast cancer, offering group therapy weekly for a year to 50 treatment patients, and administering routine oncological care both to the 50 treatment patients and to the 36 control patients. At 10-year follow-up 3 treatment patients were alive, and death records were examined for the remaining 83 patients. Mean survival for the intervention patients from time of randomization, which was also the beginning of treatment for those alive at that point, was 36.6 months, and was 18.9 months for the controls. Divergence in survival did not begin until 20 months after the entry, or 12 months after the end of the group therapy sessions. This study has been widely cited, but Spiegel properly said that it must be replicated, and as of late 1997 he was well into the conduct of such a study. It is of interest that, from the time of randomization, 14 intervention patients had either died, were too ill to participate, or had moved away, leaving 36 who were actually treated. Similarly, only 24 of the 36 controls could participate in the testing phase of the study, so the actual comparison of living subjects at the time of intervention was 36 vs. 24, not an impressive number. However, the authors, quite properly, followed the "intention to treat" paradigm, and hence all 86 patients were included in the analysis.

A second study with positive results was done on melanoma patients by Fawzy and colleagues (95), but their series of group therapy sessions lasted six weeks rather than a year. They found the death rate over the five to six years of follow-up to be 10 out of 34 for the controls, and 3 out of 34 for the treatment group, a significant difference. Neither of the death frequencies is particularly large, and one hesitates to give much weight to these findings.

Linn and colleagues (96) carried out a study using individual counselling on 120 end-stage male cancer patients, 62 randomly assigned to the counselling group and 58 to the control group. Treatment patients improved in quality of life measures, but did not differ from controls in survival over a year's time.

Another study, by Gellert and colleagues (97) on breast cancer patients, examined the effectiveness of Bernie Siegel's group therapy sessions in a follow-up study to an earlier one that showed practically no improved survival for the therapy group when compared to a control group. The earlier result had emerged after correcting for a difference in intervals between diagnosis and treatment of the two groups. The Gellert et al. study improved the selection of controls by using historical controls matched with the treatment patients on several important variables, and extended the observed survival time by 10 years. Three controls were matched to each of the 34 treatment patients, and their survival was monitored from the treatment dates (1971 through 1980) until March, 1991. No difference in ultimate survival of the two groups could be observed after matching the interval between diagnosis and entry into therapy of the two groups. If that necessary matching was not done, the treatment group spuriously showed longer survival.

Ilnyckyj and colleagues (98) studied 127 cancer patients randomly assigned to three treatment groups and a control group, the weekly psychotherapy group extending to 6 months. One treatment group ($n = 31$) was led by a professional social worker for 6 months; a second ($n = 30$) was led for 3 months, then continued to meet for 3 months without a leader; a third ($n = 35$) met for 6 months without professional leadership. The control group had no treatment other than normal oncologic care, which all groups received. Mean survival from time of randomization was 70.7 months in the professionally led group, 62.0 months in the unled groups, and 82.4 months in the control group. None of these means differed significantly from any other.

Richardson and colleagues (99) carried out a study on patient compliance and educational treatment, with positive results. Three groups experienced three educational programs (N's = 22, 23, and 24), graded in content and aimed at better compliance, and a fourth group ($N = 25$), a control, received no education. Each patient was assigned to the group that was in effect on the day of entry into the study. When entered into a Cox regression whose variables were sex, severity of illness, Karnofsky at diagnosis, appointments kept, allopurinol compliance, and presence or absence of any education, all were significant. RR for education was 0.39, CI = 0.17–0.89, control being the reference level with RR = 1.

It is clear that the issue of extension of life among cancer patients by psychotherapeutic intervention is quite unsettled. Too many differences exist in procedures, samples, disease types, stages, experimental designs, approaches to therapy, durations of treatment, etc. to allow a clear conclusion.

PREBIOPSY OR SO-CALLED QUASI-PROSPECTIVE STUDIES

These studies refer to designs in which psychosocial measures are taken from patients before biopsy, usually in the belief that knowledge of disease status will have no effect on psychosocial measures. Only two studies directly addressing this issue could be found, those of Schwarz and Geyer (100) and those of Schwarz (101). The former derived data on 76 breast tumor patients (23 malignancies); the latter derived data on 195 possible breast cancer patients (58 malignancies) and 86 suspected lung cancer patients (59 malignancies). In the earlier breast cancer study, 55/76 patients (72%) correctly predicted their biopsy outcome. In the later study 150/195 breast patients (77%) did so and 60/86 lung patients (70%) were correct. In the 1993 study both the breast patient predictions and the combined breast patient and physician predictions were correct at ($p < 0.001$, but for lung patients only the combined patient and physician predictions were correct ($p < 0.01$). These results suggest that prebiopsy studies are carried out with the correct preconception of outcome by most breast cancer patients, but not with lung cancer patients. Obviously, appropriate caution should be observed in any prebiopsy studies.

Some Considerations

How confident can one be about the state of affairs in regard to any of the psychosocial factors discussed above or, indeed, about any of the much larger number that have been associated with cancer in one or another study? In regard to initiation of cancer, we have very little information. Stress in rats and mice generally stimulates initiation of viral tumors but inhibits that of chemically induced tumors. In humans only a few, perhaps 3–4%, seem to be virus-related, the most prominent ones being cervix, liver, Burkitt's lymphoma, and nasopharyngeal carcinoma. Factors already mentioned that differentiate most rodent responses from those of humans suggest that we should not extrapolate readily to humans the tumor-stimulating findings regarding stress in animals.

As for prognosis, the theory espoused in most of the recent papers on presumably negatively acting psychosocial factors is that immune system activity may be depressed in people with such factors, and hence the cancer tends to grow faster in them. Positively acting psychosocial factors would tend to do the opposite.

But things are not so simple. The few studies looking at both immune system activity and survival have reported that even if responsiveness of one or several immune system elements (T_4 cells, T_8 cells, T_4/T_8 ratio, natural killer cells, mitogen-responsive mononuclear cells in general, etc.) declines, there has not appeared a corresponding reduction in survival time [e.g., Fawzy et al. (95)]. It is of further interest that among the few intervention studies, to my knowledge none of the psychosocial factor measures given to the treatment and control groups of patients has predicted survival differences in the groups [e.g., Speigel et al. (94) Fawzy et al. (95)].

It has been suggested from time to time [e.g., Fox (4)] that the influence of psychosocial factors might ride on top of the known influence of various carcinogens, selectively causing certain people to get cancer among all those exposed to the risk factor (which smokers get lung cancer?). It seems to me that such an interaction is very difficult to justify across the large array of psychosocial factors, the equally large array of known—and unknown—carcinogens, and the more than one hundred types of cancer, each peculiar to the cytologic, hormonal, etc., characteristics of particular cancer patients. Such a notion must remain a speculation at present, but should not be discarded out of hand.

Thus, in regard to the basic question of possible influence of psychosocial factors on cancer, the position seems fairly firm for a few factors, namely, that there is no influence (or at most, very little influence), but the position is quite uncertain in the remainder. For example, social support is unlikely to be associated with cancer incidence, but may well be associated with prognosis. After all, epidemiology is not an exact science, and studies are occasionally found to contradict each other's results. In my opinion, some people, for some cancer types, under some conditions may well be affected by psychosocial factors such that cancer is more *or less* likely to occur in them than in others, or if the people are patients, that it may progress faster *or slower* than in other patients. I feel, moreover, that such cases are probably comparatively rare, and it would be quite impossible, at present, to identify them singly.

REFERENCES

1. Baltrusch HJF. Ergebnisse klinisch-psychosomatischer Krebsforschung. (Results of clinical-psychosomatic cancer research). *Z Psychosom Med.* 1975; 5:175–208.
2. Bahnson CB, Kissen DM, eds. Psychophysiological aspects of cancer. *Ann NY Acad Sci.* 1966; 125:773–1055.
3. Crisp AH. Some psychosomatic aspects of neoplasia. *Br J Med Psychol.* 1970; 43:313–331.
4. Fox BH. Premorbid psychological factors as related to cancer incidence. *J Behav Med.* 1978; 1:45–133.
5. Cullen JW, Fox BH, Isom RN, eds. *Cancer: The Behavioral Dimensions.* New York: Raven Press; 1976.
6. Fox BH. The role of psychological factors in cancer incidence and prognosis. *Oncology.* 1995; 9:245–253.
7. Stein S, Spiegel D. Psychophysiologic effects on cancer progression. In: Goodkin K, Visser A, eds. *Psychoneuroimmunology: Stress, Mental Disorders and Health.* Washington, D.C.: American Psychiatric Press, 1998. [In press.]
8. Hagnell O. The premorbid personality of persons who develop cancer in a total population investigated in 1947 and 1957. *Ann NY Acad Sci.* 1966; 125:846–855.
9. Hagnell O. Personal communication. Division of Psychiatry, University of Lund, Sweden, 1980.
10. *Cancer Statistics Review 1973–1986.* Bethseda, MD: U.S. Department of Health and Human Services, Public Health Service, National Institutes of Health, National Cancer Institute; 1989 [NIH Publication no. 89-2789.]
11. Bernhard J, Ganz PA. Psychosocial issues in lung cancer patients (Part 1). *Chest.* 1991; 99:216–223.
12. Justice A. Review of the effects of stress on cancer in laboratory animals: importance of time of stress application and type of tumor. *Psychol Bull.* 1985; 98:108–138.
13. Riley V. Mouse mammary tumors: alteration of incidence as an apparent function of stress. *Science.* 1975; 129:465–467.
14. Newberry BH, Sengbusch L. Inhibitory effects of stress on experimental mammary tumors. *Cancer Detect Prev.* 1979; 2:225–233.
15. Goodkin K, Antoni MH, Sevin B, Fox BH. A partially testable, predictive model of psychosocial factors in the etiology of cervical cancer. I. Biological, psychological and social aspects. *Psycho-Oncology.* 1993; 2:79–98.
16. Claman HN. Corticosteroid and lymphoid cells. *N Engl J Med.* 1972; 287:388–397.
17. Kinlen LJ. Malignancy in auto-immune diseases. *J Autoimmun.* 1992; 5 (supplement A):363–371.
18. Holland JC, Rowland JH, eds. *Handbook of Psychooncology.* New York: Oxford University Press; 1990.
19. Clark DM, Teasdale JD. Diurnal variation in clinical depression and accessibility of memories of positive and negative experiences. *J Abnorm Psychol.* 1982; 91:87–95.
20. Charlson ME, Feinstein AR. A new clinical index of growth rate in the staging of breast cancer. *Am J Med.* 1980; 69:527–536.
21. Greene WA. The psychosocial setting of the development of leukemia and lymphoma. *Ann NY Acad Sci.* 1966; 125:794–801.
22. LeShan L, Worthington RE. Personality as a factor in the pathogenesis of cancer: a review of the literature. *Br J Med Psychol.* 1956; 29:49–56.
23. Schonfield J. Psychological and life experience differences between Israeli women with benign and cancerous breast lesions. *J Psychosom Res.* 1975; 19:229–234.

24. Greer S, Morris T. Psychological attributes of women who develop breast cancer. A controlled study. *J Psychosom Res.* 1975; 19:147–153.

25. Courtney JG, Longnecker MP, Theorell T, Gerhardsson de Verdier M. Stressful life events and the risk of colorectal cancer. *Epidemiology.* 1993; 4:407–414.

26. Geyer S. Life events prior to manifestation of breast cancer. A limited prospective study covering eight years before diagnosis. *J Psychosom Res.* 1991; 35:355–363.

27. Ramirez AJ, Craig TKJ, Watson JP, Fentiman IS, North WRS, Rubens RD. Stress and relapse of breast cancer. *Br Med J.* 1989; 298:291–293.

28. Edwards JR, Cooper CL, Pearl G, de Paredes ES, O'Leary T, Wilhelm MC. The relationship between psychosocial factors and breast cancer: Some unexpected results. *Behav Med.* 1990; 16:5–14.

29. Priestley TJ, Priestman SG, Bradshaw C. Stress and breast cancer. *Br J Cancer.* 1985; 51:493–498.

30. Blaney PH. Affect and memory: a review. *Psychol Rev.* 1986; 99:229–246.

31. Brett JF, Brief AP, Burke MJ, George JM, Webster J. Negative affectivity and the reporting of stressful life events. *Health Psychol.* 1990; 9:57–68.

32. Cohen L, Towbes L, Flocco R. Effects of induced mood on self-reported life events and perceived and received social support. *J Pers Soc Psychol.* 1988; 55:669–674.

33. Weinstock MA, Colditz GA, Willett WC, Stampfer MJ, Rosner B, Speizer FE. Recall (report) bias and reliability in the retrospective assessment of melanoma risk. *Am J Epidemiol.* 1991; 133:240–245.

34. Keehn RJ, Goldberg ID, Beebe GW. Twenty-four year mortality follow-up of army veterans with disability separation for psychoneurosis in 1944. *Psychosom Med.* 1974; 36:27–46.

35. Keehn RJ. Follow-up studies of World War II and Korean conflict prisoners of war. *Am J Epidemiol.* 1980; 111:194–200.

36. Joffres M, Reed DM, Nomura AMY. Psychosocial processes and cancer incidence among Japanese men in Hawaii. *Am J Epidemiol.* 1985; 121:488–500.

37. Barraclough J, Pinder P, Cruddas M, Osmond C, Taylor I, Perry M. Life events and breast cancer prognosis. *Br Med J.* 1992; 304:1078–1081.

38. Grossarth-Maticek R, Frentzel-Beyme R, Becker N. Cancer risks associated with life events and conflicts solution. *Cancer Detect Prev.* 1984; 7:201–209.

39. *Psychological Inquiry.* Whole issue. 1991; 2(3):221-323.

40. Holmes TH, Rahe RN. The social readjustment rating scale. *J Psychosom Res.* 1967; 11:213–218.7.

41. Jones DR, Goldblatt PO. Cancer mortality following widow(er)hood: Some further results from the Office of Population Censuses and Surveys Longitudinal Study. *Stress Med.* 1986; 2:129–140.

42. Kaprio J, Koskenvuo M, Rita H. Mortality after bereavement: A prospective study of 95,647 widowed persons. *Am J Public Health.* 1987; 77:283–287.

43. Helsing KJ, Comstock GW, Szklo M. Causes of death in a widowed population. *Am J Epidemiol.* 1982; 116:524–532.

44. Ewertz M. Bereavement and breast cancer. *Br J Cancer.* 1986; 53:701–703.

45. Neale AV. Racial and marital status influences on 10-year survival from breast cancer. *J Clin Epidemiol.* 1994; 47:475–483.

46. Holland JC, Zittoun R, eds. *Psychosocial Aspects of Oncology.* Berlin: Springer-Verlag; 1990.

47. Mitchell WM. Etiological factors producing neuropsychiatric syndromes in patients with malignant disease. *Int J Neuropsychiatry.* 1967; 3:464–468.

48. Shekelle RB, Raynor WJ, Ostfeld AM, et al. Psychological depression and 17-year risk of death from cancer. *Psychosom Med.* 1981; 43:117–125.

49. Persky VW, Kempthorne-Rawson J, Shekelle RB. Personality and risk of cancer: 20-year follow-up of the Western Electric Study. *Psychosom Med.* 1987; 49:435–449.

50. Kaplan GA, Reynolds P. Depression and cancer mortality and morbidity: prospective evidence from the Alameda County study. *Psychosom Med.* 1988; 11:1–13.

51. Hahn RC, Petitti DB. Minnesota Multiphasic Inventory-rated depression and the incidence of breast cancer. *Cancer.* 1988; 61:845–848.

52. Linkins RW, Comstock GW. Depressed mood and incidence of cancer. *Am J Epidemiol.* 1990; 132:962–972.

53. Zonderman AB, Costa PT, McRae RR. Depression as a risk for cancer morbidity and mortality in a nationally representatve sample. *J Am Med Assoc.* 1989; 262:1191–1195.

54. Fox BH. Depressive symptoms and risk of cancer [editorial]. *J Am Med Assoc.* 1989; 262:1231.

55. Fox BH. A hypothesis to reconcile conflicting conclusions in studies relating depressed mood to later cancer. In: Stein M, Baum A., eds. *Chronic Diseases.* Mahwah, NJ: Lawrence Erlbaum Associates, 1995.

56. Perrin GM, Pierce IR. Psychosomatic aspects of cancer: a review. *Psychosom Med.* 1959; 21:397–421.

57. Fox BH. Cancer death risk in hospitalized mental patients. *Science.* 1978; 201:966–968.

58. Tsuang MT, Woolson RF, Fleming JA. Causes of death in schizophrenia and mental depression. *Br J Psychiatry.* 1980; 136:239–242.

59. Gulbinat W, Dupont A, Jablensky A, et al. Cancer incidence of schizophrenia patients. Results of record linkage studies in three countries. *Br J Psychiatry.* 1992; 161 (suppl 18):75–85.

60. Jørgensen P, Mortensen PB. Cause of death in reactive psychosis. *Acta Psychiatr Scand.* 1992; 85:351–353.

61. Visintainer MA, Volpicelli JR, Seligman MEP. Tumor rejection in rats after inescapable and escapable shock. *Science.* 1982; 216:437–439.

62. Sklar LS, Anisman H. Stress and cancer. *Psychol Bull.* 1981; 89:369–406.

63. Fox BH. Psychogenic etiology and prognosis of cancer—current status of theory. In: Christ AE, Flomenhaft K, eds. *Childhood Cancer.* New York: Plenum Press; 1984: 3–29.

64. Faragher EB, Cooper CL. Type A stress prone behaviour and breast cancer. *Psychol Med.* 1990; 20:663–670.

65. Ragland DR, Brand, RJ, Fox BH. Type A/B behavior and cancer mortality: Confounding/mediating effect of covariates. *Psycho-Oncology.* 1992; 1:25–33.

66. Greer S, Morris T, Pettingale KW. Psychological response to breast cancer: effect on outcome. *Lancet.* 1979; 2:785–787.

67. Greer S, Morris T, Pettingale KW, Haybittle JL. Psychological response to breast cancer and 15 year outcome. *Lancet.* 1990; 1:49–50.

68. Buddeberg C, Sieber M, Wolf C, Landolt-Ritter C, Richter D, Steiner R. Are coping strategies related to disease outcome in early breast cancer? *J Psychosom Res.* 1996; 40:255–263.

69. Heim E, Augustini KF, Schaffner L, Valach L. Coping with breast cancer over time and situation. *J Psychosom Res.* 1993; 37:523–542.

70. Jensen MR. Psychobiological factors predicting the course of breast cancer. *J Pers.* 1987; 55:317–342.

71. Schmale AH, Iker H. Hopelessness as a mediator of cervical cancer. *Soc Sci Med.* 1971; 5:95–100.

72. Cassileth BR, Walsh WP, Lusk EJ. Psychosocial correlates of cancer survival: a subsequent report 3 to 8 years after cancer diagnosis. *J Clin Oncol.* 1988; 6:1753–1759.

73. Dean C, Surtees PG. Do psychological factors predict survival in breast cancer? *J Psychosom Res.* 1989; 33:561–569.

74. Ringdal GI. Correlates of hopelessness in cancer patients. *J Psychosoc Oncol.* 1995; 13:47–66.

75. Cody M, Nichols S, Brennan C, Armes J, Wilson P, Slevin M. Psychosocial factors and lung cancer prognosis [abstract]. *Psycho-Oncology.* 1994; 3:141.

76. Gross J. Emotional expression in cancer onset and progression. *Soc Sci Med.* 1989; 28:1239–1248.

77. Kune GA, Kune S, Watson LF, Bahnson CB. Personality as a risk factor in large bowel cancer: data from the Melbourne Colorectal Cancer Study. *Psychol Med.* 1991; 21:29–41.

78. Temoshok L. Personality, coping style, emotion, and cancer: towards an integrative model. *Cancer Surv.* 1987; 6:545–567.

79. Morris T, Greer S. A 'type C' for cancer? Low trait anxiety in the pathogenesis of breast cancer [abstract 102]. *Cancer Detect Prev.* 1980; 3:102.

80. Kissen D. Personality characteristics in males conducive to lung cancer. *Br J Med Psychol.* 1963; 36:27–36.

81. Greer S, Morris T. Psychological attributes of women who develop breast cancer: A controlled study. *J Psychosom Res.* 1975; 19:147–153.

82. Kreitler S, Chaitchik S, Kreitler H. Repressiveness: Cause or result of cancer? *Psycho-Oncology.* 1993; 2:43–54.

83. Servaes P, Vingerhoets A, Vreugdenhil G, Keuning J, Broekhuijsen MA. Breast cancer and nonexpression of emotions [abstract]. *Psychosom Med.* 1996; 58:67.

84. Hürny C, Piasetsky E, Bagin R, Holland J. High social desirability in patients being treated for advanced colorectal and bladder cancer: eventual impact on the assessment of quality of life. *J Psychosoc Oncol.* 1987; 5:19–29.

85. Ratcliffe MA, Dawson AA, Walker LG. Eysenck Personality Inventory L-scores in patients with Hodgkin's disease and non-Hodgkin's lymphoma. *Psycho-Oncology.* 1995; 4:39–45.

86. Reynolds P, Kaplan GA. Social connections and risk for cancer: Prospective evidence from the Alameda County study. *Behav Med.* 1990; 16:101–110.

87. Joffres M, Reed DM, Nomura AMY Psychosocial processes and cancer incidence among Japanese men in Hawaii. *Am J Epidemiol.* 1985; 121:488–500.

88. Ell K, Nishimoto R, Mediansky L, Mantell J, Hamovitch M. Social relations, social support and survival among patients with cancer. *J Psychsom Res.* 1992; 36:531–541.

89. Vogt TM, Mullooly JP, Ernst D, Pope CR, Hollis JF. Social networks as predictors of ischemic heart disease, cancer, stroke and hypertension: incidence, survival and mortality. *J Clin Epidemiol.* 1992; 45:659–666.

90. Neale AV, Tilley BC, Vernon SW. Marital status, delay in seeking treatment and survival from breast cancer. *Soc Sci Med.* 1986; 23:305–312.

91. Goodwin JS, Hunt WC, Key CR, Samet JM. The effect of marital status on stage, treatment and survival of cancer patients. *J Am Med Assoc.* 1987; 258:3125–3130.

92. Waxler-Morrison N, Hislop TG, Mears B, Kan L. Effects of social relationships on survival for women with breast cancer: a prospective study. *Soc Sci Med.* 1991; 33:177–183.

93. Funch DP, Marshall J. The role of stress, social support and age in survival from breast cancer. *J Psychosom Res.* 1983; 27:77–83.

94. Spiegel D, Bloom JR, Kraemer HC, Gottheil E. Effect of psychosocial treatment on survival of patients with metastatic breast cancer. *Lancet.* 1989; 2:888–891.

95. Fawzy F, Fawzy NW, Hyun CS, et al. Malignant melanoma. Effects of an early structured psychiatric intervention, coping, and affective state on recurrence and survival 6 years later. *Arch Gen Psychiatry.* 1993; 50:681–689.

96. Linn MW, Linn BS, Harris R. Effects of counselling for late stage cancer patients. *Cancer.* 1982; 49:1048–1055.

97. Gellert GA, Maxwell RM, Siegel BS. Survival of breast cancer patients receiving adjunctive psychosocial support therapy: A 10-year follow-up study. *J Clin Oncol.* 1993; 11:66–69.

98. Ilnyckyj A, Farber J, Cheang MC, Weinerman BH. A randomized controlled trial of psychotherapeutic intervention in cancer patients. *Ann R Coll Phys Surg Can.* 1994; 27:93–96.

99. Richardson JL, Shelton DR, Krailo M, Levine AM. The effect of compliance with treatment on survival among patients with hematologic malignancies. *J Clin Oncol.* 1990; 8:356–364.

100. Schwarz R, Geyer S. Social and psychological differences between cancer and noncancer patients: cause or consequence of the disease? *Psychother Psychosom.* 1984; 41:195–199.

101. Schwarz R. Psychosoziale Faktoren in der Karzinogenese: Zur Problematik der sogenannten Krebspersönlichkeit. (Psychosocial factors in carcinogenesis: The problem of the so-called cancer personality). *Psychother Psychosom Med Psychol.* 1993; 43:1–9.

12

Psychoneuroimmunology: Implications for Psycho-oncology

DANA H. BOVBJERG AND HEIDDIS B. VALDIMARSDOTTIR

The immune system, once widely viewed as operating as an autonomous bodily defense mechanism, is increasingly recognized to be subject to regulatory control by the central nervous system. Interdisciplinary research efforts in "psychoneuroimmunology" have provided compelling evidence of intimate connections between the brain and the immune system, as well as hints of the potential impact of such links for health and disease. This chapter briefly highlights possible implications of psychoneuroimmune interactions for psycho-oncology. The primary purpose of the chapter is to examine the "conventional view" that neural–immune interactions may provide the biologic mechanism(s) by which psychosocial factors affect the incidence and/or progression of cancer (1). We suggest alternative conceptualizations, highlighting the opportunities for further research. A secondary purpose of the chapter is to call attention to the possible impact of psychoneuroimmune interactions for infectious disease in cancer patients. These effects, which could have profound implications for morbidity and mortality, have received surprisingly little attention. The chapter concludes with a brief comment concerning the potential implications of neuroimmune interactions for oncology.

PSYCHONEUROIMMUNOLGY AND CANCER: THE CONVENTIONAL VIEW

The influences of psychological, behavioral, and social variables on the immune system are increasingly recognized by the biomedical research community, health care providers, and the lay public. As immune defenses are thought by many to play a role in preventing or slowing the progression of cancer, it has become widely accepted that psychologically induced changes in immune function are likely to provide the mechanism by which behavioral and psychosocial variables may affect neoplastic disease. The individual links in this chain of reasoning (see Fig. 12–1), which so strongly influences the thinking of both the lay public and researchers in psycho-oncology (e.g., Refs. 2–6), need to be carefully examined, as each has conceptual and methodologic difficulties often overlooked by nonspecialists (1).

Psychosocial Factors Affect the Incidence and/or Progression of Cancer

As extensively reviewed in other chapters of this book, the impact of psychological factors on the development and/or progression of cancer remains controversial. Three basic study designs have been used in this research literature: *(1)* retrospective studies, in which cancer patients are asked to recollect psychological factors from before their diagnosis; *(2)* quasi-prospective studies, in which patients with suspected cancer are assessed prior to diagnosis; and *(3)* prospective studies, in which healthy subjects are assessed and then followed for several years. Although not without exception, investigators using each of these designs have reported finding relations between psychological factors and cancer. It is important to recognize, however, that even positive findings can be difficult to interpret, as has been emphasized by Fox (7).

The most critical problem with retrospective designs is that the knowledge that one has cancer (or the presence of cancer-related symptomatology) is likely to affect recollections of past stressful events (e.g., searching after meaning), measures of current distress, and even measures thought to reflect "traits" (7). Although the quasi-prospective approach may eliminate the effects of conscious knowledge that one has cancer, the potential confounding biologic effects of the tumor itself on psychosocial factors remain an issue (7). It should also be noted that a high proportion of patients and their physicians have been found to correctly guess what the results of biopsy will be (8).

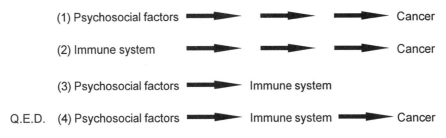

FIG. **12–1.** Psychoneuroimmunology and cancer: the conventional view.

Prospective studies provide the strongest test of the role of psychosocial factors in cancer development; however, the pattern of results in these studies has been neither consistent nor simple. Discrepant results may be due to differences between studies on several key variables, including the wide range of assessment instruments used, the types of cancer studied, the timing of the psychosocial assessment, and the lack of control for other better established risk factors (e.g., smoking) known to be related to psychosocial variables. There has also been little attention paid to the possibility that psychosocial factors may interact with other known risk factors for cancer (9). In light of the recent explosion of information on the genetics of cancer, it would be of particular interest to consider the possibility that the impact of psychosocial variables may be more profound among individuals at familial risk than in the population as a whole.

In summary, the lines of evidence noted above are consistent with the possibility that psychosocial factors may play a role in the development and/or progression of cancer. However, it is clear that there are many issues that researchers need to address before one can conclude that the biologic consequences of psychological factors are responsible for the relations between psychosocial factors and cancer. Behavioral mechanisms are also likely to play a role in these relationships. To take one obvious example, smoking is one of the strongest risk factors for certain types of cancer. For these cancers, it is distinctly possible that psychological influences on smoking behavior may thus prove to have a far greater impact than influences on biological pathways.

The Immune System Defends Against Cancer

There is now a voluminous research literature, including both preclinical (animal) and clinical studies, examining the role of the immune system in cancer. Various aspects of this multifaceted literature have been reviewed in depth elsewhere (10–17). In the brief

section that follows, we highlight a few of the key concepts and continuing controversies in this complex area of research. The history of cancer immunology over the past century has been characterized as "great expectations and bitter disappointments" (18). Clinicians have been tantalized by the potential promise of therapies designed to enhance putative immune defenses against cancer, while basic researchers have been stimulated by the possibility that the immune system may play a major role in preventing cancer by eliminating cells that have started down the pathway toward malignancy ("immune surveillance"). Overblown expectations born in the flush of initial successes have been followed by periods of disillusionment and undue pessimism when nonconfirming data emerges, a pattern that continues to the present day.

Fundamental Questions. Research in this field has largely been driven by four fundamental questions: *(1)* Are there characteristics of cancer cells (or premalignant cells) that allow them to be detected by the immune system (i.e., are transformed cells antigenic)? *(2)* Can the immune system mount a response to these cellular characteristics associated with the development of cancer (i.e., are transformed cells immunogenic)? *(3)* Can immune responses to premalignant and/or malignant cells protect the host against the development and/or progression of cancer? *(4)* Can interventions be devised to augment the immune system's capabilities to recognize, respond to, and protect against cancer?

Animal Cancer Models. The answers to these questions are much clearer in animal models than in humans. Based on one model or another among the thousands of published articles, the answer to each of these questions has been a resounding yes. To take just one well-cited example, a series of studies beginning in the 1940s demonstrated that prior immunization could protect inbred mice against the otherwise lethal effects of tumors transplanted from the same strain of mice (13). These studies provide evidence that some tumors (at least those induced by a particular carcinogen, MCA) bear antigens that can be recognized by the immune system (at least as inferred from the effect on the subsequent transplant), and can elicit specific responses (at least after vaccination of a healthy recipient) that provide protection against the lethal consequences of the identical tumor (at least when it is subsequently transplanted into the previously healthy host) in some inbred strains of mice. Although the data from this particular animal model are compelling, the parenthetical comments suggest some of the obvious limitations to the conclusions that can be drawn from even such classic studies as these. Perhaps most critically, one must question the relevance of a model based on previously primed (by immunization) specific host immune responses to the sudden appearance of a large transplanted tumor for our understanding of the responses to the development of spontaneous tumors (or even for our understanding of responses to residual tumor following surgery) (11).

Enthusiasm for the results with any particular tumor model in animals must be tempered by the recognition that other models yield other results, no doubt sometimes indicative of real biologic differences, but sometimes also indicative of experimental procedural differences. Cited out of context, results can be misleading. Findings from other well-designed studies have included tumors that failed to be antigenic; tumor antigens that failed to be immunogenic; immune responses to tumor antigens that failed to prevent the lethal consequences of tumors; the absence of specific immune effector mechanisms (e.g., cytotoxic T cells) but protective effects of nonspecific mechanisms (e.g., natural killer cells, cytokines); immune reactions to tumors that actually facilitated their growth; and so on (13,19). With regard to animal models, the literature thus suggests that the appropriate answer to the four fundamental questions we posed above is "it depends." It must also be emphasized that, while important to our understanding of our fellow species, the relevance of any animal model (including those involving "spontaneous" tumors) to our understanding of the processes involved in human cancer can be challenged on many grounds. For example, spontaneous tumors in mice often have a viral etiology and are rarely metastatic (13).

Detection of Cancer by the Immune System (Antigenicity). One important point that must be kept in mind when considering any area of research in oncology, but perhaps particularly when considering the role of the immune system, is that the term "cancer" encompasses a multitude of malignant neoplastic diseases that should not be viewed as homogeneous. Some of the differences among cancers are likely to have important implications for their interactions with the immune system (13). Some are known to have a viral etiology; such cancers would be likely to bear virus-associated determinants (antigens) that might be recognized by the immune system as "non-self" and specifically targeted for destruction (18). For example, Epstein–Barr Virus (EBV), which would typically cause a transient case of infectious mononucleosis, has been found to be related to the development of Burkitt's lymphoma, nasopharyngeal carcinoma, and immunoblastic lymphoma in individuals who are immunosuppressed (e.g., from malaria) (14). Other DNA viruses with apparent oncogenic effects, which may be exacerbated in immunosuppressed individuals, include hepatitis B virus, which is associated with hepatocellular carcinoma, and some types of human papilloma virus, which are associated with skin and urogenital cancers (e.g., cervical cancer) (4,13).

For the majority of human cancers, which are not virally induced, at least three other classes of proteins could conceivably serve as antigens that would allow the immune system to recognize the development of malignancy: *(1)* proteins encoded by one or more mutated oncogenes (e.g., p53); *(2)* unique proteins resulting from somatic mutation; *(3)* aberrantly expressed self-proteins (e.g., mucin) (18). Serologic evidence of antibodies to such proteins has been in the literature for over fifty years (13). More recently, it has been recognized that the protein need not be a constitutive part of the cell membrane. Basic research in immunology has revealed that intracellular proteins undergo a "processing" step, after which antigenic fragments are expressed on the cell surface in the peptide-binding groove of a major histocompatibility (MHC) molecule, where they are recognized by specific MHC-restricted T lymphocytes (18). In the past five years more than a dozen specific tumor antigens, all recognized by cytotoxic T lymphocytes from the patients who were the source of the tumor, have been characterized at the molecular level (16). One limitation of this approach, which focuses on patients in whom cancer has already been detected, is that one cannot tell when in the course of the multistep process of cancer development any particular antigen was first expressed; indeed, some antigens expressed early in the process of carcinogenesis may no longer be expressed by the time a tumor is large enough for clinical detection (and antigens associated with metastatic disease may not yet be expressed). It is tempting to speculate that the series of mutations in the preneoplastic cell, which are thought to be required for malignant transformation (20), may be paralleled by the sequential expression of their related proteins, which could provide the antigens needed for the immune system to detect and eliminate aberrant cells before they become malignant (i.e., immune surveillance against preneoplastic phenotypes).

Responses of the Immune System to Cancer (Immunogenicity). Consideration of the research on immune defenses against infectious disease suggests that immune defenses against cancer will similarly not be limited to one particular effector mechanism (e.g., cytotoxic T cells) (11). Although cancer researchers all too often assess only one immunologic mechanism at a time, multifactorial responses with overlapping "fields of fire" are likely to be the norm; increased activity in one domain could then compensate for deficiencies in another (11). Consistent with this view, virtually every known immune effector mechanism has been reported to be involved in the response to cancer (21). These include the highly specific responses of cytotoxic T cells and antibody-producing B cells (22). The binding of antibodies to tumor antigens, for example, has been reported to directly interfere with some cellular growth mechanisms; antibody-specific binding also classically triggers complement-mediated cell lysis, as well as antibody-dependent cellular cytotoxicity (ADCC), which is mediated by nonspecific effector cells that attach to the Fc region of the specific antibody molecule (e.g., natural killer cells, macrophages, granulocytes) (23). Although the molecular mechanisms have yet to be fully elucidated, natural killer (NK) cells are also capable of recognizing and killing tumor cells, particularly following stimulation by cytokines (e.g., interleukin-2 [IL-2]) (17). Macrophages have been reported not only to serve as antigen-presenting cells (required to activate antigen-specific helper T cells) but also to be capable of direct cytotoxic effects on tumors (although the tumor recognition mechanisms have yet to be determined) (22).

Assessment of immune responses to tumor antigens in cancer patients has typically revealed that such responses are weak or nonexistent, a finding that perhaps should be expected in individuals for whom putative immune surveillance mechanisms have obviously failed (22). Many factors have been hypothesized to contribute to this lack of immunogenicity. Although likely to differ among different types of cancer, and from individual to individual, these factors can be conceptually grouped as being either tumor-related or host-related (13). Tumor-related factors may include low expression of MHC class I molecules required for cytotoxic T cell recognition of antigen; shedding of antigen, resulting in tolerance induction; and production of factors inhibitory to immune function (13). Host-related factors may include immune suppression secondary to carcinogen exposure, infection, age, medical treatment, and stress (13,24). Surprising numbers of investigators interested in immune defenses in cancer patients fail to take into consideration the potential confounding effects of even obvious factors such as chemotherapy, which is known to have powerful, pervasive, and prolonged effects on the immune system (25). Inherited deficits in immune effector mechanisms, or intercellular amplification circuits (see below), could also contribute to poor antitumor responses (13). Reports of lower NK cell activity in individuals with family histories of cancer raise the possibility that inherited deficits in putative immune defense mechanisms may contribute to familial risk (26). On the other hand, we have argued that higher levels of stress in individuals at familial risk may contribute to their immunologic deficits (27).

Another major category of host-related factors that may contribute to poor immune defenses against cancer is deficiency in the cellular interactions within the immune system that determine whether a specific response will be generated at all (e.g., antigen presentation), and also determine the magnitude of the subsequent response (e.g., IL-2 secretion by "helper" T cells) (13). Accumulating evidence of the extensive cellular "cross-talk" required for an effective immune response suggests the difficulty of pinpointing the source of apparent deficiencies in any particular final effector mechanism (e.g., cytotoxic T cell killing of tumor cells). To take just one apposite example, basic research in immunology suggests that a signal from NK cells is necessary for the induction of cytotoxic lymphocytes (28).

Does the Immune System Protect Against the Development and/or Progression of Cancer? Investigation of the relationship between deficits in putative immune defense mechanisms and the subsequent development of cancer is difficult in humans for both ethical and pragmatic reasons. Ethically, one cannot randomly assign healthy individuals to receive immunosuppressive treatments.

Instead, investigations have focused on "natural experiments" with selected groups of individuals known to have deficits in immune function, such as congenital immune deficiencies, or chemotherapy-induced immune suppression (e.g., in transplant patients) (13). Such studies have provided little evidence of a general increase in the risk of cancer, although there is some evidence of increases in particular types of cancer (e.g., those with a viral etiology) (13). Alternative explanations for positive results are difficult to rule out. For example, the higher incidence of lymphopoietic cancers in individuals with congenital immune deficiencies may be a direct effect of the underlying genetic abnormalities; the higher incidence of some cancers in immunosuppressed chemotherapy patients may be due to the direct mutagenic/carcinogenic effects of the drugs (13).

The low incidence and slow development of cancer make it impractical to attempt to correlate results of assessments of immune function in healthy individuals with the subsequent development of disease; however, this approach has been taken in a few studies exploring the progression of cancer in previously diagnosed patients. Although controversial (again, confounding variables are a problem), there have been several reports (not without exception) of statistically significant relationships between various immune measures in cancer patients and the subsequent outcome of their disease. For example, in a study of 102 colorectal cancer patients, low levels of NK cell activity prior to surgery were found to be related to the risk of local recurrence of disease (17). In addition to differences in the activity of putative effector mechanisms (e.g., NK cell activity), assessments exploring individual differences in the strength of amplification mechanisms (e.g., IL-2 production) required for effective immune responses have also been reported to be related to the progression of disease. For example, postchemotherapy reductions in the proliferative responses of lymphocytes to in vitro challenge with the mitogen phytohemaglutinin (PHA) (an IL-2-dependent response) were reported to be related to the subsequent development of metastatic disease in a study of 90 breast cancer patients (29).

Perhaps the most compelling evidence that immune defenses can play a role in the progression of cancer has come from recent clinical studies of immunologic interventions, which have provided striking examples of clinical benefits to some patients (23,30,31). A wide range of interventions, including both nonspecific and specific strategies to augment putative immune defenses, are currently being investigated in clinical studies. Nonspecific approaches include infusions of cytokines (e.g., IL-2) (32). There is also continuing interest in the possible clinical efficacy of treatment with IL-2 in conjunction with tumor-infiltrating lymphocytes (TILs) isolated from the patient's own tumor and then expanded in vitro (22,32). Although vaccination with specific tumor antigens has generally not been found to elicit strong immune responses in patients who already have cancer, there is considerable interest in the possibility that specific responses could be effectively augmented by the addition of other non-specific stimuli (e.g., IL-2) (16).

Psychosocial Factors Affect the Immune System

As recently confirmed in a meta-analytic review (33), naturalistic studies have consistently found alterations in a number of measures of immune function in humans facing a variety of life events ("stressors"), even after controlling for behavioral variables (e.g., lack of sleep) that could affect immune function. For example, in an influential series of studies with medical student volunteers, Glaser, Kiecolt-Glaser, and colleagues have demonstrated the impact of academic examinations on a number of immune parameters, including decreased NK cell activity (34,35); lowered mitogen-induced lymphocyte proliferation (36,37); decreased mitogen-stimulated production of γ-interferon (35,37); lowered percentages of total T lymphocytes, T helper cells, and T suppressor cells (36); and increased plasma concentrations of immunoglobulin A (IgA), IgM, and IgG (34), as well as increased plasma levels of antibody to herpesviruses (interpreted as being due to reductions in cellular immune defenses to these viruses) (36,37).

Effects of Stressful Life Events. Changes in measures of immune function have also been detected following exposure to other, more major, stressful life events, such as surviving the death of a spouse (38–40). Bartrop and colleagues (38) were the first to investigate the effects of bereavement on the immune system. Comparing bereaved spouses to nonbereaved controls, they found that lymphocyte proliferation was lower in bereaved spouses. In a prospective study, Schleifer and colleagues (39) found that mitogen-induced lymphocyte proliferation was reduced in widowers during the first two months after the death of their spouse. Irwin and colleagues (41) found that, compared to nonbereaved controls, NK cell activity was lower among women whose husbands had recently died of cancer and among women whose husbands were terminally ill with cancer.

A number of other major stressful life events have also been reported to affect the immune system. These have included living close to Three-Mile Island at the time of the nuclear accident (42,43); enduring marital problems and divorce (44,45); taking care of sick relatives (46,47); being unemployed (48); and having a partner undergoing bone marrow transplantation (49). The most consistently reported immunologic changes in these studies have been reductions in in vitro measures of cell-mediated immune function (e.g, proliferative responses to T cell mitogens and natural killer (NK) cell activity) (33), but humoral immunity (antibody production) has also been reported to be affected (50). These naturalistic studies support the view that stressors can alter the activity of the immune system, but these studies have typically not examined the mechanisms responsible. Although it is generally assumed that the emotional distress elicited by the stressor represents the first step in a mechanistic pathway (which presumably includes stress-associated neuroendocrine changes), relatively little research has directly addressed this assumption. Statistical relationships between measures of affect and immune variables, however, have been reported both in naturalistic studies (51,52) and in studies of immune response to vaccinations (50).

Intervention Studies. Further support for the view that psychobehavioral variables may influence the immune system comes from psychosocial intervention studies. As has been reviewed elsewhere in more detail (53–55), immune measures in healthy individuals have been reported to be affected by a variety of behavioral intervention techniques, including relaxation (54), hypnosis (56), meditation (57), biofeedback (58), and self-disclosure (59–61). Interventions have also been conducted with patients suffering from various diseases, including cancer. For example, Fawzy and colleagues (62) have reported that a structured psychiatric intervention for newly diagnosed melanoma patients had both psychological and immunologic effects. Although not without exception (55), the literature is consistent with the view that such interventions can affect the immune system. The psychobiologic mechanisms responsible for these effects have yet to be determined. The interventions may affect various health behaviors (e.g., amount of sleep) known to influence immune function (63,64), as well as reduce subjective distress and its neuroendocrine consequences. Multiple factors may be the rule. Interestingly, following their intervention with cancer patients, Schedlowski and colleagues (65) observed increases in absolute numbers of white blood cells, which were paralleled by decreases in plasma levels of cortisol; however, statistical analyses suggested that these were not causally related.

The studies reviewed above provide strong support for the hypothesis that there are relationships between stressful life events, emotional distress, and alterations in immune function. Naturalistic studies, however, do not allow one to rule out the contribution of immunomodulatory factors such as nutrition, drug use, or sleep disturbances. There are difficulties in establishing causal relations between stress and immune changes owing to the correlational nature of the research as well as difficulties in studying the underlying biologic mechanisms (63). In an attempt to address these issues, researchers in human psychoneuorimmunology have recently turned to experimental models, long used by cardiovascular researchers (66,67). Acute changes in a number of immune measures (e.g., lymphocyte proliferation, NK cell activity, white cell counts) have been consistently reported in these studies and these have been found to be related to changes in neuroendocrine measures (e.g., plasma catecholamine levels) (68–71).

TYING IT ALL TOGETHER (MEDIATIONAL STUDIES)

The brief review of the three literatures underlying the conventional view of the role of psychoneuroimmunology and cancer suggests that the three links in the chain of reasoning (Fig. 12–1) are not individually as strong as is commonly assumed. To date, few investigators have attempted to directly examine each of the three links within the same study to determine the strength of their connection. In addition to the work of Fawzy and colleagues (see above), one must mention in this regard the early efforts of Levy, Herberman, and colleagues. These investigators examined the possibility that psychoimmune relations in early-stage breast cancer patients may play a role in prognosis (72). Using a quasi-prospective research design, these researchers found that women who were rated as well adjusted to their illness reported symptoms of fatigue, and perceived less social support had lower levels of NK cell activity. NK cell activity, in turn, was reported to be related to known prognostic variables (e.g., number of cancer-positive lymph nodes). Interestingly, at a 5-year follow up, NK cell activity predicted rate of progression, as did psychosocial factors, but the mediational influence was not established (72). Additional research along these lines is clearly needed. It is likely to prove difficult, however, given the complexity of psychobiologic interactions in cancer patients (see Fig. 12–2). To take just one example: chemotherapy treatment can increase psychological distress in cancer patients, which, as we have seen, can affect their immune systems; at the same time, chemotherapy has direct suppressive effects on the immune system, which can increase the risk of infection, which can (in turn) influence psychological and immune assessments.

THE CHUTZPAH HYPOTHESIS

As we have noted above, the evidence that the immune system is involved in the defense against cancer remains highly controversial. Until immunologists provide more compelling evidence for such immune defenses, should psychoneuroimmunology research in cancer be called to a halt? We think not. On the contrary, one can argue that relations between immune measures and cancer would become more evident if our colleagues in immunology were to take into account the effects of psychological factors on the immune system. Despite the powerful psychological consequences of cancer and its treatment, immunologic studies ignore psychological variables; indeed, published articles rarely even indicate under what circumstances blood was collected for immune assessments. Our colleagues have provoked the chutzpah hypothesis: the failure to control for the effects of psychological factors on the immune system may be one reason why the evidence for effective immune defenses against cancer is not yet compelling (1).

PSYCHONEUROIMMUNOLOGY AND CANCER: INFECTIOUS DISEASE

In all of the discussion above, the focus has been on psychological influences on putative immune defenses against cancer. Perhaps equally important, if not more so, are possible effects on immune defenses against infectious disease, which is a major source of morbidity and mortality in cancer patients. Accumulating evidence, reviewed elsewhere (73,74), supports the view that psychological stress can alter susceptibility to infectious disease, as well as the severity and duration of illness. The literature indicates that: *(1)* During periods of psychological stress, individuals *report* more upper respiratory infections and are more likely to seek medical attention. *(2)*

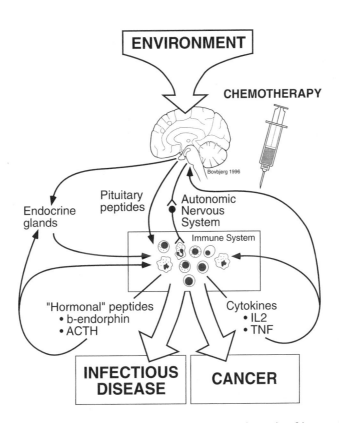

FIG. **12–2.** Psychoneuroimmunology and cancer: a schematic of interactions.

Periods of psychological stress are associated with increased numbers of *verified* upper respiratory infections. *(3)* Individuals with high levels of psychological stress have increased numbers of *verified* bacterial infections (e.g., streptococcal infections). *(4)* There is some evidence that psychological stress is associated with reactivation of latent viruses (e.g., herpes). In addition, recent experimental studies, in which volunteers were deliberately exposed to live rhinoviruses, have found relations between measures of stress and the incidence of verified infection, as well as the severity of cold symptoms (75,76).

Psychological influences on infectious disease may be particularly important in cancer patients, because these patients are likely to be emotionally distressed and to receive treatments (e.g., chemotherapy) known to suppress the immune system. This "double-whammy" may leave these patients particularly vulnerable to infectious disease, which continues to be the leading cause of cancer-related death (77). The impact of psychoimmune influences on infectious disease in cancer patients has received little research attention, although there is some initial data from our group that suggests that psychological distress on the day of patients' first chemotherapy infusion is predictive of their subsequent risk of infection (78).

PSYCHONEUROIMMUNOLOGY AND CANCER: A BROADER PERSPECTIVE

In all of the discussion above, the focus has been on the possible importance of psychological influences on the immune system. Research in psychoneuroimmunology has documented numerous pathways by which the central nervous system and the immune system may communicate with each other (see Fig. 12–2) (79). These efferent and afferent pathways provide communication loops likely to be involved in the day-to-day regulation of the immune system by the central nervous system (CNS), as well as in mediating the effects of psychological factors. Consistent with this view, both feed-back and feed-forward regulation of the immune system by the CNS have been documented (1). The possible importance of these nonpsychological aspects of research in psycho-*neuro*immunology to cancer has received little research attention. A greater understanding of these regulatory influences may suggest novel strategies to improve immune defenses against cancer (1).

CONCLUSIONS

According to the "conventional" view of the role of psychoneuroimmunogy in psycho-oncology, psychological influences on the immune system provide a mechanism for (mediate) the relationship between psychological factors and the development and/or progression of cancer. We have argued in this brief chapter that none of the links in this chain of reasoning should be accepted as well established. We have noted that greater appreciation of psychological influences on immune function might facilitate research efforts to understand the role of the immune system in cancer. We have emphasized the potential clinical significance of *psycho*immune interactions in infectious disease associated with cancer and its treatment. Finally, we have highlighted the importance of considering the potential of *neuro*immune interactions to influence immune defenses against cancer.

Psychoneuroimmunology research in oncology is in its infancy. Only additional rigorous research will determine whether the promise of its birth is fulfilled.

REFERENCES

1. Bovbjerg DH. Psychoimmunology: A critical analysis of the implications for clinical oncology in the 21st century. In: Lewis CE, O'Sullivan C, Barraclough J, eds. *The Psychoimmunology of Human Cancer*. Oxford: Oxford University Press; 1994: 417–426.
2. Chopra D. *Quantum Healing: Exploring the Frontiers of Mind/Body Medicine*. New York: Bantam Books; 1989.
3. Andersen BL, Kiecolt-Glaser JK, Glaser R. A biobehavioral model of cancer stress and disease course. *Am Psychol.* 1994; 49:389–404.
4. Goodkin K, Antoni MH, Sevin B, Fox BH. A partially testable, predictive model of psychosocial factors in the etiology of cervical cancer. II. Bioimmunological, psychoneuroimmunological, and socioimmunological aspects, critique and prospective integration. *Psycho-Oncology.* 1993; 2:99–121.
5. Berland W. Can the self affect the course of cancer? *Advances: J Mind-Body Health.* 1995; 11:5–39.
6. Block KI. The role of the self in healthy cancer survivorship: a view from the front lines of treating cancer. *Advances: J Mind-Body Health.* 1997; 13:6–26.
7. Fox BH. The role of psychological factors in cancer incidence and prognosis. *Oncology.* 1995; 9:245–255.
8. Schwartz R, Geyer S. Social and psychological differences between cancer and noncancer patients: cause or consequence of disease? *Psychother Psychosom.* 1984; 41:195–199.
9. Eysenck HJ. Synergistic interaction between psychosocial and physical factors in the causation of lung cancer. In: Lewis CE, O'Sullivan C, Barraclough J, eds. *The Psychoimmunology of Cancer.* New York: Oxford University Press; 1994: 163–178.
10. Woodruff MFA. Immunosurveillance. *Curr Opin Immunol.* 1989; 1:910–912.

11. Stutman O. Cancer. In: Nelson DS, ed. *Natural Immunity*. Boston: Academic Press; 1989: 749–794.

12. Herberman RB. Tumor immunology. *J Am Med Assoc.* 1992; 268:2935–2939.

13. Schreiber H. Tumor immunology. In: Paul WE, ed. *Fundamental Immunology*, 3d ed. New York: Raven Press; 1993:1143–1170.

14. Souberbielle B, Dalgleish A. Anti-tumour immune mechanisms. In: Lewis CE, O'Sullivan C, Barraclough J, eds. *The Psychoimmunology of Cancer*. New York: Oxford University Press; 1994: 267–290.

15. Roth C, Rochlitz C, Kourilsky P. Immune response against tumors. *Adv Immunol.* 1994; 57:281–351.

16. Cerottini J-C, Lienard D, Romero P. Recognition of tumor-associated antigens by T-lymphocytes: perspectives for peptide-based vaccines. *Ann Oncol.* 1996; 7:339–342.

17. Brittenden J, Heys SD, Ross J, Eremin O. Natural killer cells and cancer. *Cancer.* 1996; 77:1226–1243.

18. Greenberg PD, Riddell SR. Tumor-specific T-cell immunity: ready for prime time? *J Natl Cancer Inst.* 1992; 84:1059–1061.

19. Prehn RT, Prehn LM. The flip side of tumor immunity. *Arch Surg.* 1989; 124:102–106.

20. Vogelstein B, Kinzler KW. The multistep nature of cancer. *Trends Genet.* 1993; 9:138–141.

21. Roitt I. *Essential Immunology*, 8th ed. Boston: Blackwell Scientific; 1994.

22. Greenberg PD. Mechanisms of tumor immunology. In: Stites DP, Terr AI, eds. *Basic and Clinical Immunology*, 7th ed. Norwalk, CT: Appleton & Lange; 1991: 580–587.

23. Baxevanis CN, Papamichail M. Characterization of the anti-tumor immune response in human cancers and strategies for immunotherapy. *Crit Rev Oncol./Hematol.* 1994; 16:157–179.

24. Lewis CE, McGee JO. Natural killer cells in tumour biology. In: Lewis CE, McGee, JO, eds. *The Natural Immune System: The Natural Killer Cell*. Oxford: IRL Press; 1992:175–203.

25. Ehrke MJ, Mihich E, Berd D, Mastrangelo MJ. Effects of anticancer drugs on the immune system in humans. *Semin Oncol.* 1989; 16:230–253.

26. Whiteside TL, Herberman RB. Human natural killer cells in health and disease: biology and therapeutic potential. *Clin Imunother.* 1994; 1:56–66.

27. Bovbjerg DH, Valdimarsdottir H. Familial cancer, emotional distress, and low natural cytotoxic activity in healthy women. *Ann Oncol.* 1993; 4:745–752.

28. Kos FJ, Engleman EG. Immune regulation: a critical link between NK cells and CTLs. *Immunol Today.* 1996; 17:174–176.

29. Wiltschke C, Krainer M, Budinsky AC, et al. Reduced mitogenic stimulation of peripheral blood mononuclear cells as a prognostic parameter for the course of breast cancer: a prospective longitudinal study. *Br J Cancer.* 1995; 71:1292–1296.

30. Mukherji B, Chakraborty NG. The features of immune response to melanoma in vivo. *Curr Opin Oncol.* 1995; 7:175–184.

31. Goey SH, Verweij J, Stoter G. Immunotherapy of metastatic renal cell cancer. *Ann Oncol.* 1996; 7:887–900.

32. Takaku F. Clinical application of cytokines for cancer treatment. *Oncology.* 1994; 51:123–128.

33. Herbert TB, Cohen S. Stress and immunity in humans: a meta-analytic review. *Psychosom Med.* 1993; 55:364–379.

34. Kiecolt-Glaser JK, Garner W, Speicher C, Penn GM, Holliday J, Glaser R. Psychosocial modifiers of immunocompetence in medical students. *Psychosom Med.* 1984; 46:7–14.

35. Glaser R, Rice J, Speicher CE, Stout JC, Kiecolt-Glaser JK. Stress depresses interferon production by leukocytes concomitant with a decrease in natural killer cell activity. *Behav Neurosci.* 1986; 100:675–678.

36. Glaser R, Kiecolt-Glaser J, Stout J, Tarr K, Speicher C, Holliday J. Stress-related impairments in cellular immunity. *Psychiatry Res.* 1985; 16:233–239.

37. Glaser R, Rice J, Sheridan J, et al. Stress-related immune suppression: Health implications. *Brain Behav Immun.* 1987; 1:7–20.

38. Bartrop RW, Lockhurst E, Lazarus L, Kiloh LG, Penny R. Depressed lymphocyte function after bereavement. *Lancet.* 1977; 1:834–836.

39. Schleifer SJ, Keller SE, Camerino M, Thornton JC, Stein M. Suppression of lymphocyte stimulation following bereavement. *J Am Med Assoc.* 1983; 250:374–377.

40. Irwin M, Daniels M, Bloom ET, Smith TL, Weiner H. Life events, depressive symptoms, and immune function. *Am J Psychiatry.* 1987; 144:437–441.

41. Irwin M, Daniels M, Smith TL, Bloom ET, Weiner H. Impaired natural killer cell activity during bereavement. *Brain Behav Immun.* 1987; 1:98–104.

42. Baum A, Gatchel RJ, Schaeffer MA. Emotional, behavioral, and physiological effects of chronic stress at Three Mile Island. *J Consult Clin Psychol.* 1983; 5:565–572.

43. McKinnon W, Weisse CS, Reynolds CP, Bowles CA, Baum A. Chronic stress, leukocyte subpopulations, and humoral response to latent viruses. *Health Psychol.* 1989; 8:389–402.

44. Kiecolt-Glaser J, Fisher LD, Ogrocki P, Stout J, Speicher C, Glaser R. Marital quality, marital disruption, and immune function. *Psychosom Med.* 1987; 49:13–34.

45. Kiecolt-Glaser JK, Kennedy S, Malkoff S, Fisher L, Speicher CE, Glaser R. Marital discord and immunity in males. *Psychosom Med.* 1988; 50:213–229.

46. Kiecolt-Glaser JK, Glaser R, Dyer C, Shuttleworth E, Ogrocki P, Speicher CE. Chronic stress and immunity in family caregivers of Alzheimer's disease victims. *Psychosom Med.* 1987; 49:523–535.

47. Kiecolt-Glaser JK, Dura JR, Speicher CE, Trask OJ, Glaser R. Spousal caregivers of dementia victims: longitudinal changes in immunity and health. *Psychosom Med.* 1991; 53:345–362.

48. Arnetz BB, Wasserman J, Petrini B, Brenner SO, Levi L, Eneroth P. Immune function in unemployed women. *Psychosom Med.* 1987; 49:3–12.

49. Futterman AD, Wellisch DK, Zighelboim J, Luna-Raines M, Weiner H. Psychological and immunological reactions of family members to patients undergoing bone marrow transplantation. *Psychosom Med.* 1996; 58:472–489.

50. Stone AA, Bovbjerg DH. Stress and humoral immunity: a review of the human studies. *Adv Neuroimmunol.* 1994; 4:49–56.

51. Stone AA, Cox DS, Valdimarsdottir H, Jandorf L, Neale JM. Evidence that secretory IgA antibody is associated with daily mood. *J Pers Soc Psychol.* 1987; 52:988–993.

52. Valdimarsdottir H, Bovbjerg DH. Positive and negative mood: Association with natural killer cell activity. *Psychol Health.* 1997; 12:319–327.

53. Kiecolt-Glaser J, Glaser R. Psychoneuroimmunology: Can psychological intervention modulate immunity? *J Consult Clin Psychol.* 1992; 60:569–575.

54. Van Rood Y, Bogaards M, Goulmy E, van Houwelinger HC. The effects of stress and relaxation on the in vitro immune response in man: a meta-analytic study. *J Behav Med.* 1993; 16:163–181.

55. Ironson G, Antoni M, Lutgendorf S. Can psychological interventions affect immunity and survival? Present findings and suggested targets with a focus on cancer and human immunodeficiency virus. *Mind/Body Med.* 1995; 1:85–110.

56. Zachariae R, Bjerring P, Arendt-Nielsen L. Modulation of type I immediate and type IV delayed immunoreactivity using direct suggestion and guided imagery during hypnosis. *Allergy.* 1989; 44:537–542.

57. Smith GR, McKenzie JM, Marmer DJ, Steele RW. Psychologic modulation of the human immune response to varicella zoster. *Arch Intern Med.* 1985; 145:2210–2212.

58. McGrady A, Conran P, Dickey D. The effects of biofeedback-assisted relaxation on cell mediated immunity, cortisol, and white blood cell count in healthy adult subjects. *Behav Med.* 1992; 15:343–354.

59. Pennebaker JW, Kiecolt-Glaser JK, Glaser R. Disclosure of traumas and immune function: health implications for psychotherapy. *J Consult Clin Psychol.* 1988; 56:239–245.

60. Esterling BA, Antoni MH, Kumar M, Schneiderman N. Emotional repression, stress disclosure responses, and Epstein-Barr viral capsid antigen titers. *Psychosom Med.* 1990; 52:397–410.

61. Christensen AJ, Edwards DL, Wiebe JS, et al. Effect of verbal self-disclosure on natural killer cell activity: moderating influence of cynical hostility. *Psychosom Med.* 1996; 58:150–155.

62. Fawzy FI, Fawzy NW, Hyun CS. Short-term psychiatric intervention for patients with malignant melanoma: Effects on psychological state, coping, and the immune system. In: Lewis CE, O'Sullivan C, Barraclough J, eds. *The Psychoimmunology of Cancer.* New York: Oxford University Press; 1994: 292–319.

63. Kiecolt-Glaser JK, Glaser R. Methodological issues in behavioral immunology research with humans. *Brain Behav Immun.* 1988; 2:67–78.

64. Irwin M, Smith TL, Gillin JC. Electroencephalographic sleep and natural killer activity in depressed patients and control subjects. *Psychosom Med.* 1992; 54:10–21.

65. Schedlowski M, Tewes U, Schmoll HJ. The effects of psychological intervention on cortisol levels and leukocyte numbers in the peripheral blood of breast cancer patients. In: Lewis CE, O'Sullivan C, Barraclough J, eds. *The Psychoimmunology of Cancer.* New York: Oxford University Press; 1994: 336–348.

66. Kiecolt-Glaser JK, Cacioppo JT, Malarkey WB, Glaser R. Editorial comment. Acute psychological stressors and short term immune changes: What, why, for whom, and to what extent? *Psychosom Med.* 1992; 54:680–685.

67. Schneiderman N, Weiss SM, Kaufman PG. *Handbook of Research Methods in Cardiovascular Behavior Medicine.* New York: Plenum; 1989.

68. Manuck SB, Cohen S, Rabin BS, Muldoon MF. Prediction of individual differences in cellular immune response to stress. *Psychol Sci.* 1991; 2:111–115.

69. Zakowski SG, McAllister CG, Deal M, Baum A. Stress, reactivity, and immune function in healthy men. *Health Psychol.* 1992; 11:223–232.

70. Herbert TB, Cohen S, Marsland AL, et al. Cardiovascular reactivity and the course of immune response to an acute psychological stressor. *Psychosom Med.* 1994; 56:337–344.

71. Cacioppo JT. Social neuroscience: autonomic, neuroendocrine, and immune responses to stress. *Psychophysiology.* 1994; 31:113–128.

72. Levy ML, Roberts DC. Clinical significance of psychoneuroimmunology: prediction of cancer outcomes. In: Schneiderman N, McCabe P, Baum A, eds. *Stress and Disease Processes.* Hillsdale, NJ: Lawrence Erlbaum; 1992: 165–174.

73. Cohen S, Williamson GM. Stress and infectious disease in humans. *Psychol Bull.* 1991; 109:5–24.

74. Bovbjerg DH, Stone AA. Psychological stress and upper respiratory illness. In: Friedman H, Klein T, Friedman A, eds. *Psychoneuroimmunology, Stress, and Infection.* Boca Raton, FL: CRC Press; 1996: 195–213.

75. Cohen S, Tyrrell DAJ, Smith A. Psychological stress and susceptibility to the common cold. *N Engl J Med.* 1991; 325:606–612.

76. Stone AA, Bovbjerg DH, Neale JM, et al. Development of common cold symptoms following experimental rhinovirus infection is related to prior stressful life events. *Behav Med.* 1992; 18:115–120.

77. White MH. Prevention of infection in patients with neoplastic disease: use of a historical model for developmental strategies. *Clin Infect Dis.* 1993; 17:S355–358.

78. Bovbjerg DH, Valdimarsdottir HB. Stress, immune modulation, and infectious disease during chemotherapy for breast cancer. *Ann Behav Med.* 1996; 18:S63.

79. Madden KS, Felten DL. Experimental basis for neural-immune interactions. *Physiol Rev.* 1995; 75:77–106.

13

Psychoneuroendocrinology and Cancer

DOMINIQUE L. MUSSELMAN, J. STEVEN McDANIEL,
MARYFRANCES R. PORTER, AND CHARLES B. NEMEROFF

In the past thirty years, literally hundreds of reports document hypothalamic–pituitary–adrenal (HPA) axis hyperactivity in patients with major depression. Unfortunately, few of these neuroendocrine and neuroanatomical alterations have been systematically investigated in medically ill populations. Such biologic markers are potentially valuable as adjuncts in the diagnosis of depression in those patients who represent diagnostic conundrums; the medically ill are an example of such patients. Furthermore, as state-dependent variables, certain of these markers may reflect and even portend treatment response in patients with depression (1). We will briefly discuss the rationale underlying the use of neuroendocrine measures of function and structural imaging in patients with affective disorders, review the three studies of depression in patients with cancer that have utilized such markers, and discuss the interplay of mood, neuroendocrine pathophysiology, and cytokine-mediated immune alterations in a particular neoplasm, pancreatic adenocarcinoma.

BIOLOGIC MARKERS OF DEPRESSION

In the search for the underlying pathophysiology of the major psychiatric disorders, neuropeptides, in general, and hypothalamic releasing factors, in particular, have been scrutinized closely. Undoubtedly one rationale for such intensive study in patients with primary psychiatric disorders is the higher than expected psychiatric morbidity in patients with primary endocrine disorders such as Addison's disease or Cushing's syndrome. However, the "neuroendocrine window strategy" remains the essential impetus for continuing investigation of the major endocrine axes in psychiatric disorders. This so-called strategy is based on a large literature which indicates that the secretion of the target endocrine organs, e.g., the adrenal or thyroid, is largely controlled by their respective pituitary trophic hormone, which in turn is controlled primarily by the secretion of their respective hypothalamic release and/ or release-inhibiting hormone. There is now considerable evidence that the secretion of these hypothalamic hypophysiotropic hormones is controlled by many of the classical neurotransmitters such as serotonin (5-HT), acetylcholine (ACh), and norepinephrine (NE), all previously posited to play a preeminent role in the pathophysiology of affective, anxiety, and/or psychotic disorders. The hypothesis that one can infer information about higher CNS neuronal activity, as for example the activity of serotonergic neurons in a particular disease state, solely by measuring the activity of a specific endocrine axis, is, however, far from proven.

What the "neuroendocrine window strategy" has provided, however, is clear evidence for alterations of endocrine axes in psychiatric illness and an appreciation of the complexity of neuropeptidergic neuronal circuits and hypothalamic releasing factors in man. Whether alterations in peripheral hormone secretion contribute primarily to the pathogenesis of psychiatric disorders or conversely whether altered secretion of pituitary and hypothalamic hormones primarily contribute to the signs and symptoms of one or another mental illness remains a subject of considerable controversy.

Of the many neuroendocrine systems studied in depression, alterations of three endocrine axes have been the best characterized: the hypothalamic–pituitary–adrenal (HPA) axis, the hypothalamic–pituitary–thyroid (HPT) axis, and the hypothalamic–growth hormone (HGH) axis. HPA axis hyperactivity as evidenced by increased urinary free cortisol levels, cortisol nonsuppression to dexamethasone, a blunted corticotropin (ACTH) response to corticotropin-releasing factor (CRF), elevated cerebrospinal fluid (CSF) CRF concentrations, and adrenal and pituitary hypertrophy have all been reported in patients with major depression. Alterations in the HPT axis have also been reported in depression including a blunted thyrotropin (TSH) response to thyrotropin-releasing hormone (TRH), elevated CSF TRH concentrations, and an unusually high prevalence rate of symptomless autoimmune thyroiditis. Alterations of the HGH axis in patients with unipolar depression include a blunted GH response to clonidine and reduced CSF somatostatin concentrations.

Serotonergic and noradrenergic neuronal circuits have long been implicated in the pathophysiology of mood disorders. Alterations in serotonergic neurotransmission observed in patients with major depression include: reduced CSF 5-hydroxyindoleacetic acid (5HIAA) concentrations, diminished density of brain and platelet 5-HT transporter binding, increased platelet and brain 5-HT$_2$ receptor binding, and a blunted prolactin response to fenfluramine. Patients with major depression also exhibit increased brain and lymphocyte β-adrenergic receptor binding density, and decreased urinary catecholamine metabolite excretion.

Functional [positron emission tomography (PET) and single photon emission computed tomography (SPECT)] and structural [computed tomography (CT) and magnetic resonance imaging (MRI)] brain abnormalities have also been observed in depressed patients, the latter including subcortical and periventricular hyperintensities as well as decreased volume of specific cortical and subcortical (e.g. caudate, putamen) structures. Furthermore, derangements in sleep architecture as assessed by polysomnography including reduced rapid eye movement (REM) latency, redistribution of REM sleep, and decreased delta wave production have been observed in patients with primary depression. Although numerous putative biologic markers of primary depression have been identified, none has been yet validated in depressed patients with any co-morbid medical illness.

We will later review the only three investigations that have incorporated biologic markers in the study of cancer patients with depression (2–4). All of these studies examined the HPA axis, while one also evaluated the HPT axis (3). We will first discuss the most intensely scrutinized neuroendocrine system in depression, the HPA axis.

ALTERATIONS OF THE HYPOTHALAMIC–PITUITARY–ADRENAL AXIS IN DEPRESSION

Hyperactivity of the HPA axis has been documented in literally hundreds of studies of drug-free patients with primary major depression. This hyperactivity is currently thought to be due largely to hypersecretion of CRF from paraventricular hypothalamic neurons, which results in anterior pituitary ACTH hypersecretion, which in turn results in adrenocortical glucocorticoid hypersecretion. CRF-containing circuits in the CNS not only play a seminal neuroendocrine role but coordinate behavioral, autonomic, and immune responses of mammals to stress. As noted above, CRF-containing neurons within the hypothalamus project from the paraventricular nucleus to the median eminence (5) controlling the secretion of ACTH and ß-endorphin secretion from the anterior pituitary (6). Extrahypothalmic CRF neurons likely play a preeminent role in the regulation of both affective and anxiety states. When injected directly into the CNS of laboratory animals, CRF produces many effects similar to the signs and symptoms of depression, e.g., disrupted sleep, diminished libido, and decreased appetite.

Increased CSF CRF concentrations have repeatedly been observed in drug-free patients with major depression (7–11) and in depressed suicide victims (8). Moreover the elevations in CRF concentrations observed in major depression normalize with clinical recovery following treatment with electroconvulsive therapy (12) and antidepressants (13). In fact, persistently elevated CSF CRF concentrations may predict early relapse despite symptomatic improvement (14). A reduction in CSF CRF concentrations occurs in normal volunteers following treatment with the tricyclic antidepressant desipramine (15).

The CRF stimulation test is one method by which the activity of the HPA axis can be assessed. CRF is administered intravenously (usually 1 µg/kg) and the resulting ACTH (or β-endorphin) and cortisol response is measured over the next 2–to 3 h. (16,17). The ACTH and β-endorphin response to intravenously administered ovine CRF is blunted in drug-free depressed patients (18–23). This blunted response occurs in depressed patients who are dexamethasone nonsuppressors (see later) but not in those who are dexamethasone suppressors (24).

The majority of investigations of HPA axis activity in patients with depression have utilized measures of adrenocortical function, e.g., increased plasma corticosteroid concentrations (25,26) and elevated levels of cortisol metabolites (27). Moreover, increased 24 h urinary free cortisol concentrations and nonsuppression of plasma hydroxycorticosteroid levels after the administration of dexamethasone [utilizing the dexamethasone suppression test (DST)] have been reported. In the standard DST paradigm, patients ingest 1 mg of the synthetic glucocorticoid dexamethasone by mouth at 11 P.M. Blood samples for measurement of cortisol concentrations are obtained the following day at 4 P.M.

and 11 P.M.. Approximately 50%–67% of patients with major depression exhibit plasma cortisol concentrations above 5 ng/ml in contrast to that observed in virtually all normal controls who suppress plasma cortisol concentrations to levels below this concentration. Since Carroll's (28) initial report in 1968 and subsequent claims for diagnostic utility (29), the DST has generated considerable controversy (30). Most investigators agree that the rate of cortisol nonsuppression after administration of dexamethasone correlates with depression severity. Indeed, nearly all patients with major depression with psychotic features exhibit dexamethasone nonsuppression (31–34); this diagnosis is extremely rare in cancer patients. Furthermore, dexamethasone nonsuppressors exhibit not only elevated CSF CRF concentrations (see later) but, as noted above, a blunted ACTH response to intravenously administered CRF (35,36). One factor that may contribute to dexamethasone nonsuppression is the more rapid metabolism of this synthetic glucocorticoid in depressed patients when compared to normal controls (37).

Anatomical abnormalities of components of the HPA axis have been observed in depression, perhaps in part in response to hypersecretion of CRF and other hypothalamic hypophysiotropic hormones. Depressed patients have been reported to exhibit pituitary gland enlargement (38), which correlates with post-dexamethasone cortisol concentrations (39). Adrenal gland enlargement has also been reported in depressed patients utilizing computed tomography (40,41) and magnetic resonance imaging (42), as well as in postmortem suicide victims (43,44); This is likely due to chronic ACTH hypersecretion. Adrenocortical hypertrophy may explain the fact that although the ACTH and β-endorphin response to CRF is blunted, the plasma cortisol response is not significantly different in depressed patients compared to normal controls (18,19,20,21,22,45). Therefore, with each pulse of ACTH in depressed patients with enlarged adrenal cortices, greater quantities of cortisol would be secreted compared to normal controls. Adrenocortical hypertrophy would also explain the exaggerated cortisol response to pharmacologic doses of ACTH in depressed patients (20,46–49).

In summary, the multitude of studies that report HPA axis hyperactivity in depressed patients can be explained by hypersecretion of CRF during and/or immediately preceding a depressive episode with secondary pituitary and adrenal gland hypertrophy and hypersecreton of ACTH and cortisol, respectively. Dysregulation of the HPA axis as reflected by dexamethasone nonsuppression and elevated CSF CRF

concentrations usually normalizes after recovery from depression (12,13,28,33) and may help predict early relapse (14,33). Normalization of abnormal DST results, like hypercortisolemia (27), CRF hypersecretion (12), blunting of the ACTH response to CRF (21), and adrenal gland hypertrophy (42), occurs upon clinical recovery.

ALTERATIONS OF THE HYPOTHALAMIC–PITUITARY–ADRENAL AXIS IN DEPRESSED PATIENTS WITH CANCER

Three studies have studied neuroendocrine dysfunction in patients with cancer (2–4); all have utilized the standard 1 mg DST. Evans, Nemeroff, and their colleagues (2) conducted a study of 83 women with gynecological cancer (cervical, endometrial, or vaginal) Psychiatric morbidity and neuroendocrine function were scrutinized in these patients. Major depression was diagnosed in 23% ($n = 19$) of the women with cancer, and adjustment disorder with depressed mood was diagnosed in 24% ($n = 20$). Of the depressed cancer patients, 40% ($n = 8$) exhibited dexamethasone nonsuppression. Interestingly, many of the women diagnosed with adjustment disorder with depressed mood also exhibited dexamethasone nonsuppression. These investigators also performed TRH stimulation tests on their cohort; a blunted thyrotropin (TSH) response to TRH was observed in 29% ($n = 6$) of those patients with a diagnosis of major depression and in 43% ($n = 9$) of those women who fulfilled criteria for adjustment disorder with depressed mood. Of paramount importance is the finding that these rates for DST nonsuppression and the blunted TSH response to TRH are similar to rates observed in psychiatric inpatients with primary depression *without* cancer.

Joffe and colleagues (3) reported a 50% prevalence rate of major depression in patients with pancreatic cancer ($n = 9$) compared to 11% in patients with gastric cancer ($n = 11$). The DST was then administered to a subgroup of these patients (6 patients with pancreatic cancer and 6 patients with gastric cancer). Although only 1 of these 6 pancreatic cancer patients fulfilled the diagnosis of major depression, they all exhibited DST nonsuppression. Remarkably, 5 of the 6 patients with gastric cancer (none with major depression) also exhibited DST nonsuppression. These findings remain difficult to interpret because of the absence of DST testing of the depressed patients with cancer, lack of dexamethasone plasma measurements, and the small sample size of the study. Nevertheless, these results suggest that the DST may not be a useful adjunct in the diagnosis of depression in patients with gastric and pancreatic cancer.

·In our ongoing study, we are seeking to determine the rates of the psychiatric co-morbidity, particularly depression in cancer patients, with a focus on pancreatic and breast cancer (4). Thus far, in comparison to other cancers, adenocarcinoma of the pancreas is associated with the highest rate of major depression (see Chapter 45). Indeed, case studies and clinical reports indicate that depressive symptoms in patients with pancreatic cancer may *precede* the onset of physical symptoms that typically are attributed to this cancer (50). In our study, 3 of 5 patients with pancreatic cancer reported a major depressive episode in the month prior to their diagnosis of cancer, whereas only 1 of 18 other patients with cancer (11 with breast cancer, 6 with esophageal cancer, and 1 with gastric cancer) reported this phenomenon ($p = 0.002$) (4).

Furthermore, nonsuppression of plasma cortisol concentrations following dexamethasone administration occurred in 2 of the 3 patients with pancreatic cancer who were tested, whereas nearly all of the other patients with cancer (6 of 11) exhibited dexamethasone suppression. As expected, the DST discriminated between the normal controls ($n = 5$) and the depressed controls ($n = 5$). Four of five of the normal controls exhibited DST suppression, whereas all of the depressed controls (primary depression without cancer) exhibited DST nonsuppression ($p = 0.048$).

Our study essentially confirms the findings of both Joffe et al. (2) and Evans et al. (3) in that many cancer patients exhibit dysregulation of the HPA axis that is similar to that observed in depressed patients without cancer. However, considerably more data is necessary in cancer patients before firm conclusions can be drawn concerning the diagnostic utility of neuroendocrine testing in cancer patients.

THE HYPOTHALAMIC–PITUITARY–ADRENAL AXIS AND IMMUNE DYSFUNCTION IN CANCER PATIENTS

Activation of the HPA Axis by the Immune System

The immune system has the capacity not only to sense the presence of foreign molecules but also to communicate this information to the brain and neuroendocrine system via cytokines, hormones secreted by cells of the immune system, and inflammatory mediators (51). This "communication" between the immune and neuroendocrine systems (52) is embodied by the increased pituitary and adrenocortical secretion that occurs in response to infection or inflammation. Circulating cytokines such as interleukin-1 (IL-1),

interleukin-6 (IL-6), and tumor necrosis factor (TNF) account for most of the HPA axis-stimulating activity in plasma (53). Exerting one of the most powerful stimulatory influences on the HPA axis of any substance yet discovered, IL-1 is now known to induce fever, and slow-wave sleep, and to alter CNS activity (54–56). Indeed, intrahypothalamic infusion of IL-1 initiates a classic stress response by directly stimulating release of hypothalamic CRF (57), thereby elevating ACTH secretion, which in turn increases circulating glucocorticoid levels (58–61). Similarly, stimulation of the HPA cascade induced by systemic administration of IL-2 was demonstrated in a preliminary report of 30 cancer patients (62). In humans, Il-6 elevates plasma concentrations of corticotropin and cortisol well above the concentrations achieved with maximal stimulating doses of CRF (63–64). Marked elevations of plasma glucocorticoids, either by administration of exogenous steroids or by administration of substances which markedly elevate circulating steroids such as the cytokine γ-interferon (65) result in the depression in a large number of cases (66).

Stress-Related HPA Axis Hyperactivity and Tumor Growth

Syndromal major depression is believed by many to be, at least in part, a psychological stress reaction gone awry, particularly the stress related to the personal and social loss and disruption experienced by many patients with cancer (67). Whether through stress-induced (e.g., inflammation or infectious challenge) cytokine release or via CRF hypersecretion associated with major depression, HPA hyperactivity in patients with cancer may exert untoward effects on immunological function. Activation of the HPA axis subsequently reduces the intensity of the immune response, because virtually all components of the immune response are inhibited by cortisol and related glucocorticoids. Glucocorticoids not only influence the movement of circulating leukocytes but inhibit many functions of leukocytes and immune accessory cells (68–71), including the reduction of circulating T cell subsets (72). In a series of elegant studies, investigators have shown that intracerebroventricular (ICV) injection of CRF in rats reduces splenic NK cell numbers, splenic and peripheral blood NK cell activity, and lymphocyte response to mitogenic stimulation (62,73). The diminished NKA linked to ICV CRF administration may play a role in understanding the possible immunosuppressive influence of the HPA axis in patients with cancer. Particularly relevant is the observation that HPA hyperactivity induced by exposure to stress is associated with increased tumor growth in rats, particular in the aged (60).

Studies that examine in vitro immune changes linked to HPA dysregulation may offer important information about the possible in vivo interplay among the endocrine, nervous, and immune systems, particularly in depressed patients with cancer. Although numerous investigators have examined the relationship of stress and immune function, the impact of stress on the development and clinical outcome of cancer remains unknown (74). Laboratory animal studies have clearly documented the profound effects of stress on the immune system (75,76) but clinical studies have provided more conflicting findings. Numerous studies addressing the effect of depression on immune function have appeared in recent years (77–81); this literature has been difficult to interpret because of multiple and complex methodological issues including sample size, control group composition, diagnostic heterogeneity, overlapping databases, and assay techniques (77). Furthermore, even though a recent meta-analysis (82) found substantial evidence for a relationship between depression and immunity for both immunocyte population numbers and functional measures of immune function, Stein and colleagues (79) have discussed the inherent complications in conducting such a metaanalysis on a database with such methodologically diverse studies. Nonetheless, gender, age, and depression severity appear to be important variables (77,79,81). The underlying pathophysiologic mechanism(s) of how depression affects immune function in humans remain obscure, as does which patient subpopulations are affected. The findings of Levy and colleagues (83) that psychosocial variables such as depressive symptoms and lack of social support may be linked to reduced NKA in women with breast cancer clearly illuminate the need for more research in this area, including research on neuroendocrine and immune measures in patients with cancer. From a psychoneuroimmune and endocrine standpoint, such studies may help clarify the later findings of Levy and colleagues (84) that more metastatic nodes and increased NKA were associated with depressive symptoms in their patients with breast cancer, as well as the finding of Sapolsky and Donnelly (60) that stress-induced HPA hyperactivity is associated with increased tumor growth.

Tumor-Derived Factors, Depression, and Immune Dysfunction

Important factors in the relationship between certain types of cancer and depression may be the proinflammatory cytokines IL-1, IL-6, and TNF. These three inflammatory cytokines activate the HPA axis independently; however, in combination, their effects are synergistic (85–90). Such cytokines may be produced by host cells in response to cancer or may even be derived from the neoplasm itself. Certain cancer cells are known to release IL-1, e.g., renal cell carcinoma and Hodgkin's lymphoma (54). Pancreatic islet cells produce IL-6 when exposed to TNF (91), and IL-1 and IL-6 after viral infection (92). Yamaguchi and colleagues have also (93) isolated a novel cytokine from a human pancreatic tumor cell line.

Tumor-induced inflammation may be another mechanism whereby proinflammatory cytokines IL-1, IL-6, and TNF are produced. Sites of inflammation contain large amounts of immunoreactive CRF, mostly within immune accessory cells and inflammatory exudate (94). Although mild in severity, the pancreatitis associated with primary pancreatic tumors exists in approximately 10% of pancreatic cancer patients (95). Moreover, the proteolytic capacity of the pancreas has been clearly recognized since 1838 (96), as well as its capacity for autodigestion due to release and intrapancreatic activation of digestive enzymes (97). Such release of active digestive enzymes is accompanied by subsequent release of soluble mediators such as IL-1 and IL-6 by pancreatic acinar cells (98). Reflecting the severity of pancreatitis (99), IL-6 in turn induces hepatic synthesis of C-reative protein (CRP) as well as other acute-phase proteins. One study (100) found that 45% of 21 pancreatic cancer patients exhibited evidence of this inflammatory response, i.e., increased serum concentrations of CRP in comparison to healthy controls. Furthermore, those pancreatic cancer patients that exhibited this inflammatory response exhibited significantly increased secretion of TNF and IL-6 by isolated peripheral blood mononuclear cells in vitro. An integral component of any inflammatory process, enhanced secretion of cytokines and subsequent increased HPA axis hyperactivity (e.g., nonsuppression of cortisol secretion) in some patients with pancreatic cancer may together contribute to the oft-observed signs and symptoms of major depression in this population.

CONCLUSIONS AND FUTURE INVESTIGATIONS

Approximately thirty years of investigations of the physiologic alterations associated with unipolar depression have resulted in the discovery of so-called biologic markers, measures that presumably reflect the underlying pathophysiologic processes of this affective disorder. Of all of these markers, the most intensively studied and well characterized has been hyperactivity of the HPA axis. Specifically, elevated CSF concentrations of CRF, a blunted ACTH response to CRF, and dexamethasone nonsuppression reflect the HPA axis hyperactivity associated with major depression. HPA axis hyperactivity can also be induced through increased secretion or exogenous administration of cytokines. In response to stress, including infectious or inflammatory challenge, cytokine-induced hypothalamic secretion of CRF may contribute to the affective syndrome of unipolar depression in patients with and without cancer. Remarkably, dysregulation of the HPA axis as reflected by elevated CSF CRF concentrations usually normalizes after recovery with effective treatment with either electroconvulsive therapy (12) or antidepressants (13). Not only does antidepressant treatment alleviate the signs and symptoms of unipolar depression, such as abnormal sleep, but these drugs also diminish perceived levels of pain in patients with cancer. Remarkably, only two research groups have investigated antidepressant drug treatment of patients with cancer in controlled studies (101,102). Unfortunately, measurement of HPA axis activity and immune function were not investigated in either study. Treatment of depression in cancer patients with diminished risk of serious complications and intolerable side effects is now possible with the selective serotonin reuptake inhibitors (SSRIs). Because these agents are newer than the tricyclic antidepressants and monoamine oxidase inhibitors, no systematic research on their efficacy in cancer patients has been performed. Our research group has recently begun a randomized, double-blind, multicenter study of paroxetine vs. desipramine and placebo in breast cancer patients with major depression or adjustment disorder with depressed mood. The efficacy of antidepressant activity, side-effect profiles, and impact upon HPA axis activity and immune function will be compared. Future research will determine whether normalization of HPA axis activity in patients with cancer via somatic (antidepressant or electroconvulsive therapy) treatment is associated with alterations of cytokine plasma concentrations (e.g., diminution of IL-1, IL-6, or TNF). Furthermore, future inquiries must determine whether neurochemical and neuroendocrine alterations in cancer patients are due to depression and not merely an epiphenomenon of a single symptom such as pain. It will be equally important to determine that biologic alterations in depressed patients are not simply due to altered metabolism, such as altered metabolic rates, of dexamethasone, for example. Such investigations must consider the importance of utilizing standardized methods of diagnosis (with structured interviews) and assessing the effects of age, gender,

hospitalization status, tumor site, type, grade, stage, time since knowledge of diagnosis, pain, psychiatric history, genetic vulnerability to mood disorders, and measures of immune status on their outcome measures. These details of the exceedingly complex interplay between optimal immune function, neuroendocrine function, and emotional state remain to be explored.

ACKNOWLEDGMENTS

This work was supported by NIMH MH49523, NIH RR000039, and NIH DK07298.

REFERENCES

1. Ribeiro SCM, Tandon R, Grunhaus L, et al. The DST as a predictor of outcome in depression: a meta-analysis. *Am J Psychiatry.* 1993; 150:1618–1629.
2. Joffe RT, Rubinow DR, Denicoff KD, Maher M, Sindelar WF. Depression and carcinoma of the pancreas. *Gen Hosp Psychiatry.* 1986; 8:241–245.
3. Evans DL, McCartney CF, Nemeroff CB, et al. Depression in women treated for gynecological cancer: clinical and neuroendocrine assessment. *Am J Psychiatry.* 1986; 143(4):447–452.
4. Musselman DL, Nemeroff CB, McDaniel JS, et al. Cancer and depression: diagnostic considerations and biologic markers. Presented at the 32nd Annual Meeting of the American College of Neuropsychopharmacology; December 14, 1993; Honolulu, Hawaii.
5. Swanson LW, Sawchenko PE, Rivier J, Vale W. Organization of ovine corticotropin-releasing factor immunoreactive cells and fibers in the rat brain: an immunohistochemical study. *Neuroendocrinology.* 1993; 36:165–186.
6. Vale W, Spiess J, Rivier C, Rivier J. Characterization of a 41-residue ovine hypothalamic peptide that stimulates secretion of corticotropin of β-endorphin. *Science.* 1981; 213:1394–1397.
7. Nemeroff CB, Evans DL. Correlation between the dexamethasone suppression test in depressed patients and clinical response. *Am J Psychiatry.* 1984; 141:247–249.
8. Arato M, Banki CM, Nemeroff CB, Bissette G. Hypothalamic-pituitary-adrenal axis and suicide. *Ann NY Acad Sci.* 1986; 487:263–270.
9. Banki CM, Bissette G, Arato M, O'Connor L, Nemeroff CB. CSF corticotropin-releasing factor-like immunoreactivity in depression and schizophrenia. *Am J Psychiatry.* 1987; 144(7):873–877.
10. France RD, Urban B, Krishnan KR, et al. CSF corticotropin-releasing factor-like immunoreactivity in chronic pain patients with and without major depression. *Biol Psychiatry.* 1988; 23(1):86–88.
11. Risch SC, Lewine RJ, Kalin NH, et al. Limbic-hypothalamic-pituitary-adrenal axis activity and ventricular-to-brain ration studies in affective illness and schizophrenia. *Neuropsychopharmacology.* 1992; 6:95–100.
12. Nemeroff CB, Bissette G, Akil H, Fin M. Neuropeptide concentrations in the cerebrospinal fluid of depressed patients treated with electroconvulsive therapy: cortico-

tropin-releasing factor, beta-endorphin and somatostatin. *Br J Psychiatry.* 1991; 158:59–63.

13. De Bellis MD, Gold PW, Geracioti TD Jr., Listwak SJ, Kling MA. Association of fluoxetine treatment with reductions in CSF concentrations of corticotropin-releasing hormone and arginine vasopressin in patients with major depression. *Am J Psychiatry.* 1993; 150(4):656–657.

14. Banki CB, Karmacsi L, Bissette G, et al. CSF corticotropin-releasing hormone and somatostatin in major depression: response to antidepressant treatment and relapse. *Eur Neuropsychopharmacol.* 1992; 2(2):107–113.

15. Veith RC, Lewis N, Langohr JI, et al. Effect of desipramine on cerebrospinal fluid concentrations of corticotropin-releasing factor in human subjects. *Psychiatry Res.* 1992; 46:1–8.

16. Hermus AR, Pieters GF, Pesman GJ, et al. Differential effects of ovine and human corticotropin-releasing factor in human subjects. *Clin Endocrinol (Oxf).* 1984; 21(5):589–595.

17. Watson SJ, Lopez JF, Young EA, Vale W, Rivier J, Akil H. Effects of low-dose ovine corticotropin-releasing hormone in humans: endocrine relationships and beta-endorphin/ beta-lipotropin responses. *J Clin Endocrinol Metab.* 1986; 66:10–15.

18. Gold PW, Chrousos G, Kellner C, et al. Psychiatric implications of basic and clinical studies with corticotropin-releasing factor. *Am J Psychiatry.* 1984; 141(5):619–627.

19. Gold PW, Loriaux DL, Roy A, et al. Responses to corticotropin-releasing hormone in the hypercortisolism of depression and Cushing's disease: pathophysiologic and diagnostic implications. *N Engl J Med.* 1986; 314(21):1329–1335.

20. Holsboer F, von Bardeleben U, Gerken A, Stalla GK, Muller OA. Blunted corticotropin and normal cortisol response to human corticotropin-releasing factor in depression. *N Engl J Med.* 1984; 311(17):1127.

21. Amsterdam JD, Maislin G, Winokur A, Berwish N, Kling M, Gold P. The oCRH test before and after clinical recovery from depression. *J Affect Disord.* 1988; 14(3):213–222.

22. Kathol RG, Jaeckle RS, Lopez JR, Mullter WH. Consistent reduction of ACTH responses to stimulation with CRH, vasopressin and hypoglycemia in patients with depression. *Br J Psychiatry.* 1989 155:468–478.

23. Young EA, Watson SJ, Kotun J, et al. β-lipotropin–β-endorphin response to low-dose ovine corticotropin releasing factor in endogenous depression. *Arch Gen Psychiatry.* 1990; 47: 449–457.

24. Krishnan KRR, Rayasam K, Reed D, et al. The corticotropin releasing factor stimulation test in patients with major depression: relationship to dexamethasone suppression test results. *Depression.* 1993; 1:133–136.

25. Gibbons JL, McHugh PR. Plasma cortisol in depressive illness. *J Psychiatr Res.* 1962; 1:162–171.

26. Carpenter WT Jr., Bunney WE Jr. Adrenal cortical activity in depressive illness. *Am J Psychiatry.* 1971; 128(1):31–40.

27. Sachar E, Hellman L, Fukushima D, Gallagher T. Cortisol production in depressive illness. *Arch Gen Psychiatry.* 1970; 23:289–298.

28. Carroll BJ, Martin FI, Davies B. Pituitary-adrenal function in depression. *Lancet.* 1968; 1(556):1373–1374.

29. Carroll BJ. Use of the dexamethasone suppression test in depression. *J Clin Psychiatry.* 1982; 43(11 Pt 2):44–50.

30. Arana GW, Mossman D. The dexamethasone suppression test and depression: approaches to the use of a laboratory test in psychiatry. *Neurol Clin.* 1988; 6(1):21–39.

31. Evans DL, Nemeroff CB. Use of the dexamethasone suppression test using DSM-III criteria on an inpatient psychiatric unit. *Biol Psychiatry.* 1983; 18(4):505–511.

32. Schatzberg AF, Rothschild AJ, Bond TC, Cole JO. The DST in psychotic depression: diagnostic and pathophysiologic implications. *Psychopharmacol Bull.* 1984; 20:362–364.

33. Arana GW, Baldesarrini RJ, Ornsteen M. The dexamethasone suppression test for diagnosis and prognosis in psychiatry. *Arch Gen Psychiatry.* 1985; 42(12):1193–1204.

34. Krishnan KRR, France RD, Pelton S, McCann UD, Manepalli AN, Davidson JR. What does the dexamethasone suppression test identify? *Biol Psychiatry.* 1985; 20:957–964.

35. Roy A, Pickar D, Paul S, Doran A, Chrousos GP, Gold PW. CSF corticotropin-releasing hormone in depressed patients and normal control subjects. *Am J Psychiatry.* 1987; 144:641–645.

36. Pitts AF, Kathol RG, Gehris TL, et al. Elevated cerebrospinal fluid corticotropin-releasing hormone and arginine vasopressin in depressed patients with dexamethasone nonsuppression [abstract]. *Soc Neurosci Abstr.* 1990, 16: 454.

37. Ritchie JC, Belkin BM, Krishnan KRRK, Nemeroff CB, Carroll BJ. Plasma dexamethasone concentrations and the dexamethasone suppression test. *Biol Psychiatry.* 1990; 27:159–173.

38. Krishnan KRR, Doraiswamy PM, Lurie SN, et al. Pituitary size in depression. *J Clin Endocrinol Metab.* 1991; 72:256–259.

39. Axelson DA, Doraiswamy PM, Boyko OB, et al. In vivo assessment of pituitary volume with magnetic resonance imaging and systematic sterology: relationship to dexamethasone suppression test results in patients. *Psychiatry Res.* 1992; 44(1):63–70.

40. Amsterdam JD, Marinelli DL, Arger P, Winokur A. Assessment of adrenal gland volume by computed tomography in depressed patients and healthy volunteers: a pilot study. *Psychiatry Res.* 1987; 21(3):189-197.

41. Nemeroff CB, Krishnan KRR, Reed D, Leder R, Beam C, Dunnick NR. Adrenal gland enlargement in major depression: a computed tomographic study. *Arch Gen Psychiatry.* 1992; 49:384–387.

42. Rubin RT, Philips JJ, Sadow TF, et al. Adrenal gland volume in major depression: increase during the depressive episode and decrease with successful treatment. *Arch Gen Psychiatry.* 1995; 52(3):213–218.

43. Zis KD, Zis A. Increased adrenal weight in victims of violent suicide. *Am J Psychiatry.* 1987; 144:1214–1215.

44. Szigethy E, Conwell Y, Forbes NT, Cox C, Caine ED. Adrenal weight and morphology in victims of completed suicide. *Biol Psychiatry.* 1994; 36(6):374–380.

45. Amsterdam JD, Winokur A, Abelman E, Lucki I, Rickels K. Cosyntropin (ACTH alpha 1-24) stimulation test in depressed patients and healthy subjects. *Am J Psychiatry*. 1983; 140(7):907–909.

46. Kalin NH, Risch SC, Janowsky DS, Murphy DL. Plasma ACTH and cortisol concentrations before and after dexamethasone. *Psychiatry Res*. 1982; 7:87–92.

47. Linkowski P, Mendlewicz J, LeClerq R, et al. The 24-hour profile of ACTH and cortisol in major depressive illness. *J Clin Endocrinol Metab*. 1985; 61:429–438.

48. Jaeckle RS, Kathol RG, Lopez JF, Meller WH, Krummel SJ. Enhanced adrenal sensitivity to exogenous ACTH stimulation in major depression. *Arch Gen Psychiatry*. 1987; 44:233–240.

49. Krishnan KRR, Ritchie JC, Saunders WB, Nemeroff CB. Adrenocortical sensitivity to low-dose ACTH administration in depressed patients. *Biol Psychiatry*. 1990; 27:930–933.

50. Green AL, Austin CP. Psychopathology of pancreatic cancer: a psychobiological probe. *Psychosomatics*. 1993; 34(3):208–221.

51. Reichlin S. Neuroendocrine-immune interactions. *N Engl J Med*. 1993; 329:1246-1253.

52. Blalock JE. A molecular basis for bidirectional communication between the immune and neuroendocrine systems. *Physiol Rev*. 1989; 69(1):1–32.

53. Chrousos GP. The hypothalamic–pituitary–adrenal axis and immune-mediated inflammation. *N Engl J Med*. 1995; 332(20):1351–1362.

54. Dinarello CA. Interleukin-1. *Rev Infect Dis*. 1984; 6(1):51–95.

55. Krueger JM, Walter J, Dinarello CA, Wolff SM, Chedid L. Sleep-promoting effects of endogenous pyrogen (interleukin-1). *Am J Physiol*. 1984; 246(6 Pt 2):R994–999.

56. Tobler I, Borbely AA, Schwyzer M, Fontana A. Interleukin-1 derived from astrocytes enhances slow wave activity in sleep EEG of the rat. *Eur J Pharmacol*. 1984; 104(1-2):191–192.

57. Barbanel G, Ixart G, Szafarczyk A, Malaval F, Assenmacher I. Intrahypothalamic infusion of interleukin-1 beta increases the release of corticotropin-releasing hormone (CRH 41) and adrenocorticotropic hormone (ACTH) in free-moving rats bearing a push-pull cannula in the median eminence. *Brain Res*. 1990; 516(1):31–36.

58. Besedovsky H, del Rey A, Sorkin E, Dinarello CA. Immunoregulatory feedback between interleukin-1 and glucocorticoid hormones. *Science*. 1986; 233(4764):652–654.

59. Berkenbosch F, van Oers J, del Rey A, Tilders F, Besedovsky H. Corticotropin-releasing factor-producing neurons in the rat activated by interleukin-1. *Science*. 1987; 238(4826):524–526.

60. Sapolsky RM, Donnelly TM. Vulnerability to stress-induced tumor growth increases with age in rats: role of glucocorticoids. *Endocrinology*. 1985; 117:662–666.

61. Sundar SK, Becker KJ, Cierpial MA, et al. Intravcerebroventricular infusion of interleukin-1 rapidly decreases peripheral cellular immune responses. *Proc Natl Acad Sci USA*. 1989; 86(16):6398–6402.

62. Denicoff KD, Durkin TM, Lotze MT, et al. Neuroendocrine effects of interleukin-2 treatment. *J Clin Endocrinol Metab*. 1989; 69(2):402–410.

63. Mastorakos G, Chrousos GP, Weber JS. Recombinant interleukin-6 activates the hypothalamic- pituitary-adrenal axis in humans. *J Clin Endocrinol Metab*. 1993; 77:1690–1694.

64. Mastorakos G, Weber JS, Magiakou MA, Gunn H, Chrousos GP. Hypothalamic-pituitary- adrenal axis activation and stimulation of systemic vasopressin secretion by recombinant interleukin 6 in humans: potential implications for the syndrome of inappropriate vasopressin secretion. *J Clin Endocrinol Metab*. 1994; 79:934–939.

65. Holsboer F, Stalla GK, von Bardeleben U, Hammann K, Muller H, Muller OA. Acute adrenocortical stimulation by recombinant gamma interferon in human controls. *Life Sci*. 1988; 42(1):1–5.

66. Adams F, Quesada JR, Gutterman JU. Neuropsychiatric manifestations of human leucocyte interferon therapy in patients with cancer. *J Am Med Assoc*. 1984; 252(7): 938–941.

67. O'Leary A. Stress, emotion, and human immune function. *Psychol Bull*. 1990; 108:363–382.

68. Chrousos GP, Gold PW. The concepts of stress and stress system disorders: overview of physical and behavioral homeostasis. *J Am Med Assoc*. 1992; 267(9):1244–1252. [Published erratum appears in 1992; 268(2):200.]

69. Chrousos GP. Regulation and dysregulation of the hypothalamic-pituitary-adrenal axis: the corticotropin-releasing hormone perspective. *Endocrinol Metab Clin North Am*. 1992; 21(4):833–858.

70. Boumpas DT, Chrousos GP, Willder RL, Cupps TR, Balow JE. Glucocorticoid therapy for immune-mediated diseases: basic and clinical correlates. *Ann Intern Med*. 1993; 119(12):1198–1208.

71. Chrousos GP, Detera-Wadleigh SD, Karl M. Syndromes of glucocorticoid resistance. *Ann Intern Med*. 1993; 119(11):1113–1124.

72. Cupps TR, Fauci AS. Corticosteroid-mediated immunoregulation in man. *Immunol Rev*. 1982; 65:134–155.

73. Straubaugh H, Irwin M. Central corticotropin-releasing hormone reduces cellular immunity. *Brain Behav Immun*. 1992; 6:11–17.

74. Schulz KH, Schulz H. Overview of psychoneuroimmunological stress and intervention studies in humans with emphasis on the uses of immunological parameters. *Psycho-Oncology*. 1992; 1:51–70.

75. Weiss JM, Sundar S. Effects of stress on cellular immune responses in animals. In: Tasman A, Riba MB, eds. *American Psychiatric Press Review of Psychiatry*. Washington, DC: American Psychiatric Press; 1992; 11:145–168.

76. Coe CL. Psychosocial factors and immunity in nonhuman primates: a review. *Psychosom Med*. 1993; 55(3):298–308.

77. Scheifer SJ, Keller SE, Meyerson AT, Raskin MJ, Davis KL, Stein M. Lymphocyte function in major depressive disorder. *Arch Gen Psychiatry*. 1984; 41:484–486.

78. Scheifer SJ, Keller SE, Bond RN, Cohen J, Stein M. Major depressive and immunity: role of age, sex, sever-

ity, and hospitalization. *Arch Gen Psychiatry.* 1989; 46:81–87.

79. Stein M, Miller AH, Trestman RL. Depression, the immune system, and health and illness. *Arch Gen Psychiatry.* 1991; 48:171–177.

80. Rabkin JG, Williams JB, Remien RH, Gooetz R, Kertzner R, Gorman JM. Depression, distress, lymphocyte subsets, and human immunodeficiency virus symptoms on two occasions in HIV-positive homosexual men. *Arch Gen Psychiatry.* 1991; 48:111–119.

81. Evans DL, Folds JD, Petitto JM, et al. Circulating natural killer cell phenotypes in men and women with major depression: relation to cytotoxic activity and severity of depression. *Arch Gen Psychiatry.* 1992; 49(5):388–395.

82. Herbert TB, Cohen S. Depression and immunity: a meta-analytic review. *Psychol Bull.* 1993; 113(3):472–486.

83. Levy SM, Herberman RB, Lippman M, d'Angelo T. Correlation of stress factors with sustained depression of natural killer cell activity and predicted prognosis in patients with breast cancer. *J Clin Oncol.* 1987; 5:348–353.

84. Levy SM, Herberman RB, Whitside T, Sanzo K, Lee J, Kirkwood J. Perceived social support and tumor estrogen/progesterone receptor status as predictors of natural killer cell activity in breast cancer patients. *Psychosom Med.* 1990; 42:73–85.

85. Imura H, Fukata J, Mori T. Cytokines and endocrine function: an interaction between the immune and neuroendocrine systems. *Clin Endocrinol (Oxf).* 1991; 35(2):107–115.

86. Bernardini R, Kamilaris TC, Calogero AE, et al. Interactions between tumor necrosis factor-alpha, hypothalamic corticotropin-releasing hormone, and adrenocorticotropin secretion in the rat. *Endocrinology.* 1990; 126(6):2876–2881.

87. Sapolsky R, Rivier C, Yamamoto G, Plotsky P, Vale W. Interleukin-1 stimulates the secretion of hypothalamic corticotropin-releasing factor. *Science.* 1987; 238: 522–524.

88. Naitoh Y, Fukata J, Tominaga T, et al. Interleukin-6 stimulates the secretion of adrenocorticotropin hormone in conscious, free-moving rats. *Biochem Biophys Res Commun.* 1988; 155(3):1459–1463.

89. Perlstein RS, Mougey EH, Jackson WE, Neta R. Interleukin-1 and interleukin-6 act synergistically to stimulate the release of adrenocorticotropin hormone in vivo. *Lymphokine Cytokine Res.* 1991; 10:141–146.

90. Perlstein RS, Whitnall MH, Abrams JS, Mougey EH, Neta R. Synergistic roles of interleukin-6, interleukin-1, and tumor necrosis factor in adrenocorticotropin response to bacterial lipopolysaccharide in vivo. *Endocrinology.* 1993; 132: 946–952.

91. Campbell IL, Cutri A, Wilson CA, Harrison LC. Evidence for IL-6 production by and effects on the pancreatic beta cell. *J Immunol.* 1989; 143(4):1188–1191.

92. Cavallo MG, Baroni MG, Toto A, et al. Viral infection induces cytokine release by beta islet cells. *Immunology.* 1992; 75(4); 664–668.

93. Yamaguchi N, Hattori K, Masayoshi O, Kojima T, Imai N, Ochi N. A novel cytokine exhibiting megakaryocyte potentiating activity from a human pancreatic tumor cell line HPC-Y5. *J Biol Chem.* 1994; 269: 805–808.

94. Karalis K, Sano H, Redwne J, Listwak S, Wilder RL, Chrousos GP. Autocrine or paracrine inflammatory actions of corticotropin-releasing hormone in vivo. *Science.* 1991; 254:421–423.

95. Kohler H, Lankisch PG. Acute pancreatitis and hyperamylasaemia in pancreatic carcinoma. *Pancreas.* 1987; 2(1):117–119.

96. Purkinje JE, Pappenheim S. Vorlaufige Mitteilung aus einer Untersuchung uber kunstliche Verdauung. *Arch Ant Phys Wissen Med.* 1838; 1; 14–27.

97. Chiarai H. Uber die Selbstverdauung des menschlichen Pankreas. *Z Heilk.* 1896; 17; 69–96.

98. Lerch MM, Adler G. Acute pancreatitis. *Curr Opin Gastroenterol.* 1992; 8:817–823.

99. Leser HG, Gross V, Scheibenhogen C, et al. Evaluation of serum interleukin-6 concentration precedes acute phase response and reflects severity in acute pancreatitis. *Gastroenterology.* 1991; 101:782–785.

100. Falconer JS, Fearon KC, Plester CE, Ross JA, Carter DC. *Ann Surg.* 1994; 219(4):325–331.

101. Costa D, Mogos I, Toma T. Efficacy and safety of mianserin in the treatment of depression of women with cancer. *Acta Psychiatr Scand Suppl.* 1985; 320:85–92.

102. Evans DL, McCartney CF, Haggerty JJ. Treatment of depression in cancer patients is associated with better life adaptation: a pilot study. *Psychosom Med.* 1988; 50:72–76.

III

PSYCHOLOGICAL ISSUES IN CANCER SCREENING

Editor: PAUL B. JACOBSEN

14

Psychological Responses to Tumor Markers

DEBRA L. FERTIG AND DANIEL F. HAYES

Tumor markers are defined as genetic and/or biochemical changes that can be identified in association with a neoplastic deviation from normalcy. These changes can be detected using a variety of technologies, including immunologic and genetic assays. The development of these newer technologies has resulted in examples of potentially useful markers for a variety of clinical situations, including estimates of the risk, presence, status, or future behavior of malignancy. Ostensibly, marker results should allow clinicians to provide better care than if they were unaware of these data. Unfortunately, tumor marker results are often obtained without consideration of the clinical consequence that they might affect. Along with this exciting new technology comes the need to be aware of the psychological impact of conveying information about the status of these tumor markers to patients. In this review we will discuss the basic principles of tumor marker utility, and then we will place the emotional impact of tumor marker results in their proper perspective.

UTILITIES OF TUMOR MARKERS

In order to understand how the technology of tumor markers translates into clinical practice, it is helpful to place their potential use into categories representing several clinical situations (Table 14.1). For example, tumor markers might be used to identify individuals who are at high genetic risk for cancer for whom prevention and/or screening and early treatment might be effective. Tumor markers might also be helpful to screen an "at risk" population to detect clinically occult cancers at an early stage. Furthermore, in patients with established malignancy, tumor markets could be used to predict the risk of future relapse, to

predict the odds of responding to a specific type of therapy, or to monitor patients after primary therapy in order to detect occult recurrent disease prior to clinical manifestations. For those patients with clinically detectable metastases, tumor markers might be useful for monitoring clinical course during follow-up, particularly to determine benefits from and response to therapy. Standard use of a marker in routine clinical practice should only be recommended if the marker reliably adds to the clinician's judgment during clinical decision making, resulting in a more favorable clinical outcome for the patient (1). These outcomes include improved overall survival (OS), disease-free survival (DFS), and quality of life (QOL). A fourth outcome would be decreased cost of care while maintaining each of the first three outcomes (Table 14.2).

Patients with a malignancy principally hope that therapy will result in a cure or at least in a substantially longer life span than if they were not treated. In the absence of cure or OS prolongation, patients might wish to be treated in order to remain free of detectable disease for a substantial time period (DFS). Presumably, these patients will benefit from existing in a disease-free state even if OS is not prolonged because they will either not suffer from the physical effects of gross disease or not suffer from the emotional turmoil generated by knowledge of recurrence. In many instances, quality of life (QOL) assessment may be considered a more meaningful endpoint than DFS. Recent advances in the science of evaluating QOL should allow correlation between tumor marker-induced changes in clinical practice and patients' feeling of well-being.

Even if practice changes do not positively benefit the patient in terms of OS, DFS, or QOL, a reduction in cost of practice while achieving similar outcomes is a

TABLE 14.1. *Utilities of Tumor Markers*

Risk assessment
Screening of healthy individuals
Determination of prognosis
Monitoring for relapse and evaluation during course of metastatic disease

TABLE 14.2. *Outcomes to be Improved by Tumor Marker Results*

Cure rates
Overall survival
Disease-free survival
Quality of life, palliation
Decreased cost

worthwhile endeavor. Reduction in costs could occur as a result of elimination of redundant tests or more efficient use of specific therapies.

PERFORMANCE CHARACTERISTICS OF TUMOR MARKERS

For any diagnostic test, it is important to draw correlations between the result of the test and the process it is reputed to indicate. These correlations, termed "performance characteristics," include sensitivity and specificity within the known population to be tested (Table 14.3). *Sensitivity* is the proportion of people who have the disease detected and who have a positive tumor marker result. *Specificity* is the proportion of people who do not have the disease and whose assay results are negative. The performance of tumor markers in any given population is measured by a test's predictive value, which is a function of the likelihood that the predicted event will occur: *positive* (the proportion of people with positive tests found to have disease) and *negative* (the proportion of people with negative tests found not to have disease). Thus, even a very good test may be of less worth in a population of individuals not likely to suffer the event, and a test with lower sensitivity and specificity might be of great value in a population in which the disease/event is quite common. The performance characteristics for the tumor marker tests we will be discussing in this chapter depend on the disease, the marker, and the study design, and may be reviewed elsewhere (1).

POSSIBLE STATISTICAL BIASES IN TUMOR MARKER USE

Tumor marker data provide estimates of the likelihood of some event's future occurrence. In other words, one is "screening" for a possible future event with the assumption that the knowledge can be used to improve a clinical outcome. In this regard, the lessons taken from screening studies in general pertain to tumor marker use in any situation. When evaluating the clinical outcomes affected by tumor markers in any of the situations discussed earlier, one must bear in mind four biases inseparable from screening for cancer: lead time, length time, selection, and overdiagnosis (Table 14.4) (2).

Lead time bias occurs when the point of diagnosis has been advanced by the application of a screening test even if overall survival is not lengthened. Thus, if tumor marker results provide earlier detection, the time from detection to the relevant event (such as mortality) is lengthened. *Length time bias* relates to the fact that fast-growing tumors will progress rapidly through the preclinical detectable phase. Thus, tumors detected by screening tests have an inherently better prognosis than those not detected by screening. *Selection bias* relates to the inevitable self-selection for participation in screening programs. Part of this effect is offset by the self-selection of individuals with increased risk. *Overdiagnosis bias* results from the detection by screening of lesions of questionable malignancy that might never have been diagnosed in the absence of screening. Although screening-detected lesions are generally associated with a very good prognosis, it is not clear how many might actually be clinically irrelevant.

TABLE 14.3. *Performance Characteristics of Tumor Markers*

Sensitivity
Specificity
Positive predictive value
Negative predictive value

TABLE 14.4. *Possible Statistical Biases in Tumor Marker Use*

Lead time bias
Length bias
Selection bias
Overdiagnosis bias

These four biases contribute to the difficulty in assessment of the utility of a tumor marker unless a prospectively identified control group is an integral part of the study design. Evaluation of any tumor marker use, therefore, has to be performed with a methodology that avoids these biases, such as random selection of control subjects.

POTENTIAL TUMOR MARKERS FOR USE IN CLINICAL PRACTICE

Although many markers have been proposed for a variety of malignancies, few have actually been widely used clinically within the confines of the previous discussion. Table 14.5 provides a list of recently identified or commonly used markers for specific uses, and the following discussions review these in greater detail.

Identification of Risk. Identification of patients at higher risk to develop cancer has two potential utilities. First, identification of various risk factors might permit insight into the cause and biology of the disease. Second, identification of risk factors permits more efficient application of preventive and/ or screening maneuvers, if these are available. Recent studies have identified several genes that might be associated with the development of cancer. For example, members of families with the Li–Fraumeni syndrome have an extraordinarily high risk of developing multiple epithelial and mesenchymal

TABLE 14.5. *Potential Tumor Markers for Use in Clinical Practice*

RISK ASSESSMENT
BRCA1: brest and ovarian cancer
p53: Li-Fraumeni syndrome
2p (*MsH1*): colon cancer

SCREENING HEALTHY INDIVIDUALS
PSA: prostate cancer

DETERMINATION OF PROGNOSIS
PSA: prostate cancer
Estrogen and progesterone receptors: Breast cancer
CA125: ovarian cancer
CEA: colon cancer

MONITORING FOR RELAPSE AND EVALUATION DURING COURSE OF METASTATIC DISEASE
CA15-3: breast, colon, lung, and ovarian cancer
CEA: colon, lung, and breast cancer
CA125: ovarian and breast cancer
PSA: prostate cancer

cancers at very early ages (3). In about one-half of these families, affected individuals carry mutations in one allele of the tumor suppressor gene *p53* (4). Recently a gene on chromosome 17q, designated as *BRCA1*, which confers increased susceptibility to the development of early-onset breast and ovarian cancers, has been cloned (5). Although abnormalities in *BRCA1* only account for a small percentage of those patients likely to get breast cancer, the cloning of this gene has been a significant step forward in the development of tests for genetic screening of women at risk for breast cancer, as well as for research on the etiology of inherited breast cancer syndromes.

Additionally, two separate investigators have reported that mutations and/or deletions in a gene located on 2p (*MsH1*) are associated with familial colon cancers (6,7). It is estimated that individuals born with abnormalities in this gene will have a lifetime risk of colon cancer approximating 90%. Moreover, a number of other susceptibility genes have been identified for less common malignancies, such as retinoblastoma, Wilm's tumor, medullary thyroid carcinoma, medulloblastoma, and hepatoblastoma.

In summary, a rapidly increasing number of cancer susceptibility genes have been or are being identified and cloned. Commercially available tests to determine whether an individual carries an abnormality in one or more of these genes will soon be available.

Screening Healthy Individuals. One of the basic tenets of oncology has been that malignancies are, in general, more effectively treated if detected early. For example, mammographic screening trials demonstrate that early detection and treatment results in reduced mortality due to breast cancer (8–10). The dramatic decline in cervical cancer mortality in the Western world has been attributed to screening Papanicolau tests (11). Although controversial, studies suggest that early detection and treatment of colonic malignancies results in improved survival rates (12). Unfortunately, screening has not been demonstrated to effectively reduce mortality due to other common malignancies, such as lung, prostate, or ovarian cancers (13–16). It is hoped that in the future genetic or biochemical markers of early malignancy might provide inexpensive, low-risk, and potentially more effective means of monitoring for early malignant changes.

Circulating tumor markers, such as CA125, CA15-3, carcinoembryonic antigen (CEA), and prostate specific antigen (PSA), offer a particularly convenient and appealing method of screening. Unfortunately, no currently available biochemical or genetic test or circulating marker has been shown to be sufficiently sensitive or tumor-specific to be of value for wide-scale screening with the possible exception of PSA for prostate cancer (16,17).

Determination of Prognosis. Another use of tumor markers is to determine whether a patient with newly diagnosed cancer has been rendered free of malignancy after initial therapeutic efforts, or whether that patient has residual microscopic disease and is at risk for future local and/or distant relapse. Such patients might then be candidates for further local or systemic therapy. For the most part, most prognostic factors are tissue-based, although in some cases soluble and/or circulating markers might be of value.

If effective adjuvant systemic therapy is available, markers to predict distant relapse are very important. For example, in breast cancer, many putative prognostic factors have been proposed that might be more powerful than nodal status or might further divide node-positive and node-negative patients into those likely or not likely to recur. These include ER, PR, S-phase fraction and other markers of cellular turnover, certain oncogene/protooncogene abnormalities (overexpression of HER-2/*neu*, p53 mutations), neovascularization, and certain enzyme activities. However, the precise clinical utility of these markers in treatment planning has not been determined (18).

Adjuvant systemic therapy has not been proven to be as beneficial in other epithelial malignancies, although recent data indicate that patients with poor prognosis colon cancer achieve increased survival after adjuvant chemotherapy (19). Therefore, the search for prognostic factors has been less compelling in non-breast malignancies. Nonetheless, certain biologic factors have been reported to predict systemic relapse in patients with lung, colon, prostate, bladder, and ovarian cancers.

In addition to predicting growth rate and/or metastatic potential (i.e., likelihood of residual malignancy and ultimate relapse), tumor markers might also predict response to specific therapies. Indeed, it has been well established that response to hormone therapy in breast cancer patients is directly related to tissue content of both ER and PR (20). Therefore, levels of ER and PR not only predict prognosis but help guide the specific type of systemic therapy that is most appropriate for a particular patient. Likewise, elevated postoperative CA125 levels are highly predictive of recurrence, and are an indication for adjuvant chemotherapy in patients with newly diagnosed ovarian cancer (21).

Elevated levels of circulating antigens may be prognostic in solid malignancies, but even fewer studies have been published regarding detection of micrometastases. Although preoperative CEA, CA125, and CA15-3 levels may be associated with worse prognosis in colon, ovarian, and breast cancer, respectively, elevated levels are rarely independent of stage. In contrast, elevated pre- or postoperative or postradiotherapy PSA levels are predictive of subsequent relapse in men with early-stage prostate cancer, although no study has demonstrated benefit with adjuvant therapy in this disease (22–29).

Monitoring for Relapse and Evaluation of Course of Metastatic Disease. Patients with a prior history of invasive cancers might be screened for impending relapse throughout their course. Serial measurements of tumor markers during follow-up or treatment may provide an indication of current or future clinical course. Since serum (and/or plasma) and urine are easily accessible, soluble/circulating tumor markers would be ideal for such monitoring. Such information may be either reassuring or anxiety-provoking, depending on the results, the manner in which they are conveyed, and the therapeutic options that are available if the disease is progressing.

Several studies have shown that CEA, CA15-3, CA125, and PSA levels may become elevated prior to the development of symptoms or the detection of metastatic colon, lung, breast, ovarian, and prostate carcinoma by physical or radiographic findings (30–37). The sensitivity, specificity, and lead times of these assays depend on the disease, the marker, and the study design.

Although impending systemic relapse of several solid tumors can be predicted with some degree of certainty using rising tumor markers, the clinical utility of this observation is not clear. Treatment of asymptomatic metastases with potentially toxic systemic therapy has not been demonstrated to result in either increased cure or increased survival rates for any solid tumor, and treatment of patients with asymptomatic metastases is unlikely to provide improved palliation (38,39). Thus, routine screening of patients following primary therapy with serial marker levels should be considered investigational at this time for most diseases. One exception might arise in colon cancer patients who are found to have an isolated hepatic metastasis. Resection of such lesions has been reported to be associated with a prolonged DFS in approximately 25% of patients, although no prospective randomized trial has been performed (40). Nonetheless, a rising CEA may lead to the clinician to further evaluate potential candidates with CT or other liver imaging.

Palliation of patients with metastatic cancer may be accomplished with a series of treatment modalities, including surgery, radiation, hormone therapy, and chemotherapy, depending on the tumor type (41). Although each may provide benefit, the risks and toxicities of the separate therapies differ widely. Therefore, accurate knowledge of the status of a patient's disease is essential in deciding whether to continue the current therapy or proceed to an alternate regimen. For most solid tumors, serial circulating antigen such as CEA, CA15-3, CA125, and PSA levels are reasonably reliable indicators of clinical course.

THE PSYCHOLOGICAL CONSEQUENCES OF TUMOR MARKER USE

General Considerations

Little is known about how patients react specifically to tumor marker information. In recent years there has been a growing literature studying the psychological consequences of risk assessment and screening in oncology. We will be discussing some of these studies in an attempt to understand the possible psychological consequences of using tumor markers.

Tumor marker results are usually reported as part of a much larger physician–patient interchange. Hence, the relationship that the physician has with his or her patient, and how the information is communicated, will be important in determining how it is actually received by the patient. The manner in which a patient cognitively and emotionally processes medical information may likewise affect the overall physician–patient relationship, and in some cases the patient's attitude toward the health care system as a whole, thus possibly affecting compliance with future medical treatment. Psychological distress could also be long-lasting, adversely affecting overall quality of life. Indeed, recent research has even pointed toward a link between psychological stress and the immune system in patients with cancer, suggesting that psychological state may be important in determining immune status and possibly even overall survival (42,43).

Risk Assessment

Although tumor susceptibility genes are being discovered rapidly, few data are yet available for assessing the emotional aspects of their use. In this regard, the research that has been done on predictive testing for Huntington's disease might serve as a model. However, several key differences exist between these models (Table 14.6) (44). The most important of these relates

TABLE 14.6. *Comparison of Genetic Testing for Cancer Susceptibility vs. Huntington's Disease*

	Cancer Susceptibility	Huntington's Disease
Penetrance	Incomplete	Complete
Environmental factors	Present (?)	Absent
Genetic information obtained	Uncertain	Certain
Age of onset of disease	Wide variability	Relatively predictable

to the underlying cause and expression of the disease for which testing is provided. In Huntington's disease, genetic testing has been applied to a well-defined, monogenic syndrome that is inherited in a strict Mendelian fashion, whereby inheritance of the disease gene leads to expression of the disease phenotype. In contrast, inherited cancer susceptibility genes generally exhibit incomplete penetrance, suggesting that the inheritance of an altered cancer gene is not sufficient to produce the disease (45). Additional genetic events, acting in conjunction with environmental cofactors, may be necessary (46). One clinical implication is that a substantial proportion of families who provide genetic material will not receive any genetic information. Moreover, incomplete penetrance of a gene means that even when a carrier of a specific cancer gene can be identified with a high level of certainty, the individual's risk of developing the disease remains less than 100%. Expression of the phenotype (i.e., development of cancer) may be distributed widely over several decades of life. Thus, counseling, preventative strategies, and screening must be applied with less certainty and over a longer period of time than with other genetic diseases.

Do patients wish to be tested for genetic susceptibility? Before the initiation of predictive testing for Huntington's disease, about two-thirds of at-risk individuals surveyed said that they wanted to be tested. Of interest, fewer than 15% of these individuals have come forward for testing (47,48). Individuals at high risk for malignancies have also expressed interest in genetic testing. In one study, 75% of first-degree relatives of ovarian cancer patients were interested in genetic testing for *BRCA1*, and a majority consented to complete the testing process (44). In a study in Utah of random residents, 83% expressed a desire for genetic screening for colon cancer (49). It appears that perception of cancer susceptibility, rather than actual personal risk, is a key predictor in determining desire to be tested for both *BRCA1* and colon cancer susceptibility (49–51).

What are the emotional and psychological consequences of genetic susceptibility testing? Recent studies of predictive testing for Huntington's disease have provided mixed results for this disease model (52). Participants in a Dutch predictive screening program, when compared with nonparticipants prior to genetic testing, denied that a positive result might have adverse effects on personal mood, quality of life, or marriage (53). Six months after testing, they had a significantly more optimistic outlook for themselves and their futures than did nonparticipants (54). In contrast, in a prospective American study of the impact of predictive testing in Huntington's disease, carriers were found at baseline to have increased distress on all scales measured when compared to noncarriers (52). By 12 months, all measures of distress declined significantly for both carriers and noncarriers, and the two groups were nearly identical. Also included in this study were nonparticipants, who either withdrew their consent or had uninformative test results. At baseline, nonparticipants' scores on distress scales were similar to those of participant groups, but at 12-month follow-up they were found to have significantly higher levels of depression and had lower scores on general well-being than both carriers and noncarriers. Interestingly, in some studies, negative test results presented unique difficulties, such as excessive guilt, in some patients (52,55). These studies suggest that genetic testing for Huntington's disease may cause psychological sequelae in participants that can occasionally be long-lasting, but that testing may actually produce favorable outcomes in the self-selected population that chooses to undergo it (48).

Preliminary studies indicate that patient populations and subsequent emotional reactions to *BRCA1* testing may be different. For example, when asked about anticipated attitudes if they were to undergo genetic testing, more than 75% of high-risk women anticipated that they would become very depressed and anxious if they were to test positive (50). If they were to test negative, 42% said that they would still worry about cancer risk, and 25% said that they would feel guilty. High-risk women expecting a negative impact of genetic testing tended to have more vigilant, information-seeking coping styles, and be more likely to have a generalized mood disturbance. Thus, the population coming forward to *BRCA1* testing may actually be those who are most vulnerable to the adverse consequences of participation in genetic screening. Indeed, in one study, follow-up at three to six weeks revealed that many of the women identified as *BRCA1* gene carriers were experiencing some level of psychological distress: persistent worries, depression, confusion, and

sleep disturbance (44). Fifty percent of noncarriers reported that they continued to worry about their risk status.

These findings demonstrate that it is critical that genetic testing for cancer susceptibility not be initiated before establishing resources and plans for pretest and follow-up counseling. One important objective of pretest counseling is to identify individuals with psychiatric disorders or those who are psychologically vulnerable to the negative consequences of testing. In addition, preparatory counseling is critical to plan for the impact of test results and the tailoring of follow-up (48,50,56). In Huntington's disease, investigators have found it useful to identify maladaptive coping responses and to explore strategies for improving them (55). Such preparation is essential in minimizing the likelihood of adverse psychological consequences from genetic testing. Prospective studies to determine the psychological consequences of cancer susceptibility testing and counseling are increasingly critical as molecular genetics technology advances and new tests become available.

Screening of Healthy Individuals

Currently no tumor marker has been established for screening healthy individuals for cancer. Of the available candidates, the most promising are PSA and HPV (human papilloma virus) for prostate and cervical cancer. The main aim of screening for cancer in the general population is to detect diseases at a less advanced stage. A further aim is to reassure those for whom no problem is detected. Implicit in many studies of the psychological effects of screening is a stimulus–response model: negative or low-risk results are expected to predict low rates of distress, positive or high-risk results are expected to predict high rates of distress, and in some situations behavioral change (57). However, this model may be too simplistic, and the psychological costs of participation in screening programs may be more complicated (57–59).

In the absence of any widely accepted screening tumor markers, it is helpful to review those successful screening programs that use non-tumor marker indicators of malignancy: cervical and breast cancer. The lessons learned from these examples might be applicable to the use of tumor markers for screening, such as PSA. In many respects, cytologic examination of exfoliated cervical cells represents a highly successful application of a "tumor marker." The potential of annual screening to produce psychological sequelae is of particular importance because of the possible impact of such sequelae on patient compliance with subsequent screening and diagnostic follow-up (60,61). Women undergoing cervical screening tend to underestimate the likelihood of being recalled (57) and erroneously think that the test is screening for cancer (62). Given the latter misperception, women recalled after Pap screening may be extremely anxious (63). Proper education and counseling of women with positive Pap tests can improve psychological status and also enhance compliance with follow-up. Women who received informational leaflets and materials that bolster positive attitudes along with written notification of a positive Pap test were less anxious and more compliant than women who did not receive this additional information (64,65). These lessons learned from Pap smears should be remembered as better tumor markers are developed and tested for other malignancies.

Although no "tumor marker" per se exists for breast cancer screening, the success of mammographic screening in lowering mortality rates in women over 50 years of age deserves careful examination as a model for screening. In spite of this success, the psychological costs of mammography may be high if women are not properly informed of the risks and benefits involved in routine screening mammography. Some authors have questioned the validity of public health information which may give false expectations about screening, and these warnings must be heeded as new tumor markers are tested (66).

Do these lesson carry over into true tumor marker utilities? Recently, several studies have suggested that an elevated level of prostate-specific antigen (PSA) may be indicative of early prostate cancer and that screening PSA levels might be an effective and useful strategy to reduce morbidity and mortality due to prostate cancer (67). However, the medical benefits of the strategy remain controversial. Indeed, some investigators have argued that the performance characteristics of PSA are not sufficient for an effective screening program. Moreover, some studies have suggested that many men with early stage, "screening-detected" prostate cancer might never develop clinically important disease, and no prospective randomized studies have demonstrated that early detection and treatment of prostate cancer reduces mortality. Although not yet studied, the medical, economic, and especially emotional consequences of overtreatment of this common disease, resulting in both sexual and urinary dysfunction, may be enormous. Investigations of the psychological consequences of screening PSAs in general, especially as related to false negative and positive results, are essential.

In light of these potential psychological consequences of screening programs, it is helpful to review the categories of uncertainties that may exist: false and true negatives and false and true positives (Table 14.7). Individuals faced with results that represent each of these categories may have many different, perhaps damaging, emotional reactions.

False Negatives. The psychological consequences of false negative tumor marker tests are unknown. Anecdotal reports document patients developing feelings of mistrust and anger toward health care professionals as a result of false negative mammogram readings later reported as positive. Indeed, failure to diagnose breast cancer at an early stage is one of the most common reasons for malpractice suits (68). However, the long-standing psychological effects of false negative screening results have not yet been studied, and serve as an important area for future research.

True Negatives. Receipt of a negative result is not always reassuring. As discussed in the Huntington's disease model, the mere process of participating in screening for risk correlated with less psychological distress than was observed in the nonparticipating group (52). In contrast, in a study screening for cardiovascular risk, those individuals who received negative or low-risk test results had higher levels of distress after screening (57,69). In this case, screening was an anxiety-producing experience. This higher distress level may be at least in part due to the "uncertain wellness" paradigm described by Cioffi (70). She speculated that receiving an unclear diagnosis of wellness, such as a "normal" result after screening, orients an individual toward detecting possible illness, while providing only uncertain

TABLE 14.7. *Possible Psychological Consequences of Screening of Healthy Individuals*

FALSE NEGATIVES
Anger, mistrust due to delayed diagnosis
Lack of compliance with future diagnosis and treatment

TRUE NEGATIVES
Anxiety and distress of screening
Orientation toward illness

FALSE POSITIVES
Anger, mistrust due to incorrect diagnosis
Immediate anxiety and distress of screening and of positive result
Sustained worries over health

TRUE POSITIVES
Orientation toward illness
Labeling effect: impairment in mood and daily activities

information about the absence of illness. Thus, screening a healthier population may generate information about the absence of illness. Thus, screening a healthier population may generate information that is not as easily cognitively processed as information about a clearly negative outcome, which frequently induces minimization (71) or other predicted psychological responses. Therefore, in a population perceived to be at risk for a condition, such as individuals from Huntington's families, screening lowers distress; while in a population chosen at random, screening for an unexpected illness may raise it. This discrepancy may exist because individuals in healthy populations who undergo screening programs are likely to be overly optimistic that their health is good, since most people underestimate their vulnerability to adverse risks, including illness (72). Moreover, unrealistic optimism may promote many aspects of mental health (73). In other words, the mere act of screening may for some patients be sufficient to introduce doubts about one's health and affect one's overall sense of well-being.

False Positives. False positive results almost certainly raise psychological costs as well, although at present few studies have assessed the magnitude of the effect (74). For example, 6% of patients who had received false positive results in a trial of colorectal cancer screening reported continuing serious worries over their health (75).

Breast cancer may be one of the most emotionally charged of the malignant diseases. The effects of false positive screening mammography highlight the importance of understanding the performance characteristics of using tumor markers to screen for cancer. For example, three months after a suspicious but ultimately benign breast finding had been detected during screening, women reported increased and persistent cancer worries and mood disturbances (76).

The affect with which a physician communicates an ambiguous mammogram result to a patient may be a factor in how patients process the information. For example, women at risk for breast cancer who received ambiguous mammogram results from a worried physician recalled significantly less information than women receiving the same information from a nonworried physician (77). They also perceived the medical situation as significantly more severe, reported more anxiety, and were found to have higher pulse rates.

Although a subsequent negative report about a previously suspicious test may engender a feeling of relief, patients may later develop anger at having been put through the unnecessary emotional turmoil. Such negative responses may induce a loss of confidence in the health care system and may damage compliance. Investigations of the psychological effects of these tests are becoming increasingly important as technology in this area advances.

True Positives. In the case of a true positive result in other areas of health screening, psychological effects can be more extreme than expected from the seriousness of the condition. For example, Canadian steel mill workers who were detected and labeled as hypertensive had significantly greater rates of absenteeism in the year following the screening (78). This observation was not explained by any differences related directly to the disease (blood pressure levels, organ damage, drug treatment). Thus, the authors speculated that the observation might be related to the effects of labeling a previously healthy worker as hypertensive. Several subsequent studies have supported the finding that increased absenteeism (78,79), as well as lower psychological well-being, increased rates of depression, and decrements in marital adjustment occur after a diagnosis has been ascribed, even in the absence of physical morbidity (80).

Clinical experience with cancer screening suggests that people can be very disturbed by the news of any abnormality related to cancer, and may not be able to understand the subtle distinctions drawn by health professionals. It has also been suggested that psychiatric disturbance may be more common after screening-detected, compared with symptomatic, cancer has been diagnosed. Patients in whom cancer is detected by screening might feel that they should be grateful, since early diagnosis is the main goal of such a program (66). However, an individual's response to the discovery that disease was developing outside of their awareness could lead them to be fearful and mistrustful of their doctor's ability to detect recurrences (66). Such a serious threat to the self could result in special difficulties in emotional adjustment. Unfortunately, little is known about whether people respond differently to a diagnosis if it is detected during routine screening. In one study, no difference in psychological states was found between 30 women in whom breast cancer had been detected during routine screening and 30 women whose breast cancer had been diagnosed following self-referral for symptoms (81).

In conclusion, these data suggest that as tumor markers are developed to screen otherwise healthy populations for early malignancies, it is important that physicians have a working knowledge of the utility and performance characteristics of the tests that they

TABLE 14.8. *Possible Psychological Consequences of Close Monitoring for Relapse of Cancer*

ADVANTAGES

Emotional support

Reassurance for patient

Reassurance for physician

Adapting to new "disease-free" state

Illusion of control over relapse

DISADVANTAGES

Heightened awareness of possibility of relapse

Uncertain information about relapse

Decreased quality of life during otherwise asymptomatic phase by news of impending relapse

order, and that patients be counseled prior to and following screening.

Determination of Prognosis

The specific psychological effects of receiving information about tumor markers such as PSA in prostate cancer, and ER and PR levels in breast cancer, are largely unknown. In one study, ER-negative patients had significantly more anxiety and psychological distress, but this finding has not been consistently observed (82,83). As the availability of prognostic tumor markers increases, clinicians should be advised to weigh the psychological risks to their patients against the benefits (if any) of obtaining specific tumor marker levels and reporting them to their patients. The effects of knowing this information, both when it will affect treatment decisions and when it will not, is an important area for future research. Previous studies indicate that most patients with cancer receive less information and involvement in their care than they desire (84,85). As a result, a substantial proportion are inadequately informed about their diagnoses (86), about the rationale for treatment, and about the associated risks and benefits (87,88). Even when health care providers do offer extensive information to patients, many patients have problems comprehending this information (56,84,87). Lack of comprehension may occur as a result of the patient's inability to process specific details due to high levels of anxiety (89), and may subsequently affect both the ability to make decisions (90) and the level of psychological well-being. However, in many cases, increased delivery of information can increase a patient's level of psychological autonomy (91). Hence, prognostic information may produce either a stress-inducing or a stress-reducing effect (92).

What determines what effect this information will have? In fact, individual variations in coping style have been found to be a key factor in explaining the different psychological responses to receiving information (93,94). Some patients respond with avoidance of disease-related information, and others with a search for information. For patients who prefer minimal information, large amounts of information can be associated with increased psychological distress. Conversely, for patients who generally seek out more information, large amounts may be associated with less distress (93).

In conclusion, providers may be better able to reduce their patients' psychological distress related to prognostic results if individual patient coping styles are known before the medical visit. As with genetic testing for breast cancer susceptibility, it is not clear how much information should be provided to individual patients, especially when there may be no changes in treatment from this information. Thus, caregivers must be clear regarding the potential outcomes that the tumor marker results may or may not effect for that specific patient (Table 14.2). It is likely that sociodemographic characteristics, data on personality and coping styles, and ethnic and cultural differences in perceptions are all important areas for helping us to understand individual differences in receiving medical information and important areas for future study (44).

Monitoring for Relapse and Evaluation During Course of Metastatic Disease

As previously discussed, for most solid malignancies, early detection of impending recurrence may not substantially increase medical benefit. In the absence of clear-cut physical benefits of monitoring tumor markers, should they be ordered? Results of a recent survey of physician members of the American Society of Clinical Oncology demonstrated that, in following asymptomatic women with early stage breast cancer, 38% of the physicians ordered CEA levels and 21% ordered CA15-3 levels routinely in their follow-up visits one year out of treatment (95). Whether or not early detection provides enhanced physical benefits, many physicians feel that patients are reassured with sequential tumor marker analysis (96–104). This, however, is a viewpoint that requires further investigation. It may be that patients whose recurrent cancer is detected early by virtue of a rising tumor marker might actually suffer from the psychological morbidity of this diagnosis months to years before the onset of symptoms. Knowledge of an asymptomatic recurrence may possibly diminish a patient's QOL during a period when they would otherwise be emotionally secure.

Taken together, these results suggest both psychological advantages and disadvantages to intense follow-up (Table 14.8). Close regular evaluation of cancer patients after primary therapy might provide additional emotional support to them at a time when they have suffered considerable psychological stress related to the diagnosis and treatment of their disease. The perception that one is disease-free may be important in subsequent psychological adjustment (104). For some patients, close follow-up may give an illusion of control over the situation. Interestingly, in nonmedical situations, close involvement has the effect of increasing people's expectations for future success (105). On the other hand, it may be that for some individuals, close follow-up, even if results are negative, heightens awareness of the possibility of recurrence. In other words, a potentially serious threat such as a recurrent cancer may be put aside if there is no particular reason to worry about it "today" (106,107). Further, as with screening, uncertain information about wellness may be more distressing than no information at all (70). People prefer symmetry between illness labels and symptoms (108). When disease is latent, remitting or asymptomatic patients may become acutely distressed and uncertain (109).

What type of follow-up do patients prefer? In a survey of breast cancer patients, 43% of those with localized disease felt that 3- to 6-month intervals of follow-up were adequate, while 55% of those with metastatic disease felt that monthly or bimonthly intervals were adequate (102). They were also asked how valuable they thought selected tests were in detecting recurrence. The majority of patients believed that radiographs, scans, and blood tests were much more effective than the history. Further, most patients incorrectly perceived the significance of a "normal" test, interpreting it as meaning an absence of cancer cells in the organ being evaluated, rather than a threshold of detection. Of great interest is the finding that 92% of the patients interviewed believed that early detection of metastases improved long-term outlook, a chance for cure, or the chance to respond to therapy.

Other investigators have observed that although routine follow-up after potentially curative treatment of breast cancer is inefficient in the detection of recurrence, 81% of women who were recurrence-free said they felt "reassured and less anxious" when they had their follow-up visit (96). The authors concluded that reassurance rather than detection of recurrence may be the most important function of the breast cancer follow-up clinic. Furthermore, as with prognostic information, individual patient differences are important in judging the ability of follow-up to provide emotional

support (98). Some women may be reassured by extensive negative investigations, while others may view these tests as anxiety-provoking, unwelcome reminders of a disease with an uncertain future.

Importantly, prospective analysis of QOL was performed as part of a recently published randomized trial of intensive follow-up versus simple physicians' visits only for women with stage I, II, and III breast cancer (110). Intensive follow-up included physician visits and performance of bone scan, liver echography, chest roentgenography, and laboratory tests but not serum tumor markers. Over 70% of all patients said they wanted to be seen frequently by a physician and undergo diagnostic tests even if they were free of symptoms. However, overall QOL perception, health perception, and emotional well-being were nearly identical in the two follow-up groups. The authors concluded that "the intensity of diagnostic tests does not affect emotional well-being and other aspects of QOL. If anything, the real issue is to clarify whether a favorable effect of being seen by a physician exists." Further, they suggest that the benefits of the diagnostic tests may, at least in part, be for the *physicians*, who "will always seek, whenever uncertain, the support of information from a diagnostic test even though they may be aware of its limitations in terms of sensitivity, specificity, and predictive value." Thus, these results suggest that clinical use of many tumor marker tests may actually be the physicians' method of coping with their patients' uncertain health status.

Indeed, in this study, QOL was shown to decline after detection of recurrence, even if it was asymptomatic. One might infer that if early detection of asymptomatic recurrence does not prolong survival or improve palliation, it may actually decrease QOL. Thus, although a follow-up schedule appears to be reassuring and worthwhile, a program involving fewer procedures, including laboratory tests and roentgenographic studies, may prove more satisfactory. The authors conclude that "little attention is paid to the psychological distress of women waiting for the results, the anticipated consciousness of having a recurrence of the disease, anticipation of the adverse effects of treatment, and the risk of a false-positive report leading to invasive diagnostic procedures and, possibly, overtreatment."

Perhaps the most important points to remember when monitoring a patient with cancer for relapse is that patients have differing coping styles and emotional needs, as well as different reactions to receiving information. Many patients tend to overestimate the utility of diagnostic tests and incorrectly perceive the significance of a "normal" test (102). Many medical interventions provide benefits primarily to the sense of well-being of a patient seeking medical care for the sympathy, reassurance, and validation provided (90). Prospective evaluations of QOL and patients' perceptions of our diagnostic interventions are needed, as well as physician training to assess and address the specific psychological needs of patients.

CONCLUSIONS

In conclusion, the use of tumor markers in clinical practice may have a great psychological impact on patients. However, the specific effects are largely unknown. In this regard, data from studies of screening and risk assessment in oncology can provide clues into how tumor marker tests might affect patients. Clearly this is a fertile and important area for research, and one which will become increasingly important in the future as biotechnological advances proceed. In the meantime, it is critical that oncologists clarify whether the benefits of obtaining a diagnostic tumor marker result for a given patient and clinical situation outweigh the risks. As more tumor markers become available, their proper use will present new challenges to both primary clinicians and mental health care providers.

ACKNOWLEDGMENTS

This work was supported in part by NIH grant U01-CA64057 and by the Eva Brownman Fund.

REFERENCES

1. Hayes DF, Bast RC, Desch CE, et al. Tumor marker utility grading system: a framework to evaluate clinical utility of tumor markers. *J Natl Cancer Inst.* 1996; 88:1419–1420.
2. Miller AB. Early detection of breast cancer. In: Harris J, Hellman S, Henderson IC, Kinne SW, eds. *Breast Diseases.* Philadelphia: J. B. Lippincott; 1991:215–228.
3. Li F, Fraumeni J. Prospective study of a family cancer syndrome. *J Am Med Assoc.* 1990; 255:1233–1238.
4. Malkin D, Li F, Strong L, Fraumeni J, et al. Germ line p53 mutations in a familial syndrome of breast cancer. *Science.* 1990; 255:1233–1238.
5. Hall J, Lee M, Newman B, et al. Linkage of early-onset familial breast cancer to chromosome 17q21. *Science.* 1990; 250:1684–1689.
6. Fishel R, Lescoe MK, Rao MRS, et al. The human mutator gene homolog *MSH2* and its association with hereditary nonpolyposis colon cancer. *Cell.* 1993; 75:1027–1038.
7. Leach FS, Nicolaides NC, Papadopoulos N, et al. Mutations of a *mutS* homolog in hereditary nonpolyposis colorectal cancer. *Cell.* 1993; 75:1215–1225.
8. Eddy DM. Screening for breast cancer. *Ann Int Med.* 1989; 111:389–399.
9. Nyström L, Rutqvist LE, Wall S, et al. Breast cancer screening with mammography: overview of Swedish randomised trials. *Lancet.* 1993; 341:973–978.
10. Fletcher SW, Fletcher RH. The breast is close to the heart. *Ann Int Med.* 1992; 117:969–971.
11. Boring CC, Squires TS, Tong T, Montgomery S. Cancer statistics, 1994. *CA-A Cancer J Clin.* 1994; 44:7–26.
12. DeCosse JJ, Tsioulias GJ, Jacobson JS. Colorectal cancer: detection, treatment, and rehabilitation. *CA-A Cancer J Clin.* 1994; 44:27–42.
13. Fontana RS, Sanderson DR, Taylor WF. Early lung cancer detection: results of the initial (prevalence) radiologic and cytologic screening at the Mayo Clinic study. *Am Rev Respir Dis.* 1984; 130:561–565.
14. Martini N. Results of the Memorial Sloan-Kettering lung project. *Rec Res Cancer Res.* 1982; 82:174–178.
15. Levin ML, Tockman NS, Frost JK. Lung cancer mortality in males screened by chest x-ray and cytologic sputum examination: a preliminary report. *Rec Res Cancer Res.* 1982; 82:138–146.
16. Helzlsouer KJ, Bush TL, Alberg AJ, Bass KM, Zacur H, Comstock GW. Prospective study of serum Ca-125 levels as markers of ovarian cancer. *J Am Med Assoc.* 1993; 269:1123–1126.
17. Tondini C, Hayes DF, Kufe D. Circulating tumor markers in breast cancer. In: Henderson IC, eds. *Diagnosis and Therapy of Breast Cancer.* Philadelphia: W. B. Saunders; 1989: 653–674.
18. Bast Jr RC, Bates S, Bredt AB, et al. Clinnical practice guidelines for the use of tumor markers in breast and colorectal cancer. *J Clin Oncol.* 1996; 14:2843–2877.
19. Moertel CG, Fleming TR, Macdonald JS, et al. Levamisole and fluorouacil for adjuvant therapy of resected colon carcinoma. *N Engl J Med.* 1990; 322:352–358.
20. Osborne CK. Receptors. In: Harris J, Hellman S, Henderson I, Kinne D, eds. *Breast Diseases.* Philadelphia: J. B. Lippincott; 1991: 301–325.
21. Young RC, Perez CA, Hoskens WJ. Cancer of the ovary. In: DeVita VT, Hellman S, Rosenberg S, eds. *Cancer: Principles and Practice of Oncology,* 4th ed. Philadelphia: J. B. Lippincott; 1993: 1226–1255.
22. Partin AW, Carter HB, Chan DW. Prostate specific antigen in the staging of localized prostate cancer: influence of tumor differentiation, tumor volume and benign hyperplasia. *J Urol.* 1990; 149:510–515.
23. Stamey TA, Dietrick DD, Issa MM. Large, organ confined, impalpable transition zone prostate cancer: influence of tumor differentiation, tumor volume and benign hyperplasia. *J Urol.* 1993; 143:747–752.
24. Partin AW, Yoo J, Carter HB. The use of prostate specific antigen, clinical stage and Gleason score to predict pathological stage in men with localized prostate cancer. *J Urol.* 1993; 150:110–114.
25. Kleer E, Larson-Keller JJ, Zincke H, Oesterling JE. Ability of preoperative serum prostate-specific antigen value to predict pathologic stage and DNA ploidy. *J Urol.* 1993; 41:207–216.
26. Russell KJ, Dunatov C, Hafermann MD. Prostate specific antigen in the management of patients with loca-

lized adenocarcinoma of the prostate treated with primary radiation therapy. *J Urol.* 1991;146:1046–1052.

27. Ritter MA, Messing EM, Shanahan TG. Prostate-specific antigen as a predictor of radiotherapy response and patterns of failure in localized prostate cancer. *J Clin Oncol.* 1992; 10:1208–1217.

28. Zagars GK. Prostate-specific antigen as a prognostic factor for prostate cancer treated by external beam radiotherapy. *J Clin Oncol.* 1992; 23:47–53.

29. Pisansky TM, Cha SS, Earle JD, et al. Prostate-specific antigen as a pretherapy prognostic factor in patients treated with radiation therapy for clinically localized prostate cancer. *J Clin Oncol.* 1993; 11:2158–2166.

30. Sikorska HM, Fuks A, Gold P. Carcinomebryonic antigen. In: Sell S, ed. *Serological Cancer Markers.* Totowa, NJ: The Humana Press; 1992: 47–97.

31. Ruibal A, Colomer R, Genolla J. Prognostic value of CA15-3 serum levels in patients having breast cancer. *Hormones Metab.* 1987; 1:11–15.

32. Chan D, Beveridge R, Muss H, et al. Use of Truquant BR radioimmunoassay for early detection of breast cancer recurrence in patients with Stage II and III disease. *J Clin Oncol.* 1997; 15:2322–2328.

33. Maigre M, Fumoleau P, Ricolleau G, et al. CA15-3 in breast cancer. Comparison with CEA (French). *Semin Hop Paris.* 1988; 64:9–13.

34. Kallioniemi O, Oksa H, Aaran R, Hietanen T, Lehtinen M, Koivula T. Serum CA15-3 assay in the diagnosis and follow-up of breast cancer. *Br J Cancer.* 1988; 58:213–215.

35. Colomer R, Ruibal A, Genolla J, et al. Circulating CA 15-3 levels in the postsurgical follow-up of breast cancer patients and in non-malignant diseases. *Breast Cancer Res Treat.* 1989; 13:123–133.

36. Safi F, Kohler I, Rottinger E, Suhr P, Beger HG. Comparison of CA 15-3 and CEA in diagnosis and monitoring of breast cancer. *Int J Biol Markers.* 1989; 4:207–214.

37. Montz FJ. CA 125. In: Sell S, ed. *Serological Cancer Markers.* Totowa, NJ: The Humana Press; 1992: 417–427.

38. Hayes DF, Kaplan W. Evaluation of patients following primary therapy. In: Harris J, Hellman S, Henderson I, Kinne D, eds. *Breast Diseases.* Philadelphia: J. B. Lippincott; 1991: 505–525.

39. Stierer M, Rosen HR. Influence of early diagnosis on prognosis of recurrent breast cancer. *Cancer.* 1989; 64:1128–1131.

40. Malt RA. Current concepts: surgery for hepatic neoplasms. *N Engl J Med.* 1985; 313:1591–1596.

41. Hayes DF, Henderson IC, Shapiro CL. Treatment of metastatic breast cancer: present and future prospects. *Semin Oncol.* 1995; 22:5–21.

42. Fawzy FI, Fawzy NW, Arndt LA, Pasnau R. Critical review of psychosocial interventions in cancer care. *Arch Gen Psychiatry.* 1995; 52:100–113.

43. Spiegel D, Bloom JR, Kraemer MC, Gottheil E. Effect of psychosocial treatment on survival of patients with metastatic breast cancer. *Lancet.* 1989; 2:888–891.

44. Lerman C, Croyle C. Psychological issues in genetic testing for breast cancer susceptibility. *Arch Intern Med.* 1994; 154:609–616.

45. Skolnick MH, Cannon-Albright LA, Goldgar DE. Inheritance of proliferative breast disease in breast cancer kindreds. *Science.* 1990; 250:1715–1720.

46. Moolgavkar SH, Day NE, Stevens RG. Two step model for carcinogenesis: epidemiology of breast cancer in females. *J Natl Cancer Inst.* 1980; 65:59–69.

47. Craufurd D, Dodge A, Kerzin-Storrar L. Uptake of presymptomatic predictive testing for Huntington's disease. *Lancet.* 1989; 2:603–605.

48. Bloch M, Fahy M, Fox S, Hayden MR. Predictive testing for Huntington's disease, II: Demographic characteristics, life-style patterns, attitudes, and psychosocial assessments of the first fifty-one test candidates. *Am J Med Genet.* 1989; 32:217–224.

49. Croyle RT, Lerman C. Interest in genetic testing for colon cancer susceptibility: Cognitive and emotional correlates. *Prev Med.* 1993; 22:284–292.

50. Lerman C, Daly M, Masny A, Balshem A. Attitudes about genetic testing for breast-ovarian cancer susceptibility. *J Clin Oncol.* 1994; 12:843–850.

51. Becker MH, Kaback MM, Rosenstock IM. Some influences on public participation in a genetic screening program. *J Community Health.* 1975; 1:3–14.

52. Wiggins S, Whyte P, Huggins M, et al. The psychological consequences of predictive testing for Huntington's disease. *N Engl J Med.* 1992; 327:1401–1405.

53. Tibben A, Frets PG, van de Kamp JJ, et al. Presymptomatic DNA-testing for Huntington disease: pretest attitudes and expectations of applicants and their partners in the Dutch program. *Am J Med Genet.* 1993; 48:10–16.

54. Tibben A, Frets PG, van de Kamp JJ, et al. On attitudes and appreciation 6 months after predictive DNA testing for Huntington's disease in the Dutch program. *Am J Med Genet.* 1993; 48:103–111.

55. Nance MA, Leroy BS, Orr HT. Protocol for genetic testing in Huntington disease: three years experience in Minnesota. *Am J Med Genet.* 1991; 40:518–522.

56. Lerman C, Daly M, Walsh W. Communication between patients with breast cancer and health care providers: determinants and implications. *Cancer.* 1993; 72:2612–2620.

57. Marteau TM. Psychology and screening: narrowing the gap between efficacy and effectiveness. *Br J Clin Psychol.* 1994; 33:1–10.

58. McCormick J. Cervical smears: a questionable practice. *Lancet.* 1989; ii:207–209.

59. Lerman C, Miller SM, Scarborough R, Hanjani P, Nolte SDS. Adverse psychologic consequences of positive cytologic cervical screening. *Am J Obstet Gynecol.* 1991; 165:658–662.

60. Beresford JS, Gervaize PA. The emotional impact of abnormal pap smears on patients referred for colposcopy. *Colposc Gynecol Laser Surg.* 1986; 2:83–87.

61. Lerman C, Rimer B, Trock B, Balshem A, Engstrom P. Factors associated with repeat adherence to breast cancer screening. *Prev Med.* 1990; 19:279–290.

62. Schwartz M, Savage W, George J, Emohare L. Women's knowledge and experience of cervical screening: a failure of health education and medical organisation. *Community Med.* 1989; 11:279–289.

63. Marteau TM, Thwaltes S. Presenting cervical screening in primary and secondary care: practice observed. Paper

presented at the 1992 AUTGP Annual Scientific Meeting.

64. Wilkinson C, Jones JM, McBride J. Anxiety caused by abnormal result of cervical smear test: a controlled trial. *Br Med J.* 1990; 300:440.

65. Paskett ED, White E, Carter WB, Chu J. Improving follow-up after an abnormal Pap smear: a randomized controlled trial. *Prev Med.* 1990; 19:630–641.

66. Roberts MM. Breast screening: time for a rethink? *Br Med J.* 1989; 299:1153–1155.

67. Kantoff PW, Talcott JA. The prostate specific antigen: its use as a tumor marker for prostate cancer. In: Hayes DF, eds. *Hematology/Oncology Clinics of North America: Tumor Markers in Adult Solid Malignancies.* Philadelphia: W. B. Saunders; 1994: 555–572.

68. Hayes DF. Medical oncologists and risk management in breast cancer. In: Kern KA, Cady B, eds. *Surgical Oncology Clinics of North America. Medicolegal Controversies in Breast Cancer: Biologic Basis and Risk Prevention.* Philadelphia: J. B. Lippincott; 1994: 149–172.

69. Stoate H. Can health screening damage your health? *J R Coll Gen Pract.* 1989; 39:193–195.

70. Cioffi D. Asymmetry of doubt in medical self-diagnosis: the ambiguity of "uncertain wellness." *J Pers Social Psychol.* 1991; 61:969–980.

71. Taylor SE. Asymmetrical effects of positive and negative events: the mobilization-minimization hypothesis. *Psychol Bull.* 1991; 109:67–85.

72. Weinstein ND. Why it won't happen to me: perceptions of risk factors and susceptibility. *Health Psychol.* 1984. 3:431–457.

73. Taylor SE, Brown JD. Illusion and well-being: A social psychological perspective on mental health. *Psychol Bull.* 1988; 103:193–210.

74. Wardle J, Pope R. The psychological costs of screening for cancer. *J Psychosom Res.* 1992; 36:609–624.

75. Mant D, Fitzpatrick R, Hogg A, et al. The experiences of patients with false positive results from colorectal cancer screening. *Br J Gen Pract.* 1990; 40:423–425.

76. Lerman C, Trock B, Rimer BK, Jepson C, Brody D, Boyce A. Psychological side effects of breast cancer screening. *Health Psychol.* 1991; 10:259–267.

77. Shapiro DE, Boggs SR, Melamed BG, Graham-Pole J. The effect of varied physician affect on recall, anxiety, and perceptions in women at risk for breast cancer: an analogue study. *Health Psychol.* 1992; 11:61–66.

78. Haynes RB, Sackett DL, Taylor DW, Gibson ES, Johnson AL. Increased absenteeism from work after the detection and labeling of hypertensive patients. *N Engl J Med.* 1978; 299:741–744.

79. Taylor DW, Haynes RB, Sackett DL. Longterm follow-up of absenteeism among working men following the detection and treatment of hypertension. *Clin Invest Med.* 1981; 4:173–177.

80. Mossey JM. Psychological consequences of labelling in hypertension. *Clin Invest Med.* 1981; 4:201–207.

81. Farmer AJ, Payne S, Royle GT. A comparative study of psychological morbidity in women with screen detected and symptomatic breast cancer. *Br Psychol Soc Abstr.* 1992; 10.

82. Razavi D, Farvacques C, Delvaux N, et al. Psychosocial correlates of oestrogen and progsterone receptors in breast cancer. *Lancet.* 1990; 335:931–933.

83. Rosenqvist S, Berglund G, Bolund C, et al. Lack of correlation between anxiety parameters and oestrogen receptor status in early breast cancer. *Eur J Cancer.* 1993; 29A:1325–1326.

84. Cassileth B, Zupkis C, Sutton-Smith K, March V. Information and participation preferences among cancer patients. *Ann Intern Med.* 1980; 92:832–836.

85. Wiggers JH, Donovan KO, Redman S, Sanson-Fisher RW. Cancer patient satisfaction with care. *Cancer.* 1990; 66:610–616.

86. Rimer BK, Jones WL, Keintz MK, Catalano RB, Engstrom PF. Informed consent: a crucial step in patient education. *Health Educ Q.* 1984; 10(suppl):30–42.

87. Siminoff LA. Cancer patient and physician communication: progress and continuing problems. *Ann Behav Med.* 1989; 7:1192–1200.

88. Peck A, Boland J. Emotional reactions to radiation treatment. *Cancer.* 1977; 40:180–184.

89. Wine J. Test anxiety and direction of attention. *Psychol Bull.* 1971; 7:1192–1200.

90. Redelmeier DA, Rozin P, Kahneman D. Understanding patients' decisions. *J Am Med Assoc.* 1993; 270:72–76.

91. Sutherland H, Llewellyn-Thomas H, Lockwood G, Tritchler D, Till J. Cancer patients: their desire for information and participation in treatment decisions. *J R Soc Med.* 1989; 82:260–263.

92. Vernon DTA, Bigelow DA. Effect of information about a potentially stressful situation on responses to stress impact. *J Pers Social Psychol.* 1974; 29:50–59.

93. Miller SM, Mangan CE. Interacting effects of information and coping style in adapting to gynecologic stress: should the doctor tell all? *J Pers Social Psychol.* 1983; 45:223–236.

94. Feifel H, Strack S, Nagy VT. Degree of life-threat and differential use of coping modes. *J Psychosom Res.* 1987; 31:91–99.

95. Simon MS, Hoff M, Hussein M, Martino S, Walt A. An evaluation of clinical follow-up in women with early stage breast cancer among physician members of the American Society of Clinical Oncology. *Breast Cancer Res Treat.* 1993; 27:211–219.

96. Morris S, Corder AP, Taylor I. What are the benefits of routine breast cancer follow-up? *Postgrad Med J.* 1992; 68:904–907.

97. Tomiak EM, Piccart MJ. Routine follow-up of patients following primary therapy for early breast cancer: what is useful? *Acta Clin Belg Suppl.* 1993; 15:38–42.

98. Tomiak E, Piccart M. Routine follow-up of patients after primary therapy for early breast cancer: changing concepts and challenges for the future. *Ann Oncol.* 1993; 4:199–204.

99. Schapira DV. A minimalist policy for breast cancer surveillance. *J Am Med Assoc.* 1991; 265:380–382.

100. Wertheimer MD. Against minimalism in breast cancer follow-up [editorial]. *J Am Med Assoc.* 1991; 265:396–397.

101. Holli K, Hakama M. Effectiveness of routine and spontaneous follow-up visits for breast cancer. *Eur J Cancer Clin Oncol.* 1989; 25:251–254.

102. Muss HB, Tell GS, Case LD, Robertson P, Atwell BM. Perceptions of follow-up care in women with breast cancer. *Am J Clin Oncol.* 1991; 14:55–59.

103. Kagan AR, Steckel RJ. Routine imaging studies for the posttreatment surveillance of breast and colorectal carcinoma. *J Clin Oncol.* 1991; 9:837–842.

104. Hayes DF, Kaplan W. Evaluation of patients after primary therapy. In: Harris J, Lippman M, Morrow M. Hellman S, eds. *Diseases of the Breast.* Philadelphia: J. B. Lippincott; 1996: 627–645.

105. Langer EJ, Roth J. Heads I win, tails it's chance: the illusion of control as a function of the sequence of outcomes in a purely chance task. *J Pers Social Psychol.* 1975; 32:951–955.

106. Linville PW, Fischer GW. Preferences for separating and combining events. *J Pers Social Psychol.* 1991; 60:5–23.

107. Tversky A, Shafir E. Choice under conflict: the dynamics of deferred decision. *Psychol Sci.* 1992; 3:358–361.

108. Baumann LJ, Cameron LD, Zimmerman RS, Leventhal H. Illness representations and matching labels with symptoms. *Health Psychol.* 1989; 8:449–469.

109. Scheinberg LC, Holland NJ. *Multiple Sclerosis: A Guide for Patients and their Families.* New York: Raven Press; 1987.

110. GIVIO Investigators. Impact of follow-up and testing on survival and health-related quality of life in breast cancer patients: a multicenter randomized controlled trial. *J Am Med Assoc.* 1994; 271:1587–1593.

15

Psychosocial Issues in Cancer Screening

JOANNE DiPLACIDO, ANN ZAUBER, AND WILLIAM H. REDD

In the absence of effective methods of primary prevention for many cancers, there is growing appreciation of the importance of screening and early detection as means of reducing cancer incidence. The goal is to identify precancerous and/or early-stage disease and then to take steps to prevent or curb the malignancy. Although both the American Cancer Society (ACS) and National Cancer Institute (NCI) recommend some form of screening for a number of cancers, overall participation is low, especially among those at highest risk (e.g., African Americans, individuals with less income and education, and individuals with a family history for cancer). Research seeking to determine why certain individuals do not comply with screening recommendations suggests that psychosocial factors play an important role.

The purpose of this chapter is to discuss cancer screening and to consider how psychosocial factors influence participation. Of particular importance is the possible application of psychosocial intervention to increase compliance with screening recommendations. We begin by reviewing criteria used to determine those sites for which screening should be recommended. We consider why screening is appropriate for certain cancers (i.e., breast, cervical, and colorectal) and not for others. We also review specific screening methods. That discussion leads to a consideration of factors that determine who should and should not be screened. We then address psychosocial barriers and facilitators to screening and use various theoretical model as a guide. The final issue is the design and implementation of broad-scale behavioral intervention packages to promote participation in screening.

Unfortunately, our understanding of psychosocial barriers and facilitators to screening is, in many ways, primitive and efforts to investigate how to intervene are at a preliminary stage. Indeed, at this point in time there are relatively few case control studies or randomized clinical trials that have investigated the role of psychological factors in screening.

CRITERIA FOR CANCER SCREENING

To be a viable component of the fight against cancer, screening methods must be cost-effective and accepted by potential screenees. In recognition of such public health concerns, Shapiro (1) has outlined a series of criteria that should be considered in identifying those cancers for which screening is appropriate. First, the cancer should represent a serious public health problem affecting a large number of individuals. In practical terms, there must be enough cases to justify the outlay of resources that screening typically requires. Second, the disease must pass through detectable preclinical phases during which effective treatments can be initiated. That is, the specific cancer must be both detectable and treatable at an early phase of development. Third, risks associated with the actual screening procedure should be low. Fourth, the screening procedure must be reliable (i.e., identifying those who have the targeted condition). Avoiding false negatives is especially important in cancer screening and steps must be taken to prevent an individual with early-stage disease from not being unidentified (and therefore not treated). Finally, the screening tests and follow-up procedures must be acceptable to the target population.

Screening programs are typically directed to a particular segment of the population. Some are used with the general population (those at normal or average risk) while others are used with those at higher risk (such as first-degree relative of cancer patients). Screening methods often differ depending on the level of risk for the group being screened. To be cost-effective, a screening program must determine who should be screened, at what ages, and with what tests. For individuals with strong risk factors for a disease, more frequent monitoring (annual rather than biannual or triannual rescreening) or more extensive testing (e.g., sonograms for younger women at high risk for ovarian cancer) are recommended.

SCREENING RECOMMENDATIONS FOR SPECIFIC CANCERS

Professional groups (e.g., the ACS) have established screening guidelines for specific cancers. Unfortunately, the list is short and recommendations from different groups do not always agree. This confusion is explained by at least two facts. First, a number of common cancers do not meet the criteria listed for screening, making screening impossible. Second, because different professional groups do not rely on the same set of studies as the bases for their recommendations, there are inconsistencies in recommendations (reflecting differences in the results obtained in independent studies). Table 15.1 summarizes current ACS screening recommendations (2).

Although the ACS has not established screening guidelines for melanoma, recent case-control research by Berwick and her colleagues (3) found that repeated skin self-examination is associated with a reduction in lethal melanoma.

It is indeed unfortunate that screening procedures for two common cancers have not been developed. These are lung and ovarian. In the case of lung cancer, there is no screening test with proven efficacy to detect disease at a phase at which effective intervention is possible. Instead preventive measures of not smoking, stopping smoking, and avoidance of tobacco products and tobacco smoke are the only means for preventing lung cancer that can be recommended at the present time (see Chapter 3). In the case of ovarian cancer, there are tests but they are unreliable and can lead to unnecessary surgery.

HEALTH BELIEFS AND CANCER SCREENING

Interest in the possible contribution of psychosocial factors on participation in cancer screening stems, in part, from research carried out in the 1940s and 1950s by medical sociologists and educators on barriers and facilitators to participation in screening for tuberculous (4). Although a number of clinical researchers have challenged assumptions underlying the early work and have identified other additional factors influencing participation in screening, the Health Belief Model (5) (HBM) remains as a heuristic for clinical research. Janz and Becker reasoned that an individual's beliefs about his or her own health and vulnerability to disease are critical to participation in screening. They proposed the HBM, which is now the most widely used and researched theoretical model for the study of behavior change (4).

The HBM identifies four components: *perceived susceptibility* (how vulnerable to the disease the individual

TABLE 15.1 *ACS Recommendations* for the Early Detection of Cancer in Asymptomatic Average Risk People*

Cancer	Procedure	Age begin (yr)	Frequency
Breast	Breast self-examination	20	Monthly
	Breast clinical examination	20–39	Every 3 yr
		≥ 40	Annual
	Mammography	40–49	1–2 yr
Cervical	Pelvic examination	18–39	1–3 yr
	With Pap test†	≥ 40	Annual
		≥ 50	Annual
Colorectal	Flexible sigmoidoscopy	≥ 50	3–5 yr
	Stool blood	≥ 50	Annual
	Digital rectal	≥ 40	Annual
Prostate	Digital rectal examination	≥ 50	Annual
	Prostate-specific antigen (PSA) test	≥ 50	Annual

*A cancer related checkup is recommended every 3 years for people aged 20–40 and every year for people 40 years of age and older. This examination should include health counseling and examinations for cancers of the thyroid, oral cavity, skin, lymph nodes, testes, prostate, skin, oral region, and ovaries as well as for some nonmalignant diseases.

+ All women who are, or who have been, sexually active or have reached age 18 years, should have an annual Pap test and pelvic examination. After a woman has had three or more consecutive satisfactory normal annual examinations, the Pap test may be performed less frequently at the discretion of her physician.

Source: Above table is taken from *Cancer Facts and Figures–1996*, American Cancer Society, Inc. (2).

perceives himself or herself to be); *perceived severity* (how severe the individual perceives the targeted disease to be), *perceived barriers* (factors that the individual identifies as standing in the way of participating in screening); and *perceived benefits* (the benefits that the individual believes that he or she will receive by participating in screening). This model also identifies "cues to action," which are environmental cues that are believed to help initiate or "facilitate" participation in positive health behaviors. All of these factors are assumed to play significant roles in motivating participation in health prevention. The HBM has been especially used in the study of breast cancer screening practices (6–11). The HBM has also been studied with other cancers (e.g., prostate, ovarian, cervical, colorectal).

Health Beliefs among Individuals at Average Risk

According to the HBM, increased knowledge (perceived severity and perceived benefits) should be related to increased cancer screening practices. The more individuals know about cancer, including the importance of early diagnosis, and the benefits of cancer screening the more likely they should be to participate in cancer screening. Knowledge about cancer and screening procedures has been found to be a significant facilitator of cancer screening behavior for breast (12), prostate (13), and colorectal (14) cancer. Specifically, knowledge of breast cancer (15); knowledge of early warning signs for prostate cancer, and knowledge about the importance, effectiveness, and convenience of prostate cancer screening (16); knowledge of effectiveness of cervical cancer screening (17); and knowledge of benefits of colorectal cancer screening, and that colorectal cancer can be cured if detected early (18) have all been related to increased cancer screening participation. In one study the vast majority of *nonparticipants* for colorectal cancer screening saw no benefits to participating in screening; they did not perceive that a fecal occult blood test would give them peace of mind, nor did they believe it could help save their lives—the majority perceived colorectal cancer as incurable even if found early (19). These respondents clearly lacked a significant amount of knowledge to help them make an informed decision about whether or not to go through screening.

Importantly, some of the reasons reported for noncompliance for breast, cervical, and colorectal cancer screening represent a lack of appreciation for the concept of *asymptomatic illness* (14,20,21). Asymptomatic illness refers to an illness that does not display any observable symptoms. In these studies people did not come in for screening because they felt healthy; they did not realize that they could have cancer without displaying any symptoms. Hynam and colleagues (22) found that 25% of their sample did not participate because they felt well and did not see any need to be screened. Ferrand and colleagues (23) reported that only 43% of noncompliers believed in the concept of asymptomatic illness, and only 62% thought medical tests could show asymptomatic illness. Screening interventions need to teach individuals about the concept of asymptomatic illness, and the benefits of screening (22).

Not surprisingly, income and education have been found to be related to level of knowledge about cancer and cancer screening behaviors. Weinrich and colleagues (24) found that, similarly to results of research with breast and prostate cancer screening, Caucasians had more knowledge of colorectal cancer than African Americans, and persons with higher incomes had more knowledge than those with less income (24–26). Undereducated poor, because of their lack of knowledge, appear to be at more risk of not participating in screening and consequently to have cancer detected at later stages than those with more education and higher incomes.

Knowledge has also been found to be related to health beliefs and perceptions that can effect cancer screening behavior. For example, in a study of low socioeconomic status (SES) participants, those who were more knowledgeable of colorectal cancer perceived themselves as more susceptible to colorectal cancer, perceived fewer barriers of screening, and perceived more benefits of screening for colorectal cancer (19).

Previous participation in cancer screening, which increases a person's knowledge about cancer screening, is a significant predictor of subsequent participation. Lindholm and colleagues (21) found that in the process of conducting their colorectal screening study, 32 of the 97 nonattenders who were called for an interview after the first screening participated in the rescreening. Similar findings have been found by others (27–30). Moreover, first-round adherence has been found to be a strong independent predictor of participation in future screening (31). According to Myers and colleagues (31), the importance of first-round adherence may reflect greater acceptance of screening due to increased familiarity—increased knowledge and comfort with the process involved in testing, or the experience of positive feelings about prevention due to screening. Attaining high levels of initial screening participation, or at least following up with people who do not engage in prior testing, offers good intervention strategies to increase future cancer screening behavior (31).

According to the HBM, a person's perception of susceptibility, or risk of developing a disease, is believed to be an important determinant of their health-related behavior (4). In the case of cancer screening, the more a person believes they are at risk of developing cancer the more likely they should be to participate in cancer screening behavior that can detect early signs of cancer contributing to successful treatment. There has been very little research examining the influence of perceived risk on cancer screening behavior, especially among individuals at average risk for developing cancer. In general, the research indicates that those who have a greater perceived risk for cancer are more likely to have undergone screening for breast cancer (32), cervical cancer (33), and colorectal cancer (18). This relationship between perceived risk and cancer screening behavior, however, is not always so clear cut. Black, Nease, and Tosteson (34) found that women younger than 50, who were not at high risk for developing breast cancer, substantially overestimated their risk of developing breast cancer, as well as overestimating the benefits of mammography. These researchers suggest that exaggeration of risk may create unnecessary anxiety, which in some women could prevent health prevention efforts. These misperceptions of risk present a problem, because women between the ages of 40 and 50 years are expected to have a greater share of the decision making about mammography screening owing to the somewhat unclear guidelines for women in this age group. The NCI states that women need to assess their risk in order to make an informed decision about whether or not to have screening. This is a serious problem if women are not accurately perceiving their risk. Women, and all individuals, need to be educated about their real risk for cancer.

Of the four dimensions in the HBM, perceived barriers appear to be the most powerful in predicting screening behavior (4). Different barriers to cancer screening behavior (e.g., psychological, logistic, economic) have been reported for various cancers including, breast, prostate, ovarian, cervical, and colorectal.

Economic factors (lack of money or cost of screening procedures) explain noncompliance for cancer screening among a significant portion of the population. Indeed, such barriers have been reported as reasons for noncompliance for mammography screening (6,35,36), colorectal cancer screening (19,20), and cervical cancer screening (37). Moreover, higher SES and higher educational level (which is related to higher SES) have been found to be associated with increased screening adherence for breast cancer (12), cervical cancer (38,39), ovarian cancer (40), and colorectal can-

cer (24). Having health insurance has also been associated with increased cervical cancer screening (41), and being employed has been related to increased cancer screening participation for cervical (39,41) and ovarian cancer (40). However, women who have reported having to take time off from work to see a doctor in a low-income managed-care program have been found to be less likely to obtain mammograms (15). The uneducated poor without good jobs appear to be at more risk of not participating in screening and consequently to have cancer detected at later stages than those with more education and incomes.

Individuals often report logistic barriers that prevent them from following through with screening. Location of screening (i.e., transportation problems), and lack of time have been reported as barriers for mammography screening (35,42), ovarian cancer screening (40), and colorectal cancer screening (20). Inconvenience has also been reported as a common barrier (43,44).

Eardley and colleagues report health care system problems (e.g., accurate identification of women, communication problems, difficulty in arranging appointments, inconvenient locations for screening) that effect cervical cancer screening to be the most important factors affecting why women are not having screening, while personal perceptions and beliefs play a secondary role to these system barriers (17,33,45).

Numerous psychological barriers have also been reported as reasons for cancer screening noncompliance. Embarrassment, worry about radiation, anxiety, fear of pain or discomfort, fear of knowing, and fear of cancer have been perceived as barriers for breast (35,36), cervical (38,46), and colorectal (14,20) cancer screening. Procrastination and indifference have also been reported (38,43).

With colorectal cancer screening, psychological barriers involving the stool collection method of the fecal occult blood test have often been reported. Embarrassment, unpleasantness, as well as difficulty collecting specimens, and time involved in conducting the test (19–21,29,30,47) are common barriers reported for nonparticipants. Hunter and colleagues (48) found that five times as many nonparticipants as participants reported the stool collection procedure as disgusting.

It has been proposed that those who give seemingly more inocuous reasons, such as a lack of time or that they cannot be bothered (19,23,27), may not be giving real reasons for nonparticipation, and may be masking fears about cancer (22). Reasons such as unpleasantness of the screening procedure and intercurrent illness (other sickness preventing them from attending screening) may also be excuses for people who are fearful of dying from cancer; they may be worried about further hospital tests but are reluctant to admit this to the interviewer (22).

As reported earlier, cues from the environment (e.g., one's social network, health care resources) can act as initiators to participation in positive health behaviors. Having social ties has been found to be a facilitator of mammography use among low-income, older, Mexican-American women (49), and African-American women (50). Having seen a doctor within the previous two years, having a usual source of medical care (13), and presence of reminders (e.g., knowing someone with cancer, newspaper advertisements) (51) have increased prostate cancer participation. Facilitators such as personal initiation letters to screening, community-based campaigns (52), and presence of greater social ties (49,50) have been found to increase cervical cancer screening use. Similarly, living with other screening participants in the household (53), explanations by doctors, handouts received in the mail (20), and reminder letters (21) have all facilitated colorectal cancer screening behavior.

Health Beliefs among High-Risk Populations

Most of the research on health beliefs among individuals at high risk for cancer have focused on risk perception among women with a family history of breast cancer. Even though breast cancer has received the most attention, still little is known about breast cancer screening knowledge, attitudes, and behaviors among women at risk for breast cancer owing to family history (54). The research that does exist has found that some women with a family history of breast cancer have significantly overestimated their risk (55–57), while others have underestimated their risk (54,56,58). In terms of women overestimating their risk, there is a concern that, while they may know that they are at increased risk (which is accurate), many are overestimating their *actual risk* of developing breast cancer (55). Although these women know they are at increased risk, their cancer screening behavior is no different from that of women who are not at risk (57,59), and is thought to be unsatisfactory (60).

Polednak, Lane, and Burg (58) found an interesting interaction between perceived risk and family history of breast cancer. Among women with no history of breast cancer in the family, mammography use was less for those with lower perceived risk; while for women with positive history of breast cancer in the family, mammography use was less with those with higher perceived risk. Moreover, only for those with lower perceived risk was mammography use greater with knowledge of asymptomatic illness. It seems that higher perceived risk among women with a family history of breast cancer may act as a barrier to mammography screening.

In these high-risk women, psychological distress may be the mediating variable that is inhibiting them from following cancer screening guidelines. Lerman and her colleagues (55) suggest that overestimations of risk may be leading to greater psychological distress (e.g., worries and anxieties) that is somehow preventing these women from participating in screening. The relationship between psychological distress and mammography use is complex. Based on their findings, Lerman and her colleagues (55) posit a curvilinear relationship between the two; in their study, mammography adherence was reduced for women who scored higher on a clinical measure of intrusive thoughts, but was heightened among women who scored higher on a single-item measure of breast cancer worries. These researchers assert that moderate breast cancer concerns can have a motivating effect (61) but more serious psychological distress can have a deterrent effect (62) among women at increased risk for breast cancer. Lerman and Schwartz (63) have proposed that intermediate levels of anxiety may be optimal for getting high-risk women to participate in breast cancer screening, but that high levels of anxiety may actually act as a barrier to screening—perhaps immobilizing further positive health behaviors. As Lerman and colleagues (55) reported, high-risk women of all ages in their samples cited breast cancer worries as being problematic. However, women who were 29 years of age and younger showed the highest levels of global psychological distress. They assert that while serious psychological morbidity may not be prevalent in the general population of younger women at increased risk, many have breast cancer worries that have potential to compromise their daily functioning (55). According to Lerman et al. (55), there is a need to develop counseling approaches, especially for younger women at increased risk for breast cancer, that promote accurate perception of risk and reduce breast cancer worries (more extreme distress) that may compromise the quality of life of younger women.

Stefanek and Wilcox (54), based on their findings, recommend that women must be informed of their *personal* risk of developing breast cancer and be made to realize that screening can help them personally. In one study (64), women were informed of their individual risk status and those at increased risk on the basis of combinations of risk factors were invited to have a mammogram. Seventy-one percent of the high risk women came in for mammograms. The results from this study suggest that providing *personal* breast cancer risk information may encourage participation in screening—which is consistent with the HBM, which suggests that perceived vulnerability to disease should influence the likelihood of an individual undertaking preventive health behaviors.

While women with a family history of breast cancer are inaccurately perceiving their risk for breast cancer, thus experiencing greater psychological distress that can inhibit cancer screening participation, they are also reporting that their physicians have never recommended mammography to them, have never asked them about their family history, and have never given them any breast cancer risk information (54,56,59). The lack of inquiry about family history and the lack of information provided by medical professionals prevents women from making a well-informed decision about breast screening practices (54). Moreover, Vogel and colleagues (57) reported in their study that women cited lack of physician referral as a barrier to mammography screening. This lack of involvement by health care professionals poses a serious concern given how cues (cues to action from the HBM) from one's health care provider can increase participation in screening.

It appears that one's physician can also function as a barrier, because some physicians are better informed than others in regard to breast cancer risk and some may advise their patients in a manner that may not encourage screening. One study found that women usually seen by obstetrician/gynecologists, or internists, were more likely to have annual mammograms than women usually seen for breast examinations by general practitioners (59). With many Americans being insured under health maintenance organizations (HMOs), primary care physicians (general practitioners) become very important sources of information liaison between patients and the medical field. If general practitioners are taking on this role then they need to be better informed about cancer risk and screening and to pass this information along to their patients. It appears that not only does the lack of knowledge of asymptomatic illness inhibit individuals from pursuing cancer screening, it also contributes to the failure of physicians to follow established guidelines for breast cancer screening in asymptomatic women (65,66). Enhanced educational efforts that promote mammography need to target both primary health professionals and women at increased risk because of family history (59).

As indicated, among high-risk individuals, perceived risk and psychological distress may work together to influence cancer screening behavior. Research has examined other possible psychological barriers as well. Research has addressed the possible impact of

cancer and notification of results on psychological adjustment. The findings from this area of psychological research have been relatively consistent, showing moderate levels of psychological distress even when the results have been negative, or when a follow-up examination has revealed a negative result. Several studies have assessed the relationship between psychological distress and subsequent adherence to screening and have found that psychological distress is a barrier to screening adherence, particularly in high-risk women (63). Researchers have also found that, among women who have undergone mammography, false positive results lead to high levels of anxiety, fear, and breast cancer worries (61,67) which, in turn, negatively affect moods and functioning (61). Women at high risk who perceived high susceptibility and experienced elevated psychological distress (e.g., high levels of anxiety) have been found to be immobilized by their anxiety and therefore engaged in fewer health behaviors (68). This negative psychological sequelae of cancer screening notification may contribute to subsequent nonadherence to repeat screening (8). Excessive anxiety and cancer worries have been linked to reduced likelihood of repeat mammography screening (61), infrequent breast self examinations (69), and less use of ovarian cancer screening practices (70,71).

For those at increased risk because of family history, health care professionals need to recognize and acknowledge that many of these people at increased risk for cancer will have psychological effects from their experiences with their ill or deceased family members. The resultant anxieties and fears could act as a barrier to preventive health behavior, such as cancer screening.

In one ovarian cancer screening program (72) social workers were used to help women at high risk for ovarian cancer to deal with their unresolved emotions brought on by their relatives' death from cancer. Many of these high-risk women were daughters who had suffered psychological sequelae because their mothers had ovarian cancer. Smith and Schwartz (72) report that by evaluating coping skills and defense mechanisms (i.e., denial) the social worker is better able to connect with these women and encourage them to continue their participation in early detection procedures.

Unresolved grief is a major issue for those who have had to deal with a family member's fatal illness. For one participant in the aforementioned ovarian cancer screening program, for example, this distress became an impediment to her joining the study. However, once a social worker worked with her and helped her release the flood of emotions she was experiencing, she was then able to adhere to the program's guidelines (e.g., completing the questionnaire and keeping appointments).

Health Beliefs among Minority Populations

Unfortunately, African-American men and women, who are at much higher risk for many cancers, are less likely to participate in early cancer detection than other groups (73). Moreover, Lerman and colleagues (74) found that low-income minority men and women are less likely to participate in early cancer detection compared to other SES groups. As reported earlier, it is not surprising to find that the elderly, minorities, and those with lower SES, perceive more barriers to mammography screening, whereas knowledge of breast cancer, higher SES, and higher educational level were associated with screening adherence. (12). African-Americans also have less knowledge about cancer, in general, than whites (75) and do not accurately perceive their increased level of susceptibility (19), perhaps contributing to their nonparticipation in cancer screening. Michielutte and Diseker (75) have argued that differences in knowledge are due to different means of obtaining information through the media, different levels of education, and a lack of motivation of blacks to obtain knowledge about cancer owing to less access to medical care.

Price and colleagues investigated perceptions of African-American men regarding prostate cancer (19). The most common barrier reported was the cost of the examination; moreover, less education and low income were related to more perceived barriers. Various organizational and practical factors (e.g., less technically advanced physicians and facilities, lack of continuity of care, cost, travel time, and location) are all possible barriers to equal care for African Americans (76,77). Low-SES minorities also tend to delay seeking medical care after detecting symptoms, and therefore are consequently diagnosed at a later stage of the disease and have a shortened survival time (78).

In order to understand the determinants of cancer screening among African-Americans we must focus on the unique issues (e.g., racism and poverty) connected with the African-American community. In more recent years there has been a movement to emphasize the inclusion of culture, ethnicity, and race in psychological research (51), and the particular importance of studying cultural factors and health beliefs (79).

African Americans face many barriers to health care. Many lack purchasing power to obtain health care. A disproportionate number live in low-income households and many have no medical insurance (80), helping to explain the differences in the use of

the health care system between blacks and whites (81). The socioeconomic conditions promote inequality in the access to health care (80). According to Navarro (82) both race *and* class need to be considered when trying to understand health behaviors. Holliman (83) identified three barriers that affect access to health care for blacks: *(1)* Because of care being provided by non-black medical personnel, African-Americans are often reluctant to obtain early treatment for illnesses; *(2)* medical personnel can be perceived by African Americans as prejudiced against blacks; and *(3)* medical care is reduced because many doctors do not provide services in poor communities. African-Americans, lacking the ability to purchase health care, and having fewer alternative sources of care, end up having less knowledge about health promotion.

Many health beliefs and behaviors among African Americans may stem from their perception of negative biases by health care professionals (82). It has been suggested that the closing of an inequitable number of hospitals in black communities is evidence of institutional racism (80). Bailey (84) asserts that African Americans follow culturally specific health care seeking patterns that are significantly influenced by sociocultural factors. Although many barriers to health care have been slowly eliminated for blacks, many continue to have attitudes and practices that were adopted in a time when many barriers still existed (84). Living under a sociocultural system that traditionally denied equal access to health care for African-Americans has led to the holding of negative attitudes about the health care system, which in turn lead to a tendency to not seek help or delay seeking help until the condition is too serious to ignore (85).

Solely calling for individuals to change to more positive health practices may not be effective, especially among African Americans. Such a shift requires changes in roles, norms, and practices as well as access to information, facilities, and support. Development of plans to overcome barriers must focus on structural, economic, and cultural factors (86). Importantly, perceived racism becomes a very important determinant to consider.

In trying to understand sociocultural determinants of health behavior we must be careful that race as a classification does not preclude acknowledgment of ethnic or cultural differences (87). Cultural diversity among African Americans has for the most part been ignored. More recently some health professionals are emphasizing the heterogeneity of communities, and the necessity to consider differences within groups (e.g., language, values, customs, literacy levels, neighborhoods, nationality) (88–91). Persons of African descent, for example, share African history, and similar experiences based upon their racial group membership, but they also experience differences as a result of different backgrounds, cultural values, geographical location, ethnic affiliation, and subcultural beliefs (92). Barriers can arise when health professionals fail to recognize socioculturally defined subgroups (93). In order for health professionals to deliver more personalized and more culturally appropriate messages to different ethnic groups it is necessary to identify differential cultural determinants of the reluctance to obtain cancer screening within the African-American community (94).

INTERVENTIONS

Most of the work focusing on interventions has involved breast cancer screening. Moreover, in more recent years the bulk of this work has been done with community-based intervention programs designed to increase participation in breast cancer screening among poor, older, African-American women who are at highest risk. All the intervention programs (no matter what the type of screening) use the HBM as a guide, and attempt to increase knowledge, increase accurate perceptions of risk, and decrease barriers. There has been virtually no intervention work with women who are at risk for cancer due to family history.

Community-Based Interventions

Components of the Theory of Reasoned Action (TRA) have also been incorporated into the community-based intervention programs in minority communities, and have influenced health care professionals to rely on the use of models from the community to act as educators about screening. TRA contends that attitudes about the health behavior and the individual's personal (i.e., subjective) norms influence behavioral intentions, which then influence whether the health behavior in question is adopted. Subjective norms represent the individual's perceptions of whether individuals or groups of individuals think the person should or should not perform the behavior. Janz and Becker (4) have suggested adding this "social approval" component to the HBM as a refinement to the dimensions of perceived benefits and barriers. Bloom and colleagues (95) suggested that, among African American communities, in order to change factors such as knowledge of cancer warning signs, perceived susceptibility, and belief in its curability, the oral tradition of the black community should be used to desensitize cancer. For example, cancer survivors who are local residents

as well as local government and church leaders who are influential in the community can publicize the cure and control of cancer (elicit "cues to action" from the HBM). Similarly, Fisher and colleagues (96) discuss the use of modeling using government officials and clergy. In changing perceived risk, knowledge, susceptibility, and barriers to screening, family and friends become very important agents. A person will often turn to a friend or relative for advice before seeking professional help (95,96). Interventions that rely on individual communities to reach out to people with diverse cultures have met with some success.

Role models from the community who were previously diagnosed and treated with cancer have been used in programs in a church-based screening intervention for prostate cancer (97) and in a community-based intervention designed to increase mammography and cervical cancer screening in communities of Mexican-American, and African-American women (98). Suarez and colleagues had role models from the community tell their personal stories about cancer screening through the local media, including newspapers, radio, and television. In another intervention program, elderly educators were used to try to increase fecal occult blood testing among socioeconomically disadvantaged older persons (99). Family members have also been used as a resource. In the "Save Our Sisters Project," African-American women were recruited as "natural helpers" to serve the community as lay health advisors. These advisors reached older African American women through their family, friendship, and job networks (100).

Many of these programs also target individuals in culturally familiar locales in the community so that these intervention procedures are less threatening, and most likely to have the greatest impact. In one program, older African-American women in a local beauty salon were offered culturally sensitive educational pamphlets and videos to promote breast cancer screening (101). African-American and Latina women in New York City and Los Angeles received information on cervical cancer screening via culturally sensitive health education videos that were displayed in the waiting rooms of two community clinics. (102)

Other interventions include a nurse-delivered community-based intervention set up in two public clinics designed to increase breast and cervical cancer screening among poor African-American women in Chicago (103), a brief educational intervention given to female employees at various work sites (104), and a community-based project on Long Island that used a game to create a positive atmosphere to help disseminate information about breast cancer and screening (105).

Physician-Based Interventions

Given the important influence that physicians have on their patient's cancer screening behavior, and the fact that many of them are not encouraging cancer screening in their patients or performing screening practices with their patients, intervention programs have also been designed to increase physicians' (and other health professionals') knowledge and awareness about the importance of cancer screening, especially among high-risk patients. Intervention programs have been designed to increase knowledge about breast cancer and the benefits of screening for community health professionals (106); and for primary care physicians (107). In-office cancer screening education has been offered for primary care physicians and staff members (108); in one program, computerized reminders to perform fetal occult blood test (FOBT), mammography, and cervical Pap smears were given to primary care physicians (109). A metaanalysis that reviewed the effectiveness of interventions designed to enhance physician breast cancer screening behavior concluded that physician-based interventions can be effective in increasing screening behavior.

FUTURE DIRECTIONS

The primary objective of all work in the area of cancer screening is to increase participation in screening. We need to understand better why certain individuals do not participate and to determine how to address those issues so as to reduce barriers. In an effort to increase that understanding and to devise more effective interventions, researchers explore the role of psychosocial factors in screening participation. Toward that end, future research must become more sensitive to individual differences and determine how individual differences can be integrated into interventions to increase participation.

A promising strategy for understanding how to increase participation in cancer screening is Prochaska's Transtheoretical Model (TTM) of behavior change (110–112). The TTM has been successfully used in the design of interventions to promote positive health behaviors (e.g., smoking cessation and mammography screening). A major feature of the model is its emphasis on detailed assessment of attitudes and intentions of potential screenees and the individualization of intervention. TTM outlines methods for determining an individual's readiness to change ("where the person is," to use behavioral jargon) and then designing an intervention that considers that individual's level of readiness to change. In a very real sense, the TTM model represents "good" behavioral intervention strategy: It stresses the importance of careful assessment of the targeted individual's assets and deficits (in terms of readiness to change) and it focuses on individualized intervention. In light of the successful application of the TTM in interventions to change addictive behaviors and mammography participation, a new direction in cancer screening might well be to consider how to incorporate key features of the TTM into efforts to increase screening participation.

REFERENCES

1. Shapiro S, Vent W, Strax P. Ten-to fourteen year effect of screening on breast cancer mortality. *J Natl Cancer Inst*. 1982; 69:349–355.
2. American Cancer Society. *Cancer Facts and Figures*. Atlanta: American Cancer Society; 1996.
3. Berwick M, Begg CB, Fine JA, Rousch GC, Barnhill RL. Screening for cutaneous melanoma by skin self-examination. *J Natl Cancer Inst*. 1996; 88:17–23.
4. Janz NK, Becker MH. The health belief model: A decade later. *Health Educ Q*. 1984; 11:1–47.
5. Rosenstock IM. The health belief model: origins and correlates. *Health Educ Monogr*. 1974; 2:336–353.
6. Stein JA, Fox SA, Murata PJ, Morisky DE. Mammography usage and the health belief model. *Health Educ Q*. 1992; 19:447–462.
7. Champion VL. The relationship of breast self-examination to Health belief model variables. *Res Nurs Health*. 1987; 10:375–382.
8. Lerman C, Rimer B, Trock B, Balshem AM, Engstrom PF. Factors associated with repeat adherence to breast cancer screening. *Prev Med*. 1990; 19:1–12.
9. Massey V. Perceived susceptibility to breast cancer and the practice of breast self-examination. *Nurs Res*. 1986; 35:183–185.
10. Fajardo LL, Saint-Germain M, Meakem III TJ, Rose C, Hillman BJ. Factors influencing women to undergo screening mammography. *Radiology*. 1992; 184:59–63.
11. Aiken LS, West SG, Woodward CK, Reno RR. Health beliefs and compliance with mammography-screening recommendations in asymptomatic women. *Health Psychol*. 1994; 13:122–129.
12. Roetzheim RG, Van Durme DJ, Brownlee HJ, Herold AH, Woodard LJ, Blair C. Barriers to screening among participants of a media-promoted breast cancer screening project. *Cancer Detect Prev*. 1993; 17:367–377.
13. Brown ML, Potosky AL, Thompson GB, Kessler LG. The knowledge and use of screening tests for colorectal and prostate cancer: data from the 1987 National Health Interview Survey. *Prev Med*. 1990; 19:562–574.
14. Hart AR, Wicks ACB, Mayberry JF. Colorectal cancer screening in asymptomatic populations. *Gut*. 1995; 36:590–598.
15. Lantz PM, Stencil D, Lippert MT, Beversdorf S, Jaros L, Remington PL. Breast and cervical cancer screening in a low-income managed care sample: the efficacy of physician letters and phone calls. *Am J Public Health*. 1995; 85:834–836.

16. Myers RE, Ross E, Jepson C, et al. Modeling adherence to colorectal cancer screening. *Prev Med.* 1994; 23:142–151.

17. Elkind AK, Haran D, Eardley A, Spencer B. Well you can come in but I'm not having it? *Health Visitor.* 1989; 62:20–21.

18. Weller DP, Owen N, Hiller JE, Willson K, Wilson D. Colorectal cancer and its prevention: Prevalence of beliefs, attitudes, intentions and behavior. *Aust J Public Health.* 1995; 19:19–23.

19. Price JH. Perceptions of colorectal cancer in a socio-economically disadvantaged population. *J Community Health.* 1993; 18:347–362.

20. Arveux P, Durand G, Milan C, et al. Views of a general population on mass screening for colorectal cancer: the Burgundy study. *Prev Med.* 1992; 21:574–581.

21. Lindholm E, Berglund B, Haglind E, Kewenter. Factors associated with participation in screening for colorectal cancer with faecal occult blood testing. *Scand J Gastroenterol.* 1995; 30:171–176.

22. Hynam KA, Hart AR, Gay SP, Inglis A, Wicks ACB, Mayberry JF. Screening for colorectal cancer: reasons for refusal of faecal occult blood testing in a general practice in England. *J Epidemiol Community Health.* 1995; 49:84–86.

23. Ferrand PA, Hardcastle JD, Chamberlain J, Moss S. Factors affecting compliance with screening for colorectal cancer. *Community Med.* 1984; 6:12–19.

24. Weinrich SP, Weinrich MC, Boyd MD, Johnson E, Frank-Stromborg M. Knowledge of colorectal cancer among older persons. *Cancer Nurs.* 1992; 15:322–330.

25. Weinrich SP, Weinrich MC, Keenan L, Boyd MD. Cancer knowledge and health practices of homebound elderly persons. *Adv Health Educ Curr Res.* 1991; 3:191–204.

26. Weinrich SP. Predictors of occult blood screening in the elderly. *Oncol Nurs Forum.* 1990; 17:715–720.

27. Klaaborg K, Stahl Madsen M, Sondergaard K, Kronborg O. Participation in mass screening for colorectal cancer with faecal occult blood test. *Scand J Gastroenterol.* 1983; 21:1180–1184.

28. Kronborg O, Fenger C, Sondergaard O, Pedersen KM, Olsen J. Initial mass screening for colorectal cancer with faecal occult blood. *Scand J Gastroenterol.* 1987; 22:677–686.

29. Silman A, Mitchell P. Attitudes of non-participants in an occupational based programme of screening for colorectal cancer. *Community Med.* 1984; 6:8–11.

30. Box V, Nichols S, Lallemand RC, Person P, Vahil PA. Haemoccult compliance rates and reasons for non-compliance. *Public Health.* 1984; 98:16–25.

31. Myers RE, Balshem AM, Wolf TA, Ross EA, Millner L. Adherence to continuous screening for colorectal neoplasia. *Med Care.* 1993; 31:508–519.

32. Vernon SW, Vogel VG, Halabi S, Bondy ML. Factors associated with perceived risk of breast cancer among women attending a screening program. *Breast Cancer Res Treat.* 1993; 28:137–144.

33. Elkind AK, Haran D, Eardley A, Spencer B. Reasons for nonattendance for computer-managed cervical screening: pilot interviews. *Soc Sci Med.* 1988; 27:651–660.

34. Black WC, Nease RF, Tosteson AN. Perceptions of breast cancer risk and screening effectiveness in women younger than 50 years of age. *J Natl Cancer Instit.* 1995; 87:720–731.

35. Mootz AR, Glazer-Waldman H, Evans WP, Peters GN, Kirk LM. Mammography in a mobile setting: Remaining barriers. *Radiology.* 1991; 180:161

36. Rimer BK, Kasper Keintz M, Kessler HB, Engstrom PF, Rosan JR. Why women resist screening mammography: patient-related barriers. *Radiology.* 1989; 172:243–246.

37. Carney P, Dietrich AJ, Freeman DH Jr. Improving future preventive care through educational efforts at a women's community screening program. *J Community Health.* 1992; 17:167–174.

38. Harlan LC, Bernstein AB, Kessler LG. Cervical cancer screening: who is not screened and why? *Am J Public Health.* 1991; 81:885–890.

39. Goel V. Factors associated with cervical cancer screening: results from the Ontario Health Survey. *Can J Public Health.* 1994; 85:125–127.

40. Pavlik EJ, van Nagell JR Jr, et al. Participation in transvaginal ovarian cancer screening: compliance, correlation factors, and costs. *Gynecol Oncol.* 1995; 57:395–400.

41. Hayward RA, Shapiro MF, Freeman HE, Corey CR. Who ges screened for cervical and breast cancer? Results from a new national survey. *Arch Intern Med.* 1988; 148:1177–1181.

42. Rimer BK, Trock B, Engstrom PF, Lerman C, King E. Why do some women get regular mammograms? *Am J Prev Med.* 1991; 7:69–74.

43. Dent OF, Bartrop RW, Goulston KJ, Chapuis PH. Participation in faecal occult blood screening for colorectal cancer. *Soc Sci Med.* 1983; 17:17–23.

44. Myers RE, Ross EA, Wolf TA, Balshem AM, Jepson C, Millner L. Behavioral interventions to increase adherence in colorectal cancer screening. *Med Care.* 1991; 29:1039–1050.

45. Eardley A, Elkind AK, Spencer B, Hobbs P, Pendleton LL, Haran D. Attendance for cervical screening–whose problem? *Soc Sci Med.* 1985; 20:955–962.

46. Seow A, Wong ML, Smith WCS, Lee HP. Belief and attitudes as determinants of cervical cancer screening: a community-based study in Singapore. *Prev Med.* 1995; 24:134–141.

47. Macrae FA, Hill DJ, St.John JB, Ambikapathy A, Garner JF. Predicting colon cancer screening behaviour from health beliefs. *Prev Med.* 1984; 13:115–126.

48. Hunter W, Farmer A, Mant D, Verne J, Northover J, Fitzpatrick R. The effect of self-administered faecal occult blood tests on compliance with screening for colorectal cancer: results of a survey of those invited. *Family Pract.* 1991; 8:367–372.

49. Suarez L, Lloyd L, Weiss N, Rainbolt T, Pulley L. Effect of social networks on cancer-screening behavior of older Mexican-American women. *J Natl Cancer Inst.* 1994; 86(10):775–779.

50. Kang SH, Bloom R, Romano PS. Cancer screening among African-American women: their use of tests and social support. *Am J Public Health.* 1994; 84:101–103.

51. Betancourt H, Lopez SR. The study of culture, ethnicity, and race in American Psychology. *Am Psychol.* 1993; 48:629–637.

52. Mitchell H, Hirst S, Cockburn J, Reading DJ, Staples MP, Medley G. Cervical cancer screening: a comparison of recruitment strategies among older women. *Med J Aust.* 1991; 155:79–82.

53. Thomas W, White CM, Mah J, Geisser MS, Church TR, Mandel JS. Longitudinal compliance with annual screening for faecal occult blood. *Am J Epidemiol.* 1995; 142:176–182.

54. Stefanek ME, Wilcox P. First degree relatives of breast cancer patients: screening practices and provision of risk information. *Cancer Detect Prev.* 1991; 15:379–384.

55. Lerman C, Kash K, Stefanek M. Younger women at increased risk for breast cancer: perceived risk, psychological well-being, and surveillance behavior. *Monogr Natl Cancer Inst.* 1994; 16:171–176.

56. Evans DGR, Brunell LD, Hopwood P, Howell A. Perception of risk in women with a family history of breast cancer. *Br J Cancer.* 1993; 67:612–614.

57. Vogel VG, Graves DS, Vernon SW. mammographic screening of women with increased risks of breast cancer. *Cancer.* 1990; 66:1613–1620.

58. Polednak AP, Lane DS, Burg MA. Risk perception, family history, and use of breast cancer screening tests. *Cancer Detect Prev.* 1991; 15:257–263.

59. Kaplan KM, Weinberg GB, Small A, Herndon JL. Breast cancer screening among relatives of women with breast cancer. *Am J Public Health.* 1991; 81(9):1174–1179.

60. Krisher JP, Cook B, Weiner RS. Indentification and screening of women at high risk of breast cancer. *Cancer Detect Prev.* 1988; 13:65–74.

61. Lerman C, Trock B, Rimer BK, Jepson C, Brody D, Boyce A. Psychological side effects of breast cancer screening. *Health Psychol.* 1991; 10:259–267.

62. Lerman C, Daly M, Sands C, et al. Mammography adherence and psychological distress among women at risk for breast cancer. *J Natl Cancer Inst.* 1993; 85:1074–1080.

63. Lerman C, Schwartz M. Adherence and psychological adjustment among women at high risk for breast cancer. *Breast Cancer Res Treat.* 1993; 28:145–155.

64. Taplin S, Anderman C, Grothaus L. Breast cancer risk and participation in mammographic screening. *Am J Public Health.* 1989; 79:1494–1498.

65. Holleb AI. 1989 survey of physicians' attitudes and practices in early cancer detection. *CA: Cancer J Clin.* 1990; 40:77–101.

66. Holleb AI. Survey of physicians' attitudes and practices in early cancer detection. *CA: Cancer J Clin.* 1985; 35:197–213.

67. Ellman R, Angeli N, Christians A. Psychiatric morbidity associated with screening for breast cancer. *Br J Cancer.* 1989; 60:781–784.

68. Kash KM, Holland JC, Halper MS, Miller DG. Psychological distress and surveillance behaviors of women with a family history of breast cancer. *J Natl Cancer Inst.* 1992; 84:24–30.

69. Alagna SW, Morokoff PJ, Bevett JM, Reddy DM. Performance of breast self-examination by women at high risk for breast cancer. *Wom Health.* 1987; 12:29–46.

70. Schwartz M, Lerman C, Daly M, Audrain J, Masny A, Griffith K. Utilization of ovarian cancer screening by women at increased risk. *Cancer Epidemiol Biomarkers Prev.* 1995; 4:269–273.

71. Wolfe CDA, Raju KS. The attitudes of women and feasibility of screening for ovarian and endometrial cancers in inner city practices. *Eur J Obstet Gynecol.* 1994; 56:117–120.

72. Smith PM, Schwartz PE. Social work role in an early ovarian cancer detection program. *Social Work in Health Care.* 1993; 19:67–80.

73. Rimer BK. Interventions to increase breast screening. Lifespan and ethnicity issues. *Cancer.* 1994; 74:323–328.

74. Lerman C, Rimer B, Engstrom P. Reducing avoidable cancer mortality through prevention and early detection regimens. *Cancer Res.* 1989; 49:4955–4962.

75. Michielutte R, Diseker RA. Racial differences in knowledge of cancer: a pilot study. *Soc Sci Med.* 1982; 16:245–252.

76. Escarce JJ, Epstein KR, Colby DC, Schwartz JS. Racial differences in the elderly's use of medical procedures and diagnostic tests [see comments]. *Am J Public Health.* 1993; 83:948–954.

77. Lieu TA, Newacheck PW, McManus MA. Race, ethnicity, and access to ambulatory care among US adolescents [see comments]. *Am J Public Health.* 1993; 83:960–965.

78. Berg JW, Ross R, Latourette HB. Economic status and survival of cancer patients. *Cancer.* 1977; 39:467–477.

79. Landrine H, Klonoff EA. Culture and health-related schemas: A review and proposal for interdisciplinary integration. *Health Psychol.* 1992; 11:267–276.

80. Rice MF, Winn M. Black health care in America: A political perspective. *J Nat Med Assoc.* 1991; 82:429–437.

81. Cornelius LJ. Access to medical care for Black Americans with an episode of illness. *J Natl Med Assoc.* 1991; 83:617–626.

82. Navarro V. Race or class, or race and class. *Int J Health Ser.* 1989; 19:311–314.

83. Holliman JS. Access to health care. In: *Securing Access to Health Care: The Ethical Implications of Differences in Availability of Health Services,* 2d ed. Washington, DC: President's Commission for the Study of Ethical Problems in Medicine and Biomedical and Behavioral Research; 1983.

84. Bailey EJ. Sociocultural factors and health care-seeking behavior among Black Americans. *J Natl Med Assoc.* 1987; 79:389–392.

85. Neighbors H. Ambulatory medical care among adult Black Americans: The hospital emergency room. *J Natl Med Assoc.* 1986; 78:275–282.

86. Hardy RE, Hargreaves MK. Cancer prognosis in Black Americans: a mini-review. *J Natl Med Assoc.* 1992; 83:574–579.

87. Wilkinson DY, King G. Conceptual and methodological issues in the use of race as a variable: policy implications. *Milbank Q.* 1987; 65:56–71.

88. Johnson KM, Arfken CL. Individual recruitment strategies in minority-focused research. In: Becker DM, Hill DR, Jackson JS, Levine DM, Stillman FA, Weiss SM,

eds. *Health Behavior Research in Minority Populations: Access, Design, and Implementation.* NIH Publication No. 92-2965: 1992.

89. Rand C, Mebane-Sims I, Doak L, et al. Individual recruitment: task group 1. In: Becker DM, Hill DR, Jackson JS, Levine DM, Stillman FA, Weiss SM, eds. *Health Behavior Research in Minority Populations: Access, Design, and Implementation.* NIH Publication No. 92-2965; 1992.

90. Gritz ER, Berman BA, Bennett G, et al. Recruitment through school and churches: task group 2. In: Becker DM, Hill DR, Jackson JS, Levine DM, Stillman FA, Weiss SM, eds. *Health Behavior Research in Minority Populations: Access, Design, and Implementation.* NIH Publication No. 92-2965; 1992.

91. Esparaza DM. The influence of ethnic patient values on cancer nursing. In: Jones LA, ed. *Minorities and Cancer.* New York: Springer-Verlag; 1989.

92. Cross WE, Parham TA, Helms JE. Nigrescence revisited: Theory and Research. In: Jones R, ed. *Advances in Black Psychology.* Cobb & Henry; 1992.

93. Orlandi MA. Community-based substance abuse prevention: a multicultural perspective. *J Sch Health.* 1986; 56:394–401.

94. Stein JA, Fox SA, Murata PJ. The influence of ethnicity, socioeconomic status, and psychological barriers on use of mammography. *J Health Soc Behav.* 1991; 32:101–113.

95. Bloom JR, Hayes WA, Saunders F, Flatt S. Cancer awareness and secondary prevention practices in Black Americans: implications for intervention. *Fam Community Health.* 1987; 10:19–30.

96. Fisher EB, Auslander W, Sussman L, Owens N, Jackson-Thompson J. Community organization and health promotion in minority neighborhoods. In: Becker DM, Hill DR, Jackson JS, Levine DM, Stillman FA, Weiss SM, eds. *Health Behavior Research in Minority Populations: Access, Design, and Implementation.* Washington, D.C.: National Institutes of Health; 1992: 53–72.

97. Boehm S, Coleman-Burns P, Schlenk EA, Funnell MM, Parzuchowski J, Powell IJ. Prostate cancer in African American men: increasing knowledge and self-efficacy. *J Community Health Nurs.* 1995; 12:161–169.

98. Suarez L, Nichols DC, Brady CA. Use of peer role models to increase Pap smear and mammogram screening in Mexican-American and black women. *Am J Prev Med.* 1993; 9:290–296.

99. Weinrich SP, Weinrich MC, Stromborg MF, Boyd MD, Weiss HL. Using elderly educators to increase colorectal cancer screening. *Gerontologist.* 1993; 33:491–496.

100. Eng E. The Save our Sisters Project. A social network strategy for reaching rural black women. *Cancer.* 1993; 72:1071–1077.

101. Forte DA. Community-based breast cancer intervention program for older African American women in beauty salons. *Public Health Rep.* 1995; 110:179–183.

102. Yancey AK, Tanjasiri SP, Klein M, Tunder J. Increased cancer screening behavior in women of color by culturally sensitive video exposure. *Prev Med.* 1995; 24:142–148.

103. Ansell D, Lacey L, Whitman S, Chen E, Phillips C. A nurse-delivered intrvention to reduce barriers to breast and cervical cancer screening in Chicago inner city clinics. *Public Health Rep.* 1994; 109:104–111.

104. Kurtz ME, Kurtz JC, Given B, Given CC. Promotion of breast cancer screening in a work site population. *Health Care Wom Int.* 1994; 15:31–42.

105. Forsyth MC, Fulton DL, Lane DS, Burg MA, Krishna M. Changes in knowledge, attitudes and behavior of women participating in a community education program on breast cancer screening. *Patient Educ Couns.* 1992; 19:241–250.

106. Reding DJ, Huber JA, Lappe KA. Results of a rural breast health education demonstration project. *Cancer Pract.* 1995; 3:295–302.

107. Costanza ME, Zapka JG, Harris DR, et al. Impact of physician intervention program to increase breast cancer screening. *Cancer Epidemiol Biomarkers Prev.* 1992; 1:581–589.

108. Williams PT, Eckert G, Epstein A, Mourad L, Helmick F. In-office cancer-screening education of primary care physicians. *J Cancer Educ.* 1994; 9:90–95.

109. Litzelman DK, Dittus RS, Miller ME, Tierney WM. Requiring physicians to respond to computerized reminders improves their compliance with preventive care protocols. *J Gen Intern Med.* 1993; 8:311–317.

110. Prochaska JO, DiClemente CC. Stages and processes of self-change of smoking: toward an integrative model. *J Cons Clin Psychol.* 1983; 390–395.

111. Prochaska JO, DiClemente CC. Transtheoretical therapy: Toward a more integrative model of change. *Psychother Theory Res Pract.* 1982; 20:161–173.

112. Prochaska JO, DiClemente CC, Norcross JS. In search of how people change: applications to addictive behaviors. *Am Psychol.* 1992; 47:1120–1114.

IV

HIGH GENETIC RISK OF CANCER

EDITOR: JIMMIE C. HOLLAND

16

Genetics for the Psycho-oncologist

ALEXANDER KAMB AND MARK H. SKOLNICK

Our genes, or more precisely the interplay between our genes and our environment, determine to a high degree who we are. Genes affect appearance, behavior, and health. They are the most fundamental distinguishing characteristics among individual people; and, they are the biochemical signatures of kin relationships. They identify us with our parents and siblings, and to a lesser extent with our more distant relatives, our ethnic groups, our species, and so on through the evolutionary steps that connect us with all living things.

The essence of genes is the polymeric chemical DNA. The individual units of the DNA polymer, the information "bits," are the four nucleotide bases, adenine, thymine, cytosine, and guanine, denoted as A, T, C, G. The linear order of these bases specify the 100,000 or so proteins encoded within the human genome. To accommodate the large set of genes, the human genome possesses 3 billion bases organized into 23 chromosome pairs. Straightened and opposed end to end, these chromosomes would extend over 1 meter in length. The long DNA polymers must be packed within a cell nucleus, typically one millionth of a meter in diameter. Moreover, the entire stretch of DNA must replicate and segregate to daughter cells within the space of one day. The error rate of this replication process is astonishingly low.

Expression of genes that comprise the human genome in a defined spatial and temporal pattern following conception gives rise to humans in all their variety. Often, a particular gene—for example, the gene for blood group antigen—comes in multiple forms (or *alleles*) that are inherited, or segregate, independently. One familial line may segregate allele type *A*, while a different line may segregate allele *a*. Since we are diploid—that is, we inherit one set of alleles from our mother and a second set from our father—we are each heterozygous at many loci (gene locations); we

carry one allele type *A* from our mother, and a different allele *a* from our father. We are also homozygous at other loci, *A/A* or *a/a*. Differences among individual humans derive from allelic variation.

Particular alleles may behave differently in combination with one another. Individuals who are heterozygous at a particular locus (*A/a*) may have the same external characteristics (phenotype) as those who are homozygous (*A/A*). This is termed *allele dominance*. In contrast, individuals homozygous for *a* may appear different from *Aa* heterozygotes or *AA* homozygotes. Thus, allele *a* is *recessive* to allele *A*. In some instances the *Aa* heterozygotes may be intermediate between *AA* and *aa* homozygotes. In such cases, the two alleles are said to be *codominant*.

This simple pattern of genetic behavior, segregation and phenotypic expression of dominant or recessive traits, accounts to a great extent for the genetics of human disease. Syndromes that range from color blindness to cancer can be understood by application of the same genetic principles used to describe inheritance in simpler model organisms such as fruit flies. As will be discussed later, the methods are different but the genetic phenomena are similar.

Genetic analysis demonstrated several decades ago that human cancer is, in certain cases, familial (1); that is, kindreds can be identified which display significant clusters of specific tumor types. In some instances, such as xeroderma pigmentosum, cancer susceptibility is primarily recessive. In general, however, the major cancer susceptibilities are inherited in a dominant fashion. Inheritance of a single susceptibility allele from either parent is sufficient to increase risk.

The same genetic loci that contribute to familial cancer are also involved in the development of nonfamilial (also called sporadic) cancer. As normal cells evolve through various stages toward malignancy, the expres-

Sporadic

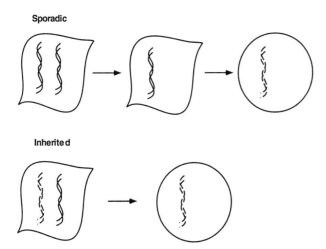

Inherited

FIG. **16–1.** Genetic changes required to inactivate a tumor suppressor gene in sporadic or familial cancer. In both cases two hits are needed, but in the familial case the first hit (indicated by the fragmented double helix) is inherited.

sion of specific genes is altered. These genes are typically associated with the cellular growth control apparatus. Such genes come in two forms: protooncogenes and tumor suppressor genes. Protooncogenes are genes whose normal function is to increase cell growth. Thus, their activity is dominant. Alteration of a single allele to generate an oncogene is sufficient to achieve a stimulatory effect on tumor growth. Tumor suppressor genes, in contrast, normally act to limit cell growth. They behave as recessive genes because inactivation of both alleles is required to affect growth. Study of genetic changes that take place during tumor cell development is part of the field termed *somatic cell genetics*, since it applies to individual somatic cells in the body. The progression to malignancy involves genetic changes in multiple protooncogenes and tumor suppressor genes. When some but not all of these changes have occurred, cells have intermediate characteristics and are called tumor precursors or benign tumors. Familial cancer predisposition syndromes can be understood as the inheritance of tumor suppressor gene mutations (or less commonly, oncogenes) which increase the likelihood that a particular cell will overcome the internal growth control mechanisms and give rise to a clonal, neoplastic mass (Fig. 16–1).

The past two decades have seen a gradual convergence of cancer research with basic studies on the mechanisms that underlie cell growth. Cell division is a process that is highly conserved through eukaryotic evolution. It involves a cycle of four steps: G_1, a phase

during which the cell prepares for DNA synthesis; S, a phase during which DNA is replicated; G_2, a phase during which preparations are made for mitosis; and M, the mitotic phase itself (Fig. 16–2). An emerging set of molecules controls the transitions in the cell cycle. Chief among these molecules are the cyclin-dependent kinases (CDKs) which, when active, drive the cell forward through the different phases. They are assisted by a group of positive regulatory factors, the cyclins, and a group of inhibitory molecules, the CDK inhibitors. The balance between these molecules, in particular the relative levels of cyclins and CDK inhibitors, determines the rate of cell growth. In cancer cells, this balance is shifted in favor of active CDK molecules due to a variety of genetic and epigenetic changes.

HUMAN GENETIC ANALYSIS

Genetic analysis often proceeds by consideration of a series of interrelated phenotypes associated with a disease. This may be straightforward, as in the genetics of

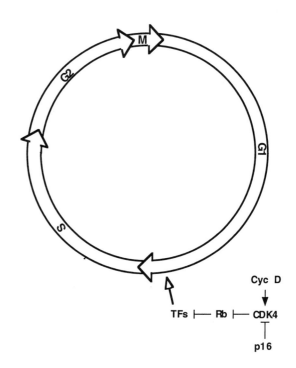

FIG. **16–2.** The cell cycle. The approximate relative duration of each phase is reflected by the relative lengths of the curved arrows. In many cycling cells, the total length of the cycle is one day. An important transition point, the G_1 checkpoint, is shown by a heavy arrow. One of the genetic/biochemical pathways that regulate the checkpoint is shown below. Arrows indicate activation; blunt-ended lines indicate inhibition. Cyc D is cyclin D, TFs are transcription factors that drive the cell from G_1 to S.

hemophilia, or it may be more complex, as in asthma. In certain cases, linkage analysis may assist in the definition of a reliable phenotype—the description and/or quantitation of a specific trait or set of traits. Linkage analysis can identify the trait(s) that segregate reliably in families.

Once the phenotype is determined, the next step is identification of kindreds that appear to segregate the trait(s) of interest. If the disease is common, this task may be easier than for rare diseases. The traditional approach to obtaining such kindreds is through family histories collected by physicians in a piecemeal fashion. In some cases, more systematic efforts toward collection of family information have been made (2,3). The larger the family and the more pronounced the clustering of disease, the simpler the genetic analysis is likely to be. Thus, large kindreds with many affected individuals are highly prized. Individuals from such kindreds, both affected and unaffected, must provide blood samples that can be used to produce DNA for subsequent genetic mapping experiments.

The genealogical records of kindred relationships and the corresponding DNA samples serve as the basis for linkage analysis. The goal is to identify a particular chromosome or chromosomal region that is more commonly shared among the affected members of the family (and not among the unaffecteds) than would be expected by chance. In the case of X-linked diseases such as hemophilia, the linkage is clear. Males are thousands of times more likely to develop the disease because the underlying genetic defect is recessive and is carried on the X chromosome. Since males have a single X chromosome, a single mutant X chromosome is sufficient to cause the disease.

For autosomal (non-X-linked) traits, linkage behavior is less obvious, but the genetic principles are the same (Fig. 16–3). The chromosomes can be tracked in the different DNA samples using molecular tags, or markers. These marker sets are chosen to cover the entire genome spaced at regular genetic intervals. For example, each chromosome might include 20–60 markers distributed evenly across its length. To distinguish the paternal and maternal chromosomes in the kindred, markers must be polymorphic; they must exist in multiple allelic forms. One must be able to assign a specific marker allele to a particular chromosome that segregates with affected individuals within the kindred. In practice, most contemporary linkage studies use short tandem repeat (STR) markers (4). These consist of tandemly repeated blocks of nucleotides averaging 15 or 20 repeated units of, for example, the (CA) dinucleotide. The exact length of the repeat varies in the population. The size thus serves as an allele that

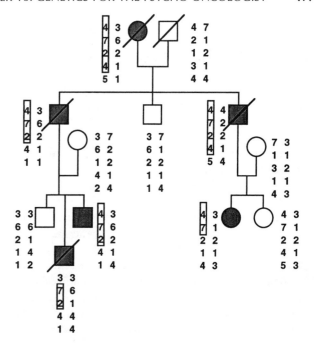

FIG. **16–3.** A hypothetical human cancer-prone pedigree. Circles are females; squares are males. The allele types for a set of genetic markers on a specific chromosome (haplotype) are shown next to each individual. Each column of numbers represents markers from one of the two homologous chromosomes, maternal or paternal. The numbers represent specific marker alleles. In boxes are the portions of the predisposing haplotype (allele set) inherited by the descendents of the founding male. Recombination through the generations trims the haplotype and allows genetic localization of the gene to a smaller chromosomal interval bounded by the external genetic markers shown.

can be followed from individual to individual in kindreds.

Although genes are transmitted on complete chromosomes from generation to generation, the allelic makeup of chromosomes is variable. This feature of genetics is due to genetic recombination, a property that leads to exchange of chromosomal segments of parental chromosomes. In humans there is on average at least one recombination event per chromosome in each fertilized egg. Thus, in time, different allelic types tend to become randomly mixed with respect to other loci on the chromosome. The measure of recombination frequency is the centiMorgan (cM) named for the great *Drosophila* geneticist Thomas Hunt Morgan. This unit reflects the rate per generation that two separate markers recombine. The rate of recombination can be viewed as a genetic distance in cM; close markers recombine infrequently, distant markers recombine often. One cM corresponds to one recombination event observed in 100 fertilized eggs.

The genetic distance between two markers corresponds in a rough way to the physical distance, the length of DNA, between them. In humans, 1 cM is approximately equivalent to one million nucleotides. Genetic recombination is extremely important in localizing genes since it allows the order of marker sets to be determined the basis of the rate at which they recombine with one another (Fig. 16–3). The more distant two markers are, the less likely they are to be inherited together through the generations.

The objective of linkage analysis is to develop strong statistical support for the physical proximity of a particular set of markers and the trait of interest. This statistical support is often expressed as the logarithm of the odds, or LOD score (5). The LOD score is simply the base-10 logarithm of a ratio of the likelihood of sharing a particular marker allele (or set of alleles) over the likelihood that the markers and the disease gene lie on separate chromosomes. Many factors influence the LOD score; for example, the rarity of the trait in the population, the density of markers in the linked region, the location of the markers with respect to the disease gene, the frequency of the marker alleles, and the allelic penetrance (see below). Sometimes the linkage assignment is unequivocal; more often it is marginal, and further effort involving more individuals and more markers is required to gain a measure of confidence.

It is possible to extract useful genetic information from more limited family studies. Comparisons of twins, both monozygotic and dizygotic, can provide estimates for the degree of heritability of particular traits. The analysis of multiple, independent sets of affected relatives can yield linkage information. However, much larger numbers of genotypes are required than in kindred studies to achieve reasonable statistical power. Finally, in situations where the trait was introduced into a relatively isolated population by a single founder several generations ago, remote ancestor analysis may be feasible. This method is very powerful, and may supply precise linkage information from a small number of affected, distant relatives. As in traditional linkage analysis in families, the goal is to identify a chromosomal region that is shared among the affected individuals, a DNA segment inherited from their common ancestor.

Owing to the complexity of human physiology, many alleles involved in human disease do not contribute in an all-or-none fashion. Rather, the inheritance of a particular allele may increase the probability of developing the disease; but this probability may be well below 100%. The likelihood that a gene carrier will develop the disease by a particular age is termed *allelic penetrance*. Penetrance can vary from disease to disease

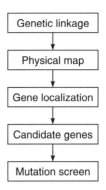

FIG. **16–4.** The steps involved in a positional cloning project.

and allele to allele. In many familial cancer syndromes, allelic penetrances fall between 30% and 90%.

Recombinant DNA methods provide the tools to go from genetic linkage to isolation of the gene itself. This process is termed *positional cloning*. The individual steps are straightforward, but labor-intensive and tedious (Fig. 16–4). First, a physical map is constructed of the relevant genetic interval using genomic clones; these clones are organized into appropriate overlapping segments such that they cover the entire region within which the genetic locus must lie. Second, new markers are generated using the ordered genomic clones to assist in further localization of the gene; this localization is generally achieved by study of recombinant chromosomes (Fig. 16–3) and/or chromosomal rearrangements in somatic tissues. Third, the refined physical interval is screened to identify as many genes as possible; each of these genes is a candidate for the genetic locus of interest. Finally, sequences of the candidate genes are screened for mutations in affected individuals from disease-prone kindreds. Proof that the sought after gene has been found follows from identification of sequence variants, linked to the appropriate carrier chromosomes, and disruptive to the function of the gene. Such sequence variants are expected to be found more frequently in diseased individuals than in normal individuals.

SOMATIC CELL GENETICS

In the area of cancer, it is particularly valuable to consider a different type of genetic analysis—the genetics of somatic cells. This discipline is relevant because somatic cells undergo a series of genetic changes as they evolve more malignant traits. Unraveling these changes has been one of the most productive fields of investigation in cancer biology. It has had ramifications for many areas of basic biology as well, especially with regard to the mechanisms that regulate cell growth and differentiation.

One of the most important applications of somatic cell genetics to cancer research has been the study of interactions between tumor-causing (transforming) viruses and cells in culture. Especially significant were experiments with acutely transforming retroviruses. These studies led to the identification of the first oncogenes (*src* and *ras*), and were the basis for the Nobel Prize in Physiology and Medicine awarded to J. Michael Bishop and Harold Varmus in 1990. An extraordinary observation followed from the molecular analysis of retroviral genomes: the oncogenes carried by several retroviruses are close relatives of normal cellular genes (6). Shortly thereafter, Robert Weinberg and Geoffrey Cooper independently showed that transformed cells that have not experienced viral infection often contain mutant, activated forms of the same oncogenes possessed by acutely transforming retroviruses (7,8). These experiments supported the line of thought that cancer traits are passed from parent to daughter cell via DNA. Subsequently, it was shown that protooncogenes, when activated to oncogenes, cause some of the changes characteristic of the cancerous state. Normal cells that are artificially engineered to contain certain oncogenes behave abnormally, especially with respect to growth control.

Since the first discoveries of oncogenes, dozens of such dominant, growth-promoting genes have been added to the list. Some of these have been identified through the study of viruses, but many have been found by somatic cell genetics directly. In most cases, oncogenes have been identified by application of cytological methods to tumor cells. Microscopic examination of tumor cells reveals that certain karyotypic abnormalities—chromosomal translocations in particular—occur frequently in specific tumor types. For example, in chronic myelogenous leukemias, a portion of chromosome 22 is often exchanged with a portion of chromosome 9, giving rise to two chimeric chromosomes (9). The junction of one of these hybrid chromosomes, the so-called Philadelphia chromosome, contains a chimeric gene that consists of the *abl* protooncogene fused to a second gene. The fused *abl* gene is active as an oncogene. There are many examples of cytological abnormalities serving to guide isolation of oncogenes. Cytological studies of tumor cells have also proved useful in the classification of tumor cells based on karyotype. A set of altered genes are presumed to underlie the grosser, karyotypic changes.

A combination of cytogenetic studies and genetic epidemiology led to the discovery of a second class of cancer genes, the tumor suppressor genes. In 1971 Strong and Knudsen proposed that retinoblastoma was caused by inactivation of both alleles (paternal and maternal) of a specific locus called *rb* (10). They based their hypothesis on the frequency of retinoblastoma in certain retinoblastoma-prone kindreds compared to the sporadic frequency. The analysis suggested that two hits were required to complete the genetic inactivation of *rb*. Knudsen's hypothesis led directly to the concept of tumor suppressor genes. Consistent with this idea, experiments involving fusions between normal and tumor cells demonstrated that normal cells contain chromosomal regions that suppress tumor growth (11,12). This independent line of investigation also suggested the existence of tumor suppressor loci.

Karyotypic studies of tumor cells show that many chromosomal regions suffer heterozygous deletions as tumors progress, a process termed loss of heterozygosity (LOH) (Fig. 16–5) (13). LOH is taken as evidence for the existence of tumor suppressor genes. In several instances, tumor suppressor genes have been identified directly with regions that exhibit LOH. In these cases, the remaining allele often contains inactivating mutations. The typical pathway of tumor suppressor gene

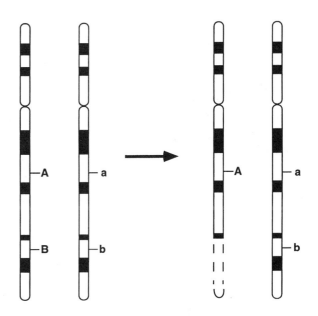

FIG. **16–5.** Cartoon of loss of heterozygosity (LOH). In this figure, one of the pair of homologous chromosomes undergoes a heterozygous deletion, losing genetic material from one end. This event removes an allele (B) from one heterozygous locus, conferring hemizygosity.

disruption involves LOH as a first step, followed by inactivation of the remaining tumor suppressor allele through mutation. The result of this process, tumor suppressor gene inactivation, confers a growth advantage on the cell.

Direct demonstration of the growth inhibitory activity of tumor suppressor genes has been obtained from gene transfer experiments. Tumor cell lines that receive wild-type copies of tumor suppressor genes can in many cases be shown to recover a measure of growth regulation (14).

A third class of cancer genes has recently been described. This class is not involved in growth control per se, but rather in the fidelity of the DNA replication and chromosome segregation process. Given the ability of tumor cells to accumulate large numbers of mutations in a relatively small number of generations, it is not surprising that so-called mutator loci participate in the process of tumorigenesis. These genes act directly in the replication process, for example, in the excision of misincorporated bases, or they regulate cell cycle checkpoints that enable the cell to monitor and respond to DNA damage.

RARE FAMILIAL CANCERS

Genetic studies have been remarkably successful in tracking down genes involved in rare forms of cancer (Table 16.1). In most of these cases, the loci contain highly penetrant, mutant tumor suppressor alleles. Gene carriers have a very high likelihood of developing tumors. These properties, high allelic penetrance and

rare occurrence, greatly simplify the genetic analysis. The preponderance of tumor suppressors among the set of familial cancer genes, as opposed to oncogenes, suggests that inheritance of dominant alleles may be strongly disfavored through evolution owing to their dominant effect on cell growth. In contrast, inheritance of a recessive tumor suppressor allele may have little effect on cell growth until function of the second allele is eliminated in a specific cell. Alternatively, tumor suppressor germline mutation may be more common because it is more likely to inactivate one copy of a gene by a single mutational event than to activate a protooncogene.

The first tumor suppressor gene to be identified, Retinoblastoma (*rb*), was isolated through a combination of kindred studies and cytogenetics (15). Cytological deletions in the 13q14 region were well known. This region was isolated in genomic clones and the target of this deletion, *rb*, proved to contain mutations in many retinoblastoma kindreds. *rb* is a target for somatic mutation in several tumor types other than retinoblastoma, including lung, breast, and bladder cancers (16). This gene encodes a 105 kDa protein that has a central role in cell cycle control. In concert with CDKs, cyclins, CDK inhibitors, and assorted transcription factors, the Rb protein appears to regulate one of the most important cell cycle transitions, the G_1 checkpoint (Fig. 16–2).

Li–Fraumeni syndrome is a rare disease characterized by multiple early onset tumors, especially breast carcinomas and soft tissue sarcomas. The spectrum of cancers in Li–Fraumeni kindreds led to consideration

TABLE 16.1. *Genes Involved in Familial Cancer Syndromes*

Syndrome	Gene	Location	Protein*	Rate (Cancer)
Familial adenomatous polyposis	*apc*	5q21	Cytoskeleton binding	High (colorectal)
Familial breast	*brca1*	17q21	RING finger	Low (breast/ovarian)
	brca2	13q13	–	Low (breast)
Hereditary nonpolyposis colo.	*hmsh2*	2p21	DNA repair	Low (colon)
	hmlh1	3p21	DNA repair	Low (colon)
Multiple endocrine neoplasia	*men2a*	10q11	RET tyrosine kinase	Medium (pituitary)
Multiple malignant melanoma	*mlm*	9p21	p16 (CDK inhibitor)	High (melanoma)
Neurofibromatosis type 1	*nf1*	17q11	GTPase	Medium (meningioma)
Neurofibromatosis type 2	*nf2*	22q12	Membrane/cytoskeleton	Medium (meningioma)
Retinoblastoma	*rb1*	13q14	Cell cycle regulator	High (retinoblastoma)
Li–Fraumeni	*tp53*	17p13	Transcription regulator	Medium (breast)
von Hippel–Lindau	*vhl*	3p25	Transcription elongation	High (renal clear cell)
Wilms's tumor	*wt1*	11p13	Transcription regulator	Low (Wilms's)

*Functions ascribed to the encoded proteins, or sequence motifs, are listed under the heading "Protein." The last column indicates approximate mutation rates in sporadic cancers (listed in parentheses): high > 50%, medium 10%–50%, low < 10%

of the *p53* gene located at 17p13 as a candidate for the Li–Fraumeni locus (17). *p53* was known to be a frequent target of mutation in sporadic tumors of many types including breast tumors and sarcomas (18). It encodes a product, *p53*, whose function appears to be transcriptional control. However, *p53* participates in several important physiological pathways including cell cycle arrest and programmed cell death. Identification of *p53* germline mutations in Li-Fraumeni kindreds demonstrated that *p53* is the underlying genetic defect. It is interesting that these germline mutations cause the appearance of limited types of tumors, despite the occurrence of *p53* mutations in nearly all types of cancer.

Another rare syndrome, adenomatous polyposis coli (APC), accounts for less than 1% of colon cancer in the United States and is characterized by the appearance of hundreds or thousands of benign polyps in the colons of predisposed individuals. APC affecteds often suffer from a series of other colonic abnormalities known collectively as Gardner's syndrome. The *apc* gene was mapped to 5q21 and then cloned through a classic positional cloning strategy, except that somatic LOH lesions were employed to help localize the gene (19). The *apc* gene encodes a protein of 2844 amino acids whose biochemical function remains obscure, but which may function as a component of the cytoskeleton (20). The gene is commonly mutated in sporadic colon cancer, but rarely in other cancer types.

A third rare familial cancer syndrome is Wilms's tumor, an embryonal malignancy of the kidney which affects roughly one in 10,000 children. The familial form of the cancer is caused by a gene, *wt1*, mapped by cytogenetic studies of small germline deletions to 11p13 (21,22). *wt1* encodes a 110 kDa protein with sequence characteristics of a transcription factor, including a zinc finger domain.

Neurofibromatosis is one of the most common highly penetrant genetic disorders, affecting about 1 in 2500 persons. It causes a variety of benign growths of neural origin, and occasionally malignancies such as Schwannomas and neurofibrosarcomas. Two separate genes, *nf1* and *nf2*, have been mapped and isolated by conventional positional cloning methods (23,24). Based on homologies to known proteins and to its GTPase activating behavior, *nf1* may participate in the growth regulatory pathway that involves the *ras* protooncogene. *nf2* protein includes several stretches of homology to known membrane-associated, cytoskeleton proteins.

Like most other familial cancer syndromes, multiple endocrine neoplasia is also dominantly inherited. However, its underlying cause is different from the other hereditary cancers. The responsible gene, *men2a*, is actually an oncogene not a tumor suppressor gene. The gene was mapped genetically to 10q11, and identified by considering the *ret* protooncogene, a tyrosine kinase, as a candidate (25). Missense mutations that affect the kinase activity are found frequently in the germlines of *men2a* families.

von Hippel–Lindau's disease is a rare familial cancer syndrome characterized by multiple, bilateral renal carcinomas and other tumor types. The responsible gene, *vhl*, was isolated through the application of positional cloning techniques and the observation of a causal translocation in 3p25 (26). *vhl* encodes a protein with little similarity to other known proteins. The *vhl* product appears to function as a transcription elongation factor, a novel function for a tumor suppressor.

Several other rare cancer syndromes of clear genetic origin have been identified. In the next few years, genes for these heritable defects will likely be unmasked (27).

COMMON HUMAN CANCERS

Many studies have provided evidence that all cancers, not just the rare forms, have genetic components. The actual fraction is difficult to estimate. Familial clustering increases both with increasing family size and frequency of the specific cancer type. Most common cancers are thought to have a genetic predisposition in about 10% of cases. However, only when the relevant predisposing genes are isolated will these proportions be known accurately. The increased risk of cancer in affected individuals is typically two- to threefold in first-degree relatives (28) and can often be shown to extend to more distant relatives (29). Even the portion of cancer that is not obviously genetic in origin may have genetic factors as an underlying influence, especially low-penetrance genes that modify risk (30). An alternative possibility is that nonfamilial cancers are merely the statistical outcome of wear and tear on our genes, with rates determined by diet and other lifestyle influences. Perhaps the most likely possibility is that both effects, genetic and environmental, are important in the vast majority of cancers .

Colon cancer is a very common neoplasm in the United States, second only to prostate and breast cancer in incidence. Insight into the molecular genetics of colon cancer has come from somatic cell genetic studies conducted principally by Vogelstein and colleagues, and from genetic studies of rarer familial forms such as APC (31). Another type of familial colon cancer, hereditary nonpolyposis colon cancer (HNPCC), has been shown by molecular analysis to account for a percentage of familial colon cancer (32). Two distinct loci appear to explain the bulk of HNPCC familial cancer (33). Interestingly, these loci, *hmlh1* and *hmsh2,* do not act as classical tumor suppressor genes. Rather, they encode proteins with significant homologies to known DNA repair enzymes from bacteria and fungi. The molecular identification of these genes, accomplished through a combination of genetics and clever biochemical intuition, neatly explains one of the characteristics of HNPCC patients: tumors from HNPCC gene carriers exhibit a high degree of genetic instability—especially in the length of short tandem repeat (STR) sequences. This cellular phenotype fits perfectly with the proposed biochemical function of the HNPCC genes as DNA mismatch repair proteins. The extent of involvement of *hmlh1* and *hmsh2* in non-HNPCC familial colon cancer remains unclear.

Breast carcinoma is the most common cancer among women. More than 1 in 10 American women will develop breast cancer by the age of 90. The familial nature of breast cancer was noted in the 1940s, but it was not until linkage was obtained in 1990, and subsequently confirmed, that the disease was put on a firm genetic basis (34). The familial component of breast cancer has been estimated at 5%–10% of the total incidence. *brca1*, the first breast cancer susceptibility locus to be identified, is responsible for roughly half of all clearly familial, early-onset breast cancer (35). For breast cancer, the age-specific risk is increased by a factor of over 30 for younger women who inherit a predisposing *brca1* allele. *brca1* also influences susceptibility to ovarian cancer, increasing the risk about 50-fold. In tumor cells, *brca1* behaves as a classical tumor suppressor gene; breast tumors from gene carriers invariably retain the inherited, predisposing chromosome and lose the wild-type allele (36). After a well-publicized race, *brca1* was isolated using standard positional cloning methods (37). The gene encodes a 1863-amino-acid protein whose biochemical function is unknown. It contains a zinc finger motif, suggestive perhaps of interactions with nucleic acids. A second locus, *brca2*, contributes to approximately the same proportion of breast cancer as *brca1* (38). *brca2* has also been isolated recently and encodes a protein roughly twice the size of that of *brca1* (39,40). Like *brca1*, the biochemical function of *brca2* is unknown.

A third locus, ataxia-telangiectasia (*at*), may also influence breast cancer incidence in a dominant fashion, though the increased risk to heterozygotes may be relatively slight (41). However, predisposing *at* alleles are more common in the population than *brca1* and *brca2*. Thus, if *at* heterozygotes are at increased risk, the overall contribution to breast cancer incidence by *at* may be significant. Interestingly, *at* homozygotes are

viable and have a vastly increased risk of cancer. The *at* gene encodes a protein with similarities to phosphoinositide kinases (42).

Melanoma, the most rapidly increasing cancer type in the United States, proved to be a difficult subject for genetic analysis, primarily owing to confusion over the phenotype. Many investigators focused on the relationship between moles (nevi) and melanoma, with misinterpretation of histological dysplasia as diagnostic of a precursor lesion. This approach confused the genetic analysis and hindered linkage assignment (43). Finally, by ignoring moles entirely and limiting the phenotype to melanoma itself, a susceptibility locus (*mlm*) was identified in chromosomal region 9p21 (44). This region was known to contain chromosome rearrangements in sporadic melanomas and cell lines. Thus, a strategy was devised to isolate *mlm* based on the assumption that the somatic rearrangements were due to inactivation of the *mlm* gene in somatic cells. Many rearrangements in 9p21 involve homozygous deletions. Therefore, *mlm* was presumed to lie within the boundaries of such homozygous deletions. A large set of melanoma cell lines was screened for deletion of 9p21 markers. The results of this analysis provided a simple picture of the location of *mlm*, because all the homozygous deletions converged on a small region encompassing one or two genes. One of these genes proved to encode the CDK inhibitor *p16*, while the other encodes its close relative *p15* (45). *p16* contains inactivating lesions in the germlines of many melanoma-prone, 9p21-linked kindreds; *p15* does not. In addition, *p16* is the target for somatic mutations in melanomas and a wide variety of other tumor types; *p15* does not appear to be a unique target for somatic mutation. Thus, it appears that *p16* is *mlm*.

Prostate cancer has a clear familial component (46). However, the common occurrence of prostate cancer (nearly half of 70-year-old males have histopathological prostate malignancy), and the late age of onset complicate the genetic analysis considerably. However, major predisposing genes have been suggested by segregation analysis (47) and linkage analysis is in progress in several laboratories. Similarly, lung cancer has an obvious environmental component. Nonetheless, there is strong evidence for a major gene effect in early-onset lung cancer (48).

INHERITED VS. SPORADIC CANCER

From first principles, genes that control the heriditary predisposition to cancer should be targets for mutation in non-heriditary type (sporadic) cancer. The reason is that mutations, when inherited, increase the likelihood of cancer by accelerating the process of tumorigenesis. In the multistep model of tumorigenesis, many individual somatic changes are required to complete the process; germline mutations obviate the need for one somatic step. Thus, the probability of completing the entire set of changes and developing cancer is increased. On average, an earlier age of cancer onset compared to the normal population results.

Consistent with this view of sporadic cancer, most familial cancer genes are mutated at high rates in nonfamilial tumors of the same type that arise in the familial predisposition syndromes (Table 16.1). The mutation frequencies range broadly. *mlm* (*p16*) is mutated at very high frequencies in sporadic melanoma and in many other tumor types. *p53* is also a frequent target. In contrast, no somatic *brca1* mutations have been found to date in sporadic breast carcinomas, while only a small number have been observed in ovarian tumors. WT1 also has a low mutation rate in sporadic Wilms's tumors.

How can this broad range of somatic mutation frequencies be explained? One possibility hinges on the concept that tumor progression depends on inactivation of multiple growth control pathways. Each pathway is composed of many genes. Inactivation of a particular pathway can be achieved through mutation of any gene in the pathway (Fig. 16–6). Thus, a specific gene, *brca1*, for example, may only rarely be a target for somatic mutation owing to the preferred inactivation of other elements in the pathway within which *brca1* functions. This idea implies differences in somatic mutation rates of various genes, the differences dependent on the effective target size of the specific genes. Genes such as *p53* may offer large targets for somatic mutation for a variety of reasons, whereas genes such as *brca1* may be smaller targets.

Another puzzle is why *mlm* (*p16*) germline mutations influence primarily melanoma rates. Inherited *mlm* mutations should cause cancers in practically all tissues, because it is a target for somatic mutation in most tumor types. An explanation for this conundrum can once again be found in the multistep nature of tumorigenesis. If *mlm* mutations are rate limiting only in formation of melanomas, inherited *mlm* mutations should not increase the incidence of other cancers. *mlm* inactivation may be necessary for progression to malignancy in many tissues, but may not be the rate-limiting step in most cell types.

DIAGNOSTIC AND THERAPEUTIC IMPLICATIONS OF GENETIC DISCOVERIES

The isolation of several genes that influence disease incidence suggests the possibility of genetic screening. The goal of such screening is to identify individuals at increased risk for disease. This information may be useful to individuals and physicians to guide prevention strategies and therapy. For example, if a predisposing *mlm* allele were discovered in someone, that person would be advised to minimize sunlight exposure, a major risk factor for melanoma. For *brca1* germline mutations, close monitoring and prophylactic surgery are options. Genetic testing for *mlm*, *brca1* and other genes provides an inexpensive method of risk assessment that many will find useful.

Genotypic analysis of tumors is a burgeoning field. Detailed knowledge of the pathways that have been inactivated in a particular tumor may assist in diagnosis and classification of cancers. Such information may also be relevant to the therapeutic choice. For instance, *p53*-deficient tumors do not respond well to many forms of chemotherapy (49). Thus, knowledge of the *p53* status of a tumor might prevent the exposure of patients to a host of noxious, futile treatments.

Conversion of research into practical therapies is always slow. Medically important genetic findings are no exception. Tumor suppressor genes offer the obvious possibility of gene therapy. Although progress

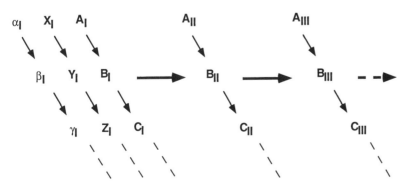

FIG. **16–6.** Hypothetical genetic pathways of growth control. Each diagonal set of three letters represents a specific pathway of regulation; each letter represents a particular gene in the pathway. A pathway can be inactivated by mutations in any gene in the pathway. Inactivation of multiple genetic pathways consitute the changes that underlie tumor progression.

in this area has been significant, gene therapy for cancer has yet to materialize. The barriers are considerable. Good gene delivery vehicles must be designed and tested thoroughly. The genes must be directed selectively to cancer cells, or delivered in a manner that is not toxic to normal cells in the body. Tumor cell variants that escape the therapy must be controlled in some other way. Although a variety of good tumor suppressor gene candidates for gene therapy exist, a workable strategy remains elusive.

Oncogenes and tumor suppressor genes offer routes for development of more traditional small-molecule-based therapies. These approaches are the strength of the major pharmaceutical houses. Thus, we may expect to see dividends from investment in a new generation of chemotherapeutic compounds based on specific biochemical targets in the cell. One example of such investigative compounds are the *ras* farnesylation inhibitors. These are designed to prevent the function of the *ras* oncogene, a common molecular constituent of human cancers.

CONCLUSION

Genetic analysis of human kindreds and tumor cells in culture is conceptually straightforward. In concert with molecular methods, it has led to discovery of numerous genes involved in predisposition to and progression of cancer. Many of these genes participate in fundamental cellular processes. Thus, they contribute to our understanding of basic biological phenomena such as growth control. These genes also provide an opportunity for genetic screening and for new therapeutic approaches to cancer.

REFERENCES

1. Lynch HT. Hereditary factors in carcinoma. In: Rentchnick P, ed. *Recent Results in Cancer Research.* New York: Springer-Verlag; 1967; 12:1–186.
2. Skolnick M. Prospects for population oncogenetics. In: Mulvihill JJ, Miller RW, Fraumeni JFJ, eds. *Genetics of Human Cancer.* New York: Raven Press; 1977:19–25.
3. Skolnick M. The Utah genealogical data base: a resource for genetic epidemiology. In: Cairns J, Lyon JL, Skolnick M, eds. *Banbury Report No 4: Cancer Incidence in Defined Populations.* New York: Cold Spring Harbor Laboratory; 1980: 285–297.
4. Weber JL, May PE. Abundant class of human DNA polymorphisms which can be typed using the polymerase chain reaction. *Am J Hum Genet.* 1989; 44:388–396.
5. Morton NE. LODs past and present. *Genetics.* 1995; 140:7–12.
6. Stehelin D, Varmus HE, Bishop JM, Vogt PK. DNA related to the transforming gene(s) of avian sarcoma viruses present in normal avian DNA. *Nature.* 1976; 260:170–173.
7. Der CJ, Drontiris TG, Cooper GM. Transforming genes of human bladder and lung carcinoma cells are homologous to the ras genes of Harvey and Kirsten sarcoma viruses. *Proc Natl Acad Sci. USA.* 1982; 79:3637–3640.
8. Parada LF, Tabin CJ, Shih C, Weinberg RA. Human EJ bladder carcinoma oncogene is a homologue of Harvey sarcoma virus ras gene. *Nature.* 1982; 297:474–478.
9. Rabbitts TH, Forster A, Matthews JG. The breakpoint of the Philadelphia chromosome 22 in chronic myeloid leukaemia is distal to the immunoglobulin lambda chain constant region genes. *Mol Biol Med.* 1983; 1:11–19.
10. Knudson AG. Mutation and cancer: Statistical study of retinoblastoma. *Proc Natl Acad Sci USA.* 1971; 68:820–823.
11. Sager R. Genetic suppression of tumor formation. *Adv Cancer Res.* 1985; 44:43–68.
12. Harris H. The analysis of malignancy by cell fusion: the position in 1988. *Cancer Res.* 1988; 48:3302–3306.
13. Vogelstein B, Fearon ER, Kern SE, et al. Allelotype of colorectal carcinomas. *Science.* 1989; 244:207–211.
14. Huang H-JS, Yee JK, Shew JY, et al. Suppression of the neoplastic phenotype by replacement of the RB gene in human cancer cells. *Science.* 1988; 242:1563–1566.
15. Friend SH, Bernards R, Sneza R, et al. A human DNA segment with properties of the gene that predisposes to retinoblastoma and osteosarcoma. *Nature.* 1986; 323:643–646.
16. Weinberg. Tumor suppressor genes. *Science.* 1991; 254:1139–1146.
17. Malkin D, Li FP, Strong LC, et al. Germline p53 mutations in familial syndrome of breast cancer, carcomas and other neoplasims. *Science.* 1990; 250:1233–1238.
18. Nigro JM, Baker SJ, Preisinger AC, et al. Mutations in the p53 gene occur in diverse human tumour types. *Nature.* 1989; 342:705–708.
19. Nishisho I, Nakamura Y, Miyoshi Y, et al. Mutations of chromosome 5q21 genes in FAP and colorectal cancer patients. *Science.* 1991; 253:665–669.
20. Munemitsu S, Souza B, Muller O, Albert I, Rubinfeld B, Polakis P. The APC gene product associates with microtubules in vivo and promotes their assembly in vitro. *Cancer Res.* 1994; 54:3676–3681.
21. Francke U, Holmes LB, Atkins L, Riccardi VM. Aniridia-Wilms' tumor association: evidence for specific deletion of 11p13. *Cytogenet Cell Genet.* 1979; 24:185–192.
22. Gessler M, Poustka A, Cavenee W, Neve RL, Orkin SH, Bruns GA. Homozygous deletion in Wilms tumours of a zinc-finger gene identified by chromosome jumping. *Nature.* 1990; 343:774–778.
23. Rouleau GA, Merel P, Lutchman M, et al. Alternation in a new gene encoding a putative membrane-organizing protein causes neuro-fibromatosis type 2. *Nature.* 1993; 363:515–521.
24. Wallace MR, Marchuk DA, Andersen LB, et al. Type 1 neurofibromatosis gene: Identification of a large transcript disrupted in three NF1 patients. *Science.* 1990; 249:181–186.
25. Mulligan LM, Kwok JBJ, Healey CS, et al. Germ-line mutations of the RET proto-oncogene in multiple endocrine neoplasia type 2A. *Nature.* 1993; 363:774–778.

26. Latif F, Tory K, Gnarra J, et al. Identification of the von Hippel–Lindau disease tumor suppressor gene. *Science.* 1993; 260:1317–1320.

27. Knudson AG. All in the (cancer) family. *Nature Genet.* 1993; 5:103–104.

28. Goldgar DE, Easton DF, Cannon-Albright LA, Skolnick MH. Systematic population-based assessment of cancer risk in first-degree relatives of cancer probands. *J Natl Cancer Inst.* 1994; 86:1600–1608.

29. Cannon-Albright LA, Thomas A, Goldgar DE, et al. Familiality of cancer in Utah. *Cancer Res.* 1994; 54:2378–2385.

30. Krontiris TG, Devlin B, Karp DD, Robert NJ, Risch N. An association between the risk of cancer and mutations in the HRAS1 minisatellite locus. *N Engl J Med.* 1993; 329:517–523.

31. Fearon ER, Vogelstein B. A genetic model for colorectal tumorigenesis. *Cell.* 1990; 61:759–767.

32. Lewis CM, Goldgar DE, Cannon-Albright LA, Skolnick MH. Genetic analysis of cancer and precursor lesions. *Ares Serono Symposia* [Submitted].

33. Liu B, Parsons R, Papadopoulos N, et al. Analysis of mismatch repair genes in hereditary non-polyposis. *Nature Med.* 1996; 2:169–174.

34. Hall JM, Lee MK, Newman B, et al. Linkage of early-onset familial breast cancer to chromosome 17q21. *Science.* 1990; 250:1684–1689.

35. Easton DF, Ford D, Bishop DT. Breast and ovarian cancer incidence in *brca1*-mutation carriers. *Am J Hum Genet.* 1995; 56:265–271.

36. Neuhausen SL, Marshall CJ. Loss of heterozygosity in familial tumors from three *brca1*-linked kindreds. *Cancer Res.* 1994; 54:6069–6072.

37. Miki Y, Swensen J, Shattuck-Eidens D, et al. A strong candidate for the breast and ovarian cancer susceptibility Gene BRCA1. *Science.* 1994; 266:66–71.

38. Wooster R, Neuhausen SL, Mangion J, et al. Localization of a breast cancer susceptibility gene, BRCA2, to chromosome 13q12-13. *Science.* 1994; 265:2088–2090.

39. Tavtigian SV, Simard J, Rommens J, et al. The complete BRCA2 gene and mutations in chromosome 13Q-linked kindreds. *Nature Genet.* 1996; 12:1–6.

40. Wooster R, Bignell G, Lancaster J, et al. Identification of the breast cancer susceptibility gene BRCA2. *Nature.* 1995; 378:789–792.

41. Shiloh Y. Ataxia-telagiectasia: closer to unraveling the mystery. *Eur J Hum Genet.* 1995; 3:116–138.

42. Lavin MF, Khanna KK, Beamish H, Spring K, Watters D, Shiloh Y. Relationship of the ataxia-telangiectasia protein ATM to phoslphoinositide 3-kinase. *Trends Biochem Sci.* 1995; 20:382–383.

43. Skolnick MH, Cannon-Albright LA, Kamb A. Genetic predisposition to melanoma. *Eur J Cancer.* 1994; 13:1991–1995.

44. Cannon-Albright LA, Goldgar DE, Meyer LJ, et al. Assignment of a locus for familial melanoma, *mlm*, to chromosome 9p 13-p22. *Science.* 1992; 258:1148–1152.

45. Kamb A, Gruis NA, Weaver-Feldhaus J, et al. A cell cycle regulator potentially involved in genesis of many tumor types. *Science.* 1994; 264:436–440.

46. Cannon L, Bishop DT, Skolnick M, Hunt S, Lyon JL, Smart CR. Genetic epidemiology of prostate cancer in the Utah Mormon genealogy. *Cancer Surv.* 1982; 1:47–69.

47. Carter BS, Bova GS, Beaty TH, et al. Hereditary prostate cancer: epidemiologic and clinical features. *J Urol.* 1993; 150:797–802.

48. Bailey-Wilson JE, Sellers TA, Elston RC, Evens CC, Rothschild H. Evidence for a major gene effect in early-onset lung cancer. *J La State Med Soc.* 1993; 145:157–162.

49. Lowe SW, Bodis S, McClatchey A, et al. p53 status and the efficacy of cancer therapy in vivo. *Science.* 1994; 266:807–810.

17

Genetic Counseling for the Oncology Patient

ELIZABETH GETTIG, JOAN H. MARKS, AND JOHN J. MULVIHILL

GENETIC COUNSELING

The definition of genetic counseling was established by an ad hoc committee of the American Society of Human Genetics in 1974 and has survived without revision over two decades. The profession of genetic counseling provided by individuals prepared with a Masters degree has evolved over its twenty-five years, moving from the specialties of obstetrics and pediatrics to general medicine. The rapid advances in the genetic bases of cancer has made the services of genetic counselors in oncology centers increasingly important.

Genetic counseling is a communication process that deals with the human problems associated with the occurrence or the risk of occurrence of a genetic disorder in a family. This process involves an attempt by one or more appropriately trained persons to help the individual or family: *(1)* comprehend the medical facts, including the diagnosis, the probable course of the disorder, and the available management; *(2)* appreciate the way heredity contributes to the disorder and the risk of recurrence in specified relatives; *(3)* understand the options for dealing with the risk of recurrence; *(4)* choose the course of action that seems appropriate to them in view of their risk and their family goals and act in accordance with that decision; and *(5)* make the best possible adjustment to the disorder in an affected family member or to the risk of recurrence of that disorder (1).

The application of genetic counseling practices to the needs of patients at risk of cancer is a constructive development in medical care. Genetic counseling is just now being applied to cancer. The model of genetic counseling is well suited to deliver to families highly charged information that is medically, genetically, and emotionally complex. Genetic counselors assist families in understanding both the medical and emotional aspects of disease while providing a connection to support services. The elements of the basic definition of genetic counseling—explaining medical facts, concepts of heredity, and recurrence risk information; working within the context of family decision making; and providing support and option for care and surveillance—are readily applied to the challenges that a diagnosis of cancer or a discovery of a cancer gene brings to an individual or family.

TRAINING AND STANDARDS OF GENETIC COUNSELING

Masters-level genetic counselors are trained in medical genetics and counseling psychology to educate patients with or at risk for a genetic disease to understand the hereditary nature of their condition, to help them cope psychologically with their risk, and to make informed decisions about their medical and reproductive choices.

Training of non-physician genetic counselors was initiated at Sarah Lawrence College in 1969. There are currently 19 accredited graduate programs in this country and four programs in foreign countries. Standards for accreditation have recently been set by the American Board of Genetic Counseling and certification of genetic counselors has been available since 1980. Training consists of two years of graduate work in medical genetics and related sciences and counseling plus at least 400 hours of supervised clinical experience counseling patients and families.

According to the patient's diagnosis, genetic counselors work with various medical specialties as members of the clinical team. The majority of counselors work in reproductive medicine or pediatrics; increasingly they have become members of oncology services as screening for inherited susceptibility to cancer has become possible.

THE ROLE OF THE GENETIC COUNSELOR IN PSYCHO-ONCOLOGY

Genetic counseling for a person with cancer or at high risk of developing cancer involves several steps, including collection of medical records, interpretation of the family history (personal, medical and extended family), recognition of precancerous syndromes, assessment of risk, and follow-up for surveillance recommendations. Genetic counseling includes information on diagnosis, prognosis, and decision making for the individual. Additional members of the extended family may wish to be counseled as well, but issues of confidentiality and possible insurance discrimination must be clearly recognized, thought out, and addressed with the client and extended family members. Discussion of possible gene testing or participation in ongoing research protocols is often part of the genetic counseling process. Issues of coercion of other family members to be tested or even to be informed of risk issues must be discussed before establishing a cancer genetics program. Policies should be established to address these issues which inevitably occur when working with families (2–5).

The diagnosis of a specific cytogenetic or Mendelian disorder is rare in cancer counseling. A counselor experienced in evaluating cancer families can sometimes offer empirical risk estimates regarding future cancer occurrence. In general, if a person develops a cancer, first-degree relatives (i.e., parents, children, brothers, sisters) have a threefold risk of developing the same type of cancer, based on old death certificate studies. Empirical risk counseling will remain imprecise, but essential, until specific genes are found for common adult cancers thereby enabling accurate risk assessment.

COMMUNICATING RISK CONCEPTS

Communication with the family is the most essential component of genetic health care delivery. Families require inordinate amounts of time to review and develop a care plan and to establish mutual communication and understanding of the disease. Families hold their own theories as to why their family has a disproportionate number of cancer cases. Simply eliciting the client's own theory of cancer causation validates the belief system of the family and may give rise to a lasting relationship. Communication can begin "on the same page" and the building of a mutually supportive relationship should evolve. Even if answers to questions are not known or if theories cannot be proven, factual information can often correct some of the misinformation or fears families have

in regard to cancer. It is important that the family members have validation of their concerns and at the same time be given factual responses to known information about their particular form of cancer.

Interaction with a genetic service can occur at several life-cycle points: the time of cancer diagnosis; following treatment; prior to or during a pregnancy; and following discussions with other family members who may be concerned about their risk status or monitoring/screening recommendations. Follow-up and monitoring of the family are essential for successful intervention by both oncologist and geneticists (6–7).

GENETICS OF CANCER

Genes play a role in the origins of most human cancers, and sometimes they are conspicuous. Certain features that suggest that a cancer has major genetic determinants, and, if found, might identify persons with cancer in themselves or in a close relative who could benefit from clinical genetics evaluation and counseling (Table 17.1).

Three categories of genetic determinants of any disease are *(1)* cytogenetics (chromosomes), *(2)* single gene (Mendelian) traits, and *(3)* familial aggregation, multifactorial inheritance, or ecogenetics (gene–environment interactions).

Cytogenetics. Although most if not all cancers and leukemias have abnormal chromosomes, they are usually *acquired* and hence seen only in the neoplastic tissues in persons with normal karyotypes. Some eight conditions with *constitutional* chromosomal abnormalities predispose to neoplasia and may, on rare occasion, account for a person's cancer, especially when it occurs in childhood in association with birth defects. Examples include Down's syndrome (trisomy 21) with leukemia, trisomy 18 with embryonal tumors, and Klinefelter (XXY) syndrome with germ cell or breast cancer.

Single Gene Traits. Of the approximately 6700 human traits that are considered to be caused by single major genes, about 420 have neoplasia as a feature, complication, or association (8). Put in other terms, 6% of known human genes influence the occurrence of human neoplasia. There are a few hereditary neoplasia traits where the chief manifestation is frank neoplasia, such as retinoblastoma, the multiple endocrine neoplasia syndromes, and the hereditary breast and ovarian cancer familial syndrome due to mutations in *BRCA1*. There are many more conditions that have

TABLE 17.1. *Identifying Patients and Families for Possible Genetic Counseling*

Criterion (Patient with a cancer that has one of these features)	Example
Bilateral, as separate primary neoplasms	Both kidneys, both breasts
Multifocal, within one organ	Multicentric colorectal cancers
An additional primary malignancy	Endometrial after colon cancer
At an atypical age	Breast cancer before 40 years
At an atypical site	Osteosarcoma of the mid-humerus
In the sex not usually affected	Breast cancer in a male
Associated with birth defects	Wilms's tumor with aniridia
Associated with a Mendelian trait	Sarcoma in neurofibromatosis I
Associated with a precursor lesion	Melanoma in dysplastic nevus syndrome
Associated with a rare disease	Lymphoma in immunodeficiency
A rare or unusual tumor type	Pheochromocytoma, sarcoma
Families with	
One first-degree relative* with a cancer with any of the above features	Siblings and children of person with pheochromocytoma or melanoma arising in a dysplastic news
Two first-degree relatives* with any cancer	Parents and siblings of a boy with sarcoma and his sister with brain tumor

*Brother, sister, parent or child.

Sources: (Parry DM, Berg K, Mulvihill JJ, et al. Strategies for controlling cancer through genetics: Reports of a workshop. *Am J Hum Genet.* 1987; 41: 63–69. Parry DM, Mulvihill JJ, Miller RW, et al. Strategies for controlling cancer through genetics. *Cancer Res.* 1987; 47: 1814–1817. Mulvihill JJ. Prospects for cancer control and prevention through genetics. *Clin Genet.* 1989; 36: 313–319.

precursor lesions, associated dysplasias, or malformations: the phakomatoses and hamartoses (e.g., neurofibromatosis 1, the nevoid basal cell carcinoma syndrome, familial adenomatous polyposes); the genodermatoses (dysplasic nevus syndrome, oculocutneous albinism, xeroderma pigmentosum); the chromosomal fragility syndromes (Fanconi's pancytopenia, Bloom's syndrome); and the genetic immunodeficiencies (agamma globulinemia; ataxia-telangiectasia).

Ecogenetics, Familial Aggregation. Twenty-two genetic conditions well illustrate the principle that each person's cancer likely arises from a complex interaction of an inborn susceptibility with a lifelong history of environmental exposures (9). Examples include Epstein–Barr virus causing lymphomas in persons with the X-linked Purtillo's lymphoproliferative syndrome, and stilbestrol causing adenosquamous endometrial carcinoma in persons with Turner's syndrome.

CANCER RISK COUNSELING

By strict definition, all cancer is genetic, involving a change at the cell level toward unregulated and uncontrolled cell division. Therefore, criteria for distinguishing the families with cancer inherited through the generations from those individuals with a cancer that is nonhereditary in terms of transmission must be established, but in general have not been. Certainly errors in the establishing of criteria will occur as molecular genetic findings evolve. The most obvious hereditary cancer families will be spotted easily by the taking of detailed family histories or pedigrees, but the interactions of environmental effects with hereditary factors will continue to be evaluated well into the twenty-first century (10).

One of every four Americans develops cancer and one of every eight or nine women develops breast cancer. Several clinical surveys subjected to independent validation have provided insights into the incidence of familial cancer. The clinical surveys indicated that 6% of persons with cancer have three or more first-degree relatives with cancer; 12% have two; 30% have one; and 50% have no relatives with cancer. Identification of the primary site of cancer was increasingly inaccurate as the number of first-degree relatives with cancer increased. In the same study, the primary site was listed correctly 83% of the time for first-degree relatives (parents, siblings and offspring), 67% for second-degree relatives (grandparents, aunts and uncles), and 60% for third-degree relatives (cousins, great grandparents, great aunts and uncles). Documentation by medical record review regarding the primary cancer site is critical for genetic risk assessment. In particular, the pathology report and surgical record are of absolute importance in determining accurate risk assessment (11).

Generally, four basic family history questions must be addressed prior to genetic counseling for cancer:

1. Is this a first cancer or did the person have a prior cancer, tumor, or growth?
2. Are there any hereditary conditions known to be in the family such as a child with a birth defect, or a recognized preneoplastic trait like dysplastic nevus syndrome?
3. Does the pathology report or description of the primary tumor suggest a genetic etiology?
4. Does any other member of the family have a history of cancer or precancerous lesions?

There are many features that suggest that a person has an inherited or genetic cancer: earlier than expected onset of a cancer, excess of bilaterality with paired organs, and a pattern of multiple primaries may be a signal of a hereditary cancer (12–17).

Less straightforward is counseling of the family with an aggregation or clustering of cancer cases but no definite mode of transmission. Empirical information may be shared with families, such as the data provided by the American Cancer Society or registries or long-term study cohorts. Since cancer is a household word and just about every person knows someone with cancer, the "true" cancer families of genetic origins are difficult to distinguish.

Environmental effects cannot be overlooked. The familial incidence of mesothelioma due to asbestos transported from the worksite to the home environment is well known, as are the associations such as tobacco use and lung cancer. Because families share their environment, sorting environmental determinants from hereditary ones is a difficult task (18).

At least two distinct patterns occur repeatedly enough to have gained the label of "cancer family syndrome." Both are inherited in an autosomal dominant fashion. One is the cancer family syndrome of Lynch (19), which is characterized by two or more generations with cancer of the colon and endometrium (and sometimes ovaries and breasts) with diagnosis at an early age and with an excess of persons with multiple primary cancers. The alternate name of the disorder is hereditary nonpolypotic colorectal cancer. Four different genes have been associated with the Lynch cancer family syndrome.

The second distinct pattern is the Li–Fraumeni cancer family syndrome or SBLA syndrome, an acronym for the tumor types seen to excess: (S) sarcomas; (B) breast, bone, and brain tumors; (L) lung cancer, laryngeal cancer, and leukemia; and (A) adrenal cortical neoplasia. Constitutional mutations of the gene *P53* on chromosome 17p have been documented in many but not all cases. The predisposition to the syndrome is clearly a Mendelian dominant trait with high penetrance (20–21).

CANCER PREVENTION COUNSELING

Genetic counseling can lead to cancer prevention. Persons identified at an increased risk for developing cancer due to genetic determinants can be offered effective cancer screening and surveillance. Prevention has been a tenet in clinical genetics in general, but unfortunately the message of the public and professional community often becomes one of "If it is genetic, nothing can be done." This myth overlooks the distinct possibility that genetic factors may be monitored and preventive action may be taken if surveillance methods are followed. The best current example is monitoring of high cholesterol levels, which are often determined by heredity but are controlled by dietary restriction of high-fat foods, regular exercise, and sometimes medication. Cancer surveillance can follow the same model. However, the cancer model would include surgical alternatives such as prophylactic surgery to remove the target organ, which may prevent cancer. Currently, prophylactic colectomy is performed for patients with a polyposis syndrome or those at risk for familial colon cancer; gonadectomy is performed for cryptochordism, familial ovarian cancer or gonadal dysgenesis; mastectomy is performed for familial breast cancer; and thyroidectomy is performed for persons with the multiple mucosal neuroma syndrome. Less invasive alternatives would affect the gene–environment interaction: Use of sun block and avoidance of sun may reduce the risk of skin cancers, especially in those at high risk because of their genes (22).

REPRODUCTIVE COUNSELING

Pregnancy at the time of diagnosis of cancer is a difficult counseling situation. Pregnancy is contraindicated during cancer therapy because most cancer therapies are teratogenics, hence directly toxic to the fetus. Part of the advice at the onset of cancer therapy of a woman of reproductive age is to avoid pregnancies, recommendation of birth control, or at least alerting the woman of the potential for teratogenicity. Radiation exposure to the developing fetus between 8 and 15 weeks of gestational age is thought to result in some loss on IQ performance, based upon studies of Japanese exposed to the atomic bombs. Microcephaly and short stature are the results of fetal exposure to higher doses of ionizing radiation. The older fetus appears radioresistant (23).

Fertility may be decreased as a result of cancer and therapy or treatment of cancer. The reproductive organs may be directly affected by chemotherapeutic agents or radiation. Surgery may also interfere with reproduction. Alternatives such as positioning the ovaries outside the radiotherapy fields or banking of sperm prior to therapy may preserve fertility.

If therapy has been inadvertently given to a woman with cancer who is later recognized to be pregnant, or if life-saving therapy for a pregnant woman with cancer must begin, it may be possible to modify therapy by use of agents that are less likely to be teratogenic than others. For the purpose of genetic counseling, a registry of pregnancies exposed to cancer therapy was established at the NCI and is maintained at the University of Pittsburgh. Because cancer treatment during pregnancy is a rare and sometimes accidental event, the exact teratogenicity of various chemotherapeutic agents may never be the subject of rigorous analytic epideimiologic study. It seems best to register the rare human experience as it accrues. The registry is available to answer immediate questions, for example, about the published and unpublished experience of vincristine given to women who are five- to six-weeks pregnant. Contrary to expectations, even substantial chemotherapy in the first trimester is not inevitably teratogenic. If a pregnancy exposed to cancer treatment is much wanted, there is some room for reassurance that gross malformations are not inevitable. However, given the experience with other human teratogens (e.g., fetal alcohol syndrome), the least apparent manifestation of toxicity to the developing fetus is often a loss of higher brain function (i.e., behavioral traits, IQ). It is best to expose no embryo or fetus to chemotherapy or radiotherapy (24,25).

Somatic and germ cell mutations are theoretical concerns which must be discussed with patients. DNA is susceptible to damage from cancer treatment as the therapies are designed to interfere with cell division. Animal studies have demonstrated mutations due to cancer treatments and therapies, but human evidence has been lacking. Even in the survivors of the atomic bombs of Japan, alteration of genetic material resulting in effects for the offspring of survivors has not been observed (26).

GENETIC TESTING—BREAST CANCER RISK COUNSELING

Breast cancer is a common disease, affecting 1 in 8 or 9 American women in their lifetime. In 1996, an esti-

mated 186,000 women and 1000 men in the United States were diagnosed with breast cancer. Approximately one-third of all individuals with breast cancer have a positive family history. Multiple individuals in the same family may be affected due to chance events or to shared environmental exposures, similar lifestyles, or predisposing genes. Approximately 5%–10% of all individuals with breast cancer are thought to have a *single*, highly penetrant, dominantly inherited predisposition gene that confers a high risk for developing breast and/or ovarian cancer (*BRCA1*) (27–29).

Two models are commonly used for breast cancer risk assessment. They are referred to as the Gail model and the Claus model (16,30,31). The Gail model incorporates age at menarche, number of breast biopsies, age at first live birth, and number of first-degree relatives with breast cancer to calculate a relative risk for developing breast cancer. Calculations are applicable to Caucasian females. The Gail model assumes no genetic model and allows point estimates of the risk of breast cancer with associated confidence intervals of the absolute probability of a woman's developing breast cancer in 10, 20, or 30 years after counseling. Individualizing the probability of developing breast cancer is the approach used in the clinical research trial of tamoxifen as a way to prevent new clinical breast cancers (Table 17.2). The Gail model is simple to use. The limitation of the model is lack of ethnic diversity and exclusion of family history beyond first-degree relatives.

Another widely used risk assessment model is that of Claus. The Claus model assumes a single-gene model and calculates breast cancer risk using a formula that considers family history of breast cancer and the age of the affected relative at the time of her diagnosis. It takes into consideration maternal and paternal relatives in the following combinations: two first degree; one first degree and one second degree; and one maternal and one paternal (16–30).

The objective of the risk counseling strategies is to inform the patient of the magnitude of her risk. The empowerment of the client may then lead to greater surveillance compliance for individuals at an increased risk. However, success of genetic counseling ought not be measured in rates of follow-up compliance but by information retained by the patient. It is a common fact that Americans, in particular, are well educated about health matters but often do not apply that knowledge to their own individual situation. Follow-up studies of women counseled about their high risk of cancer revealed a low percentage who complied with the complete recommendation for surveillance. One study showed that only 40% performed monthly

TABLE 17.2. *Gail Model: Relative Risks for Selected Risk Factors*

Risk Factor		Relative Risk
AGE AT MENARCHE (yr)		
≥ 14		1.00
12–13		1.10
< 12		1.21
NUMBER OF BREAST BIOPSIES		
Age < 50 yr		
0		1.00
1		1.70
≥ 2		2.88
Age ≥ 50 yr		
0		1.00
1		1.27
≥ 2		1.62
AGE AT FIRST TERM LIVE BIRTH (yr)	Number of first degree relatives with breast cancer	
< 20	0	1.00
	1	2.61
	≥ 2	6.80
20–24	0	1.24
	1	2.68
	2	5.78
25-29 or nulliparous	0	1.55
	1	2.76
	2	4.91
≥ 30	0	1.93
	1	2.83
	2	4.17

Source: Gail MH, Brinton LA, Byar DP, et al. Projecting individualized probabilites of developing breast cancer for white females who are being examined annually. *J Natl Cancer Inst*. 1989; 81: 1879–1886.

breast self-examination, and 69% went for clinic examinations; 94% had regular mammography (32).

Caution has been suggested in relation to breast cancer risk assessment. Clients must be informed that testing may not result in an informative result (Table 17.3). The concept of risk assessment must be clearly communicated. The individual with a seemingly increased risk may never develop cancer, and conversely, the client with a low risk may develop a cancer. Risk is a chance of an event occurring. The genes for specific cancers simply increase the likelihood of a cancer occurring. Lastly, screening for cancer has limitation in regard to prevention and early detection. There is no scheme for preventing a cancer (33–35).

TABLE 17.3. *Criteria for BRCA1 testing*

CANDIDATES

Women affected with breast or ovarian cancer who have any one of the following:

1. A personal history or premenopausal breast cancer
   (a) Autosomal dominant inheritance of breast and/or ovarian cancer susceptibility based on pedigree analysis
   (b) At least one first- or second-degree relative with early onset (premenopausal) breast or ovarian cancer
2. two primary tumors, either breast/breast or breast/ovarian

NOT CANDIDATES

3. Men with breast cancer
4. Women who do not have a family history of breast cancer
5. Women who appear to have an isolated case and late onset (postmenopausal) disease *or* women with a distant family history

Owing to these issues, there is the potential for adverse psychological consequences for the client electing risk assessment (Table 17.4). Clients entering a risk assessment counseling program must grapple with their own potential for developing cancer and concurrently must deal with the effects of cancer for extended family members. Beliefs about cancer etiology, unresolved grief, anger, fear, guilt and anxiety, and family dynamics are issues the client presenting for risk assessment has prior to an actual counseling session. The underlying motivation(s) for such counseling must be explored and resolved with the patient prior to actual evaluation. Clients must be given the option of with-

TABLE 17.4. *Genetic Breast Cancer Risk Counseling*

WHAT HAPPENS AT A GENETIC COUNSELING VISIT FOR BREAST CANCER RISK?
- Detailed review of family, medical, and life-style histories
- Documentation of cancer (individual and primary sites)
- Risk assessment and counseling
- Review of early detection and prevention options

SURVEILLANCE/EARLY DETECTION FOR BREAST CANCER
- Breast self-examination (BSE)
- Clinical breast examination (CBE)
- Mammography
- Breast ultrasound
- Breast MRI—under investigation

CANCER PREVENTION FOR BREAST CANCER
- Surgical options
- Prophylactic (preventive) mastectomies
- Breast reconstruction
- Breast biopsies

CANCER PREVENTION FOR BREAST CANCER
- Tamoxifen
- Chemoprevention

drawing from risk assessment or testing protocols. Psychological profiles may be altered by psychosocial interventions as described by Kash. Behaviors as well as psychological profiles may benefit from such intervention (36,37).

Although many clients will have heard of and seek "the cancer gene test," currently testing is appropriate and available only for rare individuals. For the occasional client who enters a gene (DNA) testing protocol, it has to be acknowledged that cancer gene testing presents several nuances not found with other genetic tests such as cytogenetics. Specifically, in the example of *BRCA1* testing, testing gene positive does not necessarily confer disease status. Only 5%–10% of all breast cancer seem to be strongly inherited. Of the inherited breast cancers, *BRCA1* accounts for half of the families; *BRCA2* accounts for an additional 35% of cases. Another challenge is to explain the concept of age-related risk in a way the patient can understand for both sporadic and inherited breast cancer. Every woman is at some risk to develop breast cancer. In the general population, a woman's risk to develop breast cancer by age 50 is 2% and her lifetime risk is 10%. The risk of a second primary breast cancer after one breast cancer has been diagnosed is about 1% per year, to about 15% overall. In comparison, if a woman has a strong family history of breast cancer and carries a mutation in *BRCA1*, her risk for developing breast cancer by age 45 is 50%. Once she has had breast cancer, the risk of a second primary 87% by age 80. Her overall lifetime risk of developing breast cancer is 85% which also means she has a 15% chance of never developing breast cancer. Therefore, in the example of *BRCA1* testing, testing positive for a mutation does not confer disease status. This is in stark contrast to Huntington's Disease, where patients know that if they live long enough and are gene positive, they will develop the diesease (38,39).

Yet another challenge is to explain the possible limitations of using genetic testing for risk assessment. For example, *BRCA1* is a large gene spanning more than 5500 base pairs of coding sequence. Mutation analysis is, therefore, time consuming. In addition, in studies of high-risk families, it has not been possible to correlate age-related risks of developing breast cancer with specific mutations or mutations in regions of the gene, which means that the same mutation in different families may cause a very different pattern of cancer. Also it is important to recognize that our understanding of risks associated with carrying a mutation in *BRCA1* is generated from studies of families in which there are multiple cases of breast cancer in several generations. Therefore, these risk figures may not be appropriate for carriers of a *BRCA1* mutation found in the general population. Population-based studies are currently underway in several laboratories to learn more about mutation frequency and disease penetrance in the population as a whole.

INFORMED CONSENT ISSUES

The experience of presymptomatic or asymptomatic testing of individuals at risk for Huntington's disease (HD) has led to a tentative code of conduct for genetic researchers that may be applied to genetic testing for cancer predisposition (40). A code related to cancer counseling issues has not been agreed upon but is currently being studied by Ethical, Legal and Social Issues (ELSI) unit of the Human Genome Project. The HD code evolved from research on families with genetic disease and from the development of new molecular tests. The proposed code of conduct intends to protect both the subject and researchers. Harper points out that most problems encountered in genetic testing are a result of not paying adequate attention to the ethics of gene testing and therapy. Huntington's disease protocols have often been examined by review committees, but with more attention given to the physical risks of the sampling procedure (dangers and discomfort of venipuncture) rather than the social, psychological, and economic consequences of the test results that can follow the detection of a genetic defect.

The proposed code also addresses the conflicts of interest between the patient's needs and the physician's or researchers' interest. Financial ties with industry, through research, personal investment in commercial ventures, or consulting fees, occur in genetics as in other fields of medicine with a dependence on high technology. Fost has written that "sometimes it is difficult to distinguish a conflict of interest from a congruence of interest. The scientist's desire of fame and fortune may drive him or her to the extra effort that results in a discovery that benefits others. The physician's desire for income may stimulate him or her to work long hours and provide beneficial services to others. But there is also evidence that self-interest can adversely affect clinical judgment, whether it be for suggesting elective surgery or for ordering expensive diagnostic tests" (41).

Disclosure statements have become commonplace to minimize the possible effects of conflicts of interest, and some groups, notably a multicenter clinical trial of treatment after coronary artery bypass graft surgery, have moved toward prohibiting ties with industry when such ties are not necessary for the practice of medicine or the advancement of science (42).

The code of conduct proposed by Harper also points to some of the difficulties that will be faced as genetic technologies developed in a research setting are applied in the clinical diagnostic or therapeutic context (43). The code states:

1. Family members "at risk" for a genetic disorder should not be sampled unless strictly necessary for the research, especially in late-onset or variable disorders. This applies particularly to children. Proposals should clearly justify the testing of unaffected subjects and should include a clear plan stating what will be done in the event that a genotypic abnormality is detected.

2. When consent is given for sampling by an unaffected person, to assist a family member in determining his/her risk status, it should be made clear that the risk status of the unaffected person will not be disclosed and the result of the test should not be expected, nor will they be sent to his/her doctor or placed in his/her medical record unless specifically requested.

3. If the sample is to be stored and used for future tests, new consent should be obtained if the implications for the person at risk resulting from the new research are likely to be considerably different—for example, if direct mutations analysis, rather than a general linkage analysis, is possible.

4. If the possibility of identifying defects in people at risk is foreseeable or inevitable, then such a sample should be coded or made anonymous for the purpose of these tests unless the person concerned has specifically requested that relevant information should be disclosed and has received information that allows him/her to fully understand the implications of such disclosure.

5. If a person at risk who gave a research sample later requests presymptomatic testing or other genetic services, a new sample should be taken and the request handled in the same way as it would be for any other person electing presymptomatic testing.

6. When a test may show a specific genetic defect in people affected by a disorder not previously known to be genetic, the possible genetic implications (as well as psychosocial implications) should be made clear and new consent obtained if samples previously obtained are being restudied.

7. Ethics committees should pay at least as much attention to the consequences of a sample being taken as to the risks attached to the sampling procedure.

The presymptomatic HD testing programs have attempted to create and preserve trust and understanding between researchers and test providers. Presymptomatic testing is a multi-step process involving numerous visits to testing centers. The HD protocols prescribe review of the subject's family history, neurologic examination, psychiatric examination, review of medical charts of extended family members for confirmation of diagnostic information, psychological testing, pre-test counseling, and disclosure of results. Follow-up both clinically and for research purposes is a standard feature of presymptomatic testing protocols (44).

The HD model sometimes limited the subject's right to privacy because of the need for extensive review of family medical data and the need for samples for linkage analysis (prior to the recent discovery of the HD gene). The protocol was born from the traditional pre-1970s model for the physician–patient relationship. It is therefore criticized for its paternalism. The protocols were neither publicly reviewed nor discussed. As individuals have "graduated" from the testing program, the protocols are being revisited. Suggestions and recommendations from participants are being sought in order to evaluate and possibly to modify the protocols. Moreover, the 1993 discovery of the gene responsible for HD has pushed the scientific community to reevaluate the protocols because extended family review is no longer necessary.

The HD model represents the first testing program that enables a person to choose to know with a high degree of certainty that he or she will die of a fatal, inherited, and presently untreatable disease. The psychiatric and social consequences of having such knowledge were anticipated and prompted the rigid protocol structure to preserve the most basic of ethical tenets—to do no harm. Experience with the HD protocols has shown that explaining genetic risks is a complex subject and that understanding comes slowly (45).

The counseling steps of the HD protocols may be adapted in future genetic testing models of testing for cancer-predisposing genes. Testing without giving information, counseling, and support is unacceptable. Concern about stigmatization and discrimination in employment, insurance, and personal relationships should provoke society to monitor and regulate the availability and use of genetic testing to ensure that abuse or coercion does not occur (43).

CONCLUSION

Genetic counseling for patients with cancer has only recently been recognized as a necessary component of quality care for cancer patients (46). Most patients and their family members have immediate concerns about their own risk of developing cancer once a relative has been diagnosed with the disease. Parents faced with the diagnosis of cancer in their family usually worry about their children's risks. These fears and concerns should be verbalized by health professionals caring for the cancer patient and his/her family. To provide the greatest benefit to the patient, risk counseling should assist patients to address their conscious and unconscious agendas and to appreciate the emotional component of their risk status.

The opportunity to consult with a specialist in genetics should be given to cancer patients and their extended families as needed. Support groups for cancer families should include discussion of the heritability of cancer and resources for obtaining genetic counseling. Counseling often informs patients that their risks are lower than anticipated and can be a positive force in reducing the family's anxiety. At the same time, patients and families need to understand that testing may not always be informative.

The provision of genetic services for familial cancer should include programs of detection, screening and counseling, at a minimum. Our understanding of the genetic basis of hereditary cancers obligates the health care system today to provide these specialized services to all cancer patients. In the final analysis, genetic counseling can lead to cancer prevention.

REFERENCES

1. Fraser FC. Genetic counseling. *Am J Hum Genet.* 1974; 26(5): 636–659.
2. Parry DM, Mulvihill JJ, Miller RW, et al. Meeting report: strategies for controlling cancer through genetics. *Cancer Res.* 1987; 47: 6814–6817.
3. Mulvihill JJ. Genetic counseling for the cancer patient. In: DeVita VT, Hellman S, Rosenberg S, eds. *Principles and Practice of Oncology*, 4th ed. Philadelphia: JB Lippincott; 1993: 2529–2537.
4. Stadler MP, Mulvihill JJ. Establishing a cancer genetics clinical program in an academic medical center. *Am J Hum Genet.* 1995; 57: A348.
5. Biesecker BB, Boehnke M, Calzone K, et al. Genetic counseling for families with inherited susceptibility to breast and ovarian cancer. *J Am Med Assoc.* 1993; 269: 1970–1974.
6. Hoskins KF, Stopfer JE, Calzone KA, et al. Assesment and counseling for women with a family history of breast cancer: a guide for clinicians. *J Am Med Assoc.* 1995; 273: 577–585.
7. Peters J. Breast cancer risk counseling. *The Genetic Resource.* 1994; 8(1): 20–25.
8. Mulvihill JJ. *Mendelian Inheritance in Man for Oncology.* Baltimore: The Johns Hopkins University Press; 1996.
9. Mulvihill JJ. Clinical ecogenetics of human cancer. *Hem/Onc Ann.* 1994; 2: 157–161.
10. Schneider KA. *Counseling about Cancer: Strategies for Genetic Counselors.* Dennisport, MA: Graphic Illusions; 1994.
11. Love RR, Evans AM, Josten DM. The accuracy of patient reports of a family history of cancer. *J Chron Dis.* 1985; 38: 289–293.
12. Offit K, Brown K. Quantitating familial cancer risk: a resource for clinical oncologists. *J Clin Oncol.* 1994; 12(8): 1724–1736.
13. Lynch HT. Cancer and the family history trail. *NY State J Med.* 1991; 91(4): 145–147.
14. Eng C, et al. Familial cancer syndromes. *Lancet.* 1994; 343: 709–713.
15. Kelly P. Breast cancer risk analysis. *J Genet Counsel.* 1992; 2: 155–167.
16. Claus EB, Risch NJ, Thompson WB. Age of onset as an indicator of familial risk of breast cancer. *Am J Epidemiol.* 1991; 131(6): 961–972.
17. Lynch HT, Hirayama T. *Genetic Epidemiology of Cancer.* Boca Raton, FL: CRC Press; 1989.
18. Li FP, Lokich J, Lapey J, Neptune WB, Wolkes WE Jr. Familial mesothelioma after intense asbestos exposure at home. *J Am Med Assoc.* 1978; 240:467.
19. Lynch HT, Lynch JF, Cristofaro G. Genetic epidemiology of colon cancer. In: Lynch HT, Hirayama T, eds. *Genetic Epidemiology of Cancer.* Boca Raton: CRC Press; 1989: 251–277.
20. Li FP, Fraumeni JF Jr., Mulvihill JJ, et al. A cancer family syndrome in twenty-four kindreds. *Cancer Res.* 1988; 48: 5358–5362.
21. Malkin D, Li FP, Strong LC, Fraumeni JF Jr., et al. Germ line p53 mutations in a familial syndrome of breast cancer, sarcomas, and other neoplasms. *Science.* 1990; 250: 1233–1238.
22. Weber W, Durig M, eds. *Hereditary Cancer and Preventive Surgery.* Basel: Karger; 1990: 1118.
23. Allen HH, Nisker JA, eds. *Cancer in Pregnancy: Therapeutic Guidelines.* Mt. Kisco, NY: Futura Publishing; 1986.
24. Mulvihill JJ, Harvery EB, Boice JD, et al. Normal findings 52 years after in utero radiation exposure. *Lancet.* 1991; 338: 1202–1203.
25. Mulvihill JJ, Stewart KR. A registry of pregnancies exposed to chemotherpeutic agents. *Teratology.* 1986; 33: 80C.
26. Neel JV, Satoh C, Goriki K, et al. Search for mutations altering protein charge and/or function in children of atomic bomb survivors: final report. *Am J Hum Genet.* 1988; 42: 663–676.
27. Houlston RS, et al. Screening and genetic counseling for relatives of patients with breast cancer in a family cancer clinic. *J Med Genet.* 1992; 29: 691–694.
28. King MC, et al. Inherited breast and ovarian cancer: What are the risks? what are the choices? *J Am Med Assoc.* 1993; 269(15): 1975–1980.
29. Hall JM, Friedman L, Guenther C, et al. Closing in on a breast cancer gene on chromosome 17q. *Am J Hum Genet.* 1992; 50: 1235–1242.
30. Claus EB, et al. Autosomal dominant inheritance of early-onset breast cancer: implications for risk prediction. *Cancer.* 1994; 73: 643–651.
31. Gail MH, Brinton LA, Byar DP, et al. Projecting individualized probabilities of developing breast cancer for white females who are being examined annually. *J Natl Cancer Inst.* 1989; 81: 1879–1886.

32. Kash KM, Holland JC, Halper MS, Miller DG. Psychological distress and surveillance behaviors of women with a family history of breast cancer. *J Natl Cancer Inst.* 1992; 84: 24–30.

33. Lerman C, Croyle R. Psychological issues of genetic testing for breast cancer susceptibility. *Arch Intern Med.* 1994; 154: 609–616.

34. Lerman C, Rimer BK, Engstrom PF. Cancer risk notification: psychosocial and ethical implications. *J Clin Oncol.* 1991; 9(7): 1275–1282.

35. Lerman CE, Rimer BK. Psychosocial impact of cancer screening. *Oncology.* 1993; 7: 67–72.

36. Breo DL. Altered fates—counseling families with inherited breast cancer. *J Am Med Assoc.* 1993; 269: 2017–2022.

37. Crowther ME, et al. Psychosexual implications of gynecological cancer. *Br Med J.* 1994; 208: 869–870.

38. Weber BL, Garber JE. Family history and breast cancer: probabilities and possibilities. *J Am Med Assoc.* 1993; 270: 1602–1603.

39. Easton DE, Narod SA, Ford D, Steel M. The genetic epidemiology of BRCA1. *Lancet.* 1994; 344: 761.

40. Harper P. Research samples from families with genetic diseases: a proposed code of conduct. *Br Med J.* 1993; 306: 1391–1394.

41. Fost N. Genetic diagnosis and treatment. *Am J Dis Child.* 1993; 146: 1190–1195.

42. Healy B. Remarks for the RAC Committee Meeting of January 14, 1993, Regarding Compassionate Use Exemption. *Hum Gene Ther.* 1993; 4: 196–197.

43. Harper P. Clinical consequences of isolating the gene for Huntington's disease. *Br Med J.* 1993; 307: 397–398.

44. Folstein S. *Huntington Disease.* Baltimore: The Johns Hopkins University Press; 1989; 177–187.

45. Murray T. Ethical issues in human genome research. *FASEB J.* 1991; 5: 55–60.

46. Thompson J, Weisner G, Sellers T, et al. Genetic services for familial cancer patients: A survey of National Cancer Institute Cancer Centers. *The National Cancer Institute Special Report.* 1995; 87: 1446–1455.

18

Psychological, Social, and Ethical Issues in Gene Testing

KATHRYN M. KASH AND CARYN LERMAN

Individuals with family histories of cancer have an excess risk of developing the disease themselves. For example, having a first-degree relative (FDR) with breast cancer imparts a twofold to fourfold excess risk of developing this disease (1). Women are considered to be at higher risk for breast cancer if they have two or more first-degree relatives with breast cancer diagnosed under age 60, a first-degree relative diagnosed with breast cancer under the age of 40, or a combination of first- and second-degree relatives diagnosed with breast or ovarian cancer that would indicate an inherited susceptibility (for example, see Fig. 18–1). These classifications are based on the model developed by Claus and colleagues (2). Men and women who have an FDR affected with colon cancer also have about a three-fold increased risk (3). Yet, research shows that many high-risk women do not adhere to breast cancer screening recommendations (4,5). The same is true for adherence to colon cancer screening among relatives of colon cancer patients (6). Furthermore, some high-risk individuals experience problems in psychological adjustment. Clinically significant psychological distress has been documented in a substantial proportion of women at risk for breast cancer (7,8). and those at risk for ovarian cancer (9). Psychosocial interventions designed to enhance adjustment and adherence in these high-risk populations are promising. Such interventions may be especially important for individuals who have inherited mutations in cancer-predisposing genes.

This chapter is devoted to these psychological and behavioral issues associated with elevated cancer risk status. First, we discuss issues of psychological adjustment in high-risk individuals. This is followed by a discussion of the implications of distress for adherence to cancer screening and for medical decision-making. The next section addresses psychosocial aspects of can-cer risk counseling and genetic testing for cancer susceptibility. The fourth section focuses on psychosocial interventions to enhance quality of life and facilitate medical decision-making. The final section focuses on the ethical issues involved in genetic testing.

PSYCHOLOGICAL ISSUES FOR INDIVIDUALS AT RISK FOR CANCER

What are the psychological issues in women at risk for breast cancer? The first and most overwhelming issue for women is their *anxiety* about developing breast cancer. Anxiety peaks at certain points in their lives, for example, when a woman reaches the age at which her mother or sister developed breast cancer. On reaching that age, a woman fears she too will develop breast cancer and die. Another peak in anxiety occurs when a woman has the same number of children as her mother had when she developed breast cancer. Some women believe if they have fewer children, they will be protected against breast cancer. One study found that over one-fourth of women at risk for breast cancer suffered sufficient psychological distress to warrant counseling (7).

A woman's *sense of vulnerability* leads to an overestimation of risk, which in turn heightens their subjective certainty of developing breast cancer. Data from other studies indicate that a substantial number of women with a family history of breast cancer have a heightened perception of risk (10,11). Underestimation most frequently occurs when a woman has a very high risk (35%–50%) and has not received risk counseling. Frequently women report that they are "100% sure" that they will get breast cancer, as well as describing themselves as "walking time bombs." In other words, women at high risk do not wonder *if* they will get breast cancer but *when* it will appear.

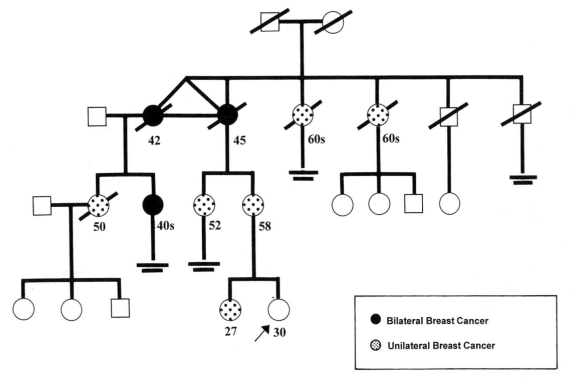

FIG. **18–1.** Family history of an inherited predisposition to breast cancer. Numbers indicate age at onset of cancer.

The *fear of disfigurement or death* is a common theme and is sometimes worse for women who were young when their grandmothers, mothers, and sisters developed the disease and died. Fears such as having "mutilating" surgery for breast cancer are prevalent in their thinking. Many women remember the radical Halstead mastectomies of 20 years ago and believe this procedure would still be used today if they developed breast cancer.

Guilt, related to several issues, is pervasive in women at high risk. Some women express guilt because they feel they did not support a family member at the time she had cancer. Other women feel guilty because they may have passed the "bad" gene to their daughters. Women who have not developed breast cancer while other relatives have, feel "survivor" guilt. And, many healthy women at risk feel guilty because they are so preoccupied and concerned about breast cancer.

The *misconceptions and myths* about breast cancer are overwhelming for many women. Some of these have been passed from one generation to the next. One myth is that "if you have a blow to the breast, you will develop breast cancer." A misconception about breast cancer is that "if you have fibrocystic breasts, this leads to breast cancer." And, stress in one's life is often feared as a factor that will increase risk of breast cancer. Yet another misconception is that "if you have surgery for breast cancer, it spreads."

Frequently, women who have strong family histories of breast cancer often feel *powerless* about the disease. They believe that they have a gene mutation, they can do nothing about it, and breast cancer is their destiny. In addition, they recall that they felt helpless when their mothers and sisters had breast cancer; they feel hopeless (and helpless) about avoiding the disease themselves. In other words, a woman's sense of self-efficacy regarding the prevention of breast cancer is lacking. This often impacts negatively on their ability to adhere to surveillance screening procedures that would lead to early detection of a curable tumor.

Another psychological issue for women at high risk is their passivity and their use of *denial* regarding breast cancer, and in particular, avoidance of breast cancer screening. Women frequently make statements, such as, "If I don't think about breast cancer, I won't get it" or "I just don't want to know if I have breast cancer." Sometimes women join a surveillance program, and after having a couple of negative mammograms and clinical breast examinations, feel protected and postpone future screening dates.

Finally, one of the major issues surrounding all the above concerns is that women feel *isolated* and alone.

They are reluctant to talk to other family members who are at risk. Generally, women feel that these closest family members often do not want to hear about how they are feeling. In addition, women feel that their friends do not understand their "obsession" with breast cancer. Thus, there are few opportunities for reflection about feelings and sharing the information in a way that would reduce their isolation.

IMPLICATIONS OF PSYCHOLOGICAL DISTRESS

Adherence to Cancer Screening

Several studies have examined the role of psychological distress on adherence to breast cancer screening in women who have a family history of breast cancer. In one study of 207 high risk women attending a surveillance program (7), the authors found lower rates of screening adherence in women who were more distressed. While 52% came in for regular clinical breast examinations (CBE), only 27% performed breast self-examination monthly. In women over age 40, less than half (46%) came in for yearly mammograms. For all three methods of early detection, greater cancer anxiety and psychological distress were significant predictors of poor adherence. They also found that younger, well-educated women were significantly less likely to perform monthly breast self-examination (BSE). Women with the highest psychological distress levels had more barriers to screening. Over 72% of these women thought that their risk for developing breast cancer was moderately likely to extremely likely. Based on family history, no woman's risk is ever greater than 50%, yet these women estimated their mean risk to be between 41% and 50%, which indicated that many overestimated their risk. In fact, 80% of this cohort of 207 women overestimated their risk for developing breast cancer, with only 15% estimating accurately, and 5% underestimating their risk status. In addition, 27% of these women had levels of psychological distress high enough to warrant counseling.

In examining the best predictors of women adhering to screening, one study found that younger, well-educated women were the least likely to perform BSE (12). Women who reported higher scores on a general anxiety scale performed BSE less often than the recommended monthly schedule. There was a significant difference on anxiety between women who performed BSE monthly versus women who performed BSE less than monthly (Fig. 18–2). In addition, the more social support and the fewer barriers they had, the more likely they were to perform BSE. In examining the best predictors of women coming in for a CBE,

again, increased levels of cancer anxiety and psychological distress interfered with frequency of CBEs. Adherence to mammography recommendations was also impaired by high levels of psychological distress. Thus, cancer anxiety or psychological distress interfere with all three screening behaviors.

Similarly, Lerman and colleagues (8) found FDRs of breast cancer patients who had intrusive breast cancer worries were significantly less likely to adhere to mammography guidelines than women without such symptoms. As shown in Figure 18–3, this was especially true for women who had less formal education. By contrast, Stefanek and Wilcox (4) found that breast cancer worries were associated positively with adherence to mammography and CBE in a similar sample of women. The differences in adherence rates to breast cancer screening may be related to the number of relatives with breast cancer. Many participants in the study of Kash and colleagues (7) had two or more first-degree relatives with breast cancer, which may have contributed to a decrease in screening behaviors. One study showed that distress in high-risk women persisted even after the receipt of the information that their mammogram was normal (13).

At the extreme end of the continuum of behaviors are women whose fears lead them to engage in excessive or inappropriate breast cancer screening. For example, in studies of younger women at high risk for breast cancer, over one-third reported practicing breast self-examination more often than the recommended monthly frequency (14). Among FDRs of recently diagnosed breast cancer patients, a study by Epstein and colleagues (15) found that 8% reported that they practiced BSE at least daily. Excessive BSE was significantly more common among women with high levels of breast cancer-related distress.

Fewer studies have examined distress and screening for other cancers. In a study of FDRs of ovarian cancer patients, those who were more worried about their cancer risks were more likely to have ovarian cancer screening tests (16). On the other hand, for younger, lower-income women, mood disturbance was shown to interfere with adherence to colposcopy following an abnormal Pap smear (17). Worry about cancer has also been found to be a barrier to colorectal cancer screening in both men and women (18).

This brief overview shows that the links between psychological distress and adherence to cancer screening in high-risk groups are very complex. To explain these divergent findings, one hypothesis is that the relationship between distress and adherence may be U-shaped, rather than linear (7,19,20). Individuals who are unconcerned about their cancer risks may not see

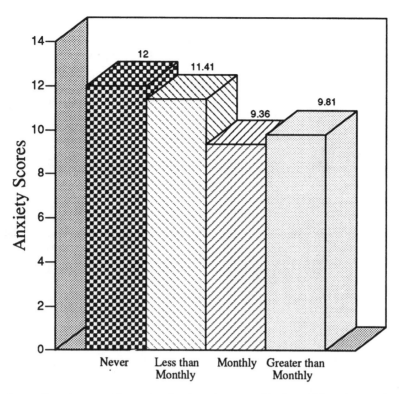

FIG. **18–2.** Women who perform breast self-examination less than monthly ($n = 190$) and never ($n = 47$) are more anxious than women ($n = 106$) who perform it monthly ($p < 0.007$).

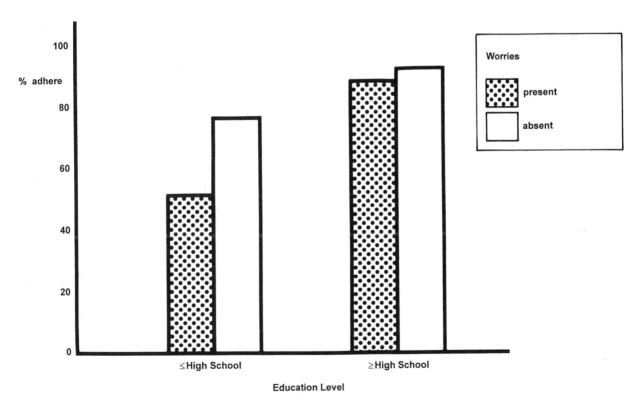

FIG. **18–3.** Breast cancer-related worries by mammography adherence, controlling for education.

the need for adhering to screening recommendations. Heightened concerns or moderate distress about cancer risk may be necessary to motivate this behavior. However, excessive distress may provoke avoidance of cancer screening. To cope with anxieties about cancer, some individuals may suppress thoughts about cancer and avoid cancer-related experiences, including screening tests. However, this U-shaped explanation of distress and adherence fails to explain the observation that heightened distress can also prompt excessive breast cancer screening. Such behavior is consistent with the presence of a psychiatric diagnosis such as generalized anxiety, obsessive-compulsive disorder, or hypochondriasis; it warrants a referral for a psychiatric evaluation (15).

To facilitate adherence to cancer screening in high-risk populations, health care providers need to pay greater attention to the fears, concerns, and psychological coping strategies of their patients. By enhancing awareness of excess cancer risk, providers may be able to motivate their high-risk patients to adhere to cancer screening recommendations. However, to avoid provoking avoidance behavior or inappropriate screening, communications that heighten perceived risk must be balanced by reassuring messages. Such messages could emphasize the benefits of continued cancer screening, including the potential for detection of early stage cancers, increased treatment options, and an increased rate of cure. In addition, providers should address psychological barriers to screening adherence, including embarrassment and anxiety about positive results (21–23).

Medical Decision-Making

Relatively little attention has focused on understanding how psychological factors influence medical decision-making. For individuals at high risk for cancer, one important decision concerns whether to participate in a cancer chemoprevention trial. For example, women with a family history of breast cancer are being targeted for enrollment in the Breast Cancer Prevention Trial (BCPT), a trial of anti-estrogen therapy for asymptomatic women (24). As yet, however, the factors that influence high-risk women's decisions about participation in the BCPT are poorly understood. A study of recruitment of high-risk women to a breast cancer health promotion trial suggests that the determinants of participation may differ for women with different levels of education (25). The timing of the recommendation may be another important determinant. In a recent study, women with more formal education were more likely to participate in a risk counseling program if they were approached within

the first two months following the breast cancer diagnosis of a close relative (26). Familial polyposis patients also were more likely to participate in a colon cancer chemoprevention program if they had been diagnosed more recently (27). During this initial period following diagnosis, heightened perceived risk and/or distress may motivate risk reduction behaviors, such as participation in a chemoprevention or health promotion trial.

In addition to decisions about chemoprevention, many high-risk women are seeking counseling about whether to obtain prophylactic mastectomies or hysterectomies. Among carriers of cancer-predisposing genes, prophylactic surgery may have psychological benefits, such as the reduction of chronic worry (28). However, there are also psychological risks (29) and the long-term efficacy of these techniques has been questioned (30,31). Thus, decisions about prophylactic surgery may be especially challenging and stressful for high risk women.

A recent unpublished study by Stefanek and Lerman suggests that breast cancer-related distress may also influence prophylactic mastectomy decisions (29). In this study, women were presented with vignettes that described a woman at high risk for breast cancer who was deciding whether to obtain a prophylactic mastectomy or to have close breast cancer follow-up. Women were asked to indicate what their choice would be in that situation. Women who had higher levels of perceived personal risk and higher levels of breast cancer worries were significantly more likely to select prophylactic mastectomy over close follow-up. Younger women and women selecting prophylactic mastectomy reported less confidence in their choices. These findings suggest that psychological support may facilitate informed decision-making for high-risk individuals faced with difficult decisions about prophylactic surgery.

CANCER RISK COUNSELING AND GENETIC TESTING

Impact of Individualized Cancer Risk Counseling

Increasingly, individuals with a family history of cancer are seeking information and counseling about their personal risks. There has been some attention to ovarian cancer risk counseling (32) and counseling for members of hereditary colon cancer families (33,34). Breast cancer risk counseling programs have been initiated in many medical centers in the United States (11,12,35).

Lerman and colleagues conducted a randomized trial to evaluate the impact of individualized breast cancer risk counseling (BCRC) for women with a family history of breast cancer (36,37). Women aged 35 and older were randomized to receive either BCRC or general health education (GHE, as the control condition). The BCRC protocol was a multicomponent intervention delivered by a nurse or health educator in a 1.5-hour visit, containing the following elements: *(1)* discussion of individual factors contributing to elevated risk; *(2)* presentation of individualized risk data based on the model developed by Gail and colleagues (38); *(3)* recommendations for annual mammography and clinical breast examination based on guidelines for women with familial risk (39); and *(4)* instruction in breast self-examination using silicone breast models.

Initial findings from the BCRC trial are promising. Women who received BCRC were significantly more likely to improve their comprehension of their personal risks compared to women in the GHE condition (36). However, in both groups, about two-thirds of women continued to substantially overestimate their lifetime risks of breast cancer. The results of this trial also showed that BCRC did not produce improved comprehension among the large proportion of women who had high precounseling levels of intrusive thoughts about breast cancer. Thus, psychological distress appeared to be a barrier to comprehension of personal risk information.

The impact of BCRC on psychological distress was also examined (37). The results of this study indicated that the psychological benefits of BCRC were greater for women with less formal education. As shown in Figure 18–4, women with a high school education or less showed significant reductions in cancer-related distress following BCRC, while those who received GHE showed no changes in distress. The women in this study are being followed for one year to evaluate the impact of GHE on adherence to mammography.

While much additional research on cancer risk counseling is needed, these data on BCRC suggest that this counseling approach may be an effective way to enhance personal risk comprehension, enhance psychological well-being, and improve adherence to cancer screening. The cancer risk counseling model has been used as the basis for the development of more complex protocols for genetic counseling and testing for cancer susceptibility.

GENETIC TESTING FOR CANCER SUSCEPTIBILITY

Several major cancer susceptibility genes have been isolated in the early 1990s. These include the *BRCA1* gene for hereditary breast-ovarian cancer (HBOC) (40), the *BRCA2* gene for site-specific breast cancer (41), and the *hMLH1*, *hMSH2*, *PMS1*, and *PMS2* genes for hereditary non-polyposis colon cancer (HNPCC) (42,43). These scientific advances offer unprecedented opportunities for high-risk members of hereditary cancer families to discover whether or not they carry a genetic mutation and have a significantly increased risk of one or more of these diseases. The pretest counseling of these individuals is very important, as well as the fact that it should be structured to contain all the elements to assist them in making an informed decision about testing. A standard protocol for genetic counseling and testing for cancer susceptibility is shown in Figure 18–5. More detailed descriptions of this process can be found in other reports (44,45).

Attitudes About and Uptake of Testing

Prior to the availability of genetic testing for cancer-predisposing genes, several surveys were conducted to examine attitudes and intentions to obtaining a genetic test. Both in the general population and among individuals at high-risk, a majority (over 75%) expressed interest in having genetic tests for colon cancer risk (46–48), breast cancer risk (49,50) and ovarian cancer risk (51). In one unpublished study by Kash and colleagues, over 1000 women who were in a national registry for familial risk for breast cancer were queried concerning their willingness to undergo genetic testing to identify factors that would influence their decision. Over 72% stated they would have genetic testing immediately and request to learn their results if the test were clinically available. Women who reported more pros for testing, reported fewer cons of testing, perceived themselves to be gene mutation carriers, and had greater breast cancer anxiety were the most likely to undergo testing (31% of variance accounted for in multiple regression analyses). In another unpublished study comparing 394 women at risk with 385 women at average risk, Kash and colleagues found that 42% of average risk women and 71% of high-risk women would have genetic testing for *BRCA1* gene mutations. While the potential uptake for high-risk women is similar to those approached for Huntington's disease (HD), it is worrisome that almost half of women at average risk would consider genetic testing for breast and ovarian cancers. However, previous studies of HD have shown that intentions to have a hypothetical genetic test often do not correspond to subsequent test utilization (52).

The notion that some individuals may not want to learn their genetic status is supported by results from a prospective study of actual *BRCA1* testing in 279

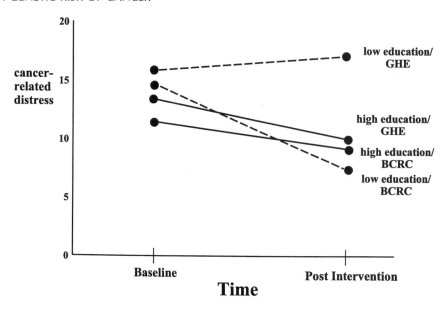

FIG. 18–4. Impact of breast cancer risk (BCRC) and general health education (GHE) on breast cancer-related distress (based on impact of events scale).

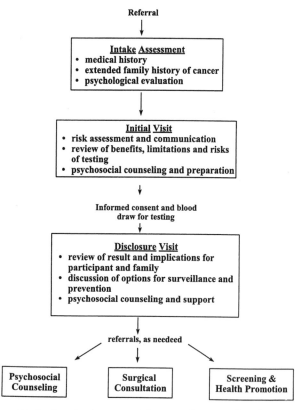

FIG. 18–5. Standard protocol for genetic counseling for cancer susceptibility.

members of hereditary breast ovarian families (53). Only 43% of individuals opted to receive their *BRCA1* test results. Individuals with health insurance, those who had a greater number of affected relatives, and those who were more knowledgeable about breast cancer genetics were more likely to participate. In addition to these factors, psychological factors also appeared to impact on decisions whether to have a *BRCA1* test. In the same sample of families, breast cancer-related distress was found to be significantly and positively related to *BRCA1* test use. This is consistent with an earlier study showing that women who reported disturbances in mood were more likely to intend to have *BRCA1* test when available (51).

The finding that cancer-related distress motivates use of genetic testing is worrisome, because is suggests that the individuals most likely to request testing may be more psychologically vulnerable. As mentioned above, distress during counseling may interfere with comprehension of risk information delivered during the counseling session. Furthermore, distressed individuals may be more vulnerable to adverse psychological consequences of learning their genetic status. A study of predictive testing for Huntington's disease showed that the presence of intrusive symptoms at baseline increased the likelihood of maladjustment following disclosure of test results (54). The HD data from the study of Wiggins and colleagues (55) showed that those who did not receive their test results were most distressed; those who did receive their results (positive or negative) were less distressed at a year post test.

In one of the first outcome studies of *BRCA1* testing, Croyle and colleagues (56) reported on the short-term (1–2 week) impact of testing on general distress and breast cancer-specific distress in high-risk women. Although *BRCA1* carriers did not evidence increases in general distress, they did report significantly higher post-test levels of intrusive thoughts. The highest levels of distress were found in carriers who had no prior cancer diagnosis or preventive surgery.

Recently, Lerman and colleagues (53) reported interim data from a prospective cohort study of members of several HBOC families in a registry maintained by Creighton University. Changes in depressive symptoms and functional impairment from baseline to one-month post testing were reported for 46 carriers of *BRCA1* mutations, 50 noncarriers, and 44 decliners of *BRCA1* testing. At baseline and one-month follow-up, all three groups scored in the normal ranges on these measures. Noncarriers of *BRCA1* mutations exhibited significant decreases in depressive symptoms and role impairment and marginally significant decreases in sexual impairment, compared to carriers and decliners. Carriers and decliners of testing did not exhibit increases in any of these distress outcomes. Unpublished six-month follow-up data from this cohort suggest that this pattern of responses is maintained over time.

While these two initial reports do not provide evidence for significant or pervasive adverse psychological effects of *BRCA1* testing, caution is warranted in generalizing these findings to other populations and settings. Participants in these studies were members of high-risk families in hereditary cancer registries, many of whom were involved in prior cancer genetics studies. These families had been included in the registries because of their unusually high cancer rates. As a consequence of witnessing cancer in many close family members, emotional responses of study participants may have been blunted. In fact, an unpublished study by Lerman, Schwartz, and colleagues found that levels of distress were lower in these HBOC families than in population-based samples of women with a family history of cancer and cancer patients. In addition, most unaffected individuals in these high-risk families reported prior to testing that they expected to be mutation carriers. Thus, receiving a positive test result may have confirmed what they believed to be true all along. In some cases, worrying about the possibility of being a mutation carrier may be no less distressing than having that belief confirmed. Individuals who have less significant family histories, and who do not expect to receive positive results, may be more vulnerable to adverse psychological sequelae of

BRCA1 testing. It should also be noted that all individuals in these studies were white (all of the Utah subjects were Mormon) and most had a high school education. In addition, all testing was provided as part of research protocols with extensive education and counseling. Such counseling may be responsible for the observed psychological benefits in the Lerman et al. study (53).

PSYCHOSOCIAL INTERVENTIONS

While little is known about the potential psychological outcomes of genetic testing for cancers, even less is understood about how to intervene with the negative sequelae. However, we can extrapolate from psychosocial interventions for coping with cancer as to how we can help individuals cope with genetic testing.

Behavioral Interventions

In the oncology field, interventions using support groups (57), individual psychotherapy (58), psychoeducational models for cancer patients (59) or those at risk for cancer (12), or behavioral modification (60) have been used to help cancer patients with their diagnosis or to foster adherence to appropriate screening practices. For example, Myers and colleagues (61) used health education interventions to increase adherence in a colorectal cancer screening program. While they found that more intensive programs increased adherence, interventions needed to be tailored in such a manner as to address the reasons for nonadherence. In an extensive overview, Andersen (62) suggested that interventions for cancer patients can help in decreasing emotional distress, improve coping, and enhance quality of life. In fact, a recent meta-analysis (63) of pyschosocial interventions found that all were beneficial, but perhaps further investigation into different treatments would be important. Certainly intervention strategies could be tailored for different populations, such as those with cancer and those at genetic risk for cancers. Kash and colleagues (12) are currently conducting psychoeducational groups for women at familial risk for breast and ovarian cancer. Preliminary data indicate that anxiety is decreased and adherence to screening is improved in women in the experimental arm.

Coping Skills Training

As Sharpe (64) has noted, "professional standards for medical genetics and genetic counseling recognize that a geneticist has a duty to provide appropriate psychological support." Promising strategies to bolster patients' coping skills have been developed and evaluated in several studies of cancer patients (62,65). For example, psychoeducational interventions designed to increase cancer patients' awareness of the possible consequences of treatment have been shown to improve psychological and physical adjustment (66). Such approaches are easily adapted to the genetic testing context. In fact, most genetic counselors currently utilize similar strategies, such as asking patients to anticipate how they would react emotionally and behaviorally to different outcomes of the testing.

By probing patients' coping plans, providers can identify maladaptive coping strategies and suggest more adaptive approaches. Denial is observed frequently among patients undergoing predictive genetic testing (54,67,68) but can be difficult to detect in brief interactions. Research conducted with breast cancer patients suggests that active behavioral coping and acceptance lead to better overall psychological adjustment than coping by avoidance or denial (69). Furthermore, if nurses provide brief coaching in specific skills, such as problem-solving or relaxation training, patients' actual coping efforts and self-confidence may be improved. Post-disclosure counseling and follow-up "booster" contacts can be used to determine how patients are actually coping with their genetic status and to reinforce strategies that are most likely to be beneficial.

Decision Counseling to Facilitate Informed Decisions about Genetic Testing and Prophylactic Surgery

In the past, counselors have taken a nondirective approach when providing genetic counseling. However, in considering genetic testing for cancers, decisions must be made and counselors must provide information not only about the risk for certain diseases but also about potential treatment options (29,70). Prophylactic surgery (mastectomy, oophorectomy, or subtotal colectomy) may be offered to mutation carriers of *BRCA1*, *BRCA2*, *hMLH1*, or *hMSH2*. Studies have shown that training individuals how to make decisions can decrease psychological distress and increase decision-making ability and problem solving (71).

ETHICAL PRINCIPLES OF GENETIC TESTING

The current ethical principles guiding risk notification and genetic testing were derived from the Canadian collaborative study of predictive testing for Huntington's disease (72) and expanded by the Institute of Medicine (73). The Canadian group was the first to look at the impact of testing for a genetic disease. While there are major differences between hereditary susceptibility for Huntington's disease and for cancers, both areas involve genetic testing and counseling, and both have similar ethical and psychological implications (73).

When one applies ethical principles to genetic testing, several principles are important. The first is respect for autonomy. This refers to the rights of those approached for testing to be fully informed as to the profound effects and implications that testing may have on their lives so that they can exercise autonomy in making a decision. They should have a discussion of all possible outcomes, positive and negative, of genetic testing. In addition, people making this decision need to know what the impact is on their lifetime risk for developing cancer. It is not just knowing the information about testing or risk analysis that is important, but also having the ability to fully understand the result of the outcomes of testing. Individuals seeking genetic testing should be free from coercion and not feel pressure from others to undergo testing.

The principle of beneficence has application in genetic testing. "First, do no harm" is a salient concept for those in genetic counseling and mental health whose role requires attention to possible adverse effects of improper counseling methods. In genetic counseling for cancer susceptibility, counselors ought to consider whether or not the testing results will do "more harm than good" rather than "more good than harm". Genetic counselors need to think about the potential for harming an individual who is under extreme emotional distress after learning about their risk level or the results of testing. Some individuals, especially those with a psychiatric history, require particular evaluation to assure that their vulnerability is taken into account.

In terms of confidentiality or privacy, it is important that testing results not be disclosed to third parties or other family members without discussion with the person and getting their approval for what will be revealed and establishing to whom the information may be disseminated. Confidentiality of data is also crucial in terms of employment and insurance (74,75). Health and life insurance could be lost or denied to individuals, and employers might not promote or hire individuals who are cancer gene carriers. Marital and sibling relationships can be strained around what other family members learn. Genetic testing becomes very complicated when some individuals in a family want to know their carrier status while others do not. Who will have access to this information needs to be discussed and resolved at the time of counseling, prior to testing.

In terms of the principle of equity or justice, there should be equal access for all to genetic testing or risk analyses. Currently, testing is being done on a research basis only and there is no financial cost to the individual, with the exception of one private company which offers testing for a fee. However, in the future when testing becomes available on a clinical level, cost will be high. One question that needs to be addressed is, who will pay for individuals whose family histories are congruent with hereditary susceptibility but who cannot pay? Will testing be offered to those who can pay but are at the lowest risk for susceptibility? Genetic testing or risk analyses should be obtainable for appropriate family members regardless of ethnicity, geographical location, or ability to pay. In this sense justice refers to fairness for all.

SUMMARY AND CONCLUSION

Psychological assessment has played an important role in examining adherence to screening practices as well as adherence to cancer treatment options. High levels of stress clearly impact negatively upon screening surveillance behaviors. Psychosocial interventions have been helpful. With the emergence of genetic testing for several types of cancer, the psychological issues are paramount and must be taken into account when an individual is considering genetic testing. The complex ethical, psychological, and social consequences can be daunting for individuals trying to become fully informed and to make a decision about having genetic testing. The role of pre- and post-testing counseling, with attention to any psychological problems, is critically important. This chapter is an overview of many of the issues involved in genetic testing and has highlighted the most salient ones within the context of testing.

REFERENCES

1. Slattery ML, Kerber RA. A comprehensive evaluation of family history and breast cancer risk. The Utah Population Database. *J Am Med Assoc.* 1993; 270:1563–1568.
2. Claus EB, Risch N, Thompson WD. Age of onset as an indicator of familial risk of breast cancer. *Am J Epidemiol.* 1992; 131: 961–972.
3. Anderson DE. Familial cancer and cancer families. *Semin Oncol.* 1978; 5:11–16.
4. Stefanek ME, Wilcox P. First degree relatives of breast cancer patients: Screening practices and provision of risk information. *Cancer Detect Prev.* 1991; 15:379–384.
5. Vogel VG, Graves DS, Vernon SW, Lord JA, Winn RJ, Peters GN. Mammographic screening of women with increased risk of breast cancer. *Cancer.* 1990; 66:1613–1620.
6. Sandler RS, DeVellis BM, Blalock SJ, Holland KL. Participation of high-risk subjects in colon cancer screening. *Cancer.* 1989; 63:2211–2215.
7. Kash KM, Holland JC, Halper MS, Miller DG. Psychological distress and surveillance behaviors of women with a family history of breast cancer. *J Natl Cancer Inst.* 1992; 84:24–30.
8. Lerman C, Daly M, Sands C, et al. Mammography adherence and psychological distress among women at risk for breast cancer. *J Natl Cancer Inst.* 1993; 85:1074–1080.
9. Schwartz MD, Lerman C, Miller SM, Daly M, Masny A. Coping disposition, perceived risk, and psychological distress among women at increased risk for ovarian cancer. *Health Psychol.* 1995; 14:232–236.
10. Evans DGR, Burnell LD, Hopwood P, Howell A. Perception of risk in women with a family history of breast cancer. *Br J Cancer.* 1993; 67: 612–614.
11. Stefanek ME. Counseling women at high-risk for breast cancer. *Oncology.* 1990; 4:27–33.
12. Kash KM, Holland JC, Osborne MP, Miller DG. Psychological counseling strategies for women at risk for breast cancer. *Monogr Natl Cancer Inst.* 1995; 17: 73–79.
13. Valdimarsdottir HB, Bovbjerg DH, Kash KM, Holland JC, Osborne MP, Miller DG. Psychological distress in women with a familial risk of breast cancer. *Psycho-Oncology.* 1995; 4:133–141.
14. Lerman C, Kash K, Stefanek M. Younger women at increased risk for breast cancer: perceived risk, psychological well-being, and surveillance behavior. *Monogr Natl Cancer Inst.* 1994; 16:171–176.
15. Epstein SA, Lin TH, Audrain J, Stefanek M, Rimer B, Lerman C, and The High Risk Cancer Consortium. Excessive breast self-examination among first-degree relatives of newly diagnosed breast cancer patients. *Psychosomatics.* 1997; 38:253–261.
16. Schwartz M, Lerman C, Daly M, Audrain J, Masny A, Griffith K. Utilization of ovarian cancer screening by women at increased risk. *Cancer Epidemiol Biomarkers Prev.* 1995; 4:269–273.
17. Lerman C, Miller SM, Scarborough R, Hanjani P, Nolte S, Smith D. Adverse psychologic consequences of positive cytologic cervical screening. *Am J Obstet Gynecol.* 1991; 165:658–662.
18. Blalock SJ, DeVellis BM, Sandler RS. Participation in fecal occult blood screening: a critical review. *Prev Med.* 1987; 16:9–18.
19. Hailey BJ. Family history of breast cancer and screening behavior: an inverted U-shaped curve? *Med Hypotheses.* 1991; 36:397–402.
20. Lerman C, Schwartz M. Adherence and psychological adjustment among women at high-risk for breast cancer. *Breast Cancer Res Treat.* 1993; 28:145–155.
21. Lerman C, Rimer B, Trock B, Balshem A, Engstrom PF. Factors associated with repeat adherence to breast cancer screening. *Prev Med.* 1990; 19:279–290.
22. Myers RE, Trock BJ, Lerman C, Wolf T, Ross E, Engstrom PF. Adherence to colorectal cancer screening in an HMO population. *Prev Med.* 1990; 19:502–514.
23. Rimer BK. Understanding the acceptance of mammography by women. *Ann Behav Med.* 1992; 14:197–203.

24. Nayfield SG, Karp JE, Ford LG, Dorr FA, Kramer BS. Potential role of Tamoxifen in prevention of breast cancer. *J Natl Cancer Inst.* 1991; 83:1450–1459.

25. Lerman C, Rimer BK, Daly M, et al. Recruiting high-risk women into a breast cancer health promotion trial. *Cancer Epidemiol Biomarkers Prev.* 1994; 3:271–276.

26. Rimer BK, Schildkraut JM, Lerman C, Lin TH, Audrain J, and the High Risk Breast Cancer Consortium. Participation in a women's breast cancer risk counseling trial: Who participates? Who declines? *Cancer.* 1996; 77:2348–2355.

27. Miller HH, Bauman LJ, Friedman DR, DeCosse JJ. Psychosocial adjustment of familial polyposis patients and participation in a chemoprevention trial. *Int J Psychiatry Med.* 1987; 16:211–230.

28. Lerman C, Croyle R. Psychological issues in genetic testing for breast cancer susceptibility. *Arch Intern Med.* 1994; 154:609–616.

29. Stefanek ME. Bilateral prophylactic mastectomy: Issues and concerns. *Monogr Natl Cancer Inst.* 1995; 17:37–42.

30. King MC, Rowell S, Love SM. Inherited breast and ovarian cancer: What are the risks? What are the choices? *J Am Med Assoc.* 1993; 269:1975–1980.

31. Struewing JP, Watson P, Easton DF, Ponder BAJ, Lynch HT, Tucker MA. Prophylactic oophorectomy in inherited breast/ovarian cancer families. *Monogr Natl Cancer Inst.* 1995; 17:33–35.

32. Daly MB, Lerman C. Ovarian cancer risk counseling: A guide for the practitioner. *Oncology.* 1993; 7:27–38.

33. Lynch HT, Smyrk T, Watson P, et al. Hereditary colorectal cancer. *Semin Oncol.* 1991; 18:337–366.

34. Houlston RS, Murday V, Harocopos C, Williams CB, Slack J. Screening and genetic counselling for relatives of patients with colorectal cancer in a family cancer clinic. *Br Med J.* 1990; 301:366–368.

35. Kelly PT. *Understanding Breast Cancer Risk.* Philadelphia, PA: Temple University Press; 1991.

36. Lerman C, Lustbader E, Rimer B, Daly M, Miller S, Sands C, Balshem A. Effects of individualized breast cancer risk counseling: a randomized trial. *J Natl Cancer Inst.* 1995; 87:286–292.

37. Lerman C, Schwartz MD, Miller SM, Daly M, Sands C, Rimer BK. A randomized trial of breast cancer risk counseling: interacting effects of counseling, educational level, and coping style. *Health Psychol.* 1996; 15:75–83.

38. Gail MH, Brinton LA, Byar DP, et al. Projecting individualized probabilities of developing breast cancer for white females who are being screened annually. *J Natl Cancer Inst.* 1989; 81:1877–1886.

39. Hayward RS, Steinberg EP, Ford DE, et al. Preventive care guidelines. *Ann Intern Med.* 1991; 114:758–772. [Published erratum appears in *Ann Intern Med.* 1991; 115:332.]

40. Miki Y, Swensen J, Shattuck-Eidens D, et al. A strong candidate for the breast and ovarian cancer susceptibility gene BRCA1. *Science.* 1994; 266:66–71.

41. Wooster R, Bignell G, Lancaster J, et al. Identification of the breast cancer susceptibility gene BRCA2. *Nature.* 1995; 378:789–792.

42. Nicolaides NC, Papadopoulos N, Liu B, et al. Mutations of two PMS homologues in hereditary nonpolyposis colon cancer. *Nature.* 1994; 271:75–78.

43. Peltomäki P, Aaltonen LA, Sistonen P, et al. Genetic mapping of a locus predisposing to human colorectal cancer. *Science.* 1993; 260:810–812.

44. Biesecker BB, Boehnke M, Calzone K, et al. Genetic counseling for families with inherited susceptibility to breast and ovarian cancer. *J Am Med Assoc.* 1993; 269: 1970–1974.

45. Peters JA, Stopfer JE. Role of the genetic counselor in familial cancer. *Oncology.* 1996; 10:159–175.

46. Croyle RT, Lerman C. Interest in genetic testing for colon cancer susceptibility: cognitive and emotional correlates. *Prev Med.* 1993; 22:284-292.

47. Croyle RT, Smith KR. Attitudes toward genetic testing for colon cancer risk. *Am J Public Health.* 1995; 85:1435–1438.

48. Lerman C, Marshall J, Audrain J, Gomez-Caminero A. Genetic testing for colon cancer susceptibility: anticipated reactions of patients and challenges to providers. *Int J Cancer (Pred Oncol).* 1996; 69:58–61.

49. Chaliki H, Loader S, Levenkron JC, Logan-Young W, Hall J, Rowley PT. Women's receptivity to testing for a genetic susceptibility to breast cancer. *Am J Public Health.* 1995; 85:1133–1135.

50. Lerman C, Seay J, Balshem A, Audrain J. Interest in genetic testing among first-degree relatives of breast cancer patients. *Am J Med Genet.* 1995; 57:385–392.

51. Lerman C, Daly M, Masny A, Balshem A. Attitudes about genetic testing for breast-ovarian cancer susceptibility. *J Clin Oncol.* 1994; 12:843–850.

52. Craufurd D, Dodge A, Kerzin-Storrar L, Harris R. Uptake of presymptomatic predictive testing for Huntington's disease. *Lancet.* 1989; 2:603–605.

53. Lerman C, Narod S, Schulman K, et al. BRCA1 testing in hereditary breast-ovarian cancer families: a prospective study of patient decision-making and outcomes. *J Am Med Assoc.* 1996; 275;1885–1892.

54. Tibben A, Duivenvoorden HJ, Vegter-van der Vlis M, et al. Presymptomatic DNA testing for Huntington disease: Identifying the need for psychological intervention. *Am J Med Genet.* 1993; 48:137–144.

55. Wiggins S, Whyte P, Huggins M, et al. The psychological consequences of predictive testing for Huntington's disease. Canadian Collaborative Study of Predictive Testing. *N Engl J Med.* 1992; 327:1401–1405.

56. Croyle RT, Smith K, Botkin J, Baty B, Nash J. Psychological responses to BRCA1 mutation testing. Preliminary findings. *Health Psychol.* 1997; 16:63–72.

57. Spiegel D, Bloom JR, Kraemer HC, Gottheil E. Effect of psychosocial treatment on survival of patients with metastatic breast cancer. *Lancet.* 1989; 2:888–891.

58. Greer S, Moorey S, Baruch JDR. Adjuvant psychological therapy for patients with cancer: a prospective randomised trial. *Br Med J.* 1992; 304:675–680.

59. Fawzy FI, Fawzy NW, Hyun CS, et al. Malignant melanoma: Effects of an early structure psychiatric intervention, coping and affective state on recurrence and survival 6 years later. *Arch Gen Psychiatry.* 1993; 50:681–689.

60. Baider L, Uziely B, De-Nour AK. Progressive muscle relaxation and guided imagery in cancer patients. *Gen Hosp Psychiatry.* 1994; 16:340–347.

61. Myers RE, Ross EA, Wolf TA, Balshem A, Jepson C, Millner L. Behavioral interventions to increase adherence

in colorectal cancer screening. *Med Care.* 1991; 29:1039–1050.

62. Andersen BL. Psychological interventions for cancer patients to enhance the quality of life. *J Consult Clin Psychol.* 1992; 60:552–568.

63. Meyer TJ, Mark MM. Effects of psychosocial interventions with adult cancer patients: a meta-analysis of randomized experiments. *Health Psychol.* 1995; 14:101–108.

64. Sharpe NF. Psychological aspects of genetic counseling: a legal perspective. *Am J Med Genet.* 1994; 50:234–238.

65. Glanz K, Lerman C. Psychosocial impact of breast cancer: a critical review. *Ann Behav Med.* 1992; 14:204–212.

66. Rainey LC. Effects of preparatory patient education on radiation oncology patients. *Cancer.* 1985; 56:1056–1061.

67. Falek A. Sequential aspects of coping and other issues in decision making in genetic counseling. In: Emery AH, Pullen IM, eds. *Psychological Aspects of Genetic Counseling.* London: Academic Press; 1984: 23–36.

68. Kessler S, ed. *Genetic Counseling: Psychological Dimensions.* New York, NY: Academic Press; 1979.

69. Carver CS, Pozo CP, Harris SD, et al. How coping mediates the effect of optimism on distress: a study of women with early stage breast cancer. *J Pers Soc Psychol.* 1993; 65:375–390.

70. Lynch HT, Watson P, Conway TA, et al. DNA screening for breast/ovarian cancer susceptibility based on linked markers. *Arch Intern Med.* 1993; 153: 1979–1987.

71. Owens RG, Ashcroft JJ, Leinster SJ, Slade PD. Informal decision analysis with breast cancer patients: an aid to psychological preparation for surgery. *J Psychosoc Oncol.* 1987; 5:23–33.

72. Huggins M, Bloch M, Kanani S, et al. Ethical and legal dilemmas arising during predictive testing for adult-onset disease: the experience of Huntington disease. *Am J Hum Genet.* 1990; 47: 4–12.

73. Andrews LB, Fullarton JE, Holtzman NA, Motulsky AG, eds. *Assessing Genetic Risks: Implications for Health and Social Policy.* Committee on Assessing Genetic Risks, Division of Health Sciences Policy, Institute of Medicine, Washington, DC: National Academy Press; 1994.

74. Billings PR, Kohn MA, de Cuevas M, et al. Discrimination as a consequence of genetic testing. *Am J Hum Genet.* 1992; 50:476–482.

75. Ostrer H, Allen W, Crandall LA, et al. Insurance and genetic testing: Where are we now? *Am J Hum Genet.* 1993; 52:565–577.

V

PSYCHOLOGICAL ADAPTATION TO CANCER

EDITOR: RUTH McCORKLE

19

Psychological and Social Factors in Adaptation

STACIE M. SPENCER, CHARLES S. CARVER, AND ALICIA A. PRICE

Although the odds of recovery from many forms of cancer have improved greatly in recent years, diagnosis and treatment of cancer still create significant distress (1). Cancer patients must cope with a sense of uncertainty about the future; noxious side effects of treatment; and feelings of isolation, stigma, and guilt (2,3). Sometimes they are deluged with information about their diagnoses (including survival statistics), and are encouraged to seek second opinions. This increase in information and the behavioral options confronting them creates additional stresses that patients did not encounter in the past (4).

In considering adaptation to treatment for cancer, a simple question concerns the pattern of distress over time. When is distress most intense? What is its time course? Distress arises with the first suspicion of cancer (5). Indeed, the diagnostic period before surgery is widely seen as the most emotional portion of the treatment period (6,7). Surgery marks an important step in dealing with the distress, in part because prognosis is known with greater certainty shortly thereafter. However, surgery and even the completion of adjuvant therapy do not mark the end of the adaptation process. Adaptation continues for a long time afterward. Indeed, adaptation remains a long-term problem for the *families* of cancer patients, as well as for the patients themselves (8,9).

Psychological distress, negative attitudes, somatic distress, and anxiety about separation and death decrease gradually over the first year following diagnosis (10,11). Still, emotions associated with having cancer often continue to be powerful for many years after treatment is complete (12). Five years and more afterward, some patients continue to report physical, emotional, and social complaints such as pain, anxiety about implants, relationship difficulties, feelings of isolation, and fear of recurrence (13). Although the literature is inconsistent on the question of whether distress levels increase or decrease with cancer-free survival time, there is general agreement that residual concern exists even after the cancer appears to have been eliminated (14,15).

In some cases, of course, patients experience a recurrence of the cancer. This is likely to be far more disturbing than the initial diagnosis (16,17), because recurrence has ominous implications for longer-term survival. For people who experience a recurrence, adjustment to the new diagnosis means adjusting to the prospect of a far more limited future.

Several further questions also arise regarding adaptation to cancer. In what *ways* do cancer patients go about coping with the stresses of diagnosis and treatment of cancer? What coping responses are most effective, or ineffective? What personal and social resources have an important impact on the adaptation process? This chapter addresses these questions (for other reviews of coping and adaptation see Refs. 18–22). Our focus here is a broad one, dealing with overall psychosocial adaptation. Adaptation will be considered here in terms of emotional distress and subjective quality of life, and in terms of social functioning at work and with friends and family. Other chapters in this volume deal with more specialized adaptations to specific problems associated with particular disease sites or specific types of medical treatment.

Our discussion is oriented within the framework of a self-regulation model of coping (23). That is, we assume that coping constitutes behavior and cognitive activity aimed at responding to and overcoming adversity. These responses may be aimed at ensuring that the cancer is completely eliminated; they may be aimed at minimizing the disruption to the other aspects of one's life from the diagnosis and treatment; they may be aimed at dealing with feelings of distress elicited by the diagnosis and treatment process. All of these are potential focuses of a person's coping efforts (24,25). All of these focuses, however, serve the ultimate function of placing the person back into the activities of his or her life, a point we return to presently. To the extent that these various coping efforts are successful in doing that, the person is adapting well to the experience of having been treated for cancer.

One way of thinking about coping effectiveness is that to cope successfully with any crisis depends on having various kinds of resources (26). When people think of a medical crisis, the first kinds of resources that usually come to mind are financial resources and access to skilled medical personnel. Other resources are also important, however, especially when the medical crisis has passed and the process of adjusting psychologically to the new identity of cancer patient has begun. These other resources are personal and social in nature. As we examine the process of coping with cancer, we will be identifying some of the personal and social resources that help some people cope better than others.

The chapter is organized as follows. We begin by briefly considering conceptual issues in coping and adaptation. We present in this section a view in which effective coping serves to foster the attainment of the person's array of life goals, and ineffective coping represents disengagement from those goals. Then we turn to research on the contextual and personal resources that appear to predict good adjustment among cancer patients. The next topic we take up is the types of coping responses that cancer patients use to deal with the stress of their situation, and evidence that some responses are more useful than others. This is followed by a brief discussion of interventions aimed at enhancing adaptive coping among cancer patients. We conclude the chapter with a brief reminder of some of the limitations on current knowledge in this area.

ISSUES IN COPING AND ADAPTATION

The approach to adaptation we are taking here incorporates some assumptions about successful coping that we should spell out before we turn to adaptation among cancer patients. One assumption is that stress depends on the psychological situation that the person experiences, rather than the objective event (24,25). The psychological situation is certainly influenced by external reality, but it is also influenced by what the individual brings to that external reality. Thus, an event that is deeply threatening to one person may be far less so to another.

There is a similar interplay between person and external reality in the determination of responses to a threat. People differ in their repertoire of coping responses. They differ in their beliefs about what responses are helpful, and in their beliefs about their abilities to adequately carry out certain responses. As a result, different people cope in different ways, even given the same level of perceived threat.

Engagement versus Giving Up
Another important issue concerns the ultimate function of coping. We said earlier that coping can be aimed at reducing distress reactions, at minimizing the impact of the stressful event on the person's life in other domains, and at removing the stressor (if possible). All these purposes of coping serve the ultimate function of returning the person to an active pursuit of his or her preexisting goals in life (cf. Refs. 27–30). This is the hallmark of successful adaptation: a full and enthusiastic return to the normal activities of life.

Sometimes, however, stresses are so severe as to cause people to doubt their ability to return to the ordinary pursuits of life. When people's doubts about moving toward their goals are strong enough, the result is a tendency to disengage effort, to withdraw from pursuit of the goal, even to give the goal up entirely (27,28,31–34). For a patient with a serious illness such as cancer, the goals that are threatened by the disease are literally the goals that define the person's very life. Feeling the desire to give up on such goals creates a very serious problem. The experience of someone in this situation combines intense distress with an inability to motivate oneself to try again. In the literature of coping with cancer, this experience has received the label "helplessness/hopelessness" (35).

As we go on to consider how cancer patients cope with their diagnosis and treatment, and the comparative success with which different people cope, we will pay special attention to this issue of continued effort versus giving up. We see this issue as critically important in people's adaptation. We also note that withdrawal or giving up can come in many guises. Those working with cancer patients either as researchers or clinicians must be aware of the possibility that the tendency to disengage may underlie certain coping acts that otherwise seem unremarkable. It is just as important to consider these potentially dysfunctional coping responses as to consider responses that are expected to be useful and functional (36–40).

Commitment and Disengagement: A Further Issue
Much of the contribution of self-regulation models of coping and adjustment concerns issues of commitment

versus disengagement. One more issue related to this disjunction should be noted. This issue concerns the avoidance tactics that people employ when they do not want to deal with problems they are facing. Such tendencies are sometimes linked to the term *denial*, though the concept of denial—which itself is notoriously hard to pin down—is usually taken to refer to a range of phenomena that extends beyond these tendencies. At a minimum, however, these tactics reflect a temporary disengagement from dealing with threatened goals.

It is sometimes argued that avoidance coping is useful because it gives the person a psychological breather, an opportunity to escape from the constant pressure of the situation (41,42). Similarly, it is often held that denial is adaptive in the short run, because it protects people from having to deal all at once with the implications of the problem they are confronting (43–45). Whether avoidance coping and denial really are useful or adaptive has long been a matter of debate (19,46–48), and a number of problems stand in the way of the debate's resolution.

One problem is that avoidance tendencies vary quite widely. A woman just diagnosed with breast cancer may literally deny the reality of the diagnosis, accept that the diagnosis is real but deny that it is problematic, or deny that the diagnosis will be life disrupting (49). Denial may also mean denial of an emotional reaction to the threat, avoidance of thinking about the situation, or active efforts at self-distraction from such thoughts or feelings of distress. Although the responses just named share some characteristics, they are also quite different in other respects.

Because of these differences, there are conceptual problems in deciding whether a person's response does or does not imply denial. If a woman says she is trying not to focus on her feelings of distress so that she can move beyond them to taking active steps forward, is this denial? If she reports trying to derive something positive from the experience of having cancer, is this denial? We believe it is not (see also Ref. 50). It should be clear, though, that these questions are hard to answer with certainty. This is a problem that permeates discussions of coping with a life-threatening illness such as cancer.

COPING WITH CANCER: WHO DOES BETTER, WHO DOES WORSE?

Let us turn now to evidence about adaptation to cancer. The focus of much research on adjustment to cancer has been on normative tendencies in a given population (51,52). This research generally indicates that the period of about a year following diagnosis and treatment represents a crisis in patients' lives, but that this crisis is usually weathered fairly well by most patients, at least among those with a good prognosis. It is clear, however, that some people adapt better than do others (18). As a number of writers have pointed out, psychosocial support services cannot yet be offered to every patient. For this reason, it is important to determine who is at greatest risk of adjustment problems, so that support services can be targeted to those in greatest need of them (18,53–56).

Many kinds of differences among people are relevant to success in adapting to cancer. Most of us think first of differences originating within the person, but some differences between people are in fact contextual (57). For example, consider the extent of surgical intervention. Among breast cancer patients, many women choose to have lumpectomies, rather than mastectomies, as surgical treatment. However, some women who might prefer lumpectomies are prevented from having this procedure by the size and placement of their tumors. Because of this, a difference comes to exist between these two groups of women in the extent of their surgery and thus the extent of their physical disfigurement. A large literature attests to the fact that this difference matters. The more extensive procedure leads to feelings of less attractiveness and less of a sense of femininity; it does not, however, lead to greater overall emotional distress (58–69).

Social Support

Another difference among people is the social context of their lives. Some patients are married or in other comparably close relationships, others are not. Some patients have a close-knit circle of family and friends, others do not. Thus, patients differ from one another in how much social support from various people is available to them. This difference in levels of social support resources can have an important impact on patients' sense of well-being when confronting the challenge of treatment for cancer.

Several studies have shown that women who perceive themselves as having adequate social support resources fare better than women who perceive their support as inadequate (5,18–19,70–75). Evidence from a recent study indicates a need to distinguish among the *sources* of the social support (76). That is, the benefit of social support in that sample derived principally from support by the woman's *partner*. Support from other sources was not an independent contributor to positive outcomes (though a tendency in that direction was seen among women without partners).

Social support is usually thought of in terms of spousal support or support from friends and family, but other social interactions may also be relevant to the broad issue of social support. For example, patients have many interactions with the physicians who diagnose and treat their cancers, and with the nurses and office staff. The tone of these various interactions probably also play a role in the degree of comfort or assurance with which the patients face the future (77). A caring medical professional who expresses support and concern for the patient will start the patient's journey through the cancer experience in a very different way than will the one who is brusque, cold, abrupt, and mechanical. The interactions between patients and their physicians is an aspect of the social nature of the cancer experience that is beginning to receive increasing research attention.

Personality

Individual differences in personality also have an important impact on how well people adjust to the diagnosis and treatment of cancer. When considering personality, we quickly enter something of a grey area, where it can be difficult to tell where personality leaves off and more circumscribed coping responses begin. That conceptual problem is encountered repeatedly in the literature of adaptation to cancer. As early as 1976, Weisman reported the clinical impression that cancer patients did better if they had an optimistic, upbeat attitude than if they were more pessimistic, and evidence consistent with this position (48,78). Cancer patients themselves similarly believe a positive outlook is important, both while in the hospital and during the subsequent recovery phase (6). But is this optimistic outlook a cancer-specific attitude—pertaining only to the cancer—or does it instead reflect a broader quality of personality? It is difficult to be sure.

Research has shown that having an optimistic outlook on life in general is related to many important outcomes. Optimists and pessimists differ in the manner in which they cope with various stresses (79,80) and in the extent to which they experience distress under conditions of adversity (81). At least two projects have now examined systematically the involvement of this broad personality variable in the experiences of cancer patients. One of these projects assessed optimism prior to biopsy for breast cancer (7). Optimism was a strong correlate of prebiopsy distress, though it was not predictive of distress following diagnosis or surgery. The other project assessed of optimism before surgery and

then followed patients for a year after surgery (82). Optimism in this sample was a significant prospective predictor of distress at each measurement point, even after controlling for the distress reported at the preceding assessment.

Another variable that is important in the adaptation of cancer patients is identified with the term "fighting spirit" (11,35). Fighting spirit is an engagement in active efforts to overcome the adversity posed by the diagnosis of cancer. It represents a determined struggle to regain one's strength and remain fully involved in the process of living life. This variable was initially conceived of as a coping response that is specific to the diagnosis and treatment of the cancer. However, there is good reason to ask whether this variable might reflect more permanent and broadly based aspects of personality. In particular, there is evidence that fighting spirit is linked to the disposition to be optimistic about life in general (83).

Another variable related to both of these is neuroticism. Neuroticism is a very broad personality trait involving such tendencies as the ready experience of distress, worrying, and pessimism about one's self-worth and one's future. At least two studies have investigated associations between this personality quality and emotional adjustment at a period of approximately two years post treatment (5,11). These studies found that higher levels of neuroticism were related to poorer emotional adjustment.

Conclusions

The studies reviewed in this section indicate that several kinds of differences among people can be expected to relate to their success in adapting to cancer. Some kinds of treatments may produce more disruption than others. Having the perception that one has a good base of social support seems to confer a resilience that makes adaptation easier. Perceptions of support from a spouse may be particularly important in this regard, but the patient's entire social matrix may play a role in the patient's well-being. Finally, personality differences help determine who does well and who does poorly in adapting to the cancer experience. People who are positive about their lives in general, and who are willing to take on and master challenges, can be expected to adapt relatively well. People who are negative about their lives, who are prone to distress in response to adversity, and who are more likely to feel helpless and hopeless when confronting adversity can be expected to have a harder time adapting effectively and moving forward with their lives.

COPING RESPONSES AMONG CANCER PATIENTS: WHICH ONES ARE HELPFUL?

We turn now to a related, but distinguishable, set of questions: In what *manner* do people go about coping with cancer? What kinds of tactics do people naturally turn to? What kinds of responses turn out to be more useful or less useful? Information on the usefulness of various coping responses comes from two kinds of studies. In cross-sectional studies, patients report at the same time the ways they have been coping and their current levels of well-being. In more complex, prospective studies, coping in a given time frame is used as a predictor of well-being later on. The latter type of study has an important advantage: it can yield a clearer picture of which variable is influencing which. That is, when all the information is collected at a single time point, there is no assurance that coping responses are influencing distress level. It could just as easily be the other way around.

Cross-Sectional Studies

With this caution in mind, we turn to cross-sectional studies. Although limited in what they can say, these studies do provide a sense of the range of coping responses used by cancer patients and a sense of which responses relate to concurrent distress. Coping responses reported by cancer patients are in fact quite diverse. The diversity ranges across acceptance of the reality of the diagnosis, acceptance of impending death, trying to forget about the diagnosis, becoming more repressive overall, engaging in positive self-talk, trying to find something positive in the situation, seeking information, seeking social support, taking a positive attitude toward the future, confronting or tackling the problem head-on, and giving up (6,12,13,84).

What kinds of coping relate to lower levels of distress? The types of coping that patients say are effective for them are, in general, those that theory predicts should be effective. Patients indicate that using their emotional support resources, confronting the situation head-on, seeking information, having a positive attitude, having a fighting spirit, and finding comfort in their religion are effective methods of coping (6,13,85). Such reponses relate to lower distress (83, 86-88) and better social functioning (85,89). Patients say that coping by being evasive or emotive, or by taking a fatalistic or helpless attitude, are the least effective strategies (13), and avoidant coping (denial, wish-fulfilling fantasy) and self-blame relate to higher levels of distress (82,87), as do avoidant activities such as eating, drinking, and sleeping (70).

Regarding denial as a coping response, there is conflicting evidence. Some of the research just cited found denial related to higher distress, other studies found the opposite. For example, Watson and colleagues (90) interviewed patients after surgery and identified them as deniers (said they chose not to think about the seriousness of the illness) or acceptors (said they accepted the implications of the diagnosis and admitted to fears for the future). Deniers reported less mood disturbance than acceptors, leading the researchers to conclude that denial may in the short term be useful. Meyerowitz similarly found cancer-specific denial to be associated with less distress (91).

To some extent, differences among findings depend on how denial is measured. As noted earlier, denial is a hard concept to pin down, and no measurement technique is free of criticism. Meyerowitz (91) assessed denial as patient reports of how much they felt upset when they thought about cancer-related issues (with low levels of upset viewed as an indication of denial). She also used a questionnaire devised to reflect minimization of the adverse consequences of cancer. Although there is a logical basis for each of these measures, each also has a problem. It might be argued that the first one is very nearly a measure of distress itself (this is also a problem in Watson et al. (90)). It might be argued that the second measure is more a measure of catastrophizing than of denial.

Although measures of denial differ in the problems they have, virtually every approach to this concept has some sort of problem. This illustrates the difficulty researchers have in studying denial, and it also explains why findings for denial are more inconsistent than those for other coping responses. In assessing the usefulness of denial in coping, observers must pay close attention to how denial is measured in a given study and use their own judgment about the meaning of various findings.

Prospective Studies

As noted earlier, the findings from these cross-sectional studies have an important limitation. It is impossible to judge the directionality of influence from measurements that are made at a single point in time. This is one important reason for conducting research prospectively.

There are other reasons, as well. Having cancer is not a single stressful event; rather, having cancer is a series of interconnected stressful events (92). Coping begins with the first suspicion of cancer, and it continues beyond treatment, for the rest of the patient's life. Success in coping with one event is likely to influence adjustment and subsequent coping with the next event, and so on. Prospective designs permit one to observe this potential cascade of influence across time points. Although there have been relatively few prospective studies of coping with cancer, the available evidence suggests that this type of study gives a far clearer picture of the experience of coping with cancer than does the single-time-point cross-sectional design.

Consider, for example, the relatively simple question of whether coping responses vary over time. Several retrospective studies found no relationship between length of illness and the extent to which various kinds of coping strategies were used, but propective studies indicate otherwise. One study found that fighting spirit was reported significantly less at two years after surgery for breast cancer than at three months and one year post surgery (11). Stoic acceptance was reported more often at the two year mark than at earlier periods. Another study found that reported use of a wide range of coping strategies decreased over the year following surgery for early-stage breast cancer (82). Only one coping response increased across time: acceptance (of the reality of the situation) rose gradually but steadily across the study period.

Heim and colleagues measured coping in breast cancer patients in a prospective study across seven illness stages, including suspicion of cancer, diagnosis, treatment, metastases, and terminal illness (92). They found different patterns across time for different sorts of coping. Reliance on attention and care and acceptance–stoicism were reported at high levels at all illness stages. Problem analysis (analysis of the illness and its consequences) was reported at all phases except times when no additional treatment was required, or when the patient had been diagnosed as terminally ill. Tackling the problem (cooperation in treatment, actively seeking information) was reported at the time of surgery, during periods of aggressive chemotherapy or radiotherapy, and at the discovery of recurrence or metastasis. Use of religion, passive cooperation, and self-validation were reported primarily at diagnosis of terminal illness. This study also found that patients reported using many different coping methods in the first year after diagnosis, but fewer methods (5 out of 26 possible) by the thirtieth month.

What kinds of coping emerge from these prospective studies as being adaptive and desirable? In an early prospective study, Penman characterized patients as good or poor copers, on the basis of their emotional well-being a week after surgery (93). She also assessed patients' self-reports of their coping responses at two time points. Patients categorized as good copers reported tackling their problems head-on, at the same measurement point. These patients also reported

a shift to rationalizing as a method of coping at four months post surgery. Patients categorized as poorer copers reported using avoidance coping and having a fatalistic outlook at the initial measurement, and they continued to do so at four months post mastectomy.

A more recent study found substantial evidence among breast cancer patients that acceptance of the reality of the situation they were confronting (as opposed to a fatalistic acceptance of the adverse implications of a cancer diagnosis) was a prospective predictor of positive emotional well-being (82). The authors argued that a willingness to accept that the situation was real and was not going to go away kept these patients life-engaged. In this view, a person has to accept the reality of a challenge before the challenge can be taken on. This seemed to be exactly what was these patients were doing.

In contrast to this finding for the positive role of acceptance, this study found little evidence of prospective benefit from other coping reactions that are often invoked in the coping literature as important. For example, subjects reported elevated use of their social support resources early in the transaction, but the data did not reveal any positive effect of doing so. Similarly, although active coping and planning were reported at high levels early in the transaction, neither response predicted less distress later on. Inasmuch as the situation these patients were facing was one that had to be endured rather than being amenable to active attempts to control it (25), it may be unreasonable to expect active coping (at least as it was measured there) to play a major role in adjustment in this context. The only other coping response that prospectively predicted lower levels of distress was the use of humor at three months post surgery, which predicted less distress three months later.

Although this study did not find benefits from the turning to social support resources, another study that focused on the period surrounding the biopsy process did find benefit, albeit limited (7). Specifically, women who engaged in the seeking of social support at prebiopsy (compared to women who did so less) reported higher levels of vigor after receiving the diagnosis. There was no effect on mood per se, however.

What kinds of responses are associated with *adverse* effects on well-being? In general, the answer seems to be that avoidance coping results in poorer adaptation. As we have noted, Penman (93) found that her poor copers were those who reported using avoidance coping and holding a fatalistic outlook about their disease. In the same vein, other research (82) found that both the giving-up reaction and denial led to higher levels of subsequent distress. The denial measure used in that study reflected an overt denial, an attempt to push the reality of the experience aside (as reflected in such items as "I've been saying to myself this isn't real"). Other evidence that avoidance coping is dysfunctional comes from a study that found cognitive avoidance at prebiopsy to be a reliable predictor of distress after diagnosis and after surgery (7). These findings complement and extend the earlier finding that an index of several aspects of avoidance coping was related to greater distress in cancer patients (70).

These various findings also appear to complement and extend those of other studies in the literature of coping more generally (36,37,39,88,94–98). The available data from other domains suggest that avoidance coping is a predictor of future distress when confronting a major stressor or chronic burden (87,99,100).

Coping and Physical Well-Being

Two other prospective projects provide evidence of a very different kind of benefit from certain kinds of coping. These studies suggest that certain kinds of coping responses may promote longer survival of patients with more severe forms of cancer. One of these projects examined recurrence and death among a group of breast cancer patients. In an initial prospective study of women with nonmetastatic breast cancer, Greer and colleagues found that those who reacted to their diagnosis and surgery with fighting spirit—a focused engagement with the struggle of living and regaining one's strength—were significantly more likely to experience recurrence-free survival at a 5-year follow-up than women who reacted with what they labeled stoic acceptance (a kind of fatalism) or feelings of hopelessness and helplessness (35). A similar pattern of results emerged at the time of a 10-year follow-up and a 15-year follow-up (101,102).

In another project, Fawzy and colleagues measured active-behavioral coping among a sample of malignant melanoma patients, while evaluating the effectiveness of a six-week structured psychiatric group intervention (103). They found that higher initial levels of active coping were related to lower rates of recurrence and death. Active-behavioral coping as assessed in that project was a style of coping with the illness characterized by behavioral engagement. Specifically, patients who showed this pattern tried to alter aspects of their disease course by activities such as exercising, using relaxation techniques, and frequent consultations with physicians.

It is of more than passing interest that there is a considerable similarity between the coping responses that lead to better vs. poorer emotional adjustment and those that seem to lead to better vs worse prog-

nosis for recurrence. For example, Carver and colleagues found that a giving-up response predicted poorer emotional well being (82), and Greer and colleagues found that helplessness and hopelessness in response to the initial diagnosis predicted later recurrence (35). Apparently, the giving up response has effects that are manifest in physical well-being as well as in emotional well-being.

Personality and Coping Responses

In an earlier section we noted that personality plays a role in who adapts better and who adapts worse. We also noted there the difficulty that researchers sometimes have in distinguishing between personality and more delimited and focused coping responses. Before leaving our discussion of coping responses, we should note that many of the coping responses in this section are also linked to broader qualities of personality. Optimism among breast cancer patients has been found to be positively tied to higher levels of acceptance, use of humor as a coping tactic, and positive reframing of the experience, particularly in the early stages surrounding surgery (82). Optimism was inversely associated with the giving-up response and with denial. Indeed, in this sample the coping differences proved to be an important mechanism by which optimism influenced distress level. That is, the evidence suggested that the effects of optimism on distress were not primarily direct, but rather indirect through coping.

A particular theme reverberates through all of the studies reviewed in this section of the chapter: People who remain engaged in the struggle to overcome the diagnosis of cancer and all its implications are the people who fare best, both emotionally and in terms of recurrence of the disease. People who cannot seem to bear to accept the reality of the problems they are facing, or who face those problems with a sense of helplessness and hopelessness, are the ones who fare poorly, both in elevated distress and in diminished physical well-being. Further, these divergences in coping appear to be rooted at least in part in individual differences in a general confidence about being able to succeed—a sense of optimism versus pessimism.

Conclusions

The studies reviewed here suggest that as distress levels experienced by cancer patients change over time, methods of coping also change with time. What is an effective method of coping at one time may be less so at another time during treatment. Coping at one time does appear to have an impact on future distress. There is evidence that avoidance coping has adverse effects, and there is also evidence that certain kinds of reality-focused and confrontive coping have beneficial effects. Finally, there is evidence that adaptive and maladaptive coping reactions rarely occur in a vacuum. Rather, these coping tendencies are determined in part by personality differences that patients bring with them to the cancer experience.

INTERVENTION STUDIES

Although knowledge of what kinds of coping lead to better outcomes is thus far rudimentary, many interventions have been developed that are intended at least in part to help cancer patients cope in more effective ways with their situations. Psychosocial interventions with cancer patients do seem to yield improvements (see Part X of this volume for more detailed treatments). Such interventions foster greater emotional well-being, better functional adjustment, and reduced disease- and treatment-related symptoms. This is the conclusion from several recent reviews of the literature, including a recent meta-analysis (55,56,104–106).

Several issues must be taken into account in developing interventions for cancer patients. It is important to assess and address the needs associated with specific cancer sites (see also Part VII of this volume), because each site is likely to raise different issues (body esteem, treatment choices, related side effects, etc.) (107). This line of reasoning has found support in findings from a number of studies (55). In this review of studies, interventions that were tailored to meet the needs of the individual patient had a greater impact on distress levels, fatigue, sexuality problems, self-concept, and health locus of control than did highly structured counseling interventions or strictly behavioral interventions targeted at specific symptoms.

Whether individualized or structured, most interventions among cancer patients are multifaceted (105,107–111). Interventions typically include an educational component—incorporating such specifics as information about cancer, information about normal emotional reactions, training in relaxation techniques, and training in communication skills. Most interventions also include an element of counseling—providing social support, opportunities to express and clarify emotions, and opportunities to do cognitive restructuring and to engage in problem solving. Some interventions also include making changes in the person's environment, for example, by making specific referrals for medical consultation.

Psychosocial interventions have been found in various studies to yield improvements in fighting spirit, and reductions in helplessness, anxiety, depression,

and anxious preoccupations (109). Patients often show improvements in affect, satisfaction with life, participation in activites, reported self-efficacy, communication, and coping with medical procedures, and a decrease in distress. There is some suggestion that psychosocial interventions are more effective if they are implemented a few months after diagnosis, rather than right away (105).

Consider, for example, an intervention study with a group of cancer patients who were having psychological difficulties (anxiety or depression, or both high helplessness and low fighting spirit) (112). This intervention focused in part on enhancing coping strategies. In particular, therapists tried to identify patients' strengths, to help them overcome their sense of helplessness and to promote fighting spirit. Participants were also taught cognitive restructuring and progressive muscle relaxation, and they were encouraged to express their feelings and communicate with their spouses. This intervention was compared to a "routine care" control group. After eight weeks, the therapy group had higher fighting spirit than the control group and less helplessness, anxious preoccupation, and fatalism. They also had less anxiety and other psychological symptoms. After four months, the therapy group continued to display lower anxiety and distress. A longer-term follow up revealed that the gains from the therapy persisted for a year afterward (113).

Many authors have suggested the importance of identifying new patients who are at risk for future psychological morbidity, and targeting intervention efforts at those patients (54–56). Important factors influencing relative risk are the person's level of personal and social support resources. Another important factor is the person's repertoire of methods readily available as coping responses during the course of the cancer experience. Presumably patients who have useful coping strategies readily at hand are at less risk than those whose coping repertoire is smaller or is more heavily weighted toward dysfunctional responses.

Work on interventions proceeds under the assumption that the coping strategies that are useful in the "natural history" of adaptation can be taught to women who do not naturally employ them as readily. It is hoped that these responses when newly acquired will work in the same way as they work in women to whom they come more naturally. To determine whether this is true, future intervention research must carefully assess patients' coping responses (as well as their psychological and social functioning) both before the intervention and afterward.

In sum, it appears that social support, personal orientations such as fighting spirit and optimism, and coping responses are all important issues for intervention and intervention research, as well as for investigations of individual differences in the natural course of adaptation. In characterizing these findings, we return to a theme that we introduced early in the chapter: The ways in which cancer patients regulate the pursuit (or abandonment) of their life goals may well be a critical determinant of how well they do in adapting to their disease.

A LIMITATION AND A CAUTION

In the preceding sections we reviewed evidence that the personal and social resources that people bring to treatment for cancer can play a major role in determining how successfully they adapt to the experience. Similarly, the manner in which people cope with the crisis can either relieve distress or exacerbate it. Finally, psychosocial interventions can help patients to cope in more effective ways and foster better adaptation.

Although this information provides some clear suggestions for applications in clinical contexts, some of the limitations of the information that is now available should be briefly noted. One limitation is the small number of prospective studies that have been carried out on the adaptation process. It should be apparent that more information is needed on the relationship between ways of coping at specific time points and subsequent distress. Assumptions are made both by patients and by health care providers about what is the best way to cope (114), and it is important to have enough information on this question to be able to provide people with the best possible answers.

Another limitation stems from the fact that most of the information comes from breast cancer patients. Obviously there is a need for information about adaptation to cancers at other sites. The focus on breast cancer also means that most of the information available pertains to women, with far less being known about adaptation among male patients. Again, there is a need for more information, to prevent inappropriate generalizations.

Another important limitation on the evidence concerns ethnicity and socioeconomic status. The studies that make up this literature have examined primarily non-Hispanic white patients. This leaves serious gaps in the knowledge base. Minority groups may use different coping methods from the samples studied thus far. Alternatively, the effectiveness of specific coping strategies may differ among ethnic groups. Low socio-economic status has been found to predict higher levels of avoidance coping (115,116), which may result in higher levels of distress. In order to be sure that the help given to various groups is appropriate, more information is needed about what coping responses are most relevant and adaptive to those groups.

Despite these limitations, the literature of studies of adaptation to cancer provides important insights into the adaptational process. Although the picture doubtless will come into clearer focus as additional research is done, its outlines are by now relatively apparent. Cancer presents a crisis with which most people can come to terms. Without question, this is easier for some people than others. However, the development of a broader research and clinical base will permit those for whom adaptation is difficult to benefit from the skills of those for whom it is less so.

ACKNOWLEDGMENTS

Preparation of this chapter was facilitated by support from the American Cancer Society (PBR-82) and the National Cancer Institute (CA-64710).

REFERENCES

1. Fallowfield LJ, Hall A, Maguire GP, Baum M. Psychological outcomes of different treatment policies in women with early breast cancer outside a clinical trial. *Br Med J.* 1990; 301:575–580.
2. Dunkel-Schetter C, Feinstein LG, Taylor SE, Falke RL. Patterns of coping with cancer. *Health Psychol.* 1992; 11:79–87.
3. Maguire P. Improving the detection of psychiatric problems in cancer patients. *Soc Sci Med.* 1985; 20:819–823.
4. Sinsheimer LM, Holland JC. Psychological issues in breast cancer. *Semin Oncol.* 1987; 14:75–82.
5. Jamison KR, Wellisch DK, Pasnau RO. Psychosocial aspects of mastectomy. I: The woman's perspective. *Am J Psychiatry.* 1978; 135:432–436.
6. Northouse LL. The impact of breast cancer on patients and husbands. *Cancer Nurs.* 1989; 12:276–284.
7. Stanton AL, Snider PR. Coping with a breast cancer diagnosis: a prospective study. *Health Psychol.* 1993; 12:16–23.
8. Cassileth BR, Lusk EJ, Strouse TB, Miller DS, Brown LL, Cross, PA. A psychological analysis of cancer patients and their next-of-kin. *Cancer.* 1985; 55:72–76.
9. Ell K, Nishimoto R, Mantell J, Hamovitch M. Longitudinal analysis of psychological adaptation among family members of patients with cancer. *J Psychosom Res.* 1988; 32:429–438.
10. Bloom JR, Cook M, Fotopoulos S, et al. Psychological response to mastectomy: a prospective comparison study. *Cancer.* 1987; 59:189–196.
11. Morris T, Greer S, White P. Psychological and social adjustment to mastectomy: a two-year follow-up. *Cancer.* 1977; 40:2381–2387.

12. Shanfield SB. On surviving cancer: Psychological considerations. *Compr Psychiatry*. 1980; 21:128–134.

13. Halstead MT, Fernsler JI. Coping strategies of long-term cancer survivors. *Cancer Nurs*. 1994; 17:94–100.

14. Derogatis LR, Abeloff MD, Melisaratos N. Psychological coping mechanisms and survival time in metastatic breast cancer. *J Am Med Assoc*. 1979; 242:1504–1508.

15. Kennedy BJ, Tellegen A, Kennedy S, Havernick N. Psychological response of patients cured of advanced cancer. *Cancer*. 1976; 38:2184–2191.

16. Mahon SM, Cella DF, Donovan MI. Psychological adjustment to recurrent cancer. *Oncol Nurs Forum*. 1990, 17: 47–54.

17. Silberfarb PM, Maurer LH, Crouthamel CS. Psychosocial aspects of neoplastic disease: I. Functional status of breast cancer patients during different treatment regimens. *Am J Psychiatry*. 1980; 137:450–455.

18. Irvine D, Brown B, Crooks D, Roberts J, Browne G. Psychosocial adjustment in women with breast cancer. *Cancer*. 1991; 67:1097–1117.

19. Meyerowitz BE. Psychosocial correlates of breast cancer and its treatments. *Psychol Bull*. 1980; 87:108–131.

20. Rowland JH. Intrapersonal resources: coping. In: Holland JC, Rowland JH, eds. *Handbook of Psychooncology: Psychological Care of the Patient with Cancer*. New York: Oxford University Press; 1989.

21. Somerfield M, Curbow B. Methodological issues and research strategies in the study of coping with cancer. *Soc Sci Med*. 1992; 34:1203–1206.

22. Welch-McCaffrey D, Hoffman B, Leigh SA, Loeschler LJ, Meyskens FL. Surviving adult cancer. Part 2: Psychosocial implications. *Ann Intern Med*. 1989; 111:517–524.

23. Carver CS, Scheier MF, Pozo C. Conceptualizing the process of coping with health problems. In Friedman HS, ed. *Hostility, Coping, and Health*. Washington, DC: American Psychological Association; 1992.

24. Lazarus RS. *Psychological Stress and the Coping Process*. New York: McGraw-Hill; 1966.

25. Lazarus RS, Folkman S. *Stress, Appraisal, and Coping*. New York: Springer; 1984.

26. Hobfoll SE. Conservation of resources: A new attempt at conceptualizing stress. *Am Psychol*. 1989; 44:513–524.

27. Carver CS, Scheier MF. Principles of self-regulation: action and emotion. In: Higgins ET, Sorrentino RM, eds. *Handbook of Motivation and Cognition: Foundations of Social Behavior*, vol. 2. New York: Guilford; 1990:3-52.

28. Carver CS, Scheier MF. *On the Self-regulation of Behavior*. New York: Cambridge University Press; 1998.

29. Pervin LA. The stasis and flow of behavior: toward a theory of goals. In: Page MM, Dienstbier R, eds. *Nebraska symposium on motivation*, vol. 31. Lincoln: University of Nebraska Press; 1983.

30. Pervin LA, ed. *Goal Concepts in Personality and Social Psychology*. Hillsdale, NJ: Erlbaum; 1989.

31. Bandura A. *Social Foundations of Thought and Action: A Social Cognitive Theory*. Englewood Cliffs, NJ: Prentice-Hall; 1986.

32. Carver CS, Scheier MF. *Attention and Self-regulation: A Control-theory Approach to Human Behavior*. New York: Springer-Verlag; 1981.

33. Kanfer FH, Hagerman SM. Behavior therapy and the information-processing paradigm. In Reiss S, Bootzin RR, eds. *Theoretical Issues in Behavior Therapy*. New York: Academic Press; 1985: 3–33.

34. Kirsch I. *Changing Expectations: A Key to Effective Psychotherapy*. Pacific Grove, CA: Brooks/Cole; 1990.

35. Greer S, Morris T, Pettingale KW. Psychological response to breast cancer: Effect on outcome. *Lancet*. 1979; 13:785–787.

36. Aldwin CM, Revenson TA. Does coping help? A reexamination of the relation between coping and mental health. *J Pers Soc Psychol*. 1987; 53:337–348.

37. Holahan CJ, Moos RH. Life stress and health: personality, coping, and family support in stress resistance. *J Pers Soc Psychol*. 1985; 49:739–747.

38. Manne SL, Zautra AJ. Spouse criticism and support: their association with coping and psychological adjustment among women with rheumatoid arthritis. *J Pers Soc Psychol*. 1989; 56:608–617.

39. Rohde P, Lewinsohn PM, Tilson M, Seeley JR. Dimensionality of coping and its relation to depression. *J Pers Soc Psychol*. 1990; 58:499–511.

40. Warner GC, Rounds JB. Stress, coping and adjustment to spinal cord injury. Paper presented at the 97th annual meeting of the American Psychological Association, New Orleans, Louisiana, 1989.

41. Miller SM. To see or not to see: cognitive informational styles in the coping process. In: Rosenbaum M, ed. *Learned Resourcefulness: On Coping Skills, Self-control, and Adaptive Behavior*. New York: Springer; 1990: 95–126.

42. Repetti RL. Social withdrawal as a short-term coping response to daily stressors. In Friedman HS, ed. *Hostility, Coping, and Health*. Washington, DC: American Psychological Association; 1992.

43. Levine J, Warrenburg S, Kerns R, et al. The role of denial in recovery from coronary heart disease. *Psychosom Med*. 1987; 49:109–117.

44. Mullen B, Suls J. The effectiveness of attention and rejection as coping styles: a meta-analysis of temporal differences. *J Psychosom Res*. 1982; 26:43–49.

45. Suls J, Fletcher B. The relative efficacy of avoidant and non-avoidant coping strategies: a meta-analysis. *Health Psychol*. 1985; 4:249–288.

46. Cohen F, Lazarus RS. Active coping processes, coping dispositions, and recovery from surgery. *Psychosom Med*. 1973; 35:375–389.

47. Klein RA. A crisis to grow on. *Cancer*. 1971; 28:1660–1665.

48. Weisman AD, Worden JW. The existential plight in cancer: significance of the first 100 days. *Int J Psychiatry Med*. 1976/1977; 7:1–15.

49. Singer JE. Some issues in the study of coping. *Cancer*. 1984; 53:2303-2315.

50. Lazarus RS. The costs and benefits of denial. In: Breznitz S, ed. *The Denial of Stress*. New York: International Universities Press; 1983.

51. Psychological aspects of breast cancer study group. (1987). Psychological response to mastectomy: a prospective comparison study. *Cancer*. 1987; 59:189–196.

52. Penman DT, Bloom JR, Fotopoulos S, et al. The impact of mastectomy on self-concept and social function: A combined cross-sectional and longitudinal study with comparison groups. *Women Health.* 1987; 11:101–130

53. Andersen BL. Psychological interventions for cancer patients to enhance the quality of life. *J Consult Clin Psychol.* 1992; 60: 552–568.

54. Carver CS, Pozo-Kaderman C, Harris SD, et al. Optimism vs. pessimism predicts the quality of women's adjustment to early stage breast cancer. *Cancer.* 1994; 73:1213–1220.

55. Trijsburg RW, van Knippenberg, CE, Rijpma SE. Effects of psychological treatment on cancer patients: a critical review. *Psychosom Med.* 1992; 54:489–517.

56. Watson M. Psychosocial intervention with cancer patients: a review. *Psychol Med.* 1983; 13:839–846.

57. Lipowski ZJ. Physical illness, the individual and the coping processes. *Psychiatry Med.* 1970; 1:91–102.

58. Bartelink H, van Dam F, van Dongen J. Psychological effects of breast conserving therapy in comparison with radical mastectomy. *Int J Radiat Oncol Biol Phys.* 1985; 11: 381–385.

59. de Haes JCJM, Welvaart K. Quality of life after breast cancer surgery. *J Surg Oncol.* 1985; 28: 123–125.

60. Kemeny MM, Wellisch DK, Schain WS. Psychosocial outcome in a randomized surgical trial for treatment of primary breast cancer. *Cancer.* 1988; 62:1231–1237.

61. Lasry JM, Margolese RG, Poisson R, et al. Depression and body image following mastectomy and lumpectomy. *J Chron Dis.* 1987; 40: 529–534.

62. Margolis GJ, Goodman RL, Rubin A. Psychological effects of breast conserving cancer treatment and mastectomy. *Psychosomatics.* 1990; 31: 33–39.

63. Pozo C, Carver CS, Noriega V, et al. Effects of mastectomy versus lumpectomy on emotional adjustment to breast cancer: a prospective study of the first year post-surgery. *J Clin Oncol.* 1992; 10: 1292–1298.

64. Sanger CK, Reznikoff M. A comparison of the psychological effects of breast-saving procedures with the modified radical mastectomy. *Cancer.* 1981; 48: 2341–2346.

65. Schain WS, d'Angelo TM, Dunn ME, Lichter AS, Pierce LJ. Mastectomy versus conservative surgery and radiation therapy: psychosocial consequences. *Cancer.* 1994; 73: 1221–1228.

66. Schain WS, Edwards BK, Gorrell CR, et al. Psychosocial and physical outcomes of primary breast cancer therapy: mastectomy vs. excisional biopsy and irradiation. *Breast Cancer Res Treat.* 1983; 3: 377–382.

67. Steinberg MD, Juliano MA, Wise L. Psychological outcome of lumpectomy versus mastectomy in the treatment of breast cancer. *Am J Psychiatry.* 1985; 142: 34–39.

68. Taylor SE, Lichtman RR, Wood JV, Bluming AZ, Dosik GM, Leibowitz RL. Illness-related and treatment-related factors in psychological adjustment to breast cancer. *Cancer.* 1985; 55:2506–2513.

69. Wellisch DK, DiMatteo R, Silverstein M, et al. Psychosocial outcomes of breast cancer therapies: Lumpectomy versus mastectomy. *Psychosomatics.* 1989; 30: 365–373.

70. Bloom JR. Social support, accommodation to stress, and adjustment to breast cancer. *Soc Sci Med.* 1982; 16:1329–1338.

71. Bloom JR. Social support and adjustment to breast cancer. In: Andersen BL, ed. *Women with Cancer: Psychological Perspectives.* New York: Springer-Verlag; 1986.

72. Funch DP, Mettlin C. The role of support in relation to recovery from breast surgery. *Soc Sci Med.* 1982; 16:91–98.

73. Northouse LL. Social support in patients' and husbands' adjustment to breast cancer. *Nurs Res.* 1988; 37:91–95.

74. Vachon ML. A comparison of the impact of breast cancer and bereavement: personality, social support, and adaptation. In Hobfall S, ed. *Stress, Social Support, and Women.* New York: Hemisphere; 1986: 187–204.

75. Wortman CB. Social support and the cancer patient: Conceptual and methodological issues. *Cancer.* 1984; 53:2339–2360.

76. Pozo C. Perceptions of social support, seeking of social support, and psychological adjustment to breast cancer surgery. Unpublished doctoral dissertation, University of Miami, Coral Gables, Florida; 1991.

77. Ruckdeschel JC, Blanchard CG, Albrecht T. Psychosocial oncology research. Where we have been, where we are going, and why we will not get there. *Cancer.* 1994; 74:1458–1463.

78. Weisman AD. Early diagnosis of vulnerability in cancer patients. *Am J Med Sci.* 1976; 271:187–196.

79. Carver CS, Scheier MF, Weintraub J. Assessing coping strategies: A theoretically based approach. *J Pers Soc Psychol.* 1989; 56:267–283.

80. Scheier MF, Weintraub JK, Carver, CS. Coping with stress: divergent strategies of optimists and pessimists. *J Pers Soc Psychol.* 1986; 51:1257–1264.

81. Scheier MF, Carver CS. Effects of optimism on psychological and physical well-being: theoretical overview and empirical update. *Cogn Ther Res.* 1992; 16:201–228.

82. Carver CS, Pozo C, Harris SD, Noriega V, Scheier MF, Robinson DS, Ketcham AS, Moffat FL, Clark KC. How coping mediates the effect of optimism on distress: A study of women with early stage breast cancer. *J Pers Soc Psychol.* 1993; 65:375–390.

83. Nelson DV, Friedman LC, Baer PE, Lane M, Smith FE. Attitudes to cancer: psychometric properties of fighting spirit and denial. *J Behav Med.* 1989; 12:341–355.

84. Kreitler S, Chaitchik S, Kreitler H. Repressiveness: cause or result of cancer? *Psycho-Oncology.* 1993; 2:43–54.

85. Watson M, Greer S, Rowden L, et al. Relationships between emotional control, adjustment to cancer and depression and anxiety in breast cancer patients. *Psychol Med.* 1991; 21:51–57.

86. Burgess C, Morris T, Pettingale KW. Psychological response to cancer diagnosis—II. Evidence for coping styles (coping styles and cancer diagnosis). *J Psychosom Res.* 1988; 32:263–272.

87. Felton BJ, Revenson TA. Coping with chronic illness: a study of illness controllability and the influence of coping strategies on psychological adjustment. *J Consult Clin Psychol.* 1984; 52:343–353.

88. Felton BJ, Revenson TA, Hinrichsen GA. Stress and coping in the explanation of psychological adjustment

among chronically ill adults. *Soc Sci Med.* 1984; 18:889–898.

89. Bloom JR, Spiegel D. The relationship of two dimensions of social support to the psychological well-being and social functioning of women with advanced breast cancer. *Soc Sci Med.* 1984; 19:831–837.

90. Watson M, Greer S, Blake S, Shrapnell K. Reaction to a diagnosis of breast cancer: relationship between denial, delay and rates of psychological morbidity. *Cancer.* 1984; 53:2008-2012.

91. Meyerowitz BE. Postmastectomy coping strategies and quality of life. *Health Psychol.* 1983; 2:117–132.

92. Heim E, Augistiny KF, Schaffner L, Valach L. Coping with breast cancer over time and situations. *J Psychosom Res.* 1993; 37:523–542.

93. Penman DT. Coping strategies in adaptation to mastectomy. *Psychosom Med.* 1982; 44:117.

94. Billings AG, Moos RH. Coping, stress, and social resources among adults with unipolar depression. *J Pers Soc Psychol.* 1984; 46:877–891.

95. Cronkite RC, Moos, RH. The role of predisposing and moderating factors in the stress-illness relationship. *J Health Soc Behav.* 1984; 25:372–393.

96. Folkman S, Lazarus RS. If it changes it must be a process: study of emotion and coping during three stages of a college examination. *J Pers Soc Psychol.* 1985; 48:150–170.

97. Vaillant GE. *Adaptation to Life.* Boston: Little, Brown; 1977.

98. Wills TA. Stress and coping in early adolescence: relationships to substance use in urban high schools. *Health Psychol.* 1986; 5:503–529.

99. Bolger N. Coping as a personality process: a prospective study. *J Pers Soc Psychol.* 1990; 59:525–537.

100. Litt MD, Tennen H, Affleck G, Klock S. Coping and cognitive factors in adaptation to in vitro fertilization failure. *J Behav Med.* 1992; 15:171–187.

101. Pettingale KW, Morris T, Greer S, Haybittle JL. Mental attitudes to cancer: an additional prognostic factor. *Lancet.* 1985; 30:747–750.

102. Greer S, Morris T, Pettingale KW, et al. Psychological response to breast cancer and 15-year outcome. *Lancet.* 1990; i: 49–50.

103. Fawzy FI, Fawzy NW, Hyun CS, et al. Malignant melanoma: effects of an early structured psychiatric intervention, coping, and affective state on recurrence and survival 6 years later. *Arch Gen Psychiatry.* 1993; 50:681–689.

104. Andersen BL. Psychological interventions for cancer patients to enhance the quality of life. *J Consult Clin Psychol.* 1992; 60:552–568.

105. Fawzy FI, Fawzy NW, Arndt LA, Pasnau RO. Critical review of psychosocial interventions in cancer care. *Arch Gen Psychiatry.* 1995; 53:100–113.

106. Meyer TJ, Mark MM. Effects of psychosocial interventions with adult cancer patients: A meta-analysis of randomized experiments. *Health Psychol.* 1995; 14:101–108.

107. Gordon WA, Freidenbergs I, Diller L, et al. Efficacy of psychosocial intervention with cancer patients. *J Consult Clin Psychol.* 1980; 48:743–759.

108. Edgar L, Rosberger Z, Nowlis D. Coping with cancer during the first year after diagnosis: assessment and intervention. *Cancer.* 1992; 69:817–828.

109. Greer S, Moorey S, Baruch JDR. Evaluation of adjuvant psychological therapy for clinically referred cancer patients. *Br J Cancer.* 1991; 63:257–260.

110. Lyles JN, Burish TG, Krozely MG, Oldham RK. Efficacy of relaxation training and guided imagery in reducing the aversiveness of cancer chemoterapy. *J Consult Clinl Psychol.* 1982; 50:509–524.

111. Telch CF, Telch MJ. Group coping skills instruction and supportive group therapy for cancer patients: a comparison of strategies. *J Consult Clin Psychol.* 1986; 54:802–808.

112. Greer S, Moorey S, Baruch JDR, et al. Adjuvant psychological therapy for patients with cancer: a prospective randomised trial. *Br Med J.* 1992; 304:675–680.

113. Moorey S, Greer S, Watson M, et al. Adjuvant psychological therapy for patients with cancer: outcome at one year. *Psycho-Oncology.* 1994; 3:39–46.

114. Wortman CB, Silver RC. The myths of coping with loss. *J Consult Clin Psychol.* 1989; 57:349–357.

115. Behen JM, Rodrigue JR. Predictors of coping strategies among adults with cancer. *Psychol Rep.* 1994; 74:43–48.

116. Feifel H, Strack S, Nagy VT. Coping strategies and associated features of medically ill patients. *Psychosom Med.* 1987; 49:616–625.

20

Psychosocial Adaptation of Cancer Survivors

ALICE B. KORNBLITH

Within the past thirty years there have been three extraordinary success stories in the treatment of cancer that have excited the oncology community by significantly increasing cancer survival for those with advanced and largely fatal disease. With the advent of the MOPP regimen (mechlorethamine, vincristine, procarbazine, prednisone) in the mid-1960s for the treatment of advanced stage Hodgkin's disease, 5-year survival dramatically increased from less than 5% to 80%, with current therapy curing 65%–75% (1–3). Similarly, effective multidrug chemotherapy for the treatment of testicular seminoma has resulted in an overall cure rate of over 90%, even for those with metastatic disease, whereas prior to 1975 it was less than 10% (4,5). Allogeneic bone marrow transplantation (BMT), introduced in the 1970s for the treatment of acute myeloid and lymphoblastic leukemia, has produced a long-term survival of 40%–70% in adults when performed during their first complete remission (6), compared to a 5-year survival of less than 5% in the early 1960s (7). In a less dramatic fashion, the widespread use of mammography and the Papanicolaou (Pap) smear has also played an important role in improved survival through early detection, reducing breast cancer mortality by approximately 25% (8), and cervical cancer by an estimated 60%–90% by the year 2000 (9,10).

As the number of cancer survivors began to increase owing to these as well as other medical advances, in the early 1980s scientific attention began to turn from the *quantity* of survival to considerations of its *quality*. Of interest now were the long-term consequences of being treated for cancer: medically, psychologically, vocationally, socially, and sexually. This chapter is dedicated to examining the literature in relation to this question, discussing clinical interventions and future lines of research suggested by the findings, as well as theoretical models of adaptation within which to better under-stand cancer survivorhood and target psychosocial interventions.

PSYCHOSOCIAL ADJUSTMENT

There is a tremendous variation in cancer treatment for the different cancer diagnoses, as well as a wide diversity of patients, in terms of their sociodemographic, personality and social characteristics. Thus, survivors' adaptation can be quite unique to their specific diagnosis and treatment, in response to the express demands placed on them. However, there is also a commonality of experience of survival from cancer that is shared by all cancer patients, of all different backgrounds, across diagnoses. The foundation of the cancer experience is built on the life-threatening character of cancer, with its range of treatments, many of which are highly toxic, often resulting in permanent physical impairment (11), and the uncertainty of knowing when one is truly cured. The survivors' need to work and function in their various roles in spite of any physical limitations, the problems with insurance that many face, and the strengths and limitations of others in responding to them all are part of forging the commonality of the survivors' experience long after treatment has been completed. Consequently, this chapter is organized in terms of the adjustment of cancer survivors as a group, with the unique medical and psychological issues posed by the different diagnoses and treatments discussed within each area of psychosocial functioning.

Methodological Considerations

In order to permit examination of the range of psychosocial issues survivors may face after overcoming their disease and resuming their lives, survivorhood has been defined as being currently free of disease and off treatment for a minimum of one year. Table 20.1 in the Appendix is a summary of empirical studies of the psychosocial adaptation of adult cancer survivors that have met the following inclusion criteria, adhering as closely as possible to the above definition: *(1)* diagnosed at 18 years old or older; *(2)* research involving either quantitative or qualitative analysis of psychosocial issues; *(3)* survivor cohorts from cross-sectional studies who were assessed, on the average, either at one year post treatment or two years post diagnosis; *(4)* patients in prospective studies with good to excellent prognoses, generally with early-stage disease, who were assessed through the first two years from diagnosis or primary treatment; *(5)* a minimum of 20 patients. While numerous studies included in Table 20.1 did not determine whether the survivors were truly free of disease, most stated that they were no longer in treatment. When multiple articles were written regarding the same data set, only the most significant article was selected for the table, unless important, different psychosocial issues appeared across several articles. All other articles relevant to adult cancer survivorhood not included in Table 20.1 are discussed in the text.

As can be seen from Table 20.1, the vast majority of studies used cross-sectional designs with identified survivor cohorts, assessed at a single point in time, long past the completion of all treatment. This in part has been a cost-effective approach to evaluating the long-term psychosocial adaptation of large cohorts of survivors; to have followed a cohort of patients prospectively from diagnosis or initial treatment would have entailed studies of much larger size and much longer duration, with smaller subsets of the sample becoming survivors. Most prospective studies to date involve the longitudinal evaluation of the impact of mastectomy and breast-conserving treatments in women with early-stage breast cancer.

Overall Psychosocial Adjustment

The overwhelming evidence from the literature across a range of studies involving survivors with different cancer diagnoses, assessed by different methods and measures at different points in their post treatment course, is that on the average the majority do very well after the initial adjustment in the first 1–2 years post treatment. However, there is also a subset of survivors whose adjustment is poor, requiring psychiatric treatment, varying in size from study to study and among the different disease sites. To a much greater extent than the prevalence of psychiatric disturbance, survivors report subsyndromal levels of psychological distress and have attributed an array of physical, social, sexual, employment, and insurance problems to having had cancer. Very clearly, cancer patients do not go through this experience unscathed.

Psychological Distress

In studies comparing survivor cohorts and healthy comparison groups, many found no significant differences between the two groups in terms of psychological distress (12–14), as well as marital and sexual adjustment (12,15), social functioning (14), and overall psychosocial functioning (16). Testis cancer survivors were even reported to have significantly less psychological distress than the comparison group (17). While the implication of these studies is that there were no long-term psychological sequelae resulting from cancer, this was not universally found to be true in studies of this kind. Breast cancer survivors were found to be significantly more depressed (15), Hodgkin's disease survivors had more avoidant thoughts concerning cancer (12), and mixed cancer survivors and BMT survivors were more psychologically distressed (18,19) than their respective comparison groups.

Elevated levels of psychological distress involving anxiety and depression not reaching diagnostic criteria for a formal psychiatric disorder have been reported in survivors of Hodgkin's disease (20), acute leukemia (21,22), and a mixed cohort of cancer survivors (18). High prevalence of symptoms of anxiety and depression have been reported in survivors of breast cancer (64%) (23), BMT (45%–63%) (24,25), colorectal (41%–44%) (26), prostate (48%–49%) (26), and lung cancer (51%–63%) (26).

With the exception of a few studies (27,28), most studies did not determine prevalence of psychiatric diagnoses through the use of clinical interviews by mental health professionals or structured clinical interviews schedules. However, estimates were made by some researchers using well-established instruments with normative data and cutoff scores suggestive of a psychiatric diagnosis, such as the Brief Symptom Inventory (BSI), Hamilton Depression Rating Scale (HDRS), the Center for Epidemiological Studies-Depression Scale (CES-D), the General Health Questionnaire (GHQ), and the Hospital Anxiety and Depression Scale (HADS). Using this approach, 18%–22% of Hodgkin's disease survivors (20,29), 14%–31% of acute leukemia survivors (21,22,30), 16% of BMT survivors (31), 22%–47% of breast cancer survivors (15,32,33), and 18% of testis cancer survivors (34) scored at levels suggestive of a psychiatric diagnosis. When clinical interviews have been used, 2% of lymphoma survivors were diagnosed with current depression and/or anxiety, and 12%, with borderline levels of these states (28). In several studies primarily involving survivors of breast cancer, 4%–10% were likely to have met criteria for a current diagnosis of post-traumatic stress disorder (27,35).

The much higher and wide range of rates of possible psychiatric disorders reported for survivors of the same cancer diagnosis based upon questionnaires may be due to a range of factors, including patients having varying disease, treatment, and sociodemographic characteristics, as well as different measures, and assessment at different points in survivors' posttreatment clinical course. Given these issues, combined with the relatively low rates of psychiatric disorders in studies based on clinical interviews, the actual prevalence of psychiatric disorders in cancer survivors remains to be established, and it may be much less than suggested by questionnaire-derived figures.

Cancer-Specific Psychological Distress

Symptoms of Post-Traumatic Stress Disorder (PSRD). Although only 4%–10% of survivors were likely to have met criteria for a diagnosis of PTSD (27,35), 48% reported a range of cancer-related PTSD symptoms, such as reexperiencing the event, avoidance of painful reminders of cancer, and re-experiencing emotional states associated with cancer (27). In Cordova and colleagues' study (35), 44% endorsed 'being superalert, watchful or on guard' as a consequence of being diagnosed and treated for breast cancer, with 4%-24% reporting other PTSD-like symptoms. PTSD symptoms involving intrusive thoughts about cancer uncontrollably appearing in one's mind, oscillating with avoidant attempts to deny or block cancer-related thoughts, have been assessed in several studies of Hodgkin's disease and leukemia survivors (12,20–22), using the Impact of Event Scale (IES) (36). Those who had finished treatment more recently were found to have significantly more intrusive and avoidant cancer-related thoughts than those who had finished all treatment for a longer time (20,21). Further, the combined effect of late-stage disease with more recent completion of treatment in Hodgkin's disease survivors resulted in significantly greater intrusive thoughts than in those with early-stage disease who had completed treatment a longer time ago (12). With higher IES scores in leukemia survivors significantly related to worse adjustment (21,22) and fears of recurrence (21), IES might serve as an indicator of maladjustment particularly in those who completed treatment a long time ago.

Fear of Recurrence. A psychological entity unique to the experience of survivorhood is the fear of disease recurrence, the "sword of Damocles" (37) that hangs over a survivor's head, threatening to fall at any point. The fear of recurrence was found to be highly prevalent in some studies, ranging from 42% to 89% among breast cancer survivors (23,33,38), and from 39% to 76% in BMT survivors (24,39). Much lower levels of fear of recurrence were reported in other studies of BMT survivors (10%) (40) and a mixed cohort (19%) (41).

Fears of recurrence, triggered by reminders of their disease or treatment, were reported to be brought on by physical symptoms in two-thirds of Hodgkin's disease survivors (12). Survivors treated for more advanced disease have realistic grounds for greater fears of disease recurrence. Breast cancer survivors, either with advanced disease or who had been treated more aggressively with adjuvant chemotherapy due to nodal involvement, were found to have significantly greater fears of recurrence than those who had not been treated with chemotherapy (32,42). Passage of time has been suggested as an important factor in decreasing cancer-related fears. Only 5% of testis cancer survivors reported fear of recurrence, a mean of 3.8 years post treatment, a decrease from 35% retrospectively reported at six months post treatment (34). Given the reported prevalence of fear of recurrence, its decline over time (34), and correlation with psychological distress (BSI, $r = 0.37$, $p < 0.0001$) and overall adjustment (PAIS, $r = 0.33$, $p < 0.0001$) in acute leukemia survivors (21), fear of recurrence could serve as an indicator of survivors' overall adjustment.

Body Image. There is considerable evidence that the wide range of surgical, chemotherapeutic, and radiation therapies can leave permanent damage to organs and physiological functioning and disfigurement, across the different cancer diagnoses (11). Consequently, body image has frequently been included in many studies of survivors in order to assess the long-term psychological impact of these injuries to the body. Given the importance of the breast to women's sense of femininity and its role in sexual relationships, mastectomy and breast-conserving treatment have been the most heavily studied treatments of all in terms of their impact upon body image and related psychosocial and sexual functioning.

Most studies have shown that by 18 months post surgery, those who had breast-conserving surgery + radiation therapy (RT) have a significantly better body image and greater satisfaction with their sexual life than those who had a mastectomy, but equivalent psychological distress, fear of recurrence, and overall psychosocial adjustment (43–48). A number of studies found that women who had a mastectomy continued to have significant problems with body image for many years after their surgery, ranging from a mean of 3.4 to 8 years (23,32,38). In one study, even 25% of women who had undergone only breast-conserving surgery had serious body image problems, with those reporting edema of the arm having significantly worse body image ($r = 0.43, p < 0.01$) (33). Distress over scars, feelings of being less sexually attractive, and being uncomfortable in more revealing clothes such as bathing suits (23,48) and therefore avoiding leisure activities that necessitated this exposure (38) were common expressions of body image problems. Not surprisingly, a poorer body image was significantly related to worse adjustment (33,42).

The effect of significant and observable disfigurement and impairments upon long-term adjustment has been studied in other patient populations. Head and neck cancer survivors' adjustment was significantly related to resultant physical dysfunction (e.g. eating, swallowing, talking, the senses) ($r = 0.56$, $p < 0.0001$), rather than the degree of facial disfigurement (49). In a small study of extremity sarcoma patients treated by amputation + chemotherapy, it had been anticipated that they would experience greater problems in adjustment than those randomized to limb-sparing surgery + RT + chemotherapy, primarily due to presumed worse physical function and greater emotional trauma. Limb-sparing survivors reported a significantly greater decrement in sexual functioning than amputees, possibly due to testicular damage from the combined effects of chemotherapy and RT. No other substantial differences were found 1–3 years post surgery on any measure of psychosocial adjustment, physical functioning or pain (50). While no measure of body image was included in the battery, indirectly this study was a test of the impact of a major alteration in the body upon long-term adjustment.

Among Hodgkin's disease survivors, a population in which there are no long-term outward changes in appearance, 26% felt that their physical attractiveness had decreased as a consequence of cancer. This perceived change was significantly related to changes in energy, sexual frequency, and depression (29). Similarly, acute leukemia survivors had a significantly poorer body image than that of a physically healthy normative group (51). In several studies of BMT survivors, who can experience treatment-related effects affecting their appearance (e.g. osteoporosis, joint contractures, changes in pigmentation), as well as physical function (e.g. neuropathy, muscle pain, cataracts, gonadal failure), 8%–46% reported dissatisfaction with their appearance (24,52,53). The findings from the above studies underscore the fundamental point that body image often reflects one's physical ability to function as well as appearance (54). Further, poorer body image appears to be broadly related to "survivors' . . . (coping) with chronic uncertainty about bodies that have to some extent failed them, and with frequent reminders of their past treatment ordeal" (55, p. 150).

Conditioned Nausea and Vomiting. Because of the intensity of the experience of diagnosis and treatment for cancer, classic conditioning of a range of stimuli associated with the treatment experience can trigger physical and emotional responses long past treatment completion. The most widely known of these has been conditioned nausea and vomiting, reported by survivors of Hodgkin's disease, leukemia, and breast cancer (20,21,23,56). Patients on emetogenic chemotherapy regimens, who experienced nausea and vomiting at the time of their treatment, reported conditioned nausea and vomiting occurring long after treatment completion: 39%–60% in Hodgkin's disease survivors (20,56), 26% in leukemia survivors (21), and 39% in breast cancer survivors (23). Much of conditioned nausea and vomiting consisted of nausea triggered primarily by smells (30%) (20) and secondarily by sights (17%) (20); vomiting was relatively rare, noted as occurring in less than 5% of survivors (21,56). Although a wide range of stimuli triggered conditioned nausea and vomiting, as indicated by as many as 81 stimuli noted by Cella and colleagues (56), many related to smells and sights associated with the hospital, such as the smell of deodorizer spray in the oncologist's office, rubbing alcohol or cleaning solutions, stepping into the elevator in the doctor's building, walking on the block of the clinic, or seeing intravenous injections on television programs (20,23,56). Hodgkin's disease survivors who had received the most highly emetogenic chemotherapy regimens, as rated by a panel of oncologists, reported more intense conditioned nausea ($p < 0.001$; Cella and Herndon, personal communication). Following the conditioning paradigm in which the conditioned response progressively declines with the continued lack of pairing of the initial stimuli and response, the most intense conditioned nausea responses in Hodgkin's disease survivors were experienced by those who had completed treatment more recently [(56); Cella and Herndon, personal communication], similar to the time gradient reported for PTSD.

Positive Psychological Consequences of Having Had Cancer. Given the life-threatening nature of cancer, with multiple late medical effects, it is not surprising that the focus of much of the literature has been on its long-term negative psychological consequences. However, a number of studies have also either assessed or anecdotally noted some unanticipated positive psychological effects of being treated for cancer. Seventy-four percent of breast cancer survivors reported that, overall, cancer had changed their lives for the better (23). BMT survivors reported significantly more positive than negative psychological changes in their lives as a result of having had cancer (53). The most frequently mentioned positive effect of having had cancer was a *change in survivors' values or philosophical approach to life*. Life was no longer experienced as infinite; survivors had been given a second chance in which to reassess priorities and values in order to have a fuller, more meaningful life (39,53). Survivors commented that they wanted there to be "more to (their) life than personal pleasures" (57, p. 158). Carter (58) suggests that the reprioritization of values, occurring midway through survivors' course of adaptation, is a necessary ingredient for healthy adjustment. A greater appreciation of life as a result of being treated for cancer was reported in several studies involving BMT, breast cancer, and Hodgkin's disease survivors (12,40,59), with Hodgkin's disease survivors reporting a significantly greater appreciation of life than a healthy comparison group (12). Second, a *strengthening of spiritual or religious beliefs* as a consequence of being treated for cancer was reported in several studies of BMT survivors (40,53,57). Last, *improved emotional state* was noted by some, expressed as an optimistic outlook concerning the future (17,39) as well as a diminished fear of death (17).

Vocational Functioning

Vocational Status. Because of the fundamental need to earn a living and obtain important employee-related benefits (e.g., health insurance), most survivors employed at the time of diagnosis were likely to be strongly motivated to return to work when physically able. Those unable to return to work have therefore been considered indicative of a gross estimate of the minimum proportion of survivors significantly adversely affected by cancer.

In two studies in which employment status of survivor cohorts was compared with that of healthy comparison groups, no differences were found between the two, the implication being that the overall impact of cancer upon employment status was negligible. Among breast cancer survivors, 31% of survivors vs. 25% of the comparison group were employed (16). Among Hodgkin's disease survivors, 64% were employed full-time and 30%, part-time, compared to 61% of the comparison group working full-time, and 33%, part-time (14).

However, much of the literature has fairly consistently demonstrated that approximately three-quarters of cancer survivors have been able to resume employment at their previous level when diagnosed, and one-quarter have not as a result of having been treated for cancer. Unemployment attributed to having had cancer varied by disease site as well as disease-related age and gender characteristics: 19% of Hodgkin's disease (20), 25% of leukemia (21), 9%–19% of BMT (25,60), 19% of breast cancer (61), 11% of prostate cancer, 22% of colon cancer, and 40% of lung cancer (26) survivors. Other studies have simply reported survivors' current employment status, letting very high percentages of those currently employed speak for themselves. Eighty-eight percent of testis cancer (17), 71% of Hodgkin's disease (29), 80% of BMT (31), 82% of blue-collar and 90% of white-collar (62,63) cancer survivors were currently employed, either full-time or part-time.

Survivors most vulnerable to becoming unemployed or working at a reduced level were those with significant cancer- and treatment-related physical problems (14,26,39) who had become disabled (40) or had highly strenuous occupations, such as blue collar workers (63). More subtle effects of physical sequelae on vocational functioning were not being able to work at their former pace (45% of Hodgkin's disease and 25% of testis cancer survivors) (64), and having to exert greater effort in carrying out activities (35% of Hodgkin's disease survivors vs. 17% of controls) (14).

Job Discrimination. In addition to cancer-related physical problems affecting continued employment, a subset of survivors reported incidents of gross discrimination in which they were fired or laid off because of their having had cancer (65,66): 4% of testis cancer (64), 5%–6% of Hodgkin's disease (20,29), and 7% of leukemia survivors (21) survivors. Other evidence of job discrimination survivors cited were: being encouraged to leave (4%-6%) (20,21); being transferred to less desirable jobs (65); denial of a deserved salary increase (65); denial of a promotion (2%) (21), not being offered a job (10%–12%) (21,29); difficulty finding a new job owing to their cancer history (25%, colon cancer survivors) (26); being demoted (1%–2%) (20,21); and work responsibilities being unnecessarily limited (4%) (21). A second category of events comprised general attitudes and interactions with those at work, which derived from discriminatory attitudes but did not affect employment status or benefits (67). These included hostile actions and statements of others (65) and conflicts with supervisors and co-workers (5%–12%, breast and testis cancer and Hodgkin's disease survivors) (23,29,64). Considering all of the above issues, 21% of leukemia survivors (21), 38% of white-collar survivors, and 45% of blue-collar survivors (65) reported one or more of the above incidents of discrimination as a result of having been treated for cancer.

None of these studies was able to provide objective evidence of job discrimination, as such cases are very difficult to prove, and most individuals do not have the financial wherewithal, legal knowledge, and/or stamina to pursue them (68). It is certainly possible that a proportion of the reported incidents were erroneous attributions of discrimination that survivors made, either to free themselves of their own responsibility or because they were unaware of the real reasons. That was indicated by a study of the Mayo Clinic, in which of 28 cases reviewed by a medical panel for cancer-related employment discrimination (6% of 473 employees with cancer), discrimination probably occurred in 17; the employer's actions were probably justified in the remaining 11 cases (69). Given that similar types of discrimination were reported across five studies and multiple cancer diagnoses, it is likely that overt acts of cancer-related discrimination existed, with a low prevalence of the worst violations (ca. $\leq$ 5%).

Hoffman (66) posited three "myths" that are primarily responsible for job discrimination against those treated for cancer: *(1)* cancer is a death sentence, and therefore there is little benefit to the employer to retain or hire those with cancer histories; *(2)* productivity of cancer patients is less than that of other employees, either owing to physical sequelae or continuous treatment demands; and *(3)* cancer is physically contagious, and therefore puts other employees at risk. Although the degree to which each of these myths continues to fuel job discrimination against the cancer patient is really not known, particularly the last one, it is probably the case that all apply, varying with the educational level of employers and co-workers. As the continuing success of cancer treatments becomes more widely known, and increasing numbers of cancer patients are either cured or have longer disease-free intervals (1), the myths that cancer is always a death sentence and that patients' productivity is suboptimal

may slowly fade, diminishing survivors' cancer-related employment problems (68).

Survivors' own personality characteristics and attitudes generated a third constellation of employment problems, such as projection of their own negative attitudes about cancer onto others, discomfort or general lack of social skills in dealing with others' sympathy or cancer prejudices, and self-imposed pressure to demonstrate independence, productivity, and self-worth (67). The degree to which these problems occurred and how they interacted with others' behavior and attitudes at the workplace are unknown.

Although many instances of discrimination were reported, not all cancer-related work experiences were negative. In Feldman's (65) studies, nearly two-thirds reported positive experiences, such as being relieved of difficult physical tasks or the modification of equipment to accommodate cancer-related physical limitations and changing of work schedules to enable the survivor to go to medical appointments. Further, 26% of BMT survivors reported positive changes in their vocational plans as a consequence of having had cancer (53), in line with the existential reprioritizing of survivors' values discussed above.

Legal Forms of Redress for Job Discrimination: The Rehabilitation Act of 1973. The Rehabilitation Act of 1973 was designed to prohibit employment discrimination based on medical conditions that did not affect an employee's qualification for the position for employers who receive federal financial assistance. In 1987 and 1988, in several landmark cases (*Arline v. School Board of Nassau County; Ritchie v. City of Houston*), the Rehabilitation Act was explicitly extended to healthy cancer survivors (66) by clarifying the "definition of 'handicapped individual' to include not only those who are actually impaired, but also those who are regarded as impaired, and who, as a result, are substantially limited in major life activity . . . " (70, p. 282–283). Survivors not covered under the Rehabilitation Act because the employer in question does not receive federal financial assistance must turn to state laws. Because state laws vary widely in their application of cancer-related discrimination, survivors may need to depend on existing state laws prohibiting employment discrimination due to disabilities (66). While legal suits of cancer survivors may be few in relation to the actual incidence of cancer-related employment discrimination, the extension of the Rehabilitation Act to cancer survivors not only provided the possibility of legal recourse but, perhaps equally as important, established the fundamental ethical principle guiding employers' treatment of cancer survivors in the workplace.

Insurance Problems Attributed to Having Had Cancer. Insurance problems survivors attributed to having had cancer have been reported across most of the cancer diagnoses reviewed in this chapter, with the magnitude of the problem ranging widely. While numerous problems were reported, the most frequent and important ones were difficulty in obtaining or denial of life and health insurance. Denial of life insurance ranged from 3% to 31% in Hodgkin's disease survivors (14,20,64), 5% in testis and breast cancer survivors (23,64), 29% in leukemia survivors (21), and 39%, in BMT survivors (71). When examined in relation to a comparison group, Hodgkin's disease survivors had significantly greater problems in obtaining life insurance (27% vs. 4%, $p < 0.01$) (14). Denial of health insurance ranged from 3% to 22% in Hodgkin's disease survivors (20,64), 4% in testis cancer survivors (64), and 21% in leukemia survivors (21).

Other insurance problems were encountered by survivors as well, including *(1)* increase of life insurance (9%) and health insurance (7%–12%) rates; *(2)* denial of health benefits (3%); *(3)* difficulty changing from a group or company to individual plan (7%); and *(4)* the need to supplement their current insurance (8%) or having no health insurance (10%) (20,21,23,62,63). Even in the Netherlands, where 68% of the population are covered by national health insurance or other compulsory forms of insurance (72), 70% of a mixed group of cancer survivors who tried to take out a life, health, or funeral insurance policy or modify an existing one encountered either refusal (80%), or higher premiums and medical reexaminations (36%) (18).

One of the most important consequences of being treated for cancer was survivors' fear concerning their future health, with the possibility of a recurrence or new primary, with yet more medical costs and the need for health insurance. Forty-four percent of breast cancer survivors reported great anxiety about their health insurance coverage in the future (23). A consequence of this anxiety has been survivors feeling "locked in" to their current job in order to retain their current insurance, as reported by 18% of leukemia survivors (21). Feldman (63) described a "pervasive" fear of medical costs and need for health insurance among blue collar survivors, causing some to stay in jobs they were no long able to perform (p. 22).

To some extent, recent legislation has helped to ease survivors' insurance problems and anxieties. The Consolidated Omnibus Reconciliation Act (COBRA) of 1986 requires employers who have 20 or more employees to continue to offer group medical insurance to their employees for a period of 18 months, and for 36 months for their dependents, if the employee is fired or laid off or resigns (66). While cancer survivors have to pay for the continued coverage, which is usually at higher rates, COBRA has provided an insurance safety net for the past 10 years where none had existed before. In addition to COBRA, the Employee Retirement and Income Security Act of 1974 (ERISA) provides legal recourse for those denied full participation in an employee benefit plan because of a cancer history (66). Violations would include dismissing an employee for the purposes of excluding him or her from a group health plan upon learning of his or her cancer history, for fear that the employer's insurance premiums would increase. If future health care reform includes "portability," with employees maintaining their health insurance from one job to the next, or elimination of insurance exclusions due to pre-existing medical conditions, then survivors' fears concerning inadequate health insurance for cancer-related medical problems will be permanently allayed.

Social Functioning: Relationships with Spouse, Family, Friends, and Social Activities

Relationships with Spouse/Partner. The resilience of the majority of cancer survivors' marriages in the face of considerable stress as a consequence of their disease has been suggested by a number of studies. Only 7% of testis cancer survivors (17) and 17% of women and 9% of men BMT survivors (73) became separated or divorced after being diagnosed with cancer. Further, no significant differences in marital status were found between breast cancer survivors and a comparison group (16), or between those who had a mastectomy vs. lumpectomy (32).

However, there was simultaneous evidence of a significant percentage of those who had become separated or divorced attributing the breakdown of their marriage to having had cancer. In Fobair and colleagues' (29) study, of 69 (of 403) Hodgkin's disease survivors who had been married at the time of their diagnosis and were currently separated or divorced, 49% ($n = 34/69$) attributed their current marital status to having had cancer. Similarly, in our Cancer and Leukemia Group B (CALGB) studies of leukemia and Hodgkin's disease survivors, of those currently separated or divorced, 33% ($n = 7/21$) of leukemia (21) and 56% ($n = 23/41$) of Hodgkin's disease survivors (74) attributed being separated or divorced to having had cancer.

For the majority of survivors who remained married or had married subsequent to their diagnosis, the question then became how the marital relationship changed in response to one of the partners having cancer. No significant differences in marital adjustment between survivors and a comparison group were reported in several studies [Hodgkin's disease (14); breast cancer survivors (15)]. Also, a number of breast cancer survivor studies reported either satisfactory marital adjustment in the vast majority (77%) (75), or that their marital relationship had not worsened as a consequence of their having cancer (85%) (33). Nor were significant differences found in the marital adjustment of leukemia survivors who had received either BMT or chemotherapy (30), suggesting that by the time of assessment, six years post diagnosis, survivors' marriages had been able to withstand stresses imposed by highly toxic regimens. In fact, of those marriages that remained intact, several studies reported a strengthening of survivors' marriages as a result of having had cancer [59% of breast cancer survivors (42); 72% of married testis cancer survivors (17)], with increased feelings of warmth and understanding [83% of Hodgkin's disease survivors (14)].

While a minority of survivors' marriages appeared to end in separation and divorce due to cancer, more common perhaps were subtle changes in the marital relationship, as indicated by survivors' reports of communication problems with their spouse. Lung cancer survivors reported difficulties in talking about their feelings (31%), their fears (29%), their future (29%), and what would happen after their death (45%) (26). Twenty-one percent of breast cancer survivors reported that their husbands did not understand what they had been through (23), a feeling commonly expressed by cancer patients with regard to their relationships with the non-cancer patient world (see section below on relationships with family and friends). Further, among head and neck cancer survivors, communication with their partner worsened over time ($p < 0.001$) (76). The result of cancer-related problems in communication, emotional support, and sexual functioning was strained relationships in a subset of survivors: 28% of testis cancer survivors (17) and 11%–23% of breast cancer survivors (23,42,75).

Relationships with Other Family Members. Outside of the survivors' relationship with his or her spouse or partner, little research has been directed toward other family members and the functioning of the family as a whole. While family adaptation has been included in some global measures of social adjustment such as the Psychosocial Adjustment to Illness Scale (PAIS) (20,21,77,78) and the Social Adjustment Scale (SAS) (75), analyses have provided insufficient detail as to what the nature of the adaptation has been.

Positive consequences of having had cancer for family relationships were found in several studies of BMT survivors. High satisfaction with the family as a whole (72%) (19) has been found, as well as the development of stronger family bonds (39) and positive changes in their relationships with siblings (53%), parents (49%), and children (17%) (53). However, other studies have reported a negative impact of having had cancer on family relationships. Forty-three percent of breast cancer survivors reported that family members did not understand well what they had experienced (23). There was a significantly greater disruption in family and extended family relationships among women leukemia survivors compared to healthy norms (22).

Family functioning was found to be one of three most pervasive problem-laden areas for head and neck cancer survivors, with the worst functioning occurring for those more recently diagnosed (6 months to 1.5 years), and also at 5 years or more since diagnosis; the best family functioning was for those in-between these times (76). Rapoport and colleagues (76) suggested that worsening family relationships with longer-term survival may be indicative of "patient burnout," that is, the chronic stress produced by having the disease, coping with health difficulties and limitations, and the "emotional strain of . . . acting 'normal and healthy' " (p. 73). Because most of the cancer survivor literature has used cross-sectional designs with single assessments, this finding would need to be verified in longitudinal studies with different cancer diagnoses, to explore whether this course of family relationships is common to many or unique to head and neck cancer survivors.

Social Activities and Relationships with Friends. The extent of the impact of being treated for cancer on social and leisure activities has varied across different populations and studies. In several studies involving Hodgkin's disease, leukemia and breast cancer survivors, no significant differences were found in their level of participation in social activities compared to community norms or healthy comparison groups (14,16,22,23). Further, fewer than 5% of breast cancer survivors reported that breast cancer led to any change in their social activities (23). In several studies of BMT survivors, 68% reported being "quite a bit" satisfied or more with their participation in leisure activities (19), and 33% noted positive changes in their relationships with friends as a consequence of having cancer (53). Only 5% of survivors with varying diagnoses stated that they received fewer visitors than they used to because of having had cancer (18).

However, a significant decline in participation in leisure activities from prior to their cancer diagnosis has been reported with lymphoma, BMT, colon, and prostate cancer survivors (26,28,53). Both physical and psychosocial factors limiting leisure activities were indicated in studies of women with mastectomies who avoided activities necessitating exposure of the body (38), head and neck cancer survivors' whose participation in leisure activities declined as their speech and eating difficulties worsened ($r = 0.44$, $p < 0.001$) (49), and Hodgkin's disease survivors whose lack of energy was significantly related to reduction in their leisure activities ($p < 0.001$) (64). BMT survivors had also anecdotally reported that lack of energy affected their pursuit of leisure activities (40,57).

Also to be considered among the factors affecting social participation is the withdrawal of family and friends from cancer survivors. Almost all of BMT survivors (96%) in Bush and colleagues' study (24) reported that people had been less supportive over time, and that this was the "single most distressing hardship of long-term survival" (p. 484). Diminished support may be partly due to friends not understanding what survivors have experienced as a result of cancer, as was reported by 45% of breast cancer survivors (23). Others' lack of ease in discussing cancer with the patient, not wishing to offend or distress him/her (40), and their own fear of the disease, with the specter of death that cancer often raises, also play a role in reduced support. The more survivors felt that being treated for cancer was a central, traumatizing experience to their life, the more barriers in communication might then develop with those who do not understand it or wish to discuss it. The diminution of support over time is not too surprising, with the passing of the crises of cancer diagnosis and treatment, and poorly understood long-term physical and psychological effects of cancer and its treatments. However, it is alarming that BMT survivors viewed diminishing support as the single most distressing aspect of survivorhood (24). While this finding may be unique to BMT survivors or the methodological characteristics of Bush and colleagues' study (24), this phenomenon has probably been underappreciated in the literature.

Sexual Functioning

Because the different aspects of psychosocial functioning are interrelated, it was expected that survivors' cancer-related physical, psychological, body image, and communication problems with their partners would spill over into their sexual lives. Disruption in sexual functioning due to cancer occurred in survivors of all diagnoses, with the nature and extent of the problems varying by disease site. Decreased sexual interest and activity, or general worsened sexual functioning attributed to having been treated for cancer ranged from 18% to 25% in Hodgkin's disease (14,20,28,29), 21% to 29% in leukemia (21), 31% to 40% in BMT (52,73,79), 35% in testis cancer (34), and 22% to 36% in breast cancer (33,38). In a mixed diagnostic group of women survivors receiving hormone replacement therapy due to premature menopause from radiation and/or chemotherapy, 38% met DSM-IV criteria for sexual dysfunction disorder (reduced sexual desire, 33%; dyspareunia, 15%), significantly more than those in a comparison group (8%) (80). Across many of the survivor groups, as body image worsened, sexual activity and functioning significantly decreased (21,29,33,42,60). Superimposed on these generic sexual functioning problems were medical and psychiatric sequelae specific to the cancer diagnosis and treatment.

Fertility. In Hodgkin's disease, testis cancer, and BMT, the primary treatment-related sexual functioning problem was infertiltiy. Because of the intrinsic association of reproduction with sexual self-image and overall self-worth, the potential for infertility creating emotional distress and marital discord was considerable, particularly if occurring in the child-bearing years (81).

The dramatic increase in survival for patients with Hodgkin's disease began with the MOPP regimen (2,3). However, owing to the inclusion of gonadally toxic alkylating agents in the MOPP regimen, nearly all men became permanently sterile, 80% of women over the age of 25 years old underwent premature menopause, and 41% of those older than 26 years of age had permanent amenorrhea (3,82). Infertility was reported in 91% of male Hodgkin's disease survivors who had been tested ($n = 20/22$) (12); 24% of 165 survivors reported that they could not conceive (29); and in our study (20), 26% reported being tested and found infertile, with an additional 27% who were untested but believed they were infertile. Consequently, significant problems in Hodgkin's disease survivors' sexual adjustment were expected.

When sexual functioning of Hodgkin's disease survivors was compared to that of a comparison group, significantly worse sexual functioning among survivors was found in one study (14), while another found no significant differences (12). However, in our study comparing the psychosocial and sexual adaptation of Hodgkin's disease and acute leukemia survivors, even when other medical and sociodemographic factors were controlled, Hodgkin's disease survivors reported significantly worse sexual functioning ($p = 0.0002$), as well as greater psychological distress ($p < 0.01$) than leukemia survivors (83). Further, as infertility in Hodgkin's disease survivors increased (based on test results or perceived infertility), overall psychosocial adjustment worsened significantly ($p < 0.05$) (78). Contrary to expectation, *no* significant differences in sexual functioning were found in Hodgkin's disease survivors treated by the less gonadally toxic regimen ABVD (doxorubicin, bleomycin, vinblastine, and dacarbazine) (84) than MOPP, an average of 2.2 years after their treatment (78). Long-term problems in sexual functioning due to infertility may possibly have been mitigated by survivors already having had children by the time of their diagnosis, and partial resolution of problems in psychosexual adjustment by one year after treatment completion, the minimum time for entry into this study (78). Further, defects in spermatogenesis that affect 30%–50% of male Hodgkin's disease patients *prior* to the initiation of any treatment (85) may obscure treatment-related sexual functioning problems.

Similarly, fertility was a treatment-related problem for survivors of testis cancer, diagnosed predominantly in younger adults when issues of fertility are more paramount. With surgical removal of the affected testicle, azoospermia or high-grade oligospermia is found in 30% of survivors. If no further treatment is given, spermatogenesis has been found to improve in the contralateral testicle over a three-year period (86). Retroperitoneal lymphadenectomy (RPLND) performed prior to 1980 for disease staging purposes produced sterility due to failure to ejaculate, while subsequent nerve-sparing modifications of this procedure have preserved ejaculatory function. Those with metastatic disease cured by multidrug chemotherapy are also at risk for diminished reproductive capacity, although, as with Hodgkin's disease survivors, a proportion (approximately 10%–15%) are rendered permanently infertile by the effects of the disease itself, prior to any chemotherapy (4).

As a consequence of these assaults, sexual satisfaction worsened in 22%–33% of testis cancer survivors (17,34). Erectile dysfunction was reported by 32% of

survivors, a significant increase from 17% retrospectively reported at the time prior to diagnosis ($p < 0.01$) (34). Problems in ejaculation (24%) and not being able to get or maintain an erection (10%) were reported significantly more often among survivors than among those in a comparison group (1%) (17). In one of the largest studies of testis cancer survivors involving 223 survivors, Rieker and colleagues (17) found that being distressed about fertility and sexual performance problems over half the time during the previous six months occurred in 22% and 30%, respectively, both significantly greater than the comparison group ($p < 0.001$). Those at greater risk of fertility distress had been diagnosed at a younger age ($p < 0.01$), treated by chemotherapy plus RPLND ($p < 0.05$), were childless ($p < 0.01$), and had a lower socioeconomic status ($p < 0.05$–0.01). Similar correlates were identified for those reporting greater sexual performance distress, with the exception that being childless was not a significant factor.

While distress about infertility was reported by a significant number of testis cancer survivors, its impact did not necessarily extend into survivors' psychological well-being, with no significant correlations found between fertility distress and measures of psychological distress (81). In a similar vein, Gritz and colleagues (87) found that only 10% of survivors felt that their infertility would create marital problems. Thus, it would appear that testis cancer survivors were able to compartmentalize their feelings about infertility as a means of protecting their overall emotional state, with factors such as already having had children, sperm-banking, and adoption offsetting the medical and psychological impact of infertility (81,87). It is also possible that current measures are not sufficiently sensitive to capture the "depth of . . . feelings" (81, p. 352) about such a highly charged area as fertility.

Infertility has been almost universally observed in both men and women bone marrow transplant survivors due to total body irradiation (TBI) and alkylating agents in chemotherapy regimens (88,89). Women treated by TBI when older than 40 years develop permanent ovarian failure, while those younger may recover gonadal function if treated with less than 20.0 Gy. Men treated with higher doses than 3.0 Gy may require 5–6 years before recovery of sperm counts and follicle-stimulating hormone (FSH) levels (89). Further, in women who received chemotherapy-based BMT regimens, ovarian atrophy, amenorrhea, damaged germinal epithelium, and an increased incidence of spontaneous abortions have all been noted (89). Given these findings, it was not surprising that sterility was the most common problem reported by BMT survivors in Wellisch and colleagues' study (30), occurring in 66%. Difficulty having erections was reported in 24%–39% of BMT survivors, and 13%–35% were unable to ejaculate (60,79).

Anticipated as a consequence of the highly toxic, prolonged treatment period required in BMT, significantly greater impotence (31) and worse sexual functioning was found in BMT than chemotherapy-treated survivors (25% vs. 0%) (90), an average of approximately three years post treatment. However, neither Wellisch and colleagues (30) nor Mumma and colleagues (51) found significant differences in overall sexual functioning between the BMT and conventional chemotherapy groups. Thus, it is possible that, as with Hodgkin's disease and testis cancer survivors, other factors may have mitigated the impact of infertility.

The Impact of Breast Surgery on Sexual Functioning. Overall, sexual functioning appeared to recover from the trauma of a mastectomy in 67%–85% of survivors (38,75). In spite of mastectomy patients' enduring body image problems commented on earlier (see 'Body Image' section), a number of breast cancer survivor studies found no significant differences in long-term sexual adjustment between those treated by mastectomy, either with or without breast reconstruction, or lumpectomy, or with benign breast disease an average of 1.5–4 years post surgery (15,42,48,91). These findings suggest that body image distress is less accessible to restorative forces operating in other areas of the survivor's life, perhaps because disfiguration due to breast surgery so visibly embodies the trauma of being treated for breast cancer, in such a psychosexually charged area. Further, in Schover and colleagues' study (42), adjuvant chemotherapy was a more significant determinant of sexual dysfunction than having had lumpectomy or mastectomy with immediate reconstruction. While this finding was confounded by chemotherapy having been given to those with more advanced disease (stage II vs. stage I), part of the constellation of sexual problems for this group was vaginal dryness and dyspareunia, side effects of chemotherapy-induced menopause. Extremely high prevalence rates of adjuvant chemotherapy-induced amenorrhea in premenopausal breast cancer patients due to CMF (cylophosphamide, methotrexate and fluouracil) treatment have been widely reported, occurring on the average in 68% of patients (92). Thus, treatment factors other than mastectomy may become more important in breast cancer survivors' sexual adjustment, particularly when breast reconstruction has diminished the psychosexual

effects of mastectomy and there have been long-term chemotherapy side effects.

Profile of Those with Adjustment Problems

In order to identify which cancer survivors were adjusting well or poorly, numerous studies have examined a range of medical, treatment, sociodemographic, and psychosocial factors as predictors or correlates of adaptation. Findings varied across different disease sites, as well as by different authors within the same disease site, partly determined by which characteristics were chosen to be examined, different measures used, a wide range in sample sizes rendering varying degrees of power, and different sample characteristics related to the cancer diagnosis and/or institution. In spite of these issues, five major factors emerged, whose interplay generally either exacerbated or diminished patients' vulnerability to the stresses imposed by cancer: *(1)* medical problems, including late effects of cancer and/or its treatment as well as co-morbid conditions; *(2)* social support; *(3)* economic resources; *(4)* intrapsychic factors, including personality traits and premorbid psychological state; and *(5)* length of time since treatment was completed.

Among testis cancer survivors, those having the lowest income and reporting sexual dysfunction were also significantly more likely to have a negative mental outlook (17). In studies of Hodgkin's disease survivors, energy level not returning to normal was significantly predictive of depression (29). In our own research, Hodgkin's disease survivors in greatest distress were those who were not married, as well as men with incomes of less than $15,000, who were currently unemployed (20). Further, the presence of other serious illnesses post treatment (of which 42% were judged by oncologists to be disease- and/or treatment-related) was significantly related to worse overall psychosocial adaptation. Leukemia survivors in greatest distress were men and those who were more highly educated (22). However, in Greenberg and colleagues' study (21), those in greatest distress were those who were less educated, who had reported anticipatory distress in relation to their chemotherapy, and had serious illness post treatment combined with poorer family functioning. In head and neck cancer survivors, the greater the physical dysfunction resulting from surgery (eating, talking, etc.) and the less social support, the worse was their psychological state and overall adjustment (49). Feeling less control over their lives (i.e. less internal control) and having more chronic illnesses were associated with greater dissatisfaction with life among melanoma survivors (93). A poorer Karnofsky Performance Status was predictive of a worse overall quality of life in prostate, colorectal and lung cancer survivors (26). In addition, co-morbid medical conditions were associated with a worse quality of life in prostate cancer survivors, while being a woman and being employed were significant predictors for a worse quality of life for colorectal cancer survivors (26). Breast cancer survivors who remained depressed for two years post mastectomy had higher preoperative levels of neuroticism and depression than those not depressed (15). In another study, younger breast cancer survivors had worse adjustment than those who were older (42).

Survivors treated by bone marrow transplantation (BMT), most involving cohorts with varying diagnoses (see Table 20.1, Appendix), have the most information concerning factors associated with psychological distress and maladjustment. Those with worse overall quality of life or greater psychological distress had the widest spectrum of medical sequelae resulting from BMT (19,24) or worse physical health (53); were older at the time of transplant (mean age of 42 years old) (52); were more recently treated (52); were less educated (52); had more conflict in their families prior to transplantation (25); and were not married (25,53). In addition, for BMT survivors who had a high number of negative changes in their lives due to BMT, a high number of positive changes "protected" their ability to remain satisfied with their life. Those with the greatest dissatisfaction had reported only a high number of negative changes (53).

As can be seen from the above findings, the likelihood of poor adjustment increased with the more cancer-related physical problems and/or co-morbid medical conditions, coupled with fewer financial resources with which to deal with them, weaker social support with which to buffer the stress, and a poorer prediagnosis adjustment. While not all the findings support this generalization, the results are clearly marshalled in this direction for cancer survivors across multiple disease sites.

Length of time since diagnosis or treatment has been widely tested as a predictor of adjustment, with better adjustment anticipated with the passage of time. This has been found to be the case in conditioned phenomena, where conditioned nausea and vomiting and PTSD symptomatology have been found to decrease significantly over time in leukemia (21) and Hodgkin's disease survivors (12,20).

However, with regard to survivors' overall psychosocial adjustment, the results are inconsistent. One study found improved adjustment of breast cancer survivors over time (75). Surprisingly, two studies involving prostate cancer (26) and BMT survivors (24) found a *worsening* adjustment over time. Further complicating the picture was that while anxiety and anger significantly increased with time in head and neck cancer survivors, a curvilinear relationship was found between their family relationships and time (described in the above section) (76). However, more commonly, numerous studies found no significant relationship between time since diagnosis or treatment and adjustment [leukemia (21); BMT (94); lung and colon cancer (26); Hodgkin's disease (12,20,95)]. In part, this may have been largely a function of the cross-sectional design of these studies, in which survivor cohorts were assessed on average 2–6 years after diagnosis or treatment, ranging from 6 months to 20 years. If most overall adjustment occurred within the first 18 months of treatment completion, as suggested by the breast cancer literature described earlier, as well as a study of BMT survivors (25), then further significant improvement in adjustment would not be found in survivors assessed farther out from treatment. These seemingly inconsistent findings indicate the need for longitudinal evaluation of survivors' adaptation in order to better understand the course of adjustment for the different survivor groups.

Disease stage, by itself was rarely found to be a significant predictor of adjustment, but rather it was the impact of cancer-related physical sequelae upon physical functioning. This issue was perhaps best exemplified by BMT (19,24) and head and neck cancer survivors (49) due to the magnitude of their physical problems and effect upon functioning. Sugarbaker and colleagues' (50) surprising finding of no substantial differences in the psychosocial adjustment of sarcoma survivors who had been treated by limb-sparing or amputation was largely due to the worse than anticipated physical functioning as well as significantly worse sexual functioning in those with limb-sparing surgery. The impact of post-surgical RT and chemotherapy upon limb-spared survivors' adjustment, possibly resulting in radiation fibrosis and testicular damage, had clearly been underestimated (50).

Sociodemographic factors of gender and age were routinely explored as correlates of survivors' adjustment; neither was consistently related to greater distress across diagnoses. The roles of gender and age in survivors' adaptation to cancer need to be understood in relation to the specific demands and characteristics of the disease site and treatment. For example, in Hodgkin's disease, the survivor population was younger and treated by alkylating agents (e.g., nitrogen mustard), causing infertility in men to a much greater extent than women (3,84). Within this context, it was therefore understandable that socioeconomically disadvantaged men were more likely to be distressed than women (20). Conversely, women survivors of colon cancer were in signifcantly greater distress than men (26). The secretiveness of colorectal cancer survivors was interpreted by Feldman (65) as related to their having had cancer of the bowel, involving bodily functions and body image changes that often give rise to feelings of embarrassment (26,96). Women colon cancer survivors may feel these problems more keenly than men, with concomitant diminishment of feeling attractive, sexual, and socially accepted. Further research would be required to elucidate the gender difference in colon cancer survivors' adjustment.

CLINICAL IMPLICATIONS AND RECOMMENDATIONS

Current Psychosocial Interventions

While the majority of survivors appear to have made a good adjustment to having being treated for cancer, a subset experienced problems in adjustment long after treatment completion and are clearly in need of some form of psychosocial intervention. Most of the well-designed, controlled psychosocial and psychoeducational interventions have been developed for cancer patients in active or palliative treatment, many consisting of supportive and educational components, with some also including problem-solving or behavioral interventions such as relaxation training. Most interventions involve 3–10 sessions beginning during diagnosis and treatment or within a few months post treatment. In general, the results have indicated that patients who received *any* intervention experienced an improvement in psychosocial adaptation, irrespective of content or whether the format was individual or group (97–99). However, while the improvement was significant, the magnitude was deemed small, approximating half of a standard deviation of standardized means (99).

There has been widespread proliferation of self-help organizations serving cancer patients and their families throughout the patients' clinical course, offering a range of information and referral services and support groups (100,101). However, similarly to the tested psychosocial interventions, the emphasis in self-help organizations has been upon patients in active or palliative treatment.

In order to provide a structure by which to foster survivorship activities, the National Coalition for Cancer Survivors (NCCS) was formed in 1986. The NCCS advocates for the psychosocial needs and legal rights of cancer survivors, serves as a national clearing house for information on topics of concern for survi-

vors (e.g., "Charting the Journey") (102), and provides technical assistance to community cancer-support organizations (100). The National Cancer Institute's newly created Office of Cancer Survivorship, established to support cancer survivorship research, was due partly to the advocacy efforts of the NCCS.

A unique, comprehensive program specifically designed for cancer survivors, the Post-Treatment Resource Program (PTRP), was developed at Memorial Sloan-Kettering Cancer Center in 1988. PTRP combines cancer support groups, individual counseling, educational seminars, and consultation on insurance problems, offered to patients upon completion of their treatment (103). Because of its breadth of services and understanding of survivorship issues, PTRP serves as a model to the field.

Clinical Recommendations

Based on the body of research on psychosocial adaptation of cancer survivors, and the current status of psychosocial interventions, the following clinical recommendations are suggested.

1. The range of problems encountered by cancer survivors strongly suggests that *programs need to be comprehensive* in nature, with the core consisting of educational and either group or individual counseling components. Problems with sexual functioning, often sidestepped owing to their highly private nature, need to be more frequently included as part of a comprehensive program, particularly given the prevalence of treatment-related infertility and surgical disfigurations of the body. Reliance on either group support (104) or education alone may not be sufficient to help the survivor cope with the array of problems presented by having been treated for cancer.

2. It is unknown exactly when the optimal time for intervention might be. However, the downward trajectory of survivors' problems in adjustment, coupled with a subset of approximately 20% with poor adjustment long after treatment completion, suggests that *psychosocial interventions applied earlier, either during treatment or soon after completing treatment* would be beneficial (98). Rooted in preventive mental health principles, Worden and Weisman (105) advocated in 1984 the need to identify *"in advance* of serious distress the patients . . . at highest risk . . . , {offering} help *before* serious emotional distress and poor coping develop" (p. 243). Twelve years later, with much more evidence as to the range and magnitude of the problems experienced by cancer survivors, this advice increasingly makes sense.

3. Information is now available about which medical, sociodemographic, social, and premorbid personality variables are associated with survivors in greater distress. Andersen (104) organized her theoretical framework of survivor adaptation in terms of these variables as risk factors for psychological morbidity, highlighting the importance of extent of disease, treatment, appearance of new health problems post treatment, and unavailable or ineffective medical treatment for post treatment medical problems. These *psychosocial morbidity factors could be used to focus efforts as to which survivors need to be targeted* for psychosocial interventions.

4. Because cancer survivors are less enmeshed in the medical system the farther out they are from treatment, it is possible that they would benefit from *closer, systematic monitoring of psychological distress between infrequently scheduled office visits,* an approach endorsed by the NCCS (106). Using a two-stage approach, monitoring could be accomplished by an initial identification of those potentially in distress, followed by further evaluation and referral (107,108). Telephone monitoring of psychological distress with follow-up for those in need has been used in patients with breast cancer (109) and stroke patients and their families (110), and has been found to be effective in identifying and reducing psychological distress in patients with ischemic heart disease (111). Occupying a key position with regard to their patients, *oncologists can serve as a fulcrum for change, by identifying those in distress and actively referring them for the appropriate mental health treatment* (112). Spitzer and colleagues' (113) approach, which directly involves primary care physicians in identifying patients in distress at the time of their clinic visit, is clearly applicable to oncologists as well. The enduring emotional bond that many patients have with their oncologists may make them more seriously consider and comply with their doctors' recommendations. The undertreatment of psychiatric disorders is a multi-determined phenomenon, most likely due to *(1)* survivors' underreporting their emotional distress to health care professionals because they want to be viewed as the "good patient," as well as the perceived stigma of needing mental health treatment; *(2)* doctors not recognizing signs and symptoms of distress, not feeling they have the time, or not liking to deal with patients' emotional problems, which some feel ought to be handled by other disciplines; and *(3)* financial limitations that make treatment financially inaccessible. Closer monitoring of patients to identify those in distress by any one of a number of methods might help to reduce or bypass some of these barriers.

5. Interventions need to focus on *reducing cancer survivors' emotional and social isolation. Patient-to-patient' relationships,* sometimes established while the patient is in treatment [e.g., Reach to Recovery; Patient-to-Patient Program (114)], but continuing well into the post treatment period, might be effective, particularly as the survivor experiences problems while regaining his or her life. However, cancer support groups or patient-to-patient programs alone will not adequately address barriers in communication with non-cancer relationships. *Educational and counseling programs involving both cancer survivors and their family members and friends,* concerning cancer-related problems told from the vantage point of *both,* might help to reduce the communication barriers between the cancer and non-cancer world. *Art therapy* (115), which has been used in diverse populations (116), might also be tested as a means for transcending the barriers.

FUTURE RESEARCH DIRECTIONS

Particular areas have been highlighted in this literature review by their virtual absence, and others are suggested as the logical next step for future research.

1. Most of the longitudinal studies of survivors have been conducted with women with breast cancer. *More longitudinal studies are needed in other survivor cohorts in order to better understand the dynamics of adaptation over time*; when cancer-related problems begin in the different areas of functioning, when they worsen and subside, how they are interrelated, and when it would be best to intervene. Cross-sectional studies can only serve as an approximation of the adaptational process. Cancer patients with a high probability of cure could be targeted for longitudinal studies beginning with their diagnosis or prior to primary treatment. Even if a proportion were to later relapse, the "yield" would still remain high.

2. *Survivors of colon, prostate and cervical cancer have gone almost completely unstudied.* Since early treatment of each of these diagnoses results in excellent prognoses, studies of these cohorts are needed to better understand the survivorship issues unique to each group.

3. *Barriers in communication between cancer survivors and their family members and friends need to be examined,* from the vantage point of both sides of the relationship. Observational methods, used in conjunction with self-report and interview methods, would enhance our understanding of what the nature of the barriers are and how they get expressed. Innovative interven-

tions designed to improve communication could then be better fashioned.

4. *Improved measurement of social adjustment and body image is needed* in order to expand our understanding of the impact of cancer on these important aspects of survivors' lives.

5. *Two subsets of cancer survivors which need to be studied in greater depth are the elderly and minorities.* In both there have been insufficient numbers included in the studies to adequately understand the cancer-related problems specific to each, and how their psychosocial adaptation differs, if at all, from other survivors with their diagnosis. This research would guide the kind of psychosocial interventions that would be needed and most effective for each.

Theoretical Framework of Psychosocial Adaptation of Cancer Survivors

It was appropriate that the initial wave of research in adaptation of cancer survivors was not theory-driven, but rather consisted of mapping the nature and extent of their problems and identifying characteristics associated with those adjusting well and poorly. However, the focus now needs to shift for the next stage of research to understanding *what the specific psychosocial mechanisms are by which cancer survivors adjust to their disease and treatment. The stress–illness vulnerability theory is proposed as a broad theoretical model for understanding patient adaptation* (117,118). In this model adapted for application to cancer patients (see Fig. 20–1) (112), cancer and its treatment are the stressors, and patient adaptation is the outcome. The conduit through which cancer and its treatments are experienced is physical functioning, with a range of mediating factors which may then further exacerbate or ameliorate the stress of having been treated for cancer, including social support, economic resources, individual characteristics (e.g., health perceptions, premorbid adjustment, and personality traits), and other stressors (e.g., concurrent stressful life events, co-morbid conditions). The complex interrelationship among the mediating variables, often reciprocally interactive, is indicated. The supportive role of the medical team to a patients' adjustment, often overlooked by researchers, is highlighted in this model. Social support is figured prominently in this proposed model, either serving as a potential "buffer" protecting patients from the impact of cancer-related stress (119) or exacerbating it (120). Goffman's (121) theory of stigma can be conceptually incorporated into the vulnerability model as a partial explanation of strained and negative interactions with others. According to stigma theory, the greater the visibility and obtrusiveness of cancer-related functional problems, the greater the likelihood of strained social interactions and restricted social functioning and, consequently, problems with psychological adjustment. When survivors incorporate others' devaluation of them, there is a

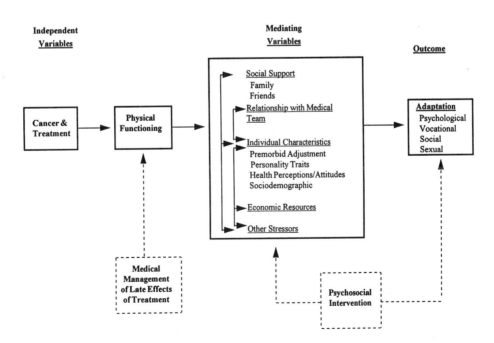

FIG. 20-1. Vulnerability model of psychosocial adaptation of cancer survivors.

resultant devaluation of their own self-worth. Individual characteristics of survivors, such as their cognitive appraisal of cancer and related health beliefs (122–125), personality traits (126), pre-morbid adjustment and sociodemographic factors (age, ethnicity) are positioned as central to their ability to marshall forces to improve their adaptation. PTSD, recently proposed as a theoretical model for understanding cancer patients' adjustment, is conceptually subsumed within the vulnerability model as a subset of psychiatric reactions that may occur as a consequence of being treated for cancer. Through the use of psychosocial interventions, adaptation is portrayed as potentially being improved either directly, or indirectly via mediating variables. Similarly, medical management of late medical effects may also indirectly improve psychosocial adaptation via improved physical functioning. Guided by the vulnerability model, longitudinal assessment of survivors would help to elucidate the complex pathway charted by these variables in relation to survivors' adaptation. With theoretically driven research, our understanding would be expanded of how to most effectively intervene with which type of survivor, at what time, and under what conditions.

ACKNOWLEDGMENTS

With deep appreciation to all cancer patients who have so graciously participated in the studies reviewed, from whom we have learned so much; Alfred M. Cohen, M.D., for his encouragement, so central to my professional life over the past five years; and the memory of my beloved mother, to whom this chapter is dedicated.

REFERENCES

1. American Cancer Society. *Cancer Facts & Figures—1996*. Atlanta, GA: American Cancer Society; 1996.
2. DeVita Jr VT. The consequences of the chemotherapy of Hodgkin's disease: The 10th David A. Karnofsky Memorial Lecture. *Cancer*. 1981; 47:1–13.
3. Urba WJ, Longo DL. Hodgkin's disease. *N Engl J Med*. 1992; 326:678–687.
4. Einhorn LH, Richie JP, Shipley WU. Cancer of the testis. In: DeVita Jr VT, Hellman S, Rosenberg SA, eds. *Cancer: Principles and Practice of Oncology*. 4th ed. Philadelphia, PA: JB Lippincott; 1993: 1126–1151.
5. Horwich A. Testicular germ cell tumours: an introductory overview. In: Horwich A, ed. *Testicular Cancer: Investigation and Management*. Baltimore, MD: Williams & Wilkins; 1991:1–13.
6. Armitage JO. Bone marrow transplantation. *N Engl J Med*. 1994; 330:827–838.
7. American Cancer Society. *Cancer Facts and Figures—1987*. New York City, NY: American Cancer Society; 1987.
8. Harris JR, Morrow M, Bonadonna G. Cancer of the breast. In DeVita Jr VT, Hellman S, Rosenberg SA, eds. *Cancer: Principles and Practice of Oncology*, 4th ed. Philadelphia, PA: JB Lippincott; 1993: 1264–1332.
9. Eddy DM. Screening for cervical cancer. *Ann Intern Med*. 1990; 113:214–226.
10. Miller AB. Cancer screening. In: DeVita Jr VT, Hellman S, Rosenberg SA, eds. *Cancer: Principles and Practice of Oncology*, 4th ed. Philadelphia, PA: JB Lippincott; 1993:564–573.
11. Loescher LJ, Welch-McCaffrey D, Leigh SA, Hoffman B, Meyskens FL. Survivng adult cancers. Part 1: Physiologic effects. *Ann Intern Med*. 1989; 111: 411–432.
12. Cella DF, Tross S. Psychological adjustment to survival from Hodgkin's disease. *J Consult Clin Psychol*. 1986; 54:616–622.
13. Schmale AH, Morrow GR, Schmitt MH, et al. Well-being of cancer survivors. *Psychosom Med*. 1983; 45:163–169.
14. van Tulder MW, Aaronson NK, Bruning PF. The quality of life of long-term survivors of Hodgkin's disease. *Ann Oncol*. 1994; 5:153–158.
15. Morris T, Greer HS, White P. Psychological and social adjustment to mastectomy: a two-year follow-up study. *Cancer*. 1977; 40:2381–2387.
16. Craig TJ, Comstock GW, Geiser PB. The quality of survival in breast cancer: a case-control comparison. *Cancer*. 1974; 33:1451–1457.
17. Rieker PP, Fitzgerald EM, Kalish LA, et al. Psychosocial factors, curative therapies, and behavioral outcomes: a comparison of testis cancer survivors and a control group of healthy men. *Cancer*. 1989; 64:2399–2407.
18. Greaves-Otte JGW, Greaves J, Kruyt PM, van Leeuwen O, van der Wouden JC, van der Does E. Problems at social reintegration of long-term cancer survivors. *Eur J Cancer*. 1991; 27:178–181.
19. Wolcott DL, Wellisch DK, Fawzy FI, Landsverk J. Adaptation of adult bone marrow transplant recipient long-term survivors. *Transplantation*. 1986; 41:478–484.
20. Kornblith AB, Anderson J, Cella DF, et al. Hodgkin's disease survivors at increased risk for problems in psychosocial adaptation. *Cancer*. 1992; 70:2214–2224.
21. Greenberg DB, Herndon JE, Kornblith AB, et al. Long-term psychosocial adaptation of survivors of acute leukemia [meeting abstract]. *Proc Am Soc Clin Oncol*. 1995; 14(A1668):508.
22. Lesko LM, Ostroff JS, Mumma GH, Mashberg DE, Holland JC. Long-term psychological adjustment of acute leukemia survivors: impact of bone marrow transplantation versus conventional chemotherapy. *Psychosom Med*. 1992; 54:30–47.
23. Polinsky ML. Functional status of long-term breast cancer survivors: demonstrating chronicity. *Health Soc Work*. 1994; 19:165–173.
24. Bush NE, Haberman M, Donaldson G, Sullivan KM. Quality of life of 125 adults surviving 6-18 years after bone marrow transplantation. *Soc Sci Med*. 1995; 40:479–490.
25. Syrjala KL, Chapko MK, Vitaliano PP, Cummings C, Sullivan KM. Recovery after allogeneic marrow transplantation: prospective study of predictors of long-term physical and psychosocial functioning. *Bone Marrow Transplant*. 1993; 11:319–327.

26. Schag CAC, Ganz PA, Wing DS, Sim MS, Lee JJ. Quality of life in adult survivors of lung, colon and prostate cancer. *Qual Life Res.* 1994; 3:127–141.

27. Alter CL, Pelcovitz D, Axelrod A, et al. The identification of PTSD in cancer survivors. *Psychosomatics.* 1996; 37:137–143.

28. Devlen J, Maguire P, Phillips P, Crowther D, Chambers H. Psychological problems associated with diagnosis and treatment of lymphomas. *Br Med J.* 1987; 295:953–954.

29. Fobair P, Hoppe RT, Bloom J, Cox R, Varghese A, Spiegel D. Psychosocial problems among survivors of Hodgkin's disease. *J Clin Oncol.* 1986; 4:805–814.

30. Wellisch DK, Centeno J, Guzman J, Belin T, Schiller GJ. Bone marrow transplantation vs. high-dose cytarabine-based consolidation chemotherapy for acute myelogenous leukemia. *Psychosomatics.* 1996; 37:144–154.

31. Molassiotis A, van den Akker OBA, Milligan DW, et al. Quality of life in long-term survivors of marrow transplantation: comparison with a matched group receiving maintenance chemotherapy. *Bone Marrow Transplant.* 1996; 17:249–258.

32. Lasry JCM, Margolese RG, Poisson R, et al. Depression and body image following mastectomy and lumpectomy. *J Chron Dis.* 1987; 40:529–534.

33. Sneeuw KCA, Aaronson NK, Yarnold JR, et al. Cosmetic and functional outcomes of breast conserving treatment for early stage breast cancer. 2: Relationship with psychosocial functioning. *Radiother Oncol.* 1992; 25:160–166.

34. Gritz ER, Wellisch DK, Landsverk JA. Psychosocial sequelae in long-term survivors of testicular cancer. *J Psychosoc Oncol.* 1988; 6 (3/4):41–63.

35. Cordova MJ, Andrykowski MA, Redd WH, Kenady DE, McGrath PC, Sloan DA. Frequency and correlates of posttraumatic-stress-disorder-like symptoms after treatment for breast cancer. *J Consult Clin Psychol.* 1995; 63:981–986.

36. Zilberg NJ, Weiss DS, Horowitz MJ. Impact of Event Scale: a cross-validation study and some empirical evidence supporting a conceptual model of stress response syndromes. *J Consult Clin Psychol.* 1982; 50:407–414.

37. Koocher GP, O'Malley JE. *The Damocles Syndrome: Psychosocial Consequences of Surviving Childhood Cancer.* New York: McGraw-Hill; 1981.

38. Meyer L, Aspegren K. Long-term psychological sequelae of mastectomy and breast conserving treatment for breast cancer. *Acta Oncol.* 1989; 28:13–18.

39. Belec RH. Quality of life: perceptions of long-term survivors of bone marrow transplantation. *Oncol Nurs Forum.* 1992; 19(1):31–37.

40. Haberman M, Bush N, Young K, Sullivan KM. Quality of life of adult long-term survivors of bone marrow transplantation: a qualitative analysis of narrative data. *Oncol Nurs Forum.* 1993; 10:1545–1553.

41. Halstead MT, Fernsler JI. Coping strategies of long-term cancer survivors. *Cancer Nurs.* 1994; 17:94–100.

42. Schover LR, Yetman RJ, Tuason LJ, et al. Partial mastectomy and breast reconstruction: a comparison of their effects on psychosocial adjustment, body image, and sexuality. *Cancer.* 1995; 75:54–64.

43. Fallowfield LJ, Hall A, Maguire GP, Baum M. Psychological outcomes of different treatment policies in women with early breast cancer outside a clinical trial. *Br Med J.* 1990; 301:575–580.

44. Kiebert GM, de Haes JCJM, van de Velde CJH. The impact of breast-conserving treatment and mastectomy on the quality of life of early-stage breast cancer patients: a review. *J Clin Oncol.* 1991; 9:1059–1070.

45. Levy SM, Haynes LT, Herberman RB, Lee H, McFeeley S, Kirkwood J. Mastectomy versus breast conservation surgery: mental health effects at long-term follow-up. *Health Psychol.* 1992; 11:349–354.

46. Maunsell E, Brisson J, Deschenes L. Psychological distress after initial treatment for breast cancer: a comparison of partial and total mastectomy. *J Clin Epidemiol.* 1989; 42:765–771.

47. Steinberg MD, Juliano MA, Wise L. Psychological outcome of lumpectomy versus mastectomy in the treatment of breast cancer. *Am J Psychiatry.* 1985; 142:34–39.

48. Wellisch DK, DiMatteo R, Silverstein M, et al. Psychosocial outcomes of breast cancer therapies: lumpectomy versus mastectomy. *Psychosomatics.* 1989; 30:365–373.

49. Baker CA. Factors associated with rehabilitation in head and neck cancer. *Cancer Nurs.* 1992; 15:395–400.

50. Sugarbaker PH, Barofsky I, Rosenberg SA, Gianola FJ. Quality of life assessment of patients in extremity sarcoma clinical trials. *Surgery.* 1982; 91:17–23.

51. Mumma GH, Mashberg D, Lesko LM. Long-term psychosexual adjustment of acute leukemia survivors: impact of marrow transplantation versus conventional chemotherapy. *Gen Hosp Psychiatry.* 1992; 14:43–55.

52. Andrykowski MA, Greiner CB, Altmaier EM, et al. Quality of life following bone marrow transplantation: findings from a multicentre study. *Br J Cancer.* 1995; 71:1322–1329.

53. Curbow B, Somerfield MR, Baker F, Wingard JR, Legro MW. Personal changes, dispositional optimism, and psychological adjustment to bone marrow transplantation. *J Behav Med.* 1993; 16:423–443.

54. Shontz FC. Body image and physical disability. In: Cash TF, Pruzinsky T, eds. *Body Images: Development, Deviance, and Change.* New York: Guilford Press; 1990:149–169.

55. Cella DF. Psychological sequelae in the cured cancer patient. In: Higby DJ, ed. *Issues in Supportive Care of Cancer Patients.* Netherlands: Martinus Nijhoff; 1986:149–171.

56. Cella DF, Pratt A, Holland JC. Persistent anticipatory nausea, vomiting, and anxiety in cured Hodgkin's disease patients after completion of chemotherapy. *Am J Psychiatry.* 1986; 143: 641–643.

57. Ferrell B, Grant M, Schmidt GM, et al. The meaning of quality of life for bone marrow transplant survivors. Part 1: The impact of bone marrow transplant on quality of life. *Cancer Nurs.* 1992; 15:153–160.

58. Carter BJ. Long-term survivors of breast cancer. *Cancer Nurs.* 1993; 16:354–361.

59. Kennedy BJ, Tellegen A, Kennedy S, Havernick N. Psychological response of patients cured of advanced cancer. *Cancer.* 1976; 38:2184–2191.

60. Wingard JR, Curbow B, Baker F, Zabora J, Piantadosi S. Sexual satisfaction in survivors of bone marrow

transplantation. *Bone Marrow Transplant.* 1992; 9:185–190.

61. Schottenfeld D, Robbins GF. Quality of survival among patients who have had radical mastectomy. *Cancer.* 1970; 26:650–655.

62. Feldman FL. *Work and Cancer Health Histories: A Study of the Experiences of Recovered Patients (White Collar Study).* Oakland, CA: American Cancer Society, California Division, 1976.

63. Feldman FL. *Work and Cancer Health Histories: Study of Experiences of Recovered Blue-Collar Workers.* Oakland, CA: American Cancer Society, California Division; September 1978.

64. Bloom JR, Hoppe RT, Fobair P, Cox RS, Varghese A, Spiegel D. Effects of treatment on the work experience of long-term survivors of Hodgkin's disease. *J Psychosoc Oncol.* 1988; 6 (3/4):65–80.

65. Feldman FL. Wellness and work. In: Cooper CL, ed. *Psychosocial Stress and Cancer.* New York: Wiley; 1984: 173–200.

66. Hoffman B. Employment discrimination against cancer survivors: multidisciplinary interventions. *Health Matrix.* 1989; 7(1):2–10.

67. Feldman FL. Inquiries into work experiences of recovered cancer patients: The California experience. In: Barofsky I, ed. *Work and Illness: The Cancer Patient.* New York: Praeger; 1989: 25–47.

68. Mellette SJ, Franco PC. Psychosocial barriers to employment of the cancer survivor. *J Psychosoc Oncol.* 1987; 5(4):97–115.

69. Vocational Insurance Committee. *A Study of Discrimination Towards Patients by Insurer, Employer, and Vocational Rehabilitation Agencies.* Rochester, MN: Mayo Clinic Rehabilitation Program; 1977.

70. Arline v. School Board of Nassau County. 480 U.S. 273, 1987.

71. Wingard JR, Curbow B, Baker F, Piantadosi S. Health, functional status, and employment of adult survivors of bone marrow transplantation. *Ann Intern Med.* 1991; 114: 113–118.

72. van Loden J. The Netherlands: Dutch health care—a study in purple. *Lancet.* 1996; 347:1229–1231.

73. Schmidt GM, Niland JC, Forman SJ, et al. Extended follow-up in 212 long-term allogeneic bone marrow transplant survivors. *Transplantation.* 1993; 55:551–557.

74. Kornblith AB, Anderson J, Cella DF, et al. Quality of life assessment of Hodgkin's disease survivors: a model for cooperative clinical trials. *Oncology.* 1990; 4 (5): 93–101.

75. Omne-Ponten M, Holmberg L, Sjoden PO. Psychosocial adjustment among women with breast cancer stages I and II: six year follow-up of consecutive patients. *J Clin Oncol.* 1994; 12:1778–1782.

76. Rapoport Y, Kreitler S, Chaitchik S, Algor R, Weissler K. Psychosocial problems in head-and-neck cancer patients and their change with time since diagnosis. *Ann Oncol.* 1993; 4:69–73.

77. Andrykowski MA, Altmaier EM, Barnett RL, Burish TG, Gingrich R, Henslee-Downey PJ. Cognitive dysfunction in adult survivors of allogeneic marrow transplantation: relationship to dose of total body irradiation. *Bone Marrow Transplant.* 1990; 6:269–276.

78. Kornblith AB, Anderson J, Cella DF, et al. Comparison of psychosocial adaptation and sexual function of survivors of advanced Hodgkin's disease treated by MOPP, ABVD, or MOPP alternating with ABVD. *Cancer.* 1992; 70: 2508–2516.

79. Vose JM, Kennedy BC, Bierman PJ, Kessinger A, Armitage JO. Long-term sequelae of autologous bone marrow or peripheral stem cell transplantation for lymphoid malignancies. *Cancer.* 1992; 69:784–789.

80. Moadel AB, Ostroff JS, Lesko LM, Bajorunas DB. Psychosexual adjustment among women receiving hormone replacement therapy for premature menopause following cancer treatment. *Psycho-Oncology.* 1995; 4:273–282.

81. Rieker PP, Fitzgerald EM, Kalish LA. Adaptive behavioral responses to potential infertility among survivors of testis cancer. *J Clin Oncol.* 1990; 8:347–355.

82. Longo DL, Young RC, Wesley M, et al. Twenty years of MOPP therapy for Hodgkin's disease. *J Clin Oncol.* 1986; 4:1295–1306.

83. Kornblith AB, Herndon J, Zuckerman E, et al. Comparison of long-term psychosocial adaptation of Hodgkin's disease and acute leukemia survivors [meeting abstract]. *Proc Am Soc Clin Oncol.* 1996; 15(1631):508.

84. Viviani S, Santoro A, Ragni G, Bonfante V, Bestetti O, Bonadonna G. Gonadal toxicity after combination chemotherapy for Hodgkin's disease. Comparative results of MOPP vs ABVD. *Eur J Cancer Clin Oncol.* 1985; 21:601–605.

85. Bookman MA, Longo DL. Concomitant illness in patients treated for Hodgkin's disease. *Cancer Treat Rev.* 1986, 13:77–111.

86. Aass N, Fossa SD, Raghavan D, Vogelzang NJ. Late toxicity after chemotherapy of testis cancer. In: Vogelzang NJ, Scardino PT, Shipley WU, Coffey DS, eds. *Comprehensive Textbook of Genitourinary Oncology.* Baltimore, MD: Williams & Wilkins; 1996: 1090–1096.

87. Gritz ER, Wellisch DK, Wang HJ, Siau J, Landsverk JA, Cosgrove MD. Long-term effects of testicular cancer on sexual functioning in married couples. *Cancer.* 1989; 64:1560–1567.

88. Negrin RS, Blume KG. Bone marrow and peripheral blood progenitor cell transplantation. In: Henderson ES, Lister TA, Greaves MF, eds. *Leukemia,* 6th ed. Baltimore, MD: W.B. Saunders; 1996: 389–418.

89. Sanders JE and the Seattle Marrow Transplant Team. The impact of marrow transplant preparative regimens on subsequent growth and development. *Semin Hematol.* 1991; 28:244–249.

90. Altmaier EM, Gingrich RD, Fyfe MA. Two-year adjustment of bone marrow transplant survivors. *Bone Marrow Transplant.* 1991; 7:311–316.

91. Kemeny MM, Wellisch DK, Schain WS. Psychosocial outcome in a randomized surgical trial for treatment of primary breast cancer. *Cancer.* 1988; 62:1231–1237.

92. Bines J, Oleske DM, Cobleigh MA. Ovarian function in premenopausal women treated with adjuvant chemotherapy for breast cancer. *J Clin Oncol.* 1996; 14:1718–1729.

93. Dirksen SR. Perceived well-being in malignant melanoma survivors. *Oncol Nurs Forum.* 1989; 16:353–358.

94. Andrykowski MA, Henslee PJ, Farrall MG. Physical and psychosocial functioning of adult survivors of allogeneic bone marrow transplantation. *Bone Marrow Transplant.* 1989; 4:75–81.

95. Carpenter PJ, Morrow GR, Schmale AH. The psychosocial status of cancer patients after cessation of treatment. *J Psychosoc Oncol.* 1989; 7 (1/2):95–103.

96. MacDonald LD, Anderson HR. Stigma in patients with rectal cancer: a community study. *J Epidemiol Commun Health.* 1984; 38:284–290.

97. Andersen BL. Psychological interventions for cancer patients to enhance the quality of life. *J Consult Clin Psychol.* 1992; 60:552–568.

98. Fawzy FI, Fawzy NW, Arndt LA, Pasnau RO. Critical review of psychosocial interventions in cancer care. *Arch Gen Psychiatry.* 1995; 52:100–113.

99. Meyer TJ, Mark MM. Effects of psychosocial interventions with adult cancer patients: a meta-analysis of randomized experiments. *Health Psychol.* 1995; 14:101–108.

100. Leigh S, Logan C. The cancer survivorship movement. *Cancer Invest.* 1991; 9:571–579.

101. Lieberman MA. The role of self-help groups in helping patients and families cope with cancer. *CA-A Cancer J Clinic.* 1988; 38:163–168.

102. Mullan F, Hoffman B, eds. *Charting the Journey: An Almanac of Practical Resources for Cancer Survivors.* Mt. Vernon, NY: Consumers Union; 1990.

103. Zampini K, Ostroff JS. The Post-Treatment Resource Program: portrait of a program for cancer survivors. *Psycho-Oncology.* 1993; 2:1–9.

104. Andersen BL. Surviving cancer. *Cancer.* 1994; 74:1484–1495.

105. Worden JW, Weisman AD. Preventive psychosocial intervention with newly diagnosed cancer patients. *Gen Hosp Psychiatry.* 1984; 6:243–249.

106. Leigh S. Cancer survivorship: a consumer movement. *Semin Oncol.* 1994; 21:783–786.

107. Burnam MA, Wells KB, Leake B, Landsverk J. Development of a brief screening instrument for detecting depressive disorders. *Med Care.* 1988; 26:775–789.

108. Shrout PE, Dohrenwend BP, Levav IA. Discriminant rule for screening cases of diverse diagnostic types: preliminary results. *J Consult Clin Psychol.* 1986; 54:314–319.

109. Polinsky ML, Fred C, Ganz PA. Quantitative and qualitative assessment of a case management program for cancer patients. *Health Soc Work.* 1991; 16:176–183.

110. Bishop D, Evans R, Maynard P, et al. *Family Intervention: Telephone Tracking (FITT).* Family Research Program, Providence, RI: Brown University; June 1993.

111. Frasure-Smith N, Price R. The ischemic heart disease life stress monitoring program: impact on mortality. *Psychosom Med.* 1985; 47:431–444.

112. Kornblith AB, Thaler HT, Wong G, et al. Quality of life of women with ovarian cancer. *Gynecol Oncol.* 1995; 59:231–242.

113. Spitzer RL, Williams JBW, Kroenke K, et al. Utility of a new procedure for diagnosing mental disorders in primary care. *J Am Med Assoc.* 1994; 272:1749–1756.

114. Mastrovito R, Moynihan R, Parsonnet L. Self-help and mutual support programs. In: Holland JC, Rowland JH, eds. *Handbook of Psychooncology: Psychological Care of the Patient with Cancer.* New York: Oxford; 1989: 502–507.

115. Birtchnell J. Art therapy as a form of psychotherapy. In: Dalley T, ed. *Art as Therapy: An Introduction to the Use of Art as a Therapeutic Technique.* London: Tavistock Publications; 1984: 30–44.

116. Wadeson H. *The Dynamics of Art Psychotherapy.* New York: Wiley; 1987.

117. Dohrenwend BS, Dohrenwend BP. Life stress and illness: formulation of the issues. In: Dohrenwend BS, Dohrenwend BP, eds. *Stressful Life Events and Their Contexts.* New York: Prodist; 1981: 1–27.

118. Holahan CJ, Moos RH. Life stressors and mental health: advances in conceptualizing stress resistance. In: Avison WR, Gotlib IH, eds. *Stress and Mental Health: Contemporary Issues and Prospects for the Future.* New York: Plenum Press; 1994: 213–238.

119. Cohen S, Syme SL. Issues in the study and application of social support. In: Cohen S, Syme SL, eds. *Social Support and Health.* Orlando, FL: Academic Press; 1985: 3–22.

120. Rook KS. The negative side of social interaction: impact on psychological well-being. *J Pers Soc Psychol.* 1984; 46:1097–1108.

121. Goffman E. *Stigma: Notes on the Management of Spoiled Identity.* Englewood Cliffs, NJ: Prentice-Hall; 1963.

122. Rodin J. Personal control through the life course. In: Abeles RP, ed. *Life-Span Perspectives and Social Psychology.* Hillsdale, NJ: Lawrence Erlbaum Associates; 1987:103–119.

123. Taylor SE. Adjustment to threatening events: a theory of cognitive adaptation. *Am Psychol.* 1983; 38:1161–1173.

124. Thompson SC, Collins MA. Applications of perceived control to cancer: an overview of theory and measurement. *J Psychosoc Oncol.* 1995; 13 (1/2):11–26.

125. Weinstein ND. Testing four competing theories of health-protective behavior. *Health Psychol.* 1993; 12:324–333.

126. Basic Behavioral Science Task Force. Basic behavioral science research for mental health: vulnerability and resilience. *Am Psychol.* 1996; 51:22–28.

TABLE 20.1. *Psychosocial Adaptation of Adult Cancer Survivors: Review of the Literature*

Disease Site/Study (Ref.)	Research Design	Sample	Method	Time since Dx or Rx Frequency Assessment	Variables	Measures	Major Results
BREAST							
Carter, 1993 (58)	Cross-sectional survivor cohort	25 breast	In-person interview; qualitative descriptive analysis	10.6 yr post-Dx (mean); 5-26 yrs [range]; single assessment	Impact of cancer on psychosocial adjustment; cancer-related beliefs	SSIG	1. "Going through", a phased, nonlinear survival process; *(1)* interpreting Dx and how it will affect their lives; *(2)* confronting mortality; *(3)* reprioritizing values; *(4)* coming to terms with cancer, including acceptance *(5)* moving on, putting cancer behind them; *(6)* flashbacks of cancer experience, with reintegration with current life.
Cordova et al., 1995 (35)	Cross-sectional survivor cohort	55 breast/ 96% stage I/II	Telephone interview	2.5 yr post-Rx (mean); 0.5-5 yr (range)	Post-traumatic stress disorder (PTSD); QOL	PCL-C; MOS-20; IES	1. 5%–10% would likely meet DSM-IV PTSD diagnostic criteria.
Craig et al., 1974 (16)	Cross-sectional survivor cohort with 2 matched comp. gr. (a) age and gender pop.; (b) neighborhood	134 breast/260 comp. gr. (139: pop.; 121: neighborhood)	Mailed Q + census data	Most 5 + yr post-Dx; single assessment	Psychosocial function; socio-demographic and SES; Physical health	Q developed by authors	1. No significant difference between survivors and comp. gr. in their SES, sociodemographic status, physical disability, and psychosocial function.
Kemeny et al., 1988 (91)	Randomized clinical trial; mastectomy vs. BCT	52 breast/ stage I/II	Mailed Q	2.3 yr post-surgery (mean); 0.5-4.0 yr (range); assessed twice	Psychological state; impact of surgery on psychological, marital, social, sexual function and body image	BSI; impact of surgery items developed by authors	1. At 1.5 yr post surgery (mean), significantly greater cancer-rel psychological distress, worse body image and greater fear of recurrence in mastectomy than BCT patients. 2. No significant difference between mastectomy and BCT groups in general psychological distress at 2.3 yr (mean) post surgery (BSI), or sexual function at 1.5 yr (mean) post surgery.
Kennedy et al., 1976 (59)	Cross-sectional survivor cohort + 3 comp. gr: college students, diabetics, noncancer patients in cancer detection program	22 mixed/ advanced disease; (59% testis; 14% breast; 18% lymph; 9% endometrial) comp. gr. 597 college; 26 diabetics; 131 cancer detection program	Taped interview + Q	9.1 yr post-Rx (mean); 5–21 yr (range)	Personality traits; impact of cancer on psychological, vocational function, values and health beliefs	Differential personality Q; SD	1. Most survivors reported positive attitudes and value changes as a result of having cancer, becoming more tolerant and appreciative of life, and continued to lead their regular life 2. Survivors valued time significantly more than all other groups (SD)

Reference	Study design	Sample	Method	Timing	Outcomes assessed	Measures	Results
Lasry et al., 1987 (32)	Randomized clinical trial (NSABP): mastectomy vs. BCT + RT vs. BCT without RT.	123 breast/non-met; patients living in Montreal only	Q	3.4 yr post-surgery (mean); 1–9 yr (range); single assessment	Depression; body image	CES-D; body image items developed by authors	1. 50% mast, 50% BCT + RT, 41% BCT without RT had CES-D scores of 15+, consistent with clinical depression. No significant differences in depression among the 3 groups 2. Mast patients had significantly worse body image than BCT + RT and BCT without RT groups
Meyer and Aspegren, 1989 (38)	Cross-sectional survivor cohort, 5 yr post-mastectomy or BCT	58 breast/stage I: (52% mast; 48% BCT)	In-person interview + Q	5 yr post-Rx; single assessment	Psychiatric and social adjustment; impact of surgery on physical symptoms, psychosocial adjustment and sexual function	Psychiatric clinical interview; Dependency items based on CPRS; anxiety and phobia items developed by Meyer	1. No significant difference between mastectomy and BCT in psychiatric state or marital adjustment. However, 28% showed clinical signs of psychiatric problems 2. Mast patients were significantly more socially isolated, avoided activities requiring exposure of body, and felt greater negative impact on female identity, than BCT patients 3. 33% of all patients had problems in sexual adaptation
Morris et al., 1977 (15)	Prospective, longitudinal study of breast cancer patients with mastectomy vs. those with benign breast disease	69 breast/early stage; 92% with mastectomy; 91 benign breast disease	In-person interview	Followed-up 2 yr post-surgery; assessed at baseline, 3, 12, 24 mo	Psychosocial adjustment; personality traits; impact of cancer and mastectomy on psychosocial adjustment	HDRS; Eysenck Personality Inventory; marital, sexual, social adjustment items developed by authors	1. At 24 mo, 22% of breast cancer patients had depression, scoring 10+ on HDRS, vs. 8% benign disease patients 2. No significant differences in marital and sexual adjustment between the 2 groups 3. By 24 mo, 71% of breast cancer patients had returned to preoperative vocational function, up from 54% at 3 mo 4. Breast cancer patients scoring high on Neuroticism [Eysenck] at baseline, were significantly likely to be depressed at 24 mo (HDRS)
Omne-Ponten et al., 1994 (75)	Prospective longitudinal study of patients having mastectomy vs. BCT	66 breast, at 6 yr follow-up/23% with recurrence stage I/II (61% mastectomy; 39% BCT)	In-person interview, at home	6 yr post-primary Rx (median); 5.8–8.1 yr (range); assessed at 4 mo, 13 mo, 6 yr post-Rx	Psychosocial adjustment; personality traits	SAS; Eysenck Personality; items developed by authors	1. No significant differences in psychosocial adjustment between mastectomy and BCT patients (SAS) 2. Overall maladjustment decreased over time; 27% had suboptimal to poor adjustment

(continued)

TABLE 20.1. *Psychosocial Adaptation of Adult Cancer Survivors: Review of the Literature — Continued*

Disease Site/Study (Ref.)	Research Design	Sample	Method	Time since Dx or Rx Frequency Assessment	Variables	Measures	Major Results
Polinsky, 1994 (23)	Cross-sectional survivor cohort	223 breast/Reach to Recovery volunteers (86% mastectomy; 14% BCT)	Mailed Q	8 yr post-surgery (mean); 1.3–32 yr (range); single assessment	Psychosocial adjustment; physical health; cond. n & v; impact of cancer on psychosocial adjustment, sexual function, body image, insurance and employment	POMS; MOS-20; BCSM	1. Minimal overall mood disturbance (POMS), but 64% reported anxiety about cancer 2. Little impact of cancer on social function (MOS), but felt that family members (43%) and friends (55%) did not understand them well enough 3. Persistent Rx-related problems: cond n & v (39%); surgery-related numbness (66%), pain (39%), and swelling (34%) in arm. 4. Scar-related body image problems (55%) 5. Dissatisfaction with frequency of sexual activity for those sexually active (44%)
Schottenfeld and Robbins, 1970 (61)	Cross-sectional survivor cohort, randomly selected from tumor registry	636 breast/primary operable breast cancer treated by radical mastectomy	Mailed Q	5–15 yr post-Rx; single assessment	Performance status; employment; mortality	Karnofsky Performance Status adapted for patient-rating by authors	1. 93% had resumed normal daily activities within 12 months 2. Of those previously employed, 19% were unable to work 5 yr post-Rx, and 3% at 10 yr post-Rx 3. Significantly worse performance status in those with regional than local disease at 5 yr post-Rx; no significant differences at 10 and 15 yr post-Rx
Schover et al., 1995 (42)	Cross-sectional; patients who had breast reconstruction vs. BCT	218 breast/99% stage 0–II (67% breast reconstruction; 33% BCT)	Mailed Q	4.1 yr post-surgery (mean); 0.4–9.5 yr (range); single assessment	Impact of cancer on psychosocial adjustment, sexual function, fertility, and body image	PAIS; Sex History Form; sexual attractiveness subscale of the BES	1. No significant differences in psychosocial adjustment (PAIS), body image (BES), or sexual function (Sex History Form) between breast reconstruction and BCT patients 2. <20% of all patients reported poor adjustment, across all measures 3. Greater maladjustment in younger patients and those who had chemotherapy (PAIS)

Study	Design	Sample	Data collection	Constructs	Timing	Measures	Findings
Sneeuw et al., 1992 (33)	Cross-sectional survivor cohort; patients who had BCT	76 breast/early stage	In-person interview at home + observer ratings in clinic	2 yr post-Rx (mean); 2–11 yr (range); single assessment	Psychosocial adjustment; physical function; impact of surgery on psychological, sexual function and body image; cosmetic and functional outcomes of BCT	GHQ-28; impact of surgery on psychological sexual function and body image items developed by Aaronson; cosmetic and functional results of BCT items developed by author	1. Problems reported: body image (c. 25%); greatly decreased frequency of sexual activity (64%); greatly decreased sexual enjoyment (20%); fear of recurrence (42%) 2. Breast cosmetic results significantly correlated with body image ($r = 0.48$). Survivors dissatisfied with breast cosmetic results were significantly more likely to report psychological (GHQ) and marital problems 3. As time since Rx increased, problems with body image, sexual and marital function worsened
Wellisch et al., 1989 (48)	Cross-sectional; patients who had mastectomy with reconstruction, mastectomy without reconstruction, and BCT	50 breast/stage I/II; (30%: mastectomy with reconstruction; 26% mastectomy without reconstruction; 44%: BCT)	Mailed Q	1.75 yr post-surgery (mean); 1–3 yr (range); single assessment	Psychosocial adjustment and sexual function; body image	Q for patients who have undergone breast surgery developed by authors; BSI	1. BCT patients had significantly better body image and felt more sexually desirable than mast patients with or without reconstruction 2. BCT patients retrospectively reported feeling significantly more attractive than those who had mastectomy without reconstruction at 6 mo post surgery; no significant differences between groups at current assessment 3. No significant differences between groups in current psych distress (BSI) or sexual function
HEAD AND NECK Baker, 1992 (49)	Cross-sectional survivor cohort	51 H&N	Q + observer rated measures	1.9 yr post-Rx (mean); 0.6–5 yr (range); single assessment	Impact of cancer on physical function and psychosocial adjustment; facial disfigurement; H&N related dysfunction; social support	SIP; PRQ (Part 2); severity of disfigurement; ladder of H&N dysfunction items developed by author (LD)	1. H&N-related dysfunction (LD) significantly related to physical function and psychosocial adjustment (SIP) 2. As perceived social support (PRQ) increased survivors' psychosocial adjustment (SIP) improved 3. Severity of facial disfigurement did not significantly relate to psychosocial adjustment (SIP)
Rapoport et al., 1993 (76)	Cross-sectional survivor cohort	55 H&N/29 partners (53% spouse; 20% child; 27% relatives and friends)	In-person interview + observer ratings	4.3 yr post-Dx (mean); 0.5–21 yr (range); single assessment	Impact of cancer on psychosocial adjustment; partner's report of patient's adjustment; psychological state	PAQ; MAACL; STPI-Anxiety, Anger	1. Most pervasive problems were communication with partner, family and social function 2. As time since Dx increased: (a) coping with health and Rx-related problems significantly improved; (b) communication with partner, sexual and social functioning significantly worsened; (c) anxiety and anger significantly increased (PAQ)

(continued)

TABLE 20.1. *Psychosocial Adaptation of Adult Cancer Survivors: Review of the Literature — Continued*

Disease Site/Study (Ref.)	Research Design	Sample	Method	Time since Dx or Rx Frequency Assessment	Variables	Measures	Major Results
LEUKEMIA Greenberg et al., 1995 (21)	Cross-sectional survivor cohort; all previously treated on CALGB protocols	206 ALL, AML	Telephone interviews	5.6 yr post-Rx (mean); 1–17 yr (range); single assessment	Psychosocial adjustment and sexual function; impact of cancer on SES, employment, insurance; cond. n & v; family functioning	BSI; POMS; PAIS; IES; Derogatis Body Image; FFS; cond. n & v; employment and insurance indices; negative SES impact; MHLC	1. 14% reported psychological distress 1.5 s.d. above non-patient norms (BSI) 2. Range of problems: employment (31%); insurance (56%); negative SES impact (39%); decreased sexual satisfaction (25%) 3. Greatest distress (BSI) in those younger, less educated with anticipatory distress at time of Rx, poorer family function + medical problems post-Rx
Lesko et al., 1992 (22)	Cross-sectional; chemotherapy vs. ABMT survivors	70 acute leukemia (49 chemotherapy; 21 ABMT)	In-person and telephone interview + Q	5 yr post-Rx (mean); 3.1 yr (s.d.); single assessment	Psychosocial adjustment; perceived Rx-related physical problems	BSI; IES; SAS; medical sequelae Q	1. No significant differences in psychological and social function between chemotherapy and ABMT survivors 2. Psychological distress of total group was 0.5–1.0 s.d. above non-patient norms (BSI); 31% exceeded cutoff suggestive of psychiatric disorder 3. Women reported heightened level of family disruption. Men had greater vocational problems and disruption in parenting (SAS) 4. Greatest distress (BSI) in men with better education; greater social maladjustment (SAS) in women who had BMT and better education
Mumma et al., 1992 (51)	Same as Lesko et al., 1992 (22)	Same as Lesko et al., 1992 (22)	Same as Lesko et al., 1992 (22)	Same as Lesko et al., 1992 (22)	Sexual function	DSFI; PAIS	1. No significant differences in psychosexual function between chemotherapy and ABMT survivors 2. Significantly poorer body image in total group than physically healthy norms (DSFI) 3. Significantly less sexual drive and sexual satisfaction among women survivors than physically healthy norms (DSFI)
Wellisch et al., 1996 (30)	Cross-sectional survivor cohort of ABMT vs. conventional chemotherapy	30 AML (37% ABMT; 63% conventional chemotherapy)	Mailed Q	6 yr post-Dx (mean)	Impact of cancer on psychosocial and sexual adjustment; psychological state; physical health and health care utilization	CARES; BSI; CES-D; current health status Q developed by authors	1. No significant differences between ABMT and conventional chemotherapy survivors in psychological distress (BSI, CES-D) and overall psychosocial and sexual adjustment (CARES) 2. 17% exceeded cutoff on CES-D suggestive of psychiatric disorder of depression

	Design	Sample	Method	Time since Dx/Rx	Variables	Measures	Findings
BMT Andrykowski et al., 1990 (77)	Cross-sectional survivor cohort	30 ABMT (ALL, AML, CML)	Mailed Q	3.9 yr post-BMT (mean); 1–8 yr (range); single assessment	Cognitive function, impact of cancer on physical function and psychosocial adjustment	POMS; PAIS; SIP	1. Dose of total body irradiation was significantly related to greater dysfunction on SIP Alertness Behavior Subscale. Areas affected: slowed reaction time, reduced attention span and concentration, difficulties reasoning and problem solving
LYMPHOMA Devlen et al., 1987 (28)	Cross-sectional survivor cohort	90 HD + NHL	In-person interview at home	2.7 yr post-Dx (mean) 0.5–6 yr (range); single assessment	Psychiatric disorder; social function; Rx-related physical problems	PSE; social interview schedule; toxicity rating scales developed by authors	1. 22% retrospectively diagnosed with depression and/or anxiety at Dx; an additional 29% had borderline depression and/or anxiety. At interview: 2% diagnosed with depression and/or anxiety & 12% with borderline depression and/or anxiety. 2. Problems reported: restriction in leisure activities (29%); fatigue (34%), loss of libido in those with active sex lives (25%); impaired thinking/short-term memory (33%).
HODGKIN'S Carpenter et al., 1989 (95)	Cross-sectional survivor cohort divided into: ≤ 2 yr and 2 yr + since Rx	43: HD/Stage I,II; all had RT; (35% ≤ 2 yr; 65% 2 yr +)	Q + in-person interview	4.7 yr post-Rx (mean); 0.5–13 yr (range); single assessment	Psychosocial adjustment; impact of cancer on psychosocial adjustment, family functioning and physical health; health care system attitudes	BDS; BPS; PAIS; SCL-90; STAI; Kaufmann Hostility Scale; items developed by authors	1. No significant effect of time since Rx completion on depression (BDS), anxiety (STAI), pessimism (BPS) and overall adjustment (PAIS) 2. Survivors completing Rx 2 yr + reported greater obsessive-compulsivity, phobic anxiety and interpersonal sensitivity (SCL-90) and rated MDs as significantly more difficult to find & less concerned about them than survivors completing Rx ≤ 2 yr 3. Survivors completing Rx 2 yr + reported significantly better vocational function than survivors completing Rx ≤ 2 yr (PAIS)
Cella and Tross, 1986 (12)	Cross-sectional survivor cohort with age-matched comp gr	60 HD men; 20 healthy male friends	Interview + Q + projective tests	2 yr post-Rx completion (median); 0.5–11.7 yr (range); single assessment	Psychosocial adjustment and sexual function; impact of cancer on physical health, psychosocial adjustment and finances	BSI; DSFI; IES; Rosenberg Self-Esteem Scale; DAQ; Problem-Oriented Record; TAT	1. No significant difference in psychological distress (BSI), DSFI, or self-esteem between survivors and healthy men 2. Significantly fewer hours worked and more avoidant thoughts concerning HD for survivors than healthy men (IES) 3. Greater death anxiety in those off Rx ≤ 2 yr vs. 2.5 yr + (DAQ) 4. HD survivor problems: somatic anxiety (67%), energy level (57%), sleep (27%), concentration (27%); infertility in those tested (91%) *(continued)*

TABLE 20.1. *Psychosocial Adaptation of Adult Cancer Survivors: Review of the Literature — Continued*

Disease Site/Study (Ref.)	Research Design	Sample	Method	Time since Dx or Rx Frequency Assessment	Variables	Measures	Major Results
Fobair et al., 1986 (29)	Cross-sectional survivor cohort	403 HD (stage I/II 60%; III/IV 40%)	Interview + Q administered in clinic	9 yr post-Rx (mean); 1–21 yr (range); single assessment	Psychological state; impact of cancer on physical health, psychosocial adjustment and sexual function	Interview developed by authors; CES-D	1. Energy level not returned to normal in 37% 2. 18% had scores consistent with clinical depression (CES-D) 3. Problems due to HD: denial of insurance (11%); less sexual activity (20%); infertility (19%); decreased physical attractiveness (26%); less vocational ambition (19%)
Kornblith et al., 1992 (20)	Cross-sectional survivor cohort	273 HD/all stage III/IV; all previously treated on CALGB protocols	Telephone interview	6.3 yr post-Rx (mean); 1–20 yr (range); single assessment	Psychosocial adjustment; impact of cancer on psychosocial adjustment, sexual function, fertility, SES, employment, insurance; cond n & v	BSI; POMS; PAIS; IES; cond n & v; sexual, employment and insurance problems indices; negative SES impact	1. Mean level of psychological distress 1 s.d. above healthy norms for both men and women; 22% exceeded cutoff suggestive of psychiatric disorder (BSI) 2. Problems due to HD: denial of life (31%) and health insurance (22%), cond n & v (39%), sexual function (37%), negative SES impact (36%) 3. Those at high risk for distress (BSI): men, income <$15,000/yr, less education, unemployed, not married, serious illnesses since end of Rx.
Kornblith et al., 1992 (78)	Cross-sectional survivor cohort; all treated on 1 CALGB protocol 8251: MOPP vs. ABVD vs. MOPP/ABVD	93 HD/all stage III/IV	Telephone interview	2.2 yr post-Rx (mean); 1–5 yr (range); single assessment	Same as Kornblith et al., 1992 (20)	Same as Kornblith et al., 1992 (20)	1. No significant differences in survivors' psychosocial adjustment or sexual function between the 3 Rx regimens MOPP, ABVD, and MOPP/ABVD
van Tulder et al., 1994 (14)	Cross-sectional survivor cohort with age-matched comp. gr.	81 HD/114 hospital visitors	Mailed Q	14 yr post-Rx (mean); 10–18 yr (range); single assessment	Psychosocial and sexual adjustment; physical function; impact of cancer on employment, insurance, obtaining mortge	MOS-SF-36; Maudsley Marital Q	1. No significant differences between survivors and comp. gr. in: psychological distress, social function, pain, vitality, intimacy, employment, obtaining health insurance (MOS-SF-36; Maudsley Marital Q) 2. Significantly worse physical function, fewer hours worked, worse sexual function and greater problems in obtaining life insurance in survivors than comp. gr. (MOS-SF-36, Maudsley Marital Q)
MELANOMA Dirksen, 1989 (93)	Cross-sectional survivor cohort	31 melanoma	Q	9 yr post-Dx (mean); 5–14 yr (range); single assessment	Locus of control; social support; self-esteem; life satisfaction	CHLC; Norbeck Social Support Q; SEI; IWB	1. Survivors most satisfied with their life (IWB) had significantly greater internal locus of control (CHLC), better self-esteem (SEI), fewer chronic illnesses, and had received immunotherapy + vitamin A 2. Social support indirectly improved life satisfaction (IWB) by improving self-esteem (SEI)

Study	Design	Sample	Method	Time	Focus	Measures	Findings
SARCOMA Sugarbaker et al., 1982 (50)	Prospective, longitudinal assessment; randomized clinical trial: amputation + chemotherapy vs. limb-sparing + RT + chemotherapy	26 extremity soft tissue sarcoma (35% amputation; 65% limb-sparing)	In-person interview + Q + observer-rated measures	1–3 yr post-Rx (range); two assessments	Impact of cancer on physical health and function; psychosocial adjustment, and SES	SIP; PAIS; Katz Activities of Daily Living Scale; Bartel Function Scale; Pain, mobility and Rx trauma; sexual function items developed by authors	1. No substantial differences in psychosocial adjustment, physical function, or economic impact of Rx between the 2 groups 2. Significantly poorer sexual function in limb-spared than amputation patients (PAIS)
TESTIS Gritz et al., 1988 (34)	Cross-sectional survivor cohort	88 testis	In-person interview; most at home	3.8 yr post-Rx (mean); 1–7.5 yr (range); single assessment	Psychological state; impact of cancer on physical, psychological, sexual function	POMS; FES; CES-D; Social Activities Scale; Social and Emotional Support Scale; Orientation to Life Scale; testicular cancer knowledge and beliefs	1. 18% had energy level that had not returned to normal 2. 18% scored above cutoff score suggestive of major depression on CES-D 3. Curvilinear relation of cancer-related distress and psychological distress with time, with current distress returning to pre-Dx levels 4. Increase in sexual dysfunction over time from pre-Dx levels
Gritz et al., 1989 (87)	Cross-sectional survivor cohort + spouse	34 testis + spouse	Same as Gritz et al., 1988 (34)	4 yr post-Rx (mean); single assessment	Sexual function and fertility of survivors and spouse	Same as Gritz et al., 1988 (34)	1. Concordance between survivors and spouse on sexual function and fertility ranged from 60% to 94%, including inability to ejaculate (91%), frequency of intercourse (62%), infertility causing a problem (94%), loss of sexual drive (67%) and worsening sexual attractiveness (62%)
Rieker et al., 1989 (17)	Cross-sectional survivor cohort with age-matched comp. gr.	223 testis/120 healthy men	Q	2–5 yr post-Dx (median); single assessment	Psychological state; impact of cancer on physical function, psychosocial adjustment and sexual function	POMS; CES; CPBS; Self-Report Q	1. Less psychological distress in survivors than comp. gr. (POMS) 2. Greater infertility and sexual performance distress in survivors than comp. gr.; desire distress equal in both groups 3. Greatest infertility and sexual performance distress in survivors with advanced disease and RPLND
Rieker et al., 1990 (81)	Cross-sectional survivor cohort	153 testis	Q	5.1 yr post-Dx (mean); single assessment	Psychosocial issues of infertility	POMS; CES; CPBS; Self-Report Q	1. Greatest infertility distress in those who were childless, had post-Rx ejaculatory dysfunction, and had RPLND 2. Greatest interest in banking sperm in survivors ≤35 yr at Dx, childless, college educated, with strained relationships

(continued)

TABLE 20.1. *Psychosocial Adaptation of Adult Cancer Survivors: Review of the Literature — Continued*

Disease Site/Study (Ref.)	Research Design	Sample	Method	Time since Dx or Rx Frequency Assessment	Variables	Measures	Major Results
MIXED							
Alter et al., 1996 (27)	Cross-sectional survivor cohort vs. healthy comp. gr.	27 mixed/all women; (81% breast; 19% other); 27 comp. gr.	In-person interview at home or clinic + Q	4.6 yr post-Rx (mean); 1.7 yr (s.d.)	Post-traumatic stress disorder (PTSD); psychological distress	PTSD module of SCID; SCL-90	1. 4% of survivors vs. none of comp. gr. met criteria for current PTSD 2. Survivors had significantly greater levels of PTSD symptoms of reexperience, avoidance, and arousal than comp. gr.
Feldman, 1976, 1978 (62,63)	Cross-sectional cohort	203 mixed/all employed at Dx; (breast, H&N, colorectal; 45% white-collar (WC); 55% blue-collar (BC)) + 101 employers, 37 MDs, 13 union representatives	Q + in-person interview of patients; in-person interview of employers and union reps.; telephone interview of MDs	1.5–2.5 yr post-Dx (range); single assessment	Impact of cancer on vocational function; employer and union attitudes and practices; MD role in patients' vocational function	Interview developed by author	1. 90% WC and 82% BC patients were currently employed; 71% WC and 58% BC remained with precancer employer. Unemployment in most BC patients due to physical limitations from cancer 2. Nearly two-thirds reported some positive impact of cancer on work life. 55% WC and 84% BC patients reported negative impact. 38% WC and 45% BC reported instances of job discrimination due to cancer 3. BC survivors reported "pervasive fear" of medical costs and need for health insurance, causing some to stay in jobs they were not able to perform due to cancer
Greaves-Otte et al., 1991 (18)	Cross-sectional survivor cohort from Netherlands	649 mixed (33% breast; 24% GYN; 10% H&N; 33% other)	Mailed Q	7–9 yr post-Dx (range); single assessment	SES; psychological state; impact of cancer on physical health and function, social function, employment and insurance	Dutch health survey; ABS	1. Significantly greater psychological distress in survivors vs. Dutch norms (ABS) 2. 62% survivors had the same employment status at time of Dx. 22% survivors reported physical limitations and 13% were disabled or had retired due to cancer 3. 70% survivors who tried to take out insurance or modify existing policy met with problems (n = 100/142) 4. 50% survivors reported physical sequelae of cancer Rx
Halstead and Fernsler, 1994 (41)	Cross-sectional survivor cohort	59 mixed (51% breast; 10% melanoma; 12% lymph; 27% other)	Mailed Q	13.0 yr post-Dx (mean); 5–48 yr (range); single assessment	Coping strategies	JCS	1. 48% survivors reported changes in coping strategies since Dx. Strategies reported frequently and effectively used since Dx: optimistic thinking; greater use of social, emotional, and spiritual supports; greater use of problem-solving methods; distraction ("keeping busy") (JCS)

250

Study	Design	Sample	Method of assessment	Timing	Domains assessed	Measures	Findings
Moadel et al., 1995 (80)	Cross-sectional survivor cohort on hormone replacement therapy vs. comp. gr.	34 mixed (53% HD; 24% leukemia; 15% NHL; 8% other) 24 comp. gr., healthy premenopausal women	Survivors: in-person interview in private office Comp. gr: Telephone interview	6.5 yr post-Rx (mean); 0.67–16 yr (range)	Sexual function; menopausal symptoms; marital relationship; psychological distress	SHSI; DSFI; BSI; Dyadic Adjustment Scale; menopausal symptom checklist	1. 38% met DSM-IV criteria for sexual dysfunction: hypoactive sexual desire (32%), dyspareunia (15%), sexual arousal disorder (12%) (SHSI) 2. Significantly greater sexual dysfunction disorder (SHSI) ($p < 0.01$) and psychological distress (BSI) ($p < 0.05$) in hormone replacement therapy survivors than comp. gr.
Schag et al., 1994 (26)	Cross-sectional survivor cohorts, stratified by length of time from Dx: < 2 yrs, 2–5 yr, 5 yr +	278 mixed (42% colon; 37% prostate; 21% lung)	Q given to patient in clinic and returned by mail	3.4 yr post-Dx (mean); single assessment	Physical function; pyschosocial adjustment and sexual function; relationship with health care professionals	CARES; QOL linear analog scale	1. Length of time since Dx not significantly related to QOL in lung and colon survivors. QOL worsened in long-term prostate survivors owing to worsening health and marital relations (CARES) 2. Lung survivors reported more serious problems with physical function, pain, and marital relation than colon and prostate survivors (CARES) 3. Highly prevalent but less severe problems across all 3 groups: psychological distress, physical and sexual function (CARES)
MIXED/BMT Schmale et al., 1983 (13)	Cross-sectional survivor cohort with age, gender and education matched comp. gr.	104 mixed/104 health-matched comp. gr.	Q administered in clinic	3 yr post-Rx (mean) 1–8 yr (range); single assessment	Psychological status	GWB	1. No significant differences between survivors and comp. gr. in psychological distress or positive affect (GWB) 2. Significantly greater physical health concerns among survivors than comp. gr. (GWB)
Andrykowski et al., 1989 (94)	Cross-sectional survivor cohort	23 ABMT (78% ALL, AML, CML; 22% other)	Telephone or in-person interview + mailed Q	2.2 yr post-BMT (mean); 0.25–4.3 yr (range); single assessment	Psychosocial adjustment; physical symptoms and function	FLIC; POMS	1. Survivors <30 yr old at BMT had significantly better physical and social function and less nausea than those 30+ (FLIC)
Andrykowski et al., 1995 (52)	Cross-sectional survivor cohort	200 BMT/54% autologous; 46%: ABMT (24% AL; 22% CL; 26% HD; 28% NHL)	Mailed Q	3.4 yr post-BMT (mean); 1.0–10.6 yr (range); single assessment	Psychosocial adjustment; physical symptoms	POMS; PAIS; SIP; ROF; Perceived Health Q; SER	1. Functional areas survivors rated as not normal: employment (28%), vigorous physical activity (43%), sexual activity (31%) (ROF) 2. Significantly better vocational function and personal appearance (ROF) and less physical symptoms (SER) in autologous than ABMT survivors 3. Survivors who were older at BMT, less educated and were more recently treated, had significantly worse psychosocial adjustment (SIP, ROF, PAIS Sexual Rel subscale)

(continued)

TABLE 20.1. *Psychosocial Adaptation of Adult Cancer Survivors: Review of the Literature — Continued*

Disease Site/Study (Ref.)	Research Design	Sample	Method	Time since Dx or Rx Frequency Assessment	Variables	Measures	Major Results
Belec, 1992 (39)	Cross-sectional survivor cohort	24 BMT/96% ABMT (67% AML, CML, CLL; 17% NHL, HD; 17% other)	In-person interview + Q	1.9 yr post-BMT (mean); 1–3.2 yr (range); single assessment	Psychosocial adjustment; impact of BMT on psychosocial adjustment, physical health and values	Quality of Life Index (QLI); interview developed by author	1. BMT led to a positive impact on their lives, with a reassessment of priorities and values for 90% 2. Physical health was a major concern for 75%, with fears of recurrence and maintaining health. Half reported fatigue 3. 38% reported cancer had negative impact on employment
Bush et al., 1995 (24)	Cross-sectional survivor cohort	125 BMT/98% ABMT; (60% AL, CL; 34% AA; 6%: other)	Mailed Q	10.1 yr post-BMT (mean); 6–18.4 yr (range); single assessment	Physical symptoms and function; psychological and vocational status; impact of BMT on psychosocial adjustment; health perceptions	EORTC-QLQ-C30 + BMT module; Demands of Bone Marrow Recovery Inventory (DBMRI); POMS; Ware's Health Perceptions Q; Long-term Recovery Q	1. 74% reported same or better QOL as before BMT (DBMRI). Significantly less psychological distress in survivors than other cancer patient groups (POMS) 2. QOL declined over 10 yr post-BMT, followed by a return to normalcy (EORTC, POMS, DBMRI) 3. Most frequent reported problems: psychological distress (63%) and fatigue (56%) (EORTC) 4. 96% reported single most distressing hardship of survival was people being less supportive over time (DBMRI)
Curbow et al, 1993 (53)	Same as Wingard et al., 1992 (60)	Same as Wingard et al., 1992 (60)	Same as Wingard et al., 1992 (60)	Same as Wingard et al., 1992 (60)	Impact of BMT on psychosocial adjustment	Same as Wingard et al., 1992 (60)	1. 61% of life changes due to BMT were positive and 37% negative 2. Significantly more positive than negative changes in relationship and psychological domains. Significantly more negative than positive changes in physical domain 3. High number of positive changes protected those with high number of negative changes against dissatisfaction with future life
Schmidt et al., 1993 (73)	Cross-sectional adult + pediatric survivor cohort	162 adult ABMT (83% ALL, ANLL, CML; 17% AA, HD, MDS, other)	Telephone interview	3–4 yr post-BMT (median); 1–5 yr + (range); single assessment	Rx-related physical symptoms; vocational and marital status; body image; sexual function; overall QOL	Interview developed by authors	1. 74% had resumed full-time employment or school 2. Of those married at time of BMT, 83% remained married; 17% became separated or divorced (8/48) 3. 31% had chronic GVHD and 60% were on regular medication for physical problems

Reference	Study design	Sample	Method	Timing	Variables	Measures	Results
Syrjala et al., 1993	Prospective longitudinal assessment ABMT cohort	67 ABMT (91% ALL, ANLL, CML; 7% HD, NHL)	Q + telephone interview	4.5–6 yr post-BMT; assessed at baseline, 90 days, 1 yr 4.5–6 yr	Impact of cancer on physical function and psychosocial adjustment; psychological state; family function	SIP; BDS; BSI; FES; Ways of Coping Checklist	1. Significant worsening adjustment at 90 days, with most returning to baseline levels at 1 yr (SIP) 2. 35% remained impaired in physical and social function at 1 yr (SIP) 3. Of 23 survivors over 4 yr post-Rx 91% had returned to full-time work or homemaking by 4 yr post-BMT 4. Family conflict (FES) significantly predicted worse physical function (SIP) and psychological distress (BSI) at 1 yr
Wingard et al., 1992 (60)	Cross-sectional BMT survivor cohort	135 BMT (64% ALL, AML, CML; 36% AA, lymph, HD, neuroblastoma)	Mailed Q	3.9 yr post-BMT (mean); 0.6–3.9 yr (range); single assessment	Psychosocial adjustment and sexual function; gonadal physiology; life satisfaction; self-esteem; optimism	SLDS-C; Faces Life Satis; Cantril's Ladder; Rosenberg's Self Esteem Scale; PERI Life Events; LOT; MOS	1. 53% had high sexual satisfaction; 22% sexual dissatisfaction 2. Sexual dissatisfaction in men related to problems with erections or ejaculation. Sexual dissatisfaction in women related to loss of menses 3. Greater sexual satisfaction in those who were: younger at BMT; Dx of AA vs. cancer; satisfied with appearance; satisfactory relationship with partner
Wolcott et al., 1986 (19)	Cross-sectional BMT survivor cohort	26 ABMT (50% ALL, AML, CML; 50%: AA); 18 donors	Mailed Q	3.5 yr post-BMT (mean); 1.6–7.6 yr (range); single assessment	Psychosocial adjustment; self-esteem; Rx-related physical problems; medical care utilization; relationship with donors	POMS; SAS; Simmons Scale; medical status Q	1. 19%–28% frequently experience dry mouth, mouth soreness, abdominal cramps/pain, itching skin 2. Women survivors had significantly higher distress than donors (POMS)

Disease/treatment

AA	=	aplastic anemia
ABMT	=	allogeneic bone marrow transplant
ABVD	=	doxorubicin, bleomycin, vinblastine, dacarbazine
AL	=	acute leukemia
ALL	=	acute lymphocytic leukemia
AML	=	acute myelogenous leukemia
ANLL	=	acute nonlymphocytic leukemia
BCT	=	breast-conserving treatment
BMT	=	bone marrow transplantation
CALGB	=	Cancer and Leukemia Group B
CL	=	chronic leukemia
CLL	=	chronic lymphocytic leukemia
CML	=	chronic myelogenous leukemia
GVHD	=	graft vs. host disease
GYN	=	gynecological
HD	=	Hodgkin's disease
H&N	=	head and neck
HRT	=	hormone replacement therapy
Lymph	=	lymphoma
MDS	=	myelodysplastic syndrome
MOPP	=	mechlorethamine, vincristine, procarbazine, prednisone
Neurobl	=	neuroblastoma
NHL	=	non-Hodgkin's lymphoma
RPLND	=	retroperitoneal lymph node dissection
RT	=	radiation therapy

Measures

ABS	=	Affect Balance Scale (Bradburn)
BCSM	=	Breast Cancer Specific Measure (Polinsky)
BDS	=	Beck Depression Scale
BES	=	Body Esteem Scale (Franzoi and Shields)
BPS	=	Beck Pessimism Scale
BSI	=	Brief Symptom Inventory (Derogatis)
CARES	=	Cancer Rehabilitation Evaluation System (Schag and Heinrich)
CES	=	Concealing Emotions Scale (Brannon)
CES-D	=	Center for Epidemiologic Studies—Depression Scale (Radloff)
CHLC	=	Cancer Health Locus of Control (Dickson et al.)
Cond N & V	=	Conditioned Nausea and Vomiting Index (Cella)
CPBS	=	Cancer Patient Behavior Scale (Ross)
CPRS	=	Comprehensive Psychopathological Rating Scale (Montgomery and Asberg)
DAQ	=	Death Anxiety Questionnaire (Conte)
DBMRI	=	Demands of Bone Marrow Recovery Inventory (Haberman)
DSFI	=	Derogatis Sexual Functioning Inventory
DSM-IV	=	Diagnostic and Statistical Manual—IV
EORTC-QLQ-C30	=	EORTC Quality of Life Core Questionnaire—30 items (Aaronson et al.)
FES	=	Family Environment Scale (Moos)
FFS	=	Family Functioning Scale (Kornblith et al.)
FLIC	=	Functional Living Index—Cancer (Schipper)
GHQ-28	=	General Health Questionnaire—28 item version (Goldberg)

253

TABLE 20.1. *Psychosocial Adaptation of Adult Cancer Survivors: Review of the Literature — Continued*

GWB	= General Well-Being (Brook et al.)	PRQ	= Personal Resources Questionnaire (Weinert)	STAI	= State-Trait Anxiety Inventory (Spielberger)
HDRS	= Hamilton Depression Rating Scale	PSE	= Present State Examination (Wing)	STPI	= State-Trait Personality Inventory (Spielberger)
IES	= Impact of Event Scale (Horowitz et al.)	QLI	= Quality of Life Index (Ferrans and Powers)	TAT	= Thematic Apperception Test
IWB	= Index of Well-Being (Campbell et al.)	ROF	= Recovery of Function Scale (Andrykowski)	Testic Cancer Knowl	= Survey of Men's Knowledge and Beliefs about Testicular Cancer (Cummings)
JCS	= Jalowiec Coping Scale	SAS	= Social Adjustment Scale (Weissman)		
LD	= Ladder of H&N Disfigurement (Baker)	SCID	= Structured Clinical Interview for DSM	*Miscellaneous abbreviations*	
LOT	= Life Orientation Test (Scheier and Carver)	SCL-90-R	= Symptom Check List-90-R (Derogatis)	BC	= blue collar
MAACL	= Multiple Affect Adjective Check List (Zuckerman et al.)	SD	= Semantic Differential	Comp. gr.	= comparison group
MHLC	= Multidimensional Health Locus of Control (Wallston and Wallston)	SEI	= Self-Esteem Inventory (Coopersmith)	Dx	= diagnosis
MOS-20	= Medical Outcomes Scale, Short Form—20 items (Stewart et al.)	SER	= Symptom Experience Report (Andrykowski)	NSABP	= National Surgical Adjuvant Breast and Bowel Project
MOS-SF-36	= Medical Outcomes Scale, Short Form—36 items (Ware)	SHSI	= Sexual History Structured Interview (Schover and Jensen)	pop.	= population
Neg SES Impact	= Negative Socioeconomic Impact Index (Kornblith et al.)	SIP	= Sickness Impact Profile (Bergner et al.)	PTSD	= post-traumatic stress disorder
PAIS	= Psychosocial Adjustment of Illness Scale (Derogatis)	SLDS-C	= Satisfaction with Life Domains Scale for Cancer (Baker)	Q	= questionnaire
PAQ	= Patient Adjustment Questionnaire (Rapoport et al.)	Social Act S	= Social Activities Scale (Donald and Ware)	QOL	= quality of life
PCL-C	= PTSD Checklist—Civilian Version (Weathers et al.)	Soc & Emot Supp S	= Social & Emotional Supports Scale (Schaeffer)	Rx	= treatment
POMS	= Profile of Mood States (McNair et al.)	SSIG	= Semi-Structured Interview Guide (Carter)	s.d.	= standard deviation
				SES	= socioeconomic status
				WC	= white collar

VI

PSYCHOLOGICAL RESPONSES TO TREATMENT

EDITOR: RUTH McCORKLE

21

Surgery

PAUL B. JACOBSEN, ANDREW J. ROTH, AND JIMMIE C. HOLLAND

Surgery is the oldest recorded form of cancer treatment. Egyptian papyruses dating from 1600 B.C. show evidence of tumors being cut out (1). The modern history of cancer surgery can be traced to the early nineteenth century (2). Following the introduction of ether anesthesia by Warren in 1846, surgical removal of tumors became increasingly common. The subsequent introduction of antisepsis by Lister in 1867 reduced the high frequency of postoperative infections and deaths. These events paved the way for the development of new procedures that allowed for radical excision of previously inoperable neoplasms: gastrectomy, laryngectomy, mastectomy, and hysterectomy (2) (see Table 21.1). Over the course of the twentieth century, primary surgical treatment has been complemented first by radiotherapy and, since the 1960s, by chemotherapy. The combined-modality approach came about as the result of better understanding of tumor biology, which made it clear that increasingly radical surgery could not deal with the micrometastases that were already present in 70% of solid tumors at the time of presentation (3).

Current surgical interventions in cancer are not limited to tumor removal. Far more accurate histological diagnosis can be obtained today through use of bronchoscopy, mediastinoscopy, and laparoscopy. Debulking procedures help in the management of recurrent disease. Solitary metastatic lesions in the liver, lungs, and brain are treated surgically with curative outcome. In cases of advanced disease, palliative surgical procedures are used to provide pain relief and symptom control. Increasingly sophisticated reconstructive procedures have been developed for patients who have previously undergone facial and breast surgery (4). Surgery also plays a role in prevention of cancer (2) (see Table 21.2). With certain familial conditions that are associated with a high incidence of subsequent cancer, prophylactic removal of an organ can prevent the development of a predictable malignancy.

Surgery today continues to play a central role in treatment of cancer. Yet it cannot be applied effectively without attention to possible psychological influences on the person's ability to understand the procedure proposed, recognize its necessity, and tolerate the associated stress and discomfort in order to reap the benefits. In most instances the surgeon, through interaction with the patient, is aware of the patient's psychological needs. Several issues, however, may require outside intervention: a disturbed relationship to the surgeon or staff, inability to give consent, severe preoperative anxiety, refusal to undergo surgery, exacerbation of preexisting psychiatric disorders, postoperative delirium, and poor compliance with rehabilitation. It is here that knowledge of the common types of psychiatric disturbance that occur in surgical patients and their management becomes important.

This chapter describes the range of normal and abnormal psychological reactions that occur in patients undergoing cancer surgery. In addition to describing these general reactions, specific emotional problems that relate to procedures for breast, head and neck, genitourinary, and colon cancer are described. Rehabilitation of patients after cancer surgery, which depends heavily on the individual's psychological state, commitment, and perseverance, is also reviewed.

PSYCHOLOGICAL RESPONSES TO IMPENDING SURGERY

Strain and Grossman (5) described several concerns that are commonly evoked by impending surgery. These include threat to the sense of personal invulnerability; concern that one's life is being entrusted largely to strangers; separation from the familiar

TABLE 21.1. *Selected Historical Milestones in Surgical Oncology*

Year	Surgeon	Event
1809	Ephraim McDowell	Elective abdominal surgery (excised ovarian tumor)
1846	John Collins Warren	Use of ether anesthesia (excised submaxillary gland)
1867	Joseph Lister	Introduction of antisepsis
1860–1880	Albert Theodore Billroth	First gastrectomy, laryngectomy, and esophagectomy
1878	Richard von Volkmann	Excision of cancerous rectum
1880s	Theodore Kocher	Development of thyroid surgery
1890	William Stewart Halsted	Radical mastectomy
1896	G.T. Beatson	Oophorectomy for breast cancer
1904	Hugh H. Young	Radical prostatectomy
1906	Ernest Wertheim	Radical hysterectomy
1908	W. Ernest Miles	Abdomenoperineal resection for rectal cancer
1912	E. Martin	Cordotomy for the treatment of pain
1910–1930	Harvey Cushing	Development of surgery for brain tumors
1913	Franz Torek	Successful resection of cancer of the thoracic esophagus
1927	G. Divis	Successful resection of pulmonary metastases
1933	Evarts Graham	Pneumonectomy
1935	A.O. Whipple	Pancreaticoduodenectomy
1945	Charles B. Huggins	Adrenalectomy for prostate cancer

Source: Reprinted with permission from S.A. Rosenberg. Principles of surgical oncology. In: V.T. DeVita, Jr., S. Hellman, and S.A. Rosenberg, eds, *Cancer: Principles and Practice of Oncology*, 4th ed. Philadelphia: Lippincott, 1993.

environment of home and family members; fears of loss of control or death while under anesthesia; fears of being partially awake during surgery, and fears of damage to body parts. Although these preoperative reactions occur to some degree in all surgical patients, there is a significantly greater stress involved when cancer is the suspected diagnosis or the condition for which surgery is being performed (6). These normal concerns, heightened in cancer, should be addressed by all members of the surgical team, but the surgeon who will perform the procedure is central.

When one considers the stresses surgery presents, it is not surprising that the surgeon is invested with strong emotions that come from entrusting one's life to another. By virtue of this fact, however, the surgeon may elicit reactions similar to those associated with authority figures in the individual's past (7). This accounts for some of the special feelings of affection and admiration patients develop for the surgeon, as

TABLE 21.2. *Surgery That Can Prevent Cancer*

Underlying Condition	Associated Cancer	Prophylactic Surgery
Cryptorchidism	Testicular	Orchiopexy
Polyposis coli	Colon	Colectomy
Familial colon cancer	Colon	Colectomy
Ulcerative colitis	Colon	Colectomy
Multiple endocrine neoplasia, types II and III	Medullary cancer of the thyroid	Thyroidectomy
Familial breast cancer	Breast	Mastectomy
Familial ovarian cancer	Ovary	Oophorectomy

Source: Reprinted with permission from S.A. Rosenberg. Principles of surgical oncology. In: V.T. DeVita, Jr., S. Hellman, and S.A. Rosenberg, eds. *Cancer: Principles and Practice of Oncology*, 4th ed. Philadelphia: Lippincott, 1993.

well as for some of the unwarranted hostile and angry responses. These reactions can complicate the relationship and impede good cooperation and optimal surgical outcome. Surgeons who are alert to such responses try to avoid a personal response, but at times the subtlety of the response, or its extreme nature, may require evaluation and intervention.

Ideally, psychological management begins with the doctor who refers the patient to the surgeon. The patient should arrive at the surgeon's office with some explanation of the reason for the consideration of an operation. This preparation provides a sense of security about the continuity of care. The preoperative consultation visit with the surgeon is a critically important opportunity for the surgeon to assess the patient's emotional stability and to begin psychological preparation for the procedure. It is in this conversation that a sense of respect and trust develops and a positive doctor–patient relationship is established, which makes it easier for the patient to face the anticipated procedure. It is most important that the patient be given an adequate explanation of all aspects of the proposed procedure: the type of anesthesia to be administered, the nature of the surgical procedure itself, the expected length of time in the recovery room and in the hospital, the body part(s) that may be removed, the functions that may be temporarily or permanently lost, and the corrective and rehabilitative procedures that are available. It is also important that the surgeon develop a relationship with the patient, rather than with some self-designated relative spokesperson who has decided to protect the patient from any bad news, with such an attitude as "We know she will give up if she knows she has cancer," or "Don't tell her what's wrong, doctor." In addition to providing information, preoperative discussions should also be used to clarify misconceptions or unrealistic expectations. This point is particularly important with children, who are prone to misunderstand information about medical procedures and who therefore experience greater distress (8). Because all patients are anxious, explanations must be given clearly, in nonmedical terms, and with adequate opportunity to ask questions. Drawings that depict the procedure may aid the patient in understanding what will be done. Having a relative present allows for later discussion at home. Tape-recording the interview allows the patient and relative to listen together at home when they are less stressed. Moreover, because the patient is anxious, the information the surgeon has conveyed may not be "heard," and may need to be repeated at more than one visit. Patients will sometimes have no recall months later of the preoperative discussion for informed consent.

PSYCHOLOGICAL PREPARATION FOR SURGERY

Empirical research on psychological preparation for surgery initially focused on the role of the anesthesiologist. Anesthesiologists are traditionally seen as technicians administering anesthesia and as having little interaction with patients. However, they typically visit the patient preoperatively to explain the anesthetic procedures. In 1964, Egbert and colleagues at the Massachusetts General Hospital conducted a study in which the anesthesiologist did or did not prepare patients scheduled to undergo intraabdominal surgery for the experience of postoperative pain. More than half the patients in the study underwent gastrectomy, colectomy, or bowel resection; it is likely that these procedures were largely done for cancerous disease, although it is not reported. For patients randomized to the experimental condition, the anesthesiologist described the pain that patients would have after surgery and the pain medications they would receive and encouraged the use of deep breathing to relieve painful muscle spasms. The anesthesiologist continued to make daily visits after surgery, giving encouragement and reassurance. Results indicated that, compared to a control group that received no information or reassurance about pain, the experimental group used significantly fewer analgesics. They also went home an average of three days earlier. The study by Egbert and colleagues (9) demonstrating that preoperative reassurance by the anesthesiologist reduced postoperative narcotics requirements was a landmark; unfortunately, it still has not led to changes in clinical practice in many settings. Other studies have confirmed that such interventions can reduce hospital stay and the use of analgesics (10,11). However, the multifaceted nature of the interventions employed by Egbert and others prevents a clear understanding of how psychological considerations affect recovery. Later efforts have tried to isolate and examine the principal determinants: psychological support, provision of information, and skills training.

Several studies in the 1970s examined the psychological effects of providing patients with detailed information about the procedure(s) to be performed (12–14). Two major reviews of these studies (15,16) concluded that providing such information had only a modest effect on postoperative adjustment and recovery. Subsequent research examined the efficacy of information about the specific physical sensations patients would experience before and after the operation (17–21). The addition of sensory information has been found to yield more beneficial effects, perhaps because sensory information permitted patients to form more accurate expectations of postoperative sensations, including those that are uncomfortable.

Several studies have examined the effects of behavioral interventions such as active and passive relaxation training and stress inoculation training. The active form of relaxation training involves teaching patients to tense and relax muscle groups progressively as a means of inducing relaxation. The passive form of relaxation training is similar to self-hypnosis or meditation, and typically involves calming self-statements and the use of pleasant mental imagery (see Chapter 62 on cognitive-behavioral interventions for more information on these techniques). In controlled studies, passive relaxation training was found to reduce intraoperative and postoperative anxiety in outpatients undergoing skin cancer surgery (22). Active relaxation training reduced length of stay and the use of analgesics in abdominal surgery patients (20). In both studies, patients received training in relaxation techniques by use of audiocassette tapes, an inexpensive and simple intervention. In an interesting exploratory study, Rapkin and colleagues (23) examined the impact of passive relaxation training on recovery from head and neck cancer surgery. Patients who received preoperative instruction in passive relaxation techniques were found to go home an average of four days sooner than a comparison group of patients who received standard care.

Another behavioral technique that has been evaluated is stress inoculation training (24). Wells and colleagues (25) developed a stress inoculation procedure for general surgical patients that was administered during a one-hour training session the day before surgery. During this session, patients received instruction in monitoring themselves for cognitive and physiological signs of stress, deep breathing, muscle relaxation, induction of pleasant imagery, and substitution of coping self-statements for negative self-statements. In addition to experiencing less preoperative anxiety, the patients who underwent stress inoculation training experienced less postoperative anxiety and pain than a control group of patients receiving standard hospital care. Moreover, patients who received training went home an average of 3.5 days earlier than their control group counterparts. The effectiveness of stress inoculation training for cancer surgery patients has yet to be evaluated.

In summary, there is considerable evidence that psychological preparation for surgery facilitates postoperative emotional adjustment and recovery.

Indeed, two metaanalyses of research in this area have demonstrated that brief psychological interventions are superior to standard hospital care in reducing postoperative pain and in increasing satisfaction with care and psychological well-being (26,27). These analyses also indicated that psychological interventions possess cost-saving effects; patients who received psychological preparation were discharged an average of two days sooner than patients who received standard care (26).

PSYCHIATRIC SYNDROMES IN SURGICAL PATIENTS

Several psychological problems and psychiatric disorders can lead to distress in surgical patients that exceeds normal limits. These are reviewed in order of likely appearance, from the period before to that after the operation.

Patients Receiving Psychotropic Drugs

Patients who are receiving psychotropic drugs pose a particularly difficult problem when they are awaiting surgery that raises the possibility of cancer. Their known vulnerability to the exacerbation of symptoms of schizophrenia, major depression, anxiety disorders, or manic-depressive illness in a stressful situation makes the psychiatrist reluctant to stop medication for a lengthy period in advance of major surgery. Although some psychiatrists and anesthesiologists suggest the conservative approach of suspending the use of all psychotropic drugs two weeks before surgery (28), our experience has not supported such a blanket guideline for management of this problem. In fact, in a survey of 50 patients with severe psychiatric illness who were studied for prevalence of psychiatric complications in their postoperative hospital course (29), both chronic schizophrenics and chronic depressives tolerated surgery well without exacerbation of symptoms. Only those who had acute symptoms in the preoperative period tended to have significant postoperative psychiatric difficulties. Flexibility is possible when the psychiatrist and the anesthesiologist coordinate their care. The guidelines we suggest are as follows.

1. At the time that a patient who is receiving a serotonin specific reuptake inhibitor (SSRI), a tricyclic antidepressant, a monoamine oxidase inhibitor (MAOI), lithium, or a major tranquilizer is referred for surgery, a consultation between the anesthesiologist and the psychiatrist should take place in order to develop a coordinated plan based on the particular patient's needs and the drug involved.

2. The drugs that are of most concern are the MAOIs, because their metabolism alters the sympathetic amines serotonin, norepinephrine, and dopamine. Narcotics interact with an MAOI to cause an exaggerated response to the usual dose, thus producing possible hypotension and apnea. The narcotic chosen is important. Meperidine is contraindicated because of its interaction with MAOIs to produce hyperpyrexia and hypertension. A hypertensive crisis, should it occur, is treated by an α-adrenergic blocker such as chlorpromazine. As some MAOIs may enhance the neuromuscular blocking effect of succinylcholine, their administration should be stopped well in advance of surgery.

3. SSRIs or tricyclic antidepressants can be continued until the day before surgery if the anesthesiologist is aware of the situation and can plan anesthesia with that in mind. It should be recalled that SSRIs are highly protein bound and can interact with medications such as phenytoin, cimetidine, and coumadin. The half-lives of these SSRIs are such that the drugs will stay in a patient's system from one week (sertraline and paroxetine) to six to eight weeks (fluoxetine).

4. Minor tranquilizers used for anxiety disorders should not be discontinued abruptly in those patients who have been using them regularly for more than a few weeks at a time. They can be administered intravenously if needed to prevent benzodiazepine withdrawal. Clinical judgment should focus on a risk/benefit balance in those patients who have respiratory compromise, which may be exacerbated by these drugs.

5. Major tranquilizers block the dopamine receptor, and the low-potency drugs (e.g., thioridazine and chlorpromazine) produce hypotension by central and peripheral anticholinergic action. They also increase the risk of postoperative delirium when other drugs (e.g., scopolamine) are used (28).

6. Lithium carbonate can be continued until the time of surgery and poses few difficulties that cannot be anticipated. Muscle relaxants such as succinylcholine may be potentiated by lithium, and this should be taken into account in the dosage.

7. All of the preceding medications can be resumed at the time that the patient resumes taking liquids orally. Starting the drug again must take into account the patient's needs for the drug and any possible contraindications that result from the surgery, as with bowel resection.

Inability to Understand and Give Consent

Some patients appear for surgery who are unable to understand the nature and consequences of the procedure proposed. When it is lifesaving and relatives are absent, the surgery may be performed with a note from the psychiatrist and agreement of the hospital to accept responsibility. If the surgery is elective or palliative, and there is need for a guardian to be appointed for the individual, one is justified in requesting a legal test of competency and the appointment of a legal guardian is indicated. This procedure is usually followed for dementia and does not occur often in oncology situations. More common are cases that involve a patient with an alcoholic history who understands in part the need for a major resection, but whose ability to cooperate after surgery is minimal. These cases require thoughtful evaluation.

CASE REPORT

Mr. P. was a 66-year-old widow, recently retired man who underwent resection of an esophageal tumor. He had a long history of alcohol use and gave different reports of his daily intake. He lived alone and no one was available to confirm his report. The patient was given a low dose of lorazepam as prophylaxis against alcohol withdrawal prior to surgery. Forty-eight hours after surgery the patient had a change in mental status with disorientation, paranoid ideation, and agitation. Treatment with a neuroleptic and a benzodiazepine for presumptive alcohol withdrawal, and a change in his pain medication regimen cleared his sensorium. An organic evaluation, including a CT scan of the brain, was negative. Discussion with the family about the patient's preoperative mental state noted a slow decline of the patient's cognitive functioning over the previous three months with loss of memory and impairment in concentration. The patient had refused to undergo neurologic evaluation. When the family visited his apartment they found it in disarray with several empty liquor bottles strewn about. Although the delirium resolved, mild cognitive impairment, poor ability to understand the postoperative and self-care instructions persisted. Though the patient initially protested discharge plans that precluded him from returning home, he agreed to stay with his daughter for two weeks.

Preoperative Panic and Refusal of Surgery

Paralyzing anxiety or panic prior to surgery is most likely to occur in patients with a preexisting anxiety disorder (e.g., panic disorder; generalized anxiety disorder). In many patients, the anxiety or panic takes the form of a fear of being alone in an unfamiliar environment, of losing control under anesthesia, or of dying during the operation. Clinical experience with both general and cancer surgery settings suggests that these reactions are relatively uncommon, occurring in less than 5% of surgical patients (30,31). Nevertheless, these unusual cases present challenging management problems as surgical cases.

CASE REPORT

Ms. R. a 39-year old married white female with metastatic breast cancer was referred for psychiatric consultation owing to her refusal to undergo surgery for placement of a central line catheter. The patient related that she disliked the experience of being rendered unconscious by anesthesia and was preoccupied with the idea that she would "never wake up." Although she recognized that the risk of death was extremely remote and that placement of the central line was necessary for subsequent chemotherapy treatment, she felt unable to provide consent. Intervention focused on ways to assist the patient in gaining control of her fear. A treatment plan was developed that consisted of *(1)* allowing the patient's spouse to room in that evening to provide emotional support; *(2)* instructing the patient in a brief relaxation exercise designed to provide a means of regaining emotional control; and *(3)* prescribing a low-dose benzodiazepine to alleviate acute symptoms of anxiety. Once this plan was developed and implemented, the patient, though still hesitant, agreed to proceed with the procedure. The patient underwent the procedure the following day without incident and subsequently reported that she appreciated the opportunity to participate in her own care.

Postoperative Delirium

The postoperative period is a time when acute confusional states (i.e., delirium or cognitive disorders due to general medical condition) frequently occur. These states usually appear within 3–4 days after surgery. The initial signs are often subtle, with slight loss of memory, changes in behavior, irritability, or misinterpretation of sights or sounds. It is important that the mental status change be recognized early and that a psychiatric consultation be called to assist in determining etiology and management. The delirium, when unrecognized, usually becomes worse, with disruptive behavior (e.g., pulling out tubes) and fatigue resulting from agitation and lack of rest. (See Chapter 48 on delirium for additional information).

The common causes of postoperative cognitive disorders include: response to anesthesia or analgesics; anticholinergic syndrome based on the additive effects of several drugs with anticholinergic side effects; electrolyte, fluid, or metabolic imbalance; delirium tremens caused by alcohol withdrawal; CNS complications; and loss of circadian pattern and the stress of an unfamiliar environment (especially in the elderly). An understanding of these issues helps identify those patients who may be at risk and therefore may help in preventing these untoward events (32). Older individuals are at greater risk, as are those with any preexisting mild dementia, particularly alcohol-related.

One of the most common examples of postoperative delirium seen in oncology settings occurs in patients with head and neck cancer who have an alcoholic history, transient hypoxia, and cerebral anoxia. Many of these patients are in the older age group and are habituated to excessive alcohol use (33). They often drink until admission, undergo surgery, and develop withdrawal reactions with delirium tremens on the second

or third postoperative day. Treatment of withdrawal with the newer benzodiazepines such as lorazepam and midazolam has become more widespread, and mortality rates from severe alcohol withdrawal have decreased in recent years (34).

Depression and Suicide Risk

Major depression most often occurs following surgery for cancer when the results are particularly ominous, for example, when a tumor is found unresectable and the prognosis is poor, when a limb or breast is amputated, or when gynecological or urological surgery is known to result in sterility or sexual dysfunction. The postoperative period then is one of recovery from the procedure but also of confrontation with and adaption to loss and possible death. This process resembles anticipatory grieving. The initial shock is usually followed by emotional turmoil, and resolution may be difficult. Suicidal ideation is not uncommon. "Why put my family through more?" "What do I have to live for?" "My life is over, I might as well end it." These patients require urgent attention because they sometimes attempt suicide, usually after discharge. Families need help in planning care at home, and referral for help from a mental health professional is important.

PSYCHOSOCIAL ISSUES RELATED TO THE SITE OF SURGERY

In addition to the common postoperative reactions already described, there are psychological reactions that are largely related to the site of surgery and the functional loss sustained. Adverse emotional reactions correlate with the psychological significance of the loss, especially with the face, breast, genitals, or colon. Site-specific problems also arise when surgery results in a major loss of a particular function. Loss of normal bowel function following colostomy and loss of normal speech following laryngectomy are the two most notable examples. This section briefly reviews the site-specific problems that occur following breast surgery, colostomy, head and neck surgery, and genitourinary surgery. More detailed discussion can be found in the chapters on each site (see Chapter 32 on breast cancer, Chapter 27 on gastrointestinal cancer, and Chapter 26 on head and neck cancer).

Breast Surgery

In the 1950s, Sutherland and colleagues (35) at Memorial Hospital conducted one of the first studies of psychosocial reactions to radical mastectomy. A majority of the women studied were found to be experiencing significant postoperative depression, anxiety, and low self-esteem along with prolonged impairments in physical and sexual functioning. For many of the women, the loss of a breast signified the loss of an organ intimately associated with their sense of self-esteem, sexuality, and femininity. Subsequent studies indicate that approximately 25% of women who undergo radical or modified radical mastectomies experience significant psychological distress in the year following surgery (36,37). Among the variables that appear to determine the severity of the patient's reaction are the point in the life cycle during which breast surgery occurs and the social tasks that are threatened or interrupted. Threats to femininity and self-esteem occur in all women, but may be more pronounced in younger women for whom attractiveness and reproductive functioning are major life issues (38–40). Other factors associated with more severe postmastectomy reactions include a history of psychiatric disorder, problems with body image, a history of unsatisfying or negative sexual experiences, and difficulty discussing personal, especially sexual, problems (41).

During the past two decades, several important changes have occurred in the surgical treatment of breast cancer. Depending on such factors as the size and location of the tumor, many women today may be offered the choice of undergoing either a mastectomy or a lumpectomy, a surgical technique designed to conserve breast tissue. A major impetus for developing breast-conserving techniques was to reduce the presumed psychological impact of mastectomy. In general, studies have found few differences in emotional well-being or sexual functioning in the months after surgery based on whether patients underwent mastectomy or lumpectomy (42–48). The only consistent difference to emerge across studies is that women who undergo lumpectomy generally report less body image disturbance than women who undergo mastectomy (44–45).

Another important change in the surgical treatment of breast cancer is the increase in the percentage of women who undergo reconstructive procedures. Epidemiologic data suggest that the number of women who undergo mastectomy and reconstruction has increased from 10% to 30% over a ten-year period (49). Among the many different methods used in breast reconstruction, insertion of silicone implants is one of the more common methods. Recently, there has been a highly publicized debate concerning the safety of silicone breast implants (50). Survey data suggest that relatively few women who received silicone implants following mastectomy and who are aware of the con-

troversy regret their decision. Winer and colleagues (51) found that, while 55% of the women were worried about potential health problems, only 13% considered having their silicone implants removed. The overwhelming majority of the women (77%) believed that reconstruction with silicone implants had helped them cope with breast cancer.

Colostomy

In oncology, the colostomy procedure is performed chiefly for treatment of colorectal cancer. This procedure results in the loss of normal bowel function, which is replaced by fecal elimination through a surgically constructed stoma. For some patients, the diversion of their fecal stream to an observable stoma violates their sense of cleanliness. In the first days following surgery it is not uncommon for patients to refuse to look at the stoma. Even thoughts about it evoke feelings of disgust, anger, embarrassment, and shame. When the colostomy starts to work, patients may be embarrassed by the gas and noise that cannot be controlled. In one of the first psychosocial studies of cancer patients who had undergone colostomy, Sutherland and colleagues (52) surveyed patients who had survived disease-free for five or more years from rectal cancer. In general, these patients were significantly impaired in both their sexual and social functioning. Among patients who were employed prior to surgery, the majority had experienced decreases in their work status and earning capacity. Difficulties with practical management of the colostomy were common, as were depression, chronic anxiety, and a sense of social isolation. In the years since this study was completed, a number of changes have been made aimed at improving the adjustment of cancer patients undergoing colostomy. Perhaps the most important advance has been the development of improved equipment, which virtually eliminates problems with odor and spillage of feces. In addition, the location of the stoma site has been given more attention preoperatively to take into account skin folds, patient preference, and style of dress.

It is generally felt that improvements in patient care have resulted in less distress and better postoperative adjustment (53). However, one study (54) of patients who had undergone stoma surgery for a variety of diseases, including bowel cancer, found that 22% of the subjects had moderate or severe psychiatric symptoms one year postoperatively. Most of these patients had shown similar disturbance at a three-month assessment, suggesting that their problems were relatively chronic. Ability to perform housework and to engage in leisure and sexual activities was affected in a number of subjects (54). Using a longitudinal research design, Barsevick and colleagues (55) examined patient adjustment from diagnosis of colorectal cancer through the first three months of treatment. Results indicated that having an ostomy, undergoing additional treatment, and having depressive symptoms preoperatively predicted greater dependency three months after surgery.

Head and Neck Surgery

Although all parts of the body have psychological significance, the head and neck areas are central. Attractiveness, social interaction, and emotional expression all depend to a great extent on the integrity of facial features. For most persons, the disfigurement of the head and neck from cancer surgery is difficult to contemplate (56). Suicidal thoughts are not uncommon preoperatively, especially if the patient is to undergo extensive surgery. Following surgery many patients are concerned about the reactions of others and express fears of isolation and rejection. Unlike the mastectomy and colostomy patient, head and neck surgery cannot be hidden. It has a strong negative impact on self-esteem and self-confidence (57). In addition to the stress of an altered facial appearance, many patients must also cope with the loss or impairment of speech, sight, taste, or smell. The psychological impact of surgery appears to be directly related to the extent of disfigurement and sensory impairment. More severe structural and functional loss has been shown to be associated with a slower recovery, more prolonged social isolation, lower self-esteem, and more severe postoperative depression (58,59).

Genitourinary Surgery

Malignant tumors of the genitourinary tract arise in men in the prostate, bladder, and testis. In women, the uterus, cervix, bladder, and ovaries are the common sites of genitourinary neoplasms. This group of diseases share at least two major features. First, treatment typically involves surgery for localized disease, either alone or in conjunction with chemotherapy and radiotherapy. Second, both the disease and the treatments can result in disturbances in sexual functioning. The physiological effects of the disease and side effects of treatment often affect the patient's sexual desire and capacity for stimulation and orgasm. These same aspects of sexual functioning can also be disrupted by the patient's psychological reactions to the disease and its treatment. The partner's usual sexual function may also be impaired by the psychological impact of the meaning of cancer in the genital organs, or fears aroused by its treatment. The reader is referred

to Chapter 42 for a more detailed discussion of sexual problems in cancer patients and their management.

In men, the prostate is the most common site of genitourinary cancer. In cases where the tumor is localized, treatment generally involves radical prostatectomy (removal of the prostate gland) or radiotherapy. The development of a nerve-sparing surgical technique has significantly reduced the prevalence of postoperative impotence and is generally felt to improve overall quality of life (60–63). Currently, research in this area is focused on examining the relative benefits of prostatectomy versus nonsurgical techniques such as radiotherapy, cryotherapy, or "watchful-waiting." Preliminary findings suggest that overall quality of life does not differ among patients undergoing these different forms of treatment. However, treatment-specific complications do impact on specific quality of life domains such as sexual functioning and urinary continence, and may lead patients to choose one form of therapy over another (64–69). For patients who do not recover full erectile function postoperatively, implantation of a penile prosthesis, use of a vacuum pump, or injection with vasoactive substances (e.g., papaverine) offer rehabilitative options. In assessing the impact of surgery on sexual functioning, it is essential to take into account preoperative sexual activity (70). In fact, Libman and colleagues (71) found that psychosexual consequences of prostatectomy for benign prostatic hypertrophy and inguinal hernia repair did not differ significantly; sexual difficulties related more to the general stress of undergoing surgery.

Radical cystectomy for bladder cancer in men can also effect sexual functioning. In addition to possible problems with erectile function, all radical cystectomy patients must contend with impact of the ostomy appliance on sexual activity. A recent study showed that health-related quality of life is retained to a greater degree after bladder substitution when compared with the standard method of diversion after cystectomy via ileal conduits (72). Urostomy patients often benefit from brief counseling on more comfortable positions for lovemaking and on ways of keeping the appliance as unobtrusive as possible (73).

Cancer of the testes is the second most common tumor in men between the ages of 20 and 34. Treatment for localized disease typically involves only unilateral orchiectomy. The procedure does not produce impairment in fertility or in endocrine function; however, it can result in psychologically based sexual problems (74). Retroperitoneal lymph node dissection is often performed in conjunction with orchiectomy. This procedure can result in dry ejaculation and loss of fertility. (See Chapter 20 on cancer survivors and Chapter 42 on sexual dysfunction).

As stated previously, the major genitourinary cancers in women arise in the uterus, cervix, ovaries, and bladder. In women, surgery for genitourinary cancer may also include hysterectomy and bilateral salpingo-oophorectomy. Sexual dysfunction is relatively common following radical pelvic surgery, and education, support, and sexual counseling are important in the treatment of these women. The full impact of these malignancies on psychological and sexual functioning is reviewed in Chapter 42.

In any patient with genitourinary cancer it is important that the surgeon explain preoperatively to the patient and his or her partner the expected impact of surgery on sexual functioning (75). At the same time, the available rehabilitative options for the expected sexual dysfunction should also be discussed. This discussion by the surgeon serves to dispel common misconceptions and may thereby prevent the development of certain psychologically based postoperative sexual problems (e.g., avoidance of sexual activity for fear of transmitting cancer).

REHABILITATION FOLLOWING CANCER SURGERY

Cancer rehabilitation is that part of treatment that assists patients in attaining maximal physical, social, psychological, and vocational functioning with the limits imposed by their disease and its treatment (76). In order to provide comprehensive rehabilitation, professionals from many disciplines must collaborate in a team approach to patient care, including the psychological aspects. The role of the mental health professional in the interdisciplinary rehabilitation team is reviewed here.

Ideally, the plan to begin rehabilitation as soon as possible after surgery is reviewed with the patient before the procedure is undertaken. The preoperative discussion of available rehabilitative options can serve to reduce the patient's fears of surgery and strengthen motivation to begin rehabilitation in the immediate postoperative period. As part of the preoperative evaluation, it is also important to determine whether there are any psychosocial determinants present that could lead to a poor rehabilitation outcome. Compliance could be limited by a previous psychiatric disorder, alcoholism, a chaotic family situation, or circumstances that could limit access to treatment, such as limited finances and geographic distance. With the identification of potential problems preoperatively, it is possible to anticipate and prevent them rather than wait until they arise and impede rehabilitation.

There is general agreement that the sooner rehabilitation is initiated after surgery, the more successful the outcome will be. However, the readiness to learn, the ability to work in physical therapy, and the willingness to make life-style changes are all dependent on the patient's psychological state. Patients who have not come to terms with the loss of body parts or functions may not be ready to begin rehabilitation. A number of psychological interventions can be employed in the immediate postoperative period to motivate the patient to engage in rehabilitation. These include individual counseling, couples counseling, and group meetings with other patients who have undergone similar procedures (77). Visits by previously rehabilitated patients are also very beneficial. This form of peer support is the basis of many self-help programs, such as the American Cancer Society's Reach to Recovery (78). An individual whose experience is close to that of the patient provides an effective role model for coping and is an important source of emotional support during the stressful postoperative period.

Following hospital discharge, most patients continue to recuperate from their cancer surgery at home. Given the trend toward shorter hospital stays, patients often require considerable physical care in the period immediately following discharge. Providing this level of care and mobilizing the patient to resume activities of daily living can place severe burdens on family members. Oberst and James (53) have shown that spouses typically suffer an increase in somatic complaints and emotional problems after the cancer surgery patient comes home. The demands placed on the spouse frequently lead to physical complaints (e.g., diffuse aches and pains as well as upper respiratory infections) and emotional responses (e.g., irritability and dysphoria) associated with exhaustion. In a novel approach to this problem, Heinrich and Schag (79) developed a stress and activity management group for ambulatory cancer patients and their spouses. Over a 6-week period, patients and their spouses received information about coping with cancer, a relaxation and exercise program, and reviewed strategies for solving cancer-related problems. Participation in the group was found to increase the level of knowledge about cancer and coping for both the patient and the spouse. Moreover, spouses who completed the program had a more positive attitude toward the patient's health care team and felt better able to handle stressful situations. Almost all participants said that they would recommend the group to other patients and spouses.

CONCLUSIONS

The psychological problems associated with cancer surgery represent those of surgery in general, with the added meaning of cancer and its threat to life. Understanding patients' normal reactions to surgery and to rehabilitation will help the clinician recognize abnormal responses which may require psychiatric or psychological intervention. Attention to psychosocial issues, especially in the preoperative period, can have a positive impact on postoperative recovery, adjustment, and rehabilitation. Thus, optimal care of the surgical oncology patient is likely to require a multidisciplinary team approach in which mental health professionals contribute to the treatment effort both before and after surgery.

REFERENCES

1. Shimkin MB. *Contrary to Nature.* DHEW Publ. No. (NIH) 79-720. Washington, DC: U.S. Government Printing Office; 1977.
2. Rosenberg SA. Principles of surgical oncology. In: DeVita VT Jr, Hellman S, Rosenberg SA, eds. *Cancer: Principles and Practice of Oncology,* 4th ed. Philadelphia: Lippincott; 1993: 238–247.
3. Fisher B, Barboni P. Breast cancer. In: Holland JF, Frei E III, eds. *Cancer Medicine,* 2d ed. Philadelphia: Lea and Febiger; 1982: 2025–2056.
4. Patterson WB. Surgical interventions that can improve quality of life for older cancer patients. *Oncology.* 1992; 6:81–85.
5. Strain JJ, Grossman S. *Psychological Care of the Medically Ill.* New York: Appleton-Century-Crofts; 1975.
6. Gottesman D, Lewis MS. Differences in crisis reactions among cancer and surgery patients. *J Consult Clin Psychol.* 1982;50:381–388.
7. Small SM. Psychological and psychiatric problems in aged and high-risk surgical patients. In: Siegel JH, Chodoff PD, eds. *The Aged and High Risk Surgical Patient: Medical, Surgical and Anesthetic Management.* Orlando, FL: Grune & Stratton; 1976: 307–328.
8. Seeman RG, Rockoff MA. Preoperative anxiety: the pediatric patient. *Int Anesthesiol Clin.* 1986; 24:1–15.
9. Egbert LD, Battit GE, Welch CE, Bartlett MK. Reduction of postoperative pain by encouragement and instruction of patients. *N Engl J Med.* 1964; 270:825–827.
10. Lindeman CA, Van Aernam B. Nursing intervention with the presurgical patient: The effects of structured and unstructured pre-operative teaching. *Nurs Res.* 1971; 20:319–332.
11. Schmitt FE, Woolridge PJ. Psychological preparation of surgical patients. *Nurs. Res.* 1973; 22:108–116.
12. Andrew JM. Recovery from surgery, with and without preparatory instruction, for three coping styles. *J Pers Soc Psychol.* 1970; 15:223–226.
13. Chapman CR, Cox GB. Anxiety, pain, and depression surrounding elective surgery: a multivariate comparison of abdominal surgery patients with kidney donors and recipients. *J Psychosom Res.* 1977; 21:1–15.
14. Vernon DTW, Bigelow DW. Effect of information about a potentially stressful situation on responses to stress impact. *J Pers Soc Psychol.* 1974; 29:50–59.
15. Anderson KO, Masur FT. Preoperative preparation for cardiac surgery facilitates recovery, reduces psychological distress, and reduces the incidence of acute postoperative hypertension. *J Consult Clin Psychol.* 1983; 55:513–520.
16. Ludwick-Rosenthal R, Neufeld RWJ. Stress management during noxious medical procedures: an evaluative review of outcome studies. *Psychol Bull.* 1988;104: 326–342.
17. Kendall PC, Williams L, Pechacek TF, Graham LE, Sisslak C, Herzoff N. Cognitive-behavioral and patient education interventions in cardiac catheterization procedures: The Palo Alto Medical Psychology Project. *J Consult Clin Psychol.* 1979; 47:49–58.
18. Johnson JE, Leventhal H. Effects of accurate expectations and behavioral instructions on reactions during a noxious medical examination. *J Pers Soc Psychol.* 1974; 29:710–718.
19. Johnson JE. The effect of accurate expectations about sensations on the sensory and distress components of pain. *J Pers Soc Psychol.* 1973; 27:261–275.
20. Wilson JF. Behavioral preparation for surgery: benefit or harm. *J Behav Med.* 1981; 4:79–102.
21. Anderson EA. Preoperative preparation for cardiac surgery facilitates recovery, reduces psychological distress, and reduces the incidence of acute postoperative hypertension. *J Consult Clin Psychol.* 1987; 55: 513–520.
22. Domar AD, Noe JM, Benson H. The preoperative use of the relaxation response with ambulatory surgery patients. *J Hum Stress.* 1987; 13:101–107.
23. Rapkin DA, Straubling M, Holroyd JC. Guided imagery, hypnosis and recovery from head and neck cancer surgery: an exploratory study. *Int J Clin Exp Hypnosis.* 1991; 39:215–226.
24. Turk DC, Meichenbaum D, Genest M. *Pain and Behavioral Medicine: A Cognitive-Behavioral Perspective.* New York: Guilford Press; 1983.
25. Wells JK, Howard GS, Nowlin WF, Vargas MJ. Presurgical anxiety and postsurgical pain and adjustment: effects of a stress inoculation procedure. *J Consult Clin Psychol.* 1986; 54:831–835.
26. Mumford E, Schlesinger HJ, Glass GV. The effects of psychological intervention on recovery from surgery and heart attacks: an analysis of the literature. *Am J Public Health.* 1982; 72:141–151.
27. Devine EC, Cook TD. Clinical and cost-saving effects of psychoeducational interventions with surgical patients: a meta-analysis. *Res Nurs Health.* 1986; 9:89–105.
28. DiGiacomo JN. Preoperative considerations concerning psychotropic drugs. *Med Psychiatry.* 1985; 2:4–6.
29. Solomon S, McCartney JR, Saravay SM, Katz E. Postoperative hospital course of patients with history of severe psychiatric illness. *Gen Hosp Psychiatry.* 1987; 9:376-3-82.
30. Massie MJ, Holland JC. The cancer patient with pain: psychiatric complications and their management. *Med Clin N Am.* 1987; 71:243–258.

31. Strain JJ. The surgical patient. In: Michels R, Cavenar JO Jr, Brodie HKH, et al, eds. *Psychiatry*. vol. 2. Philadelphia: Lippincott; 1985.

32. Weed HG, Lutman CV, Young DC, Schuller DE. Preoperative identification of patients at risk for delirium after major head and neck cancer surgery. *Laryngoscope*. 1995; 105:1066–1068.

33. Golden WE, Lavender RC. Perioperative medical considerations in head and neck cancer. In: Myers EN, Suen JU, eds. *Cancer of the Head and Neck*, 2d ed. New York: Churchill Livingstone; 1989:101–120.

34. Newman JP, Terris DJ, Moore M. Trends in the management of alcohol withdrawal syndrome. *Laryngoscope*. 1995; 105:1–7.

35. Sutherland AM, Orbach CE. Psychological impact of cancer and cancer surgery: II. Depressive reactions associated with surgery for cancer. *Cancer*. 1953; 6:958–962.

36. Morris T, Greer HS, White P. Psychological and social adjustment to mastectomy. *Cancer*. 1977;40:2381–2387.

37. Maguire GP, Lee EG, Bevington DJ, Kuchemann CS, Crabtree RJ, Cornell CE. Psychiatric problems in the first year after mastectomy. *Br Med J*. 1978;1:963–965.

38. Jamison KR, Wellisch DK, Pasnau RO. Psychosocial aspects of mastectomy: I. The woman's perspective. *Am J Psychiatry*. 1978;135:432–436.

39. Metzger LF, Rogers TF, Bauman LJ. Effects of age and marital status on emotional distress after a mastectomy. *J Psychosoc Oncol*. 1983;1:17–33.

40. Northouse LL, Swain MA. Adjustment of patients and husbands to the initial impact of breast cancer. *Nurs Res*. 1987; 36:221–225.

41. Holland JC, Rowland JH. Psychological reactions to breast cancer and its treatment. In: Harris JR, Hellman S, Henderson IC, Kinne DW, eds. *Breast Diseases*. Philadelphia: Lippincott; 1987: 632–647.

42. Fallowfield LJ, Baum M, Maguire GP. Effects of breast conservation on psychological morbidity associated with diagnosis and treatment of early breast cancer. *Br Med J*. 1986;293:1331–1334.

43. Steinberg MD, Juliano MA, Wise L. Psychological outcome of lumpectomy versus mastectomy in the treatment of breast cancer. *Am J Psychiatry*. 1985;142:34–39.

44. Ganz PA, Schag AC, Lee JJ, Polinsky ML, Tan SJ. Breast conservation versus mastectomy: is there a difference in psychological adjustment or quality of life in the year after surgery? *Cancer*. 1992;69:1729–1738.

45. Schain WS, d'Angelo TM, Dunn ME, Lichter AS, Pierce LJ. Mastectomy versus conservative surgery and radiation therapy: psychosocial consequences. *Cancer*. 1994;73:1221–1228.

46. Wellisch DK, DiMatteo R, Silverstein M, et al. Psychosocial outcomes of breast cancer therapies: lumpectomy versus mastectomy. *Psychosomatics*. 1989; 30:365–373.

47. Wolberg WH, Romsaas EP, Tanner MA, Malec JF. Psychosexual adaptation to breast cancer surgery. *Cancer*. 1989;63:1645–1655.

48. Kemeny MM, Wellisch DK, Schain WS. Psychosocial outcome in a randomized surgical trial for treatment of primary breast cancer. *Cancer*. 1988; 62:1231–1237.

49. Rowland JH, Holland JC, Chaglassian T, Kinne D. Psychological response to breast reconstruction: expectations for and impact on postmastectomy functioning. *Psychosomatics*. 1993; 34:241–250.

50. Fisher JC. The silicone controversy: When will science prevail? *N Engl J Med*. 1992; 326:1696–1698.

51. Winer EP, Fee-Fulkerson K, Fulkerson CC, et al. Silicone controversy: a survey of women with breast cancer and silicone implants. *J Natl Cancer Inst*. 1993; 85:1407–1411.

52. Sutherland AM, Orbach CE, Dyk RB, Bard M. The psychological impact of cancer and cancer surgery: I. Adaptation to the dry colostomy: preliminary report and summary of findings. *Cancer*. 1952; 5:857–872.

53. Oberst MT, James R. Going home: Patient and spouse adjustment following cancer surgery. *Top Clin Nurs*. 1985; 7:46–57.

54. Madden TC, Jehu D. Psychological effects of stomas–I. Psychosocial morbidity one year after surgery. *J Psychosom Res*. 1987; 31:311–316.

55. Barsevick AM, Pasacreta J, Orsi A. Psychological distress and functional dependency in colorectal cancer patients. *Cancer Pract*. 1995; 3:105–110.

56. Dropkin MJ. Coping with disfigurement and dysfunction after head and neck cancer surgery: a conceptual framework. *Semin Oncol Nurs*. 1989;5:213–219.

57. Scott DW, Oberst MT, Dropkin MJ. A stress-coping model. *Adv Nurs Sci*. 1980; 3:9–23.

58. Gamba A, Romano M, Grosso IM, et al. Psychosocial adjustment of patients surgically treated for head and neck cancer. *Head & Neck*. 1992;14:218–223.

59. Krouse JH, Krouse HJ, Fabian RL. Adaptation to surgery for head and neck cancer. *Laryngoscope*. 1989;99:789–794.

60. Walsh PC, Lepar H. The role of radical prostatectomy in the management of prostatic cancer. *Cancer*. 1987; 60:526–537.

61. Walsh PC, Partin AW, Epstein JI. Cancer control and quality of life following anatomical radical retropubic prostatectomy: results at 10 years. *J Urol*. 1994; 152:1831–1836.

62. Leandri P, Rossignol G, Gautier JR, Ramon J. Radical retropubic prostatectomy: morbidity and quality of life. *J Urol*. 1992; 147:883–887.

63. Pedersen KV, Carlsson BP, Rahmquist M, Varenhorst E. Quality of life after radical retropubic prostatectomy for carcinoma of the prostate. *Eur Urol*. 1993; 24:7–11.

64. Fowler FJ. Patient reports of symptoms and quality of life following prostate surgery. *Eur Urol*. 1991; 1:44–49.

65. Herr HW. Quality of life of incontinent men after radical prostatectomy. *J Urol*. 1994; 151: 652–654.

66. Litwin MS, Hays RD, Fink A, et al. Quality of life outcomes in men treated for localized prostate cancer. *J Am Med Assoc*. 1995; 273:129–135.

67. Baslis KG, Santa-Cruz C, Brickman AL, Soloway MS. Quality of life 12 months after radical prostatectomy. *Br J Urol*. 1995; 75:48–53.

68. Lim AJ, Brandon AH, Fiedler J, et al. Quality of life: radical prostatectomy versus radiation therapy for prostate cancer. *J Urol*. 1995; 154:1420–1425.

69. Fowler FJ, Barry MJ, Lu-Yao G, et al. Effect of radical prostatectomy for prostate cancer on patient quality of life: results from a Medicare survey. *Urology*. 1995; 45: 1007–1013.

70. Fichten CS, Libman E, Amsel R, et al. Evaluation of the sexual consequences of surgery: retrospective and prospective strategies. *J Behav Med.* 1991; 14:267–285.

71. Libman E, Fichten CS, Rothenberg P, et al. Prostatectomy and inguinal hernia repair: a comparison of the sexual consequences. *J Sex Marital Ther.* 1991; 17:27–34.

72. Bjerre BD, Johansen C, Steven K. Health-related quality of life after cystectomy: bladder substitution compared with ilead conduit diversion. A questionnaire survey. *Br J Urol.* 1995; 75:200–205.

73. Schover LR. Sexuality and fertility in urologic cancer patients. *Cancer.* 1987; 60:553–558.

74. Thachil JV, Jewitt MAS, Rider WD. The effects of cancer and cancer therapy on male fertility. *J Urol.* 1981; 126:141–145.

75. Corney RH, Everett H, Howells A, Crowther ME. Psychosocial adjustment following major gynecological surgery for carcinoma of the cervix and vulva. *J Psychosom Res.* 1992; 36:561–568.

76. Cromes GF Jr. Implementation of interdisciplinary cancer rehabilitation. *Rehab Couns Bull.* 1978; 21:230–237.

77. Shea B, Kleban R, Knauer CJ. Breast cancer rehabilitation. *Semin Surg Oncol.* 1991; 7:326–330.

78. Willits M. Role of "Reach to Recovery" in breast cancer. *Cancer.* 1994; 74:2172–2173.

79. Heinrich RL, Schag CC. Stress and activity management: group treatment for cancer patients and spouses. *J Consult Clin Psychol.* 1985; 53:439–446.

22

Radiotherapy

DONNA B. GREENBERG

Patients encounter radiation therapy as a first-line potentially curative treatment, for instance, for Hodgkin's disease, throat cancer, or prostate cancer; or as one component of the treatment with surgery or chemotherapy, as in sarcomas, breast cancer, lung or cervical cancer (1). If the tumor recurs or progresses, radiation will target the local problem to reduce tumor size or fracture risk in a palliative strategy. Radiation oncology has a palliative role for relief of pain, hemorrhage, fungation and ulceration, dyspnea, blockage of hollow viscera, nerve root infiltration, cerebral metastases that raise intracranial pressure, and shrinkage of tumors that injure by taking up space (2). It is an emergency treatment for spinal cord compression, airway compromise, and superior vena cava obstruction. Radiation can be prophylactic, to prevent brain metastases in the setting of acute lymphoblastic leukemia or small cell lung cancer, or adjuvant to prevent local recurrence as in breast cancer.

Because of its highly technological nature, the large machines, and general fears of radiation energy, patients often approach treatment with apprehension. Detailed preparation for treatment makes a clinical difference in their anxiety. Since a patient must be able to cooperate, to lie still in one position briefly in isolation, patients with anxiety about closed spaces, other phobias, or inadequate pain relief require special attention. Anxiety disorders, then, are the most likely to require psychiatric intervention. High-dose corticosteroids used to prevent edema during central nervous system irradiation can also provoke significant psychiatric complications (see Table 22.1). Daily hospital visits for radiation therapy also allow an opportunity to screen for clinical depression and to engage patients in supportive psychotherapy. Furthermore, acute somatic side effects of fatigue and nausea require medical management but may have a psychological dimension. Many of the delayed side effects of radiation such as hypothyroidism after neck radiation or sterility after radiation to ovaries have psychological ramifications.

PRINCIPLES OF RADIATION

Radiation oncologists use high-energy electromagnetic radiation or high-speed particles to injure cancer cells (3). Radiation activates molecules to an unstable, ionized state. These molecules become chemically reactive free atoms, free radicals (molecules with unpaired electrons), and distinct stable molecules. This reaction directly or indirectly disrupts the chemical bonds of DNA and the conformation of proteins and other cell components. Cells can recover from potentially lethal radiation. Repair is more likely if the dose is low or if more time elapses before the next dose. The biological effect of radiation varies with dose and volume and inversely with time.

Cells in mitotic phase are most sensitive to radiation; erythroblasts, intestinal crypt cells, and germinal epidermal cells are thus most sensitive while nerve and muscle cells have the least sensitivity. The microvascular structure of tissues has intermediate sensitivity to radiation. Damage to the small blood vessels and supporting connective tissue may ultimately limit tissue viability.

The challenge of the radiation oncologist is to target tumor cells and spare healthy tissue. Telecobalt units and linear accelerators produce megavoltage beams that release energy spatially such that skin and superficial tissues are spared and more energy is released at the target tumor in the body. Electron beams facilitate treatment of superficial cancers without injuring deeper tissue (4).

The planned dose to any tissue depends on the risk/benefit ratio of cure compared to complications. Normal tissues recover faster than tumors. The determination of the dose-limiting tolerance of any organ

TABLE 22.1. *Psychiatric Side Effects of Steroids*

Insomnia

Nervousness

Lability

Depression

Psychosis

depends on the radiosensitivity of the tissue and the general health of the patient. Curative treatment is less likely with larger tumors or tumors composed of more radioresistant cells. While seminomas, lymphomas, and dysgerminomas are radiosensitive, osteogenic sarcomas, melanomas, and thyroid cancers are relatively insensitive to radiation. Squamous cell carcinoma of cervix or head and neck as well as breast and ovarian cancer are intermediate.

The plan for radiation delivery takes into account the size and stage of the tumor, proximity of normal structures, and dose-limiting vital tissues like liver, kidney, and spinal cord. Each plan requires individualized computer-assisted dosimetry. The process is simulated by a radiographic unit that delineates the field of the megavoltage treatment unit. Small tattoos facilitate consistent positioning for each treatment. This simulation treatment occurs in the radiation oncology department in one session prior to the start of radiation treatments.

With external-beam or teletherapy, the total treatment is divided into fractions delivered Monday through Friday over six weeks for curative or two weeks for palliative treatment. Patients come for evaluation, simulation, and explanation, and then return each weekday for the several minutes they must stay carefully in one same position on the table.

Brachytherapy implies that the source of radiation has been implanted temporarily in the patient. An applicator or tube is positioned in the patient while he is in the operating room. The isotope is afterloaded in the radiology suite or hospital room. Then the patient is isolated in a hospital room for several days until the desired dose is reached. Sometimes, patients are released with permanent low-energy seeds in the tumor.

ADJUSTMENT TO RADIATION TREATMENT

Patients undergoing radiotherapy have significant apprehension, sadness, anger, and social withdrawal as they respond to the diagnosis of malignancy (5–8). Depressive symptoms were not as severe in 200 radio-

therapy patients studied by Forester and colleagues as they were in psychiatric patients, but anorexia, insomnia, and fatigue were similarly severe in both groups (5). Systematic interviews (7,8) of 50 radiotherapy patients revealed a dominant coping strategy of denial, not denying the diagnosis but the likelihood of death due to cancer. Patients equated their cancer with a less dreaded disease. They focused on concerns for others, identified with the doctor's fight, and depended on the physician and treatment. Patients were found to be unprepared for treatment and pessimistic about its benefit. Treatment side effects were misinterpreted as permanent damage.

While these patients coped with the larger issues of life-threatening illness, radiation itself arouses anxiety (see Table 22.2). Radiation conjured up associations with the atomic bomb, nuclear accidents, radiation sickness, and ionizing radiation in the atomosphere. To those who would have preferred for the tumor to be cut out, radiation treatment seemed to be a less aggressive, palliative procedure. Some patients feared that the machine would not accurately release radiation, or that the toxicity of radiation burns would be too great. Most were concerned about disrobing, type of machine, and being alone in the room. Others worried about the duration of exposure and the danger of coughing, breathing, or moving during an exposure.

Many patients find the waiting room experience difficult but appreciate the support and attention of radiotherapy staff. Patients have anticipatory anxiety awaiting real or sham radiation (9). By clinical observation and projective analysis of interview samples of 20 breast cancer patients referred for radiotherapy, Holland found that patients were most anxious at the outset of treatment (6). At the end of treatment, they were more angry, depressed, and less hopeful. Their mood reflected in part the malaise of radiation side effects as treatment progressed. However, separation anxiety increased at the end of treatment. Women felt that they would be more vulnerable to tumor recurrence when they were no longer monitored closely by radiotherapy staff. Forester and colleagues believed

TABLE 22.2. *Anxiety in the Setting of Radiation*

Fears about radiation energy

Anticipatory anxiety

Fears of isolation

Claustrophobia

Conditioned nausea induced by chemotherapy

Poor pain control

that decreased dysphoria over the time of treatment could be attributed to the supportive staff (5).

Brachytherapy for gynecological cancer provoked physiological arousal and agitation in women before treatment (10). The anxiety persisted afterward and continued with the second treatment, although physicians saw them as less anxious the second time. Brachytherapy required 48–72 hours of isolation after an applicator was positioned and loaded with radioactive pellets. The most anxious group remained most anxious after treatment.

Those least anxious before treatment had the most disruption after treatment. Anderson and Tewflik suggested that the "work of worry" at the outset allowed better adaptation as Janis's concept of anxiety would suggest (11). The highest anxiety and lowest anxiety groups were more angry at the end of treatment. The moderately anxious group had the lowest hostility scores.

Brachytherapy in isolated hospital rooms is difficult for patients who are claustrophobic or frightened about being alone. Staying mostly in one position for an extended period of time can be a challenge. Delirium or poor pain control can complicate care if not given close attention. Staff of all sorts and visitors will tend to maintain a distance from the patient and visit less frequently because of lead shields and the fear of radiation exposure. With brachytherapy and prolonged isolation, it is helpful for staff to consider that radiation energy decreases by the inverse square of distance from the source (3). Staff can anticipate that the patient will be more isolated, and can plan to visit the room proactively, using shields as appropriate.

High trait anxiety, history of claustrophobia, chronic pain, and preconditioned nausea all heighten the risk of anxiety syndromes with radiation treatment. Those patients with high levels of anxiety will be more prone to anticipatory anxiety and anxiety during isolation. Those who come to radiation with anticipatory nausea already conditioned by previous emetic chemotherapy will be more apt to vomit on entering the hospital, before and after radiation treatment. Patients in pain are already physiologically aroused and on guard. They will naturally worry about lying in position if they do not have adequate analgesia and be more apt to develop aversive conditioning from radiation treatment.

PREPARATION FOR TREATMENT

Radiotherapy patients wish more information from the physician (12) (see Table 22.3). The referring physician

TABLE 22.3. *Strategies to Prepare Patients*

Orientation by radiation oncologist
Extension of information by nurses
Videotape or tape/slides with time for questions
Relaxation and imagery techniques
Preparation for posttreatment worries
Opportunity to call staff after treatment ends

cannot prepare patients adequately for radiotherapy or clarify the specific radiotherapy plan (13). The patient looks to the radiation oncologist for clarification of medical factors, treatment plan, and side effects. The value of orientation to the treatment area by the radiotherapist was documented by Holland (6). The physician introduced the patient to the room, the machine, and the technician. The half-hour concluded with an opportunity to discuss patient concerns. Women who received the orientation were less anxious at the first visit than the control group.

Nurses typically have one-to-one sessions to extend information offered by the physician, particularly aiding in management of side effects (14). Since most patients are anxious on the first visit, they often will not remember what was said. Some questions do not arise until later. Nurses are available to answer these questions. Preparations for side effects with guidelines depending on specific site, for mouth care, skin care, and diet add to a patient's sense of control and make strict compliance more likely (14–15).

To meet the need for more preparation, Rainey and colleagues developed an educational intervention (16). Patients assigned to the high-information group were individually shown a 12-minute slide–tape program that introduced the staff, machines, and procedure. The program included information about what the patient would see, hear, and feel, and a discussion of common misconceptions about treatment. Staff were available to answer questions. Irrespective of coping style, patients who had the educational intervention rather than a booklet introduction were less anxious at the first and last visit.

Detailed sensory information was a key to an educational intervention which reduced the amount of disruption of usual activities for men with prostate cancer during and after radiation treatment (17). The experimental group listened to 4–7 minute informational tapes addressing issues derived from interviews with other patients. At simulation the tape described the treatment planning session. Patients were advised that they would "see red lights coming from the walls of the room" and would hear a whirring and buzzing sound as a machine moved." Prior to the first treatment, the experience of receiving radiation treatment was described. At the fifth treatment, discussion focused on side effects that might occur as treatment continued. During the last week of treatment, the patients heard what to expect after treatment. Neither group expressed emotional distress; their main concern was function. Relaxation training and imagery techniques for stress reduction benefited radiotherapy patients in comparison to a counseling and education intervention. Decker and colleagues found in a randomized controlled trial of 82 patients that those who had relaxation training reported less tension, depression, fatigue, and anger on the Profile of Mood States (18).

PSYCHIATRIC CONSULTATION

Since patients do not generally feel that the radiation oncologist is a physician to speak with about emotional needs (13), psychological distress is often dealt with privately (19). Forester and colleagues randomized 100 patients to a ten-week course of supportive–educative psychotherapy or a control group 20. They found that the psychotherapy group had a greater reduction of emotional and physical symptoms of distress compared to the control group during and after treatment. The patients were told that these sessions were meant to facilitate coping with feelings, but many were hesitant to talk about feelings for a number of sessions. Gradually, over 10 sessions, they were more forthcoming with the guidance of the therapist. The style of treatment was educative, supportive, with opportunity for interpretive clarification and catharsis. The authors believed that the opportunity for psychotherapy allowed them not to be alone with their emotional distress.

The most likely reason for psychiatric referral among radiation patients is management of mood disorder or psychiatric side effects of steroids. Major depressive disorder is a serious, treatable diagnosis. The daily interaction with patients in treatment provides an opportunity for identificatin of patients with high likelihood of emotional problems. Patients with a history of depression or with somatic complaints more severe than expected may have depression. All pains are worse through its prism. Since fatigue is a central symptom of depression, patients with undiagnosed depression may have persistent fatigue after radiation. Steroids, commonly prescribed for central nervous system radiation, can cause insomnia, agitation, lability, depression, or psychosis.

Radiation treatment requires commitment and cooperation by the patient. Patients with chronic psychosis like schizophrenia may be competent and able to cooperate if explanations and medications are appropriate. Since many physicians are not comfortable talking to patients with chronic mental illness, psychiatrists can facilitate communication and refine treatment medications to get the job done.

ACUTE SIDE EFFECTS

Acute side effects of radiation treatment depend on the site, dose, and volume of treatment. Tissues with rapidly dividing cells show acute injury more rapidly: skin, hair follicles, and intestinal lining. Leukopenia and thrombocytopenia may develop. Skin may suffer dry or moist desquamation and darking. Nausea, diarrhea, fatigue, dysuria, sore throat, and anorexia are typical. Lung radiation may lead to dry cough, dyspnea, and pneumonitis. Late effects are related to small-vessel changes and fibrosis.

Nausea

Nausea is likely in about 60% of cases after treatments including total body radiation, upper hemibody, total nodal, and abdominal bed radiation; it is less likely (30%) in upper abdominal, lower thorax, pelvis, and least likely with head and neck and extremities (20). Nausea in patients with brain radiation may signal increased central nervous system pressure.

The mechanism that produces nausea is thought to be related to the release of serotonin in the gut as intestinal mucosal cells are injured. Gastric emptying may also be delayed. Both serotonin and other toxins provoke nausea via the chemoreceptor trigger zone. Antiemetics, dopamine antagonists like perphenazine, have some benefit; ondansetron, granisetron, and other 5HT3 antagonists prevent nausea associated with total body irradiation (21) and radiation directed at the gastrointestinal tract (22).

The expectation of nausea or fatigue, once patients are told about side effects, leads to nausea and fatigue even when radiation is only sham. With sham radiation, 75% of subjects developed symptoms of nausea and fatigue (23). Conditioned nausea after previous emetic chemotherapy or previous radiation-induced nausea may augment the direct toxic effect and provoke nausea before treatment. Benzodiazepines may prevent the conditioned component of nausea (24).

Anorexia with radiotherapy may be ameliorated by megestrol acetate 40 mg four times a day or prednisolone 10 mg three times a day. Megestrol led to greater improvement in appetite in a prospective, randomized trial (25).

Fatigue

Fatigue is a systemic effect of radiation treatment that may also be related to the consequences of cell injury (26). Separate from nausea, dyspnea, or weariness from daily trips to the hospital, sequential radiation treatments are associated with fatigue and an increased tendency to sleep. This symptom varies with site. In the study of King and colleagues 14 of 15 patients with chest radiation reported fatigue by the third week, initially intermittent then continuous (27). Fatigue remained mild to moderate throughout treatment and persisted over several months. In head and neck, gynecologic, and genitourinary patients, 65%–72% of 25–30 patients had fatigue by the latter part of the treatment. Fatigue was more severe in the head and neck group, least severe in the genitourinary group. Fatigue was generally worse in the afternoon and evening; afternoon naps were helpful. Nausea, which itself is fatiguing, was present in half the gynecological group but not the others.

In studies of fatigue from localized radiation to breast and prostate, fatigue increased at about 17 fractions, on average in the fourth week, and plateaued (28,29). Fatigue was not associated with clinical depression or nausea. There was no significant improvement on the weekend in this study, but weekend improvement did occur in a similar study (30).

Since fatigue is a core symptom of major depressive disorder, fatigue from radiation may be amplified by depression, panic attacks, or generalized anxiety. Classically, the fatigue of mood disorder has a different character, associated with dread of the day, broken sleep, early morning wakening, and morning exacerbation. Hypothyroidism should be considered in a patient who has had head or neck radiation.

Brain Edema

Acutely, swelling of the central nervous system secondary to radiation is a threat. The somnolence syndrome that occurs in children with acute lymphocytic leukemia 3–8 weeks after cranial radiation is not well understood (31). Alopecia is temporary unless the dose to treat a primary brain tumor is extremely high.

Dexamethasone during brain and spinal cord radiation prevents brain swelling. This treatment exposes patients to the psychiatric side effects of steroids in addition to the neurologic compromise of the cancer. These range from mild to moderate hyperactivity and insomnia to lability, anxiety, and agitation (32). A blatant psychosis with variable manic symptoms can occur suddenly. A clinically significant depressive disorder may develop with steroids or with their withdrawal. The tendency to psychiatric manifestation is dose related. Manic symptoms may be more likely when the patient is already on antidepressants, which can also lead to a manic reaction.

These psychiatric syndromes sometimes occur when discontinuation of steroids cannot be stopped. Even if steroids are discontinued, remission of psychosis or depression does not occur immediately without psychotropic treatment. Psychosis should be treated acutely with antipsychotic medications. Antianxiety and hypnotic benzodiazepines may reduce anxiety and insomnia. Lability may be reduced by perphenazine or haloperidol.

Discontinuation of steroids may be associated with dysphoria or a persistent depression which requires antidepressant treatment.

DELAYED EFFECTS

Patients undergoing radiation (34) treatment do risk delayed adverse effects. These include secondary tumors, cognitive impairment, hypothyroidism, growth retardation, pulmonary fibrosis, enteritis, and sterility. General quality of life after definitive radiotherapy is good (33), but a general evaluation may not call attention to specific, more uncommon losses.

Brain

Neuropsychiatric side effects of radiation (34) are described in Chapter 43. Cranial radiation can cause leukoencephalopathy. Children with acute lymphocytic leukemia, who have both cranial radiation and intrathecal methotrexate suffer neurotoxicity. In one study this meant a mean 10-point drop in IQ, with greater impairment in those treated at the youngest age (35). The injury is dose related and occurs with 18–19 Gy as well as 24 Gy (36). Deficits were noted in nondominant hemisphere function, perceptual localization, nondominant hand motor skills, visual–motor integration, and tendency to distraction.

In adults who receive prophylactic cranial radiation as treatment for small-cell lung cancer with chemotherapy and chest radiation, three-fourths of long-term survivors had diminished mental acuity (17). There is a poor correlation between the leukoencephalopathy which appears on magnetic resonance scan and intellectual dysfunction (37). Radiation-induced dementia can occur with radionecrosis, with edematous white matter and cortical atrophy (38).

Endocrine

Patients treated with neck or head radiation are at risk for pituitary failure or hypothyroidism. After radiation for head and neck cancer, 40% had thyroid dysfunction after five years (39). When the hypothalamic–pituitary axis has been in the radiation field, inadequate growth hormone, thyroid-stimulating hormone, or adrenocorticostimulating hormone (ACTH), or hyperprolactinemia may occur later (40). The effect is dose related. Growth may be retarded (41).

Nutritional

Treatment of head and neck cancer may leave changes in taste and a very dry mouth due to lack of saliva production. Dental and nutritional difficulties may result. Radiation in pelvis or abdomen may cause persistent diarrhea.

Sterility and Sexual Dysfunction

Radiation treatment for prostate cancer is associated with a decrease in erectile capacity, smaller ejaculate volume, and a decrease in orgasmic pleaure (42). Erectile dysfunction after pelvic irradiation has been attributed to development of arterial fibrosis, accelerated arteriosclerosis, and microvascular damage (43), although one researcher could not confirm this (44).

In planning radiation to other areas, radiotherapists shield ovaries and testes. After orchiectomy for seminoma, radiation to pelvic and paraaortic fields, even with shielding of the remaining testicle, produces acute azospermia. Spermatogenesis usually returns after after 1–5 years. In a series of survivors of seminoma, the most common problems were reduced semen volume and reduced intensity of orgasm. Patients remained concerned about fertility and sexual dysfunction (45).

Consideration of sperm banking must be discussed with the patient prior to a treatment that could jeopardize fertility. Children who were treated for Hodgkin's disease did not know their fertility status when they became sexually active. Their parents had never found the right time to discuss the consequences of treatment (46). Children cured of leukemia by bone marrow transplantation that requires total body radiation and chemotherapy will face this adjustment.

Radiation to the ovary will cause sterility depending on the age and dose. Restriction of the vagina can occur after pelvic irradiation, and pelvic irradiation may limit the ability for congestion with excitement in women. (See Chapter 42 on sexuality.)

CONCLUSIONS

While radiation treatment may be one aspect of an overall oncologic treatment, the referring physician cannot adequately prepare the patient for the radiation treatment. Patients are apt to have fears of radiation itself and to misconstrue side effects of treatment as progressive weakness due to disease. The patient looks to the radiotherapist for clarification of the plan specific to his or her case. Orientation to the treatment and time to answer questions, offered by the radiotherapist and extended by nurses, have documented benefit. A creative addition is video tapes with specific sensory information describing what acute side effects patients should expect during the procedure. Nurses monitor side effects, suggest treatment strategies, and continue to answer questions.

Proven antianxiety techniques include pretreatment benzodiazepines and systematic relaxation training. Attention to the ambience of the waiting room area can alleviate the anxiety of daily waiting. A friend or relative with the patient, a bidirectional intercom, and a television monitor will alleviate the sense of isolation. Patients isolated for brachytherapy require optimal treatment for anxiety, cognitive clarity, and pain control. Patients trust the staff and become anxious about coping with side effects without their help after the last session. Benzodiazepines and relaxation training are appropriate for patients with persistent anxiety, claustrophobia, panic attacks, and anticipatory nausea.

Psychiatric consultation is particularly appropriate for diagnosing and treating depression, managing anxiety syndromes, or coordinating treatment of patients with chronic mental illness. The patients' daily visits to receive radiation provide an opportunity for support from social service or psychiatry. Educative supportive psychotherapy has documented advantages. Preparation for the weeks after treatment and the continuous option of telephone advice helps the transition.

REFERENCES

1. Perez CA, Brady LW. Overview. In: Perez CA, Brady LW, eds. *Principles and Practice of Radiation Oncology,* 2d ed. Philadelphia, JB Lippincott; 1992: 1–63.
2. Ashby M. The role of radiotherapy in palliative care. *J Pain Symptom Manage.* 1991; 6:380–383.
3. Rubin P, Siemann D. Basic concepts of radiation oncology and cancer radiotherapy. In: Rubin P, ed. *Clinical Oncology: A Multidisciplinary Approach.* New York: American Cancer Society; 1983: 58–71

4. Keller BE, Rubin P. Basic concepts of radiation physics. In: Rubin P, ed. *Clinical Oncology: A Multidisciplinary Approach.* New York: American Cancer Society; 1983: 72–81.

5. Forester BM, Kornfeld DS, Fleiss J. Psychiatric aspects of radiotherapy. *Am J Psychiatry.* 1978; 135:960–965.

6. Holland JC, Rowland J, Lebovitz A, Rusalem R. Reactions to cancer treatment: assessment of emotional response to adjuvant radiotherapy as a guide to planned intervention. *Psychiatr Clin North Am.* 1979; 347–358.

7. Peck A. Emotional reactions to having cancer. *Am J Roentgenol Radiat Ther Nucl Med.* 1972; 114:591–599.

8. Peck A, Boland J. Emotional ractions to radiation treatment. *Cancer.* 1977; 40:180–184.

9. Gottschalk LA, Kunkal R, Wohl TH, et al. Total and half body irradiation: effect on cognitive and emotional processes. *Arch Gen Psychiatry.* 1969; 21:574–580.

10. Anderson BL, Karlsson JA, Anderson B, Tewfik. Anxiety and cancer treatment: response to stressful radiotherapy. *Health Psychol.* 1984; 3:535–551.

11. Anderson BL, Tewfik HH. Psychological reactions to radiation therapy: reconsideration of the adaptive aspects of anxiety. *J Pers Soc Psychol.* 1985; 48:1024–1032.

12. Cassileth BR, Volckmar D, Goodman RL. The effect of experience on radiation therapy patients' desire for information. *Int J Radiat Oncol Biol Phys.* 1980; 6:493–496.

13. Mitchell GW, Glicksman AS. Cancer patients' knowledge and attitudes. *Cancer.* 1977; 40:61–66.

14. Strohl RA. The nursing role in radiation oncology: symptom management of acute and chronic reaction. *Oncol Nurs Forum.* 1988; 15:429–434.

15. Herbert D, The assessment ofthe clinical significance of noncompliance with prescribed schedules of irradiation. *Int J Radiat Oncol Biol Phys.* 1977; 2:763–772.

16. Rainey LC. Effects of preparatory patient education for radiation oncology patients. *Cancer.* 1985; 56:1056–1061.

17. Johnson JE, Nail LM, Lauver D, et al. Reducing the negative impact of radiation therapy on functional status. *Cancer.* 1988; 61:46–51.

18. Decker TW, Cline EJ, Gallagher M. Relaxation therapy as an adjunct in radiation oncology. *J Clin Psychol.* 1992; 48:388–393.

19. Forester B, Kornfeld DS, Fleiss JL. Psychotherapy during radiotherapy: effects on emotional and physical distress. *Am J Psychiatry.* 1985; 142:22–27.

20. Feyer P, Titlbach O, Fiola M, et al. Gastrointestinal reactions in radiotherapy. *Support Care Cancer.* 1996; 4:249. [Abst #100.]

21. Spitzer TR, Bryson JC, Cirenza E, et al. Randomized double-blind, placebo-controlled evaluation of oral ondansetron in the prevention of nausea and vomiting associated with fractionated total body irradiation. *J Clin Oncol.* 1994; 12:2432–2438.

22. Priestman TJ. Roberts JT, Lucraft H, et al. Results of a randomized, double-blind comparative study of ondansetron an metoclopramide in the prevention of nausea and vomiting following high-dose upper abdominal irradiation. *Clin Oncol.* 1990; 2:71–75.

23. Parsons JA, Webster JH. Evaluation of the placebo effect in the treatment of radiation sickness. *Acta Radiol.* 1961; 56:129–140.

24. Greenberg DB, Surman OS, Clarke J, Baer L. Alprazolam for phobic nausea and vomiting related to cancer chemotherapy. *Cancer Treat Rep.* 1987; 71: 549–550.

25. Lai YL, Fang FM, Yeh CY. Mangement of anorexic patients in radiotherapy: a prospective randomized comparison of megestrol and prednisolone. *J Pain Symptom Manage.* 1994; 9:265–268.

26. Anno GH, Baum SJ, Withers HR, Young RW. Symptomatology of acute radiation effects in humans after exposure to doses of 0.5–30 Gy. *Health Phys.* 1989, 56:821–838.

27. King KB, Nail LM, Kreamer K, et al. Patients' descriptions of the experience of receiving radiation therapy. *Oncol Nurs Forum.* 1985; 12:55–61.

28. Greenberg DB, Sawicka J, Eisenthal S, Ross D. Fatigue syndrome due to localized radiation *J Pain Symptom Manage.* 1992; 7:38–45.

29. Greenberg DB, Gray JL, Mannix SM, Eisenthal S, Carey M. Treatment-related fatigue and serum interleukin-1 levels in patients during external beam irradiation for prostate cancer. *J Pain Symptom Manage.* 1993; 8: 196–199.

30. Haylock PJ, Hart LK. Fatigue in patients receiving localized radiation. *Cancer Nurs.* 1979; 2:461–467.

31. Freeman JE, Johnston PG, Voke JM. Somnolence after prophylactic cranial irradiation in children with acute lymphocytic leukemia. *Br Med J.* 1973; 4:523–525.

32. Ling MHM, Perry PJ, Tsuang MT. Side effect of corticosteroid therapy: psychiatric aspects. *Arch Gen Psychiatry.* 1981; 38:471–477.

33. Danoff B, Kramer S, Irwin P, Gottlieb A. Assessment of quality of life in long-term survivors after definitive radiotherapy. *Am J Clin Oncol.* 1983; 6:339–345.

34. Schultheiss TE, Kun LE, Ang KK, Stephens LC. Radiation response of the central nervous system. *Int J Radiat Oncol Biol Phys.* 1995; 31:1093–1112.

35. Rowland JH, Glidewell OJ, Sibley RF, et al. for the Cancer and Leukemia Group B. Effects of different forms of central nervous prophylaxis on neuropsychologic function in childhood leukemia. *J Clin Oncol.* 1984; 2:1327–1336.

36. Butler RW, Hill JM, Steinherz PG, Meyers PA, Finlay JL, Neuropsychologic effects of cranial irradiation, intrathecal methotrexate, and systemic methotrexate in childhood cancer. *J Clin Oncol.* 1994; 12:2621–2629.

37. Roman DD, Sperduto PW. Neuropsychiatric effects of intracranial radiation: current knowledge and future directions. *Int J Radiat Oncol Biol Phys.* 1995; 31: 983–998.

38. DeAngelis LM, Delattre J-Y, Posner JB. Radiation-induced dementia in patients cured of brain metastases. *Neurology.* 1989; 39:789–796.

39. Turner SL, Tiver FW, Bayage SC. Thyroid dysfunction following radiotherapy for head and neck cancer. *Int J Radiat Oncol Biol Phys.* 1995; 31:279–283.

40. Sklar CA, Constine LS. Neuroendocrinological sequelae of radiation therapy. *Int J Radiat Oncol Biol Phys.* 1995; 31:1113–1121.

41. Duffner PK, Cohen NE, Voorhees ML, et al. Long-term effects of cranial irradiation on endocrine function in children with brain tumors: a prospective study. *Cancer.* 1985; 56:189–193.

42. Helgason AR, Fredrikson M, Adolfsson J, Steineck G. Decreased sexual capacity after external radiation therapy for prostate cancer impairs quality of life. *Int J Radiat Oncol Biol Phys.* 1995; 32:33–39

43. Goldstein I, Feldman MI, Deckers PJ, et al. Radiation-associated impotence: a clinical study of its mechanism *J Am Med Assoc.* 1984; 251:903–910.

44. Mittal BA. A study of penile circulation before and after radiation in patients with prostate cancer and its effect on impotence. *Int J Radiat Oncol Biol Phys.* 1984; 11:1122–1125.

45. Schover LR, Gonzales M, von Eschenbach AC. Sexual and marital relationships after radiotherapy for seminoma. *Urology.* 1986; 27:117–123.

46. Cella DF, Cherin EA. Measuring quality of life in patients with cancer. Paper presented at the American Cancer Society Fifth National Conference on Human Values and Cancer, San Francisco, March, 1987.

23

Chemotherapy, Hormonal Therapy, and Immunotherapy

M. TISH KNOBF, JEANNIE V. PASACRETA, ALAN VALENTINE, AND
RUTH McCORKLE

Systemic forms of cancer treatment include chemotherapy, biologicals, and hormonal therapies. The goals associated with each of these treatments may be to cure, to extend life, or to provide palliation. In any case, the general public has limited knowledge regarding the various forms of systemic therapy. Their knowledge is often derived from personal experiences and from the media, whose content may be outdated and/or dramatized. These limited sources of information coupled with society's fear of cancer have led to many negative attitudes, irrational fears, and misperceptions about cancer therapy among the general public and health care professionals alike. Misconceptions and fears about systemic cancer therapies (particularly chemotherapy because it is the most common and best-known treatment) have lead to several commonly held, but erroneous, beliefs. For example, treatments are often viewed as experimental rather than conventional. Concern about being a "guinea pig" is common among patients and their families as well as the anticipation of severe and toxic side effects from all treatment agents. In light of these issues, emotional distress for individuals anticipating, receiving, or completing a course of therapy is often universal. There is a need to understand and distinguish "normal" responses to treatment from those responses that are more severe and may warrant a referral to a psychiatric specialist. This chapter will review the various forms of systemic cancer therapies, their goals, and common psychological accompaniments to various stages of treatment. In recent years, with the advent of aggressive new therapies, the varied goals of treatment have been highlighted and have directed clinicians and researchers to address the risk/benefit ratio of therapy and to explore quality of life issues for the patient and family. This chapter will also address these issues.

CANCER CHEMOTHERAPY

The first dose of chemotherapy was administered nearly fifty years ago to a patient with lymphoma (1). The early years of chemotherapy research concentrated on treatment of the hematologic malignancies, focusing on cell cycle kinetics, combination of drugs, and the pharmacokinetics of drug therapy. By the 1970s, the success of chemotherapy in inducing remissions and producing long-term responses was established for acute childhood leukemia and Hodgkin's lymphoma. Over the next three decades, the subspecialty of medical oncology evolved with significant scientific advances in the biologic understanding of cancer, results from controlled randomized clinical drug trials, new drug development, understanding of the mechanisms of drug resistance, and the use of biologicals. During this time, chemotherapy, alone or in combination with other modalities, resulted in the reality of long-term survival for selected patients (e.g., testicular cancer, sarcoma in children) and dramatically improved the survival of other patients. The progress of oncology research has also helped us to understand the outcomes of treatment, such as why we can cure late-stage Hodgkin's disease with chemotherapy alone or fail to impact survival of patients with lung cancer even with multimodality therapy.

Combination Chemotherapy

Chemotherapeutic drugs are classified by their cell cycle activity and presumed mechanism of action (2). The classifications include alkylating agents, antimetabolites, antitumor antibiotics, and plant alkaloids/ natural products, with a few drugs falling into a "miscellaneous" category. Combination drug therapy is the cornerstone of treatment because of superiority over single drug therapy in response rates, durability of response, and survival outcomes. The basis for combining drugs includes synergy of drugs, cell cycle specificity, modes of action, varied toxicities and effectiveness of the individual drugs for a specific disease site. Combination chemotherapy also has the potential of producing a wide range of side effects and toxicity, as drugs are included with different mechanisms of action and often, different organ system toxicity (Table 23.1). (See also Chapter 55 on psychiatric side effects of chemotherapeutic agents.)

Goals of Therapy

The goal of standard chemotherapy ranges from cure to prolonged survival to palliation of symptoms. Chemotherapy can be used *(1)* alone as primary therapy with a curative intent (e.g., Hodgkin's disease); *(2)* as adjuvant therapy (adjunct to primary therapy modality) with a curative or long-term survival intent (e.g., stage I and II breast cancer); *(3)* as neoadjuvant (administered prior to surgery or radiotherapy) to reduce tumor burden or spare an organ (e.g., stage IIb or III breast cancer, bone sarcoma); *(4)* as therapy for advanced disease with intent to prolong survival (e.g., stage IV breast cancer, small-cell lung cancer); and *(5)* as palliative therapy for advanced disease (e.g., late-stage ovarian cancer, large-cell lung cancer).

Clinical trials provide the scientific mechanism to test new drug therapies and the effectiveness of therapeutic approaches. The scientific integrity related to the conduct of multisite clinical trials has received much attention in the past years, but, despite criticisms of either design or conduct, the clinical trial is the vehicle to answer important clinical questions with the least amount of bias in a reasonable period of time (2). Clinical trials present challenges to the oncologist and the patient, requiring more time for discussion, detailed explanations, decision-making and often, more frequent monitoring. Less than 5% of eligible patients in the United States are enrolled in clinical trials. Some reasons cited by physicians for not enrolling patients reflect those challenges mentioned, such as dislike of open discussions about uncertainty, extra time involved in discussing protocol, concern of harm to the doctor–patient relationship, and difficulty with informed consent (3). Well-informed patients may inquire about the standard therapy recommended and seek information about clinical trials, but this does not represent the majority of patients in the United States. Unfortunately, the challenges cited by physicians for not enrolling patients in clinical trials involve basic issues of communication skills and time. The end result is that patients do not always get adequate information about available options that may impact on their ability to make informed decisions about their treatment.

TABLE 23.1. *Potential Outcomes by Systems Associated with Cancer Chemotherapy Toxicity*

Systems	Potential Outcomes
Hematologic	Anemia, thrombocytopenia and neutropenia. May be associated with fatigue, risk or actual infection, need for supportive care, functional alterations and dependency on health care system
Gastrointestinal	Nausea, vomiting, anorexia, taste changes, stomatitis, diarrhea, and constipation
Dermatologic	Alopecia, local skin reactions, hyperpigmentation, dermatitis and nail changes
Urologic	Alterations in renal function; cystitis, electrolyte imbalance
Cardiopulmonary	Uncommon: pneumonitis, pulmonary fibrosis which may result in dyspnea and respiratory distress syndrome; cardiomyopathy
Neurotoxicity	Alterations in mental status and peripheral neuropathy
Gonadal	Infertility, inadequate sperm counts, amenorrhea associated with menopausal symptoms
Other	Drug dependent and uncommon: hepatic and ocular toxicities; allergic reactions

ENDOCRINE THERAPY

The efficacy of hormonal therapy in hormone-responsive tumors is well established. The major hormonal agents and their disease indications include estrogens, gonadotropin-releasing hormone agonists, and antiandrogens for prostate cancer; antiestrogens, aromatase inhibitors, and androgens for breast cancer; progestins for endometrial and breast carcinomas; and glucocorticoids for leukemia, lymphoma, and breast cancer (4). Glucocorticoids are also used as adjuncts to antiemetic regimens or to treat complications of cancer. Hormonal agents are associated with a wide spectrum of side effects, which include depression and irritability and confusion associated with glucocorticoids. Mood can also be impacted indirectly as a response to a treatment-related side effect such as impotence or infertility.

BIOTHERAPY

Biotherapy is a global term for use of biologic agents that have multiple actions. Because of this pleiotropic characteristic of biologics, they may augment or modulate the immune system, produce direct cytotoxic or antiproliferative activity, be influential in differentiation or maturation of cells, or interfere with tumor cell metastases of transformation (5,6). While there is no one classification system for biologics because of their diverse spectrum of action, there are accepted major categories: interferons, interleukins, hemato-

poietic growth factors, monoclonal antibodies, tumor necrosis factor and immunomodulators, differentiating agents, and vaccines (7). There is a wide range of clinical indications (8) and an equally wide range of clinical side effects of biologics. Interferon-α (IFN-α) is employed as a single agent or in combination therapy against several malignant diseases, including chronic myelogenous leukemia (CML), renal cell carcinoma, and melanoma. In addition, it is now employed as a primary therapy against hepatitis C. Interleukin-2 (IL-2) is currently used in combination therapy of solid tumors, including melanomas, sarcomas, and renal cell carcinomas, and also in intraventricular therapy for leptomeningeal disease.

Many of the biologics produce a systemic effect, often described as a flulike syndrome, but most toxicity is influenced by the specific agent, route, dose, and duration of treatment. Side effects of the major categories of biologics have been described in detail and a brief summary of the major effects is presented in Table 23.2 (9–14). Of particular note with biologics are neurotoxic effects, which are usually acute and reversible but may produce significant alterations in mental status (Table 23.3) and impair the patient's ability to function (15). Serious neurotoxic side effects are associated with only a small number of the many biologics. However, these few include agents which are now commonly employed in clinical oncology, and may complicate the treatment of large numbers of patients. These side effects will be discussed later in the chapter.

TABLE 23.2. *Side Effects of Biologics*

Category	Side Effects
Interferons	Flulike syndrome (fatigue, chills, fever, myalgias, headache, anorexia), leukopenia, anemia, thrombocytopenia, and alteration in mental status
Interleukins	Flulike syndrome, vascular leak syndrome, diffuse rash, pruritus, dry skin, universal organ system toxicity, and alteration in mental status
Hemaotpoietic growth factors	
Epo	Flulike syndrome
G-CSF	Bone pain
GM-CSF	Fever, dose-related fluid retention, dyspnea, myalgias, joint and bone pain
Monoclonal antibodies	Chills, rigors, urticaria, nausea, diarrhea, myalgias, anaphylaxis, mucosal congestion
Tumor necrosis factor	Dose- and route-dependent hypotension, chills, rigors, focal neurological deficits, flulike syndrome, local skin reaction, and alteration in mental status
Immunomodulators, differentiating agents	
BCG	Intravesicular: dysuria, frequency, hematuria, flu-like syndrome
Retinoids	Headaches, visual disturbances, dizziness, lethargy, teratogenesis, acute hypervitaminosis A
Levamisole	Flulike syndrome, nausea, vomiting, diarrhea

TABLE 23.3. *Neurological Side Effects Associated with Biologic Agents**

INTERFERON

Confusion

Depression†

Hypersomnia

Difficulty concentrating†

Memory problems†

Trouble with calculations

Slowed thinking†

Impaired motor coordination†

Impaired visual-motor skills

Impaired frontal lobe functioning†

Paraesthesias

INTERLEUKIN-2

Confusion†

Hypersomnolence†

Difficulty concentrating†

Agitation

Withdrawal from social contact

Irritability†

Depression

Bizarre dreams

Paranoia

Delusions

Hallucinations

TUMOR NECROSIS FACTOR

Confusion

Somnolence

Lethargy

*The occurrence and severity of side effects tend to increase as the dose is increased. Most side effects are readily reversible when therapy is discontinued. However, some may persist or progress off treatment.

†More frequently seen.

Source: Meyers (15), reproduced with permission.

PSYCHOLOGICAL ISSUES

Before Treatment

Patients have identified the period following diagnosis and before definitive therapy as very stressful (16). Patients continue with their emotional responses to the diagnosis and are further challenged by the need to choose a systemic therapy, all in a relatively short period of time (17). The patient's and family's understanding of the treatment and perceptions of side effects and purpose of therapy (primary/curative, adjuvant or for advanced disease) are factors that influence their coping abilities and level of emotional distress. Information and support are the predominant needs for the patient and family. This period is characterized by anxiety, related to uncertainty and unpredictability of the disease, its treatment, the scheduling of treatments, and the complicated decision making and often inadequate information (18–21). However, patients vary in terms of how much information they want. Patients who are information seekers and who actively participate in the decisions, weighing all available information, are more emotionally distressed than those who are less active in the decision making (22). Difficulty falling asleep, wakefulness during the night, tiredness after waking, and subjective reports of feeling upset, nervous, and tense are common manifestations of anxiety during this diagnostic and pretreatment period (23–25).

In clinical practice, coping strategies, information processing, and psychological adjustment are thought to be influenced by moderate to high levels of anxiety, although few data exist on the association of pretreatment anxiety and treatment outcomes (26). Subjectively, most patients dislike feeling anxious (27) and interventions are generally aimed at anxiety reduction by giving information and support (28–31). These interventions are important for all patients and families, but particularly for those in the decision-making phase of treatment.

During Treatment

Emotional distress is almost universal in patients receiving active systemic treatment. The etiology of this distress, however, is complex, influenced by the incidence and severity of side effects, individual characteristics (e.g. personality, coping style), age, diagnosis, disease status, and intent and type of therapy. Every bodily system has the potential of being affected by systemic therapy. Treatment may result in subjective symptom distress or produce toxicity that interferes with the patient's functional abilities and level of independence. Anxiety may be related to expectations of side effects, knowledge of actual side effects, uncertainty, and inadequacy of information about the experience of treatment (27,32). Procedures such as intravenous access, dependency on the health care provider for scheduling of treatment, and unpredictable needs for supportive care are also sources of anxiety that persists throughout treatment courses (27).

Symptoms are frequently rated by patients regarding their incidence and level of distress they cause; both are associated with emotional distress. Likert type scales are often used to rate symptom distress subjectively by the patient on scales of 0–5 or 0–10. The outcome is typically categorized into mild, moderate, or severe distress. In contrast, ratings used in clinical trials, such as the NIH Common Toxicity Criteria, objectively rate side effects and do not assess subjective distress. Moderate to severe drug toxicity is obviously important clinical information; however, mild to moderate symptom distress may be equally important with significant implications for the patient. Nerenz, Leventhal and Love (33) reported that vague long-term side effects were reported as more emotionally distressing than acute short-term side effects. Symptom distress was also reported as the most consistent predictor of adaptation in women treated with systemic therapy for breast cancer (34).

The most common distressing physical and nonphysical symptoms reported by patients who receive systemic chemotherapy are fatigue, nausea, vomiting, alopecia, anticipation of having treatment, insomnia, anorexia, weight changes, taste alterations, anxiety, and depressed mood (25,35–38). Many of these symptoms rated as mild to moderate have a more severe impact on the patient's daily function, body image, family relationships, sexual relationship, and overall psychological distress (37,39–43). Anxiety and symptom distress also often increase over the cycles of chemotherapy, resulting in higher levels of emotional distress (27,44). Patients comment that it becomes harder to come in for treatment. However, they are fearful of ending treatment as well, since implications are that, without treatment and close monitoring, they are at greater risk of recurrence.

In assessing psychological responses of a patient, it is important to determine whether they relate to a drug side effect, since organic mental status changes are associated with CNS effects of several chemotherapeutic agents (see Chapter 55). Clinicians should be mindful of drug toxicities that are associated with neuropsychiatric side effects, resulting from cerebral and cerebellar dysfunction, central nervous system toxicity, and encephalopathy. Symptoms which occur are delirium, confusion, poor concentration, depression, hallucinations, disorientation, somnolence, irritability, agitation, impaired memory, or alterations in cognition (45).

Neurotoxic side effects are a major dose-limiting toxicity of IFN-a therapy. This toxicity can take several forms, including simple fatigue, dementia, and affective syndromes. Formal thought disorder and frank neurologic presentations (usually Parkinson's syndrome symptoms) are encountered rarely. The neurotoxicity of IFN-a is largely dose-dependent, with a prevalence of approximately 17% in patients treated for hepatitis C (46). In the oncology setting, where patients are treated with significantly higher doses, the prevalence of neurotoxicity is 50%–70% in certain subpopulations (47,48). Combination treatment with other agents or modalities appears to increase the risk of severe neurotoxicity (49).

The acute toxicity of IFN-a resembles an influenza syndrome. Within hours of initiation of therapy, patients usually experience fever, malaise, myalgias, nausea, and headache (50,51). This syndrome is usually self-limited, though fatigue may persist (52,53). Patients who discontinue IFN-a therapy for even a few days will (typically) experience symptoms on resumption of treatment. The acute toxicity is generally well tolerated, and is treated symptomatically. Patients with poorer performance status have more difficulty, and the syndrome occasionally becomes a compliance issue in therapy.

Impairment of intellectual function can pose major problems for cancer patients treated with IFN-a. Deficits can be subtle and may easily be missed. They may be considered relatively unimportant in the context of attempts to cure or control a disease. For those who are seriously ill with aggressive tumors (renal cell carcinomas, melanomas) impairment of memory and concentration interferes with participation in treatment and family interaction. Patients with hematologic malignancies (e.g., chronic myelogenous leukemia) are often sufficiently well that they are able to work and participate in everyday life for years, yet cognitive side effects can significantly impair function.

Intellectual function may become impaired with initiation of interferon therapy. In the healthy volunteer, reaction time is slowed within hours of a single IFN injection at pharmacologic doses (51). Within days, patients complain of feeling mentally "slow" and lethargic. Word-finding difficulties, apathy, and confusion are reported (50). At IFN doses encountered in the oncology setting ($>5\,\mathrm{MU/day}$), up to 33% of patients experience such symptoms, and up to 10% request discontinuation of treatment within days after it is initiated (54).

IFN-α neurotoxicity appears to become more pronounced (or more difficult to tolerate) over time (47,55). In current practice, patients with hematologic malignancies are particularly vulnerable to long-term effects of IFN therapy. In evaluation of patients with CML, up to 70% have been shown to suffer impairment of motor coordination, frontal lobe executive function and depression (47), a pattern consistent with mild subcortical dementia (56). Memory and verbal reasoning were spared in these patients. Resolution of neurotoxic side effects is expected after discontinuation of IFN therapy, usually within days to weeks (52,57). However, persistence of cognitive dysfunction (similar to that described above) has been documented in patients up to three years post treatment (48).

Subjective depression is a frequently encountered, but poorly understood, side effect of IFN-α therapy. The prevalence of IFN-α-induced depression as an isolated entity is not known. The onset of symptoms can be quite sudden. On rare occasions patients may become acutely dysphoric and actively suicidal within hours or days of initiation of therapy. More often, the presentation is less intense, and of a chronic nature during treatment. Patients complain of sadness and lack of motivation. Vegetative symptoms, including insomnia or hypersomnia, anorexia, poor memory and concentration, and (especially) decreased libido are common. The difficulties in diagnosing IFN-α-induced depression are similar to those encountered in other cancer patients. Some symptoms may be accounted for on the basis of expected systemic effects of the primary neoplastic process or IFN treatment. Depressive syndromes may be a manifestation of neurotoxicity, and may be detected, with cognitive deficits, during neuropychological assessment. At other times depression appears to be a reactive phenomenon independent of cognitive status, as the patient deals with the implications either of an acute life-threatening illness or the prospect of long-term treatment with unpleasant side effects. As is the case with cognitive side effects, depression may be sufficiently severe that a patient will decline therapy.

While affective and cognitive disorders are most common, other neurologic and psychiatric complications may be encountered. Organic personality syndromes have been described (52), as have visual hallucinations and delirium (58–60). Patients treated with IFN-α may develop Parkinsonism (48,60) paresthesias, or peripheral neuropathy (61).

Compared to the interferons, the neurotoxicity of IL-2 is more pervasive and more severe. In addition to constitutional symptoms, the clinician should expect to encounter patients with acute onset dementia, delirium, as well as paranoia and other delusional disorders (55,62). Affective (depressive) disorders, while encountered relatively less often than with IFN-α, tend to be of acute onset and may require emergent intervention. Like IFN-α, the neurotoxicity of IL-2 is dose related, with serious neuropsychiatric syndromes encountered in up to 50% of patients (62). The severe systemic side effects of this agent, including fever and hypotension, place the patient at additional risk for neuropsychiatric complications, as does the fact that IL-2 is used with other biologics (63,64). Though acute IL-2 neurotoxicity usually resolves completely (8), acute neuropsychiatric syndromes may persist for days after IL-2 therapy is discontinued, and it is not clear whether subtle cognitive symptoms persist (49,64).

Chronic or severe neuropsychiatric side effects of biological agents can be very problematic for clinician and patient. An otherwise effective therapy may be compromised. Especially in the case of IFN-α and IL-2, poor understanding of the etiology of the toxicity has impeded attempts to intervene. Preexisting neurologic disorder may be a risk factor for some forms of biologic neurotoxicity (60), as may past psychiatric history (62). While not formally studied to date, clinical experience suggests that biologic neurotoxicity and current psychosocial stress may exacerbate each other. Despite these problems, interventions are possible.

It is first necessary to recognize the possibility of biologic-induced neurotoxicity. Especially in the community setting, clinicians are relatively poorly informed of potential side effects of biologics. Constitutional, affective, and cognitive symptoms are easy to overlook or may be attributed to a primary psychiatric disorder or to the malignancy itself. Given the prevalence of these side effects, neurotoxicity should always be considered when patients treated with biologics present with behavioral symptoms. Formal neuropsychologic assessment can be very useful in evaluation of subtle deficits or symptoms of uncertain etiology (Table 23.4). Psychiatric consultation may also be indicated. In the context of life-threatening disease, the importance of neuropsychiatric side-effects may be minimized or overlooked. As biologic agents may be used for long periods of time, it is especially important that the possibility of neurotoxicity be discussed before treatment is started. Given the stigma that remains associated with psychiatric illness, patients may be reluctant to admit to symptoms. They may feel that they are the only ones experiencing such problems. Even if a remedy is not immediately available, patients are often relieved to know that symptoms may be due to treatment-induced neurotoxicity.

As noted, much of the neurotoxicity of biotherapy is dose related. Consequently, the most reliable way to minimize or eliminate symptoms is to reduce the dose of the agent in question. Obviously this can compromise an otherwise effective, perhaps life-sustaining therapy. Under these circumstances, most patients are willing to "endure" neurotoxicity, while others are not, citing a preference for quality of life. In some cases it may be possible (or necessary) to allow some time off from therapy.

Pharmacologic intervention may be helpful. The constitutional side effects of biologics may be successfully treated with hydration, antipyretics, antiemetics, and analgesics. Corticosteroids have also proven effective in this setting and may allow patients to tolerate higher, more effective doses of interferon (65,66),

TABLE 23.4. *Neuropsychological Assessment of Cognitive Functioning*

INTELLECTUAL FUNCTIONS
Attentional abilities
Abstract reasoning
Problem solving

MEMORY
Verbal learning and recall
Visual and spatial memory
Remote memory

LANGUAGE
Naming
Fluency
Comprehension
Reading
Writing

VISUAL PERCEPTION
Scanning
Discrimination

MOTOR FUNCTIONS
Strength
Motor speed
Coordination and dexterity

EXECUTIVE (FRONTAL LOBE) FUNCTIONS
Cognitive flexibility (shifting mental set)
Motivation
Social judgement
Planning
Learning from experience
Insight and self-awareness

MOOD
Depression
Anxiety
Agitation
Withdrawal

Source: Meyers (15), reproduced with permission.

though they have their own well-known psychiatric complications. Acute delusional or hallucinatory presentations put the patient at great risk and require emergent intervention with antipsychotic medications.

The appropriate treatment of cognitive and affective symptoms has not been determined. Successful use of fluoxetine (67) and nortriptyline (68) has been reported in single case reports of IFN-α-induced depression, though the former drug appears to be used quite often by those who treat this problem. The opiate antagonist naltrexone has also been used to palliate IFN-α neurotoxicity in a small series of patients (69).

Studies of other pharmacologic and behavioral interventions are in progress. Mental status assessment is indicated for all patients who receive biologicals and there are subsets of patients for whom a very careful neuropsychological assessment is indicated (Table 23.4).

The physical and psychosocial responses of individuals receiving cancer treatment are complex and multifaceted. The majority of patients are managed in the ambulatory care setting, which is being challenged by increasing patient volume, more complicated treatment regimens, higher patient acuity, and diminishing resources. Many outpatient oncology facilities do not have the supportive care resources that previously existed in the acute care hospital setting such as social workers, dietitians, advanced practice nurses, psychiatrists, and psychologists. It becomes even more important to have routine assessments in order to recognize patients' problems in the physical, psychological, and social spheres. Subtle changes in the patient's physical condition or mild symptom distress may have significant implications for the patient and family at home. Persistent or delayed postchemotherapy nausea, diarrhea, cognitive changes or anorexia can result in dehydration, weight loss, time lost from work, depressed mood, and family disruption. In today's health care climate, assessments need to be succinct but sensitive enough to capture variability in symptoms related to the disease, treatment, psychological response and impact on the patient and family. Patient self-report forms or flow sheets for health care providers are two examples of approaches for enhancing routine, yet comprehensive assessments.

At the End of and After Treatment

There are many systemic treatments which are designed with a definitive endpoint. Most are those with a curative intent, such as combination chemotherapy for stage IV Hodgkin's disease or adjuvant therapy for breast or colorectal cancer. For those patients who achieve a remission or receive adjuvant therapy, there is no evidence of cancer present following cessation of treatment. The lack of measurable disease, less contact with the health care providers, and persistence of symptoms are three major factors which help explain patient responses to the end of treatment. Anxiety, depression, sadness, general emotional distress, concern over finances, increased fear of recurrence, and uncertainty have been associated with ending treatment (25,36,70,71). Patients experience loss: loss of regular medical surveillance, loss of the security of treatment, described as losing one's "safety net"; and loss of support related to ongoing communication and with availability of health care providers (70,71). Symptom distress can also accentuate the psychological responses at the end of therapy. Persistent fatigue is a salient example of distress for patients, which may have physical, psychological, and functional implications. For patients who receive aggressive therapy, or ablative therapy with autologous or allogeneic transplantation, the degree of physical symptoms or complications from therapy may result in significant persistent physical symptoms and psychological distress. Visual impairment, steroid-induced diabetes, infertility, respiratory compromise, and limited functional ability are examples of physical complaints of survivors of bone marrow transplantation (72,73). The recovery process following ablative therapy and marrow transplantation does not necessarily reflect a gradual improvement, but is characterized by periods of decline, improvement, or stability related to a range of physical, psychological, family, or social issues that are a consequence of therapy (72).

For treatments that have an endpoint, such as adjuvant therapy or curative primary chemotherapy, most family and friends expect the patient to rally. It is often very difficult for patients to explain their lack of psychological and physical resilience. Employers may have similar expectations and lack understanding that subtle symptoms persist. Additionally, patients may be inadequately informed regarding the prevalence of persistent symptoms. Furthermore, patients are frequently instructed to return to see their physician after one month or even three months and are often given a jubilant message of "You're all done, I don't need to see you for a while." These messages leave the patient feeling uncertain, fearful, and insecure. An increase in the number of telephone calls from patients following cessation of therapy is common, for any physical symptoms, since their first thought is that it represents recurrence. Fear of recurrence and the uncertainty of being truly disease free underlie much of the anxiety and emotional distress. By this point in time, patients are usually aware of the limitations of diagnostic technology and the lack of guarantees of scans or tests that the cancer is not there or will not return. Yet, they desperately hope for such guarantees and may request frequent or even inappropriate tests from their care providers in an attempt to gain some level of certainty (see Chapter 20 on cancer survivors).

Once treatment is completed, patients are in the "follow-up" mode. Time from treatment, persistence of symptoms, known risk of recurrence or development of complications from therapy will contribute to the level of the patient's psychological adjustment.

The first year is the most stressful, adapting to the impact of the diagnosis, treatment and anxiety of follow-up visits and tests. Although patients describe improvement in emotional distress over the subsequent years, annual reevaluation continues to be associated with anxiety and fear of recurrence. While some level of anxiety is reality-based, related to risk of recurrence, even small variations within the normal limit range of laboratory tests may disproportionately heighten anxiety.

Ambulatory cancer patients who had been diagnosed for an average of 28 months, and who had completed therapy an average of 4–18 months previously, were surveyed to determine the physical and psychosocial changes in their lives since diagnosis (74). Of the entire sample, only 10% had metastatic disease and 78% had received chemotherapy. Three physical parameters were reported as changed: physical activity, sleep patterns, and weight. Changes in financial status and self-image were reported by 46% of subjects. Communication with family and friends was explored and 27% of subjects reported not discussing illness or responses to illness with friends and family because they thought they did not understand, did not want to burden them, or felt that communication with them was meaningless and superficial. These comments are frequently heard from support group members who are cancer survivors and are cited as reasons for attending the group. Family and friends are often criticized by patients for expecting the patient to act "normal" now that treatment is over, and the patients struggle with the reality of the risk of recurrence and possible mortality. Knowledge of other patients who have had recurrence and died may exacerbate a patient's anxiety or may help put the reality in perspective that everyone's risk is different and each is unpredictable.

It is clear that there is a wide spectrum of psychological responses after systemic therapy. This fact strengthens the argument for individualized and routine assessment for patients who are being followed, regardless of time of follow-up. Although there is likely philosophical agreement with this statement, the reality in practice is incongruent. Ambulatory practice is being challenged today to do more with less. Yet, it is plagued with inadequate comprehensive resources for patients and families, such as advanced practice nurses, social workers, and psychiatric clinicians. Creative and innovative assessment strategies must be developed, such as patient-completed assessments that can be briefly reviewed by the health care providers. This is one approach that would allow identification of high-risk patients in need of interventions and promote the best utilization of existing resources.

TREATMENT CONSIDERATIONS IN CASES OF PROGRESSIVE DISEASE

An issue that repeatedly surfaces among patients, family members, and professional care providers deals with the use of aggressive treatment protocols in the presence of disseminated disease. Often patients and families request to participate in experimental protocols even when there is little likelihood of extending survival. Controversy continues about the efficacy of such therapies, their sometimes devastating impact on quality of life, and the role health professionals can play in facilitating patients' choices about participating.

The establishment of structured dialogue with patients, family members, and care providers regarding treatment goals and expectations is essential. The idea that certain individuals may respond to investigational treatments with increased hope and quality of life despite the existence of progressive illness should be a consideration in treatment planning. The need to separate and clarify the values, thoughts, and emotional reactions of care providers, patients, and families to these delicate issues is important if individualized care, with attention to the patients' psychosocial needs, is to be provided. These issues are discussed in detail in Chapter 37.

QUALITY OF LIFE CONSIDERATIONS

Since the mid 1980s a proliferation of powerful new cancer treatment agents as well as increasingly aggressive protocols using maximum dosages and combined modalities have been added to a growing anticancer arsenal. Although the benefits associated with these new treatment agents and strategies are at times unclear, their enhanced toxicity and side effect profiles are not. Within this context, in 1985, the Food and Drug Administration, clearly stated that two requirements for approval of new anti cancer treatments were improved survival and benefit to quality of life (75).

The most common purposes for measuring quality of life that are cited in the literature include (*1*) a means to select and justify treatment including the superiority of one treatment over another; (*2*) a means of documenting sequelae to cancer illness and treatment so that therapeutic interventions can be developed; and (*3*) to provide a basis for allocation of health care resources where quality of life is considered along with survival in the cost-effectiveness equation (76).

Because there has been an increase in the use of promising but toxic chemotherapies, there has been growing attention to the subjective experience of treatment on quality of life. Quality of life evaluations are needed in both curative and palliative treatment approaches, because the information obtained can guide the selection of therapeutic strategies leading to a more normal life and can help clinicians to deliver care aimed at enhancing those aspects of quality of life that have been disrupted secondary to illness and treatment. Obviously, since some cancers as well as many other chronic diseases are not curable, quality of life becomes a primary concern, particularly when palliation and symptom control are the issues at hand. According to Goodinson and Singleton (77) the precept of *primum non nocere* that has served as the ethical basis of therapeutics can be translated to mean that the benefits of treatment must be greater than the potential suffering. When there is a choice for a therapy that confers increased survival time or one that provides a better quality of life, an informed, autonomous decision of the patient must be respected.

A number of researchers (78–81) have studied the impact of various cancers and/or cancer treatments on aspects of quality of life. The goal of these studies has been to identify characteristic problem profiles so that therapeutic interventions to alleviate them can be systematically tested and developed. The alleviation of illness and treatment side effects is exceedingly important, as failure to do so may impinge on an individual's ability to make informed autonomous medical decisions (see Chapter 99 on quality of life assessment).

One major problem in evaluating quality of life in the clinical setting is the lack of standardized quality of life measures. The most common proxy measure of quality of life has been the physician/nurse-rated measure of performance status, Karnofsky Performance Status (KPS); however, this measure reveals physical performance only and thus provides limited information regarding other key aspects of functioning. Historically, indices of quality of life used with patients with cancer have included performance status, weight, general well-being, subjective improvement, and decrease of disease-related symptom distress such as cough, pain, and hemoptysis. There has also been an appeal to extend the response criteria measuring impact of quality of life during treatment to include the family as the unit of assessment (82). The importance of assessing multidimensional quality of life cannot be underestimated, including function in physical, psychological, and social domains.

ADDRESSING PATIENT CONCERNS ABOUT QUALITY HEALTH CARE DELIVERY

In 1994, potentially fatal overdoses of anticancer drugs were administered to two breast cancer patients at a well known cancer center in the United States. One of the patients died as a result of the incident and the other sustained irreversible heart damage. The federal Health Care Financing Administration (HCFA) found serious deficiencies in patient care and poor supervision of physicians and nurses at the cancer center (83). Additionally, it was reported that both patients had complained of extraordinary side effects while they were receiving high dosages of chemotherapy and that their complaints were unheeded. These unfortunate and tragic events were widely and sensationally publicized by the national media and struck a universal note as they appealed to a growing skepticism regarding health care delivery among increasingly wary consumers. Based on the preceding incidents, professional organizations and individual cancer centers across the country have established guidelines for monitoring scientific integrity and clinical practice to prevent potential future incidents and address allegations of scientific and procedural misconduct.

Concurrent with these widely publicized "treatment mistakes" is a rapid proliferation of anticancer agents, coupled with a growing responsibility being placed on patients and caregivers to choose among a range of treatments and to more carefully monitor their own health care. These demands are placed on patients and caregivers at a time of unparalleled stress in terms of the need to assimilate a new or recurrent cancer diagnosis and all the real or imagined threats that it entails.

In light of these issues, clinicians should be mindful of potential concerns and assist patients and families as much as possible to participate in treatment planning and decision making. Additionally, patient complaints should be fully heard and investigated and every attempt should be made to reassure patients and families that their concerns and complaints are taken seriously. Patient fears and concerns about procedural issues regarding treatment administration should be taken seriously and questions openly encouraged. While the prevailing attitude in health care supports open discussion and active involvement of patients in decisions that affect them, the actual behavior of health care providers is not always consistent with those values. Securing assistance from alternate providers to assist patients with issues and concerns that primary clinicians do not feel prepared or comfortable dealing with is a useful strategy for ensuring maximum support for patients and families faced with the complex decisions inherent in cancer treatment.

SUMMARY

Ongoing advances in the development of new anticancer drugs are rendering previously untreatable cancers treatable and are extending the lives of countless individuals. The goals of treatment should always be clear to health care providers, patients and families and the desired effects, side effects, risks, and benefits should be considered. Accompanying the various stages of treatment are psychological and neuropsychiatric sequelae that are vital to recognize and manage. Education, supportive care in managing side effects, and emotional support are essential for the patient undergoing chemotherapy. Ongoing awareness and monitoring of patients who experience psychological problems that extend beyond the usual is important so that more intensive assistance can be obtained. The efficacy of hormonal therapies in hormone-responsive tumors is well established and is associated with a range of psychological side effects such as depression and irritability. The neurotoxic effects of many of the biologic therapies extend from mild mood changes to severe symptoms of delirium and depression. These neurotoxic side effects deserve careful attention, monitoring, and ongoing management. The physical and psychosocial responses of individuals receiving systemic cancer treatments are complex and multifaceted. The changing health care environment is seriously challenging the ability to address these important problems, with an overall reduction in resources along with increased acuity of patients in all settings.

Systemic treatment agents often produce short-term and long-term consequences that impact upon quality of life of patients and their families. Quality of life is a substantial issue that must be considered when decisions are made about cancer treatment and its potential risks and benefits. Another important consideration is the increased responsibility that patients have in their health care decisions. The stress that this places on individuals who are already dealing with the stress of managing a cancer diagnosis cannot be overestimated and should be an important consideration in all phases of the treatment process.

REFERENCES
1. Gilman A. The initial clinical trial of nitrogen mustard. *Am J Surg.* 1963; 105:574–578.

2. Fisher D, Knobf MT, Durivage H. *The Cancer Chemotherapy Handbook*, 5th ed. St Louis: Mosby-Yearbook; 1997.

3. Taylor KM, Margolese RG, Soskoline CL. Physicians' reasons for not entering eligible patients in a randomized clinical trial of surgery for breast cancer. *N Engl J Med.* 1984; 310:1363–1367.

4. Allegra JC, Hamm JT. Hormonal therapy for cancer. In: Wittes R, ed. *Manual of Oncologic Therapeutics.* Philadelphia: Lippincott; 1989: 170–176.

5. Jassak P. An overview of biotherapy. In: Reiger PT, ed. *Biotherapy. A Comprehensive Overview.* Boston: Jones & Bartlett; 1995: 3–14.

6. Krown S. Biologic response modifiers. In: Wittes R, ed. *Manual of Oncologic Therapeutics.* Philadelphia: Lippincott; 1989: 177–185.

7. Reiger PT, ed. *Biotherapy. A Comprehensive Overview.* Boston: Jones & Bartlett; 1995.

8. Rosenberg SA. Principles and application of biologic therapy. In: DeVita VT, Hellman S, Rosenberg SA, eds. *Cancer Principles and Practice*, 4th ed. Philadelphia: Lippincott; 1993: 293–339.

9. Moldawer NP, Figlin RA. The interferons. In: Reiger PT, ed. *Biotherapy. A Comprehensive Overview.* Boston: Jones & Barlett; 1995: 67–92.

10. Sharp, E. The interleukins. In: Reiger PT, ed. *Biotherapy. A Comprehensive Overview.* Boston: Jones & Bartlett; 1995: 92–112.

11. Wujcik, D. Hematopoietic growth factors. In: Reiger PT, ed. *Biotherapy. A Comprehensive Overview.* Boston: Jones & Bartlett; 1995: 113–134.

12. DiJulio JE, Liles TM. Monoclonal antibodies. In Reiger PT, ed. *Biotherapy: A Comprehensive Overview.* Boston: Jones & Bartlett; 1995: 135–156.

13. Brophy L. Tumor necrosis factor. In Reiger PT, ed. *Biotherapy: A Comprehensive Overview.* Boston: Jones & Bartlett; 1995: 161–176.

14. Dean GE. Immunomodulators, differentiation agents and vaccines. In Reiger PT, ed. *Biotherapy. A Comprehensive Overview.* Boston: Jones & Bartlett; 1995: 177–192.

15. Meyers CA. Mental status changes. In Reiger PT, ed. *Biotherapy. A Comprehensive Overview.* Boston: Jones & Bartlett; 1995: 259–270.

16. Cella DF, Tross S, Orav EJ, et al. Mood states of patients after the diagnosis of cancer. *J Psychosoc Oncol.* 1989; 7:45–54.

17. Sinsheimer L, Holland JC. Psychosocial issues in breast cancer. *Semin Oncol.* 1987; 14(1):75–82.

18. Edgar L, Rosenberger Z, Nowlis D. Coping with cancer during the first year after diagnosis. *Cancer.* 1992; 69(3):817–828.

19. Northouse LL. A longitudinal study of adjustment of patients and husbands to breast cancer. *Oncol Nurs Forum.* 1989; 16(4):511–516.

20. Tringali CA. The needs of family members. *Oncol Nurs Forum.* 1986; 13(4):65–70.

21. Wells ME, McQuellon RP, Hinkle JS, Cruz JM. Reducing anxiety in newly diagnosed cancer patients. *Cancer Pract.* 1995; 3(2):100–104.

22. Pierce P. Deciding on breast cancer treatment: a description of decision behavior. *Nurs Res.* 1982; 42(1) 22–28.

23. Lamb M. The sleeping patterns of patients with malignant and non-malignant disease. *Cancer Nurs.* 1982; 5:389–396.

24. Holland JC. Anxiety and cancer: the patient and the family. *J Clin Psychiatry.* 1989; 50(11S):20–25.

25. Lenox R. Adjuvant therapy for breast cancer: a longitudinal quality of life study. Masters' thesis. Yale University School of Nursing; 1995.

26. Clark J. Psychosocial responses of the patient. In: Groenwald S, Frogge M, Goodman M, Yarbro C, eds. *Cancer Nursing Principles and Practice*, 3d ed. Boston: Jones & Bartlett; 1993; 449–467.

27. Buckalew PG. On the opposite side of the bed: a nurse clinician's experiences with anxiety during chemotherapy. *Cancer Nurs.* 1982; 5(6):435–439.

28. Brody DS. The patient's role in clinical decision making. *Ann Intern Med.* 1980; 93:718–722.

29. Johnson J. The effects of patient education course on persons with a chronic illness. *Cancer Nurs.* 1982; 5: 117–123.

30. McHugh NG, Christman NJ, Johnson J. Preparatory information: what helps and why. *Am J Nurs.* 1982; 82:780–782.

31. Messerli ML, Garamedi C, Romano J. Breast cancer: information as a crisis intervention. *Am J Orthopsychiatry.* 1980; 50:728–731.

32. Rhodes VA, Watson PM, McDaniel RW, et al. Expectation and occurrence of postchemotherapy side effects. *Cancer Pract.* 1995; 3(4):247–253

33. Nerenz DR, Leventhal H, Love R. Factors contributing to emotional distress during cancer chemotherapy. *Cancer.* 1982; 50:1020–1027.

34. Kinsey RD. Predictors of psychosocial adaptation among women with breast cancer. *Proc Third American Cancer Society Nurs Research Conference.* Newport Beach, CA; 1994. [Abstract.]

35. Blesch KS, Paice J, Wickham R, et al. Correlates of fatigue in people with breast or lung cancer. *Oncol Nurs Forum.* 1991; 18(1):81–87.

36. Knobf MT. Physical and psychological distress associated with adjuvant chemotherapy in women with breast cancer. *J Clin Oncol.* 1986; 4(5):678–684.

37. Greene D, Nail LM, Fieler VK, et al. A comparison of patient-reported side effects among three chemotherapy regimens for breast cancer. *Cancer Pract.* 1994; 29(1):57–62.

38. Coates A, Abraham S, Kaye SB, et al. On the receiving end-patient perception of the side effects of cancer chemotherapy. *Eur J Cancer.* 1983; 19(2): 203–208.

39. Winningham ML, Nail L, Burke MB, et al. Fatigue and the cancer experience: the state of the knowledge. *Oncol Nurs Forum.* 1994; 21(1):23–36.

40. Irvine D, Vincent L, Graydon J, et al. The prevalence and correlates of fatigue in patients receiving treatent with chemotherapy and radiotherapy. *Cancer Nurs.* 1994; 17(5):367–378.

41. Freedman T. Social and cultural dimensions of hair loss in women treated for breast cancer. *Cancer Nurs.* 1994; 17(4):334–341.

42. Lamb M. Effects of cancer on sexuality and fertility of women. *Semin Oncol Nurs.* 1995; 11(2):120–127.

43. Young-McCaughan S. Sexual functioning in women with breast cancer after treatment with adjuvant therapy. *Cancer Nurs.* 1996; 19:308–319

44. Love RR, Leventhal H, Easterling DV, Nerenz D. Side effects and emotional distress during cancer chemotherapy. *Cancer.* 1989; 63:604–612.

45. Meehan J, Johnson BL. The neurotoxicity of antineoplastic agents. In: Hubbard S, Knobf MT, Greene P, eds. *Current Issues in Cancer Nursing Practice.* Philadelphia: Lippincott; 1991: 1–11.

46. Renault PF, Hoofnagle JH, Park Y, et al. Psychiatric complications of long term interferon alfa therapy. *Arch Intern Med.* 1987; 147:1577–1580.

47. Pavol MA, Meyers CA, Rexer JL, et al. Pattern of neurobehavioral deficits associated with interferon alfa therapy for leukemia. *Neurology.* 1995; 45:947–950.

48. Meyers CA, Scheibel RS, Forman AD. Persistent neurotoxicity of systemically administered interferon-alpha. *Neurology.* 1991; 41:672–676.

49. Meyers CA, Valentine AD. Neurologic and psychiatric adverse effects of immunologic therapy. *CNS Drugs.* 11995; 3:56–68.

50. Fent K, Zbinden, G. Toxicity of interferon and interleukin. *Trends Pharmacol Res.* 1987; 8:100–105.

51. Smith A, Tyrrell D, Coyle K, et al. Effects of interferon alpha on performance in man: a preliminary report. *Psychopharmacology.* 1988; 96:414–416.

52. Adams F, Quesada JR, Gutterman JU. Neuropsychiatric manifestations of human leukocyte interferon in patients with cancer. *J Am Med Assoc.* 1984; 252:938–941.

53. Piper BF, Rieger PT, Brophy L, et al. Recent advances in the management of biotherapy-related side effects: fatigue. *Oncol Nurs Forum.* 1989; 16(4 suppl):27–34.

54. Spiegel RJ. The alpha interferons: clinical overview. *Urology.* 1989; 4(4 suppl):75–79.

55. Triozzi PL, Kinney P, Rinehart JJ. Central nervous system toxicity of biological response modifiers. *Ann NY Acad Sci.* 1990; 594:347–354.

56. Cummings JL, ed. *Subcortical Dementia.* New York: Oxford University Press; 1990.

57. Bocci V. Central nervous system toxicity of interferons and other cytokines. *J Biol Regul Homeostat Agents.* 1988; 3:107–118.

58. Renault PF, Adams F, Fernadez F, Mavligit G. Interferon-induced organic mental disorders associated with unsuspected pre-existing neurologic abnormalities. *J Neurooncol.* 1988; 6:355–359.

59. Rohatiner AZ, Prior PF, Burton AC, et al. Central nervous system toxicity of interferon. *Br J Cancer.* 1983; 47:419–422.

60. Adams F, Fernadez F, Mavligit G. Interferon-induced organic mental disorders associated with unsuspected pre-existing neurologic abnormalities. *J Neurooncol.* 1988; 6:355–359.

61. Quesada JR, Talpaz M, Rios A, et al. Clinical toxicity of interferons in cancer patients: a review. *J Clin Oncol.* 1986; 4:234–243.

62. Denicoff KD, Rubinow DR, Papa MZ, et al. The neuropsychiatric effects of treatment with interleukin-2 and lymphokine-activated killer cells. *Ann Intern Med.* 1987; 107:293–300.

63. Kriegel RL, Padavic-Shaller KA, Rudolph AR, et al. A phase I study of recombinant interleukin 2 plus recombinant B-interferon. *Cancer Res.* 1988; 48:3875–3881.

64. Smith MJ, Khayat D. Residual acute confusional and hallucinatory syndromes induces by interleukin-2/α-interferon treatment. *Psycho-Oncology.* 1992; 1:115–118.

65. Abdi EA. Combination of interferon and prednisone in human cancer. *Eur J Cancer Clin Oncol.* 1988; 24:723–724.

66. Fossa SD, Gunderson R, Moe B. Recombinant interferon-alpha combined with prednisone in metastatic renal cell carcinoma. *Cancer.* 1990; 65:2451–2454.

67. Levenson J, Fallon H. Fluoxetine treatment of depression caused by interferon-α *Am J Gastroenterol.* 1993; 88:760–761.

68. Goldman LS. Successful treatment of interferon-alpha-induced mood disorder with nortriptyline. *Psychosomatics.* 1994; 35:412–413.

69. Valentine AD, Meyers CA, Talpaz M. Treatment of neurotoxic side effects of interferon-α with naltrexone. *Cancer Invest.* 1995; 13:561–566.

70. Hart GJ, McQuellon RP, Barrett RJ. After treatment ends. *Cancer Pract.* 1994; 2(6):417–420.

71. Ward SE, Viergutz G, Tormey D, et al. Patients' reactions to completion of adjuvant breast cancer therapy. *Nursing Res.* 1992; 41(6):362–366.

72. Haberman M, Bush N, Young K, Sullivan KM. Quality of life of adult long-term survivors of bone marrow transplantation: a qualitative analysis of narrative data. *Oncol Nurs Forum.* 1993; 20(10):1545–1553.

73. Ferrell B, Grant M, Schmidt GM, et al. The meaning of quality of life for bone marrow transplant survivors. Part i. The impact of bone marrow transplant on quality of life. *Cancer Nurs.* 1992; 15:153–160.

74. Frank-Stromborg M, Wright P. Ambulatory cancer patients' perception of the physical and psychosocial changes in their lives since the diagnosis of cancer. *Cancer Nurs.* 1984; 7:117–130.

75. Johnson JR, Temple R. Food and Drug Administration requirements for approval of new anticancer drugs. *Cancer Treat Rep.* 1985; 69:1155–1157.

76. LaPuma J, Lawlor EF. Quality adjusted life years: ethical implications for physicians and policy makers. *J Am Med Assoc.* 1990; 263:2917–2921.

77. Goodinson SM, Singleton J. Quality of life: a critical review of current concepts, measures and their clinical implications. *Int J Nurs Stud.* 1989; 26:327–332.

78. Clark A, Fallowfield LJ. Quality of life measurements in patients with malignant disease: a review. *J Soc Med.* 1986; 79:165–169.

79. Holmes S, Dickerson JWT. The quality of life: design and evaluation of a self assessment instrument for use with cancer patients. *Int J Nurs Stud.* 1987; 24:15–24.

80. Kornblith AB, Anderson J, Cella D, et al. Quality of life assessment of Hodgkin's disease survivors: A model for cooperative clinical trials. *Oncology.* 1990; 4, 93–101.

81. McCorkle R, Quint-Benoliel J. Symptom distress, current concerns and mood disturbance after diagnosis of life threatening disease. *Soc Sci Med.* 1983; 17, 431–438.

82. Aaronson NK. Quality of life research in cancer clinical trials: a need for common rules and language. *Oncology.* 1990; 4, 59–66.

83. Altman L. Federal officials cite deficiencies at Harvard hospital. *New York Times.* 1995 May 31: A-16.

24

Bone Marrow Transplantation

MICHAEL A. ANDRYKOWSKI AND RICHARD P. McQUELLON

Bone marrow transplantation (BMT) is a complex medical procedure in which blood cells (hematopoietic progenitor cells) in bone marrow are infused into a patient following high-dose chemotherapy and/or radiotherapy. Because BMT is associated with life-threatening physical morbidity, lengthy convalescence, and social isolation, the potential for significant psychosocial morbidity is high. In this chapter, we provide: *(1)* a history of the development of BMT; *(2)* an overview of the medical procedures used in BMT; and *(3)* a review of psychosocial and behavioral issues relevant to BMT. (See Chapter 34 by Lesko for overview of hematologic dyscrasias.)

HISTORICAL OVERVIEW

The roots of modern BMT in humans can be traced to the 1930s (1). While initial attempts at marrow transplantation in humans were mostly unsuccessful (2), these studies initiated a series of necessary discoveries leading to successful BMT in humans (3). In 1959, two patients given a supralethal dose of total-body irradiation (TBI) and a marrow infusion from an identical twin recovered hematologic function in two weeks. This demonstrated that a compatible marrow graft could protect against lethal marrow aplasia. Second, description of the human histocompatibility system led to the discovery that matching at the major histocompatibility complex could predict a successful outcome of the marrow graft. This expanded the potential pool of marrow donors to include genetically similar individuals, both related as well as unrelated. Finally, the development of platelet collection and transfusion technology, more effective isolation techniques, and broad-spectrum antibiotics to treat infections, resulted in improved supportive care critical to immmunocompromised patients. These developments set the stage for the beginning of the modern era of BMT. In 1968 the first successful marrow graft was performed

in an infant with severe immunological insufficiency (4). Since then the use of BMT has expanded dramatically (5,6).

MEDICAL OVERVIEW

There are three types of BMT: allogeneic, syngeneic, and autologous. Allogeneic BMT involves the transfer of bone marrow from a genetically similar donor to the patient. Human leukocyte antigen (HLA)-matched family members are the best candidates for this procedure since they are not only phenotypically identical (share the same tissue type) but are at least partially genotypically identical (at the DNA level). Allogeneic BMT with unrelated, but phenotypically identical, donors is also possible and is becoming more common. Syngeneic BMT involves marrow donation from an identical twin. Finally, in autologous BMT, the patient is both donor and recipient. Reinfusion of the patient's own disease-free bone marrow or peripheral blood progenitor (i.e., stem) cells occurs following administration of high-dose chemotherapy.

BMT is indicated in both nonmalignant and malignant diseases as well as genetic anomalies. Indications for both allogeneic and autologous BMT are shown in Table 24.1. (Indications for syngeneic BMT are identical to those for allogeneic BMT.) While not exhaustive, this list includes diseases for which BMT is most commonly employed. In general, allogeneic and syngeneic BMT are indicated when the bone marrow itself is diseased (e.g., leukemias) whereas autologous BMT is used when marrow is disease-free.

Medically, BMT can be viewed as a sequence of six steps. These steps vary slightly from one BMT center to another and with the type of BMT performed. First, potential recipients are referred to a BMT center where their medical history is evaluated; the selection and consent process begins here. Once a decision for treatment has been made, the second step involves several

TABLE 24.1. *Indications for Bone Marrow Transplantation*

Allogeneic	Autologous
Severe aplastic anemia	Acute leukemias in complete remission
Acute myeloid leukemia	Some non-Hodgkin's lymphomas
Acute lymphoblastic luekemia	Hodgkin's disease
Chronic myeloid leukemia	Brain tumors
Severe combined immunodeficiency disease	Breast cancer
Myelodysplastic syndromes with leukemic transformation	Ovarian and testicular cancer
Acute osteomyeolofibrosis	Small-cell lung cancer
Thalassemia major	Multiple myeloma
Fanconi's anemia	Sarcomas

days of laboratory and diagnostic tests. Patients may be deemed ineligible for BMT on the basis of these tests. At this time, or later, at the time of hospital admission, a Hickman catheter may be placed in a large vein in the chest. The catheter is used for drawing blood samples, administering blood or blood products, antibiotics, other drugs, or nutritional support, and for transplanting the new marrow. Generally, one end of the catheter remains outside the chest and must be kept clean to prevent infection. The catheter remains in place for several weeks to several months. While a catheter may limit the patient's lifestyle, the number of venipunctures necessary during treatment is dramatically reduced.

Step three involves the marrow harvest and differs depending upon whether allogeneic or autologous BMT is involved. In allogeneic BMT, the marrow donor is hospitalized and marrow is removed from the pelvic bone or iliac crest. This procedure requires approximately one hour. The harvested marrow is then processed to remove blood and bone fragments. Allogeneic marrow may be treated to remove T lymphocytes (T cell depletion) to reduce the likelihood of graft rejection.

In autologous BMT, bone marrow or peripheral blood progenitor cells are harvested from the patient. Marrow harvest procedures are similar to those for allogeneic donors. In some instances, marrow may be treated, or purged, to remove or destroy cancer cells. Blood progenitor cells are harvested from peripheral blood by apheresis or leukophoresis. In this outpatient procedure, blood is removed though an intravenous catheter and passed through a machine that collects white blood cells, which contain progenitor cell function. The remainder of the blood is then returned to the patient. Blood growth factors (e.g., colony-stimulating factors and interleukins) may be used to stimulate white blood cell production prior to progenitor cell harvest.

In step four, a conditioning regimen of high-dose chemotherapy with or without radiation therapy is administered over a period of 3–10 days. The intensive doses of radiation and chemotherapy employed during pre-BMT conditioning result in more effective elimination of cancer cells throughout the body than is possible through conventional doses of these therapies. Pre-BMT conditioning also suppresses the immune system in allogeneic recipients, thus reducing the likelihood of graft rejection. Pre-BMT conditioning regimens vary according to the patient's disease and medical condition.

Step five is the rescue process. Bone marrow or peripheral blood progenitor cells are infused into the recipient after completion of conditioning. The procedure resembles a blood transfusion. The marrow or progenitor cells travel through the bloodstream to the bone marrow, where they begin to produce new white blood cells, red blood cells, and platelets. Blood cell production from transplanted stem cells, called engraftment, begins 2–4 weeks after BMT. Complete recovery of the immune system can require several months in autologous recipients or 1–2 years in allogeneic recipients.

Step six consists of provision of supportive care during hospitalization, convalescence, and follow-up. The goal at this time is to prevent or manage the side effects of pre-BMT conditioning as well as to monitor and manage reactions to antibiotics, steroids, cyclosporins, and other medications. Common physical complications of pre-BMT conditioning include hair loss, severe nausea, mucositis (i.e., mouth sores), loss of appetite, and diarrhea. Less common, yet more serious, side effects include malfunction of the lungs, liver, kidneys and the heart. Mouth sores may make eating difficult. Nutritional support, called total parenteral nutrition, is often necessary and also allows the gastrointestinal tract to heal following pre-BMT conditioning.

The most serious side effect of pre-BMT conditioning is marked immunosuppression. Supportive care includes protective isolation, in which patients are confined to a small area and must wear masks and latex gloves when out of their rooms. Rooms are protected by special filters. Medical staff and visitors are required to wash their hands before entering patient rooms and may be required to wear masks and gowns as well. Patients may receive antibiotics, antiviral agents, and antifungal agents as precautionary measures to prevent infection. Blood growth factors may also be used to speed engraftment, decrease the risk of infection, and reduce the likelihood of engraftment failure. Patients usually need periodic blood transfusions to treat anemia and thrombocytopenia. Finally, patients are carefully monitored for signs of graft-versus-host disease (GVHD). This potentially life-threatening complication occurs when allogeneic donor marrow attacks the recipient or host's body. Symptoms include skin rash, jaundice, liver disease, and diarrhea and can develop within days (acute GVHD) or as long as three years after BMT (chronic GVHD). GVHD can be rapidly fatal or a life-long management problem.

Patients are discharged from the hospital when their blood cell counts reach a certain level, infections have been managed, and their general physical condition is good. This may be anywhere from two weeks to several months following BMT. In general, hospitalization following autologous BMT is shorter than that following allogeneic BMT. Outpatient follow-up care initially requires frequent visits to monitor the patient's potentially unstable physical condition.

The BMT procedure itself is associated with a 0%–36% mortality rate (7–8). One-year survival rates may exceed 90% for autologous BMT (5,9,10) with 70%–80% survival for allogeneic BMT from a related donor (10–11) and approximately 50% survival for allogeneic BMT from an unrelated donor (11,12). While the length and likelihood of disease-free survival varies, it is generally believed that younger age, better general health, limited disease, and earlier stage of disease at BMT are predictive of positive outcome. However, these are very general prognostic factors which may vary in importance depending upon disease type. Finally, attempts to identify psychosocial factors predictive of post-BMT survival have been made (13,14), but these efforts are preliminary.

PSYCHOSOCIAL AND BEHAVIORAL ISSUES

The BMT setting is populated by several classes of individuals. These include the BMT recipient as well as the recipient's family, the marrow donor, and the BMT medical staff. While the focus of our discussion will be upon the BMT patient, we will also provide an overview of the psychosocial and behavioral issues relevant to families, donors, and medical staff.

The BMT Patient

Much has been written about the BMT patient. The myriad physical and psychosocial challenges confronted by the patient throughout the course of BMT have been catalogued, the range of normal and abnormal responses to these stressors has been described, and recommendations for management of the BMT patient to minimize distress associated with BMT have been advanced (15–21). This literature has been largely clinical or anecdotal in nature, consisting of discussions of case studies or small series of cases. While lacking the methodological rigor necessary to draw firm conclusions, this literature is a rich source of both clinical insights as well as testable hypotheses.

Early discussions of psychosocial and behavioral issues associated with BMT were organized by various "stages" of BMT (22,23). For example, Brown and Kelly (22) described eight stages of BMT beginning with the decision to undergo BMT and concluding with the patient's adaptation outside the hospital. This "stage" approach suggests that, as the BMT treatment process unfolds, patients are confronted with a predictable sequence of physical and psychosocial stressors. Although the specific time line and sequence of events may vary somewhat in contemporary BMT, the stage approach is a useful heuristic. We will organize our discussion around five stages of BMT: *(1)* the decision to undergo BMT; *(2)* pre-BMT preparation; *(3)* post-BMT hospitalization; *(4)* hospital discharge and early post-BMT recovery; and *(5)* long-term recovery.

The Decision to Undergo BMT. The decision to undergo BMT is the culmination of a series of prior decisions. These include the decision by the patient's physician to consider BMT as a treatment option and refer the patient to a BMT center for evaluation, as well as the BMT center's decision to offer the patient the opportunity to undergo BMT. While little is known about how patients are initially referred to a BMT center for evaluation, the final decision to offer BMT as a treatment option is based primarily upon medical and insurance considerations. While psychosocial considerations, such as a history of alcohol or substance abuse or a history of medical noncompliance, may be used to screen candidates for solid organ transplantation (24–26), it is very rare for an individual to be refused BMT solely on the basis of psychosocial considerations. While many BMT centers include a psychosocial "work-up" in their pre-BMT evaluation, the information obtained is typically used to plan for the care of the patient during and following BMT.

The decision to undergo BMT is formalized by the provision of consent. At this time, a lengthy discussion takes place between medical staff and the BMT recipient, often accompanied by family members. The medical procedures involved in BMT are specified, available alternative courses of treatment are indicated, and the risks, benefits, and likely short-term and long-term outcomes of both BMT and alternative courses of action are described to the extent possible. Provision of this information should, in theory, allow the patient (or parents) to make an informed and uncoerced decision whether to proceed with BMT (27). In reality, however, several factors mitigate against this idealization. First, the consent process is likely to occur in the context of considerable distress (28,29). This is not surprising given the arduousness and life-threatening nature of the BMT procedure and the uncertainty associated with whether the right choice is being made. As a result, communication between the patient and medical staff might be hindered and rational consideration of the costs and benefits of BMT limited. Indeed, BMT physicians perceive many patients (or parents) as wishing to avoid the seriousness of consent discussions (30). Second, it is likely that the patient's decision to undergo BMT has been made long before initiation of the consent process (31,32). Many patients decide to pursue BMT when the option is introduced. This is likely when BMT is the lone potentially curative treatment option. By the time patients present at a BMT center for evaluation, they may already be committed to the procedure without fully understanding the potential hazards.

In sum, several factors combine to increase the likelihood that patients (or parents) will deny, distort, or avoid consideration of threatening information provided during the consent process. While such behavior may be characterized as irrational or maladaptive, avoidance of threatening information about an arduous, life-threatening course of action that one is already committed to may be a reasonable means by which patients (or parents) muster the psychological strength required to cope with the adversity posed by BMT. In light of this, it is advised that BMT staff view informed consent as a process rather than as a discrete event. While patients (or parents) might resist threatening information presented prior to BMT, this same information might be acknowledged and accepted later in the course of BMT. For example, information about long-term post-BMT complications might be

reintroduced and discussed at discharge or later during the first year post-BMT. Patients may be more receptive to this information at these times since the acute threat posed by BMT is diminished. The importance of promoting realistic expectations for post-BMT outcomes is underscored by research suggesting that poorer long-term psychological adjustment is associated not with poorer post-BMT outcomes but with *unrealized* post-BMT outcome expectations (31).

Pre-BMT Preparation. Following provision of consent, the patient begins pre-BMT conditioning therapy. The side effects of conditioning are typically severe. Depending upon the conditioning regimen, nausea peaks during administration of conditioning and tapers off as conditioning concludes (33). Pain due to mucositis begins a few days prior to BMT and peaks 7–14 days post BMT. While pharmacologic therapy is typically employed in the management of pain and nausea, behavioral therapy may be a useful adjunct. In a well-controlled study, training in hypnosis was found to be effective in reducing oral pain during BMT hospitalization (34).

In addition to initiation of pre-BMT conditioning and management of its side effects, the period prior to BMT should be devoted to planning for the psychosocial management of the patient. A detailed psychosocial or psychiatric evaluation should be completed at this time. Futterman and colleagues (35) have identified key content areas to be assessed, including prior psychiatric history, quality of support, coping history, history of coping with disease and treatment, quality of affect, past and present mental status, and proneness to anticipatory anxiety. Using this information, patients can be classified with regard to potential level of psychosocial adjustment. Benefits of this "psychosocial levels system" include: *(1)* anticipation of psychosocial management needs and BMT staff stress levels at any point in time; *(2)* the ability to communicate in "shorthand" about patient problems; and *(3)* the ability to develop interventions that are appropriate for patients classified at different psychosocial levels (21,35). While it has not been subjected to extensive empirical evaluation, this system appears to have much to recommend it. Regardless of the specific system used in the psychosocial evaluation of BMT patients, however, it is recommended that the approach to psychosocial or psychiatric management in the BMT setting be proactive rather than reactive.

Post-BMT Hospitalization. Following completion of pre-BMT conditioning, the marrow transplant occurs. Compared to solid organ transplantation, the marrow transplant itself is anticlimatic. Donor marrow (allogeneic or syngeneic BMT) or the patient's own previously harvested marrow (autologous BMT) is simply infused into the BMT recipient. A period of waiting follows during which blood counts are monitored for evidence of engraftment and immune system reconstitution. Patients are observed closely for evidence of life-threatening post-BMT complications. During the first few weeks after BMT and following resolution of any nausea and pain associated with conditioning, the patient may feel relatively good, although quite weak. This state of quiescence can change markedly, however, should medical complications arise. Not only is distress then likely to rise precipitously, but the presence of medical complications often increases the length of hospitalization required. Prolonged hospitalization, particularly if a tentative discharge date had already been set, can be profoundly demoralizing. Many patients react with depression and lethargy; others become agitated and angry, stating that their tolerance has been reached and demanding to be discharged.

Neurocognitive symptoms are likely to become evident during hospitalization. Episodes of delirium, often lasting several hours to several days, may occur, particularly in allogeneic recipients. Symptoms include alterations in level of consciousness or sensory/perceptual function (e.g., hallucinations), impaired concentration, memory, and higher cognitive processes, sleep disturbance, mood swings, and impaired social judgment (21). Symptoms are typically multifactorial in nature. Potential pathophysiological mechanisms include CNS disease, infection, intoxication or withdrawal associated with a psychoactive substance, interstitial pneumonia with respiratory compromise, immunosuppressive medications (e.g., cyclosporin, steroids), or metabolic imbalance or liver/renal dysfunction associated with GVHD (21). Management is based upon early symptom recognition and treatment of the underlying pathophysiology.

Unfortunately, sound empirical investigations of the psychosocial and psychiatric difficulties encountered during post-BMT hospitalization are lacking. Extant studies typically involve small samples and less than rigorous methods (17,18). There is need for additional research in this area, particularly studies investigating the: *(1)* the prevalence of various difficulties, whether psychosocial or organic in origin; *(2)* the psychosocial and biological factors associated with the occurrence of these difficulties; and *(3)* the utility of interventions for managing these difficulties.

Hospital Discharge and Early Post-BMT Recovery. Hospital discharge occurs when white cell counts indicate an adequately functioning immune system, any acute GVHD is managed, the patient is eating regularly, and no serious medical problems are present. Initially, patients may be discharged to temporary quarters in the vicinity of the BMT center, rather than to their homes. This allows for frequent clinic follow-up during the first 70 to 100 days post BMT. The patient's condition is still unstable and it is critical that medical assistance be readily available. During this time, chronic GVHD may emerge in allogeneic recipients. Once this 70- to 100-day period is completed, and if no serious uncontrolled medical complications exist, the patient can return home and begin the process of recovery and life reintegration.

While hospital discharge is typically an eagerly anticipated milestone, it can be distressing. Patients may experience anxiety at the realization that they will no longer be under the constant care of the BMT medical staff and may fear that life-threatening difficulties might arise when medical assistance is not immediately available. In addition, patients may remain physically compromised. Fatigue and weakness, often profound, are typically present at discharge and may persist throughout the first 6–12 months post BMT (36,37). These symptoms can impose functional limitations that limit resumption of a premorbid lifestyle. While most patients expect and tolerate some limitations following discharge, frustration, depression, and anger can develop if weakness or fatigue persist. This is especially true if friends or family members do not appreciate the debilitation that can result after BMT and pressure the patient to "get on with life."

Both before and after BMT, patients are responsible for performing a variety of self-care behaviors and observing behavioral restrictions intended to reduce the risk of infection and promote functional recovery. Some of these behaviors include mouth and Hickman catheter care, administration of medication, getting adequate physical exercise, and avoiding crowds or individuals who might be infectious. While adherence to these recommendations is important during hospitalization, adherence assumes critical importance after discharge. Despite its importance, only one study has investigated nonadherence in BMT patients (38). Retrospective examination of nursing records during hospitalization found reports of significant noncompliance in 52% of pediatric patients studied. While no research has examined nonadherence after discharge, clinical experience suggests that adherence to self-care behaviors and restrictions is problematic. In some instances, nonadherence can be attributed to knowledge or skill deficits. In these cases, nonadherence can be managed through patient or family education and training. In other cases, motivational deficits might underlie the failure to follow self-care recommendations. Patients have an understandable need to feel that they are no longer sick and are essentially "normal" following BMT. The need to perform self-care behaviors or observe various restrictions may imply otherwise. Similarly, patients may decide to abandon portions of their self-care regimen to "test" whether certain restrictions are necessary. In these cases, management of nonadherence requires education and attention to the patient's perceptions of the costs and benefits of adherence, as well as flexibility on the part of medical staff.

Long-Term Recovery. Successful transition from BMT patient to a functioning, healthy individual is a significant task during post-BMT recovery. For some patients, however, cure or control of their disease is not accompanied by a full restoration of health. Indeed, while BMT can be a life-saving therapy, it is associated with significant risk for long-term physical and psychosocial morbidity. Various physical "late effects" of BMT are recognized, including pulmonary problems, cataracts, sterility, chronic GVHD of the skin, gut, or liver, weakness and fatigue, and disease relapse or development of a secondary malignancy (39–41). These can negatively impact upon performance of daily activities and a patient's sense of well-being.

In recognition of this, quality of life (QOL) has received increasing attention as a significant post-BMT clinical endpoint. QOL is a multidimensional construct, incorporating information regarding individuals' current physical symptoms and general health perceptions, as well as information regarding physical, occupational, emotional, and interpersonal functioning (42–44). While QOL is important to consider throughout the course of BMT, it is particularly significant during the long-term recovery phase when the disease process has been controlled and acute stresses associated with medical treatment have subsided.

Several large-scale studies of post-BMT QOL exist (31,37,45–51). These studies are summarized in Table 24.2. This research has demonstrated that many adult BMT recipients report an essentially "normal" QOL. However, other recipients report various QOL deficits, including low self-esteem and psychological distress, occupational disability, impaired social relationships, limitations upon performance of routine household tasks or recreational activities, sexual dysfunction, cog-

nitive impairment, and sleep difficulties. Efforts to identify disease, demographic, treatment, and psychosocial variables associated with differences in post-BMT QOL have met with only modest success. While no one variable is consistently associated with poorer status across all QOL domains, some likely "risk" factors for poorer post-BMT QOL include older age at BMT, less education, chronic GVHD, and higher doses of total body irradiation (TBI) during conditioning.

While evidence suggests that QOL in BMT survivors is likely to be compromised to a degree, whether QOL deficits are due wholly or in part to BMT itself is not known. None of the large scale studies cited above collected QOL data from appropriately matched comparison groups of other medically ill or healthy individuals. Additionally, only the study by Syrjala and colleagues (37) collected measures of pre-BMT QOL. For many patients, BMT is only part of a long, arduous process of adaptation to disease and treatment. Consequently, QOL may be impaired even prior to BMT. In the absence of appropriate comparison groups and pre-BMT assessments of QOL, it is difficult to gauge the specific negative impact that BMT itself might have on QOL. Regardless of cause, research suggests that the majority of BMT recipients do not experience a complete restoration of health following BMT. Thus, efforts to enhance psychological adaptation and promote functional rehabilitation are integral to the long-term management of BMT recipients. Enhancement of post-BMT QOL is predicated upon knowing: *(1)* likely deficits experienced by BMT patients; *(2)* risk factors associated with specific deficits; and *(3)* when specific deficits are likely to emerge and become salient to the patient. At the moment, understanding of the latter two considerations is limited.

The BMT Patient's Family

According to Wellisch and Wolcott (21), "BMT is a biomedical experience for patients, but a psychological experience for the whole family unit" (p. 556). Mental health professionals who counsel families of BMT recipients and the BMT medical team are familiar with the many stressors facing the family: geographic dislocation when a patient must travel long distances to be treated; financial burden due to the high costs of BMT and loss of income; disrupted marital communication and sexual behavior; the burden of providing daily care for a very ill patient; shifting of parental roles required when a spouse is unable to care for children; and the griefwork and readjustment necessary if the patient dies. There is considerable research on cancer's

TABLE 24.2. *Summary of Methods and Findings of Large-Scale Reports of Post-BMT Quality of Life in Adults*

Authors and Ref.	BMT Type*	Samples Size	Disease	Mean Time Post BMT (Range) (Months)	Mean Age (Range) (Years)	Design/Methods	Findings†
Andrykowski et al. (1995) (31)	Allo + auto	172	100% malignant	43.5 (12–124)	39.1 (19–70)	Retrospective/ Cross section, questionnaire + interview	32% "not back to normal"; sexual activity (32%) and physical activity (43%) most likely to be "not normal"
Andrykowski et al. (1995) (45)	Allo + auto	200	100% malignant	41.0 (12–127)	38.5 (19–70)	Retrospective/ Cross section, questionnaire	Allo QOL < auto QOL; age at BMT, education, less advanced diseases at BMT, and time since BMT positively related to QOL
Baker et al. (1991) (46)	Allo + auto + syng	135	81% malignant	47.0 (6–149)	30.6 (18–53)	Retrospective/ Cross section; questionnaire	Role retention post BMT positively related to QOL and negatively related to mood disturbance
Baker et al. (1994) (47)	Allo + auto + syng	135	81% malignant	47.0 (6–149)	30.6 (18–53)	Retrospective/ Cross section; questionnaire	Majority report high QOL across multiple domains; least satisfied with bodies, physical strength, and sexual satisfaction; previous GVHD and older age at BMT related to poorer QOL
Bush et al. (1995) (48)	Allo + auto	125	66% malignant	121 (72–220)	38.1 (??)	Retrospective/ Cross section; questionnaire	Current QOL same or better than pre-BMT in 74%; current health and QOL good to excellent in 80%; some problems with fatigue and problems with fatigue and sex, sleep, and cognitive dysfunction
Chao et al. (1992) (49)	Auto	58	100% malignant	(3–12)	36 [median] (19–53)	Retrospective/ Longitudinal; questionnaire 3 and 12 mo post BMT	QOL improved between 3 and 12 mo assessments; 78% employed at 12 mo; sexual difficulties in 14%; above-average to excellent QOL in 88% at 12 mo post BMT
Schmidt et al. (1993) (50)	Allo	162	89% malignant	60 [median] (12–156)	32 [median] (19–50)	Retrospective/ Cross section; interview	Median QOL score of 9 on 10-point scale; 26% not returned to pre-BMT school or work activities; sexual dissatisfaction related to poor QOL
Syrjala et al. (1993) (37)	Allo	67	100% malignant	(Pre-BMT to 72)	32 (19–60)	Prospective/ Longitudinal; questionnaire pre-BMT and 3, 12 mo, and 4.5–6 yr post BMT	Physical function most impaired at 3 mo with return to pre-BMT levels at 12 mo; 68% return to full-time work at 12 mo; poor physical recovery at 12 mo related to severe chronic GVHD
Wingard et al. (1991) (51)	Allo + auto + syng	135	81% malignant	47.0 (6–149)	30.6 (18–53)	Retrospective/ Cross section; questionnaire	Global health good to excellent in 67%; 65% returned to work; social activities (80%) or physical function (67%) unimpaired or slightly affected

*Allo = allogeneic; auto = autologous; syng = syngeneic.
†QOL = quality of life.

295

impact upon the family in general (52–56) but only a modest, yet expanding, literature on BMT families in particular (16,21,57,58). These literatures overlap and much that has been learned regarding cancer's impact upon the family can be extended to the BMT setting.

Wellisch and Wolcott (21) identify various family subsystems that can be affected by BMT. We will highlight three: *(1)* the relationship between the patient and their spouse or significant other; *(2)* the patient–child relationship; and *(3)* the patient–parent relationship.

BMT places definite stresses upon the patient–spouse relationship. The spouse or significant other may face a leave of absence from work to care for the patient or other family members. Consequently, increased parental and caregiver role demands during hospitalization and during convalescence at home can sap the partner both physically and psychologically. BMT is also likely to disrupt the normal pattern and rhythm of the patient–spouse relationship. Marital communication and sexual behavior are likely to be disrupted, particularly in couples characterized by greater inflexibility in their relationship. In order to care for their partner, many spouses choose to "stay in" with the patient. This prolonged propinquity, however, exposes them to small hospital rooms, sleep deprivation, and first-hand observation of suffering that their partner experiences in the way of nausea, vomiting, diarrhea, or other side-effects of treatment.

The relationship between BMT patients and their children can also be adversely affected during hospitalization and convalescence. Specific difficulties vary markedly with the disposition and developmental stage of the child. Young children may experience anxiety and apprehension that accompanies enforced separation from parents. Adolescents, involved in their own activities at school or with friends, may appear indifferent to the situation. In fact, however, they are typically quite concerned yet unable to express their anxieties verbally. Advance preparation and opportunities for discussion and visitation can be effective in reducing the distress of children and adolescents.

Finally, BMT can strain the relationship between patients and their parents. The adolescent or young adult patient may find their need for autonomy conflicts with the enforced dependency required by BMT. This can manifest in rebellion against required health care behaviors, resulting in treatment noncompliance. Both parents and patients may encounter conflict around the need to control a medical situation that is often simply not controllable. If the BMT patient is an older adult with children, grandparents may assume increased responsibility for caring for grandchildren.

This, of course, can result in conflict regarding child care. Depending upon the BMT outcome, this could be a prolonged responsibility, ultimately greatly interfering with other life demands of these older parents.

The specific impact of BMT upon each of the subsystems described above varies as a function of the family's support resources, the developmental and life cycle stage of the family and family members, and the course of the BMT recipient's disease and BMT. In general, the majority of families adapt well and recover their equilibrium as the patient's medical recovery progresses. In fact, it is not uncommon for patients and family members to report that the BMT experience has had a positive, salutary impact upon family relationships. Psychosocial factors that pre-date BMT, such as poor communication, lack of social support, and maladaptive responses to previous stressors are likely to be critical to identifying families at risk for poor adaptation. There is a clear need for more quality research in this area.

The Marrow Donor

The experience of the marrow donor has received little empirical attention. Two areas of interest can be identified: *(1)* impact of marrow donation upon the donor, and *(2)* the process leading to the decision to donate marrow.

Marrow donation involves removal of marrow cells from the donor's iliac crest or sternum. The procedure is performed while the donor is hospitalized under general anesthesia. Despite the risks and discomforts inherent in donation, and despite frequent anecdotal discussions of potential psychosocial problems following donation (e.g., donor guilt), few studies have examined the physical and psychosocial sequelae of marrow donation. While pain is often reported, only one study has investigated post-donation pain in any detail (59). Results indicated that many donors reported mild to moderate pain despite use of analgesic medication, suggesting that more attention should be devoted to post-donation pain management. Two other studies examined a broader range of post-donation outcomes. In one study (60), the physical and psychosocial impact of donation was assessed in 20 adult unrelated donors 1–36 days post donation. While no serious aftereffects were reported, about 25% indicated that the donation experience was more negative than anticipated, suggesting the need for better donor preparation. Finally, the impact of donation was assessed 18–89 months post BMT in 18 adult related donors (61). In general, donors reported little change in the donor–recipient relationship and little distress. However, some donors reported negative experiences (e.g., estrangement from the recipient) associated with their donation.

Existing studies suggest that serious psychological and physical complications following marrow donation are rare. While research has focused upon potential negative sequelae of donation, it is also important to examine potential positive sequelae such as increased self-esteem or positive mood and enhancement of family relationships. Understanding of the positive sequelae of donation might be critical to efforts to recruit unrelated volunteer marrow donors. The occurrence of GVHD, graft rejection, or death following BMT might also be critical determinants of donor adjustment, and for unrelated volunteer donors could affect willingness to donate again in the future.

The process leading to the decision to become a marrow donor differs depending upon whether the donor is a relative of the BMT recipient or an unrelated volunteer donor. In the former instance, the decision to donate marrow evolves in the context of an existing network of family relationships (21). In many instances, testing might have identified a single relative as the only suitable donor. Even when more than one relative is identified as a suitable donor, a potential donor is likely to experience pressure to donate. While most potential donors are genuinely eager to serve as the marrow donor, medical staff must be aware that the pressure to donate can limit the donor's expression of any ambivalence regarding donation. The potential donor should be given the opportunity to discreetly discuss their views regarding marrow donation with a member of the medical staff before the decision to donate has been formalized. This predonation conference can also provide a forum for establishing realistic expectations for the transplant outcome as well as educating the donor regarding likely postdonation psychological sequelae.

Medical Staff

While there has been some research on the stresses experienced by medical care providers in the oncology setting in general (62,63), there are few or no data on the impact of BMT upon medical staff in the BMT setting. It is generally assumed, however, that work on a BMT unit is highly stressful. Medical staff are in continuous contact with patients and can develop strong emotional attachments to patients and families. Establishment of such attachments is facilitated by the often lengthy period of hospitalization and the use of nursing approaches that discourage "rotating off" patients. Given this bond, it is difficult to observe patients' progress from a state of relative health and vitality to serious illness and even death within a few

weeks. Medical staff can also serve as the focus of patients' and families' anger and hostility when difficulties arise. Finally, medical staff must also strive to maintain patients' and families' realistic hopes, even when obstacles are overwhelming. In light of this, recommendations for supporting the psychosocially demanding work of the transplantation team have been advanced (64,65).

Several key dynamics have been observed among medical staff treating BMT patients (21). First, staff may experience guilt at being the agents of treatment that often produces suffering and death. Second, the attachments formed by medical staff can lead to intense grief following the death of a patient. Many BMT units function as a family of sorts and experience a patient's death as if a family member had died. This bereavement may be a key issue in any burnout experienced by BMT staff. Again, this is an area where further research could prove fruitful.

Psychosocial and Behavioral Issues: Summary

The BMT setting consists of a complex network of human relationships embedded in a context of multiple physical and psychosocial stressors associated with the treatment of life-threatening disease. This chapter has provided an overview of the medical procedures as well as principal actors and issues associated with the BMT setting. Interested readers are encouraged to refer to other excellent discussions of the psychosocial, psychiatric, and behavioral issues associated with BMT (15–21,66).

REFERENCES

1. Armitage JO. Bone marrow transplantation. *N Engl J Med.* 1994; 330:827–838.
2. Thomas ED, Lochte HL Jr, Lu WC, Ferrebee JW. Intravenous infusion of bone marrow in patients receiving radiation and chemotherapy. *N Engl J Med.* 1957; 257:491–496.
3. Thomas ED. The evolution of the scientific foundation of marrow transplantation based on human studies. In: Forman SJ, Blume KG, Thomas ED, eds. *Bone Marrow Transplantation.* Boston: Blackwell Scientific 1994:12–15.
4. Gatti RA, Meuwissen HJ, Allen HD, Hong R, Good RA. Immunological reconstitution of sex-linked lymphogenic immunological deficiency. *Lancet.* 1968; 2:1366–1369.
5. Bortin MM, Horowitz MM, Rimm AA. Increasing utilization of allogeneic bone marrow transplantation: results of the 1988-1990 survey. *Ann Intern Med.* 1992; 116:505–512.
6. Bortin MM, Rimm AA. Increasing utilization of bone marrow transplantation II: results of the 1985–1987 survey. *Transplantation.* 1989; 48:453–458.

7. Cohen SC, Krigel RL. High-dose therapy with stem cell infusion in lymphoma. *Semin Oncol.* 1995; 22:218–229.

8. Coiffier B, Philip T, Burnett AK, Symann ML. Consensus conference on intensive chemotherapy plus hematopoietic stem cell transplantation in malignancies: Lyon, France, June 4–6, 1993. *J Clin Oncol.* 1994; 12:226–231.

9. Advisory Committee of the International Autologous Bone Marrow Transplant Registry. Autologous bone marrow transplants: different indications in Europe and America. *Lancet.* 1989; 2:317–318.

10. Horowitz MM. New IBMTR/ABMTR slides summarize current use and outcome of allogeneic and autologous transplants. *IBMTR Newsletter.* 1995; 2:1, 3–8.

11. Marks DI, Cullis JO, Ward KN, et al. Allogeneic bone marrow transplantation for chronic myeloid leukemia using sibling and volunteer unrelated donors: a comparison of complications in the first 2 years. *Ann Intern Med.* 1993; 119:207–214.

12. McGlave P, Bartsch G, Anasetti C, et al. Unrelated donor marrow transplantation therapy for chronic myelogenous leukemia: initial experience of the National Marrow Donor Program. *Blood.* 1993; 81:543–550.

13. Andrykowski MA, Brady MJ, Henslee-Downey PJ. Psychosocial factors predictive of survival following allogeneic bone marrow transplantation for leukemia. *Psychosom Med.* 1994; 56:432–439.

14. Colon EA, Callies AL, Popkin MK, McGlave PB. Depressed mood and other variables related to bone marrow transplant survival in acute leukemia. *Psychosomatics.* 1991; 32:420–425.

15. Abramowitz LZ. Perspectives on pediatric bone marrow transplantation. In: Whedon MB, ed. *Bone Marrow Transplantation: Principles, Practice, and Nursing Insights.* Boston: Jones and Bartlett; 1991:70–104.

16. Ahles TA, Shedd P. Psychosocial impact of bone marrow transplantation in adult patients: Prehospitalization and hospitalization phases. In: Whedon MB, ed. *Bone Marrow Transplantation: Principles, Practice, and Nursing Insights.* Boston: Jones and Bartlett; 1991:280–292.

17. Andrykowski MA. Psychiatric and psychosocial aspects of bone marrow transplantation. *Psychosomatics.* 1994; 35:13–24.

18. Andrykowski MA. Psychosocial factors in bone marrow transplantation: a review and recommendations for research. *Bone Marrow Transplant.* 1994; 13:357–375.

19. Lesko LM. Bone marrow transplantation. In: Holland JC, Rowland JH, eds. *Handbook of Psychooncology: Psychological Care of the Patient with Cancer.* New York: Oxford University Press; 1989:163–173.

20. Rodrigue JR, Greene AF, Boggs SR. Current status of psychological research in organ transplantation. *J Clin Psychol Med Settings.* 1994; 1:41–70.

21. Wellisch DK, Wolcott DL. Psychological issues in bone marrow transplantation. In: Forman SJ, Blume KG, Thomas ED, eds. *Bone Marrow Transplantation.* Boston: Blackwell Scientific 1994: 556–571.

22. Brown HN, Kelly MJ. Stages of bone marrow transplantation: a psychiatric perspective. *Psychosom Med.* 1976; 38:439–446.

23. Pfefferbaum B, Lindamood MM, Wiley FM. Stages in pediatric bone marrow transplantation. *Pediatrics.* 1978; 61:625–628.

24. Frierson RL, Lippman SB. Heart transplantation patients rejected on psychiatric considerations. *Psychosomatics.* 1987; 28:347–355.

25. Mai FM, McKenzie FN, Kostuk WJ. Psychiatric aspects of heart transplantation: preoperative evaluation and postoperative sequelae. *Br Med J.* 1986; 292:311–313.

26. Schroeder JS, Hunt S. Cardiac transplantation update 1987. *J Am Med Assoc.* 1987; 258:3142–3145.

27. Annas GJ. Informed consent. *Ann Rev Med.* 1978; 29:9–14.

28. Dermatis H, Lesko LM. Psychological distress in parents consenting to child's bone marrow transplantation. *Bone Marrow Transplant.* 1990; 6:411–417.

29. Dermatis H, Lesko LM. Psychosocial correlates of physician-patient communication at time of informed consent for bone marrow transplantation. *Cancer Invest.* 1991; 9:621–628.

30. Lesko LM, Dermatis H, Penman D, Holland JC. Patients', parents' and oncologists' perceptions of informed consent for bone marrow transplantation. *Med Pediatr Oncol.* 1989; 17:181–187.

31. Andrykowski MA, Brady MJ, Greiner CB, et al. "Returning to normal" following bone marrow transplantation: outcomes expectations, and informed consent. *Bone Marrow Transplant.* 1995; 15:573–581.

32. Patenaude AF, Rappeport JM, Smith BR. The physician's influence on informed consent for bone marrow transplantation. *Theor Med.* 1986; 7:165–179.

33. Chapko MK, Syrjala KL, Schilter L, Cummings C, Sullivan KM. Chemoradiotherapy toxicity during bone marrow transplantation: time course and variation in pain and nausea. *Bone Marrow Transplant.* 1989; 4:181–186.

34. Syrjala KL, Cummings C, Donaldson GW. Hypnosis or cognitive behavioral training for the reduction of pain and nausea during cancer treatment: a controlled clinical trial. *Pain.* 1992; 48:137–146.

35. Futterman AD, Wellisch DK, Bond G, Carr CR. The psychosocial levels system: a new rating scale to identify and assess emotional difficulties during bone marrow transplantation. *Psychosomatics.* 1991; 32:177–186.

36. Andrykowski MA, Brady MJ, Bruehl S, Henslee-Downey PJ. Physical and psychosocial status of adults one year following bone marrow transplantation: a prospective study. *Bone Marrow Transplant.* 1995; 15: 837–844.

37. Syrjala KL, Chapko MK, Vitaliano PP, Cummings C, Sullivan KM. Recovery after allogeneic marrow transplantation: prospective study of predictors of long-term physical and psychosocial functioning. *Bone Marrow Transplant.* 1993; 11:319–327.

38. Phipps S, DeCuir-Whalley S. Adherence issues in pediatric bone marrow transplantation. *J Pediatr Psychol.* 1990; 15:459–476.

39. Deeg HJ. Bone marrow transplantation: a review of delayed complications. *Br J Haematol.* 1984; 57:185–208.

40. Kolb HJ, Bender-Gotze C. Late complications after allogeneic bone marrow transplantation for leukaemia. *Bone Marrow Transplant.* 1990; 6:61–72.

41. Vose JM, Kennedy BC, Bierman PJ, Kessinger A, Armitage JO. Long-term sequelae of autologous bone marrow or peripheral stem cell transplantation for lymphoid malignancies. *Cancer.* 1992; 69:784–789.

42. Cella DF, Tulsky DS. Quality of life in cancer: definition, purpose, and method of measurement. *Cancer Invest.* 1993; 11:327–336.

43. Ware JE. Conceptualizing disease impact and treatment outcomes. *Cancer.* 1984; 53(3, suppl):2316–2323.

44. Moinpour CM, Feigl P, Metch B, Hayden KA, Meyskens FL Jr, Crowley J. Quality of life end points in cancer clinical trials: review and recommendations. *J Natl Cancer Inst.* 1989; 81:485–495.

45. Andrykowski MA, Greiner CB, Altmaier EM, et al. Quality of life following bone marrow transplantation: findings from a multicentre study. *Br J Cancer.* 1995; 71:1322–1329.

46. Baker F, Curbow B, Wingard JR. Role retention and quality of life of bone marrow transplant survivors. *Soc Sci Med.* 1991; 32:697–704.

47. Baker F, Wingard JR, Curbow B. Quality of life of bone marrow transplant long-term survivors. *Bone Marrow Transplant.* 1994; 13:589-596.

48. Bush NE, Haberman M, Sullivan KM. Quality of life of 125 adults surviving 6–18 years after bone marrow transplantation. *Soc Sci Med.* 1995; 40:479–490.

49. Chao NJ, Tierney DK, Bloom JR. Dynamic assessment of quality of life after autologous bone marrow transplantation. *Blood.* 1992; 80:825–830.

50. Schmidt GM, Niland JC, Forman SJ. Extended follow-up in 212 long-term allogeneic bone marrow transplant survivors: issues of quality of life. *Transplantation.* 1993; 55:551–557.

51. Wingard JR, Curbow B, Baker F, Piantadosi S. Health functional status and employment of adult survivors of bone marrow transplantation. *Ann Intern Med.* 1991; 114:113–118.

52. Baider L, De-Nour AK. Impact of cancer on couples. *Cancer Invest.* 1993; 11:706–713.

53. Houts PS, Rusenas I, Simmonds MA, Hufford DL. Information needs of families of cancer patients: a literature review and recommendations. *J Cancer Educ.* 1991; 6:255–261.

54. Kristjanson LJ, Ashcroft T. The family's cancer journey: a literature review. *Cancer Nurs.* 1994; 17:1–17.

55. Mor V, Allen S, Malin M. The psychosocial impact of cancer on older versus younger patients and their families. *Cancer.* 1994; 74:2118–2127.

56. Rait D, Lederberg MS. The family of the cancer patient. In: Holland JC, Rowland JH, eds. *Handbook of Psychooncology: Psychological Care of the Patient with Cancer.* New York: Oxford University Press; 1989: 585–597.

57. Lesko LM. Bone marrow transplantation: support of the patient and his/her family. *Support Care Cancer.* 1994; 2:35–49.

58. Zabora JR, Smith ED, Baker F, Wingard JR, Curbow B. The family: the other side of bone marrow transplantation. *J Psychosoc Oncol.* 1992; 10:35–46.

59. Hill HF, Chapman CR, Jackson TL, Sullivan KM. Assessment and management of donor pain following marrow harvest for allogeneic bone marrow transplantation. *Bone Marrow Transplant.* 1989; 4:157–161.

60. Stroncek D, Strand R, Scott E, et al. Attitudes and physical condition of unrelated bone marrow donors immediately after donation. *Transfusion.* 1989; 29:317–322.

61. Wolcott DL, Wellisch DK, Fawzy FI, Landsverk J. Psychological adjustment of adult bone marrow transplant donors whose recipient survives. *Transplantation.* 1986; 4:484–488.

62. Whippen DA, Canellos GP. Burnout syndrome in the practice of oncology: results of a random survey of 1,000 oncologists. *J Clin Oncol.* 1991; 9:1916–1920.

63. Cohen MZ. The meaning of cancer and oncology nursing: link to effective care. *Semin Oncol Nurs.* 1995; 11:59–67.

64. Sarantos S. Innovations in psychosocial staff support: a model program for the transplant nurse. *Semin Oncol Nurs.* 1983; 4:69–73.

65. Kris A. Support of the transplant team. *Support Care Cancer.* 1994; 2:56–60.

66. Wolcott DL, Fawzy FI, Wellisch DK. Psychiatric aspects of bone marrow transplantation: a review and current issues. *Psychiatr Med.* 1987; 4:299–317.

VII

PSYCHOLOGICAL ISSUES
RELATED TO SITE OF CANCER

EDITOR: RUTH McCORKLE

25

Central Nervous System Tumors

STEVEN D. PASSIK AND PATRICIA L. RICKETTS

Cancers of the central nervous system (CNS), whether primary or metastatic, are devastating forms of illness that take a dramatic toll on patients, their families, and caregivers. CNS cancers directly affect the mind, self, and memory of the patient and thereby pose special problems. Patients with CNS tumors are particularly vulnerable to a range of psychosocial difficulties due to a disease course characterized by incipient decline and mounting neurologic deficits. The typical psychological problems of people with cancer are compounded by the cognitive problems accompanying CNS cancers. In this chapter we provide medical information about the presentation and treatment of CNS cancers, the range of psychiatric difficulties seen in CNS cancer patients, and discuss psychopharmacologic and psychotherapeutic interventions for patients, family, and staff.

THE SPECTRUM OF NEURO-ONCOLOGIC ILLNESSES: PREVALENCE AND PRESENTATION

All CNS cancers have been increasing in prevalence in the United States. CNS metastases, the most prevalent form of CNS cancer, are affecting growing numbers of patients who are living longer with systemic cancers (1). Between 25% and 45% of all brain tumors are metastatic (2). The CNS may serve as a "sanctuary" for cancer cells affected elsewhere by chemotherapies that do not cross the blood–brain barrier (3). Of patients with systemic cancer, 24% are found to have intracranial metastases on autopsy (4). Presently in the United States, 125,000 patients die per year with brain metastases (2). Of these, approximately 80,000 (64%) manifest significant neurologic symptomatology during their lives. Brain metastases are present in 5% of all fatal cancers (2,5). Common neurological symptoms of brain metastases found in a series of 363 patients were hemiparesis, which affected 59% of patients; impaired cognitive function (32%); followed by unilateral sensory loss (21%); gait disturbance (19%); and aphasia (12%) (5).

Solid tumors carry different degrees of risk for the development of CNS metastases. Lung cancers have the highest degree of associated risk, with 65%–70% of these patients going on to develop brain metastases. Breast cancer (5%–20%), kidney cancer (5%–10%), gastrointestinal tract cancers (5%), and melanoma (less than 5%) follow lung in terms of associated risk for the development of brain metastases (6).

Primary brain tumors such as glioblastoma multiforme (GBM) are also becoming increasingly prevalent in the United States. While still relatively rare, accounting for approximately 1% of all primary cancers in this country, there are on average 17,600 new cases per year (7). The largest increase has been in older patients (1,8). Primary CNS lymphomas are also increasing in prevalence. In one setting these tumors increased from 1% to 15% of CNS tumors (9).

Common signs and symptoms of primary brain tumors and CNS lymphoma include change in mental function, headache, vomiting, seizures, and focal deficits, such as problems in speech comprehension or production. As tumors progress or as damage to the brain increases (as a result of radiation necrosis, dementia, or other insults) loss of cognitive functions tends to worsen. In the latter stages of illness, patients tend to become barely responsive and their need for nursing care increases dramatically.

Paraneoplastic syndromes are distant, nonmetastatic effects of systemic cancers on the brain. These syndromes are quite rare and include a number of neurologic complications not due to direct tumor invasion or metastases of the nervous system. Their cause is unknown, although an autoimmune etiology is speculated (3). Paraneoplastic syndromes affecting the brain and nervous system present with a range of symptoms including mimicking psychiatric disturbances (particularly organic mental disorders such as dementia and organic mood disorder-depressed). Limbic encephalitis (3) can present with dementia, memory loss, mood change, hallucinations, or delusions. Bulbar and brainstem encephalitis can also present with cognitive and memory deficits that are accompanied by vertigo, nystagmus, ataxia, dysphagia, ophthalmoplegia and extensor plantar reflexes. Subacute cerebellar degeneration often presents with symmetrical ataxia of the arms and legs, dysarthria, diplopia, vertigo, and occasionally nystagmus. Dementia is often an associated finding. These rare effects often appear (50%–66% of cases) before the primary cancer and their diagnosis can lead to early treatment of occult tumor (3).

TREATMENT APPROACHES TO NEURO-ONCOLOGIC ILLNESSES

Primary Brain Tumors

The standard treatment of primary brain tumors varies depending on tumor type but generally involves surgery in some combination with radiation therapy and/or chemotherapy. This combined approach has lengthened the median survival of patients with glioblastoma multiforme (GBM) from less than 6 months to approximately 18 months (10). Primary brain tumors usually recur in the area of their initial site and rarely metastasize outside of the brain. Before the development of radiation and chemotherapies, this recurrence generally began soon after surgery and often proved fatal. At present treatment begins with the surgical removal of the tumor, followed by radiation and chemotherapies. The degree of residual tumor following surgery has been shown to predict survival, as patients with less than $1\,cm^2$ have been found to survive longer (10). Age has been demonstrated to be the single best predictor of survival, with younger patients outliving older ones (10). Neurosurgery accelerates the growth rate of remaining tumor cells, rendering them more vulnerable to the antineoplastic effects of chemotherapy. Radiation therapy (RT) for primary brain tumors has been used widely since the 1970s when it was found to double survival (from 17 to 24 weeks) for patients who received postoperative RT following surgery (11,12). Recent advances in the use of RT for primary brain tumors generally involve more focused delivery of the radiation (13,14). Such approaches minimize damage done to surrounding tissue and neurologic consequences of treatment.

Chemotherapy can extend survival of patients with primary brain tumors. Two studies have demonstrated that the use of either BCNU (carmustine) or vincristine with radiation therapy lengthens the median survival of patients to 50 weeks as compared to only 35 weeks

for patients receiving radiation therapy alone. BCNU continues to be the most widely used chemotherapy treatment for primary brain tumors (15). One new area of inquiry in the chemotherapeutic approach to the treatment of primary brain tumors is experimenting with means of enhancing the permeability of the blood–brain barrier (e.g., the bradykinin analog RMP-7) (16). Such attempts are aimed at making chemotherapy a more powerful tool in the treatment of these tumors.

Brain Metastases

Brain metastases are serious complications of many systemic cancers. The standard approach to patients with brain metastases is combined treatment drawing upon surgical extirpation (when possible), whole brain radiation therapy, and/or chemotherapy. The location and number of brain metastases, the patient's overall functional status, extent of illness, and site of primary tumor will all influence the application of these available treatments.

A study of combined treatment for brain metastases demonstrated that 75% of patients neurologically improved and 6% worsened (17). After 2 months follow-up, CT studies showed that in 25% of cases (in those patients who were still alive) the lesions had disappeared; in 35% of cases there was shrinkage of the lesion by greater than 50% of original size; and in 40% of cases there was no change in the original lesion. Surgical extirpation offers many patients with brain metastases a chance of cure. Further, debulking of the tumor serves as an adjuvant to chemotherapy and radiation therapy, and offers improvement in neurologic symptoms (18) . Fifty percent of patients are found to have single brain metastases upon presentation and are therefore candidates for surgical intervention (6,19). Occasionally, patients who are found to have two and even three brain metastases (and who are otherwise functional) will be considered for surgical intervention. Another important factor in the consideration of surgical intervention is accessibility of the lesion(s). Lesions deep within the brain (i.e., in the basal ganglia) or too close to major blood vessels are generally not considered for surgical extirpation.

Glucocorticoids (steroids) are widely prescribed in the neuro-oncology setting for patients with brain metastases and primary tumors. At Memorial Sloan-Kettering, 70% of neuro-oncology patients receive treatment with steroids as compared to only 33% of general neurology patients or 15% of general oncology patients (3). Seventy to eighty percent of patients with brain metastases demonstrate neurologic improvement on steroids (3). This improvement is most pronounced in patients with generalized neurologic dysfunction as compared to focal deficits. The psychiatric side effects of steroids include insomnia, agitation, anxiety, depression, mania, and delirium and are described in greater detail below.

Whole-brain radiation therapy (WBRT) is the standard form of radiation therapy for brain metastases. The median survival of patients with brain metastases treated with WBRT is 3–6 months, with 10% to 15% of patients surviving up to one year (2). Better functional status at the outset of WBRT is the best predictor of survival. The side effects of WBRT, especially high-dose therapy, include headache, worsening of neurologic symptoms, cerebral herniation, and death. Greater than 10% of patients, if they live longer than a one year, will have WBRT-induced brain damage due to radiation necrosis (2,20).

All of the treatments described above can lead to the development of neuropsychiatric complications. In the section to follow, the psychiatric and psychosocial aspects of neuro-oncologic illness and its treatments will be detailed.

PSYCHIATRIC AND PSYCHOSOCIAL ASPECTS OF CNS TUMORS

In contrast to the spectrum of psychiatric disorders in non-CNS cancers where the predominant diagnoses are adjustment disorders, when the psychiatric diagnoses of CNS cancer patients referred for psychiatric consultations at Memorial Sloan-Kettering Cancer Center were reviewed, the usual proportion of adjustment disorders to organic mental disorders was reversed. In this sample, 41% of patients were diagnosed with organic mental disorders, 11% with major depressions, and only 26% were diagnosed with adjustment disorders. Thus, it is crucial for the psycho-oncologist to be able to differentially diagnose the range of organic mental disorders seen in this population.

Delirium

Delirium is a common psychiatric complication of CNS cancers and their treatment. It presents a significant, but often reversible, problem that can intensify the impact of the disease on the patient and add to the already burdensome task of caregiving. CNS cancer patients are more vulnerable to delirium than are other cancer patients because their disease and treatments directly damage the brain and can alter its functioning. The main causes of delirium in neuro-oncology patients are CNS insults, medications (especially corticosteroids), and metabolic changes. (See Chapter 48 on delirium for a description of signs and symptoms of this and other cognitive disorders.)

In its early stages or mild forms, delirium can be misdiagnosed as dementia or depression in patients with CNS tumors. While this is true in psychiatric oncology as a whole, in neuro-oncology, where patients are often unable to articulate their experience, the symptoms of delirium can be missed. Differences in onset, course, and symptomatology help with differential diagnosis of delirium, dementia, and depression. Delirium can be superimposed on an underlying dementia. The early stages of a delirium often are marked more by decreased level of awareness, withdrawal, somnolence, lethargy, and mood changes than the more dramatic types of symptomatology (e.g., hallucinations; confusion). Not surprisingly then, a patient with poor prognosis and devastating symptoms who suddenly becomes withdrawn will often be thought of as depressed. Family members may believe that even very severe symptoms such as hallucinations are part of a psychological reaction to these circumstances and feel that the stress of the illness has "driven the patient crazy." The psycho-oncologist must be careful to assess for the time course of the mood change; to take into account organic factors such as new drugs or treatments; and most importantly, to assess for the full range of depressive versus delirious symptoms. Once the diagnosis is made, education of caregivers is essential to ensure appropriate treatment and to reassure family.

Dementia

Dementia appears in relatively alert individuals with little or no clouding of consciousness. Unlike delirium, the temporal onset of symptoms in dementia is subacute or chronic and the sleep–wake cycle is less impaired. The neurologic deficits and dementia associated with CNS metastases or tumors can be focal or global in nature. Focal deficits are those caused by tumor or radiation damage to areas of the brain responsible for specific intellectual, motor, or speech functions. Global deficits are caused by more diffuse effects of the tumor or treatment such as increased intracranial pressure and edema, which can cause gait disturbances, loss of bowel and bladder control, and profound dementia. DeAngelis and colleagues (20) reviewed 370 cases and reported on 12 cases (3%) of radiation-induced dementia in patients cured of their brain metastases. Within 5–36 months these patients developed a severe and progressive dementia accompanied by ataxia and urinary incontinence. This syndrome appeared similar to a subcortical dementia and was fatal in 7 out of the 12 patients.

As a result of their disease or treatment, patients with CNS cancer often develop mood syndromes that meet the DSM-IV criteria for major mood or anxiety disorders (major depression, bipolar disorder, or panic disorder). The key diagnostic distinction between these syndromes and endogenous versions of them is the assumption that etiology can be traced to some aspect of the disease or treatment. Additionally, these syndromes are often accompanied by subtle cognitive abnormalities. Their treatments differ considerably, both in terms of the likely decreased utility of psychotherapy alone, in the more organic syndromes, and in differing psychopharmacologic approaches. The standard treatment for nonorganic panic attacks, for example, is a combination of the short-term use of benzodiazepines (such as alprazolam or lorazepam) and cognitive behavioral psychotherapy with relaxation training. If the disorder persists, tricyclic antidepressants or specific serotonin reuptake inhibitors are usually used to replace the benzodiazepines. Therapy is quite different in the case of the patient with CNS cancer who develops panic attacks and anxiety from a combination of tumor and/or medication effects. The use of cognitive behavioral therapy—requiring focused attention—may be impossible, depending upon the extent of cognitive difficulty the patient manifests. Further, the benzodiazepines can have paradoxical effects on patients with brain disease. As will be described in more detail below, the treatment of organic anxiety, mood, or other mental syndromes in the neurooncology population generally begins with a trial of low-dose neuroleptic medications.

One of the main causes of these mood and anxiety syndromes in the neurooncology population are the glucocorticoids (such as decadron and prednisone). Breitbart and colleagues (21,22) studied cancer patients with epidural spinal cord compression (ESCC). These patients are treated with very high doses of steroids. Twenty-four percent of the patients were diagnosed with delirium (as compared to 10% in a non-ESCC control group), with the tendency to develop delirium being slightly higher for female patients. Twenty-two percent of the patients in the ESCC group were found to have major depressive disorders (organic mood syndrome and major depression), compared to only 4% in the non-ESCC control group. Estimates of the prevalence of severe psychiatric disorders caused by steroids vary widely. The development of psychotic reactions, including delusions and hallucinations, has been reported to be as high as 92% (23) and as low as 3% of patients (24).

WBRT, used to treat primary as well as metastatic lesions of the brain, can be complicated by a radiation-induced organic mental syndrome. Three types of organic mental syndromes have been described: acute (seen immediately after first radiation treatment); early-delayed (beginning 6–16 weeks after treatment); and late-delayed (seen 6 months to several years later) (3). Acute organic mental syndrome can occur during the immediate course of high-dose radiation therapy. Patients can become lethargic; and complain of headache, nausea, vomiting, and fever. It is thought that this type of acute reaction is due to increased intracranial pressure secondary to radiation-induced changes in the blood–brain barrier. Left untreated it can lead to worsening of neurologic deficits and even brain herniation. An early-delayed organic mental syndrome can begin 1–4 months after radiation treatment but has been reported earlier or later. Symptoms consist of lethargy, headache, nausea, and vomiting. Patients who receive more focal RT to the brain can present with symptoms of focal neurologic disease suggestive of recurrence of tumor. The cause of early-delayed radiation organic mental syndromes is unknown, but may be related to radiation-induced edema or demyelination. Improvement in symptoms usually occurs spontaneously in 1–6 weeks. A late-delayed organic mental syndrome (usually severe and permanent) may develop 6 months to 3 years (average 12 months) after radiation therapy. This syndrome is characterized by symptoms that suggest a focal neurological lesion, accompanied by personality change and headache. Seizures can also complicate the picture.

Seizure Disorders

For patients with brain metastases, seizures are the presenting symptom in 20% of cases (25). Additionally, 30%–40% of patients will experience seizures at some point after the development of brain metastases (25). The management of seizure disorders in patients with compromised cognitive capacities and serious systemic cancers is difficult. For this and several reasons to be described below, the initiation of prophylactic phenytoin (Dilantin) treatment is controversial. This is especially true for patients who have experienced a single seizure as the presenting symptom of a brain metastasis. Of these patients, only between 10 and 15% will experience a second seizure (3). Moreover, phenytoin may interfere with the beneficial effects of steroids and may not interact well with other forms of chemotherapy. Patients with memory or other cognitive deficits may not be able to comply with instructions for taking their anticonvulsants. This problem can lead to difficulty in maintaining proper blood levels of these medicines and/or the development of toxicity from overdose. The occurrence of a seizure for a patient who has never experienced them before is a frightening and mysterious development. Patients fear the loss of control of their behavior signaled by the onset of a seizure disorder. Seizures can be a frightening event for inexperienced family members. The fear of further seizures often places the burden for the proper administration of the anticonvulsant medicines squarely upon the family, compounding their other caretaking responsibilities.

Management of organic mental disorders in the CNS cancer patient begins with attention directed toward determination of the etiologic factors. In addition to the treatment of underlying medical problems, there are a range of useful environmental interventions (see Chapter 48).

Antipsychotic medications given orally are the preferred medications to use in mild organic mental disorders. Benzodiazepines, sedative-hypnotics or barbiturates may be effective over the first few hours or days, but may make organic mental disorders worse (see below).

PSYCHOTHERAPEUTIC AND PSYCHOPHARMACOLOGIC INTERVENTIONS FOR PATIENTS, FAMILIES, AND STAFF

Psychotherapy can help patients with neuro-oncologic illnesses cope with the often grim realities of their disease and treatment. The key issues of concern to cancer patients (26)—disability, dependency, disruption, disfigurement, and death—are all part of the reality of neuro-oncologic illnesses. The grim prognosis associated with these diseases moves preparation for death to the forefront of psychological issues facing the patient. Many patients with cancers arising outside of the CNS adjust quite well prior to development of brain metastases. Upon the development of neurologic symptomatology, they find themselves in unchartered psychological waters and the fear of loss of control and of losing their minds (27) can be profound.

Patients with brain metastases often find that they can no longer exert the same mastery over their illness that they once achieved. The awareness of cognitive deficits for patients with primary or metastatic neurologic disease can be a frightening and frustrating experience for the patient. For example, the patient with an expressive or receptive aphasia caused by CNS disease often presents with a pathetic struggle to speak and communicate. The resulting isolation can be profound, as the illness decreases the ability of the patient to interact with supportive family members. It is very common for neuro-oncology patients to begin to feel that they have become terribly burden-

some to their family members. This realization can be so intolerable that it is accompanied by suicidal thoughts.

Psychotherapy with neuro-oncology patients is generally supportive in nature (psychotherapy that begins in a expressive or dynamic vein is likely to become supportive as illness progresses), drawing upon crisis intervention and psychoeducational techniques. The principles that guide crisis intervention therapy are useful for the therapist to bear in mind when helping the patient confront the overwhelming nature of neuro-oncologic illness. These principles involve the adoption of an active and involved stance on the part of the therapist, an emphasis on providing specific information for coping with specific and solvable problems, the goal of returning the patient to psychological baseline (as opposed to aiming for personal change or growth); and stress on the importance of symptom control as an aid to adaptation. Despite the grave nature of CNS cancers and their symptomatology, the therapist need not be overly solemn in his approach to the patient. Often, as the illness has undermined normal modes of relating to family and friends, it will be the therapist alone who is able to engage the patient in more light-hearted forms of communication (28). The therapist can help to normalize the patient's reactions to the illness and help the patient to prepare for the typical disease course.

Finally, in crisis intervention psychotherapy, successful adaptation is seen as highly dependent upon symptom control. It is crucial that the therapist working with the neuro-oncology patient keep relief of distressing physical and psychological symptoms at the center of an ongoing dialogue with the patient. The simple act of engaging in such a dialogue communicates care and concern on the part of the therapist, and the mental health professional or team can play a very important role in the provision of symptom relief (29). CNS cancer patients can benefit from the judicious use of psychotropic medicines (see below) and, if not too impaired in attention and concentration, can benefit from the use of relaxation therapy and other cognitive behavioral techniques. Pain, especially in the form of headache, is common in neuro-oncology patients. The problem of pain and its impact on quality of life is often overlooked in this population and its assessment can be difficult in those patients with severe communication problems. It is often helpful in the application of cognitive-behavioral and relaxation techniques to enlist the spouse or a family member as a cotherapist. The cotherapist can then augment the patient's memory and aid the practice and application of techniques learned with the therapist outside of sessions. This is one of the many ways in which psychotherapy with neuro-oncology patients must take account of and augment failing memory and cognitive abilities on the part of the patient. Techniques that we have used for this purpose include having patients keep a therapy diary. It can be useful for patients with memory problems to write down one or two key points during each session. Ideally, the diary should be kept in a book that is small enough for the patient to keep with them at all times. Thus, by consulting the diary, the patient can both remember content aspects of the therapy and also evoke a sense of support to decrease isolation. The scheduling of sessions must also be altered to accommodate the neuro-oncology patient. Sessions should be short, generally not longer than 20–30 minutes, so as not to overwhelm or fatigue the patient. Additionally, sessions should be frequent, to provide a sense of continuity.

Anticipatory bereavement and preparation for death is often the focus of psychotherapy with neuro-oncology patients. We have found it helpful to encourage patients to think about and give advance directives about treatment alternatives and resuscitation early in the course of illness. Making such wishes known early can mitigate the sense of burden that patients feel is imposed on their families and grants patients a modicum of control over an illness course that is often overwhelming. Nonverbal techniques such as music and art therapy can help patients learn to communicate and express themselves when the illness has made verbal expression difficult or impossible. We know of several brain tumor patients who realized their artistic abilities only after their diagnosis of cancer. One patient became a talented sculptor (after the diagnosis of his tumor) and during the course of his illness filled his home with extraordinary works of art. This patient expressed to the therapist his desire to help his wife cope with his death by filling their home with reminders of him for her to have after he was gone. Another patient had been a talented painter but could no longer paint because of his tumor. He sought self-expression by arranging and rearranging books on his bookshelves.

An interesting phenomenon involving singing (and whispering) should be kept in mind by therapists working with aphasic patients. Patients who cannot speak, can sometimes sing or whisper, as these abilities are not controlled by exactly the same areas within the brain. The spouse of a brain tumor patient who suffered with abulia—the inability to initiate speech—due to a frontal lobe tumor told us of how she had not heard her husband's voice from not long after the onset of his illness. One day, while working in the kitchen, she had left her husband sitting in the living room listening to the radio. Suddenly, during the playing of a Beatles' song, he began to sing along with the record! The therapist encouraged the spouse to find more old records that her husband knew (and was likely to have memorized) for him to sing along with. The patient seemed to enjoy this enhancement to his self-expression, and the spouse was comforted by the sound of her husband's voice. On occasion, she was able to "converse" with the patient by addressing him in a sing-song voice. Therapists should take note of this phenomenon and not give up on the possibility of verbal interaction with neuro-oncologic patients until trying these types of vocal patterns. Speech disorders induced by neuro-oncologic illnesses may also affect second and third languages acquired later by patients but not their primary or "mother tongue." Thus, the ability of the patient to speak their first language should be investigated as this too can be useful in the service of the therapy and to increase quality of life in general.

Finally, professionals working in neurologic rehabilitation, in both the physical and cognitive domains, have begun to pay increased attention to neuro-oncology patients. Referral of patients for these types of intervention can augment psychotherapy in powerful ways. Cognitive rehabilitation strategies can teach patients how to improve concentration and assist memory. Small gains in these areas can pay big dividends in psychotherapy and in enhancing quality of life. Additionally, physical therapy can be used to increase ambulation and thereby decrease dependency and increase self-esteem.

PSYCHOPHARMACOLOGY FOR NEURO-ONCOLOGY PATIENTS

The use of psychotropic medications can lead to important enhancements of quality of life and symptom control. Some general guidelines for the use of psychotropic medications in the neuro-oncology population have arisen from clinical experience as psychiatry service liaison with the neuro-oncology service. So far, the data that supports these guidelines have emerged mainly from anecdotal and clinical experiences as there have been few published reports and no placebo-control studies of these medications in neuro-oncology patients.

The treatment of neuro-oncology patients with psychotropic medications must be initiated at low doses. Owing to the often extensive brain insults caused by the illness and its treatment, such patients often respond to low doses of centrally acting medications, and can be vulnerable to drug reactions. Short-acting drugs that do not produce active metabolites are preferable to longer acting drugs. Bearing these initial caveats in mind, the treatment of choice for most psychiatric complications of neurologic cancers are the neuroleptic drugs. As in other populations, these medications should be the first choice for the treatment of delirium or confusion associated with dementia or organic mood and anxiety syndromes. Because of the difficulty in identifying major depression as distinct from organic mood syndrome-depressed in such patients, we often initiate the treatment of depressive syndromes in this population with the use of a neuroleptic at bedtime as well.

Often, with treatment of insomnia and communication difficulties, patients begin to show improvement in their mood. If this is to be so, it is generally clinically evident considerably more quickly than an antidepressant would demonstrate its benefit. Other symptoms, such as fatigue, anhedonia, or social withdrawal can then be treated concomitantly with a psychostimulant (see below). Sedating neuroleptics can be used to relieve anxiety or confusion for procedures such as brain scans or lumbar punctures. The benzodiazepines should be used with caution in this population. As when treating other patients with brain injuries, neuro-oncology patients can be vulnerable to paradoxical reactions or disinhibition caused by these drugs. Their main use in the neuro-oncology population is as an adjunct to neuroleptics when emergency sedation is needed for the acutely agitated or delirious patient or for their anticonvulsant effects. Patients who do not respond to neuroleptics for the relief of anxiety can benefit from a trial of short-acting benzodiazepines such as lorazepam in low doses.

The tricyclic antidepressants can be useful in this population for the treatment of major depression. Neuro-oncology patients, like other cancer patients, tend to respond to lower doses than healthy patients. As will be discussed below, these drugs can be selected so as to maximize the benefits of their side effects. Finally, the psychostimulants, also in low doses, can be useful for the treatment of mood syndromes, the lethargy, withdrawal, and anhedonia associated with dementia, to improve the patient's ability to pay attention and therefore to augment memory. A series of case reports demonstrated beneficial effects of psychostimulants (e.g., methylphenidate) on cognitive slowing in primary and metastatic brain tumors (30).

Neuroleptics

The use of psychotropic medications for neuro-oncology patients begins with the neuroleptic medications because these drugs are safe, effective, and, most importantly, do not worsen confusion. Low doses of neuroleptic medications can be useful in the treatment of confusion, anxiety, and organic mood disorders. The high-potency neuroleptics such as haloperidol can be used to treat confusion, anxiety, and agitation (i.e., 0.5 to 2.0 mg orally once or twice daily) without sedating the patient. If sedation is desired, the lower potency medications (such as thioridazine, in doses of 10 to 50 mg orally once or twice daily) can also be used in low doses and are highly effective for these same indications.

As noted above, we often initiate the treatment of organic mood syndrome-depressed in our neuro-oncology patients with neuroleptic medications, sometimes in combination with a psychostimulant. The addition of a psychostimulant is often helpful in alleviating fatigue and attention problems after the neuroleptic has been started. Such a symptomatic approach to depressive syndromes in this population often works more quickly than through the use of other approaches and is unlikely to cause the patient problems with serious medication side effects.

There are, however, several side effects that the clinician should be concerned with when treating the CNS cancer patient. Neuroleptics can lower the seizure threshold and so must be used with certain cautions. The lowering of the seizure threshold does not often provide too great an obstacle to the use of neuroleptics if these drugs are initiated after the patient's seizure disorder has been well-controlled on anticonvulsants. Additionally, among the neuroleptics there are several agents that have less effect upon the seizure threshold. Molindone, a medium potency neuroleptic, and thioridazine, a low-potency one, have the least effect on the seizure threshold and should be chosen for patients in whom seizures are a concern. Chlorpromazine, which has the greatest potential to lower the seizure threshold, should be avoided.

Owing to the short-term exposure and low doses that characterize neuroleptic use in CNS cancer patients, concerns about neuroleptic malignant syndrome (NMS) or tardive dyskinesia (TD) are rarely a factor in considering treatment with these medications. There are, however, other less severe but uncomfortable side effects of neuroleptics that should be monitored. Akathisia, a movement disorder that involves motor restlessness, can cause great discomfort and even agitation in patients who cannot communicate well. The risk for development of akathisia is greatest when the patient is being treated with a high-potency neuroleptic, and especially for patients who are receiving other neuroleptics for nausea and vomiting concomitantly such as prochlorperazine and metachlo-promide. Lowering the dose of the neuroleptic or switching the patient to a low-potency agent can often relieve akathisia. Finally, for patients with nausea and vomiting, one agent with both antiemetic and antipsychotic effects (i.e., haloperidol) can be used and can help to avoid the development of neuroleptic side effects.

Psychostimulants

The psychostimulants are a useful class of medications for symptom control in the neuro-oncology population. These medicines, used in low, divided doses, can improve attention, mood, activity level, and cognitive function, and decrease social withdrawal while being safe and effective. A typical treatment with methylphenidate begins with 2.5 mg, orally at 8 A.M. and 12 noon, and is slowly titrated up to approximately 10–15 mg at 8 A.M. and 12 noon. Pemoline is a chewable tablet that can be dissolved in the mouth for patients who cannot swallow. A similar pattern of upward titration is used with this medication, for example, 18.75 mg orally at 8 A.M. and 12 noon titrated up to approximately 75 mg orally at 8 A.M. and 12 noon. Side effects that should be monitored carefully are psychotomimetic, such as paranoia or hallucinations. These side effects are generally only seen in patients receiving very high doses and rarely complicate treatment. These medicines can, however, have the effect of revealing a delirium in a somnolent patient. In such cases, the stimulant should be temporarily discontinued while the patient is started on a neuroleptic. When the patient is no longer confused, and the sleep–wake cycle has returned to or approaches normal, the stimulant can be restarted if needed.

Two additional cautions apply to the use of stimulants in neuro-oncology patients. First, patients' hepatic functions should be assessed before initiation of treatment. Pemoline can cause an elevation in hepatic enzymes. Routine monitoring of hepatic enzymes should accompany treatment with pemoline. Second, the psychostimulants should not be used when patients are receiving procarbazine (a mild monoamine oxidase inhibitor) as a chemotherapeutic agents owing to possible serious drug interactions.

The Tricyclic Antidepressants and Specific Serotonin Reuptake Inhibitors (SSRIs)

The tricyclic antidepressant medications can be effective in low doses for the treatment of depression in neuro-oncology patients. These medications have been most efficacious in our experience for patients who are not confused, are taking a minimum of other medicines and/or who have a prior personal or familial history of major depression. These medications can be selected so that the patient can benefit from their side effects. Thus, for example, sinequan is highly antihistaminic and can increase appetite for patients who are not eating well; amitriptyline is highly anticholinergic and sedating, and can be especially useful for the treatment of depressed patients with insomnia; finally, nortriptyline and desipramine have few side-effects and should be chosen for patients in whom sedation and other side effects should be minimized so as to make treatment most tolerable for the patient.

The use of the SSRIs (fluoxetine, paroxetine, and sertraline) is becoming more common in the clinical treatment of mood and anxiety syndromes in patients with CNS tumors. Anecdotal experience suggests that they too are safe and effective in low doses for this population. They are often first-line treatments in patients with cardiac histories or in whom sedation, weight gain, and anticholinergic side effects are undesirable. They should be dosed cautiously in patients being treated with certain anticonvulsants (e.g., valproic acid) owing to the possibility of drug interactions. Anticonvulsant levels should be checked frequently to avoid toxicity when patients are taking SSRIs. SSRIs should not be given to patients taking procarbazine.

PSYCHOSOCIAL IMPACT OF CNS TUMORS ON FAMILIES

The families of patients with neuro-oncologic illnesses face many unique stressors related to CNS disease. Feelings of loss and of being overwhelmed and angry are common reactions to neuro-oncologic illnesses. Family members must be prepared for often intense and conflicting emotional responses to the disease and treatment course. Anger at the patient for behavior that he/she cannot control is common and is often followed by feelings of guilt. Ambivalence about providing high levels of care while watching one's loved ones suffer with poor quality of life can be difficult to endure. It is not unusual for family members to experience the painful wish that the disease would simply run its course and take the life of the patient. Spouses often take on the complete care of the patient to avoid exposing others to the stark realities of the illness (motivated by the desire to protect the patient's waning dignity). The disease can have a terribly isolating effect on caregivers.

The role and relationship changes that characterize neuro-oncologic illnesses tend to be more profound than those seen in other forms of cancer. The rapid deterioration into a completely dependent position requires that family members perform complete, intimate, physical care for the patient. The spouse in particular, is called upon to adopt a parental-like role assuming responsibility for the total well-being of the patient.

The mode of communication between the patient and family changes dramatically as a result of brain tumors or metastases. Family members and patients must often adopt the most rudimentary and basic form of interaction, in which family members must rely heavily upon nonverbal cues as to what the patient's needs are. This is often an exhausting and frustrating process for both parties. With limited communication, family members often find themselves struggling to discern the patient's thoughts and feelings from the effects of the disease or treatments. The dementia and withdrawal caused by destruction of the brain is often interpreted by family members as an exclusively psychological event signaling depression and the loss of the desire to "fight the illness." Additionally, patients' behaviors caused by organic factors can also be viewed as volitional by family members. Complicating this process is the fact that, as in the case of most organic mental phenomena, the degree of impairment or withdrawal can tend to wax and wane. Thus, the patient may have moments of extraordinary clarity and normality. Many family members are comforted if they can come to realize that these moments are not necessarily characteristic of the ongoing insight and understanding that the patient possesses. Another possibility that offers solace to some distressed families is that the effects of the illness may be more distressing when viewed from "the outside" by an observer with intact cognitive ability than as it is experienced by the patient.

In recognition of the unique stressors faced by spouses of brain tumor patients, the neuro-oncology treatment team at Memorial Hospital organized a psychoeducational support program for the spouses of brain tumor patients. Horowitz, Passik, and Malkin describe the format, dynamics, goals, and outcome of this group experience (31).

PSYCHOSOCIAL IMPACT OF NEURO-ONCOLOGIC ILLNESSES ON STAFF

The nursing and medical care of patients with neuro-oncologic illnesses is demanding, exhausting, and complex. Grief has a tremendous impact upon staff members in a cancer hospital generally; it is even more problematic in a neuro-oncology service for many rea-

sons. Patients with primary cancers that are outside of the CNS are often admitted to the neuro-oncology service with CNS complications of their diseases that mark the beginnings of the terminal stages of illness.

Health care providers who work in the neuro-oncology setting often face frequent and multiple losses of their patients. As in the treatment of family members, the psycho-oncologist must know how to detect pathological grief reactions (32) in staff members. Manifestation in staff members of a high degree of somatic distress, a preoccupation with images of a recently deceased patient, guilt about their actions during the care of the patient, or hostile reactions to the actions of other staff, or even adoption of traits of the deceased patient, are signs of pathologic reaction which should result in referral for individual counseling.

Other typical problems are focused on the ethical dilemmas encountered in neuro-oncology, such as those surrounding "Do Not Resuscitate" (DNR) status. Patients whose disease affects their ability to communicate may not have had the opportunity to indicate their wishes regarding resuscitation and other aspects of treatment. Family members and staff can become quite divided about the patient's wishes. Staff members knowing more about the typical course of many neuro-oncologic illnesses (and wanting to avoid futile efforts to revive a dying patient) can pressure families to make patients DNR. The resulting breach between family and staff can be stressful as it creates hostility between them. Another common dilemma regards refusal of treatment. Often it is unclear whether a patient would have wanted to have a potentially terminal complication of their illness treated (e.g., a pneumonia) while they are slowly dying of a brain tumor or metastasis. These issues can be very divisive for staff.

There are various ways in which the stresses of working on a neuro-oncology service can be mitigated. For nurses, rotation of demanding patients or difficult families is essential. Physicians in training can benefit from the close supervision by more senior doctors and briefer rotations (usually reserved for latter stages of training) on neuro-oncology services. Several years ago at Memorial Sloan-Kettering, in recognition of the high level of stress encountered on neuro-oncology, a weekly multidisciplinary staff support group was started on the neuro-oncology service. Horowitz and colleagues (33) described the format and approach of this successful staff intervention. The group has been enormously successful in generating a sense of unity among the staff working in this high-pressure environment.

FUTURE DIRECTIONS: QUALITY OF LIFE RESEARCH IN CNS CANCERS

To date there has been a paucity of research focusing on quality of life in patients with primary and metastatic cancers of the CNS. As the prevalence of all of these problems continues to rise, interest in the quality of life of these patients will hopefully expand. More recent work (34) has been completed on the validation of a brain tumor subscale for the Functional Assessment of Cancer Therapy [FACT: Cella et al. (35)] that has demonstrated sound psychometric qualities. Preliminary findings on a series of 50 patients with primary brain tumors has suggested that quality of life is worse for female patients and for those who are divorced, have bilateral tumor involvement, have received chemotherapy, and have a poor performance status (36). Further studies with larger samples are needed to help identify patients at risk for poor quality of life and to describe the problems that arise for them. This will allow for improved palliative care for these patients.

CONCLUSION

The psychiatric and psychosocial issues in neuro-oncology are highly complex. Working in this area as a mental health professional can be difficult but it is also consistently important, interesting, and enriching. The nature of the issues faced in neuro-oncology test the clinician's flexibility and understanding of organic and psychological disorders and require that the focus of treatment go beyond patients to include those around them.

REFERENCES

1. Levin VA, Gutin PH, Leibel S. Neoplasms of the central nervous system. In: Devita VT, Hellman S, Rosenberg SA, eds. *Cancer: Principles and Practice of Oncology.* 4th ed. Philadelphia: JB Lippincott; 1993.
2. DeAngelis LM. Management of brain metastases. *Cancer Invest.* 1994; 12 (2):156–165.
3. Posner JB. *Neurologic Complications of Cancer.* Philadelphia: FA Davis; 1995.
4. Posner JB, Chernik NL. Intracranial metastases from systemic cancer. *Adv Neurol.* 1978; 19: 575–587.
5. Cairncross JG, Kim JH, Posner JB. Radiation therapy of brain metastases. *Ann Neurol.* 7:529–534.
6. Delattre J-Y, Krol G, Thaler HT, et al. Distribution of brain metastases. *Arch Neurol.* 1988; 45:741–744.
7. American Cancer Society: *Cancer Facts and Figures.* Atlanta, GA: American Cancer Society; 1997.
8. Mahaley MS, Mettlin C, Natarajan N, et al. National survey of patterns of care for brain tumor patients. *J Neurosurg.* 1989; 71(6):826–836.
9. DeAngelis LM, Yahalom J, Thaler HT, et al. Combined modality therapy for primary CNS lymphoma. *J Clin Oncol.* 1992; 10(4):636–643.
10. Shapiro WR. Therapy of adult malignant brain tumors: What have the clinical trials taught us? *Semin Oncol.* 1986; 13(1):38–45.
11. Nelson DF, Urtasun RC, Saunders WM, et al. Recent and current investigations of radiation therapy of malignant gliomas. *Semin Oncol.* 1986; 13(1):46–55.
12. Loeffler JS, Alexander E, Shea WM, et al. Radiosurgery as part of the initial management of patients with malignant gliomas. *J Clin Oncol.* 1992; 10(9):1379–1385.
13. Fontanesi J, Clark WC, Weir A, et al. Interstitial iodine 125 and concomitant cisplatin followed by hyperfractionated external beam irradiation for malignant supratentorial glioma. *Am J Clin Oncol.* 1993; 16(5):412–417.
14. Scharfen CO, Sneed PK, Wara WM, et al. High activity iodine 125 interstitial implant for gliomas. *Int J Radiat Oncol Biol Phys.* 1992; 24(1):583–591.
15. Brain Tumor Collaborative Group. *Semin Oncol.* Brain Tumors. 1986; 13(1).
16. Inamura T, Nomura T, Bartus RT, Black. Intracarotid infusion of RMP-7, a bradykinin analog: a method for selective drug delivery to brain tumors. *J Neurosurg.* 1994; 81:752–758.
17. Rosner D, Nemoto T, Lane WW. Chemotherapy induces regression of brain metastases in breast carcinoma. *Cancer.* 1986; 58:832–839.
18. Adler JR, Cox RS, Kaplan I, et al. Stereotactic radiosurgical treatment of brain metastases. *J Neurosurg.* 1992; 76:444–449.
19. Posner JB: Surgery for metastases to the brain [editorial]. *N Engl J Med.* 1990; 322:544–545.
20. DeAngelis LM, Delattre J-Y, Posner JB. Radiation-induced dementia in patients cured of brain metastases. *Neurology.* 1989; 39:789–796.
21. Steifel FC, Breitbart WS, Holland JC. Corticosteroids in cancer: neuropsychiatric complications. *Cancer Invest.* 1989; 7:479–491.
22. Breitbart WS, Steifel FC, Kornblith A, et al. Neuropsychiatric disturbance in cancer patients with epidural spinal cord compression receiving high dose corticosterids: a prospective comparison study. *Psycho-Oncology.* 1993; 2: 233–245.
23. Wolkowitz OM, Reus VI, Weingartner H, et al. Cognitive effects of corticosteroids. *Am J Psychol.* 1990; 147:1297–1303.
24. Boston Collaborative Drug Surveillance Program. Acute adverse reactions to prednisone in relation to dosage. *Clin Pharm Ther.* 1972; 13:694–698.
25. Paillas JE, Pellet W. Brain metastases. In: Vinken PJ, Bruyn GW, eds. *Handbook of Clinical Neurology,* vol 18. New York: Elsevier; 1975.
26. Holland JCB. Psychological aspects of cancer. In: Holland JF, Frei E, eds. *Cancer Medicine.* Philadelphia: Lea and Febiger; 1996.
27. Strohl RA. Review of Wegman JA: CNS tumors: Supportive management of the patient and family. *Oncology.* 1991; 11:109–113.
28. Cassem NH. The dying patient. In: Hackett TP, Cassem NH, eds. *Massachusetts General Handbook of General Hospital Psychiatry.* Littleton, MA: PSG Publishing; 1987.

29. Breitbart WS, Passik SD. Psychiatric aspects of palliative care. In: Doyle D, Hanks GWC, Macdonald I, eds. *Oxford Textbook of Palliative Medicine*. New York: Oxford University Press; 1993.

30. Weitzner MA, Meyers CA, Valentine AD. Methylphenidate in the treatment of neurobehavioral slowing associated with cancer and cancer treatment. *J Neuropsychiatry*. 1995; 7:347–350.

31. Horowitz SA, Passik SD, Malkin MG. "In sickness and in health": A group intervention for spouses caring for patients with brain tumors. *J Psychosoc Oncol*. 1996; 14:43–56.

32. Chochinov HM. Management of grief in the cancer setting. In: Breitbart WS, Holland JCB, eds. *Psychiatric Aspects of Symptom Management in Cancer Patients*. Littleton, MA: PSG Publishing; 1992.

33. Horowitz SA, Passik SD, Brish M, Breitbart WS. A group intervention for staff on a neuro-oncology service. *Psycho-Oncology*. 1994; 3:329–332.

34. Weitzner MA, Meyers CA, Gelke CK, et al. The Functional Assessment of Cancer Therapy (FACT) scale: development of a brain subscale and revalidation of the general version (FACT-G) in patients with primary brain tumors. *Cancer*. 1995; 75:1151–1161.

35. Cella DF, Tulsky DS, Gray G, et al. The functional assessment of cancer therapy scale: development and validation of the general measure. *J Clin Oncol*. 1993; 11:570–579.

36. Weitzner MA, Meyers CA, Byrne K. Psychosocial functioning and quality of life in patients with primary brain tumors. *J Neurosurg*. 1996; 84: 29–34.

26

Head and Neck Cancer

ALYSON B. MOADEL, JAMIE S. OSTROFF, AND
STIMSON P. SCHANTZ

Head and neck cancer most commonly refers to cancers of the oral cavity, pharynx, and larynx. In the United States, there are approximately 41,000 new annual cases of head and neck cancer, the majority of which are men over the age of 50 (1). Overall, 52% of head and neck cancer patients survive five years after diagnosis. Among patients who are diagnosed with local or regionally advanced disease (stage III or IV), tumor recurrence poses the greatest threat to long-term survival (2). Etiology is strongly linked to environmental pathogens, with major risk factors being tobacco and alcohol use (3). As a consequence of their smoking and drinking history, the disease course of many head and neck cancer patients often includes additional second primary cancers typically diagnosed in tobacco-exposed organs (e.g. lung, esophagus, bladder, kidney) (4).

Currently, the standard treatment for local head and neck cancer consists of surgery and/or radiotherapy. Chemotherapy is typically included in the case of laryngeal cancer and recurrent or metastatic disease (5). Advances in nonsurgical treatment strategies and reconstructive surgical techniques have greatly reduced treatment-related physical disfigurement and dysfunction. For example, organ preservation protocols have enabled many patients with laryngeal cancer to maintain their larynx, and hence their speech (6,7). Similarly, the use of cutaneous, myocutaneous, and microvascular free flap reconstructive techniques has improved cosmetic rehabilitation (8). A common course of treatment may consist of repeated surgical resections and radiation therapy protocols, followed by reconstructive surgery and/or physical rehabilitation. Owing to the risk of recurrence, second primary cancers, and treatment-related morbidity, frequent medical follow-up examinations are required.

In this chapter, we will highlight four main topics pertinent to the psychological care of the patient with head and neck cancer. First, we will describe patterns of psychosocial impairment among head and neck cancer patients throughout the course of illness. Second, we will describe the factors that affect psychosocial adjustment in this patient population. Third, specific strategies and interventions in the rehabilitation of the head and neck cancer patient will be discussed. Finally, we will address the stresses of staff working with head and neck cancer patients and offer recommendations in how best to cope with these stresses.

PSYCHOSOCIAL ADJUSTMENT

Overview

At various points in the course of their illness and treatment, head and neck cancer patients are likely to experience and exhibit strong emotional and social responses. As attempts to adapt to the stress of cancer and treatment, these reactions are normal at certain levels. However, some patients will experience extreme reactions that not only cause the patient and his or her family discomfort and distress but can interfere with the patient's cooperation with his medical care as well. The specific type and range of responses head and neck cancer patients experience at each point in their illness are described below.

The psychosocial challenges to the head and neck cancer patient begin at diagnosis. Like all patients faced with a diagnosis of cancer, they are confronted with the fears of death, loss, and pain (9–11). In response, most patients will experience shock, numbness, or overt distress. In others, the crisis of diagnosis, compounded by the anticipation of the disfiguring and disabling treatments that lie ahead, can trigger a severe emotional reaction. Such an intense grief reaction may manifest in regressive behavior, depression, and suicidal ideation for which intensive psychological intervention is needed. Concomitant with the patient's emotional adjustment to diagnosis, a pattern of social response may become established. For example, some patients may begin to retreat socially, and become withdrawn and noninteractive. Others, exhibiting greater dependency needs, may place excessive emotional and physical demands on family and medical staff (e.g., requesting nursing assistance frequently). At each stage of the illness, psychological and social adjustment affect each other as well as the patient's ability to participate in the demands of their recovery.

The period between initial diagnosis and treatment is often wrought with feelings of anxiety, sadness, and despair associated with the anticipated loss of valued physical attributes and functions. As patients prepare for surgery, fear and anxiety are typically heightened. In a significant proportion of hospitalized head and neck patients, psychiatric levels of reactive depression and anxiety have been reported with adjustment disorders diagnosed in as high as 36% to 50% of patients (12,13). Compared to other cancer sites, head and neck cancer patients have also been found to be at increased risk for suicide (14–17). The numerous factors that contribute to this increased risk, including personality, treatment sequelae, and alcoholism, will be discussed in detail in the subsequent section.

During the postsurgical hospitalization period, a number of psychiatric issues may arise. For example, alcohol withdrawal, metabolic instability, and other medical complications can lead to delirium and dementia (18,19). There are several psychiatric and behavioral symptoms associated with these organic mental disorders, including disturbances in memory, thinking, judgment, and orientation. In addition, poor response to treatment, or terminal stage disease, presents issues related to symptom control (e.g., pain), deterioration of function, anticipatory grieving, and fears about dying. The prevalence of depression is higher among cancer patients with advanced disease, with estimates between 23% and 58% (20). In response to severe physical and psychological morbidity, the dying head and neck cancer patient may become noncompliant with palliative treatment, become irritable and angry, and alienate supportive family, friends, and hospital staff.

For those successfully treated and released from the hospital, high levels of distress are often replaced by a feeling of relief associated with believing that one may be cured from a life-threatening condition (21). Over time, the majority of head and neck cancer patients adjust well both psychologically and socially to having been treated for head and neck cancer. In one large-scale study into the quality of life of 1533 long-term head and neck cancer survivors, three-quarters of patients reported having returned to their normal (pre-morbid) lifestyle within a year after treatment (22). For some patients, however, psychosocial sequelae related to the illness and its treatment may present months or even years after treatment has ended (23,24). In one study, nearly one-third of patients continued to experience psychiatric levels of distress following treatment (25). Negative changes in self-image, including loss of self-esteem and self-perceptions of diminished attractiveness, have been reported following treatment (26).

This vulnerable subgroup of head and neck cancer patients tend to have particular difficulties in the area of social and interpersonal adjustment (10,11,23,27–29). Social withdrawal and avoidance are commonly observed, although the range of response is quite variable. While many patients reduce such activities as eating in restaurants, visiting with friends and relatives, and participating in social functions (e.g., church, clubs), others resign themselves to a solely reclusive life. Similarly, changes in family relationships and roles may result in interpersonal conflict or distancing in the home. In particular, among patients and their significant others, sexual activity and satisfaction are often disrupted (24,30). Occupational functioning can become limited in some patients following treatment, making reemployment difficult (28). Various problems encountered by patients include a loss of previous employment, reduced opportunities for new employment, and work-place discrimination (11,26).

FACTORS AFFECTING PSYCHOSOCIAL ADJUSTMENT

A number of factors influence the psychosocial adjustment of patients treated for head and neck cancer (see Table 26.1). In particular, physical disfigurement and

TABLE 26.1. *Factors Associated with Positive Adaptation to Head and Neck Surgery*

1. Preoperative teaching
2. Postoperative rehabilitation
3. Strong social support
4. Absence of postoperative radiation therapy
5. Absence of a high level of physical symptoms (e.g., pain, emesis, fatigue)
6. Absence of persistent major speech defects
7. Absence of definite premorbid character disorder
8. Absence of substance abuse
9. Absence of organic mental disorder
10. Early postoperative psychiatric treatment of individuals at risk

Source: Adapted from Bronheim H, Strain JJ, Biller HF. Psychiatric aspects of head and neck surgery. Part I: New surgical techniques and psychiatric consequences. *Gen Hosp Psychiatry*. 1991; 13:165–176.

dysfunction, tobacco/alcohol use, personality and social factors are important to understanding psychosocial responses in these patients. These four factors are examined individually in relation to their unique impact on adaptation.

Physical Disfigurement and Dysfunction

In addition to the threat to life, a diagnosis of head and neck cancer carries with it unique significance related to the site of the disease. Given that the head and neck area plays a critical role in identity and self-expression, head and neck cancer can impose a direct challenge to a patient's sense of self. Not surprisingly, the majority of these patients view cancer of the head and neck as more threatening than cancer to any other part of the body (31). As the cancer and its treatment affect visible aspects of the patient's head and face, self-image and self-esteem often suffer as well. These psychological effects are best understood in the context of the vast physical effects these patients can experience. Surgical disfigurement of the face often results from removal of significant portions of bony structure and soft tissue, including for example, the mandible, eye, ear, tongue, or larynx. As such, surgery, radiotherapy, and chemotherapy can lead to or exacerbate impairment of highly valued physical functions such as sight, hearing, speech, taste, smell, breathing, and eating. In addition, a host of physical symptoms, such as dry mouth, bleeding, coughing, sensitivity to heat and cold, hoarseness, nasal discharge, belching, fatigue, and pain, may become a persistent hindrance to quality of life after treatment (32–34).

Head and neck cancer patients most at risk for psychological and social problems are those with the greatest levels of disfigurement (i.e., facial deformity), dysfunction (i.e., impairment in speech, swallowing, eating), and physical symptoms (i.e., pain, fatigue) (10,24,29,35–37). Given the nature and site of these physical sequelae, issues around *body image* alteration are at the center of the patient's psychological response and rehabilitation (38). The degrees of body image alteration related to various structural and functional losses following head and neck surgery are delineated in Table 26.2. The nurse evaluations from which this table was derived indicate that the psychological impact of operative treatment for head and neck cancer is twofold: severity of the disfigurement and severity of the associated dysfunction each contribute to body image disturbance independently (38). This is illustrated by the patient who, following total laryngectomy, must adjust to the disfiguring effects of a stoma as well as the loss of speech prior to reconstruction and rehabilitation.

Redefining one's self-concept following disfigurement to the head and neck area is a formidable task and requires a high degree of coping resources. At first, some patients may experience great difficulty in acknowledging and accepting their physical appearance and may engage in nonadaptive behavior, including avoiding looking in mirrors or touching the postoperative site. Such behavior is likely to reinforce negative self-evaluations, including disgust and shame, which in turn may increase emotional distress and social discomfort (24). Patients who express strong feelings of unattractiveness are most likely to withdraw from social activity and interaction and avoid intimate sexual contact (39).

In addition to disfigurement, the reduced ability to perform normal activities of daily living, such as speaking, eating, or swallowing, provides one of the greatest sources of distress among head and neck cancer patients. Even six months following total laryngectomy, one study found that clinician-rated diet and understandability of speech did not return to normal for 40% of patients, and eating in public was an avoided activity among 20% of patients (40).

Communication difficulties are a significant barrier to the psychosocial adjustment of the head and neck cancer patient. Impairment or loss of speech is one of the most pervasive sequelae of treatment affecting these patients. Surgical resection of many parts of the head and neck area including the larynx, oral cavity (e.g., tongue, floor of mouth, mandible, hard/soft palate), or hypoglossal nerve can lead to disrupted speech production (41,42). Although numerous rehabilitative methods are used to restore verbal communication, including use of an electrolarynx, esophageal speech, tracheo-esophageal punctures, or maxillofacial prostheses, abnormal voice quality, reduced speech intelligibility, and impaired articulation are commonly reported. The implications of "losing one's voice" for self-esteem and identity are obvious and may extend into many domains of adjustment. For example, maxillectomy patients who had not acquired optimal speech function were more apt to experience greater psychological distress, employment difficulties, and diminished family, social, and sexual functioning (43).

The enjoyment of eating is particularly vulnerable to the effects of disease and treatment. Removal of oral tissue, oral pain, and xerostomia can result in impaired ability to taste, smell, chew, or swallow. For some, the level of impairment may be so severe as to preclude typical eating behavior, in which case either liquid nutritional supplements or, in most severe cases, a feeding tube may be substituted. Persistent drooling and chewing difficulties may interfere not only with

TABLE 26.2. *Clinical Derivation of Nursing Diagnoses Based on the Disfigurement/Dysfunction Scale*

Surgical Procedure	Degree of Body Image Alteration	Related to
LARYNGECTOMY		
Hemilaryngectomy	None	–
Supraglottic	Moderate	Difficulty swallowing
Total	Severe	Aphonia
	Moderate	Stoma
	Minor	Decreased smell
NECK DISSECTION		
Radical	Minor	Neck contour
Bilateral radical	Moderate	Neck contour
Modified	None	–
Supraomohyoid	None	–
PAROTIDECTOMY		
Facial nerve sacrifice	Minor	Facial droop (unilateral)
GLOSSECTOMY		
Base of tongue	Moderate	Speech impairment and/or difficulty swallowing
Partial	Moderate	
Hemiglossectomy		
Subtotal	Moderate	Speech impairment and/or
	Moderate	difficulty swallowing,
	Moderate	salivary drooling,
	Moderate	impaired mastication
MAXILLECTOMY		
Partial	None	–
Radical	None	–
Radical and orbital exenteration	Severe	Facial defect
	Moderate	Unilateral vision
MANDIBULECTOMY		
Marginal	None	–
Segmental + RND*	Severe	Facial contour
	Moderate	Impaired mastication
	Moderate	Salivary drooling
Anterior Partial	Severe	Facial contour
	Moderate	Difficulty swallowing
	Moderate	Impaired mastication
	Moderate	Speech impairment
Hemimandibulectomy + RND*	Moderate	Facial contour
	Moderate	Impaired mastication
Mandibulotomy	Moderate	Difficulty swallowing
	Moderate	Impaired mastication

Source: Reprinted with permission from Dropkin MJ. Coping with disfigurement and dysfunction after head and neck cancer surgery: a conceptual framework. *Sem Oncol Nurs*. 1989; 5:213–219.
*RND, radical neck dissection.

eating pleasure but with social behavior as well. These patients may feel ashamed and uncomfortable in public places, leading them to withdraw socially. Poor diet and malnutrition, common signs of eating difficulties, have been associated with depression among head and neck cancer patients (37).

Psychological care providers should be aware of a number of additional physical issues that can contribute to psychosocial distress in this patient population. For example, radiation therapy disrupts thyroid function in 30%–40% of patients (2), a condition that can lead to hormonally induced symptoms of depression (44). Similarly, with inadequate pain control, patients may become depressed, irritable or even suicidal (44). Treatments that disrupt normal breathing, such as tracheotomies, neck dissections, or resections of the pharynx, may be particularly anxiety-provoking for patients. Constantly faced with the task of airway care and prevention of obstruction, patients may become obsessively concerned about suffocation and death. Other wound management problems have also been known to raise fears in patients. For example, one middle-aged male patient who experienced excessive wound bleeding expressed fears of being alone and dying by hemorrhage (39).

Tobacco/Alcohol Use

The majority of head and neck cancer patients have a history of heavy tobacco and alcohol use (3). These health risk behaviors can impact upon psychosocial adjustment following cancer diagnosis and treatment in a number of ways. First, patients may engage in self-blame and guilt related to their disease and the suffering it may cause loved ones. Second, acting as ineffectual coping behaviors, these addictions themselves may result in increased psychosocial problems. That is, as the patient turns to cigarettes and alcohol to cope with illness-related concerns, continued health risk behavior serves to further compound the patient's fears, self-blame, and guilt. In addition, interpersonal conflict at home centering around the patient's smoking and alcohol use often arises due to the resentment of family members that the patient is not taking better care of his or her health. Third, patients are confronted with strong incentives to quitting smoking/drinking, including physicians' advice to quit, hospital restrictions, and physical discomfort. While these barriers may provide the added motivation needed for those who have been contemplating and preparing to change their smoking and drinking habits, they may raise distress in others who feel forced into abstaining prior to being ready to make that commitment. Lacking alternative coping resources, patients may experience great anxiety related to abstaining from a behavior that has been used for coping with stress, and may be prone to relapse into smoking and drinking again. Fourth, tobacco and alcohol withdrawal may lead to acute physical and emotional symptoms. For example, among highly nicotine- and alcohol-dependent patients, forced abstinence during hospitalization can result in a variety of withdrawal symptoms including irritability, anger, cravings, anxiety, depression, insomnia, and delirium (19,45). These patients are also at risk for post-surgical complications related to severe alcohol withdrawal such as delirium tremens and Wernicke's encephalitis (46). Fifth, the existence of co-morbid alcohol- and tobacco-related conditions such as liver damage, heart disease, diabetes, or chronic obstructive pulmonary disease (2,47,48) provides additional health concerns and potential medical complications that further tax the patient's psychological coping resources. As a result, these patients are particular vulnerable to psychiatric problems including depression. Finally, approximately one-third of patients will continue to smoke and drink excessively following diagnosis and treatment (49–52). Despite the fact that these patients are generally characterized by early-stage disease, their continued health risk behaviors place them at risk for greater treatment-related morbidity, increased risk of recurrence, and mortality.

Personality

Premorbid personality plays a critical role in the psychosocial response and rehabilitation to medical illness and treatment. Given that life-style patterns are predisposing factors in head and neck cancer, these patients tend to share certain personality traits that are influential to their adjustment. Concomitant with a history of heavy tobacco and alcohol use, many head and neck cancer patients tend to have poorly developed coping skills (53). As a result they often face diagnosis with limited psychological, social, physical, and financial resources. Personality disorders have been diagnosed in 18% of head and neck cancer patients (13). With the added stress of cancer, these maladaptive personality traits become more pronounced. For example, patients with dependent personalities will often demand care far beyond their objective needs, while avoidant personality types are likely to exhibit self-neglect and noncompliance. Often, these patients are experienced as angry, covertly hostile, and manipulative among hospital staff (48). As can be seen, these personality-based coping responses can result in a number of management problems, adjustment difficulties, and obstacles to optimal recovery.

Social Factors

With oral expression and one's physical integrity severely altered, immense psychosocial resources are called upon in these patients. Successful adaptation following head and neck cancer depends as much on the patient's coping resources as it does on the response of his or her social network. Positive reassurance and acceptance toward the patient by immediate family and friends is important to the patient's ultimate acceptance of the physical sequelae of treatment (31,54). Patients' sexual adjustment is particularly vulnerable to the reactions of others. Spouses' responses to the patient's disfigurement have a profound impact on the return to sexual intimacy and expression. For example, kissing and eye-gazing are sometimes avoided by partners unable to look past the mutilative consequences of facial surgery.

Casual social reactions can also affect the head and neck cancer patient's psychosocial adjustment. In a culture where appearance and verbal expression are highly valued aspects of attractiveness and popularity, head and neck cancer and its treatment can profoundly impact the return to one's social role. Even among those patients who are well-adapted to their physical changes, social reintegration can be hampered by social stigma and avoidance (11). For example, a return to one's occupational role may be hindered by unsupportive responses at the work place including a changed work atmosphere, a demotion, and a reduction in salary (11,26). Similarly, other less obvious physical sequelae, such as subtle changes in facial muscle movement and facial expression, can interfere with important social cues. In such cases, patients may experience confusing and frustrating social interchanges as a result of being misunderstood.

REHABILITATION

Through all stages of the disease course, including diagnosis, treatment, recovery, or impending death, the goal of psychological rehabilitation is to maximize the patient's physical, psychological, and social resources and functioning. In order to do so, rehabilitation of the head and neck patient involves two primary strategies: *(1)* promotion of psychosocial adaptation following treatment; and *(2)* reducing health risk behaviors (i.e., tobacco and alcohol use).

Promoting Psychosocial Adjustment

Rehabilitation is guided by the knowledge that physical, psychological, and social adaptation are integrally related. Most patients who have difficulties in one area experience difficulties in one or both of the other areas as well. Given the multiple factors associated with psychosocial adaptation, a thorough *pretreatment* psychosocial evaluation is an essential first step in ensuring optimal posttreatment rehabilitation. This evaluation should obtain information on the patient's medical history, psychiatric history, personality, life-style, health risk behaviors, social support network, and coping resources. The patient's level of knowledge about and preparation for treatment should also be assessed at this time, as such information can mitigate feelings of shock and loss following treatment (11,31). In addition, one study found that patients who were better informed about their illness and its treatment were more apt to have spouses who understood their illness-related attitudes and experiences better (55). This awareness may be the stepping stone toward improving family support and reintegration following treatment.

Similar to other tumor sites, the focus of psychological rehabilitation is physical and psychiatric symptom control. Both supportive psychotherapy and pharmacotherapy are useful treatments of anxiety, depression, delirium, and pain, common complications of advanced disease (56). Specific pharmacologic treatments include antidepressants, anxiolytics, opioid analgesics for pain, and correction of underlying physiological causes of delirium (56). Assessment of suicide ideation is critical in this population, and should be addressed with crisis intervention and treatment of psychiatric symptomatology. Pretreatment psychological intervention may be needed to manage distress, offer supportive care, reinforce preoperative teaching and preparation, and advise patients on smoking and alcohol cessation.

The immediate postoperative recovery period is a critical time in which to intensify efforts to address initial reactions to cosmetic and functional changes. Pain, intravenous/gastric tubing, head and neck bandaging, nicotine and alcohol withdrawal, and temporary alterations in normal eating, speaking, swallowing, breathing, and seeing, can result in discomfort and heightened anxiety. In response, patients may exhibit avoidance of the surgical site, feelings of dependency, and regressive behaviors. Since self-care behaviors figure prominently in the postoperative care of head and neck cancer, promoting adaptation to physical deficits is an important strategy in the rehabilitation process. Reinforcing self-care practices, such as oral cleansing, wound irrigation, or prosthesis care, allows patients to gain a sense of control in their recovery and begin to accept a new body-image, and may counter nonadaptive coping responses (57).

Following treatment, patients may anticipate surgical reconstruction, permanent prostheses, and speech devices/therapy aimed at reducing the severity of disfigurement and dysfunction. The effectiveness of these interventions, however, is contingent upon the patient's participation in his or her physical rehabilitation. Fortunately, most patients learn and adapt to new ways of communicating and eating (32,54,58). One of the major impediments to physical rehabilitation, however, is depression. Self-neglect, lack of motivation, or noncompliance may signal an underlying depression. Both pharmacologic and psychological interventions can be effective in treating depression in these patients (e.g., 12,59). In addition, patient support groups may promote physical and psychosocial adjustment by providing emotional and instrumental support from similar others, enhancing patients' morale, improving compliance with treatment, and encouraging self-care behavior (60).

When the psychological demands of the initial recovery period remit, concerns about self-image, impaired communication, threatened employment, changing family roles, interpersonal problems, and illness recurrence become the critical focus of intervention (47). Referrals to hospital or community-based support services, such as MSKCC's Post Treatment Resource Program, Lost Cord Society, or Support for People with Oral Head & Neck Cancer, should be offered to all patients and their families. Like patients, family members of head and neck cancer patients are clearly affected by the disease and treatment and many express concerns about changes in family roles and responsibilities (27,36). Family, couples, or individual therapy is effective in helping families address the complex issues they face following head and neck cancer.

Reducing Health Risk Behaviors

Health risk behaviors include those behaviors that affect the patient's disease course, risk of recurrence, and compliance with treatment. For head and neck cancer patients, tobacco and alcohol use are of particular importance. Research shows that continued tobacco and alcohol use among patients diagnosed with tobacco-related malignancies is associated with increased risk of secondary or primary cancers, disease recurrence, complications of surgery, radiation therapy and chemotherapy, and development or exacerbation of other noncancer smoking-related diseases (61–67).

Among head and neck cancer patients, approximately one-third report continued tobacco use following treatment (49,50). Similarly, substance abuse disorders have been diagnosed in 18% of head and neck cancer patients (13). Given the deleterious impact of tobacco and alcohol use on physical, psychological, and social recovery following head and neck cancer treatment, specific intervention should be directed toward smoking and alcohol cessation with these patients. Since many of these patients do not comply with their physician's advice to quit smoking/drinking, psychologists and psychiatrists play an important role in reinforcing physicians' messages.

At Memorial, we have adopted a stepped-care approach (68) to managing symptoms of nicotine dependency and promoting smoking and alcohol cessation and maintenance. This clinical service delivery model emphasizes a facilitative (tobacco/alcohol-free) environment, and psychoeducational treatment to achieve initial cessation and sustained abstinence. Intervention should begin early, optimally at diagnosis, with strategies based on a thorough tobacco and alcohol history and motivation to quit. Tailoring interventions to the patient's illness-related concerns and readiness to change will facilitate health behavior change (69). In addition, there are a number of specific ways to assist patients in quitting. Advising patients to quit, providing education about the deleterious effects of continued smoking/drinking on the course of their disease and the benefits of quitting, setting a quit date, encouraging family support and involvement, providing written material on smoking/drinking cessation, offering nicotine replacement, and providing appropriate referrals and follow-up sessions with the patient are intervention strategies that should be included in the rehabilitation of patients who smoke and drink.

STAFF ISSUES

For medical and psychological staff, facial deformity, head and neck dysfunction (e.g. speech impairment, salivary drooling), and malodorous necrotic tissue may trigger uncomfortable feelings and reactions toward the head and neck cancer patient that include pity and repugnance (47). In addition, resentment and anger may develop among staff members towards *difficult* (i.e., demanding or uncooperative) patients. The way in which staff members deal with their feelings can affect the patient's psychosocial adjustment. For example, staff may engage in avoidant behaviors ranging from diverting one's vision away from the patient's disfigurement to minimizing/avoiding interactions with the patient. Staff members play an important role in body image reintegration by encouraging patients to view and care for their postsurgical defects. They also provide a safe base in which patients can begin to practice new socialization skills. However, in order to best provide the modeling and support that facilitate the patient's psychosocial recovery, staff members may need to receive support themselves. Provider-support groups, individual therapy, and supervision may be necessary for staff working with head and neck cancer patients. Through these services a number of important issues can be addressed, including emotional reactions to disfigurement, pain management, enhancing communication, dealing with acting-out behavior, interactions with family members, and grief (70).

The views of one terminal head and neck cancer patient looking back on her experience with the health care system make a poignant statement about the important role health care providers play in the patient's psychosocial rehabilitation:

Reflecting on the course of my disease and its treatment, I have often considered the medical profession's power to affect people's lives. Their caring attitudes sustained me through the most daunting procedures. Clearly, I could not have reached this far without the encouragement of physicians, nurses, secretaries, and technicians who have given me their love and concern.

These professionals entered into a relationship with me, their patient, a relationship that plays a powerful role in the healing partnership. Amidst the pain, agonizing decisions, and changing self-image, the one constancy I had was the bond tying healer and afflicted together . . . Beyond what machines and medicines and procedures can do for the patient, the act of caring remains a powerful weapon in the fight against disease. It is the one thing that medical technology can never replace. When everything is done that can be done, compassion is the only thing that remains . . . It is the irreplaceable gift. (71)

SUMMARY

The goal of this chapter was to provide information that could be used to maximize the patient's, family's and staff's resources in dealing with these issues. Head and neck cancer patients face numerous medical, psychological, and social challenges. In addition to dealing with the trauma of a life-threatening diagnosis, these patients must cope with one of the most daunting of cancer treatments. Despite its often curative results, head and neck surgery can be synonymous with facial disfigurement and physical disability that may profoundly challenge psychosocial functioning. Loss of speech and facial integrity threaten the core of one's identity. Stigmatizing reactions from the social world, substance abuse, and poor coping resources predispose

these patients to a host of psychological and social problems, many of which can be prevented or alleviated with appropriate psychosocial intervention. By understanding the specific issues of these patients, the unique medical and psychosocial challenges they face, and the rehabilitative approaches to these challenges, the goal of improving quality of life can be achieved.

REFERENCES

1. American Cancer Society. *Cancer Facts & Figures—1996*. Atlanta, GA: American Cancer Society; 1996.
2. Vokes EE, Weichselbaum RR, Lippman SM, Hong WK. Head and neck cancer. *N Engl J Med*. 1993; 328:184–194.
3. Maier H, Dietz A, Gewelke U, Heller WD, Weidauer H. Tobacco and alcohol and the risk of head and neck cancer. *Clin Invest*. 1992; 70:320–327.
4. Begg CB, Zhang ZF, Sun M, Herr HW, Schantz SP. Methodology for evaluating incidence of second primary cancers with application to smoking-related cancers from SEER. *Am J Epidemiol*. 1995; 142:653–665.
5. Liggett W, Forastiere AA. Chemotherapy advances in head and neck oncology. *Semin Surg Oncol*. 1995; 11:265–271.
6. Dibb CR, Urba S, Wolf GT. Organ preservation in advanced head and neck cancer. In: Hong WK, Weber RS, eds. *Head and Neck Cancer*. Norwell, MA: Kluwer Academic; 1995: 199–219.
7. Kraus DH, Pfister DG, Harrison LB, et al. Larynx preservation with combined chemotherapy and radiation therapy in advanced hypopharynx cancer. *Otolaryngol Head Neck Surg*. 1994; 111:31–37.
8. Droughton ML, Krech RL. Head and neck cancer resection and reconstruction: from past to present. *Today's OR Nurse*. 1992; Sep 12:25–34.
9. Weisman A, Worden J. The existential plight in cancer: significance of the first 100 days. *Int J Psychiatry*. 1976-77; 7:1–15.
10. Krouse JH, Krouse HJ, Fabian RL. Adaptation to surgery for head and neck cancer. *Laryngoscope*. 1989; 99:789–794.
11. Strauss RP. Psychosocial responses to oral and maxillofacial surgery for head and neck cancer. *J Oral Maxillofac Surg*. 1989; 47:343–348.
12. Breitbart W, Holland JC. Head and neck cancer. In: Holland JC, Rowland JH, eds. *Handbook of Psychooncology: Psychological Care of the Patient with Cancer*. New York: Oxford University Press; 1989: 232–239.
13. Bronheim H, Strain JJ, Biller HF. Psychiatric aspects of head and neck surgery Part I: New surgical techniques and psychiatric consequences. *Gen Hosp Psychiatry*. 1991; 13:165–176.
14. Bolund C. Suicide and cancer: II. Medical and care factors in suicides by cancer patients in Sweden, 1973–1976. *J Psychosoc Oncol*. 1985; 3:31–52.
15. Breitbart W. Identifying patients at risk for, and treatment of major complications of cancer. *Support Care Cancer*. 1995; 3:45–60.
16. Farberow NL, Shneidman ES, Leonard CB. Suicide among general medical and surgical hospital patients

with malignant neoplasms. Medical Bulletin of the Department of Medical Surgery Veterans Administration (Washington). Washington, D.C.: U.S. Veterans Administration; 1963: MB-9, 1–11.

17. Weisman AD. Coping behavior and suicide in cancer. In: Cullen JW, Fox BH, Isom RN, eds. *Cancer: The Behavioral Dimensions*. DHEW publ. No. (NIH) 76-1074. Washington, D.C.: National Cancer Institute; 1976; 3:105–118.

18. Fleishman SB, Lesko LM, Breitbart W. Treatment of organic mental disorders in cancer patients. In: Breitbart W, Holland JC, eds. *Psychiatric Aspects of Symptom Management in Cancer Patients*. Washington, DC: American Psyciatric Press; 1993: 23–47.

19. Lundberg JC, Passik SD. Alcohol and cancer: a review for psychooncologists. [Submitted.]

20. Breitbart W, Bruera E, Chochinov H, Lynch M. Neuropsychiatric syndromes and psychological symptoms in patients with advanced disease. *J Pain Symptom Manage*. 1995; 19:131–141.

21. Kelly R. Post-discharge care: head and neck surgery. Community Outlook 1990; Nov.: 19–22.

22. Argerakis GP. Psychosocial considerations of the post-treatment of head and neck cancer patients. *Maxillofac Prosthodon*. 1990; 34:285–305.

23. Rapoport Y, Kreitler S, Chaitchik S, Algor R, Weissler K. Psychosocial problems in head-and-neck cancer patients and their change with time since diagnosis. *Ann Oncol*. 1993; 4:69–73.

24. Gamba A, Romano M, Grosso IM, et al. Psychosocial adjustment of patients surgically treated for head and neck cancer. *Head Neck*. 1992; 14:218–223.

25. Espie CA, Freedlander E, Campsie LM, Soutar DS, Robertson AG. Psychological distress at follow-up after major surgery for intraoral cancer. *J Psychosom Res*. 1989; 33:441–448.

26. Pruyn JFA, deJong PC, Bosman LJ, et al. Psychosocial aspects of head and neck cancer—a review of the literature. *Clin Otolaryngol*. 1986; 11:469–474.

27. Mah MA, Johnston C. Concerns of family members in which one member has head and neck cancer. *Cancer Nurs*. 1993; 16:382–387.

28. Devins GM, Henderikus JS, Koopmans JP. Psychosocial impact of laryngectomy mediated by perceived stigma and illness intrusiveness. *Can J Psychiatry*. 1994; 39:608–625.

29. Langius A, Bjrvell H, Lind MG. Functional status and coping in patients with oral and pharyngeal cancer before and after surgery. *Head Neck*. 1994; 16:559–568.

30. Metcalfe MC, Fischman SH. Factors affecting the sexuality of patients with head and neck cancer. *Oncol Nurs Forum*. 1985; 12:21–25.

31. van Doorne JM, van Wass MAJ, Bergsma J. Facial disfigurement after cancer resection: a problem with an extra dimension. *J Invest Surg*. 1994; 7:321–326.

32. Ackerstaff AH, Hilgers FJM, Aaronson NK, Balm AJM. Communication, functional disorders and lifestyle changes after total laryngectomy. *Clin Otolaryngol*. 1994; 19:295–300.

33. Jones E, Lund VJ, Howard DJ, Greenberg MP, McCarthy M. Quality of life of patients treated surgically for head and neck cancer. *J Laryngol Otol*. 1992; 106:238–242.

34. Bjordal K, Kaasa S, Mastekaasa A. Quality of life in patients treated for head and neck cancer: a follow-up study 7 to 11 years after radiotherapy. *Int J Radiat Oncol Biol Phys*. 1994; 28:847–856.

35. Bjordal K, Kaasa S. Psychological distress in head and neck cancer patients 7–11 years after curative treatment. *Br J Cancer*. 1995; 71:592–597.

36. Watt-Watson J, Graydon J. Impact of surgery on head and neck cancer patients and their caregivers. *Nurs Clin N Am*. 1995; 30:659–671.

37. Westin T, Jansson A, Zenckert C, Hällström T, Edström S. Mental depression is associated with malnutrition in patients with head and neck cancer. *Arch Otolaryngol Head Neck Surg*. 1988; 114:1449–1453.

38. Dropkin MJ. Coping with disfigurement and dysfunction after head and neck cancer surgery: a conceptual framework. *Semin Oncol Nurs*.1989; 5:213–219.

39. Droughton ML. Head and neck carcinomas. *J Palliative Care*. 1990; 6:43–46.

40. List MA, Ritter-Sterr CA, Baker TM, et al. Longitudinal assessment of quality of life in laryngeal cancer patients. *Head Neck*. 1996; 18:1–10.

41. Fletcher SG, Jacob RF, Kelly DH, et al. Speech Production. *Head Neck*. 1991; 13:8–9.

42. Jacobs JR, Pearson BW, Singer M, Hamaker R, Blum E, Tucker H. Rehabilitation of the patient following total laryngectomy. *Head Neck*. 1991; 13:5–6.

43. Kornblith AB, Zlotolow IM, Gooen J, et al. Quality of life of maxillectomy patients using an obturator prosthesis. *Head Neck*. 1996; 18:323–334.

44. Massie MJ, Gagnon P, Holland JC. Depression and suicide in patients with cancer. *J Pain Symptom Manage*. 1994; 9:325–340.

45. Hughes JR, Higgins ST, Bickel WK. Nicotine withdrawal versus other drug withdrawal syndromes: Similarities and dissimilarities. *Addiction*. 1994; 89:1461–1470.

46. Hybels RL. Medical complications of head and neck surgery. In: Eisele DW, ed. *Complications in Head and Neck Surgery*. St. Louis, MO: Mosby–Year Book; 1993: 49–50.

47. Petrucci RJ, Harwick RD. Role of the psychologist on a radical head and neck surgical service team. *Prof Psychol Res Pract*. 1984; 15:538–543.

48. Fine R, Krell W, Ranella K, Sessions D, Williams M. Respiratory problems and rehabilitation in the head and neck cancer patient. *Head Neck*. 1991; 13:12–13.

49. Ostroff JS, Jacobsen PB, Moadel AB, et al. Prevalence and predictors of continued tobacco use after treatment of patients with head and neck cancer. *Cancer*. 1995; 75:569–576.

50. Ostroff J, Moadel A, Jacobsen P, Schantz S, Abate M, McKiernan J. Smoking cessation following diagnosis of head and neck cancer. Presented at the 20th Annual Meeting of the American Society of Preventive Oncology 1996. [Abstract.]

51. Gritz ER, Carr CR, Rapkin D, et al. Predictors of long-term smoking cessation in head and neck cancer patients. *Cancer Epidemiol Biomarkers Prev*. 1993; 2:261–270.

52. Spitz MR, Fueger JJ, Chamberlain RM, Goepfert H, Newell GR. Cigarette smoking patterns in patients after treatment of upper aerodigestive tract cancers. *J Cancer Educ*. 1990; 5:109–113.

53. Burgess L. Facing the reality of head and neck cancer. *Nurs Standard*. 1994; 8:30–34.

54. Baker CA. Factors associated with rehabilitation in head and neck cancer. *Cancer Nurs.* 1992; 15:395–400.

55. Chaitchik S, Kreitler S, Rapoport Y, Algor R. What do cancer patients' spouses know about the patients? *Cancer Nurs.* 1992; 15:353–362.

56. Breitbart W, Levenson JA, Passik SD. Terminally ill cancer patients. In: Breitbart W, Holland JC, eds. *Psychiatric Aspects of Symptom Management in Cancer Patients.* Washington, DC: American Psychiatric Press; 1993: 173–230.

57. Dropkin MJ. Rehabilitation after disfigurative facial surgery. *Plast Surg Nurs.* 1985; Winter:130–134.

58. Wilson PR, Herman J, Chubon SJ. Eating strategies used by persons with head and neck cancer during and after radiotherapy. *Cancer Nurs.* 1991; 14:98–104.

59. Fernandez F, Adams F. Methylphenidate treatment of patients with head and neck cancer. *Head Neck Surg.* 1986; 8:296–300.

60. Harris LL, Vogtsberger KN, Mattox DE. Group psychotherapy for head and neck cancer patients. *Laryngoscope.* 1985; 95:585–587.

61. Browman GP, Wong G, Hodson I, et al. Influence of cigarette smoking on the efficacy of radiation therapy in head and neck cancer. *N Engl J Med.* 1993; 328: 159–164.

62. Day GL, Blot WJ, Shore RE, et al. Second cancers following oral and pharyngeal cancers: Role of tobacco and alcohol. *J Natl Cancer Inst.* 1994; 86:131–137.

63. Deleyiannis FWB, Thomas DB, Vaughan TL, Davis S. Alcoholism: independent predictor of survival in patients with head and neck cancer. *J Natl Cancer Inst.* 1996; 88:542–549.

64 Eriksen M, Kondo, A. Smoking cessation for cancer patients: rationale and approaches. *Health Educ Res.* 1989; 4:489–494.

65. Hiyama T, Sato T, Yoshino K, Tsukuma H, Hanai A, Fujimoto I. Second primary cancer following laryngeal cancer with special reference to smoking habits. *Jpn J Cancer Res.* 1992; 83:334–339.

66. Johnston WD, Ballantyne AJ. Prognostic effect of tobacco and alcohol use in patients with oral tongue cancer. *Am J Surg.* 1977; 134:444–447.

67. U.S. Department of Health and Human Services. The Health Benefits of Smoking Cessation. U.S. Department of Health and Human Services, Public Health Service, Centers for Disease Control, Center for Chronic Disease Prevention and Health Promotion, Office on Smoking and Health. DHHS Publication No. (CDC) 90-8416; 1990.

68. Orleans CT. Treating nicotine dependence in medical settings: a stepped care model. In: Orleans CT, Slade J, eds. *Nicotine Addiction: Principles and Management.* New York: Oxford Unversity Press; 1993: 145–161.

69. Prochaska JO, DiClemente CC. Stages and processes of self-change of smoking: toward an integrative model of change. *J Consult Clin Psychol.* 1983; 51:390–395.

70. Shapiro PA, Kornfeld DS. Psychiatric aspects of head and neck cancer surgery. *Psychiatric Clin N Am.* 1987; 10:87–100.

71. Theisen A. The irreplaceable gift. *J Am Med Assoc.* 1991; 266:1283.

27

Gastrointestinal Cancer

JÜRG BERNHARD AND CHRISTOPH HÜRNY

Overall, gastrointestinal (GI) tumors are the most frequent malignancies and rank top as cause of cancer mortality in Western countries. A common feature is their nonspecific initial symptoms, frequently overlooked or misinterpreted. Accordingly, patients are often diagnosed with locally advanced disease or distant metastases. This circumstance limits the possibility of curative treatment and has a major impact not just on survival but also on quality of life. Surgery is by far the most important intervention with regard to both curative and palliative intention.

Special problems in psychosocial adjustment are posed when tumors develop in the GI tract. Both patient and family may have to cope with a severe eating disorder, significant weight loss, nausea and vomiting, abdominal discomfort, diarrhea or constipation, as well as other disease-related events that are difficult to manage and often a challenge for multidisciplinary diagnostic procedures and interventions. The psychological characteristics of GI symptoms need further consideration.

Relating a sense of well-being to normal GI function is common. Loss of appetite, inability to taste or eat food, nausea, abdominal discomfort, diarrhea, or constipation result in immediate emotional distress and concern. Care for healthy digestion may be observed in all affluent countries and is reflected in the many over-the-counter nostrums available for appetite control, dyspepsia, and regular elimination. From earliest childhood, eating and GI function are intimately tied to key relationships and psychological state; emotional distress produces eating problems and a range of GI symptoms. These known intimate interrelations require that physician and nurse be particularly attuned to the emotional component of disease and treatment sequelae. For example, anorexia or difficulty in eating may develop from pathophysiological changes related to cancer but also from anxiety about the status of the tumor.

Guidelines by cancer societies and research councils recommend specific dietary modifications to reduce cancer risk, in particular in the GI tract, emphasizing the role of diet in health and cancer. The current enthusiasm for holistic health, focused on diet, spirituality, and exercise, further reflects the concept of personal responsibility in this area. Thus, the social and cultural context in which patients and their families must cope with GI cancer is of high clinical relevance. Besides general preoccupation with the site, the cause of disease is often perceived as being within personal control.

In patients with certain traits, habits and beliefs, body image is intimately related to their self-esteem. They are particularly vulnerable and need special attention in adjusting emotionally to surgical sequelae. For example, those who place high value on a healthy appearance will be especially disturbed by mutilating surgery or by the weight loss that may occur. Those who are meticulous in their concern for normal body function and bowel control may be exceptionally distressed when a colostomy or ileostomy is required.

The psychosocial sequelae of colorectal and pancreatic cancer were investigated decades before psychooncology became an accepted field within the medical community. Arthur Sutherland's pioneering group at the Memorial Sloan-Kettering Cancer Center in the early 1950s evaluated patients with colostomies and their families [1,2]. This is in contrast to the historical development in other cancer sites (e.g., lung cancer), where psychosocial research began with ideas about the cause of cancer, and questions of quality of life evolved later.

A consequent integration of psychosocial concerns into clinical practice and research is of particular importance in those sites with limited and poor survival. Regarding the uncommon primary sites of hepatobiliary, small-bowel and anal cancer, no systematic psychosocial data are currently available.

In several advanced GI malignancies, palliative chemotherapy has been standard practice, but only recently has the goal of best supportive care become an explicit endpoint of clinical trials in these patients (3). A recent shift of emphasis toward a comprehensive view of patients with GI tumors can be observed in the literature and hopefully will contribute to patient care.[1]

CANCER OF THE ESOPHAGUS AND STOMACH

Tumors of these two sites have been studied in relation to eating behavior and cultural habits owing to their particular epidemiology. Cancer of the esophagus shows the greatest variation in geographical distribution of any malignancy, with the highest incidence in China (Lin Xian County), Puerto Rico, and Singapore (6). In contrast, in the United States it is a less common disease, with a much higher incidence in blacks, elderly men (sex ratio about 3:1), and those with history of excessive alcohol intake and smoking.

Until 1988, adenocarcinoma of the stomach was the leading cause of cancer death worldwide (7). In the United States and other Western countries, the incidence has constantly been decreasing for the last sixty years. However, there is evidence, that the percentage of patients with proximal gastric and gastro-esophageal adenocarcinomas (i.e., with poorer prognosis) has substantially increased. In contrast, in Japan, Eastern Europe, and South America, gastric cancer is epidemic. In Japan, stomach cancer is the leading cause of cancer deaths; gastric cancer screening is the most common screening program in this country and has contributed to a decreasing mortality (8). Stomach cancer is more frequent in men (sex ratio about 2:1). The incidence increases after the age of 40 years, reaching a peak in the seventh decade for men and slightly later for women. Various nutritional, environmental, social (low socioeconomic status), and medical risk factors for developing stomach cancer have been identified (7).

Initial Symptoms, Diagnosis, and Surgery

Many patients with esophageal and stomach tumors have a poor prognosis because the tumor has metastasized before diagnosis. They have often experienced vague symptoms of discomfort, fatigue, pain and difficulty in swallowing, and regurgitation, vomiting, or ulcerlike symptoms. Difficulties in passing solid food is the key complaint in patients with esophagus cancer.

1. Parts of this chapter are based on previous reviews by Hürny and Holland (4) and Holland (5) with the authors' approval.

Common in middle age and often ascribed to "stress" or "eating the wrong foods," these symptoms are frequently ignored until they become troublesome. These individuals have usually been treated initially without suspicion of cancer by an antacid, often with symptomatic relief in the early stages. Patients with upper gastrointestinal lesions often have symptoms of both organic and psychosomatic origin (9).

Diagnostic esophagoscopy and gastroscopy for a suspected neoplasm that results in a positive biopsy leads to an exploratory operation. Different types of gastric resection can have a different impact not just on patient's appetite and eating behavior but also on physical and emotional functioning (10,11); quality of life after total gastrectomy has been suggested to be better in patients with a pouch reconstruction compared to those without (11). Especially in the elderly, a usually reduced performance status after gastrectomy needs to be considered (12). Finding evidence of metastatic spread at the time of exploration commonly results in symptoms of anxiety and depression. Patients have to decide about further use of radiotherapy and/or chemotherapy (see Chapters 22 and 23). Finally, premorbid alcohol dependence (risk factor) is often observed in patients with esophagus cancer and preoperative withdrawal may be overlooked in case of anxiety and agitation.

The emotional impact during this period is troublesome for the patient and family because each phase requires major decisions and new adjustments. Patients sometimes feel "numb" in the two to three weeks before surgery, and it is only after surgery that the impact of the diagnosis and treatment begins to be felt and distress experienced (see Chapter 21).

Recovery after Surgery and Rehabilitation

The surgical procedure itself is usually followed by a rapid postoperative recovery. However, the presence of diminished stamina for some time is an unexpected, though common, consequence for many patients. After surgery, patients are apprehensive about recurrence and each minor symptom is viewed as a possible return of the disease. Many minor discomforts and pains are experienced as the patient resumes a normal diet and as the pattern of meals becomes regular. Sometimes these are similar to or the same as symptoms that appeared as the first signs of illness. There are also occasionally persistent postoperative pain syndromes that require careful work-up to rule out cancer recurrence, and efforts to control the chronic pain problems.

During this time patients may need particular reassurance about eating. Sometimes anorexia and nausea reflect fears about being able to eat sufficient amounts to maintain weight (see Chapters 39 and 40). In turn, weight loss triggers fears of recurrence, creating a vicious cycle of concerns. A significant weight loss should prompt both physical (e.g., metabolic abnormalities) and psychological (e.g., depression) examination. Eating habits and taste of food may be different after surgery. In stomach cancer, postsurgery nutrition and body weight are closely associated with quality of life (11). Concerns about "healthy food," not fostering cancer spread, are common. In regard to cause and onset of disease, questions concerning diet and eating habits may express doubts and feelings of guilt about past life style.

As *esophagus* cancer often progresses after surgical resection, effective symptom control and quality of life are the main goals of treatment. Dysphagia, often with pain, is the principal symptom; it can be a burden also for patient's caring partner (alteration in patient's nutrition). A successful treatment, such as with laser therapy and intubation, has a substantial positive impact on patient's quality of life (13,14). Implantation of self-expanding metal stents is a further possibility. They are relatively well tolerated and show promising results (15). With progressive disease in the terminal phase, the burden of this symptom increases again.

Knippenberg and colleagues have suggested astonishingly, that overall, swallowing and eating difficulties play a subordinate role in these patients' perception of their psychological distress and quality of life (16). A frequent major stressor is impaired social functioning (17). Although to some extent related to physical symptoms (e.g., loss of energy secondary to anorexia), it may reflect difficulties in psychosocial adjustment or even indicate symptoms of depression. Major improvements in physical symptoms and functional performance have been reported after curative resection (18). A frequent long-term experience in these patients is a sensation of early fullness (19).

Similarly, in *stomach* cancer, surgery is the only curative treatment and the major approach for palliation. After curative surgery, approximately 50%–70% of these patients survive five years. Despite the possibility of early detection of relapse, combination chemotherapy usually has little impact on survival in advanced disease. However, considering quality of life and survival as combined endpoints, some regimens are definitely superior to others. Thus, patients' quality of life in terms of their subjective experience is a key endpoint both for clinical trials and patient care (20); the conventional focus on performance status and physical symptoms in these patients has to be expanded. Frequently reported symptoms are abdominal pain and lasting fatigue (see Chapters 38 and 41). The latter may be a direct cause of surgery, chemotherapy, or radiotherapy, as well as advanced disease or anorexia, but can also be an indicator of depression and requires psychiatric evaluation. Many of these patients respond well to a psychostimulant.

It is important for the patient whose esophagus or stomach cancer has been resected with curative intention to have access to the surgeon when questions about symptoms arise, in addition to regularly scheduled check-ups during which an explanation about the course and management of distressing symptoms is provided. Usually, this is accomplished with antacids and mild sedation. It may be helpful to have the patient meet another patient who has undergone the same surgery. Enlisting the support of the family is crucial in all phases of treatment in assisting the patient's emotional and social rehabilitation as well as the family's adjustment to rapid and fundamental changes in everyday life. In the case of severe emotional distress, psychiatric consultation is wanted to provide diagnosis and management by psychotherapeutic and pharmacological intervention. Behavioral means are helpful at times for control of nausea and anorexia, particularly when it is related to anxiety (see Chapter 62). Rehabilitation is often fully achieved within a few months, but the return to work may take longer.

Management of advanced disease is outlined in Chapter 37.

CANCER OF THE COLON AND RECTUM

The large bowel is the most common site of GI tumors. In contrast to gastric cancer, colorectal cancer is more frequent in North America, Australia, New Zealand, and parts of northern and western Europe compared to Japan; in the United States, the incidence of colorectal cancer ranks second for men and third for women. There is an almost equal incidence in men and women (21). Two thirds of affected patients are over 50 years of age. Overall, the 5-year survival in both colon and rectal cancer patients has been increased to over 50% of all patients; a key issue is early diagnosis and control of micrometastases. Nutritional risk factors and predisposing diseases (familial polyposis, chronic ulcerative colitis, familial cancer syndrome) for development of colorectal cancer have been identified (21). Cigarette smoking has shown a significant association with the formation of colorectal adenomas and carcinomas (22).

Prevention and Early Detection

Recent advances in biology and molecular genetics of colorectal cancer have an increasing impact on prevention, early detection and treatment of this disease; most colorectal carcinomas arise from preexisting adenomas. Colorectal cancer can be viewed as a model for studying the etiology and pathogenesis of a common tumor and its complex multistage process of carcinogenesis. Its mortality can significantly be reduced by identifying and removing premalignant lesions or diagnosing malignancies at a curable stage.

An illustrative example is familial polyposis, a rare, genetically transmitted (autosomal dominant) disease. It may be recognized in an early, asymptomatic stage by corresponding family history only. In affected individuals, adenomas begin to form usually in adolescence or early adulthood and are very likely to become malignant. Siblings and parents of patients with adenomatous polyps are also at increased risk for colorectal cancer (23). Concerning long-term adaptation, three main stressors have been described in individuals with this disease: fear about future health owing to the high risk for cancer, guilt about transmitting this disease to one's children; and physical disfigurement resulting from prophylactic surgery (24).

It is a common observation that early diagnosis of colorectal cancer is delayed by several months because of the wide prevalence of GI symptoms in the general population (25). These symptoms are even more frequent in the elderly (26). Change in bowel habit, rectal bleeding, anorexia, weight loss, and abdominal pain are the most discriminatory symptoms for colorectal cancer. Education concerning their early report is an important public health issue. As described for rectal bleeding, such education should concentrate on simple factual information to increase symptom awareness and to prompt medical check-up (27).

There are two preventive strategies in colorectal cancer: screening and surveillance (28). The first refers to testing asymptomatic individuals to assess their risk for the development of this disease; the second implies following a population known to be at high risk for this disease. Fecal occult blood test, sigmoidoscopy, and colonoscopy are currently the main screening and diagnostic techniques. The contribution of psychooncology is significant for both screening and surveillance of colorectal cancer (see also Chapter 15).

For the majority of people with a family history of colorectal cancer, especially after the age of 60, the excess risk of this disease is not large (29). In contrast, younger people with this family history are at increased risk and therefore a target population for early screening. For designing intervention strategies it is crucial to understand the facilitators of and barriers to participation in a preventive program; for example, perceived risk for colon cancer was an important but only modestly associated factor with level of interest in genetic testing (30).

Genetic counseling for these individuals requires a long-term follow-up. Continuing support is important for counsellees and their families for both preventive and psychological purposes (e.g., increased anxiety) (31). As has been shown in a controlled trial in women with increased risk for breast cancer, successful genetic counseling is not likely to be effective unless their breast cancer anxieties are also appropriately addressed (32) — from a psychooncological perspective an obvious finding (see also Chapters 17 and 18).

How to approach the targeted individuals for mass screening or check-up, and how to achieve a good compliance, depend on the specific population, test procedure, and setting, and therefore needs systematic evaluation. Cultural factors, including different attitudes and local health care systems, also need to be considered. As pointed out by Arveux and colleagues (33), the active involvement of general practitioners and occupational doctors appeared to be particularly important in southern European countries, and compliance by selective mailings was low, whereas studies in northern European countries indicated a high compliance by the latter approach. "Subjective" barriers, such as personal concerns related to the screening procedure, generally play a key role. A fecal occult blood test to detect early-stage colorectal cancer may be viewed as unpleasant. Changing this response by public intervention is difficult, but health information provided by health care professionals is an effective factor in patients' motivation. Adherence to screening is influenced strongly by the extent to which the corresponding behavior is judged to make sense in everyday life (34).

In contrast to biomedical end economic endpoints, psychological consequences of screening programs are in general much less frequently and systematically assessed. In regard to fecal occult blood test, screening does not seem to have an impact on patients' post-intervention quality of life (35). Patients with false positive results found this procedure as acceptable as those with negative results (36). However, long-term effects of colorectal cancer screening, such as false reassurance in case of negative tests or increased distress in anxious individuals, have not been studied.

Treatment and Rehabilitation

The only curative treatment is surgical resection of the primary tumor and regional mesenteric lymph nodes.

If the tumor involves adjacent (e.g., bladder) or distant organs (e.g., liver), partial or total resection of these organs may be indicated, which additionally impacts on patient's functioning and well-being. Adjuvant and palliative chemotherapy and radiotherapy play an important role in colorectal cancer. A major advance in the treatment of colorectal cancer is the modulation of 5-fluorouracil by leucovorin, which has been shown to have a significant impact on both quality of life and survival, compared to 5-fluorouracil alone in advanced colorectal cancer (37). A randomized comparison in patients with metastatic or locally recurrent disease between combination chemotherapy plus supportive care and supportive care alone revealed an improved survival in the chemotherapy group with no significant impairment in quality of life (38). Similarly, in patients with liver metastases, prolongation of survival by chemotherapy has been reported with no impairment in physical symptoms or anxiety or depression (39).

The psychological problems relate primarily to concerns about the cancer itself and the impact of treatment on bowel function in relation to social and sexual activity. Impotence is observed in a high percentage of men, although those who have anterior resection alone, increasingly used today, generally retain sexual potency. Women undergoing this procedure remain sexually responsive, but many experience significant discomfort during intercourse for considerable periods after surgery, resulting in diminished interest and arousal; interventions for dealing with the sexual sequelae after pelvic surgery are covered in Chapter 42.

In general, a patient's adjustment is closely related to her or his partner's adjustment. The impact on the spouse has been reported to be as strong as on the patient, with a better adjustment for male patients than for females (40). The husbands' adjustment has been reported to be worse than that of wives (40). Regardless, if these findings may be generalized in terms of a gender bias, they are opposing the conventional view of the spouse as primary source of support. Correspondingly, psychosocial interventions should be designed for couples rather than individual patients.

Patients with predisposing conditions are diagnosed with colorectal cancer at younger age and warrant special attention. Those with preceding ulcerative colitis may have more emotional difficulties than patients without prior medical history. This is due to both the added emotional effects of a long-standing chronic illness, often dating to childhood, and the fact that some patients with ulcerative colitis have a history of psychological difficulties. A second group of patients with special psychological needs are those who come from a family with high genetic risk of colon cancer. The spec-

ter of being at high genetic risk and the fact of having seen family members die of the same tumor add to the fear, depression, and distress. Prophylactic colectomy with colostomy or restorative proctocolectomy, respectively, recommended at an early age to prevent colon cancer, is a common decision faced by these individuals. It has been suggested that a majority of patients are satisfied with the latter procedure, despite the presence of postoperative symptoms (41).

Sphincter Saving versus Sacrificing Surgical Procedures

For patients whose bowel is reanastomosed after surgery, in general with a tumor above 5–8 cm from the anal verge, the problems are little different psychologically from those described above for gastric and esophageal cancer. A lower located tumor is in general treated by abdominoperineal resection, which results in a permanent colostomy. As vulnerability to surgical sequelae varies considerably among individuals, and as it is impossible to predict postsurgery outcome, careful presurgery information and evaluation of patient's values (i.e., utilities) in regard to benefits and risks are crucial. The choice of treatment may be influenced strongly by the value assigned to life with a colostomy (42). However, once patients are having a colostomy and getting adjusted to it, they often change their attitude. In addition, the fact of being confronted with life-threatening illness fosters this process.

Sprangers and colleagues (43) comprehensively reviewed 17 studies that compared patient-reported quality-of-life aspects in those with sphincter saving or sacrificing surgical procedures. Both groups were troubled by frequent or irregular bowel movements and diarrhea, which often prevent patients from leaving their home. Those with stoma suffered more from gas and urinary problems (e.g., incontinence), and those without stoma more from constipation. Stoma patients reported higher level of psychological distress (e.g., low self-esteem), including a more negative body image. In general, younger female patients showed more impairment than older male patients; however, there was a broad spectrum in all age groups. Both groups showed impairment in social functioning (e.g., leisure activities) but this was more prevalent in stoma patients; in general, activities at home are less affected by presence of a stoma.

Similarly, sexual functioning was more impaired in both female and male stoma patients. Age, tumor size, location and spread, surgical damage of pelvic nerves, as well as the patient's and the partner's emotional coping, are the most important factors that contribute to the large range of dysfunction reported across all studies. For example, only 2 of 21 (9.5%) men with rectal excision and coloanal anastomosis reported an absence of erection, but 90% had no ejaculation six months after surgery (44); in contrast, 45% of patients with abdominoperineal surgery reported an absence of erection and 50% of ejaculation ($n = 20$, 2 year follow-up) (45). In summary, both patients with sphincter saving and those with sphincter sacrificing procedures had a broad range of substantial impairment in all main domains of quality of life. Patients with no stoma reported a better quality of life but also suffered from physical impairments (e.g., impaired bowel and sexual function).

The stigma of having rectal cancer was assessed in an early study by McDonald and Anderson ($n = 420$) (46). They defined stigma as damaging social influences perceived by the patient. Half the patients reported signs of feeling stigmatized, as reflected in increased self-consciousness (31%), decreased attractiveness (27%), avoidance of other people (14%), and feeling different (11%). More symptoms were seen in younger patients and in those with a colostomy. Feeling stigmatized correlated positively with poorer physical health and greater emotional distress. Although family interactions were retained, social isolation was a result in some cases, suggesting a need for preparation both before and after the operation to diminish this negative influence on interpersonal relationships.

With the introduction in the early 1980s of modified abdominoperineal procedures, less than 15%–20% of patients with colorectal cancer (mainly rectal) undergo permanent colostomy, and this figure will further decrease with improvement of surgical techniques (i.e., ultralow anastomosis). Psychosocial problems of a permanent colostomy are reviewed below in the context of other ostomies, which are less frequently performed but which have similar sequelae.

Patients with Ostomies

It is estimated that 100,000 ostomies per year are performed in the United States, representing a number similar to that of mastectomies (124,000) (47). Approximately half are permanent. By far the most common stoma is colostomy for colorectal cancer. In general, 57% are colostomies, 16% ileostomies, and 27% other enterostomies; of these, less than 2% of the patients have both a colostomy and an urostomy. Table 27.1 outlines the types of ostomies, the diseases with which they are associated, and the sequelae and complications (4).

Once the diagnosis of colorectal cancer is established and resection with possible ostomy is recommended, the patient has to deal with both the threat of life posed by the cancer and the threat to body integrity raised by the specter of ostomy and its consequences. The shock, anxiety, hopelessness, and helplessness are reduced by sharing the crisis with a close relative, friend, or veteran patient. The patient who is unable to decide to undergo surgery will be helped by meeting and talking with an ostomate (48). The extra time needed to make a decision is often valuable. The postoperative period is smoother and emotionally less distressing when it follows adequate preoperative preparation (49,50). An individual assessment (e.g., misconceptions) and teaching on practical issues are essential (51). The important strategies to help manage

TABLE 27.1. *Types of Ostomies and Possible Sequelae and Complications*

	Disease	Procedure	Excreta	Continence	Physical Impairment of Sexual Function	Other Complications
Colostomy	Colorectal cancer	Abdomino-perineal resection	± Formed stool	± With irrigation	+	Skin irratation, bowel obstruction, prolapse or retraction of stoma, stenosis of stoma
Ileostomy	Inflammatory bowel diseases (ulcerative colitis, Crohn's disease)	Total colectomy	Fluid stool	— With conventional care + With Kock pouch	±	Renal stone formation* and the above
Urostomy (ileal conduit)	Bladder cancer	Radical cystectomy	Urine	—	+	Urinary infections and all the above
Colostomy and urostomy (ileal conduit)	Gynecological cancer (advanced and recurrent)	Pelvic exenteration	± Formed stool Urine	± With irrigation —	++	Combination of all the above

*Due to chronic asymptomatic water and salt depletion.
Key: —, absent in all patients; ±, present in half; ++, present in all patients; + present in majority.

the patient with an ostomy at different phases of recovery are outlined in Table 27.2 (4).

The psychological and social effects of stoma surgery have often been described in terms of significant *loss* (52,53). Patients' and next-of-kins' emotional responses reflect a grief process, including mainly feelings of anger, despondency, and sadness, but any emotion is possible in such situations. From this point of view, it becomes evident, that psychological recovery usually takes longer than physical recovery. Table 27.3 reveals the physical, emotional and interpersonal problems that these patients are confronted with (4).

Thomas and colleagues reported in about 20% of stoma patients with mixed diagnosis a serious level of psychiatric disturbance during the first year (54). The vast majority occurred during postoperative recovery. Difficulty coping with the stoma initially and at three months after surgery was a greater determinant of psychiatric disturbance over the first year than difficulty in coping with the illness (55). Factors associated with increased risk of psychiatric disturbance were past psychiatric history, postoperative physical symptoms and

TABLE 27.2. *Management of the Cancer Patient with an Ostomy*

PREOPERATIVE PHASE
1. Adequate explanation of the actual medical situation, the needed surgical procedure, and possible (especially sexual) sequelae is crucial. Simple drawings are often of great help. Due to patient's anxiety, explanations may have to be given more than once. Include spouse or "significant other" in the discussions.
2. Preoperative visit by a veteran patient with an ostomy and/or an enterostomal therapist, who functions as part of physician's team.
3. Physician should take time to listen to questions and concerns from patient and family.

POSTOPERATIVE PHASE
4. Postoperative care directed by enterostomal therapist or experienced surgical nurse. Self-care must be learned before discharge. Inclusion of significant other who will care for the patient at home is important, with adequate counseling of both by physician.

DISCHARGE HOME
5. Detailed information to family physician about medical and emotional state of the patient.
6. Offer of continued contact with patient and availability by phone of one team member, e.g., enterostomal therapist.

LONG-TERM ADJUSTMENT
7. At clinic visits after discharge, questions about emotional state and sexual function have to be addressed.
8. Coping of the patient's significant other should be explored.
9. Immediate referral to proper experts for care when emotional or sexual function is impaired and is of concern to the patient but cannot be handled by the family physician.
10. Information about ostomy groups in patient's community.

TABLE 27.3. *Common Psychological Problems in Ostomy Patients*

PHYSICAL
Practical problems of handling the stoma and bowel/urinary function: irrigation, changing bags, finding the adequate appliance, leakage.

EMOTIONAL
Impaired self-esteem and psychological dysfunction with depression and anxiety; anxiety in social situations; fears of sexual undesirability.

INTERPERSONAL
Impaired sexual function or fears about sexual function, even if function is actually unimpaired.
Strain on key relationships (partner, family, friends).
Strain in work situation imposed by stoma care and concerns about odors.
Social isolation resulting from sense of stigma, low self-esteem, withdrawal due to depression/anxiety.

complications, perceived inadequate advice after surgery regarding the stoma and its functioning, as well as traits of neuroticism, anxiety, and obsessionality (56). In another study, patients' physical state (e.g., fatigue, pain, smell) was also closely related to the prevalence of anxiety and depression, and single and widowed males reported better emotional adjustment than married men (57).

From a historical perspective, an impressive development in patient care has taken place, noted in a summary by Hürny and Holland (4). Until the late 1940s, patients were largely left on their own to adjust to both the practical and emotional problems resulting from colostomy. Toward the end of that decade, the American Cancer Society's visitor programs began to help ostomy patients by having other cured patients visit the new patients. Individual surgeons began to ask particularly well-adjusted patients to provide practical advice to the new patient with an ostomy. In 1947, Dukes, a British surgeon and pathologist whose classification of colorectal cancer is still used, reported on practical, social, psychological, and sexual problems of "expert patients" who had been living with a colostomy, some for more than 30 years (58). He suggested new or future patients be counseled by these "expert patients," matching for age and social class.

The first in-depth study was done in the early 1950s by Sutherland (1,2). Patients who had survived disease-free from rectal cancer for five or more years showed considerable impairment in both social (work, community, and family) and sexual (of both neurologic and psychological origin) function. Depression, chronic anxiety, and a sense of social isolation were frequently observed. Patients also had difficulties in the practical management of the colostomy associated with the use of clumsy belts and cumbersome dressings to cover the colostomy. Significant problems occurred with spillage and odor despite lengthy irrigation procedures. Today, patients have vastly improved equipment available to manage the stoma. In addition, the placement of the stoma is given attention to take into account skinfolds and patient preference (e.g., with regard to bathing suits).

Practical Management. The practical management problems of early ostomy patients led to the formation of patient self-help groups in the early 1950s. The groups were supported by surgeons who performed the procedure often and understood the psychological and practical problems. In the late 1950s, enterostomal therapy emerged as a nursing specialty. Most of the first enterostomal therapists themselves had ostomies. In addition, local and later national ostomy groups formed and created ostomy newsletters as a platform for mutual exchange of experience between ostomates. The International Ostomy Association (IOA) now serves a worldwide advocacy role for these individuals.

All patients are concerned about the possibility of diversion of the fecal stream to the abdominal wall. Fears of spillage, noises, and odors often inhibit return to social and work settings, and concern about being sexually unacceptable is frequently significant in men and women. Advice and counseling from other patients who have been through the experience, practical suggestions about covering the stoma, use of deodorants and perfumes, and routine care to prevent spillage have all been shown to be major methods of increasing self-confidence and in promoting return to normal activity.

Practical management of the ostomy centers on learning to handle the stoma well. This often leads to development of a sense of mastery and even pride. A special problem may be phantom rectum sensations following removal of the rectum, often with the sensation of an urge to defecate, which continues for some time. Common emotional issues involve loss of self-esteem and depression and their consequences as well as anxiety about ability to function adequately in social and sexual situations. The interpersonal impairment is often the most difficult to overcome, with persistent self-consciousness in the presence of others and avoidance and withdrawal being common problems. Patient care is mainly provided and coordinated by the stoma nurse. The patient's individual perspective and needs (59), including those of the partner, are the focus of care. Guidelines for management of the cancer patients with an ostomy at each stage are given in Table 27.2 (4).

Ostomy patients may initially refuse to look at the stoma; even thoughts about it evoke disgust, anger, embarrassment, and shame. The nurse may have to encourage participation in care. When the colostomy starts to work, the surgeon is pleased because normal bowel function has begun; the patient, however, is embarrassed. The guidance of an experienced nurse or enterostomal therapist helps the patient to become accustomed to the sight of the stoma and to learn to maintain it, even eventually being able to use humor in dealing with the stoma and the problems it produces.

Caregivers have to be aware of cross-cultural issues. A comparison of attitudes of Asian migrants and the indigenous population in England toward abdominal surgery and stomas showed similar anxieties among different ethnic groups in both patients and healthy individuals (60). In patients' coping and practical management, however, important differences can be

TABLE 27.4. *Sexual Function after Radical Surgery for Colorectal, Bladder, and Gynecological Cancer*

	Men					Women			
	Drive	Erection	Ejaculation	Orgasm	Fertility	Drive	Lubrication	Orgasm	Fertility
Abdomino-perineal resection (colostomy)	+	±	−	+	−	+	+	+	−
Radical cystectomy (ileal conduit)	+	−	—	±	—	?	?	?	?
Pelvic exenteration (colostomy and ileal conduit)	(No data; very rarely performed in men)					−	—	−	—

Key: —, absent in all patients; ?, no systematic data available;
¬, absent in majority; +, present in majority;
±, present in half; ++, present in all patients.

observed. A significant example concerns religious practice, such as bodily cleansing before prayer and keeping one hand clean in Muslims.

Coping with a newly placed stoma in the hospital, where professional help is available, is one thing; coping at home is another. This is true not only for the patient, but even more so for the spouse or others close to the patient, who are confronted with the burden of care that has previously been taken by the hospital staff. For the first two months, concerns about the stoma have been suggested to be the main issue (61). Life and death concerns begin to surface later, when the patient has mastered the stoma management. Although stoma patients nowadays cope better with their experience, their level of anxiety has been observed to rise constantly from the day they leave the hospital through the first two months (61).

The pattern for the partner is quite different. The spouse of an ostomy patient often experiences even more distress and anxiety than the patient at home. After ten days back at home, when the patient begins to cope relatively well, the spouse's ability to cope effectively may diminish and, by two months after discharge, his or her anxiety level is often observed to be above that recorded for hospitalized psychiatric inpatients. Typical partners' comments include: "Nobody understands what I'm going through"; "He is feeling better and I keep feeling worse"; "Everyone is patting him on the back and says how well he is managing, but no one asks about me, and no one [including the patient] says thanks." It is evident that it is not only the patients who need assistance to cope; the closest relatives and friends need it as well. As Oberst stated, "learning to live with someone else's cancer (and stoma) may be even more difficult, precisely because no one recognizes just how hard it really is" (61). Helpless family members represent one end of the spectrum; on the other are those who become overprotective and keep patients dependent.

Sexuality. The sexual taboo is an additional problem confronted by the cancer patient who undergoes stoma surgery. Surgeons and nurses sometimes fail to invite open discussion, and patients and partners discover these problems alone.

It is still difficult for many caregivers and patients to address the question that both are reluctant to ask. For example, it is important to know why patients completely stop sexual activity after diagnosis, many with no physical impairment of sexual function. Their response is likely related to psychological problems. Common misconceptions are that sex is not important if one is older or if one is physically ill, especially with cancer

(62). Patients may have rewarding means of sexual expression despite physical limitations and often in the absence of intercourse. This is helpful to know in dispelling the myth that intercourse is necessary for satisfaction and serves to caution against its use as a sole criterion for assessing satisfactory sexual adaptation.

It has been recognized since the early 1950s that major surgical procedures in men that involve the pelvic area may lead to disturbance in sexual function (63). This occurs secondarily to damage to the pelvic sympathetic nerves (L1, L2, L3: responsible for ejaculation) and parasympathetic nerves (S2, S3, S4: responsible for erection). The main effects on sexual function of abdominoperineal resection are summarized in Table 27.4 (4). Although some information on women is provided, the majority of the studies have involved men; one reason for this limited view is that the effects are more clearcut and easier to describe in men.

A broad range of prevalence of symptoms of sexual impairment and dysfunction has been reported across studies. Overall, it is safe to conclude that there is a 30% to 50% risk of impotence and a 50% to 75% risk of sterility after excision of the rectum. After total colectomy for inflammatory bowel disease (usually done in younger individuals with less damage to the pelvic nerves), the prevalence of sexual disfunction is lower, reported as 15% in men under the age of 35; this increases to 53% in those over 45 years of age (64). Radical cystectomy (including prostatectomy and vesiculectomy) for bladder cancer has a much higher prevalence of complete impotence (65). Inability to have an erection after pelvic surgery can be reversed by surgical implantation of a prosthesis, using either a rigid or an inflatable implant (see also Chapter 42).

Considerably less attention has been paid to physiological changes after abdominoperineal resection in women. One study described decreased libido, vaginal lubrication, and frequency of orgasm after abdominoperineal resection for rectal cancer (65); others reported dyspareunia, diminished orgasm, and less frequent or cessation of intercourse in more than half of the patients (43). As with males, sexual disturbance seems to be less frequent in women treated with ileostomy after colectomy for inflammatory bowel disease (65).

Sometimes the problems of physical and psychological dysfunction are so intertwined that they are difficult to separate. Impotence and decreased libido may be symptoms of depression rather than the sequelae of the operation. Shame and embarrassment may interfere with pleasurable sex. For example, a 53-year-old man was completely impotent two years after cystectomy, but was able to enjoy orgasm through oral stimulation. He said that he could not expose his ileal conduit bag and covered it by wearing a shirt. Covering it was important to him, but not to his wife (4). Besides burdensome emotions, such as the feeling in women with a stoma of having being assaulted, the stoma can become eroticized in both sexes; patients may then feel embarrassed about autoerotic sensations.

In summary, much has been done to improve the quality of life for patients with ostomies through better surgical techniques with fewer sequelae, improved technical devices for practical management of the stoma, better understanding of the accompanying psychosocial and sexual problems, and more available support through ostomy groups and enterostomal therapists. However, it still is a difficult experience to face the diagnosis of colorectal cancer and to have a stoma. The period of adjustment to the many difficulties may exceed one year. These patients need considerable support by all involved caregivers (nurse, enterostomal therapist, surgeon, ostomate). Family-oriented psycho-oncologic interventions are especially indicated.

Rehabilitation and Psychosocial Adaptation from a Long-Term Perspective

Rehabilitation needs and quality of life issues in long-term survivors have received only little attention. Given the relatively good prognosis for many patients with colorectal cancer, the question of long-term adaptation, in particular concerning surgical sequelae, is of high clinical relevance. An increasing psychosocial well-being with length of survival time has been reported in these patients (66). However, impairment in sexuality appears to be stable. Not surprisingly, an improving performance status was associated with better overall quality of life. In agreement with clinical experience, other predicting factors in this study (type of hospital, gender, work status) indicate the importance of an *individualized* approach for long-term rehabilitation.

In particular for the patients with a stoma, there is a range of possible psychological outcomes. At one end of the spectrum is the patient who actually gets more out of life after the ostomy experience. This occurs with patients who have been chronically sick with inflammatory bowel disease, for whom the placement of an ileostomy marks the end of being chronically ill and makes the start of a healthier life. Such a positive response is also likely to occur when the ostomy is performed in an attempt to cure cancer in someone

in previously good health. A similar adjustment is seen in patients with a temporary stoma whose bowel is reanastomosed. At the other end of the spectrum is the stoma patient, who actually is cured of cancer and physically healthy, but who becomes disabled for psychological reasons.

PANCREATIC CANCER

The pancreas is the second most common site of GI tumors and the fourth leading cause of cancer death in adults in the United States. The incidence is increasing after the age of 30, reaching a peak in the seventh decade for men and slightly later for women (67). The male to female ratio differs according to age (approximately overall ratio 1.3:1). The incidence varies across countries and immigrant groups within countries; overall, it is increasing. Relatively unspecific environmental, social (low socioeconomic status), nutritional, and medical risk factors for developing pancreatic cancer have been identified (67); cigarette smoking has also shown to be associated with an increased risk.

The vast majority of these tumors are ductal adenocarcinomas (about 80%). It is a tumor with an extremely grim prognosis. The median survival is between 4 and 6 months with no major improvement in the past decades; less than 5% survival at 5 years is currently obtained by any treatment. This is largely because a majority of patients have locally advanced or metastatic disease at diagnosis, only a minority of patients are candidates for curative resection. Patients with one of the rare endocrine tumors have a much better outlook; concerning these tumors no systematic psychosocial data are currently available.

Pain and Symptoms of Depression

The clinical features, mainly weight loss, anorexia, pain in the abdomen (often boring through to the back), and jaundice, are generally nonspecific. Of particular interest are symptoms of depression. There has been a long held belief among clinicians that pancreatic cancer patients at times have a history of unexplained depression and distress that preceded the appearance of physical symptoms (68–74). Most early clinical case reports, beginning in the 1920s, described a triad of depression, anxiety, and premonition of impending doom. From a historical perspective it is worth noting that melancholia was thought to originate in the pancreas in antiquity and in the Middle Ages.

Whether this phenomenon is medical folklore or a psychiatric syndrome associated specifically with pancreatic cancer has been debated at length (75–78).

Most attention has focused on symptoms of depression, even though many accounts also reported anxiety as a prominent part of the mental disturbance. Green and Austin (78) psychiatrically classified 21 of 52 patients of published case reports, who had pathologically documented pancreas cancer and were described in sufficient detail to allow a retrospective DSM-III-R classification. Seventy-one percent of these patients had symptoms of a depression-related disorder, 48% of a anxiety-related disorder, and 29% had symptoms of both.

In the first prospective study, Fras and colleagues (79) asked patients to fill in the Minnesota Multiphasic Personality Inventory (MMPI) when they were admitted with symptoms suggestive of an abdominal neoplasm. Depression, anxiety, and loss of ambition were present in 76% of patients who subsequently received the diagnosis of pancreatic cancer at surgery as compared to 20% of patients who were found to have another abdominal neoplasm. Half of all patients with pancreatic cancer reported that psychiatric symptoms appeared on average 6 months before physical symptoms.

The largest controlled study concerning this issue was part of a Cancer and Leukemia group B (CALGB) controlled clinical trial. The question of presence of psychiatric morbidity in pancreatic cancer patients was addressed by comparing a cohort of patients with advanced pancreatic carcinoma ($n = 107$) to a group of patients with advanced gastric cancer ($n = 111$) who were about to undergo chemotherapy on one of two nearly identical chemotherapy protocols (80). All patients were stratified for medical and sociodemographic variables; pain was not controlled for. Patients were assessed using the Profile of Mood States (POMS) before beginning of treatment. Their self-ratings of depression, tension-anxiety, fatigue, confusion-bewilderment, and total mood disturbance were significantly greater for the pancreatic cancer patients than for the gastric cancer group, providing evidence for greater psychiatric disturbance in pancreatic cancer patients compared to those with other intraabdominal malignancies.

Symptoms of psychological distress are confounded by pain, as pain is a key symptom over the whole course of disease. Pain in pancreatic cancer has mainly been assessed in retrospective investigations. Saltzburg and Foley (81) concluded from their review that most studies reported pain at diagnosis in at least 80% of the patients. Overall, pain prevalence increased by up to 97% during disease course. Despite these high figures, a considerable range can be observed. This may partly be explained by the specific location and stage of the tumor, as indicated by two prospective studies (82, 83); various different pain syndromes in pancreatic cancer patients are discussed elsewhere (81).

Kelsen and colleagues (83) investigated pain and psychological distress prospectively in patients with newly diagnosed pancreatic cancer. A quarter of these patients reported moderate, strong, or severe pain i.e., a lower prevalence than expected from earlier reports. Patients scheduled for chemotherapy reported significantly more intense pain than did those about to undergo surgery. Most patients described diffuse abdominal pain which was exacerbated by change in position or ingestion of food. About one-third of all patients reported symptoms of depression by the Beck Depression Inventory (BDI) and the Beck Hopelessness Scale (BHS). These symptoms were more frequent in chemotherapy patients. As expected, measures for pain intensity, symptoms of depression, functional activity, and quality of life showed different degrees of association in various subgroups.

In summary, a significant proportion of these patients show pain and symptoms of depression and anxiety, and a majority of them report psychological symptoms before the physical ones. Prevalence rates vary substantially among these investigations, owing to differences in design (i.e., retrospective versus prospective assessment) and sampling methods (84), measures for distress (self-report versus psychiatric assessment), and patient characteristics (tumor location and stage). Still, there is evidence that symptoms of depression and to a lesser degree of anxiety are more frequent in patients with pancreatic cancer compared to those with other intraabdominal malignancies. Both prevalence and course over time suggest a tumor-induced biologic pathogenesis of the mental disturbance.

However, several other explanations must be considered. The greater disturbance in the pancreatic cancer patients may reflect the psychological response to the knowledge of having a tumor whose extremely poor prognosis is well known. Moreover, the person may have had several months of unexplained systemic and rather vague but distressing symptoms. When finally diagnosed through more definite symptoms, the person is told a diagnosis, often of advanced disease, for which depression and anxiety are well known responses.

Possible Biologic Pathways of Mental Disturbance

As pointed out above, the other more intriguing explanation for greater psychological distress in patients with this disease is that a biologic, tumor-mediated paraneoplastic syndrome exists, similar to the unusual manifestations described by Schnider and Manolo (85), that may alter mood in patients with advanced cancer through the production of a false neurotransmitter. The extensive presence of neuropeptides in the GI tract and brain suggest a range of possible interactions.

Brown and Paraskevas (77) proposed that some cases of depression in cancer could be caused by immunologic interference with the activity of serotonin. They postulated a model in which serotonin, possibly mediated by an antibody induced against a protein released by the tumor, could cross react with CNS tissue, bind to serotonin receptors, and block them. An alternative explanation could be antibody production that stimulates anti-idiotypic antibodies that act as an alternative receptor for serotonin and reduce its synaptic availability.

Green and Austin (78) put forward several hypotheses regarding neuroendocrine mechanisms. Since pancreatic cancers can secrete ACTH (adrenocorticotropic hormone), and/or CRH (corticotropin-releasing hormone) resulting in mild hypercortisolemia and DST (dexamethasone suppression test) nonsuppression, as in subsets of patients with major depression, this mechanism could explain the symptoms of anxiety and depression. Another possible mechanism is the paraneoplastic secretion of PHT (parathormone) or a PHT-like factor resulting in mild hypercalcemia, leading to depression, anhedonia, irascibility, and emotional lability.

Thyroid dysfunction is linked to both anxiety and depression. Since TRH (thyroxin-releasing hormone) has been found within the islets of the pancreas and since a history of thyrotoxicosis seems to be more frequent in patients with pancreatic cancer, a disturbance of the thyroid axis is another, although less likely, pathway. Further proposed endocrine mechanisms are glucagon and insulin dysregulation.

Finally, a metabolic imbalance due to an increased bicarbonate load, emanating from obstructed pancreatic ducts, is postulated as a cause for the anxiety-related symptoms in analogy to the induction of panic attacks by infusion of sodium lactate and bicarbonate in individuals prone to panic.

In summary, these proposed immunologic, neuroendocrine, and metabolic mechanisms are speculative but testable. As pointed out by Green and Austin (78), further research is needed. It might be relevant for early detection of pancreatic cancer and improvement of patient care, as well as for our understanding of the biology of emotional dysfunction.

Diagnosis and Management

Individuals who are middle-aged or older and who have affective symptoms without a clear precipitant, particularly when vegetative symptoms predominate, should be thoroughly worked up medically for an occult neoplasm of the pancreas. Clinically, patients may show anxiety and agitation along with depression that respond poorly to all interventions including psychological support or psychopharmacologic treatment.

The more common situation is one in which a patient shows depression and distress in the context of increasing physical symptoms, where inadequately controlled pain may be a predominant feature. This pain is of visceral nature, often constant and only relieved by high doses of narcotic analgesics. Although opioid analgesics in most cases are effective, it has to be assumed that underdosing still is common (83). Nerve blocks of the celiac plexus may be required and give good relief in some patients. A comprehensive overview of pain treatment modalities in these patients is given by Saltzburg and Foley (81).

Few systematic data are currently available concerning patients' distress over the course of disease. In addition to tumor-related pain, GI symptoms, for example anorexia, nausea, and vomiting, as well as narcotic-induced constipation and fatigue, have a major impact on patients' psychological well-being. In two controlled trials, patients with inoperable pancreatic carcinoma estimated their distress by the Hospital Anxiety and Depression Scale (HADS). Comparing tamoxifen ($n = 22$) with double-blind placebo ($n = 22$) showed no effect on anxiety and depression, or on survival (86). In contrast, in the second trial (87), patients receiving chemotherapy (5-fluorouracil, adriamycin, mitomycin) survived significantly longer than the untreated group. They also showed significantly less depression but not anxiety after randomization and following two months of chemotherapy; HADS data were available for 18 patients under treatment and 13 in the control group. This effect may reflect palliation through chemotherapy. However, it also sheds light on the common observation that active treatment is usually associated with hope and supports particular patients in coping with fatal outlook. Although no final conclusion can be drawn from these small trials, they illustrate the need to include patients' subjective experience as endpoint in clinical trials.

Given the poor outlook in terms of survival and the burden of increasing symptoms, management should focus on maximum comfort and symptom control. The need for a multidisciplinary approach is highlighted by the fact that physical and emotional components of psychological burden are inextricably mingled in these patients. The staff should be aware also of subtle symptoms of distress, such as social withdrawal and reduced self-esteem that may occur in the early phase of disease.

In the infrequent case of total pancreatectomy, the daily diagnostic, dietetic, and therapeutic measures are a traumatic experience for many of these patients; their burden and coping are comparable to those with a resection due to chronic pancreatitis (88). Comparison of partial versus total resection shows similar psychosocial consequences, with depression, aggressive irritability, and withdrawal as known features. Partial pancreatectomy often results in lasting pain (inflammation) (88). The lost endocrine and exocrine function can produce alterations in insulin secretion and cause nausea, reduction in appetite, and most importantly, severe diarrhea.

Supportive care at home can be very meaningful to the patient and family (see also Chapter 87). Psychotropic drugs are used as adjuvant for control of psychological symptoms and often insomnia. Low-dose psychostimulants may enhance poor appetite. Pancreatic cancer patients and their families require active and aggressive support programs to cope with hopelessness and a sense of helplessness in altering the disease course and a patient's rapid decline.

RECOMMENDATIONS FOR FUTURE INVESTIGATIONS

Delay and knowledge of early warning signs are key issues in all GI tumors. In particular in colorectal cancer, the importance of strategies for prevention and early detection are clear cut. The questions of how to approach the targeted individuals for screening and surveillance, and how they assimilate the medical information, have promoted an alliance between health professionals and social and behavioral scientists. This integrative biopsychosocial approach should also be the perspective for further research in the growing area of molecular genetics. For example, more information on long-term adjustment of individuals with the familial cancer syndrome is important for all health care providers engaged in any phase of disease development.

The predictive value of psychosocial factors for onset (89,90) and survival (91) has also been investigated in colorectal cancer. Similar methods with similar methodological pitfalls were used as in other sites, although less frequently and with no conclusive results. The new understanding of the biological pathogenesis of these malignancies offers new opportunities to investigate biopsychosocial interactions in a more sophisticated and clinically meaningful way.

So far, formal quality of life assessment has received little attention in GI cancer clinical trials. In particular cases, this may be of relevance also in small phase II trials (92). In patients with a poor prognosis, such as unresectable pancreatic cancer, methodologically sound benefit–risk evaluation is difficult. Highly symptomatic diseases and rapid deterioration of health status require an adapted, specifically tailored quality-of-life assessment, feasible for patients and staff. This concern has received only minimal attention by quality-of-life methodologists. Considering the generally poor prognosis in advanced GI tumors, supportive interventions should be included in future trials. To compare the findings of those trials, it would be helpful to have standardized measures for specific symptoms, such as dysphagia in patients with esophagus cancer (93).

In addition to the existential threat of a GI cancer diagnosis, there are many everyday problems and practical needs that patients and their families will experience; for example, persistent fatigue in the patient and corresponding helplessness in the partner. Providing timely specific information and support will encourage them in their adjustment. Despite the high prevalence of GI tumors, many clinical questions have not yet been addressed systematically. More specific assessment of patients' needs are required, for example, of sexual rehabilitation in colorectal cancer, particularly in female patients.

Furthermore, quality of life should be investigated more in terms of an adaptation process (94). Also, in patients with poor survival we need to learn more about contributing factors and possibilities for improvement of comfort. There are several behavioral and other types of psychosocial interventions available for use within the clinical routine as an adjunct to oncological and psychopharmacologic treatment. Finally, partner, family, and even social network are an important focus of many multidisciplinary interventions in these patients. However, from our literature review we have to conclude that the social domains so far have received only marginal attention in care and research.

In conclusion, the trend followed in recent years clearly stresses the importance for *integrating* psychosocial aspects into routine medical care. Without multidisciplinary efforts it is not possible to implement goals of psycho-oncology, palliative care, and "quality of life" into routine care. This shift defines the research agenda for the near future in patients with GI cancer.

ACKNOWLEDGMENTS

The authors thank Ruth McCorkle, PhD, FAAN, and Markus Borner, MD, for their helpful comments.

REFERENCES

1. Sutherland AM, Orbach CE, Dyk RB, Bard M. The psychological impact of cancer and cancer surgery: I. Adaptation to the dry colostomy: preliminary report and summary of findings. *Cancer.* 1952; 5:857–872.

2. Dyk RB, Sutherland AM. Adaptation of the spouse and other family members to the colostomy patient. *Cancer.* 1956; 9:123–138.

3. Glimelius B, Hoffman K, Graf W, et al. Cost-effectiveness of palliative chemotherapy in advanced gastrointestinal cancer. *Ann Oncol.* 1995; 6:267–274.

4. Hürny C, Holland JC. Psychosocial sequelae of ostomies in cancer patients. *CA.* 1985; 35:170–183.

5. Holland JC. Gastrointestinal cancer. In: Holland JC, Rowland JH, eds. *Handbook of Psychooncology. Psychological Care of the Patient with Cancer.* Oxford: Oxford University Press; 1989: 208–217.

6. Roth JA, Lichter AS, Putnam JB, Forastiere AA. Cancer of the esophagus. In: DeVita VT, Hellman S, Rosenberg SA, eds. *Cancer. Principles and Practice of Oncology*, 4th ed. Philadelphia: J. B. Lippincott; 1993: 776–817.

7. Alexander HR, Kelsen DP, Tepper JE. Cancer of the stomach. In: DeVita VT, Hellman S, Rosenberg SA, eds. *Cancer. Principles and Practice of Oncology*, 4th ed. Philadelphia: J. B. Lippincott; 1993: 818–848.

8. Wang B, Yanagawa H, Sakata K. Gastric cancer screening programme in Japan: how to improve its implementation in the community. *J Epidemiol Community Health.* 1994; 48:182–187.

9. Vatn MH, Mogstad TE, Gjone E. A prospective study of patients with uncharacteristic abdominal disorders. *Scand J Gastroenterol.* 1985; 20:407–414.

10. Buhl K, Schlag P, Herfarth C. Quality of life and functional results following different types of resection for gastric carcinoma. *Eur J Surg Oncol.* 1990; 16: 404–409.

11. Roder JD, Herschbach P, Henrich G, Nagel M, Böttcher K, Siewert JR. Lebensqualität nach totaler Gastrektomie wegen Magenkarzinoms. Ösophagojejunoplication mit pouch versus Ösophagojejunostomie ohne pouch. *Dtsch Med Wschr.* 1992; 117:241–247.

12. Habu H, Saito N, Sato Y, Takeshita K, Sunagawa M, Endo M. Quality of postoperative life in gastric cancer patients seventy years of age and over. *Int Surg.* 1988; 73:82–86.

13. Barr H, Krasner N. Prospective quality-of-life analysis after palliative photoablation for the treatment of malignant dysphagia. *Cancer.* 1991; 68:1660–1664.

14. Loizou LA, Rampton D, Atkinson M, Robertson C, Bown SG. A prospective assessment of quality of life after endoscopic intubation and laser therapy for malignant dysphagia. *Cancer.* 1992; 70:386–391.

15. Neuhaus H, Hoffmann W, Dittler HJ, Niedermeyer HP, Classen M. Implantation of self-expanding esophageal metal stents for palliation of malignant dysphagia. *Endoscopy.* 1992; 24:405–410.

16. van Knippenberg FCE, Out JJ, Tilanus HW, Mud HJ, Hop WCJ, Verhage F. Quality of life in patients with resected oesophageal cancer. *Soc Sci Med.* 1992; 35:139–145.

17. Roder JD, Herschbach P, Ritter M, Kohn MM, Sellschopp A, Siewert JR. "Lebensqualität" nach Ösophagektomie. *Dtsch Med Wschr.* 1990; 115:570–574.

18. Sugimachi K, Maekawa S, Koga Y, Ueo H, Inokuchi K. The quality of life is sustained after operation for carcinoma of the esophagus. *Surg Gynaecol Obstet.* 1986; 62:544–546.

19. Collar JM, Otte JB, Reynaert M, Kestens PJ. Quality of life three years or more after esophagectomy for cancer. *J Thorac Cardiovasc Surg.* 1992; 104:391–394.

20. Delbrück H, Aghabi E. Subjektive Befindlichkeitsstörungen bei Magenkarzinom- und Ösophaguskarzinompatienten in der Nachsorge. *Rehabilitation.* 1993; 32:232–235.

21. Cohen AM, Minsky BD, Schilsky RL. Colon cancer. In: DeVita VT, Hellman S, Rosenberg SA, eds. *Cancer. Principles and Practice of Oncology*, 4th ed. Philadelphia: J. B. Lippincott; 1993: 929–977.

22. Giovannucci E, Rimm EB, Stampfer MJ, et al. A prospective study of cigarette smoking and risk of colorectal adenoma and colorectal cancer in U.S. men. *J Natl Cancer Inst.* 1994; 86:183–191.

23. Winawer SJ, Zauber AG, Gerdes H, et al. Risk of colorectal cancer in the families of patients with adenomatous polyps. *N Engl J Med.* 1996; 334:82–87.

24. Miller HH, Bauman LJ, Friedman DR, DeCosse JJ. Psychosocial adjustment of familial polyposis patients and participation in a chemoprevention trial. *Int J Psychiatry Med.* 1986; 16:211–230.

25. Hollyday HW, Hardcastle JD. Delay in diagnosis and treatment of symptomatic colorectal cancer. *Lancet.* 1979; I, 309–311.

26. Curless R, French J, Williams GV, James OF. Comparison of gastrointestinal symptoms in colorectal carcinoma patients and community controls with respect to age. *Gut.* 1994; 35:1267–1270.

27. Dent OF, Goulston KJ, Tennant CC, et al. Rectal Bleeding. Patient delay in presentation. *Dis Colon Rectum.* 1990; 33:851–857.

28. Toribara NW, Sleisenger MH. Screening for colorectal cancer. *N Engl J Med.* 1995; 332:861–867.

29. Fuchs CS, Giovannucci EL, Colditz GA, Hunter DJ, Speizer FE, Willett WC. A prospective study of family history and the risk of colorectal cancer. *N Engl J Med.* 1994, 331:1669–1674.

30. Croyle RT, Lerman C. Interest in genetic testing for colon cancer susceptibility: cognitive and emotional correlates. *Prev Med.* 1993; 22:284–292.

31. Müller H, Scott R, Weber W, Meier R. Colorectal cancer: lessons for genetic counselling and care for families. *Clin Genet.* 1994; 46:106–114.

32. Lerman C, Lustbader E, Rimer B, et al. Effects of individualized breast cancer risk counseling: a randomized trial. *J Natl Cancer Inst.* 1995; 87:286–292.

33. Arveux P, Durand G, Milan C, et al. Views of a general population on mass screening for colorectal cancer: The Burgundy study. *Prev Med.* 1992; 21:574–581.

34. Myers RE, Ross E, Jepson C, et al. Modeling adherence to colorectal cancer screening. *Prev Med.* 1994; 23:142–151.

35. Whynes DK, Neilson AR, Robinson MHE, Hardcastle JD. Colorectal cancer screening and quality of life. *Qual Life Res.* 1994; 3:191–98

36. Mant D, Fitzpatrick R, Hogg A, et al. Experiences of patients with false positive results from colorectal cancer screening. *Br J Gen Pract.* 1990; 40:423–425.

37. Poon MA, O'Connell MJ, Moertel CG, et al. Biochemical modulation of fluorouracil: evidence of significant improvement of survival and quality of life in patients with advanced colorectal carcinoma. *J Clin Oncol.* 1989; 7:1407–1417.

38. Scheithauer W, Rosen H, Kornek GV, Sebesta C, Depisch D. Randomised comparison of combination chemotherapy plus supportive care with supportive care alone in patients with metastatic coloretal cancer. *Br Med J.* 1993; 306:752–755.

39. Allen-Mersh TG, Earlam S, Fordy C, Abrams K, Houghton J. Quality of life and survival with continuous hepatic-artery floxuridine infusion for colorectal liver metastases. *Lancet.* 1994; 344:1255–1260.

40. Baider L, Perez T, Kaplan De-Nour A. Gender and adjustment to chronic disease. A study of couples with colon cancer. *Gen Hosp Psychiatry.* 1989; 11:1–8.

41. Anseline PF. Quality of life after restorative proctocolectomy. *Aust NZ J Surg.* 1990; 60:683–688.

42. Boyd NF, Sutherland HJ, Heasman KZ, Tritchler DL, Cummings BJ. Whose utilites for decision analysis? *Med Decis Making.* 1990;10:58–67.

43. Sprangers MAG, Taal BG, Aaronson NK, te Velde A. Quality of life in colorectal cancer. Stoma vs. nonstoma patients. *Dis Colon Rectum.* 1995; 38:361–369.

44. Filiberti A, Audisio RA, Gangeri L, et al. Prevalence of sexual dysfunction in male cancer patients treated with rectal excision and coloanal anastomosis. *Eur J Surg Oncol.* 1994; 20:43–46.

45. Koukouras D, Spiliotis J, Scopa CD, et al. Radical consequence in the sexuality of male patients operated for colorectal carcinoma. *Eur J Surg Oncol.* 1991; 17:285–288.

46. MacDonald LD, Anderson HR. Stigma in patients with rectal cancer: a community study. *J Epidemiol Community Health.* 1984; 38:284–290.

47. Centers for Disease Control and Prevention/National Center for Health Statistics. *Vital and Health Statistics: Detailed Diagnosis and Procedures, National Hospital Discharge Survey.* Washington DC: U.S. Department of Health and Human Services; 1993:Series 13, No. 122.

48. Genzdilov AV, Alexandrin GP, Simonov NN, Evtjuhin AI, Bobrov UF. The role of stress factors in the postoperative course of patients with rectal cancer. *J Surg Oncol.* 1977; 9:517–523.

49. Kelly MP, Henry T. A thirst for practical knowledge: Stoma patients' opinions of the services they receive. *Profess Nurse.* 1992; 7:350–356.

50. Barsevick AM, Pasacreta J, Orsi A. Psychological distress and functional dependency in colorectal cancer patients. *Cancer Pract.* 1995; 3:105–110.

51. Jeter K. Perioperative teaching and counseling. *Cancer.* 1992; 70:1346–1349.

52. Model G. A new image to accept: psychological aspects of stoma care. *Profess Nurse.* 1990; 5:310–316.

53. Kelly MP, Henry P. Open discussion can lead to acceptance. The psychosocial effects of stoma surgery. *Profess Nurse.* 1993; 9:101–106.

54. Thomas C, Madden F, Jehu D. Psychological effects of stomas - I. Psychosocial morbidity one year after surgery. *J Psychosom Res.* 1987; 31:311–316.

55. Thomas C, Turner P, Madden F. Coping and the outcome of stoma surgery. *J Psychosom Res.* 1988; 32:457–467.

56. Thomas C, Madden F, Jehu D. Psychological effects of stomas - II. Factors influencing outcome. *J Psychosom Res.* 1987; 31:317–323.

57. Wade BE. Colostomy patients: psychological adjustment at 10 weeks and 1 year after surgery in districts which employed stomacare nurses and districts which did not. *J Adv Nurs.* 1990; 15:1297–1304.

58. Dukes CE. Management of a permanent colostomy: study of 100 patients at home. *Lancet.* 1947; 2:12–14.

59. Deeny P, McCrea H. Stoma care: the patient's perspective. *J Adv Nurs.* 1991; 16:39–46.

60. Bhakta P, Probert CSJ, Jayanthi V, Mayberry JF. Stoma anxieties: a comparison of the attitudes of Asian migrants and the indigenous population in the United Kingdom towards abdominal surgery and the role of intestinal stomas. *Int J Colorect Dis.* 1992; 7:1–3.

61. Oberst MT, James RH. Going home: patient and spouse adjustment following cancer surgery. *Top Clin Nurs.* 1985; 7: 46–57.

62. Leiber L, Plumb MM, Gerstenzang ML, Holland JC. The communication of affection between cancer patients and their spouses. *Psychosom Med.* 1976; 38:379–389.

63. Goligher JC. Sexual function after excision of the rectum. *Proc R Soc Med.* 1951; 44:819–828.

64. Burnham WR, Lennard-Jones JE, Brooke BN. Sexual problems among married ileostomists. Survey conducted by the Ileostomy Association of Great Britain and Ireland. *Gut.* 1977; 18:673–677.

65. Bergman B, Nilsson S, Petersen I. The effect on erection and orgasm of cystectomy, prostatectomy and vesiculectomy of cancer of the bladder: a clinical and eletromyographic study. *Br J Urol.* 1979; 51:114–120.

66. Schag CAC, Ganz PA, Wing DS, Sim MS, Lee JJ. Quality of life in adult survivors of lung, colon and prostate cancer. *Qual Life Res.* 1994; 3:127–141.

67. Brennan MF, Kinsella TJ, Casper ES. Cancer of the pancreas. In: DeVita VT, Hellman S, Rosenberg SA, eds. *Cancer. Principles and Practice of Oncology*, 4th ed. Philadelphia: J. B. Lippincott; 1993: 849–882.

68. Scholz T, Pfeiffer F. Roentgenologic diagnosis of carcinoma of the tail of the pancreas. *J Am Med Assoc.* 1923; 81:275–277.

69. Yaskin JD. Nervous symptoms at earliest manifestations of carcinoma of the pancreas. *J Am Med Assoc.* 1931; 96:1664–1668.

70. Latter KA, Wilbur DL. Psychic and neurological manifestations of carcinoma of the pancreas. *Mayo Clinic Proc.* 1937; 12:457–462.

71. Savage C, Butcher W, Noble D. Psychiatric manifestations in pancreatic disease. *J Clin Psychopathol.* 1952; 13:9–16.

72. Savage C, Noble D. Cancer of the pancreas: two cases simulating psychogenic illness. *J Nerv Ment Dis.* 1954; 120:62–65.

73. Perlas AP, Faillace LA. Case report: psychiatric manifestations of carcinoma of the pancreas. *Am J Psychiatry*. 1964; 121:182.

74. Karlinger W. Psychiatric manifestations of cancer of the pancreas. *N Engl J Med*. 1967; 56:2251–2252.

75. Jacobsen L, Ottoson JO. Initial mental disorder in carcinoma of the pancreas and stomach. *Acta Psychiatr Scand*. 1971; 220:120–127.

76. Sachar E. Evaluating depression in the medical patient. In: Strain J, Grossman S, eds. *Psychological Care of the Medically Ill: A Primer in Liaison Psychiatry*. New York: Appleton-Century-Crofts; 1975:64–75.

77. Brown JH, Paraskevas F. Cancer and depression: Cancer presenting with depressive illness: an autoimmune disease? *Br J Psychiatry*. 1982; 141:227–232.

78. Green AI, Austin CP. Psychopathology of pancreatic cancer. A psychobiologic probe. *Psychosomatics*. 1993; 34:208–221.

79. Fras I, Litin EM, Pearson JS. Comparison of psychiatric symptoms in carcinoma of the pancreas with those in some other intraabdominal neoplasms. *Am J Psychiatry*. 1967; 123:1553–1562.

80. Holland JC, Hughes AH, Tross S, et al. Comparative psychological disturbance in patients with pancreatic and gastric cancer. *Am J Psychiatry*. 1986; 143: 982–986.

81. Saltzburg D, Foley KM. Management of pain in pancreatic cancer. *Surg Clin North Am*. 1989; 69: 629–649.

82. Krech RL, Walsh D. Symptoms of pancreatic cancer. *J Pain Symptom Manage*. 1991; 6:360–367.

83. Kelsen DP, Portenoy RK, Thaler HT, et al. Pain and depression in patients with newly diagnosed pancreas cancer. *J Clin Oncol*. 1995; 13:748–755.

84. Joffe RT, Rubinow DR, Denicoff KD, Maher M, Sindelar WF. Depression and carcinoma of the pancreas. *Gen Hosp Psychiatry*. 1986; 8:241–245.

85. Schnider B, Manolo A. Paraneoplastic syndrome's unusual manifestations of malignant disease. *Disease-a-Month*. 1979; 25:1–59.

86. Taylor OM, Benson EA, McMahon MJ, Yorkshire Gastrointestinal Tumour Group. Clinical trial of tamoxifen in patients with irresectable pancreatic adenocarcinoma. *Br J Surg*. 1993; 80:384–386.

87. Palmer KR, Kerr M, Knowles G, Cull A, Carter DC, Leonard RCF. Chemotherapy prolongs survival in inoperable pancreatic carcinoma. *Br J Surg*. 1994; 81:882–885.

88. Lang H, Faller H. Coping and adaptation in pancreatectomized patients: a somatopsychic perspective. *Psychother Psychosom*. 1992; 57:17–28.

89. Kune GA, Kune S, Watson LF, Bahnson CB. Personality as a risk factor in large bowel cancer: data from the Melbourne Colorectal Cancer Study. *Psychol Med*. 1991; 21:29–41.

90. Kavan MG, Engdahl BE, Kay S. Colon cancer: personality factors predictive of onset and stage of presentation. *J Psychosom Res*. 1995; 39:1031–1039.

91. Richardson JL, Zarnegar Z, Bisno B, Levine A. Psychosocial status at initiation of cancer treatment and survival. *J Psychosom Res*. 1990; 34:189–201.

92. Hill M, Norman A, Cunningham D, et al. Royal Marsden phase III trial of fluorouracil with or without interferon Alfa-2b in advanced colorectal cancer. *J Clin Oncol*. 1995; 13:1297–1302.

93. Gelfand GAJ, Finley RJ. Quality of life with carcinoma of the esophagus. *World J Surg*. 1994; 18:399–405.

94. Padilla GV, Grant MM, Lipsett J, Anderson PR, Rhiner M, Bogen C. Health quality of life and colorectal cancer. *Cancer*. 1992; 70:1450–1456.

28

Lung Cancer

LINDA SARNA

Lung cancer is a disease of the twentieth century; deaths due to lung cancer were almost unheard of prior to the epidemic of smoking. As the most common cause of cancer-related death among men and women in the United States, a diagnosis of lung cancer engenders multiple and complex psychosocial phenomena. Patients with progressive lung cancer commonly experience symptom distress and decline in physical function status related to disease and treatment. The impact of these phenomena can be reflected in assessments of emotional well-being and overall quality of life. Symptom palliation is often a key component to any psychotherapeutic intervention.

OVERVIEW OF LUNG CANCER

Approximately 178,100 new cases of lung cancer and 160,400 deaths due to lung cancer are projected for 1997. Lung cancer is estimated to account for 13% of all cancers diagnosed in men and women (1). Lung cancer is the number one cause of cancer death for men aged 35 years and older, and it comprises almost a third (32%) of all male cancer-related deaths. Lung cancer is the number one cause of cancer death among U.S. women (25% of all female cancer deaths). This gives U.S. women the highest death rate from lung cancer in the world (1). Lung cancer deaths appear to be declining in men, but continue to increase among women (6.4% increment in the past five years) (2). Tobacco is the primary risk factor, with over 80% of all cases linked to smoking history; an additional 1000 cases a year are the result of exposure to environmental tobacco smoke (3). The prolonged lag time of 20–40 years between smoking initiation and a diagnosis of lung cancer is often misunderstood by patients (3). This fact complicates primary prevention efforts. Recent studies have suggested that women with a shorter smoking history may be at even higher risk for lung cancer than men (4). Currently the average age at diagnoses is in the mid-sixties, but diagnosis may come earlier based on age at initiation of smoking (5).

One of the reasons lung cancer is associated with a high mortality is that it is difficult to diagnose early. This allows it to grow substantially before it becomes symptomatic. Unlike the case for breast, cervical, and colorectal cancers, there are no effective screening procedures. As a result, carcinoma of the lung is often diagnosed in advanced stages (26% with regional disease beyond local control, 44% with distant metastasis), for which treatment is largely of palliative not of curative intent (5). The five-year survival for all patients diagnosed is only 13% (1,5). However, survival rates for those with limited disease are more hopeful (over 50% five-year survival) (5). Because of the poor prognosis, apathy and treatment nihilism may affect clinical care. There are indications that despite modest advances in treatment benefits, attitudes among clinicians have not altered substantially (6). This may be another factor affecting the psychosocial impact of lung cancer.

Because of patterns of clinical and treatment characterics, lung cancers can be grouped into two major categories: non-small-cell (adenocarcinoma, squamous cell carcinoma, and large-cell carcinoma) and small-cell lung cancer. Small cell lung cancers comprise 25% of all lung cancers (5). They are rapidly growing but, at least initially, are very responsive to chemotherapy and radiation treatment. They are generally treated with chemotherapy as a systemic disease, regardless of apparent extent at diagnosis. Because central nervous system involvement is common, brain irradiation therapy may used. Patients with small-cell lung cancer usually require six months to one year of intensive treatment, most of which is given on an out-patient basis.

The most common lung cancers (non-small-cell, 75%) are usually diagnosed in advanced stages. Even

340

in early-stage disease (stage I and II), despite attempts at surgical cure, recurrent disease may occur. Palliation rather than cure is often the goal of treatment, with attention to symptom management as well as prolonged survival. Involvement of the chest beyond the primary and regional lymph nodes and metastasis to brain and bone are common. Recent clinical trials have shown temporary responses to treatment in 20%–60% of patients with advanced disease, but the cost-effectiveness of such therapy as well as the impact of therapy on the patient's quality of life continues to make such treatment ultimately inadequate (6–8). The quality as well as the quantity of survival comes into question, but patients may be willing to accept treatment toxicity with hope for longer survival and palliation of disease symptomatology (9). In addition, recent reviews of treatment have indicated a lack of consensus regarding the wide range of strategies used to treat locally advanced (stage IIIA and B) lung cancer (including how best to integrate radiation therapy, chemotherapy, and surgery) (6). The use of neoadjuvant chemotherapy to reduce tumor size before surgery or radiation therapy has improved survival (18–27 months) for some patients with previously unresectable or marginally resectable lung cancer (10).

EMOTIONAL DISTRESS AND LUNG CANCER

In their classic study documenting the psychosocial impact of cancer, Weisman and Worden (11) reported that patients with lung cancer experienced greater emotional distress than patients with other advanced cancers. Since that time, numerous studies and reviews have described the psychological disruptions experienced by people with lung cancer (12,13). A review of the major findings of these studies as they focus on emotional distress in lung cancer is presented in Table 28.1. More recent papers (1992–1996) were defined through MEDLINE and CANCERLIT searches using MeSH topics including "psychological, psychosocial, quality of life, and lung neoplasms." After review, articles related to psychosocial causes of lung cancer (including psychosocial risks for smoking) and articles in which instrument development was a primary focus without distinct lung cancer data were eliminated. Additional studies known by the author through prior searches were added. In studies with more than one tumor type, only the findings for lung cancer are reported. Findings reported are limited to those related to emotional distress.

Research in this debilitated population is challenging and sample sizes of research studies are generally small. Even when quality of life or psychosocial assess-ments are included in clinical trials, there are often missing data, and in general longitudinal data, especially after treatment cessation, are rare. Findings of these studies reveal a relatively low prevalence of psychiatric disorders, including anxiety and depression, given the seriousness of the disease. Emotional distress appears to peak after diagnosis, abate during the course of treatment, especially if a response is achieved, and increase again with disease progression and elevated symptom distress. Disease-related symptoms (pain, fatigue, dyspnea) appear to affect emotional well-being more profoundly than short-term symptoms (nausea, vomiting) related to treatment (8).

For rare patients, the occurrence of psychiatric disorders/personality changes due to brain metastases may be the first indication of lung cancer. Although disease- and treatment-related symptoms of lung cancer such as fatigue, anorexia, and sleep disturbances may mask symptoms of depression, they do not necessarily indicate serious psychological problems. Some symptoms, such as the alterations in sleep patterns noted in patients with lung cancer, may contribute to, if not directly affect, levels of psychological well-being (28). Because of the symptomatology of lung cancer, traditional measures of depression which include these somatic symptoms may not be valid. Similar to other populations of people with cancer, women with lung cancer have been noted to have a higher prevalence of psychological symptoms (18–19). There is limited information about the impact of nicotine withdrawal on psychological sequelae such as anxiety and depression in patients with lung cancer who stop smoking at diagnosis (29–30). Although symptom distress has been related to disruptions in psychological well-being in many studies, the presence of symptoms such as shortness of breath and pain are often not analyzed in investigations focused on emotional well-being.

COGNITIVE DISORDERS

Cognitive impairment, particularly in small-cell lung cancer, has been associated with the diagnosis and treatment of lung cancer. This contributes to difficulties in both the assessment and treatment of psychological distress. Cognitive impairment may result from brain metastases or other effects of the disease or treatment. Paraneoplastic syndromes (sometimes resulting from ectopic production of hormones), and treatment of the central nervous system with whole-brain irradiation or with drugs (systemic or intrathecal) have been linked with cognitive dysfunction and encephalopathy (31–34). For example, memory loss associated with

TABLE 28.1. *Research Documenting Emotional Distress and Lung Cancer*

Author	Sample Size	Major Findings
Ahles et al., 1994 (14)	57	Increased psychological distress in patients receiving combination chemotherapy/radiation therapy, but increased survival as compared to chemotherapy alone
Abratt and Viljoen, 1995 (15)	40	Anxiety (17.5%) and depression (22.5%) noted in a clinic setting
Anderson et al., 1993 (16)	37	Anxiety and depression were reduced during treatment despite no change in physical symptoms; depression (18%) and anxiety (20%) were present pretreatment
Benedict, 1989 (17)	30	More suffering due to symptom distress than emotional distress
Bleehen et al., 1989 (18)	96	Moderate depression (10%, 1% severe) and anxiety (17%, 8% severe) prior to treatment with decline in anxiety, but minimal change in depression over time; depression and anxiety more common in females
Bleehen et al., 1993 (19)	458	Anxiety (14% moderate, 5% severe) and depression (24% mild, 1% severe) decreased during treatment; more prevalent and severe distress among women but improvement in mood was similar over time
Ganz et al., 1991 (20)	40	Lower quality of life associated with poorer survival for those unmarried
Ginsburg et al., 1995 (21)	71	Affective disorder (4%), adjustment disorder (12%), suicidal ideation (13%) noted in newly diagnosed patients; 52% had insomnia, and 48% loss of libido
Hopwood and Thatcher, 1990 (22)	102	A third of the sample had significant anxiety and depression
Hughes, 1985 (23)	134	16% of newly diagnosed had clinical depression
Hughes, 1985 (24)	50	Depression correlated with severe disability; patients undergoing treatment less depressed than those on palliative care
Klemm, 1994 (25)	56	Physical and psychosocial demands of illness in newly diagnosed patients were associated with adjustment to illness
McCorkle and Benoliel, 1983 (26)	56	Improvement in mood over time after diagnosis; more distress than those with a heart attack
Sarna, 1993 (27)	69	Symptom distress and poverty associated with lower quality of life

limbic encephalopathy may be a consequence of anti-neural antibodies (34). In some cases, cognitive dysfunction may be the first sign of disease. Although neuropsychological deficits in lung cancer patients without central nervous system metastases have generally been attributed to treatments, such as systemic chemotherapy and brain irradiation, a study of cognitive deficits in patients with newly diagnosed small cell lung cancer ($n = 46$) found that verbal memory alterations (70%–80%), motor coordination (33%), and frontal lobe executive dysfunction (38%) existed prior to treatment and did not increase or decrease after chemotherapy and radiation (34). Such neurological alterations may not be clinically obvious unless routine neuropsychiatric testing is performed (32). Not unique to treatment of lung cancer patients, the use of narcotics, sedatives, steroids, and antiemetics used in symptom palliation also may affect cognitive function.

SYMPTOM DISTRESS

A number of studies have linked symptom distress and functional decline with psychological distress in lung cancer. Rather than a precursor, psychological distress is often the sequela of uncontrolled symptomatology. Thus the key to alleviation of distress for many of these patients may lie first in effective symptom management. Symptoms of lung cancer may be directly related to the disease or to manifestations of treatment. Symptoms related to the disease may differ in individuals depending on the location of the cancer, the extent of the disease, and response to treatment.

Symptoms may be relieved with treatment, but some may be refractory to medical interventions. Kukull and colleagues (35) found that postdiagnosis symptom distress was an important predictor of survival after controlling for age, functional status, and personality traits. These findings have been confirmed by others (20,36,37). Symptoms such as fatigue and malaise have been used as proxy indicators of quality of life (38).

Less than 20% of lung cancer clinical trials in locally advanced disease have included symptom distress as an outcome variable (7). However, symptom distress has been the focus of or a part of an increasing number of recent investigations (8). These studies are reviewed in Table 28.2. Only findings related to symptom distress are included and, in studies with heterogeneous samples, only findings related to lung cancer patients are reported.

These data describe a variety of disease- and treatment-related symptoms that can have an impact on emotional well-being. Although there are some differences among symptoms by treatment status, there are no clear distinctions. Pain, dyspnea, fatigue, functional decline, anorexia, and alterations in sleep are common.

TABLE 28.2. *Lung Cancer and Symptom Distress*

Author	Sample Size	Major Findings
Bergman et al., 1994 (39)	735	Dyspnea, cough, and pain common symptoms; advanced disease and poor performance status related to worsened symptoms
Bergman et al., 1992 (40)	62	Pain control and improved appetite linked to better quality of life
Bleehen et al., 1993 (19)	448	Regardless of chemotherapy regimen, disease-related symptoms were palliated in 63% of subjects
Fayers et al., 1991 (41)	196	Chemotherapy and radiation therapy associated with greater symptom distress compared with no treatment
Ganz et al., 1989 (42)	48	Functional status not significantly better for those on chemotherapy as compared to those on supportive care only
Geddes et al., 1990 (43)	53	Mood, sleep, activity and well-being seriously affected during and following treatment; prolonged treatment group had greater mood disturbances
Hurny et al., 1993 (38)	127	Fatigue/malaise most frequent symptoms (over 1/3 during treatment); symptoms and side effects contributors to psychological distress.
Hopwood and Stephens, 1995 (44)	650	Symptoms at diagnosis similar for both small-cell and non-small-cell types; worry, anxiety, tiredness, lack of energy, lack of appetite, difficulty sleeping, shortness of breath and cough were most common; symptoms increased with decline in functional status; females reported more severe psychological symptoms
Kaasa et al., 1988 (45)	95	Patients on chemotherapy had worse quality of life than those on radiation therapy
Kaasa et al., 1988 (46)	102	Symptom distress and well-being predictors of survival
Kaasa et al., 1988 (33)	95	Sleep disturbances, pain, fatigue and lack of appetite common symptoms during treatment
Kukull et al., 1986 (35)	54	Degree of symptom distress predictive of survival
McCorkle et al., 1989 (47)	166	Patients receiving home nursing care had less symptom distress and better functional status
Maasilita et al., 1990 (48)	55	Increasing doses of chemotherapy linked to decrease in quality of life
Munro and Potter, 1996 (49)	24	Most serious symptoms one month after a course radiation therapy include shortness of breath on stair climbing, cough, feeling tired, weakness, family worry, and constipation; more distress than those with breast or head and neck cancer
Sarna, 1993 (50)	69	Fatigue, difficulty with household chores were serious problems for women patients

Rarely are solitary symptoms experienced. Some symptoms thought to be treatment-specific, such as anorexia, may persist long after the treatment ends. In many cases, symptoms are inextricably linked to quality of life.

FUNCTIONAL DECLINE

Historically, performance status (often as assessed by the doctor) was the primary indicator of quality life in this population (8,51). Disruptions in the capacity to engage in a variety of physical activities (functional status) are common, especially as the disease progresses. This physical compromise can be linked to subsequent emotional decline (52–55). Weight loss can contribute to fatigue and decreased functional performance during the course of progressive disease (56). Clinicians can play a vital role in the early identification of those vulnerable patients at greatest risk for psychological distress at diagnosis and closely reassess psychological stress during the course of the disease. Those patients can be referred, evaluated, and followed by mental health clinicians.

Other than therapeutic clinical trials, there have been very few intervention studies which have sought to diminish the suffering experienced by adults with lung cancer and their families. McCorkle (47) intervention of home nursing care diminished symptom distress and prolonged independent functioning six weeks longer than seen in a standard office care comparison group. Patients were targeted early after the diagnosis of advanced disease and followed for six months. Other studies that focused on symptom control have reported a beneficial outcome on psychological well-being. The weight loss that accompanies progressive lung cancer and functional decline may be a result of lack of eating due to depression, but more likely depression is one of the consequences of the metabolic process of cachexia and may contribute to increased symptom distress (56). Nutritional replacement has been found to improve overall sense of well-being and quality of life in some studies (57,58). Pain is a prominent symptom for many with advanced lung cancer and affects physical function directly and indirectly (59,60). Symptom relief is essential to facilitate physical and emotional well-being.

The prevalence of co-morbid conditions contributing to decline in functional status, particularly those causing physical impairment in the face of lung cancer, is not defined. Because of the relationship of smoking to lung cancer, the co-incidence of concurrent pulmonary and cardiovascular disease is not unusual. Those at highest risk for co-morbid disease, those over 65 years

of age, have been underrepresented in lung cancer clinical trials in proportion to the prevalence (61). Thus, current data describing functional status may not be generalizable to an older, more frail population. Multiple health problems may be important factors contributing to additional psychological distress.

FAMILY IMPACT

The distressing symptoms experienced by those with lung cancer—dyspnea, cognitive impairment, pain, profound anorexia and weight loss—cannot but impact the family and affect the emotional well-being of the caregiver (62). Spouses of patients with lung cancer have been reported to suffer profound emotional distress (63). Particularly with the increase of lung cancers in women, traditional housekeeping and caretaking roles may be disrupted and the subsequent family burden substantially increased.

QUALITY OF LIFE AS AN OUTCOME

Psychosocial well-being is a key component in health-related conceptions of quality of life (8). Current medical treatments with multimodal therapies for lung cancer have raised profound issues affecting the quality of life of adults with advanced lung cancer (6,8,51,64,65). In Splinter's (51) review of 142 clinical trials in non-small-cell lung cancer, few studies addressed issues related to quality of life other than physician-rated performance status. However, a number of tools modified for or specific to the quality of life concerns of people with lung cancer have been developed, tested, and incorporated into clinical trials. The Symptom Distress Scale (66) has been used in many clinical trials of patients with lung cancer and includes items "outlook" and "concentration" relevant to screening for emotional distress in addition to items evaluating disease and treatment-related symptoms (8). Another instrument, the Lung Cancer Symptom Scale (67,68), was developed specifically for lung cancer patients. It includes professional as well as patient appraisal of symptoms (appetite, fatigue, cough, dyspnea, hemoptysis, and pain), but it does not assess psychological or social dimensions of the impact of illness. The FACT-L ("L" for Lung) (69) scale is a measure of quality of life, with specific questions related to lung cancer symptoms added to core questions for all cancer patients (the FACT). Emotional well-being is briefly assessed in six questions, with one overall assessment of the impact of emotional well-being on quality of life. Similarly, the EORTC Quality of Life Questionnaire (QLQ-C30) now includes an additional module relevant to people with lung cancer (8,19,70). Lung cancer symptoms have been added to core cancer disease and treatment assessments. The use of a daily diary card has been shown to be another way of detecting day-to-day variations in symptom distress and well-being and of assessing the impact of palliative care (8,41,48,70). These tools, as well as other generic instruments, provide reliable and valid methods for use in the clinical setting to screen for disruptions and focus more on intensive assessment and intervention. Most of the instruments used to measure quality of life are self-reports and as such may vary from the clinician's assessment.

GUILT AND TOBACCO USE

Despite the encouraging findings of a decrease in smoking prevalence in the United States, 26.8% of adult men and 21.8% of adult women still smoke (approximately 46 million Americans) (71). Tobacco-related diseases will become the number one cause of preventable death throughout the world in the next century, and lung cancer will continue to be a major health problem (3). Despite the importance of ongoing tobacco use as a risk factor, there is limited information about smoking patterns or withdrawal symptoms experienced by patients with lung cancer (29). There are limited data about the impact of a smoking history on emotional distress of patients with lung cancer. Anger and resentment may be exhibited by patients who do not have a smoking history (almost 25% of women with lung cancer) (4), but who may have been exposed to second-hand smoke in the work place or the home. On the other hand, because of the lag time for risk after smoking initiation, and the length of time before reduction of risk after cessation, patients who have quit smoking a number of years before diagnosis may experience additional frustration. Cella has included one item assessing regret for smoking as part of the lung cancer module in his FACT-L (69). Several studies have included patient's causal attributions regarding lung cancer. Patients' history of smoking correlated with greater emotional distress (72,73). However, not all patients acknowledge a regret for previous smoking. In a study by Sell and colleagues ($n = 50$), only 42% of recently diagnosed patients with lung cancer with a smoking history experienced a sense of guilt (74).

The lung cancer experience can be used as a "teachable moment" for relatives of patients with lung cancer who smoke (29). Unfortunately, not even a diagnosis of potentially curable lung cancer will necessarily result in permanent tobacco cessation. Further psychological

support, skills training, and nicotine replacement may be warranted. Sarna reported that although most women ceased smoking soon after diagnosis with lung cancer, many family members continued to smoke (30). A recent study targeting family members of patients with cancer ($n = 103$ patients, including 23% with lung cancer) reported that 9% (17/198) of relatives quit smoking for six months after receiving written advice and materials from the patient's physicians (75). The recent guidelines for the most effective strategies for smoking cessation may be applied to the patient setting (76). However, there are no data testing their use in this population. Smoking cessation advice for patients with incurable disease is questionable. Smoking cessation may promote weight gain and decrease symptom distress in some cases, but in others psychological and physiological withdrawal may be untenable. Further studies regarding smoking cessation in lung cancer are needed in both curable and incurable situations In some cases, guilt and blame by family members toward a smoker (or former smoker) can complicate adjustment to the diagnosis and may require psychological intervention.

LONG-TERM SURVIVORS AND EMOTIONAL WELL-BEING

There are limited data about long-term survivors of lung cancer. Schag and colleagues report that in comparison with survivors of colon cancer and prostate cancer, lung cancer survivors ($n = 57$, 44% female) had more problems (77). Difficulty in working and disruptions in activities of daily living were severe and continuing problems. Psychological distress was greatest among those with lung cancer (63% with frequent anxiety, 51% frequently depressed), including continued difficulties with cognition (63% with memory difficulties, 32% with difficulty concentrating). Lung cancer patients also expressed more difficulties with sexual functioning (79% decrease in intercourse, 56% difficulties with arousal). Interestingly, there was no difference in overall quality of life between the long-term survivors (five years or longer) and the shorter term survivors (less than two years). Functional status was the best predictor of quality of life. Even for these survivors, 58% expressed worry that the cancer was progressing.

ECONOMIC CONSEQUENCES AND PSYCHOSOCIAL DISTRESS

Recently, a number of investigations have pursued the financial trade-offs for lung cancer treatment protocols and many have included dimensions reflecting psychosocial well-being and quality of life (78–80). Jaakimainen et al reported that supportive care for lung cancer was not necessarily less costly than treatment (80). Supportive care was associated with increased use of radiation for symptom control and increased hospitalization. As protocols have been compared for efficacy (disease response and survival) along with quality of life and symptom improvement, the cost for that improvement may be another consideration. As health care moves increasingly to the home, the cost of care may shift to the family with, at times, unanticipated consequences. Along with the cost of treatment, the cost of care, particularly the nonfinancial cost of care for the family, needs to be a consideration.

CONCLUSIONS

Despite the grim prognoses, the majority of people with lung cancer do not have serious psychological disorders. However, many comparative studies have suggested that people with lung cancer have more emotional distress than other people with different types of cancer. Routine, systematic screening for anxiety and depression along with symptom distress should be included as part of the therapeutic plan of care to detect individuals who require more detailed assessment and perhaps more intensive psycho-oncology intervention. In addition to the traditional "red flags" for psychological morbidity, increased symptom distress (including weight loss) and impaired functional status may portend increased risk for emotional distress. An interdisciplinary approach focused on therapeutic treatment and symptom management can be a part of effective psychological treatment, although clinical trials in this area are pointedly lacking. Women appear to be at greater risk for psychological distress, but further study is needed as the percentage of women with lung cancer increases. Very limited data are available to differentiate cross-cultural and ethnic/racial psychosocial responses to lung cancer, although lung cancer is the most common cause of cancer death among African Americans (26.1% of cancer deaths), Asian and Pacific Islanders (22.3%), Native Americans (26.8%), Hispanics (17.9%), as well as whites (28.4%) (1). Access to care, influenced by socioeconomic status, is not a unique issue for patients with lung cancer, but the need for symptom relief as well as for treatment may make this a critical factor for emotional well-being.

REFERENCES

1. Parker SL, Tong T, Bolden S, Wingo PA. Cancer statistics, 1997. *CA Cancer J Clin.* 1997; 47:5–27.
2. Cole P, Rodu B. Declining cancer mortality in the United States. *Cancer.* 1996; 78:2045–2048.
3. Peto R, Lopez, AD, Boreham J, et al. *Mortality in Relation to Smoking in Developed Countries, 1950–2000: Indirect Estimates from National Vital Statistics, 1994.* New York: Oxford University Press; 1994.
4. Zang EA, Wynder EL. Differences in lung cancer risk between men and women. examination of the evidence. *J Natl Cancer Inst.* 1996; 88:183–192.
5. Ries KAG, Miller BA, Hankey BF, Kosay CL, Harras A, Edwards BK, eds. Lung and bronchus. In: *SEER Cancer Statistics Review, 1973–1991: Tables and Graphs.* Bethesda, MD: National Cancer Institute; NIH Pub. No 94-2789; 1994: 263–286.
6. McVie JG. Non-small lung cancer. meta-analysis of efficacy of chemotherapy. *Semin Oncol.* 1996; 23(3 Suppl 7):12–16.
7. Brundage MD, Mackillop WJ. Locally advanced non-small cell lung cancer: do we know the questions? Survey of randomized trials from 1966-1993. *J Clin Epidemiol.* 1996; 49:183-92.
8. Moinpour CM. Measuring quality of life. an emerging science. *Semin Oncol.* 1994; 21 (Suppl):48-63.
9. Thatcher N, Niven RM, Anderson H. Aggressive vs non-aggressive therapy for metastatic NSCLL. *Chest.* 1996; 109:87S–92S.
10. Tonato M. The role of neoadjuvant chemotherapy in NSCLC. *Chest.* 1996;109:93S–95S.
11. Weisman AD & Worden JW. The existential plight in cancer: significance of the first 100 days. *Int J Psychiatr Med.* 1976–1977; 7:1–15.
12. Bernhard J, Ganz PA. Psychosocial issues in lung cancer patients (part 1). *Chest.* 1991; 99:216–223.
13. Bernhard J & Ganz PA. Psychosocial issues in lung cancer patients (part 2). *Chest.* 1991; 99:480–485.
14. Ahles TA, Silberfab PM, Rundle AC, et al. Quality of life in patients with limited small-cell carcinoma of the lung receiving chemotherapy with or without radiation therapy, for cancer and leukemia group B. *Psychother Psychosom.* 1994; 62:193–199.
15. Abratt R, Viljoen G. Assessment of quality of life by clinicians—experience of a practical method in lung cancer patients. *S Afr Med J.* 1995;85:896–898.
16. Anderson H, Hopwood P, Prendville J, Radford JA, Thatcher N, Ashcroft L. A randomised study of bolus vs continuous pump infusion of ifosfamide and doxorubicin with oral etoposide for small cell lung cancer. *Br J Cancer.* 1993; 67:1385–1390.
17. Benedict S. The suffering associated with lung cancer. *Cancer Nurs.* 1989; 12:34–40.
18. Bleehen NM, Fayers PM, Girling DJ, Stephen RJ. Survival, adverse reactions and quality of life during combination chemotherapy compared with selective palliative treatment for small-cell lung cancer. *Respir Med.* 1989; 83:51–58.
19. Bleehen NM, Girling DJ, Machin D, Stephens RJ. A randomised trial of three or six courses of etoposide cyclophosphamide methotrexate and vincristine or six courses of etoposide and ifosfamide in small cell lung

cancer (SCLC). II. Quality of life. *Br J Cancer*. 1993; 68:1157–1166.

20. Ganz PA, Lee JJ, & Siau J. Quality of life assessment: an independent prognostic variable for survival in lung cancer. *Cancer*. 1991; 67:3131–3135.

21. Ginsburg, ML, Quirt, C, Ginsburg, AD, MacKillop WJ. Psychiatric illness and psychosocial concerns of patients with newly diagnosed lung cancer. *Can Med Assoc J*. 1995. 152:701–708

22. Hopwood P & Thatcher N. Preliminary experience with quality of life evaluation in patients with lung cancer. *Oncol Williston Park*. 1990; 4:158–162.

23. Hughes JE. Depressive illness and lung cancer. I. Depression before diagnosis. *Eur J Surg Oncol*. 1985; 11:15–20.

24. Hughes JE. Depressive illness and lung cancer. II. Follow-up of inoperable patients. *Eur J Surg Oncol*. 1985; 11:21–24.

25. Klemm PR. Variables influencing psychosocial adjustment in lung cancer. a preliminary study. *Oncol Nurs Forum*. 1994;21:1059–1062.

26. McCorkle R, Benoliel JQ. Symptom distress, current concerns and mood disturbance after diagnosis of life-threatening disease. *Soc Sci Med*. 1983; 17:431–438.

27. Sarna L. Women with lung cancer. impact on quality of life. *Qual Life Res*. 1993; 2:13–22.

28. Silberfarb PM, Hauri PJ, Oxman TE, Schnurr P. Assessment of sleep in patients with lung cancer and breast cancer. *J Clin Oncol*. 1993:11:997–1004

29. Gritz ER. Smoking and smoking cessation in cancer patients. *Br J Addict*. 1991; 86:549–554.

30. Sarna L. Smoking behaviors of women after diagnosis with lung cancer. *Image*. 1995; 27:35–41.

31. Van Oosterhout AG; Ganzevles PG; Wilmink JT, et al. Sequelae in long-term survivors of small cell lung cancer. *Int J Radiat Oncol Biol Phys*. 1996; 34:1037–1044.

32. Cull A, Gregor A, Hopwood P, et al. Neurological and cognitive impairment in long-term survivors of small cell lung cancer. *Eur J Cancer*. 1994; 30A:1067–1074,

33. Kaasa S, Olsnes BT, Mastekaasa A. Neuropsychological evaluation of patients with inoperable non-small cell lung cancer treated with combination chemotherapy or radiotherapy. *Acta Oncol*. 1988; 27:241–246.

34. Meyers CA, Byrne KS, Komaki R. Cognitive deficits in patients with small cell lung cancer before and after chemotherapy. *Lung Cancer*. 1995; 12:231–235.

35. Kukull WA, McCorkle R, Driever M. Symptom distress, psychosocial variables and lung cancer survival. *J Psychosoc Oncol*. 1986; 4:91–104.

36. Kaasa S, Mastekaasa A, & Lund E. Prognostic factors for patients with inoperable non-small cell lung cancer, limited disease. The importance of patients' subjective experience of disease and psychosocial well being. *Radiother Oncol*. 1989; 15:235–242.

37. Buccheri GF, Ferrigno D, Tamburni M, Brunelli C. The patient's perception of his own quality of life might have an adjunctive prognostic significance in lung cancer. *Lung Cancer*. 1995; 12:45–52.

38. Hurny C, Bernhard J, Joss R, et al. "Fatigue and malaise" as a quality-of-life indicator in small-cell lung cancer patients. *Support Care Cancer*. 1993; 1:316–320.

39. Bergman B, Aaronson NK, Ahmedzai S, Kaasa S. Sullivan M, for the EORTC Study Group on Quality of Life. The EORTC QLQ- LC13. a modular supplement to the EORTC core quality of life questionnaire (QLQ-C30) for use in lung cancer clinical trials. *Eur J Cancer*. 1994; 30A:635–642.

40. Bergman B, Sullivan M, & Sorenson S. Quality of life during chemotherapy for small cell lung cancer. II. A longitudinal study of the EORTC Core Quality of Life Questionnaire and comparison with the Sickness Impact Profile. *Acta Oncol*. 1992; 31:19–28.

41. Fayers PM, Bleehen NM, Girling DJ, et al. Assessment of quality of life in small-cell lung cancer using a Daily Diary Card developed by the Medical Research Council Lung Cancer Working Party. *Br J Cancer*. 1991; 64:299–306.

42. Ganz PA, Figlin RA, Haskell CM, La Soto N, Siau J. Supportive care versus supportive care and combination chemotherapy in metastatic non-small cell lung cancer. Does chemotherapy make a difference? *Cancer*. 1989; 63:1271–1278.

43. Geddes DM, Dones L, Hill E, et al. Quality of life during chemotherapy for small cell lung cancer. Assessment and use of a daily diary card in a randomized trial. *Eur J Cancer*. 1990; 26:484–492.

44. Hopwood P, Stephens RJ. Symptoms at presentation for treatment in patients with lung cancer. implications for the evaluation of palliative treatment. *Br J Cancer*. 1995; 71:633–636.

45. Kaasa S, Mastekaasa A. Psychosocial well-being of patients with inoperable non-small cell lung cancer. *Acta Oncol*. 1988; 27:342.

46. Kaasa S, Mastekaasa A, Naess S. Quality of life of lung cancer patients in a randomized clinical trial evaluated by a psychosocial well-being questionnaire. *Acta Oncol*. 1988; 27:335–342.

47. McCorkle R, Benoliel JQ, Donaldson G, Georgiadou F, Moinpour C, Goodell B. A randomized clinical trial of home nursing care for lung cancer patients. *Cancer*. 1989; 64:199–206.

48. Maasilta PK, Rautonen JK, Mattson MT, Mattson KV. Quality of life assessment during chemotherapy for non-small cell lung cancer. *Eur J Cancer*. 1990; 26:706–708.

49. Munro AJ, Potter S. A quantitative approach to the distress caused by symptoms in patients treated with radical radiotherapy. *Br J Cancer*. 1996; 74:640–647.

50. Sarna L. Correlates of symptom distress in women with lung cancer. *Cancer Pract*. 1993; 1:21–28.

51. Splinter TAW. Chemotherapy in advanced lung cancer. *Eur J Cancer*. 1990; 26:1093–1099.

52. Kaasa S, Mastekaasa A, Thorud E. Toxicity, physical function and everyday activity reported by patients with inoperable non-small cell lung cancer in a randomized trial (chemotherapy versus radiotherapy). *Acta Oncol*. 1988; 27:343–349.

53. Cella DF, Orofiamma B, Holland JC, et al. The relationship of psychological distress, extent of disease, and performance status in patients with lung cancer. *Cancer*. 1987; 60:1661–1667.

54. Sarna L. Functional status in women with lung cancer. *Cancer Nurs*. 1994; 17:87–93.

55. Hyde L, Wolf J, McCracken S, & Yesner R. Natural course of inoperable lung cancer. *Chest*. 1973; 64: 309–312.

56. Sarna L, Lindsey AM, Dean H, Brecht ML, McCorkle R. Weight change and lung cancer: relationships with symptom distress, functional status, and smoking. *Res Nurs Health.* 1994; 17:371–379.

57. Chelbowski RT. Nutritional support of the medical oncology patient. *Hematol/Oncol Clin North Am.* 1991; 5:147–160.

58. Tchekmedyian NS, Hickman M, Siau J, et al. Treatment of cancer cachexia with megesterol acetate: impact on quality of life. *Oncology.* 1990; 4:185–192.

59. Madison JL, Wilkie DJ. Family members' perceptions of cancer pain. Comparisons with patient sensory report and by patient psychological status. *Nurs Clin North Am.* 1995; 30:625–645.

60. Mercadante S, Armata M, Salvaggio L. Pain characteristics of advanced lung cancer patients referred to a palliative care service. *Pain.* 94; 59:141–145.

61. Trimble EL, Carter CL, Cain D, Friedlin B, Ungerleider RS, Friedman MA. Representation of older patients in cancer treatment trials. *Cancer.* 1994; 74:2208–2214.

62. Sarna L, McCorkle R. Burden of care and lung cancer. *Cancer Pract.* 1996; 4:245–251.

63. Wellisch D, Fawzy F, Landsverk J, et. al. Evaluation of psychosocial problems of the home-bound cancer patient: the relationship of disease and the sociodemographic variables of patients to family problems. *J Psychosoc Oncol.* 1983; 1:1–15.

64. Evans WK. Combination chemotherapy confers modest survival advantage in patients with advanced non-small cell lung cancer. Report of a Canadian multicenter randomized trial. *Semin Oncol.* 1988; 15:42–45.

65. Ferugusson RJ, Cull A. Quality of life measurement for patients undergoing treatment for lung cancer. *Thorax.* 1991; 46:671–675.

66. McCorkle R. The measurement of symptom distress. *Semin Oncol Nurs.* 1987; 3:234–256.

67. Hollen PJ, Gralla RJ, Kris MG, Potanovich LM. Quality of life assessment in individuals with lung cancer. testing the Lung Cancer Symptom Scale (LCSS). *Eur J Cancer.* 1993; 29A:S51–S58.

68. Hollen PJ, Gralla RJ. Comparison of instruments for measuring quality of life in patients with lung cancer. *Semin Oncol.* 1996; 23 (Suppl 5):31–40.

69. Cella DF, Bonomi AE, Lloyd SR, Tulsky DS, Kaplan E, Bonomi P. Reliability and validity of the Functional Assessment of Cancer Therapy—Lung (FACT-L) quality of life instrument. *Lung Cancer.* 1995;12:199–220.

70. Hopwood P, Stephens RJ, Machin D. Approaches to the analysis of quality of life data: experiences gained from a Medical Research Council Lung Cancer Working Party palliative chemotherapy trial. *Qual Life Res.* 1994; 3: 339–352.

71. Shopland DR, Hartman AM, Gibson JT, Mueller MD, Kessler LG, Lynn WR. Cigarette smoking among U.S. adults by state and region. estimates from the current population survey. *J Natl Cancer Inst.* 1996; 23:1748–1758.

72. Berckman KL, Austin JK. Causal attribution, perceived control, and adjustment in patients with lung cancer. *Oncol Nurs Forum.* 1993;20:23–30.

73. Faller H, Schilling S, Lang H. Causal attribution and adaptation among lung cancer patients. *J Psychsom Res.* 1995; 39:619–627.

74. Sell L, Devlin B, Bourke SJ, et al. Communicating the diagnosis of lung cancer. *Respir Med.* 1993; 87:61–63.

75. Schilling A, Conaway MR, Wingate PJ, et al. Recruiting cancer patients to participate in motivating their relatives to quit smoking. *Cancer.* 1997; 79:152–160.

76. Fiore MC, Bailey WC, Cohen SJ, et al. *Smoking Cessation.* Clinical Practice Guideline No. 18. Rockville, MD: U.S. Department of Health and Human Services, Public Health Service, Agency for Health Care Policy and Research. AHCPR Publication No. 96-0692. 60; 1996.

77. Schag CAC, Ganz PA, Wing DS, Sim MS, Lee JJ. Quality of life in adult survivors of lung, colon and prostate cancer. *Qual Life Res.* 1994; 3:127–141.

78. Bergman B, Aaronson NK. Quality-of-life and cost-effectiveness assessment in lung cancer. *Curr Opin Oncol.* 1995; 7:138–143.

79. Vergnenegre A; Perol M; Pham E. Cost analysis of hospital treatment–two chemotherapeutic regimens for non-surgical non-small cell lung cancer. *Lung Cancer.* 1996; 14:31–44.

80. Jaakkimainen L, Goodwin PJ, Pater J, Warde P, Murray N, Edna R. Counting the costs of chemotherapy in a National Cancer Institute of Canada randomized trial in non-small-cell lung cancer. *J Clin Oncol.* 1990; 8: 1301–1309.

29

Genitourinary Malignancies

ANDREW J. ROTH AND HOWARD I. SCHER

Genitourinary (GU) cancers represent the most common cancers in American men, and the second most common cause of cancer death in males (1). The effect of treatment on quality of life of patients has become more significant as survival has improved for many cancers, and as more cancers are diagnosed at an asymptomatic, curable stage. With the exception of testicular cancer, the GU cancers increase in incidence with advancing age. Thus, recognition of other life phase characteristics is important in understanding the ability of each individual patient to cope with his illness.

There are common elements to the consequences of therapy for illnesses that effect the genitalia and urinary organs. Psychosocial areas affected include body image and integrity changes, degrees of sexual dysfunction, and infertility. These compound the generic difficulties of coping with cancer, such as dealing with pain and other side effects of treatment, interruption of daily functioning, and career uncertainty. It has been estimated that 60%–75% of patients with genitourinary cancer, experience pain (2). Survivorship issues are particularly important for men with testicular cancer who are usually younger. They have to deal with various fears such as the cancer returning, the effects of having cancer on job and health insurance opportunities, and potential effects on future social and sexual relationships.

This chapter gives an overview of the medical and psychosocial aspects and their management in patients and their families as they cope with genitourinary cancers. We have placed primary attention on prostate cancer as it is the most common of these cancers, and there is more controversy over its treatment options. Discussions about coping with various aspects of prostate cancer such as sexuality are applicable to the other cancers as well.

PROSTATE CANCER

Epidemiology

Prostate cancer is the most common site of cancer in males in the United States, with an estimated 316,000 new cases in 1996, 80% of which will occur in men over 65 years old (55). This compares to 106,000 new cases in 1990. It is the most common non-skin cancer in men and the second leading cause of cancer death in men. Prostate cancer incidence rates are 32% higher for black men than white men, and the mortality rates are twice as high. This generally older population of men has particular needs determined by their specific life phases. The psychological reactions will depend on psychiatric history, and other significant life changes or events such as recent widowhood, recent or impending retirement, loss of friends or family to cancer or prostate cancer in particular, and available supports.

Nine percent of all prostate cancers are believed to be hereditary; 40% of these occur in men under the age of 55. The frequency of latent cancers is the same in Japanese and American males, but the clinical incidence increases as Japanese men move to the United States, leading some to speculate about environmental factors. Other risk factors reported include occupational exposure to different substances such as cadmium oxide, rubber, and sheet metals (3). Some nutritional factors have also been correlated with increased incidence of prostate cancer. These include caffeine, vitamin A, red meat, and a diet high in saturated fat (4).

Screening Guidelines

American Cancer Society guidelines recommend a yearly digital rectal examination (DRE) for men 40 years of age and older. After age 50, DRE should be performed along with an annual prostate specific antigen (PSA) test. Men who are at high risk, such as African Americans or those with a strong family history of prostate cancer, are advised to begin testing starting at age 40 (55). Other than self-examination for testicular cancer, it is the only GU cancer that has a reliable tool for early detection.

Diagnosis and Medical Work-up

This illness has received much publicity in the last few years because of the increased numbers of men diagnosed with it and numbers of celebrities who are making public their experiences with prostate cancer. The increased incidence of the disease is directly related to improved detection afforded by the serum prostate specific antigen test. There are many uncertainties that arise about the early detection and treatment of prostate cancer, that have implications for the psychological well-being of these men and their families. There are currently attempts to increase the availability of the PSA. However, it is controversial whether an earlier diagnosis of prostate cancer is always necessary. There are forms of prostate cancer that are relatively indolent, and will not impact on the quality or quantity of a patient's survival. However, it is difficult to distinguish these from more lethal varieties at an early stage. In the past many men would die of another cause, never knowing they had prostate cancer, with detection only occurring at autopsy. Those who were diagnosed with the disease often presented with signs of metastatic disease, such as pain and urinary problems. It is unclear whether early detection and treatment of these indolent forms is beneficial when the distress and impairment of quality of life from these treatments is taken into account (5,6). On the other hand, if one could identify a lethal variety, there would be little question that an earlier diagnosis might be beneficial.

PSA is a glycoprotein in prostatic epithelial cells needed for liquification of semen. As it leaks out into the serum, it can be measured (1). Although the test is the most sensitive assay available, it remains somewhat controversial as a broad screening tool (7). A PSA level can be normal even in the presence of cancer. It is also not cancer specific. False positive results can be seen with prostatitis, with benign prostatic hypertrophy, and with manipulation of the prostate as with transrectal ultrasound and needle biopsies (3). Improvement in the specificity of this test by evaluating the percentage of free serum PSA will help to rule out many of these false positives (8). In general, a PSA reading of less than 4 is normal, 4–10 is questionable, and greater than 10 is worrisome for cancer. However, these numbers may vary with the age of patient as well as other medical factors (9). One of the psychological distresses oncologists have noted in patients is the degree of anxiety surrounding each PSA test, and the anticipation before getting the result. This has been termed "PSA anxiety." Some men put great significance on each test and even on minuscule changes within the normal range, leading themselves and their families to needless worry. This screening test represents a symbolic totem on which many patients and their families base their futures. Some men will go to multiple laboratories to get "the best reading," which usually increases confusion and distress rather than relieving it.

CASE REPORT

A 70-year-old man who had a radical prostatectomy two years ago, was referred for psychiatric evaluation of anxiety. For the last year he would experience significant restlessness, insomnia, and anxiety for three weeks preceding his PSA test and the days before getting the results. Each test would come back in the low normal range, indicating no evidence of progressive disease. He remarked that the waiting period reminded him of his combat experience in World War II, seeing and hearing bullets fly over his head. He wondered then "How long can I beat the odds and dodge the bullets?", and now wondered similarly "When will I be hit by the PSA bullet?"

Some men feel they cope better by making graphs of their PSA scores. They put "worry time" into graph-making. For others, their charts are more reflections of how anxious they are, and become daily visual reminders of their disease, thus increasing their anxiety.

An elevated PSA or suspicious digital rectal examination for prostate cancer necessitates the following medical evaluation: transrectal ultrasound; guided needle biopsy to determine the presence of cancer, stage of disease and Gleason score (a measurement of tumor differentiation and growth pattern, ranging from 2 to 10); bone scan; and imaging for metastases.

Management/Treatment

Guidelines are currently being created to determine proper treatment for prostate cancer. To date there has not been a definitive comparative analysis of the major primary treatment options. Thus, there is still some controversy about selection of primary treatments. Differences of opinion often trickle down to patients, creating uncertainty and making their decision about treatment difficult. Primary treatment options vary from "watchful waiting" or "expectant monitoring," to surgery, radiation, and cryotherapy (10). Watchful waiting (deferred therapy) is often recommended for those with significant co-morbid illness, low-grade indolent cancers, and less than ten years life expectancy (11,12). The definitive treatment choice in the past was surgery, the radical prostatectomy. Not all urologists perform the newer "nerve-sparing" procedure that has decreased the rate of complications of impotence and urinary incontinence (13). Radiation therapy, either conventional or by seed implants (also not available in many locales), yields less incidence of impotence and urinary problems; however, there are difficulties with bowel function depending on factors of technique and total dose delivered (14).Three-dimensional conformal external radiation therapy has decreased the incidence of local complications and has increased the ability to control these cancers. Cryosurgery is another option for early-stage disease, but it has not yet been sufficiently studied against the more standard methods of treatment to be recommended on a routine basis.

One study found no difference in overall quality of life among patients receiving the surgical, radiation, or "watchful waiting" options (15). There were, understandably, compromises in quality of life when considering specific treatment-related side effects. Another study found no difference in survival among patients with low-grade prostate cancer treated with "watchful waiting" when compared to those of similar age in the general population (16). It must be emphasized that patients offered deferred therapy were highly selected and may have included men who were more able to manage the uncertainty of a nondefinitive treatment option. Tumor histologic findings and patient co-morbidities were powerful independent predictors of survival. Earlier studies had shown higher rates of progression-free survival with the surgical option, yet the data have been criticized on the basis of biased sample selection (12). There has been some experience with giving men neoadjuvant hormonal therapy prior to surgery (17) or radiation therapy, but the long-term benefits, if any, are unknown.

For more advanced disease, hormonal manipulations are used to decrease the synthesis of testosterone or its action on prostate cancer cell growth. This can be done with gonadotropin releasing hormone (GnRH) agonists such as leuprolide; with estrogenic substances such as diethylstilbestrol; with antiandrogenic agents that reduce production of testosterone in the adrenal glands, such as flutamide, or bicalutamide; or by orchiectomy (9). Equally effective in slowing tumor growth, with similar side effects profiles, medical hormonal therapy may be preferred over orchiectomy by patients because of improved body image and therefore improved quality of life (18). There are recent findings that show that antiandrogens will initially reduce tumor burden, but through an uncertain mechanism, possibly genetic mutation, may later fuel tumor growth (56). Chemotherapeutic agents are used for more advanced tumors as palliative measures.

Management of Psychological Distress

Many of the psychological issues present in men with prostate cancer are similar to those for cancer in general. Distress about choice of treatment options, including the uncertainty of watchful waiting and the potential sexual dysfunction, urinary incontinence, weakness, fatigue, pain, and other side effects of the disease or treatment, can have profound effects on mood, irritability, and anxiety. Many men often entertain multiple second opinions regarding their primary therapy, while others look to one physician to make the decision for them. Though men may often prefer to defer to the doctor, they do want to be informed and have their opinions considered by their doctors (19). Treatment choices and decisions may vary based on extent of disease, age of patient, life expectancy, specialty bias of physician, side effect risk profile acceptable to a patient, expense, and geography (20). Some men feel more comfortable with a watchful waiting approach, so that they can avoid potential side effects of surgery or radiation such as sexual or urinary dysfunction. For others whose anxiety is high, or who may come with a "take charge" attitude, and who cannot tolerate "doing nothing," the watchful waiting approach would be too difficult to tolerate. Side effects of medications used for prostate cancer, such as hormonal therapy, steroids, and pain medications, cause distress as well. The side effects of hormonal therapies can be particularly distressing for asymptomatic males, and has led to the use of intermittent hormonal therapy to decrease the morbidity of therapy.

An awareness of these problems and attempts at resolving them, or helping patients cope better with them, can significantly reduce psychological tension. However, there may be considerable variations between the patient's and doctor's evaluation of performance status, pain, and pain relief that reduce optimal symptom control (12). Most physicians do not ask how a couple is coping and fail to recognize when men or their spouses are having problems.

DIFFICULTIES WITH SEXUAL FUNCTIONING. This occurs from aging, the cancer itself and treatments by surgery, radiation, and hormonal therapy (22). Hormonal therapy, in particular, eliminates libido, though newer drugs are available that are equally effective yet less disruptive to the intimacy of relations. Coupled with impotence, feelings of being emasculated occur. Often the degree of distress about sexual difficulties after treatment is correlated with sexual functioning before treatment. Therefore, an honest or realistic discussion of prior sexual functioning may assist a man in choosing a treatment option.

CASE REPORT

A 75-year-old retired physician, married for 43 years, was quite proud of his sex life. Within months of starting hormonal treatment he could no longer get a full erection, which upset him very much. He suddenly felt like a failure in his relationship, despite having a very supportive and understanding wife. He canceled an annual trip to Europe with his wife, because he felt the trip could not be as romantic as it was in the past, and he did not want to ruin the memories. He was referred for a consultation with a urologist, who recommended injection of a vasoactive substance, papavarine. He was quite satisfied with the results.

URINARY INCONTINENCE. This occurs as a complication of surgery and radiation (9). Loss of urinary continence leads men to shun social contact. The fear of urine leaking, of smelling of urine, and of having to use diapers is humiliating.

CASE REPORT

A 68-year-old retired attorney was referred to the psychiatrist for depression. His wife noted that as his urinary incontinence worsened, he refused to go out socially with friends. He had been an active tennis player, and enjoyed theater, however a few leakage accidents led him to spend so much time making preparations and contingency plans before he would go outside that he eventually felt it was not worth the effort. To his family and friends, he looked depressed as he stopped doing the activities he had enjoyed so much. His anxiety was relieved with several psychotherapy visits, and paroxetine 10 mg per day improved his mood and social withdrawal.

Urologists and their staffs can work with patients to identify etiologies of incontinence, to educate patients and families about the incontinence, and to offer suggestions to alleviate or reduce symptoms. Three types of urinary incontinence following prostatectomy are stress, urge, and mixed varieties (24). Interventions depend on the type of incontinence. They include pelvic muscle reeducation, bladder training, and anticholinergic medications.

PAIN. Pain is often a symptom of advanced disease which can be difficult to control. Pain syndromes result from local expansion and inflammation of the prostate gland; pain referred to the back, lower extremities, and abdominal area from local tumor growth; and distant bone pain from long bone, vertebral, and skull metastases. Pain not only impairs mobility but also accompanies neurologic impairments such as cranial nerve deficits, paralysis, incontinence of bowel and bladder, and impotence (25). Patients with pain are significantly more depressed or anxious when compared with patients without pain; these mood changes may not be related to extent of disease (26–28). However, older men are often reluctant to take pain medications or dosages adequate to truly help. It is not clear to what degree this relates to a fear of side effects, such as constipation and fatigue, that may inhibit functioning or to a machismo attitude of feeling compelled to endure the pain.

CASE REPORT

A 72-year-old man was evaluated for suicidal ideation. After living with his cancer for 11 years, he told us "Life is not worth suffering through, putting up with the kind of pain I face daily." He was taking only a small amount of morphine because he did not like the sedated feeling he got from it. Increase of his opioid dose with long-acting oral morphine 30 mg twice daily and rescues of Dilaudid 2 mg as needed led to control of the pain. Suicidal ideation disappeared.

WEAKNESS AND FATIGUE. These symptoms are particularly upsetting to men who have led active and independent lives. They usually result in increased dependence on family or friends, which are further reminders of the contrast with how they were before the cancer. Fatigue and weakness can be caused by the illness, hormonal therapy, pain medication, steroids, and other factors (29). Helping the patient to reorganize his schedule and set realistic goals may result in less distress. A psychostimulant, such as pemoline titrated from 37.5 mg per day or ritalin titrated from 5 mg per day in two divided doses early in the day, may counter the sedating effects of opioids, increase motivation, enhance appetite, and elevate a patient's mood. If a depression is present, activating antidepressants such as fluoxetine or buproprion can be used.

HOT FLASHES. In men, hot flashes are caused by many of the hormonal therapies, including orchiectomy. They are the result of increased vasomotor activity that leads to diaphoresis, feelings of intense heat, and chills, similar to symptoms that women have during menopause. At times hormonal therapy must be stopped because of the effect these flashes cause in terms of drenching sweat and discomfort. This has led to a strategy of intermittent hormonal use to decrease the side effect burden, although it is unclear how this may affect tumor progression. Megestrol acetate and other medications have helped relieve many of these symptoms (30,31); however, some oncologists will not use megestrol fearing that the same paradoxical result seen with other hormones may at some point fuel the growth of the tumor, similar to the effect seen with antiandrogens.

There have been anecdotal reports of antidepressants, particularly the serotonin reuptake inhibitors, reducing the frequency and intensity of hot flashes, but this has not been studied in a systematic way. It is not clear whether they relieve the distress of having the hot flash symptoms or work in some way to alleviate the flashes themselves. Changes in habits that stimulate onset of the hot flashes, such as decreasing caffeine, alcohol, and hot fluid intake may be useful.

CASE REPORT

A.A. was a 64-year-old businessman with prostate cancer treated with leuprolide and flutamide for three years. He noted some time after his hormonal therapy began that his mood became depressed and his energy decreased. Although never a good sleeper, he had worsening of his insomnia as well as mild anhedonia. He described mild, intermittent periods of anxiety related to his work. He had significant distress from hot flashes five to ten times per day and night. He had no past family or personal history of psychiatric disorder. His medical history was significant for hypertension, for which he took nifedipine. The patient was started on sertraline 25 mg per day and titrated to 100 mg over six weeks. His mood improved as did his energy. The patient noted a significant decrease in the frequency and intensity of his hot flashes with decreased duration of each flash.

In general, men with prostate cancer respond to education and various kinds of brief psychotherapy, including supportive, cognitive-behavioral, and insight-oriented therapies. Unfortunately, some men are reluctant to participate in therapy, particularly if they have never done so previously. There are support groups available specifically for men with prostate cancer. Two of the national support groups available to men are "Us Too" and "Man to Man."

At a time when a couple's communication needs to be at its best, it is often at its worst because of the stress of the situation.

CASE REPORT

A 78-year-old retired teacher with late-stage prostate cancer and atrial fibrillation was asked by his wife to see a psychiatrist for depression. The wife was concerned because the husband did not feel like doing anything pleasurable anymore: "I know he's tired, but there are some things that don't take much energy." Husband and wife were seen together by the psychiatrist. The wife continued, "He used to play the piano, but in the last few months he stopped." The husband added, "Actually I do still play, but I wait for you to leave the house." The wife was surprised and hurt, and her eyes begged an explanation. He continued, "I don't play as well as I used to and I'm ashamed of that. I just feel too tired." The wife answered, "The truth is you were never that great a pianist, but it really was a pleasure for me to listen to you. However you play, I know it's a sign that you're alive and have life." This was an important breakthrough for the couple, as was fluoxetine to counter the depressed mood and fatigue.

Older men tend to be uncomfortable sharing emotions. They often have a need to be seen as the protector and provider for the family, however incompatible this is with the reality of their physical deterioration. It has been noted that spouses suffer significant distress coping with their husbands' cancer (28). Family members are often concerned when they see the suffering

and pain in the movements of these patients, yet often feel powerless to change the course of events. For those men who are particularly bothered by sexual dysfunction, sex therapy with a trained therapist can help a man express the feelings engendered by this dysfunction, and also to help a couple learn alternative ways of sharing sexual intimacy. Couple's counseling can improve the ability of spouses to cope with the cancer together. These options are also useful for those with other genitourinary cancers that affect sexuality.

TESTICULAR CANCER

Epidemiology

Testicular cancer is the most common cancer in American men between the ages of 20 and 34, though it accounts for only about 1% of all male cancers (32). It is considerably more common in Caucasian than African-American men, with intermediate rates for Hispanics, Native Americans, and Asians.

The causes of testicular cancer are still not well understood. One major known risk factor is cryptorchidism, the congenital failure of one or both testes to descend into the scrotal sac (33). This risk factor is overcome if surgical repair of the condition is performed before the age of 6 years. Other congenital conditions that have been associated with testicular cancer are Klinefelter's syndrome, gonadal aplasia, and various forms of hermaphroditism. Other associative factors that have been suggested, but not confirmed, include infections of testicular tissue; incidence of unusual bleeding or spotting during mothers' pregnancies; exposure of mothers to exogenous estrogens, alcohol, or X-rays during pregnancy; and history of testicular cancer in the family.

Diagnosis and Medical Work-up

Testicular self-examination is the most common form of detection of this cancer, usually with the presence of a small, hard lump in either testicle, an enlarged testicle, a collection of fluid, or unusual pain. However, most patients will first seek medical attention because of development of a painless, swollen testis. The most frequent symptom from metastatic disease is back pain from tumor in the retroperitoneum. Pulmonary complaints such as shortness of breath, chest pain, or hemoptysis occur due to advanced lung metastases (33). The latter are rare and more men are detected early!

The standard diagnostic procedure, after ruling out infection or other disease by urinalysis and urine culture, is to remove the affected testis via inguinal orchiectomy. Biopsy is not possible in this disease because of the fear of spread of cancer cells during the procedure. Orchiectomy also prevents further growth of the primary tumor. Germ cell cancers, seminomas and nonseminomas account for the bulk of these tumors. Staging of the extent of disease to develop a treatment plan is accomplished by several methods. Imaging techniques, such as X-rays, computed tomography, magnetic resonance imaging scans, ultrasonography, and intravenous pyelography, can locate disease throughout the body. The tumor markers α-fetoprotein (AFP), β-human chorionic gonadotropin (B-HCG), and lactate dehydrogenase (LDH), are used for detection of small tumors, and for comparison over time to see response to treatment. Retroperitoneal lymph node dissection (RPLND) is used to examine nonseminomatous tumor spread to lymphatic tissue. This procedure is often associated with ejaculatory dysfunction, though newer nerve sparing procedures may preserve normal ejaculation.

Medical Management/Treatment

Survival in this population has significantly improved in recent years owing to improved diagnostic and treatment techniques. Cure rates for seminomas exceed 95 percent. Cure rates of nonseminomas have increased to between 75% and 95%, depending on the stage of disease. It is felt that approximately 75% of men with advanced testicular cancer can be cured. Treatment differs for seminomatous and nonseminomatous tumors, as well as stage of disease. Early-stage seminomatous disease is treated with orchiectomy and radiation therapy. Treatment of moderate disease will combine orchiectomy with either radiation or chemotherapy. More advanced disease is treated with orchiectomy and multidrug chemotherapy. Common regimens of chemotherapies include *(1)* bleomycin, etoposide, and cisplatin (BEP); or *(2)* etoposide and cisplatin (EP).

Nonseminomas have often metastasized at the time of clinical presentation. Early and moderate stage disease can be treated with orchiectomy alone, or followed by chemotherapy. Chemotherapy regimens similar to those used in seminoma tumors may be used in advanced-stage nonseminoma treatment.

High-dose chemotherapy with autologous bone marrow transplantation is currently being investigated for refractory germ cell cancer and has been found to improve survival for some patients (34).

Management of Psychosocial Issues

As with prostate cancer, many of the psychosocial stressors are related to coping with side effects of the cancer therapy. However, this tumor occurs in young men when sexuality, fertility, and intimacy are critically important. Although unilateral orchiectomy does not lead to infertility or sexual dysfunction, men are often concerned about their appearance. Artificial testicular implants have been successful in helping men cope with this issue. Retroperitoneal lymph node dissection can lead to infertility by causing retrograde ejaculation, though sexual desire and ability to have erections and orgasms are not affected. However, a pattern of sexual avoidance and decreased sexual interest can develop related to the distress of the cancer treatment in general. Couple's therapy can address these issues. It can help a couple develop understanding of these problems and new coping mechanisms for them. It can also help the couple gain some perspective on how their relationship has been changed by cancer.

Infertility can be related to surgery, with retroperitoneal lymph node dissection posing the greatest threat by interfering with ejaculation. Infertility can also be due to radiotherapy or chemotherapy. Many men with testicular cancer have been found to have low sperm counts even prior to diagnosis, perhaps due to an autoimmune process. This process is probably confined to the few months just prior to diagnosis. Unfortunately, this can limit the usefulness of sperm banking at the time of diagnosis. Antegrade ejaculation may return spontaneously over the months or years following surgery. If it does not, administration of sympathomimetic drugs can convert retrograde to antegrade ejaculation. Sperm production can also be affected by radiation therapy. Infertility from this degree of radiation is temporary in most patients.

Chemotherapeutic agents such as cyclophosphamide can also cause infertility, though this may last for a transient period of 2–3 years after completing chemotherapy. However, this is not used as a primary therapy very much in the United States. One study showed that at least one-third of patients treated with chemotherapy alone have been able to successfully father children without increased evidence of congenital anomalies (35).

Psychologically, the impact of this illness can affect key aspects of a young man's life or a young couple's relationship. Its presentation at the peak of a young male adult's development leads to heightened risk of depression, anxiety, anticipation of pain, bodily trauma, and death. Apart from infertility, fears about the effects on sexual functioning need to be addressed, especially before a young man has been involved in a long-term sexual relationship. Decreased sexual activity and diminished intensity of orgasm have been most often noted (36,37). Thorough sexual histories should include questions about frequency and intensity of sexual activity, desire, erection, orgasm, and satisfaction (38).

Surviving patients have to be concerned with late complications of curative therapy, as is seen in other malignancies, as well as fears of recurrence (39). (See Chapter 20 by Kornblith on cancer survivors.) Compromised renal function from cisplatin nephrotoxicity, Raynaud's phenomenon following combinations of vinblastine and bleomycin, and neuropathy and ototoxicity attributable to cisplatin and vinblastine leave patients with secondary deficits that challenge their daily living. Though there is concern about the possibility of therapy-related second malignancies, the risk does not seem to increase with administration of short course, intensive chemotherapy (33).

BLADDER CANCER

Epidemiology

There will be an estimated 50,500 new cases of bladder cancer diagnosed in 1996 (55). The majority of these cases will occur in men (38,300 vs. 14,600). The incidence is greater in whites than in blacks.

The largest known risk factor is tobacco smoking, leading to twice the number of cases relative to those who do not smoke. Other risk factors include exposure to dyes, rubber, or leather. There are no good tests for early detection of bladder cancer. Most of these cancers are detected because they cause grossly visible or microscopic hematuria. It is usually diagnosed with cystoscopy. The vast majority of these cancers are transitional cell carcinomas (TCC) (1). Unlike prostate cancer, bladder cancer is unlikely to be found incidentally at autopsy, indicating that it is likely to cause symptoms or other significant problems at some time during a patient's life. Disease stage has been shown to be the single best predictor of outcome for TCC of the bladder (40).

Diagnosis and Management

There is more of a consensus about the diagnostic work-up and treatment plan for bladder cancer than for other GU cancers. Transurethral resection is the primary modality for diagnosis of these tumors and is also the definitive treatment for low-grade and superficial tumors. Surgery, alone or in combination with other treatments, is used in over 90% of cases. Preoperative chemotherapy alone or with radiation before cystectomy has improved some treatment results for more advanced tumors. Although radiotherapy is controversial in some patients with bladder cancer, one study found no difference in the quality of life of patients after radical radiotherapy versus a similar

control group (41). There is an attempt to avoid or postpone cystectomy for localized, noninvasive bladder cancers with treatment by local means, though this may require long-term follow up with repeated cystoscopies. It remains to be seen what effect the presence of the *P53* gene with bladder cancer will have upon treatment options. If detected at an early stage, the 5-year survival rate is 93%. For more advanced disease, the survival rates are between 6% and 49%, depending on extent of disease (55).

Radical cystectomy impacts sexual and urinary functioning in men in a similar fashion to radical prostatectomy. A large proportion of men have suffered erectile impotence, though the incidence is decreasing with nerve sparing techniques. Testosterone secretion is unimpaired, so sexual desire remains unchanged. Ileal loop diversion with creation of a permanent stoma necessitates consideration of concerns about odor, leakage, spills, and embarrassment (42). These concerns impact patients' feelings about their sexuality as well as their sexual partners. Patients have reported significant impact on their lives outside the home, impeding social and occupational functioning (43,44). Again, reactions such as anxiety, depressed mood, and social isolation are similar to patients with prostate cancer who face similar disruptions in their lives. Many patients have been helped by the internal development of urinary reservoirs constructed from bowel. These can be anastomosed to either the skin or urethra. When attached to the urethra, continence can be maintained. This has permitted the creation of the neobladder, with which almost all patients achieve daytime urinary continence (1,45). Although complications are higher than with the conduit, these procedures obviate the need for an appliance.

Women make a better adjustment to the presence of a stoma than do men; this is perhaps related to their being more independent in their stoma care than men. Radical cystectomy in women also includes hysterectomy and oophorectomy and resection of the anterior wall of the vagina. The major sexual side effect for women is genital pain, particularly during intercourse. Use of vaginal dilators, lubricants, and estrogen creams can help women become more comfortable during sexual activity by overcoming the consequences of scarring and premature menopause (46).

Agents used for bladder carcinomas are the immune modulator Bacillus Calmette-Guerin (BCG), and chemotherapeutic agents such as thiotepa, mutamycin, adriamycin, and epodyl, usually given by the intravesical route. Cystitis is often an uncomfortable side effect of these treatments. Advanced-disease transitional cell carcinoma is usually treated with systemic chemotherapy, usually a combination of cisplatin, methotrexate, and vinblastine with or without adriamycin; or a taxol-based combination.

RENAL CARCINOMA

Epidemiology

Renal cell carcinoma is the most common neoplastic lesion of the kidney. Often the diagnosis is made incidentally at the time of radiographic procedures such as ultrasonography or a CT scan for nonneurologic problems (47). About 28,000 patients will be diagnosed with this cancer per year, and more than 11,500 will die of the disease (48). The incidence rises with age, as with transitional cell carcinoma of the bladder and prostate cancer. Renal cell carcinoma is almost twice as common in men as in women. There does not appear to be strong evidence of environmental or racial factors that increase the incidence of these cancers, though there has been some association with cigarette smoking, obesity, and exposure to lead phosphate, dimethyl nitrosamine, and aflatoxins. Von Hippel–Lindau disease is also associated with renal cell carcinoma (47). A large percentage of these cancers may remain undiagnosed during life as for prostate cancer; however, with renal cancers a significant proportion of those found incidentally at autopsy actually cause death (1).

Twenty-five percent of new cases have overt metastatic disease at the time of diagnosis (49). Prognosis of these patients is bleak, with a median survival of 10 months. For the remaining cases, in whom the disease appears to be localized, the treatment of choice is radical nephrectomy. However, one-third of these patients (25% of the total) will later manifest metastatic disease and ultimately succumb to their cancer (50).

Diagnosis and Management

Patients' presentations may range from the infrequent triad of hematuria, pain, and palpable renal mass, to more obscure paraneoplastic syndromes, fever, anemia, or polycythemia. Diagnosis is made by IVP, ultrasound, renal arteriography, CT scans, and MRI. Initial evaluations include chest X-rays to evaluate potential sites of pulmonary metastases. Pathologic staging is the most important determinant of prognosis.

The treatment of choice is surgical removal of the affected kidney, with regional lymphadenectomy. Five-year survival for stage I disease ranges from 60% to 75%, and from 40% to 65% in those with stage II disease (47). Survival is greatly diminished with lymph node involvement, as there is no effective treatment for metastatic renal cell carcinoma. Renal preser-

vation with only partial excision of renal tissue has become more widely accepted, though there is still controversy about long-term prognosis. Postoperative pain can be distressing. Its treatment can provide challenges because of compromised renal function.

To date, chemotherapeutic agents have not demonstrated sufficient antitumor activity to prolong the survival of patients with metastatic disease. Many drugs have been evaluated, yet all have demonstrated poor response rates (50). Development of new diagnostic and therapeutic modalities is therefore of utmost importance.

There is hope for immunotherapy, autolymphocyte therapy, vaccines, and nonspecific immunomodulators prolonging survival in patients with metastatic renal disease (51). Interferon and interleukin-2 in particular have been used with some success in treating advanced renal cancer (52,53). However, these two agents can cause depression and anxiety, which may be mediated through physical or somatic side effects such as fatigue and fever. Delirium may also be seen as an independent effect on the central nervous system (54).

The poor prognosis for this illness is cause for much psychological distress experienced by many patients and their families after diagnosis. Later stages of disease are highlighted by metastases to bone, lungs, and brain, and necessitates coping with pain, shortness of breath, concentration deficits, and other cognitive difficulties. As the disease progresses, anticipatory bereavement becomes a pertinent challenge. It is complicated by the fact that there may be periods when the person is free of disease after surgery but has the knowledge that recurrence is likely. The conflict of maintaining hope for successful treatment, while understanding discouraging odds, can be burdensome and can lead to various degrees of anxiety and depression.

SUMMARY

The genitourinary neoplasms are affecting a larger proportion of our population as detection methods are improving. The illnesses and treatments affect patients' quality of life in multiple spheres. Physical symptoms such as pain, fatigue, sexual dysfunction, and anorexia as a result of these cancers lead to psychological distress and irritability as with other cancers. Most prominent issues in this population include coping with changes in sexuality, bladder and bowel function, body image, relationships, and lifestyle. Assessment of these problems is not easy, particularly in distinguishing between physical and psychological etiologies of distress. Discomfort and beliefs about stigma on the part of the patient, the family, and the health care provider in discussing these issues provide formidable barriers to evaluation and resolution of distress. Although there are fears that acknowledging and addressing psychological issues will make these symptoms worse, psychological interventions provide avenues for decreased stress and improved quality of living. This may be especially true for those people dealing with survivorship issued as they attempt to reintegrate into a world after cancer. Avoiding these issues leads to increased suffering, major psychiatric disorders and feelings of despair, isolation, hopelessness, and suicidal ideation.

Medical caregivers should have a low threshold for assessment of these problems as well as referral to mental health practitioners. Once assessed, management of these areas includes a spectrum of psychologic and psychiatric interventions that includes education, individual and group psychotherapy, couples therapy, behavioral interventions, and medications. These referrals may be facilitated by increased knowledge on the part of the mental health practitioner about the illness and treatment-specific stressors, as well as a physically closer liaison with the genitourinary oncology clinic.

REFERENCES

1. Bossinger SO, Messing EM. Genitourinary cancer: early stage cancers of the prostate, bladder and kidney. In: Brain MC, Carbone P, eds. *Current Therapy in Hematology-Oncology*. 1995: 423–436.

2. Twycross R, Lack S. *Symptoms Central in Far Advanced Cancer*. London: Pitman; 1983: 3–14.

3. Vaughan ED, Girardi SK. Current approaches to the diagnosis and treatment of prostate cancer. *Dir Psychiatry*. 1994; 14.

4. Wang Y, Corr JG, Thaler HT, et al. Decreased growth of established human prostate LNCap tumors in nude mice fed a low-fat diet. *J Nat Cancer Inst*. 1995; 87:1456–1462.

5. Mokulis J, Thompson I. Screening for prostate cancer: pros, cons, and reality. *Cancer Control*. 1995; Jan/Feb:15–21.

6. Krahn MD, Mahoney JE, Eckman MH, et al. Screening for prostate cancer, a decision analytic view. *J Am Med Assoc*. 1994; 272:773–780.

7. Garnick MB. Prostate cancer: screening, diagnosis, and management. *Ann Intern Med*. 1993; 118:804–818.

8. Catalona, WJ, Smith DS, Wolfert RL, et al. Evaluation of percentage of free serum prostate-specific antigen to improve specificity of prostate cancer screening, *J Am Med Assoc*. 1995; 274:1214–1220.

9. Trump DL, Robertson CN. Neoplasms of the prostate. In: Holland JF, Frei E III, Bast RL Jr, et al., eds. *Cancer Medicine*. 3d ed. Philadelphia: Lea & Febiger; 1993; 1562–1585.

10. Kelly WK, Scher HI. Prostate cancer: how can a common disease be so controversial? *Curr Sci*. 1994; 318–331.

11. Whitmore WF, Warner JA, Thompson IM. Expectant monitoring of localized prostatic cancer. *Cancer*. 1991; 67:1091–1096.

12. Catalona WJ. Management of cancer of the prostate. *N Engl J Med*. 1994; 331:996–1004.

13. Garnick MB. The dilemmas of prostate cancer. *Sci Am*. 1994; 72–81.

14. Leibel SA, Zelefsky MJ, Kutcher GJ, et al. The biological basis and clinical application of three-dimensional conformal external beam radiation therapy in carcinoma of the prostate. *Semin Oncol*. 1994; 21:580–597.

15. Litwin MS, Hays RD, Fink A, et al. Quality of life outcomes in men treated for localized prostate cancer. *J Am Med Assoc*. 1995; 273:129–135.

16. Albertsen PC, Gryback DG, Storer BE, et al. Long-term survival among men with conservatively treated localized prostate cancer. *J Am Med Assoc*. 1995; 274:626–631.

17. Fair WR, Cookson MS, Stroumbakis N, et al. Update on neoadjuvant androgen deprivation therapy and radical prostatectomy in localized prostate cancer. *Proc Am Urol Assoc*. 1996; 155:667A.

18. Cassileth BR, Soloway MS, Vogelzang NJ, et al. Quality of life and psychosocial status in stage D prostate cancer. *Qual Life Res*. 1992; 1:323–329.

19. Davison, BJ, Degner LF, Morgan TR. Information and decision-making preferences of men with prostate cancer. *Oncol Nurs Forum*. 1995; 22:1401–1408.

20. Harlan L, Brawley O, Pommerenke F, et al. Geographic, age, and racial variation in the treatment of local/regional carcinoma of the prostate. *J Clin Oncol*. 1995; 13:93–100.

21. Fossa SD, Aaronson NK, Newling D, et al. Quality of life and treatment of hormone resistant metastatic prostatic cancer. *Eur J Cancer*. 1990; 26:1133–1136.

22. Ofman, US. Sexual quality of life in men with prostate cancer. *Cancer (Suppl)*. 1994; 75:1949–1953.

23. Singer PA, Tasch ES, Stocking C, et al. Sex or survival: trade-offs between quality and quantity or life. *J Clin Oncol*. 1991; 9:328–334.

24. Pickett M, Cooley ME, Patterson J, McCorkle R. Needs of newly diagnosed prostate cancer patients and their spouses: recommendations for postsurgical care at home. *Home HealthCare Consult*. 1996; 3:1A–12A.

25. Payne R. Pain management in the patient with prostate cancer. *Cancer (Suppl)*. 1993; 71:1131–1137.

26. Heim HM, Oei TPS. Comparison of prostate cancer patients with and without pain. *Pain*. 1993; 53:159–162.

27. Daut RL, Cleeland CS. The prevalance and severity of pain in cancer. *Cancer*. 1982; 50:1913–1918.

28. Kornblith AB, Herr HW, et al. Quality of life of patients with prostate cancer and their spouses. *Cancer*. 1994; 73:2791–2802.

29. da Silva FC, Reis E, Costa T, et al. Quality of life in patients with prostate cancer. *Cancer*. 1993; 71:1138–1142.

30. Loprinzi CL. Michalak JC, et al. Megestrol acetate for the prevention of hot flashes. *N Engl J Med*. 1994; 331:347–352.

31. Smith JA Jr. A prospective comparison of treatments for symptomatic hot flushes following endocrine therapy for carcinoma of the prostate. *J Urol*. 1994; 152:132–134.

32. Frank IN, Graham SD Jr, Nabors WL. Urologic and male genital cancers. In: Holleb AJ, Fink DJ, Murphy

GP, eds. *American Cancer Society Textbook of Clinical Oncology.* American Cancer Society; 1991.

33. Roth BJ, Nichols Cr, Einhorn LH. Neoplasms of the testis. In: Holland JF, Frei E III, Bast RL Jr, et al, eds. *Cancer Medicine.* 3d ed. Philadelphia: Lea & Febiger; 1993: 1592–1619.

34. Broun ER, Nichols CR, Turns MA, et al. Early salvage therapy for germ cell cancer using high dose chemotherapy with autologous bone marrow support. *Cancer.* 1994; 73:1716–1720.

35. Roth B, Greist A, Kubilis P, et al. Cis-platin based combination chemotherapy for disseminated germ cell tumors: long term follow-up. *J Clin Oncol.* 1988; 6:1239.

36. Rieker P, Edbril SD, Garnick MB. Curative testis cancer therapy: psychosocial sequelae. *J Clin Oncol.* 1985; 3:1117–1126.

37. Schover LR, Gonzalez M, von Eschenbach AC. Sexual and marital relationship after radiotherapy for seminoma. *Urology.* 1986; 27:117–123.

38. Tross S. Psychological adjustment in testicular cancer. In: Holland JC, Rowland JH, eds. *Handbook of Psychooncology.* New York: Oxford University Press; 1989: 240–245.

39. Gorzynski G, Holland JC. Psychological aspects of testicular cancer. *Semin Oncol.* 1979; 6:25–29.

40. Macfarlane MT, Figlin RA, de Kernion JB. Neoplasms of the bladder. In: Holland JF, Frei E III, Bast RL Jr, et al, eds. *Cancer Medicine.* 3d ed. Philadelphia: Lea & Febiger; 1993: 1546–1558.

41. Lynch WJ, Jenkins BJ, Fowler CG, et al. The quality of life after radical radiotherapy for bladder cancer. *Br J Urol.* 1992; 70:519–521.

42. Schover LR, Von Eschenbach AC. Sexual function and female radical cystectomy: a case series. *J Urol.* 1985; 134:465–468.

43. Mansson A, Johnson G, Mansson W. Psychosocial adjustment to cystectomy for bladder carcinoma and effects on interpersonal relationships. *Scand J Caring Sci.* 1991; 5:129–134.

44. Fossa SD, Reitan JB, Ous S, Kaalhus O. Life with an ileal conduit in cystectomized bladder cancer patients: expectation and experience. *Scand J Urol Nephrol.* 1987; 21:97–101.

45. Ganz P. Long-range effect of clinical trial interventions on quality of life. *Cancer (Suppl).* 1994; 74:2620–2624.

46. Ofman U. Preservation of function in genitourinary cancers: psychosexual and psychological issues. *Cancer Invest.* 1995; 13:125–131.

47. Richie JP. Renal cell carcinoma. In: Holland JF, Frei E III, Bast RL Jr, et al. *Cancer Medicine.* 3d ed. Philadelphia: Lea & Febiger; 1993: 1529–1538.

48. Parker SL, Tong T, Bolden S, Wingo PA. Cancer statistics. *CA Cancer J Clin.* 1996; 46:5–27.

49. Novick AC. Current surgical approaches, nephron-sparing surgery, and the role of surgery in the integrated immunologic approach to renal cell carcinoma. *Semin Oncol.* 1995; 22:29–33.

50. Yagoda A, Abi-Rached B, petrylak D. Chemotherapy for advanced renal cell carcinoma. *Semin Oncol.* 1995; 22:42–60.

51. Osband ME, Lavin PT, Babayan RK, et al. Effect of autolymphocyte therapy on survival and quality of life in patients with metastatic renal-cell carcinoma. *Lancet.* 1990; 335:994–998.

52. Rosenberg SA, Lotze MT, Yang JC, et al. Combination therapy with interleukin-2 and alpha-interferon for the treatment of patients with advanced cancer. *J Clin Oncol.* 1989; 7:1863–1874.

53. Linehan WM, Shipley WU, Parkinson DR. Cancer of the kidney and ureter. In: DeVita VT Jr, Hellman S, Rosenberg SA, eds. *Cancer.* Cancer: Principles and Practice of Oncology, 4th ed Philadelphia: Lippincott; 1993: 1023–1049.

54. Smith MJ, Mouawad R, Vuillemin E, et al. Psychological side effects induced by interleukin-2/alpha interferon treatment. *Psycho-Oncology.* 1994; 3:289–298.

55. American Cancer Society. *Cancer Facts & Figures—1996.* Atlanta, GA: American Cancer Society; 1996.

56. Kelly WK, Scher HI. Prostate specific antigen decline after antiandrogen withdrawal: the flutamide withdrawal syndrome. *J Urol.* 1993; 149:607–609.

30

Gynecologic Cancer

SARAH S. AUCHINCLOSS AND CHERYL F. McCARTNEY

Gynecologic cancer is diagnosed in approximately 80,000 women a year (1), and includes cancer of the ovary, fallopian tube, uterine corpus, cervix, vagina, and vulva. The gynecologic cancers as a group most commonly present in older women, but may be diagnosed at any time in the life cycle. This group of tumors has long held the deep respect of oncology professionals, as effective treatment and significant cure rates were difficult to establish. Of the gynecologic cancers, a screening test is available only for early cervix cancer. Many gynecologic cancers produce few or no symptoms until the tumor is advanced. Symptoms may include abdominal discomfort, distention, vaginal bleeding between menses or after menopause, abdominal or low back pain, pain during sex (dyspareunia), or changed bowel or bladder function. Women often delay seeking evaluation because the initial symptoms may be mild, or familiar from another context; for example, the early mild abdominal discomfort or bloating of ovarian cancer may be mistaken for constipation or premenstrual tension, or a small amount of intermenstrual bleeding may be thought to be innocuous, even over a period of months. Physicians or health care givers who are unfamiliar with the signs and symptoms of gynecologic cancer, or who have a low index of suspicion with an otherwise healthy younger patient, may defer a work-up, suggesting observation, or miss early signs on examination. As a result, the natural tendency of the gynecologic cancers to present late is compounded by reluctance to seek care in some cases and reluctance to pursue diagnosis aggressively in others; treatment starting with diagnosis of advanced-stage cancer is a common clinical challenge in this area.

Treatment of ovarian cancer ordinarily includes initial surgery followed by chemotherapy, and/or radiation. Uterine and cervix cancer utilize surgery and radiation therapy, though chemotherapy is becoming more important. Vulvar cancer is still primarily treated with surgery. The woman with gynecologic cancer often receives multiple treatment modalities; her treatment is often a sequence of treatments. She then lives with side effects not just of surgery, but cumulatively of chemotherapy and/or radiation therapy as well. The cancer and its treatment effects will ordinarily change her hormonal, sexual, reproductive, and often bowel and bladder function as well as her psychological state and social ties. Her relationship to the oncology team and their understanding and support are crucial to her recovery.

Advances in the treatment of gynecologic cancer during the 1980s and 1990s now offer women an improved chance of a good outcome, and further advances and refinements are evolving steadily. Still, the experience of the diagnosis and treatment of gynecologic cancer remains an enormous physical and psychological challenge for the individual woman and for those who care about her. Oncology clinicians have always been aware of the special needs of these women, although specialized support resources within the oncology field have been limited in the past and, with the advent of managed care, may continue to be so. However, in the past few years more psychosocial research has been devoted to the impact of this group of cancers. Grassroots and lay support organizations for gynecologic cancer patients and survivors have begun to develop, using various formats (group, newsletter, audio cassette, Internet) to link women with gynecologic cancer through treatment information, supports, and referral services. More media attention has focused on the gynecologic cancers as more women with public stature acknowledge their experience with the disease. All this serves to improve the psychological experience of a woman with gynecologic cancer by diminishing her experience of loneliness and increasing the information and support available to her, as well as improving the knowledge of gynecologic cancer in people around her.

This chapter will offer first a brief review of the issues that affect all women with gynecologic cancer and their care givers. Each tumor site will then be discussed, with reference to the recent medical literature in each site, and with clinical vignettes to illustrate specific clinical issues. The use of the various psychosocial interventions will then be reviewed: psychotherapy, groups, self-help, couple counseling, and sexual counseling, with resources provided. Finally, new research directions in gynecologic oncology will be explored.

Cancer treatment creates many challenges for patient and care giver which are universal across cancer types, and not specific to the experience of gynecologic cancer. These include the crisis of diagnosis; the inception, carrying out, and completion of treatment; cancer survivorship; the painful dilemmas of recurrence; advancing illness and palliative care; dying, death, and bereavement. The management of the common clinical concerns of these phases, and the psychosocial issues that accompany them, is covered elsewhere in this text.

GYNECOLOGIC CANCER: ISSUES ACROSS ALL SITES

Stigma and Loneliness

Gynecologic cancer carries a measure of social stigma, probably related to its historically poor prognosis and to its presence in the site of female sexual response and reproduction. While the perception of breast cancer has modified in past years, the gynecologic tumors remain little understood and much feared by the lay public; the diagnosis of gynecologic cancer may still be equated with a death sentence. Women with gynecologic cancer often refrain from openly discussing their treatment, speaking only to family or a few close friends; irrational feelings of shame, embarrassment, and guilt may remain powerful for years. Even a woman who feels no shame may not wish anyone to speculate about her cancer's effect on her sexuality or reproductive future.

As a result, the woman treated for gynecologic cancer is often keenly lonely. She may know no other woman who has been treated, except those she meets in a treatment setting. She may try to find support resources for gynecologic cancer and come up empty-handed. Groups for cancer patients may not address her concerns with menopause, sexuality, or fertility; breast cancer patients have more varied resources. She will indubitably experience estranging social responses to her illness and treatment ("Ovarian? Like Gilda Radner?"); this confirms her isolation.

She will need encouragement from gynecologic oncology professionals and mental health professionals in her search for local cancer support groups, networks, and supportive connections, including newsletters or audio cassette series (Voices in the Night); these formats are of great value in reducing loneliness and helping women come to terms with their new realities with strength, grace, and humor.

In addition to medical knowledge and expertise, the oncology professional tries to provide for his or her patients steady support, emotional sensitivity, good humor, clear explanations, strength, toughness, and patience. All these qualities are in fact needed each day, and the cumulative drain for the oncology professional is immense. The special concerns for the oncology professional working with gynecologic cancer are that this tumor type combines a number of keenly distressing elements above and beyond its malignant nature: the often difficult prognostic situation, the complex, ever-evolving treatment protocols, the lost fertility, the damaged sexual response, the acute onset of menopause, the continued power of stigma and avoidance, the rarity and accompanying sense of profound isolation that women with gynecologic cancer feel, and the extensive ripple effect on their emotional ties to others. This combination of elements creates around gynecologic cancer treatment what can be described as a highly charged emotional field which adds to the challenge of doing the job (see Chapter 89).

For both men and women working with gynecologic cancer patients, identification with the woman patient is a natural response; one sees oneself and one's own family connections in the patient's experience. The patient may remind the care giver of a grandmother, mother, sister, wife, daughter, or oneself. Because of the inherent emotional elements, in the absence of some thought or discussion there will be a constant tendency for the identification to intensify. Further, some clinical situations tax even the most experienced professional. All oncology care givers have known the frustrations of treating a patient who cannot be pleased, plays staff off against one another, or cannot cooperate reasonably with treatment. Some deaths are harder to care for than others; with gynecologic cancer, death from a slow obstructive intraabdominal process is not an unusual event; comfort may be difficult to accomplish and the distress of patient and family may be painful to witness. The relationships of the women treated on the unit are highlighted by the cancer; both deep love and affection, and painful estrangement between a woman and her partner will affect staff in unspoken ways.

It is helpful for staff to have a regular psychosocial rounds to discuss and review the psychological issues and management of patients on the unit or in the clinic, to recognize the demands placed on staff in an emotionally charged treatment arena, to identify patterns of interaction, to facilitate referral to mental health professionals when needed, and to offer the relief of shared perception, insight, and reactions.

Physical Changes

Loss of ovarian function often accompanies treatment for gynecologic cancer. For premenopausal women treated for gynecologic cancer, treatment-related menopause is one of the less obvious but still bitterly difficult aspects of life after cancer. The woman treated for gynecologic cancer loses the ordinary cycles and milestones with which female life is measured out: menstruation, pregnancy, delivery. She moves immediately to the "end of the line"—menopause. Onset of hot flashes, vaginal dryness, hair and skin changes, and mood disturbance related to lack of estrogen may occur quite abruptly after treatment, augmenting the sense of premature aging. As the patient is well aware, menopause requires continuing management both symptomatically and as a long-term health concern; estrogen replacement may be contraindicated, depending on type of cancer and other factors. It is essential for the oncology professional to remain attentive to the patient's care from other medical professionals, who may be insufficiently aware of the risks that follow from a cancer diagnosis.

Careful medical attention and support to this area is invaluable in assisting the patient in feeling as healthy and vital as she can, despite the reality of these physiologic changes. A careful gynecologic examination to determine the status of the vaginal mucosa is helpful for the woman with vaginal dryness; a vaginal moisturizer (such as Replens) may be used every other day when estrogen cream is contraindicated, and a vaginal lubricant (Astroglide, and others) may help alleviate discomfort with sexual experiences. Talking over the symptoms and management of menopause is very helpful, especially for the younger gynecologic cancer patient for whom the transition to menopause is both abrupt and asynchronous with her point in the life cycle. Cancer support groups for women often offer discussion of menopausal symptoms and their management without estrogen; such groups may be located through the American Cancer Society local chapters.

Treatment ordinarily brings about other physical changes, and much time and emotional energy is given over in the first two years of survivorship to accommodating these changes and learning to live with them. In the early stages of survivorship, fatigue management may be a primary concern. A woman's response to her surgical scars (or other body change) may include repulsion if the scar is very extensive or misshapen, sadness over the lost body integrity or youthful appearance, outrage and resentment that the cancer occurred at all, appreciation of the surgeon's skill, curiosity about wound healing, and guarded respect for the mark of a victorious battle.

Radiation to the pelvis may alter gastrointestinal, bladder and sexual function. Significant changes in bladder function such as pain, frequency, or leakage may require considerable medical attention that may have great impact on daily living. Urostomy and colostomy care requires mastery of the entire range of issues in this area: use of appliances, maintenance of cleanliness, fear of accidents, issues of clothing and appearance, and gradual acceptance of a major body change. Patients after vulvectomy and some radiation treatments may have discomfort sitting for any duration or directing the flow of urine. The gynecologic oncology patient is often dealing with more than one of these concerns, and staff may need to follow closely the evolution of her progress in dealing with each of them as she recovers after treatment.

It is useful to bear in mind that even a small physical change may require a significant process of adaptation on the part of the patient. Abdominal scars, skin changes from radiation, and changes in hair thickness or texture after chemotherapy all alter a woman's sense of who she is, and particularly how acceptable she is as an attractive romantic and sexual partner in the eyes of the world. It is important that oncology staff, though perhaps affected by years of exposure to greater physical losses, remain sensitive to the meaning of smaller changes to the woman who experiences them.

For a woman dealing with any more extensive body changes, such as ostomies, changes due to radiation, or surgical changes, a referral to a mental health professional with competence in counseling in this area can be invaluable; even a small number of sessions may be very helpful in easing the process of adjustment. The patient may be referred preoperatively to help with preparation, after surgery to help with adjustment and recovery, or at any time during the period after treatment ends, as part of a more gradual effort to restore a sense of body acceptance and comfort with one's body, often a common area of concern after cancer treatment. A cancer support group may help the woman become more familiar with the many ways in which people work to accept their changed bodies after cancer, and offer a safe place to explore one's own reactions. Women who undergo radical surgical procedures such as pelvic exenteration or vulvectomy should always be offered the opportunity to talk over their feelings about their bodies, and changes in both sexuality and elimination, that must be gradually worked through in order for the woman to arrive at a sense of herself as vigorous and worthwhile; clinical reports show that women who receive such counseling fare better than those who do not (2).

Sexuality and Sexual Dysfunction

Difficulties with sexual desire, response, and communication arise frequently after cancer treatment; for an overview of these issues see Chapter 42. Women with gynecologic cancer are particularly vulnerable to problems with sexuality: the cancer arises in the pelvic site of sexual response, treatment modalities may adversely affect sexual function in several ways, and emotional, relationship, and fertility concerns are closely tied to sexual expression for these women. Women often experience loss of sexual desire and dyspareunia, resulting in decreased frequency of sexual experiences and at times culminating in complete sexual abstinence.

Dyspareunia (painful intercourse) requires a careful gynecologic evaluation. Contributing factors may be surgical change or shortening of the vagina; radiation change with scar tissue formation and narrowing of the vagina; lack of estrogen after surgery, chemotherapy, or radiation, resulting in atrophic vaginal mucosa; and anxiety resulting in impaired excitement response. It is not uncommon for patients who are understandably anxious about painful sex to try to minimize pain by "hurrying through"; the excitement phase response of engorgement and lubrication, probably already slowed by treatment effects, then has even less time to evolve. The evaluation offers the opportunity to clarify and explain to the woman what the physical components of her discomfort appear to be. Treatment of physical factors is essential to improving the situation. When not contraindicated, the use of an estrogen cream such as Premarin is most effective for vaginal atrophy due to lack of estrogen. A nonestrogen vaginal moisturizer (Replens) used three times a week regardless of sexual activity will improve vaginal comfort, and a vaginal lubricant (Astroglide, others) used with each sexual experience will improve lubrication. Reestablishing the possibility of comfortable sex is the first step, and good medical care is essential to this. Some excellent booklets on sexuality and cancer for the patient have been prepared by Schover (3,4).

The psychologic factors bearing on sexual desire and response after cancer are very powerful. Many women struggle to find a way to see themselves as vital, lively, strong, attractive, female, sensual, and sexual after treatment. The role models are few; each woman feels as though she must reinvent the wheel in this area. The process of re-learning how to be able to be relaxed and, gradually, responsive in a sexual situation takes time and support. The role of the partner is crucial; the partner must be attentive and supportive to this effort. The woman herself must be clear about what she would like, with herself and with her partner. At first this is hard, as the woman herself may be hesitant, confused, and worried about sex. Many women find initially that the sexual experience after cancer is full of opportunities for sad reflection on what has occurred, what has been lost and changed, as well as concern about discomfort. Given time to talk these feelings through and explore ways to rediscover themselves as sexual persons, most survivors find that it is ultimately very gratifying and renewing to learn again how to enjoy all aspects of sexuality. When the woman is sure of what she can do to ensure comfortable sex, and can rely on the support of her partner in this rediscovery process, she is likeliest to find ways to feel relaxed and responsive sexually; even so, most find this is a very gradual process.

The concerns of the partner are often overlooked. Whether male or female, the partner is often preoccupied with concern about in any way hurting the woman who was treated, whether by expressing sexual interest and being seen as demanding, or physically during a sexual experience. The partner's desire may be dampened by this worry, and silence on both sides often leads to misunderstanding. It is also normal for the patient to be deeply concerned with physical changes which are far less concerning to the partner. Taking time, first to talk through some of these concerns, and later to relax in a special, intimate setting, is the first step toward re-learning how to connect after treatment, accommodating whatever changes the treatment has brought.

The effect of gynecologic cancer treatment on sexuality has received ongoing research attention over the past several decades. Published data confirm what is seen clinically: after treatment most women find satisfaction in their lives and relationships, but a high proportion experience persisting problems with sexual functioning (5). Andersen (6,7), studying sexual dysfunction in post-cancer-treatment women not limited to gynecologic cancer, reported that while there was no evidence of impaired social adjustment in this group, approximately 30% of women treated for cancer were diagnosed with sexual dysfunction, most frequently decreased frequency and decreased excitement response, often secondary to pain, treatment-related menopause, and side effects of cancer therapy. Sichel (8) studied a group of 58 women, combining gynecologic cancer subtypes including cervix, endometrial, ovarian, and vulvar cancers. Of 42 patients ultimately studied, half were not sexually active, and of the half that were sexually active some confined sexual activity to masturbation; this author reaffirms that decreased sexual activity is not exclusively linked to the degree of surgical mutilation.

Identification of risk factors predicting difficulty in the psychosexual or quality-of-life realms has received attention. Andersen (9) has argued generally that the magnitude of treatment is the primary determinant of whether sexual difficulties will develop after treatment; her ALARM model for risk prediction also considers other factors. Meanwhile, Schover (10,11) has argued cogently for the primary role of the patient's relationship and prior sexual function in the development of posttreatment sexual problems. In her view, a patient with a smaller treatment but a troubled relationship or poor prior sexual functioning might be at greater risk for impaired sexual functioning than one with a treatment of some greater magnitude but with a strong relationship and a history of good sexual functioning.

Weijmar Schultz, van de Wiel and colleagues (12) are in accord with Schover, suggesting that the relationship may be the best place to intervene to support sexual recovery after gynecologic cancer treatment. In their reviews of the literature on sexual functioning after gynecologic cancer, these authors reconfirm that *(1)* the time frame receiving most research attention is the symptomatic period preceding diagnosis, and the period surrounding diagnosis and treatment; *(2)* gynecologic cancer frequently has a deleterious effect on sexual function; and *(3)* methodologic problems include incomplete data, patient selection, different treatment modalities, and diverse times of assessment (13). They encourage physicians to reduce radical treatment in order to lower sexual complication rates, and psychologists to reduce patient sexual morbidity by pursuing further study of gynecologic cancer, focusing on premorbid sexual and relationship issues, couple interventions, and the psychological effects of additive medical interventions in gynecologic cancer (14). These researchers have also studied partners of women treated for gynecologic cancer, interviewing 16 men one year after their partners' treatment, and describing the crisis nature of the experience of gynecologic cancer for the partner, with attendant stress, self-doubt, and sexual problems for the partner (15).

The nursing literature offers clinical reviews and further suggestions regarding clinical interventions with gynecologic cancer patients. Shell (16) and Lamb (17) have provided thoughtful reviews of the issues relating to sexual recovery in this population.

In recent years, sexuality research methodology has improved and the volume of clinical reports continues to grow. The magnitude of treatment impact in gynecologic cancer makes study of the psychological and sexual outcome essential in order to design optimal therapeutic interventions, as Andersen (18) and others (13,14) have affirmed.

Infertility

The premenopausal woman who wished to become pregnant but has had gynecologic cancer instead must contend with both cancer and infertility on a continuing basis. Some defer dealing with the infertility for a year or two and focus on the cancer issues primarily; others remain largely focused on the effort to make a family and absorb the cancer experience as a postponement rather than a cancellation of those plans. The loss of the capacity to become pregnant is a devastating development to most women, so great that any technological intercession that preserves even partial fertility receives the closest attention. Possible concerns include wanting to harvest ova for fertilization and storage after the cancer diagnosis but before starting treatment, and researching partial ovarian removal for later reimplantation. Single women, of course, share these concerns; the impact of fertility impairment may be greater when it is not buffered by the support of a solid ongoing relationship. Decisions about making a family are best undertaken after the cancer experience has been sorted through emotionally to a fair degree. Adoption, egg donation, or surrogacy may be considered and carried out. As with other infertility patients, dealing during this time with other women's questions about one's cancer, as well as their pregnancies, births, and small children, is often tremendously painful for the gynecologic cancer survivor. Egg donation and surrogacy procedures may catalyze feelings about the precipitous loss of fertility. Support and information from infertility organizations may be helpful; having the opportunity to talk, in therapy, in a support group, or with friends, helps many women the most.

Although infertility is a common consequence of gynecologic cancer treatment, the oncology specialist is often unfamiliar with the experience of working actively with infertility issues and decisions; until recently, cancer treatment always came first, reproductive concerns second. Many oncology staff members may continue to feel that this is the only appropriate prioritization; others may be sensitive to the concerns of the younger women they see, whose desire for children may be backed up by a willingness to consider taking real risks that cannot yet be precisely ascertained. Location of infertility specialists may be accomplished through the nearest medical school departments of urology, obstetrics-gynecology, and endocrinology, as well as infertility clinics and national organizations.

Special Populations

For each patient the experience of gynecologic cancer is filtered through a personal lens of individual characteristics and situational factors that give the illness its special meaning for that patient. Maintaining an awareness of this can clarify the early interactions between staff and patient, and help again in the recovery period after treatment. The adolescent or young adult patient is diagnosed with pelvic cancer before a firm sense of self is established and while sexual identity and familiarity with dating relationships are being created. Adaptation to the mortality and fertility aspects of gynecologic cancer will affect the developmental process, and referral to a dextrous mental health professional can be invaluable in helping the teenager or young woman to begin the process of coming to terms with what life has dealt her. Referrals may be obtained by contacting the nearest hospital department of child psychiatry, adolescent medicine, adult psychiatry, psychology, or social work.

Single patients often have concerns about loneliness and feel keenly the lack of a strong, supportive relationship during and after treatment. Single women must contend with special challenges in meeting people and dating, such as when to talk about the treatment, how much to tell, how to describe the fertility and hormonal impact, bearing rejection if it occurs, and maintaining hope when ordinary stretches of singledom seem prolonged by the cancer aspect. Support groups form an excellent setting for patients to share these frustrations, lessen the loneliness, and gain strength to "rejoin the fray."

Patients in many situations will try to "contain" the impact of the cancer treatment and not lean on their support system. Women of any age in new relationships will have heightened concern about the impact of the cancer on the relationship, and may try somehow to spare the new partner the brunt of this terrifying new problem, or the many later nuances that affect life together: checkup fears, recurrence scares, working out solutions to vaginal dryness without estrogen, baby shower invitations. Women in troubled or unstable relationships may try to avoid

further stressing the relationship, and deal with the cancer and its effects as much as possible on their own or with other, safer supports such as family and friends. When the partner appears to be stressed, whether by unemployment, alcoholism, mental illness, or other factors, help should be made available to the patient and her partner, so that the woman gets some of the help she needs.

Mothers of young children have special concerns about how their own cancer treatment will affect their families, and benefit from special support and counseling in addressing these issues at home. Children usually possess great sensitivity to the goings-on in the household, and as a result should be included in simple, clear family discussions of the cancer, its treatment, and the ways in which this affects daily life in the home. Their questions need direct answers, appropriate to their age and level of understanding. It is easier for both adults and children to continue family life in an atmosphere of trust and clarity than in one of mystery and denial, even when difficult realities must be faced. Support groups of parents dealing with adult cancers while raising children can be very helpful.

During the course of treatment and after, many patients will find themselves dealing with further life crises, such as job loss or change, aging or ill parents, or family problems with alcohol or drugs or violence. The multiplicity of crises will overwhelm even the strongest person at times, and the need for support from different sources and of different kinds is undeniable. Adult women who are at the age when gynecologic cancer is likeliest to arise are often emotional or actual caretakers for children, partners, parents, friends, and other family members, as well as often working full time. For these women, the therapeutic effort is often to obtain the information needed in order to deal with the immediate crisis, and then to set up some sort of ongoing support to help the woman stabilize and restructure her life, both to accommodate the evolving demands she faces and to provide some nourishment to her own hopes and needs.

The cancer experience for the woman who is aging may upset the delicate balance of needs and supports in her life or crystallize the obviousness of the need for change. The same is true for any woman with a fragile or poor support system, and these problems may present first with great clarity to oncology staff. The availability to the oncology staff of a capable social work service is invaluable in these settings.

GYNECOLOGIC CANCER: SITE-SPECIFIC ISSUES

Cervix Cancer

There are an estimated 15,800 cases of invasive cervix cancer diagnosed yearly, and 65,000 cases of cervix cancer in situ (1). Largely because an excellent screening test is available for early disease (in contrast to ovarian cancer), this tumor is associated with 4800 deaths a year. Considerably more information has developed about factors that contribute to risk: exposure to sexually transmitted diseases, early and frequent unprotected sexual contacts that expose to the human papilloma virus. Smoking, substance abuse, and immunosuppression are additional factors that contribute to risk. How these factors interact is an important area of study. For example, women with HIV who are immunosuppressed have a 15-fold to 20-fold increase in risk, suggesting greater vulnerability to this virally related tumor.

Reports comparing sexual outcome in cervix cancer after surgery with the outcome after surgery combined with radiation indicate that radiation has greater capacity to impair sexual response. Schover (5), comparing these two groups, found that the radiation group at one year had increased complaints of dyspareunia, and of decreased quality of life. Further, the entire group had decreased sexual function over the first year post-treatment, but marital stability and happiness were not affected by the modality of treatment. Overall, the question of which treatments create the least sexual dysfunction, or in which settings the least sexual dysfunction occurs, including partner support, education, and therapeutic interventions by oncology staff, deserves further study.

Corney (19–21) studied a group of 105 patients with carcinoma of the cervix or vulva. Many patients were still depressed and anxious and described chronic sexual problems as long as five years after surgery. Examining the role of age in return of sexual function in women, Corney found that 40% of women under 50 years of age had intercourse less frequently, and over 50 years of age, most patients had intercourse less frequently or not at all. The most commonly reported sexual dysfunction was loss of desire. A high proportion of patients wanted more information, and many younger patients preferred that the partner be included.

Cervix cancer is widely seen as a preventable cancer either by behavior or by early diagnosis, since cervical dysplasia progresses to carcinoma over a period of months to years. Women diagnosed with invasive cervix cancer often contend with the perception that they failed to take care of themselves. Increasingly, women are learning that the human papilloma virus, which is sexually transmitted, is a major etiologic factor. They struggle with the fact that cervix cancer is related to sexually transmissible viruses. Lay understanding of the evolving medical exploration of the role of papilloma viruses in cervix cancer is highly variable, and many women with cervix cancer fear being thought to have been promiscuous.

Information, support, and education are essential to minimize the impact of radiation. A vaginal dilator should be provided to every woman who receives pelvic radiation, regardless of her partner or sexual status, and she should be educated about why and how it is used. A simple schedule of insertions is helpful, and follow-up support is essential. The availability of a partner is nice, but women are happier when they can separate the medical care needed for maintenance of a healthy vagina from the sexual experiences most people need and enjoy in order to feel fulfilled in life. Having a vaginal dilator available and being dexterous in its use enables most women to provide good care for themselves, to identify problems themselves (outside of sexual situations, which advantages both the patient and her partner), and then to seek care as appropriate. Women who feel in control of this part of their care are better able to approach sexual situations with a relaxed attitude. The woman's relationship with her physician is improved when she has been taught to provide her own care to her vagina; the physician is then not so often confronted with a perplexing blend of medical and relationship issues regarding sex or dyspareunia, and counseling referrals to deal with relationship or sexuality issues are made easier.

Other more difficult sequelae of radiotherapy such as fistulas and bowel or urinary obstructive episodes present the patient with the reality of further hospitalizations and surgery to treat the consequences of what may well have been a successful cancer therapy. Women may struggle with anger and frustration over this course of events, questioning their choice of physicians, and their treatment, and feeling trapped in a medical universe they had hoped to leave behind, in part by agreeing to an aggressive treatment in the first place. Brief counseling in hospital or in support groups may be helpful in assisting women in coming to terms with these new challenges, which may include ostomy and other self-care developments, as well as dilemmas of personal and support system exhaustion and the need to regroup in order to carry on in life.

Pelvic exenteration is a surgical procedure entailing the removal of the bladder, vagina, uterus, ovaries, and rectum, with urinary and fecal diversion. It is performed when a tumor has advanced locally but may be removed en bloc with realistic hope of cure. Patients who undergo exenteration need special counseling in order to recover psychologically, manage their ostomy care, and regain a measure of sexual comfort (2). The creation of a new vagina remains a reconstructive challenge; various techniques are available, but the combination of sexual usefulness, comfort, and acceptability to the patient remains an elusive outcome.

Uterine Cancer

Endometrial cancer is diagnosed in approximately 32,800 women each year, and is associated with 5900 deaths (1). This type of gynecologic cancer is diagnosed primarily in postmenopausal women, but 25% are premenopausal, and 5% are less than 40 years old (22). The use of preoperative radiation has been studied over the past twenty years; however, current treatment approaches favor initial surgical staging, with further treatment as determined by the staging outcome. Adjunctive therapy ordinarily includes radiation, as effective chemotherapeutic agents for this disease have yet to be established. Current endometrial cancer treatment offers a favorable prognosis; an uncorrected five-year survival for this disease is 75% (22).

Women who are treated for endometrial cancer often have some sense that, relative to other gynecologic cancers, theirs has a reasonable prognosis. As a result, the intense awareness of mortality risk that is so often a first consideration with women with ovarian cancer is somewhat attenuated among women with endometrial cancer, and attention may turn somewhat sooner to issues of hormonal status, fertility, and sexuality impact. Younger women with endometrial cancer, on the other hand, often have a distinct awareness of the rareness of this tumor type in their age range, and may feel especially lonely. One young women in a support group of women with gynecologic cancer went around the room checking what type of gynecologic cancer each had; when each had answered, and all had cervical or ovarian cancer, she sat back and said quietly, "I'm the only one."

The younger woman treated for early endometrial cancer may be able to retain her ovaries, and so may avoid a treatment-related menopause, as well as being able to use her own ova for reproduction. When this is not possible, she faces both menopause and loss of her own fertility. Because endometrial cancer is more frequently diagnosed in postmenopausal women, fertility issues may not be a primary concern; and with surgical treatment alone, sexual response and comfort may not be adversely affected as much as with radiation or chemotherapy.

Ovarian Cancer

At present, approximately 26,000 cases of ovarian cancer are diagnosed each year, and 14,000 deaths result from this tumor annually; ovarian cancer represents 5% of all cancers in women (1). Approximately 1 woman in 70 will develop ovarian cancer in her lifetime, and 1 in 100 will die of this disease (22). The incidence of ovarian cancer increases with age. Factors associated with increased risk are a history of breast cancer or family history of ovarian cancer; factors associated with decreased risk include parity and history of oral contraceptive use. Because early stages of the disease may present few or mild symptoms (mild abdominal fullness, bloating, bowel changes), ovarian cancer is often diagnosed at an advanced stage. Initial treatment includes surgical staging and debulking; removal of as much tumor bulk as possible improves the outcome of chemotherapy. Chemotherapy regimens for ovarian cancer continue to evolve steadily; cisplatin, carboplatin, taxol, and newer agents offer evidence of improved survival. Because of its silent onset, the need for an accurate marker is critically important in achieving detection.

The advent of improved surgical and chemotherapeutic regimens for ovarian cancer and resulting improved prognosis have increased interest in the psychosocial, sexual, and quality of life impact of this disease. Mitchell (23) contrasted 43 patients with ovarian dysgerminoma treated with radiation therapy with 55 controls, querying sexual as well as bowel, bladder, thyroid, and menstrual sequelae. While 23% of patients versus 6% of controls reported dyspareunia, this author found that most patients were satisfied with their sexual function after radiation therapy, again raising the same questions framed by Weijmar Schultz about the elements of sexual interaction that form the basis for the perception of pleasure and satisfaction in this population. As surgery and chemotherapy constitute the primary therapy for most ovarian cancers at present, quality of life studies of larger cohorts of women treated with these modalities for ovarian cancer are needed; Kornblith and colleagues have undertaken this work (24).

In the eyes of the general public, this illness retains an aura of danger and lethality; the best-known people who have had it have died. Any woman diagnosed with ovarian cancer faces both a true medical challenge and a clear awareness that when she shares her diagnosis with anyone she changes dramatically how she is perceived. Women with ovarian cancer may receive unmistakable messages that their situation frightens others; friends may be supportive, or may respond with shock, silence, and abandonment. Family may understand, or minimize and deny the seriousness of the illness. Women describe being treated as if they were heroines, or written off as if they were already dead. This type of gynecologic cancer seems to bring with it an extra burden of social challenge; the patient must learn to know when she is ready to talk about her condition, ready to deal with the many possible responses, to educate her support system about the disease and its treatment. Loneliness is, not surprisingly, a common dilemma for these women. Each woman needs to determine who in her life is truly supportive of her during her illness; many women benefit from counseling, a cancer support group, or other supports (newsletter, audio cassettes) during treatment and afterwards. Not the least important, the black humor and pithy observations that sustain women through many life stresses can be freely expressed in these settings.

Women with ovarian cancer must also deal with risk of recurrence, the need for second-look surgery, and re-treatment extending over months and years, utilizing chemotherapeutic agents with strong acute and long-term toxicities. Palliative care issues are often complex in terms of pain management, fatigue, nausea, and depression which are concerns for every cancer patient.

Other Gynecologic Cancers

Vulvar, vaginal, and fallopian tube cancers are diagnosed in approximately 5700 women a year, and are associated with 1200 deaths a year (1). Treatment for these rarer tumors varies according to cell type; new treatment approaches are continually being sought for these challenging disease entities.

Vulvar cancer is a rare form of gynecologic cancer, usually diagnosed in postmenopausal women, which may present as a painless itching or sore on the vulva. The original treatment of vulvar cancer with radical vulvectomy, a highly effective but physically mutilating procedure associated with a bilateral lymphedema and a high incidence of sexual dysfunction, is now being reconsidered in light of these quality of life concerns, and partial vulvectomy or local excision are more commonly performed. Radical vulvectomy entails the removal of the labia majora, minora, and clitoris, as well as bilateral lymph node dissection; the effectiveness of surgical approaches that preserve vulvar structures has become a primary focus of research in this area. However, the possibility of surgical cure in this condition is the hallmark of treatment. Management of locally advanced disease or recurrence remains a therapeutic challenge, as effective radiation

or chemotherapeutic regimens have not been established.

Psychosocial and sexual response to vulvectomy has drawn research attention in recent years. Thuesen (25), studying 18 women with vulvar cancer who received local excision, reported that less than one-third reported postoperative sexual problems, in contrast with one-half of vulvectomy patients in another series; further, 14 of the 18 expressed satisfaction with the cosmetic result. Weijmar Schultz and van de Wiel (12) described a well-constructed two-year study of 10 couples wherein the women had been treated for vulvar cancer with radical or partial vulvectomy, contrasted with a group of controls. The women were studied physiologically and, with spouses, psychometrically; sexual function was assessed at 6, 12, and 24 months. With longer follow-up, the women patients' satisfaction with sexual function was not different from pretreatment levels or from controls, despite continued perception of impaired genital sensation during lovemaking. These researchers found psychological and social variables more crucial for rehabilitation than physical variables.

With regard to other, less frequently encountered gynecologic cancers, Wenzel (26) studied 76 patients treated for gestational trophoblastic disease (GTD), and observed that across disease subtypes GTD patients experienced anxiety, anger, fatigue, and sexual problems and were affected by pregnancy concerns for protracted periods of time.

Women who have had radical vulvectomy often have slow initial wound healing over weeks; dismay and depression are common. When bilateral lymph node dissection has been performed, lymphedema is often extreme; this condition is both uncomfortable and unsightly, and requires daily management with surgical support stockings and other measures. The woman may experience difficulty sitting for prolonged periods, or directing the flow of urine. Her sexual response may take time to return; while the vagina remains intact, the clitoral area, once healed, retains variable sexual sensitivity, and masturbation to orgasm may be relearned. Rediscovering what is possible and comfortable sexually should be undertaken gradually; counseling may be invaluable in restoring the patient's self-esteem as a woman and as a potential sexual partner. While this is primarily a disease of older women, the emphasis on surgical treatment means that hormonal status is not altered by treatment; in the younger woman, fertility is preserved and pregnancy and vaginal delivery are possible.

NEW RESEARCH

New research areas are related to quality of life (24), psychoimmune function in gynecologic cancer (27), and psychological issues for those at increased risk (28–30). Psychosocial research in gynecologic cancer faces the same challenges across cancer subtypes: allocation of funding for research on psychosocial issues; access to staff to carry out research projects of significant magnitude; developing cohort size sufficiently to clarify psychosocial questions; and development of valid research instruments relating to issues of psychosocial adjustment, sexual functioning, immune status, and quality of life.

Quality of Life in Gynecologic Cancer

A small number of studies have been done examining measures of quality of life in gynecologic cancer, introducing the hope of greater clinical usefulness of this body of work to the gynecologic oncologist. de Haes and colleagues (31) studied quality of life in women with advanced ovarian cancer treated with combination chemotherapy, and found different assessments of psychological state by physicians and by patients. She underscored the need for careful research implementation, notably the need to measure quality of life at different points in the treatment cycle and over different cycles. Willemse and colleagues (32) applied quality of life measures to the use of cisplatin chemotherapy in 52 patients with stage III–IV ovarian cancer and found that, although duration of treatment was limited (six cycles), about 28% of the cumulative period of progression-free survival was consumed by the treatment and its side effects. Similarly, Guidozzi (33) found decreased quality of life in those with persistent ovarian cancer compared with treatment responders.

Kornblith (24), studying 151 women with advanced ovarian cancer, found that 33% had high levels of psychological distress suggesting need for psychological evaluation and therapy, while 23% were "resilient" and required no psychological intervention. In the same cohort, Portenoy (34) found that frequent and persistent pain occurred in 42%, undermining function in two-thirds of this group. Padilla and colleagues (35), studying the impact of uncertainty in illness outcome on quality of life in 100 women in treatment for gynecologic cancer, reported that health-related quality of life scores were predicted by mood states, mastery beliefs, appraisal of situation, and ambiguity in illness, but not by coping strategies.

McCartney (36) discussed the usefulness of reliable measurement of quality of life across several dimensions in making decisions regarding treatment: at diagnosis, during curative treatment, during palliative treatment, in terminal illness, and for the gynecologic cancer survivor. Andersen (9) presented a model to predict the risk in women who might have more difficult posttreatment outcomes than others: younger patients; single patients with less well-established support systems, and patients choosing aggressive treatment being among them. Roberts and co-workers (37) studied 32 women treated for gynecologic cancer, and found that while most reported a good quality of life, younger patients appeared to be more at risk for psychological problems after gynecologic surgery. Further studies in this area might simplify the process of identifying which patients with gynecologic cancer are at risk for psychological distress, pain and lowered quality of life, in an effort to expedite needed help. Bovbjerg, Redd, and co-workers (27) described conditioned nausea and immune responses during cyclic chemotherapy for ovarian cancer. Women experienced anticipatory nausea and vomiting prior to receiving their chemotherapy treatment, which was accompanied by immunosuppressive responses. (See Chapter 12 on psychoimmune function.)

Psychosocial Aspects of Increased Risk

The issues of women who are at increased risk for gynecologic cancer are receiving attention. Schwartz and colleagues (28) studied 103 women with at least one first-degree relative with ovarian cancer, and found moderately high levels of psychological distress. A social work program for women at increased risk is helpful in women completing the screening process, making use of the clinic's medical resources, and moving into stages of medical intervention (29). Wardle and colleagues (30) studied 43 women with false positive findings at ovarian cancer screening and found no long-term psychiatric morbidity, although women with a monitoring coping style appeared to be more vulnerable to worry about cancer in the aftermath of a false positive finding. This will become increasingly important in terms of genetic testing and use of markers that engender anxiety.

CONCLUSION

In gynecologic psycho-oncology, several areas in particular merit further study: the effect of staff training in psychosocial and sexual issues upon patient outcomes; the use of support groups; and the use of print materials, audiocassettes, and video or computer materials in supplementing or replacing one-to-one counseling. Couple-based interventions should figure more prominently for study. The nature, duration, and treatment of sexual dysfunction after gynecologic cancer treatment deserves further study, with emphasis on effective treatment strategies. The psychological and sexual issues of the ovarian cancer patient remain very little studied, even as this population gains greater voice in the lay media. The special nature and clinical management of fertility issues in gynecologic cancer survivors deserve greater attention, with attention to issues of medical risk and relationship impact, in addition to loss and grief over treatment-related infertility. Finally, the nature and treatment of staff stresses and concerns particular to gynecologic cancer merit further study.

REFERENCES

1. American Cancer Society. *Cancer Facts and Figures—1995*. Atlanta, GA: American Cancer Society; 1995: 1–29.
2. Lamont, JA, DePetrillo AD, Sargent ES. Psychosexual rehabilitation and exenterative surgery. *Gynecol Oncol.* 1978; 6:236–242.
3. Schover LR. *Sexuality and Cancer: For the Woman Who Has Cancer, and Her Partner.* New York: American Cancer Society; 1988.
4. Schover LR. *Sexuality and Fertility after Cancer.* New York: John Wiley; 1997.
5. Schover LR, Fife M, Gershenson D. Sexual dysfunction and treatment for early stage cervical cancer. *Cancer.* 1989; 63(1):204–212.
6. Andersen B, Anderson B, deProsse C. Controlled prospective longitudinal study of women with cancer: I. Sexual functioning outcomes. *J Consult Clin Psychol.* 1989; 75(6):683–691.
7. Andersen BL, Anderson B, deProsse C. Controlled prospective longitudinal study of women with cancer: II. Psychological outcomes. *J Consult Clin Psychol.* 1989; 57(6):692–697.
8. Sichel M. Quality of life and gynecological cancers. *Eur J Gynecol Oncol.* 1990; 11(6):485–488.
9. Andersen BL. Predicting sexual and psychologic morbidity and improving the quality of life for women with gynecologic cancer. *Cancer.* 1993; 71(4 Suppl): 1678–1690.
10. Schover LR, Evans RB, von Eschenbach AC. Sexual rehabilitation in a cancer center: diagnosis and outcome in 384 consultations. *Arch Sexual Behav.* 1987; 16(6):445–461.
11. Schover LR. The impact of breast cancer on sexuality, body image, and intimate relationships. *CA: Cancer J Clin.* 1991; 41(2):112–120.
12. Weijmar Schultz WCM, van de Wiel HBM, Bouma J, Janssens J, Littlewood J. Psychosexual functioning after the treatment of cancer of the vulva: a longitudinal study. *Cancer.* 1990; 66(2):402–407.
13. Weijmar Schultz WC, Bransfield DD, van de Wiel HB, Bouma J. Sexual outcome following female genital cancer treatment: a critical review of methods of investigation and results. *Sexual Marital Ther.* 1992; 7(1):29–64.
14. Weijmar Schultz W, van de Wiel H. Sexual rehabilitation after gynecologic cancer treatment. *J Sex Educ Ther.* 1992; 18(4):286–293.
15. van de Wiel HB, Weijmar Schultz WC, Wouda J, Bouma J. Sexual functioning of partners of gynaecological oncology patients: a pilot study on involvement, support, sexuality, and relationship. *Sexual Marital Ther.* 1990; 5(2):123–130.
16. Shell JA. Sexuality for patients with gynecologic cancer. *NAACOGS Clin Issues Perinat Wom Health Nurs.* 1990; 1(4):479–494.
17. Lamb MA. Psychosexual issues: the woman with gynecologic cancer. *Semin Oncol Nurs.* 1990; 6(3):237–243.
18. Berek JS, Andersen BL. Sexual rehabilitation: surgical and psychological approaches. In: Hoskins WJ, Perez CA, Young RC, eds. *Principles and Practice of Gynecologic Oncology.* Philadelphia: JB Lippincott; 1992: 401–416.
19. Corney RH, Everett H, Howells A, Crowther ME. Psychosocial adjustment following major gynaecological surgery for carcinoma of the cervix and vulva. *J Psychosom Res.* 1992; 36(6):561–568.
20. Corney R, Everett H, Howells A, Crowther M. The care of patients undergoing surgery for gynaecological cancer: the need for information, emotional support and counselling. *J Adv Nurs.* 1992; 17(6):667–671.
21. Corney RH, Crowther ME, Howells A. Psychosexual dysfunction in women with gynaecologic cancer following radical pelvic surgery. *Br J Obstet Gynaecol.* 1993; 100:73–78.
22. Hoskins WJ, Perez CA, Young RC. *Principles and Practice of Gynecologic Oncology.* Philadelphia: JB Lippincott; 1992.
23. Mitchell MF, Gershenson DM, Soeters R, Eifel P, Delclos L, Wharton JT. The long-term effects of radiation therapy on patients with ovarian dysgerminoma. *Cancer.* 1991; 67(4):1084–1090.
24. Kornblith AB, Thaler H, Wong G, et al. Quality of life of women with ovarian cancer. *Gynecol Oncol.* 1995; 59:231–242.
25. Thuesen B, Anreasson B, Bock J. Sexual function and somatopsychic reactions after local excision of vulvar intra-epithelial neoplasia. *Acta Obstet Gynecol Scand.* 1992; 71(22):126–128.
26. Wenzel L, Berkowitz R, Robinson S, Bernstein M, Goldstein D. The psychological, social and sexual consequences of gestational trophoblastic disease. *Gynecol Oncol.* 1992; 46:74–81.
27. Bovbjerg DH, Redd WH, Maier LA, Holland JC. Anticipatory immune suppression and nausea in women receiving cyclic chemotherapy for ovarian cancer. *J Consult Clin Psychol.* 1990; 58(2):153–157.
28. Schwartz MD, Lerman C, Miller SM, Daly M. Coping disposition, perceived risk, and psychological distress among women at increased risk for ovarian cancer. *Health Psychol.* 1995; 14(3):232–235.
29. Smith PM, Schwartz PE. Social work role in an early ovarian cancer detection program. *Soc Work Health Care.* 1993; 19(2):67–80.
30. Wardle J, Pernet A, Collins W, Bourne T. False positive reports in ovarian cancer screening: one year followup of psychological status. *Psychol Health.* 1994; 10(1):33–40.

31. de Haes JCJM, Raatgever JW, van der Burg MEL, Els H, Neijt JP. Evaluation of the quality of life of patients with advanced ovarian cancer treated with combination chemotherapy. In: Aaronson NK, Beckman J, eds. *The Quality of Life of Cancer Patients.* New York: Raven Press; 1987: 215–225.

32. Willemse PHB, Van Lith J, Mulder NH, et al. Risks and benefits of cisplatin in ovarian cancer. A quality-adjusted survival analysis. *Eur J Cancer.* 1990; 26(3):345–352.

33. Guidozzi F. Living with ovarian cancer. *Gynecol Oncol.* 1993; 50:202–207.

34. Portenoy RK, Kornblith AB, Wong G, et al. Pain in ovarian cancer: prevalence, characteristics, and associated symptoms. *Cancer.* 1994; 74:907–915.

35. Padilla GV, Mishel MH, Grant MM. Uncertainty, appraisal, and quality of life. *Qual Life Res.* 1992; 1(3):155–165.

36. McCartney C, Larson D. Quality of life in patients with gynecologic cancer. *Cancer.* 1987; 60:2129–2136.

37. Roberts CS, Rossetti K, Cone D, Cavanaugh D. Psychosocial impact of gynecologic cancer: a descriptive study. *J Psychosoc Oncol.* 1992; 10(1):99–109.

31

Skin Neoplasms and Malignant Melanoma

FAWZY I. FAWZY AND NANCY W. FAWZY

Skin cancer is the most common site of cancer yet it is also the most highly curable, with the overall rate exceeding 95% (1). The outermost layer of skin, the epidermis, is mainly comprised of flat squamous cells. The lower part of the skin, the dermis, contains basal cells and melanocytes. Melanocytes contain melanin, which is responsible for skin color.

The three types of skin cancer fall into two very distinct categories. The first category contains basal cell and squamous cell carcinomas. Most people are familiar with these kinds of skin cancer. Since they are commonly and accurately felt to be easily treatable and highly curable, they have never carried the same degree of fear or stigma associated with other cancers. The second category of skin cancer contains the rarer and more serious malignant melanoma. It has been the authors' clinical experience that reactions to melanoma usually fall into one of two extremes. Lay people initially view it benignly as "just skin cancer" while most community professionals consider it a guaranteed death sentence. Reality lies somewhere in between. The medical aspects of these two categories of skin cancer will be discussed separately, followed by a discussion of psychological factors.

BASAL CELL AND SQUAMOUS CELL CARCINOMA

Description

Basal cell carcinomas usually present as nontender, pale, waxlike, pearly nodules, which may ulcerate. They occur most frequently on the head, neck, and trunk. Squamous cell carcinomas look more like red, scaly, outlined patches and are seen most on areas that receive high degrees of sun exposure such as the backs of hands, ears, nose, and lower lips. Neither of these skin cancers is prone to distant metastases, but they spread by local invasion into surrounding bone and nerve tissue and blood vessels.

Incidence and Mortality

Over 3 million cases of nonmelanoma skin cancer (basal cell and squamous cell carcinoma) occur worldwide each year, with 900,000 diagnosed in the United States. Incidence varies tremendously geographically and racially, with the lowest rates in Asian populations and the highest in white Australians (2). If found early and treated appropriately, nonmelanoma skin cancers are almost 100% curable. However, 2190 people a year do die from these skin cancers in the United States alone (1).

Etiology

The first etiologic factor was identified as early as 1775, when it was observed that chimney sweeps developed scrotal tumors after chronic exposure to soot. Other high risk factors include occupational exposure to coal tar, pitch, creosote, arsenic compounds, or radium. Ultraviolet radiation acts as both an initiator and a promoter of these tumors and is divided into three bands: UVC, UVB, and UVA. UVC waves which are the shortest (200–294 nm) rarely reach the earth's surface. UVB consists of slightly longer waves (295–319 nm) and are the principal cause of sunburn. UVB can also damage DNA and converts 7-dehydrocholesterol in the skin to vitamin D_3. Five to ten percent of UV light reaching the earth is UVB. Only 14% of that UVB passes through the outer layers of the skin and reaches the level of the melanocytes. Ninety to ninety five percent of the ultraviolet light that reaches the earth is in the UVA range. Indoor tanning booths use UVA light. UVA are the longer waves (320–400 nm) and 50% or more penetrate down to the level of the melanocytes. UVA contributes to the loss of skin elasticity, speeds up aging and wrinkling, and may interfere with the immune system. (See Chapter 6 by Berwick on sun exposure.)

The relationship of ultraviolet light to cancer is extremely complex and is still being explored.

Animals exposed to UVB alone developed squamous cell carcinoma but not basal cell carcinoma or malignant melanoma. When the same type of animals were exposed to a combination of UVB and UVA, the rate of squamous cell carcinoma rose dramatically and basal cell carcinoma and malignant melanoma also developed (3).

Prevention

Prevention involves reducing exposure to occupational hazards, decreasing UV radiation exposure by staying out of the sun as much as possible, and wearing sun-protective clothing and broad-spectrum sunscreens when in the sun.

It is advisable to stay out of the sun as much as possible between the hours of 11 A.M. to 3 P.M. when the amount of radiation reaching the earth is most intense. Sitting in the shade may not protect from reflected rays. Pale areas rarely exposed to the sun such as underarms and chins are especially vulnerable to reflected sunlight. In addition, 80% of the sun's rays can pass through clouds and result in sunburn. Geographic location is also a factor; the closer to the equator and/or the higher altitude, the greater the intensity of the sun's rays. Many people have been sunburned while skiing high in the mountains in the middle of winter on a cloudy day!

When in the sun, protective clothing should be worn. Not all clothing is equally protective. Darker colors are better than white; tightly woven fabrics are better than looser ones (e.g., nylon is better than cotton.) Several companies are now producing special lines of clothing that are sun-protective. Hats and sunglasses rated as blocking both UVA and UVB are also effective measures.

Sunscreens protect the skin by absorbing, reflecting, and scattering radiation. The SPF or sun protection factor number that appears on every sunscreen reflects that product's ability to block only UVB and is regulated by the Food and Drug Administration (FDA). Para-aminobenzoic acid or (PABA) and PABA-related compounds such as Padimate-O (octyl *p*-dimethylaminobenzoate) are the most common UVB radiation blockers. Non-PABA sunscreens are titanium dioxide, cinnamates, and benzophenes.

There is a controversy over the use of only UVB sun screens. UVB sunscreens prevent the skin from normally adapting to sun exposure, and because they prevent burning, people may actually spend more time in the sun thereby increasing exposure to UVA which has been implicated in basal cell carcinoma and malignant melanoma. Some individuals who do not drink vitamin D-fortified milk and who use UVB sunscreens regularly have been shown to be vitamin D deficient. Some vitamin D metabolites have actually been shown to inhibit the growth of melanoma cells. In addition, there is the very remote possibility that the sunscreens themselves may, in some way, promote melanoma or basal cell carcinoma (3).

As of November 1, 1997, there are no federal standards or SPF for protection against UVA. While some products claim to give broad-spectrum protection, their ingredients provide only partial UVA protection. There is only one ingredient, PARSOL 1789 (avobenzone), which has been FDA approved for providing adequate protection throughout the UVA range (i.e., from 320 to 400 nm).

There is confusion regarding which SPF number to use. The SPF indicates how long an individual can stay in the sun without beginning to turn red. If it normally takes an hour to burn then it will take 15 hours with an SPF of 15. In general, an SPF of 15 gives an adequate amount of protection without unnecessary levels of chemicals. Using a higher SPF only increases the time it takes to burn, it does not substantially increase the degree of protection at a given point in time.

Sunscreen must be applied liberally 15–30 minutes before sun exposure to allow time for bonding to the skin and must be reapplied frequently if swimming or sweating. Waterproof sunscreens last 80 minutes and water-resistant sunscreens last 40 minutes in the water. Reapplying the sunscreen does not extend the amount of time you can stay in the sun, it just reestablishes the original SPF time (4).

Diagnosis

Early diagnosis and treatment are critical to positive outcome. Most tumors are self-diagnosed and individuals should practice skin self-examination once a month. The American Cancer Society provides a simple guide for such an examination. The appearance of new growths or a sudden or progressive change in existing growths should be a warning signal. Any suspicious lesions should be evaluated promptly. It should be noted that there are many skin conditions that could initially mimic these cancers. An excisional biopsy and pathological tissue examination are, at present, the best way to form a definitive diagnosis (4).

Treatment

In 90% of cases treatment is by surgical removal (2). In early-diagnosed cases, the surgery is rather minor. However, in advanced or progressive cases more radical and sometimes disfiguring surgeries are required. Advances in plastic surgery have helped tremendously in the physical rehabilitation of such patients (5,6).

Radiation therapy, electrodessication, or cryosurgery are sometimes used.

Prognosis

Again, if found early, these carcinomas are almost 100% curable.

MALIGNANT MELANOMA

Description

There are three major clinical categories and one group of unclassified melanoma. Accounting for 75% of all melanomas, superficial spreading melanoma usually develops between the ages of 40 and 50 and may be large (i.e., >2 mm.) It may grow horizontally for many years before growing vertically. Nodular malignant melanoma (15% of melanomas) usually develops between the ages of 40 and 50, grows rapidly in a vertical direction, and invades the dermis. It is a particularly malignant tumor with a characteristically blue-black color. Lentigo malignant melanoma (5% of melanomas) usually develops between the ages of 60 and 70, develops slowly, tends to be a chronic lesion on the face, and presents as large and flat with irregular borders. The remaining 5% of melanomas are unclassified and include subungual, amelanotic, ocular, giant hairy nevus, and malignant blue nevus (7,8).

Incidence and Mortality

Melanoma is much rarer than other skin cancers. In 1997, over 100,000 cases will be diagnosed worldwide, with 40,300 invasive melanomas diagnosed in the United States. However, approximately 7500 people in the United States will die of melanoma in 1997, indicating a higher death rate than for nonmelanoma skin cancers (1,2). Of significant concern is the fact that the rate of increase in melanoma is between 15% and 50% in northern Europe and between 30% and 50% in white populations in North America and Hawaii *every five years*. Although not as high, there have also been substantial increases in populations where melanoma was previously much less common, such as in Cuba and Puerto Rico and in Jews in Israel (9).

Etiology

As for the other skin cancers, exposure to ultraviolet light is believed to be a major factor in the development of malignant melanoma. The latency period between sun exposure and melanoma development has been shown to be as little as 2 years and as great as 20 years. As discussed earlier, UVA may be particularly culpable. Additional evidence for the role of UVA can be found in the fact that as UVB sunscreens began to be commonly used in the early 1960s an increased incidence of melanoma would be expected to begin in the mid 1960s and 1970s. This is exactly what happened (3). There is also evidence of a hormonal relationship. More women than men get melanoma; prepubescent children rarely develop the disease, pregnancy may increase incidence and exacerbate growth; and 40% of melanomas have estrogen and progesterone receptors. Genetics may also play a role, since there are some families with a strong history of melanoma and, although it is rare in black Americans, there is a high incidence in the Bantu of southern Africa (7–10).

Prevention

The same recommendations presented for basal cell and squamous cell carcinoma apply for malignant melanoma. Stay out of the sun and when necessary wear protective clothing and use a true broad-spectrum sunscreen.

Diagnosis

Many, but not all, melanomas arise from a new or existing mole. There are eight cancer warning signs in a mole (11) (see Table 31.1).

Once a diagnosis is confirmed, staging occurs. Melanomas are described by Clark Level which is a measure of the depth of a melanoma in terms of the anatomic layers of skin involved. There are five levels measuring from the superficial surface of the skin (Clark I) to subcutaneous fatty tissue (Clark V.) Melanomas are also measured by Breslow Depth which is a measure of the vertical depth of a lesion in terms of millimeters. It is written as a decimal (e.g., 1.2 mm). The combination of Clark Level, Breslow Depth, and the degree of spread (e.g., regional or distant lymph nodes, organ sites) is used to determine the stage of the disease. Several staging systems exist for melanoma, but the current standard is that recommended by the American Joint Commission of Cancer (see Table 31.2) (11,12). Stages I and II represent local disease. Stage III indicates regional lymph node metastasis and/or in-transit disease. Stage IV refers to distant metastatic spread.

Treatment

Primary growths must be adequately removed along with surrounding tissues (i.e., wide excisions), although the amount of tissue that needs to be removed remains controversial (13–15). The single most important prognostic indicator is the presence of tumor in regional lymph nodes. The standard for determining nodal status has been complete lymphadenectomy followed by

TABLE 31.1. *Warning Signs of Skin Cancer*

Look for any one or more of the following changes in moles:

1. *Size* (sudden or continuous enlargement from side to side or elevation)
2. *Color* (darkening, multiple colors, spread of color)
3. *Shape* (irregular border or notching)
4. *Surface characteristics* (roughness, scaliness, crusting, oozing)
5. *Surrounding skin* (inflammation, redness, swelling, satellite pigmentation)
6. *Consistency* (softening, friability);
7. *Sensation* (itchiness, tingling, tenderness, pain)
8. *Sudden appearance* of a new mole.

Monthly self examinations using mirrors to examine the back should be done. Those at high risk should have someone else examine the back area as well.

Source: Johnson et al. (11).

TABLE 31.2. *TNM Classification System: Malignant Melanoma of the Skin*

DEFINITION OF TNM

- Both the level of invasion (Clark Level) and the maximum thickness (Breslow Depth) determine the T classification and should be recorded. In case of discrepancy between tumor thickness and level, pT category is based on the less favorable finding.
- Satellite lesions or subcutaneous nodules more than 2 cm from the primary tumor but not beyond the site of the primary lymph node drainage are considered in-transit metastases* and are listed under the N categories.
- The extent of tumor is classified after excision.

PRIMARY TUMOR (pT)

pTX	Primary tumor cannot be assessed
pT0	No evidence of primary tumor
pTis	Melanoma in situ (atypical melanocytic hyperplasia, severe melanocytic dysplasia), not an invasive lesion (Clark Level 1)
pT1	Tumor 0.75 mm or less in thickness and invading the papillary dermis (Clark Level II)
pT2	Tumor more than 0.75 mm but not more than 1.5 mm in thickness and/or invades to the papillary-reticular dermal interface (Clark Level III)
pT3	Tumor more than 1.5 mm but not more than 4 mm in thickness and/or invades the reticular dermis (Clark Level IV)
	pT3a Tumor more than 1.5 mm but not more than 3 mm in thickness
	pT3b Tumor more than 3 mm but not more than 1 mm in thickness
pT4	Tumor more than 4 mm in thickness and/or invades the subcutaneous tissue (Clark Level V) and/or satellite(s) within 2 cm of the primary tumor
	pT4a Tumor more than 4 mm in thickness and/or invades the subcutaneous tissue
	pT4b Satellites within 2 cm of the primary tumor

REGIONAL LYMPH NODES (N)

NX	Regional lymph nodes cannot be assessed
N0	No regional lymph nodes metastasis
N1	Metastasis 3 cm or less in greatest dimension in any regional lymph node(s)
N2	Metastasis more than 3 cm in greatest dimension in any regional lymph node(s) and/or in- transit metastasis
	N2a Metastasis more than 3 cm in greatest dimension in any regional lymph node
	N2b In-transit metastasis
	N2c Both (N2a and N2b)

DISTANT METASTASIS (M)

MX	Presence of distant metastasis cannot be assessed
M0	No distant metastasis
M1	Distant metastasis
	M1a Metastasis in skin or subcutaneous tissue or lymph node(s) beyond the regional lymph nodes
	M1b Visceral metastasis

*In-transit metastasis involves skin or subcutaneous tissue more than 2 cm from the primary tumor not beyond the regional lymph nodes.
Source: Ref. 12.

pathological examination using hematoxylin and eosin (H&E) staining. However, a new system has been developed utilizing preoperative lymphoscintigraphy, intraoperative lymphatic mapping, and a selective lymph node dissection followed by the standard H&E staining. All negative results are verified by immunohistochemical staining (i.e., HMB-45 and S-100). This program has resulted in less extensive surgical procedures for many patients and more accurate staging (16). Although most melanomas are radioresistant, some will respond. A number of different immunotherapy approaches are being tested alone and in combinations that show some promise for slowing the disease and/or preventing recurrence. These include local and systemic use of BCG (bacillus Calmette-Guerin), melanoma vaccines, systemic cytokines (e.g. interleukin-2 , interferon, and tumor necrosis factor), and monoclonal antibodies. Historically, the use of chemotherapy has been disappointing, but new combinations of several types of chemotherapy with an antihormonal agent show some promise. The Dartmouth regimen combining dacarbazine (DTIC), carmustine (BCNU), cisplatin, and tamoxifen reports response rates of 20% to 30%. Trials combining interferon-α, interleukin-2, and cytostatic drugs have also shown promising preliminary responses of 50% to 60% (11,17).

Prognosis—Recurrence and Survival

Small, thin melanomas that are removed promptly have a 95% to 100% cure rate. However, as the stage of the disease increases, the survival statistics drop precipitously (see Table 31.3).

PSYCHOLOGICAL FACTORS

Etiology

Most people are now aware that sun exposure plays a significant role in the development of skin cancer. However, many continue to "sun bathe" on a regular basis. Phrases such as "I'm going to work on getting a good tan" or "I feel so sickly white, I need to get a healthy tan" are commonly heard. Several factors have contributed to this paradox. Historically, the epitome of social beauty was defined as "milky white skin." In the 1930s, several haute couture designers began promoting a tan as a high fashion statement. When fears about skin cancer surfaced, various drug and cosmetic companies promoted the concept of a "safe tan" via the use of UVB-blocking sunscreens. Tanning parlors then began advertising their UVA sunbeds as a way to get a "healthy tan without the risk of sunburn." In addition, the lay press continues to promote the myth of a safe and healthy tan with numerous articles appearing every spring and summer. Finally, many people state that lying in the warmth of the sun is psychologically comforting and physically relaxing.

Many melanoma patients report greater than average major life stressors such as marital separation (via divorce or death), bankruptcy, and unemployment, within the five years prior to their diagnosis (18,19). It has been suggested that there is a type C personality that predisposes individuals to getting cancer and, in particular, melanoma (20). This personality type is characterized by emotional repression and high social desirability. There were, however, major methodological flaws associated with the data supporting these findings, including poor validity and reliability of measures and/or retrospective designs.

Prevention

Especially, most people do not believe they will get skin cancer and that even if they do it is "no big deal." Patients with basal cell carcinoma, in contrast to other kinds of non-skin cancer, show no more psychosocial problems than members of the general population (21). Education is paramount in the prevention of skin cancers. People need to learn about the true nature of these diseases, which are highly preventable and are curable if diagnosed and treated early but can

TABLE 31.3. *Staging and Prognosis of Malignant Melanoma*

Stage	Breslow Depth (mm)	Clark Level	Primary Tumor (pT)	Regional Lymph Nodes (N)	Distant Metastasis (M)	Percentage 5-year Survival
I	< 0.75	CII	pT1	N0	M0	95–99
	0.76–1.49	CIII	pT2	N0	M0	80–95
II	1.5–3.99	CIV	pT3	N0	M0	60–78
	>4.0	CV	pT4	N0	M0	< 50
III	NA	NA	Any pT	N1	M0	13–45
	NA	NA	Any pT	N2	M0	25
IV	NA	NA	Any pT	Any N	M1	10

Source: Refs 11 and 12.

be disfiguring and even deadly if ignored. Society needs to overcome the "healthy tan" syndrome and adopt a new psychological perspective toward prevention of all kinds of skin cancer, but especially malignant melanoma.

For those who will not accept the concept of "pale is beautiful," the new self-tanners may be a solution. These contain a synthetic compound called dihydroxyacetone or DHA. DHA binds with certain amino acids in the stratum corneum, or the top, dead layer of the skin. A real tan is caused by an increase in melanin released by the melanocytes. Since the DHA is only in the dead cells, the "tan" it produces lasts only as long as it takes to shed these cells. The new self-tanners produce a natural color and are generally considered safe (22).

Diagnosis

While the majority of people who develop skin cancer are diagnosed and treated appropriately, there are those who delay such action. First, are those who feel that it is "just skin cancer" and, therefore, not to be taken too seriously. At the opposite end of the spectrum are those who are so cancer phobic that they cannot contemplate the idea that they have any kind of cancer. Their fear is so great that they can only cope by using major denial. This is exemplified by reports of two unrelated elderly women who developed squamous cell carcinoma after loved ones died of cancer and chose to ignore the lesions despite disfiguring evidence. They took evasive measures to prevent others from noticing and finally died from their disease (23).

Delay in diagnosis of malignant melanoma has been associated with greater tumor thickness, which in turn is associated with poorer prognosis. Longer delays in diagnosis have been found in patients with lesions on the back, less previous knowledge about melanoma, and less understanding about treatment. Interestingly, patients who minimized the seriousness of their disease actually had shorter delays in seeking treatment. This may mean that patients who appraise their disease as very serious may be so emotionally overwhelmed that they are immobilized and can only cope by denial (24,25).

Treatment

Primary surgical treatment could range from a five-minute office procedure under local anesthesia to prolonged hospitalization and general anesthesia. Treatment decisions can be influenced by a number of psychological factors including fear of disfigurement, structural changes, pain, anesthesia, and death. These issues need to be explored with patients pre-

operatively and may include consultations with oncologic and plastic surgeons, speech therapists, dentists, and mental health professionals. A clear description of the nature of the disease, including prognosis, is necessary. The exact plan of treatment and expected outcome should be presented. Pertinent knowledge about major advances in microsurgery and reconstructive plastic surgery, skin grafts and facial prostheses, as well as improvements in anesthesia and pain control, may help to alleviate many patient concerns. Patients who were prepared for the both the length and depth of their surgical excision faired better psychologically than those were not adequately informed (26). Patients whose anxiety is interfering with decision making and/or rehabilitation should be referred for psychological help. Postoperative problems are most likely to develop in those who have had major surgery, and include impaired self-esteem, fear of negative responses from others, and social withdrawal.

The physical signs and symptoms of melanoma range along a continuum from none at all to those denoting multiple organ system impairment and correlate with stage of disease. Patients with no physical symptoms may also have no psychological symptoms, while others struggle with the uncertainty and anxiety regarding possible recurrence and metastasis. As the disease progresses, the severity of treatments also increases and psychological symptoms increase in both number and severity.

The majority of these patients will benefit from ongoing education, symptom management (psychological as well as physical), and emotional support. Psychiatric referral may be indicated for a number of reasons including: *(1)* management of reactive anxiety and depression; *(2)* pain management; *(3)* diagnosis of psychological versus organic syndromes; and *(4)* management of other psychiatric symptoms.

Prognosis

Little has been reported on the role that psychological factors play in the prognosis of squamous or basal cell carcinoma. This is probably due to the fact the majority of these skin cancers are rapidly removed and not allowed to progress. One study found that 5-year survival rates were not related to the subjects' reports of the duration of the lesions before treatment but suggested that individual stress responses could account for the differences (27).

Both high and low psychological distress levels in patients with malignant melanoma correlate positively with recurrence and survival (28–30). These contradictory findings may have to do with the degree of illness symptoms being experienced, the timing of the measurements (i.e., the specific point in the diagnosis/disease process), and the coping measures that are subsequently employed. In general, the fewer the symptoms the lower the level of distress. Patients with malignant melanoma who are diagnosed early usually do not have any major physical symptoms. Once the mole is removed, many patients feel that they are cured and that they truly have nothing to worry about. However,

TABLE 31.4. *Melanoma and Nonmelanoma Skin Cancer (NMSC): Psychosocial Studies*

	Author, Year (Ref.)	Variables Measured or Reviewed
MELANOMA		
Review	Pensiero, 1995 (31)	Stage IV malignant melanoma characteristics
	Servodidio, 1995 (32)	Choroidal melanoma: nursing care
	Perkins, 1993 (33)	Psychosocial support
	Servodidio, 1992 (34)	Choroidal melanoma: patient response
	Servodidio and Abramson, 1992 (35)	Choroidal melanoma: nursing interventions
	Lickiss, 1992 (36)	Symptom management
	Servodidio, 1991 (37)	Teaching aids for choroidal melanoma patients
	Temoshok, 1991 (38)	Psychological factors of cancer outcomes
	Holland, 1989 (39)	Psychological care
Research: *Identification of* *Psychosocial* *Variables*	Kelly et al. 1995 (40)	Post-traumatic stress response
	Brandberg et al. 1995 (41)	Psychosomatic complaints, depression
	Bunston et al., 1994 (42)	Nonmedical needs of ocular melanoma patients
	Brandberg et al., 1993 (43)	Cognitive and emotional responses to skin examination
	Sigurdardottir et al., 1993 (44)	Quality of life, depression prior to chemotherapy
	Gibertini et al., 1992 (19)	Stress, coping, psychiatric disturbance
	Havlik et al., 1992 (18)	Impact of stress on presentation of melanoma
	Cassileth et al., 1988 (28)	Cosmetic impact of melanoma resection
	Temoshok et al., 1985 (20)	Depression, mood, medical, demographic data
	Temoshok, 1985 (45)	Psychosocial factors, psychophysiology
	Kneier and Temoshok, 1984 (46)	Repressive coping reactions
	Temoshok et al., 1984 (24)	Delay in diagnosis
	Cassileth et al., 1983 (26)	Cosmetic impact of malignant melanoma resection
	Friedenbergs, 1981 (25)	Psychosocial management
	Rogentine et al., 1979 (29)	Psychosocial factors and prognosis
Research: *Interventions*	Fawzy, 1995 (47)	Coping, affective state
	Brandberg et al., 1994 (48)	Knowledge, satisfaction with knowledge
	Fawzy et al., 1993 (30)	Coping, affective state, recurrence, survival
	Brandberg et al., 1992 (49)	Prevention, early detection, emotional response
	Fawzy et al., 1990 (50)	Coping, affective state
	Fawzy et al., 1990 (51)	Immunological measures
	Levy et al., 1990 (52)	Mood, cognitive and immunological functioning
	LeBaron, 1989 (53)	Case history: image therapy for depression
NMSC		
Review	Mortimer, 1991 (54)	Nonmelanoma skin cancer
	Holland, 1989 (39)	Psychological care
Research: *Psychosocial* *Variables*	Zervas et al., 1993 (23)	Patient delay in diagnosis: crisis model
	Holfeld et al., 1990 (21)	Psychosocial assessment of patients with basal cell cancer
Research: *Interventions*	Robinson and Rademaker, 1995 (55)	Patient and care giver knowledge
	Robinson, 1992 (56)	Patient knowledge, sun protection behavior

melanoma may remain dormant for long periods of time and then recur, often after periods of high stress (18). In these cases, baseline measurements of distress may not have any relationship to later disease recurrence or survival.

A negative correlation between the emotional expression of sadness and anger (considered effective coping behavior) and the mitotic rate of tumors (a negative prognostic indicator) as well as a positive correlation between emotional expression and tumor-specific immune responses (a positive prognostic indicator) have been found (19). Patients who give a low estimate of the amount of adjustment needed to cope with their malignant melanoma, suggesting denial, have shown a greater rate of recurrence within the first year (29). Patients with a more realistic understanding of this disease, who experience high distress early on but also use effective behavioral and cognitive coping techniques, have been shown to have better 5-year recurrence and survival rates than those who do not express such distress or who do not employ effective coping (30). These data suggest that high levels of distress contribute to the progression of melanoma but that effectively coping with this distress, especially by expression of emotion, may buffer the otherwise negative effects.

Psychological Interventions

Numerous interventions for cancer patients, many of them using patients with malignant melanoma, have been proposed and tested and most have been of some psychological value. In general, the interventions providing a combination of education, coping skills training, and group emotional support seem to provide the most benefit. A complete review of interventions for cancer patients may be found in Chapter 59.

The dramatic rise in both nonmelanoma and melanoma skin cancers over the last few decades has resulted in a rapidly increasing population of patients whose unique psychosocial issues need to be identified and addressed. Although they have been slow in appearing, the number of psychosocial studies involving patients with skin cancer is now increasing. Psychosocial characteristics of specific skin cancer populations are being identified and therapeutic modalities are being suggested and tested (see Table 31.4).

REFERENCES

1. American Cancer Society. *Cancer Facts & Figures—1997.* Atlanta, GA: American Cancer Society, 1997.
2. Armstrong BK, Kricker A. Skin cancer. *Dermatol Clin.* 1995; 13:583–594.
3. Garland CF, Garland FC, Gorham ED. Rising trends in melanoma: an hypothesis concerning sunscreen effectiveness. *Ann Epidemiol.* 1993; 3:103–110.
4. Johnson EY, Lookingbill DP. Sunscreen use and sun exposure. *Arch Dermatol.* 1984; 120:727–731.
5. Ianetti G, Belli E, Spallacia F, Cicconetti A, Cavallaro A, Cisternino S. The use of the jejunum free flap in the reconstruction of the oral cavity. *Acta Otorhinolaryngol Ital.* 1994; 14:167–183.
6. Papadopoulos ON, Gamatsi IE. Use of the latissimus dorsi flap in head and neck reconstructive microsurgery. *Microsurgery.* 1994; 15:492–495.
7. Nathanson I. Melanoma and other skin malignancies. In: Skeel RT, ed. *Handbook of Cancer Chemotherapy*, 2d ed. Boston: Little, Brown; 1987: 182–191.
8. Nixon DW. Melanoma. In: Nixon DW, ed. *Diagnosis and Management of Cancer*, Ch. 18. Menlo Park, CA: Addison-Wesley; 1982: 237–248.
9. Coleman MP, Esteve J, Damiecki P, Arslan A, Renard H. Melanoma of the Skin. In: *Trends in Cancer Incidence and Mortality*, Ch. 18. IARC Scientific Publications No. 121. Lyon: IARC; 1993: 379–410.
10. Runkle GP, Zaloznik AJ. Malignant melanoma. *Am Fam Physician.* 1994; 49:91–98.
11. Johnson TM, Smith JW, Nelseon BR, Chang AC. Current therapy for cutaneous melanoma. *J Am Acad Dermatol.* 1995; 32:689–707.
12. Malignant melanoma of the skin (excluding eyelid). In: Beahrs OH, Henson DE, Hutter RVP, et al., eds. *American Joint Committee on Cancer Manual for Staging of Cancer*, 4th ed. Philadelphia: JB Lippincott; 1992:143–148.
13. Brown CD, Zitelli JA. The prognosis and treatment of true local cutaneous recurrent malignant melanoma. *Dermatol Surg.* 1995; 21:285–290.
14. Jakowitz JG, Meyskens FL Jr. Evaluation and treatment of the patient with early melanoma. *Compr Ther.* 1995; 21:46–50.
15. Dzubow LM. Malignant melanoma: treatment in evolution. *Dermatol Surg.* 1995; 21:924.
16. Morton D. Intraoperative lymphatic mapping and sentinel lymphadenectomy: community standard care or clinical investigation? *Cancer J Sci Am.* 1997; 3(6)1–3.
17. Marks R, Motley RJ. Skin cancer: recognition and treatment. *Drugs.* 1995; 50:48–61.
18. Havlik RJ, Vukasin AP, Ariyan S. The impact of stress on the clinical presentation of melanoma. *Plast Reconst Surg.* 1992; 90:57–61.
19. Gibertini M, Reintgen DS, Baile WF. Psychosocial aspects of melanoma. *Annals Plast Surg.* 1992; 28:17–21.
20. Temoshok L. Biopsychosocial studies on cutaneous malignant melanoma: psychosocial factors associated with prognostic indicators, progression, psychophysiology and tumor-host response. *Soc Sci Med.* 1985; 20:833–840.
21. Holfeld KI, Hogan DJ, Eldemire M, Lane PR. A psychosocial assessment of patients with basal cell carcinoma. *J Dermatol Surg Oncol.* 1990; 16:750–753.
22. Levy SD. Dihydroxyacetone-containing sunless or self-tanning lotions. *J Am Acad Dermatol.* 1992; 27(6, pt.1):989–993.

23. Zervas IM, Augustine A, Fricchione GL. Patient delay in cancer: a view from the crisis model. *Gen Hosp Psychiatry*. 1993; 15:9–13.

24. Temoshok L, DiClemente RJ, Sweet DM, Blois MS, Sagebiel RW. Factors related to patient delay in seeking medical attention for cutaneous malignant melanoma. *Cancer*. 1984; 54:3048–3053.

25. Freidenbergs I. Psychosocial management of patients with cutaneous cancers: a preliminary report. *J Dermatol Surg Oncol*. 1981; 7:828–830.

26. Cassileth BR, Lusk EJ, Tenaglia A. Patient's perceptions of the cosmetic impact of melanoma resection. *Plast Reconstruct Surg*. 1983; 71:73–75.

27. Sutton PR. Prognosis of carcinoma of the lip or tongue in relation to mental stress: speculation on an anomalous finding. *Med J Aust*. 1968; 2:312–313.

28. Cassileth BR, Walsh WP, Lusk EJ. Psychosocial correlates of cancer survival: a subsequent report 3 to 8 years after cancer diagnosis. *J Clin Oncol*. 1988; 6: 1753–1759.

29. Rogentine GW, Van Kammen DP, Fox BH, et al. Psychosocial factors in the prognosis of malignant melanoma: a prospective study. *Psychosom Med*. 1979; 41:647–655.

30. Fawzy FI, Fawzy NW, Hyun CS, et al. Malignant melanoma: effects of an early structured intervention, coping, and affective state on recurrence and survival 6 years later. *Arch Gen Psychiatry*. 1993; 50:681–689.

31. Pensiero L. Stage IV malignant melanoma. Psychosocial issues. *Cancer*. 1995; 75:742–747.

32. Servodidio CA. Nursing care of the choroidal melanoma patient. *Semin Perioperative Nurs*. 1995; 4:211–219.

33. Perkins PJ. Psychosocial support and malignant melanoma. *Eur J Cancer*. 1993; 2:161–164.

34. Servodidio CA. Human responses to the diagnosis of choroidal melanoma. *J Ophthal Nurs Technol*. 1992; 11:247–249.

35. Servodidio CA, Abramson DH. Choroidal melanoma. *Nurs Clin N Am*. 1992; 27:777–791.

36. Lickiss JN. Palliative care and melanoma: the care of the patient with progressive disease. *World J Surg*. 1992; 16:282–286.

37. Servodidio CA. Teaching aids for patients diagnosed with choroidal melanoma. *Insight*. 1991; 16:21–23.

38. Temoshok L. Malignant melanoma, AIDS, and the complex search for psychosocial mechanisms. Symington Foundation Symposium: New directions in cancer care (1990; Stanford, California). *Advances*. 1991; 7:20–28.

39. Holland JC. Skin cancer and melanoma. In: Holland JC, Rowland JH, eds. *Handbook of Psychooncology: Psychological Care of the Patient with Cancer*. New York: Oxford University Press; 1989: 246–249.

40. Kelly B, Raphael B, Smithers M, et al. Psychological responses to malignant melanoma. An investigation of traumatic stress reactions to life-threatening illness. *Gen Hosp Psychiatry*. 1995; 17:126–134.

41. Brandberg Y, Mansson-Brahme E, Ringborg U, Sjoden PO. Psychological reactions in patients with malignant melanoma. *Eur J Cancer*. 1995; 31A:157–162.

42. Bunston T, Mackie A, Jones D, Mings D. Identifying the nonmedical concerns of patients with ocular melanoma. *J Ophthal Nurs Technol*. 1994; 13:227–237.

43. Brandberg Y, Bolund C, Michelson H, Mansson-Brahme E, Ringborg U, Sjoden PO. Psychological reactions in public melanoma screening. *Eur J Cancer*. 1993; 29A:860–863.

44. Sigurdardottir V, Bolund C, Brandberg Y, Sullivan M. The impact of generalized malignant melanoma on quality of life evaluated by the EORTC questionnaire technique. *Qual Life Res*. 1993; 2:193–203.

45. Temoshok L. Biopsychosocial studies on cutaneous malignant melanoma: psychosocial factors associated with prognostic indicators, progression, psychophysiology and tumor-host response. *Social Sci Med*. 1985; 20:833–840.

46. Kneier AW, Temoshok L. Repressive coping reactions in patients with malignant melanoma as compared to cardiovascular disease patients. *J Psychosom Res*. 1984; 28:145–155.

47. Fawzy NW. A psychoeducational nursing intervention to enhance coping and affective state in newly diagnosed malignant melanoma patients. *Cancer Nurs*. 1995; 18:427–438.

48. Brandberg, Y, Bergenmar M, Bolund C, et al. Information to patients with malignant melanoma: a randomized group study. *Patient Educ Couns* 1994; 23:97–105.

49. Brandberg Y, Bergenmar M, Bolund C, Mansson-Brahme E, Ringborg U, Sjoden PO. Psychological effects of participation in a prevention programme for individuals with increased risk for malignant melanoma. *Eur J Cancer*. 1992; 28A:1334–1338.

50. Fawzy FI, Cousins N, Fawzy NW, et al. A structured psychiatric intervention for cancer patients: I. Changes over time in methods of coping and affective disturbance. *Arch Gen Psychiatry*. 1990; 47:720–725.

51. Fawzy FI, Kemeny ME, Fawzy NW, et al. A structured psychiatric intervention for cancer patients: II. Changes over time in immunological measures. *Arch Gen Psychiatry*. 1990; 47:729–735.

52. Levy S, Herberman RB, Rodin J, Seligman M. Psychological and immunological effects of a randomized psychosocial treatment trial for colon cancer and malignant melanoma patients. In Balner H, van Rood Y, eds. *Conceptual and Methodological Issues in Cancer Psychotherapy Intervention Studies*. Publications of the Helen Dowling Institute for Biopsychosocial Medicine, 3. Lisse: Swets & Zeitlinger; 1990: 75–88.

53. LeBaron, S. The role of imagery in the treatment of a patient with malignant melanoma. *Hospice J*. 1989; 5:13–23.

54. Mortimer P. Squamous cell and basal cell skin carcinoma and rarer histologic types of skin cancer. *Curr Opin Oncol*. 1991; 3:349–354.

55. Robinson JK, Rademaker AW. Skin cancer risk and sun protection learning by helpers of patients with nonmelanoma skin cancer. *Prev Med*. 1995; 24:333–341.

56. Robinson JK. Compensation strategies in sun protection behaviors by a population with nonmelanoma skin cancer. *Prev Med*. 1992; 21:754–765.

32

Breast Cancer

JULIA H. ROWLAND AND MARY JANE MASSIE

Breast cancer, the most common form of cancer among American women, will be diagnosed in over 184,300 women in 1996, and an estimated 44,300 women will die of the disease (1). While an exact understanding of the causes and control of breast cancer continues to elude researchers, rapid advances in detection and treatment have led to increases in the disease-free survival among women diagnosed with breast cancer (1–3). The majority of women diagnosed today, can expect to be cured of or live for long periods with their disease. However, unlike treatment for other chronic diseases such as diabetes and heart disease, the treatments for cancer are both more toxic and intensive. The result is increasing demands not only on patients' physical reserves, but also on their psychological and social resources to survive and manage illness.

Specific developments in breast cancer care have drawn attention to the key role of psychosocial factors in prevention, detection, treatment, and outcome (4). Improvements in and broader use of screening mammography have led not only to an increase in numbers of women whose cancers are diagnosed at earlier stages, but also to questions of who gets screened and who does not. The greater availability of options for surgical management (e.g., lumpectomy plus radiation versus mastectomy with or without breast reconstruction with implants and/or autologous tissue) has expanded women's role in the decision-making process. More extensive use of aggressive multimodal treatment regimens has increased sensitivity to issues of patient–doctor and family communication and of patient adherence. Finally, identification of genetic markers of breast cancer risk and the evaluation of chemopreventive agents has raised awareness of the psychological toll on unaffected women who are at increased risk for this disease, sometimes referred to as the "worried well" (5).

All of these changes have occurred in the context of greater demand by patients for involvement in their own care, consumer activism, attention to ethical and informed consent issues, use of quality of life assessment in treatment outcomes, and, most recently, emphasis on cost efficacy in care. The consequence of these changes is a growing demand for medical professionals to recognize and address the psychosocial impact of breast cancer across the course of care.

While breast cancer is a major stress for any woman, there is great variability in women's psychological responses. This chapter outlines the normal as well as abnormal responses to breast cancer and those factors that may increase a woman's risk for poor adaptation. In addition, because of their growing importance, the role of family in women's adaptation and special concerns related to sexual functioning will be addressed.

FACTORS AFFECTING PSYCHOLOGICAL IMPACT

Three sets of factors contribute to psychological response: the sociocultural context in which treatment options are offered, the psychological and psychosocial factors that the woman and her environment bring to the situation, and the medical factors or physical facts the woman must confront in terms of disease stage, treatment, response, and clinical course (Table 32.1). To provide comprehensive care to every woman, each of these areas must be assessed and, when encountered, problems must be addressed across the illness trajectory.

Sociocultural Context

To understand—and interpret—the data on women's responses to breast cancer, it is critical to appreciate the context within which diagnosis and treatment occur, both medically and socially. Several specific changes that have taken place in the scientific under-

TABLE 32.1. *Factors Contributing to the Psychological Responses of Women to Breast Cancer*

CURRENT SOCIOCULTURAL CONTEXT, TREATMENT OPTIONS, AND DECISION-MAKING

Changes in surgical management from a uniform approach

- Breast-conserving management; more acknowledged uncertainty

Social attitudes

- Public figures disclose having had breast cancer
- Autobiographic accounts of and "how to" guides for treatment of breast cancer in popular press

Ethical imperative for patient participation in treatment issues; legal imperative for knowledge of treatment options

Variations in care by ethnicity, location, age

Public awareness of treatment and research controversies; advocacy for more funding and lay oversight

PSYCHOLOGICAL AND PSYCHOSOCIAL FACTORS

Type and degree of disruption in life cycle tasks caused by breast cancer (e.g. marital, childbearing)

Psychological stability and ability to cope with stress

Prior psychiatric history

Availability of psychological and social support (partner, family, friends)

MEDICAL FACTORS

Stage of cancer at diagnosis

Treatment(s) received: mastectomy/lumpectomy and radiation, adjuvant chemotherapy, hormonal therapy, bone marrow transplant

Availability of rehabilitation

- Psychological (partner, support groups)
- Physical (reconstruction)

Psychological support provided by physicians and staff

Source: Rowland JH, Massie MJ, Psychologic reactions to breast cancer diagnosis, treatment and survival. In Harris JR Lippman ME, Morrow M, Hellman S, eds., *Diseases of the Breast*, Philadelphia: Lippincott–Raven, 1996.

standing of and medical approach to breast cancer in the last decade have had a significant impact on how this disease is viewed by the public. Primary among these changes have been growing attention to the patient's role in decision making across the course of cancer care, increased demand for and greater public involvement in the assessment of research into the prevention and treatment of breast cancer in particular, and more federal support for research on the psychosocial and behavioral aspects of cancer.

Decision-Making. The importance of patient involvement in treatment choices is the result both of the broader range of options offered at time of diagnosis and greater intensity of treatments recommended for the majority of women, even those with early-stage disease, as well as increased public demand for informed consent. Today, women with a diagnosis of breast cancer are aware of the plurality of views about primary breast cancer treatment. Most recognize that no "best" treatment exists, that they have options, and that their preference can be considered in the decision. Women are often provided with survival statistics associated with each mode of treatment, although physicians may vary in

the emphasis placed on them. The increased dialogue between physician and patient about treatment reduces some of the stresses formerly faced by women in an earlier period when there was little discussion about management of the disease. However, the new psychological burden of responsibility for making the right choice can increase anxiety when it is already great.

Over the course of initial care, women face three major decision points. The first of these is at the time of initial discovery of the lump. Most women consult their gynecologist or a trusted and accessible physician when they find a lump (64%–70% of which are found by women themselves) (6). How quickly a woman decides to seek evaluation of her lump or to follow up on a recommended course of action depends on a number of variables including sociodemographic status; knowledge, attitudes, and beliefs about cancer; personality and coping styles; and the nature of the existing doctor–patient relationship (7). It is well established that the earlier her tumor is detected, the more likely a woman's breast cancer is to be curable. However, presence of advanced disease does not always imply delay (8). Further, responsibility for delay may rest with the physician, the woman, or both. In cases where delay has occurred, a woman's response, including feelings of guilt over her role in the delay, anger at her physician's role, or both, can interfere with her ability to adapt to treatment. Helping her to focus on the fact that she is receiving care now and deferring until after treatment is commenced exploration of what impact, if any, delaying diagnosis may have had can be important in enabling a woman to engage in the recovery process.

At the time of consultation with a surgeon, the woman is faced with her second set of decisions: whether to accept a one-step or a two-step procedure; if given a choice, whether to undergo mastectomy or lumpectomy plus irradiation; and whether to seek a second opinion or care elsewhere. In 18 states the law and clinical practice dictate that the surgeon must inform the woman that she has the option of a two-stage surgical procedure, which separates the diagnostic biopsy from the primary treatment procedure. In these states, the two treatment options of mastectomy or lumpectomy with irradiation must be presented as well, although how this is done varies widely by state (9). Some insurance carriers mandate a second opinion before the performance of any elective procedure. Research has shown that these laws make a difference; in those states that mandate informed decision-making, more women receive lumpectomy (10,11). At the same time, while these policies provide a valuable impetus for women to obtain thorough medical evaluation and information, they also serve to introduce other sets of opinions. The woman whose second, or third opinion differs dramatically has the difficult task of deciding which physician she trusts and which treatment plan to accept. Meanwhile, considerable time can be lost.

In the past few years, a number of cancer centers across the country have developed multidisciplinary breast clinics to address the need for women to seek opinions from diverse specialists. In these centers, women are usually seen after their initial biopsy and meet with a surgeon, medical oncologist, and radiation oncologist, and, in some centers, other breast specialists including a pathologist, a radiologist, a plastic surgeon, a mental health professional, and a clinical research nurse. The concept behind this one-stop visit is to provide the woman with information about all of her treatment options in a comprehensive setting and to outline for her treatment that can be tailored to her specific cancer as well as personal needs. Clinical experience suggests that such programs are helpful in reducing the stress experienced by women around decision-making and facilitating information gathering.

During the diagnostic work-up period, the woman must cope simultaneously with the need to keep her distressing emotions of anxiety and fear within tolerable limits while making the difficult decision about treatment for a potentially fatal disease. To accomplish this, she must assimilate new medical information that, in itself, produces anxiety. One study has shown that before and after breast biopsy, anxiety and information overload compromise some women's decision-making ability, making informed decisions difficult, even at best (12). Valanis and Rumpler noted that a woman's previous experiences and her personal and demographic characteristics, as well as those of her social support network (family and friends) and her physician influence her treatment selection (13).

The current legal climate that dictates that full and complete disclosure of information be given by the doctor, in a uniform manner to all women, fails to take into account the wide variation in women's reactions to the information and the range of ways of dealing with the decisions about treatment. Ideally, the method of giving information should be individualized for each patient. Emphasis on informed decision-making places a heavy responsibility on the physician to be cognizant of the individual patient's physical and psychological needs and to tailor the discussion and recommendations with that in mind. At times it may mean tempering a woman's demands for unrealistic treatment, acquiescing to another woman's desire to defer a final decision to her physician or significant other, or in some cases, reassuring a woman that she need not reach a decision instantly but has a few days to research her options and come to an appropriate choice. [A broader review of women's response styles and physician–patient communication issues is provided elsewhere (14–16).]

Some women when faced with breast cancer find themselves emotionally paralyzed by the decision making process. They may be overwhelmed by the knowledge that they have breast cancer and by its potential threat to their lives. For these women, even the options are too painful to consider. They often benefit from referral for psychiatric consultation. It is helpful for them to have the pressure temporarily removed by postponement of surgery and to be able to review the events and possible treatments in a setting in which they can express concerns and fears and identify the reasons for their response. A useful procedure is for the mental health consultant or specially trained nurse clinician to take them, step by step, through each treatment option, asking at each juncture "How would you respond to that?" By this method, with reduced anxiety, it usually becomes clear that certain aspects of one or the other treatment are more acceptable to the patient. These women can then return to their surgeon ready to proceed with treatment.

While many women report the decision-making process as highly stressful, research indicates that women who are given a choice about treatment do better than those who are not (17–20). Other studies show that the quality of physician communication during this phase is a critical determinant of subsequent psychological well-being in breast cancer patients (21). Finally, although most women when confronted with breast cancer want to have information, clinicians need to be aware that not all women wish to make the final decision about treatment (22). A woman's need for information must be assessed separately from her desire to participate in or delegate treatment choice.

Public Attitudes. Recent years have seen a growing sense of public distrust toward the medical community in general and cancer research in particular. Some of this arises from confusion about the state of progress in the war on cancer (23). In addition, the public and some researchers remain uncertain about the attributable risk of a variety of epidemiologic factors (e.g., use of exogenous hormones such as oral contraceptives and hormone replacement; exposure to environmental carcinogens such as pesticides; dietary risks) (24). Finally, several specific events have fueled public concern. These include questions raised at the Food and Drug Administration hearings about silicone and saline implant safety, publication of early reports that tamoxifen may have more serious long-term effects than anticipated (25), and media reports challenging the results of clinical trials whose outcomes have influenced the course of breast cancer care.

While at times creating fear, rage, and confusion for women who felt their treatment or lives were affected, disclosure of this information has served to empower a sector of the population to become more vocal advocates for better breast cancer prevention and treatment research. The Breast Cancer Coalition, represented largely by breast cancer survivors and the health care professionals caring for them, was successful in lobbying substantial funds from the Department of Defense earmarked for breast cancer research. More recently, lay advocates have been specifically included in clinical trials oversight committees. The net effect of this movement is growing attention to the need for more research on prevention as well as methods to increase survival. Included in this is emphasis on the role that psycho-

social factors play in breast cancer risk, detection, and survival.

Psychological Variables

In her now classic review, Meyerowitz (26) delineated the psychosocial impact of breast cancer in three broad areas: psychological discomfort (anxiety, depression and anger); changes in life patterns (consequent to physical discomfort, marital, or sexual disruption, and altered activity level); and fears and concerns (mastectomy/loss of breast, recurrence and death) (26). Although women diagnosed today may have many more treatment options, the psychological concerns remain the same. In addition to these variables, the life stage at which the cancer occurs, previous emotional stability (personality and coping style), and the presence of interpersonal support should be included.

Age, or the point in the life cycle at which breast cancer occurs, and what social tasks are threatened or interrupted, are of prime importance. The threat to a sense of femininity and self-esteem occurs in all women, but it may be more difficult for a young woman whose attractiveness and fertility are paramount, especially for those who are single and without a partner. In their review, Mor and colleagues (27) highlight several factors that may put younger women at greater risk for problems in adapting. These include the "off-timedness" of a diagnosis in the younger patient; disruption of primary role as caregiver and, increasingly, as "breadwinner"; and their perception of having more to lose (including careers and chance to see offspring grow up). At the other end of the spectrum, breast cancer diagnosed in a woman over 65 years old may be experienced in the presence of other major losses, particularly of spouse, which means that she must adjust to concurrent life stresses. Fotopoulos and Cook, reporting from a multicenter psychological study of breast cancer, noted a high level of distress in older women (28). Such reports, coupled with recent findings that indicate that older women are significantly less likely to receive appropriate surgical care or rehabilitation (29), suggest that women at both ends of the developmental continuum are at particular risk for problems in adapting to breast cancer.

The second variable contributing to adaptation relates to the patient herself, that is, her personality and coping patterns. Studies of breast cancer patients suggest that women who use an active, problem-solving approach to the stresses of illness exhibit less distressed mood and better adaptation (30–32). In addition, because adaptation to illness is necessarily a dynamic process, those who exhibit flexibility in their efforts cope better. For example, Glanz and Lerman note that while information-seeking and problem-solving skills may be critical during treatment planning, use of denial and avoidant coping strategies during active chemotherapy or radiation may be more helpful in reducing or minimizing treatment side effects (4). The relative efficacy of each style thus may be situation-specific (33). Finally, women who are able to draw upon and use available social resources and support adapt better as well (34). By contrast, women at risk for poor coping are those who exhibit a passive, helpless, hopeless, or pessimistic stance in the face of illness, are rigid in their use of coping strategies, and tend to be socially isolated or to reject help when offered. Further studies suggest that women who exhibit a pattern of active "fighting spirit" to their disease not only have better quality of life but may also survive longer than women who appear to "give up" (35).

In the context of any discussion of coping responses, it is important to note that the relationship between attitudes and cancer survival, as well as risk, has become a growing area of public interest and psycho-oncologic research. Because breast cancer is a prevalent neoplasm and one with great psychological impact, the possible role of psychological variables in risk and survival has been explored extensively. The question of a potential role for emotions in vulnerability to breast cancer and its progression has received much attention in the public press. Many women express concern that they "brought it on themselves," or that their attitude is bad and that they or their lifestyle may be making the cancer worse. In a study of what women attributed to having caused their breast cancer, Taylor and colleagues found that 41% of their well-educated sample felt that they were responsible for the development of the disease and that stress was a major contributor to its development (31). In our own research at Georgetown University among women 4–12 months after treatment for node-negative breast cancer, 44 of 151 women interviewed (29%) indicated that they felt stress and/or emotions contributed to their illness; 21% felt such factors played a major role in disease onset (36).

The belief that they may be responsible for their own illness and its outcome has become an added psychological burden for many women with breast cancer. Indeed, it is a hazard for those who, based on these beliefs, seek questionable and unproved therapies as primary treatment for their breast cancer, either never starting or discontinuing conventional treatments. Publication in the public media of early and controversial findings about emotions in breast cancer is a growing concern. For these reasons, it is important

that oncologists are familiar with the status of psychological research in breast cancer risk and survival so as to be able to answer their patients' questions on the subject and provide clarification and reassurance. For an extensive review of the research on psychological factors in cancer risk and survival, the reader is referred to Chapters 11 and 12 in this text, as well as reviews by Levenson and Bemis (37), and Spiegel (38).

Prior personal association with breast cancer can also influence adjustment. The memory of a mother's, sister's or grandmother's death from breast cancer, or that of a close friend, makes the diagnosis seem far more ominous and may result in greater levels of psychological distress during and after treatment. Some women with a high investment in their bodies cannot tolerate even the idea of loss or damage to a breast. Such women are at risk for delay in seeking consultation when a symptom occurs; they may also be at risk for problems in adaptation following treatment, particularly if hoped-for attempts to preserve cosmetic appearance are less successful than expected or must be abandoned owing to the extent of disease.

Finally, adjustment depends on the response from other significant people—first and foremost from spouse or partner, but also from family and friends. Because of the importance of social support to women's adaptation, this is addressed at greater length under the section on family adaptation.

It is important to note that prolonged anxiety or depression is not an expected reaction to a cancer diagnosis. Of 50 studies of the prevalence of depression in individuals with cancer published between 1967 and 1993, 17 included women with breast cancer (39). Reported rates of depression in these 17 studies range from 1.5% to 50%. Most of this variance can be attributed to the lack of standardization of methodology and diagnostic criteria. The common stress reactions around the time of diagnosis and during early treatment can be quickly evaluated and managed by the patient's physician, nurse, or specially designated cancer counselor. However, some women have greater problems and will benefit from psychological management by psychiatrists and psychologists who often are collaborating members of the treatment team (see Table 32.2).

Consultation is usually requested for women who are at high genetic risk for breast cancer and request prophylactic mastectomy; for women who are cancer-phobic and are considering prophylactic mastectomy; for those unable to make a decision about treatment; and for those with a psychiatric history of an anxiety or depressive disorder, substance abuse, or other mental illness. The patient who presents as a management

TABLE 32.2. *Women with Breast Cancer Who Should be Considered for Psychiatric Evaluation*

- Those who present with current symptoms or a history of:

  depression or anxiety

  suicidal thinking (attempt)

  substance or alcohol abuse

  confusional state (delirium or encephalopathy)

  akathisia from neuroleptic antiemetics

  mood swings, insomnia or irritability from steroids

- Those who:

  have a family history of breast cancer;

  are very young, old, pregnant, nursing, single or alone;

  are adjusting to multiple losses and managing multiple life stresses;

  seem paralyzed with cancer treatment decisions;

  fear death during surgery or are terrified by loss of control under anesthesia;

  request euthanasia;

  seem unable to provide informed consent.

Source: Rowland JH, Massie MJ, Psychologic reactions to breast cancer diagnosis, treatment and survival. In Harris JR, Lippman ME, Morrow M, Hellman S, eds., *Diseases of the Breast*, Philadelphia: Lippincott–Raven, 1996.

problem for the physician and his or her staff, or who is unable to comply with hospital rules, also needs psychiatric consultation. Rarely are patients so depressed that they are frankly suicidal during evaluation and treatment. However, if suicidal thinking is expressed, a formal psychiatric evaluation should be requested.

Medical Variables

The stage of breast cancer at diagnosis, the treatment required, the prognosis, and the rehabilitative opportunities available constitute the medical variables that influence psychological adjustment. Central, however, is the relationship to the supportive surgeon, radiotherapist, or oncologist, who, ideally, is sensitive to the concerns of the patient, communicates clearly, and monitors emotional as well as physical well-being. Both the expanded length and intensity of treatments and the recognition that women treated for breast cancer must be followed for the remainder of their lives have placed an added burden on health care providers who are expected to provide support across the course of care, often involving years of follow-up. The office or clinic nurse and treatment staff become the patient's "second family." Receptionists as well as radiotherapy technicians additionally contribute actively to the social environment that the patient experiences. While some clinicians and staff welcome this added demand, others may not be comfortable with the expected intimacy and care, particularly around psychosocial issues.

Mastectomy. Because it was for so long the standard treatment for breast cancer, and still continues to be recommended for large numbers of women, there is considerable research on the impact of loss of one or both breasts on women's physical, social, and emotional functioning. Among the effects documented are feelings of mutilation and altered body image, diminished self-worth, loss of a sense of femininity, decrease in sexual attractiveness and function, anxiety, depression, hopelessness, guilt, shame, and fear of recurrence, abandonment, and death (26,40). While mourning for the loss of a cherished body part and the threat to life are universal, the extent to which other sequelae are experienced appears variable. Early research indicated that anywhere from 10% to 56% of women studied one to two years after mastectomy experienced some degree of social or emotional impairment (41,42). However, a large prospective study found that women who are well adjusted before they have a mastectomy, and whose disease is in an early stage, can expect at one year to have a quality of life equal to that of unaffected peers, a finding since replicated in other controlled studies (43,44). In addition to more advanced disease, other predictors of poorer adaptation in this study were additional concurrent illness or stress, expectation of poor support from others, and a tendency to perceive events in life as less under one's own control. More recently, research suggests that while most women report improvement in emotional and physical well-being over time, for a significant minority (20%–

25%) problems may persist beyond two years post treatment (45).

There has been a dramatic shift away from more radical surgical approaches to breast cancer based on scientific evidence that systemic versus more extensive local management therapy was more critical to survival (46). This also has been advanced by the hope that, by sparing breast tissue, much of the psychosocial morbidity associated with the disease could be reduced.

Lumpectomy and Irradiation. Since 1980, more than two dozen studies have examined the differences on social and emotional as well as sexual functioning among women undergoing mastectomy or lumpectomy with irradiation (Table 32.3) (47–57). Despite the variability in methods employed, the early pattern of results was very consistent: women who received breast-sparing surgery were less self-conscious, had a better body image, reported greater satisfaction with sexual activity, and manifested a somewhat better overall adjustment. In particular, women in the conservation group felt they were less sexually inhibited, had sex more frequently, and reported that their husbands were more sexual and affectionate than did women undergoing mastectomy.

While the overall data suggest that women receiving lumpectomy and irradiation have, as a group, adapted well (58,59), three important criticisms have been leveled at this research. First, most of these studies evaluated women within the first year and often the first few months of their treatment. Thus it was not known whether these early differences would persist over time. Indeed, there is some evidence to suggest that women in the conservation group fare no differently from (60,61), or may do worse than their mastectomy peers in the long term (62).

There is also the concern that the populations of women undergoing each option were self-selected and perhaps differed before surgery. Of the studies reviewed, all were conducted after surgery was completed, and in most cases women or their physicians had chosen between one or the other option. The four exceptions to this were the studies by Schain and colleagues (48), de Haes and Welvaart (51), Fallowfield and colleagues (53), and Lasry and colleagues (55). In each of these studies the women were randomized to receive either mastectomy or limited resection and irradiation. Both Schain's and the de Haes and Welvaart's data demonstrated more positive feelings about body image among the lumpectomy and irradiation group but little difference with respect to the other parameters measured. In contrast, Fallowfield found no significant differences between the groups; if anything,

the lumpectomy group appeared to do somewhat worse. The data of Lasry and colleagues data fell in between: lumpectomy patients had a better body image than mastectomy patients, but women receiving irradiation exhibited higher levels of depression. A further confounder to interpretation of the results of the studies is that younger women, already at increased risk for psychosocial problems in adaptation to breast cancer by virtue of age and developmental stage disruption, tend to select breast conservation.

Given the expected dramatic emotional benefit that saving the breast was expected to provide women, the differences seen are less than might have been predicted (63,64). In some cases, while statistically significant, the differences observed do not appear to be clinically significant. It is important to be aware that breast conservation is not a psychosocial panacea (62); rather, it serves to provide a woman with options in her care that may facilitate her particular adaptation.

Two critical factors that continue to influence the surgical decision-making process are attitudes about cancer and irradiation. The thought of leaving tumor cells in the breast is intolerable for some women, who feel more secure with mastectomy. Other women fear irradiation or are unable to devote six weeks to daily radiation therapy treatments because of family or work demands or distance from a treatment center. Personality characteristics also influence a woman's decision. Women selecting lumpectomy plus irradiation over mastectomy have been found to be more concerned about insult to body-image, to be more dependent on their breasts for self-esteem, and to believe that they would have difficulty adjusting to loss of the breast to mastectomy (17,65,66). In contrast, patients choosing mastectomy perceived the breast containing cancer as an offending part that should be removed, and they were more fearful of the side effects of irradiation. While it has been suggested that older women may be more likely to select mastectomy (66), there is some concern that this may reflect as much a bias in the provision of treatment options as personal preference (67). Although it is not clear what percentage of women nationally are *offered* a choice, figures suggest that approximately 50% of women with early-stage breast cancer undergo breast conservation (68).

It is important to remember that it is only in the last decade that American women have routinely been given a choice between lumpectomy or mastectomy; even today this is mandated by fewer than half the states. Little is understood about *how* women make their decisions. It is likely that a significant proportion of decisions are made on the nature of the care that is

TABLE 32.3 *Controlled Studies of Psychological Response to Mastectomy (M) versus Limited Resection and Radiation (L-R)*

Study	Subjects L–R	Subjects M	Satisfaction with Body Image	Marital Adjustment	Satisfaction with Sexual Function	Psychological Adjustment	Fear of Recurrence
Sanger and Reznikoff (47)	20	20 modified	L-R more positive feelings	Equal	—	Equal	—
Schain et al. (48)	18	20 modified	L-R less negative feelings	Equal	Equal	Equal	Equal (M = 80%; L-R = 83%)
Steinberg et al. (49)	21	46 modified	L-R more positive feelings	Equal	L-R report husbands more sexual	Equal depression, anxiety; L-R better in general	Equal
Bartelink et al. (50)	114	58 modified	L-R less self-conscious	—	L-R less sexually inhibited	—	M greater
Taylor et al. (31)	26	31 simple/modified 9 radical	L-R less concern about disfigurement	Equal	L-R report more frequent sex, more affectionate husbands	L-R best overall adjustment	—
de Haes and Welvaart (51)	21	18 radical	L-R less negative feelings	Equal	Equal	Equal	Equal (older patients less fearful)
Baider et al. (52)	32	32 modified	—	M slightly less conflict than L-R	Equal	Equal	—
Fallowfield et al. (53)	48	53 modified	—	—	Equal	M slightly fewer problems (32% vs. 38% for L-R)	L-R more?
Ganz et al. (54)	19	31 modified	L-R less uncomfortable with changes	Equal	Equal	Equal; but more M (42%) than L-R (18%) report decrease over all quality of life	Equal
Lasry et al. (55)	36 L-R 44 L only	43 total	L-R and L less negative feelings	—	—	Equal (LR slightly lower than L or M)	Equal
Wellisch et al. (56)	11 L-R 14 L only	27 total	L-R more positive feelings	Equal	Equal; however within M significant decrease in libido	Equal	M more worried
Margolis et al. (57)	32	20 modified 2 modified + reconstruction	L-R more positive feelings (esp. in nude)	—	L-R report higher quality of relationship	M higher report of transient suicidal thoughts	—

available (10,11,29). For women diagnosed in communities that are removed from major medical centers, mastectomy may simply be a more practical and safe treatment choice. Another deciding factor may be the availability of high-quality radiation therapy. Restricted access to implants as well as to plastic surgeons having extensive experience with TRAM flap reconstruction have already limited the availability of reconstructive options. Cultural and ethnic values may also direct or even dictate choice, although the role of these is poorly understood. Research and clinical experience suggest that physician recommendation continues to exert the most significant influence on treatment choice for the majority of women (17,65).

Clinical experience indicates that many women who are treated by breast conservation may not feel the emotional effect of the experience until they begin the daily routine of radiotherapy. Spared the loss of their breast, these women often feel they should be grateful and not complain. There is evidence that they elicit, or at least perceive themselves as receiving, less emotional support from others than women undergoing mastectomy (62). It is often only when the irradiation starts, with daily visits to the clinic, exposure to others with cancer, cumulative fatigue, and realization of what they have gone through that patients react with distress. Physicians and staff should be aware of these delayed reactions, since they too may perceive these women as having less severe psychological trauma. It has become clear that women undergoing radiation are at higher risk of psychological disturbance than has been assumed, in particular depressive symptoms (55,69). Although these may be due to the side effects of irradiation, which may vary widely in the degree of discomfort and fatigue produced, mood states need to be monitored.

Women undergoing radiation therapy experience initial anxiety, which is usually allayed after a few treatments. It often returns, however, as end of treatment is approaching because of fear of regrowth of tumor without treatment, as well as in anticipation of the loss of close observation and frequent visits with the doctor and staff. To ease the transition, patients should be made aware of when treatment will end, and the common paradoxical increase in distress. Reassurance should be provided about staff availability by telephone contact and by systematic scheduling of follow-up appointments. Fears of disease recurrence remain high in many women and reach distressing levels before follow-up visits and scans and while waiting for test results. Anxiety returns to usual levels with news of normal findings.

Reconstruction. The FDA hearings, opened in November 1991, on the safety of silicone gel-filled breast implants brought to the attention of the public and the medical community several important questions: How many women seek implants, what are the benefits of their use, and what are the medical risks associated with these devices? These questions were no more keenly felt than among the estimated half a million breast cancer survivors with implants. While some feel the medical questions have been answered (70), other questions remain.

It is uncertain what percentage of women choosing or undergoing mastectomy do so with the intention of seeking reconstruction. Prior to the implant hearings, national figures suggested that as many as 30% of eligible patients might pursue breast reconstruction (71). The American Society of Plastic and Reconstructive Surgeons reported that a total of 42,888 breast reconstructions were performed by their 3000 members in 1990; this represented a 25% increase over figures gathered in 1988 and a 114% increase from 1981 (72). Despite the controversy, post-mastectomy breast reconstruction continues to be an important cosmetic and rehabilitative option pursued by a subset of women undergoing mastectomy.

Although breast reconstruction for cancer has been available much longer than breast conservation, few studies have systematically examined the psychosocial impact of mastectomy alone compared with mastectomy plus reconstruction. There have been only three studies to date in which women selecting each of the three different surgical options (lumpectomy vs. mastectomy alone vs. mastectomy with reconstruction) were compared (57,59,73). All of this research involved implant populations and in only one were women undergoing reconstruction evaluated separately from those receiving mastectomy. In this latter study, which looked only at body image and self-esteem, breast conservation patients reported more positive body image than either mastectomy or immediate reconstruction groups (73). Interestingly, this difference was not significant for the delayed reconstruction group, suggesting that these women may use a different standard for comparison. No differences were seen between groups on self-esteem, which was uniformly high.

Three empirical studies have appeared comparing women receiving conservation versus those undergoing mastectomy with reconstruction. The first of these included a very small sample ($n = 9$) and found no differences between groups in quality of life, mood, and marital or sexual satisfaction one year after surgery (74). A Japanese study compared 42 women with breast conservation to 48 women undergoing immediate reconstruction with myocutaneous flaps (75). No differences in sexual satisfaction or fear of recurrence were found between groups an average of three years post surgery. Conservation group members were less self-conscious about their appearance and stated that they would be more likely to choose the same treatment again than women in the reconstruction group. In a recent retrospective study, 72 women who had partial mastectomy were compared with 146 women who had undergone immediate reconstruction, predominantly with implants, an average of four years after surgery (76). No differences were observed between groups in overall psychosocial adjustment to illness, body image, or satisfaction with relationships or sexual life. However, women who had breast reconstruction reported less frequent breast caressing and more loss of pleasure with this activity. They also tended to be less likely to achieve orgasm with noncoital sexual stimulation. Factors predictive of greater psychosocial distress included a conflicted marriage, feeling unattractive, sexual dissatisfaction, less education, and treatment with chemotherapy.

In the largest prospective study to date, the psychological variables associated with who does and does not seek reconstruction, and women's response to reconstruction, were examined. A total of 150 women seeking consultation for reconstruction after mastectomy were evaluated along surgical and psychological parameters; 83 of the 117 women undergoing reconstruction were reassessed postoperatively (77). In addition, a matched comparison sample of 50 women who had not sought reconstruction was studied (78). The results of this research can be summarized as follows. First, women seeking consultation for reconstruction were psychologically well adjusted, high functioning, and, importantly, looked no different from their peers not seeking this surgery. Second, for women undergoing breast reconstruction, the net effect of the surgery was to increase both observed and stated satisfaction with levels of psychological, social, and sexual function. More than 80% stated that they were happy or absolutely delighted with the overall results, and most found that the surgical results met or surpassed their expectations. However, women who pursued reconstruction primarily to please others, or with the expectation of improving sexual and social relations, were at risk of disappointment. Time since cancer surgery also modified response, such that the longer the woman was since mastectomy, the greater her satisfaction with the overall results. Third, comparisons between women who consulted and went on to have reconstruction and those who sought consulta-

tion but opted *not* to pursue additional surgery suggested that women who are at increased risk for subsequent emotional or surgical disappointment following reconstructive procedures may select themselves out at the time of consultation. Similar findings have been reported in other study samples (79–85). This study was helpful in dispelling some of the myths about who seeks reconstruction and why. As reflected in age range of women interviewed (28 to 68 years), it also brought attention to the fact that attractiveness is not primarily a concern of younger women; older women may reacts as strongly as younger to breast loss.

It should be noted that because most of the extant research among women undergoing reconstruction was conducted at a time when mastectomy was still the primary treatment of choice, it is not clear how many of these women might have selected breast conservation had it been available to them. At the same time, many women today may select mastectomy precisely because they feel reconstruction will provide an acceptable cosmetic outcome, while avoiding the more limited surgery and irradiation. Clearly, these studies need to be replicated in the context of more recent treatment changes, including the shift to use of saline versus silicone implants (86). They also need to be expanded to address cultural and ethnic issues as it is clear that cultural beliefs and practices influence women's choice of options as well as outcomes (87–89).

Further, limited research has been done evaluating the psychosocial outcomes for women undergoing reconstruction using abdominal flaps (TRAM surgery) (90). Use of autologous tissue for reconstruction has the advantage of eliminating many of the medical (e.g. rejection, encapsulation, altered mammographic imaging) as well as device-related (e.g., rupture, deflation, leakage) problems associated with implants. The cosmetic outcomes can also be as good as or better than implant. On the negative side, these procedures require lengthy exposure to anesthesia, major abdominal surgery, and, although it is reportedly low, risk for failure. As long term follow-up data on the cosmetic or physical sequelae associated with such reconstruction are as yet unavailable, it is difficult to provide women with information upon which to make their decision.

Key concerns of women about reconstruction include the cost of the surgery, the length of time under anesthesia, number of procedures required, the safety of the techniques used in both, potential for complications, and, in the case of implants, risk of masking recurrent cancer or promoting recurrent autoimmune disease, and cosmetic results achievable (91). Surgeons differ in their approach to this latter concern.

Some prefer to use written materials only, others show pictures of reconstructed breasts, whereas many use some combination of these approaches and, at times, may refer a woman to a previously reconstructed patient for more details. In our own research and that of others, several additional issues appeared of importance in counseling women considering or undergoing these procedures (92,93). These include the need for discussion of all facets of the surgical steps (including number and length of hospitalizations), a thorough review of the surgical procedures planned to achieve symmetry of the breasts and to create a nipple, and consideration of timing of the procedure. The psychological impact of the timing of reconstruction has been the focus of additional studies.

IMMEDIATE VERSUS DELAYED RECONSTRUCTION. Physician support for immediate reconstruction (versus delayed, i.e., that performed more than a week after mastectomy) is based on the perception of the absence of medical contraindications to immediate reconstruction and anticipation of significant benefits to the woman in sparing her the pain of disfigurement and loss that accompany mastectomy (94). The American Society of Plastic and Reconstructive surgeons reported that of reconstructions performed in 1990 by member surgeons, 38% were immediate and 62% delayed (81). In a more recent retrospective sample of women treated in two large metropolitan areas (L.A. and D.C.), 75% of reconstructions were done in the immediate context (95).

Research with women undergoing immediate reconstruction has shown not only high levels of patient satisfaction with surgical results but also significantly less psychosocial morbidity than in those who undergo mastectomy alone (94,96–99). Patients undergoing immediate reconstruction were less depressed and suffered less impairment of their sense of femininity, self-esteem, and sexual attractiveness than their peers who delayed or did not seek reconstruction. However, as with findings on lumpectomy versus mastectomy, researchers have noted that initial differences in adjustment may be minimal and disappear over time (98). In addition, although Schain and colleagues suggested that immediate reconstruction does not interfere with the necessary mourning process associated with threat to life and breast loss (98), clinicians have reported this as a problem in long-term follow-up of these patients. It is an issue that warrants further study.

Adjuvant Chemotherapy. The news that adjuvant chemotherapy is needed demands psychological adjustment to yet another treatment modality. This involves a lengthened treatment period, and awareness of the threat to life implicit in the need for systemic therapy. Some women in this group describe their early weeks of treatment as having been characterized by "one piece of bad news after another." Deciding whether or not to undergo adjuvant treatment, and if more than one treatment is proposed choosing which drugs or protocol, constitutes the third decision point in the course of cancer.

Anticipation of chemotherapy can be difficult. Women's fears of the side effects arise from knowledge of the distressing sequelae of chemotherapy. Since many women with node-negative early stage breast cancer now receive some form of adjuvant therapy, the association of these treatments with "more serious disease" has diminished. Women anticipating and undergoing adjuvant therapy are told the specific drugs they will receive, and the transient nature of drug side effects. Despite having fears, few women refuse treatment, and most comply with their regimen (100). Reactive anxiety and depression identified should be treated to assist in the woman's adjustment.

Meyerowitz and colleagues studied women with breast cancer during chemotherapy and two years after completing it (101). Among those disease free at two years, 23% reported difficulty with personal and family relationships during treatment, and 44% had continuing physical problems two years later. Despite this, 89% stated they would recommend adjuvant chemotherapy to friends in a similar situation. Many reported that they had coped with treatment by "staying busy," "getting information about the treatment," and "keeping a positive, hopeful outlook." In this study, 41% of women reported that the treatment had been easier than they expected. Clinical experience suggests that some women cope with the short-term adverse psychological effects by focusing on delayed benefits (e.g. reassurance that they have done everything possible to eradicate their disease).

Nausea and vomiting, once common side effects of adjuvant chemotherapy, feared and dreaded by patients, are now well-controlled with pharmacologic and behavioral interventions (see Chapters 60 and 62). However, three additional troublesome side effects of adjuvant therapy that have psychological consequences have received less attention. These include hair loss, weight gain, and problems with concentration. While anticipated, the impact of alopecia for women undergoing chemotherapy is often devastating. Some women report this as more distressing than the breast surgery itself, in part because it is a visible indicator of disease but also because it is overtly disfiguring. In our own research, women rated hair loss as distressing as learning of their diagnosis. Early discussion of the expected changes, information about wigs, and referral to the American Cancer Society sponsored *Look Good . . . Feel Better* program can all help reduce distress caused by hair loss (102).

The cause of weight gain remains unclear (103). A study by Huntington revealed that 50% of patients gained more than 10 lb (104). No difference was found by treatment regimen (CMF versus CMF plus vincristine and prednisone), estrogen receptor status, age or menopausal status, although a decrease in activity level was found in those who experienced weight gain. At least one study has shown that weight may be negatively associated with mortality (105). The added insult to self-esteem posed by significant weight gain suggests that more attention should be paid to this problem. The introduction of exercise programs during chemotherapy is increasingly being considered, along with nutritional guidance.

Difficulty with concentration and memory are also reported by many women undergoing chemotherapy. Not well researched or clearly documented, these symptoms may be associated with the stress of illness, antiemetic drugs, and the chemotherapy itself, and possibly with hormonal changes secondary to chemotherapy-induced menopause (106).

A final troublesome effect of chemotherapy in younger women is premature menopause (107). The threatened or actual loss of fertility and acute onset of menopause anticipated with adjuvant treatment often causes distress in the woman who is premenopausal at diagnosis. The hot flashes, nightsweats, and vaginal dryness and atrophy caused by chemotherapy-induced menopause produce severe discomfort. The latter symptoms may lead to dyspareunia. While instruction in the use of vaginal lubricants is helpful, thinning of the vaginal mucosa may still result in irritation on intercourse. A further effect of chemotherapy is loss of libido likely associated with a reduction in circulating androgens (108). For many women loss of desire is the most difficult sequela to treat. In these cases, use of androgen supplements may be considered (108,109).

Although longitudinal data are lacking, it can be expected that early loss of ovarian function also increases the risk in these young patients of later morbidity associated with osteoporosis and cardiovascular disease (110,111). In a randomly selected survey of 224 breast cancer survivors, differences were found in women's concerns about these health issues by menopausal status (112). Premenopausal women were more concerned about osteoporosis (82% vs. 66% for post-

menopausal), and heart disease (92% vs. 73%), and that estrogen replacement therapy (ERT) might precipitate cancer recurrence (98% vs. 73%). At the same time, they were more willing to consider ERT under medical supervision (59% vs. 40%). Discussion of these issues early in the course of care and referral for evaluation for risk and intervention is appropriate. While estrogen replacement in these women remains controversial, it is currently being investigated (113).

Psychological preparation for chemotherapy is essential and should incorporate patient educational materials, nursing input, and an outline by the physician of the disease-related and treatment-related expectations. It is equally important to anticipate and plan for emotional reactions to ending treatment when, as with radiotherapy, fears of recurrence peak. Our clinical experience suggests that women experience more severe reactive anxiety and depression during this part of the treatment than at an earlier period, perhaps because of their greater awareness of prognosis. One symptom in particular that may continue to distress patients long after treatment has ended is fatigue. Noted clinically, the prevalence and etiology of post-treatment fatigue is not well studied. In one sample of 60 women, 87.5% reported fatigue as a serious and unexpected side effect of chemotherapy (114). While careful work-up to rule out underlying depression or any medical cause of persistent fatigue is warranted, many women benefit from reassurance that it may take months, not weeks, before they feel their energy level is back to pre-illness levels.

Adjuvant Hormonal Therapy. Increasing use of tamoxifen in the adjuvant setting has drawn attention to the psychological as well as sexual impact of hormonal therapies. While used most often with postmenopausal patients, tamoxifen may also be given to premenopausal women as part of their adjuvant therapy. Although it is an antiestrogen, research has shown that tamoxifen may have weak estrogenic effects on the vaginal mucosa. Some older women find that the associated increase in hot flashes with use of this drug are a side limiting factor. By contrast, we have had some younger patients report that tamoxifen provides relief from their vaginal dryness and loss of libido that accompany chemotherapy-induced premature menopause. Reports of a small, but unexpected number of deaths due to tamoxifen-related uterine cancer as well as concern over ocular toxicities with prolonged use have made many patients and physicians anxious about continued or long-term use of this drug (25,115). The outcome has been recommendation by many of careful gynecologic monitoring. However, whether this should include endometrial biopsy and/or transvaginal ultrasound, and at what intervals, remains unclear (116). A variety of hormonal manipulations are given for recurrent disease, including tamoxifen, megestrol acetate, progestins, aminoglutethimide, luteinizing hormone releasing hormone (LHRH) analogues, and estrogens. Aminoglutethimide has been associated with severe vaginal atrophy (117). Megace increases appetite and results in significant weight gain for many women. As noted earlier, alterations in appearance due to hormonal therapy may result in embarrassment and loss of self-esteem. Counseling around expected changes is important.

Bone Marrow Transplantation. The most recent application of bone marrow transplantation (BMT) has been in the area of solid tumors such as ovarian and breast cancer. While much has been written about the psychological stages in, and patients' adaptation to BMT (see Chapter 24), this research has focused largely on samples of patients treated for hematologic cancers, with allogeneic transplants (118–120). Long-term follow-up of patients undergoing BMT suggests that, while most patients do well, 15%–20% may continue to experience distress and might benefit from psychological or psychiatric intervention. At least one study reports that, despite the additional strain and longer hospitalization associated with BMT, no difference could be seen in psychological or social functioning between BMT survivors and those treated with conventional chemotherapy alone (121). It is not known to what extent this will be true for women with breast cancer undergoing these procedures with the benefit of less invasive stem cell transfer procedures, growth factor support, effective antiemetics and shorter hospitalization. What is clear is that, as with other intensive therapies, the toll on quality of life is often high. Ensuring that psychological support is provided across the course of transplantation and follow-up is critical. Regardless of whether psychiatric problems alter survival, they can dramatically impact quality of survival and should be rapidly diagnosed and treated (122).

Advanced Disease

Supportive care for patients with advanced breast cancer is aimed at comfort and control of symptoms. Different metastatic sites, especially bone, lung and brain, present special supportive problems. Bone pain is often difficult to control (see Chapter 38), and confusional states must be monitored and treated (see Chapter 48). As discussed in Chapter 61, the use of support groups may influence quantity as well as quality of survival significantly in this group of women.

Today, advanced care can be provided at home with support from the family or, in a hospice setting (see Chapter 87). Central to the success of a supportive program is a sense of continuity of care with physicians and staff and continued support of family and friends. Psychiatric consultation should be considered when distress (anxiety and depression) is not responsive to the usual supportive measures (see Chapter 60).

Because it is such a prevalent concern in more advanced stages of disease, attention to pain is important in the management of care (123,124). Cancer patients who experience pain are more likely to exhibit higher levels of mood disturbance and functional disability than those who have little or no pain (125). Spiegel and Bloom found that for women with metastatic breast cancer, beliefs about the meaning of the pain in relation to the illness predicted level of pain better than site of metastasis (126). Glajchen and colleagues found that 64% of patients surveyed cited communication barriers as an impediment to pain relief (127). Attitudinal barriers to compliance with medical treatment were cited by over half the respondents, including stoicism and fear of narcotic addiction. Thus, addressing the meaning of and response to pain from the perspective of the patient is as important as an explanation of proposed control techniques.

INTERVENTIONS

The last decade has seen rapid growth in the use and variety of psychosocial interventions applied in the cancer setting in general, and in breast cancer care in particular (128–130). Although varying greatly by the type (e.g., individual versus group), orientation (e.g., behavioral versus cognitive versus supportive), duration (time-limited versus open-ended), and timing (e.g., before, during, or after treatment), as well as target populations served (early vs. advanced, under 40 vs. older, partnered vs. single, or mixed), the fundamental purpose of interventions developed has been the same: to provide each woman with the skills or resources necessary to cope with her illness and improve the quality of her life. The various types of educational and supportive interventions currently in use in the breast cancer setting are reviewed in Chapter 59. However, three points need to be made regarding their use in the overall care of breast cancer patients and families.

First, taken as a whole, researchers have found that patients who received an intervention designed to improve knowledge or coping or to reduce distress do better than those who do not. Specifically, patients provided or randomized to some form of individual or group intervention experienced less anxiety and depression (131,132), had an increased sense of control (133), and improved body image (134), reported greater satisfaction with care (135) and better sexual function (136,137), and exhibited improved adherence to medication (138). Importantly, in no studies to date have women who received additional help done worse than their "standard care" peers.

Second, utilization of psychosocial interventions is increasing (139,140). This reflects not only patient demand for supportive care but growing recognition that addressing psychosocial issues may improve outcomes for patients. In their seminal study, Spiegel and colleagues found that women with metastatic breast cancer who participated in a year of weekly supportive group therapy with self-hypnosis for pain ($n = 50$), survived an average of 18 months longer from time of randomization, compared with a control group ($n = 36$)(141).

Third, while it might be argued that an individually tailored invention should result in the best outcome for any given patient, this may not be suitable or even desirable in all cases. Most cancer patients resist being singled out for individual therapy and feel burdened by any label that might suggest that they are mentally ill and not simply medically ill. Further, there is increasing evidence that participation in group activity offers a uniquely supportive and normalizing experience for many cancer patients struggling to deal with the realities of their new or continued status as cancer survivors. In studies that have specifically compared use of individual to group interventions, groups were as effective as individual counseling or support in reducing patient distress (134,135). Krupnick and co-workers have developed a model that uses groups to educate and support patients across the course of care that can be tailored to the needs of the oncology community being served (142).

Key to the development of an effective intervention is the recognition that cancer represents for many women a transitional event. As defined by Andrykowski and colleagues (143), this is "a traumatic event that alters an individual's assumptive world with the potential to produce long-lasting changes of both a positive as well as negative nature" (p. 827). As such, the primary goal in any intervention is to use this teachable moment to help minimize the negative and enhance the positive impact of illness on recovery and well-being.

SPECIAL ISSUES

Three changes in the way breast cancer is diagnosed and treated have important ramifications for clinicians in their management of patients. These include increased awareness of the familial nature of breast cancer, greater involvement of family in patient care, and growing attention to the impact of breast cancer treatment on women's sexual functioning. Psychological issues related to being at genetic risk for breast cancer are covered in Chapter 18. In the remaining two sections the special issues related to the care of other family members, and to the role of sexual quality of life in rehabilitation will be reviewed.

Role and Care of the Family

Research into the impact of social support and health has blossomed in the last decade (144–147). That a positive relationship exists between social support and health or illness outcome is a consistent finding (148). This has been no more dramatically illustrated than in the context of cancer, where adequate social support has been found to be integral not only to positive adjustment (149), but also to length of survival (141,150). For most patients, primary support comes from the family. At the same time, however, new stresses have taxed this resource. Greater demands on family decision-making, the lengthened course of treatment with more aggressive therapies, and shift of care into the outpatient setting have all served to place renewed focus on the family in the management of care.

When people are ill, they tend to feel less in control, less powerful, and more inferior, especially when they must rely on others. At the same time, serious illness of any kind increases the ill person's need for closeness to others to counteract feelings of insecurity and vulnerability. The need for love and support often heightens in patients over time, both as a reaction to the effects of disease and treatment and from the fear that they will no longer be loved or cared for. Fears of abandonment and rejection, experienced by other critically ill patients, are often keenly felt by the cancer patient. Absence of social support, or loss of a significant person who withdraws during the patient's illness becomes an additional stressor that may be more emotionally painful than the illness itself (151).

Active involvement of the family clearly serves a range of patient needs—from the most basic, namely, provision of emotional support (the "psychic fuel" that keeps a patient going), to the practical (e.g., transportation to therapy sessions and financial resources to support these services), to the more abstract (e.g., providing meaningful roles and hence functional goals toward which the patient can strive). For their part, the oncology team may count on the family member to be an advocate, a care provider, and a one-person cheering section on behalf of the patient.

Despite their recognized importance, the role of partners and family in caring for women with breast cancer has been the focus of few studies. Work by Wellisch and colleagues indicated that involvement of the husband in the decision-making process, hospital visitation, early viewing of scars, and early resumption of sexual activity were important for optimal couples' functioning (152). Open dialogue would appear critical to this process. Sabo and colleagues found that the tendency for some men to assume a "protective guardian" stance was sometimes a deterrent to effective and open communication (153). Maguire found that husbands of mastectomy patients reported more distress than a control group of husbands whose wives had benign breast disease up to a year after surgery (154). Similarly, Baider and Kaplan-DeNour reported that both patients and partners reported moderate degrees of emotional distress related to mastectomy (155). Further, they found that patients' and husbands' levels of adjustment were significantly related; if one partner was experiencing difficulties adjusting, the other was also likely to be having problems. Northouse reported that when asked what helped them cope with illness during hospitalization and one month later, both patients and husbands identified emotional support, information, attitude, and religion as important factors (156). In her research, patients and partners who reported higher levels of social support reported fewer adjustment difficulties at both 3 days and 30 days post surgery. However, younger couples may be at particular risk for problems (157).

The vital nature and complexity of the relationship of spouse or partner and family to patient well-being is no more obvious than when this system goes awry. When such situations occur, it is critical to remember that support is a two-way street; the source of the problem may arise in the provider of support (family member) as well as in the recipient and commonly involves both (158). The impact of cancer can be as devastating to a family member as to the patient herself. Spouses may feel angry, ashamed, and vulnerable to illness themselves. Clinicians working with families of cancer patients suggest that they may at times need to be viewed as second-order patients. Further, their needs may vary across the course of illness and recovery (159). Seeing that partners have a support network and the chance to air conflicting emotions can be critical to ensuring that they will be available to patients when needed. Toward this end it is helpful for staff to acknowledge the difficult task faced by family members, to provide opportunities for them to talk about questions and reactions both with the patient and alone, and to ensure that backup supports are available and provision is made to give family members relief, especially if care is going to be complex or long term. It is also important to permit family members to limit care to those areas in which they are most comfortable and effective.

The traumatic effect on children, both sons and daughters, is great when the mother develops breast cancer. Behavioral disorders, conflicts with parents, and regressive and acting-out behaviors in children have been seen to increase during a parental illness (160–164). Lichtman and colleagues noted deterioration of the mother–child relationship in 12% of women with breast cancer whom they studied (165). Problems were more likely to arise in those situation in which the mother had a poor prognosis, extensive surgery, poor psychological adjustment, or, to a smaller extent, difficulty adjusting to chemotherapy or radiotherapy. A prior history of parent–child conflicts also placed the relationship at risk during the mother's illness. Mothers' relationships with their daughters were significantly more stressed than those with their sons. Daughters were more likely to show signs of fearfulness, withdrawal, and hostility, emanating, perhaps, from their greater fears of developing the disease and the greater demands placed on the daughters. These findings parallel those reported by Litman (161) and Wellisch (166), who noted that mothers rely more often on daughters than on sons during illness and that adolescent daughters may be particularly vulnerable to disruption in their lives.

The monitoring of all children, especially when the mother's breast cancer is advanced, is important. The opportunity for parents to discuss how and what to tell their children about the mother's illness early in the course of care is also important, and should include advice on tailoring these conversations to meet appropriate developmental needs of their offspring. Two books by Harpham (167) and LeShan (168), as well as a publication put out by the National Cancer Institute, *When Someone in Your Family Has Cancer*, may be useful in this process.

Finally, concern about what impact breast cancer may have on a mother's survival may be complicated by worry about its meaning for an offspring's future well-being. As 70% of women diagnosed have no known risk factors for developing breast cancer, they will be the first in their family to have the disease. Many of these women report feeling guilty at having "brought the disease into the family." At the same time, adult offspring, in particular daughters, may feel angry about or frightened by the potential implications of their mother's illness on their risk of disease. Recently, attention has focused on the overall psychological adjustment and quality of life of female first-degree relatives (FDRs) of patients. These patterns of response in female family members warrant special attention, as excessive psychological distress can potentially interfere not only with family function but also adherence to subsequent breast cancer screenings, an issue addressed in greater detail in Chapter 15.

A number of books are now available that may be helpful to both women and their families dealing with the challenges imposed by breast cancer. These include *Dr. Susan Love's Breast Book*, Kathy LaTour's *Breast Cancer Companion*, Wendy Harpham's *After Cancer*, and Andy Murcia and Bob Stewart's book *Man to Man*. Each is thoughtfully written, highlights the problems families can expect, and provides resources for dealing with these. In addition, the National Coalition for Cancer Survivorship, based in Silver Spring, Maryland, has produced a useful volume with Consumer Reports entitled, *Charting the Journey*, which, as its title implies, discusses the practical problems that arise from diagnosis through survivorship, and solutions to each.

Quality of Life and Sexual Functioning
Although there has been extensive research on the psychosocial consequences of breast cancer, little of this work addressed the impact of disease and treatment on sexual functioning. Early studies focused on loss of breast and its impact on sexual relationships. These older, longitudinal studies, conducted among women treated with radical or modified radical mastectomy, reported significant sexual problems in 30%–40% of samples assessed (41,42). However, more recent studies have shown that the sexual disruption that occurs is independent of type of surgical treatment (58,62,67). In her review of breast cancer on sexuality, body image, and intimate relationships, Schover notes the lack of detail and specificity of available data on sexuality after breast cancer treatment, with most studies limiting the assessment to overall satisfaction or information on the frequency of intercourse (169). She observes that the premature and severe menopausal impact of systemic therapy may be the "most common culprit in causing sexual dysfunction." As noted earlier, with increasing numbers of women receiving chemotherapy or hormonal therapy, this less-explored area of sexual morbidity needs attention.

In their review of sexuality and cancer in women, Schultz and colleagues have described the range of psychological reactions to cancer that threaten sexual function, including threats to *(1)* sexual identity and self-esteem, such as disturbances of mood, gender, and sexual identity and body image; *(2)* personal control over body functions, such as disease-related symptoms (e.g. pain, fatigue, nausea) that interfere with or inhibit sexual functioning; *(3)* intimacy, such as loss of social contacts that have potential for intimate physical expression, or the disintegration of established patterns of achieving physical pleasure and intimacy, or myths related to contagion; *(4)* reproductive function, such as the direct impairment of fertility or the fear of recurrence with pregnancy (170). In addition to these psychological reactions, some women experience less joy and vigor, as well as an underlying uncertainty about their health, and the vulnerability of their bodies to further assault (171). All of these factors affect the sexual response in the breast cancer survivor.

In research conducted by Ganz and colleagues, 227 early-stage breast cancer patients were assessed at four points in time during the first year after surgery; some of these women were reassessed at two years ($n = 69$) or 3 years ($n = 70$) post surgery (172,173). Their data suggest that a subset of women may be at risk for psychosexual distress following treatment. Specifically, one-year problems and frequencies for the at-risk group included not feeling sexually attractive (54%), not being interested in having sex (44%), decreased frequency of sexual intercourse (58%), difficulty becoming sexually aroused (42%), difficulty with lubrication (50%), and difficulty achieving orgasm (41% low risk and 56% at risk). Of the 70 women assessed at three years, 43% continued to be uncomfortable with body changes, 47% reported disinterest in sex, and many continued to experience specific sexual dysfunction including difficulty with arousal (48%), lubrication (64%), and orgasm (52%). Important in their research was the finding that survivors appear to attain maximum recovery from the physical and emotional trauma by one year after surgery. Further, in spite of relatively good physical and emotional recovery achieved, a number of problems persist beyond one year, in particular those associated with sexual rehabilitation.

The emotional distress, pain, fatigue, and insult to the patient's body image and self-esteem caused by the diagnosis and treatment of breast cancer can damage sexual functioning, even among individuals who had a strong and satisfying sexual relationship prior to illness. When illness occurs in the context of preexisting problems or before relationships are fully established, the outcome may be devastating. Despite heightened sensitivity to sexual issues, in practice, provision of effective sexual interventions remains highly variable, in part because of staff avoidance. (See Chapter 42 for a more in depth discussion of these issues.)

It is beyond the scope of this chapter to go into the particular types of problems that may occur or their treatment. What is important is to recognize is that sexual rehabilitation starts ideally before treatment (174). Raising the topic of sexual function early, by letting the patient know that it is an appropriate focus of concern and that the health care provider is willing to discuss it, opens the door for future dialogue in this area and helps to ensure that problems with sexual function will be addressed. There are a number of excellent resources in the growing field of sexual rehabilitation of cancer patients (175–177). An excellent manual for patients entitled *Sexuality and the Woman Who Has Cancer and Her Partner* is available through the American Cancer Society. In addition, there are a small number of programs around the country that train sex counselors and therapists. For women with more difficult sexual problems, or long-standing issues further compounded by treatment, referral to a qualified sex therapist should be considered. Names of trained professionals for referral or workshop purposes can be obtained from the American Association of Sex Educators, Counselors and Therapists, based in Washington, D.C.

SUMMARY

Breast cancer remains the most common tumor in women; it has a unique and, at times, complex psychological impact, but one to which psychologically healthy women respond well without developing serious psychological symptoms. Increased use in primary treatment of breast-conserving and reconstructive procedures is reducing the negative effect on self-image and body image. However, current ethical and legal constraints relating to treatment options have added substantially to decision-making dilemmas and to fears of recurrence, which may persist for an indefinite period. As newer therapies such as intensive chemotherapy and bone marrow transplantation are introduced, research on their immediate and delayed psychosocial impact is needed. Broader dissemination of information from the psychological studies of adaptation to the available treatment options will help in efforts to determine the best treatment to meet patients' physical and emotional needs. Currently, suf-

ficient data exists to indicate that addressing the psychosocial and psychosexual needs of breast cancer patients improves quality of survival, and may even enhance length of survival. Finally, with the increasing demand for their involvement in care, special attention must be directed to the psychological well-being of the immediate relatives of women with breast cancer, especially their partners and offspring.

ACKNOWLEDGMENTS
This chapter represents an adaptation of one appearing in J. R. Harris, M. E. Lippman, M. Morrow and S. Hellman (eds.), *Diseases of the Breast*, Philadelphia: J. B. Lippincott–Raven, 1996.

REFERENCES
1. Parker SL, Tong T, Bolden F, Wingo PA. Cancer Statistics, 1996. *CA Cancer J Clin*. 1996; 46:5.
2. Hankey BF, Miller B, Curtis R, Kosary C. Trends in breast cancer in younger women in contrast to older women. *Mongr Natl Cancer Inst*. 1994; 16:7.
3. Early Breast Cancer Trialists' Collaborative Group. *Treatment of Early Breast Cancer, Vol. 1: Worldwide Evidence 1985–1990*. Oxford: Oxford University Press; 1990.
4. Glanz K, Lerman C. Psychosocial impact of breast cancer. A critical review. *Ann Behav Med*. 1992; 14:204.
5. Lerman C, Rimer BK, Engstrom PF: Cancer risk notification: psychosocial and ethical implications. *J Clin Oncol*. 1991; 9:1275.
6. Rosato FE, Rosenberg AL. Examination techniques: role of the physician and patient in evaluating breast diseases. In: Bland KI, Copeland EM III, eds. *The Breast. Comprehensive Management of Benign and Malignant Diseases*. Philadelphia: W.B. Saunders; 1991: 409.
7. Holland JC. Fears and abnormal reactions to cancer in physically healthy individuals. In: Holland JC, Rowland JH, eds. *Handbook of Psychooncology: Psychological Care of the Patient with Cancer*. New York: Oxford University Press; 1989: 18.
8. Robinson E, Mohilever J, Zidan J, Sapir D. Delay in diagnosis of cancer. Possible effects on the stage of disease and survival. *Cancer*. 1984; 54:1454.
9. Nayfield SG, Bongiovanni CG, Alciati MH, Fischer RA, Bergner L. Statutory requirements for disclosure of breast cancer treatment alternatives. *J Natl Cancer Inst*. 1994; 86:1202.
10. Nattinger AB, Gottlieb MS, Veum J, Yahnke D, Goodwin JS. Geographic variation in the use of breast-conserving treatment for breast cancer. *N Engl J Med*. 1992; 326:1102.
11. Farrow DC, Hunt WC, Samet JM. Geographic variation in the treatment of localized breast cancer. *N Engl J Med*. 1992; 326:1097
12. Scott DW. Anxiety, critical thinking and information processing during and after breast biopsy. *Nurs Res*. 1983; 32:24.
13. Valanis BG, Rumpler CH. Helping women to choose breast cancer treatment alternatives. *Cancer Nurs*. 1985; 8:167.

14. Hack TF, Degner LF, Dyck DG. Relationship between preferences for decisional control and illness information among women with breast cancer: a quantitative and qualitative analysis. *Soc Sci Med.* 1994; 39:249.

15. Emanuel EJ, Emanuel LL. Four models of the physician-patient relationship. *J Am Med Assoc.* 1992; 267:2221.

16. Siminoff LA. Cancer patient and physician communication: progress and continuing problems. *Ann Behav Med.* 1989; 11:108.

17. Ashcroft JJ, Leinster SJ, Slade PA. Breast cancer-patient choice of treatment: preliminary communication. *J Royal Soc Med.* 1985; 78:43.

18. Morris J, Royle GT. Offering patients a choice of surgery for early breast cancer: A reduction in anxiety and depression in patients and their husbands. *Soc Sci Med.* 1988; 26:583.

19. Glynn Owens R, Ashcroft JJ, Leinster SJ, Slade PD. Informal decision analysis with breast cancer patients: an aid to psychological preparation for surgery. *J Psychosoc Oncol.* 1987; 5:23.

20. Fallowfield LJ, Hall A, Maguire GP, Baum M. Psychological outcomes of different treatment policies in women with early breast cancer outside a clinical trial. *Br Med J.* 1990; 301:575.

21. Lerman C, Daly M, Walsh WP, et al. Communication between patients with breast cancer and health care providers. Determinants and implications. *Cancer.* 1993; 72:2612.

22. Cassileth BR, Zupkis RV, Sutton-Smith K, March V. Information and participation preferences among cancer patients. *Ann Intern Med.* 1980; 92:832.

23. Weiss R. How goes the war on cancer? Are cases going up? Are death rates going down? *Washington Post Health,* 1995; Feb. 14:12.

24. Velentgas P, Daling JR: Risk factors for breast cancer in younger women. *Monogr Natl Cancer Inst.* 1994; 16: 15–22.

25. van Leeuwen FE, Benraadt J, Coebergh JW, et al. Risk of endometrial cancer after tamoxifen treatment of breast cancer. *Lancet.* 1994; 343:448.

26. Meyerowitz BE. Psychosocial correlates of breast cancer and its treatment. *Psychol Bull.* 1980; 87:108.

27. Mor V, Malin M, Allen S. Age differences in the psychosocial problems encountered by breast cancer patients. *Monogr Natl Cancer Inst.* 1994; 16:191.

28. Fotopoulos S, Cook MR. Psychological aspects of breast cancer: age. Presented at the American Psychological Association Meetings, Montreal, Quebec, Canada, Sept. 1980.

29. Hynes DM. The quality of breast cancer care in local communities: implications for health care reform. *Med Care.* 1994; 32:328.

30. Penman DT. Coping strategies in adaptation to mastectomy. Doctoral dissertation. New York: Yehshiva University; 1979.

31. Taylor SE, Lichtman RR, Wood JV, Bluming AZ, Dosik GM, Leibowitz RL. Illness-related and treatment-related factors in psychological adjustment to breast cancer. *Cancer.* 1985; 55:2506.

32. Hilton BA. The relationship of uncertainty, control, commitment, and threat of recurrence to coping strategies used by women diagnosed with breast cancer. *J Behav Med.* 1989; 12:39.

33. Suls J, Feltcher B. The relative efficacy of avoidant and non-avoidant coping strategies: a meta-analysis. *Health Psychol.* 1985; 4:249.

34. Rowland JH. Interpersonal resources: social support. In: Holland JC, Rowland JH, eds. *Handbook of Psychooncology: Psychological Care of the Patient with Cancer.* New York: Oxford University Press; 1989: 58.

35. Pettingale KW, Morris T, Greer S, Haybittle JL. Mental attitudes to cancer: an additional prognostic factor. *Lancet.* 1985; 1:750.

36. Green BL, Rowland JH, Krupnick JL, et al. Prevalence of posttraumatic stress disorder (PTSD) in women with breast cancer. *Psychosomatics.* [In press.]

37. Levenson JL, Bemis C. The role of psychological factors in cancer onset and progression. *Psychosomatics.* 1991; 32:124.

38. Spiegel D. Psychosocial aspects of cancer. *Curr Opin Psychiatry.* 1991; 4:889.

39. DeFlorio M, Massie MJ. A review of depression in cancer: gender differences. *Depression.* 1995; 3:66.

40. Lewis FM, Bloom JR. Psychosocial adjustment to breast cancer: A review of selected literature. *Int J Psychiatr Med.* 1978–79; 9:1.

41. Maguire GP, Lee EG, Bevington DJ, et al. Psychiatric problems in the first year after mastectomy. *Br Med J.* 1978; 279:963.

42. Morris T, Greer HS, White P. Psychological and social adjustment to mastectomy: A two-year follow-up study. *Cancer.* 1977; 77:2381.

43. Psychological Aspects of Breast Cancer Study Group. Psychological response to mastectomy: a prospective comparison study. *Cancer.* 1987; 59:189.

44. Hughson AV, Cooper AF, McArdle CS, et al. Psychosocial consequences of mastectomy: levels of morbidity and associated factors. *J Psychosom Med.* 1988; 32:383.

45. Irvine D, Brown B, Crooks D, Roberts J, Browne G. Psychosocial adjustment in women with breast cancer. *Cancer.* 1991; 67:1097.

46. General Accounting Office. *Breast Conservation versus Mastectomy: Patient Survival in Day-to-Day Medical Practice and in Randomized Studies.* Washington, DC: U.S. Govt. Printing Office; Nov. 15, 1994.

47. Sanger CK, Reznikoff M. A comparison of the psychological effects of breast-saving procedures with the modified mastectomy. *Cancer.* 1981; 48:2341.

48. Schain W, Edwards BK, Gorrell EV, et al. Psychosocial and physical outcomes of primary breast cancer therapy: mastectomy vs. excisional biopsy and irradiation. *Breast Cancer Res Treat.* 1983; 3:377.

49. Steinberg MD, Juliano MA, Wise L. Psychological outcome of lumpectomy versus mastectomy in the treatment of breast cancer. *Am J Psychiatry.* 1985; 142:34.

50. Bartelink H, van Dam F, van Dongen J. Psychological effects of breast conserving therapy in comparison with radical mastectomy. *Int J Radiat Oncol Biol Phys.* 1985; 11:381.

51. de Haes JCJM, Welvaart K. Quality of life after breast cancer surgery. *J Surg Oncol.* 1985; 28:123.

52. Baider L, Rizel S, Kaplan-DeNour A. Comparison of couples adjustment to lumpectomy and mastectomy. *Gen Hosp Psychiatry.* 1986; 8:251.

53. Fallowfield LJ, Baum M, Maguire GP. Effects of breast conservation on psychological morbidity associated with diagnosis and treatment of early breast cancer. *Br Med J.* 1986; 293:1331.

54. Ganz PA, Schag CC, Polinsky ML, Heinrich RL, Flack VF. Rehabilitation needs and breast cancer: the first month after primary therapy. *Breast Cancer Res Treat.* 1987; 10:243.

55. Lasry J-CM, Margolese RG, Poisson R, et al. Depression and body image following mastectomy and lumpectomy. *J Chron Dis.* 1987; 40:529.

56. Wellisch DK, DiMatteo R, Silverstein M, et al. Psychosocial outcomes of breast cancer therapies: lumpectomy versus mastectomy. *Psychosomatics.* 1989; 30:365.

57. Margolis G, Goodman RL, Rubin A. Psychological effects of breast-conserving cancer treatment and mastectomy. *Psychosomatics.* 1990; 31:33.

58. Keibert GM, de Haes JCJM, van de Velde CJH. The impact of breast-conserving treatment and mastectomy on the quality-of-life of early-stage breast cancer patients: a review. *J Clin Oncol.* 1991; 9:1059.

59. Fallowfield LJ. Psychosocial adjustment after treatment for early breast cancer. *Oncology.* 1990; 4:89.

60. Maunsell E, Brisson J, Deschenes L. Psychological distress after initial treatment for breast cancer: a comparison of partial and total mastectomy. *J Clin Epidemiol.* 1989; 42:765.

61. Omne-Ponten M, Holmberg L, Sjoden P-O. Psychosocial adjustment among women with breast cancer stages I and II: six-year follow-up of consecutive patients. *J Clin Oncol.* 1994; 12:1778.

62. Levy SM, Haynes LT, Herberman RB, Lee J, McFeeley S, Kirkwood J. Mastectomy versus breast conservation surgery: mental health effects at long-term follow-up. *Health Psychol.* 1992; 11:349.

63. Zevon MA, Rounds JB, Karr J. Psychological outcomes associated with breast conserving surgery: a meta-analysis. Paper presented at the Eighth Annual Meeting of the Society of Behavioral Medicine, Washington, D.C., March, 1987.

64. Fallowfield LJ, Hall A. Psychosocial and sexual impact of diagnosis and treatment of breast cancer. *Br Med Bull.* 1991; 47:388.

65. Margolis GJ, Goodman RL, Rubin A, Pajac TF. Psychological factors in the choice of treatment for breast cancer. *Psychosomatics.* 1989; 30:192.

66. Wolberg WH, Tanner MA, Romsaas EP, et al. Factors influencing options in primary breast cancer treatment. *J Clin Oncol.* 1987; 5:68.

67. Ganz PA. Treatment options for breast cancer—beyond survival. *N Engl J Med.* 1992; 326:1147.

68. Wolberg WH. Surgical options in 424 patients with primary breast cancer without systemic metastases. *Arch Surg.* 1991; 126:817.

69. Monroe AJ, Biruls R, Griffin AV, Thomas H, Vallis KA. Distress associated with radiotherapy for malignant disease: a quantitative analysis based on patients' perceptions. *Br J Cancer.* 1989; 60:370.

70. Angell M. Shattuck Lecture: Evaluating the health risks of breast implants: the interplay of medical science, the law, and public opinion. *N Engl J Med.* 1996; 334:1513.

71. Miller BA, Ries LAG, Hankey BF, et al. (eds). *Cancer Statistics Review: 1973–1989.* Bethesda, MD: National Cancer Institute; 1992 NIH Publication No. 92-2789.

72. American Society of Plastic and Reconstructive Surgeons (ASPRS). *1990 Statistics.* Arlington Heights, IL: ASPRS; 1991.

73. Mock V. Body image in women treated for breast cancer. *Nurs Res.* 1993; 42:153.

74. Pozo C, Carver CS, Noriega V, et al. Effects of mastectomy versus lumpectomy on emotional adjustment to breast cancer: a prospective study of the first year post-surgery. *J Clin Oncol.* 1992; 10:1292.

75. Noguchi M, Kitagawa H, Kinoshita K, et al. Psychologic and cosmetic self-assessments of breast conserving therapy compared with mastectomy and immediate breast reconstruction. *J Surg Oncol.* 1993; 54:260.

76. Schover LR, Yetman RJ, Tuason LJ, et al. Partial mastectomy and breast reconstruction: a comparison of their effects on psychosocial adjustment, body image, and sexuality. *Cancer.* 1995; 75:54.

77. Rowland JH, Holland JC, Chaglassian T, Kinne D. Psychological response to breast reconstruction. Expectations for and impact on postmastectomy functioning. *Psychosomatics.* 1993; 34:241.

78. Rowland JH, Dioso J, Holland JC, Chaglassian T, Kinne D. Breast reconstruction after mastectomy: who seeks it, who refuses? *Plast Reconstr Surg.* 1995; 95:812.

79. Goin JM, Goin MK. Breast reconstruction after mastectomy. In: Goin JM, Goin MK. *Changing the Body: Psychological Effects of Plastic Surgery.* Baltimore: Williams & Wilkins; 1981: 163.

80. Clifford E. The reconstruction experience: The search for restitution. In: Georgiade NG, ed. *Breast Reconstruction Following Mastectomy.* St.Louis: CV Mosby; 1979: 22.

81. Houpt P, Dijkstra R, Storm van Leeuwen JB. The result of breast reconstruction after mastectomy for breast cancer in 109 patients. *Ann Plast Surg.* 1988; 21:517.

82. Gilboa D, Borenstein A, Floro S, Shafir R, Falach H, Tsur H. Emotional and psychosocial adjustment of women to breast reconstruction and detection of subgroups at risk for psychological morbidity. *Ann Plast Surg.* 1990; 25: 397.

83. Teimourian B, Adham M: Survey of patients' response to breast reconstruction. *Ann Plast Surg.* 1982; 9: 321–325.

84. Gerard D. Sexual functioning after mastectomy: life vs. lab. *J Sex Marital Ther.* 1982; 8:305–315.

85. Goin MK, Goi, JM. Midlife reactions to mastectomy and subsequent breast reconstruction. *Arch Gen Psychiatry.* 1981; 38:225–227.

86. Fee-Fulkerson K, Conaway MR, Winer EP, Fulkerson CC, Rimer BK, Georgiade G. Factors contributing to patient satisfaction with breast reconstruction using silicone implants. *Plast Reconst Surg.* 1996; 97:1420.

87. Filiberti A, Tamburini M, Murru L, et al. Psychologic effects and esthetic results of breast reconstruction after mastectomy. *Tumori.* 1986; 72:585.

88. Mueller SC, Cioroiu M, LaRaja RD, Rothenberg RE. Postmastectomy breast reconstruction: a survey of general and plastic surgeons. *Plast Reconstr Surg.* 1988; 82:555.

89. van Dam FSAM, Bergman RB. Psychosocial and surgical aspects of breast reconstruction. *Eur J Surg Oncol.* 1988; 14:141.

90. Cederna PS, Yates WR, Chang P, Cram AE, Ricciardelli EJ. Postmastectomy reconstruction: comparative analysis of the psychosocial, and cosmetic effects of transverse rectus abdominus musculocutaneous flap versus breast implant reconstruction. *Ann Plast Surg.* 1995; 35:458.

91. Schain WS, Jacobs E, Wellisch DK. Psychosocial issues in breast reconstruction: Intrapsychic, interpersonal, and practical concerns. *Clin Plast Surg.* 1984; 11:237.

92. Winder AE, Winder BD. Patient counseling. Clarifying a woman's choice for breast reconstruction. *Patient Educ Couns.* 1985; 7:65.

93. Matheson G, Drever JM. Psychological preparation of the patient for breast reconstruction. *Ann Plast Surg.* 1990; 24:238.

94. Noone R B, Frazier TG, Hayward CZ, Skiles MS. Patient acceptance of immediate reconstruction following mastectomy. *Plast Reconstr Surg.* 1982; 69:632–640. Rowland J, Meyerowitz B, Ganz P, Wyatt G, Desmond K, Honig S. Body image and sexual functioning following reconstructive surgery in breast cancer survivors. *Proc ASCO.* 1996; 15:24. [Abstract].

95. Ganz PA, Rowland JH, Desmond K, Meyerowitz BE, Wyatt GE. Life after breast cancer: understanding women's health-related quality of life and sexual functioning. *J Clin Oncol.* [In press.]

96. Dean C, Chetty U, Forrest APM. Effects of immediate breast reconstruction on psychosocial morbidity after mastectomy. *Lancet.* 1983; 1:459-462.

97. Stevens LA, McGrath MH, Druss RG, Kister SJ, Gump FE, Forde KA. The psychological impact of immediate breast reconstruction for women with early breast cancer. *Plast Reconstr Surg.* 1984; 73:619.

98. Schain WS, Wellisch DK, Pasnau RO, Landsverk J. The sooner the better: a study of psychological factors in women undergoing immediate versus delayed breast reconstruction. *Am J Psychiatry.* 1985; 142:40.

99. Wellisch DK, Schain WS, Noone BR, Little JW. Psychosocial correlates of immediate versus delayed reconstruction of the breast. *Plast Reconstr Surg.* 1985; 76:713.

100. Taylor SE, Lichtman RR, Wood JV. Compliance with chemotherapy among breast cancer patients. *Health Psychol.* 1984; 3:553.

101. Meyerowitz BE, Watkins IK, Sparks FC. Psychosocial implications of adjuvant chemotherapy: a two year follow-up. *Cancer.* 1983; 52:1541.

102. Manne SL, Girasek D, Ambrosino J. An evaluation of the impact of a cosmetics class on breast cancer patients. *J Psychosoc Oncol.* 1994; 12:83.

103. Denmark-Wahnefried W, Winer EP, Rimer BK. Why women gain weight with adjuvant chemotherapy for breast cancer. *J Clin Oncol.* 1993; 11:1418.

104. Huntington M. Weight gain in patients receiving adjuvant chemotherapy for carcinoma of the breast. *Cancer.* 1985; 65:572.

105. Senie RT, Rosen PP, Rhodes P, Lesser ML, Kinne DW. Obesity at diagnosis of breast carcinoma influences duration of disease-free survival. *Ann Intern Med.* 1992; 116:26.

106. Wieneke MH, Dienst ER. Neuropsychologic assessment of cognitive functioning following chemotherapy for breast cancer. *Psycho-Oncology.* 1995; 4:61.

107. Schover LR. Sexuality and body image in younger women with breast cancer. *Monogr Natl Cancer Inst.* 1994; 16:177.

108. Kaplan JS. A neglected issue: the sexual side effects of current treatments for breast cancer. *J Sex Marital Ther.* 1992; 18:3.

109. Sherwin BB. A comparative analysis of the role of androgen in human male and female sexual behavior: behavioral specificity, critical thresholds, and sensitivity. *Psychobiology.* 1988; 16:416.

110. Henderson BE, Paganini-Hill A, Ross RK. Decreased mortality in users of estrogen replacement therapy. *Arch Intern Med.* 1991; 151:75.

111. Dupont WD, Page DL. Menopausal estrogen replacement therapy and breast cancer. *Arch Intern Med.* 1991; 151:67.

112. Vassilopoulou-Sellin R, Zolinski C. Estrogen replacement therapy in women with breast cancer: a survey of patient attitudes. *Am J Med Sci.* 1992; 304:145.

113. Vassilopoulou-Sellin R, Theriault RL. Randomized prospective trial of estrogen-replacement therapy in women with a history of breast cancer. *Monogr Natl Cancer Inst.* 1994; 16:153.

114. Tierney A, Leonard R, Taylor J, et al. Side effects expected and experienced by women receiving chemotherapy for breast cancer. *Br Med J.* 1991; 302:272.

115. Pavlidis NA, Petris C, Briassoulis E, et al. Clear evidence that long-term, low-dose tamoxifen treatment can induce ocular toxicity. *Cancer.* 1992; 69:2961-2964.

116. Uziely B, Lewin A, Brufman G, Dorembus D, Mor-Yosef S. The effect of tamoxifen on the endometrium. *Breast Cancer Res Treat.* 1993; 26:101.

117. *Physician's Desk Reference*, 49th ed. Oradell, NJ: Medical Economics Company; 1995: 878.

118. Winer EP, Sutton LM. Quality of life after bone marrow transplantation. *Oncology* 1994; 8:19.

119. Wolcott DL, Fawzy FI, Wellisch DK. Psychiatric aspects of bone marrow transplantation: a review and current issues. *Psychiatr Med.* 1987; 4:299.

120. Andrykowski MA. Psychosocial factors in bone marrow transplantation: a review and recommendations for research. *Bone Marrow Transplant.* 1994; 13:357.

121. Lesko LM, Ostroff JS, Mumma GH, Mashberg DE, Holland JC. Long-term psychological adjustment of acute leukemia survivors: impact of bone marrow transplantation versus conventional chemotherapy. *Psychosom Med.* 1992; 54:30.

122. Jenkins PL, Lester H, Alexander J, Whittaker J. A prospective study of psychosocial morbidity in adult bone marrow transplant recipients. *Psychosomatics.* 1994; 35:361.

123. Portenoy RK, Foley KM. Management of cancer pain. In: Holland JC, Rowland JH, eds. *Handbook of Psychooncology: Psychological Care of the Patient with Cancer.* New York: Oxford University Press; 1989: 369.

124. Breitbart W. Psychotropic adjuvant analgesics for cancer pain. *Psycho-Oncology.* 1992; 1:133.

125. Massie MJ, Holland JC. The cancer patient with pain: psychiatric complications and their management. *J Pain Symptom Manage.* 1992; 7:99.

126. Spiegel D, Bloom JR. Group therapy and hypnosis reduce metastatic breast carcinoma pain. *Psychosom Med.* 1983; 4:333.

127. Glajchen M, Fitzmartin RD, Blum D, Swanton R. Psychosocial barriers to cancer pain relief. *Cancer Practice.* 1995; 3:76.

128. Massie MJ, Holland JC, Straker N. Psychotherapeutic interventions. In: Holland JC, Rowland JH, eds. *Handbook of Psychooncology: Psychological Care of the Patient with Cancer.* New York: Oxford University Press; 1989: 455.

129. Andersen BL. Psychological interventions for cancer patients to enhance the quality of life. *J Consult Clin Psychol.* 1992; 60:552.

130. Fawzy FI, Fawzy NW, Arndt LA, Pasnau RO. Critical review of psychosocial interventions in cancer care. *Arch Gen Psychiatry.* 1995; 52:100.

131. Maguire P, Tait A, Brooke M, Thomas C, Sellwood R. The effects of counseling on the psychiatric morbidity associated with mastectomy. *Br Med J.* 1980; 281:1454.

132. Spiegel D, Bloom JR, Yalom I. Group support for patients with metastatic cancer. *Arch Gen Psychiatry.* 1981; 38:527.

133. Bloom JR, Ross RD, Burnell G. The effect of social support on patient adjustment after breast surgery. *Patient Couns Health Educ.* 1978; 1:50.

134. Farash JL. Effects of counseling on resolution of loss and body image disturbance following mastectomy. *Dissertation Abstracts Int.* 1979; 39:4027.

135. Cain EN, Kohorn EI, Quinlan DM, Latimer K, Schwartz PE. Psychosocial benefits of a cancer support group. *Cancer.* 1986; 57:183.

136. Capone MA, Good RS, Westie KS, Jacobson AF. Psychosocial rehabilitation of gynecologic oncology patients. *Arch Phys Med Rehabil.* 1980; 61:128.

137. Telch CF, Telch MJ. Group coping skills instruction and supportive group therapy for cancer patients: a comparison of strategies. *J Consult Clin Psychol.* 1986; 54:802.

138. Richardson JL, Shelton DR, Krailo M, Levine AM. The effect of compliance with treatment on survival among patients with hematologic malignancies. *J Clin Oncol.* 1990; 8:356.

139. Pressberg BA, Levenson JL. A survey of cancer support groups provided by National Cancer Institute clinical and comprehensive centers. *Psycho-Oncology.* 1993; 2:215.

140. Coluzzi PH, Grant M, Doroshow JH, Rhiner M, Ferrell B, Rivera L. Survey of the provision of supportive care services at National Cancer Institute-designated cancer centers. *J Clin Oncol.* 1995; 13:756.

141. Spiegel DS, Bloom JR, Kraemer HC, Gottheil E. Effect of psychosocial treatment on survival of patients with metastatic breast cancer. *Lancet.* 1989; 2:888.

142. Krupnick JL, Rowland JH, Goldberg RL, Daniel UV. Professionally-led support groups for cancer patients: an intervention in search of a model. *Int J Psychiatry Med.* 1993; 23:275.

143. Andrykowski MA, Curran SL, Studts JL, et al. Psychosocial adjustment and quality of life in women with breast cancer and benign breast problems: a controlled comparison. *J Clin Epidemiol.* 1996; 49:827.

144. Wortman CB. Social support and the cancer patient. Conceptual and methodologic issues. *Cancer.* 1984; 53:2339.

145. House J, Landis NR, Umberson D. Social relationships and health. *Science.* 1988; 241:540.

146. Cohen S, Syme SL (eds). *Social Support and Health.* New York: Academic Press; 1985.

147. Reifman A. Social relationships, recovering from illness, and survival: a literature review. *Ann Behav Med.* 1995; 17:124.

148. Wallston BS, Alagna SW, DeVellis BM, DeVellis RF. Social support and physical health. *Health Psychol.* 1983; 2:367.

149. Nelles WB, McCaffrey RJ, Blanchard CG, Ruckdeschel JC. Social supports and breast cancer: a review. *J Psychosoc Oncol.* 1991; 9:21.

150. Funch DP, Marshall J. The role of stress, social support and age in survival from breast cancer. *J Psychosom Res.* 1983; 27:77.

151. Dunkel-Schetter C, Wortman C. The interpersonal dynamics of cancer: problems in social relationships and their impact on the patients. In: Friedman JS, DiMatteo RM, eds. *Interpers Issues Health Care.* New York: Academic Press; 1982: 69.

152. Wellisch DK, Jamison KR, Pasnau RO. Psychosocial aspects of mastectomy. II. The man's perspective. *Am J Psychiatry.* 1978; 135:543.

153. Sabo D, Brown J, Smith C. The male role and mastectomy: support groups and men's adjustment. *J Psychosoc Oncol.* 1986; 4:19.

154. Maguire P. The repercussions of mastectomy on the family. *Int J Fam Psychiatry.* 1981; 1:485.

155. Baider L, Kaplan-DeNour A. Couples' reactions and adjustment to mastectomy: a preliminary report. *Int J Psychiatry Med.* 1984; 14:265.

156. Northouse LL. The impact of breast cancer on patients and husbands. *Cancer Nurs.* 1989; 12:276-284.

157. Northouse LL. Breast cancer in younger women: effects on interpersonal and family relations. *Monogr Natl Cancer Inst.* 1994; 16:183.

158. Fisher JD, Nadler A, Whitcher-Alagna S. Recipient reactions to aid. *Psychol Bull.* 1982; 91:27.

159. Hoskins CN, Baker S, Budin W, et al. Adjustment among husbands of women with breast cancer. *J Psychosoc Oncol.* 1996; 14:41.

160. Wellisch DK. Family relationships of the mastectomy patient: interactions with the spouse and children. *Isr J Med Sci.* 1981; 17:993.

161. Litman TJ. The family as a basic unit in health and medical care: a social behavioral overview. *Soc Sci Med.* 1974; 8:495.

162. Lewis FM. The impact of cancer on the family: a critical analysis of the research literature. *Patient Educ Couns.* 1986; 11:269.

163. Howes MJ, Hoke L, Winterbottom M, Delafield D. Psychosocial effects of breast cancer on a patient's children. *J Psychosoc Oncol.* 1994; 12:1.

164. Lewis FM, Hammond MA, Woods NF. The family's functioning with newly diagnosed breast cancer in the

mother: the development of an explanatory model. *J Behav Med.* 1993; 16:351.

165. Lichtman RR, Taylor SE, Wood JV, Bluming AZ, Dosik GM, Leibowitz RL. Relations with children after breast cancer: the mother–daughter relationship at risk. *J Psychosoc Oncol.* 1984; 2:1.

166. Wellisch DK. Adolescent acting out when a parent has cancer. *Int J Fam Ther.* 1979; 1:238.

167. Harpham WS. *When a Parent Has Cancer. A Guide to Caring for Your Children.* New York: Harper Collins; 1997.

168. Leshan E. *When a Parent Is Very Sick.* Boston: Little, Brown; 1986.

169. Schover LR. The impact of breast cancer on sexuality, body image, and intimate relationships. *CA Cancer J Clin.* 1991; 41:112.

170. Schultz WCMW, Van de Wiel HBM, Hahn DEE, et al. Sexuality and cancer in women. *Annu Rev Sexual Res.* 1992; 3:151.

171. Quigley KM. The adult cancer survivor: psychosocial consequences of cure. *Semin Oncol Nurs.* 1989; 5:63.

172. Ganz PA, Hirji K, Sim M-S, Schag CAC, Fred C, Polinsky ML. Predicting psychosocial risk in patients with breast cancer. *Med Care.* 1993; 31:419.

173. Ganz PA, Coscarelli A, Fred C, Kahn B, Polinsky ML, Petersen L. Breast cancer survivors: Psychosocial concerns and quality of life. [Submitted].

174. Auchincloss SS. Sexual dysfunction in cancer patients: issues in evaluation and treatment. In: Holland JC, Rowland JH, eds. *Handbook of Psychooncology: Psychological Care of the Patient with Cancer.* New York: Oxford University Press; 1989: 383.

175. Schover LR. *Sexuality and Fertility after Cancer.* New York: John Wiley; 1997.

176. Vaeth JM, ed. *Body Image, Self-Esteem, and Sexuality in Cancer Patients*, 2d ed. Basel: Karger; 1986.

177. Anderson BL, Cyranowski JM. Women's sexuality: behaviors, responses, and individual differences. *J Consult Clin Psychol.* 1995; 63:891.

33

Sarcoma

DAVID K. PAYNE AND JEREMY C. LUNDBERG

Sarcomas are rare but highly aggressive neoplasms that occur in bone and soft tissue. Sarcomas of the bone occur primarily in adolescents, whereas soft-tissue sarcomas most often arise in either the second or sixth decade. Both types of sarcoma are associated with significant morbidity as well as mortality. This chapter reviews sarcomas of the bone and soft tissue and the psychological issues associated with each.

SARCOMAS OF THE BONE

Sarcomas of the bone include osteosarcoma, Ewing's sarcoma, chondrosarcoma, and parosteal sarcoma, but the most common are osteosarcoma and Ewing's sarcoma. These tumors are virtually unknown in childhood and have their peak incidence in the teens; there are, however, 4000 new cases of bone cancer every year in the United States (1). Although these tumors develop most commonly during the adolescent growth spurt between the ages of 10 and 20, they may occur later as a complication from Paget's disease or as a sequela of radiation therapy (2). The primary sites are usually femur, tibia, and humerus; metastases are found in 23% of patients at the time of diagnosis; the majority of these (85%) are in the lung (3). Originally, surgical amputation was the only treatment, resulting in a survival rate of 20%. In the 1970s, two modifications in treatment were introduced: limb-sparing surgery as an alternative to amputation, and adjuvant chemotherapy. With the use of doxorubicin and high-dose methotrexate with leucovorin, a 5-year relapse-free survival rate of 59% has been obtained along with an overall survival rate of 78% (4). A six-agent chemotherapeutic protocol has resulted in a 5-year survival rate of greater than 80% for patients (5).

Ewing's sarcoma is the second most frequent tumor in the teenage group, rarely occuring above the age of 25 years. Most Ewing's tumors arise in the shaft of a long bone such as the femur, humerus, and ribs, or in the pelvis, more commonly in boys. As with osteosarcoma, Ewing's sarcoma was originally treated solely with surgical resection, which resulted in a 5-year survival rate of less than 5%–10% (6). The use of multidrug chemotherapy with radiation, surgery, or bone marrow transplantation has increased the 5-year survival rates for localized disease to better than 50% and for patients with metastatic disease, between 20%–50% (7).

Psychological Issues

Despite the psychic trauma engendered by the diagnosis of cancer in adolescent patients, several studies have supported the view that the prognosis for healthy emotional adaptation in adolescent cancer survivors is quite good (2,8–10). In understanding the adolescent cancer patient, several issues related to normal development must be considered. An important goal of adolescence is developing an ability to deal with the external demands of the social environment while also beginning to gain greater understanding and mastery of the emotions engendered by the complexities and uncertainties of adult living. In the social arena, the adolescent's growing sense of self as a social and sexual being is developing. The effort toward mastery of these goals is often manifested in the sense of invincibility that healthy adolescents feel as they negotiate their way toward adulthood. The sense of vulnerability engendered by cancer frequently curtails this development of the sense of self and the adolescent's emerging social roles. Adolescents face not only the psychological distress associated with cancer diagnosis and treatment but also the physical impact of surgery, chemotherapy, and potential disability (11). These stressors frequently reverse the developmental trend and return adolescents to a state of both psychological and physical dependence.

The news that amputation for treatment of sarcoma may be required not uncommonly throws adolescents into a period of mourning. They fear that they may lose the best years of their life as a result of undergoing cancer treatment and may withdraw from their peer groups feeling that they are "different" from their age-mates because of the cancer. The psychological adaptation to amputation is not unlike that of grieving after the loss of a loved one or following the traumatic loss of a body part. Following the surgery, the increased dependency resulting from amputation may thwart the naturally growing sense of autonomy. Whether resulting from amputation or from limb salvage, the physical disfigurement may interfere with the adolescent's sense of body image and sexuality. As adolescents begin the journey toward intimacy which, if successful, culminates in pair-bonding, the loss of a limb or the disfigurement resulting from limb salvage may impede this process (12).

Although sarcoma patients who underwent limb-saving surgeries would be expected to have a quality of life advantage as compared to patients treated with amputation, the research does not support this advantage (13,14). For both amputation and limb salvage, however, patients are typically faced with issues of autonomy and body image.

The ability to form healthy relationships may be jeopardized for sarcoma patients. Sammallahti and colleagues found that, compared to normal controls, survivors of osteosarcoma more often feel a lack of support from significant others and a sense of disappointment that others are not trustworthy (15). These findings are consistent with that noted for adolescent survivors of other cancers in that one of the core interpersonal areas affected by cancer is the ability to be understood by and to feel supported by both peers and adults (16).

Psychological interventions may be helpful for adolescents facing treatment for sarcoma with either limb salvage or amputation. A thorough psychosocial assessment of the adolescent, their family, and significant relationships sets the stage for a comprehensive understanding of the impact of treatment on the adolescent and also can be used to assist the adolescent in capitalizing on their strengths in the rehabilitative period following surgery. Information about the nature of the cancer and treatment plans should be presented, avoiding talking to parents alone and treating the adolescent as a younger child. Given the risk for increased dependency and regression following surgery, it is essential to involve the adolescent as an active member of the treatment team who assists in decision making. Psychotherapeutic interventions are needed which focus on helping the adolescent to learn new coping strategies while shoring up existing adaptive defenses

and social skills (see Chapter 65 on telephone counseling).

SOFT-TISSUE SARCOMAS

Soft-tissue sarcomas occur in the extraskeletal connective tissues of the body that join, support, and surround other anatomic structures. This portion of the body mass comprises more than 50% of the body weight (17). Soft-tissue sarcomas occur primarily in the lower extremities (37%), trunk (9%), upper extremities (15%), retroperitoneum (14%), and head/neck (5%) (18). Brennan and colleagues developed a grading system for soft-tissue sarcomas that classifies the tumors into low-grade lesions (well-differentiated) or high-grade lesions (poorly differentiated) (19). Soft-tissue sarcomas develop primarily in the second and sixth decade. Although soft-tissue sarcomas account for a relatively small percentage of annual cancer diagnoses (1%) they comprise approximately 2% of all cancer-related deaths. While surgical resection remains the most effective treatment, an increasing number of patients now receive adjuvant radiation and multiple drug chemotherapy (18). Estimated 5-year survival rates are 79% (stage I), 65% (stage II), 45% (stage III), and 10% (stage IV) (20). Despite the effectiveness of current treatment modalities, however, sarcoma patients face better than a 25% likelihood that their cancer will recur (13). The treatment of recurrent soft-tissue sarcoma utilizing radiation and chemotherapy is ineffective.

Psychological Issues

The psychological impact of the diagnosis of soft-tissue sarcoma and surgical resection is heightened by knowledge of the daunting statistic that 25% of tumors will recur. In a study of the psychosocial issues faced by patients with soft-tissue sarcoma, in patients who were on average 2.6 years post initial treatment, 45% had a significant level of distress consistent with the diagnosis of a psychiatric disorder (21). In order of prevalence, these diagnoses were alcoholism, major depression, dysthymia, panic disorder, and phobia.

The authors have conducted support groups with soft-tissue sarcoma patients over two years and several themes common to this population have been noted (22). In these groups, sarcoma patients reported that family members, friends, and even patients with other types of cancer fail to appreciate the stresses on those who have a soft-tissue sarcoma diagnosis. The burden they bear is that while they appear well and healthy, they live in fear because they face a high likelihood of recurrence of tumor and death. Unlike the experience of patients with more visible neoplasms, this phenomenon has also been noted in patients with melanoma that, although resected, has left patients with the fear of recurrence. As a result of their apparent wellness, they experience less support from family and friends as compared to patients with other types of neoplasms who have visible signs of their illness or treatment. Their paradoxical look of good health also made it difficult to discuss their cancer diagnosis with others. Since they did not manifest the typical visible signs of cancer or cancer treatment, they felt that others did not regard their situation as serious or life-threatening.

Younger patients in the study expressed the concern about forming intimate relationships. They felt that it was unfair to prospective partners to establish an intimate relationship when their future was so uncertain. Also, despite being told that soft-tissue sarcoma had no known genetic basis, the concern about genetic risk of sarcoma to potential children was frequently voiced.

All the patients surveyed described devastating changes in their lives since their diagnosis. Fifty percent had been divorced since their diagnosis and the remainder reported major interpersonal disruptions attributable to cancer. They related the presence of significant financial and employment problems since their diagnosis; for many, these problems persisted.

The level of psychological distress in these soft-tissue sarcoma patients was high despite the fact that they had no evidence of disease. Many of the patients reported that they had been initially misdiagnosed and expressed fear that many physicians' lack of knowledge about sarcoma would lead mismanagement of the disease. They had difficulty understanding why they developed sarcoma and struggled to find ways to avoid recurrence by engaging in life-style changes such as avoiding stress and changing diet. They also reported feeling confused about the treatments they received. They compared their treatment with that of other patients, wondering whether differences in initial treatment had had an impact upon the course of their disease. Finally, the fear of relapse led most patients to fear follow-up examinations. Like other patients, anxiety rises in anticipation of routine check-ups. It continues until they are informed that they have no evidence of disease. In summary, patients with sarcoma often suffer psychological, interpersonal, and financial problems as a result of their illness. They may frequently feel isolated and misunderstood, and may worry that others do not recognize or appreciate the gravity of their circumstances.

PSYCHOLOGICAL INTERVENTIONS

Sarcoma patients have several needs: information, support, and treatment of any significant distress or psychiatric disorder that complicates their treatment. Most patients find that their local health care providers know little about sarcoma and that there is a dearth of written information available to them. Although patients will benefit from traditional supportive psychotherapy, alternative approaches may include psychoeducational interventions focused on providing information about sarcoma and teaching them cognitive-behavioral tools for dealing with the psychological distress associated with the diagnosis. Groups may be especially useful for this population since many sarcoma patients have never known another patient with their diagnosis. Although groups may not be possible, telephone counseling may prove to be a viable alternative for many patients. Whatever intervention is deemed most appropriate, one of the goals should be to offer patients consistent information. There is now a Sarcoma Newsletter available through Memorial Sloan-Kettering Cancer Center (contact David Payne at payned@mskcc.org on the Internet).

SUMMARY

Although sarcomas represent one of the less common cancer diagnoses, their impact on adolescents and adults is often devastating. Whether patients are treated with limb-salvage or amputation, their passage through developmental tasks associated with developing relationships is frequently impeded and the diagnosis has a negative impact on most spheres of functioning. Knowledge of both developmental tasks and the impact of treatment for sarcoma on these tasks, as well as an understanding of fears experienced by adults with sarcoma, provide the clinician with a framework out of which they can assist the patient with sarcoma. The assessment of psychological distress followed by the appropriate psychological intervention, whether individual psychotherapy, support groups, or telephone counseling, can enhance the quality of life of the sarcoma patient.

REFERENCES

1. Mankin HJ, Willett CG, Harmon DC. Malignant tumors of the bone. In: Holleb A, Fink D, Murphy G, eds. *American Cancer Society Textbook of Clinical Oncology*. Atlanta GA: American Cancer Society; 1991: 355–358.
2. Greenberg D, Goorin A, Gebhardt M, et al. Quality of life in osteosarcoma survivors. *Oncology*. 1994; 8:19–25.

3. Goorin AM, Abelson HT, Frei E. Osteosarcoma: fifteen years later. *N Engl J Med*. 1985; 313:1637–1643.

4. Goorin AM, Perez-Atayde A, Gebhardt M, et al. Weekly high-dose methotrexate and doxorubicin for osteosarcoma: The Dana Farber Cancer Institute/The Children's Hospital—Study III. *J Clin Oncol*. 1987; 5:1178–1184.

5. Goorin A, Rinsky R, Libsitz S, et al. New plateau in cure rate for patients with non-metastatic osteosarcoma: experience of the Dana Farber Cancer Institute and Stanford [Abstract 1256]. *Proc Am Soc Clin Oncol*. 1992; 11:365.

6. Glaubiger GL, Mackuch RW, Schwarz J. Influence of prognostic factors in Ewing's sarcoma. *Monogr Natl Cancer Inst*. 1981; 56:285–288.

7. Rosen G, Caparros B, Nirenberg A, et al. Ewing's sarcoma: ten-year experience with adjuvant chemotherapy. *Cancer*. 1981; 47:2204–2213.

8. Byrne J, Fears T, Whittley C, Parry D. Survival after retinoblastoma: long-term consequences and family history of cancer. *Med Pediatr Oncol*. 1995; 24:160–165.

9. Nicholson H, Mulvihill J, Byrne J. Late effects of therapy in adult survivors of osteosarcoma and Ewing's sarcoma. *Med Pediatr Oncol*. 1992; 20:6–12.

10. Redd VH. Advances in psychosocial oncology in pediatrics. *Cancer*. 1994; 74:1496–1502.

11. Zeltzer LK The adolescent with cancer. In: Kellerman J, ed. *Psychological Aspects of Childhood Cancer*. Springfield, IL: Charles Thomas; 1989: 70–99.

12. Heiligenstein E, Holland JC. Malignant bone tumors. In: Holland J, Rowland J, eds. *Handbook of Psychooncology: Care of the Patient with Cancer*. New York: Oxford University Press; 1989: 250–253.

13. Sugarbaker PH, Barofsky I, Rosenberg S, Gianola F. Quality of life assessment of patients in extremity sarcoma trials. *J Surg*. 1982; 91:17–23.

14. Weddington WW, Segraves KB, Simon MA. Psychological outcome of extremity sarcoma survivors undergoing amputation or limb salvage. *J Clin Oncol*. 1985; 3:1393–1399.

15. Sammallahti P, Lehto-Salo P, Maenpaa H, et al. Psychological defenses of young osteosarcoma survivors. *Psycho-Oncology*. 1995; 4:283–287.

16. Varni J, Katz E, Colegrove R, Dolgin M. Perceived social support and adjustment of children with newly diagnosed cancer. *J Dev Behav Pediatr*. 1995; 22:321–326.

17. Yang J, Glatstein E, Rosenberg S, Antman K. Sarcomas of soft tissues. In: Devita VT Jr, Hellman S, Rosenberg S, eds. *Cancer: Principles and Practice of Oncology*. 4th ed. Philadelphia, PA: JB Lippincott; 1995: 1436–1488.

18. Conlon K, Brennan M. Soft tissue sarcoma. In: Murphy G, Lawarence W, Lenard R, eds. *American Cancer Society Textbook of Clinical Oncology*. 2nd ed. Atlanta, GA: American Cancer Society; 1990: 435–450.

19. Brennan M. Managemrent of extremity soft-tissue sarcoma. *Am J Surg*. 1993; 158:71–78.

20. Lawrence W Jr, Donegan WL, Nachimuth J, et al. Adult soft tissue sarcoma. A pattern of care survey of the American College of Surgeons. *Ann Surg*. 1987; 205:349–359.

21. Weddington WW, Segraves KB, Simon MA. Current and lifetime incidence of psychiatric disorders among a group of extremity sarcoma survivors. *J Psychosom Res*. 1986; 30:121–125.

22. Payne D, Lundberg J, Holland J, Brennan M. A psychosocial intervention for patients with soft tissue sarcoma. *Psycho-Oncology*. 1997; 6:65–71.

34

Hematopoietic Dyscrasias

LYNNA M. LESKO

Despite the dramatic advances made in treatment and prognosis of hematologic malignancies over the past two decades with the advent of bone marrow transplantation (BMT), the diagnosis of leukemia is still equated with fear and hopelessness. Leukemia as a "curable disease" is a concept difficult to accept in the "community practice of medicine"; consequently, undue pessimism about treatment options is often shared by the patient, the family, and even the health care team. Psychological responses of all three must be considered in order to deliver optimal care.

Currently, coping with leukemia is a very different experience than it was twenty years ago. Once considered a universally fatal disease with a survival of barely a few months, leukemia is now regularly arrested and often cured, particularly in childhood. Accordingly, therapy is aimed at long-term remission rather than immediate comfort and palliative care and may involve treatments offered very early in the course of one's illness. Consent for innovative treatment is often requested at a time when patients and families have just begun to "digest" the cancer vocabulary, the impact of the illness, and its treatment.

A diagnosis of leukemia produces psychological stresses due to the actual symptoms of the disease, the partient's and family's perceptions of the disease, and its social stigma. The fear of death; dependency on family, spouse, and physician; disfigurement and change of self-image (sometimes resulting in loss or changes in sexual functioning); disability that interferes with age-appropriate tasks in work, school, or leisure roles; disruption in interpersonal relationships; and lastly discomfort and pain in later stages of illness are all issues that must be faced and, if possible, overcome. As successful treatments are introduced and survival becomes a more reasonable expectation, disengagement from the cancer illness and "reentry" into a near normal life-style becomes an added challenge.

The patient's ability to manage these normal stresses depends on factors determined by medical, psychological, and social issues. These include: *(1)* the disease itself (i.e., severity of illness, symptoms, clinical course, and type of treatment required); *(2)* the threat that leukemia poses in attaining age-appropriate development tasks and goals (i.e., adapting to adolescence, school, career, and family); *(3)* level of adjustment and coping strategies, especially to previous medical illness; *(4)* cultural and religious attitudes; *(5)* the patient's own personality and coping style; *(6)* the patient's potential for physical and pyschological rehabilitation; and finally *(7)* the presence of emotionally supportive persons in the patient's environment (hospital, clinic, home, and community).

Health care professionals are now beginning to focus on the psychological concerns of patients with hematologic malignancies. As a clear and impressive decline in leukemia mortality for patients under 20 years of age has occurred, and those under 60 years of age show a plateau, optimism about patient outcome has increased. More rigorous treatment, however, requires a high level of patient participation and responsbility. With that responsibility and with greater dialogue between patients and families resulting from more frank disclosure of disease and treatment, patients have become more interested in psychosocial and quality of life issues. patients no longer accept statemsn such as "you should be grateful just to be alive." In addition, patients surviving longer may be susceptible to the delayed effects of treatment. Consequently, attention has turned from death and dying to the emotional, physical, and behavioral consequences of rigorous treatment regimens. Delayed side effects of treatment and quality of life during terminal illness have also become important clinical and research issues.

DISEASE CLASSIFICATIONS

Leukemia

The reader is encouraged to review the article by Preisler (1) for a medical update of the leukemias. Since its first description by Donne in 1839, leukemia has been equated with hopelessness and a rapidly fatal outcome. The untreated median survival time is less than 2 months for acute leukemia; survival is longer with chronic leukemia, but it is also eventually fatal. Leukemias are classified according to the type of aberrant hematopoietic cell: lymphocytic leukemia, and the nonlymphocytic leukemias comprising myeloid monocytic, and erythroid cell types.

In the United States, 24,000 new cases of leukemia are diagnosed each year. The 16,000 deaths due to leukemia each year constitute 9% of all deaths related to cancer (2). Whereas many think of leukemia as a disease of childhood or adolesence, 89% of cases are adults over the age of 60.

Pediatric leukemia peaks at 7 cases per 100,000 in children under 5 years of age. Even though it is rare in children, it is the second most common cause of death after accidents. Acute lymphocytic leukemia is most common form in children and accounts for 75% of all cases, with the acute nonlymphocytic forms making up the remainder.

Chronic and acute nonlymphocytic leukemia are the most common forms of the disease among adults (see Table 34.1). In the population of young adults from 15 to 35 years of age, leukemia is the leading cause of cancer death in men and the second in women after breast cancer. Although the cause of leukemia is unknown, chemotherapeutic agents, used to treat

TABLE 34.1 *Approximate Annual Incidence of Leukemia*

Types of leukemia*	Age group		Total
	Children	Adults	
ALL	1,700	1,600	3,300
ANLL	250	8,000	8,250
CLL	rare	9,600	9,600
CML	50	4,600	4,650
Total	2,000	23,800	25,800

Source: Leukemia Society of America (1994). Facts about leukemia. National Office, 733 Third Avenue, New York, NY 10017, USA.

*ALL, Acute lymphocytic; ANLL, acute nonlymphocytic; CLL, chronic lymphocytic; CML, chornic myelongenous.

TABLE 34.2. *Lymphoma Statistics*

Lymphoma	Annual Incidence per 100,000*
Hodgkin's lymphoma	3.3 (male) 2.8 (female)
Non-Hodgkin's lymphoma	14.7 (male) 12.3 (female)

Source: Fact Sheet: Hodgkin's Disease and Non-Hodgkin's Lymphoma. National Cancer Institute, Office of Cancer Communication, Washington D.C.; 1985.

*Approximately 30,000 new cases diagnosed per year for all age groups.

other cancers, can cause acute leukemia as one of the delayed effects.

Lymphoma

Lymphoma is general term for the group of neoplastic disorders involving the lymphorecticular tissue. First described by Hodgkin in 1832, the lymphomas were classified early in the twentieth century by Kundral-Brill. The cause or causes of this lymph node tumor are still unknown; however, histological, serological, and epidemiological evidence strongly suggest a viral or infectious origin. The lymphomas are usually separated into Hodgkin's lymphoma and the non-Hodgkin's lymphomas; the numerous subtypes within each group are identified by histopathologic characteristics.

Lymphomas represent a relatively common form of malignancy in the United States. The incidence of Hodgkin's disease is approximately 3 cases per 100,000 per year (Table 34.2). Although rare in children under the age of 5 years, it is the most common form of lymphoma in children and has a bimodal age incidence with peaks between the ages of 15 and 34 and after age 50 years. Survival in the younger group is better than in the older. Currently, 80% of all patients under age 35 years with Hodgkin's disease are alive five years or more after treatment, making it one of the significant successes in cancer treatment. The incidence of non-Hodgkin's lymphoma is close to 13 cases per 100,000 per year in the United States, with a peak between the ages of 40 and 70 years. For the non-Hodgkin's lymphomas, 5-year survival is only 43% with current treatment.

CLINICAL COURSE AND TREATMENT OF HEMATOLOGIC MALIGNANCIES

Clinical Course

Figure 34–1 outlines the several clinical courses that leukemia or lymphomas may follow. They determine the patient's psychological concerns and contribute to

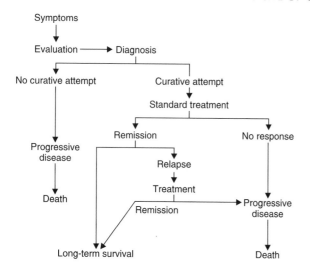

FIG. **34–1.** Chemical courses that leukemia and lymphomas may follow.

the adjustment to illness and treatment. The first stage begins often with seemingly minor symptoms. The presenting symptoms of leukemia vary but may include anemia with weakness and pallor, fatigue, dyspnea, palpitations, bleeding from gums, gastrointestinal tract, uterus, or bladder, petechiae, ecchymoses, increased susceptibility to infections, low-grade fever, and lymphadenopathy. In the case of lymphoma, similar symptoms of fatigue and lymphadenopathy appear. Loss of appetite and weight loss, accompanied by night sweats and pruritus, are more common with lymphoma. Usually the person seeks medical advice when these symptoms persist or worsen. People with leukemia usually seek medical attention earlier than those with lymphoma. Occasionally a patient may present with a chronic anemia and neutropenia that may herald a preleukemic syndrome. These myelodysplasias need little treatment until they develop into an acute phase but are often resistant to treatment.

Leukemia is diagnosed by bone marrow aspiration. A histopathologic diagnosis is made by subjecting the aspirate to cytochemical staining and identification of cell surface markers. To diagnose lymphoma, a pathologic diagnosis is made from a lymph node biopsy. Staging of disease is done by physical examination to determine all involved lymph nodes, lung tomograms (to identify pulmonary involvement, hilar, or mediastinal adenopathy), and/or lymphangiography to outline nodes further. An exploratory laparotomy is often also necessary for staging in lymphomas. Later stages reflect more extensive disease, which necessitates lengthier treatment and more intense cycles of drugs.

Discussing the diagnosis and treatment plan to the patient and family may take several sessions, because patients have such high anxiety that their recall of the facts is poor. Decisions must be made quickly, especially in patients with acute leukemia in whom rapid disease progression may occur if chemotherapy is delayed, even by a few days. Very few patients and families choose to accept *no* treatment. When this occurs, it is usually because of religious convictions about use of blood products, commitment to an alternative treatment, or the opinion that the treatment is too arduous for an older individual. However, most patients accept the treatment offered them, often participating in controlled clinical trials when treatment is in a cancer center. In fact, one study showed that children who participated in clinical research trials had better survival rates than children who were treated without a protocol.

In leukemia, induction chemotherapy is the first phase of treatment, followed by consolidation and possibly maintenance chemotherapy; the three phases may require 2–3 years to complete. The lengthy treatment involves many painful procedures and requires dedication and a high level of compliance on the part of patients. Cranial irradiation, intrathecal chemotherapy via an Ommaya shunt, venipunctures, bone marrow aspirations, and biopsies occur during clinic visits and hospitalizations. Neutropenia and sepsis are frequent serious complications in the first few months of treatment. Some adults with acute leukemia do not respond to initial treatment; others go on to remission and then relapse.

At times of relapse or failure of conventional frontline treatment, families sometimes engage in frenetic efforts to find other treatments, second opinions, or alternative therapies. These are not their only options, however; they can also seek out other conventional approaches such as second-line chemotherapy, or participation in clinical investigative research trials. For the patient who does not relapse after initial treatment, uncertainty about outcome and adjustment to the side effects of chemotherapy or irradiation are continuing problems.

TREATMENT

More effective treatments for leukemia and lymphoma have occurred because of improved techniques in identifying pathologic and histologic subtypes of cells in leukemia, more precise staging of extent of disease in lymphoma, more effective supportive measures (antibiotics, antifungal and antiviral agents, blood products, protected environments, and intensive care units), and multimodal cytoreductive regimens along with allogeneic, autologous, or mismatched bone marrow transplantation (BMT) procedures.

Leukemia

The treatment of leukemia aims to eradicate all abnormal cells and to promote regeneration of normal cells. However, treatment often accomplishes only reduction of the cell population, and relapse follows as the remaining malignant cells regrow. Chemotherapy is the primary treatment; in select cases of young individuals, irradiation supplements intensive chemotherapy to eradicate a major sanctuary for leukemia cells.

The treatment of acute leukemia begins with *induction* chemotherapy, given in the hospital. It is a multiagent regimen aimed at inducing a complete remission, defined as no clinical evidence of disease or less than 4% blast cells in the marrow. It usually requires 4–6 weeks of hospitalization at a cost of $50,000 or more. Only partial remissions are often achieved in older patients. Relapse can occur within weeks and is treated by chemotherapy again to accomplish reinduction. Chemotherapy, continuing into remission, is given in two phases: consolidation, possibly followed by maintenance. *Consolidation* chemotherapy requires hospitalization for one or two cycles, employing the same cytoreductive agents used in the induction phase. *Maintenance* therapy, however, is given in the clinic or office over 1–2 years; lower doses of the same agents are used to prevent regrowth of residual leukemic cells. *Intensification* therapy is occasionally given after maintenance and involves administration of high doses of antileukemic drugs for six months. The optimal length of maintenance treatment is not known and its impact on survival is debated. Most ALL treatment schedules rely on vincristine, prednisone, and L-asparaginase, whereas those for ANLL use a combination of cytarabine and an anthracycline (3).

Children and adults with ALL are at risk of developing leukemia in the central nervous system (CNS), even while in remission. This is because the CNS serves as a sanctuary for leukemic cells that are not destroyed by systemic chemotherapy, which does not effectively cross the blood–brain barrier. To reach these leukemic cells, intrathercal methotrexate, with or without cranial irradiation, is given as prophylaxis. Use of such therapy has reduced meningeal leukemia from greater than 40% to less than 10% incidence.

BMT is increasingly being used for acute and chronic leukemia and, more recently, for lymphoma (4) and multiple myeloma. Currently the four types of transplants used are syngeneic (bone marrow from a twin), allogeneic (bone marrow from a histocompatible sibling or parent), autologous (the individual's own bone marrow that has been "purged" of neoplastic ells by chemotherapeutic agents and later reinfused), or mismatched (donated from an unrelated or HLA mismatched donor). In the 1970s, BMT was an experimental therapy reserved for end-stage disease. Experience suggests that better results are obtained when transplantations are done in the first or second remission of leukemia, while patients are medically stable, and when they are done early in the course of the disease (i.e., the chronic phase of CML, first remission of ANLL, and second or third remission of ALL). Unfortunately, BMT is an appropriate treatment for only 25% of patients, that is, for those under the age of 60 and those who have a histocompatible donor. Morbidity from this procedure may be as high as 50%, but BMT produces a disease-free survival in at least 75% of patients for periods of as long as 2–10 years. In contrast, standard chemotherapy results in 5-year disease-free survival in 20% of the adults with ANLL. long-term sequelae of BMT are significant and include sterility, endocrine dysfunction, graft-versus-host disease (GVHD), interstitial pneumonitis, cardiomyopathy, cataracts, and immunosuppression.

Lymphomas

The histopathological diagnosis and sites of involved lymph nodes—above or below the diaphragm—determine the type and stage of lymphoma, from which treatment is determined. The sites of disease are also used to monitor response to treatment and to estimate prognosis. Treatment begins immediately after staging. Limited, localized, or early stages of disease are treated by radiotherapy alone to involved areas and regional lymph nodes. More extensive disease is treated by multiagent combination chemotherapies [MOPP (nitrogen mustard, vincristine, procarbazine, and prednisone) or ABVD (adriamycin, bleomycin, vinblastine, and dacarbazine) which is thought to produce less sterility]. Six to eight cycles of the multiagents are usually given over six months. Adjuvant multiagent chemotherapy is used with radiotherapy in later stages of disease, in children, and in patients with large mediastinal tumors. Several classes of agents are employed, including vinca alkaloids, procarbazine, alkylating agents, nitrosoureas, bleomycin, doxorubicin, and corticosteroids (5).

PSYCHOLOGICAL CONCERNS ASSOCIATED WITH DIAGNOSIS AND TREATMENT

Hematologic malignancies are widely known to be rapidly fatal when untreated. Thus, when patients or parents learn that leukemia or lymphoma has been diagnosed, the word alone strikes fear in their hearts. The psychosocial concerns associated with all cancers are intensified in these patients. The "five Ds" of psychosocial concerns are particularly poignant in these diseases.

Death—Death is a central fear, as is fear of discomfort from the medical procedures (bone marrow aspirations and lumbar pucture) as well as from the disease itself (pain secondary to leukemia infiltrates in joints or enlarged retroperitoneal nodes).

Dependence—Dependence on family and physician is necessary during long hospitalizations for induction treatment and years of follow-up treatment.

Disfigurement—A sense of disfigurement is consequent to changes in body appearance and function (hair loss, Broviac catheters, and infertility with lymphoma).

Disruption—Disruption occurs in relationships during long and numerous hospitalization.

Disability—Disability interferes with achievement of age-appropriate school, career, and personal goals.

Patients realize from the outset that the prognosis may be guarded. Especially in adults, leukemia is generally known to be a "worse" diagnosis than lymphoma. The survival statistics, the physicians' tone during treatment discussions, and the rigors of treatment outlined all convey "bad news." It is during this period that patients and their families find the appearance of a "veteran" patient so helpful. The reassuring words that someone has "been there before" and "made it" are invaluable.

The supportive measures just described require the patient and family to assume a heavy responsibility for their maintenance, which adds an additional burden. Lengthy periods in germ-free environments are particularly difficult because of the fluctuation between isolation and overstimulation produced by such environments. Broviac or Hickman line catherization, providing access to the right atrium via the subclavian vein, is used for the administration of chemotherapy, blood products, antibiotics, and nutrition, and for obtaining blood samples for study (thus eliminating multiple venipunctures). patients adjust well to these catheters, which are in place over months. However, they require daily care by patients, including sterile dressing changes and flushing with heparinized solutions. Because the most common complication of indwelling catheters is infection, they require careful monitoring. Psychological issues that arise include overdependence on nurses for sterile techniques, the

high level of mandatory technical self-care at home (a problem that may be particularly stressful for the adolescent or older individual), negative body image (an issue most apparent in young adults, who are often embarrassed in their intimate relationships by the presence of a catheter), and chronic loss of the ability to eat when total parenteral nutrition (TPN) is used for long periods. The impact on appetite makes it difficult to discontinue TPN at times and to reinstate normal feeding.

FACTORS IN PSYCHOLOGICAL ADJUSTMENT TO DISEASE

As with other forms of cancer, the variables that contribute to psychological adjustment to leukemia or lymphoma are medical and psychosocial. The medical variables are particularly important in leukemia, in which the clinical course is uncertain. The relapses, episodes of sepsis, hospitalizations, isolation, and treatment side effects can wear thin even strong psychological defences. Emotional exhaustion and demoralization are common. Different treatment modalities (Ommaya shunts, intrathecal chemotherapy, and multiple bone marrow aspirates) increase the stress; however, other measures can substantially reduce it, such as the use of Broviac catheter access to eliminate painful venipuncutres. Profound fatigue and diminished stamina continue for long periods after treatment.

Young children adapt better psychologically than adults to long hospitalization and germ-free environments, although extra time and assistance from parents and staff are often needed to reinforce precautions and instructions. Emotional stability of patient and family, as well as positive support from social and interpersonal resources, assist the patient in weathering the disappointments that are frequent throughout the course of the illness and in adjusting to the extensive treatment.

The financial burden of a catastrophic illness is an additional silent and unexpected problem. "Out-of-pocket" medical expenses—those not reimbursed by health insurance—are high with the longer hospitalizations required in leukemia. Specialized home care, administration of chemotherapy by infusion pumps, skilled nursing care, and TPN, are often not covered by insurance plans. The financial burden of nonmedical costs to the family of a child with leukemia is great and well documented. Other hidden expenses with an afflicted child are wages lost as a result of need for child care of siblings and money spent on convenience foods, transportation to and from the physician's office or medical center, lodging for the parent or family member to stay near the hospital, wigs, clothing of several sizes to accommodate weight changes, baby-sitters, housekeepers, and supportive supplies for Broviac catheter care. Miscellaneous expenses that are often overlooked include telephone calls, special gifts, flowers, posters for the patient's room, toys, VCRs, air conditioners, and tutors for educational needs. According to Cairns and colleagues (6), out-of-pocket costs can average 15% or more of a family's annual salary. The financial burden is felt long after the child has been cured or has died. Difficult choices about the use of financial resources must be made by parents when the education or financial needs of other children or the family are compromized.

Giving consent for the treatment when it involves potentially fatal doses of radiation and chemotherapy that are countered only in BMT is a difficult decision for patients and their families, especially parents. The consent process has been studied for both chemotherapy and BMT. Both studies confirm the value of the discussion with the doctor, as compared to the use of the informed-consent form only. The latter was helpful in investigational treatments, reaffirming the right to withdraw. It also appeared that better-informed patients adjusted more positively to treatment.

Some patients adjust poorly to illness because they enter treatment with poor coping strategies. Poor coping is seen in the patient who does not confront these problems, assumes a passive "what will be, will be" stance, and employs abnormal levels of denial. Patients with psychiatric disorder find it difficult to balance the self-care requirements with the need to be compliant and to relinquish overall care to others. Drug abuse and alcoholism are apt to be associated with noncompliance with treatment, in particular among those who must be involved in home administration of antibiotics, chemotherapy, or TPN.

Those patients who have good coping ability seem to adjust well to the treatment regimen. They become well-informed about illness and treatment; they see illness as a challenge and solve problems one at a time, accepting limitations on their activities as well as their transiently altered appearance. In one of the studies on coping mechanisms, in leukemic patients in remission, Sanders and Kardinal (7) reported moderate levels of denial of illness as well as a strong identification with fellow patients and staff from the "hospital family." Grief over deaths of fellow patients was common.

Isolation

Acute leukemia and chronic myelocytic leukemia (CML) treatment with aggressive chemotherapy and bone marrow transplantation (BMT) may require iso-lation in a germ-free protected environment. Although therapeutically useful, these environments (whether reverse isolation or sterile laminar airflow units) impose upon the patient prolonged physical and psychological isolation from family and staff. The consequences of such protected environments have been reviewed extensively (8). Initially, clinicians and researchers hypothesized that responses to such isolation would be similar, perhaps identical, to behavior and responses associated with sensory deprivation, social isolation, and parent–child separation paradigms. This has not been borne out. Pyschopathologic behavior, when it occurs, is more often a consequence of the underlying physical illness rather than an effect of the environment. Very rarely is it mandatory to discontinue isolation therapy for psychological reasons; few patients require psychiatric medication. Most authors agree that a protected environment gives most patients a positive feeling of being attentively cared for and, for some, promotes feelings of becoming a privileged, "special" patient during the hospitalization. The hypothesis that isolation environments are psychologically adverse more likely reflects the medical staff's reaction to this environment rather than consequences of it to the patient. The patient's primary psychological difficulty is in adjusting to the diagnosis and treatment of a life-threatening illness with all its accompanying physical complications. Germ-free environments may aggravate or attenuate these psychological difficulties. Guidelines listed below offer ways to minimize any adverse psychological sequelae of isolation.

Patient Education. Knowledge about one's illness, its severity, and treatment fosters emotional stability and cooperation in such a restricted environment. The physician's relationship with patient and family members is an important key in preparing the patient for isolation. A close, frank relationship allows the patient to gather more information about his illness and at the same time affords the physician an opportunity to obtain more information about the patient's character, psychological functioning, modes of coping with illness in the past, and capacity for dealing with stress.

Preparation. It is recommended that all patients and family members tour the isolation unit prior to admission, especially if siolation will be for many months or is in a sterile laminar airflow unit. Meeting the unit's personnel, especially the nursing staff, can be comforting to children and will also provide an opportunity for family members to ask questions about items that they can bring from home for the patient. Many units develop an orientation booklet which includes procedural as well as psychological preparation for one's stay.

Environmental Manipulation. Environmental and behavioral manipulation are suggested from the pediatric and adult isolation and ICU literature. Patients are encouraged to bring personal belongings (books, hobbies, paintings, posters, pictures, stereos, radios, stuffed animals, albums, and clothes) to brighten up the isolation area and promote a sense of familiarity. Access to windows, clocks, calendars, TVs, and natural light are helpful in orienting patients and in helping them maintain a daily routine and diurnal rhythm. Psychological regression, due to pscyhological stress and physical illness, can be reduced by encouraging patients to participate in their own care and to remain as self-sufficient as possible (e.g., managing their own hygiene, operating radios and televisions, exercising).

Psychological Support. Ample visiting privileges for families assist in maintaining necessary object ties and contacts with the outside world. Support from the staff is a more valuable tool than psychotropic drugs in improving a patient's and family's capacity to cope with illness, physical concerns, and the stress of isolation. Preparation for leaving the isolation unit should take place a few days before actual discharge. Patients should be encouraged to talk about feelings of "going home," since patients often develop anxiety about being out of the hospital and their special environment. Patients in protected environments have been accustomed to being monitored and supervised very closely; every change in their daily functions is brought to their attention. Upon discharge, minor aches and pains can produce acute anxiety, and for a period some patients may need constant reassurance that they are progressing as expected. Paradoxically, some patients become unconcerned about their medical condition when they return home, becoming careless about aspects of their care and noncompliant about taking medication. This may be a form of rebellion against the hospital routine with which they needed to comply for so long. Others view their protective environments as "special" and they become "special" because of their care.

Medication. Anxiolytics can be used to modulate excessive anxiety, relieve insomnia, and serve as an adjunct in the management of pain. Major tranquilizers (neuroleptics) are rarely indicated and could mask recognition of an acute confusional state secondary to metabolic abnormalities.

Survivorship

The problems of cancer survivors are reviewed in Chapter 20. Those medical and pyschological concerns specific to leukemia and lymphoma are outlined here (Table 34.3). Of considerable interest are the persistent problems with associations that remind the individual of the chemotherapy. In studies by Cella and colleagues (9,10) and Lesko and colleagues (11), Hodgkin's disease and leukemia survivors were found to have conditioned nausea and anxiety as long as 12–17 years after chemotherapy had been completed when exposed to a reminder of their chemotherapy treatment.

Medical Concerns. In the first major report on a large group of children with survival of 10 years or more treated at St. Jude's, half were survivors of Hodgkin's disease or leukemia. Although 90% judged that they had a good quality of life and social function, about 30% had problems specific to treatment, including infertility in the Hodgkin's patients and a decrease in IQ among the leukemia patients who received cranial irradiation (12).

Neurological Problems. Neurological toxicity from chemotherapy regimens has increased as toxicity from chemotherapy has increased, as more drugs are

---

TABLE 34.3. *Common Concerns in Survivors of Hematologic Malignancies*

MEDICAL CONCERNS

Neurological and CNS dysfunction

Occurrence of a second malignancy

Organ failure (cardiovascular, pulmonary, renal, hepatic)

Retardation or failure of maturation and growth

Decreased stamina

Relapse

PSYCHOLOGICAL CONCERNS

Fears of minor physical symptoms

Fears of termination of treatment

Adjustment to accepting normal responsibilities; difficulty being on their own

Difficulties in transition from being a patient to becoming healthy (Lazarus syndrome)

Problem in revealing diagnosis when seeking jobs

Awareness of job and health insurance discrimination

Sense of vulnerability to illness and death (Damocles syndrome)

used together, and as they are more often combined in high doses with radiation. Intrathecal routes and aggressive treatment of relapses add to toxicity. In addition, as children and young adults treated for cancer survive longer, there is more opportunity for delayed CNS side effects to become apparent.

Immediate CNS side effects of chemotherapeutic agents include transient nausea, vomiting, anorexia, fatigue and weakness, confusion, and irritability. Immediate side effects are seen transiently primarily with intrathecal administration of methotrexate in acute leukemia. Cognitive dysfunction and neurologic impairment occur largely in children treated for acute leukemia by intrathecal methotrexate and cranial irradiation. Seizures, motor abnormalities, and language and behavioral difficulties have been reported. Other studies found largely normal psychological and neurologic development in spite of evidence of cerebral atrophy on CT scan. The clinical significance of CT scan abnormalities in children receiving various forms of CNS prophylaxis is unclear. Subsequent research has revealed both structural abnormalities and cognitive deficits in 25%–30% of childhood ALL survivors.

Relapse and Second Malignancies. Patients with leukemia usually relapse because leukemia cells find sanctuary from chemoterhapy in the CNS, tesis, and ovary. Even though there have been improvements in the prevention of CNS relapse, testicular relapse still occurs in between 5% and 16% of males during initial remission and up to 30%–40% after treatment is discontinued. Often early testicular relapse heralds subsequent (within 3 months) bone marrow relapse of drug-resistant leukemia.

Second malignant neoplasms (SMN) as a result of treatment are rare in leukemia; they most often appear as a secondary lymphoma or another type of leukemia (13). More often, SMN occur in patients with Hodgkin's disease treated with alkylating agents, with or without radiation. The review of the large cohort of children treated at St. Jude's 10 or more years after treatment identified SMN in only 2% of the children. Sarcomas, thyroid carcinomas, and ANLL have developed as SMN in children with Hodgkin's disease 3 months to 21 years after termination of treatment. Solid tumors appear at a mean of 9.5 years after treatment in leukemia and 5.5 years after treatment for lymphoma in adults and children (14). Hodgkin's disease adult patients are at increased risk for lung and breast cancer and secondary ALL, incidence of which may be as high as 10%.

Growth and Organ Failure. Most children with hemoatologic malignancies grow and mature normally, although patterns of growth and growth hormone (GH) levels in children with acute leukemia who receive cranial irradiation along with chemotherapy are at greater risk of growth abnormalities. Impaired GH responses to provocative tests of GH release has been reported in children with acute leukemia treated with cranial irradiation for CNS prophylaxis. Later, others noted only temporary impairment of growth in children receiving chemotherapy and cranial irradiation, with symmetrical loss in height. Unfortunately, there are conflicting studies about GH concentration, GH stimulation after provocative testing, and linear growth patterns in children with acute leukemia after treatment by CNS prophylaxis. Voorhess and colleagues (15) studied the hypothalamic-pituitary function of 93 children receiving CNS prophylaxis (intrathecal methotrexate (IT-MTX), IT-MTX and 2400 rad cranial irradiation, or IT MTX and intravenous intermediate dose MTX. Eleven patients had subnormal GH responses after pharmacologic stimulation of the pituitary; however, long-term linear growth patterns were unaffected. Children who are subsequently treated by bone marrow transplantation with additional high-dose chemotherapy and total body irradiation appear to be at particularly high risk of endocrine abnormalities that adversely affect growth and development.

Children with Hodgkin's disease and non-Hodgkin's lymphoma who received irradiation to specific sites (e.g., thoracic and pelvic areas), especially during rapid growth periods, experience maturation loss in the irradiated area. Unilateral irradiation of the thoracic area of growth centers of the long bones produces scoliosis and short stature.

Survivors may also experience delayed toxicity to the cardiovascular, endocrine, pulmonary, hepatic, renal, and peripheral nervous systems. Patients may have permanent vincristine-associated peripheral neuropathy, anthracycline-related cardiomyopathy, hepatic fibrosis secondary to methotrexate, and antibiotic-related renal failure. Occasionally, when chemotherapy is given with irradiation, organ damage is enhanced. Some agents, such as methotrexate, are "radiation reactivators" and, when given weeks to months later, reactivate the radiation effects. Radiotherapy for Hodgkin's disease in the thorax can result in delayed pneumonitis, pericarditis, pleurisy, and thyroid dysfunction.

The delayed sequelae of hematologic malignancy treatment on fertility and sexual function have been a particular focus of psychological studies. Young men who undergo chemotherapy and pelvic irradiation for Hodgkin's disease or rigorous induction leukemia chemotherapy often become aspermic and remain sterile. Sperm-banking is important to allow a later possibility of a natural child. Fertility in men with acute leukemia treated with standard chemotherapy is less well studied. Evenson and colleagues (16) noted that men treated at Memorial Sloan-Kettering on the L-10 protocol for this disease remained fertile. Treatment consisted of a minimum of 3.5 years of continuous chemotherapy using adriamycin, vincristine, prednisone, intrathecal methotrexate, cytosine arabinoside (Ara-C), BCNU, and dactinomycin. The fertility may have been spared by the use of intrathecal methotrexate rather than cranial irradiation as CNS prophylaxis, thereby sparing the hypothalamic–pituitary–gonadal axis.

Chemotherapy-related ovarian failure and subsequent amenorrhea, diminished libido, and sexual dysfunction have occurred in a number of young women who are Hodgkin's disease survivors (17,18). Radiation of less than 2000 rad and/or relocation of the ovaries during treatment for lymphoma may prevent reproductive damage. Siris and colleagues found that most young women aggressively treated for leukemia in childhood have a relatively good prognosis for normal CNS-controlled ovarian function (19). On a more optimistic note, it appears that for fertile couples in whom one survives cancers, neither chemotherapy nor radiation has an oncogenic or mutagenic effect on progeny. However, many young adult survivors are unaware of or are unprepared for possible treatment-related sexual dysfunction, adding further stress and problems in adjustment.

Psychological Concerns. Most early psychological studies of cancer survivors were retrospective reviews of children with leukemia and Hodgkin's disease. The need for longitudinal studies of adults and children was noted by several investigators who identified problems of survivors. These studies highlighted several important psychological areas of concern that related in large part to the medical concerns of physical damage, risk of a second neoplasm, relapse, survival, and psychological function (20,21). Remissions brings a return to near-nromal appearance, but stamina is slow to return. Consequently, there can be a precarious balance between elation at achieving cure and fears of future disease. Depressive mood, anxiety, and a sense of diminished self-worth and control over events are frequently seen (22). Cure itself imposes a difficult task—that of discarding the patient role in separating from the hospital-family and reentering into job or school and actual family while continuing regular, if less frequent, clinic visits. Patients with hematologic malignancies often have a transient enhanced level of psychological distress related to the uncertainty of how long maintenance treatment should continue: "How many cycles of treatment are enough?" Patients at this time are often concerned about the loss of close monitoring of their physical condition and experience a sense of increased vulnerability to relapse.

Follow-up visits with bone marrow aspirations or development of minor physical symptoms result in increased anxiety. As time goes by, anniversaries of diagnosis and treatment are reminders that cause transient distress. In a survey of 70 leukemia patients, they outlined issues that made their clinic visits difficult. Dislike of returning to the clinic enviroment and the discomfort of the examination and diagnostic procedure were noted. Further sources of complaint were that clinic visits served to remind patients of the lack of certainty about cure, coupled with interference with work or school caused by the visits.

The inability to ignore everyday aches and pains adds to the survivors' preoccupation with physical symptoms and loss of control over their health and future. This is particularly evident in leukemia because relapse may occur without any warning, becoming apparent only by an abnormal bone marrow test result or development of frequent infections. Finally, these malignancies are "visible" upon completion of therapy, leaving no physical manifestations. The invisibility of physical damage can aid in the patient's denial of being chronically ill and diminish the sense of being only precariously in good health. Other psychological sequelae of survivorship (e.g., Lazarus and Damocles syndromes, survivor guilt, job and insurance discrimination) are described in research by Koocher and O'Malley (23).

Systematic studies on the psychological adaptation of adults surviving hematologic malignancies are increasing in numbers. Wolcott and colleagues (24) reported on the adaptation of 26 patients with leukemia and aplastic anemia who were treated with BMT. At an average of 3.6 years after treatment, only 2.5% had some physiological sequelae secondary to disease or treatment. These authors reported that 25% or less of patients reported low self-esteem, less than optimal life satisfaction, and significant emotional distress.

The psychological profile of survivors and the long-term psychological impact of disease and treatment on patients are under active study. At Memorial Sloan-Kettering, research was conducted among young adults with acute leukemia and Hodgkin's disease. Data from these studies reveal that survival is achieved without impairment of quality of life and psychological well-being of survivors. Survivors in both studies were at least 6–12 months off treatment. No differences were found between survivors and healthy controls. However, depending on the patient population, the cancer survivor demonstrated lower intimacy motivation, increased avoidant thinking about illness, numerous illness-related concerns, and prolonged difficulty returning to premorbid work status. Such data suggest that cancer and its diagnosis and treatment have some residual psychological effects.

Over the past five years, research in the area of quality of life in BMT survivors has burgeoned. Many issues of such patients are similar to those of patients with hematologic malignancies undergoing conventional chemotherapy (25). However in some patients a BMT procedure may mean an extensive hospitalization, longer convalesence and more long-term sequelae. The clinical issues surrounding BMT and the research in evaluating the quality of life of such patients are reviewed in Chapter 24.

CONCLUSION

The hematologic malignancies have been among the first to respond to treatment, which has produced cures initially among children and young adults. However, to achieve a cure from leukemia or lymphoma, the required chemotherapy, irradiation, and bone marrow transplantation cause psychological stresses that are predictable on the basis of the treatment side effects. Transplantation particularly requires an intensive treatment regimen and long hospitalization in a germ-free environment. Maladaptive responses often require psychiatric evaluation and intervention to prevent inability to continue treatment. Because the hematologic malignancies occur at all ages, it is necessary to have knowledge of the disease and treatment, as well as having an understanding of the common psychological responses. Optimal patient and family care for these diseases is best done in a center where a team of specialists who work together can maximize the patient's chance for the best physical and emotional outcome.

REFERENCES

1. Preisler HD. The leukemias. *Disease a Month.* 1994; 40(10):525–579.
2. Margolis CP, McCredie KB. *Understanding Leukemia.* New York: Scribner's; 1983.
3. Clarkson BS, Ellis C, Little T, et al. Acute lymphoblastic leukemia in adults. *Semin Oncol.* 1985; 12:160–179.
4. O'Reilly RJ. Allogenic bone marrow transplantation: current status and future directions. *Blood.* 1983; 62:941–964.
5. Straus DJ, Gaynor JJ, Lieberman PH, et al. Non-Hodgkin's lymphomas: characteristics of long-term survivors follow conservative treatment. *Am J Med.* 1987; 75:1058–1062.
6. Cairns NV, Clark GM, Black J, Lansky SB. Childhood cancer: non-medical costs of illness. *Cancer.* 1979; 43:403–408.
7. Sanders JB, Kardinal CG. Adaptive coping mechanisms in adult acute leukemia patients in remission. *J Am Med Assoc.* 1977; 238:952–954.
8. Lesko L, Kern J, Hawkins DR. Psychological aspects of patients in germ-free isolation: a review of child, adult and patient management literature. *Med Pediatr Oncol.* 1983; 12:43–49.
9. Cella DF, Pratt A, Holland JC. Persistent anticipatory nausea, vomiting, and anxiety in cured Hodgkin's disease patients after completion of chemotherapy. *Am J Psychiatry.* 1986; 143:641–643.
10. Cella DF, Tross S. Psychological adjustment to survival from Hodgkin's disease. *J Consult Clin Psychol.* 1986; 54:618–622.
11. Lesko L, Mumma G, Mashberg D. Psychosocial functioning of acute leukemia survivors treatment with bone marrow transplantation or standard chemotherapy. *Proc Am Soc Clin Oncol.* 1987b; 6:255. [Abstract no. 1002.]
12. Moss H, Nannis ED, Poplack DG. The effects of prophylactic treatment of the central nervous system on the intellectual functioning of children with acute lymphocyti leukemia. *Am J Med.* 1981; 71:47–52.
13. Mosijczuk AD, Ruymann FB. Second malignancy in acute lymphocytic leukemia. *Am J Dis Child.* 1981; 135:313–316.
14. Meadows AT, Baum E, Fossati-Bellani F, et al. Second malignant neoplasms in children: an update from the late effects study group. *J Clin Oncol.* 1985; 4:432–538.
15. Voorhess ML, Breacher ML, Glicksman AS, et al. Hypothalamic-pituitary function of children with acute lymphocytic leukemia after three forms of central nervous system prophylaxis. *Cancer.* 1986; 57:1287–1291.
16. Evenson D, Avlin Z, Welt S, Claps M, Melamed M. Male reproductive capacity may recover following drug treatment with the L-10 protocol for acute lymphocytic leukemia. *Cancer.* 1984; 53:30–36.
17. Chapman RM, Sutcliff SB, Malpas JS. Cytotoxix-induced ovarian failure in women with Hodgkin's disease: I. Hormone function. *J Am Med Assoc.* 1979a; 242:1877–1881.
18. Chapman RM, Sutcliffe SB, Malpas JS. Cytotoxic-induced ovarian failure in women with Hodgkin's disease: II. Effects on sexual function. *J Am Med Assoc.* 1979b; 242:1882–1889.
19. Siris ES, Leventhal BG, Vaitukaitis JL. Effects of childhood leukemia and chemotherapy on puberty and repro-

ductive function in girls. *N Engl J Med.* 1976; 294: 1143–1146.

20. Bartolucci AAQ, Liu C, Durant JR, Gams RA. Acute myelogenous leukemia as a second malignant neoplasm following the successful treatment of advanced Hodgkin's disease. *Cancer.* 1983; 52:2209–2213.

21. Kushner B, Zauber A, Tan CTC. Second malignancies after childhood Hodgkin's disease. *Cancer.* 1988; 62:1364–1370.

22. Lesko L, Mumma G, Mashberg D, Holland JC. Psychosocial adjustment and sexual functioning of acute leukemia survivors: a preliminary report, The

Third National Symposium of the Leukemia Society of America. *Leukemia.* 1987; 1(3):278. [Abstract no. 23.]

23. Koocher G, O'Malley J. *The Damocles Syndrome: Psychosocial Consequences of Surviving Childhood Cancer.* New York: McGraw-Hill; 1981.

24. Wolcott DL, Wellisch DK, Fawzy FI, Lansverk J. Adaptation of adult bone marrow transplant recipient long-term survivors. *Transplantation.* 1986; 41(4):478–483.

25. Lesko L, Ostroff J, Mumma G, et al. Longer term psychological adjustment of acute leukemia survivors: impact of bone marrow transplantation vs conventional chemotherapy. *Psychosom Med.* 1992; 54(1):30–39.

35

HIV Infection and AIDS-Associated Neoplasms

BARRY ROSENFELD

Human immunodeficiency virus (HIV) and acquired immunodeficiency syndrome (AIDS) have emerged as a leading cause of death among young men and women, and a significant national health care problem. Epidemiological estimates indicate that nearly 500,000 people have been diagnosed with AIDS in the United States since the initial recognition of the HIV virus (1). Worlwide, more than 1.25 million cases of AIDS have been reported to the World Health Organization, with documented cases of AIDS in 193 countries (2). Despite increased awareness of the risk factors for HIV transmission, the onset of HIV and AIDS continues to grow in many countries and among many population subgroups.

The classification of HIV disease incorporates information regarding CD4$^+$ lymphocyte measurements as well as the presence or absence of clinical conditions associated with HIV (Table 35.1). The current CDC classification system categorizes CD4$^+$ lymphocyte functioning into three categories, and these categories have clinical implications regarding the pharmacologic management of HIV disease (3). Patients with a CD4$^+$ cell count of 500 or more are classified into CD4 category 1, patients with CD4$^+$ cell counts between 200 and 499 are classified into CD4 category 2, and patients with CD4$^+$ cell counts under 200 are classifed into CD4 category 3. A second level of classification incorporates the patients' medical history, and specifically, the presence or absence of HIV-related medical conditions. Patients with no history of HIV-associated medical conditions are classified into clinical category "A," patients with HIV-related medical disorders not considered AIDS-defining conditions are classified into clinical category "B" (previously termed AIDS-related complex or ARC), and patients with a history of specific AIDS-defining medical conditions (Table 35.1) are classified into clinical category "C."

Under current CDC guidelines, all patients with either a history of an AIDS-defining condition (clinical category "C") or CD4$^+$ cell count below 200 (CD4 category 3) are classified as having AIDS.

Shortly after the initial recognition of HIV and AIDS, the impact of this illness on social and psychological functioning became apparent. Since that time, various psychological and psychiatric sequelae have been identified, studied, and treated. The most common psychological and psychiatric conditions identified as associated with HIV and AIDS include depression, suicidal ideation, adjustment disorders with mixed depressive and anxious features, dementia, and delirium (4–13), although anxiety disorders, mania, and psychotic disorders have also been reported (Table 35.2). A comprehensive review of all psychosocial research and psychological disorders associated with HIV is beyond the scope of this chapter. Instead, this chapter will attempt to first provide an overview of the primary psychological and psychiatric complications associated with HIV and AIDS in general, and then identify sequelae associated with specific HIV-related malignancies (i.e., Kaposi's sarcoma, lymphoma, cervical cancer).

DEPRESSION IN HIV

Perhaps the most frequently cited mental health concern identified among HIV-infected persons is depression. As with any terminal illness, a common assumption among experienced mental health clinicians as well as the lay public is that depression is an inevitable consequence of an HIV$^+$ diagnosis (8–14). Self-report data have tended to support this assumption, demonstrating high levels of depressive symptoms and overall psychological distress among HIV-infected patients, and a tendency for these symptoms to

TABLE 35.1. *Medical Conditions Included in the 1993 AIDS Surveillance Case Definition*

Candidiasis of bronchi, trachea, or lungs

Candidiasis, esophageal

Cervical Cancer, invasive

Coccidiodomycosis, disseminated or extrapulmonary

Cryptococcosis, extrapulmonary

Crytposporidiosis, chronic intestinal (> 1 month duration)

Cytomegalovirus disease (other than liver, spleen, or nodes)

Cytomegalovirus retinitis (with loss of vision)

Encephalopathy, HIV-related

Herpes simplex, chronic ulcer(s) (> 1 month duration); or bronchitis, pneumonitis, or esophagitis

Histoplasmosis, disseminated or extrapulmonary

Isoporiasis, chronic intestinal (> 1 month duration)

Kaposi's sarcoma

Lymphoma, Burkitt's (or equivalent term)

Lymphoma, immunoblastic (or equivalent term)

Lymphoma, primary, of brain

Mycobacterium avavium complex or *M. kansasii*, disseminated or extrapulmonary

Mycobacterium tuberculosis, any site (pulmonary or extrapulmonary)

Mycobacterium, other species or unidentified species, disseminated or extrapulmonary

Pneumocystis carinii pneumonia

Pneumonia, recurrent

Progressive multifocal leukoencephalopathy

Salmonella septicemia, recurrent

Toxoplasmosis of brain

Wasting syndrome due to HIV

increase with disease progression (15–18). The research on depression in HIV, however, has generally failed to distinguish between major depressive episodes, chronic, mild depression (e.g., dysthymia); and brief, mild depressive episodes (e.g., adjustment disorders with depressive features). Several researchers have assessed the frequency of major depressive episodes among HIV-infected persons using standardized diagnostic interviews. These studies have contradicted earlier conclusions, reporting between 6% and 20% of patients meeting diagnostic criteria for a major depressive disorder, with the vast majority of depressed HIV$^+$ patients being more accurately diagnosed as having adjustment disorders with depressive features (14). These findings reflect the relatively mild and often transient nature of depressive symptoms typically found among HIV-infected patients. The prevalence studies of depression in HIV, however, are not without limitations, including reliance on relatively small samples that often underrepresent injecting drug users and

women infected with HIV, both groups that are at a higher risk for depression regardless of HIV infection. Another methodological problem frequent in studies of depression in HIV is the confounding influence of somatic symptoms that may be related to disease rather than depression (fatigue, weight loss, diminished appetite, concentration problems, and sleep disturbance). Focusing on cognitive symptoms of depression (e.g., hopelessness, guilt, anhedonia, preoccupation with thoughts of death) may provide a more accurate index of clinical depression in HIV-infected patients. Despite methodological limitations, a general conclusion reached by most clinicians and researchers is that major depressive episodes are not a typical response to HIV and warrant clinical intervention and treatment.

A related concern regarding HIV-infected patients is that of potential for suicide. Early reports found the rate of suicide among patients with HIV/AIDS to be 36 times greater than that of the general population (19,20); however, other more recent research has not supported these findings (21,22). Comparison of patients with AIDS with the general public also obscures potentially confounding influences of sexual identity and/or history of injecting drug use on depression and suicidal ideation. Recent studies have demonstrated comparable levels of depressive symptoms and suicidal ideation among gay males (23,24) and injecting drug users (25) with and without HIV$^+$/AIDS, along with relatively low rates of suicide attempts in the HIV-infected population (22). Other research has suggested that suicidal ideation is more pronounced immediately prior to HIV testing, and after a seropositive HIV test finding, but is not necessarily increased during other periods (23). Nearly 30% of at-risk individuals awaiting HIV testing acknowledged suicidal ideation; however, this rate dropped to 16% for patients who tested HIV seronegative, yet remained at pretest levels for patients who tested HIV seropositive. During the 8 weeks following HIV testing, the rate of suicidal ideation among HIV$^+$ patients fell to a level comparable to HIV seronegative controls. These findings have led many clinicians and researchers to conclude that depression and suicidal ideation may be an atypical response to HIV infection other than in the period immediately following HIV testing, and may be minimized by adequate pretest and posttest counselling.

Given the relative infrequency of depression and suicidal ideation among HIV-infected patients, considerable empirical attention has been paid to identifying risk factors for developing depression and suicidal ideation in patients with HIV. These studies have typically suggested that risk factors for depression in HIV

TABLE 35.2. *Psychiatric Disorders among Patients with HIV/AIDS*. Data are percentages*

Study	Perry and Tross, 1984	Atkinson et al., 1988			Perry et al., 1990
Reference	(8)	(9)			(11)
Method	Chart Review	DIS Interview			SCID Interview
Population	52 Hospitalized AIDS Patients	45 Homosexual Men with HIV, ARC, AIDS†			31 HIV⁺ Men
Adjustment D/O	65.4‡				
Major depression	17.3	17.6	7.7	6.7	6.5
Dysthymia					9.7
Bipolar disorder					0
Generalized Anxiety		17.6	38.5	26.7	9.7
Panic D/O		11.8	7.7	0	
Simple phobia		0	7.7	6.7	
Delirium	28.8				
Dementia	11.5				
Alcohol abuse					9.7
Substance abuse		5.9	38.5	6.7	6.5
Schizophrenia	1.9				

Study	Pace et al., 1990	O'Dowd and McKegney 1990	Treisman et al., 1994
Reference	(10)	(12)	(13)
Method	Clinical Evaluation	Clinical Evaluation	Clinical Evaluation
Population	95 US Air Force Personnel	67 Hospitalized AIDS Patients	50 Consecutive HIV⁺ Clinic Patients
Adjustment D/O		42	18
Major depression	17.9	3	20
Dysthymia	0		
Bipolar disorder	0		2
Generalized anxiety	1.1		
Panic D/O	2.1		
Simple phobia	18.9		
Delirium		27	
Dementia		22	12
Alcohol abuse		3	
Substance abuse		18	44
Schizophrenia	0		

*All diagnoses based on DSM-III-R criteria except Perry and Tross, 1984 (DSM-III)
† Percentages are for HIV⁺ asymptomatic, ARC, and AIDS patients respectively
‡Described as "possible depressive symptoms."

are similar to risk factors for depression in the general population, including history of depression, diagnosis of personality disorders, and poor social support (22, 23,26). A number of risk factors specific to HIV have been found as well, including stage of disease, increasing symptom severity, pain, and loss of friends or family due to HIV (15,24,26–28). With regard to stage of disease, HIV⁺ patients appear particularly vulnerable to depressive symptoms and suicidal ideation at two distinct points during the illness: immediately following HIV diagnosis, and after the onset of serious physical symptoms [e.g., hospitalization (18)]. Many patients have an immediate, extreme reaction to learning of an HIV⁺ diagnosis characterized by a preoccupation with thoughts of death, concerns about ability to cope with the illness, and fear of others' reactions to learning of the diagnosis. Interestingly, no relationship has been observed between the amount or type of information disclosed to patients (i.e., their knowledge of the course of disease, risks and benefits of treatments) and depression, despite frequent apprehension among medical professionals and the lay public that increased awareness of the disease will inevitably lead to increased depression (14,15).

Treatment of depression, a topic which has also received considerable empirical attention will be discussed only briefly here (see Chapter 45 in this volume). A general consensus among clinicians is that, as with depression in HIV seronegative persons, both psychotherapy and antidepressant medications are beneficial. Recent research studies have demonstrated the efficacy of individual cognitive-behavioral and interpersonal psychotherapy for the treatment of depression, although these studies have typically included only patients with relatively mild depressive disorders such as dysthymia or adjustment disorders with depressed features (29–31). For patients suffering from a major depressive episode, randomized trials have demonstrated several antidepressant medications (e.g., imipramine, fluoxetine) that are both safe and effective in treating HIV-infected patients (32,33). Serotonin-specific reuptake inhibitors (SSRIs) are considered the antidepressants of choice among the medically ill because of their apparent efficacy, relatively mild side effect profiles, and minimal interactions with other medications (32). Tricyclic antidepressants and ECT have also been used for treating depression in HIV-infected patients, although these interventions are used less frequently because of the fragile health status of many HIV-infected patients (33,34). Psychostimulants may also be beneficial as primary or adjuvant interventions for depression in HIV-infected patients, and have demonstrated efficacy with cognitive as well as somatic aspects of depression (35). The recommendation generally made with regard to prescribing any of these medications is to begin at doses lower than those typically used for non-medically-ill adults, and titrate the dosage upward slowly.

ANXIETY

Another common reaction to an HIV$^+$ diagnosis is anxiety. Anxiety symptoms in HIV commonly include a pervasive worry about health, physical function, uncertainties related to the course of HIV disease, and fear of death (18). Although phobic avoidance of situations or objects, and obsessive-compulsive behaviors centering around physical symptoms and health-related behaviors may occur in HIV$^+$ patients, these disorders are far less common than generalized anxiety disorders or adjustment disorders with anxious features. Atkinson and colleages found more than 25% of HIV$^+$ patients and nearly 40% of patients with AIDS met DSM-III-R criteria for a generalized anxiety disorder (9). Pace and colleagues found that nearly one-fourth of HIV$^+$ Air Force personnel met diagnostic criteria for an anxiety disorder and nearly one-fifth experienced simple phobias (10). Ostrow described compulsive checking and palpating for symptoms of

disease progression (e.g., swelling, blemishes, or other physical changes) as an aspect of anxiety related to HIV disease, but did not assess the prevalence of such symptoms (36). As with depression, however, many HIV$^+$ patients experience relatively mild, transient anxiety symptoms more consistent with a diagnosis of an adjustment disorder, and infrequently experience the disabling levels of anxiety typical of an anxiety disorder.

Treatment of anxiety symptoms in medically ill patients generally involves sedative and anxiolytic medications. Among persons with HIV/AIDS, however, such interventions are often complicated by the high frequency of substance abuse among this population. Although benzodiazepines are the agents typically used for alleviation of anxiety symptoms among medically ill patients in general, many clinicians are reluctant to prescribe these medications in patients with a history of substance abuse. Instead, clinicians may rely on psychotherapy as the sole treatment option. Psychotherapy, and in particular, cognitive and behavioral psychotherapies are often effective in anxious patients; however, the length of time necessary to achieve clinical benefits and the physical and psychological distress associated with anxiety symptoms (e.g., sleep disturbance) often justify the addition of pharmacologic interventions. No clear guidelines are available for alleviating concern about possible substance abuse, although careful monitoring of medications prescribed, and switching to alternative medications rather than titrating up with a single medication, may help minimize potential for substance abuse. Other possible treatment alternatives include the use of non-benzodiazapine anxiolytic medications (e.g., buspirone), which are less susceptible to abuse. More detailed recommendations regarding the management of patients with past or present substance abuse disorders, as well as additional information regarding the treatment of anxiety disorders among medically ill patients are available elsewhere in this volume (see Chapter 47).

COGNITIVE DISORDERS AND DEMENTIA

Another area that has received considerable mental health attention is the neurologic complications of AIDS. While the HIV virus impairs cognitive functioning directly (e.g., dementia and delirium), cognitive impairment can also occur as a consequence of central nervous system opportunistic infections to which HIV-infected individuals are susceptible (e.g., toxoplasmosis, CNS lymphoma, cytomegalovirus). Epidemiological projections have estimated that over half of all HIV-infected patients will experience some degree of cognitive deterioration during the course of their illness, and cognitive symptoms are the presenting symptoms of HIV in approximately 10% of patients (37–39). Early studies suggested that dementia symptoms may arise in the beginning phases of HIV infection, while patients were otherwise asymptomatic (39). After considerable debate regarding this issue in the empirical literature, recent longitudinal data have indicated that dementia symptoms are in fact associated with later stages of HIV infection and reflect disease progression (37). The Multicenter AIDS Cohort Study (MACS), a large, longitudinal study of dementia in HIV-infected patients, found the prevalence of HIV dementia to be less than 1% among asymptomatic HIV-infected patients, and overall severity of dementia symptoms in asymptomatic HIV$^+$ patients were no more severe than in HIV seronegative controls (37).

The most common manifestations of HIV-associated dementia (HIV-ADC, a term recommended by the American Acadamy of Neurology) reflect the predominantly subcortical nature of the impairment, although the actual clinical presentation of HIV-ADC is often quite heterogeneous. Typical symptoms include memory loss (particularly with retrieval and information integration problems), psychomotor and cognitive slowing, and personality changes, including apathy, inertia, irritability and depressive symptoms. In patients with more advanced cognitive symptoms, there is considerable difficulty in learning information and forming new memories along with increased psychomotor retardation. Clinicians have also noted the adverse impact of dementia on HIV-infected patients' mood, citing dementia as a possible correlate of depression and suicide, as well as noting the reverse, that depression may exacerbate HIV-infected patients' cognitive symptoms (40–42).

Diagnosis of HIV-ADC (or HIV-associated cognitive/motor complex for patients with only minor cognitive difficulties) is made primarily on the basis of observable symptoms, and different staging criteria have been suggested (e.g., Ref. 43). The most widely utilized guidelines for diagnosis and staging of HIV-ADC are those published by the American Academy of Neurology (42). These criteria, summarized in Table 35.3, require the presence of deterioration in at least

TABLE 35.3. *American Academy of Neurology Criteria for Diagnosis of HIV-Associated Dementia Complex*

PROBABLE DEMENTIA DIAGNOSIS (must have *each* of the following):

1. Acquired abnormality in at least two of the following cognitive abilities (present for at least 1 month): attention/concentration, speed of processing information, abstraction/reasoning, visuospatial skills, memory/learning, and speech/language. The decline should be verified by reliable history and mental status examination. In all cases, when possible, history should be obtained from an informant, and examination should be supplemented by neuropsychological testing.

   Cognitive dysfunction causing impairment of work or activities of daily living (objectively verifiable or by report of a key informant) should not be attributable solely to severe systemic illness.

2. At least one of the following:

   (a) Acquired abnormality in motor functioning or performance verified by clinical examination (e.g., slowed rapid movements, abnormal gait, limb incoordination, hyperflecis, hypertonia, or weakness), neuropsychological tests (e.g., fine motor speed, manual dexterity, perceptual motor skills), or both.

   (b) Decline in motivation or emotional control or change in social behavior. This may be characterized by any of the following: change in personality with apathy, inertia, irritability, emotional lability, or new onset of impaired judgment characterized by socially inappropriate behavior or disinhibition.

3. Absence of clouding of consciousness during a period long enough to establish the presence of # 1.

4. Evidence of another etiology, including active CNS opportunistic infection or malignancy, psychiatric disorders (e.g., depressive disorders), active alcohol or substance use, or acute or chronic substance withdrawal, must be sought from history, physical and psychiatric examinations, and appropriate laboratory and radiologic investigation (e.g., lumbar puncture, neuroimaging). If another potential etiology (e.g., major depression) is present, it is *not* the cause of the above cognitive, motor, or behavioral symptoms and signs.

POSSIBLE DEMENTIA DIAGNOSIS (must have *one* of the following):

1. Other potential etiology present (must have *each* of the following):

   (a) As above (see "Probable") # 1, 2, and 3.

   (b) Other potential etiology is present but the cause of the myelopathy is uncertain

2. Incomplete clinical evaluation (must have *each* of the following):

   (a) As above (see "Probable") # 1, 2, and 3.

   (b) Etiology cannot be determined (appropriate laboratory or radiologic investigations are not performed).

two areas of cognitive functioning (attention/concentration, information processing speed, reasoning, visual-spatial skills, memory/learning, and speech/language abilities), coupled with abnormal motor functioning (either observed or evidenced in neuropsychological test performance), or personality changes (e.g., apathy, irritability, mood lability). These symptoms must be present, in the absence of any other possible etiology which may account for the symptoms (e.g., delirium). Neuropsychological test batteries have also been utilized as screening measures to determine the existence of psychomotor deficits (e.g., to assess the need for more thorough neurologic evaluation), as well as to quantify the degree of impairment for use in assessing the efficacy or impact of treatments. The neuropsychological tests most sensitive to HIV dementia focus on psychomotor speed, information processing speed, and attention/concentration abilities [e.g., Trail Making Test, Grooved Pegboard, Finger Tapping Test, Digit Symbol Test; (38,44,45)].

The treatment of HIV-ADC has also received considerable attention, with several case reports and uncontrolled research studies suggesting that the antiretroviral medication zidovudine (AZT) may be effective in either improving cognitive functioning or preventing cognitive deterioration (37,46,47). More recently, however, a placebo-controlled trial of antiretroviral treatment of HIV-ADC indicated that cognitive improvement occurred only in patients treated with very high doses of AZT (2000 mg/day) (48). Similarly, preliminary research has suggested that high-dose AZT may help prevent the onset of HIV-ADC symptoms, but other studies have found no such benefit (37). More traditional interventions for dementia focus on symptom management, with low-dose antipsychotic medications occasionally recommended for agitation often associated with dementia, and psychostimulants for improving attention and concentration and reducing cognitive and psychomotor slowing (47,49,50). Although considerable behavioral/rehabilitative efforts have been focused on remediation and/or compensation for cognitive impairments among individuals with brain damage, such techniques have rarely been systematically adopted for treatment of cognitive deterioration related to HIV. Behavioral interventions (e.g., increased use of reminders and notepads, medication alarms, environmental changes to simplify the person's living situation) are effective in helping patients with various forms of dementia compensate for their disabilities, and may be useful, despite a lack of empirical support, for patients with HIV-ADC (e.g., 47,51).

Delirium, a rapid onset of cognitive impairment and arousal disturbance (confusion, hallucinations, somnolence, etc.), is another common cognitive disorder among HIV-infected patients (52,53). Estimates of the prevalence of delirium in hospitalized patients with AIDS have ranged from 30% to 40% (54,55). Unlike HIV-associated dementia, delirium in HIV-infected patients does not appear to be distinguishable from delirium related to other medical disorders. Similarly, the treatment of HIV-associated delirium is comparable to treatment of delirium associated with other medical disorders, with the primary pharmacologic strategy involving low-dose neuroleptic medications (48,54). In a recent double-blind, randomized comparison trial of neuroleptic (haloperidol, chlorpromazine) and sedative (lorazapam) medications in hospitalized AIDS patients with delirium, both neuroleptics studied proved to be highly effective in resolving the behavioral and cognitive symptoms of delirium, while lorazapam alone was ineffective (54). The evaluation and treatment of delirium is described in greater detail elsewhere in this volume (see Chapter 48).

OTHER MENTAL DISORDERS ASSOCIATED WITH HIV

A number of case reports have described psychotic symptoms and/or manic episodes among HIV-infected patients, although these reports have been relatively infrequent. Psychotic episodes (e.g., brief psychotic reaction, psychotic disorder due to medical condition, psychotic disorder not otherwise specified) in patients without a history of psychosis or mood disorder have been reported, albeit infrequently, and are typically associated with later stages of disease progression (11,14,56). Because of the lack of attention paid to psychotic disorders resulting from HIV infection, little is known about the cause, frequency, or course of such disorders, although organic processes (e.g., CNS disease) are often suspected. Interventions for psychotic disorders typically rely on antipsychotic medications, although the effectiveness of these medications in patients with HIV is quite variable. In addition, many patients may experience the rapid onset of mood disorder symptoms or sudden personality changes suggestive of an organic mood disorder or organic personality disorder. For example, reports of HIV-related thyroid abnormalities have been documented, and typically present as symptoms of a mood disorder. Although some patients with organic mood disorders respond to mood stabilizing (e.g., lithium, anticonvulsant agents) or antidepressant medications, there is considerable variability in patients' response to these medications. Additional research is clearly necessary before reliable treatment recommendations can be made regarding new-onset psychotic disorders and organic mood or personality disorders among HIV-infected persons.

PSYCHOLOGICAL ISSUES RELATED TO OPPORTUNISTIC CANCERS IN HIV DISEASE

In addition to psychiatric symptoms associated with HIV infection, specific consequences of particular HIV-related malignancies or treatments have also been noted. This literature is limited, however, by the frequent failure of investigators to specifically address correlates of individual illness to which HIV-infected patients are susceptible and the converse failure, in studying specific diseases, to differentiate patients whose illness is related to HIV infection from those whose illness is unrelated (e.g., cervical cancer or lymphoma).

Kaposi's sarcoma (KS) was previously a rare malignancy found primarily among older individuals of eastern European and Italian descent (57). The occurrence of purple blemishes among otherwise healthy young gay men led to the diagnosis of AIDS long before tests for HIV infection were developed. Currently, KS is estimated to be 20,000 times more likely in HIV-infected patients than in non-HIV-infected patients, and 300 times more likely than among immunocompromised patients with other medical diagnoses (58). Because KS is found almost exclusively among men, many researchers speculate that the malignancy is sexual transmitted. The disease typically appears as purple blemishes, often on the nose, feet, genitalia, or retroauricular or periorbital areas, but has been found (often on autopsy) in most organs. Particularly distressing expressions of KS include oral lesions that may interfere with eating or speech, severe, painful lymphedema of legs and arms, and CNS lesions that can result in specific or diffuse cognitive deficits. Because of the diverse presentation of KS and the lack of specific markers that correspond to prognosis, the disease is not staged in the same manner as other malignancies. Patients are classified as "good risk" or "bad risk" depending on their overall health status.

Although little research has been devoted to the psychological and psychiatric implications of KS, several areas of concern have been identified. The primary aspects of KS that impact on psychological well-being include the occurrence of visible blemishes, cognitive changes due to CNS lesions, and mood disorders resulting from pain related to KS lesions or side effects

of chemotherapeutic treatment of KS. Recent research with HIV-infected gay men demonstrated an adverse impact of visible lesions on patients' mood and overall psychological adjustment (59). Patients with visible lesions (typically resulting from KS) reported higher levels of psychological distress on a self-report measure. There are several reasons why visible symptoms may cause or exacerbate psychological distress, including the potential for unwanted disclosure of HIV status, increased likelihood of discrimination or stigma, and an increased sense of helplessness or lack of control over the disease. These possible explanations for the adverse impact of KS on psychological functioning, however, have not been studied systematically.

A second aspect of KS that impacts of HIV-infected patients psychological functioning is the pain associated with KS lesions. KS lesions are often quite painful, particularly when the lesions are located in sensitive areas (e.g., face, soles of feet, genital area). Recent research has demonstrated a substantial, adverse impact of pain on HIV-infected patients' psychological well-being (depression and suicidal ideation, psychological distress) and overall quality of life (26). These data suggest that KS may interfere with HIV-infected patients' mood because of the painful nature of KS lesions, in addition to psychological factors related to KS itself. Changes in mood, and depression in particular, have also been cited as common sequelae of interferon-α, a chemotherapeutic agent used in the treatment of KS (60) (see Chapter 23). A frequently noted side-effect of interferon-α treatment is the onset of depressive symptoms, and fatigue in particular, which often necessitates treatment with antidepressant and/or psychostimulant medications. Another possible, although less common source of depression resulting from KS is related to destruction of the thyroid gland. Case reports have indicated that severe, progressive depressive symptoms that are unresponsive to traditional antidepressant therapies can result from hypothyroidism related to KS infiltration of the thyroid (61). Similarly, KS infiltration of the central nervous system has been reported, although cognitive/dementia symptoms resulting from KS are also relatively rare (62).

Several other malignancies have been found to be associated with human immunodeficiency virus (HIV-1), and are classified by the CDC as AIDS-defining conditions, including central nervous system (CNS) lymphoma, high-grade non-Hodgkin's lymphoma, and most recently cervical cancer (3). Unfortunately, little empirical attention has been paid to whether differences exist in psychological adjustment or psychiatric sequelae between individuals who are diagnosed with these cancers without an HIV^+ diagnosis and those for whom the cancer is a manifestation of HIV infection. One frequently observed distinction between cancers related to HIV and those same cancers in patients without HIV is that the diagnosis of cancer is far less stigmatizing and easier for patients to disclose to family or friends than is an HIV diagnosis.

With regard to HIV-related lymphomas, the most commonly noted psychiatric syndromes are delirium and dementia, typically arising with central nervous system lymphomas. The clinical presentation of dementias resulting from HIV-associated lymphomas have been described somewhat differently from dementia associated with HIV infection per se (HIV-ADC). Cognitive symptoms associated with lymphoma generally result in more localized, or focal cognitive deficits, and the onset of these neurologic deficits is typically more rapid than the gradual deterioration common in HIV-ADC. Delirium symptoms are also common in patients with HIV-related CNS lymphomas, and these symptoms are treated similarly to delirium symptoms that are the product of other medical conditions.

Some empirical research has also addressed the psychological sequelae of cervical cancer, although this research has generally been conducted with patients who are not HIV^+ and is discussed in greater detail elsewhere in this volume (see Chapter 30). This literature has suggested that women with cervical cancers are particularly prone to anxiety, depression, and sexual dysfunction, but these studies have typically relied on self-report data rather than clinical diagnoses (63, 64). Although it is certainly plausible that women whose cervical cancer is related to HIV infection will experience more profound psychological difficulties, and sexual difficulties in particular, given the sexual transmission of HIV, no research has addressed this supposition.

One aspect of cervical cancer that has frequently been noted in women with HIV is the difficulty in obtaining accurate diagnosis and adequate treatment. Until recently, cervical cancer was not acknowledged as a sequela of HIV infection, in part because potential indicators of cervical disease (e.g., abnormal Pap smear) were attributed to HIV rather than cancer. As a result, many HIV-infected women are not treated for their cancer until the disease has reached a relatively advanced stage and therefore is difficult to treat effectively. This issue is compounded by the apparent aggressive nature of cervical cancer among women with AIDS. Conversely, because many women are treated primarily by gynecologists, a diagnosis of HIV^+ may be delayed, and possibly even treated less aggressively after diagnosis (65). These factors (delays in HIV^+ or cervical cancer diagnosis) complicate any attempt to assess the impact of cervical cancer on the psychological functioning of women with HIV, and must be considered in any such research.

SUMMARY

The psychological and psychiatric sequelae associated with HIV infection are frequent and varied. Although many patients report depressive and anxious symptoms, the prevalence of major depressive disorders or anxiety disorders is relatively low. More commonly, patients are diagnosed with adjustment disorders with depressive, anxious, or mixed features and these patients are usually treated effectively with both psychotherapy and psychotropic medications. In particular, interventions focused around periods typically associated with adverse psychological reactions (i.e., pretest and posttest counseling around the time of HIV testing and following the onset of opportunistic infections) may be helpful in minimizing the psychological distress often associated with HIV. In addition, rehabilitative efforts focused on minimizing difficulties due to HIV-associated dementia may help improve the quality of life for patients experiencing these symptoms.

REFERENCES

1. Centers for Disease Control and Prevention. *HIV/AIDS Surveillance Report*, 1995.
2. World Health Organization. *Weekly Epidemiol Rec*, 1995: no. 50.
3. Centers for Disease Control and Prevention. 1993 revised classification system for HIV infection and expanded surveillance case definition for AIDS among adolescents and adults. *Morbid Mortal Weekly Rep*. 1992; 41(RR-17):6.
4. Holland JC, Tross S: The psychosocial and neuropsychiatric sequelae of the acquired immunodeficiency syndrome and related disorders. *Ann Intern Med*. 1985; 103:760–764.
5. Williams JBW, Rabkin JG, Remien RH, Gorman JM, Ehrhardt AA: Multidisciplinary baseline assessment of homosexual men with and without human immunodeficiency virus: a controlled study. *Arch Gen Psychiatry*. 1991; 48:124–130.
6. Perry S, Jacobsen P. Neuropsychiatric manifestations of AIDS-spectrum disorders. *Hosp Community Psychiatry*. 1986; 37:135–142.
7. Tross S, Hirsch DA, Rabkin B, Berry C, Holland J: Determinants of current psychiatric disorder in AIDS spectrum patients. *Proceedings Third International Conference Acquired Immunodeficiency Syndrome (AIDS)*. Washington D.C.: Courtesy Associates 1987. [Abstract T.10.5.]

8. Perry SW, Tross S. Psychiatric problems of AIDS inpatients at the New York hospital: Preliminary report. *Public Health Rep.* 1984; 99:200–205.

9. Atkinson JH, Grant I, Kennedy CJ, Richman DD, Spector SA, McCutchan JA. Prevalance of psychaitric disorders among men infected with human immunodeficiency virus. *Arch Gen Psychiatry.* 1988; 45:859–864.

10. Pace J, Brown GR, Rundell JR, Paolucci S, Drexler K, Mcmanis S. Prevalence of psychiatric disorders in a mandatory screening program for infection with human immunodeficiency virus: a pilot study. *Mil Med.* 1990; 155:76–80.

11. Perry SW, Jacobsberg L, Fishman B, Frances A, Bobo J, Jacobsberg BK. Psychiatric diagnoses before serological testing for the human immunodeficiency virus. *Am J Psychiatry.* 1990; 147:89–95.

12. O'Dowd MA,McKegney FP. AIDS patients compared with others seen in psychiatric consultation. *Gen Hosp Psychiatry.* 1990; 12:50–55.

13. Treisman G, Fishman M, Lyketsos C, McHugh PR. Evaluation and treatment of psychiatric disorders associated with HIV infection. In: Price RW, Perry SW, eds. *HIV, AIDS, and the Brain.* New York: Raven Press; 1994: 238–250.

14. Perry SW. HIV-related depression. In: Price RW, Perry SW, eds. *HIV, AIDS, and the Brain.* New York: Raven Press; 1994: 223–238.

15. Hays RB, Turner H, Coates TJ. Social support, AIDS-related symptoms, and depression among gay men. *J Consult Clin Psychol.* 1992; 60:463–469

16. Perry S, Fishman B. Depression and HIV: how does one affect the other? *J Am Med Assoc.* 1993; 270:2609–2610.

17. Rabkin JG, Williams JBW, Remien RH, et al. Depression, distress, lymphocyte subsets, and himan immunodeficientcy virus symptoms on two occasions in HIV-positive homosexual men. *Arch Gen Psychiatry.* 1991; 48:111–119.

18. Kalichman SC, Sikkema KJ. Psychological sequelae of HIV infection and AIDS: review of empirical findings. *Clin Psychol Rev.* 1994; 14:611–632.

19. Marzuk PM, Tierney H, Tardiff K, et al. Increased risk of suicide in persons with AIDS. *J Am Med Assoc.* 1988; 259:1333–1337.

20. Marzuk PM. Suicidal behavior and HIV illness. *Int Rev Psychiatry.* 1991; 3:365–371.

21. O'Dowd MA, Biderman DJ, McKegney FP. Incidence of suicidality in AIDS and HIV-positive patients attending a psychiatry outpatient program. *Psychosomatics.* 1993; 34:33–40.

22. Rabkin JG, Remien R, Katoff L, Williams JB. Suicidality in AIDS long-term survivors: what is the evidence? *AIDS Care.* 1993; 5:401–411.

23. Perry SW, Jacobsberg L, Fishman B: Suicidal ideation in HIV testing. *J Am Med Assoc.* 1990; 263:679–682.

24. Lipsitz JD, Williams JBW, Rabkin JG, et al. Psychopathology in male and female intravenous drug users with and without HIV infection. *Am J Psychiatry.* 1994; 151:1662–1668.

25. Kelly JA, Murphy DA, Bahr GR, Koob JJ, et al. Factors associated with severity of depression and high-risk sexual behavior among persons diagnosed with human immunodeficiency virus (HIV) infection. *Health Psychol.* 1993; 12:215–219.

26. Rosenfeld, B, Breitbart W, McDonald MV, Passik SD, Thaler H, Portenoy RK. Pain experience in ambulatory aids patients—II. Impact on psychological well-being and quality of life. *Pain.* 1996; 68:323–328.

27. Schneider SG, Taylow SE, Hammen C, et al. Factors influencing suicide intent in gay and bisexual suicide ideators: differing models for men with and without human immunodeficiency virus. *J Pers Soc Psychol.* 1991; 61:776–788.

28. Martin JL, Dean L. Effects of AIDS-related bereavement and HIV-related illness on psychological distress among gay men: a 7-year longitudinal study, 1985–1991. *J Consult Clin Psychol.* 1993; 61:94–103.

29. Chesney MA, Folkman S. Psychological impact of HIV disease and implications for intervention. *Psychiatr Clin N Am.* 1994; 17:163–182.

30. Markowitz JC, Klerman GL, Perry SW. Interpersonal psychotherapy of depressed HIV-seropositive patients. *Hosp Community Psychiatry.* 1992; 43:885–890.

31. Perry S, Fishman B, Jacobsberg L, Young J, Frances A. Effectiveness of psychoeducational interventions in reducing emotional distress after human immunodeficiency virus antibody testing. *Arch Gen Psychiatry.* 1991; 48:143–147.

32. Rabkin JG, Rabkin R, Wagner G. Effects of fluoxetine on mood and immune status in depressed men with HIV illness. *J Clin Psychiatry.* 1994; 55:92–97.

33. Rabkin JG, Harrison WM. Effect of imipramine on depression and immune status in a sample of men with HIV infection. *Am J Psychiatry.* 1990; 147:495–497.

34. Schaerf FW, Miller RR, Lipsey JR, et al. ECT for major depression in four patients with human immunodeficiency virus. *Am J Psychiatry.* 1989; 146:782–284.

35. Fernandez F, Levy JK, Galizzi H. Response of HIV-related depression to psychostimulants. case reports. *Hosp Community Psychiatry.* 1988; 39:628–631.

36. Ostrow D. Psychiatric aspects of AIDS. an overview. In: Ostrow D, ed. *Behavioral Aspects of AIDS.* New York. Plenum Press; 1991: 9–18.

37. McArthur JC, Selnes OA, Glass JD, Hoover DR, Bacellar H. HIV dementia. Incidence and risk factors. In: Price RW, Perry SW, eds. *HIV, AIDS, and the Brain.* New York: Raven Press; 1994: 251–272.

38. Levy MR, Bredsen DE. Central nervous system dysfunction in acquired immunodeficiency syndrome. *J Acquired Immune Defic Syndr.* 1988; 1:41–64.

39. Grant I, Atkinson JH, Hesselink JR, et al. Evidence for early central nervous system involvement in the acquired immunodeficiency syndrome (AIDS) and other human immunodeficiency virus (HIV) infections. *Ann Int Med.* 1987; 107:828–836.

40. Alfonso CA, Cohen MA. HIV-dementia and suicide. *Gen Hosp Psychiatry.* 1994; 16:45–46.

41. Krikorian R, Wrobel AJ. Cognitive impairment in HIV infection. *AIDS.* 1991:5(12):1501–1507.

42. Janssen RS, Cornblath DR, Epstein LG, Fox RP, McArthur JP, Price RM. Nomenclature and research case definitions for neurological manifestatinos of human immunodeficiency virus type-1 (HIV-1) infection. Report of a working group of the American Academy of Neurology AIDS task force. *Neurology.* 1991; 41:778–785.

43. Price RW, Brew BJ. The AIDS dementia complex. *J Infect Dis.* 1988; 158:1079–1083.

44. Maruff P, Currie J, Malone V, et al. Neuropsychological characterization of the AIDS dementia complex and rationalization of a test battery. *Arch Neurol.* 1994; 51:689–695.

45. Sidtis JJ. Evaluation of the AIDS dementia complex in adults. In: Price RW, Perry SW, eds. *HIV, AIDS, and the Brain.* New York: Raven Press; 1994: 273–287.

46. Schmitt FA, Bigley JW, McKinnis R, et al. Neuropsychological outcome of zidovudine (AZT) treatment in patients with AIDS and AIDS-related complex. *N Engl J Med.* 1987; 317:1573–1578.

47. Singer EJ. HIV-associated neurological disease. *J Physicians Assoc AIDS Care.* 1994; 19–25.

48. Sidtis JJ, Gatsonis C, Price RW, et al. Zidovudine treatment of the AIDS dementia complex. results of a placebo-controlled trial. *Ann Neurol.* 1993; 51:134–140.

49. Platt MM, Breitbart W, Smith M, Marotta R, Weisman H, Jacobsen PB. Efficacy of neuroleptics for hypoactive delirium. *J Neuropsychiatry Clin Neurosci.* 1994; 6:66–67.

50. Holmes VF, Fernandez F, Levy JK. Psychostimulant response in AIDS-related complex patients. *J Clin Psychiatry.* 1989; 50:5–8.

51. Fisher JE, Carstensen LI. Behavior management of the dementias. *Clin Psychol Rev.* 1990; 10:611–629.

52. Perriens JH, Mussa M, Luabeya MK, et al. Neurological complications of HIV-1 seropositive internal medicine inpatients in Kinshasa, Zaire. *J Acquired Immune Defic Syndr.* 1992; 5:333–340.

53. World Health Organization. World Health Organization consultation on the neuropsychiatric aspects of HIV-1 infection. *AIDS.* 1990; 4:935–936.

54. Breitbart W, Marotta R, Platt M, et al. A randomized, double-blind comparison trial of haloperidol, chlorpromazine, and lorazapam in the treatment of delirium in hospitalized AIDS patients. *Am J Psychiatry.* 1996; 153:231–237.

55. Perry SW. Organic mental disorders caused by HIV. update on early diagnosis and treatment. *Am J Psychiatry* 1990;47:696–710.

56. Harris MJ, Jeste DV, Gleghorn A, Sewell DD. New-onset psychosis in HIV-infected patients. *J Clin Psychiatry.* 1991; 52:369–376.

57. Safai B, Schwartz JJ. Kaposi's sarcoma and the acquired immunodeficiency syndrome. In: DeVita VT, Hellman S, Rosenberg SA, eds. *AIDS: Etiology, Diagnosis, Treatment and Prevention*, 3rd ed. Philadelphia: JB Lippincott; 1992: 209–223.

58. Jahnke L, Von Roenn JH. HIV-related malignencies. In: Brain MC, Carbone PP, eds. *Current Therapy in Hematology-Oncology*, 5th ed. St. Louis: Mosby; 1995: 558–563.

59. Grummon KL. Biopsychosocial factors in homosexual men with AIDS. a study of psychological distress, body image, physical symptoms, and social support. Unpublished doctoral dissertation; 1995.

60. Darko DF, McCutchen JA, Kripke DF, Gillin JC, Golshan S. Fatigue, sleep disturbance, disability and indices of progression of HIV infection. *Am J Psychiatry.* 1992, 149;514–520.

61. Mollison LC, Mijch A, McBride G, Dwyer B. Hypohydrism due to destruction of the thyroid by Kaposi's sarcoma. *Rev Infect Dis.* 1991, 13:826–827.

62. Mathiessen L, Marche C, Labrousse F, et al. Neuropathology of the brain in 174 patients who died of AIDS in a Paris hospital 1982-1988. *Ann Med Intern (Paris).* 1992; 143:43–49.

63. Cull A, Cowie VJ, Farquharson DI, Livingstone JR, Smart GE, Elton RA. Early stage cervical cancer. psychosocial and sexual outcomes of treatment. *Br J Cancer.* 1993; 68:1216–1220.

64. Golden RN, McCartney CF, Haggerty JJ Jr., et al. The detection of depression by patient self-report in women with gynecological cancer. *Int J Psychiatry Med.* 1991; 21:17–21.

65. Hellinger FJ. The use of health services by women with HIV infection. *Health Services Res.* 1993; 28:543–561.

36

Tumor of Unknown Primary Site

LEONARD B. SALTZ, STEVEN D. PASSIK, AND JEREMY C. LUNDBERG

Cancer of unknown primary (CUP) represents a complex diagnostic challenge to the practice of medical oncology. Research suggests that a diagnosis of unknown primary cancer represents 0.5% to 7% of annual cancer cases (1). In general, cancer of unknown primary implies a poor prognosis with extremely limited therapeutic options and an overall median survival of 4–10 months. (2–5). Favorable clinical outcomes are typically limited to those patients in more treatable subgroups of CUP or to instances where a more favorable histologic diagnosis can be identified (6–9). Oncologic management of CUP consists of: (*1*) reasonable attempts to establish the CUP diagnosis; (*2*) a search for alternative diagnoses with better prognoses; and (*3*) attempts to identify factors that would establish the patient as a member of one of the more treatable subgroups of unknown primary cancer. In this chapter, we will provide background medical information that will serve to highlight some of the more salient psychological and psychosocial issues that arise within this patient population. Psycho-oncologists need to acknowledge that patients with CUP contend with even higher levels of uncertainty than those that most cancer patients face. Also, owing to the fact that an unknown primary cancer is by definition metastatic, and therefore advanced, at the time of initial diagnosis, issues reflective of the advanced stage of disease must be confronted quite early in the patient's adjustment to the illness.

DEFINITION OF "CANCER OF UNKNOWN PRIMARY"

The term "cancer of unknown primary" lacks a strict, universally accepted definition and is frequently also referred to as carcinoma of unknown primary, adenocarcinoma of unknown primary, or anaplastic tumor of unknown primary. The lack of strictly defined criteria makes interpretation of the literature regarding unknown primary cancers difficult. In light of the more advanced techniques presently available, many tumors included in previously published series would quite likely be categorized as other diagnoses. It is therefore difficult to ascertain how this inaccuracy has affected the interpretability of survival data and other pertinent information. A reasonable criterion for establishing the diagnosis includes a thorough medical history, physical examination, chest X-ray, and other appropriate diagnostic evaluations that histologically confirm a cancer diagnosis from a metastatic tumor mass in a patient in whom no primary cancer site has been identified.

In a large number of CUP patients, the primary site of the tumor will never be found. Even in autopsy series, 15% to 27% of patients will not have a discernible origin of their disease (2,3,4,10), possibly attributable to either extensive carcinomatosis that obscures the primary or to the immunological destruction of the original primary tumor. Primary sites of lung, pancreas, and colon have been most commonly identified during post-mortem investigation, while primary sites of the liver, ovary, prostate, kidney, and bile duct account for the primary to a lesser extent.

THE DIAGNOSTIC EVALUATION OF CANCER OF UNKNOWN PRIMARY

As mentioned above, the evaluation of the patient with cancer of unknown primary begins with a detailed medical history and physical examination. Laboratory evaluation includes a complete blood count and biochemical screening profile to assess hepatic and renal function. Since lung cancer is a common source of unknown primary cancer, a chest X-ray is obtained.

The use of computer tomographic (CT) scanning in unknown primary patients remains controversial, owing to the lack of genuinely useful information that is likely to be obtained that will influence treatment. An abdominal CT scan is frequently ordered to evaluate the extent of liver involvement and to search for a pancreatic primary. However, useful therapies for metastatic cancer to the liver and for pancreatic cancer are extremely limited. Therefore, information obtained from these studies may be of little true benefit. A CT scan of the chest contributes virtually nothing over a routine X-ray of a patient with biopsy-proven metastatic disease. In the absence of specific indications, a pelvic CT is not likely to provide useful diagnostic data either. However, women with abdominal carcinomatosis and/or ascites, in whom visualization of the ovaries, is appropriate should be evaluated with a pelvic examination and ultrasonograpy, either external or transvaginal.

In the absence of symptoms or signs suggesting a gastrointestinal primary (blood in the stool, microcytic anemia, abdominal pain, etc.), an evaluation of the gastrointestinal tract is not routinely indicated in the work-up of unknown primary cancers. Such work-ups rarely identify the primary. Furthermore, the treatment of metastatic digestive tract cancers is generally unsuccessful. The rediagnosis from metastatic cancer of unknown primary to metastatic gastric or colorectal cancer does not improve the patient's prognosis or the efficacy of treatment. An exception would be in a patient with potentially resectable metastatic disease confined only to the liver (i.e., no nodal, mesenteric, or extraabdominal disease). In such a patient, identification of a colon primary could open up a possible surgical treatment option with the potential for cure.

Pathologic Evaluation

Following the initial clinical diagnosis of CUP, expert pathologic evaluation and detailed histologic evaluation are required to ensure that the tumor is indeed a carcinoma and does not represent a more treatable form of malignancy. Adenocarcinoma of the moderately or well differentiated variety represent a majority of cases reviewed. If indicated, the pathologist may employ specific immunohistochemical stains to confirm this diagnosis. Further pathologic characterization is rarely indicated should the pathologic evaluation reveal a moderately to well differentiated adenocarcinoma. However, further study is warranted should the tumor display a poorly differentiated or anaplastic appearance. Specific immunohistochemical studies may be employed to confirm or exclude a lymphoma, a far more treatable malignancy with a signifi-

cantly more favorable prognosis (11). Although not specific, the leukocyte common antigen (LCA) is a highly sensitive marker for lymphoma and is frequently employed in this type of evaluation. A diagnosis of lymphoma is essentially excluded in the presence of a negative LCA and a positive cytokeratin, the hallmark of carcinomas. Within the cytokeratin-positive carcinomas, a thyroglobulin stain should be sought to rule out a thyroid primary. Markers for neuroendocrine differentiation, such as chromogranin, synaptophytin, or a Gremelius stain are used to rule out the presence of neuroendocrine tumor of unknown primary (12).

Cytogenetics

Cytogenetic evaluation has recently been employed to facilitate the identification of the origin of poorly differentiated tumors. A study at Memorial Sloan-Kettering Cancer Center examined 40 patients who presented with a poorly differentiated carcinoma (13). Using a Southern blot analysis and florescence in situ hybridization for the identification of an isochromosome 12p abnormality in a midline tumor distribution, which is a chromosomal aberration associated with germ cell tumors, a specific diagnosis of germ cell tumor was suggested in 30% of patients. This group of patients achieved a 75% response rate to cisplatin therapy as compared to a response rate of 18% in the larger group of patients who presented with a carcinoma. Cytogenetics can also be used in identifying mutations suggestive of Ewing's sarcoma, or lymphomas, both of which have specific chemotherapeutic treatment options.

Tumor Markers

In contrast to patients with moderately to well differentiated cancers, the evaluation of germ cell tumor markers is indicated when evaluating a male patient with a poorly differentiated unknown primary cancer. An elevated prostate-specific antigen may open the option for hormonal therapy and should be obtained in appropriate older male patients. A serum thyroglobulin can be used to rule out a thyroid primary. Other serum tumor markers are of less usefulness. Markers such as carcinoembryonic antigen (CEA), CA-125, and CA 19-9 are not specific enough for any particular tumor to be used for diagnostic purposes. Considering the high cost of these markers and the lack of useful information provided to the management of the patient, they are not appropriate for the work-up of an unknown primary cancer.

TREATABLE TYPES OF CARCINOMA

Except in cases where the primary being sought is responsive to available treatments or will otherwise change the patient's clinical management, costly radiographic studies and invasive diagnostic procedures do not benefit the patient and may heighten anxiety. Therefore, the work-up should be geared toward ruling in or out identifiable primaries or histologies that will convey either a specific therapy or a more favorable prognosis. In men, germ cell cancers, either extragonadal or gonadal, are highly curable with chemotherapy and should not be overlooked. Thus, testicular ultrasound is performed and serum levels of tumor markers α-fetal protein (AFP) and human β-choriogonadotropin (βHCG) are drawn in male patients with a histology consistent with either a germ cell tumor or poorly differentiated carcinoma. Similarly, a diagnosis of prostate carcinoma would result in specific therapy. Many prostate cancers are hormonally sensitive and respond well initially to androgen-ablative therapy. Therefore, a serum prostate-specific antigen (PSA) is drawn in male patients, especially in the presence of bone metastases.

In women, breast carcinomas are frequently hormonally responsive and amenable to systemic chemotherapy. Thus, a careful breast examination and mammography are performed in female patients with unknown primary cancers. Ovarian cancer, especially when confined to the abdomen, carries a more favorable prognosis and also responds to specific therapy. A gynecologic evaluation of this possibility through a careful pelvic examination (with transvaginal ultrasound if indicated) is performed. Because the ovary is frequently the site of metastasis from other tumors, the presence of an ovarian mass does not necessarily identify that mass as the primary.

Finally, thyroid carcinomas may be treatable with radioactive iodine and should, therefore, be taken into diagnostic consideration in CUP patients as well. A serum thyroglobulin level or stain of the tumor tissue for thyroglobulin may be helpful.

The Identification of Treatable Subgroups within the CUP Population

In cases where the work-up outlined above fails to redefine the diagnosis beyond that of unknown primary, the oncologist is then obligated to look for specific subgroups within this diagnostic category that may carry a more favorable prognosis. Several such subgroups have been identified.

Male patients, typically under the age of 50, who have a poorly differentiated histology and a tumor distribution more or less symmetrical about the midline (retroperitoneal or mediastinal adenopathy, bilateral multiple lung masses, cervical adenopathy, etc.) are felt potentially to have an unrecognized extragonadal germ cell tumor and represent one such subgroup. Careful testicular examination and testicular ultrasound are obtained, but cisplatin-based therapy along the lines of a testicular regimen is indicated even in the absence of an identified primary. One study of 71 such patients demonstrated a partial response rate of 54%, complete response rate of 22%, and a 5-year disease-free survival rate of 13% (14).

Solitary Site of Disease

Several small series and anecdotes have suggested that patients with a solitary site of disease inconsistent with a primary site (i.e., carcinoma in a lymph node or cluster of lymph nodes) carry a superior prognosis compared to patients with multiple sites of disease. Definitive local management including surgical resection, localized radiation therapy, or a combination of the two, has resulted in prolonged disease-free survival and some apparent cures. These data cannot be extrapolated to patients with more than one site of disease. Surgical debulking of unknown primary cancers and the administration of adjuvant postoperative chemotherapy should not be undertaken routinely.

Axillary Mass

The presentation of an isolated lymph node containing carcinoma in an axilla of a female patient represents a specific and prognostically favorable subgroup of CUP. Such patients are considered to have stage II breast cancer until/unless proven otherwise. Mammography and careful examination of the ipsilateral breast may reveal the primary and remove the patient from the category of unknown primary. Even if this work-up is negative, evidence suggests that a primary tumor of the breast will be identified in greater than 50% of mastectomy specimens in patients who undergo this procedure. Modified radical mastectomy with axillary dissection has been recommended as initial management for otherwise healthy patients (15,16). The option of axillary dissection and whole-breast radiotherapy has also been advocated (17). While at least short-term follow-up appears favorable, there is potential concern regarding the risk of local recurrence in the breast, since the exact site in the breast is unknown, and localized excision or "lumpectomy" with a radiation cone-down or "boost" to the primary site is not possible.

Since the disease has been clinically defined as stage II, adjuvant chemotherapy routinely used for stage II breast cancer would be appropriate. An investigation for estrogen and progesterone receptors of the tumor in patients with an axillary mass/unknown primary, with subsequent hormonal therapy for receptor-positive tumors, is also indicated.

Neuroendocrine Differentiation

Investigations have shown that poorly differentiated tumors of unknown primary that demonstrate immunohistochemical evidence of neuroendocrine differentiation have a high clinical response rate to cisplatin-based chemotherapy. In a study of 29 such patients, 24% had a partial response and 48% achieved a complete response, with 13% alive and disease-free at 2 years (18). Chromogranin, synaptophytin, or Gremelius stains should be utilized to investigate for neuroendocrine differentiation.

ONCOLOGIC THERAPY OF UNKNOWN PRIMARY CANCERS

The therapy for more favorable prognostic subgroups of unknown primary cancers has been outlined above. Such therapies frequently involve aggressive treatments such as high-dose cisplatin-based chemotherapy, surgery, or combined modality approaches. Patients with unknown primary cancers who do not fall into one of these specific favorable subgroups have, in general, a poor prognosis, and available data do not suggest that systemic chemotherapy or other aggressive measures are capable of conferring a survival advantage to treated patients. Therefore, any therapy undertaken in these patients should be regarded as strictly palliative. For this reason, patients who are relatively asymptomatic may achieve no discernible benefit from palliative chemotherapy, and expectant observation and supportive care are often the most appropriate initial treatment options for these patients. The oncologist must remain cognizant that there are both limited benefits and potential toxicity involved with chemotherapeutic treatments in this group of patients with CUP.

A trial of systemic chemotherapy may be justified in patients who have or who develop symptoms attributable to their malignant disease if there is reason to believe that a decrease in tumor size or bulk will result in the improvement of such symptoms. Patients with rapidly progressing disease under observation may also be appropriate candidates for treatment, since such patients could be expected to imminently develop symptoms.

The choice of chemotherapy for unknown primary cancers, other than in patients with better prognostic

subgroups, has not been well defined. In the absence of demonstrated efficacious therapy, enrollment in a clinical trial of investigational agents may be appropriately considered. In the absence of a clinical trial, treatments have frequently been recommended on the basis of predominant tumor location site. Tumors predominantly above the diaphragm are often treated with a relatively well tolerated lung cancer regimen such as mitomycin plus vinblastine. Tumors predominantly below the diaphragm are presumed to be more likely of gastrointestinal origin. Fluorouracil, either alone or modulated with leucovorin, is the typical chemotherapeutic agent employed. Whether or not combined use of cytotoxic agents are more efficacious than single agents in the CUP population is unclear at this time. Outside of a clinical trial, one must be cautiously aware of the increased toxicity associated with such combinations.

Several trials have reported the use of various chemotherapy regimens for unknown primary cancer patients (1–3,5). It is important to remember that, to enter these trials, patients were required to have sufficient renal, hepatic, and bone marrow function, as well as high enough performance status to meet the study's eligibility criteria. Performance status (a measure of the patient's overall energy level and state of well-being) is a strong prognostic indicator. Patients with a good performance status, who are up and about most of the day and who are not actively losing weight, have a much higher response rate and lower toxicty rate for chemotherapies than do more debilitated patients. Thus, results of clincal trials may not be generalizable to more debilitated patients. Nonambulatory or otherwise severely debilitated patients with unknown primary cancer are therefore usually poor candidates for cytotoxic therapy. In these patients, supportive care should be strongly considered as the primary mode of treatment.

PSYCHIATRIC AND PSYCHOSOCIAL ASPECTS OF CANCER OF UNKNOWN PRIMARY SITES

Unlike in cases of cancers of known primary sites, such as prostrate or breast cancer, the CUP diagnosis implies to patients and their families a general lack of information among oncologists about their disease and higher than typical levels of uncertainty. Patients generally need and desire an understanding of most or all aspects of their disease. Patients who are better educated about the various aspects of their illness generally have an increased sense of mastery and control, and thus adjust more successfully. Because of the uncertainty that is engendered by a diagnosis of

CUP, clinical experience suggests that this patient population is at elevated risk for problems of adjustment and the development of psychiatric symptoms. They are a diverse patient population and are poorly studied group from the vantage point of quality of life and psychosocial adjustment.

Psychological Adjustment

In contrast to the somewhat homogeneous populations of patients with cancer of common sites and the homogeneity of some of the accompanying psychosocial issues that correspond to these illnesses, patients with CUP comprise a population more highly diverse in age and gender and lack some of the important commonalities that other groups of patients share. The most salient psychosocial aspects that this unfortunate group of patients share are: (*1*) the guarded to poor prognosis that results from the diagnosis of metastatic disease at initial presentation; (*2*) the liability to psychological problems that is associated with the inability to traverse a process of adjustment to illness that accompanies the initial diagnosis being made in advanced stages of disease; (*3*) the uncertainty that is conveyed by the inability to locate a primary site of disease and, thus, limited disease-related information; and (*4*) the psychological difficulties associated with expectant observation as a primary therapeutic approach and the failure to understand the oncology team's lack of aggressiveness toward further diagnostic evaluation and treatment. Research that identifies and better describes the psychiatric and qaulity of life issues in the CUP population is greatly needed. Given the grim prognosis and presence of advanced illness, psychosocial interventions for these patients are generally brief, supportive and psychoeducational in nature, and focused upon issues common to patients with advanced illness (see Chapter 37 on palliative care).

A diagnosis of CUP often represents the presence of advanced, metastatic disease. Unlike patients with localized disease and a more favorable prognosis, CUP patients are denied the opportunity to acclimate to the reality of having cancer prior to being confronted with issues of advanced, sometimes terminal illness. The oncologist and psycho-oncologist share the formidable task of engaging the patient in open and frank discussions regarding what, if any, treatment approaches are available and reaffirming their commitment to the total care for the patient. The typical levels of denial and disbelief common to the initial stages of adjustment to all cancer crises are sometimes more pronounced in CUP patients. These reactions often "crystallize" in the patient's failure to understand the futility of seeking out the primary cancer and the desire to initiate "psychological" chemotherapy (i.e., chemotherapy that is unlikely to benefit them other than to provide a sense of "doing something"). The recommendation of expectant observation to the aymsptomatic patient who has metastatic cancer can be a difficult one for the patient to accept. Offering the patient emotional support and mobilizing them to utilize support groups and make positive changes in lifestyle (smoking cessation, healthful diet, stress management, exercise, if possible) will permit the patient to retain a sense of control, hope, and optimism. When this disbelief gives way, patients generally need assistance with anticipatory grief.

The overwhelmingly mysterious nature of CUP may contribute to the patient's poor emotional adjustment to illness. Certain levels of depression and anxiety are to be expected in newly diagnosed CUP patients; however, prolonged symptoms of anxiety and depression can unnecessarily diminish the patient's quality of life and should be the focus of care. Clinicians must take into consideration issues common to patients with advanced disease, such as communication with family and contemplation of one's mortality. Psychiatric consultation should be utilized to evaluate and treat psychiatric co-morbidity. The use of brief psychotherapy that reinforces positive coping skills is beneficial in helping patients face advanced stages of illness. Pharmacological interventions may be utilized to treat distressing symptoms such as fatigue, sleep disturbances, and more formal psychiatric syndromes, much as they are in other patients with advanced cancer. It is important to recognize the significant role of psychiatric treatment in the palliative care of CUP patients, since untreated psychiatric conditions such as depression, mistakenly viewed as normal consequences of such difficult situations, may be quite debilitating and worsen problems of patient and family adjustment.

Quality of Life Issues and the Continuation of Treatment

A diagnosis of CUP presents a multitude of complex issues to the patient, family, and staff. Decision-making about treatment can be highly emotional and draining and a source of family disagreement. Patients diagnosed with CUP frequently believe that further diagnostic evaluation will increase the likelihood of identifying the primary tumor and improve their prognosis. Unfortunately, this is generally not the case and may unnecessarily contribute to anxiety and psychological distress on the part of the patient. Once the more treatable subtypes of unknown primary cancer are ruled out, identification of the primary is often not important: other possible diagnoses carry an equally poor prognosis and limited number of therapeutic options. Therefore, it is crucial for the oncologist and other physicians involved to carefully communicate to the patient and family the insignificance of identification of the primary tumor. Futile attempts by both the oncologist and patient to locate the primary tumor will subject the patient to an exhaustive and costly series of diagnostic tests that will ultimately increase the risk of complications and psychological distress.

Consultation by psycho-oncologists may assist the CUP patient in evaluating impact of continuing diagnostic work-ups to locate the primary tumor and subsequent treatment options on their quality of life. The patient's age, family and social structure, religious beliefs, and value system should be taken into consideration when evaluating the patient with CUP who is considering various treatment options, as the two vignettes below illustrate:

A 35-year-old married father of two young children and a 75-year-old male, also married with two adult children, both patients with CUP, are given the opportunity to participate in a experimental protocol involving the administration of a combination chemotherapy modality. Both patients are informed by researchers of the potential for serious toxicity and the limited benefits to be expected from this treatment. A psycho-oncologist is requested for consultation with both patients. During consultation, the 35-year old CUP patient insists upon receiving the experimental chemotherapy regimen, regardless of the poor prognosis and high toxicity. The patient states to the clinician that the decision not to participate in the protocol would represent his "giving up" and subsequent "abandonment" of his family. He notes that even if he dies, he would have gone to his grave "knowing that (he) fought for (his) kids." In contrast, the older patient decides that, given the low likelihood of receiving benefits from the experimental chemotherapy, he would rather "be in my own home and spend the time I have left with my family."

The above situation represents how similar cases can differ greatly when issues regarding quality of life are taken into consideration. Psycho-oncologists can be instrumental in helping the CUP patient evaluate the continuation of treatment and the subsequent effects on their quality of life and fit the options to their value system. Even if the continuation of treatment is thought to be somewhat futile, the role of the clinician is not to discourage outright further treatment. Instead, the psycho-oncologist should assist the patient in evaluating the impact of further treatment on their quality of life. Discussion of issues regarding quality of life should proceed in a nonjudgmental and empathetic manner and respect the patient's wishes. If the patient agrees, family members should be included in all discussion of treatment options and quality of life to minimize the chance for miscommunication and allow for open exploration of differences of opinion among family members.

Dealing with Anticipatory Grief

The diagnosis of advanced cancer, such as CUP, is overwhelming and emotionally exhausting for both patient and family. Frequently, patients are aware of the seriousness of their disease, but are hesitant to discuss their approaching death with their family, because they do not wish to upset the family or appear to be "giving up the fight" against their cancer. Family members may try to protect the patient from the burden of their fears and take the same approach when talking with the patient. Unfortunately, this approach may lead to isolation of the patient. The psycho-oncologist can be instrumental in facilitating open communication between the patient and family. After meeting with the family and patient separately, the clinician may feel it appropriate to hold a group discussion with the patient and family together to discuss the emotional issues of anticipatory grief. Such an approach may significantly improve the patient's quality of life in the terminal stage of illness and subsequently contribute to a healthier period of bereavement for family members.

ALTERNATIVE THERAPIES

Because of the limited therapeutic options available to treat cancer of unknown primary, clinicians should not be surprised to learn that the patient has begun to experiment with different alternative therapies (see Chapter 70 on alternative and complementary therapies). Alternative therapies are any treatments that either have not undergone clinical evaluation and/or have not been shown to demonstrate any medicinal value. The use of alternative approaches to therapy may reflect the patient's loss of hope and/or disillusionment with conventional medicine or simply the desire to mobilize all options for a sense of control over the unknown. Patients who utilize alternative therapies are frequently thought of as having psychological problems. However, they are typically well-adjusted, educated, and desire a sense of control over stressful situations. Psycho-oncologists can be helpful in conveying to the medical staff the patient's motives for taking an alternative approach to treatment. In addition, staff should be permitted to discuss their interpretations and feelings toward the patient's actions in an attempt to minimize any resentments that may be present. The clinician should also confer with the patient and family about the use of alternative therapies in a nonjudgmental and empathetic manner, recognizing its psychological significance, while trying to dissuade patients from the use of dangerous alternatives and possibly very costly ones. Patients should be advised that the continued use of alternative therapies may interact negatively with medications they are receiving and could interfere with medical treatment.

CONCLUSION

Cancer of unknown primary constitutes a heterogeneous group of metastatic cancers. With a few notable exceptions, these patients carry a poor prognosis, and therapy is strictly palliative. Proper clinical management includes a careful evaluation to rule out the more treatable possible primaries and histologies, and to rule out those specific subgroups of unknown primary carcinoma patients in whom specific aggressive therapies have been shown to be efficacious. If the clinical and pathological evaluation fails to identify a favorable prognostic histology or subgroup, then the team has an obligation to try to protect the patient from unwarranted exhaustive searches for the primary, and to communicate effectively to the patient the lack of utility of such searches. The potential for toxicities that may be encountered from chemotherapy must be carefully weighed against the limited possibility of clinical benefit in this patient population when deciding upon the appropriateness of therapy.

Psycho-oncologists must be cognizant of the patient's perception and the potential psychological impact of the term "unknown" on CUP patients and their families. Patients may experience many negative emotions (anger, frustration, anxiety, depression) that are a part of and but interfere with normal adjustment. Given the uncertainty that constitutes CUP, the psycho-oncologist should act to improve communication between the patient and physician regarding the insignificance of locating an unknown primary when other subtypes have been excluded. Research is needed to further identify psychosocial issues, including the prevalence of psychiatric disorders and the development of interventions designed specifically for patients with CUP. Cancer of unknown primary presents a difficult challenge to the psycho-oncologist and medical staff in helping both the patient and family adjust to this frightening group of diseases.

REFERENCES

1. Kambhu SA, Kelsen DP, Fiore J. Metastatic adenocarcinomas of unknown primary site: prognostic variables and treatment results. *Am J Clin Oncol.* 1990; 13:55–60.

2. Schildt RA Lennedy PS, Chen TT, et al. Management of patients with metastatic carcinoma of unknown origin: a Southwest Oncology Group study. *Cancer Treat Rep.* 1983; 67:77–9.

3. Jordan WE III, Shildt RA. Adenocarcinoma of unknown primary site. The Brooke Army Medical Center experience. *Cancer.* 1985; 55:857–860.

4. Nystrom JS, Weiner JM, Heffelfinger-Juttner J, et al. Metastatic and histologic presentations in unknown primary cancer. *Semin Oncol.* 1977; 4:53–58.

5. Moertel CG, Reitemeier RJ, Schutt AJ, Hahn RG. Treatment of the patient with adenocarcinoma of unknown origin. *Cancer* 1972; 30:1469–72.

6. Greco FA, Hainsworth JD. The management of patients with adenocarcinoma and poorly differentiated carcinoma of unknown primary site. *Semin Oncol.* 1989; 16 (suppl 6):116–122.

7. Greco FA, Hainsworth JD. Cancer of unknown primary site. In: Devita VT, Hellman S, Rosenberg SA, eds. *Cancer: Principals and Practices of Oncology*, 4th ed. Philadelphia: JB Lippincott; 1993: 2072–2092.

8. Raber MN. Cancers of unknown primary origin. In MacDonald JS, Haller DG, Mayer RJ, eds. *Manual of Oncologic Therapeutics*, 3rd ed. Philadelphia: JB Lippincott; 1995: 308–311.

9. Sporn JR, Greenberg BR. Empirical chemotherapy in patients with carcinoma of unknown primary. *Am J Med.* 1990: 88:49–54.

10. Didolkar MS, Fanous N, Elias EG, Moore RH. Metastatic carcinomas from occult primary tumors. A study of 254 patients. *Am Surg.* 1997; 186:625–630.

11. Horning SJ, Carrier EK, Rouse RV, et al. Lymphomas presenting as histologically unclassified neoplasms: characteristics and response to treatment. *J Clin Oncol.* 1989, 7:1281–1287.

12. Mackay B, Ordonez NG. Pathologicalevaluation of neoplasms with unknown primary site. *Semin Oncol.* 1993, 20:206–229.

13. Ilson DH, Motzer RS, Rodreguez ES, et al. Genetic analysis in the diagnosis of neoplasm of unknown primary tumor site. *Semin Oncol.* 1993; 20, 229–237.

14. Greco FA, Vaughn WK, Hainsworth JD. Advanced poorly differentiated carcinoma of unknown primary site: recognition of a treatable syndrome. *Ann Intern Med.* 1986; 104:547–556.

15. Ashikari R, Rosen PP, Urban JA, Senoo T. Breast cancer presenting as an axillary mass. *Ann Surg.* 1976; 183:415–417.

16. Patel J, Nemoto T, Rosner D, et al. Axillary lymph node metastasis from an occult breast cancer. *Cancer.* 1981; 47:2923–2927.

17. Ellerbroek N, Holmes F, Singletary E, et al. Treatment of patients with isolated axillary nodal metastases from an occult primary carcinoma consistent with breast origin. *Cancer.* 1990; 66:1461–1467.

18. Hainsworth JD, Johnson DH, Greco FA. Poorly differentiated neuroendocrine carcinoma of unknown primary site: a newly recognized clinicopathological entity. *Ann Intern Med.* 1988; 109:364–371.

VIII

MANAGEMENT OF SPECIFIC SYMPTOMS

EDITOR: WILLIAM BREITBART

37

Palliative and Terminal Care

WILLIAM BREITBART, JUAN R. JARAMILLO, AND HARVEY M. CHOCHINOV

The World Health Organization defines *palliative care* as "the active total care of patients whose disease is not responsive to curative treatment" (1) (see Table 37.1). Unresolved physical and psychiatric symptoms often interact in patients receiving palliative care and impact negatively on their quality of life. Their prompt recognition and effective treatment become critically important. In general, palliative care specialists are expert at managing the spectrum of physical symptoms. Managing psychiatric complications and difficult psychosocial issues facing patients with terminal illness and their families can test the limits of the most skilled palliative medicine practitioner. It is for this reason that an interdisciplinary approach is recommended that includes a mental health expert. Assessment and treatment of the psychiatric complications of terminal illness and the application of psychological and psychiatric techniques to the management of physical symptoms requires such an expert.

Part of the palliative care approach is the need to acknowledge death as a more imminent reality.

TABLE 37.1. *Some Basic Principles of Palliative Medicine*

Listen to the patient.

Make a diagnosis before you treat.

Know the drugs you use and know them well.

Whenever possible use portmanteau medications, that is, medications that will accomplish more than one objective.

Keep treatment regimens as simple as possible.

Not everything that hurts can be treated with analgesics.

Palliative care is intensive care.

Learn to enjoy small accomplishments.

There is always something that can be done.

Learn something new from every patient.

Source: Adapted from Waller and Alexander (2).

Surveys indicate that 50%–80% of terminally ill patients experience troubling thoughts or concerns about death (3). The mental health professional must be able to discuss death issues with patients while respecting their comfort with the topic. The concept of an "appropriate death," described by Weisman and his colleagues (4), outlines several points: (*1*) Internal conflicts, such as fears about loss of control, should be reduced as much as possible. (*2*) The individual's personal sense of identity should be sustained. (*3*) Critical relationships should be enhanced or at least maintained; conflicts should be resolved if possible. (*4*) The person should be encouraged to set and attempt to reach meaningful goals — even though limited — such as attending a graduation, marriage, or birth of a child, as a way to provide a sense of continuity into the future.

The traditional role of the mental health professional is broadened in the care of the dying patient (5). Assistance with the existential crisis, advocacy for the patient, conflict management, psychotherapy for anticipated bereavement and bereavement of survivors, dealing with ethical issues in end-of-life decisions, and teaching the medical staff about psychological issues regarding dying patients are essential parts of the role of the mental health professional in this setting. This chapter outlines the principles of the management of psychiatric issues in the terminally ill cancer patient.

PREVALENCE OF PSYCHIATRIC DISORDERS

The patient with advanced disease faces many stressors during the course of illness. While such stressors are universal, the level of psychological distress is variable depending on personality, coping ability, social support, and medical factors. Cancer patients with advanced disease are a particularly vulnerable group

(7,8). The incidences of pain, depression, and delirium all increase with greater debilitation and advanced illness (11,13). Approximately 25% of all cancer patients experience severe depressive symptoms, with the prevalence increasing to 77% in those with advanced illness (12). The prevalence of organic mental disorders (delirium) among cancer patients requiring psychiatric consultation has been found to range from 25% to 40% and as high as 85% during the terminal stages of illness (13). A recent study of psychiatric morbidity of patients at the time of admission to a palliative care unit showed delirium as the most common diagnosis (28%), followed by dementia (10.7%), adjustment disorders (7.5%), amnestic disorder (3.2%), major depression (3.2), and generalized anxiety disorder (1.1%) (9). Bruera and colleagues, in a prospective study and with repeated assessments, found that 47 out of 61 patients experienced a total of 66 episodes of cognitive failure (10). In a study with 321 patients, this same group found cognitive impairment in 44% of patients upon admission, and this number rose to 62.1% prior to death (14).

Cancer patients who have pain are twice as likely to have a psychiatric diagnosis associated with it as patients who have no pain. Of the patients who received a psychiatric diagnosis in a study by the Psychosocial Collaborative Oncology Group (PSYCOG), 39% reported significant pain. Of those without a psychiatric diagnosis, only 19% had significant pain (6). The most common psychiatric symptom in patients with pain was predominantly depression, though anxiety was also common. Therefore, the mental health practitioner has to feel comfortable in assessing pain and its management since in many cases the main recommendation will be "more aggressive pain control."

CONTROLLING PSYCHIATRIC SYMPTOMS

Anxiety

The terminally ill patient presents with a complex mixture of physical and psychological symptoms in the context of a frightening reality. Thus, the recognition of anxious symptoms is challenging. Patients with anxiety may show tension, restlessness, jitteriness, autonomic hyperactivity, vigilance, insomnia, distractibility, shortness of breath, numbness, apprehension, worry, or rumination. Often the physical manifestations overshadow the psychological (16). The consultant must often use the physical symptoms as a cue to inquire about their patient's psychological state, which is apt to be described as fear, worry, or apprehension.

The patient's subjective level of distress is the primary factor determining initiation of treatment. Other considerations include problematic patient behavior such as noncompliance due to anxiety, family and staff reactions to the patient's distress, and the balancing of the risks and benefits of treatment (17).

Anxiety may be seen as part of an adjustment disorder, panic disorder, generalized anxiety disorder, phobia, or agitated depression. In the terminally ill cancer patient, symptoms of anxiety are most likely to arise from some medical complication of the illness or treatment such as mental disorders (anxiety, delirium, etc.) secondary to medical conditions. (11,16, 17). Hypoxia, sepsis, electrolyte imbalances, poorly controlled pain, adverse drug reactions such as akathisia, or withdrawal states are specific entities that often present as anxiety. Patients who have been managed for long periods of time with relatively high doses of benzodiazepines or opioid analgesics for the control of anxiety or pain often become tolerant of or physically dependent upon these drugs, which may be inadvertently stopped, resulting in withdrawal. Also, when patients become less alert, there is a tendency to minimize the use of sedating medications. Benzodiazepines and opioid analgesics must be tapered slowly to prevent acute withdrawal states. Withdrawal states in terminally ill patients often present first as agitation or anxiety and, owing to altered metabolism, become clinically evident days later than might be expected in younger, healthier patients.

Despite the fact that anxiety in terminal illness commonly results from medical complications, it is important not to forget that psychological factors related to death and dying or existential issues play a role in anxiety, particularly in patients who are alert and not confused (16). Patients frequently fear the isolation and separation of death. Claustrophobic patients may be afraid of the idea of being confined and buried in a coffin. These issues can be disconcerting to consultants, who may find themselves at a loss for words that are consoling to the patient. Nonetheless, one should not avoid eliciting these concerns, listening empathically to them, and enlisting pastoral involvement where appropriate.

The specific treatment of anxiety in the terminally ill often depends on its etiology, presentation, and setting. Anxiety associated with hypoxia and dyspnea in a patient with diffuse lung metastases is most responsive to treatment with oxygen and opioid analgesics. If the same patient's presentation included hallucinations and agitation, a neuroleptic might be added to the regimen.

Pharmacologic Treatment. The pharmacotherapy of anxiety in terminal illness (see Table 37.2) involves the judicious use of benzodiazepines, neuroleptics, antihistamines, antidepressants, and opioid analgesics (11,16,17). Benzodiazepines are the mainstay of the pharmacologic treatment of anxiety in the terminally ill. The shorter acting benzodiazepines, such as lorazepam, alprazolam, and oxazepam, are safest. The selection of these drugs avoids toxic accumulation due to impaired metabolism in debilitated individuals. Lorazepam, oxazepam, and temazepam are metabolized by conjugation in the liver and are therefore safest in patients with hepatic disease. This is in contrast to alprazolam and other benzodiazepines that are metabolized through oxidative pathways in the liver that are more vulnerable to interference with hepatic damage. The disadvantage of using short-acting benzodiazepines is that patients often experience breakthrough anxiety. Such patients benefit from switching to longer acting benzodiazepines such as diazepam or clonazepam. Dosage regimens are: lorazepam 0.5–2.0 mg, p.o., i.v., or i.m., q3–6h; alprazolam 0.25–1.0 mg., p.o.,

t.i.d.–q.i.d.; diazepam 2.5–10 mg., p.o., p.r., i.m. or i.v., q3–6h; clonazepam 1–2 mg., p.o., b.i.d.–t.i.d. Dying patients can be administered diazepam intravenously or rectally when no other route is available: dosage is equivalent to oral. Rectal diazepam has been used widely in the palliative care field to control anxiety, restlessness and agitation associated with the final days of life.

Midazolam, a very short acting, water-soluble benzodiazepine, is usually administered as an intravenous infusion in critical care settings where sedation is the goal in an agitated or anxious patient on a respirator. Midazolam may also prove useful in controlling anxiety and agitation in terminal phases of illness (15). It has a short duration of action and is less irritating to subcutaneous tissues when given by subcutaneous injection. Since it is several times more potent than diazepam, starting doses should be low with careful monitoring. Doses ranging from 2 to 10 mg per day have been found to be safe and effective for most patients. However, doses as high as 30–60 mg per day have been reported. Clonazepam, a longer acting benzodiazepine, is extremely useful in the palliative

TABLE 37.2 *Anxiolytic Medications Used in Patients with Advanced Disease*

Generic Name	Approximate Daily Dosage Range (mg)	Route†
BENZODIAZEPINES		
Very short acting	10–60 per 24 h	i.v., s.c.
Midazolam		
Short acting		
Alprazolam	0.25–2.0 t.i.d.-q.i.d.	p.o., s.l.
Oxazepam	10–15 t.i.d.-q.i.d.	p.o.
Lorazepam	0.5–2.0 t.i.d.-q.i.d.	p.o., s.l., i.v., i.m.
Intermediate acting		
Chlordiazepoxide	10–50 t.i.d.-q.i.d.	p.o., i.m.
Long acting		
Diazepam	5–10 b.i.d.-q.i.d.	p.o., i.m., i.v., p.r.
Clorazepate	7.5–15 b.i.d.-q.i.d.	p.o.
Clonazepam	0.5–2 b.i.d.-q.i.d.	p.o.
NON-BENZODIAZEPINES		
Buspirone	5–20 t.i.d.	p.o.
NEUROLEPTICS		
Haloperidol	0.5–5 q2–12 h	p.o., i.v., s.c., i.m.
Methotrimeprazine	10–20 q4–8h	i.v., s.c., p.o.
Thioridazine	10–75 t.i.d.-q.i.d.	p.o.
Chlorpromazine	12.5–50 q4–12 h	p.o., i.m., i.v.
ANTIHISTAMINE		
Hydroxyzine	25-50 q4–6 h	p.o., i.v., s.c.
TRICYCLIC ANTIDEPRESSANTS		
Imipramine	12.5–150 hs	p.o., i.m.
Clomipramine	10–150 hs	p.o.

*b.i.d., two times a day; t.i.d., three times a day; q.i.d., four times a day.
† p.o., peroral; i.m., intramuscular; p.r., per rectum; i.v., intravenous; s.c., subcutaneous; s.l., sublingual. Parenteral doses are generally twice as potent as oral doses; intravenous bolus injections or infusions should be administered slowly.

care setting for the treatment of anxiety, depersonalization or derealization in patients with seizure disorders, brain tumors, and mild mental disorders due to a medical condition. Clonazepam, for example, is useful in patients with mood disorders with symptoms of mania. It is also useful as an adjuvant analgesic in patients with neuropathic pain (19).

Fears of causing respiratory depression should not prevent the clinician from using adequate dosages of benzodiazepines to control anxiety. The likelihood of respiratory depression is minimized when one utilizes shorter acting drugs, increases the dosages in small increments, and ultimately switches to longer acting drugs. In the patient with high pCO_2 retention, an extra amount of care is advised, since these patients' ventilatory drive may be more compromised by benzodiazepines (50).

NON-BENZODIAZEPINE ANXIOLYTICS. Neuroleptics, such as thioridazine and haloperidol, are useful in the treatment of anxiety when benzodiazepines are not sufficient for symptom control (17). They are also indicated when the anxiety is secondary to medical problems or when psychotic symptoms such as delusions or hallucinations accompany the anxiety. Typically, haloperidol 0.5 mg - 5 mg., p.o., i.v. or s.c., q2–12h is sufficient to control anxious symptoms and avoid excessive sedation. Low-potency neuroleptics such as thioridazine (10 mg.–25 mg., p.o., t.i.d.) are effective anxiolytics and can help with insomnia and agitation. Neuroleptics are the safest class of anxiolytics in patients where there is legitimate concern regarding respiratory depression or compromise. Methotrimeprazine (10 mg–20 mg, every 4–8 h, i.m., i.v. or s.c.) is a phenothiazine with unique analgesic and anxiolytic properties that is often used for the treatment of pain and anxiety in the dying patient (20). Its side effects are sedation, anticholinergic symptoms, and hypotension. Intravenous administration by slow infusion is preferable to avoid problems with hypotension. Chlorpromazine (12.5 mg–50 mg, p.o., i.m. or i.v., q 4–12 h) has similar side effects that limit its application in this setting. However, it can be useful in patients where sedation is desirable. With this class of drugs in general, one must be aware of extrapyramidal side effects (particularly when patients are taking additional neuroleptics for antiemetic purposes) and the remote possibility of neuroleptic malignant syndrome.

Hydroxyzine is an antihistamine with mild anxiolytic, sedative, and analgesic properties. It is particularly useful when treating anxious, terminally ill cancer patients with pain. Hydroxyzine 100 mg given parenterally has analgesic potency equivalent to 8 mg of morphine and potentiates the analgesic effects of morphine (21). As an anxiolytic, 25 mg –50 mg of hydroxyzine q4–6 h p.o., i.v. or s.c. is effective.

Tricyclic, heterocyclic, and second-generation antidepressants are the most effective treatment for anxiety accompanying depression and are helpful in treating panic disorder (22). Guidelines for their use are discussed in the section on depression below. Their usefulness is limited in the dying patient, owing to anticholinergic and sedative side effects.

Opioid drugs are effective in the relief of dyspnea and anxiety due to cardio-pulmonary compromise (23). Continuous intravenous infusions of morphine or other narcotic analgesics allow for careful titration. Occasionally one must maintain the patient in a state of unresponsiveness in order to maximize comfort. When respiratory distress is not a major problem, it is preferable to use the opioid drugs solely for analgesic purposes and to add more specific anxiolytics (such as the benzodiazepines) to control concomitant anxiety.

Nonpharmacologic Treatment. Nonpharmacologic interventions for anxiety and distress are supportive psychotherapy and behavioral interventions. Brief supportive psychotherapy is often useful in dealing with both crisis-related issues as well as existential issues confronted by the terminally ill (24). (See Chapter 60.) Psychotherapeutic interventions should include both the patient and family. Mental health professionals should advocate for meeting the emotional needs of patients and families, such as updated information regarding the disease status and the treatment options available. This information must be delivered repeatedly and with sensitivity as to what they are currently prepared to hear and able to absorb. Families, especially, require a great deal of reassurance that they and the medical staff have done everything possible for the patient. The goals of psychotherapy with the patient are to establish a bond that decreases the sense of isolation experienced with terminal illness; to help the patient face death with a sense of self-worth; to correct misconceptions about the past and present; to integrate the present illness into a continuum of life experiences; and to explore issues of separation, loss, and the unknown that lies ahead. The therapist should emphasize past strengths and support previously successful ways of coping. This helps the patient mobilize inner resources, modify plans for the future, and perhaps even accept the inevitability of death.

It is during the terminal phase of illness that we have the greatest opportunity to effect the process of adaptation to loss. Mental health professionals must extend their supportive stance to include both the patient and the family. Anticipatory bereavement is a common experience which allows patients, loved ones, and health care providers the opportunity to prepare mentally for the impending death (25). Patients and family members should be encouraged to use this period to reconcile differences, extend important final communications, and reaffirm feelings and wishes. It is a time is of vital importance that can often set the tone for the subsequent bereavement course.

Relaxation, guided imagery, and hypnosis are useful behavioral techniques despite patients' physical debilitation (See Chapter 62 on behavioral techniques.)

Depression

The somatic symptoms of depression, e.g., anorexia, insomnia, fatigue, and weight loss, can be unreliable and lack specificity in the cancer patient (26). Thus, the psychological symptoms of depression take on greater diagnostic value: dysphoric mood, hopelessness, worthlessness, guilt, and suicidal ideation (12). Chochinov and colleagues studied the prevalence of depression in a cohort of 130 terminally ill patients in a palliative care facility (80). They reported that 9.2% met Research Diagnostic Criteria (RDC) for major depression when using high-severity thresholds for RDC criterion A symptoms (equivalent to the symptom threshold in DSM IV). This approach yielded the identical prevalence of major depression whether or not one included somatic symptoms in the diagnostic criteria or used Endicott revised criteria (28) (replacement of somatic symptoms with nonsomatic alternatives) (see Table 37.3). While concern has been raised about the nonspecificity of somatic symptoms in the medically ill, these results—along with those of other recent investigations—indicate that their inclusion may not overly influence the diagnostic classification of major depression (29,30).

Evaluation of depression must include an examination of medications such as corticosteroids, chemotherapeutic agents (vincristine, vinblastine, asparaginase, intrathecal methotrexate, interferon, interleukin), amphotericin, whole-brain radiation, central nervous system metabolic–endocrine complications, and paraneoplastic syndromes that may be etiologic (31–42).

Management of Depression. Depression in advanced disease is managed with a combination of supportive psychotherapy, cognitive-behavioral techniques, and antidepressant medications (see Table 37.4) (26,43–45). Factors such as prognosis and the time frame for treatment play a role in determining the

TABLE 37.3 *Endicott Substitution Criteria*

Physical/Somatic Symptom	Psychological Symptom Substitute
1. Change in appetite, weight	1. Tearfulness, depressed appearance
2. Sleep disturbance	2. Social withdrawal, decreased talkativeness
3. Fatigue, loss of energy	3. Brooding, self-pity, pessimism
4. Diminished ability to think or concentrate, indecisiveness	4. Lack of reactivity

Source: Breitbart and Passik (48).

pharmacotherapy for depression. Tricyclics require 2–4 weeks for effect; psychostimulants have a rapid onset of action. Patients who are within hours to days of death and in distress benefit most from sedatives or narcotic analgesic infusions.

Tricyclic antidepressant (TCA) application in the terminally ill requires a careful risk–benefit ratio analysis. Although nearly 70% of patients treated with a tricyclic for nonpsychotic depression can anticipate a positive response, these medications are associated with a side effect profile that can be particularly troublesome for terminally ill patients, owing to blockade of muscarinic cholinergic receptors, α-adrenoreceptor blockade, and H_1 histamine receptor blockade (46). The tertiary amines (amitriptyline, doxepin, imipramine) have a greater propensity to cause side effects than do secondary amines (nortriptyline, desipramine) (47).

The anticholinergic side effects are constipation, dry mouth, and urinary retention. To avoid exacerbating symptoms associated with genitourinary outlet obstruction, decreased gastric motility, or stomatitis, a relatively nonanticholinergic tricyclic such as desipramine or nortriptyline is best. Patients receiving medication with anticholinergic properties (such as pethidine, atropine, diphenhydramine, phenothiazines) should not receive tricyclics because of risk of an anticholinergic delirium (48). The anticholinergic actions of TCAs can also cause serious tachycardia; the quinidine-like effects can lead to arrhythmias in those with preexisting conduction problems, by virtue of their ability to delay conduction via the His–Purkinje system (associated with nonspecific ST-T changes and T waves on the electrocardiograph) (49).

α_1-Blockade, causing postural hypotension and dizziness, is of concern for the frail, volume-depleted patient. Nortriptyline and protriptyline are the TCAs least associated with α_1-blockade. H_1 histamine receptor blockage is associated with sedation and drowsiness. For dying patients already exposed to a variety of sedating agents (e.g., opioid analgesics, antiemetics,

TABLE 37.4 *Antidepressant Medications Used in Patients with Advanced Disease*

Generic Name	Approximate Daily Dosage Range (mg)*	Route†
TRICYCLIC ANTIDEPRESSANTS		
Amitriptyline	10–150	p.o., i.m., p.r.
Doxepin	12.5–150	p.o., i.m.
Imipramine	12.5–150	p.o., i.m.
Desipramine	12.5–150	p.o., i.m.
Nortriptyline	10–125	p.o.
Clomipramine	10–150	p.o.
SECOND GENERATION ANTIDEPRESSANTS		
Buproprion	200–450	p.o.
Fluoxetine	10–60	p.o.
Paroxetine	10–60	p.o.
Fluvoxamine	50–300	p.o.
Sertraline	50–200	p.o.
Nefazodone	100–500	p.o.
Venlafaxine	37.5–225	p.o.
Trazodone	25–300	p.o.
HETEROCYCLIC ANTIDEPRESSANTS		
Maprotiline	50–75	p.o.
Amoxapine	100–150	p.o.
MONOAMINE OXIDASE INHIBITORS		
Isocarboxazid	20–40	p.o.
Phenelzine	30–60	p.o.
Tranylcypromine	20–40	p.o.
Meclobomide	150–600	p.o.
PSYCHOSTIMULANTS		
Dextroamphetamine	2.5–20 b.i.d.	p.o.
Methylphenidate	2.5–20 b.i.d.	p.o.
Pemoline	37.5–75 b.i.d.	p.o., s.l.‡
BENZODIAZEPINES		
Alprazolam	0.25–2.0 t.i.d.	p.o.
Lithium carbonate	600–1200	p.o.

Source: Adapted from Massie MJ and Holland JC: Depression and the cancer patient. *J Clin Psychiatry*. 1990, 51:12-17.
* b.i.d., two times a day; t.i.d., three times a day.
† p.o., peroral; i.m., intramuscular; p.r., per rectum. Intravenous infusions of a number of tricyclic antidepressants are utilized outside of the United States. This route is, however, not FDA approved.
‡ Comes in chewable tablet form that can be absorbed without swallowing.

anxiolytics, neuroleptics), TCAs such as amitriptyline and doxepin are the most likely to contribute to sedation.

Tricyclic antidepressants should be started at low doses (10–25 mg at bedtime q.h.s.) and increased in 10–25 mg) increments every 2–4 days until a therapeutic dose is attained or side effects become a limiting factor. Depressed cancer patients often achieve a therapeutic response at significantly lower doses of TCAs (25–125 mg) than are necessary in the physically well (150–300 mg). There is also evidence to suggest that patients with advanced cancer achieve higher serum tricyclic levels at modest doses (48). In order to minimize drug toxicity and more carefully guide the process of drug titration, prescribing tricyclics (desipramine, nortriptyline, amitriptyline, imipramine) with well-established therapeutic plasma levels may be advantageous. Desipramine and nortriptyline are generally better tolerated in this population than amitriptyline or imipramine.

Newer antidepressant agents, often with fewer side effects and simplified dosage regimens have become available and may have important applications in the treatment of depression in patients with advanced disease. Among these agents are the selective serotonin reuptake inhibitors (SSRIs) and serotonin- norepinephrine reuptake inhibitors.

Selective Serotonin Reuptake Inhibitors (SSRIs). The SSRIs are an important addition to the available anti-depressant medications. They have been found to be as effective as the tricyclics in the treatment of depression and have a number of features that may be particularly advantageous for the terminally ill. The SSRIs have a very low affinity for adrenergic, cholinergic, and histamine receptors, thus accounting for negligible orthostatic hypotension, urinary retention, memory impairment, sedation or reduced awareness. They have not been found to cause clinically significant alterations in cardiac conduction and are generally favorably tolerated along with a wider margin of safety than the TCAs in the event of an overdose. They therefore do not require therapeutic drug level monitoring.

Most of the side effects of SSRIs result from their selective central and peripheral serotonin reuptake. These include increased intestinal motility, nausea, vomiting, insomnia, headaches and sexual dysfunction. Some patients may experience anxiety, tremor, restlessness, and akathisia. These side effects tend to be dose related and may be problematic for patients with advanced disease.

There are five SSRIs currently being marketed namely, sertraline, fluoxetine, paroxetine, nefazodone, and fluvoxamine. With the exception of fluoxetine, whose elimination half-life is 2–4 days, the SSRIs have an elimination half-life of about 24 hours. Fluoxetine is the only SSRI with a potent active metabolite (norfluoxetine), whose elimination half-life is 7–14 days. Fluoxetine can cause mild nausea and a brief period of increased anxiety as well as appetite suppression that usually lasts for a period of several weeks. The anorectic properties of fluoxetine has not been a limiting factor in the use of this drug in cancer patients. Fluoxetine and norfluoxetine do not reach a steady state for 5–6 weeks, compared with 4–14 days for paroxetine, fluvoxamine and sertraline. These differences are important, especially for the terminally patient in whom a switch from an SSRI to another antidepressant is being considered. If a switch to a monamine oxidase inhibitor is required, the washout period for fluoxetine will be at least 5 weeks, given the potential drug interactions between these two agents. Since fluoxetine has entered the market, there have been several reports of significant drug–drug interactions (51, 52). Until it has been studied further in the medically ill, it should be used cautiously in the debilitated dying patient. Paroxetine, fluvoxamine, and sertraline, on the other hand, require considerably shorter washout periods (10–14 days) under similar circumstances.

All the SSRIs have the ability to inhibit the hepatic isoenzyme P4502D6, with sertraline (and, according to some sources, fluvoxamine) being least potent in this regard. This is important with respect to dose/plasma level ratios and drug interactions, since the SSRIs are dependent upon hepatic metabolism. For the elderly patient with advanced disease, the dose–response curve for sertraline appears to be relatively linear. On the other hand, particularly for paroxetine (which appears to most potently inhibit cytochrome P4502D6), small dosage increases can result in dramatic elevations in plasma levels. Paroxetine, and to a somewhat lesser extent fluoxetine, appear to inhibit the hepatic enzymes responsible for their own clearance. The coadministration of these medications with other drugs that are dependent on this enzyme system for their catabolism (e.g., tricyclics, phenothiazines, type IC antiarrhythmics and quinidine) should be done cautiously. Luvox has been shown in some instances to elevate the blood levels of propranolol and warfarin by as much as twofold, and should thus not be prescribed together with these agents.

SSRIs can generally be started at their minimally effective doses. For the terminally ill, this usually means initiating therapy at approximately half the usual starting dose used in an otherwise healthy patient. For fluoxetine, patients can begin on 5 mg (available in liquid form) given once daily (preferably in the morning) with a range of 10–40 mg per day; given its long half-life, some patients may only require this drug every second day. Paroxetine can be started at 10 mg once daily (either morning or evening) for the patient with advanced disease, and has a therapeutic range of 10-40 per day. Sertraline can be initiated at 50 mg, morning or evening and titrated within a range of 50–200 mg per day. Nefazodone can be started at 50 mg b.i.d. and titrated within a range of 100–500 mg per day. If patients experience activating effects on SSRIs, they should be given earlier into the day. Gastrointestinal upset can be reduced by ensuring the patient does not take medication on an empty stomach.

Serotonin-Norephinephrine Reuptake Inhibitors (SNRIs). Venlafaxine (Effexor) is a potent inhibitor of neuronal serotonin and norephinephrine reuptake and appears to have no significant affinity for muscarinic, histamine or α_1-adrenergic receptors. Some patients may experience a modest sustained increase in blood pressure, especially at doses above the recommended initiating dose. Compared with the SSRIs, its protein binding ($< 35\%$) is very low. Few protein binding-induced drug interactions are thus expected. Like other antidepressants, venlafaxine should not be used in patients receiving monamine oxidase inhibitors. Its side effect profile tends to generally be well tolerated. While there are currently no data addressing its use in the terminally ill depressed patient, its pharmacokinetic properties and side effect profile suggest it may have a role to play.

Trazodone. Although its anticholinergic profile is almost negligible, trazodone has considerable affinity for α_1-adrenoreceptors and may thus predispose patients to orthostatic hypotension and its problematic sequelae (i.e., falls, fractures, head injuries). Trazodone is very sedating and in low doses (100 mg at bedtime q.h.s.) is helpful in the treatment of the depressed cancer patient with insomnia. It is highly serotonergic and its use should be considered when the patient requires adjunct analgesics effect in addition to antidepressant effects. Trazodone has little effect on cardiac conduction but can cause arrhythmias in patients with premorbid cardiac disease. Male patients have to be warned about the possibility of priapism.

Bupropion. At present, bupropion is not the first drug of choice for depressed patients with cancer. However, one might consider prescribing bupropion if patients have a poor response to a reasonable trial of other antidepressants. Bupropion may have a role in the treatment of the psychomotor-retarded, depressed, terminally ill patient as it has energizing effects similar to those of the stimulant drugs. However, because of the increased incidence of seizures in patients with CNS disorders, bupropion has a limited role in the oncology population.

Psychostimulants. The psychostimulants (dextroamphetamine, methylphenidate, and pemoline) offer an alternative and effective pharmacologic approach to the treatment of depression in the terminally ill (53–55). These drugs have a more rapid onset of action than the tricyclics and are often energizing. They are most helpful in the treatment of depression in cancer patients with advanced disease and those where dysphoric mood is associated with severe psychomotor slowing and even mild cognitive impairment. Psychostimulants have been shown to improve attention, concentration, and overall performance on neuropsychological testing in the medically ill. In cancer, specifically, this has been shown in double-blind, crossover trials. In relatively low doses, psychostimulants stimulate appetite, promote a sense of well-being, and improve feelings of weakness and fatigue in cancer patients. Treatment with dextroamphetamine or methylphenidate usually begins with a dose of 2.5 mg at 8:00 a.m. and at noon. The dosage is slowly increased over several days until a desired effect is achieved or side effects (overstimulation, anxiety, insomnia, paranoia, confusion) intervene. Typically a dose greater than 30 mg per day is not necessary,

although occasionally patients require up to 60 mg per day. Patients are usually maintained on methylphenidate for one to two months, and approximately two-thirds will be able to be withdrawn from methylphenidate without a recurrence of depressive symptoms. Those who do have recurrence can be maintained on a psychostimulant for up to one year without significant abuse problems. Tolerance will develop and adjustment of dose may be necessary. An additional benefit of such stimulants as methylphenidate and dextroamphetamine are that they have been shown to reduce sedation secondary to opioid analgesics and provide adjuvant analgesics in cancer patients (56). Common side effects of stimulants include nervousness, overstimulation, mild increase in blood pressure and pulse rate, and tremor. More rare side effects include dyskinesias or motor tics as well as a paranoid psychosis or exacerbation of an underlying and unrecognized confusional state.

Pemoline is a unique psychostimulant chemically unrelated to amphetamine. Advantages of pemoline as a psychostimulant in cancer patients include the lack of abuse potential, the lack of federal regulation through special triplicate prescriptions, the mild sympathomimetic effects, and the fact that it comes in a chewable tablet form that can be absorbed through the buccal mucosa and can be used by cancer patients who have difficulty swallowing or have intestinal obstruction. Pemoline appears to be as effective as methylphenidate or dextroamphetamine in the treatment of depressive symptoms in terminally ill cancer patients (57). Pemoline can be started at a dose of 18.75 mg in the morning and at noon, and increased gradually over days. Typically patients require 75 mg a day or less. Pemoline should be used with caution in patients with liver impairment, and liver function tests should be monitored periodically with longer term treatment (58).

Benzodiazepines. The triazolobenzodiazepine alprazolam has been shown to be a mildly effective antidepressant as well as an anxiolytic. Alprazolam is particularly useful in cancer patients who have mixed symptoms of anxiety and depression (62). Starting dose is 0.25 mg three times a day, effective doses are usually in the range of 4–6 mg daily.

Electroconvulsive Therapy. Occasionally, it is necessary to consider electroconvulsive therapy (ECT) for depressed cancer patients who have depression with psychotic features or in whom treatment with antidepressants pose unacceptable side effects. The safe, effective use of ECT in the medically ill has been reviewed by others (79).

Nonpharmacologic Treatment of Depression in Terminally Ill Patients. Supportive psychotherapy is a useful treatment approach to depression in the terminally ill patient. Psychotherapy with the dying patient consists of active listening with supportive verbal interventions and the occasional interpretation (59). A group format may be used as well (60). Despite the seriousness of the patient's plight, it is not necessary for the psychiatrist or psychologist to appear overly solemn or emotionally restrained. Often it is only the psychotherapist, of all the patient's care givers, who is comfortable enough to converse lightheartedly and allow the patient to talk about their life and experiences, rather than focus solely on impending death. The dying patient who wishes to talk or ask questions about death should be allowed to do so freely, with the therapist maintaining an interested, interactive stance. It is not uncommon for the dying patient to benefit from pastoral counseling. If a chaplaincy service is available, it should be offered to the patient and family (5).

Another nonpharmacologic method is light therapy. A 1994 article reports its successful use in three terminally ill cancer patients (61).

Delirium

Delirium is common in patients with far advanced cancer. Between 15% and 20% of hospitalized cancer patients have organic mental disorders (64). The Japanese study mentioned earlier (9) found delirium in 28% of the patients. Massie and Holland (8) found delirium in more than 75% of terminally ill cancer patients they studied. Delirium can be due either to the direct effects of cancer on the central nervous system (CNS), or to indirect CNS effects of the disease or treatments (Table 37.5) (medications, electrolyte imbalance, failure of a vital organ or system, infection, vascular complications, and preexisting cognitive impairment or dementia). Early symptoms of delirium can be misdiagnosed as anxiety, anger, depression, or psychosis. In any patient showing acute onset of agitation, impaired cognitive function, altered attention span, or a fluctuating level of consciousness, a diagnosis of delirium should be considered. A common error among medical and nursing staff is to conclude that a new psychological symptom is functional without completely ruling out all possible organic etiologies. Given the large numbers of drugs

TABLE 37.5 *Causes of Delirium in Patients with Advanced Disease*

DIRECT CENTRAL NERVOUS SYSTEM (CNS) CAUSES
Primary brain tumor
Metastatic spread to CNS
Seizures

INDIRECT CAUSES
Metabolic encephalopathy due to organ failure
Electrolyte imbalance
Treatment side effects from
  chemotherapeutic agents
  steroids
  radiation
  opioids
  anticholinergics
  antiemetics
  antivirals
Infection
Hematologic abnormalities
Nutritional deficiencies
Paraneoplastic syndromes

Source: Adapted from Fleishman SB, Lesko LM, Delirium and dementia. In: Holland J, Rowland J, eds. *Handbook of Psychooncology: Psychological Care of the Patient with Cancer.* New York: Oxford University Press, 1989:342–355.

cancer patients require, and the fragile state of their physiologic functioning, even routinely ordered hypnotics are enough to tip patients over into a delirium. Narcotic analgesics such as levorphanol, morphine sulfate, and meperidine, are common causes of confusional states, particularly in the elderly and terminally ill (65). Chemotherapeutic agents known to cause delirium include methotrexate, fluorouracil, vincristine, vinblastine, bleomycin, BCNU, cisplatin, asparaginase, procarbazine, and the glucocorticosteroids (31–36). Except for steroids, most patients receiving these agents will not develop prominent CNS effects. The spectrum of mental disturbances related to steroids includes minor mood lability, affective disorders (mania or depression), cognitive impairment (reversible dementia), and delirium (steroid psychosis). (See Chapter 48 on delirium.)

Management of Delirium in the Terminally Ill

The treatment of delirium in the dying cancer patient is unique because: (*1*) the etiology of terminal delirium is often multifactorial or may not be found; (*2*) when a distinct cause is found, it is often irreversible (such as hepatic failure or brain metastases); (*3*) work-up may be limited by the setting (home, hospice); and (*4*) the consultant's focus is usually on the patient's comfort and diagnostic procedures are avoided. Bruera (10) reported that an etiology was discovered in less than 50% of terminally ill patients with cognitive failure.

Symptomatic and supportive therapies are important (67). In fact, they may be the only steps which can be taken. Measures to help reduce anxiety and disorientation (i.e. structure and familiarity) are treatment in a quiet, well-lit room with familiar objects, a visible clock or calendar, and the presence of family. One-to-one nursing observation is useful, with restraints only as required to prevent injury. Sedation with neuroleptics or sedative drugs may be necessary to relieve severe agitation or insomnia (63) (Table 37.6.)

Haloperidol, a neuroleptic agent that is a potent dopamine blocker, is the drug of choice in the treatment of delirium in the terminally ill (63,67,68). Haloperidol in low doses, 1–3 mg, is usually effective in targeting agitation, paranoia, and fear. Typically 0.5 mg to 1.0 mg haloperidol (p.o., i.v., i.m., s.c.) is administered, with repeat doses every 45–60 minutes titrated against target symptoms (13). An intravenous route facilitates rapid onset of effects. If intravenous access is unavailable, intramuscular or subcutaneous administration can be used and switched to the oral route when possible. The majority of delirious patients are managed with oral haloperidol. Parenteral doses are approximately twice as potent as oral doses. In general, doses need not exceed 20 mg of haloperidol in a 24 hour period; however, there are those who advocate high doses (up to 250 mg/24 h of haloperidol usually intravenously) in selected cases (67). A common strategy in the management of symptoms related to delirium is to add parenteral lorazepam to a regimen of haloperidol. Lorazepam (0.5–1.0 mg q1-2h p.o. or i.v.), along with haloperidol may be more effective in rapidly sedating the agitated delirious patient. In a double blind, randomized comparison trial of haloperidol vs. chlorpromazine vs. lorazepam, Breitbart and colleagues demonstrated that lorazepam alone, in doses up to 8 mg in a 12 hour period, was ineffective in the treatment of delirium and in fact contributed to worsening delirium and cognitive impairment (78). Both neuroleptic drugs, however, in low doses (approximately 2 mg of haloperidol equivalent/per 24 h), were highly effective in controlling symptoms and improving cognitive function.

Methotrimeprazine (i.v. or s.c.) is utilized to control confusion and agitation in terminal delirium (20). Dosages range from 12.5 mg to 50 mg every 4–8 h up to 300 mg per 24 h for most patients. Hypotension and excessive sedation are problematic limitations of this drug. Midazolam, given by subcutaneous or intravenous infusion in doses ranging from 30 mg to 100 mg/per 24 h are also used to control agitation related to delirium in the terminal stages (15). The goal of treatment with midazolam, and to some extent with methotrimeprazine, is quiet sedation only. Propofol, a short-acting anesthetic agent, presents several advantages: the level of sedation can be titrated by modifying the infusion rate, it does not accumulate, and communication with the staff is possible (18). As opposed to neuroleptic drugs like haloperidol, a midazolam infusion does not clear a delirious patient's sensorium or improve cognition. These clinical differences may be due to the underlying pathophysiology of delirium. One hypothesis postulates that an imbalance of central cholinergic and adrenergic mechanisms underlies delirium, and so a dopamine blocking drug may initiate a re-balancing of these systems (66). While neuroleptic drugs are most effective in diminishing agitation, clearing the sensorium and improving cognition in the delirious patient, this is not always possible in the last days of

TABLE 37.6 *Medications Useful in Managing Delirium in Patients with Advanced Disease*

Generic Name	Approximate Daily Dosage Range (mg)	Route*
NEUROLEPTICS		
Haloperidol	0.5–5 q2-12h 4–8h	p.o., i.v., s.c., i.m.
Thioridazine	10–75 q	p.o.
Chlorpromazine	12.5–50 q4–12h	p.o., i.v., i.m.
Methotrimeprazine	12.5–50 q4–8h	i.v., s.c., p.o.
BENZODIAZEPINES		
Lorazepam	0.5–2.0 q1–4h	p.o., i.v., i.m.
Midazolam	30–100 per 24 h	i.v., s.c.

* Parenteral doses are generally twice as potent as oral doses; i.v., intravenous infusions or bolus injections should be administered slowly; i.m., intramuscular injections should be avoided if repeated use becomes necessary; p.o., oral forms of medication are preferred; s.c., subcutaneous infusions are generally accepted modes of drug administration in the terminally ill.

life. Ventafridda and colleagues (69) and Fainsinger and colleagues (70) reported that 10%–20% of terminally ill patients have a delirium that can only be controlled by sedation to the point of a significantly decreased level of consciousness.

The use of neuroleptics in the management of delirium in the dying patient remains controversial in some circles. Some have argued that pharmacologic interventions with neuroleptics or benzodiazepines are inappropriate in the dying patient. Clinical experience in managing delirium in dying cancer patients suggests that the use of neuroleptics for agitation, paranoia, hallucinations, and altered sensorium is safe and effective. The agitated, delirious, dying patient should probably be given neuroleptics to help restore calm. A "wait and see" approach may be most appropriate with patients who have a lethargic or somnolent delirium.

FAMILY ISSUES

The family of the terminal patient obviously undergoes a tremendously sustained, traumatic experience. Most of them cope well (71). One of the roles of the mental health expert is to evaluate families who are referred for what someone else (nurses, doctors, social workers, even families themselves) considers coping that merits a psychiatric intervention. Basic functions that the mental health expert can provide include a basic family assessment, supportive therapy for the family members (listening, clarifications, answering questions that the family has or facilitating the communication between the family and the medical team, eliciting fears and concerns, and providing reasonable reassurance whenever possible) and determining which families are at risk for complicated grief (73).

In terms of the last point, a practical approach is that presented by the group of Bloch and Kissane (73). Basically continuing the work of Lieberman, Bowlby, and others in trying to identify maladaptive patterns of family response, they have conducted their research about the family of the terminal patient. The well-functioning family is described, following pretty much the description of Raphael (74). Then, based on three basic characteristics (cohesiveness, expressiveness, and conflict resolution), five clusters of families are described: supportive, conflict resolving, intermediate, hostile, and sullen. The three latter are at increased risk for complicated grief and should be proactively identified and approached by the staff in order to facilitate interventions that may decrease that risk. As described by Kissane (71), the interventions should be done tactfully, not in a forced way, and perhaps not too soon after the death of the patient. The interested reader is referred to the original work of Kissane and colleagues (72,73) and to Chapter 88 on bereavement in this textbook.

There is also research that points to the difficulties that different parts of the family of the terminally ill may experience. For example, a research project conducted at Memorial Sloan-Kettering Cancer Center suggests that a large proportion of well spouses of patients with cancer who are also the parents of school-aged children may experience significant depressive distress during the terminal phase of their spouse's illness (75). Christ and colleagues have also published on the impact of parental terminal cancer on latency-age children (76) and adolescents (77). Research like this will help elucidate what happens with this families and their individual components and will facilitate the development of therapeutic interventions.

CONCLUSION

In the care of the patient with advanced cancer, the focus of treatment is upon symptom control and quality of life. These patients experience both significant physical symptoms and distressing psychiatric complications. The high prevalence of distressing physical symptoms such as pain makes the assessment of psychiatric symptoms difficult. Additionally, both groups of symptoms can interact and potentiate each other. Psychiatrists and psychologists need to be available in the team caring for the terminally ill patient, for symptom control and integration of the physical, psychological, and spiritual dimensions.

REFERENCES

1. WHO Expert Committee. *Cancer Pain Relief and Palliative Care.* Geneva: World Health Organization. 1990.
2. Alexander W, Caroline NL. *Handbook of Palliative Care in Cancer.* Boston: Butterworth- Heinemann, 1996.
3. Cherny NI, Coyle N, Foley KM. Suffering in the advanced cancer patient: a definition and taxonomy. *J Palliative Care.* 1994; 10:57–70.
4. Weisman AD. *On Dying and Denying. A Psychiatric Study of Terminality.* New York: Behavioral Publications; 1972.
5. Wiener I, Breitbart W, Holland J. Psychiatric issues in the care of dying patients. In: Rundel JR, Wise MG, ed. *Textbook of Consultation-Liaison Psychiatry.* Washington D.C.; American Psychiatric Press, 1996. 805–831.
6. Derogatis LR, Marrow GR, Fetting J, et al. The prevalence of psychiatric disorders among cancer patients. *J Am Med Assoc.* 1983; 249:751–757.

7. Breitbart W. Psychiatric management of cancer pain. *Cancer*. 1989; 63:2336–2342.

8. Massie MJ, Holland JC. The cancer patient with pain: psychiatric complications and their management. *Med Clin N Am*. 1987; 71:243–258.

9. Minagawa H, Uchitomi Y, Yamawaki S, et al. Psychiatric morbidity in terminally ill cancer patients: prospective study. *Cancer*. 1996; 78(5):1131–1137.

10. Bruera E, Miller MJ, McCallion J, et al. Cognitive failure in patients with terminal cancer: a prospective study. *J Pain Symptom Manage*. 1992; 7(4):192–195.

11. Foley KM: The treatment of cancer pain. *N Engl J Med*. 1985; 313:84-95.

12. Bukberg J, Penman D, Holland J. Depression in hospitalized cancer patients. *Psychosom Med*. 1984; 43:199–212.

13. Massie MJ, Holland JC, Glass E. Delirium in terminally ill cancer patients. *Am J Psychiatry*. 1983; 140:1048–1050.

14. Pereira J, Hanson J, Bruera E. The frequency and clinical course of cognitive impairment in patients with terminal cancer. *Cancer*. 1997; (79)4:835–841.

15. Bottomley DM, Hanks GW Subcutaneous midazolam infusion in palliative care. *J Pain Symptom Manage*. 1990; 5:259–261.

16. Holland JC. Anxiety and cancer: the patient and family. *J Clin Psychiatry*. 1989; 50:20–25.

17. Massie MJ. Anxiety, panic and phobias. In: Holland JC, Rowland J, eds. *Handbook of Psychooncology: Psychological Care of the Patient with Cancer*. New York: Oxford University Press; 1989:300–309.

18. Moyle J. The use of propofol in palliative medicine. *J Pain Symptom Manage*. 1995; 10(8):643–646.

19. Keck P, McElroy S, Nemeroff, C. Anticonvulsants in the treatment of bipolar disorder. *J Neuropsychiatry Clin Neurosci*. 1992; 4:395–405.

20. Oliver DJ. The use of methotrimeprazine in terminal care. *Br J Clin Pract*. 1985; 39:339–340.

21. Beaver WT, Feise G. Comparison of the analgesic effects of morphine, hydroxyzine and their combination in patients with post-operative pain. In: Bonica JJ, Albe-Fessard, eds. *Advances in Pain Research and Therapy*. New York: Raven Press, 1976: 553–557.

22. Mavissakalian, M. Combined behavioral and pharmacological treatment of anxiety disorders. In: *American Psychiatric Press Review of Psychiatry*, vol. 12. Washington, DC: American Psychiatry Press; 1993.

23. Bruera E, MacMillan K, Pither J, MacDonald RN. Effects of morphine on the dyspnea of terminal cancer patients. *J Pain Symptom Manage*. 1990; 5:341–344.

24. Massie MJ, Holland JC, Straker N. Psychotherapeutic interventions. In: Holland JC, Rowland JH, eds. *Handbook of Psychooncology: Psychological Care of the Patient with Cancer*. New York: Oxford University Press, 1989:455–469.

25. Chochinov HM, Holland JC. Bereavement. In: Holland JC, Rowland JH, eds. *Handbook of Psychooncology: Psychological Care of the Patient with Cancer*. New York: Oxford University Press, 1989: 612–627.

26. Massie MJ, Holland JC. Depression and the cancer patient. *J Clin Psychiatry*. 1990; 51:12–17.

27. Green A, Austin, C. *Psychopathology of Pancreatic Cancer*. Washington DC: American Psychiatric Press, 1994–5; Vol. 34.3.

28. Endicott J. Measurement of depression patients with cancer. *Cancer*. 1983; 53:2243–2248.

29. Kathol RG, Mutgi A, Williams J, Clamon G, Noyes R Jr. Diagnosis of major depression in cancer patients according to four sets of criteria. *Am J Psychiatry*. 1990; 147:1021–1024.

30. Zimmerman M, Coryell WH, Black DW. Variability in the application of contemporary diagnostic criteria: endogenous depression as an example. *Am J Psychiatry*. 1990; 147:1173–1179.

31. Stiefel FC, Breitbart W, Holland JC. Corticosteroids in cancer: neuropsychiatric complications. *Cancer Invest*. 1989; 7:479–491.

32. Young DF. Neurological complications of cancer chemotherapy. In: Silverstein A, ed. *Neurological Complications of Therapy: Selected Topics*. New York: Futura Publishing, 1982:57–113.

33. Holland JC, Fassanellos, Ohnuma T. Psychiatric symptoms associated with L-asparaginase administration. *J Psychiatry Res*. 1974; 10:165.

34. Adams F, Quesada JR, Gutterman JU. Neuropsychiatric manifestations of human leukocyte interferon therapy in patients with cancer. *J Am Med Assoc*. 1984; 252:938–941.

35. Denicoff KD, Rubinow DR, Papa M, et al. The neuropsychiatric effects of treatment with interleukin-1 and lymphokine-activated killer cells. *Ann Intern Med*. 1987; 107(3):293–300.

36. Weddington WW. Delirium and depression associated with amphotericin B. *Psychosomatics*. 1982; 23:1076–1078.

37. DeAngelis LM, Delattre J, Posner JB. Radiation-induced dementia in patients cured of brain metastases. *Neurology*. 1989; 39:789–796.

38. Breitbart WB. Endocrine-related psychiatric disorders. In: Holland JC, Rowland JH, eds. *Handbook of Psychooncology: Psychological Care of Patient with Cancer*. New York: Oxford University Press, 1989: 356–366.

39. Posner JB. Nonmetastatic effects of cancer on the nervous system. In: Wyngaarden JB and Smith LH, eds. *Cecil's Textbook of Medicine*. Philadelphia: WB Saunders, 1988:1104–1107.

40. Patchell RA, Posner JB. Cancer and the nervous system. In: Holland JC, Rowland JH, eds. *Handbook of Psychooncology: Psychological Care of the Patient with Cancer*. New York: Oxford University Press; 1989: 327–341.

41. Breitbart W. Cancer pain and suicide. In: Foley K, ed. *Advances in Pain Research and Therapy*, vol. 16. New York: Raven Press, 1990; 399–412.

42. Breitbart W. Suicide in cancer patients. *Oncology*. 1987; 1:49-53.

43. Spiegel D, Bloom JR. Group therapy and hypnosis reduce metastatic breast carcinoma pain. *Psychosom Med*. 1983; 4:333–339.

44. Purohit DR, Navlakha PL, Modi RS, et al. The role of antidepressants in hospitalized cancer patients. *J Assoc Physicians India*. 1978; 26:245–248.

45. Costa D, Mogos I, Toma T: Efficacy and safety of mianserin in the treatment of depression of women with cancer. *Acta Psychiatr Grand*. 1985; 72:85–92.

46. Davis JM, Glassman AH. Anti-depressant drugs. In: Kaplan HI, Sadock BJ, eds. *Comprehensive Textbook of Psychiatry*. Baltimore: Williams and Wilkins; 1989.

47. Preskorn SH. Recent pharmacologic advances in antidepressant therapy for the elderly. *Am J Med.* 1993; 94(5A):2S–12S.

48. Breitbart W, Passik SD. Psychiatric aspects of palliative care. In: Doyle D, Hanks GW, MacDonald N, eds. *Oxford Textbook of Palliative Medicine*. New York: Oxford University Press; 1993:609–626.

49. LeMelledo MJ, Bradweijn J. Pharmacotherapy of depression. *Pharmanual*. 1993; 25–46.

50. Stoudemire A, Fogel BS. Psychopharmacology in the medically ill. In: Stoudemire A, Fogel BS, eds. *Principles of Medical Psychiatry*. Orlando: Grune and Stratton: 1987:79–112.

51. Ciraulo DA, Shader RI. Fluoxetine drug-drug interactions: I. Antidepressants and antipsychotics. *J Clin Psychopharmacol*. 1990; 10:48–50.

52. Pearson HJ. Interaction of fluoxetine with carbamazepine. *J Clin Psychiatry*. 1990; 51:126.

53. Fernandez F, Adams F, Holmes VF, et al. Methylphenidate for depressive disorders in cancer patients. *Psychosomatics*. 1987; 28:455–461.

54. Satel SL, Nelson CJ. Stimulants in the treatment of depression: a critical overview. *J Clin Psychiatry*. 1989; 50:241–249.

55. Burns MM, Eisendrath SJ. Dextroamphetamine treatment for depression in terminally ill patients. *Psychosomatics*. 1994 (Jan.-Feb.); 35(11):80–82.

56. Bruera E. Chadwick S, Brennels C, et al. Methylphenidate associated with narcotics for the treatment of cancer pain. *Cancer Treat Rep*. 1987; 71:67–70.

57. Breitbart W, Mermelstein H. Pemoline: an alternative psychostimulant for the management of depressive disorders in cancer patients. *Psychosomatics*. 1992; 33(3): 352–356.

58. Nehra A, et al. Pemoline associated hepatic injury. *Gastroenterology*. 1990; 99:1517–1519.

59. Cassem NH. The dying patient. In: Hackett TP, Cassem NH, eds. *Massachusetts General Hospital Handbook of General Hospital Psychiatry*. Littleton: PSG Publishing; 1987:332–352.

60. Presberg BA, Kibel HD. Confronting death: Group psychotherapy with terminally ill individuals. *Group*. 1994; 18(1):19–28.

61. Cohen S, et al. Phototherapy in the treatment of depression in the terminally ill. *J Pain Symptom Manage*. 1994; 9(8):534–536.

62. Holland JC, Morrow G, Schmale A, Derogatis L, et al. A randomized clinical trial of alprazolam vs. progressive muscle relaxation in cancer patients with anxiety and depression symptoms. *J Clin Oncol*. 1991; 32:407–412.

63. Lipowski ZJ. Delirium (acute confusional states). *J Am Med Assoc*. 1987; 285:1789–1792.

64. Levine PM, Silverfarb PM, Lipowski ZJ. Mental disorders in cancer patients: a study of 100 psychiatric referrals. *Cancer*. 1978; 42:1385–1391.

65. Bruera E, MacMillan K, Kuchn N, et al. The cognitive effects of the administration of narcotics. *Pain*. 1989; 39:13-16.

66. Trzepacz P. The neuropathogenesis of delirium. *Psychosomatics*. 1994; 35(4):374–391.

67. Murray GB. Confusion, delirium, and dementia. In: Hackett TP and Cassem NH, eds. *Massachusetts General Hospital Handbook of General Hospital Psychiatry*. Littleton: PSG Publishing; 1987:84–115.

68. Fernandez F, Holmes VF, Adams F, Kavanaugh JJ. Treatment of severe refractory agitation with a haloperidol drip. *J Clin Psychiatry*. 1988; 49:239–241.

69. Ventafridda V, Ripamonti C, DeConno F, et al. Symptom prevalence and control during cancer patients last days of life. *J Palliative Care*. 1990; 6:7–11.

70. Fainsinger R, MacEachern T, Hanson J, et al. Symptom control during the last week of life in a palliative care unit. *J Palliative Care*. 1991; 7:5–11.

71. Kissane DW. Grief and the Family. In: Bloch S, Hafner J, Harari E, Szmukler GI, eds. *The Family in Clinical Psychiatry*. Melbourne: Oxford Medical Publications; 1994:102–126.

72. Kissane DW et al. The Melbourne family grief study: I. Perceptions of family functioning in bereavement. *Am J Psychiatry*. 1996; 153(5):650-658.

73. Kissane DW, et al.The Melbourne family grief study: II. Psychosocial morbidity and grief in bereaved families. *Am J Psychiatry*. 1996; 153(5):659–666.

74. Raphael B. *The Anatomy of Bereavement*. London: Hutchinson; 1984.

75. Siegel K, et al. Depressive distress among the spouses of terminally ill cancer patients. *Cancer Pract*. 1996; 4(1): 25–30.

76. Christ GH. Impact of parental terminal cancer on adolescents. *Am J Orthopsychiatry*. 1994; 64(4):604–613.

77. Christ GH. Impact of parental terminal cancer on latency-age children. *Am J Orthopsychiatry*. 1993; 63 (3):417–425.

78. Breitbart W, Marotta R, Platt M, et al. A double-blind trial of haloperidol, chlorpromazine and lorazepam in the treatment of delirium in hospitalized AIDS patients. *Am J Psychiatry*. 1996; 231–237.

79. Wiener RD, Coffey CE. ECT in the medically ill. In: Stoudmire A, Fogel BS, ed. *Psychiatric Care of the Medical Patient*. New York: Oxford University Press; 1993:223–240.

80. Chochinov HM, Wilson W, Ends M, et al. The prevalence of depression in the terminally ill: effects of diagnostic criteria and symptom threshold judgments. *Am J Psychiatry*. 1994; 51:537–540.

38

Pain

WILLIAM BREITBART AND DAVID K. PAYNE

Effective management of pain in patients with cancer requires a multidisciplinary approach, enlisting expertise from a wide variety of clinical groups (1–3). Given the important interaction between the pain experience and psychological distress, clinicians who treat cancer patients need to be knowledgeable about major issues in pain assessment and treatment. This chapter reviews the prevalence of pain in cancer, pain syndromes, pain assessment issues, as well as pharmacologic and non-pharmacologic interventions for pain. Psychiatric and psychological interventions in the treatment of cancer pain have now become an integral part of a comprehensive approach to pain management and are highlighted in this review (4,5).

PREVALENCE OF PAIN IN CANCER

Pain is a common problem for cancer patients, with approximately 70% of patients experiencing severe pain at some time in the course of their illness (2). It has been suggested that nearly 75% of patients in the United States with advanced cancer have pain (6) and that 25% of cancer patients die in severe pain despite the fact that current methods if applied could substantially reduce that number (7). There is considerable variability in the prevalence of pain amongst different types of cancer. For example, approximately 5% of leukemia patients experience pain during the course of their illness as compared to 50%–75% of patients with neoplasms of the lung, gastrointestinal tract, or genitourinary system. Patients with cancers of the bone or cervix have the highest prevalence of pain, with as many as 85% experiencing significant pain during the course of their illness (1). Yet, despite its prevalence, studies have shown that pain is frequently under-diagnosed and inadequately treated (2,8).

PAIN SYNDROMES

A number of well defined pain syndromes have been identified in cancer patients. Most are directly related to tumor involvement; this accounted for 78% of inpatient and 62% of outpatient pain complaints. (1). Tumor invasion of bone, compression or infiltration of nerves, and obstruction of hollow viscus are the most common causes. Stretching of fascia or periosteum, tumor infiltration or occlusion of blood vessels, and damage to mucous membranes or other soft tissues is a less common cause of pain.

The second pain syndrome occurring in 19% of inpatients and 25% of outpatients is related to cancer treatment. (1). Surgery, chemotherapy, and radiation therapy can each have pain sequelae. Postsurgical syndromes include postthoracotomy syndrome, postmastectomy syndrome, postradical neck syndrome, and phantom limb. Chemotherapy can result in peripheral neuropathy, aseptic necrosis of femoral head, steroid pseudoheumatism, and postherpetic neuralgia. Finally, radiation therapy can result in radiation fibrosis or brachial and lumbar plexus, radiation myelopathy, radiation-induced second primary tumors, and radiation necrosis of the bone.

Less than 10% of cancer patients have pain syndromes that are unrelated to the disease or therapy. These syndromes include cervical or lumbar osteroarthritis, thoracic and abdominal aneurysms, and diabetic neuropathy.

MULTIDIMENSIONAL CONCEPT OF PAIN IN CANCER

Pain, and especially pain in cancer is not a purely physical experience, but involves complex aspects of human functioning including personality, affect, cognition, behavior, and social relations (9,10). An enlightened description of the pain in terminal illness by

Cecily Saunders (11) is "total pain," a label that attempts to describe its encompassing nature. It is important to note that the use of analgesic drugs alone does not always lead to pain relief (12). In a recent study (13) it has been demonstrated that psychological factors play a modest but important role in pain intensity. The interaction of cognitive, emotional, socioenvironmental, and physical aspects of pain shown in Figure 38–1 illustrates the multidimensional nature of pain in terminal illness and provides a model for multi modal intervention (3). The challenge of untangling and addressing both the physical and psychological issues involved in pain is essential to developing rational and effective management strategies. Therapies directed primarily at psychological variables have profound impact on nociception, while somatic therapies directed at nociception have beneficial effects on the psychological aspects of pain. Ideally such somatic and psychosocial therapies are used simultaneously in the multidisciplinary approach to pain management in the terminally ill (4).

PSYCHOLOGICAL FACTORS IN PAIN

The cancer patient faces several universal fears during the course of illness: dependency, disability, and fear of painful death. The level of psychological distress, however, is variable and depends on medical factors, social supports, coping capacities, and personality. Pain has profound effects on psychological distress in cancer patients. and psychological factors, particularly the meaning of pain, anxiety, and depression intensify the pain. Daut and Cleeland (14) showed that cancer patients who attributed a new pain to an unrelated

benign cause reported less interference with their activity and pleasure than cancer patients who believed their pain represented progression of disease. Spiegel and Bloom (15) found that women with metastatic breast cancer experienced more intense pain if they believed their pain represented spread of their cancer, and if they were depressed.

In an attempt to define the potential relationships between pain and psychosocial variables, Padilla and colleagues. (16) found that there were pain-related quality of life variables in three domains: (*1*) physical well being; (*2*) psychological well-being consisting of affective factors, cognitive factors, spiritual factors, communication, coping, and meaning of pain or cancer; and (*3*) interpersonal well-being, focusing on social support or role functioning. The perception of marked impairment in activities of daily living also is associated with increased pain intensity (17). Measures of emotional disturbance have been reported to be predictors of pain in late stages of cancer, and cancer patients with less anxiety and depression were less likely to report pain (18,19). Patients who reported negative thoughts about their personal or social competence report increased pain intensity and emotional distress (17). In a prospective study of cancer patients, it was found that maladaptive coping strategies, lower levels of self-efficacy, and distress specific to the treatment or disease progression were modest but significant predictors of reports of pain intensity (13).

All too frequently, however, psychological variables are proposed to explain continued pain or lack of response to therapy when etiologic medical factors have not been adequately evaluated. Often, the psychiatrist is consulted late in the assessment of a patient with pain. An accurate pain diagnosis must be made and medical analgesic management outlined and implemented. Psychological distress in terminally ill patients with pain must initially be assumed to be the consequence of uncontrolled pain. Psychological and personality factors are distorted by the presence of pain, and relief of pain often results in the disappearance of a perceived psychiatric disorder (8,20).

PSYCHIATRIC DISORDERS AND PAIN

There is an increased frequency of psychiatric disorders found in cancer patients with pain. In the Psychosocial Collaborative Oncology Group study (21) on the prevalence of psychiatric disorders in cancer patients, 39% of patients who received a psychiatric diagnosis (see Table 38.1), reported significant pain, while only 19% of patients without a psychiatric diagnosis had significant pain. The psychiatric disor-

Multidimensional Concept of Pain

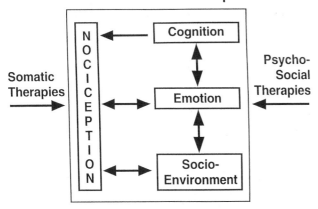

FIG. **38–1.** Schematic presentation of the concept of pain and the impact of therapies.

TABLE 38.1. *Rates of DSM-III Psychiatric Disorders and Prevalence of Pain Observed in 215 Cancer Patients from Three Cancer Centers*

Diagnostic Category	Number Diagnostic Class	Percentage of Psychiatric Diagnoses	Number with Significant Pain*
Adjustment disorders	69 (32%)	68%	
Major affective disorders	13 (6%)	13%	
Organic mental disorders	8 (4%)	8%	
Personality disorders	7 (3%)	7%	
Anxiety disorders	4 (2%)	4%	
Total with psychiatric Dx	101 (47%)		39 (39%)
Total with no psychiatric Dx	114 (53%)		21 (19%)
Total patient population	215 (100%)		60 (28%)

Source: Adapted from Deragotis LR, et al. The prevalence of psychiatric disorders among cancer patients. *J Am Med Assoc.* 1983; 249:754.
* Score greater than 50 mm on a 100 mm VAS for pain severity.

ders seen in cancer patients with pain include primarily adjustment disorder with depressed or anxious mood (69%) and major depression (15%).

CANCER PAIN AND SUICIDE

Uncontrolled pain is a major factor in suicide and suicidal ideation in cancer patients (22,23). Cancer is feared by the public as a disease associated with pain. In Wisconsin, a study revealed that 69% of the public agreed that cancer pain could cause a person to consider suicide (24). The majority of suicides reported among patients with cancer were in those who had severe pain which was often inadequately controlled or tolerated poorly (23). Although relatively few cancer patients commit suicide, they are at increased risk (25, 26). Patients with advanced illness are at highest risk and are the most likely to have the pain, depression, delirium, and deficit symptoms. Psychiatric disorders are frequently present in hospitalized cancer patients who attempt suicide. A review of the psychiatric consultation data at Memorial Sloan-Kettering Cancer Center showed that one-third of cancer patients who were seen for evaluation of suicide risk received a diagnosis of major depression; approximately 20% met criteria for delirium, and more than 50% were diagnosed with an adjustment disorder (27). In the 71 cancer patients who had suicidal ideation with serious intent, significant pain was a factor in only 30% of cases. In striking contrast virtually all 71 suicidal cancer patients had a psychiatric disorder (mood disturbance or organic mental disorder) at the time of evaluation (27).

The role of pain in suicidal ideation was examined by assessing 185 patients with pain, revealing that suicidal ideation occurred in 17% of the population, with

the majority of this group reporting suicidal ideation without intent to act. Interestingly, in these patients who had significant pain, suicidal ideation was not directly related to pain intensity but was strongly related to degree of depression and mood disturbance. Pain was related to suicidal ideation indirectly in that patients' perception of poor pain relief was associated with suicidal ideation. Perceptions of pain relief may have more to do with aspects of hopelessness than pain itself. Pain plays an important role in vulnerability to suicide, however, associated psychological distress and mood disturbance seem to be essential cofactors in raising the risk of suicide in cancer patients. Pain has adverse effects on patients' quality of life and sense of control and impairs the family's ability to provide support. Factors, other than pain, such as mood disturbance, delirium, loss of control, and hopelessness contribute to cancer suicide risk (23).

ASSESSMENT ISSUES

The initial step in pain management is a comprehensive assessment of pain symptoms. The health professional working in the cancer setting must have a working knowledge of the etiology and treatment of cancer-related pain. This includes an understanding of the different types of pain syndromes, as well as a familiarity with the parameters of appropriate pharmacologic treatment. A close collaboration of the health care team is optimal when attempting to adequately manage pain in the cancer patient.

A careful history and physical examination may disclose an identifiable syndrome (e.g., herpes zoster, bacterial infection, or neuropathy) that can be treated in a standard fashion (2). A standard pain history may provide valuable clues to the nature of the underlying process and indeed may disclose other treatable disorders. A description of the qualitative features of the pain, its time course and any maneuvers that increase or decrease pain intensity should be obtained. Pain intensity (current, average, at best, at worst) should be assessed to determine the need for weak versus potent analgesics and as a means to serially evaluate the effectiveness of ongoing treatment. Pain descriptors (e.g., burning, shooting, dull, or sharp) will help determine the mechanism of pain (somatic, nociceptive, visceral nociceptive, or neuropathic) and may suggest the likelihood of response to various classes of traditional and adjuvant analgesics (nonsteroidal anti-inflammatory drugs, opioids, antidepressants, anticonvulsants, oral local anesthetics, corticosteroids, etc.) (28,29). Additionally, detailed medical, neurological and psychosocial assessments (including a history of substance use or abuse) must be conducted. Where possible, family members or partners should be interviewed. During the assessment phase, pain should be aggressively treated while pain complaints and psychosocial issues are subject to an ongoing process of re-evaluation.

An important element in assessment of pain is the concept that assessment is continuous and needs to be repeated over the course of pain treatment. There are essentially four aspects of pain experience in cancer that require ongoing evaluation including (1) pain intensity; (2) pain relief; (3) pain-related functional interference (e.g., mood state, general and specific activities); and (4) monitoring of intervention effects (analgesic drug side effects, abuse) (30). The Memorial Pain Assessment Card (MPAC) (31) is a helpful clinical tool that allows patients to report their pain experience. The MPAC consists of visual analogue scales that measure pain intensity, pain relief, and mood. Patients can complete the MPAC in less than 30 seconds. The patient's report of pain intensity, pain relief, and present mood state provides the essential information required to help guide their pain management. The Brief Pain Inventory (32) is another pain assessment tool that has useful clinical and research applications.

The principles mentioned above have been described by Foley (2) and include (1) believe the patient's complaint of pain; (2) take a detailed history; (3) assess the psychosocial status of the patient; (4) perform a careful medical and neurological examination; (5) order and personally review the appropriate diagnostic procedures; (6) evaluate the patient's extent of pain; (7) treat the pain to facilitate the diagnostic work-up; (8) consider the alternative methods of pain control during the initial evaluation; and (9) reassess the pain complaint during the prescribed therapy.

INADEQUATE PAIN MANAGEMENT: BARRIERS TO TREATMENT

Recent studies suggest that pain in cancer is still being under treated (33). Inadequate management of pain is often due to the inability to properly assess pain in all its dimensions (2,4,7). Other causes of inadequate pain management include lack of knowledge of current pharmacotherapeutic or psychotherapeutic approaches; focus on prolonging life to the exclusion of alleviating suffering; poor communication between doctor and patient; limited expectations of patients to achieve pain relief; limited capacity of patients who are impaired by organic mental disorders to communicate; unavailability of opioids, doctors' fear of causing respiratory depression, and, most importantly, doctors' fear of amplifying addiction and substance abuse. In advanced cancer, several factors have been noted to predict the undermanagement of pain: a discrepancy between physician and patient in judging the severity of pain; the presence of pain that physicians did not attribute to cancer; better performance status, age of 70 or over; and female sex (33).

Fear of addiction affects both patient compliance and physician management of narcotic analgesics, leading to undermedication of pain in cancer patients (3,7,34). Studies of the patterns of chronic narcotic analgesic use in patients with cancer have demonstrated that, although tolerance and physical dependence commonly occur, addiction (psychological dependence) is rare and almost never occurs in an individual without a history of drug abuse prior to cancer illness (35) (see Chapter 49). Escalation of use of narcotic analgesics by cancer patients is usually due to progression of cancer or the development of tolerance.

Tolerance means that a larger dose of narcotic analgesic is required to maintain an original analgesic effect. Physical dependence is characterized by the onset of signs and symptoms of withdrawal if the opioid is suddenly stopped or a opioid antagonist is administered. Tolerance usually occurs in association with physical dependence but does not imply psychological dependence. Psychological dependence or addiction, is not equivalent to physical dependence or tolerance and is a behavioral pattern of compulsive drug abuse characterized by a craving for the drug and overwhelming involvement in obtaining and using it for effects other than pain relief. The cancer pain patient with a history of intravenous opioid abuse presents an often unnecessarily difficult management problem. Macaluso and colleagues (35) reported on 468 inpatient cancer pain consultations. Only 8 (1.7%) had a history of intravenous drug abuse, but none had been actively abusing drugs in the previous year. All eight of these patients had inadequate pain control and more than half were intentionally undermedicated because of concern by staff that drug abuse was active or would recur. Adequate pain control was ultimately achieved in these patients by using appropriate analgesic dosages and intensive staff education.

Physicians who believe they are being manipulated by drug-seeking individuals are hesitant to use opioids in appropriate dosages for adequate control of pain, often leading to undermedication. Most clinicians experienced in working with substance abusing patients recommend clear and direct limit setting (see Chapter 49). While this is an important aspect of the care of patients with a history of using drugs, it is by no means the whole answer. As much as possible, clinicians should attempt to eliminate the issue of drug abuse as an obstacle to pain management by dealing directly with the problems of opiate withdrawal and drug abuse treatment. Avoid making the analgesic drugs the focus of a battle for control between the patient and physician, especially in terminal stages of illness. Err on the side of believing patients' complaints of pain, utilizing knowledge of the specific pain syndromes seen in cancer patients to corroborate the patient's report if it appears to be unreliable.

The risk of inducing respiratory depression is too often overestimated and can limit appropriate use of narcotic analgesics for pain and symptom control. Bruera and co-workers (36) demonstrated that, in a population of terminally ill cancer patients with respiratory failure and dyspnea, administration of subcutaneous morphine actually improved dyspnea without causing a significant deterioration in respiratory function. The adequacy of cancer pain management can be influenced by the lack of concordance between patient ratings or complaints of their pain and those made by care givers. Persistent cancer pain is often ascribed to a psychological cause when it does not respond to treatment attempts. In our clinical experience we have noted that patients who report their pain as "severe" are quite likely to be viewed as having a psychological contribution to their complaints. Staff members' ability to empathize with a patient's pain complaint may be limited by the intensity of the pain complaint. Grossman and colleagues (37) found that while there is a high degree of concordance between patient and care giver ratings of patient pain intensity at the low and moderate levels, this concordance breaks down at high levels. Thus, a clinician's ability

to assess a patient's level of pain becomes unreliable once a patient's report of pain intensity rises above 7 on a visual analogue rating scale of 0 to 10. Physicians must be educated as to the limitations of their ability to objectively assess the severity of a subjective pain experience. Additionally, patient education is often a useful intervention in such cases. Patients are more likely to be believed and adequately treated if they are taught to request pain relief in a straightforward fashion (38).

PHARMACOTHERAPIES FOR PAIN

Although the management of analgesic medications is more often undertaken by the oncologist or palliative care specialist, it is essential that the psycho-oncologist have a thorough understanding of the analgesic medications used in the management of cancer related pain. The World Health Organization (28) devised guidelines for analgesic management of cancer pain that the Agency for Health Care Policy and Research (AHCPR) has endorsed for the management of pain related to cancer (29). These guidelines, also known widely as the "WHO Analgesic Ladder" (Figure 38–2), have been well validated (39). This approach advocates selection of analgesics based on severity of pain. For mild to moderate severity pain, nonopioid analgesics such as non steroidal anti-inflammatory drugs (NSAIDs) and acetaminophen are recommended. For pain that is persistent and moderate to severe in intensity, opioid analgesics of increasing potency (such as morphine) should be utilized. Adjuvant agents, such as laxatives and psychostimulants, are useful in preventing as well as treating opioid side effects such as constipation or sedation, respectively. Adjuvant analgesic drugs, such as the antidepressant analgesics, along with opioids and NSAIDs, are used in all stages of the analgesic ladder (mild, moderate, or severe pain).

Foley (2) has described the indications for and use of three classes of analgesic drugs that have applications in the management of cancer patients with pain: (1) nonopioid analgesics (acetaminophen, aspirin, and other nonsteroidal anti-inflammatory drugs); (2) opioid analgesics (of which morphine is the standard); and (3) adjuvant analgesics (antidepressants and anticonvulsants).

NONOPIOID ANALGESICS

The nonopioid analgesics (Table 38.2) are prescribed principally for mild to moderate pain or to augment the analgesic effects of opioid analgesics in the treatment of severe pain. The analgesic effects of the

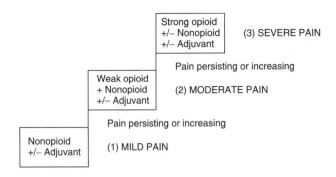

Strong opioid
+/– Nonopioid
+/– Adjuvant   (3) SEVERE PAIN

Pain persisting or increasing

Weak opioid
+ Nonopioid
+/– Adjuvant   (2) MODERATE PAIN

Pain persisting or increasing

Nonopioid
+/– Adjuvant   (1) MILD PAIN

FIG. **38–2.** WHO analgesic ladder of the management of pain in cancer. [From Ref. 28.]

NSAIDs result from their inhibition of cyclooxygenase and the subsequent reduction of Prostaglandins in the tissues (40). The concurrent use of NSAIDs or acetaminophen and opioids provides more analgesia than does either of the drug classes alone (29). In contrast to opioids, NSAIDs have a ceiling effect in their efficacy, do not produce tolerance or dependence , have antipyretic effects, and have a spectrum of side effects including renal failure, hepatic dysfunction, bleeding, and gastric toxicities.

The physiochemical properties of the NSAIDs, mechanisms of action, pharmacokinetics, and pharmacodynamics influence the analgesic response. The selection of the NSAID should take into account the etiology and severity of the pain, concurrent medical conditions which may be relative contraindications (e.g., bleeding diathesis), associated symptoms, and favorable experience by the patient as well as physician. From a practical point of view, an NSAID should be titrated to analgesic efficacy as well as to side effects. There is also variability in patient response to both relief and adverse reactions; so if the results are not favorable, an alternative NSAID should be tried.

The major adverse effects associated with NSAIDs are gastric ulceration, renal failure, hepatic dysfunction, and bleeding. The use of NSAIDs also causes gastrointestinal toxicities, including minor dyspepsia and heartburn, as well as major gastric erosion, peptic ulcer formation, and gastrointestinal hemorrhage. The nonacetylated salicylates, such as salsalate, sodium salicylate, and choline magnesium salicylate, theoretically have less gastrointestinal (GI) side effects and might be considered in cases where GI distress is an issue. Prophylaxis for NSAID-associated GI symptoms include H_2 antagonist drugs (cimetidine 300 mg t.i.d.–q.i.d. or ranitidine 150 mg b.i.d.); misoprostal 200 mg q.i.d.; omeprazole 20 mg q.d.; or an antacid. Patients should be informed of these symptoms, issued guaiac cards with reagent, and taught to check their stool weekly.

NSAIDs affect kidney function and should therefore be used with caution in patients with renal dysfunction. Prostaglandins are involved in the autoregulation of renal blood flow, glomerular filtration, and the tubular transport of water and ions. In patients with renal impairment, NSAIDs should be used with caution, since many (i.e., ketoprofen, feroprofen, naproxen, and carpofen) are highly dependent on renal function for clearance. The risk of renal dysfunction is greatest in patients with advanced age, preexisting renal impairment, hypovolemia, concomitant therapy with nephrotoxic drugs, and heart failure. Caution should be used in patients receiving β-adrenergic antagonists, diuretics, or angiotensin-converting enzyme inhibitors. Several studies have suggested that there is substantial biliary excretion of several NSAIDs, including indomethacin and sulindac. In patients with hepatic dysfunction, these drugs should be used with caution. NSAIDs, with the exception of the nonacetylated salicylates (e.g., sodium salicylate, choline magnesium trisalicylate), produce inhibition of platelet aggregation (usually reversible, but irreversible with aspirin). NSAIDs should be used with extreme caution, or

TABLE **38.2.** *Nonsteroidal Oral Analgesics for Mild to Moderate Pain in Cancer*

Analgesic	Starting Dose (mg)	Duration (h)	Plasma Half-life (h)	Comments
Aspirin	650	4–6	4–6	The standard for comparison among nonopioid analgesics
Ibuprofen	400–600	—	—	Like aspirin, can inhibit platelet function
Choline magnesium trisalicylate	700–1500	—	—	Essentially no hematologic or gastrointestinal side effects

avoided, in patients who are thrombocytopenic or who have clotting impairment.

The use of NSAIDs in patients with cancer must be accompanied by awareness of toxicity and adverse effects. NSAIDs are highly protein-bound, and the free fraction of available drug is increased in cancer patients who are cachectic, wasted, and hypoalbuminic, often resulting in toxicities and adverse effects. Patients with cancer are frequently hypovolemic and are on concurrent nephrotoxic drugs, and so are at increased risk for renal toxicity related to NSAIDs. Finally, the antipyretic effects of the NSAIDs may interfere with early detection of infection in patients with cancer.

OPIOID ANALGESICS

Opioid analgesics are the mainstay of pharmacotherapy of moderate to severe intensity pain in the patient with pain (Table 38.3). Principles that are useful in

TABLE 38.3 *Opioid Analgesics for Moderate to Severe Pain in Cancer*

Analgesic	Equi-analgesic Route*	Dose (mg)	Analgesic onset (h)	Duration (h)	Plasma Half-life (h)	Comments
Morphine (e.g., Roxonal)	p.o. i.m., i.v., s.c.	30–60* 10	1–1½ ½ –1	4–6 3–6	2–3	Standard of comparison for the narcotic analgesics. 30 mg for repeat around-the-clock dosing; 60 mg for single dose or intermittent dosing
Morphine Sustained-release (e.g., MS Contin, Oramorph SR)	p.o.	90–120	1–1½	8–12	–	Now available in long-acting sustained-release forms.
Oxycodone (e.g., Roxicodone, also in Percocet, Percodan, Tylox, others)	p.o.	20–30	1	3–6	2–3	In combination with aspirin or acetaminaphen it is considered a weaker opioid, as a single agent it is comparable to the strong opioids, like morphine. Available in immediate release and sustained-release preparation
Oxycodone sustained-release (e.g., Oxycontin)	p.o.	20–40	1	8–12	2–3	
Hydromophone (e.g., Dilaudid)	p.o. i.m., i.m.	7.5 1.5	½–1 1¼–½	3–4 3–4	2–3 2–3	Short half-life; ideal for elderly patients. Comes in suppository and injectable forms
Methadone (e.g., Dolophine, others)	p.o. i.m., i.v.	20 10	½–1 ½–1	4–8 –	15–30 15–30	Long half-life; tends to accumulate with initial dosing, requires careful titration. Good oral potency
Levorphanol (e.g., Levo-Dromoran)	p.o. i.m.	4 2	½–1½ ½–1	3–6	12–16 12–16	Long half-life; requires careful dose titration in first week. Note that analgesic duration is only 4 h
Meperidine (e.g., Demerol)	p.o. i.m.	300 75	½–1½ ½–1	3–6 3–4	3–4	Active toxic metabolite, ormeperidine, tends to accumulate (plasma half-life is 12-16 h), especially with renal impairment and in elderly patients causing delerium, myoclonus and seizures
Fentanyl Transdermal System (e.g., Duragesic)	t.d. i.v.	0.1 00.1	12–18	48–72 –	20–22 –	Transdermal patch is convenient, bypassing GI analgesia until depot is formed. Not suitable for rapid titration

*p.o. = per oral; i.m. = intramuscular; i.v. = intravenous; s.c. = subcutaneous; t.d. = transdermal.

guiding the appropriate use of opioid analgesics for pain (41) include the following: (*1*) Choose an appropriate drug; (*2*) start with lowest dose possible; (*3*) titrate dose; (*4*) use "as needed" doses selectively; (*5*) use an appropriate route of administration; (*6*) be aware of equivalent analgesic doses; (*7*) use a combination of opioid, nonopioid, and adjuvant drugs; (*8*) be aware of tolerance; and (*9*) understand physical and psychological dependence.

In choosing the appropriate opioid analgesic for cancer pain, Portenoy (29) noted several important considerations: (*1*) opioid class; (*2*) "weak" versus "strong" opioids; (*3*) pharmacokinetic characteristics; (*4*) duration of analgesic effect; (*5*) favorable prior response; and (*6*) opioid side effects. Opioid analgesics are divided into two classes, the agonists and the agonist-antagonists, based on their affinity for opioid receptors. Pentazocine, butorphanol, and nalbuphine are examples of opioid analgesics with mixed agonist-antagonist properties. These drugs can reverse opioid effects and precipitate an opioid withdrawal syndrome in patients who are opioid-tolerant or dependent. They are of limited use in the management of chronic pain in cancer. Oxycodone (in combination with either aspirin or acetaminophen), hydrocodone, and codeine are the so-called "weaker" opioid analgesics and are indicated for use in step 2 of the WHO ladder for mild-to-moderate intensity pain. More severe pain is best managed with morphine or another of the stronger opioid analgesics, such as hydromorphone, methadone, levorphanol, or fentanyl. Oxycodone, as a single agent without aspirin or acetaminophen, is available in immediate and sustained-release forms and is considered a "stronger" opioid in these forms.

A basic understanding of the pharmacokinetics of the opioid analgesics (42) is important. Opioid analgesics with long half-lives, such as methadone and levorphanol, require approximately five days to achieve a steady state. Despite their long half-lives, the duration of analgesia that they provide is considerably shorter (i.e., most patients will require administration of the drug every 4–6 hours). As both methadone and levorphanol tend to accumulate with early initial dosing, delayed effects of toxicity can develop (primarily sedation and, more rarely, respiratory depression).

The duration of analgesic effects of opioid analgesics varies considerably. Immediate-release of morphine, hydromorphone, or oxycodone will often provide only three hours of relief, and it must be prescribed on an every-three-hours, around-the-clock basis (not as needed). Methadone and levorphanol may provide up to six hours of analgesia. There is individual variation in the metabolism of opioid analgesics, and there

can be significant differences between individuals in drug absorption and disposition. These differences lead to a need for alterations in dosing, route of administration, and scheduling for maximum analgesia in individual patients. While parenteral administration (intravenous, intramuscular, subcutaneous) will yield a faster onset of pain relief, the duration of analgesia is shorter unless a continuous infusion of opioid is instituted. The use of continuous subcutaneous or intravenous infusions of opioids, with or without patient-controlled analgesia (PCA) devices, has become commonplace in caring for cancer patients with escalating pain and in hospice and home settings during late stages of disease.

It is important to note that opioids can be administered through a variety of routes: oral, rectal, transdermal, intravenous, subcutaneous, intraspinal, and even intraventricuarly (43). There are advantages and disad-vantages, as well as indications for use of these various routes. Further discussion of such alternative delivery routes as the intraspinal route are beyond the scope of this chapter; interested readers are directed to the Agency for Health Care Policy and Research Clinical Practice Guideline: Management of Cancer Pain (30) available free of charge through 1-800-4 cancer.

The oral route is often the preferred route of administration of opioid analgesics from the perspectives of convenience and cost. Longer-acting, sustained-release oral morphine preparations (MS Contin, Oramorph SR) and oxycodone preparations (Oxycontin) are now available that provide up to 8–12 hours of analgesia, minimizing the number of daily doses required for the control of persistent pain. Rescue doses of immediate-release, short-acting opioid are often necessary to supplement the use of sustained-release morphine or oxycodone, particularly during periods of titration or pain escalation.

The transdermal fentanyl patch system (Duragesic) also has applications in the management of severe pain in cancer (43). Each transdermal fentanyl patch contains a 48–72 hour supply of fenatanyl which is absorbed from a depot in the skin. Levels in the plasma rise slowly over 12–18 hours after patch placement; so with the initial placement of a patch, alternative opioid analgesia (oral, rectal, or parenteral) must be provided until adequate levels of fentanyl are attained. The elimination half-life of this form of fentanyl is long (21 hours), and so it must be noted that significant levels of fentanyl will remain in the plasma for about 24 hours after the removal of a transdermal patch. The transdermal system is not optimal for rapid dose titration of acute pain; however, a range of doses is available. As with sustained release morphine preparations, all patients should be provided with oral or parenteral rapid-acting short duration opioids to manage breakthrough pain. The transdermal system is convenient and eliminates the reminders of pain associated with repeated oral dosing of analgesics. In cancer patients, it should be noted that the absorption of transdermal fentanyl can be increased with fever, resulting in increased plasma levels and shorter duration of analgesia from the patch.

The adequate treatment of pain in cancer also requires consideration of the equianalgesic doses of opioid drugs, which are calculated using morphine as a standard. Cross-tolerance is not complete among these drugs. Therefore, one half to two thirds of the equianalgesic dose of the new drug should be given as the starting dose when switching from one opioid to another (42). For example, if a patient receiving 20 mg of parenteral morphine is to be switched to hydromorphone, the equianalgesic dose of parenteral hydromorphone would be 3.0 mg. Thus, the starting dose of parenteral hydromorphone should be approximately 1.5 to 2 mg. There is also considerable variability in the parenteral to oral ratios amongst the opioid analgesics. Both levorphanol and methadone have 1:2 intramuscular/oral ratios, whereas morphine has a 1:6 and hydromorphone a 1:5 intramuscular/oral ratio. Failure to appreciate these dosage differences in route of administration can lead to inadequate pain control.

Regular ("standing") scheduling of the opioid analgesics is the foundation of adequate pain control. It is preferable to prevent the return of pain as opposed to treating pain as it reoccurs. "As needed" orders for chronic pain often create a struggle between patient, family and staff that is easily avoided by regular administration of opioid analgesics.

Opioid Side Effects

While the opioids are extremely effective analgesics, their side effects are common and can be minimized, if anticipated in advance. Sedation is a common CNS side effect, especially during the initiation of treatment, but usually resolves after the patient has achieved a steady dose. Persistent sedation can be alleviated with a psychostimulant, such as dextroamphetamine, pernoline, or methylphenidate. All are prescribed in divided doses in early morning and at noon. Additionally, psychostimulants can improve depressed mood and enhance analgesia (44,45).

Delirium, of an either agitated or somnolent variety, can also occur while on opioid analgesics and is usually accompanied by attentional deficits, disorientation, and perceptual disturbances (visual hallucinations and more commonly illusions). Myoclonus and asterixis are often early signs of neurotoxicity that accompany the course of opioid-induced delirium. Meperidine (Demerol), when administered chronically in patients with renal impairment, can lead to a delirium due to accumulation of the neuroexcitatory metabolite normeperidine (46). Opioid-induced delirium can be alleviated through three strategies: (1) lowering the dose of the opioid drug presently in use; (2) changing to a different opioid; or (3) treating the delirium with low doses of high potency neuroleptics, such as haloperidol. The third strategy is especially useful for agitation and tends to clear the sensorium (4). For agitated states, intravenous haloperidol in doses starting at between 1 mg and 2 mg is useful, with rapid escalation of dose if no effect is noted.

Gastrointestinal side effects of opioid analgesics are common (29). The most prevalent are nausea, vomiting, and constipation. Concomitant therapy with prochlorperazine for nausea is sometimes effective. Since opioid analgesics are not all tolerated in the same manner, switching to another narcotic can be helpful if an antiemetic regimen fails to control nausea. Constipation caused by narcotic effects on gut receptors is a frequently encountered problem, and it tends to be responsive to the use of senna derivatives. Patients need to be aware that constipation will occur and to be instructed about laxatives. A careful review of medications is imperative, since anticholinergic drugs such as the tricyclic antidepressants can worsen opioid-induced constipation and can cause bowel obstruction.

Respiratory depression is a worrisome but rare side effect of the opioid analgesics. Respiratory difficulties can almost always be avoided if two general principles are adhered to: (1) Start opioid analgesics in low doses in opioid-naive patients; and (2) be cognizant of relative potencies when switching opioid analgesics, routes of administration or both.

ADJUVANT PSYCHOTROPIC ANALGESICS FOR PATIENTS WITH CANCER

Although opioid and nonopioid analgesics are the mainstay of management of pain associated with cancer, adjuvant analgesics are another class of medications frequently prescribed for the treatment of chronic pain and have important applications in the management of pain in cancer. Adjuvant analgesic drugs are used to enhance the analgesic efficacy of opioids, treat concurrent symptoms that exacerbate pain, and provide independent analgesia. They may be used in all stages of the analgesic ladder. Commonly used adjuvant drugs include antidepressants, neuroleptics, psychostimulants, anticonvulsants, corticosteroids and oral anesthetics (29,45,47) (Table 38.4).

Antidepressants

The current literature supports the use of antidepressants as adjuvant analgesic agents in the management of a wide variety of chronic pain syndromes, including cancer pain, postherpetic neuralgia, diabetic neuropathy, fibrornyalgia, headache, and low back pain (48–53). The antidepressants are analgesic through a number of mechanisms that include: antidepressant activity (49), potentiation or enhancement of opioid analgesia (54–56), and direct analgesic effects (57). The leading hypothesis suggests that both serotonergic and noradrenergic properties of the antidepressants are probably important and that variations among indivi-

TABLE 38.4. *Psychotropic Adjuvant Analgesic Drugs for Cancer Pain*

Generic Name	Trade Name	Approximate Daily Dosage Range (mg)*	Route†
TRICYCLIC ANTIDEPRESSANTS			
Amitriptyline	Elavil	10–150	p.o., i.m.
Nortriptyline	Pamelir, Aventyl	10–150	p.o.
Imipramine	Tofranil	15.5–150	p.o., i.m.
Desipramine	Norpramin	10–150	p.o.
Clomipramine	Anafranil	10–150	p.o.
Doxepin	Sinequan	12–150	p.o., i.m.
HETEROCYCLIC AND NONCYCLIC ANTIDEPRESSANTS			
Trazodone	Desyrel	125–300	p.o.
Maprotiline	Luidiomil	50–300	p.o.
SEROTONIN REUPTAKE INHIBITORS			
Fluoxetine		20–80	p.o.
Paroxetine		0–60	p.o.
Sertraline		50–200	p.o.
NEWER AGENTS			
Nefazodone	Serzone	100–500	p.o.
Venlafaxine	Effexor	75–300	p.o.
PSYCHOSTIMULANTS			
Methylphenidate	Ritalin	2.5–20 b.i.d.	p.o.
Dextroamphetamine	Dexedrine	2.5–20 b.i.d.	p.o.
Pemoline	Cylert	13.75–75 b.i.d.	p.o.
PHENOTHIAZINES			
Fluphenazine	Prolixin	1–3	p.o., i.m.
Methotri.m.eprazine	Levoprome	10–20 q6h	i.m., i.v.
BUTYROPHENONES			
Haloperidol	Haldon	1–3	p.o., i.v.
Pi.m.ozide	Orap	2–6 b.i.d.	p.o.
ANTIHISTAMINES			
Hydroxyzine	Vistaril	50 q4h-q6h	p.o.
CORTICOSTEROIDS			
Dexamethasone	Decadron	4–16	p.o., i.v.
BENZODIAZEPINES			
Alparazolam	Xanex	0.25–2.0 t.i.d.	p.o.
Clonazepan	Klonopin	0.5–4 b.i.d.	p.o.

*b.i.d. = two ti.m.es a day; q6h = every 6 hours.
†p.o. = per oral; i.m. = intramuscular; i.v. = intravenous.

duals in pain (as to the status of their own neurotransmitter systems) is an important variable (58). Other possible mechanisms of antidepressant analgesic activity that have been proposed include adrenergic and serotonin receptor effects (59), adenosinergic effects (60), antihistaminic effects (59), and direct neuronal effects, such as inhibition of paroxysmal neuronal discharge and decreasing sensitivity of adrenergic receptors on injured nerve sprouts (61). There is substantial evidence that the tricyclic antidepressants in particular are analgesic and are useful in the management of chronic neuropathic and nonneuropathic pain syndromes. Amitriptyline is the tricyclic antidepressant most studied and has been proved effective as an analgesic in a large number of clinical trials addressing a wide variety of chronic pain syndromes, including neuropathy, cancer pain, fibromyalgia, and others (49,50,62–65). Other tricyclics that have been shown to have efficacy as analgesics include imipramine (66–68), desipramine (69,70), nortriptyline (71), clomipramine (72,73), and doxepin (74).

The heterocyclic and noncyclic antidepressant drugs, such as trazadone, mianserin, and maprotiline, and the newer serotonin-specific reuptake inhibitors (SSRIs) fluoxetine and paroxetine may also be useful as adjuvant analgesics for chronic pain syndromes (45,50,57, 58,70,75–80). Fluoxetine, a potent antidepressant with specific serotonin reuptake inhibition activity (78), has been shown to have analgesic properties in experimental animal pain models (79) but failed to show analgesic effects in a clinical trial for neuropathy (70). Several case reports suggest that fluoxetine may be a useful adjuvant analgesic in the management of headache (81) and fibrositis (82). Paroxetine, a newer SSRI, is the first antidepressant of this class shown to be a highly effective analgesic in a controlled trial for the treatment of diabetic neuropathy (80). Newer antidepressants such as sertraline, venlafaxine, and nefazodone may also eventually prove to be clinically useful as adjuvant analgesics. Nefazodone, for instance, has been demonstrated to potentiate opioid analgesics in an animal model (83).

Given the diversity of clinical syndromes in which the antidepressants have been demonstrated to be analgesic, trials of these drugs can be justified in the treatment of virtually every type of chronic pain (47). The established benefit of several of the antidepressants in patients with neuropathic pains (64,68,80, 84), however, suggests that these drugs may be particularly useful in populations, such as cancer patients, where an underlying neuropathic component to the pain(s) often exists (47).

While antidepressant drugs are analgesic in both neuropathic and nonneuropathic pain models, their clinical use is most commonly in combination with opioid drugs, particularly for moderate to severe pain. Antidepressant adjuvant analgesics have their broadest application as "co-analgesics," potentiating the analgesic effects of opioid drugs (29). The "opioid sparing" effects of antidepressant analgesics has been demonstrated in a number of trials, especially in cancer patients with neuropathic and nonneuropathic pain syndromes (50,85). In a placebo-controlled study, Walsh (85) demonstrated that imipramine was a potent co-analgesic when used along with morphine in the treatment of cancer-related pain, allowing for a reduction in morphine consumption of greater than 25%. Similar co-analgesic and opioid sparing effects were demonstrated for amitriptyline and other antidepressants in two multicenter clinical trials for cancer pain (50,52).

The dose and time course of onset of analgesia for antidepressants appears to be similar to those for their use as antidepressants. There are those who have initially advocated a low-dose regimen of amitriptyline (10–30 mg) as being as equally analgesic as a high-dose regimen (75–150 mg) (65). However, Zitman (86) demonstrated only modest analgesic results from low-dose amitriptyline. Watson (63) felt that there was a "therapeutic window" (20–100 mg) for the analgesic effects of amitriptyline. More recently, there is compelling evidence that the therapeutic analgesic effects of amitriptyline are correlated with serum levels, as are the antidepressant effects, and that analgesic treatment failure is due to low serum levels (64,87). A high-dose regimen of up to 150 mg of amitriptyline or higher is suggested (64,87). The proper analgesic dose for paroxetine is likely in the 40–60 mg range, with the major analgesic trial utilizing a fixed dose of 40 mg (80). There is anecdotal evidence to suggest that the debilitated medically ill (cancer, AIDS patients) often respond (re: depression or pain) to lower doses of antidepressant than are usually required in the physically healthy, probably because of impaired metabolism of these drugs (45). As to the time course of onset of analgesia, a biphasic process appears to occur. There are immediate or early analgesic effects that occur within hours or days, and these are probably mediated through inhibition of synaptic reuptake of catecholamines. In addition, there are later, longer analgesic effects that peak over a 2 to 4 week period that are probably due to receptor effects of the antidepressants (62,64,87).

Psychostimulants

The psychostimulants dextroamphetamine, methylphenidate, and pemoline are useful antidepressants in patients with cancer who are cognitively impaired (44,88). Psychostimulants also enhance the analgesic effects of the opioid drugs (89). They diminish sedation secondary to narcotic analgesics, and they are potent adjuvant analgesics. Bruera (44) demonstrated that a regimen of 10 mg methylphenidate with breakfast and 5 mg with lunch significantly decreased sedation and potentiated the effect of narcotics in patients with cancer pain. Methylphenidate has also been demonstrated to improve functioning on a number neuropsychological tests, including tests of memory, speed, and concentration, in patients receiving continuous infusions of opioids for cancer pain (90). Dextroamphetamine has also been reported to have additive analgesic effects when used with morphine in postoperative pain (91). In relatively low doses, psychostimulants stimulate appetite, promote a sense of well-being, and improve feelings of weakness and fatigue in cancer patients.

Pemoline is a unique alternative psychostimulant that is chemically unrelated to amphetamine but has similar usefulness as an antidepressant and adjuvant analgesic in cancer patients (92). Advantages of pernoline as a psychostimulant in patients with cancer-related pain include the lack of abuse potential, the lack of federal regulation requiring special triplicate prescriptions, the mild sympathornimetic effects, and the fact that it comes in a chewable tablet form that can be absorbed through the buccal mucosa. It can be used by cancer patients who have difficulty swallowing or who have intestinal obstruction. Clinically, pernoline is as effective as methylphenidate or dextroarnphetarnine in the treatment of depressive symptoms and in countering the sedating effects of opioid analgesics. There are no studies of pernoline's capacity to potentiate the analgesic properties of opioids. Pernoline should be used with caution in patients with liver impairment, and liver function tests should be monitored periodically with longer term treatment.

Neuroleptics

Neuroleptic drugs, such as methotrimeprazine, fluphenazine, haloperidol, and pimozide, may play a role as adjuvant analgesics (20,93–95) in cancer patients with pain; however, their use must be weighed against what appears to be an increased sensitivity to the extrapyramidal side effects of these drugs in cancer patients with neurological complications. Anxiolytics, such as alprazolam and clonazepram, may also be useful as adjuvant analgesics, particularly in the management of neuropathic pains (96–98).

Placebo

A mention of the placebo response is important in order to highlight the misunderstandings and relative harm of this phenomenon. The placebo response is common, and analgesia is mediated through endogenous opioids. The deceptive use of placebo response to distinguish psychogenic pain from "real" pain should be avoided. Placebos are effective in a portion of patients for a short period of time only and are not indicated in the management of cancer pain (2).

PSYCHIATRIC AND PSYCHOLOGICAL MANAGEMENT OF PAIN IN CANCER

Optimal treatment of pain associated with advanced disease is multi modal and includes pharmacologic, psychotherapeutic, cognitive-behavioral, anesthetic, neuro stimulatory, and rehabilitative approaches. Psychiatric participation in pain management involves the use of psychotherapeutic, cognitive-behavioral, and psychopharmacologic interventions, usually in combination, which are described below.

Psychotherapy and Pain

The goals of psychotherapy with medically ill patients with pain are to provide support, knowledge, and coping skills. Utilizing short-term supportive psychotherapy focused on the crisis created by the medical illness, the therapist provides emotional support, continuity, and information, and assists in adaptation. The therapist has a role in emphasizing past strengths, supporting previously successful coping strategies, and teaching new coping skills such as relaxation, cognitive coping, information about use of analgesics, self-observation, documentation, assertiveness, and communication. Communication skills are of paramount importance for both patient and family, particularly around pain and analgesic issues.

Psychotherapy with the patient in pain consists of active listening with supportive verbal interventions and an occasional clarification (99). Despite the seriousness of the patient's plight, it is not necessary for the psychiatrist or psychologist to appear overly solemn or emotionally restrained. The psychotherapist should allow the patient to talk about any aspect of his or her life and experiences or talk and ask questions about death and pain if the patient wishes to do so. The therapist maintains an interested, interactive stance. It is not uncommon for the dying patient to benefit from pastoral counseling, which should be offered. As the disease process progresses, psychotherapy with the individual patient may become limited by cognitive and speech deficits. Visits, already short, may become briefer. It is at this point that the focus of supportive psychotherapeutic interventions shifts primarily to the family. In our experience, a very common concern for family members at this point is the level of alertness of the patient and their concern that the patient is not in pain. The trade-off between sedation and pain control may need to be explained, as well as the fact that confusion and hallucinations are related to medication. This sometimes becomes a source of conflict, with some family members disagreeing among themselves or with the patient about what constitutes an appropriate balance between comfort and alertness. It can be helpful for the physician to clarify the patient's preferences as they relate to these issues early so that conflict can be avoided and work related to bereavement can begin.

Group interventions with individual patients (even in advanced stages of disease), spouses, couples, and families are a powerful means of sharing experiences and identifying successful coping strategies. The limitations of using group interventions for patients with advanced disease are primarily pragmatic. The patient must be physically comfortable enough to participate and have the cognitive capacity to be aware of group discussion. It is often helpful for family members to attend support groups during the terminal phases of the patient's illness. Passik and colleagues (100) have worked with spouses of brain tumor patients in a psychoeducational group that has included spouses at all phases of the patient's illness. They have demonstrated how bereavement issues are often a focus of such interventions from the time of diagnosis on. The group members have benefit from one another's support into widowhood. The leaders have been impressed by the increased quality of patient care that can be given at home by the spouse (including pain management and all forms of nursing care) when spouses engage in such support.

Psychotherapeutic interventions that have multiple foci may be most useful. Based upon a prospective study of cancer pain, cognitive behavioral and psychoeducational techniques based upon increasing support, self-efficacy, and providing education may prove to be helpful in assisting patients in dealing with increased pain (99). Results of an evaluation of patients with cancer pain indicate that psychological and social variables are significant predictors of pain. More specifically, distress specific to the illness, self-efficacy, and coping styles were predictors of increased pain.

Utilizing psychotherapy to diminish symptoms of anxiety and depression, factors that can intensify pain, empirically has beneficial effects on pain control. Spiegel and Bloom (101) demonstrated, in a controlled randomized prospective study, both the effect of supportive group therapy for metastatic breast cancer patients in general and, in particular, the effect of hypnotic pain control exercises. Their support group focused not on interpersonal processes or self-exploration, but rather on a series of themes related to the practical and existential problems of living with cancer. Patients receiving group psychotherapy experienced significantly less psychological distress and pain compared to patients who did not participate in group therapy.

Cognitive-Behavioral Techniques

Cognitive-behavioral techniques can be useful as adjuncts to the management of pain in cancer patients. Such techniques include passive relaxation with mental imagery, cognitive distraction or focusing, progressive muscle relaxation, biofeedback, hypnosis, and music therapy (20,102–104). The goal of treatment is to guide the patient toward a sense of control over pain. Some techniques are primarily cognitive in nature, focusing on perceptual and thought processes, and others are directed at modifying patterns of behavior that help cancer patients cope with pain. Behavioral techniques for pain control seek to modify physiologic pain reactions, respondent pain behaviors, and operant pain behaviors.

Primarily cognitive techniques for coping with pain are aimed at reducing the intensity and distress that are part of the pain experience. This may be accomplished by the utilization of techniques including the modification of thoughts patients have about their pain or psychological distress, introduction of more adaptive coping strategies, and instruction in relaxation techniques. Cognitive modification (cognitive restructuring) is an approach derived from cognitive therapy for depression or anxiety and is based on how one interprets events and bodily sensation. It is assumed that patients have dysfunctional automatic thoughts that are consistent with underlying assumptions and beliefs. In cancer pain populations, negative thoughts about pain have been shown to be significantly related to pain intensity, degree of psychological distress, and level of interference in functional activities (17). By identifying and challenging dysfunctional automatic thoughts and underlying beliefs by restructuring or modifying thought processes, a more rational response to pain can be achieved (103). Examples of such automatic thoughts that have been shown to worsen pain experience include: "The intensity of my pain will never diminish" or "Because my pain limits my activities, I am completely helpless." Patients can be taught to recognize and interrupt such thoughts and proceed to develop a view of the pain experience as time-limited and themselves as functional despite periods in which they are limited.

Although cognitive restructuring may be a useful technique in the earlier stages of cancer, the goals change in the palliative care context. In this setting the goal is not necessarily to change the patient's maladaptive thoughts but to utilize techniques designed to diminish frustration, anxiety, and anger. Helping patients to employ more adaptive coping strategies, i.e. the avoidance of catastrophizing and encouragement an increase in problem solving skills, may be helpful at this stage (99,103,105).

Aside from modifying dysfunctional thoughts and attitudes, the most fundamental behavioral technique is self-monitoring. The development of the ability to monitor one's behaviors allows patients to notice their dysfunctional reactions to the pain experience and learn to control them. Systematic desensitization is useful in extinguishing anticipatory anxiety that leads to avoidant behaviors and in remobilizing inactive patients. Graded task assignment is essentially systematic desensitization as it is applied to patients who are encouraged to take small steps gradually so as to perform activities more readily.

Cognitive-behavioral interventions that are useful in the setting of advanced illness include a variety of techniques that range from preparatory information and self-monitoring to systematic desensitization and methods of distraction and relaxation (106) (see Chapter 62). Most often, techniques such as hypnosis, biofeedback, or systematic desensitization utilize both cognitive and behavioral elements such as muscular relaxation and cognitive distraction.

Relaxation Techniques

Several techniques can be used to achieve a mental and physical state of relaxation. Muscular tension, autonomic arousal, and mental distress exacerbate pain (103,104,107). Some specific relaxation techniques include (*1*) passive relaxation focusing attention on sensations of warmth and decreased tension in various parts of the body, (*2*) progressive muscle relaxation involving active tensing and relaxing of muscles, and (*3*) meditation (see Chapter 62). Other techniques that employ both relaxation and cognitive techniques include hypnosis, biofeeback, and music therapy and are discussed later in this chapter.

Passive relaxation, focused breathing, and passive muscle relaxation exercises involve the focusing of attention systematically on breathing, on sensations of warmth and relaxation, or on release of muscular tension in various body parts. Verbal suggestions and imagery are used to help promote relaxation. Muscle relaxation is an important component of the relaxation response and can augment the benefits of simple focused breathing exercises, leading to a deeper experience of relaxation and self-control.

Progressive or active muscle relaxation involves the active tensing and relaxing of various muscle groups in the body, focusing attention on the sensations of tension and relaxation. Clinically, in the hospital setting, relaxation is most commonly achieved through the use of a combination of focused breathing and progressive muscle relaxation exercises. Once patients are in a relaxed state, imagery techniques can then be used to induce deeper relaxation and facilitate distraction from or manipulation of a variety of cancer-related symptoms.

Imagery/Distraction Techniques

Clinically, relaxation techniques are most helpful in managing pain when combined with some distracting or pleasant imagery. The use of distraction or focusing involves control over the focus of attention and can be used to make the patient less aware of the noxious stimuli (108). One can employ imaginative inattention by picturing oneself on a beach. Mental distraction can be used and is similar to the practice of counting sheep to aid sleep. Keeping oneself busy is a form of behavioral distraction, Imagery, i.e., using one's imagination while in a relaxed state, can be used to transform pain into a warm or cold sensation. One can also imaginatively transform the context of pain, i.e., imagining oneself in battle on the football field instead of the hospital bed. Disassociated somatization can be employed by some patients, whereby they imagine that a painful body part is no longer part of their body (3,4,103,104). It is important to note that not every patient finds these techniques acceptable, and the therapist must try out a number of approaches to determine which are consistent with the patient's style.

Imagery (often referred to as guided imagery) is most effective when the specific image is chosen by the patient. The clinician may ask the patient to close his or her eyes and think of a place, an activity, or an experience where the patient felt most safe and secure. The clinician may provide suggestions for the patient such as a favorite beach scene, or a room in a house, or riding a bicycle in a park. Once the patient identifies the scene, the clinician may ask the patient to elaborate upon the scene, asking for specific details such as the temperature, season, time of day, type of ocean (calm, or with big waves). The clinician then utilizes this information and describes an image for the patient in detail. The skill is for the clinician to be as flexible and as creative as possible, and to elaborate upon the scene, utilizing all aspects of the senses and bodily sensations such as "Feel the suns rays touch your skin, allow your skin to feel warm and tingly all over" or, "Breathe in the fresh, clear air, allow it to fill your lungs with its freshness" or, "Feel the fresh dew of the grass under your feet." The clinician can focus on "aromas in the garden" or the "sounds of birds singing," always reminding the patient to breathe evenly and steadily as he or she feels more and more relaxed and more and more in control. If possible, the clinician should avoid volunteering an image or scene for the patient because the clinician is unaware of the association or meaning the image may have for the patient. For example, a patient may have a fear of the water, and therefore a beach scene may invoke feelings of fear and loss of control.

Hypnosis

Hypnosis can be a useful adjunct in the management of cancer pain (71,109–112). In a controlled trial comparing hypnosis with cognitive behavioral therapy in relieving mucositis following a bone marrow transplant, patients utilizing hypnosis reported a significant reduction in pain compared to patients who used cognitive behavioral techniques (99). The hypnotic trance is essentially a state of heightened and focused concentration, and thus it can be used to manipulate the perception of pain. The depth of hypnotizability may determine the effectiveness as well as the strategies employed during hypnosis. One-third of cancer patients, as is the case with the general population, are not hypnotizable, and it is recommended that other techniques be employed for them. Of the two-thirds of patients who are identified as being less, moderately, and highly hypnotizable, three principles underlie the use of hypnosis in controlling pain (111): use self-hypnosis; relax, do not fight the pain, and use a mental filter to ease the hurt in pain. Patients who are moderately and highly hypnotizable can often alter sensations in a painful area by changing temperature sensation or experiencing tingling. Less hypnotizable patients can often utilize an alternative focus by concentrating on a sensation in a nonaffected body part or on a mental image of a pleasant scene. The main disadvantage of hypnosis for cancer patients is that the technique frequently requires more attentional capacity than these patients generally have.

Biofeedback

Fotopoulos and colleagues (113) noted significant pain relief in a group of cancer patients who were taught electromyographic (EIVIG) and electroencephalographic (EEG) biofeedback-assisted relaxation. Only 2 of 17 were able to maintain analgesia after the treatment ended. A lack of generalization of effect can be a problem with biofeedback techniques. Although physical condition may make a prolonged training period impossible, especially for the seriously ill, most cancer patients who are motivated to try it can utilize EMG and temperature biofeedback techniques for learning relaxation-assisted pain control (103).

Music, Aroma, and Art Therapies

Munro and Mount (114) have written extensively on the use of music therapy with cancer patients, documenting clinical examples and suggesting mechanisms of action. Music can capture the focus of attention like no other stimulus, offers patients a new form of expression, and helps distract from perceptions of pain, while enhancing expression in meaningful ways (115).

Aromas have been shown to have innate relaxing and stimulating qualities. Manne and colleagues (116) have explored the use of aroma therapy for the treatment of procedure-related anxiety (i.e., anxiety related to MRI scans). Utilizing the scent heliotropin, they reported that two thirds of the patients found the scent especially pleasant and reported much less anxiety than those who were not exposed to the scent during MRI. As a general relaxation technique, aroma therapy may have an application for pain management that should be studied.

Art therapy allows adults or children who have trouble with verbal expression to express their fears and concerns, being able to depict pain and fears using visual images. Luzzatto is exploring art therapy to help patients modify and modulate their experience of pain (see Chapter 64). The creative experience is both an important means of providing support and also, an avenue for providing patients with psychological insights into their experience (117).

SUMMARY

The management of the pain associated with cancer represents a significant challenge for the psycho-oncologist. A thorough familiarity with both the pharmacologic and nonpharmacologic management of cancer pain offers the possibility of decreasing psychological distress for patients as well as improving overall quality of life.

REFERENCES

1. Foley KM. Pain syndromes in patients with cancer. In: Bonica JJ, Ventafriddi V, Fink RB, Jones LE, Loeser JD, eds. *Advances in Pain Research and Therapy,* vol. 2. New York: Raven Press; 1975:59–75.

2. Foley KM. The treatment of cancer pain. *N Engl J Med.* 1985; 313:845.

3. Breitbart W, Holland J. Psychiatric aspects of cancer pain. In: Foley KM, et al., eds. *Advances in Pain Research and Therapy*, vol. 16. New York: Raven Press; 1990:73–87.

4. Breitbart W. Psychiatric management of cancer pain. *Cancer.* 1989; 63:2336–2342.

5. Massie MJ, Holland JC. The cancer patient with pain: psychiatric complications and their management. *Med Clin North Am.* 1987; 71:243–258.

6. Bonica JJ. Cancer pain. In: Bonica JJ, ed. *The Management of Pain*, 2d ed, vol 1. Philadelphia: Lea and Febiger; 1987:400–460.

7. Twycross RG, Lack SA. *Symptom Control in Far Advanced Cancer: Pain Relief.* London: Pitman Books; 1983.

8. Marks RM, Sachar EJ. Undertreatment of medical inpatients with narcotic analgesics. *Ann Intern Med.* 1973; 78:173–181.

9. Ahles TA, Blanchard EB, Ruckdeschel JC. The multidimensional nature of cancer related pain. *Pain.* 1983; 17:277–288.

10. Stiefel, F. Psychosocial aspects of cancer pain. *Support Care Cancer.* 1 993; 1:130–134.

11. Saunders, C M. *The Management of Terminal Illness.* London: Hospital Medicine Publications; 1967.

12. Hanks, G W. Opioid responsive and opioid non-responsive pain in cancer. *Br Med Bull.* 1991; 47:718–731.

13. Syrjala, K, Chapko, M. Evidence for a biophysical model of cancer treatment-related pain. *Pain.* 1995; 61:69–79.

14. Daut RL, Cleeland CS. The prevalence and severity of pain in cancer. *Cancer.* 1982; 50:1913–1918.

15. Spiegel D, Bloom JR. Pain in metastatic breast cancer. *Cancer.* 1983; 52:341–345.

16. Padilla G, Ferrell B, Grant M, Rhiner M. Defining the content domain of quality of life for cancer patients with pain. *Cancer Nurs.* 1990; 13:108–115.

17. Payne, D. Cognition in cancer pain. University of Louisville, Louisville KY: unpublished dissertation; 1995.

18. McKegney FP, Bailey CR, Yates JW. Prediction and management of pain in patients with advanced cancer. *Gen Hosp Psychiatry.* 1981; 3:95–101.

19. Bond MR, Pearson IB. Psychological aspects of pain in women with advanced cancer of the cervix. *J Psychosom Res.* 1969; 13:13–19.

20. Cleeland CS, Tearnan BH. Behavioral control of cancer pain. In: Holzman D, Turk D., eds. *Pain Management.* New York: Pergamon Press; 1986:193–212.

21. Derogatis LR, Morrow GR, Fetting J, et al. The prevalence of psychiatric disorders among cancer patients. *J Am Med Assoc.* 1983; 249:751–757.

22. Breitbart W. Cancer pain and suicide. In: Foley K, et al., eds. *Advances in Pain Research and Therapy*, vol. 16. Raven Press, New York: 1990:399–412.

23. Massie M, Gagnon P, Holland J. Depression and suicide in patients with cancer. *J Pain Symptom Manage.* 1994; 9: 325–331.

24. Levin DN, Cleeland CS, Dan R. Public attitudes toward cancer pain. *Cancer.* 1985; 56:2337–2339.

25. Bolund C. Suicide and cancer: 11. Medical and care factors in suicide by cancer patients in Sweden, 1973–1976. *J Psychosoc Oncol.* 1985; 3:17–30.

26. Farberow NL, Schneidman ES, Leonard CV. *Suicide among General Medical and Surgical Hospital Patients with Malignant Neoplasms.* Medical Bulletin 9. Washington D.C., U.S. Veterans Administration, 1963.

27. Breitbart W. Suicide in cancer patients. *Oncology.* 1987; 1:49–53.

28. World Health Organization. *Cancer Pain Relief.* Geneva: World Health Organization; 1986.

29. Portenoy RK. Pharmacologic approaches to the control of cancer pain. *J Psychosoc Oncol.* 1990; 8:75–107.

30. Jacox A, Carr D, Payne R, et al. *Clinical Practice Guideline Number 9: Management of Cancer Pain.* U.S. Department of Health and Human Services, Public Health Service, Agency for Health Care Policy and Research. AHCPR Publication No. 94-0592:139–41; 1994.

31. Fishman B, Pasternak S, Wallenstein SL, et al. The Memorial Pain Assessment Care: a valid instrument for the evaluation of cancer pain. *Cancer.* 1987; 60:1151–1158.

32. Daut RL, Cleeland CS, Flanery RC. Development of the Wisconsin Brief Pain Questionnaire to assess pain in cancer and other diseases. *Pain.* 1983; 17:197–210.

33. Cleeland C, Gonin R, Hatfield A. Pain and its treatment in outpatients with metastatic cancer. *N Engl J Med.* 1994; 330:592–596.

34. Kanner RM, Foley KM. Patterns of narcotic use in a cancer pain clinic. *Ann NY Acad Sci.* 1981; 362:161–172.

35. Macaluso C, Weinberg D, Foley KM. Opioid abuse and misuse in a cancer pain population. [Abstract]. Second International Congress on Cancer Pain, July 14-17, Rye, New York; 1988.

36. Bruera E, MacMillan K, Pither J, MacDonald RN. Effects of morphine on the dyspnea of terminal cancer patients. *J Pain Symptom Manage.* 1990; 5:341–344.

37. Grossman SA, Sheidler VR, Sweden K, Mucenski J, Piantadosi S. Correlations of patient and caregivers ratings of cancer pain. *J Pain Symptom Manage.* 1991; 6:53–57.

38. Charap, AD. The knowledge, attitudes, and experience of medical personnel treating pain in the terminally ill. *Mt Sinai J Med.* 1978; 45:561–501.

39. Ventrafridda V, Caraceni A, Gamba A. Field testing of the WHO Guidelines for Cancer Pain Relief: Summary report of demonstration projects. In: Foley KM, Bonica JJ, Ventrafridda V, eds. *Advances in Pain Research and Therapy*, vol. 16. New York: Raven Press; 1990:155–165.

40. Brooks MP, Day OR. Nonsteroidal anti-inflammatory drugs differences and similarities. *N Engl J Med.* 1985; 24:1716–1725.

41. American Pain Society. *Principles of Analgesic Use in the Treatment of Acute Pain and Cancer Pain.* Skokie, IL: American Pain Society; 1992.

42. Foley KM, Intturrisi CE. Analgesic drug therapy in cancer pain: principles and practice. In: Payne R, Foley KM, eds. *Cancer Pain Medical Clinics of North America.* Philadelphia: WB Saunders; 1987:207–232.

43. Patt RB, Reddy SR. Pain and the opioid analgesics: alternate routes of administration. *PAACNOTES*. 1993; Nov:453–458.

44. Bruera E, Chadwick S, Brennels C, Hanson J, MacDonald RN. Methylphenidate associated with narcotics for the treatment of cancer pain. *Cancer Treat Rep.* 1987; 71:67–70.

45. Breitbart W. Psychotropic adjuvant analgesics for cancer pain. *Psycho-Oncology*. 1992; 1:133–145.

46. Kaiko R, Foley K, Grabinski P, et al. Central nervous system excitation effects of meperidine in cancer patients. *Ann Neurol.* 1983; 13:180–183.

47. Portenoy RK. Adjuvant analgesics in pain management. In D Doyle, GWC Hanks, N MacDonald, eds. *Oxford Textbook of Palliative Medicine.* New York: Oxford University Press; 1993:187–203.

48. Butler S. Present status of tricyclic antidepressants in chronic pain therapy. In: Foley M, Bonica JJ, Ventafridda V, eds. *Advances in Pain Research and Therapy*, vol 7. New York: Raven Press; 1984:173–196.

49. France RD. The future for antidepressants: treatment of pain. *Psychopathology*. 1987; 20:99–113.

50. Ventafridda V, Bonezzi C, Caraceni A, et al. Antidepressants for cancer pain and other painful syndromes with deafferentation component: comparison of amitriptyline and trazodone. *Ital J Neurol Sci.* 1987; 8:579–587.

51. Getto CJ, Sorkness CA, Howell T. Antidepressants and chronic nonmalignant pain: a review. *J Pain Symptom Control.* 1987; 2:9–18.

52. Magni G, Arsie D, DeLeo D. Antidepressants in the treatment of cancer pain. A survey in Italy. *Pain.* 1987; 29:347–353.

53. Walsh TD. Adjuvant analgesic therapy in cancer pain. In: Foley KM, ed. *Advances in Pain Research and Therapy*, vol. 16. New York: Raven Press; 1990:155–165.

54. Botney M, Fields HC. Amitriptyline potentiates morphine analgesia by direct action on the central nervous system. *Ann Neurol.* 1983; 13:160–164.

55. Malseed RT, Goldstein FJ. Enhancement of morphine analgesics by tricyclic antidepressants. *Neuropharmacology.* 1979; 18:827–829.

56. Ventafridda V, Bianchi M, Ripamonti C, et al. Studies on the effects of antidepressant drugs on the antinociceptive action of morphine and on plasma morphine in rat and man. *Pain.* 1990; 43:155–162.

57. Spiegel K, Kalb R, Pasternak GW. Analgesic activity of tricyclic antidepressants. *Ann Neurol.* 1983; 13:462–465.

58. Watson C, Chipan M, Reed K, Evans R, Birket N. Amitriptyline versus maprotiline in postherpetic neuralgia: a randomized double-blind crossover trial. *Pain.* 1992; 48:29–36.

59. Gram LF. Receptors, pharmacokinetics and clinical effects. In Burrows GD, ed. *Antidepressants.* Amsterdam: Elsevier; 1983:81–95.

60. Mersky H, Hamilton JT. An open trial of possible analgesic effects of dipyridamole. *J Symptom Manage.* 1989; 4:34–37.

61. Devor M. Nerve pathophysiology and mechanisms of pain in causalgia. *J Auton Nerv System.* 1983; 7:371–384.

62. Pilowsky I, Hallett EC, Bassett DL, Thomas PG, Penhall RK. A controlled study of amitriptyline in the treatment of chronic pain. *Pain.* 1982; 14:169–179.

63. Watson CP, Evans RJ, Reed K, Merskey H, Goldsmith L, Warsh J. Amitriptyline versus placebo in post herpetic neuralgia. *Neurology.* 1982; 32:671–673.

64. Max MB, Culnane M, Schafer SC, et al. Amitriptyline relieves diabetic-neuropathy pain in patients with normal and depressed mood. *Neurology.* 1987; 37:589–596.

65. Sharav Y, Singer E, Schmidt E, Dione RA, Dubner R. The analgesic effect of amitriptyline on chronic facial pain. *Pain.* 1987; 31:199–209.

66. Kvindesal B, Molin J, Froland A, Gram LF. Imipramine treatment of painful diabetic neuropathy. *J Am Med Assoc.* 1984; 251:1727–1730.

67. Young RJ, Clarke BF. Pain relief in diabetic neuropathy: the effectiveness of imipramine and related drugs. *Diabetic Med.* 1985; 2:363–366.

68. Sindrup SH, Ejlertsen B, Froland A, et al. Imipramine treatment in diabetic neuropathy: relief of subjective symptoms without changes in peripheral and autonomic nerve function. *Eur J Clin Pharmacol.* 1989; 37:151–153.

69. Kishore-Kumar R, Max MB, Scafer SC, et al. Desipramine relieves post-herpetic neuralgia. *Clin Pharmacol Ther.* 1990; 47:305–312.

70. Max MB, Lynch SA, Muir J, Shoaf SE, Smoller, B, Dubner, R. Effects of desipramine, amitriptyline, and fluoxetine on pain in diabetic neuropathy. *N Engl J Med.* 1992; 326:1250–1256.

71. Gomez-Perez FJ, Rull JA, Dies H, et al. Nortriptyline and fluphenazine in the symptomatic treatment of diabetic neuropathy. A double-blind cross-over study. *Pain.* 1985; 23:395–400.

72. Langohr HD, Stohr M, Petruch F. An open and double-blind crossover study on the efficacy of clorniipramine (anafranil) in patients with painful mono- and polyneuropathies. *Eur Neurol.* 1982; 21:309–315.

73. Tiegno M, Pagnoni B, Calmi A, Rigoli M, Braga PC, Panerai AE. Chlorimipramine compared to pentazocine as a unique treatment in post-operative pain. *Int J Clin Pharmacol Res.* 1987; 7:141–143.

74. Hammeroff SR, Cork RC, Scherer K, et al. Doxepin effects on chronic pain, depression and plasma opioids. *J Clin Psychiatry.* 1982; 2:22–26.

75. Davidoff, G, Guarracini M, Roth E, et al. Trazodone hydrochloride in the treatment of dysesthetic pain in traumatic myelopathy: a randomized, double-blind, placebo-controlled study. *Pain.* 1987; 29:151–161.

76. Costa D, Mogos 1, Toma T. Efficacy and safety of mianserin in the treatment of depression of woman with cancer. *Acta Psychiatr Scand.* 1985; 72:85–92.

77. Eberhard G, et al. A double-blind randomized study of clorniipramine versus maprotiline in patients with idiopathic pain syndromes. *Neuropsychobiology.* 1988; 19:25–32.

78. Feighner JP. A comparative trial of fluoxetine and amitriptyline in patients with major depressive disorder. *J Clin Psychiatry.* 1985; 46:369–372.

79. Hynes MD, Lochner MA, Bemis K, et al. Fluoxetine, a selective inhibitor of serotonin uptake, potentiates morphine analgesia without altering its descriminative stimulus properties or affinity for opioid receptors. *Life Sci.* 1985; 36:2317–2323.

80. Sindrup SH, Gram LF, Brosen K, Eshoj O, Mogenson EF. The selective serotonin reuptake inhibitor paroxetine

is effective in the treatment of diabetic neuropathy symptoms. *Pain*. 1990; 42:135–144.

81. Diamond S, Frietag FG. The use of fluoxetine in the treatment of headache. *Clin J Pain*. 989; 5:200–201.

82. Geller SA. Treatment of fibrositis with fluoxetine hydrochloride (Prozac). *Am J Med*. 1989; 87:594–595.

83. Pick CG, Paul D, Eison MS, Pasternak G, Potentiation of opioid analgesia by the antidepressant nefazodone. *Eur J Pharmacol*. 1992:375–381.

84. Max MB, Kishore-Kumar R, Schafer SC, et al. Efficacy of desipramine in painful diabetic neuropathy: a placebo-controlled trial. *Pain*. 1991; 45:3–10.

85. Walsh TD. Adjuvant analgesic therapy in cancer pain. In Foley KM, Bonica SJ, Ventafridda V, eds. *Advances in Pain Research and Therapy*. New York: Raven Press; 1990; 16:155–165.

86. Zitman FG, Linssen ACG, Edelbroek PM, Stijnen T. Low dose amitriptyline in chronic pain: the gain is modest. *Pain*. 1990; 42:35–42.

87. Max MB, Schafer SC, Culnane M, Smollen B, Dubner R, Gracel RH. Amitriptyline, but not lorazepam, relieves postherpetic neuralgia. *Neurology*. 1988; 38:427–1432.

88. Fernandez F, Adams F, Holmes VF, et al. Methylphenidate for depressive disorders in cancer patients. *Psychosomatics*. 1987; 28:455–461.

89. Bruera E, Brenneis C, Paterson AH, MacDonald RN. Use of Methylphenidate as an adjuvant to narcotic analgesics in patients with advanced cancer: *J Pain Symptom Manage*. 1989; 4:3–6.

90. Bruera E, Fainsinger R, MacEachern T, Hanson J. The use of methylphenidate in patients with incident cancer pain receiving regular opiates: a preliminary report. *Pain*. 1992; 50:75–77.

91. Forrest WH, et al. Dextroamphetamine with morphine for the treatment of post-operative pain. *N Engl J Med*. 1977; 296:712–715.

92. Breitbart W, Mermelstein H. Pemoline: an alternative psychostimulant in the management of depressive disorders in cancer patients. *Psychosomatics*. 1991; 24:125–137.

93. Beaver WT, Wallenstein SL, Houde RW, et al. A comparison of the analgesic effect of methotrimeprazine and morphine in patients with cancer. *Clin Pharmacol Ther*. 1966; 7:436–446.

94. Maltbie AA, Cavenar JO, Sullivan JL, et al. Analgesia and haloperidol: a hypothesis. *J Clin Psychiatry*. 1979; 40:323–326.

95. Lechin F, et al. Pimozide therapy for trigeminal neuralgia. *Arch Neurol*. 1989; 9:960–964.

96. Fernandez F, Adams F, Holmes VF. Analgesic effect of alprazolam in patients with chronic, organic pain of malignant origin. *J Clin Psychopharmacol*. 1987; 3:167–169.

97. Swerdlow M, Cundill JG. Anticonvulsant drugs used in the treatment of lancinating pains: a comparison. *Anesthesia*. 1981; 36:1129–1134.

98. Caccia MR. Clonazepam in facial neuralgia and cluster headache: clinical and electrophysiological study. *Eur Neurol*. 1975; 13:560–563.

99. Fishman B, Loscalzo M. Cognitive-behavioral interventions in the management of cancer pain: principles and applications. *Med Clin North Am*. 1987; 71:271–287.

100. Passik S, Horowitz S, Malkin M, Gargan R. A psychoeducational support program for spouses of brain tumor patients [Abstract]. Symposium on New Trends in the Psychological Support of the Cancer Patient. American Psychiatric Association Annual Meeting, New Orleans, May 7–12, 1991.

101. Spiegel D, Bloom JR. Group therapy and hypnosis reduce metastatic breast carcinoma pain. *Psychosom Med*. 1983; 4:333-339.

102. Cleeland CS. Nonpharmacologic management of cancer pain. *J Pain Symptom Control*. 1987; 2:523–528.

103. Loscalzo M, Jacobsen PB. Practical behavioral approaches to the effective management of pain and distress. *J Psychosoc Oncol*. 1990; 8:139–169.

104. Fishman B. The treatment of suffering in patients with cancer pain. In: Foley K, Bonica J. Ventafridda V, eds. *Advances in Pain Research and Therapy*, vol. 16. New York: Raven Press; 1990:301–316.

105. Jensen M, Turner J, Romano J, Karoly J. Coping with chronic pain: a critical review of the literature. *Pain*. 1990; 47:249–283.

106. Syrajala K. Cummings C., Donaldson G. Hypnosis or cognitive behavioral training for the reduction of pain and nausea during cancer treatment: a controlled trial. *Pain*. 1992; 48:137–146.

107. Turk D, Fernandez E. On the putative uniqueness of cancer pain: Do psychological principles apply? *Behav Res Ther*. 1990; 28:1–13.

108. Broome M, Lillis P, McGahhe T, Bates T. The use of distraction and imagery with children during painful procedures. *Oncol Nurs Forum*. 19: 1992:499–502.

109. Spiegel D. The use of hypnosis in controlling cancer pain. *CA Cancer J Clin*. 1985; 4:221–231.

110. Redd WB, Reeves JL, Storm FK, Minagawa RY. Hypnosis in the control of pain during hyperthermia treatment of cancer. In: Bonica JJ, ed. *Advances in Pain Research and Therapy*, vol. 5. New York: Raven Press; 1982:857–861.

111. Barber J, Gitelson J. Cancer pain: psychological management using hypnosis. *CA Cancer J Clin*. 1980; 3:130–136.

112. Levitan A. The use of hypnosis with cancer patients. *Psychiatry Med*. 1992; 10:119–131.

113. Fotopoulos SS, Graham C, Cook MR. Psychophysiologic control of cancer pain. In: Bonica JJ, Ventafridda V, eds. *Advances in Pain Research and Therapy*, vol 2. New York: Raven Press; 1979:231–244.

114. Munro SM, Mount B. Music therapy in palliative care. *Can Med Assoc J*. 1978; 119:1029–1034.

115. Schroeder-Sheker T. Music for the dying: a personal account of the new field of music thanatology history, theories, and clinical narratives. *Advances*. 1993; 9:36–48.

116. Manne S, Redd W, Jacobsen P, Georgiades I. Aroma for treatment of anxiety during MRI scans [Abstract]. Symposium on New Trends in the Psychological Support of the Cancer Patient. American Psychiatric Association Annual Meeting, New Orleans, May 7–12, 1991.

117. Connell C. Art therapy as part of a palliative cancer program. *Palliat Med*. 1992; 6:18–25.

39

Cancer Cachexia

STEWART B. FLEISHMAN

Although the understanding of the causes of and treatments for cancer-related cachexia receives less attention than the diagnosis and definitive treatment for cancer itself, cachexia remains the single most documented cause of death in cancer. Between 30% and 87% of cancer patients develop cachexia before death (1). It is a significant contribution to approximately 22% of cancer deaths (2).

Nutritional considerations are part of a comprehensive treatment approach in both the curative and palliative care provided by the oncology team. Understanding all of the causes and interventions available to prevent and treat cancer cachexia should be paramount to those mental health professionals working in the oncology setting. The cancer cachexia syndrome is a paradigm of a syndrome with biopsychosocial determinants. Two of the available treatment regimens are of the behavioral and pharmacologic nature. Many of the drugs used to treat cachexia have psychoactive properties familiar to most general psychiatrists, even those who lack the subspecialists' experience working with cancer patients. It is those clinicians who have the background to best advise other members of the oncology care team how to use them to best effect. Differentiating cancer cachexia from depression is a challenging diagnostic endeavor best done by those clinicians familiar with *both* disorders. On the surface, it may seem that patients are depressed, or "just don't eat," but further inquiry reveals a complex set of intertwined physiologic and behavioral factors for consideration.

The term *cachexia* is derived from two roots: *kakos* meaning "bad," and *hexis* meaning "condition" (3). It is best defined as the advanced state of starvation resulting from both decreased food intake and hormonal/metabolic abnormalities characteristic of the interaction between the tumor and host. In the cachexia syndrome, there is a failure of spontaneous food intake to keep up with the extraordinarily high energy requirements imposed on the body by the tumor. It is defined as a hypermetabolic state in which the body requires a large amount of energy, and uses it faster than it can be replaced. Most of this energy is redirected by the malignant tissue for self-maintenance, diverting it from the patient himself or herself, who feels fatigued. Cachexia is far different from other hypermetabolic states seen in clinical practice such as pregnancy, exercise, cold exposure, and thyrotoxicosis. In the other hypermetabolic states, the increased energy requirements are coupled with an ability to concomitantly increase food intake. It is culturally acceptable, and often the source of much joking, for pregnant women to eat greater quantities of food, even in unusual combinations. Runners or cold-weather skiers celebrate special meals, usually high in carbohydrate, before an event. Patients with thyrotoxicosis report increased appetite and food intake. In cancer cachexia, the opposite phenomenon occurs. Psychological, social, mechanical, and physiologic changes all preclude the patients' ability to increase their food consumption.

The term "cancer cachexia" is habitually used interchangeably, and mistakenly, with the term "anorexia." *Anorexia* refers only to the diminished appetite or an aversion for food, from a physiologic and/or psychological cause. Unfortunately, use of the term anorexia in the context of cancer is often mistaken with anorexia nervosa. Anorexia nervosa is primarily a psychiatric disorder in which emotional conflicts manifest themselves as a refusal to maintain body weight by restricting food intake. Although it has psychological determinants, the cancer cachexia syndrome is not solely due to *anorexia*, or a patient's refusal to eat, but the synonymous use of terms may lead to that erroneous assumption. The overlap in this terminology may lead less sophisticated clinicians or family members and caregivers to reach the erroneous conclusion that anorexia or cachexia secondary to cancer has its roots in a refusal to eat because the patient emotionally suffers from cancer.

Another difference between these syndromes involves the concept of "body image." A patient with anorexia nervosa (who are overwhelmingly female) sees herself as "too fat" no matter how underweight she is, but a patient with cancer cachexia is quite aware of the weight loss, and is often embarrassed by it.

SYSTEMIC EFFECTS

The cachexia syndrome effects practically every organ system in the body. Cachectic patients are often anemic, with significant electrolyte imbalance. Sodium, potassium, magnesium, or calcium are often affected by the poor nutritional state. These abnormalities are largely responsible for the cancer-associated morbidity and mortality.

A cachectic patient appears ill. His skin is atrophic, and often shiny. It appears translucent. The body habitus is often described as "sunken in." This is noticeable especially in the face, with shrunken temporal fossae and cheeks with protuberant zygomata. Periorbital edema contributes to this change physiognomy. Bony protuberances are evident over the rest of the body. Usually muscular areas seem poorly toned.

Such a cachectic state puts the patient at increased risk for pneumonia, thromboemboli, heart failure, and death (4). Quality of life during this time is greatly affected. Patients describe themselves as feeling quite ill, unable to keep up with even limited social or vocational activities and unable to complete the most passive of diversionary activities. The sleep/wake cycle is often disrupted, with patients up at night, often worrying and making up for the lost sleep by dosing during the day, missing mealtimes.

CLINICAL FEATURES

Proper food intake depends upon a hearty appetite and a well-functioning gastrointestinal system. Appetite is the desire or longing to satisfy hunger. Having a good appetite and eating well is thought to a pleasurable experience. Good appetite relies on the ability to smell and taste properly. Cultural, social, and psychological factors can either encourage or discourage good eating.

Gastrointestinal System

Cancer itself, and surgery, chemotherapy, or radiation therapy affect optimal functioning of the gastrointestinal system. Good intake is stimulated by the body's ability to smell, taste, and see food. Head and neck cancers, or their treatment with chemotherapy and/or radiation, can cause a dryness of the mouth and nose, rendering the taste buds unable to detect the smells and tastes of food. Systemic chemotherapy commonly causes a change in the taste thresholds, often decreasing the tolerance for bitter foods and increasing the tolerance for sweet foods. Chemotherapy drugs themselves, or the dryness from the accompanying antiemetics, have been implicated in imparting a metallic taste in the mouth and to food. Mucositis and stomatitis from chemotherapy may render it difficult or painful to chew. This may extend further down the esophagus, further discouraging swallowing. Dryness can also result from parotid gland tumors. Esophageal dyskinesias are rare but known side effects of dopamine-blocking antiemetics, such as prochlorperazine or metoclopromide (5). They may interfere with proper swallowing or breathing.

Chewing and swallowing take a certain degree of effort, but are usually accomplished involuntarily, without much notice. This effort to chew and swallow seems magnified in debilitated patients. It is the beginning of the spiral in which one become more tired and fatigued as a result of not eating, then eats less, and less.

Early satiety, or a fullness after eating even a small meal, is a classic sign of pancreatic cancer and reported by many patients to a lesser degree during treatment for other types of cancer. Weakened peristalsis from debility slows gastric emptying. Autonomic failure and chronic nausea can delay transit even further. Corticosteroids, used as part of a treatment regimen or as an antiemetic, are known irritants to the gastric mucosa and further discourage eating. Steroids, as well as antibiotics, change the normal flora of the intestines, causing bacterial overgrowth and malabsorption. (At first, steroids may actually improve appetite, but the effect is mostly transient.) Narcotic analgesics, as well as anticholinergic drugs, slow peristalsis and may predispose a patient to an ileus. Obstruction along the GI tract from tumor, lymphadenopathy, or impacted stool may impede substances traveling through the lower gastrointestinal tract and make evacuation painful. This may further discourage eating of the necessary amount of food to maintain oneself in a hypermetabolic state.

It has been speculated that accumulation of trypto-phan and serotonin precursors in the brain may also downregulate appetite.

Learned Food Aversions

Aversions to favorite foods given immediately prior to emetogenic chemotherapy create a powerful association of those foods with the unpleasant gastrointestinal side effects. This learned aversion is a strong and quickly learned behavior. Bernstein (6) constructed an experimental model that paired a previously non-existent flavor of ice cream with emetogenic chemotherapy in children. These pediatric patients were less likely to eat the novel flavor weeks later, compared to those children exposed to the ice cream alone and chemotherapy alone, but not both.

Associations of certain foods with pungent tastes or smells may give the sensation of nausea upon even remembering the offensive stimulus without its presence. This subtle but known phenomenon further discourages eating of adequate amounts of food. Avoidance of one's "favorite" foods prior to therapy, or even eating a low-protein, high-carbohydrate disliked food will minimize the contribution of learned aversions and minimize its effect on the patient's general nutrition.

Social and Cultural Factors

In addition to the profound fatigue that can discourage eating, the social milieu and individual psychological traits lend a complex overlay to this process. Among the many cultures that make up the world's population, gathering and preparation of foodstuffs, as well as eating and enjoying them, is a universal element of our social and family lives. Patients who find they are unable to eat the same variety of foods as usual or eat without the usual gusto, may find themselves excluded or feel sidelined from the social activities associated with food.

Family members and care givers who comprise the social network sense this and continue to encourage a patient to eat. By doing so, the social milieu is perpetuated, and the effect of the patient's illness on the group is minimized. With the reliance on more technological cancer treatment, family members feel excluded, playing a less active role in the day-to-day treatments. Often, one of their only remaining contributions involves encouraging a patient to eat, even after the patient is unable to do so. Patients respond by saying, or indicating in some way, that they are "too tired" to eat. Intuitively, care givers are reasonably concerned by the appearance of someone with cancer cachexia, and realize that a malnourished state is a bad prognostic sign. The concerned observer, emotionally attached to the patient, often sees this as a sign that the patient is "giving up," and wants to do what is necessary to retain an optimistic stance. Eating and food become the natural arena for this divergence and a difficult scenario often results. The more a care giver wants the patient to eat, the more frustrated and angry they may get with a patient too tired or too distressed to eat, or when eating becomes uncomfortable. Well meaning care givers may go so far as to chide a patient and insist that they eat, beyond the individual's capabilities. It is not unusual to see care givers at the bedside, haranguing patients to eat, or even "force-feeding" the patient as one would when an infant is being switched from liquid formula to solid food. It is not a surprise that this strategy often backfires when the coercion stimulates the patient to be oppositional. The fear of losing the patient at all or prematurely is a powerful, emotionally charged incentive, and can stimulate strong, driven actions. The patient experiences eating as a chore, rather than a pleasurable experience.

Adventuresome patients or care givers and those patients who reject traditional medical approaches to cancer treatment may turn to "alternative" treatments in an effort to gain control over unresponsive cancer. These approaches include high doses of vitamins and minerals, or special diets needing extensive preparation. These plans frequently necessitate ingesting large quantities of protein or vegetable-based foods and success is also limited by cachexia. At times, this may frustrate a patient even more and further discourage adequate nutrition.

Psychological Factors

As part of the "usual and expectable" reaction to cancer, patients often feel angry and begin to anticipate the disability brought on by illness. During the initial period after diagnosis, and even before treatment, patients describe a drop-off in appetite and interest in food. Discouragement and fear lessen participation and enjoyment in usually pleasurable activities, including eating. For most patients, this is transient and the motivation to eat returns as a treatment course is defined and some degree of hopefulness is attained. Depending upon the tumor load and treatment regimen, this level of motivation to eat well continues throughout the course of cancer illness until its late stages. Patients frequently comment that they need to maintain or even increase their weight and appetite, in case they do not respond to treatment, when they expect to lose weight. Some patients will imply or say that they are fearful to lose weight because it is a "bad" sign.

Patients themselves often suffer emotionally if or when they experience a diminished ability to exert control over the physiologic factors that overpower their desire. Control is ceded to chemotherapy or radiation scheduling and routines. Those used to being active at work or home find that they cannot keep up with their usual schedule, reinforcing the sense of loss of control.

Patients who report that they are too tired to eat are often thought to be suffering from a depressive disorder, from expectable dysphoria to major depression. Poor appetite and weight loss are usual signs and symptoms of at least a moderately depressed mood in the physically healthy. Poor appetite and intake are common systemic effects of cancer. It is often difficult to differentiate whether the symptoms are due to cancer, its treatment, or a treatable adjustment disorder or major depression, or a combination of these factors. Certain cancers, such as pancreatic cancer or gastric cancer, have historically been associated with depression (7).

No standard exists to make this differential diagnosis. What may help to differentiate the etiology of poor appetite and low oral intake is assessment of the patient's motivation to eat, and the level of enjoyment associated with eating. Patients who *want* to eat more but cannot because of fatigue, GI disturbance, or sensory changes are *less* likely to have a depression responsive to antidepressants than patients who have the ability to eat but lack the desire or motivation to do so. Inquiring about the patient's motivational state, differentiating it from the ability to eat, may provide another piece of data. Asking a patient, "Is it that you don't *want* to eat, or just *can't?*" or asking the patient to name his or her favorite food prepared in the favorite way and then imagine it in front of them and noting the reaction (excitement, interest, disgust, nausea, retching) may also help assess motivational factors. The presence of motivation to eat speaks *against* depression as a significant determining cause. A history of "affective" disorders such as major depression or substance abuse in oneself or closely related blood relatives is an additional historical fact that would sway the clinician toward treatment of depression when it is hard to determine its contribution to the patient's weight loss.

Assessing the ability to eat, without the desire to do so, is a way to differentiate the constitutional effects of illness or treatment from a depression likely to improve with pharmacologic and/or psychotherapeutic treatment.

Anxiety beyond what is part of the usual and expectable reaction to cancer illness and treatment may also provide a further diagnostic dilemma. Dysphagia and dyspepsia are often symptoms of anxiety in physically healthy patients. In cancer illness, physiologically driven symptoms may be worsened by generalized or situational anxiety. Anxiolytics, particularly short-acting benzodiazepines given 30 minutes preprandially, can offer a modicum of relaxation, allowing a patient to eat with less distress. Cisapride (Propulsid) is a prokinetic drug (an agent that restores, normalizes, and facilitates mobility throughout the length of the gastrointestinal tract) (8). It is a substituted piperidinyl benzamide, chemically related to metoclopramide, with significant cholinergic activity. Unlike metoclopramide, cisapride does not have any dopamine-blocking activity and is largely devoid of central depressant effects. The usual adult dose is 10–20 mg q.i.d., 15 minutes before meals and bedtime. Although it may cause cramps, flatulence, and dry mouth, it has not been associated with extrapyramidal side effects as has metoclopramide (9). Its cholinergic properties account for its usefulness in gastric stasis and, secondarily, it speeds food transit when anxiety subjectively delays movement of food through the gastrointestinal system.

MECHANISMS OF CACHEXIA

A multitude of metabolic changes, as well as the effects of hormones and cytokines, are implicated in the development of cancer cachexia (10–12).

Our nutritional needs are met by combinations of three major classes of nutrients: carbohydrates, proteins, and fats. Their metabolism is aided by certain vitamins and minerals as cofactors. "Simple" carbohydrates come in the form of natural or synthetic sugars, such as glucose. "Complex" carbohydrates in the form of starches, together with simple sugars, provide the main source of energy for the body once metabolized. As the common unit of energy, glucose is stored as glycogen in the liver and muscle cells. Proteins are stored in the body as their building blocks, amino acids. The small amount of stored glucose is supplemented by glucose created from proteins, through an energy-demanding process called gluconeogenesis. This takes place in the liver, but uses proteins from other tissues, such as muscle and lung. They form a secondary energy source. Lastly, our bodies use fats as an energy source. Fats require the most work to break down, so they are the last to be accessed. The energy needed for this process comes mostly from freeing the building blocks of body fat, which is an energy inefficient system. In cachexia the body expends such a great deal of energy perpetuating these process that it has little energy left for contraction of voluntary muscle and digestion, further decreasing the amount of food the body can take in to replace the nutrients it is using up.

When needed by the body, glycogen is turned into glucose in both brain and red blood cells to supply each part of the body. Both tumor cells and healthy cells can get energy from glycogen to make glucose. When glycogen stores are depleted, protein sources are accessed next. Proteins can also be used by healthy tissue and tumor cells. Fats, digested through an extended metabolic loop, are more useful to healthy tissue than tumor cells. This observation could account for the lack of muscle and poor tone of a patient with advanced cancer. Control of this system has been owed to a variety of substances. Hormonal control depends on the actions of thyroid hormone (13), growth hormone, somatostatin, and an altered insulin response (14). Metabolic control has also been ascribed to tumor necrosis factor (15), cachectin (16), interleukin-1 and interleukin-6 (17), somatostatin, vasopressin, and prostaglandin E_2 (18). The neurotransmitter serotonin has also been implicated in the control of hunger and feeding (19).

The body's normal response to insulin is also changed by cancer and its treatment. A decreased insulin response to dietary load of carbohydrate further exacerbates the energy lost in sustaining both healthy and cancer tissues (20), Because, for most patients, the longest food-free interval is at night, patients have a relative hyperglycemia except in the morning. The daytime, minor increase in blood sugar further discourages appetite. This phenomenon correlates with the usual clinical observation that breakfast is the most desirable meal of the day for patients with advanced disease.

HIV-Related Cachexia

Recent attention has been given to the cachexia syndrome associated with the human immunodeficiency virus (HIV). Often called the "AIDS wasting syndrome," it has also been attributed, until recently, to elevated levels of resting energy expenditure, occurring during episodes of active viremia or viral latency (21). Weight loss is not automatic with HIV infection, and is most prominent with active secondary (opportunistic) infections. Cachexia can be the most disabling symptom of HIV, and has only recently qualified a patient for federal disability benefits, after a much publicized political struggle.

Wasting with HIV has most recently been associated with the cytokine, tumor necrosis factor (TNF), also known as "cachectin." This catabolic substance is thought to cause HIV cachexia. The most recently developed theory concludes, in contrast to models of cancer cachexia, that the total energy expenditure is actually *reduced*, not elevated. The prime determinant of weight loss in HIV-associated wasting is a direct result of diminished food consumption.

Two drug treatments routinely used for cancer patients, megestrol acetate and dronabinol, are formally approved by the Food and Drug Administration to be used in HIV wasting to improve appetite.

TREATMENT

Making small quantities of food, including nutritional supplements, available throughout the day and night, is the simplest intervention for this vexing situation, but may not be a sufficient solution.

Treatment of cancer cachexia has centered around three modalities: pharmacologic, nutritional supplementation (enteral and parenteral), and behavioral.

Pharmacologic Treatment

Various drugs are used to stimulate appetite and forestall weight loss in cancer cachexia (22–24). None has been uniquely developed or has cancer cachexia as its primary indication, but they are commonly used for this purpose. The use of each drug capitalizes on the normally unwanted side effect of weight gain or appetite stimulation. Two of the medications have undergone controlled trials and have received formal approval for HIV-related cachexia and anorexia. The medications that are commonly used include progestational agents (megestrol acetate, Megace®) cannaboids (dronabinol, Marinol®) corticosteroids (prednisone, dexamethasone and others), and serotonin antagonist (cyproheptadine, Periactin®). Less often used are tricyclic antidepressants and neuroleptic/antipsychotic agents.

Megestrol acetate has been tested in clinical trials in cancer (25). Originally prescribed in patients to oppose the estrogenic promotion of breast cancer, the weight gain it induced discouraged continued use in some women. In tests by the Cancer and Leukemia Group B and others (26–28) in a dose-escalation trial, doses between 160 mg and 800 mg per day provided an increase in weight, and sense of well-being that improved general quality of life. Reformulated as a liquid concentrate of 800 mg/20 ml, its use avoids swallowing up to twenty 40 mg tablets, a difficult task for a cachectic patient. Vascular side effects of pulmonary embolus or arterial thrombosis are known but rare. Peripheral fluid retention may limit long term use in some patients. Both male and postmenopausal female patients with hormone-insensitive tumors such as lung or colon tumors, may benefit from its use. Surprisingly, men do not develop female secondary sex characteristics of consequence. It may suppress the action of cachectin (or tumor necrosis factor) in its action.

Dronabinol, a congener of cannabis, has been swathed in the political controversy to license drugs considered illicit and with a high potential for abuse. It is approved for use in refractory nausea and vomiting caused by cancer chemotherapy and to stimulate appetite in HIV wasting. Likewise, it is purported to decrease intraocular pressure in refractory glaucoma. Dose ranges of 2.5 to 10 mg p.o. t.i.d. have been used in cachexia. Those patients who previously avoided the recreational use of cannabis because of its disinhibiting properties similarly dislike its effects when therapeutically prescribed. Concomitant mood improvement has been reported, and this effect is probably responsible for its action.

Corticosteroids, such as prednisone and dexamethasone, are routinely used in cancer treatment as adjuvant analgesics and antiemetics. Most patients feel a sense of well being, increased appetite and strength, and insomnia during the initial few days of use. Prolonged use of corticosteroids has resulted in delirium, mood change (depression or mania) or psychosis, osteoporosis, weakness of the proximal muscle groups, and immunosuppression. Its mechanism of action is undetermined, but the effect is speculated to be a change in prostaglandin modulation. Dosages used are small, such as 10–20 mg per day of prednisone or methylprednisolone, or 4–6 mg per day of dexamethasone. A randomized double-blind cross-over trial by Bruera confirmed its efficacy, but others (29) believe that the improvement in oral intake may not be seen in patients with cancer as it is with other underlying diseases, and that the muscle deterioration from exaggerated protein requirements that it imposes on the body negates its beneficial effects.

Another drug, hydrazine sulfate has been tested in three randomized trials sponsored by the National Cancer Institute. Hydrazine, often mistaken for the homonymous antihypertensive hydralazine hydrochloride, inhibits phosphoenolpyruvate carboxykinase an enzyme in the gluconeogenic pathway, preventing the breakdown of glycogen to glucose. First used as a cytotoxic agent itself in Russia, it had never been shown to be effective in U.S. trials. Recent trials (30–33) found no survival advantage or appetite or weight gain, and increased fatigue and neuropathy. There was likewise no improvement in quality of life with the drug's use.

Cyproheptadine has been tested in healthy, underweight adults. Blocking both histamine and serotonin,

it is effective for allergic and anaphylactoid states. On the theory that 5-hydroxytryptamine (5-HT, or serotonin) agonists decrease hunger and food intake, a 5HT antagonists should encourage appetite and intake (34). Noble (35) reported a 5%–7% increase in weight and a significant increase in appetite after 42 days' use. In patients with primary anorexia nervosa, both Carroll (36) and Halmi (37) reported beneficial effects of up to 32 mg/day for 3 days and 8 weeks, respectively. In this group, sedation was reported as a transient side effect, but in patients with cancer, who are more fatigued, the sedation has been the most common reason to discontinue the drug when used off protocol for cachexia.

Other medications with the untoward effect of weight gain have not been tested in clinical trials. For both neuroleptics and tricyclic antidepressants, weight gain has been one of the main factors that limited compliance in the treatment of primary psychiatric disorders (38,39). A 28 pound weight gain was reported with an unspecified dose of amitriptyline, as well as a mean weight gain of 5.5 pounds at the mean dose of 123 mg per day through 9 months of treatment (40,41). Carbohydrate craving was also reported (42).

Weight gain has also been reported with depot fluphenazine (43), oral chlorpromazine, (44) and the "novel" antipsychotics clozapine and risperidone (45).

Use of these agents seems limited by a lack of experience and safety in patients with cancer without a comorbid psychotic or depressive disorder. Patients are often started on a tricyclic antidepressant, such as amitriptyline, as an adjuvant analgesic or for neuropathic pain from chemotherapy or herpes zoster, so these "side" effects may be helpful to those patients.

Pentoxifylline (Trental®) is a substituted methylxanthine similar to both caffeine and aminophylline and is licensed for use as a vasodilator in intermittent claudication. It has been reported to suppress tumor necrosis factor, postulated to be excessive in 50% of patients with cancer who exhibit clinically active disease (46). Trials in HIV cachexia are being conducted.

Nutritional Supplementation (Enteral and Parenteral)
Supplementation can be achieved orally, via enteral tube feedings (nasogastric, nasojejunal, feeding gastrostomy or "peg"), or via a parenteral route (via a central or peripherally inserted catheter.

Parenteral Feedings. Tube feedings are delivered by gravity or with the aid of a computer-controlled pump. Special, more dilute preparations are used. Volume of the feedings is increased gradually as tolerance builds.

The introduction of artificial parenteral nutritional supplementation in the 1970s brought new optimism to treatment of cancer cachexia (47). It was hoped that the ability to feed patients without relying on appetite and bypassing the mouth and upper GI tract would afford new options for improved survival. Smaller nasogastric and gastrostomy tubes, and computer-directed intravenous delivery systems have been developed and are currently in use. Despite more than 50 prospective randomized trials, the benefits of parenteral nutrition have yet to be proven (48). Total parenteral nutrition seems best indicated when there is a good response to cancer treatment and patients cannot provide themselves with adequate calories by the traditional routes, resulting in life-threatening complications from the cachexia rather than the cancer illness itself (49). The high incidence of infection systemically or at the entrance site of the catheter, as well as cost and availability, has precluded its widespread use (50).

Oral Route. Patients unable to consume the standard hospital food are frequently given "full liquid" or "clear liquid" diets. These are used temporarily before tests or procedures, but lack adequate calories and protein for sustained use. Commercially prepared oral supplements are used at mealtimes or in between. Most of these preparations contain carbohydrates, proteins, and easily digested lipids, vitamins, and minerals. Many are "hydrolyzed" or predigested, lactose-free, and have low residue or bulk, so they are easy to metabolize but could worsen diarrhea.

Behavioral Treatment

Behavioral interventions have also been used to encourage patients to eat a wider variety of foods and in larger quantities to slow down the development of cachexia.

An optimal approach is to prepare small meals to be eaten or snacked often through the course of the day, keeping food and oral nutritional supplements within easy reach, and reinforcing the patient with gentle reminders. This tactic seems to preserve whatever attraction remains associated with eating.

Respecting the powerful influence of learned food aversions, avoiding foods associated with chemotherapy, radiation therapy, or any related experience the patient has found disturbing will eliminate its influence. "Indulging" in previously avoided foods, if a patient had been on a low-cholesterol or fat-free diet, will further augment oral intake, unless there is a remote medical contraindication. Including patients

in mealtime activities, perhaps sitting with others while they are eating, or even in meal preparation if their stamina permits, maintains the social aspects of eating rituals.

REFERENCES

1. Nixon DW, Heymsfield SB, Cohen AE, et al. Protein-calorie undernutrition in hospitalized cancer patients. *Am J Med.* 1980; 68:683–690.
2. Warren S. The immediate cause of death in cancer. *Am J Med Sci.* 1932; 184:610–613.
3. Nelson KA, Walsh D, Sheehan FA. The cancer anorexia–cachexia syndrome. *J Clin Oncol.* 1994; 12:213–225.
4. Stein K, Mastekaasa A, Lund E. Prognostic factors for patients with inoperable non-small lung cancer, limited disease. *Radiother Oncol.* 1989; 15:235–242.
5. Breitbart W. Tardive dyskinesia associated with high-dose intravenous metoclopramide. *N Engl J Med.* 1986; 315(8): 518–519.
6. Bernstein IL. Etiology of anorexia in cancer. *Cancer.* 1986; 58:1881–1886.
7. Holland JC, Korzun AH, Tross S, Silberfarb P, Perry M, Comis R, Oster M. Comparative psychological disturbance in patients with pancreatic and gastric cancer. *Am J Psychiatry* 1986; 143(8):982–986.
8. Van Nuelen JM, Leysen JE, et al. Cholingeric vs dopaminergic properties of prokinetic substituted benzamides with gastrointestinal prokinetic activity. *Gastroenterology.* 1985; 88:1623.
9. Fleishman SB, Lavin MR, Sattler M, Szarka H. Antiemetic-induced akathisia in cancer patients receiving chemotherapy. *Am J Psychiatry.* 1994; 151(5):763–765.
10. Heber D, Byerley LO, Chi J, et al. Pathophysiology of malnutrition in the adult cancer patient. *Cancer.* 1986; 58:1867–1873.
11. Theologidis, A. Cancer cachexia. *Cancer.* 1979; 43:2004–2012.
12. Dills, WL Jr. Nutritional and physiological consequences of tumor glycolysis. *Parasitology.* 1993; 107: Suppl S177–S186.
13. Perrson H, Bennegard K, Lundberg P, Svaninger G, Lundholm K. Thyroid hormones in conditions of chronic malnutrition. *Ann Surg.* 1985; 1(201):45–52.
14. Bartlett DL, Charland S, Torosian MH. Growth hormone, insulin, and somatostatin therapy of cancer cachexia. *Cancer.* 1994; 73(5):1499–1504.
15. Parks RR, Yan S-D, Huang C-C. Tumor necrosis factor-alpha production in human head and neck squamous cell carcinoma. *Laryngoscope.* 1994; 104:860.
16. Beutler B, Cerami A. Cachectin: more than a tumor necrosis factor. *N Engl J Med.* 1987; 316:379–385.
17. Keller U. Pathophysiology of cancer cachexia. *Support Care Cancer.* 1993; 1:290–294.
18. Siddiqui RA, Williams JF. Tentative identification of the toxohormones of cancer cachexia: roles of vasopressin, prostaglandin E2 and cachectin-TNF. *Biochem Int.* 1990; 20(4):787–797.
19. Silverstone T, Goodall E. Serotoninergic mechanisms in human feeding: the pharmacological evidence. *Appetite Supplement.* 1986; 7:85–97.

20. Rofe AM, Bourgeois CS, Coyle P. Altered insulin response to glucose in weight-losing cancer patients. *Anticancer Res.* 1994; 14(2B):647–650.
21. Bell SJ, Mascioli EA, Forse RA. Nutrition support and the human immunodeficiency virus (HIV). *Parasitology.* 1993; 107:S53–S67.
22. Bruera E. Current pharmacological management of anorexia in cancer patients. *Oncology.* 1992; 6(1):125–137.
23. Delmore G. Fighting cancer cachexia—what about today's armory? *Support Care Cancer.* 1993; 1:283–284.
24. Bruera E. Is the pharmacological treatment of cancer cachexia possible? *Support Care Cancer.* 1993; 1:298–304.
25. Aisner J, Simon Tchekmedyian N, Tait N, Parnes H, Novak M. Studies of high-dose megestrol acetate: potential applications in cachexia. *Semin Oncol.* 15(2 pt. 1):68–75.
26. Abrams JS, Cirrincione C, Aisner J, et al., for the Cancer and Leukemia Group B (CALGB). A phase III dose-response trial of megestrol acetate (MA) in metastatic breast cancer (MBC). *Proc. ASCO.* 1992; 11:56 [Abstract no. 50].
27. Kornblith AB, Hollis D, Phillips CA, et al., for the Cancer and Leukemia Group B (CALGB). Effect of megestrol acetate upon quality of life in advanced breast cancer patients in a dose response trial. *Proc. ASCO.* 1992; 11:377 [Abstract no. 1305]
28. Simon Tchekmedyian N, Tait N, Moody M, Aisner J. High dose megestrol acetate a possible treatment for cachexia. *J Am Med Assoc.* 1987; 257(a):1195–1198.
29. Ottery FD. Cancer cachexia: prevention, early diagnosis, and management. *Cancer Pract.* 1994; 2(2):123–131.
30. Herbert V. Three stakes in hydrazine sulfate's heart, but questionable cancer remedies, like vampires, always rise again. *J Clin Oncol.* 1994; 12(6):1107–1108.
31. Kosty MP, Fleishman SB, Herndon II JE, et al. Cisplatin, vinblastine, and hydrazine sulfate in advanced non-small-cell lung cancer: a randomized placebo-controlled, double-blind phase III study of the cancer and leukemia group B. *J Clin Oncol.* 1994; 12:1113–1120.
32. Loprinzi CL, Goldberg RM, Su JQ et al. Placebo-controlled trial of hydrazine sulfate in patients with newly diagnosed non-small-cell lung cancer. *J Clin Oncol.* 1994; 12:1126–1129.
33. Loprinzi CL, Kuross SA, O'Fallon JR, et al. Randomized placebo-controlled evaluation of hydrazine sulfate in patients with advanced colorectal cancer. *J Clin Oncol.* 1994; 12:1121–1125.
34. Bond WS, Crabbe S, Sanders MC. Pharmacotherapy of eating disorders: a critical review. *Drug Intell Clin Pharm.* 1986; 20:659–665.
35. Noble RE. Effect of cyproheptadine on appetite and weight gain. *J Am Med Assoc.* 1969; 209(13):2054–2055.
36. Carroll BJ. Effects of cyproheptadine anorexia nervosa. *Psychopharm Bull.* 1980; 16(2):29–30.
37. Halmi KA, Eckert E, Falik JR. Cypropheptadine, An antidepressant and weight-inducing drug for anorexia nervosa. *Psychoparm Bull.* 1983; 19(1):103–105.
38. Balon R, et al. Changes in appetite and weight during the pharmacological treatment of patients with panic disorder from Lafayette Clinic, Detroit Mich. *Can J Psychol.* 1993 (Feb.); 38:19–22.
39. Lawson WB, Karson CN. Clinical correlates of body weight changes in schizophrenia. *J Neuropsychiatry.* 1994; 6:187–188.
40. Arenillas L. Amitriptyline and body-weight. *Lancet.* 1994(Feb. 22); 432–433.
41. Winston F, McCann ML. Antidepressant drugs and excessive weight gain. *Br J Psychiatry.* 1972; 120: 693–697.
42. Paykel ES, Mueller PS, De La Vergne PM. Amitriptyline, weight gain and carbohydrate craving: a side effect. *Br J Psychiatry.* 1973; 123:501–507.
43. Marriott P, Pansa M, Hiep A. Depot fluphenazine maintenance treatment and associated weight changes. *Comp Psychol.* 1981; 22(3): 320–325.
44. Cookson JC. *Current Approaches to Psychoses.* Amsterdam: Excerpta Medica Communications; 1995: 9–10.
45. Ames D, Harmon L, Berisford MA, et al. Weight gain with atypical antipsychotics. *Biol Ther Psychiatry Newsletter.* 1995 (Jan.): 3–4.
46. Dezube BJ, Sherman ML, Fridovich-Keil JL, Allen-Ryan J, Pardee AB. Down-regulation of tumor necrosis factor expression by pentoxifylline in cancer patients: A pilot study. *Cancer Immunol Immunother.* 1993; 36:57–60.
47. Keymling M. Technical aspects of enteral nutrition. *Gut Supplement.* 1994; 1:S77–S80.
48. Bloch AS. Feeding the cancer patient: where have we come from, where are we going? *Nutr Clin Pract.* 1994; 9(3):87–89.
49. The Veterans Affairs Total Parenteral Nutrition Cooperative Study Group. Perioperative total parenteral nutrition in surgical patients. *N Engl J Med.* 1991; 325:525–532.
50. Ziegler TR, Wilmore DW. Enteral and parenteral nutrition in hospital patients. In Dale DC, Federman DD eds. *Scientific American Medicine.* New York: Scientific American, 1995; 4-XIII-17.

40

Nausea and Vomiting

GARY R. MORROW, JOSEPH A. ROSCOE, AND JANE T. HICKOK

Nausea and vomiting (NV) are among the most frequently reported as well as the most troublesome adverse effects of cancer chemotherapy, and have remained prevalent despite the use of increasingly potent antiemetic medications (1,2). Approximately 60% of patients develop nausea and 50% report vomiting following chemotherapy. Patients with cancer may postpone chemotherapy or refuse it completely because of fear of these side effects, and those who initiate treatment may be unable or unwilling to tolerate their full course because of NV (3–14). Problems associated with NV extend beyond discomfort and embarrassment and can include physical complications such as fatigue, muscle strain, esophageal tears and the occurrence of metabolic alkalosis caused by the loss of sodium, potassium, or gastric acid. Psychologic disabilities may also result, including the development of anticipatory nausea and vomiting (ANV), food aversions, disruption of ability to function on a daily basis, lessening of emotional well-being, and impairment of overall quality of life. Inadequate caloric intake resulting from NV can also aggravate the cachexia, lethargy, fatigue, and weakness often caused by the disease process (6,11,12,15,16).

PATTERNS OF CHEMOTHERAPY-RELATED NAUSEA AND VOMITING

Nausea and vomiting are separate entities and should not be considered as a single side effect of cancer chemotherapy. We have shown that nausea, like retching, can occur independently of vomiting, and its frequency, severity, and duration are separable phenomena (17). Nausea is a subjective, unpleasant feeling that may signal imminent vomiting. Patients view nausea control as more important than control of emesis (18,19), while physicians and nurses judge emesis control more important to antiemetic efficacy than nausea control (19). Nausea is accompanied by changes in

autonomic nervous system activity, particularly parasympathetic activity, diminished gastric tone and reduced peristalsis. Subsequently, the contents of the intestines reflux into the stomach as a result of retrograde duodenal peristalsis (20). Retching is a synchronized movement of the diaphragm and chest wall and abdominal muscles that occurs before or after vomiting. While nausea is entirely subjective, emesis is entirely objective since it is the forceful emptying of the gastric contents via the sustained action of abdominal muscles and the opening of the gastric cardia (21).

Chemotherapy-related NV may occur prior to chemotherapy as ANV or immediately following chemotherapy as acute symptoms, or it may first present a substantial time after treatment (22). Acute nausea and vomiting usually occur within 1–4 hours of treatment and may resolve within 24 hours (Fig. 40–1). Delayed nausea and vomiting first occur at least 24 hours and sometimes even days after cytotoxic therapy. Careful examination of the pattern of emesis after chemotherapy with cisplatin suggests that delayed emesis may occur as two separate phases that follow the initial acute phase (23). These have been termed the intermediate and late phases of delayed emesis.

NV symptoms that develop during or after chemotherapy are generally assumed to be caused by the pharmacologic action of chemotherapy agents. However, nausea, vomiting, and anxiety are also known to develop in patients owing to a conditioned or learned response to chemotherapy. These conditioned responses can manifest prior to treatments as ANV and also during or after chemotherapy treatments, when the conditioned symptoms cannot be distinguished clinically from those due to the pharmacologic effects of the drugs (7,9,24–29). Among the data supporting this view is the rather curious fact that NV symptoms generally increase as the number of chemotherapy treatments increases. This finding runs counter to the usual physiologic response

476

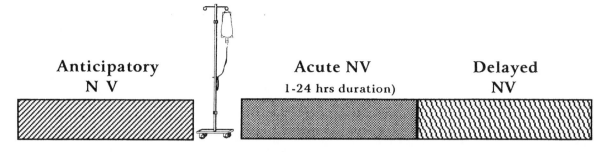

FIG. **40-1.** Phases of nausea and vomiting (NV) associated with chemotherapy.

pattern in which repeated stimulation generally leads over time to a decreased response.

PHYSIOLOGY OF NAUSEA AND VOMITING

While the sensory and motor pathways for vomiting are becoming better delineated, the mechanisms of nausea remain not well understood (30,31). Nausea is mediated by the autonomic nervous system and is accompanied by flushing, perspiration, pallor, gastric stasis, and tachycardia (32). Retching and vomiting, on the other hand, are coordinated through the somatic nervous system. A variety of anatomical systems and organs contribute to the expression of NV through a coordinating center or common pathway. A likely candidate for this coordinating center is a topographically distinct area in the lateral reticular formation in the floor of the fourth ventricle, which has been called "the emetic center" (33).

This final coordinating area receives input from a variety of "systems." There are neuropathways from the limbic system and the cerebrum, that may be involved in the mechanism by which some people experience NV in response to psychological stimuli like stress or emotional upset. The pathway also makes possible the psychological development of anticipatory symptoms. The emetic center also receives input from the vestibular system — a potent input most familiar to those sensitive to motion sickness from cars, planes, boats, or amusement park rides. A third input is from the area postrema located bilaterally in the floor of the fourth ventricle. This unique neural structure is exposed to both cerebrospinal fluid and circulating blood and thus has been implicated as a sensor for chemotherapeutic agents (34).

The two elements at the bottom of the diagram may be involved both in the stimulation of NV and in some type of feedback activity. There are neuroreceptors in the gastrointestinal tract with afferents to the emetic center. Several chemotherapeutic agents may achieve

their primary stimulation through this route. Further connections with the periphery may facilitate the expression of some of the autonomic characteristics associated with nausea and vomiting — skin pallor, temperature changes, and alterations in heart rate and respiration.

Early research showed that antiemetics (typically phenothiazines and butyrophenones) blocked dopamine receptors (7,35,36). Metoclopramide, a substituted benzamide, has been widely used as an antiemetic drug for more than 27 years and was originally believed to act solely by blocking dopamine receptors in the chemoreceptor trigger zone (CTZ) (37–39). However, its efficacy against the severe emetogenic effects of chemotherapeutic agents such as cisplatin was very limited. As a consequence, high-dose metoclopramide was introduced and proved to be more effective against cisplatin-induced emesis (40). This important development led to the conclusion that some mechanism other than dopamine receptor blockade might be producing the antiemetic effect. Within five years it was shown that high-dose metoclopramide exerted an additional antiemetic effect by its action on 5-hydroxytryptamine (5-HT$_3$) receptors located on gut neurons (41). This discovery of the role of 5-HT$_3$ receptors in the emetic response to cytotoxic drugs eventually led to the introduction of the highly specific 5-HT$_3$ receptor antagonists, which are increasingly used for the treatment of chemotherapy-induced emesis (7).

The mechanisms of antiemetic action of the 5-HT$_3$ receptor antagonists are currently being investigated (42). In early studies, two distinct areas of the central nervous system, the emetic center and the CTZ (7), appeared to mediate vomiting. However, the lack of antiemetic effect of the 5-HT$_3$ receptor antagonists against emesis induced by dopamine and opiate receptor agonists, which act via the area postrema, argues against any mechanism of action involving the emetic center (42). Recent studies in the ferret model suggest that the major site of antiemetic activity of 5-HT$_3$ receptor antagonists is on vagal afferent terminals in the upper small intestine, although central vagal sites may also be involved (43,44).

PATIENT CHARACTERISTICS AFFECTING NAUSEA AND VOMITING

Anticipatory Nausea and Vomiting

Approximately one in three cancer patients receiving chemotherapy develops anticipatory nausea, usually by the 4th treatment session (2,5,7,9,11,16,26,28, 45–49). By contrast, anticipatory emesis develops in only about 10% of patients (16,45,46,49,50). ANV does not occur without the prior development of post-chemotherapy NV (5,7,8,9,15,16,29,45,48,49,51). It is thought to be a conditioned response provoked by such factors as the sight, sound and smell of the clinic or the presence of the chemotherapy nurse (2,3,7,9,11,16,28,32,45,48,52,53). Anxiety may act as a mediating factor to facilitate conditioning (1–3,16,28,29,49,50,54–56). Although these effects are common, most patients are noticeably reluctant to mention them spontaneously, since they typically feel they are "losing their minds."

Antiemetics do not control ANV once it has developed, and indeed have been found by some investigators to paradoxically increase symptoms (7,11,16,28,46,50), perhaps by acting as conditioned stimuli themselves (46). Once developed, ANV does not appear to improve spontaneously (11,46).

Patients with fewer than three of the eight characteristics listed in Table 40.1 have been found unlikely to develop ANV (2,16,57). These characteristics may help screen patients following their first chemotherapy treatment to determine their potential to develop anticipatory side effects. Enhanced efforts at emetic control along with early intervention with behavioral techniques may be warranted for patients considered to be particularly at risk (1,3,45,50,58,59).

Posttreatment Nausea and Vomiting

A number of factors other than the emetogenicity of the drug itself (14) can influence the incidence and severity of both acute and delayed NV following chemotherapy. The degree of acute emesis observed is influenced by the patient's susceptibility to emesis (57,60), previous experience of drug-induced emesis (61), patient age (16,62), and history of alcohol abuse (63,64) (Table 40.2). Similar factors are implicated in the etiology of delayed emesis, but the mechanisms responsible may be different. Research has suggested that patients who expect chemotherapy to produce nausea are also more likely to report it as a side effect than those who do not (65–67).

CHEMOTHERAPEUTIC AGENTS AND NAUSEA AND VOMITING

There is a generally held belief that severe NV symptoms are inevitable consequences of cancer chemotherapy. This is clearly not true; the emetogenic potential of chemotherapeutic agents varies widely. Cisplatin, for example, is severely emetogenic, whereas bleomycin causes very few emetogenic effects (68). Table 40.3 summarizes the emetogenic potential of several commonly used chemotherapeutic agents.

The dosage of the chemotherapeutic agent significantly affects its emetogenicity. In the case of cisplatin, for example, the emetic effects of low doses of the drug may be prevented with certain traditional antiemetics, but higher doses are often refractory to even the most potent traditional antiemetics. The route of administration may also have an effect. Unfortunately, the emetogenic potential of combinations of chemotherapeutic agents is frequently greater than that of any single agent. Modern cancer chemotherapy regimens almost invariably contain several agents.

TABLE 40.1. *Patient Characteristics Associated with the Development of Anticipatory Nausea and Vomiting*

Age less than 50

Nausea/vomiting after last chemotherapy session

Posttreatment nausea described as "moderate, severe, or intolerable"

Posttreatment vomiting described as "moderate, severe, or intolerable"

Feeling warm or hot all over after last chemotherapy session

Susceptibility to motion sickness

Sweating after last chemotherapy session

Generalized weakness after last chemotherapy session

Source: Morrow (7).

TABLE 40.2. *Characters Affecting Nausea and Vomiting*

History of heavy alcohol intake decreases nausea and vomiting

Susceptibility to motion sickness increases nausea and vomiting

Poor previous emetic control increases nausea and vomiting

Expectations that treatments will cause nausea increases nausea

Younger patients have increased anticipatory nausea and vomiting and increased incidence of dystonic reactions

Source: Adapted from Morrow (7).

TABLE 40.3. *Relative Emetogenic Potential of Chemotherapeutic Agents (potency based on usual doses)*

Mild	Moderate	Severe
Bleomycin	Mitomycin C	Cisplatin
Vincristine	Duxorubicin (bolus)	Dacarbazine
Vinblastine	5-Fluorouracil (bolus)	Streptozotocin
Daunorubicin	Cyclophosphamide	Carmustine
6-Mercaptopurine	Cytarabine	Procarbazine
Melphalan		
5-Fluorouracil (infusion)		
Duxorubicin (infusion)		
Methotrexate		

Source: Morrow et al. (84).

NV symptoms occur at different times following the administration of different agents. In the case of cisplatin, for example, nausea and vomiting usually begin within the first 4 hours following chemotherapy, reach a peak between 4 and 10 hours, and subside by 24 hours (69). Emetic effects of some drugs (e.g. carmustine) can begin within 30 minutes, whereas others, such as cyclophosphamide, produce maximum NV 12–24 hours after administration. Emesis can persist for days after administration. Although tolerance to the adverse effects of chemotherapy can develop with some drugs, the intermittent schedule of most chemotherapy programs means that patients tend to experience repetitive bouts of NV at the start of each course of treatment (69).

Antiemetics

Pharmacologic agents have been the mainstay of treatment for chemotherapy-induced emesis for. Table 40.4 lists the major classes of antiemetics currently in use.

Phenothiazines have been used as treatment for post-chemotherapy NV for 30 years or more. They are available in oral, rectal, and parenteral forms. Their antiemetic activity is primarily attributed to blockade of dopamine receptors. Although phenothiazines are effective antiemetic agents, their widespread use has been limited by a number of side effects. Given at high doses orally or parenterally, they may cause hypotension as well as extrapyramidal symptoms, akathisia, and drowsiness (70). *Butyrophenones* are structurally related to phenothiazines but not as widely used (35). They are major tranquilizers that also act as potent blockers of dopamine receptors. Their principal side effects are sedation, anxiety, and extrapyramidal symptoms.

Low-dose *metoclopramide* (0.15–0.3 mg/kg) is ineffective as an antiemetic against cisplatin-induced NV (69). In 1981, however, the finding that high-dose metoclopramide (1–3 mg/kg) could effectively counter the severe emetogenic action of cisplatin (40), led to the discovery that it acted as a weak antagonist at 5-HT^3 receptor sites (71,72). One of the major disadvantages of high-dose metoclopramide is the extrapyramidal reactions caused by all dopamine antagonists. Intravenous diphenhydramine (50 mg), given simultaneously with high-dose metoclopramide usually prevents or ameliorates these extrapyramidal effects (69).

The *corticosteroids* dexamethasone and methylprednisolone are active antiemetics both orally and parenterally (73–75), but the mechanisms by which they act are not understood. Some reports dispute the efficacy of steroids as antiemetics (32), but on the whole they appear to be suitable for use in combination antiemetic regimes. They have generally mild side effects (13). *Cannabinoids* have been used as antiemetics for a number of years, with varying degrees of success (76–78). Dronabinol is only available orally, and it is relatively expensive. Side effects are CNS-related and are reported to be more severe than those found with the phenothiazines (13). The *benzodiazepines*, especially lorazepam, have been used in combination for the treatment of drug-induced emesis. Lorazepam, administered sublingually or parenterally, exhibits mild antiemetic activity, and its anxiolytic and amnesic properties can have a beneficial effect on anxiety (79). Its main side effects are sedation and amnesia. Lorazepam is often used in combination antiemetic therapy (69).

Only approximately 40% of all patients receiving highly emetogenic chemotherapy have their ensuing nausea and vomiting controlled by single-agent therapy using any of the aforementioned antiemetics (32).

TABLE 40.4. *Antimetics Used for Chemotherapy-Induced NV*

Drug class	Examples
Phenothiazines	Prochlorperazine; thiethylperazine
Butyrophenones	Haloperidol; droperidol
Substituted benzamides	Metoclopramide
Corticosteroids	Dexamethasone; methylprednisolone
Cannabinoids	Dronabinol
Benzodiazepines	Lorazepam; diazepam
Serotonin antagonists	Granisetron; ondansetron; tropisetron

Source: Morrow et al. (84).

However, many investigators have reported better control with combination antiemetic regimens (14,32,69,80). Agents selected for use in combination should have different modes of action, different sites of activity, and nonadditive toxicities (80). Overall, combination antiemetic therapy is more effective than use of single agents. Combinations containing metoclopramide plus dexamethasone appear to be particularly effective (14).

A large step forward in the control of chemotherapy-induced emesis came with the discovery in 1986 that *serotonin (5-HT3) receptor antagonists* which bind at the type 3 receptor had antiemetic properties (41,81–83). A new generation of antiemetic agents that included granisetron, ondansetron, and tropisetron was introduced into the clinic. Current research shows the following trends (84–90):

- The 5-HT$_3$ antiemetic agents have been shown to be clinically more effective in the control of nausea and emesis than previously used agents.
- No one of the three has demonstrated consistently greater efficacy.
- The drugs are well tolerated; side effects include headaches and constipation with only rare extrapyramidal reactions.
- Efficacy appears to be more pronounced for cisplatin-containing regimens than for moderately or less emetogenic chemotherapy regimens.
- 5-HT$_3$ agents appear to be more effective for acute symptoms of NV than for delayed ones. Potential control of ANV has not been investigated.
- Control over nausea appears to be significantly less than control over emesis. In the studies in which it has been measured, nausea control remains incomplete for approximately half the patients given 5-HT$_3$ agents.
- The efficacy of the agents appears to diminish across repeated days and, perhaps, across repeated chemotherapy cycles.
- The addition of a steroid such as dexamethasone increases the efficacy of both 5-HT$_3$ and other antiemetic agents. This effect also seems to apply to delayed nausea and emesis.

BEHAVIORAL MANAGEMENT OF NAUSEA AND VOMITING

Research on the behavioral treatment of conditioned adverse effects of chemotherapy has centered on four principal approaches: progressive muscle relaxation training, systematic desensitization, hypnosis, and cognitive distraction.

These techniques have been shown to produce greater control over nausea and vomiting than the use of standard antiemetics alone. Relaxation is a component of most of these approaches. However, if this were the primary mode of action, one would not expect additional benefit over that of those antiemetics that produce a relaxed state. Distraction is also a component of most techniques, although most of the distraction used has been of a relaxing nature (3).

Teaching patients behavioral techniques such as systemic desensitization or relaxation also has other psychological benefits. For example, anxiety, hostility, and depression may be diminished. In addition, patients report an increased sense of control by being able to do something active to aid their treatment process and, perhaps successfully, combat unwelcomed side effects.

Progressive Muscle Relaxation Training

Progressive muscle relaxation training (PMRT) enables individuals to achieve a state of muscle relaxation in anticipation of, or in response to, a variety of specific situations that may produce tension or anxiety, such as receipt of chemotherapy. The technique involves learning to relax by actively tensing and then relaxing specific muscle groups in a progressive manner. It is often combined with guided imagery in which the individual visualizes pleasant, soothing images or scenes while relaxed. PMRT is generally taught to individual patients by a trained therapist, following which the subject is requested to practice the technique at home using an audiotape made during the training session or a set of written instructions.

A number of case reports and controlled studies have indicated that PMRT can decrease postchemotherapy NV as well as reduce depression, anxiety, and physiologic arousal in cancer patients undergoing chemotherapy (15–17,32). PMRT appears to exert its greatest effects against adverse events that develop after administration of chemotherapy, including nausea, vomiting, anxiety, and physiologic (autonomic) arousal; it has been less effective against anticipatory symptoms (1,25,26,91,92). PMRT plus guided imagery also results in less nausea during chemotherapy, can prevent the development of conditioned side effects, and can also decrease the frequency and severity of conditioned side effects that have already developed (92,93).

Possible mechanisms of action of PMRT plus guided imagery include: (*1*) direct reduction of anxiety, physiologic arousal, and muscle tension, including decreased gastrointestinal contractions, and direct action on the autonomic nervous system to decrease sympathetic activity; (2) cognitive distraction to direct the patient's attention away from the clinic setting with its attendant possible conditioned stimuli; and (3) increasing the patient's sense of control over the illness and course of treatment thereby decreasing feelings of helplessness, anger, depression, and anxiety (24–26,50,94).

Systematic Desensitization

Systematic desensitization (SD), or counterconditioning, is a well-developed, standardized behavioral technique that has been found to be effective against ANV associated with cancer chemotherapy (11,50,91,95,96). A key element of SD is to construct a hierarchy of events related to the original stimulus that elicit the maladaptive response in each patient. This hierarchy might include events related to receipt of chemotherapy, such as driving to the clinic, entering the treatment room, and seeing the clinic nurse. Following this, the patient is trained to associate an alternative response (for example, deep muscle relaxation) with these events (1,11,50). SD can be taught to patients in about 20 minutes, and properly trained nurses and oncologists can use clinically SD with about the same effectiveness as can trained behavioral consultants (11).

Hypnosis

Hypnosis, also known as suggestive therapy or trance therapy, is a self-control technique in which patients learn to invoke a physiologic state incompatible with NV (97). In the method usually used to produce the altered state of consciousness, induction of total body relaxation is followed by presentation of restful psychic imagery. Suggestions for specific treatment objectives, such as increasing food intake, can then be made (98,99), and patients can undergo chemotherapy while hypnotized (97). Furthermore, while in the trance, subjects can be led to visualize a series of events (for example, those associated with ANV), a technique similar to SD (97).

Although hypnosis was one of the first psychological techniques used clinically to attempt to control ANV, few controlled studies have been done. It has been most often been used with children and adolescents (28,99–101). PMRT with guided imagery and hypnosis differ mainly in the way that relaxation is induced. Patient attitudes concerning hypnosis, the experience and expertise of the therapist, and the physical condition of the patient may serve to guide the choice between these two techniques (3).

Cognitive Distraction

It has been suggested that cognitive distraction (CD) is the common element responsible for the success of both relaxation training and hypnosis in decreasing conditioned nausea in adult patients receiving chemotherapy (102,103). CD is presumed to act by focusing patients' attention away from NV or the stimuli associated with these phenomena (103). Redd and colleagues (1987) investigated this hypothesis in two experiments in pediatric patients with documented ANV from cancer chemotherapy using commercially available video games to distract patients. In both experiments, patients had significant reductions in conditioned nausea (103). CD may be especially attractive for pediatric patients who sometimes have difficulty mastering relaxation and hypnosis (103). Video games in particular are inexpensive, effective distractors that can result in sustained distraction (102). However, the effects have been noted to decrease over successive chemotherapy sessions (104).

CONCLUSION

Currently available pharmacologic agents are unable to provide complete protection from either anticipatory or posttreatment nausea and emesis associated with cancer treatments. A multidisciplinary approach, ideally given prophylactically to prevent the occurrence of conditioned symptoms, is therefore advocated. Such an approach would include the best possible pharmacologic control of postchemothreapy NV, adequate information to modify patient expectations and anxiety, meditation to decrease anxiety, and adjunctive behavioral treatment (7,10,12,16,99,105). Since ANV is caused by a behavioral process (i.e. classical conditioning), behavioral methods of treatment may be particularly appropriate (3,26,45,50). In addition, behavioral interventions that prevent the development of or decrease the severity of postchemotherapy NV may prevent the occurrence of ANV (50).

ACKNOWLEDGMENTS

This work was supported by research grant NR01905 from the National Center for Nursing Research, NIH research grant CA37420, and grants from the Cummings Foundation and Glaxo/Welcome.

REFERENCES

1. Morrow GR, Dobkin PL. Anticipatory nausea and vomiting in cancer patients undergoing chemotherapy treatment: prevalence, etiology, and behavioral interventions. *Clin Psychol Rev.* 1988; 8:517–556.

2. Morrow GR. Behavioral factors influencing the development and expression of chemotherapy induced side effects. *Br J Cancer*. 1992; 66(Suppl XIX):S54–S61.

3. Redd WH, Andrykowski MA. Behavioral intervention in cancer treatment: Controlling aversion reactions to chemotherapy. *J Consult Clin Psychol*. 1982; 50(6): 1018–1029.

4. Zeltzer L, Kellerman J, Ellenberg L, et al. Hypnosis for reduction of vomiting associated with chemotherapy and disease in adolescents with cancer. *J Adolesc Health Care*. 1983; 4:77–84.

5. Nerenz DR, Leventhal H, Easterling DV, et al. Anxiety and drug taste as predictors of anticipatory nausea in cancer chemotherapy. *J Clin Oncol*. 1986; 4:224–233.

6. Love RR, Leventhal H, Easterling DV, et al. Side effects and emotional distress during cancer chemotherapy. *Cancer*. 1989; 63:604–612.

7. Morrow, GR. Chemotherapy-related nausea and vomiting: etiology and management. *CA Cancer J Clin*. 1989; 39:89–104.

8. Redd WH, Jacobsen PB, Andrykowski MA. Behavioral side effects of adjuvant chemotherapy. *Recent Results Cancer Res*. 1989; 115:272–278.

9. Morrow GR, Lindke JL, Black PM. Anticipatory nausea development in cancer patients: replication and extension of a learning model. *Br J Psychol*. 1991; 82:61–72.

10. Fallowfield LJ. Behavioral interventions and psychological aspects of care during chemotherapy. *Eur J Cancer*. 1992; 28A(Suppl 1):S39–S41.

11. Morrow GR, Asbury R, Hammon S, et al. Comparing the effectiveness of behavioral treatment for chemotherapy-induced nausea and vomiting when administered by oncologists, oncology nurses, and clinical psychologists. *Health Psychol*. 1992; 11(4):250–256.

12. Andrews PLR, Sanger GJ. The problem of emesis in anti-cancer therapy: an introduction. In: Andrews PLR, Sanger GJ, eds. *Emesis in Anti-Cancer Therapy: Mechanisms and Treatment*. London: Chapman and Hall; 1993.

13. Hickok, JT, Morrow, GR. A biobehavioral model of patient-reported nausea: Implications for clinical practice. *Adv Med Psychother*. 1993; 6:227–240.

14. Stewart DJ. Cancer therapy, vomiting, and antiemetics. *Can J Physiol Pharmacol*. 1990; 68:304–313.

15. Wilcox PM, Fetting JH, Nettesheim KM, et al. Anticipatory vomiting in women receiving cyclophosphamide, methotrexate, and 5-FU (CMF) adjuvant chemotherapy for breast carcinoma. *Cancer Treat Rep*. 1982; 66:1601–1604.

16. Morrow GR. Clinical characteristics associated with the development of anticipatory nausea and vomiting in cancer patients undergoing chemotherapy treatment. *J Clin Oncol*. 1984; 2(10):1170–1176.

17. Morrow GR. The assessment of nausea and vomiting: post problems, current issues, and suggestions for future research. *Cancer*. 1984; 53:2267–2278.

18. Lecomte S, Lemnager M, Duquenne I, Crépin G, Bonneterre J. Quality of life in breast cancer patients receiving adjuvant chemotherapy. *Proc ASCO*. 1995; 14:900.

19. Bonneterre B, Hecquet B, Atenis A, Fournier C, Pion JM. How do patients and physicians decide which antiemetic is the best in a cross-over study? [abstract]. *Proc Am Soc Clin Oncol*. 1991; 10:323.

20. Allan SG. Mechanisms and management of chemotherapy-induced nausea and vomiting. *Blood Rev*. 1987; 1:50-7.

21. Craig JB, Powell BL. Review. The management of nausea and vomiting in clinical oncology. *Am J Med Sci*. 1987; 293:34–44.

22. Fiore JJ, Gralla RJ. Pharmacologic treatment of chemotherapy-induced nausea and vomiting. *Cancer Invest*. 1984; 2:351-361.

23. Smyth J. Delayed emesis after high-dose cisplatin—the residual problem. Presented at the XVIIth of the European Society for Medical Oncology, Lyon, France, November 8, 1992.

24. Burish TG, Lyles JN. Effectiveness of relaxation training in reducing the aversiveness of chemotherapy in the treatment of cancer. *J Behav Ther Exp Psychiatry*. 1979; 10:357-361.

25. Lyles JN, Burish TG, Krozely MG, et al. Efficacy of relaxation training and guided imagery in reducing the aversiveness of cancer chemotherapy. *J Consult Clin Psychol*. 1982; 50:509–524.

26. Burish TG, Carey MP, Krozely MG, et al. Conditioned side effects induced by cancer chemotherapy: prevention through behavioral treatment. *J Consult Clin Psychol*. 1987; 55:42–48.

27. Burish TG, Snyder SL, Jenkins RA. Preparing patients for cancer chemotherapy: effect of coping preparation and relaxation interventions. *J Consult Clin Psychol*. 1991; 59:518–525.

28. Carey MP, Burish TG. Etiology and treatment of the psychological side effects associated with cancer chemotherapy: a critical review and discussion. *Psychol Bull*. 1988; 104(3) 307–325.

29. Burish TG, Tope DM. Psychological techniques for controlling the adverse side effects of cancer chemotherapy: findings from a decade of research. *J Pain Symptom Manage*. 1992; 7287–7301.

30. Kucharczyk J, Miller AD. Mechanisms of nausea and emesis: introduction and retrospective. In: Kucharczyk J, Stwart DJ, Miller AD, eds. *Nausea and Vomiting: Recent Reviews and Clinical Advances*. Boca Raton, FL: CRC Press; 1991:1–13.

31. Andrews PLR, Davis CJ. The mechanism of emesis induced by anti-cancer therapies. In: Andrews PLR, Sanger GJ, eds. *Emesis in Anti-Cancer Therapy*. London: Chapman & Hall, 1993:113–155.

32. Wickham R. Managing chemotherapy-related nausea and vomiting: the state of the art. *Oncology Nurs Forum*. 1989; 16:563–574.

33. Tonato M, Roila F, Del Favero A, Ballatori E. Antiemetics in cancer chemotherapy: historical perspective and current state of the art. *Support Care Cancer*. 1994; 2(3):150–60.

34. Borison HL, Borison R, McCarthy LE. Role of the area postrema in vomiting and related functions. *Fed Proc*. 1984; 43:2955–2958.

35. Wampler G. The pharmacology and clinical effectiveness of phenothiazines and related drugs for managing chemotherapy-induced emesis. *Drugs*. 1983; 25(Suppl 1): 35-51.

36. Neidhart JA, Gagen M, Young D, Wilson HE. Specific antiemetics for specific cancer chemotherapeutic agents: haloperidol versus benzquinamide. *Cancer.* 1981; 47(6):1439–1443.

37. Day MD, Blower PR. Cardiovascular dopamine receptor stimulation antagonized by metoclopramide. *J Pharm Pharmacol.* 1975; 27:276–278.

38. Perrot J, Nahas G, Laville C, Debay Y. Substituted benzamides as anti-emetics. In: Poster DS, Penta JS, Bruno S, eds. *Treatment of Cancer Chemotherapy-Induced Nausea and Vomiting.* Masson; New York: 1982:195–207.

39. Harrington RA, Hamilton CW, Brogden RN, Linkewich JA, Romankiewicz JA, Heel RC. Metoclopramide, an updated review of its pharmacological properties and clinical use. *Drugs.* 1983; 25:451–94.

40. Gralla RJ, Itri LM, Pisko SE, et al. Anti-emetic efficacy of high dose metoclopramide: Randomized trials with placebo and prochlorperazine in patients with chemotherapy-induced nausea and vomiting. *N Engl J Med.* 1981; 305:905–909.

41. Miner WD, Sanger GJ. Inhibition of cisplatin-induced vomiting by selective 5-hydroxytryptamine M-receptor antagonism. *Br J Pharmacol.* 1986; 88:497–499.

42. Andrews PLR, Bhandari P. The 5-hydroxytryptamine receptor antagonists as antiemetics: Preclinical evaluation and mechanism of action. *Eur J Cancer Clin Oncol.* 1993; 29A(Suppl 1):S11–S16.

43. Andrews PLR, Davidson HIM. Activation of vagal afferent terminals by 5-hydroxytryptamine is mediated by the 5-HT)3) receptor in the anaesthetized ferret. *J Physiol.* 1990; 422:92P.

44. Higgins GA, Kilpatrick GJ, Bunce KT, Jones BJ, Tyers MB. 5-HT)3) receptor antagonists injected into the area postrema inhibit cisplatin-induced emesis in the ferret. *Br J Pharmacol.* 1989; 97:247–55

45. Morrow GR. Prevalence and correlates of anticipatory nausea and vomiting in chemotherapy patients. *J Natl Cancer Inst.* 1982; 68(4):585–588.

46. Morrow GR, Arseneau JC, Asbury RF, et al. Anticipatory nausea and vomiting with chemotherapy [letter]. *N Engl J Med.* 1982; 306:431–432.

47. Morrow GR. The assessment of nausea and vomiting: Past problems, current issues and suggestions for future research. *Cancer.* 1984b; 53(10; Suppl):2267–2278.

48. Andrykowski MA, Redd WH, Hatfield AK. Development of anticipatory nausea: a prospective analysis. *J Consult Clin Psychol.* 1985; 53:447–454.

49. Van Komen RW, Redd WH. Personality factors associated with anticipatory nausea and vomiting in patients receiving cancer chemotherapy. *Health Psychol.* 1985; 4:189–202.

50. Morrow GR, Morrell C. Behavioral treatment for the anticipatory nausea and vomiting induced by cancer chemotherapy. *N Engl J Med.* 1982; 307:1476–1480.

51. Chin SBY, Kocuk O, Peterson R et al. Variables contributing to anticipatory nausea and vomiting in cancer chemotherapy. *Am J Clin Oncol.* 1992; 15(3):262–267.

52. Coons HL, Levanthal H, Nerenz DR, Love RR, Larson S. Anticipatory nausea and emotional distress in patients receiving cisplatin-based chemotherapy. *Oncol Nurs Forum.* 1987; 14(4):31–35.

53. Gralla RJ, Tyson LB, Kris MG, Clark RA. The management of chemotherapy-induced nausea and vomiting. *Med Clin North Am.* 1987; 71(2):289–301.

54. Morrow GR, Barry MJ, Jiang W, et al. Pre-chemotherapy total autonomic activity assessed via heart rate spectral analysis as a predictor of chemotherapy induced self-reported nausea. In: Bianchi AL, Grelot L, Miller AD, King GL, eds. *Mechanisms and Control of Emesis.* Colloque INSERM/John Libbey Eurotext; 1992.

55. Blasco T. Anticipatory nausea and vomiting: are psychological factors adequately investigated? *Br J Clin Psychol.* 1994 (Feb); 33 (Pt 1):85–100.

56. Andrykowski MA, Gregg ME. The role of psychological variables in post-chemotherapy nausea: anxiety and expectation. *Psychosom Med.* 1992; 54:48–58.

57. Morrow GR. Susceptibility to motion sickness and the development of anticipatory nausea and vomiting in cancer patients undergoing chemotherapy. *Cancer Treat Rep.* 1984; 68: 1177–1178.

58. Burnish TG, Carey MP, Redd WH, Krozely MG. Efficacy of behavioral relaxation techniques in reducing the distress of cancer chemotherapy patients. *Oncol Nurs Forum.* 1983; 10:32-35.

59. Morrow GR. Behavioral management of chemotherapy-induced nausea and vomiting in the cancer patient. *Clin Oncol.* 1986; 1:3,11–14.

60. Morrow GR. The effect of susceptibility to motion sickness on the side effects of cancer chemotherapy. *Cancer.* 1985; 55:2766–2770.

61. Gralla RJ, Braun TJ, Squillante A, et al. Metoclopramide: initial clinical studies of high dosage regimens in cisplatin-induced emesis, In: Poster D, ed: *The Treatment of Nausea and Vomiting Induced by Cancer Chemotherapy.* New York: Masson; 1981: 167–176.

62. Fetting JH, Wilcox PM, Iwata BA, et al. Anticipatory nausea and vomiting in a medical oncology clinic. *Proc Am Soc Clin Oncol.* 1983; 2:62.

63. D'Acquisto RW , Tyson LB, Gralla RJ, et al. The influence of a chronic high alcohol intake on chemotherapy-induced nausea and vomiting. *Proc Am Soc Clin Oncol.* 1986; 5:257.

64. Sullivan JR. Leyden MJ, Bell R. Decreased cisplatin-induced nausea and vomiting with chronic alcohol ingestion. *N Engl J Med.* 1983; 309:796.

65. Andrykowski MA, Jacobsen PB, Marks E, et al. Prevalence, predictors, and course of anticipatory nausea in women receiving adjuvant chemotherapy for breast cancer. *Cancer.* 1988; 62:2607–2613.

66. Jacobsen PB, Andrykowski MA, Redd WH, et al. Nonpharmacologic factors in the development of post-treatment nausea with adjuvant chemotherapy for breast cancer. *Cancer.* 1988; 61:379–385.

67. Haut MW, Beckwith BE, Laurie JA, Klatt N. Postchemotherapy nausea and vomiting in cancer patients receiving outpatient chemotherapy. *J Psychosoc Oncol.* 1991; 9(1):117–130.

68. Grunberg SM. Making chemotherapy easier. *N Engl J Med.* 1990; 322:840–848.

69. Triozzi PL, Laszlo J. Optimum management of nausea and vomiting in cancer chemotherapy. *Drugs.* 1987; 34:136–149.

70. Merrifield KR, Chafee BJ. Recent advances in the management of nausea and vomiting caused by antineoplastic agents. *Clin Pharm.* 1989; 8:187–199.

71. Sanger GJ, King FD. From metoclopramide to selective gut motility stimulants and 5-HT)3) antagonists. *Drug Design Deliv.* 1988; 3:273–295.

72. Fozard JR. Neuronal 5-HT receptors in the periphery. *Neuropharmacology.* 1984; 231:473–486.

73. Lee B. Methylprednisolone as an antiemetic. *N Engl J Med.* 1981; 304:486.

74. Cassileth PA, Lusk EJ, Torri S, DiNubile N, Gerson SL. Antiemetic efficacy of dexamethasone therapy in patients receiving cancer chemotherapy. *Arch Intern Med.* 1983; 143:1347–1349.

75. Aapro MS, Alberts DS. High-dose dexamethasone for prevention of cisplatin-induced vomiting. *Cancer Chemother Pharmacol.* 1981; 7:11–14.

76. Sallan SE, Cornin C, Zelen M, Zinberg NE. Antiemetics in patients receiving chemotherapy for cancer. A randomized comparison of delta-9-tetrahydrocannabinol and prochlorperazine. *N Engl J Med.* 1980; 302(3):135–138.

77. Carey MP, Burish TG, Brenner DE. Delta-9-tetrahydrocannabinol in cancer chemotherapy: research problems and issues. *Ann Intern Med.* 1983; 99(1):106–114.

78. Chang AE, Shilling DJ, Stillman RC, et al. A prospective evaluation of delta-9-tetrahydrocannabinol as an antiemetic in patients receiving adriamycin and cytoxan chemotherapy. *Cancer.* 1981; 47(1):1746–1751.

79. Laszlo J, Clerk RA, Hanson L, Tyson L, Crumpler L, Gralla R. Lorazepam in cancer patients treated with cisplatin: a drug having antiemetic amnesic, and anxiolytic effects. *J Clin Oncol.* 1985; 3(6):864–869.

80. Triozzi PL, Laszlo J. Recent advances in the control of nausea and vomiting. *Primary Care Cancer.* 1990; 25–32.

81. Richardson BP, Engel G, Donatsch P: Identification of serotonin M-receptor subtypes and their specific blockage by a new class of drugs. *Nature.* 1985; 31:126–131.

82. Butler A, Hill JM, Ireland SJ, Jordan CC, Tyers MB. Pharmacological properties of GR38032F, a novel antagonist at 5-HT3 receptors. *Br J Pharmacol.* 1988; 94:397–412.

83. Fake CS, King FD, Sanger GJ. BRL43694: a potent and novel 5-HT)3) receptor antagonist. *Br J Pharmacol.* 1987; 91:335P.

84. Morrow GR, Hickok JT, Rosenthal SN. Progress in reducing nausea and emesis: comparisons of ondansetron (Zofran), granisetron (Kytril), and Topisetron (Navoban). *Cancer.* 1995; 76(3):343–357.

85. Currow DC, Noble PD, Stuart-Harris RC. The clinical use of ondansetron. New South Wales Therapeutic Assessment Group. *Med J Aust.* 1995; 162(3):145–149.

86. Dilly S. Granisetron (Kytril) clinical safety and tolerance. *Semin Oncol.* 1994; (3 Suppl 5):10–14.

87. Soukop M, McQuade B, Hunter E, et al. Ondansetron compared with metoclopramide in the control of emesis and quality of life during repeated chemotherapy for breast cancer. *Oncology.* 1992; 49(4):295–304.

88. Perez EA, Gandara DR. The clinical role of granisetron (Kytril) in the prevention of chemotherapy-induced emesis. *Semin Oncol.* 1994; (3 Suppl 5):15–21.

89. Clavel M, Soukop M, Greenstreet YL. Improved control of emesis and quality of life with ondansetron in breast cancer. *Oncology.* 1993; 50(3):180–185.

90. Yarker YE. McTavish D. Granisetron. An update of its therapeutic use in nausea and vomiting induced by antineoplastic therapy. *Drugs.* 1994; 48(5):761–793.

91. Morrow GR. Effect of the cognitive hierarchy in the systematic desensitization treatment of anticipatory nausea in cancer patients: a component comparison with relaxation only, counseling, and no treatment. *Cogn Ther Res.* 1986 10:421–446.

92. Burish TG, Jenkins RA. Effectiveness of biofeedback and relaxation training in reducing the side effects of cancer chemotherapy. *Health Psychol.* 1992; 11(1):17–23.

93. Burish TG, Vasterling JJ, Carey MP, et al. Posttreatment use of relaxation training by cancer patients. *Hospice J.* 1988; 4(2):1–8.

94. Burish TG, Lyles JN. Effectiveness of relaxation training in reducing adverse reactions to cancer chemotherapy. *J Behav Med.* 1981; 4:65–78.

95. Hailey BJ, White JG. Systematic desensitization for anticipatory nausea associated with chemotherapy. *Psychosomatics.* 1983; 24:287, 290–291.

96. Hoffman ML. Hypnotic desensitization for the management of anticipatory emesis in chemotherapy. *Am J Clin Hypn.* 1983; 25:173–176.

97. Redd WH, Andresen GV, Minagawa RY. Hypnotic control of anticipatory emesis in patients receiving cancer chemotherapy. *J Consult Clin Psychol.* 1982; 50(1):14–19.

98. Fredrikson M, Hursti T, Salmi P, et al. Conditioned nausea after cancer chemotherapy and autonomic nervous system conditionability. *Scand J Psychol.* 1993; 34(4):318–327.

99. LaBaw W, Holton C, Tewell K, et al. The use of self-hypnosis by children with cancer. *Am J Clin Hypn.* 1975; 17(4):233–238.

100. Cotanch P, Hockenberry M, Herman S. Self-hypnosis antiemetic therapy in children receiving chemotherapy. *Oncol Nurs Forum.* 1985; 12(4):41–46.

101. Zeltzer L, LeBaron S, Zeltzer PM. The effectiveness of behavioral intervention for reduction of nausea and vomiting in children and adolescents receiving chemotherapy. *J Clin Oncol.* 1984; 2(6):683–690.

102. Kolko DJ, Rickard-Figueroa JL. Effects of video games on the adverse corollaries of chemotherapy in pediatric oncology patients: a single-case analysis. *J Consult Clin Psychol.* 1985; 53:223–228.

103. Redd WH, Jacobsen PB, Die-Trill M, et al. Cognitive-attentional distraction in the control of conditioned nausea in pediatric cancer patients receiving chemotherapy. *J Consult Clin Psychol.* 1987; 55(3):391–395.

104. Vasterling J, Jenkins RA, Tope DM, et al. Cognitive distraction and relaxation training for the control of side effects due to cancer chemotherapy. *J Behav Med.* 1993; 16(1):65–80.

105. Billet AL, Sallan SE. Antiemetics in children receiving cancer chemotherapy. *Support Care Cancer.* 1994; 2(5):279–285.

41

Fatigue

DONNA B. GREENBERG

The challenge of cancer treatment is to prevent cancer from subduing the life force. Fatigue stands in counterpoint, a medical symptom, a sensation that keeps the patient from moving forward fully with life. In health, we take for granted the normal energy of our temperament: sleeping well at night; waking with spontaneity to activity in the morning; accelerating for athletics, enjoyment, creativity, commitment; and resting for satisfied relief. During treatment, the patient hopes that limited energy is a temporary cost of the battle to cure the tumor. At intermediate points, fatigue engenders fear that cancer will be victorious. Declining endurance symbolizes progressive debility and waning of life.

To the physician, fatigue means a clue to cancer, a treatment side effect, the emotional strain of the predicament, progressive disease, or the residual physical change after treatment. This chapter focuses on psychological and medical causes of fatigue in cancer patients, differential diagnosis, and strategies for treatment.

CHARACTER AND MEANING OF THE SYMPTOM

To evaluate a specific patient, both the subjective sensations and behavior must be described; like pain, fatigue has a sensory character and meaning.

What takes more effort? What time of day is worst? What are precipitating factors? What is the quality and quantity of sleep pattern? What aspects are mental or physical? When a patient says that he is tired, he may mean that he is grief-stricken, cannot climb stairs without dyspnea, cannot concentrate, or feels sedated most of the day. Trouble getting started is typical of the fatigue of major depressive disorder or the stiffness of Parkinsonian syndromes. Exertional fatigue comes with low blood count, heart, lung, or muscle defects, or aerobic deconditioning. Fever, inflammation, and tumor burden cause systemic malaise: mental clouding,

more resistance to action as the day goes on, and the need to sit or lay down. Sedation is a common side effect of medications, particularly narcotics; lack of sleep from pain, depression, poor breathing, or sleep apnea can also cause daytime sleepiness.

To say, "I'm too tired," implies that the patient has the desire but not the stamina. If desire is absent, apathy or depression may be a more accurate description of the condition. Apathy occurs with frontal lobe dysfunction or chronic narcotic abuse. Depression is characterized by dysphoria, loss of interest, and fatigue.

As in Melzack's pain measure, the McGill Pain Questionnaire, both dysphoria and personal meaning color the intensity of the fatigue symptom (1). For some patients, strength and productivity may be most central to their self-image. How the patient reports his tiredness depends on how he remembers his previous capacity, whether he continues some physical activity, whether he wants to get stronger, and how great is the necessity to function.

In cancer patients, fatigue rarely comes as an isolated symptom. The words, "I'm tired," signify a feeling with multiple dimensions and multiple causative factors (2,3). We may be most interested in a generalized sensation of fatigue which occurs after major injury from tumor or treatment, which alters behavior against our will, and remains distinct from depression or discrete weakness in muscle, lung, or heart. Little is known about the physiological perception of that sensation of fatigue. Piper's definition of fatigue, "an overwhelming sustained sense of exhaustion and decreased capacity for physical and mental work," is an attempt to describe the core symptom—the subjective sensation as well as behavior (4,5). One goal of palliative medicine is to treat that symptom when it is the dominant restrictor of quality of life.

MEASUREMENT OF FATIGUE

Quality of life measurements, the composite measures of comfort, function, mood, and side effects, always include a measure of fatigue. In cancer patients, activity status and symptom distress are key predictors of quality of life (6). Positive affect correlates with subjective perception of both mental and physical energy in normal volunteers (7). Dysphoria and lack of function correlate with fatigue in cancer patients. This symptom is tightly related to self-image; sense of fatigue scored on a scale of 1 to 10 is one of only five parameters in a recent measure of self-regard (8).

Fatigue, rated by intensity, is often a one- or two-item measure in larger scales. Fatigue and insomnia are two from the Symptom Distress Scale (9). The Memorial Symptom Assessment Scale includes lack of energy, feeling drowsy, and difficulty sleeping (10). The Functional Assessment of Cancer Therapy Scale (11) includes lack of energy and time spent in bed as components of physical well-being; and ability to work, play, and sleep as components of functional well-being.

Fatigue scales, developed for a variety of testing purposes (airplane pilot endurance, industrial productivity, and the nature of chronic fatigue syndrome), have used adjective lists, visual analogue scales, and multiple dimensions. The Pearson–Byars Fatigue Feeling Checklist (12) and the fatigue/vigor scales of the Profile of Mood States use a series of endorsed descriptors (13). Anchored visual analogue scales are practical measures of fatigue and vigor (7,14). The Physical Activity Scale (PAS), a measurement of an individual's activity pattern, ergonomically derived, rating leisure and work activities, has been used with breast cancer patients and survivors of Hodgkin's disease (15,16). Piper has been developing a Fatigue Self-Report Scale with multiple dimensions: temporal, severity, affect, sensory, relief, and associated symptoms (17,18). Wessely and Powell described both mental and physical fatigue in one fatigue questionnaire (19). The subscale factors highlight operational and clinical meanings of the symptom. Schwartz and colleagues found factors of severity, pervasiveness vs. situation-specificity, consequences of fatigue, and response to rest or sleep (20). Vercoulen and colleagues defined nine dimensions: psychological well-being, functional impairment in daily life, sleep disturbance, avoidance of physical activity, neuropsychological impairment, causal attribution related to complaints, social functioning, self-efficacy expectations, and subjective experience of the personal situation (21).

Chalder and colleagues developed a 14-item scale to measure fatigue severity (22).

MEDICAL PRESENTATIONS OF FATIGUE

Fatigue can be the first clue to cancer and cancer recurrence. Fatigue is prominent in B symptoms of lymphoma (fever, sweats, weight loss greater than 10% body weight) and it is characteristic of systemic Hodgkin's disease and non-Hodgkin's lymphoma. Fatigue may call attention to anemia if the blood count has dropped gradually. Lack of endurance because of dyspnea on exertion may signal malignant pericardial effusion, lymphangitic spread of tumor, or diffuse lung metastases. Hypercalcemia, a classic oncologic emergency associated with bone metastases or paraneoplastic hormones, is characterized by fatigue, nausea, thirst, urinary frequency, and clouded sensorium. Liver dysfunction with metastases can present as general fatigue. Both infection and tumor burden, associated with cachexia and increased cytokines, cause generalized fatigue. Proximal myopathy, difficulty walking upstairs, from paraneoplastic peripheral neuromuscular weakness, associated with autoimmune antineuronal antibodies or paraneoplastic steroid production, may be interpreted by the patient as fatigue.

TREATMENT-RELATED FATIGUE

Chemotherapy

Chemotherapy begins after a number of challenges: the diagnosis of cancer, a surgical procedure, and many trips to the hospital. Most chemotherapy protocols are associated with fatigue. Specific anticancer drugs cause fatigue by distinct mechanisms (see Table 41.1). If chemotherapy works to reduce tumor-related symptoms of dyspnea, pain, or fever, the patient gains strength. The experience of chemotherapy infusion, often associated with sedating medications and nausea, may require suffering a day or two of fatigue. In combination regimens, fatigue occurs at the nadir of marrow function, 14 days after combined chemotherapy (23). As the body recovers from each cycle of treatment, energy returns. With each additional cycle of adjuvant chemotherapy, fatigue tends to increase. Women undergoing chemotherapy find sleep and exercise the most effective strategies to minimize fatigue, but these are most effective at the outset. Only a minority exercise. Later, distraction and the structure of work help (24–26).

The specific side effects of chemotherapy affect the presentation of fatigue. Biological treatments like interferon (27) and interleukin-2 (IL-2) (28) cause flu-

TABLE 41.I. *Mechanisms of Fatigue Related to Chemotherapy*

TRANSIENT ENCEPHALOPATHY

Methotrexate, ifosfamide, cytarabine

L-Asparaginase

Hexamethylmelamine—extrapyramidal side effects

Procarbazine—transient somnolence; delayed metabolism of sedatives

DIRECT SIDE EFFECT

5-Fluorouracil

Vincristine,vinblastine, vinorelbine

NEUROTOXICITY OF BIOLOGICAL TREATMENT

Flu-like malaise, secondary affective syndromes

Interferon, interleukin-2

HORMONE-INDUCED

Aminoglutethimide—sedation initially, dose related

Tamoxifen—sleep disorder related to hot flashes

Corticosteroids—fatigue associated with cessation of treatment

Type II muscle fiber atrophy, myopathy

Megestrol—fatigue

PERIPHERAL NEUROPATHY

Etoposide, cisplatin, cytarabine

Vincristine,vinorelbine

Paclitaxel, doclitaxel

HYPOMAGNESEMIA

Cisplatin

like malaise and fatigue as the drug is given. Later, interferon can induce a dose-related syndrome of fatigue, general disinterest, poor concentration, nightmares, and psychomotor retardation. Organic affective syndromes, depression, irritability, and encephalopathy may occur with time. Thyroid function may diminish during treatment.

Fatigue has been attributed to 5-fluorouracil, vincristine, vinblastine, and vinorelbine (29). Other agents associated with organic brain syndromes—methotrexate, cytosine arabinoside, hexamethylmelamine, ifosfamide—also cause fatigue (29).

Corticosteroids (30) cause lability and insomnia with treatment, but muscle aches and fatigue with cessation. Those patients who take steroids for longer periods, for instance, for cerebral edema, will develop Type II muscle fiber atrophy and proximal myopathy. Hyperphagia, weight gain, and insomnia may give way to depression and lassitude when steroids are discontinued. Aminoglutethimide causes malaise in the first weeks, but it dissipates with time. Tamoxifen, usually well tolerated, can cause hot flashes and sleep disruption. Medroxyprogesterone can also cause fatigue and depression, depending on dose, although its increase in appetite has been associated with enhanced well-being.

Hypomagnesemia in cancer patients (31), which results from renal toxicity by cisplatin and poor oral intake, adds a contribution to fatigue (32).

Postural hypotension, resulting from autonomic neuropathy of cisplatin or etoposide (29), may be interpreted as fatigue. Patients feel faint on rising, exhausted on lifting their arms to read the paper, and tend to the supine position. Anemia, deconditioning due to bedrest or anorexia, or long-term antihypertensive medications which were not readjusted in the setting of acute treatment, may all exacerbate postural hypotension.

Anemia and low white counts limit energy. Myelosuppressive anticancer agents exacerbate anemia of chronic disease. Erythropoietin production is inappropriately low for the level of anemia. Repeated chemotherapy treatments may limit recovery of marrow and erythropoietin level. A placebo-controlled double-blind trial of human erythropoietin infusions was directed at a goal hematocrit of 38%–40% in more than 150 patients with solid tumors receiving multidrug regimens who had hemoglobin less than 10.5 g/dl (33). Compared to the placebo group, the group treated with 150 U/kg three times per week had a 6% higher hematocrit at the end of the study. The patients with higher blood counts described a higher energy level and ability to perform daily tasks. A small change in hematocrit (mean 27.6% to 29.3%), brought a better sense of overall well-being in one randomized trial of 413 patients (34). A subjective benefit was also noted in patients treated for myeloma (35). About half of cancer patients with anemia of chronic disease are responsive to recombinant human erythropoietin (r-HuEPO) injections (36). Denton and colleagues discuss human and societal costs of treatment of anemia (37), but encourage decision analysis on an indivudual basis that takes into consideration fatigue and impaired physical activity as well as dyspnea on exertion. The choice between recombinant erythropoietin and transfusion also depends on clinical considerations and cost.

Radiation Treatment

Radiation treatment causes fatigue because it injures cells. The sensitivity to radiation is related to dose, time–dose fractionation, tissue volume, and the proliferative capacity of the cells. Total body irradiation causes profound fatigue. Lethargy follows brain irradiation as grade I to II toxicity; and radiation to the liver leads to lassitude. Almost all patients receiving lung irradiation experience fatigue, first intermittent then continuous by the third week (38). Fatigue and dyspnea on exertion may be acute signs of radiation pneumonitis. Two-thirds of patients (65%–72%) who have head and neck, gynecologic, and genitourinary radiation therapy experience fatigue. The severity is greater for those receiving head and neck radiation treatment. It is worse later in the day, and naps are some help (38). Fatigue after radiation to the head may reflect late hypopituitarism; radiation to the chest or neck may later result in hypothyroidism (39).

During localized irradiation, the tendency to fatigue increases for four weeks, then plateaus (40). The tendency to sleep increases in the latter part of radiation treatment (41,42). Whether there is actually less fatigue on weekend days without treatment is unclear (40,43). It is possible that the cumulative effect over weeks obscures the benefit of a one- to two-day reprieve. Despite continued visits to the hospital for electron boosts, recovery seems to begin when the conventional radiation treatment is complete. The fatigue after lumpectomy and radiation to the breast is not usually sufficient to change function at the end of seven weeks. Reports of fatigue have greater intensity in patients with more systemic symptoms and the poorest function (44). Nausea, dyspnea, depression, or anxiety would augment symptoms attributed to radiation.

Surgery

Surgery alone is associated with postoperative fatigue (45). Response to injury and repair, after-effects of general anesthesia, deconditioning by bedrest, resolution of pain, and relative anemia may all play a role.

EMOTIONAL COMPONENTS OF FATIGUE

Worry, grief, and sadness weigh on the soul. Adjustment to the diagnosis of life-threatening illness requires effort. Initial bursts of anxiety, arousal, and numbness give way to a complex commitment to treatment and recovery. As with other stresses in life, patients establish an equilibrium, a plateau that allows for daily function. Every setback and every further clinical assault provides an opportunity for weariness and demoralization (46). Uncertainty and the vigilance for disappointment keep the patient on guard without any real rest from threat. Indignity, inconvenience, and dashed hopes, must be faced. The most reliable coping strategies fail at times. Grief alone is characterized by fatigue, tearfulness, sighing, and poor concentration. Anger can energize or exhaust.

The psychological apects of energy management depend on personal meaning, values, and flexibility. The activities that take priority come first. Keep in balance what is required and what would offer energy by way of pleasure. Healing is the first assignment. Small spurts of energy do not always come when the patient wishes them, so any plan must allow for its unpredictability.

Let others help. Delegate. Allow care givers flexibility, respite, change, so that their energy is not also depleted (47). A steady plan for good nutrition, fluids, and physical movement makes sense in rehabilitation, but struggle with family who preempt patients' wishes about eating and effort can also be costly. The best strategy for management of anger is to mobilize that energy for treatment against the illness and to minimize its expression against benign care givers.

Specific diagnosis of psychiatric syndromes that cause fatigue must be distinguished from the stress of adjustment to cancer and the fatigue due to illness and treatment. This is critically important to care. Specific psychiatric syndromes determine specific treatments.

Mood Disorder

Major depressive disorder is the most important specific psychiatric diagnosis that causes fatigue in cancer patients. Loss of energy is a criterion for the diagnosis. It would be uncommon to have clinical depression and not be tired. Motivation and pleasure are absent, so there is no ignition to action. Morning dread and delay in getting out of bed are common. As in Parkinson's disease, movement is effortful. Insomnia or the tendency to sleep too much are also criteria. Those who sleep too much have atypical depression and the sensation of leaden legs, the feeling of walking through molasses (48). To overlook the diagnosis of major depressive disorder in the midst of cancer treatment, to think that this neurobiologic disorder is merely due to the sadness of coping with cancer, is a tragic loss. Depression itself is common without cancer and may pre-date the diagnosis. A life-threatening disease makes each good day count all the more. This cause of fatigue should be treated aggressively first with antidepressants. Cognitive, behavioral, and group stratgies augment emotional and physical recovery (see Chapter 62).

Anxiety Syndromes

Anxiety syndromes also sap energy. Cancer treatment provides many opportunities for anticipatory anxiety: the next procedure, the next checkup, the possibility of relapse. Anxiety conditioned by chemotherapy-induced nausea may precede each treatment. Panic attacks, sudden episodes of anxiety, can occur autonomously in the setting of panic disorder, grief, or depression. These episodes of psychic and somatic alarm are often followed by fatigue and avoidance of sites where an attack happened. Sometimes patients will speak of fatigue or effort when they mean phobic avoidance. Antianxiety medications such as benzodiazepines may be used strategically before treatment or before situations that may provoke anxiety (49,50). Antidepressant medication may be more useful for chronic, recurrent panic attacks, which may in fact have come with the onset of depression. A variety of cognitive, behavioral, systematic desensitization, and hypnotic techniques treat anticipatory symptoms and panic attacks.

Chronic, persistent pain exhausts and depresses as it jangles limbic components of the nervous system. Pain intensity and duration correlate with fatigue and total mood disturbance in cancer patients (51,52). Pain disrupts sleep and limits endurance and mobility. With severe cancer-related pain, patients are often forced to bargain between total pain relief and the sedation of narcotics. The greater the extent to which they can titrate medications and control the level of pain to manage rest and activity, the greater their function.

Poor sleep adds to fatigue. Dyspnea, chronic lung disease, lung cancer, and pain compromise sleep. One group of patients with lung cancer who were tested in a sleep laboratory slept as poorly as insomniacs but underreported their difficulties (53). Restless legs (akathisia), from dopamine-blocking antiemetics such as perphenazine, prevents rest. Sedating medications may disrupt sleep architecture and promote daytime sleepiness.

ADVANCED CANCER

In advanced cancer, fatiguing easily is one of three most common and most severe symptoms. Lack of energy, weakness, and fatiguing easily were rated by 60%–80% of patients as clinically important (53–56). Asthenia and an anticipatory subjective sensation of difficulty getting started (57) occur with anorexia and cachexia. Wasting brings loss of muscle mass, more specifically, type II muscle atrophy (58). Cytokines, tumor necrosis factor, interleukin-6, and interferons, are thought to synergistically mediate cachexia (59). Tumor necrosis factor alone is not increased in cancer patients with cachexia (60).

Fatigue may function in sickness as part of a complex immune defense that conserves energy. In sickness, humans have weakness, malaise, listlessness, inability to concentrate, hypersomnia, and reduction of social activity (61,62). Sickness behavior in animals implies anorexia, depressed activity, loss of interest in usual activities, and disappearance of grooming activities. Cytokines appear to elicit sickness behavior and to prolong slow-wave sleep. Sickness behavior may be seen as an all-out attempt to limit energy output and exhaustion in a life and death struggle.

In the setting of cancer treatment, the rules may change. Treatment itself causes some fatigue. Recovery may no longer depend on the sensation of fatigue any more than fever is a requirement to subdue infection. Treatment of fatigue in the same way as pain then becomes a goal of palliative care (Table 41.2).

Stimulants increase arousal, concentration, mood, and sometimes appetite by acting as catecholamine agonists. Methylphenidate improves attention in normal volunteers (63). Stimulants are used to treat depression in medically ill patients (64,65), reduce neurological slowing associated with encephalopathy, and counteract narcotic-mediated sedation. When patients have advanced cancer and depression, psychostimulants improve alertness, mood, and appetite more rapidly than other antidepressants. Better concentration and mood mean less pervasive fatigue. Neurobehavioral slowing, a state of Parkinsonian-like psychomotor retardation noted in patients with frontal apathy due to primary brain tumors or radiation treatment, may respond to 5–10 mg methylphenidate at 7 a.m. and 1 p.m. with better attention, arousal, and ability to initiate (66). Dextroamphetamine has increased arousal and augmented pain relief in those sedated by morphine (67,68).

Corticosteroid treatment has temporarily increased well-being in advanced cancer patients (69). One study (70) found that methylprednisolone 32 mg each day led to increased daily activity, appetite, and mood in approximately 70% of 30 patients with advanced cancer. Mood improved within 5 days but deteriorated somewhat by 33 days. The actual performance status did not change significantly over a month, nor did it differ from that of the placebo group. Dexamethasone 0.75 mg and 1.5 mg four times per day led to improvement in patients with advanced cancer after two weeks, but that improvement in strength was not sustained at four weeks (71).

More recently, synthetic progesterone, megestrol acetate, has improved appetite and sense of well-being in cachectic patients with breast cancer (72) and other cancers (73,74). It is in part an analogue of corticosteroids (75).

Because of the contribution of tumor necrosis factor (TNF) and other cytokines to malaise, cytokine antagonists could reduce sickness behavior. Pentoxifylline, which was reported to decrease TNF mRNA levels in cancer patients (76), was evaluated against placebo for anorexia/cachexia. No benefit

TABLE 41.2. *To Minimize Fatigue*

Titrate analgesia and other medications to relieve pain and to minimize sedation—Use short-acting narcotics to target activities of movement and greater personal control. Long-acting agents have the advantage of continuous relief, unbroken pain relief at night, but may be more sedating. Use adjuvant psychostimulants if necessary.

Advocate economy in emotional energy—The patient will need to set priorities, delegate, consider what brings pleasure. Allow care givers flexibility.

Diagnose and treat mood disorder.

Target anxiety syndromes with antianxiety techniques and medications to reduce anxiety again without sedation.

Attend to sleep hygiene—Pain relief. Short acting hypnotics. The best environment for sleep. Naps may be helpful if they do not preclude night-time sleep. Consider differential diagnosis of sleep disorder.

Consider other medical diagnoses—
    Hypothyroidism after radiation to head or neck
    Low cortisol after corticosteroids or high dose megestrol (84,85)
    Low magnesium with cisplatin-induced renal impairment compounded by diuretics or anorexia.

Monitor postural blood pressure change—
    Keep physical conditioning in mind. Sit if possible; stand if possible; walk if possible.
    Reduce antihypertensive medications, so that blood pressure is not overtreated during illness and cancer treatment.
    Monitor hematocit, and treat anemia as needed.
    Treat autonomic neuropathy secondary to chemotherapy; consider fluorocortisone, or stimulants.

was found in a study of 70 patients. It was not clear that TNF levels were altered.

FATIGUE IN SURVIVORS

When cancer survivors complete treatment they return to the developmental challenges of their lives, but they carry fear of recurrence and physical losses of treatment, e.g. a portion of lung or a leg may have been lost. Lingering side effects of fatigue and sleep disturbance have been reported to limit full life in survivors of bone marrow transplantation (77), Hodgkin's disease (78), or breast cancer (15).

Some complications of treatment would clearly diminish stamina. After bone marrow transplantation, some are coping with graft-versus-host disease. Subclinical cardiac compromise due to anthracycline toxicity might limit peak exercise capacity. Subclinical abnormalities of left ventricular structure and function due to anthracycline are common and progressive in survivors of childhood malignancy. While the physiological mechanism of injury in unclear, a relative restrictive cardiomyopathy with less left ventricular compliance and a small thin left ventricle may describe the course (79). The peripheral neuropathy of paclitaxel or type II muscle atrophy of corticosteroids may prolong specific muscle weakness. The tendency of bleomycin to cause pulmonary fibrosis and alveolar damage may be documented in impaired

ventilation following exercise (80). Deficits in pulmonary function tests may remain even when clinical improvement occurs (81).

If a high level of fatigue perists in survivors following treatment, hypothyroidism should be considered. It is a risk for those who had radiation near the thyroid or radiation to the sinuses or head, suppressing pituitary thyrotropin function (82,83).

CONCLUSIONS

The complaint of fatigue must be described specifically in order for the different etiologies to be explored. The meaning of the symptom must be understood in the context of the patient's values and beliefs. It may be a symptom directly related to the malignancy. The patient will appreciate knowing the course of treatment-related fatigue, so that he can plan appropriately and not worry that weakness is a sign of progressive disease. Sleep, exercise, and budgeting of energy can be helpful. When fatigue has a distinct medical cause, treatment will be specific. Since psychiatric syndromes cause profound fatigue without cancer, diagnosis of mood disorder and treatment of anxiety syndromes are essential for specific alleviating treatments. When fatigue is one aspect of advancing cancer, palliative treatments like stimulants may improve quality of life. Palliative treatment is still difficult and is an open field for research.

REFERENCES

1. Melzack R. The McGill Pain Questionnaire: major properties and scoring methods. *Pain*. 1975; 1:277–299.

2. Smets EMA, Garssen B, Schuster-Uitterhoeve ALJ, de Haes JCJM. Fatigue in cancer patients. *Br J Cancer*. 1993; 68:220–224.

3. Winningham M, Nail LM, Burke MB, Brophy L, et al. Fatigue and the cancer experience: the state of the knowledge. *Oncol Nurs Forum*. 1994; 21:23–36.

4. Barofsky I, Legro MW. Definition and measurement of fatigue. *Rev Infec Dis*. 1991; 13(1 suppl):S94–S97.

5. Piper BF. Fatigue: current bases for practice. In: Funk SG, Tornquist EM, Champagne MT, Copp LA, Wiese RA, eds. *Key Aspects of Comfort: Management of Pain, Fatigue, and Nausea*. New York: Springer; 1989:189–198.

6. Hollen PJ, Gralla RJ, Kris MG, Cox C. Quality of life during clinical trials: conceptual model for the Lung Cancer Symptom Scale (LCSS) (Review). *Support Care Cancer*. 1994; 2(4):213–222.

7. Wood C, Magnello ME, Jewell T. Measuring vitality. *Proc R Soc Med*. 1990; 83:486–489.

8. Horowitz M, Soneborn D, Sugahara C, Maercker A. Self-regard: a new measure. *Am J Pyschiatry*. 1996; 153:382–385.

9. McCorkle R, Young K. Development of a symptom distress scale. *Cancer Nurs*. 1978; 10:373–378.

10. Portenoy RK, Thaler HT, Kornblith AB, et al. The Memorial symptom assessment scale: an instrument for the evaluation of symptom prevalence, characteristics, and distress. *Eur J Cancer*. 1994; 30A:1326–1336.

11. Cella DF, Tulsky DS, Gray G, et al. The functional assessment of cancer therapy scale: development and validation of the general measure. *J Clin Oncol*. 1993; 11:570–579.

12. Pearson RG, Byars GE Jr. The development and validation of a checklist for measuring subjective fatigue. Air University, School of Aviation Medicine, US Air Force, Randolph Air Force Base, Texas; Dec 1956. Document no. 56115.

13. McNair DM, Lorr M, Droppeman LF. *Profile of Mood States*. San Diego CA: Educational and Industrial Testing Service; 1971.

14. Rhoten D. Fatigue and the postsurgical patients. In: Norris CM, ed. *Concept Clarification in Nursing*. Rockville, MD: Aspen; 1982:277–300.

15. Schag CAC, Ganz PA, Polinsky ML, et al. Characterisitics of women at risk for psychosocial distress in the year after breast cancer. *J Clin Oncol*. 1993; 11:783–793.

16. Bloom JR, Gorsky RD, Fobair P, et al. Physical performance at work and at leisure: validation of a measure of biological energy in survivors of Hodgkin's disease. *J Psychosoc Oncol*. 1990; 8:49–63.

17. Piper BF, Dibble S, Dodd MJ, Weiss M, Slaughter R, Paul S. The revised Piper Fatigue Scale: confirmation of its mutidimensionality and reduction in number of items in women with breast cancer. *Oncol Nurs Forum*. In press.

18. Piper BF. Fatigue and cancer: inevitable companions? [Editorial]. (Comment on *Support Care Cancer*. 1993; 1(6):305–315.) *Support Care Cancer*. 1993; 1(6):285–286.

19. Wessely S, Powell R. Fatigue syndromes: a comparison of chronic post-viral fatigue with neuromuscular and affective disorders. *J Neurol Neurosurg Psychiatry*. 1989; 52:940–948.

20. Schwartz JE, Jandorf L, Krupp LB. The measurement of fatigue: a new instrument. *J Psychosom Res*. 1993; 37:753-762.

21. Vercoulen JHMM, Swanink CMA, Fennis JFM, Galama JMD, van der Meer JWM, Bleijenberg G. Dimensional assessment of chronic fatigue syndrome. *J Psychosom Res*. 1994; 38:383–392.

22. Chalder T, Berelowitz G, Pawlikowska T, et al. Development of a fatigue scale. *J Psychosom Res*. 1993; 37:147–153.

23. Irvine D, Vincent L, Graydon JE, Bubela N, Thompson L. The prevalence and correlates of fatigue in patients receiving treatment with chemotherapy and radiotherapy. A comparison with the fatigue experienced by healthy individuals. *Cancer Nurs*. 1994; 17(5):367–378.

24. MacVicar MG, Winningham ML, Nickel JL. Effects of interval training on cancer patients' functional capacity. *Cancer Nurs Res*. 1989; 38:348–351.

25. Winningham ML. Walking program for people with trouble getting started. *Cancer Nurs*. 1991; 14:270–276.

26. Graydon JE, Bubela N, Irvine D, Vincent L. Fatigue reducing strategies used by patients receiving treatment for cancer. *Cancer Nurs*. 1995; 18(1):23–28.

27. Quesada Jr, Talpaz M, Rios A, et al. Clinical toxicity of interferons in cancer patients: a review. *J Clin Oncol*. 1986; 4:234–243.

28. Denicoff KD, Rubinow DR, Papa M, et al. The neuropsychiatric effects of interleukin-2/lymphokine activated killer cell treatment. *Ann Intern Med*. 1987; 107:293–300.

29. MacDonald DR. Neurotoxicity of chemotherapeutic agents. In: Perry MC, ed. *The Chemotherapy Sourcebook*. Baltimore: Williams and Wilkins; 1992:666–679.

30. Ling MHM, Perr PJ, Tsuang MT. Side effect of corticosteroid therapy. Psychiatric aspects. *Arch Gen Psychiatry*. 1981; 38:471–477.

31. D'Erasmo E, Celi FS, Acca M, et al. Hypocalcemia and hypomagnesemia in cancer patients. *Biomed Pharmacother*. 1991; 45:315–317.

32. Reinhart RA. Magnesium metabolism. *Arch Intern Med*. 1988; 148:2415–2420.

33. Case DC,Jr, Bukowski RM, Carey RW, et al. Recombinant human erythropoietin therapy for anemic cancer patients on combination chemotherapy. *J Natl Cancer Inst*. 1993; 85:801-806.

34. Abels RI. Use of recombinant human erythropoietin in the treatment of anemia in patients who have cancer. *Semin Oncol*. 1992; 19(suppl 8):29–35.

35. Oster W, Herrmann F, Gamm H, et al. Erythropoietin for the treatment of anemia of malignancy associated with neoplastic bone marrow infiltration. *J Clin Oncol*. 1990; 8:956–962.

36. Ludwig H. Erythropoietin for anemia of cancer. *Cancer*. 1995; 76:2319–2329.

37. Denton TA, Diamond GA, Matloff JM, Gray RJ. Anemia therapy: individual benefit and societal cost. *Semin Oncol*. 1994; 21:(suppl 3):29–35.

38. King K, Nail L, Kreamer K, Strohl R, Johnson J. Patients' descriptions of the experience of receiving radiation therapy. *Oncol Nurs Forum*. 1985; 12:55–61

39. Perez CA, Brady LW. Overview. In: Perez CA, Brady LW, eds. *Principles and Practice in Radiation Oncology*, 2d ed. Philadelphia: JB Lippincott; 1992:1–63.

40. Greenberg DB, Sawicka J, Eisenthal S, Ross D. Fatigue syndrome due to localized radiation. *J Pain Symptom Manage*. 1992; 7:38–44.

41. Irvine D, Vincent L, Graydon JE, Bubela N, Thompson L. The prevalence and correlates of fatigue in patients receiving treatment with chemotherapy and radiotherapy. A comparison with the fatigue experienced by healthy individuals. *Cancer Nurs*. 1994; 17(5):367–378.

42. Greenberg DB, Gray JL, Mannix CM, Eisenthal S, Carey M. Treatment-related fatigue and serum interleukin-1 levels in patients during external beam irradiation for prostate cancer. *J Pain Symptom Manage*. 1993; 8:196–200.

43. Haylock P, Hart L. Fatigue in patients receiving localized radiation. *Cancer Nurs*. 1979; 2:461–467.

44. Graydon JE. Women with breast cancer: their quality of life following a course of radiation therapy. *J Adv Nurs*. 1994; 19(4):617–622.

45. Christensen T, Bendix T, Kehlet H. Fatigue and cardio-respiratory function following abdominal surgery. *Br J Surg*. 1982; 69:417–419.

46. Weisman AD. *The Coping Capacity on the Nature of Being Mortal*. New York: Human Sciences Press; 1984.

47. Greenberg DB. Neurasthenia in the 1980s: Chronic mononucleosis, chronic fatigue syndrome, depression and anxiety. *Psychosymatics*. 1990; 31:129–137.

48. Greenberg DB, Eisenthal S, Tesar G, et al. Linking panic disorder and depression: the fatigue dimension. *Ann Clin Psychiatry*. 1991; 3:1–4.

49. Greenberg DB. Strategic use of benzodiazepines in cancer patients. *Oncology*. 1991; 5:83–88.

50. Spiegel D, Sands S, Koopman C. Pain and depression in patients with cancer. *Cancer*. 1994; 74:2570–2578.

51. Glover J, Dibble SL, Dodd MJ, Miaskowski C. Mood states of oncology outpatients: does pain make a difference? *J Pain Symptom Manage*. 1995; 10(2):120–128.

52. Silberfarb PM, Hauri PJ, Oxman TE, Schnurr P. Assessment of sleep in patients with lung cancer and breast cancer. *J Clin Oncol*. 1993; 11:997–1004.

53. Donnelly S, Walsh D. The symptoms of advanced cancer. *Semin. Oncol*. 1995; 22(2 Suppl 3):67–72.

54. Donnelly S, Walsh D, Rybicki L. The symptoms of advanced cancer; identification of clinical and research priorities by assessment of prevalence and severity. *J Palliat Care*. 1995; 11:27–32.

55. Bruera E, MacDonald RN. Asthenia in patients with advanced cancer. *J Pain Symptom Manage*. 1988; 3:9–14.

56. Breitbart W, Bruera E, Chochinov H. Neuropsychiatric syndromes and psychological symptoms in patients with advance cancer. *J Pain Symptom Manage*. 1995; 10(2):131–141.

57. Warmolts J, Petek K, Lewis R, et al. Type II muscle fibre atrophy—an early systemic effect of cancer. *Neurology*. 1975; 25:374.

58. Grunfeld C, Feingold KR. Metabolic disturbances and wasting in the acquired immunodeficiency syndrome. *N Engl J Med*. 1992; 327:329–337.

59. Socher SH, Martinez D, Craig JB, Kuhn JG, Oliff A. Tumor necrosis factor not detectable in patients with clinical cancer cachexia. *J Natl Cancer Inst*. 1988; 80:595–598.

60. Hart BL. Biological basis of the behavior of sick animals. *Neurosci Biobehav Rev*. 1988; 12:123–137.

61. Rothwell NJ, Hopkins SJ. Cytokines and the nervous system II: actions and mechanisms of action. *Trends Neurosci*. 1995; 18:130–136.

62. Clark CR, Geffen GM, Geffen LB. Catecholamines and attention, II: pharmacological studies in normal humans. *Neurosci Biobehav Rev*. 1987; 353–364.

63. Katon W, Raskind M. Treatment of depression in the medically ill with methylphenidate. *Am J Psychiatry*. 1980; 137:963.

64. Kaufmann MW, Murray GB, Cassem NH. Use of psychostimulants in medically ill depressed patients. *Psychosomatics*. 1982; 23:817.

65. Weitzner MA, Meyers CA, Valentine AD, Methylphenidate in the treatment of neurobehavioral slowing associated with cancer and cancer treatment. *J Neuropsychiatry*. 1995; 7:347–350.

66. Forrest W, Brown B, Brown C, et al. Dextroamphetamine with morphine for the treatment of postoperative pain. *N Engl J Med*. 1977; 296:712–715.

67. Bruera E, Brenneis C, Paterson A, et al. Use of methylphenidate as an adjuvant to narcotic analgesics in patients with advanced cancer. *J Pain Symptom Manage*. 1989; 4:3–6.

68. Willox M, Corr J, Shaw J, et al. Prednisolone as an appetite stimulant in patients with cancer *Br Med J*. 1984; 200:37.

69. Bruera E, Roca E, Cedaro L, Carraro S, Chacon R. Action of oral methylprednisolone in terminal cancer patients: a prospective randomized double blind study. *Cancer Treat Rep*. 1985; 69:751–754.

70. Moertel C, Shutte A, Reitemeier R, et al. Corticosteroid therapy of preterminal gastrointestinal cancer. *Cancer*. 1974; 33:1607–1609.

71. Bruera E, Macmillan K, Kuehn N, et al. A controlled trial of megestrol acetate on appetite, caloric intake, nutritional status, and other symptoms in patients with advanced cancer. *Cancer*. 1990; 66:1279–1282.

72. Loprinzi CL, Michalak JC, Schaid DJ, et al. Phase III evaluation of four doses of megestrol acetate as therapy for patients with cancer anorexia and/or cachexia. *J Clin Oncol*. 1993; 11:762–767.

73. Tchekmedyian NS, Hickman M, Siau J, et al. Megestrol acetate in cancer anorexia and weight loss. *Cancer*. 1992; 69:1268–74.

74. Loprinzi CL, Jensen MD, Jiang NS, Schaid DJ. Effect of megestrol acetate on the human pituitary-adrenal axis. *Mayo Clin Proc*. 1992; 67:1160–1162.

75. Dezube BJ, Sherman ML, Fridovich-Keil JL, et al. Down regulation of tumor necrosis factor expression by pentoxifylline in cancer patients: a pilot study. *Cancer Immunol Immunother*. 1993; 36:57–60.

76. Bush NE, Habarman M, Donaldson G, Sullivan KM. Quality of life of 125 adults surviving 6–18 yr after bone marrow transplantation. *Soc Sci Med* 1995; 40(4):479–490.

77. Fobair P, Hoppe RT, Bloom J, et al. Psychosocial problems among survivors of Hodgkin's disease. *J Clin Oncol*. 1976; 4:805–814.

78. Lipshultz SE. Dexrazoxane for protection againt cardio-toxic effects of anthracyclines in children. *J Clin Oncol.* 1996; 14:328–331 (editorial).

79. Piotti P, Genitoni V, Comazzi R, et al. Relationship between pulmonary function tests and morphologic changes in the lung in bleomycin-treated patients. *Tumori.* 1984; 70:439–444.

80. Luursema PB, Star-Kroesen MA, Van Der Mark THW, et al. Bleomycin-induced changes in the carbon monoxide transfer factor of the lungs and its components. *Am Rev Respir Dis.* 1983; 128:880–883.

81. Constine LS, Woolf PD, Conn D, et al. Hypothalamic-pituitary dysfunction after radiation for brain tumors. *N Engl J Med.* 1992; 328:87–94.

82. Hancock SL, Cox RS, McDougall R. Thyroid diseases after treatment of Hodgkin's disease. *N Engl J Med.* 1991; 325:599–604.

83. Jensen S, Given B. Fatigue affecting family caregivers of cancer patients. Comment in: *Support Care Cancer.* 1993; 1(6):321–325.

84. Loprinzi CL, Fonseca R, Jensen MD. Induction of adrenal suppression by megestrol acetate. *Ann Intern Med.* 1996; 124:613; discussion 614.

85. Leinung MC, Liporace R, Miller CH. Induction of adrenal suppression by megestrol acetate in patients with AIDS. *Ann Intern Med.* 1995; 122:843–845.

42

Sexual Dysfunction

LESLIE R. SCHOVER

THE IMPORTANCE OF SEXUAL PROBLEMS TO CANCER PATIENTS

Although sexual dysfunction is a frequent problem for men and women with cancer, it has received a good deal less attention than other sequelae of cancer treatment discussed in this part. Despite the focus on sexuality in our society, an attitude remains that sexual function is less important than other daily life activities, such as returning to work, doing household chores, or socializing with family. Yet, a recent survey about sexuality among Americans aged 18 to 59 demonstrated that those who have more frequent sex rate themselves as happier. Sexual dysfunctions were associated both with poorer health and personal unhappiness (1). Even after age 60, most Americans remain sexually active unless ill health or loss of a partner interrupts their sex lives (2). Thus, for many cancer patients, loss of the ability to enjoy sex, whether transient or permanent, has a significant impact.

Predicting Patient Distress about Sexual Issues

Minimal research is available to help clinicians predict which cancer patients are at risk for strong distress when their treatment causes sexual problems. Clinical experience suggests some obvious factors, however. Younger patients experience more distress over sexual dysfunction (3). They have not yet faced the changes of aging that slow or mute sexual responding and sex is likely to be an important force in their primary relationship. A profound change in sexual function, such as loss of erectile capacity or the sexual impact of premature ovarian failure, may also be accompanied by loss of fertility.

Being unmarried may also increase risk for distress over sexual dysfunction. Americans have their most frequent and enjoyable sex in monogamous relationships (1). Those who are single often view a sexual problem as a handicap in finding an appropriate partner. Men and women in less committed relationships,

i.e., dating or living together but not legally married, have less confidence that a partner will continue to love them despite the impact of the cancer. Whether married or not, people who have a pattern of multiple casual sexual relationships that will be interrupted by a sexual dysfunction are often highly distressed. In clinical experience, this patient group is almost exclusively male. In the recent survey on sexual behavior (1) cited above, 33% of men, but only 9% of women reported having had more than 10 sexual partners since age 18.

Another factor is the duration of the previous relationship. Even married couples who have only recently wed show more distress over sexual difficulties after cancer than those who have had a long history together. The recency of marriage can be an issue for older couples who have remarried after being divorced or widowed. The spouse with cancer may feel that he or she is burdening the new mate with an unexpected illness and loss of sexual pleasure. For younger couples who are newly married, a complicating factor occurs if not only sexual function but fertility has been impaired.

Men or women who have had a history of sexual failure or trauma in the past are often more upset when cancer interferes with sex than are those who enjoy confidence and pleasure in their sexuality. Women who have histories of sexual abuse often perceive the cancer treatment as another uncontrollable assault on their body, especially if the tumor affects the genitals or breasts. Men or women who already have sexual problems such as erectile dysfunction or pain with intercourse may dread the double burden of coping with the sexual impact of cancer treatment.

Some patients are unlikely to care a good deal about cancer-related sexual dysfunction. These include patients who have already ceased sexual activity because of aging, ill health, preexisting sexual dysfunction, or lack of a partner.

494

THE HISTORY OF PSYCHO-ONCOLOGY AND SEXUAL ISSUES

Breast Cancer: The Earliest Focus

Mental health researchers first studied sexuality as an aspect of quality of life 40 years ago, when the psychologist Morton Bard and his colleagues focused on women's efforts to cope with the mutilation of radical mastectomy (4). Sexual issues in women with breast cancer were studied further in the 1970s and 1980s by Dr. Wendy Schain and colleagues (5), who produced studies demonstrating sexual problems after mastectomy, with advantages for breast conservation or breast reconstruction in preserving sexual satisfaction. As the literature comparing breast conservation or mastectomy with reconstruction grew, however, a whole series of studies cast doubt on the idea that choice of local treatment was a crucial determinant of sexual function after breast cancer (6,7).

Gynecologic Cancers

Just as the trauma of breast loss led researchers to focus on sexuality after breast cancer, concerns about women's ability to cope with loss of the vagina, vulva, or uterus were the focus of projects to examine sexual satisfaction and function after gynecologic cancers. As it became clear that women in these diagnostic groups had sexual problems quite commonly after cancer treatment (8), efforts were made to compare the impact of different cancer therapies in women with favorable disease. Radical surgery appeared less damaging than definitive radiotherapy for women with early-stage cervical cancer (9). Wide local excision was superior to radical vulvectomy in preserving sexual function in women with in situ vulvar cancer (10).

Sexual Problems in Men after Cancer

In men, attention to sexual issues was increased as surgical techniques promised to spare damage to nerves crucial to erection and ejaculation. Increased recovery of erections has been documented after nerve sparing radical prostatectomy and cystectomy (11) as well as colorectal resection (12). In young men with testicular cancer, efforts to preserve antegrade ejaculation by limiting the extent of retroperitoneal lymphadenectomy have also been successful (13). Psychologically oriented researchers broadened their focus to demonstrate a relationship between sexual dysfunction and poor individual or couple psychological adjustment (3,14).

Sexual Problems with Other Cancer Sites

Sexual problems in patients with cancer not involving the genitals, pelvis, or breasts have more rarely been assessed. Psychological distress related to sexuality has been documented after treatment for leukemia (15) and Hodgkin's disease (16), however.

Outcome of Sexual Rehabilitation

Despite many studies documenting the prevalence and types of sexual problems after cancer treatment, research on the outcome of interventions to alleviate sexual dysfunction has been sadly lacking. A case series from M. D. Anderson Cancer Center suggested that brief counseling was the most frequently used mode of sexual rehabilitation, but that success in reversing problems increased with the number of sessions of treatment (3). A brief therapy group specifically designed to help women resume sex comfortably after gynecologic cancer treatment demonstrated some success (17).

CLINICAL UPDATE ON SEXUAL PROBLEMS OF CANCER PATIENTS

Assessing Sexual Problems Related to Cancer

The cornerstone of assessing sexual function and satisfaction remains the interview (18). In most settings, sexuality assessment will take place within the context of assessing psychological adjustment and quality of life. Although it is preferable to gather information and discuss anticipated changes in sexual function at the time of treatment disposition (18), in practice most sexual counseling takes place after cancer treatment is over, when patients complain of a problem (3).

No matter when the interaction occurs, it is important to establish rapport with the patient before asking detailed questions about sensitive sexual matters. The interviewer may begin by reviewing demographic information and eliciting the patient's emotional reactions to cancer diagnosis and treatment. Questions about the patient's social support network and the quality of the current marriage or dating relationship often lead smoothly into a discussion about sexuality. If the patient is married or living with a partner, it is quite useful to include the significant other in the interview. In asking about a committed relationship, the couple's communication, support offered by the partner during the experience of illness, expression of anger, and expression of nonsexual affection are important topics. If both partners are present, the interviewer ideally should take a few minutes to interview each individually, to make sure that no important information is being concealed, such as an extramarital affair, domestic violence, or substance abuse.

The interviewer should have a sophisticated knowledge of sexual physiology, including the medical influence of cancer treatments on sexual function (19) and the impact of other chronic illnesses and medications (18).

Table 42.1 lists sexual issues that should be assessed. Another helpful guide for the interview, and a self-report questionnaire in its own right, is the Sex History Form. In a 46-item multiple-choice questionnaire, each item can be used as a measure of an aspect of sexual function or satisfaction; alternatively, a global scale comprising 12 items can be calculated to estimate Global Sexual Functioning (20).

The Sex History Form is an appropriate research instrument when a multifaceted, detailed picture of sexual function is desired. If only a brief sexuality assessment is needed for research, the sexuality subscales of the Psychosocial Adjustment to Illness Scale (21) or the Cancer Rehabilitation Evaluation System (22) may be used.

Managing Sexual Problems across the Timeline of Cancer Treatment

Treatment Disposition.   Concerns about preserving sexual function can influence the choices men and women make about their cancer treatment. A prime example is the controversy over whether to use watchful waiting, radical prostatectomy, or radiation therapy to treat localized prostate cancer. Fear of losing erectile capacity is the most common reason that men themselves may reject the most effective treatment (23). Yet, many concerns can be alleviated by discussion, tailored to the patient's particular concerns, not only of the risks of different treatment options in terms of loss of rigid erections but the fact that across options, sexual desire and the ability to experience pleasure and orgasm will not be damaged. Men can also benefit from information on medical treatments to restore erections, including vacuum constriction devices, injection therapy, and penile prostheses (24).

For women, treatment decisions such as whether to have adjuvant chemotherapy after node-negative breast cancer are often made without adequate information on the sexual impact of premature ovarian failure (6). Preliminary data suggest that undergoing chemotherapy may be a more powerful factor in causing sexual dysfunction than the choice of local treatment for breast cancer (7). More information on normal female sexual function and the influence of cancer treatments on it can be made available (25).

Problems during Cancer Treatment.   The most common problems during treatment involve the interruption of sexual activity because of the acute effects of surgery, pelvic irradiation, or chemo-

TABLE 42.1. *Assessing Sexual Issues*

Sexual Practices, Comparing Before and After Cancer
Frequency of sexual activity with a partner
Frequency of masturbation and attitudes about it
Who initiates partner sex and how does initiation happen?
Duration and types of noncoital sexual stimulation
Activities involving penetration, positions and types
Use of contraception and safer sex precautions

Sexual Function, Comparing Before and After Cancer	
Function in Men	Function in Women
Sexual desire, frequency and triggers	Sexual desire, frequency and triggers
Ability to achieve and maintain erections; Firmness of erections; erections on waking from sleep or in masturbation; changes with aging if relevant	Vaginal expansion and lubrication; changes with menopause if relevant
Trouble reaching orgasm; premature ejaculation; ability to ejaculate semen at orgasm	Ability to reach orgasm in masturbation, with noncoital stimulation from a partner, and with penetration
Pain with sex, location, triggers, descriptors, and duration	Pain with sex, location, triggers, descriptors, and duration

Treatment Planning
What changes in sexual life are desired?
What is the partner's perspective on the sexual problem?
What knowledge does the patient have of available treatments?

therapy. Most older men and women are able to tolerate a hiatus in sexual activity without much distress. Younger patients, especially those in new or shaky relationships, however, may fear losing their partner if sexual satisfaction is reduced. A helpful intervention is to interview both partners together, reassuring them that sexual rehabilitation is possible, and previewing techniques that can be used once treatment is finished. An additional strategy is to promote more relaxed, sensual touching instead of goal-oriented, penetrative sex. Structured sensate focus exercises can be suggested (24,25).

The Year after Treatment. The first year after cancer treatment is the time when most sexual dysfunctions caused by cancer therapy will appear. Anxiety about resolving these problems also rises, as men and women return to other normal daily life activities and recover from the miseries of their illness. The routine medical follow-up appointments during this period offer an excellent opportunity for brief sexual assessment and identification of problems that require intervention.

Loss of sexual desire is one of the most frequent complaints in both men and women after cancer treatment. In men, lack of testosterone is rarely a major factor, except with hormonal treatment for metastatic prostate cancer (26). In that patient group, where testosterone replacement is anything but desirable, the only recourse is to try to enhance sexual fantasy and physical stimulation with erotic materials, prolonged and varied lovemaking, and vibrator stimulation. Occasionally, young men who have had systemic chemotherapy or treatment for testicular cancer become hypogonadal and can respond well to hormonal replacement (27). Premenopausal women whose ovaries are surgically removed, or who experience ovarian failure after pelvic irradiation or systemic chemotherapy, may also have loss of sexual desire related to deprivation of ovarian androgens (28). Although some mental health professionals advocate replacement testosterone, it is unknown how often serum androgen levels in these women are below normal and whether this biochemical change routinely translates into a subjective loss of sexual function.

More commonly, loss of sexual desire does not have a direct hormonal cause but is a concomitant of major depression; loss of physical well-being; use of medications such as opiates, serotonergic antidepressants, antihypertensives, or antiemetics; or the emotional impact of lost attractiveness or sexual function (19). Management may involve sex therapy techniques such as training in focusing on erotic images, practice in initiating sex, and specific interventions to decrease sexual problems interfering with arousal or orgasm. Changing medications that may reduce desire or alleviating chronic pain and fatigue can also be of help.

Erectile dysfunction is the most common male sexual problem related to cancer treatment. After radical pelvic surgery, especially if nerve sparing techniques were used, there is typically a 6- to 12-month waiting period to see how much erections will recover in rigidity. During that time, men who are anxious to resume sex that involves penetration may use vacuum constriction devices or injections of medication into the penis. There is even some speculation that promoting erections by artificial means during this recovery period may increase the chance that rigidity will return, probably by preventing formation of collagen deposits that render the penile tissue less elastic (29). Men who have had definitive pelvic irradiation, especially from an external beam, may develop a gradual and permanent loss of rigid erections during the first year after finishing treatment (26). Encouraging a couple to resume sex despite an erection problem helps a man to explore how strong his sexual desire, penile sensation, and ability to enjoy orgasm have remained. If these other elements of sexual function are normal, he may be more motivated to pursue a medical or surgical treatment to restore erections.

In women, pain during sexual activity, or dyspareunia, is one of the most common postcancer sexual problems. Many physical causes of dyspareunia are linked to cancer treatment (19), including loss of genital tissue or pelvic organs in radical surgery, the impact of radiotherapy on the vagina and surrounding tissue, and vaginal atrophy related to untreated menopause. Women need advice on using water-based lubricants such as Astroglide (Biofilm, Inc., Vista, CA) or the vaginal moisturizer, Replens (Columbia Laboratories, Inc., Miami, FL). Women can learn to use more comfortable positions for lovemaking, and to relax their pelvic muscles, sometimes with the aid of vaginal dilators (19,25). Women whose malignancy did not involve the breast are typically good candidates for estrogen replacement therapy, which can quickly reverse the loss of vaginal elasticity and lubrication caused by menopause. Women may be frightened to take estrogen because they know it is associated with cancer risk. The risks verus the benefits of estrogen replacement should be explored in detail with each patient, based on her own health and family history.

Trouble in reaching orgasm is usually not a direct result of cancer treatment. Even after total penectomy, many men learn to have orgasms through fantasy or caressing of remaining penile tissue (19). Women have had orgasms after total vulvectomy (30). Trouble with attaining orgasm is often a secondary problem related to lack of sexual desire and arousal, or pain interfering with sexual pleasure. When men have erection problems, they often do not try extensive noncoital stimulation to discover whether they could experience an orgasm without achieving a firm erection. The newer serotonergic antidepressants also frequently delay or prevent orgasm in both men and women. Sex therapy techniques that increase sexual pleasure and arousal are often helpful in promoting orgasm (24,25). Premature ejaculation is one sexual dysfunction that does not appear to increase after cancer treatment (3).

Long-Term Survivors. Unfortunately, many long-term cancer survivors have ongoing sexual problems that were never identified or addressed in interactions with the health care system. Sometimes the problems are brought to light because a particular practitioner takes an interest in quality of life, or because a change in relationship status makes the problem so distressing that the patient seeks professional help. It is rarely too late to treat a sexual complaint, but the years of misery already endured cannot be undone. Organizations that reach out to cancer survivors need to include information on sexual problems and their treatments in their public education programs. Rather than waiting for men and women to mention their concerns, education on causes and treatments of sexual dysfunctions after cancer should be proactive.

NEEDS FOR RESEARCH ON SEXUAL PROBLEMS

Although our knowledge about the sexual impact of varying cancer therapies has increased greatly, particularly in the past 15 years, several areas are in need of urgent attention. The sexual aftermath of systemic treatment in women needs to be much better understood (6). Is the dyspareunia and loss of sexual desire often seen after chemotherapy solely a result of ovarian failure, or do drugs have a direct and lasting impact on vaginal expansion and lubrication? How does weight gain or loss after chemotherapy influence women's body image? What percentage of women become deficient in androgens, and what is the typical impact on sexuality? The sexual side effects of tamoxifen (Nolvadex) have been poorly defined (6). In most respects, tamoxifen acts as a weak estrogen, and its effects on the vagina are to promote lubrication. Its influence on sexual desire is unexplored, although there are reports of both enhancement and impairment in the literature. The impact of bone marrow trans-

plantation or rescue on sexual function has also not been well defined (15).

Although some questions remain about the causes of sexual dysfunction related to cancer treatment, the most important need is for research on brief, economic, and effective intervention programs that provide education on sexual function after cancer, advice on resuming sex, and assign patients to more intensive interventions when necessary. In this era of managed care, many patients have little or no insurance coverage for psychotherapy or sex therapy. Cancer survivors are often struggling with high medical bills and cannot afford to pay out-of-pocket treatment costs. Clinicians in major cancer centers can design short-term group interventions tailored to a particular category of patient. Men and women treated outside of large, urban hospitals, however, rarely get any kind of information about sexuality. A self-help book may bridge this gap, however (31). Programs designed to reach out to ethnic minorities, with built-in sensitivity to cultural norms about sexuality, have not even been piloted. Use of the Internet or other computer technology to give educational information is another avenue. Although some bulletin boards include the topic of sex and cancer, nobody has studied the demographics of participants, the accuracy of information presented, or the impact on patients' lives.

Ultimately, managing sexual problems related to cancer treatment should be a routine aspect of oncology care.

REFERENCES

1. Laumann EO, Gagnon JH, Michael RT, Michaels S. *The Social Organization of Sexuality: Sexual Practices in the United States.* Chicago, IL: University of Chicago Press; 1994.
2. George LK, Weiler SJ. Sexuality in middle and late life: the effects of age, cohort and gender. *Arch Gen Psychiatry.* 1981; 38:919–923.
3. Schover LR, Evans RB, von Eschenbach AC. Sexual rehabilitation in a cancer center: diagnosis and outcome in 384 consultations. *Arch Sex Behav.* 1987; 16:445–461.
4. Bard M, Sutherland AM. Psychological impact of cancer and its treatment: IV. adaptation to radical mastectomy. *Cancer.* 1955; 8:656–672.
5. Schain WS. The sexual and intimate consequences of breast cancer treatment. *CA.* 1988; 38:154–161.
6. Schover LR. Sexuality and body image in younger women with breast cancer. *Monogr J Natl Cancer Inst.* 1994; 16:177–182.
7. Schover LR, Yetman RJ, Tuason LJ, et al. Comparison of partial mastectomy with breast reconstruction on psychosocial adjustment, body image, and sexuality. *Cancer.* 1995; 75:54–64.
8. Andersen BL, Anderson B, deProsse C. Controlled prospective longitudinal study of women with cancer: I.

Sexual functioning outcomes. *J Consult Clin Psychol.* 1989; 57:683–691.

9. Schover LR, Fife M, Gershenson DM. Sexual dysfunction and treatment for early stage cervical cancer. *Cancer.* 1989; 63:204–212.

10. Andersen Bl, Turnquist D, LoPolla J, Turner D. Sexual functioning after treatment of in situ vulvar cancer: preliminary report. *Obstet Gynecol.* 1988; 71:15–19.

11. Murphy GP, Mettlin C, Menck H, Winchester DP, Davidson AM. National patterns of prostate cancer treatment by radical prostatectomy: results of a survey by the American College of Surgeons Commission on Cancer. *J Urol.* 1994; 152:1817–1819.

12. Enker WE. Potency, cure, and local control in the operative treatment of rectal cancer. *Arch Surg.* 1992; 127:1396–1402.

13. Recker F, Tscholl R. Monitoring of emission as direct intraoperative control for nerve sparing retroperitoneal lymphadenectomy. *J Urol.* 1993; 150:1360–1364.

14. Gritz ER, Wellisch DK, Wang H, Siau J, Landsverk JA, Cosgrove MD. Long-term effects of testicular cancer on sexual functioning in married couples. *Cancer.* 1989; 64:15601–15567.

15. Mumma GH, Mashberg D, Lesko LM. Long-term psychosexual adjustment of acute leukemia survivors: impact of marrow transplantations versus conventional chemotherapy. *Gen Hosp Psychiatry.* 1992; 14:43–55.

16. Kornblith AB, Anderson J, Cella DF, et al. Comparison of psychosocial adaptation and sexual function of survivors of advanced Hodgkin disease treated by MOPP, ABVD, or MOPP alternating with ABVD. *Cancer.* 1992; 70:2508–2516.

17. Capone MA, Good RS, Westie KS, Jacobson F. Psychosocial rehabilitation of gynecologic oncology patients. *Arch Phys Med Rehabil.* 1980; 61:128–132.

18. Schover LR, Jensen SB. *Sexuality and Chronic Illness: A Comprehensive Approach.* New York: Guilford Press; 1988.

19. Schover LR, Montague DK, Schain WS. Supportive care and the quality of life of the cancer patient: sexual problems. In: DeVita VT, Hellman S, Rosenberg SA, eds. *Cancer: Principles and Practice of Oncology*, 4th ed. Philadelphia, PA: J. B. Lippincott; 1993:2464–2480.

20. Creti L, Fichten CS, Brender W, et al. Global sexual functioning: a single summary score for Nowinski and LoPiccolo's Sexual History Form (SHF). In: Davis CM, Yarber WH, Bauserman R, Schreer G, Davis SL, eds. *Sexuality-related Measures: a Compendium*, 2d ed. New York: Sage Publications. [In press].

21. Derogatis LR. Psychosocial Adjustment to Illness Scale (PAIS and PAIS-SR): administration, scoring and procedures manual. Baltimore, MD: Clinical Psychometric Research; 1983.

22. Schag CAC, Heinrich RL. Development of a comprehensive quality of life measurement tool: CARES. *Oncology.* 1990; 4:135–147.

23. Flemming C, Wasson JH, Albertsen PC, Barry MJ, Wennberg JE. A decision analysis of alternative treatment strategies for clinically localized prostate cancer. *J Am Med Assoc.* 1993; 269:2650.

24. Schover LR. *Sexuality and Cancer: For the Man Who Has Cancer, and His Partner.* New York: American Cancer Society; 1988.

25. Schover LR. *Sexuality and Cancer: For the Woman Who Has Cancer, and Her Partner.* New York: American Cancer Society; 1988.

26. Schover LR. Sexual rehabilitation after treatment for prostate cancer. *Cancer (Supplement).* 1993; 71:1024–1030.

27. Gradishar WJ, Schilsky RL. Effects of cancer treatment on the reproductive system. *Crit Rev Oncol Hematol.* 1988; 8:153–171.

28. Kaplan HS, Owett T. The female androgen deficiency syndrome. *J Sex Marital Ther.* 1993; 19:3–24.

29. Kim ED, Blackburn D, McVary KT. Post-radical prostatectomy penile blood flow: assessment with color flow Doppler ultrasound. *J Urol.* 1994; 152:2276–2279.

30. Weijmar Schultz WCM, van de Weil HBM, Bouma J, Janssens J, Littlewood J. Psychosexual functioning after the treatment of cancer of the vulva. *Cancer.* 1990; 66:402–407.

31. Schover LR. *Sexuality and Fertility after Cancer.* New York: John Wiley; 1997.

43

Neuropsychological Impact of Cancer and Cancer Treatments

SUSAN E. WALCH, TIM A. AHLES, AND ANDREW J. SAYKIN

Cognitive functioning plays an important role in quality of life. Normal cognitive functioning is critical for intellectual and academic development, occupational achievement, development and maintenance of social relationships, and appropriate self-care. Cognitive impairment can have a profound impact upon the quality of life of pediatric and adult cancer patients. Although the incidence and nature of cognitive impairment in cancer patients are still unclear, there is increasing information on these topics. Cognitive impairment can be subtle or dramatic, temporary or permanent, stable or progressive. Cognitive deficits in cancer patients have a multifactorial etiology. "Cognitive deficits are common in cancer patients who have experienced metastases to the central nervous system. However, primary central nervous system tumors or cerebral metastases from other sites need not be present in order for deficits in cognition to occur" (1; p. 100). Central nervous system tumors, cerebral metastases, and antineoplastic therapies that are directed at the central nervous system may cause cognitive impairment. Additionally, infections, fevers, nutritional deficiencies, metabolic/endocrinologic abnormalities, medications, and advancing age may also adversely impact cognitive functioning (2).

Interest in the neuropsychological impact of cancer treatment in adults dates back to the early 1980s, with studies suggesting that patients treated with chemotherapy experience measurable cognitive deficits on standard neuropsychological tests of verbal memory, psychomotor speed, sustained attention, fine motor coordination, and higher cognitive processing (3). Since that time, a growing body of research has demonstrated that adults treated with CNS radiation and/or chemotherapy show selective deficits on tasks assessing memory and other higher cognitive functions (4–9). Folstein and colleagues (10) found that between 14% and 29% of hospitalized cancer patients scored in the impaired range on a standardized mental status examination, suggesting some level of delirium or dementia. While cognitive impairment associated with cancer and its treatment in adults may not have the same developmental implications as for children, even subtle cognitive impairment can adversely impact the adult patient's quality of life. Subtle or mild dysfunction is frequently misdiagnosed as psychological reactions such as anxiety and depression (2). Cognitive disorder is associated with poorer prognosis and creates patient management problems (10). Although the neuropsychological impact of cancer and cancer therapies has been less frequently studied in adults than in children, there is mounting evidence suggesting risk for neurocognitive impairment in adults treated with conventional anticancer therapies. This chapter reviews the literature examining the neuropsychological and cognitive functioning of pediatric and adult cancer patients.

PRIMARY BRAIN TUMORS

Intuitively, primary brain tumors appear to pose a high potential for neurological and neurocognitive deficits in adults because of the inherent involvement of brain tissue; however, few systematic studies of the neurocognitive functioning of adults with brain tumors exist in the recent literature (11). This is due, at least in part, to the low frequency of certain types of brain tumors (12). As with the pediatric brain tumor literature, the small sizes of samples of patients preclude the multivariate analyses that would be required of such study because of such influential variables as location, mass effects, histology, and extent of surgery, radiation, and chemotherapy. A few systematic studies of neurocognitive functioning of adult patients with brain tumors have been performed that suggest that both focal and diffuse neurocognitive impairment may result from primary brain tumors in adults and their treatment.

Hochberg and Slotnick (13) reported diffuse deficits in all patients (13 astrocytoma patients suriving at least one year following diagnosis) tested by a neuropsychological battery, suggesting generalized cortical dysfunction. These diffuse deficits were in addition to the focal deficits compatible with the original tumor site. Meyers (14) reached similar conclusions: Patients with right hemispheric tumors demonstrated more difficulty on a task of visual perception, while patients with left hemispheric tumors demonstrated more difficulty on a verbal fluency task. In addition, impairment on a task of nonverbal reasoning and analytic ability was associated with more extensive treatment, suggesting that extensive treatment may cause more diffuse cortical dysfunction. Horn and Reitan (15) found that patients with rapidly growing tumors (e.g., glioblastoma multiforme, astrocytoma, grade III or IV) experienced greater neuropsychological and intellectual impairment than patients with slowly growing tumors (e.g., ogliodendroglioma, astrocytoma, grade I or II). Lateralization of the tumor also predicted functional outcome: Left hemisphere tumors were associated with deficits in verbal tests while right hemisphere tumors were associated with deficits in performance tests. Maire and colleague's (16) assessed the intellectual functioning of a sample of 49 patients treated for a variety of brain tumors. These authors reported that only 14 patients (28%) had full-scale IQ scores in the normal range. Impaired intellectual functioning was correlated with time elapsed since treatment: after a 4- to 5-month interval, significant intellectual deterioration was observed. However, subsequent testing of a subset of the initial sample revealed that some of the patients may demonstrate eventual improvement.

These studies indicate that primary brain tumors are often associated with diffuse cognitive dysfunction as well as focal deficits that may be related to the site of the tumor. Although the association between tumor location and specific neurocognitive/behavioral symptoms is generally modest, some relatively common symptom constellations have been described for lobular tumors (11). Frontal lobe tumors have been associated with several behavioral syndromes, characterized by the following symptom clusters: (*1*) behavioral disinhibition, emotional lability, socially inappropriate behavior, poor judgment, and lack of insight; (*2*) apathy, indifference, psychomotor retardation, attentional and/or perseveration problems; and (*3*) akinesia (motor inhibition), mutism, and failure to respond to commands. Temporal lobe tumors have been associated with episodic mood swings (including depressed mood, irritability, mania, hypomania, and anxiety); visual, olfactory, tactile, and auditory hallucinations, seizures, and memory impairment. Tumors located in the parietal lobe have been associated with sensory and motor abnormalities, including astereognosis and agraphesthesia (tactile recognition difficulties), apraxias (motor difficulties) anosognosia (unawareness of one's deficits), acalculia, and dysgraphia. Occipital tumors have been associated with visual phenomena, homonymous hemianopsia (loss of half of the visual field of both eyes), and visual recognition difficulties (e.g., agnosia, prosopagnosia). Detailed discussion of the localization effects of brain tumors is beyond the scope of this chapter; the reader is referred to other sources (11,17,18) for further discussion of the neuropsychiatric and neurocognitive impact of primary brain tumors.

RADIATION THERAPY

Radiation to the central nervous system can be used therapeutically to treat CNS malignancies or prophylactically to prevent CNS metastasis. Both forms of CNS radiation treatment have been implicated as a principal risk factor for neurocognitive impairment in children treated for brain tumors and leukemia. Several variables may influence the level of neurotoxicity from radiation to the central nervous system, including total dose of radiation, overall time of administration, volume of tissue irradiated, size of the individual fraction of radiation given, total number of fractions given, and the integrity of the blood supply in the irradiated area (19,20). Acute reactions (i.e., cerebral edema), early delayed reactions (i.e., demyelination), and late delayed reactions (e.g., leukoencephalopathy, radiation necrosis) can occur; late delayed reactions constitute the major hazard because these are generally irreversible and progressive, and may be fatal (21). Radiation encephalopathy appears to be more common than overt radiation necrosis; in fact, a comprehensive review of 47 studies of the neurobehavioral sequelae of therapuetic and prophylactic cranial irradiation including over 1100 patients concluded that 28% of patients will demonstrate encephalopathy secondary to radiation (20). Interestingly, only eight of the 47 studies utilized formal neuropsychological testing as part of the evaluation; four of these eight studies examined patients with primary brain tumors (see previous section) and one other study included only two patients.

Prophylactic cranial irradiation has frequently been used in the treatment of patients with small-cell lung cancer. Because of the high potential for neurotoxicity in patients so treated and the relatively low incidence of CNS recurrence in patients not treated with cranial irradiation, the use of this prophylaxis has been called into question (22). However, several reports have been published that describe the neurologic complications associated with prophylactic cranial irradiation in adults with small-cell lung cancer and these may be useful in understanding the impact of radiation to the adult central nervous system. Although few studies have documented neuropsychological outcomes, the neurologic impact has been carefully described. Lishner and colleagues (23) retrospectively found delayed neurologic complications in only 19% of long-term survivors of small-cell lung cancer who received prophylactic cranial irradiation, and the authors attributed most of these neurologic complications to chemotherapy or underlying disease rather than to the irradiation. Another retrospective study of similarly treated long-term survivors reported CT abnormalities (e.g., mild cerebral atrophy in 8/13 patients) but detected "no significant clinical abnormalities" as measured by clinical neurologic examination (24).

In contrast to retrospective accounts of neurologic abnormalities, Craig and colleagues (25) reported an "extraordinarily high" frequency of computed cranial tomography abnormalities in patients treated with prophylactic cranial irradiation and combination chemotherapy (cyclophosphamide, adriamycin, and vincristine) for small-cell lung cancer. Prospective, serial imaging of a small sample of patients revealed cerebral atrophy in 100%, ventricular dilation in 70%, and decreased attenuation coefficients in 15% of the sample post treatment. The relative contribution of each of the therapies could not be determined. Unfortunately, the neuropsychological impact of these abnormalities was not assessed and no control or comparison group was included.

Studies using more detailed assessment of functioning, such as neuropsychological testing and standardized mental status examinations, may find higher incidences of disturbance, however. Johnson and colleagues (5) examined the neurologic, neuropsychological, and computed cranial tomography/MRI functioning of long-term survivors of small-cell lung cancer, reporting neurologic, mental status, and neuropsychological abnormalities in 60%–65% and abnormal CT scans in 75% of survivors at two to ten years following treatment. While detailed discussion of the results of standardized neuropsychological

testing was not provided, the authors reported that memory scores were frequently impaired and that the mean performance IQ score was approximately nine points lower than the mean verbal IQ score. Patients receiving higher doses of cranial irradiation and those receiving high-dose chemotherapy concomitant with cranial irradiation tended to fare the worst. A follow-up of the same sample revealed no significant improvement in functioning four years later (6). In fact, more patients showed a decline in mental status and neuropsychological functioning than those who demonstrated improvement, suggesting the possibility of slow progression of impairment in a subsample of patients. A prospective study of patients receiving prophylactic cranial irradiation for small-cell lung cancer demonstrated significantly lower pretreatment neuropsychological performance scores (mental control, information processing speed, verbal and visual memory, visuomotor speed) for patients than those of age-, education-, and gender-matched controls, suggesting that these impairments were disease related (26). Deterioration following chemotherapy and irradiation was not detected; however, the follow-up period was limited to five months post treatment.

While these reports suggest that cranial irradiation is associated with adverse neurologic and neurocognitive outcomes in adult patients, the studies have been limited primarily to patients with small-cell lung cancer receiving prophylactic cranial irradiation and chemotherapy. The relative impact of the disease itself and the various chemotherapeutic agents used in addition to radiation are not well understood from these studies.

CONVENTIONAL CHEMOTHERAPY

The neurologic and neuropsychological impact of conventional chemotherapy has received much less attention than CNS irradiation in the published literature. While the studies described above have focused on cranial irradiation as a risk factor for impairment, most of the patients studied received chemotherapy as well as radiation to the CNS. Little information about the contribution of chemotherapy was provided by these studies. While the majority of chemotherapeutic agents are believed to be unable to pass the blood–brain barrier (27), nonetheless, "it is fair to say that there is often gross evidence of cognitive impairment sporadically reported for almost all of the commonly used chemotherapeutic agents" (3). Reviews of the neurotoxic effects of frequently used antineoplastic agents support this assertion, describing a variety of clinical syndromes that may adversely impact cognitive or neuropsychological functioning, such as central and peripheral neuropathy, encephalopathy, leukoencephalopathy, ototoxicity, and cerebellar symptoms (1, 28,29).

One study to date has focused on the neuropsychological impact of adjuvant chemotherapy for women with stage I and stage II breast cancer (30). These investigators reported that 75% of patients (tested on average of six months post chemotherapy) were greater than one standard deviation below test norms (a common indication of clinical impairment) on at least one test from the assessment battery. The deficits were most commonly seen on measures of memory and cognitive flexibility and were not associated with level of depression, type of chemotherapy, or time since treatment. However, cognitive impairment was positively associated with lengh of chemotherapy treatment. Unfortunately, patients were only tested following treatment; therefore, changes from baseline level of functioning could not be assessed.

Another study examining the neuropsychological impact of chemotherapy compared pretreatment and posttreatment neuropsychological test scores of patients who were randomly assigned to receive either local/regional irradiation (non-CNS irradiation) or combination chemotherapy (cisplatin and etoposide) for inoperable non-small-cell lung cancer (7). While patients receiving chemotherapy tended to have lower scores on almost all of the tests in the limited neuropsychological test battery, the differences were small and nonsignificant. The authors concluded that, while the trend may be the consequence of organic impairment as a function of the chemotherapeutic agents, these may also have been attributable to the time elapsed since completion of treatment (both groups were tested before treatment and 14 weeks later; radiation-treated patients were tested on average of 11 weeks following treatment completion, while chemotherapy-treated patients were tested an average of only five weeks post treatment). In this study, as well as the former, late delayed effects were not assessed because of the short time interval between treatment and assessment of patients.

Limited information is available regarding the neurocognitive impact of chemotherapy. Few studies have been performed and limited conclusions can be drawn from these. Drawing conclusions about the neurocognitive impact of chemotherapy will be inherently difficult because of the fact that there are a great number of chemotherapeutic agents, used in varying combinations and schedules, for a wide variety of neoplastic diseases. Separating all of these factors from each other will prove challenging.

BONE MARROW TRANSPLANTATION

Bone marrow transplantation typically consists of high-dose chemotherapy and/or radiation therapy, followed by replacement of bone marrow or peripheral stem cells. Allogeneic transplants (unrelated, matched donor) usually produce chronic immunosuppression and neurologic complications (including cerebral infarct, cerebral hemorrhage, hypoxia/ischemia, CNS infections, metabolic encephalopathy, seizures, leukoencephalopathy, and CNS recurrence of malignancy) occur in 60%–70% of recipients (31). Although less frequent, neurologic complications follow autologous bone marrow transplantation as well (32). Early complications (within six weeks of transplantation; including encephalopathy, seizures, psychiatric symptoms, and cerebral hemorrhage) occurred in 39% of patients receiving autologous BMT for Hodgkin's disease. Late complications (after six weeks following transplantation; including encephalopathy, peripheral neuropathy, cerebral hemorrhage, and spinal cord compression) occurred in 21% of patients. White-matter changes on MRI scans have also been noted in a small sample of patients treated with autologous bone marrow support (33).

Neuropsychological investigations of patients undergoing bone marrow transplantation have suggested cognitive impairments following this form of treatment. A cross-sectional study of 30 survivors of allogeneic transplantation for leukemia found that self-report of cognitive dysfunction (slowed reaction time, reduced attention/concentration, difficulty with reasoning/problem solving) was related to dose of total body irradiation used in the preparative regimen (34). Studies utilizing serial, prospective, standardized assessments of cognitive functioning have also demonstrated selective cognitive deficits in BMT recipients. Ahles and colleagues (35) found that higher order cognitive functioning (executive functioning) tended to worsen over the course of hospitalization for autologous BMT, while depression and anxiety improved. Parth and colleagues (8) found significant decreases from before treatment to following hospitalization (50 and 100 days, and 12 months) in performance on measures of associative memory, perceptual speed, logical reasoning, and verbal processing in a sample of patients receiving allogeneic bone marrow transplantation for hematological disorders. Meyers and colleagues (9) found that the percentage of patients demonstrating short-term memory deficits nearly doubled from before treatment (11%) to eight-month follow-up (19%) in a sample of patients receiving allo-

geneic or autologous transplant for a variety of neoplastic disorders. No association between memory
impairment and emotional distress, psychoactive
drug administration, or psychiatric disturbance was
found. While decrements in cognitive functioning following BMT have been documented prospectively, it
should also be noted that cognitive impairment as a
consequence of prior treatment history may pre-date
BMT regimens (4).

BIOLOGIC RESPONSE MODIFIERS

Biologic response modifiers are a relatively newer class
of antineoplastic therapies representing an immunotherapy approach to metastatic disease. Several
reports have described the acute neurobehavioral
effects of interferon-α, interleukin-2, and lymphokine-activated killer cells (36–39). One study of
patients receiving interleukin-2 and lymphokine-activated killer cells reported a 50% incidence of severe,
dose-related cognitive changes (including, but not limited to, disorientation, impaired attention, psychomotor slowing, and aphasia) during therapy, which
reverted to baseline by 2–4 weeks after therapy (36).
Clinical reports of small samples of patients treated
with interferon-α suggest a 50% or higher incidence
of the following acute neurocognitive impairments:
psychomotor slowing, impaired memory, impaired
concentration, and speech impairment (37,39). While
it is generally believed that these impairments resolve
after cessation of therapy (37), there is some evidence
to suggest that interferon neurotoxicity, including deficits in memory, motor coordination, and frontal lobe
executive functions, does not fully resolve in some
cases (40,41) and that preexisting neurologic abnormalities (i.e., cerebral atrophy, brain metastases, previous head injury) may place patients at increased
risk for severe neurotoxicity (38).

SUMMARY

Reports of the multiple adverse neurologic consequences of cancer treatments for adults are abundant,
suggesting high risk for cognitive impairment. In contrast, research regarding the neuropsychological
impact of cancer and cancer treatment in adults is
notably sparse. Only a handful of studies have utilized
standardized neuropsychological testing in their evaluation of adult cancer patients and these have been
limited by other methodological factors such as small
sample sizes and cross-sectional designs. Conclusions
regarding the neurocognitive impact of cancer treatments in adults are therefore highly speculative.

Overall, each of the major forms of cancer therapies
(radiation, conventional chemotherapy, bone marrow
transplantation, and biologic response modifiers)
appear to pose risk for neuropsychological impairment
because of the relatively high incidence of neurological
complications that have been reported for each. The
exact incidence, characterization, severity, and chronicity of neurocognitive impairment associated with each
of the anticancer therapies for adults are virtually
unknown and suggest the importance of systematic
research in this area. Careful, controlled prospective
neuropsychological studies, ideally coupled with
brain imaging, would help to address this knowledge
gap. Functional MRI represents a new and promising
noninvasive method with high spatial and temporal
resolution that would likely enhance knowledge of
underlying neural mechanisms of the cognitive sequelae of cancer treatments (42). Finally, little work in the
cognitive rehabilitation of cancer patients has been
reported; however, an important future direction for
this area of research is the application of cognitive
rehabilitation interventions (43,44), developed in
other patient groups, to the cancer population.

REFERENCES

1. Oxman TE, Schnurr PP, Silberfarb PS. Assessment of
cognitive function in cancer patients. *Psychosoc Assess
Terminal Care.* 1986; 2:99–128.
2. Silberfarb PS, Oxman TE. The effects of cancer therapies
on the central nervous system. *Adv Psychosom Med.*
1988; 18:13–25.
3. Silberfarb PS. Chemotherapy and cognitive defects in
cancer patients. *Annu Rev Med.* 1983; 34:35–46.
4. Andrykowski MA, Schmitt FA, Gregg ME, Brady MJ,
Lamb DG, Henslee-Downey PJ. Neuropsychologic
impairment in adult bone manrrow transplant candidates. *Cancer.* 1992; 70:2288–2297.
5. Johnson BE, Becker B, Goff WB, et al. Neurologic, neuropsychologic, and computed cranial tomography scan
abnormalities in 2- to 10-year survivors of small-cell
lung cancer. *J Clin Oncol.* 1985; 3:1659–1667.
6. Johnson BE, Patronas N, Hayes W, et al. Neurologic,
computed cranial tomographic, and magnetic resonance
imaging abnormalities in patients with small-cell lung
cancer: further follow-up of 6- to 13-year survivors. *J
Clin Oncol.* 1990; 8:48–56.
7. Kaasa S, Olsnes BT, Mastekaasa A. Neuropsychological
evaluation of patients with inoperable non-small cell lung
cancer treated with combination chemotherapy or radiotherapy. *Acta Oncol.* 1988; 27:241–246.
8. Parth P, Dunlap WP, Kennedy RS, Lane NE, Ordy JM.
Motor and cognitive testing of bone marrow transplant
patients after chemoradiotherapy. *Percept Motor Skills.*
1989; 68:1227–1241.
9. Meyers CA, Weitzner M, Byrne K, Valentine A,
Champlin RE, Przepiorka D. Evaluation of the neurobehavioral functioning of patients before, during, and

after bone marrow transplantation. *J Clin Oncol.* 1994; 12:820–826.

10. Folstein MF, Fetting JH, Lobo A, Niaz U, Capozzoli KD. Cognitive assessment of cancer patients. *Cancer.* 1984; 15:2250–2257.

11. Price TR, Goetz KL, Lovell MR. Neuropsychiatric aspects of brain tumors. In: Yudofsky SC, Hales RE, eds. *The American Psychiatric Press Textbook of Neuropsychiatry.* Washington DC: American Psychiatric Press: 1992:473–498.

12. Fisk JL, Del Dotto JE. Neuropsychological sequelae of brain tumors. *Henry Ford Hosp Med J.* 1990; 38:213–218.

13. Hochberg FH, Slotnick B. Neuropsychologic impairment in astrocytoma survivors. *Neurology.* 1980; 30:172–177.

14. Meyers CA. Neuropsychologic deficits in brain-tumor patients: effects of location, chronicity, and treatment. *Cancer Bull.* 1986; 38:30–32.

15. Horn J, Reitan RM. Neuropsychological correlates of rapidly vs. slowly growing intrinsic cerebral neoplasms. *J Clin Neuropsychol.* 1984; 6:309–324.

16. Maire JP, Coudin B, Guerin J, Caudry M. Neuropsychologic impairment in adults with brain tumors. *Am J Clin Oncol.* 1987; 10:156–162.

17. Heilman KM, Valenstein E. *Clinical Neuropsychology.* New York: Oxford University Press; 1993.

18. Lezak MD. *Neuropsychological Assessment,* 3d ed. New York: Oxford University Press; 1995.

19. Kramer S. The hazards of therapeutic irradiation of the central nervous system. *Clin Neurosurg.* 1968; 15:301–318.

20. Crossen JR, Garwood D, Glatstein E, Neuwelt EA. Neurobehavioral sequelae of cranial irradiation in adults: a review of radiation-induced encephalopathy. *J Clin Oncol.* 1994; 12:627–642.

21. Sheline GE, Wara WM, Smith V. Therapeutic irradiation and brain injury. *Int J Radiat Oncol Biol Phys.* 1980; 6:1215–1228.

22. Fleck JF, Einhorn LH, Lauer RC, Schultz SM, Miller ME. Is prophylactic cranial irradiation indicated in small-cell lung cancer? *J Clin. Oncol.* 1990; 8:209–214.

23. Lishner M, Feld R, Payne DG, et al. Late neurological complications after prophylactic cranial irradiation in patients with small-cell lung cancer: the Toronto experience. *J Clin Oncol.* 1990; 8:215–221.

24. Catane R, Schwade JG, Yarr I, et al. Follow-up neurological evaluation in paitents with small cell lung carcinoma treated with prophylactic cranial irradiation and chemotherapy. *Int J Radiat Oncol Biol Phys.* 1981; 7:105–109.

25. Craig JB, Jackson DV, Moody D, et al. Prospective evaluation of changes in computed cranial tomography in patients with small cell lung carcinoma treated with chemotherapy and prophylactic cranial irradiation. *J Clin Oncol.* 1984; 2:1151–1156.

26. van Oosterhout AG, Boon PJ, Houx PJ, ten Velde GP, Twijnstra A. Follow-up of cognitive functioning in patients with small cell lung cancer. *Int J Radiat Oncol Biol Phys.* 1995; 31:911–914.

27. Lesser GJ, Grossman SA. The chemotherapy of adult primary brain tumors. *Cancer Treat Rev.* 1993; 19:261–281.

28. Weiss HD, Walker MD, Wiernik PH. Neurotoxicity of commonly used antineoplastic agents. *N Engl J Med.* 1974; 291:127–133.

29. Tuxen MK, Hansen SW. Neurotoxicity secondary to antineoplastic drugs. *Cancer Treat Rev.* 1994; 20:191–214.

30. Wieneke MH, Dienst ER. Neuropsychological assessment of cognitive functioning following chemotherapy for breast cancer. *Psycho-Oncology.* 1995; 4:61–66.

31. Patchell RA. Neurological complications of organ transplantation. *Ann Neurol.* 1994; 36:688–703.

32. Snider S, Bashir R, Bierman P. Neurologic complications after high-dose chemotherapy and autologous bone marrow transplantation for Hodgkin's disease. *Neurology.* 1994; 44:681–684.

33. Stemmer SM, Stears JC, Burton BS, Jones RB, Simon JH. White matter changes in patients with breast cancer treated with high-dose chemotherapy and autologous bone marrow support. *Am J Neuroradiol.* 1994; 15:1267–1273.

34. Andrykowski MA, Altmaier EM, Barnett RL, Burish TG, Gingrich R, Henslee-Downey PJ. Cognitive dysfunction in adult survivors of allogeneic marrow transplantation: relationship to dose of total body irradiation. *Bone Marrow Transplant.* 1990; 6:269–276.

35. Ahles TA, Tope DM, Furstenberg C, Hann D, Mills L. Psychologic and neuropsychologic impact of autologous bone marrow transplantation. *J Clin Oncol.* 1996; 14 1457–1462.

36. Denicoff KD, Rubinow DR, Papa MZ, et al. The neuropsychiatric effects of treatment with interleukin-2 and lymphokine-activated killer cells. *Ann Intern Med.* 1987; 107:293–300.

37. Adams F, Quesada JR, Gutterman JU. Neuropsychiatric manifestations of human leukocyte interferon therapy in patients with cancer. *J Am Med Assoc.* 1984; 252:938–941.

38. Adams F, Fernandez F, Mavligit G. Interferon-induced organic mental disorders associated with unsuspected pre-existing neurologic abnormalities. *J Neuro-Oncol.* 1988; 6:355–359.

39. Niiranen A, Laaksonen R, Iivanainen, Mattson K, Farkkila M, Cantell K. Behavioral assesment of patients treated with alpha-interferon. *Acta Psychiatr Scand.* 1988; 78; 622–626.

40. Meyers C, Scheibel RS, Forman AD. Persistent neurotoxicity of systemically administered interferon-alpha. *Neurology.* 1991; 41:672–676.

41. Meyers C, Abbruzzese JL. Cognitive functioning in cancer patients: effect of previous treatment. *Neurology.* 1992; 42:434–436.

42. Saykin AJ, Riordan HJ, Burr RB, et al. Clinical application of functional MRI: studies of memory in normals and neurological and psychiatric patients. In: Bigler E, ed. *The Handbook of Human Brain Function: Neuroimaging,* vol. 2. New York: Raven Press. [In press].

43. Sohlberg MM, Mateer CA. *Introduction to Cognitive Rehabilitation: Theory and Practice.* New York: The Guilford Press; 1989.

44. Wilson, BA. *Rehabilitation of Memory.* New York: The Guilford Press; 1987.

IX

PSYCHIATRIC DISORDERS

EDITOR: MARY JANE MASSIE

44

Adjustment Disorders

JAMES J. STRAIN

The cancer patient is prone to the psychosocial stresses of a serious, perhaps chronic, and at times a fatal illness. In all phases of the disorder of cancer—anticipation, assessment, diagnosis, treatment, remission, exacerbation—patients and their significant others are confronted with stresses of enormous moment. In addition, the stigma, the fears, and the misconceptions about cancer—its cure—all leave the patient with concerns and worries. Patients may experience a frank psychiatric disorder in response to the fear or knowledge that they have cancer (e.g., major affective disorder, anxiety disorder, panic attacks) and need explicit treatment for this major psychiatric disturbance.

Patients could experience a "normal" reaction to learning that they have cancer, require treatment, and that their future life may have uncertainty. They manifest an understandable disturbance of mood, invoke "normal" coping patterns, and continue life's trajectory without overt manifestations of functional or psychological maladaptation or impairment.

The *adjustment disorders (AD)* are an intermediary psychological state between frank psychiatric pathology—major mental disorders—and normal coping under stress. Their hallmarks are clinical indicators denoting maladaptation in any one or several psychosocial spheres: work, interpersonal relationships, avocational activities, enjoyment of life, including sex. Succinctly, patients' quality of life has been impaired by maladaptation in important life endeavors.

This chapter will focus on the AD—their definition, epidemiology, etiology, problems in diagnosis, their course, and treatment. The AD are not uniquely different in the cancer patient, since most medical/surgical patients have the stress of illness with which to cope. However, the bias, prejudice, and fear elicited by cancer often augment the stresses of medical illness, which can force a maladaptive response and reaction.

CRITERIA DEFINING THE ADJUSTMENT DISORDERS

DSM-IV (1994) (1) states:

Criterion A. The essential feature of the adjustment disorder (AD) is the development of clinically significant emotional or behavioral symptoms in response to an identifiable psychosocial stressor (s). The symptoms must develop within 3 months after the onset of the stressor(s).

Criterion B. The clinical significance of the reaction is indicated either by marked distress that is in excess of what would be expected given the nature of the stressor, or by significant impairment in social or occupational (academic) functioning.

Criterion C. This disorder should not be used if the emotional and cognitive disturbances meet the criteria for *another* specific Axis I disorder (e.g., a specific anxiety or mood disorder) or is merely an exacerbation of a preexisting Axis I or II disorder. AD may be diagnosed if the latter does not account for the pattern of symptoms that have occurred in response to the stressor.

Criterion D. The diagnosis of AD does not apply when the symptoms represent Bereavement.

Criterion E. By definition, AD must resolve within 6 months of the termination of the stressor (or its consequences). However, the symptoms may persist for a prolonged period (i.e., longer than 6 months) if they occur in response to a chronic stressor (e.g., a chronic, disabling general medical condition) or to a stressor that has enduring consequences (e.g., the financial and emotional difficulties resulting from a divorce).

The criteria for the AD lack specificity—e.g., a list of symptoms, described in both qualitative and quantitative terms—in contrast to the major mental disorders—e.g., affective disorders, the organic mental disorders, the panic disorders, etc., where symptoms are exactly defined. This vagueness, however, permits the identification of early or temporary mental states where the psychiatric morbidity is greater than expected to the events at hand—usually stress—and where some treatment is indicated. This lack of specificity allows subthreshold clinical symptoms to be acknowledged. Thus, the AD are a unique and essential component in the psychiatric taxonomic hierarchical spectrum: *(1)* major disorders; *(2)* disorders not otherwise specified (NOS); *(3)* AD; *(4)* problem-level diagnoses (V-Codes, DSM-III-R) (F-Codes, DSM-IV); and, *(5)* normal fluctuations of mental states. "AD would 'trump' problem-level disorders, but be 'trumped' by a specific diagnosis, even if it were in the NOS category (2)." The AD are a linch-pin between normality and pathology.

The AD allow the labeling of mental states that are subthreshold. Also, such early identification of psychopathology and treatment diminishes not only current dysfunction, but may forestall the further erosion of mental capacity, and the emergence of more pernicious depressive or anxiety psychiatric symptomatology. It is in the gray area of the subthreshold disorders where the role of the AD become an essential diagnostic category to demarcate normality from morbidity: an important task for those who work with the cancer patient.

Cancer patients encounter an enormous stressor in receiving the news of their disease, its impending treatment, and prognosis. There is no question about the presence of a stressor: there is only a question of the kind and amount of the maladaptation the cancer patient is experiencing. Does a patient's reaction qualify for the diagnosis of an AD? Are patients maladapting in the important areas of their life? Is cancer interfering with functioning on the basis of its psychological impact on the patient?

The AD have had a major evolution since the original DSM of 1952 (Table 44.1). The committee charged with reexamining this disorder, and to propose necessary alterations for the diagnosis of AD for DSM-IV, observed two fundamental concerns for researchers and clinical care personnel. First, since the diagnosis of this entity lacks behavioral or operational criteria (e.g., a symptom checklist), the issue of reliability and validity is raised. Second, the classification of syndromes that do not fulfill the criteria for a major men-

TABLE 44.1. *Diagnostic Categories of Adjustment Disorder*

DSM-I (1952) TRANSIENT SITUATIONAL PERSONALITY DISORDER	DSM-II (1968) TRANSIENT SITUATIONAL DISTURBANCE
Gross stress reaction	Adjustment reaction of infancy
Adult situational reaction	Adjustment reaction of childhood
Adjustment reaction of infancy	Adjustment reaction of adolescence
Adjustment reaction of childhood	Adjustment reaction of adult life
Adjustment reaction of adolescence	Adjustment reaction of late life
Adjustment reaction of late life	
Other transient situational personality disturbance	

DSM-III (1980) ADJUSTMENT DISORDER	DSM-III-R (1987) ADJUSTMENT DISORDER
Adjustment disorder with depressed mood	Adjustment disorder with depressed mood
Adjustment disorder with anxious mood	Adjustment disorder with anxious mood
Adjustment disorder with mixed emotional features	Adjustment disorder with mixed emotional features
Adjustment disorder with disturbance of conduct	Adjustment disorder with disturbance of conduct
Adjustment disorder with mixed disturbance of emotions and conduct	Adjustment disorder with mixed disturbance of emotions and conduct
Adjustment disorder with work (or academic) inhibition	Adjustment disorder with work (or academic) inhibition
Adjustment disorder with withdrawal	Adjustment disorder with withdrawal
Adjustment disorder with atypical features	Adjustment disorder with physical complaints
	Adjustment disorder not otherwise specified (NOS)

DSM-IV (1994) ADJUSTMENT DISORDER	
Adjustment disorder with depressed mood	
Adjustment disorder with anxiety	
Adjustment disorder with mixed anxiety and depressed mood	
Adjustment disorder with disturbance of conduct	
Adjustment disorder with mixed disturbance of emotions and conduct	
Adjustment disorder unspecified	

tal illness, but which present with serious symptomatology that requires intervention and/or treatment, by default, may be viewed as "subthreshold," and afforded a subthreshold interest by health care workers and third party payers. In some settings, mental health workers were not reimbursed for the V-code diagnoses, and were often questioned about their use of the AD as a "legitimate" billing diagnostic category, even when the behavior in question is suicidal ideation or action. Research and payment for needed mental health care is thereby compromised with subthreshold diagnoses. Another taxonomic consideration is the relationship of the DSM-IV criteria as compared with that of the International Classification of Diseases, and how the world community views this subthreshold disorder.

Relationship to International Classification of Disease-10 (ICD-10)

It is incumbent for those working with cancer patients to also be familiar with the ICD-10 classification schema for mental disorders (3), since many colleagues in foreign countries use it in preference to the DSM-IV. A category analogous to AD exists in ICD-10, which has a similar construct, but different defining characteristics. In the ICD-10: *(1)* the onset of the disorder must occur within 1 month of the occurrence of the stressor; *(2)* some of the subtypes are defined differently and are so named (brief depressive reaction, prolonged depressive reaction, mixed anxiety and depressive reaction, disturbance of other emotions, disturbance of conduct, mixed disturbance of emotions and conduct, other specific predominant symptoms); *(3)* the subtype *prolonged depressive reaction* may last as long as 2 years. Since international collaborators rely upon the ICD-10 criteria for their diagnoses, it is critical that those who combine data sets, or review studies from disparate continents, understand the classificatory differences.

EPIDEMIOLOGY

Only one published prospective epidemiologic study which included the AD diagnosis and which was conducted in children and adolescents in Puerto Rico has been published (4). In children and youth the prevalence of adjustment disorders was 3.4–4.2 using the DSM-III diagnostic criteria and the Children's Global Assessment Scale. The Epidemiological Catchment Area Survey using the Diagnostic Instrument Scale did not examine the study cohorts for AD (5,6). The Razavi study screened for AD and major depressive disorders in cancer inpatients (7). Andreasen and Hoenk observed the outcome of assign-

ment of the diagnosis of AD and observed that youth and adolescents were more likely to have a more serious psychiatric disorder 5 years later than adults (8). In general hospital psychiatric consultation populations AD was diagnosed as 21.5% and 11.5% (9,10).

A little over 2% of the patients at Western Psychiatric Institute (Pittsburgh) evaluation ambulatory clinic who were diagnosed AD had no other diagnoses on Axis I or Axis II (11); 20% of the patient cohort had AD with other Axis I diagnoses (12,13). Males were half as likely to be given the AD diagnosis as females. Evaluations of psychiatric emergency room cohorts revealed 13% of adults and 42% of adolescents were diagnosed AD (14). By examining in- and outpatient psychiatric populations Andreasen and Wasek observed that 5% received the diagnosis of AD (15).

Mezzich et al. (16) and Fabrega et al. (17) employed a structured 64 symptom rating to examine specific psychiatric diagnoses (SD), AD, and those not ill (NI) (16,17). Vegetative, substance use, and characterologic symptoms were greatest in SD, intermediate with the AD, and least in the NI. Mood and affect, general appearance, behavior, disturbance in speech and thought pattern, and cognitive functioning, had a similar distribution: $SD > AD > NI$. The AD were significantly different from the NI with regard to more "depressed mood" and "low self-esteem" ($p > 0.0001$). However, AD and NI had minimal pathology of thought content and perception. On the suicide indicators, 29% of the AD versus 9.0% of the NI had a positive response. For those working with cancer patients it is important to note that the three cohorts did not differ on the frequency of Axis III disorders; the specific Axis III diagnoses did not affect the distribution of symptoms observed on the checklist.

MECHANISM(S) PRECIPITATING THE AD

The AD are a stress-related etiologically based phenomenon where the stressor has resulted in maladaptation and symptoms which remain until the stressor is removed or a new state of adaptation has occurred. However, there are other stress-related disorders: *posttraumatic stress disorder* and *acute stress disorder* (the latter newly described in DSM-IV (1)) are those stress reactions that follow immediately after a disaster or cataclysmic personal event. Therefore, stress alone is not sufficient for a diagnosis of AD.

It is important to note that stress disorders defy an atheoretical approach espoused by DSM-IV which is to be a phenomenologically based taxonomy on manifest symptoms alone. Etiology is not a component of the construct of a diagnosis. The stress-related disorders have a known etiology, which is critical to their diagnosis. The stress-related disorders require the diagnostician to impute etiological significance to a life event—a stressor—and relate its effect in clinical (symptomatic) terms to the patient. Another conundrum of the AD diagnosis is that, although they are stress-related disorders, they are not placed in the classification domains of the others—namely, the anxiety disorders. The importance of this discussion for the cancer patient is self-evident: the diagnosis, treatment, and management of a neoplastic illness is a critical life stressor for the patient, and thereby becomes a significant etiological source for the occurrence of stress disorders in this population.

It may help the reader to understand the debate that ensues for the stress-related disorders by examining the confounds that the current models of stress and disease present. Since the relationship between stress and a psychiatric disorder is admittedly complex, many researchers question the theoretical basis of the AD altogether (18,19). The linear model of stress–disease interaction serving as the template for AD in DSM-III, DSM-III-R, and DSM-IV has been questioned (20). This model presupposes that a direct and clearly identifiable pathological–morbid reaction follows a stressful event—a course which occurs in some individuals with AD. However, many alternative explanations and modifiers prevail to account for the relationship of stress to psychiatric illness which are not accounted for by this model.

For example, there may be multiple stressors, insidious or chronic as opposed to discrete events, and/or a multiplicity of possible stress–disease interactions, in which relatively minor precipitating events may generate pathology in an individual who has previously been sensitized to stress. This is a common occurrence in patients with cancer who have experienced a series of stressors—e.g., initial symptomatology; assessment (sometimes invasive); diagnosis (often with pernicious implications); treatment (which can result in substantial bodily changes, and somatic discomfort); alteration of relationships with loved ones, with the work place, or the management of one's personal affairs—so that it is this concatenation of stresses which may in the end adversely impact on the cancer patient's coping capacity. In fact, a minor stressor may be the "straw which breaks the camel's back," and precipitates the outbreak of a frank stress disorder.

Our ability to properly classify individuals with chronic disturbance and/or chronic stress—that observed in chronic disease like some cancers—has been particularly difficult because psychopathology in these individuals may be related to, but distinct from, the intended construct in AD. Are patients with AD unusually sensitive to psychosocial events that are unlikely to result in mental disturbances in others? Are they individuals who have been exposed to high levels of stress, the severity and/or accumulation of which would likely produce negative consequences in most people?

The use of the AD classification also demands a careful documentation of the timing of the stressor to the adverse psychological sequelae which transpire. Until the DSM-IV, a time limit was imposed on how long this diagnosis could be employed after the stressor had ceased. It was a transitory diagnoses that should not exceed 6 months, after which time another psychiatric diagnosis had to be employed or the AD diagnosis dropped. Because the 6 months limitation criteria did not conform with the course of medical illness, this was amended in DSM-IV to *acute* (less than 6 months) and *chronic* (6 months or longer). The stress of a cancer illness does not necessarily go away in 6 months, and therefore a stress-related psychiatric disorder (e.g., AD) may continue indefinitely.

STRESS(ES) AND CANCER

Because of the nature of neoplastic diseases, it is important to be able to differentiate different kinds of stressful experience the cancer patient may encounter. Cohen (21) argues that: *(1)* acute stresses are different from chronic ones in both psychological and physiological terms; *(2)* the meaning of the stress is affected by "modifiers"—ego strengths, support systems, prior mastery; and *(3)* one must differentiate the manifest and the latent meaning of the stress(ors)—e.g., loss of employment may be a relief or a catastrophe. An objectively overwhelming stress could have little impact on one individual, whereas a minor one could be regarded as cataclysmic by another. In summary, with regard to the stress etiology of the AD, the neoplastic disorders elicit all levels of stress, and for many patients over a prolonged period of time.

The vulnerability of the individual with cancer—e.g., ego strengths, support system, underlying personality disorders, the timing and concatenation of the stress(ors)—and the issue of control over the stressor need to be assessed to ascertain the import of the stressful event on the individual. A limited attempt was made in this direction by the addition of Axis IV to the diagnostic schema in DSM-III to allow the clinician to assess the presence of stress, but the value of Axis IV has been mitigated by its validity and reliability in clinical studies (22–24).

There was a significant difference in the amount of stressors reported in various patient cohorts: the group with AD compared with the SD and NI patients were overrepresented in the "higher stress" categories (16). In their evaluation of medically/surgically ill psychiatric consultation patients, Popkin et al. observed that 68.6% of the cases were judged to have their medical illness as the primary psychosocial stressor (9). Snyder and Strain described that the assessment of stressors on Axis IV was significantly higher ($p = 0.0001$) for medical/surgical consultation patients with AD compared with other psychiatric diagnostic disorders (10). These are important observations for those who care for cancer patients.

DIAGNOSIS OF THE AD

Every attribute of the diagnostic construct for the AD constitutes a problem for assessment: *(1)* The stressor; *(2)* the maladaptive reaction to the stressor; *(3)* the accompanying mood and clinical features; *(4)* the time and relationship between the stressor and the psychological response. None of these components of the diagnosis has been operationalized, which, as said earlier, contributes to the limited validity and reliability of the diagnosis.

MALADAPTATION

First, with regard to the "maladaptive reaction," it is unclear how this concept can or should be operationalized. The social, vocational, and relationship dysfunctions which are unspecified qualitatively or quantitatively neither lend themselves to reliability or to validity, or even to agreement when this clinical situation obtains. It is further confounded by the elements of culture—the expectable reactions within a specific cultural environment, gender responses, developmental level differences, and the "meaning" of events and reactions to them by an individual.

The concepts of "average expectable environment" and the "patient's explanatory belief model" are examples of where an attempt is made to weigh cultural and subjective differences in the assessment of an individual's mental state and reaction (25,26).

The patient's functional status evaluation (Axis V) is not linked via an algorithm to enhance internal consistency in the AD construct in DSM-IV. Fabrega and Mezzich state that both subjective symptoms and decrement in social function can be considered "maladaptive," and that the severity of either of these is subject to great individual variation (27). They could not conclude that the level of psychopathology correlates with impaired functioning utilizing data from either Axis V or their "new" Axis VI—a more specific functional status Axis developed for their Initial Evaluation Form (16), which assessed patients on three dimensions: occupational, with family, with other individuals and groups on seven levels of impairment.

STRESSORS

No criteria or guidelines are offered in DSM-IV to quantify stressors for the AD for a particular individual. Many of the statements regarding the problem of assessing maladaptation described above apply to the assessment of stressors as well (21,28,29). Mezzich et al attempted to classify and quantify the psychosocial stressors in 13 domains—i.e., health, bereavement, love and marriage, parental, family stressors for children and adolescents, other familial relationships, work, school, financial, legal, housing, miscellaneous (16). The "measurement" of the severity of the stressor and its temporal and causal relationship to demonstrate symptoms is often uncertain and at times impossible.

Even serious symptomatology (e.g., suicidal behavior, which is not regarded as part of a major mental disorder) needs treatment and a "diagnosis" under which it can be placed. DeLeo et al. have described that AD and suicidality are often associated (30). What is regarded as a subthreshold diagnosis—AD—does not necessarily imply the presence of symptomatology within its domain! Snyder and Strain observed that 25% of patients referred for psychiatric consultation in the general hospital were not assigned any psychiatric diagnoses, not even AD (10).

Finally, the issue of boundaries between the major syndromes, depression NOS, anxiety NOS, and the AD remains problematic with regard to the presence of a stressor. How often are the major syndromes associated with a stressor? How different are the symptom profiles of depression and anxiety NOS from those of AD? Research is needed to carefully demarcate the boundaries among the problem level, subthreshold, minor, and major disorders, and, in particular, with regard to the role of stressors as etiological precipitants, concomitants, or essentially unrelated to the psychiatric diagnoses.

EVOLUTION AND COURSE OF THE AD

Andreasen and Hoenk observed at a 5-year follow-up that there was a difference in how adolescents and adults recovered from their adjustment disorders (31). The AD were different illnesses in these two age cohorts with regard to prognosis over time. It would be important to extend this long-term observational approach to cohorts of the elderly and the "old elderly" (those older than 75 years). Most adult patients with AD were symptom-free at 5 years (71% were completely well; 8% had an intervening problem; 21% developed a major depressive disorder or alcoholism). Adolescents had a far different outcome: at follow-up, 43% had developed a major psychiatric disorder (e.g., schizophrenia, schizoaffective disorder, major depression, substance abuse, personality disorders); 13% had an intervening psychiatric illness; and 44% had no psychiatric diagnosis (31).

Although there are no operationally defined threshold criteria for assigning the diagnosis of AD, there are definitive "ceiling" threshold symptoms when a patient has moved through the subthreshold diagnosis and reaches the criteria for a major mental disorder. Snyder and Strain observed that in the acute care inpatient hospital setting, many of the psychiatric consultation patients initially thought to have an AD did not maintain that diagnosis at the time of discharge (32). Many patients initially diagnosed as having major depressive disorders were reclassified AD at discharge.

It remains to be seen if either the major depressive disorder or the AD diagnoses are significantly altered at 6 weeks follow-up and, in particular, when the patient has left the hospital. This evolution of psychiatric morbidity within the acute care general medical setting cautions the clinician to go slowly, prescribing psychotropic drug treatment only when there is sufficient psychiatric morbidity to justify this intervention. This is especially true in cancer patients, who will in many cases be on chemotherapeutic agents for their neoplastic disorders and who might have less disordered mood states when they adjust to their diagnosis and its treatment.

Attempting to diagnose disorders in an early state, or before there is a full-blown syndrome or disorder, often means that a patient will qualify for the AD criteria or subsyndromal disorder. But, just as it is difficult to know when a patient has crossed the diagnostic line from normal, but disturbed behavior, it is difficult to know how quickly the symptoms will remit, with a remission of the stressor(s): *(1)* an acute hospitalization; *(2)* uncertain medical diagnosis; *(3)* pain; *(4)* medications; *(5)* separation; *(6)* lack of ability to

function, or contain emotions. The AD must be looked at as a *transitory state* for most patients, in that symptoms may subside, respond with treatment, evolve to another diagnosis, or be maintained as the stressor continues. Some patients cannot adapt to a chronic stressor and will need ongoing treatment to assist in coping with the stressor.

TREATMENT

There are no reported randomized control trials (RCTs) regarding the psychological, social, or pharmacological treatments of the AD (33–35). Although *Index Medicus* has been searched as well as *Psychological Abstracts*, the Cochrane Collaboration (Oxford, England) has demonstrated that all RCTs may not be reported in these two primary sources (C. Adams, personal communication, 1994).

RCTs employ a variety of treatments—cognitive behavioral treatment (CBT), interpersonal therapy (ITP), behavioral therapy (BT), psychodynamic, group therapy, self-help, and pharmacotherapy trials—that take into account the predominant mood which specifies the subtype of AD. RCTs would need to compare the treatments with each other, combinations of treatment (psychological and chemotherapy), and no treatment (placebo), because of the common occurrence of spontaneous remission.

One of the major methodological difficulties in undertaking RCTs with any treatment modality is the certainty and the validity of the diagnosis—a major dilemma with the AD. These essential studies to guide a scientific treatment approach are further confounded by the limits assessing outcome and the appropriate time frame within which to do the study. Furthermore, RCTs are needed in discreet age cohorts (adolescents, adults, elderly); in homogenous medical illnesses (congestive heart failure, breast cancer), and during time intervals when the diagnosis is stabilized (e.g., the stressor(s) is not increasing or decreasing). Three additional major problems with the stressor(s) are their: *(1)* nature (quality); *(2)* severity (quantity); *(3)* acuteness (less than 6 months) or chronicity (more than 6 months). Also, studies need to be done with the co-occurence of physical illness (e.g., cancer).

In lieu of any substantive RCTs to guide treatment, the choice of intervention remains a clinical decision. The Institute of Medicine has developed *Guidelines for Clinical Practice: From Development to Use* (36). A critical attribute of a guideline is the *strength of the evidence*. Therefore, with no RCT evidence, the treatment recommendations for the AD remain on the basis of *consensus* rather than evidence. But, there has not been an official *consensus conference* on the optimal way to treat AD. And recommendations of clinical experts may differ with the results from meta-analyses of RCTs (37).

Therefore, treatment today is based upon the understanding that this disorder emanates from an overwhelming psychological reaction to a stressor. The stressor needs to be identified, described, shared with the patient, and plans made to mitigate it, if possible. The abnormal response may be attenuated if the stressor can be eliminated, or reduced. In the case of cancer patients, the major stressor may be their fears, and misconceptions. Therefore, the initial approach to treatment is to identify the stressor, and where possible diminish its impact. As said above, Popkin et al. (9) have shown that, in the medically ill, the most common stressor is the medical illness itself (e.g., having cancer).

COUNSELING/PSYCHOTHERAPY

The treatment of AD rests primarily upon psychotherapeutic measures that enable the reduction of the stressor, enhance coping to the stressor that cannot be reduced or removed, and the establishment of a mental state and support system to maximize adaptation. The first goal of psychotherapy is to analyze the stressor(ors) affecting the patient, to see if they may be avoided or minimized: for example, assuming excessive responsibility out of keeping with realistic achievements, putting oneself at risk (e.g., dietary indiscretions for a Type I diabetic, not taking recommended chemotherapeutic agents for cancer, etc.).

It is necessary to clarify and interpret the meaning of the stressor for the patient. For example, an amputation of the leg following osteogenic sarcoma may have devastated a patient's feelings about him/herself, especially if he/she was a runner. It is necessary to clarify that the patient still has enormous residual capacity, that he/she can engage in much meaningful work, does not have to lose valued relationships, can still be sexually active, and that it doesn't necessarily mean that further body parts will be lost. Otherwise, the patient's pernicious fantasies—"all is lost"—may make the patient dysfunctional at work, sex, etc., and precipitate a painful dysphoria.

Some stressors may elicit an overreaction: for example, the patient's attempted suicide or homicide after the abandonment by a lover, after learning that the patient has a cancer with a life-thourseatening prognosis. In such instances of overreaction with feelings, emotions, or behaviors, the therapist would help the patient put his or her feelings and rage into words, rather than into destructive actions. The role of verba-

lization, and the joining of affects and conflicts cannot be overestimated in an attempt to reduce the pressure of the stressor and enhance coping.

Psychotherapy, medical crisis counseling (38), crisis intervention, family therapy, group treatment, cognitive behavioral treatment (CBT), interpersonal therapy (ITP), all encourage the patient to express affects, fears, anxiety, rage, helplessness, and hopelessness to the stressors imposed. Sifneos maintains that patients with AD can profit most from brief psychotherapy (39). The psychotherapy should attempt to reframe the meaning of the stress, find ways to minimize it, and to diminish the psychological deficit secondary to its occurrence. The treatment should expose the concerns and conflicts which the patient is experiencing, identify means to reduce the stress(ors), enhance the patient's coping skills, help the patient gain perspective on the adversity, and establish relationships, attend support groups/self-help groups, to assist in the management of the stressor and the self.

Wise, drawing from military psychiatry, emphasizes the variables of brevity, immediacy, centrality, expectance, proximity, and simplicity (BICEPS principles) (40). The treatment approach is brief—usually no more than 72 hours (41).

ITP was applied to depressed HIV-positive outpatients and found to be useful (42). Psycho-education about the sick role, a here-and-now framework, formulation of the problems from an interpersonal perspective, exploration of options for changing dysfunctional behavior patterns, and identification of focused interpersonal problem areas are some of the attributes of ITP. Lazarus describes a seven-pronged approach in the treatment of minor depression (43). The therapy includes assertiveness training, a "sensate focus" of enjoyable events, coping, imagery, time projection, cognitive disputation, role-playing, desensitization, family therapy, and biological prophylaxis.

Support groups have been demonstrated not only to help patients adjust and enhance their coping mechanisms, but that they may also prolong life as well, as shown in the important study by Spiegel, that women with Stage IV breast cancer live longer after ongoing group therapy than those with standard cancer care (44).

PHARMACOTHERAPY

Stewart et al. emphasize the need to consider psychopharmacological interventions as well as psychotherapy for the treatment of minor depression: "We, therefore, advocate successive trials with antidepressants in any depressed patient, particularly if they have failed to benefit from psychotherapy or other supportive measures for thoursee months (45)." The authors would include the AD with depressed mood in the cohort who sometimes deserve drug treatment.

The following summary is of a patient who did not respond to counseling and was sufficiently distressed by her mood disorder to require pharmacotherapeutic intervention:

A 35-year-old married woman, mother of thoursee children, was desperate when she learned she had cancer and would need a mastectomy followed by chemotherapy and radiation. She was convinced that she would not recover, that her body would be forever distorted and ugly, that her husband would no longer find her attractive, and that her children would be ashamed of her baldness and the fact that she had cancer. She wondered if anyone would ever want to touch her again. Because her mother and sister had also experienced breast cancer, the patient felt she was fated to an empty future. Despite several sessions to deal with her feelings, the patient's dysphoria remained quite profound. It was decided to add antidepressant chemotherapy (fluoxetine, 20 mg daily) in addition to her psychotherapy sessions to decrease the patient's continuing unpleasant symptoms. Two weeks later the patient reported that she was feeling less despondent and less concerned about the future, and that she had a desire to start resuming her former activities with her family. As the patient came to terms with the overwhelming stressor, and assisted with antidepressant agents, her depressed mood improved, and her ability to employ more adequate coping strategies to handle her serious medical illness were mobilized.

Psychotropic medication has been used in the medically ill, the terminally ill, and in patients who have been refractory to verbal therapies. Rosenberg et al. reported that, in the medically ill with unspecified depressive disorders, 55% (16/29) improved within 2 days of treatment with the maximal dose of amphetamine derivatives (46). The presence of delirium was associated with a decreased response. Whether methylphenidate would be useful in AD with depressed mood remains to be examined. Schatzberg recommends that the therapist consider both psychotherapy and pharmacotherapy in the AD with anxious mood, and that the anxiolytics should be part of the psychiatrist's treatment (47).

However, when AD is diagnosed, as said before, the physician should be aware that the patient may be in an incipient phase of a more serious mental disorder. The therapeutic plan requires sufficient follow-up and the need to be "on guard" for the development of a more pernicious mental state—e.g., a major depressive disorder, a generalized anxiety disorder. The Agency for Health Care Policy and Research has developed guidelines for the treatment of depression in primary care (48).

Appropriate and timely treatment is essential for cancer patients with AD so that their symptoms do not worsen, they do not impair important relationships, or compromise their capacity to work, study, or be active in their interpersonal pursuits more than their physical symptoms impose. Treatment must attempt to forestall further erosion of the cancer patient's capacity to function that could ultimately have grave and untoward consequences. Maladaptation may impede the patient to overcome irreversible losses in important sectors of his/her life. Although this diagnosis lacks rigorous specificity, its treatment is no less challenging or less important for those who struggle with the stresses of cancer.

REFERENCES

1. American Psychiatric Association. *Diagnostic and Statistical Manual*, 4th ed. Washington, D.C.: American Psychiatric Press; 1994.
2. Strain JJ, Newcorn J, Wolf D, Fulop G, eds. Adjustment disorder. In: *Textbook of Psychiatry*, 2d ed. Washington, D.C.: American Psychiatric Press; 1994.
3. World Health Organization. *International Classification of Diseases*, 10th ed. Geneva: World Health Organization; 1995.
4. Bird HR, Canina G, Rubio-Stipec M, et al. Estimates of the prevalence of childhood maladjustment in a community survey in Puerto Rico: the use of combined measures. *Arch Gen Psychiatry.* 1988; 45:1120–1126.
5. Regier DA, Myers JK, Kramer M, et al. The NIMH epidemiologic catchment area program. *Arch Gen Psychiatry.* 1984; 41:934–941.
6. Robins LN. National Institute of Mental Health Diagnostic Interview Schedule: its history, characteristics and validity. *Arch Gen Psychiatry.* 1981; 38:381–389.
7. Razavi D. Screening for adjustment disorders and major depression disorders in cancer in-patients. *Br J Psychiatry.* 1990; 156:79–83.
8. Andreasen NC, Hoenk PR. The predictive value of adjustment disorders: a follow-up study. *J Psychiatry.* 1982; 139:584–590.
9. Popkin MK, Callies AL, Colon EA, et al. Adjustment disorders in medically ill patients referred for consultation in a university hospital. *Psychosomatics.* 1990; 31:410–414.
10. Snyder S, Strain JJ. Somatoform disorders in the general hospital inpatient setting. *Gen Hosp Psychiatry.* 1989; 11:288–293.
11. Fabrega H. Jr, Mezzich J. Adjustment disorder as a marginal or transitional illness category in DSM-III. *Arch Gen Psychiatry.* 1987; 44:567–572.
12. Fabrega H. Jr, Mezzich JE, Mezzich AC, Coffman GA. Descriptive validity of DSM-III depressions. *J Nerv Ment Dis.* 1986; 174:573–584.

13. Kovacs M, Feinberg TL, Crouse-Novak MA, et al. Depressive disorders in childhood I. A longitudinal prospective study of characteristics and recovery. *Arch Gen Psychiatry.* 1984; 41:229–237.

14. Newcorn JH, Strain JJ. Adjustment disorder in children and adolescents. *J Am Acad Child Adolesc Psychiatry.* 1992; 31:318–326.

15. Andreasen NC, Wasek P. Adjustment disorders in adolescents and adults. *Arch Gen Psychiatry.* 1980; 37:1166–1170.

16. Mezzic JE, Dow JT, Rich CL, et al. Developing an efficient clinical information system for a comprehensive psychiatric institute: II. Initial evaluation form. *Behav Res Methods Instrum.* 1981; 13:464–478.

17. Fabrega H Jr, Mezzich J, Ulrich RF. Interpreting the structure of diagnosis in initial evaluations: primary, auxiliary and rule out patterns. *J Psychiatr Res.* 1989; 23:169–86.

18. Depue RA, Monroe SM. Conceptualization and measurement of human disorder in life stress research: the problem of choursonic disturbance. *Psychol Bull.* 1986; 99:36–51.

19. Vinokur A, Caplan RD. Cognitive and affective components of life events. Their relations and effects on well-being. *Am J Commun Psychol.* 1986; 14:351–371.

20. Miller TW. Advances in understanding the impact of stressful life events on health. *Hosp Commun Psychiatry.* 1988; 39:615–622.

21. Cohen F. Stress and bodily illness. *Psychiatr Clin N Am.* 1981; 4:269–286.

22. Spitzer RL, Williams JBW. DSM-III field trials: II. Initial experience with the multi axial system. *Am J Psychiatry.* 1979; 136(6):818–820.

23. Zimmerman M, Pfohl B, Coryell W, Stangl D. The prognostic validity of DSM-III Axis IV in depressed patients. *Am J Psychiatry.* 1987; 144 (1):102–106.

24. Rey JM, Stewart GW, Plapp JM, et al. DSM-III Axis IV revisited. *Am J Psychiatry.* 1988; 145(3):286–292.

25. Hartmann H. Notes on the reality principle. *Psychoanal Study Child.* 1956; 11:31–53.

26. Kleinerman A. *Patients and Healers in the Context of Culture. An Explanation of the Borderline Between Anthoursopology, Medicine and Psychiatry.* Berkeley: University of California Press; 1980.

27. Fabrega H Jr., Mezzich J. Adjustment disorder and psychiatric practice: cultural and historical aspects. *Psychiatry.* 1987; 50:31–49.

28. Zilberg NJ, Weiss DS, Horowitz MJ. Impact of Event Scale. cross-validation study and some empirical evidence supporting a conceptual model of stress response syndromes. *J Consult Clin Psychol.* 1982; 50 (3):407–414.

29. Perris H, von Knorring L, Oreland L, Perris C. Life events and biological vulnerability. A study of life events and platelet MAO activity in depressed patients. *Psychiatry Res.* 1984; 12:111–120.

30. De Leo D, Pellagrin C, Cerate L. Adjustment disorders and suicidality. *Psychol Rep.* 1986; 59:355–358.

31. Andreasen NC, Honk PR. The predictive value of adjustment disorders. a follow-up study. *Am J Psychiatry.* 1982; 139:584–590.

32. Snyder S, Strain JJ. Diagnostic instability in psychiatric consultations. *Hosp Commun Psychiatry.* 1990; 41:10–13.

33. Adams C, Gelder M. The case for establishing a register of randomized controlled trials of mental health care. *Br J Psychiatry.* 1994; 164:433–436.

34. Chalmers I, Dickersin K, Chalmers TC. Getting to grips with Archie Cochoursane's agenda. *Br Med J.* 1992; 305:786–788.

35. Conte HR and Karasu TB. A review of treatment studies of minor depression. 1980-1991. *Am J Psychother.* 1992; 46 (1):58–74.

36. Field M, Lohours KN. *Guidelines for Clinical Practice. From Development to Use.* Washington, D.C.: National Academy Press; 1992.

37. Antman EM, Lau J, Kupelnick B, et al. A comparison of results of meta-analyses of randomized control trials and recommendations of clinical experts. *J Am Med Assoc.* 1992; 268 (2):240–248.

38. Pollin IS, Holland J. A model for counseling the medically ill: the Linda Pollin Foundation Approach. *Gen Hosp Psychiatry.* 1992; 14 (6S):11–24.

39. Sifneos PE. Brief dynamic and crisis therapy. In: Kaplan HI, Sadock BJ, eds. *Comprehensive Textbook of Psychiatry*, vol. 2, 5th ed. Baltimore: Williams & Wilkins; 1989: 1562–1567.

40. Wise MG. Adjustment disorders and impulse disorders not otherwise classified. In: Talbott JA, Hales RE, Yudofsky SC, eds. *The American Psychiatric Press Textbook of Psychiatry*, 2d ed. Washington, DC: American Psychiatric Press; 1994: ch. 19.

41. True PK and Benway MW. Treatment of stress reaction prior to combat using the 'BICEPS' model. *Mil Med.* 1992; 157 (7):380–381.

42. Markowitz JC, Lerman GL, Perry SW. Interpersonal psychotherapy of depressed HIV-positive outpatients. *Hosp Commun Psychiatry.* 1992; 43 (9):885–890.

43. Lazarus AA. The multi modal approach to the treatment of minor depression. *Am J Psychother.* 1992; 46 (1):50–57.

44. Spiegel D. Group support for patients with metastatic cancer. A randomized outcome study. *Arch Gen Psychiatry.* 1981; 38:527–533.

45. Stewart JW, Quitkin FM, Klein DF. The pharmacotherapy of minor depression. *Am J Psychother.* 1992; 46 (1):23–36.

46. Rosenberg PB, Ahmed I, Hurwitz S. Methylphenidate in depressed medically ill patients. *J Clin Psychiatry.* 1991; 52 (6):263–267.

47. Schatzberg AF. Anxiety and adjustment disorder. a treatment approach. *J Clin Psychiatry.* 1990; 511(Suppl):20–24.

48. Agency for Health Care Policy Research. *Depression in Primary Care*: vol 1. *Detection and Diagnosis.* AHCPR Publ. No. 93-0550. Rockville, MD: U.S. Department of Health and Human Services, Public Health Service, 1993. AHCPR Publ. No. 93-0550.

45

Depressive Disorders

MARY JANE MASSIE AND MICHAEL K. POPKIN

Emotional distress is a normal response to the catastrophic event that a cancer diagnosis represents. The diagnosis of cancer induces stresses that are caused by the patient's perceptions of the disease, its manifestations, and by the stigma commonly attached to this disease. For most individuals, the primary fear is of a painful death. In addition, all cancer patients fear becoming disabled and dependent, having altered appearance and changed body function, and losing the company of those close to them. Although such fears are similar in all patients, the level of psychological distress that accompanies these fears is highly variable. This variability is related to medical factors (i.e., site and stage of illness at the time of diagnosis, treatment(s) offered, course of the cancer, and the presence of pain); psychologic factors (i.e., prior adjustment, coping ability, emotional maturity, the disruption of life goals, and the ability to modify plans); and social factors (availability of financial support and emotional support from family, friends and coworkers) (1).

By understanding the factors outlined above, the clinician can better predict and manage the distress that exceeds what is arbitrarily defined as "normal." The presence of intolerable distress that compromises the usual function of the patient requires evaluation, diagnosis and management.

NORMAL RESPONSES TO THE STRESS OF CANCER

Individuals who receive a diagnosis of cancer, learn that relapse has occurred, or treatment has failed show a characteristic emotional response: a period of initial shock and disbelief, followed by a period of turmoil with mixed symptoms of anxiety and depression, irritability and disruption of appetite and sleep. The ability to concentrate and carry out usual daily patterns of life is impaired, and thoughts about the diagnosis and fears about the future may intrude (2).

These normal responses to crisis or transitional points in cancer resemble the response to stress that has been described in relation to other threatened or actual losses (3–6).

These symptoms usually begin to resolve over several weeks with support from family and friends, and from the physician who outlines a treatment plan that offers hope. Interventions beyond those provided by physicians, nurses, social workers and clergy are generally not required unless symptoms of emotional distress interfere with function or are prolonged or intolerable. Prescribing a hypnotic (e.g., zolpidem or triazolam) to permit normal sleep and a daytime sedative (e.g., a benzodiazepine, such as alprazolam or lorazepam) to reduce anxiety can help the patient through this crisis period.

Some patients continue to have high levels of depression and anxiety (both are usually present, although one may predominate) that persist for weeks or months. This persistent reactive distress is not adaptive and frequently requires psychiatric treatment. These disorders are classified in the current *Diagnostic and Statistical Manual of Mental Disorders* (7) as Adjustment Disorders with Depressed Mood, Anxiety, or Mixed Anxiety and Depressed Mood depending on the major symptoms. For these patients, psychiatrists working in oncology utilize short-term supportive psychotherapy based on a crisis-intervention model. This approach offers emotional support, provides information to help the patient to adapt to the crisis, emphasizes past strengths, and supports previously successful ways of coping. Patients and their families are seen at least weekly, and anxiolytic or antidepressant drugs are prescribed as indicated. As symptoms improve, medication can be reduced and discontinued. Having the patient talk with a "veteran patient," who has been through the same treatment, is often a helpful adjunct (8).

PREVALENCE OF PSYCHIATRIC DISORDERS IN PATIENTS WITH CANCER

One of the first efforts in the new field of psycho-oncology was to obtain objective data on the type and frequency of psychological problems in cancer patients. Using criteria from the DSM-III (9) classification of psychiatric disorders, the Psychosocial Collaborative Oncology Group (PSYCOG) determined the psychiatric disorders in 215 randomly selected hospitalized and ambulatory adult cancer patients in three cancer centers (10). Slightly over one-half (53%) of the patients evaluated were adjusting normally to stress; the remainder (47%) had clinically apparent psychiatric disorders. Of this 47% with psychiatric disorders, over two-thirds (68%) had "reactive" or situational anxiety and depression (Adjustment Disorders with Depressed or Anxious Mood), 13% had a major depression, 8% had an organic mental disorder, 7% had a personality disorder, and 4% had a preexisting anxiety disorder. In this study nearly 90% of the psychiatric disorders observed were reactions to or manifestations of disease or treatment. Only 11% represented prior psychiatric problems, such as personality disorders or anxiety disorders. Comparable research in children is lacking, but clinical data appear to reflect a similar spectrum of problems. The physician who treats patients with cancer can expect, for the most part, to find a group of psychologically healthy individuals who are responding to the stresses posed by cancer and its treatment.

Disorders in Cancer Patients with Pain

In the Psychosocial Collaborative Oncology Group study (10), 39% of those who received a psychiatric diagnosis experienced significant pain. In contrast, only 19% of patients who did not receive a psychiatric diagnosis had significant pain. The psychiatric diagnosis of the patients with pain was predominately Adjustment Disorder with Depressed or Mixed Mood (69%), but, of note, 15% of patients with significant pain had symptoms of a major depression.

Both data and clinical observation show that the psychiatric symptoms of patients who are in pain must initially be considered a consequence of uncontrolled pain. Acute anxiety, depression with despair (especially when the patient believes the pain means disease progression), agitation, irritability, uncooperative behavior, anger and inability to sleep may be the emotional or behavioral concomitants or sequele (11) of pain. These symptoms are not labeled as a psychiatric disorder unless they persist after pain is adequately controlled. Clinicians should first assist in pain control (12) and then reassess the patient's mental state after pain is controlled to determine whether the patient has a psychiatric disorder.

MEASURING DEPRESSION IN CANCER

Depression is challenging to study because depressive symptoms occur on a spectrum that ranges from sadness to major affective disorder, and mood change may be difficult to evaluate when a patient is confronted by a major threat to life by cancer. Depression has been studied in patients with cancer using a range of assessment methods. In general, the more narrowly the term is defined, the lower the prevalence of depression that is reported.

Cohen-Cole et al. (13) reviewed four approaches to evaluating depression in the medically ill. An *inclusive* approach counts all symptoms of depression whether or not they may be secondary to a physical illness. This method has high sensitivity, low specificity, and does not focus on etiology. In contrast, the *etiologic* approach counts a depressive symptom only if it is presumed not secondary to physical illness. This system was used in the Structured Clinical Interview for DSM-IIIR (14) and Diagnostic Interview Schedule (15). The *substitutive* approach replaces indeterminate symptoms such as fatigue, which is frequently secondary to physical illness, with cognitive symptoms such as indecisiveness, brooding and hopelessness (16). The *exclusive* approach eliminates symptoms such as anorexia and fatigue, which can be secondary to an illness such as cancer, and employs other depression criteria. This method increases specificity, which is useful in research but lowers sensitivity, which can result in lower prevalence and missed cases (13).

Kathol et al. (17) found a 13% difference (25% versus 38%) in the prevalence of depression depending on the diagnostic system used in a study of 152 oncology patients. Although the research diagnostic criteria (RDC), DSM-III and DSM-IIIR (18) criteria exclude the diagnosis of major depression if organic factors are involved, Kathol did not use this exclusionary criteria in this sample since all the subjects had cancer. An 8% higher rate of depression was found when using the DSM-III criteria (38%) as compared with DSM-IIIR (30%) criteria, which excludes symptoms if they are definitely related to a physical condition. The Endicott criteria, which substitute cognitive for physical symptoms, demonstrated a 36% prevalence of depression approximating the DSM-III system. Using the most stringent criteria, the RDC, the lowest prevalence was found (25%). Kathol suggests that different criteria identify different subsets of depressed individuals; the RDC identifies those with the most severe depression.

Using both DSM-III criteria that were modified to eliminate physical symptoms characteristic of cancer and validated observer rating scales (Hamilton Rating Scales and Beck Depression Inventory), Bukberg et al. (19) found a 42% (24% severe, 18% moderate) prevalence among 62 (30 F, 32 M) patients hospitalized on oncology units, and Plumb and Holland (20) found a 33% prevalence of depression among 80 (40 F, 40 M) hospitalized patients with advanced cancer. Bukberg's finding of 42% prevalence of depression approximates Kathol's finding of 38% using the DSM-III criteria.

Biological Markers in Depression

McDaniel and Nemeroff (21) discussed the importance of the use of biological markers when studying depression in the medically ill to attempt to address the lack of standardization in diagnostic criteria. The major biological markers that might be used are: neuroendocrine alterations, changes in serotonergic neurotransmission, alterations in sleep architecture, and structural brain abnormalities associated with mood disorders (21). McDaniel and Nemeroff reviewed 22 prevalence studies of depression in cancer covering a 25 year period and found that biological markers were used in only two of the studies. Joffe et al. (22) compared the prevalence of depression in individuals (6 F, 15 M) with pancreatic and gastric cancer. Depression was often a presenting symptom of pancreatic cancer. The authors found rates of 50% of major depression in patients with pancreatic cancer, and all of these patients were nonsuppressors of the dexamethasone suppression test (DST). Evans et al. (23) found a 40% rate of DST nonsuppression in depressed patients with gynecological cancer. We have identified one additional study which utilized the DST. Grandi et al. (24) evaluated 18 women with Stage II or III breast cancer after mastectomy or lumpectomy using DSM-III criteria and found that 22% were depressed. The DST was positive in both depressed and nondepressed patients. To date, there are no studies of serotonin metabolites in the cerebral spinal fluid, of alterations in sleep architecture, or of structural brain abnormalities of depressed individuals with cancer.

PREVALENCE OF DEPRESSION IN MEDICALLY ILL PATIENTS

To place depression in cancer in context, it is helpful to consider the broader problem of depression occurring in association with other medical illnesses. This area

has drawn increasing attention in recent years (25). Early studies of "depression in the medically ill" were drawn from hospital consultation samples with a heterogeneous mix of medical and surgical illnesses. Using varied methodologies, investigators such as Schwab et al. (26), Stewart et al. (27) and Moffic and Paykel (28) reported prevalence rates for depression in the medically ill ranging from 20% to 30%. Wallen et al. (29) reviewed data on 263,000 patients from 327 hospitals and reported 24% of those receiving a psychiatric consultation were diagnosed as having depression. Subsequently, efforts to unravel the complexities of what DSM-IV calls "mood disorder due to a general medical condition" have focused on prevalence rates in specific medical or neurological disorders. Such homogeneous samples, which may be eventually compared with one another, have generally been based on structured psychiatric interviews rather than the use of symptom rating scales such as the Beck Depression Inventory and Hamilton Depression Scale.

Using a different approach, Wells et al. (30) examined Epidemiological Catchment Area Study data regarding psychiatric disorders and eight chronic medical conditions. Six month and lifetime prevalence rates of psychiatric disorder were increased in the medically ill (25% and 42% versus 17% and 33%). In the chronically medically ill, 13% had a lifetime diagnosis of affective disorder versus 8% of those free from medical illness.

Led by studies from Johns Hopkins (31,32), work on depression in various neurological diseases has shown surprisingly consistent findings (Table 45.1). In five major neurologic conditions, lifetime rates of depression have been found to range from 30% to 50%. The only exception involves multiple sclerosis in which such rates of depression are observed in patients with cortical rather than only spinal involvement. Depression in the latter group is no greater than in the general population. These depressive disturbances have been shown to be independent of the severity of the given neurologic condition and largely independent of demographics. Lesion location appears to be a critical factor.

In contrast to neurological disease, prevalence rates of depression in patients with medical or systemic illnesses show a variable picture (Table 45.2). The highest rates have been observed in association with endocrine disturbances such as Cushing's disease. Rates for coronary artery disease and diabetes mellitus have been reported in the 19%–33% range. Surprisingly low rates of depression have been documented in end-stage renal disease.

TABLE 45.1. *Secondary Depressive Disorders in Selected Neurological Diseases*

Disease	Lifetime Prevalence of Depression	Risk Factors for Depression	Key Clinical Features of Depression
Parkinson's disease	40%–50%	Low 5-HIAA in CSF Subgroup with younger age of onset of motor symptoms, family history of affective disorder, and depression episode prior to Parkinson's disease	Independent of motor impairment; cognitive impairment frequent in late stages
Huntington's disease (HD)	≈ 40%	Confined to "certain" HD families (subgroup)	Depression may antedate chorea by years; mania also occurs
Cerebrovascular accidents	30%–50% (includes major and minor depressions)	Lesion location (left frontal, left basal ganglia); independent of demographics	Not associated with severity of impairment; major and minor constellations; mania also occurs
Multiple sclerosis (MS)	10%–50%	Cerebral involvement (versus spinal); temporal lobe involvement; family history of depression; depressive episode prior to onset of MS	Euphoria in ≈ 25%; often associated with cognitive impairment
Alzheimer's disease	15%–55%	Prior psychiatric history; younger onset of Alzheimer's; subgroup with "genetic" risk?	Psychomotor retardation, early morning awakening; ideas of worthlessness; increased cognitive dysfunction; decreased activities of daily living; greater neuronal loss in locus ceruleus

5-HIAA, 5-hydroxyindoleacetic acid; CSF, cerebrospinal fluid.
Source: Reprinted with permission from Popkin and Tucker (81).

TABLE 45.2. *Secondary (Comorbid?) Depressive Disorders in Selected Medical Illnesses*

Illness	Lifetime Prevalance of Depression	Risk Factors for Depression	Key Clinical Features of Depression
Cushing's syndrome	33%–67%	?	Often preceding hirsutism, striae Anergia, anhedonia, decreased concentration
Type I/Type II diabetes mellitus	19%–33%	Independent of gender, severity of complications	Refractory to traditional treatment (?)
End-stage renal disease	5%–8% (18% minor depression)	Drugs (steroids)	Presence of a death wish, suicidal intent Decreased concentration
Coronary heart disease (CAD)	26%	Drugs (?)	Predictive of increased combined mortality and morbidity in 1-year follow-up; effect independent of severity of CAD
Cancer (heterogeneous and single disease status types)	6%–42% (current prevalence only)	Decreased physical performance status; poor social support; drugs (chemotherapy); radiation	Seldom psychotic or melancholic; suicide risk varies by malignancy "Reactive in nature"

Source: Reprinted with permission from Popkin and Tucker (81).

Overall, rates of depression in medical illness appear to be lower than those encountered in neurological illness. This may be a function of the extent of the direct structural compromise of the central nervous system in the neurological conditions as opposed to the medical illnesses (including cancer).

To what extent depression in the medically ill is a discrete entity, separate from depression arising in patients without comorbid physical illness, remains a point of discourse. Factors including the absence of the usual female preponderance in affective disorder, no indication of genetic loading, treatment outcome and long-term course all favor the idea these disorders are "different" (25).

PREVALENCE OF DEPRESSION IN PATIENTS WITH CANCER REFERRED FOR PSYCHIATRIC CONSULTATION

Studies of the prevalence of depression in cancer patients referred for psychiatric consultation (Table 45.3) are another source of information about depression in cancer patients. Although one might expect to find a higher rate of depression in those noted to be distressed and referred for psychiatric evaluation, the five studies of depression in oncology patients referred for psychiatric consultation (33–37) report a prevalence of major depression ranging from 9% (36) to 58% (33). The high prevalence in Hinton's very early study (58%) may be reflective of the terminal status of the patients and lack of standardized instruments or diagnostic criteria utilized. Although Massie and Holland (36) report a low prevalence of depression (9%), an additional 26% of the patients had adjustment disorder with depressed mood according to DSM-III. Unlike Hinton's patients, the sample included both hospitalized and ambulatory patients. Lack of standardization in terms of population studied, disease site and stage, sample size, assessment instruments, cutoff score utilized, type of interview, and diagnostic criteria employed, including major depression versus adjustment disorder with depressed mood versus depressive symptoms, all contribute to the large variance.

PREVALENCE OF DEPRESSION IN PATIENTS WITH CANCER

In a recent review of 49 studies of the prevalence of depression in patients with cancer, DeFlorio and Massie (38) found the reported rates of depression range from 1% to 53% (Table 45.4). Most of this variance was attributed to the lack of standardization of methodology and diagnostic criteria.

Questions commonly asked about the prevalence of depression in patients with cancer include: *(1)* Are there gender differences? *(2)* Are hospitalized patients more depressed than ambulatory patients? *(3)* Are those with advanced disease more depressed? Among the 49 studies of the prevalence of depression in cancer reviewed by DeFlorio and Massie, 29 included both males and females (38). Six of these research groups did not examine or report gender differences; the remaining 23 studies found no gender differences in the prevalence of depression at a significance level of $p < .05$. However, ten of these research groups found gender differences in subsets of patients, non-significant trends, or differences in other parameters such as anxiety, psychiatric morbidity, and denial. Many clinicians have believed that hospitalized patients with advanced cancer are more depressed than ambulatory patients. However, as more studies have been done over time, hospitalization status explains little of the large variance. Now, because of insurance restrictions, many seriously ill cancer patients who would have been hospitalized are treated in ambulatory settings.

Advanced disease stage has been correlated with a higher prevalence of depression in several studies. The reported prevalence of depression in patients with advanced cancer ranges from 23% (20) to 53% (39). Bukberg et al. found that greater physical disability measured by the Karnofsky Rating Scale (the lower the score, the greater the disability) was associated with depression in their study of 62 patients with cancer (19). They found a 42% overall prevalence of depression, but a range of 23% (in those with Karnofsky scores greater than 60) to 77% (in those with Karnofsky scores less than 40).

Consultation data provides another source of information about depression in patients with cancer. Massie and Holland have reviewed data on 546 patients referred for psychiatric consultation at Memorial Sloan-Kettering Cancer Center (36). Fifty-nine percent of consultations had been requested for evaluation of depression, or suicidal risk, or both. When the consultant's actual impressions were reviewed, depressive symptoms were by far the most common; Adjustment Disorders with Depressed Mood accounted for 54% of diagnoses, and Major Depression accounted for 9%. Breitbart reviewed data on 1080 consultation requests to the Psychiatry Service at Memorial Sloan-Kettering Cancer Center and observed that evaluation of suicidal risk was the reason for referral in nearly 9% of referrals; suicide

TABLE 45.3. *Psychiatric Consultation Studies of Depression in Cancer Patients*

Reference	N	F/M	Patients	Method	Percent Depressed	Specific Findings	Gender Difference
Hinton (33)	50	36 F, 14 M	Hospitalized; terminally ill; mixed neoplasms, one collagen-vascular	Interview	58%	42% anxious; 34% adjustment reaction; 10% confusional state	Not cited for depression; more psychiatric referrals for breast cancer; fewer men with lung cancer referred; low referrals for digestive neoplasms
Levine et al. (34)	100	51 F, 49 M	Hospitalized; all stages and sites	Interview; DSM-III criteria	56%	40% OBS; 26% OBS misdiagnosed as depressed by referring physician; 58% of depressed had metastases	2:1 female to male ratio of psychiatric referrals; NS* trend of more OBS in males than females in under 60
Massie et al. (35)	334	189 F, 145 M	Hospitalized and ambulatory; all stages and sites	Interview; DSM-II criteria	49%; 5% extreme; 24% severe; 71% mild to moderate	15% organic; all patients with severe or extreme depression had advanced cancer	Women referrals higher than men; 1:1.3 M:F
Massie and Holland (35)	546	Not cited	Hospitalized and ambulatory; all stages; all sites; referred for psychiatric consultation	Interview; DSM-III criteria	9% major depression; 26% adjustment disorder with depressed mood	59% of referrals depressed or suicidal; good premorbid functioning with only 11% psychiatric history	Not cited
Razavi et al. (37)	128	Not cited	Hospitalized; mixed; 88 psychiatric referral out of total of 210 (141 F, 69 M)	Semistructured interview from the Diagnostic Interview Schedule; HADS	26% major depression; 46% adjustment disorder	Depression higher in preterminal or terminal	Not cited

OBS, organic brain syndrome; HADS, Hospital Anxiety and Depression Scale.
*NS, not significant at $p = 0.05$ level.

TABLE 45.4. *Prevalence of Depression in Cancer Patients*

Reference	N	F/M	Patients	Method	Percent Depressed	Specific Findings	Gender Difference
Koeng et al. (82)	36	18 F, 18 M	Hospitalized; advanced bowel	MMPI	25%	Cancer patients less psychopathology than depressed psychiatric inpatients	None
Fras et al. (83)	110	Not cited	Pancreatic and colon cancer	Semi-structured interview; MMPI	50% (pancreas); 13% (colon)	76% psychiatric symptoms in those with pancreatic cancer; psychiatric symptoms appeared first in half of pancreatic cancer patients	Not cited
Peck and Boland (84)	50	27 F, 23 M	Ambulataory radiotherapy: all sites; all stages	Clinical interview	MDNC 74% affective symptoms	10% severe depression; 32% moderate depression; 32% mild depression	Not cited
Craig and Abeloff (39)	30	19 F, 11 M	Hospitalized; all sites, advanced	SCL-90	53%	13% severe depression; 40% moderate depression; 30% anxious	Gender differences not significant but trend for white females, younger, and higher socioeconomic level patients to have more psychological symptoms
Plumb and Holland (20)	97	50 F, 47 M	Hospitalized, all sites, advanced; compared to 99 psychiatric inpatients with recent suicide attempt	BDI	23% cancer patients depressed; 54% psychiatric patients depressed	19% moderate severity; 4% severe; cancer patients and their next of kin were less depressed than physically healthy suicide attempt patients	None
Morris et al. (85)	160	160 F	Breast biopsy and mastectomy patients	Interview; HRSD	22% depression in mastectomy	Mastectomy patients had persistent depression (22%) at 2 yr compared to benign patients (8%)	All female
Maguire et al. (86)	201	201 F	117 ambulatory breast cancer patients, 89 benign disease	Clinical interview	26% moderate or severe depression after mastectomy	Control benign patients had 12% depression	All female
Silberfarb et al. (87)	146	146 F	Hospitalization status not inidcated; 34% primary disease; 36% recurrent; 30% advanced, all breast cancer	Structured interview; open-ended questions; modified psychiataric status scale	10% depression in primary cancer diagnosis; 15% in recurrent; 4.5% advanced cancer	Physical disability did not relate to emotional disturbances; first recurrence of breast cancer most disturbing time; advanced patients had the least depression	All female

Study	N	Sex/No.	Population	Measures	Prevalence	Findings	Sex differences
Krouse and Krouse (88)	21	21 F	Hospitalized for mastectomy, hysterectomy, or breast biopsy and assessed during hospitalization and ambulatory follow-up at 4 wk to 2 mo	BDI: Rotter Incomplete Sentences; Body Image Questionnaire	DNC; average BDI	More severe depression and poor body image among gynecologic patients; most mastectomy patients were not depressed and did not have severe body image disturbance	All female
Plumb and Holland (20)	80	40 F, 40 M	Hospitalized; all sites; advanced	Structured interview; CAPPS excluding certain physical symptoms	33%; 1% extreme; 20% severe; 24% moderate; 33% mild; 16% minimal	Cancer patients less depressed than comparative group of psychiatric patients	More men than women (12 versus 5) were severely depressed; overall depression ratings equal between men and women; males had more history of poor impulse control; females had more history of phobic symptoms
Derogatis et al. (10)	215	110 F, 105 M	Half hospitalized; half ambulatory; all stages	DSM-III criteria; SCL-90; RDS; GAIS; Karnofsky Rating Scale	6% major depression; 12% adjustment disorder with depressed mood; 13% adjustment disorder with mixed emotional features	Excluded severely ill (Karnofsky <50); 47% received DSM-III diagnosis; 68% of these diagnoses were adjustment disorder	None
Bukberg et al. (19)	62	30 F, 32 M	Hospitalized on medical oncology units	Modified DSM-III criteria eliminating physical symptoms; DACL; IIRSD; Karnofsky Rating Scale; BDI; Magill Pain Questionnaire	42% depressed; 24% severe; 18% moderate; 14% mild; 44% none	Greater physical disability, negative life events, and poor quality of social support associated with depression	None
Farber et al. (89)	141	101 F, 40 M	Ambulatory; primarily breast cancer	SCL-90	19% severe; 21% moderate; 14% mild	A comparison of males and females with clinical and global scales of the SCL-90 showed no significant differences	None
Morton et al. (90)	48	48 M	Largely ambulatory oropharyngeal, geriatric	DSM-III criteria	40%	Function disability lower in those treated with radiation alone rather than surgery or combination; no significant difference in depression among three treatment groups	All male

(continued)

TABLE 45.4. *Prevalence of Depression in Cancer Patients (continued)*

Reference	N	F/M	Patients	Method	Percent Depressed	Specific Findings	Gender Difference
Lloyd et al. (91)	40	15 F, 25 M	Hospitalized and ambulatory; Hodgkin's or non-Hodgkin's lymphoma; all stages and isles	Semistructured interview; EQP; VAS	MDNC; 38% psychiatric morbidity	26% psychiatric morbidity at 6 mo; one-third patients dissatisfied with information received about illness	Women had significantly higher psychiatric morbidity
Hughes (92)	134	30 F, 104 M	Lung cancer	Structured clinical interview	16%	Most of the depressed patients were depressed before physical symptoms began	Not cited
Robinson et al. (93)	57	33 F, 24 M	Hospitalized and ambulatory	Semistructured interview; social adjustment self-repsort; symptom questionnaire	25% both depressed and anxious; 60% depressed or anxious current or past	30% depressed or anxious current or past "not due to cancer"; 12% due to cancer; 58% "normal"; depression and anxiety more severe and in noncancer relatives	Not cited
Starkman et al. (94)	17	4 F, 13 M	Hospitalized pheochromocytoma patients compared to 52 patients with primary anxiety disorder	DSM-III criteria; STAI; SCL-90R	12%	No increased prevalence of anxiety disorder in pheochromocytoma	None
Lansky et al. (95)	500	500 F	85% ambulatory; 43% survivors with no evidence of disease; 34% early stage	DSM-III, organic brain syndrome section of the PDI; HRSD; Zung Self-rating Depression Scale; visual pain analog line	5.3% (using HDRS and Zung); 4.5% (using DSM-III criteria)	High degree of survivors; HDRS ≥ 20 and Zung ≥ 50	All female
Davies et al. (96)	72	29 F, 46 M	Hospitalized; oropharyngeal cancer	Leeds Scale for Self-assessment of Depression; General Health Questionnaire	22%	Patients and investigators were blind to biopsy results; more depression (29% versus 15%) in those with positive biopsy	None
Evans et al. (23)	83	83 F	All hospitalized women with gynecological cancer (excluding ovarian)	DSM-III; HRSD	23% major depression; 24% adjustment disorder with depressed mood	DST 40% sensitivity; 80% specificity	All female

Study	N	Sex	Population	Measure	Results	Notes	Gender
Holland et al. (97)	218	78 F, 140 M	Ambulatory; 107 advanced pancreatic, 111 advanced gastric	POMS	MDNC; 21% median POMS gastric; 38% median POMS pancreatic	Pancreatic cancer patients had higher depression than gastric cancer among men only	Male depression and distress scores equal or slightly higher than female (NS)*
Joffe et al. (22)	21	6 F, 15 M	Hospitalized; pancreas 12, gastric 9	SADS-L; SCL-90 R; BDI, STAI, RDC criteria	Major depression: 33% pancreas; 0% gastric; major depression and adjustment disorder; 50% pancreas, 11% gastric	19% of new pancreatic cancer patients had a history of major depression in the year prior to diagnosis; DST: pancreas 6 of 6 nonsuppression (1 major depression); gastric: 5 of 6 nonsuppression (0 major depression)	None
Grandi et al. (24)	18	18 F	Hospitalized; Stage II or III breast cancer postmastectomy or lumpectomy	Paykel's clinical interview for depression; DSM-III criteria	22% depression; 22% anxious	Dexamethasone stimulation test positive in both depressed and nondepressed patients	All female
Devlen et al. (98)	90	43 F, 47 M	Ambulatory; Hodgkin's disease and non–Hodgkin's lymphoma	Semistructured interview	19% depressed; 27% borderline depression	Retrospective study; with interviews conducted a mean of 32 months after diagnosis	Not cited
Devlen et al. (99)	120	56 F, 64 M	Ambulatory; Hodgkin's disease and non–Hodgkin's lymphoma	Semistructured interview	8% depressed in year after treatment	Prospective study with interviews at baseline, 2, 6, and 12 mo after diagnosis	Not cited
Friedrich et al. (100)	46	22 F, 24 M	Hospitalized; 23 twin patients, one with hematologic malignancy, the other a bone marrow donor	MMPI	MDNC; 62% mean depression MMPI score patients; 54% mean depression score donors; 50% mastectomy; 50% lumpectomy	No difference in depression in male twins	Female cancer patients showed more depression and repression of feelings than their nonpatient twins
Stefanek et al. (101)	126	71 F, 55 M	Ambulatory; mixed	BSI	33% depressed; 9% severe; 24% moderate	20% high psychiatric distress in general	None

(continued)

527

TABLE 45.4. *Prevalence of Depression in Cancer Patients (continued)*

Reference	N	F/M	Patients	Method	Percent Depressed	Specific Findings	Gender Difference
Pettingale et al. (102)	168	Not cited	Hospitalized early breast cancer and lymphoma; all stages	Interview: STAI; Wakefield	MDNC	In lymphoma patients, the more advanced the disease, the higher the depression; no correlation with disease state and depression in breast cancer	Breast patients more anxious at 12 mo; women more anxious than men at 3 and 12 mo; men more likely to believe their illness not under their control; women with lymphoma more anxious and tendency (NS*) for more depression than either men with lymphoma or women with breast cancer
Grassi et al. (103)	196	151 F, 45 M	Hospitalized and ambulatory; recent diagnosis or cancer; mixed, 18–70 yr	HRSD; IBQ; interview	24%–38%	38% depression with HDRS cutoff of 17%–24% with HDRS of 21	Higher levels of denial in women on IBQ
Hardman et al. (104)	126	54 F, 72 M	Hospitalized; mixed	Structured interview (ICD); General Health Questionnaire	3% depression; 23% anxiety and depression	Psychiatric symptoms related to feeling moderately or severely ill and previous psychiatric illness, but not with awareness of having cancer	None
Meyer and Aspergren (105)	58	58 F	Ambulatory breast cancer patients in Sweden, 5 yr after treatment	Clinical interview; CPRS depression scale	MDNC; 30% anxiety or depressive symptoms postmastectomy	5 yr posttreatment anxiety and depression persisted in 30% mastectomy and 29% partial mastectomy	All female
Fallowfield et al.	269	269 F	Stage I and II breast cancer assessed 2 wk, 3 mo, 12 mo after surgery	Interview	21% mastectomy; 19% lumpectomy	Less depression in mastectomy and lumpectomy patients given treatment choice	All female
Kathol et al. (17)	808	89 F, 63 M	Mixed; 152 depressed patients	DSM-III and DSM-IIIR criteria; RDC; Endicott Substitution criteria; HRSD; BDI	25%–38% major depression, depending on diagnostic system; 19% (depressive symptoms)	Authors concluded that self- and observer-rated scales are sufficient to screen at risk patients but not to diagnose	Women had more depression than men on RDC but not DSM-III criteria
Jenkins et al. (107)	22	22 F	Ambulatory breast cancer patients diagnosed with recent local recurrence	DSM-III; EPQ; HAS; MADRS; CIDI	32% depressed; 27% anxiety and depression; 45% depressed or anxious	46% previous major depression; previous psychiatric illness and trait neuroticism predictive of psychiatric morbidity	All female

Study	N	Sample	Setting	Measure	Prevalence	Comments	Gender
Golden et al. (108)	83	83 F	Hospitalized; cervical, endometrial, and vaginal cancer	DSM-III criteria; CRS	23% major depression according to DSM-III criteria	—	All female
Colon et al. (109)	100	35 F, 65 M	Hospitalized acute leukemia prior to BMT	DSM-III-R criteria	1% major depression; 2% organic affective syndrome; 8% adjustment disorder	Illness criteria, depressed mood and perceived social support independently affected outcome; depressed patients had poorer outcome	None
Hopwood et al. (110)	81	81 F	Ambulatory; advanced breast cancer	HADS; RSCL; Clinical Interview Schedule; DSM-III criteria	20% depression; 15% anxiety	21% of "normal" patients misclassified by RSCL and 26% by HADS; 75% sensitivity of HADS and RSCL together	All female
Hopwood et al. (111)	222	222 F	Ambulatory; advanced breast cancer	HADS; RSCL	9% depression and 9% anxiety using HADS; combined anxiety or depression: 33% (HADS), 22% RSCL; 40% depressed	HADS and RSCL detected different groups of cases; one-third of depressed patients persisted for 1–3 mo	All female
Baile et al. (112)	45	28 F, 37 M	Ambulatory; head and neck	Semistructured interview; MCAI; MAST; GARS	40%	Found no relationship between tumor stage and depression	More depression among early stage females and late stage males
Goldberg et al. (113)	320	320 F	Hospitalized for newly diagnosed breast cancer surgery	Modified RSCL; preoperative, 6 and 12 mo postoperatively	32% depressed malignant; 24% depressed benign biopsy	At 1 yr depression had decreased (21% depressed)	All female
Maraste et al. (114)	133	133 F	Ambulatory; adjuvant radiotherapy; breast cancer	HADS	1.5% depressed; 14% anxiety	Age and surgery related anxiety; anxiety in ages 50–59 yr was 44% in mastectomy versus 4% in conservative surgery	All female
Sneed et al. (115)	133	89 F, 44 M	Hospitalized; newly diagnosed; mixed sites and stages	BSI; HIS-GWB	MDNC	Women with gynecological and breast cancer had less depression, anxiety, hostility, somatization, psychological distress than men and women with other cancers	None

(continued)

TABLE 45.4. *Prevalence of Depression in Cancer Patients* (*continued*)

Reference	N	F/M	Patients	Method	Percent Depressed	Specific Findings	Gender Difference
Cathcart et al. (116)	257	257 F	Ambulatory; women with node negative breast cancer; 155 women received tamoxifen; 102 received no tamoxifen	Clinical interview	15% in tamoxifen treated group; 3% in those not receiving tamoxifen	4.5% of 155 women receiving tamoxifen had to discontinue it secondary to depression	All female
Alexander et al. (117)	60	24 F, 26 M	Hospitalized on oncology unit in India; mixed sites and stages	DSM-III-R; clinical interview	13% depressed; 20% adjustment disorder; 40% psychiatric disorder	Those who were unaware of cancer diagnosis (33%) or considered the treatment curative (82%) had less psychiatric morbidity	None
Pinder et al. (118)	139	139 F	86 Hospitalized; 53 ambulatory advanced breast cancer	HADS interview	13% depressed; 25% anxiety or depression	Depression more prevalent in low socioeconomic class, in poor performance states, and closer proximity to death	All female
Sneeuw et al. (119)	556	556 F	Ambulatory Stage I and II breast cancer; interviewed at 1½ yr after treatment	DSM-III criteria; DIS; CES-D; SCL-25	4.5% depressed; 6.3% generalized anxiety disorder; 8.8% phobic disorder	Depressive symptoms 1½ yr after treatment and longer; no significant differences in patients who had mastectomy versus conservative treatment	All female
Rapaport et al. (120)	55	15 F, 40 M	Ambulatory head and neck, all stages, who had completed treatment	Interview with opne-ended questions; PAQ	MDNC; 24% anxious	Psychological problems increased over time	None

BDI, Beck Depression Inventory; BSI Brief Symptom Inventory; CIDI, Composite International Diagnostic Interview; CPRS, Copenhagen Psychiatric Rating Scale; CRS, Carroll Rating Scale for Depression; CAPPS, Current and Past Psychiatric Adjustment Scale; CES-D, Center for Epidemiology Self-report Depression Scale; DACL, Lubin Depression Adjective Check List-form E; EPQ, Eysenck Personality Questionnaire; GAIS, Global Adjustment to Illness Sclae; GARS, Global Assessment of Recent Stress; HRSD, Hamilton Rating Scale for Depression; HAS, Hamilton Anxiety Scale; HADS, Hospital Anxiety and Depression Scale; HIS-GWB, Rand Health Insurance Study-General Well-Being Schedule; IBQ, Illness Behavior Questionnaire; MADRS, Montogmery Asberg Depression Rating Scales; MAST, Michigan Alcohol Screen Test; MCAI, Million Clinical Multiaxial Inventory; MMPI, Minnesota Multiphasic Personality Inventory; PAQ, Patient Adjustment Questionnaire; PDI, Psychiatric Checklist; SADS, Schedule for Affective Disorders and Schizophrenia; SCL-25, SCL-90, SCL-90R, Hopkins Symptom Checklist 25, 90, and 90-Revised; STAI, State-Trait Anxiety Inventory; BAS, Visual analog scales; MDNC; major depression not cited.
*NS, not significant at $p = 0.05$ level.

risk was found in 71 patients (6.5%) (40). One-third of the suicidal patients had a Major Depression, more than half had an Adjustment Disorder, and nearly 20% had a delirium.

The following sections outline the clinical presentation of depression and management approaches. The practice guidelines for depression developed both by the American Psychiatric Association (41) and the Agency for Health Care Policy and Research (42) are practical guides to the management of depression in adults and provide an overview of depression in both physically healthy and medically ill patients.

DIAGNOSIS OF DEPRESSION IN PATIENTS WITH CANCER

The diagnosis of depression in physically healthy patients depends heavily on the presence of somatic symptoms of anorexia, fatigue, insomnia, and weight loss. These indicators are of little value as diagnostic criteria for depression in cancer patients, as they are common to both cancer and depression. In cancer patients, the diagnosis of depression must depend on psychological, not somatic, symptoms. These psychological symptoms are dysphoric mood, feelings of helplessness and hopelessness, loss of self-esteem, feelings of worthlessness or guilt, anhedonia, and thoughts of "wishing for death" or suicide (43).

Mood Disorder with Depressive Features due to Cancer, Other Medical Conditions or Substances

When evaluating depressed patients, it is imperative to attempt to determine whether organic factors underlie the depressive syndrome. Depressive syndromes which are caused by the direct physiologic effects of cancer are called Mood Disorder with Depressive Features Due to Cancer in DSM-IV. The key feature of these disorders is a prominent and persistent depressed mood that resembles a Major Depression. The presence of delirium (encephalopathy) must be ruled out and, if present, precludes the diagnosis of Mood Disorder with Depressive Features unless the patient had been diagnosed as being depressed before confusional symptoms developed. The patient may have some mild cognitive deficits, such as poor memory or decreased concentration, and may have decreased control over sexual or aggressive impulses. Tumor involvement of the central nervous system and carcinoma of the pancreas may cause a Mood Disorder with Depressive Features Due to Cancer. Determining the cause of depression in individuals with pancreatic carcinoma represents a special problem in psychooncology. It is often unclear whether depressive symptoms

TABLE 45.5. *Medical Conditions Presenting with Depressive Constellations*

ENDOCRINE DISORDERS
Thyroid dysfunction (hypothyroidsim or hyperthyroidsim), adrenal dysfunction or syndrome (Cushing's disease or Addison's disease), diebetes mellitus, insulinoma, acromegaly, hypoparathyroidism, hypopituitarism

NEUROLOGICAL DISORDERS
Parkinson's disease, Huntington's disease, multiple sclerosis, Alzheimer's disease, cerebrovascular diseases

METABOLIC DISORDERS
Hypomagnesemia, hyponatremia, hypokalemia, hyperkalemia, uremia, Wilson's disease, pernicious anemia, pellagra, folic acid deficiency, pyridoxine deficiency

NEOPLASIAS
Oat cell carcinoma, pancreatic carcinoma, tumors of the central nervous system, lymphoma, leukema

COLLAGEN-VASCULAR DISEASE
Systemic lupus erythematosus, giant cell arteritis, rheumatoid arthritis

INFECTIOUS DISORDERS
Infectous mononucleosis, hepatitis, influenza, syphilis, tuberculosis, acquired immune deficiency syndrome (AIDS), encephalitis

are due to an indirect effect of the cancer on the brain (possibly alteration of serotonergic function) or due to a psychological reaction to this devastating illness (44).

The roster of "medical causes" of mood disorder is extensive (see Tables 45.5, 45.6). DSM-IV defines disturbances in mood due to the direct physiologic effects

TABLE 45.6. *What Medical Conditions Cause Depression in Cancer Patients?*

Uncontrolled pain

Metabolic abnormalities
    Hypercalcemia
    Sodium, potassium imbalance
    Anemia
    Deficient vitamin B_{12} or folate

Endocrinologic abnormalities
    Hyper- or hypothyroidism
    Adrenal insufficiency

Medicine
    Steroids
    Interferon and interleukin 2
    Methyldopa
    Reserpine
    Barbiturates
    Propranolol
    Some antibiotics (amphotericin B)
    Some chemotherapeutic agents
        Vincristine
        Vinblastine
        Procarbazine
        L-Asparaginase

of a substance (i.e., a drug of abuse or a medication) as a Substance-Induced Mood Disorder. Drugs such as β-adrenergic antagonists (45) (Table 45.7), and some anticancer drugs, particularly corticosteroids, vinblastine, vincristine, procarbazine, asparaginase (46), tamoxifen (47), and interferon, can cause depression (46) (Table 45.8).

The evaluation of every depressed individual with cancer must include consideration of medical, endocrinologic and neurologic factors. A cognitive evaluation must be performed. Many clinicians prefer to use at least one easily reproducible instrument (e.g., the Mini-Mental Status Examination) (48) to document the mental status at the time of the initial evaluation and subsequent evaluations. All such brief instruments

TABLE 45.8. *Anticancer Drugs Associated with Depression*

Drug	Cancer
Corticosteroids	
Vinblastine	Breast, lung
Vincristine	ALL, brain
Interferon	Renal, KS
Procarbazine	Brain
Asparaginase	ALL
Tamoxifen	Breast
Cyproterone	Prostate

KS, Kaposi's sarcoma.
Source: Adapted from Ref. 46.

have limitations because they assess only selected aspects of cognition.

If the depressive disorder is believed to be caused by a medical condition or by a drug, the clinician first attempts to treat the disorder or change the drug. Often, antidepressants are started concurrently in an effort to alleviate the patient's suffering more quickly or because the clinician anticipates that the depression that complicates the underlying disorder will not be relieved by addressing the medical condition alone. When the primary cause of the depression cannot be "corrected" (e.g., the chemotherapeutic agent must be continued, as it usually must), antidepressant therapy is also initiated.

Depression with Psychotic Features

Although rare, depression accompanied by delusions, hallucinations or grossly disorganized behavior is sometimes encountered in cancer patients. In the medically ill, the presence of depressive symptoms (e.g., flat affect, lack of interest in daily activities), coupled with psychotic symptoms, may more often be reflective of a delirium. Before the diagnosis of depression with psychotic features is made, the presence of underlying organic causes for these mental status changes should be explored. When psychotic features are present, an antipsychotic and an antidepressant are started concurrently. High-potency neuroleptics (e.g., haloperidol, trifluoperazine and fluphenazine) are usually preferred because of their low anticholinergic potential, which reduces the risk of delirium and other anticholinergic side effects (e.g., cardiac arrhythmias, constipation, urinary retention, and blurred vision). These high-potency neuroleptics also lower seizure threshold less than low-potency neuroleptics (e.g., chlorpromazine and thioridazine) and are preferable when the risk of seizures is a concern. Molindone, an intermediate-potency neuroleptic, has been reported to have the lowest epileptogenic potential, and may also be a good choice for a patient with psychotic symptoms

TABLE 45.7. *Drugs That Cause Depression*

Generic Name	Brand Name
Acyclovir	
Amphetamine-like drugs	
Anabolic steroids	
Anticonvulsants	
Baclofen	Lioresal
Barbiturates	
Benzodiazepines	
β-Adrenergic blockers	
Bromocriptine	Parlodex
Clonidine	Catapres
Cycloserine	Seromycin
Dapson	
Digitalis glycosides	
Diltiazem	Cardizem
Disopyramide	Norprace
Disulfiram	Antabuse
Ethionamide	Trecator-SC
Etretinate	Tegison
HMG-CoA reductase inhibitors	
Isoniazid	INH
Isosorbide dinitrate	Isordil
Isotretinoin	Accutance
Levodopa	Dopar
Mefloquine	Lariam
Methylpoda	Aldomet
Metoclopramide	Reglan
Metrizamide	Amipaque
Metronidazole	Flagyl
Nalidixic acid	NegGram
Narcotics	
Nifedipine	Procardia
Nonsteroidal anti-inflammatory drugs	
Norflaxacin	Noroxin
Ofloxacin	Floxin
Phenylephrine	NeoSynephrine
Procaine derivatives	
Reserpine	Serpasil
Sulfonamides	
Thiaziades	
Thyroid hormones	
Trimethoprim-sulfamethoxazole	Bactrim

HMG-CoA, 3-hydroxy-3-methylglutaryl coenzyme A.
Source: Adapted from Ref. 45.

and seizures that are difficult to control with anticonvulsants (49).

Depression in the Elderly

Older individuals are at greater risk for depression and suicidal acts whether they are physically healthy or not. In addition to the loss of good health, the elderly cancer patient often has sustained other losses, including physical ability (e.g., hearing loss), financial stability, death of a spouse or partner and friends, or self-esteem through retirement or changed social standing. Sometimes the clinical presentation of depression is similar to that described for younger adult patients, but other presentations are more typical of this phase of life (50). Sometimes the patient's chief complaints are cognitive, such as poor memory or concentration. By taking a thorough history and by interviewing relatives or friends to document the patient's history, the clinician learns that depressive features may antedate the cognitive complaints. When asked specific questions, the patient often responds "I don't know" instead of attempting to answer. Objective testing (e.g., with the Mini-Mental Status Examination) often reveals better results than those expected based on subjective complaints.

Suicide

Suicidal ideation requires careful assessment to determine whether the patient has a depressive illness or is expressing a wish to have ultimate control over intolerable symptoms. Thoughtful clinical judgment is required to make this differentiation, especially in the patient with advanced disease. Factors which place a cancer patient at a high risk for suicide are poor prognosis and advanced illness, depression and hopelessness, uncontrolled pain, delirium, prior psychiatric history, history of previous suicide attempts or family history of suicide, history of recent death of friends or spouse, history of alcohol abuse, and few social supports (40,51–53). Other risk factors include male sex, advanced age (sixth and seventh decades), presence of fatigue, and oral, pharyngeal, lung, gastrointestinal, urogenital, and breast cancers (Table 45.9). Cancer patients have twice the risk of committing suicide as the "general population" (54,55). Many factors, such as poor prognosis, delirium, uncontrolled pain, depression, and hopelessness, are often present in a patient with advanced disease, increasing the risk of suicide. Hopelessness is even a stronger predictive factor than depression itself (56). Cancer patients usually commit suicide by overdosage with analgesics or sedative drugs prescribed by their doctors. Men use violent means, such as hanging or gunshot, more often than women.

TABLE 45.9. *Suicide Risk Factors in Cancer Patients*

Related to mental status
    Suicidal ideation
    Lethal plans (medications)
    Depression and hopelessness
    Delirium and disinhibition
    Psychotic features (hallucinations and delusions)
    Loss of control and impulsivity
    Irrational thinking

Related to cancer
    Uncontrolled pain
    Advanced disease and poor prognosis
    Site (oral pharyngeal, lung, gastrointestinal, urogenital, breast)
    Exhaustion and fatigue
    Use of steroids (mood changes)

Related to history
    Prior suicidal attempts
    Psychopathology
    Substance abuse (alcohol)
    Recent loss (spouse or friends)
    Poor social support
    Older male
    Family history of suicide

The management of the suicidal cancer patient includes: maintaining a supportive therapeutic relationship; conveying the attitude that much can be done to improve the quality, if not the quantity, of life even if the prognosis is poor; and actively eliciting and treating specific symptoms (e.g., pain, nausea, insomnia, anxiety, and depression). The most useful psychotherapeutic modalities are based on a crisis-intervention model using cognitive techniques (e.g., giving back a sense of control by helping the patient to focus on that which can still be controlled) and supportive methods, usually involving family and friends. One should keep in mind that the spouse and other family members of the person with cancer are also at increased risk for suicide and that they also often require evaluation and support (1).

At Memorial Sloan-Kettering Cancer Center, virtually all hospitalized patients who have attempted suicide have had poorly controlled pain, mild encephalopathy, disinhibition secondary to drugs, and hopelessness combined with distress about the inability to communicate their concerns about their discomfort to care givers. If a patient is suicidal, a 24-hour companion should be provided to establish constant observation, monitor the suicidal risk and reassure the patient. Need for observation is evaluated daily; companions are discontinued when the patient is no longer suicidal and is judged to be in control and able to act rationally.

TREATMENT WITH DEPRESSION

Before planning an intervention, the psychiatrist should obtain a history of previous depressive episodes and substance (including alcohol and cocaine) abuse, family history of depression and suicide, concurrent life stresses, losses secondary to cancer (e.g., financial, social, and occupational), in addition to loss of good health and the availability of social support. An assessment of the meaning of illness to the patient and his or her understanding of the medical situation (including prognosis) is essential. Depressed patients with cancer are usually treated with a combination of supportive psychotherapy and antidepressants (8,43); electroconvulsive therapy is less often utilized.

Psychological Treatment

The goals of psychotherapy are to reduce emotional distress and to improve morale, coping ability, self-esteem, sense of control and resolution of problems (57). Cancer patients are often referred for, or request, psychiatric consultation at times of crisis in illness: at the time of diagnosis or diagnosis of recurrence, at the beginning of any new treatment, when standard or experimental treatments fail, or when patients perceive themselves as "terminal." The referral is often an "emergency" and, because of the acute crisis, the patient often readily accepts an intervention. Various models of intervention for the acutely or chronically medically ill have been described, including time-limited dynamic psychotherapy or short-term dynamic therapy (58) and cognitive-behavioral therapy (59). Often 4–15 sessions are required to treat the acute problem. The patient considers his recent losses (good health, body integrity, self-esteem, family support, presumed longevity, financial security, and opportunity for job satisfaction) in the context of his past history of loss or success and is helped to chart a future direction incorporating life and body alterations brought on by the diagnosis of a chronic life-threatening illness. As mentioned above, the model we find most useful is based on a crisis-intervention model that involves an active therapeutic role. Educational interventions, such as clarifying information and explaining emotional reactions to the patient, family and staff, are useful. Cognitive techniques are also useful to help the patient correct misconceptions and exaggerated fears. Patients are encouraged to consider an array of different possible explanations or outcomes for their situation and then to determine which aspects they can still improve. This approach provides the patient with a sense of control over his or her situation and helps the individual to avoid focusing only on the worst eventualities.

Emotional support is also provided. Listening to the patient carefully and allowing him or her to express all feelings, fears and anger in a nonjudgmental setting is often therapeutic in itself. Legitimization of the difficulty of the situation and of the "right" to be upset reduces the fear of being perceived as "weak" or "inappropriate." Reassurances should be realistic and consistent with the available knowledge of the situation. The desire of patients to maintain hope is, of course, respected, as are the defense mechanisms of denial, repression, and regression, as long as these do not interfere with diagnostic or therapeutic processes or with important personal matters that must be addressed. As we explore the patient's history of loss, we identify and reinforce his or her successful ways of coping. At the "termination" of psychotherapy, patients are reassured to hear that their psychiatrist is available for future visits if symptoms recur or if the disease worsens (1).

Another important aspect of the treatment of the depressed cancer patient is social support provided by family, friends and community or religious groups. We try to enlist relatives to provide emotional support; however, we advise family members to minimize family conflicts, which add an additional emotional burden and can be addressed more appropriately after the depression has resolved. In addition, we identify vulnerable family members who cannot provide emotional support and, indeed, may also need psychosocial help. These family members are encouraged to seek individual or group support for themselves.

Somatic Therapies

Antidepressants. Although there are many reports of the efficacy of antidepressants in depressed patients with cancer (60,61), there is only one double-blind placebo-controlled study (62) demonstrating efficacy. It is difficult to conduct controlled studies of drugs in cancer patients; patients refuse to enter such studies because they already feel like "research subjects" and, when depressed, want individualized attention. Dropout rates from such studies are high because patients may tolerate drug side effects poorly or undergo worsening of their medical condition. Nonetheless, there is much clinical experience with antidepressant drugs in this population. The antidepressant agents that can be considered for use in cancer patients are: *(1)* the newer agents, including selective serotonin reuptake inhibitors (SSRIs); *(2)* the tricyclic antidepressants (TCAs); *(3)* the psychostimulants; *(4)* lithium carbonate; and *(5)* the monoamine oxidase inhibitors (MAOIs) (63) (Table 45.10).

NEWER ANTIDEPRESSANTS. The SSRIs, fluoxetine, sertraline and paroxetine are the antidepressants prescribed first in our setting because they have fewer sedative and autonomic effects than the TCAs. The most common side effects are mild nausea, headache, somnolence or insomnia, and a brief period of increased anxiety; hyponatremia is an uncommon adverse effect (64). These drugs can cause appetite suppression that usually lasts a period of several weeks. Some cancer patients experience transient weight loss, but weight usually returns to baseline level, and the anorectic properties of these drugs have not been a limiting factor in this population. Paroxetine has no active metabolites and sertraline has fewer active metabolites than fluoxetine, and both have a short half-life, characteristics that are important if one wants to avoid accumulation of the drug and more precise titration.

Bupropion, trazodone, maprotiline and amoxapine are prescribed less frequently than the SSRIs for individuals with cancer. Bupropion is considered if patients have a poor response to a reasonable trial of other antidepressants. It may be somewhat activating in medically ill patients, and should be avoided in patients with seizure disorders and brain tumors and in those who are malnourished. Trazodone is strongly sedating and in low doses (100 mg at bedtime) is helpful in the treatment of the depressed cancer patient with insomnia. Effective antidepressant doses are often 300 mg per day. Trazodone has been associated with priapism and should, therefore, be used with caution in male patients. Maprotiline should be avoided in patients who are at high risk for seizures, as the incidence of seizures can be increased with this medication. Amoxapine has strong dopamine-blocking activity. Hence, patients who are taking other dopamine blockers (e.g., antiemetics) have an increased risk of developing extrapyramidal symptoms and dyskinesias.

When treating depression in the elderly, medications are started at a low dose, and the dosage is increased more slowly than with a younger adult patient. Also, drugs with few anticholinergic effects are preferred due

TABLE 45.10. *Antidepressant Medications Used in Cancer Patients*

Drug	Starting Daily Dosage mg (PO)	Therapeutic Daily Dosage mg (PO)
Newer agents		
Serotonin reuptake inhibitors		
Fluoxetine	10	20–60
Sertraline	25	50–200
Paroxetine	10	10–40
Others		
Amoxapine	25	100–150
Maprotiline	25	75–150
Trazodone	50	150–300
Buproprin	75	200–300
Venlafaxine	18.75	75–225
Tricyclic antidepressants		
Amitriptyline	25	50–150
Doxepin	25	50–200
Imipramine	25	50–200
Desipramine	25	50–150
Nortriptyline	25	25–100
Protriptyline	20	10–30
Psychostimulants		
Dextroamphetamine	2.5 at 8:00 A.M. and noon	5–30
Methylphenidate	2.5 at 8:00 A.M. and noon	5–30
Pemoline	18.75 in morning and noon	37.5–150
Monoamine oxidase inhibitors		
Isocarboxazid	10	20–40
Phenelzine	15	30–60
Tranylcypromine	10	20–40
Lithium carbonate	300	600–1200
Benzodiazepine		
Alprazolam	0.25–1.00	0.75–6.00

PO, orally.

to greater sensitivity of the elderly to anticholinergic complications (e.g., delirium, urinary retention and cardiac arrythmias) (65).

In contrast to the pharmacologic management of adults, there are no clear data to support the efficacy of antidepressants in children (66). Nevertheless, clinicians often find it helpful to prescribe antidepressants to treat specific symptoms associated with depression. When the target symptoms are insomnia, poor appetite or anxiety, a sedative tricyclic antidepressant (e.g., amitriptyline or doxepin) is usually prescribed. When the clinical picture is dominated by lack of energy or motivation, a serotonin reuptake inhibitor or an "energizing" tricyclic, such as desipramine, may be selected. As in the elderly, these drugs are started at a low dose.

TRICYCLIC ANTIDEPRESSANTS (AMITRIPTYLINE, IMIPRAMINE, DOXEPIN, ETC.).
TCAs are still used in the oncology setting for both adults and children with cancer. Dosing is initiated at 10–25 mg at bedtime, especially in debilitated patients, and the dose is increased by 25 mg every 1–2 days until beneficial effect is achieved. For reasons that are unclear, depressed cancer patients often show a therapeutic response to a tricyclic at much lower doses (75–125 mg daily) than are usually required in physically healthy depressed patients (150–300 mg daily). Patients are usually maintained on a TCA for 4–6 months after symptoms improve, after which time the dose is gradually lowered and discontinued (63). The effects on appetite and sleep are frequently immediate; the effects on mood may be delayed. One study observed that one-third of trials of tricyclic antidepressants in medical/surgical inpatients were terminted due to side effects (67). Half of these discontinuations were secondary to delirium.

The choice of TCA depends on the nature of the depressive symptoms, medical problems present, and side effects of the specific drug. The depressed patient who is agitated and has insomnia will benefit from the use of a TCA that has sedating effects, such as amitriptyline or doxepin. Patients with psychomotor slowing will benefit from use of the compounds with the least sedating effects, such as protriptyline or desipramine. The patient who has stomatitis secondary to chemotherapy or radiotherapy, or who has slow intestinal motility or urinary retention, should receive a TCA with the least anticholinergic effects, such as desipramine or nortriptyline.

Patients who are unable to swallow pills may be able to take an antidepressant in an elixir (amitriptyline, nortriptyline or doxepin), or in an intramuscular form (amitriptyline or imipramine). Hospital pharmacies can prepare some TCAs (e.g., amitriptyline) in

rectal suppository form, but absorption by this route has not been studied in cancer patients. Intramuscular administration causes discomfort because of the volume of the vehicle; hence, 50 mg is usually the maximum dosage that can be delivered per intramuscular injection. Parenteral administration of TCAs may be considered for the cancer patient who is unable to tolerate oral administration because of the absence of a swallowing reflex, the presence of gastric or jejunal drainage tubes or intestinal obstruction. Although three TCAs (amitriptyline, imipramine and clomipramine) are available in injectable form, the US Food and Drug Administration has approved imipramine and amitriptyline for oral and muscular administration and clomipramine for oral use only. Formal informed consent and close monitoring of cardiac conduction by electrocardiogram is recommended when these medications are used intravenously. Santos et al. have reviewed the few studies of parenteral TCA use (68) and have observed that therapeutic serum levels are more rapidly attained due to the lack of first-pass metabolism. A dose of imipramine administered intramuscularly yields twice the plasma concentration of the same dose administered orally. Route of administration also affects the pharmacologic action. With oral administration of imipramine, the demethylated metabolite (desipramine), a potent inhibitor of norepinephrine uptake, predominates in the plasma, whereas intramuscular imipramine administration yields a preponderance of imipramine, a serotonergic drug, in the plasma.

Imipramine, doxepin, amitriptyline, desipramine, and nortriptyline are used frequently in the management of neuropathic pain in cancer patients. Dosing is similar to the treatment of depression. Analgesic efficacy, if it occurs, is usually observed at a dose of 50–150 mg daily; higher doses are needed occasionally. While the initial assumption was that analgesic effect resulted indirectly from the effect on depression, it is now clear that these tricyclics have a separate specific analgesic action, which is probably mediated through several neurotransmitters, most prominently norepinephrine and serotonin (69). SSRIs are also being utilized in this regard.

In 1992, Brandes et al. (70) suggested that antidepressant drugs (amitriptyline and fluoxetine) might have a role in tumor promotion at "clinically relevant doses." Disagreements on the implications of this work in a mouse model have emerged. In an editorial, Miller (71) concluded that the evidence for such an association remains "limited." He did not advise at present changing criteria for prescribing these agents in patients with malignancies. However, he calls for additional research in the area.

LITHIUM CARBONATE. Patients who have been receiving lithium carbonate for bipolar affective disorder prior to cancer should be maintained on it throughout cancer treatment, although close monitoring is necessary when the intake of fluids and electrolytes is restricted, such as during the preoperative and postoperative periods. The maintenance dose of lithium may need reduction in seriously ill patients. Lithium should be prescribed with caution in patients receiving cisplatin due to potential nephrotoxicity of both drugs.

Although several authors have reported that the leukocytosis produced by lithium could be beneficial in neutropenic cancer patients (72,73) the functional capabilities of these leukocytes have not been determined. The bone marrow stimulation appears to be transient; no mood changes have been noted in these patients.

MONOAMINE OXIDASE INHIBITORS. If a patient has responded well to a MAOI for depression prior to treatment for cancer, its continued use is warranted. Most psychiatrists, however, are reluctant to start depressed cancer patients on MAOIs because the need for dietary restriction is poorly received by patients who already have dietary limitations and nutritional deficiencies secondary to cancer illness and treatment.

PSYCHOSTIMULANTS. In cancer patients, the psychostimulants (i.e., dextroamphetamine, methylphenidate and pemoline) promote a sense of well-being, decrease fatigue and stimulate appetite (74–76). An advantage of these drugs is a rapid onset of antidepressant action, compared with the TCAs. Psychostimulants can potentiate the analgesic effects of opioid analgesics and are commonly used to counteract opioid-induced sedation. Occasionally they can produce nightmares, insomnia, and even psychosis.

Treatment with dextroamphetamine and methylphenidate is usually initiated at a dose of 2.5 mg at 8:00 A.M. and noon. Pemoline, a chewable and a less-potent psychostimulant, is usually initiated at a dose of 18.75 mg at 8:00 A.M. Typically, patients are maintained on a psychostimulant for 1–2 months, after which time approximately two-thirds will be able to be withdrawn without a recurrence of depressive symptoms (77). Those who develop recurrence of depressive symptoms can be maintained for long periods of time (e.g., up to 1 year). Tolerance may develop, and adjustment of the dose may be necessary. Pemoline should be used with caution in patients with renal impairment; liver function tests should be monitored periodically with longer term treatment (78).

Electroconvulsive Therapy

Occasionally, it is necessary to consider ECT for patients who are depressed and are refractory to antidepressants, and for depressed cancer patients who have depression with psychotic or dangerously suicidal features or significant contraindications to treatment with antidepressant drugs. The safe and effective use of ECT in the medically ill has been reviewed by others (79). Data at present suggest ECT may achieve more favorable responses than pharmacotherapy in the medical setting (80).

SUMMARY

Depression is a common symptom in cancer patients. These symptoms warrant evaluation and the use of pharmacologic, psychological, and social interventions to relieve suffering. Suffering should not be regarded as an "unavoidable" consequence of cancer.

REFERENCES

1. Massie MJ, Gagnon P, Holland JC. Depression and suicide in patients with cancer. *J Pain Symptom Manage.* 1994; 9:325–340.
2. Massie MJ, Holland JC. Overview of normal reactions and prevalence of psychiatric disorders. In: Holland JC, Rowland JH, eds. *Handbook of Psychooncology: Psychological Care of the Patient with Cancer.* New York: Oxford University Press; 1989:273–282.
3. Hamburg D, Hamburg B, de Goza S. Adaptive problems and mechanisms in severely burned patients. *Psychiatry.* 1953; 16:1–20.
4. Horowitz M. *Stress response syndromes.* New York: Janson Aronson; 1976.
5. Lifton RJ. *Death in Life: Survivors of Hiroshima.* New York: Random House; 1967.
6. Lindemann L. Symptomatology and management of acute grief. *Am J Psychiatry.* 1944; 101:141–148.
7. American Psychiatric Association. *Diagnostic and Statistical Manual of Mental Disorders.* 4th ed. Washington, DC: American Psychiatric Association; 1994.
8. Massie MJ, Holland JC, Straker N. Psychotherapeutic interventions. In: Holland JC, Rowland JH, eds. *Handbook of Psychooncology: Psychological Care of the Patient with Cancer.* New York: Oxford University Press; 1989: 455–469.
9. American Psychiatric Association. *Diagnostic and Statistical Manual of Mental Disorders.* 3rd ed. Washington, DC: American Psychiatric Association; 1980.
10. Derogatis LR, Morrow GR, Fetting J. The prevalence of psychiatric disorders among cancer patients. *JAMA* 1983; 249:751–757.

11. Spiegel D, Saud S, Koopman C. Pain and depression in patients with cancer. *Cancer*. 1994; 74:2570–2578.

12. American Pain Society. Principles of analgesic use in the treatment of acute pain and cancer pain. *Clin Pharm*. 1990; 9:601–611.

13. Cohen-Cole SA, Brown FW, McDaniel JS. Assessment of depression and grief reactions in the medically ill. In: Stoudemire A, Fogel BS, eds. *Psychiatric Care of the Medical patient*. New York: Oxford University Press; 1993: 53–69.

14. Spitzer RL, Endicott J, Robins E. Research diagnostic criteria. *Arch Gen Psychiatry*. 1978; 35:773–782.

15. Robins LN, Helzer JE, Croughan J. National Institute of Mental Health Diagnostic Interview Schedule. *Arch Gen Psychiatry*. 1981; 38:381–389.

16. Endicott J. Measurement of depression in patients with cancer. *Cancer*. 1984; 53:2243–2249.

17. Kathol R, Mutgi A, Williams J, et al. Diagnosis of major depression according to four sets of criteria. *Am J Psychiatry*. 1990; 147:1021–1024.

18. American Psychiatric Association. *Diagnostic and Statistical Manual of Mental Disorders*. 3rd ed, rev. Washington, DC: American Psychiatric Association; 1987.

19. Bukberg J, Penman D, Holland JC. Depression in hospitalized cancer patients. *Psychosom Med*. 1984; 46:199–212.

20. Plumb M, Holland JC. Comparative studies of psychological function in patients with advanced cancer. 1. Self-reported depressive symptoms. *Psychosom Med*. 1977; 39:264–276.

21. McDaniel JS, Nemeroff CB. Depression in the cancer patient. Diagnostic, biological, and treatment aspects. In: Chapman CR, Foley KM eds. *Current and Emerging Issues in Cancer Pain: Research and Practice*. New York: Raven Press; 1993: 1–19.

22. Joffe RT, Rubinow DR, Denicoff KD, et al. Depression and carcinoma of the pancreas. *Gen Hosp Psychiatry*. 1986; 8:241–245.

23. Evans DL, McCartney CF, Nemeroff CB, et al. Depression in women treated for gynecological cancer: clinical and neuroendocrine assessment. *Am J Psychiatry*. 1986; 143:447–451.

24. Grandi S, Fava GA, Cunsolo A, et al. Major depression associated with mastectomy. *Med Sci Res*. 1987; 15:283–284.

25. Popkin MK, Tucker GJ. Mental disorders due to a general medical condition and substance-induced disorders; mood anxiety, psychotic, and personality disorders. *DSM-IV Sourcebook*. Washington, DC: APA Office of Research; 1994: 243–276.

26. Schwab JJ, Bialow M, Brown JM, Holzer CE. Diagnosing depression in medical inpatients. *Ann Intern Med*. 1967; 67:695–707.

27. Stewart JA, Drake F, Winokur G. Depression among medically ill patients. *Dis Nerv Syst*. 1965; 26:479–485.

28. Moffic HS, Paykel ES. Depression in medical inpatients. *Br J Psychiatry*. 1975; 126:346–353.

29. Wallen J, Pincus HA, Goldman HH, Marcus SE. Psychiatric consultations in short term general hospitals. *Arch Gen Psychiatry*. 1987; 44:163–168.

30. Wells KB, Golding JM, Burham MA. Psychiatric disorder in a sample of the general population with and without chronic medical conditions. *Am J Psychiatry*. 1988; 145:976–981.

31. Starkstein SE, Robinson RG. Depression and Parkinson's disease in aging and clinical practice. In: Robinson RG, Rabins PV, eds. *Depression and Co-existing Disease*. New York: Igaku-Shoin; 1989: 213–225.

32. Robinson RG, Starkstein SE. Current research in affective disorders following stroke. *J Neuropsychiatr Clin Neurosci*. 1990; 2:1–14.

33. Hinton JM. The psychiatry of terminal illness in adults and children. *Proc R Soc Med*. 1972; 65:1035–1040.

34. Levine PM, Silberfarb PM, Lipowski ZJ. Mental disorders in cancer patients. *Cancer*. 1978; 42:1385–1391.

35. Massie MJ, Gorzynski JG, Mastrovito R, et al. The diagnosis of depression in hospitalized patients with cancer. [abstract.] *Proc Am Soc Clin Oncol*. 1979; 20:432.

36. Massie MJ, Holland JC. Consultation and liaison issues in cancer care. *Psychiatr Med*. 1987; 5:343–359.

37. Razavi D, Delvaux N, Farvacques C, Robaye E. Screening for adjustment disorders and major depressive disorders in cancer in-patients. *Br J Psychiatry*. 1990; 156:79–83.

38. DeFlorio M, Massie MJ. Review of depression in cancer: gender differences. *Depression*. 1995; 3:66–80.

39. Craig TJ, Abeloff MD. Psychiatric symptomatology among hospitalized cancer patients. *Am J Psychiatry*. 1974; 131:1323–1327.

40. Breitbart W. Suicide in cancer patients. *Oncology*. 1987; 1:49–53.

41. American Psychiatric Association. Practice guideline for major depressive disorders in adults. *Am J Psychiatry* 1993; 150:4.

42. Depression Guideline Panel. *Depression in Primary Care*: vol. 2. *Treatment of Major Depression*. AHCPR Publ. 93-0551. Rockville, MD: US Department of Health and Human Services, Public Health Service, Agency for Health Care Policy and Research, 1993.

43. Massie MJ. Depression. In: Holland JC, Rowland JH, eds. *Handbook of Psychooncology: Psychological Care of the Patient with Cancer*. New York: Oxford University Press; 1989:283–290.

44. Green AI, Austin PC. Psychopathology of pancreatic cancer: a psychobiologic probe. *Psychosomatics*. 1993; 34:208–221.

45. Medical Letter. Drugs that cause psychiatric symptoms. *Med Lett*. 1993; 35:65–70.

46. Medical Letter. Drugs of choice for cancer chemotherapy. *Med Lett*. 1993; 35:43–50.

47. Jones S, Cathcart C, Pumroy S. Frequency, severity and management of tamoxifen-induced depression in women with node-negative breast cancer. *Proc Am Soc Clin Oncol*. 1993; 12:78.

48. Folstein MF, Folstein S, McHugh PR. Minimental state: a practical method for grading the cognitive state of patients for the clinician. *J Psychiatr Res*. 1975; 12:189–198.

49. Oliver AP, Luckins DJ, Wyett RJ. Neuroleptic induced seizures. *Arch Gen Psychiatry*. 1982; 39:206–209.

50. Magni G. Assessments of depression in an elderly medical population. *J Affect Dis*. 1986; 11:121.

51. Breitbart W. Suicide in cancer patients. In: Holland JC, Rowland JH, eds. *Handbook of Psychooncology:*

Psychological Care of the Patient with Cancer. New York: Oxford University Press; 1989:291–299.

52. MacKenzie TB, Popkin MK. Medical illness and suicide. In: Blumenthas S, Kupfer D, eds. *Suicide Over the Life Cycle, Understanding Risk Factors, Assessment and Treatment of Suicide Patients.* Washington, DC: APA Press; 1990:205–232.

53. Conwell Y, Caine ED, Else K. Suicide and cancer in late life. *Hosp Commun Psychiatry.* 1990; 41:1334–1339.

54. Fox BH, Stanek EJ, Boyd SC, Flannery JT. Suicide rates among women patients in Connecticut. *J Chron Dis.* 1982; 35:85–100.

55. Louhivuori KA, Hakama M. Risk of suicide among cancer patients. *Am J Epidemiol.* 1979; 109:59.

56. Kovacs M, Beck AT, Weissman A. Hopelessness: an indication of suicide risks. *Suicide.* 1975; 5:98–103.

57. Worden JW, Weisman AD. Preventive psychosocial intervention with newly diagnosed cancer patients. *Gen Hosp Psychiatry.* 1984; 6:243–249.

58. Levenson H, Hales RE. Brief psychodynamically informed therapy for medically ill patients. In: Stoudemire A, Fogel BS, eds. Medical psychiatric practice, vol 2. Washington, DC: American Psychiatric Press; 1993:3–37.

59. Beck A, Rush AJ. Cognitive approaches to depression and suicide. In: Serban G, ed. *Cognitive Defects in the Development of Mental Ilness.* New York: Brunner/Mazel; 1978:235.

60. Rifkin A, Reardon G, Siris S, et al. Trimipramine in physical illness with depression. *J Clin Psychiatry.* 1985; 46:4–8.

61. Purohit DR, Navlakha PL, Modi RS, Eshpumiyani R. The role of antidepressants in hospitalized cancer patients. *J Assoc Phys India.* 1978; 26:245–248.

62. Costa D, Mogos I, Toma T. Efficacy and safety of mianserin in the treatment of depression of women with cancer. *Acta Psychiatr Scand.* 1985; 72:85–92.

63. Massie MJ, Lesko L. Psychopharmacological management. In: Holland JC, Rowland JH, eds. *Handbook of Psychooncology: Psychological Care of the Patient with Cancer.* New York: Oxford University Press; 1989: 470–491.

64. Vishwanath BM, Navalgund AA, Cusano W, Navalgund KA. Fluoxetine as a cause if SIADH. *Am J Psychiatry.* 1991; 148:542–543.

65. Salzman C. Practical considerations on the pharmacological treatment of depression and anxiety in the elderly. *J. Clin Psychiatry.* 1990; 51:40–43.

66. Ambrosini PJ, Bianchi MD, Rabinovich HD, Elia J. Antidepressant treatments in children and adolescents: affective disorders. *J Am Acad Child Adolesc Psychiatry.* 1993; 32:1.

67. Popkin MK, Callies AL, MacKenzie TB. The outcome of antidepressant use in the medically ill. *Arch Gen Psychiatry.* 1985; 42:1160–1163.

68. Santos AB, Beliles KE, Arana GW. Parental use of psychotropic agents. In: Stoudemire A, Fogel BS, eds. *Medical Psychiatric Practice*, vol. 2. Washington, DC: American Psychiatric Press; 1993: 113–137.

69. France RD. The future for antidepressants: treatment of pain. *Psychopathology.* 1987; 20:99–113.

70. Brandes LJ, Arron RJ, Boganovic RP. Stimulation of malignant growth in rodents by antidepressant drugs at clinically relevant doses. *Cancer Res.* 1992; 52:3796–3800.

71. Miller LG. Psychopharmacologic agents and cancer; a progress report [editorial]. *J Clin Psychopharmacol.* 1995; 15:160–161.

72. Cantane RL, Kaufman J, Mittelman A, Murphy GP. Attenuation of myelosuppression with lithium. *N Engl J Med.* 1977; 297:452–453.

73. Lyman GH, Williams CC, Preston D. The use of lithium carbonate to reduce infection and leukopenia during systemic chemotherapy. *N Engl J Med.* 1980; 302: 257–260.

74. Woods SW, Tesar GE, Murray GB, Cassem NH. Psychostimulant treatment of depressive disorders secondary to medical illness. *J Clin Psychiatry.* 1986; 47:12–15.

75. Fernandez F, Adams F, Holmes VF, *et al.* Methylphenidate for depressive disorders in cancer patients. *Psychosomatics.* 1987; 28:455–461.

76. Bruera E. Use of methylphenidate as an adjuvant to narcotic analgesics in patients with advanced cancer. *J Pain Symptom Manage.* 1989; 1:3–6.

77. Chiarello RJ, Cole JO. The use of psychostimulants in general psychiatry: a reconsideration. *Arch Gen Psychiatry.* 1987; 44:286–295.

78. Breitbart W, Mermelstein H. Pemoline, an alternative psychostimulant for the management of depressive disorders in cancer patients. *Psychosomatics.* 1992; 33:352–356.

79. Weiner RD, Caffey CE. Electroconvulsive therapy in the medical and neurologic patient. In: Stoudemire A, Fogel BS, eds. *Psychiatric Care of the Medical Patient.* New York: Oxford University Press; 1993:207–224.

80. Popkin MK. Syndromes of brain dysfunction. In: Clayton T, Winokeu G, eds. *Medical Basis of Psychiatry.* New York: WB Saunders; 1994:17–37.

81. Popkin MK, Tucker GJ. "Secondary" and drug-induced mood, anxiety, psychotic, catatonic, and personality disorders: a review of the literature. *J Neuropsychiatr Clin Neurosci.* 1992; 4:369–385.

82. Koenig R, Levin S, Brennan MJ. The emotional status of cancer patients as measured by a psychological test. *J Chron Dis.* 1967; 20:923–930.

83. Fras I, Litin EM, Pearson JS. Comparison of psychiatric symptoms in carcinoma of the pancreas with those in some other intra-abdominal neoplasms. *Am J Psychiatry.* 1967; 123:1553–1562.

84. Peck A, Boland L. Emotional reactions to having cancer. *Am J Roentgenol Rad Ther Nucl Med.* 1972; 114:591–599.

85. Morris T, Greer HS, White P. Psychological and social adjustment to mastectomy. *Cancer.* 1977; 40:2381.

86. Maguire GP, Lee E, Bevington D, et al. Psychiatric problems in the first year after mastectomy. *Br Med J.* 1978; 1:963–965.

87. Silberfarb PM, Maurer LH, Crouthamel CS. Psychological aspects of neoplastic disease: I. Functional status of breast cancer patients during different treatment regimens. *Am J Psychiatry.* 1980; 137:450–455.

88. Krouse HJ, Krouse JH. Pschological factors in post-mastectomy adjustment. *Psychol Rep.* 1981; 48:275–278.

89. Farber JM, Weinerman BH, Kuypers JA. Psychosocial distress in oncology outpatients. *J Psychosoc Oncol.* 1984; 2:109–118.

90. Morton RP, Davies ADM, Baker J, et al. Quality of life in treated head and neck cancer patients: a preliminary report. *Clin Otolaryngol.* 1984; 9:181–185.

91. Lloyd GG, Parker AC, Ludlam CA, McGuire RJ. Emotional impact of diagnosis and early treatment of lymphomas. *J Psychosom Res.* 1984; 28:157–162.

92. Hughes JE. Depressive illness and lung cancer. I. Depression before diagnosis. *Eur J Surg Oncol.* 1985; 11:15–20.

93. Robinson JK, Boshier ML, Dansak DA. Depression and anxiety in cancer patients: evidence for different causes. *J Psychosom Res.* 1985; 29:133–138.

94. Starkman M, Zelnik T, Nesse R. Anxiety in patients with pheochromocytomas. *Arch Intern Med.* 1985; 145:248–252.

95. Lansky SB, List MA, Herrmann CA, et al. Absence of major depressive disorder in female cancer patients. *J Clin Oncol.* 1985; 3:1553–1560.

96. Davies ADM, Davies C, Delpo MC. Depression and anxiety in patients undergoing diagnostic investigations for head and neck cancers. *Br J Psychiatry.* 1986; 149:491–493.

97. Holland J, Hughes A, Korzan AH, et al. Comparative psychological disturbance in patients with pancreatic and gastric cancer. *Am J Psychiatry.* 1986; 143:982–986.

98. Devlen J, Maguire P, Phillips et al. Psychological problems associated with diagnosis and treatment of lymphomas. I: Retrospective study. *Br Med J.* 1987; 295:953–954.

99. Develn J, Maguire P, Phillips P, Crowther D. Psychological problems associated with diagnosis and treatment of lymphoma. II: Prospective study. *Br Med J.* 1987; 295:955–957.

100. Friedrich WN, Smith CK, Harrison SD, et al. MMPI study of identical twins: cancer patients and bone marrow donors. *Psychol Rep.* 1987; 61:127–130.

101. Stefanek ME, Derogatis LP, Shaw A. Psychological distress among oncology outpatients. *Psychosomatics.* 1987; 28:530–539.

102. Pettingale KW, Burgess C, Greer S. Psychological response to cancer diagnosis-I. Correlations with prognostic variables. *J Psychosom Res.* 1987; 23:255–261.

103. Grassi L, Rosti G, Albieri G, Marangolo M. Depression and abnormal illness behavior in cancer patients. *Gen Hosp Psychiatry.* 1989; 11:404–411.

104. Hardman A, Maguire P, Crowther D. The recognition of psychiatric morbidity on a medical oncology ward. *J Psychosom Res.* 1989; 33:235–239.

105. Meyer L, Aspergren K. Long-term psychological sequelae of mastectomy and breast conserving treatment for breast cancer. *Acta Oncol.* 189; 28:13–18.

106. Fallowfield LJ, Hall A, Maguire GP, Baum M. Psychological outcomes of different treatment policies in women with early breast cancer outside of a clinical trial. *Br Med J.* 1990; 301:575–580.

107. Jenkins PL, May VE, Hughes LE. Psychological morbidity associated with local recurrence of breast cancer. *Int J Psychiatr Med.* 1991; 21:149–155.

108. Golden RN, McCartney CF, Haggerty JJ, et al. The detection of depression by patient self-report in women with gynecologic cancer. *Int J Psychiatry Med.* 1991; 21:17–27.

109. Colon EA, Callies AL, Popkin MK, McGlave PB. Depressed mood and other variables related to bone marrow transplantation survival in acute leukemia. *Psychosomatics.* 1991; 32:420–425.

110. Hopwood P, Howell A, Maguire P. Screening for psychiatric morbidity in patients with advanced breast cancer: validation of two self-report questionnaires. *Br J Cancer.* 1991; 64:353–356.

111. Hopwood P, Howell A, Maguire P. Psychiatric morbidity in patients with advanced cancer of the breast; prevalence measured to two self-rating questionnaires. *Br J Cancer.* 1991; 64:349–352.

112. Baile WF, Gilbertini M, Scott L, Endicott J. Depression and tumor state in cancer of the head and neck. *Psycho-Oncology.* 1992; 1:15–24.

113. Goldberg JA, Scott RN, Davidson PM. Psychological morbidity in the first year after breast surgery. *Eur J Surg Oncol.* 1992; 18:327–331.

114. Maraste R, Brandt L, Olsson H, Ryde-Brandt B. Anxiety and depression in breast cancer patients at start of adjuvant radiotherapy. *Acta Oncol.* 1992; 31:641–643.

115. Sneed NV, Edlund B, Dias JK. Adjustment of gynecological and breast cancer patients to the cancer diagnosis: comparisons with males and females having other cancer sites. *Health Care Women Int.* 1992; 13:11–22.

116. Cathcart CK, Jones SE, Pumroy CS, et al. Clinical recognition and management of depression in node negative breast cancer patients treated with tamoxifen. *Breast Cancer Res Treat.* 1993; 27:277–281.

117. Alexander PJ, Dinesh N, Vidyasagar MS. Psychiatric morbidity among cancer patients and its relationship with awareness of illness and expectations about treatment outcome. *Acta Oncol.* 1993; 32:623–626.

118. Pinder KL, Ramirez AJ, Black ME. Psychiatric disorder in patients with advanced breast cancer: prevalence and associated factors. *Eur J Cancer.* 1993; 29A:524–527.

119. Sneeuw KCA, Aaronson NK, van Wouwe MCC, et al. Prevalence and screening of psychiatric disorder in patients with early stage breast cancer [abstract]. [Presented at the International Congress of Psychosocial Oncology, 12–14 October 1992, Beaune, France.] *Qual Life Res.* 1993; 2:50–51.

120. Rapaport Y, Kreitler S, Chaitchik S, et al. Psychosocial problems in head-and-neck cancer patients and their change with time since diagnosis. *Ann Oncol.* 1993; 4:69–73.

46

Suicide

WILLIAM BREITBART AND SUZANNE KRIVO

The health care professional in the oncology setting faces a dilemma when confronting the issue of suicide in the cancer patient. From the medical perspective, professional training reinforces the view of suicidal ideation as a symptom of psychiatric disturbance. However, from a philosophical perspective, many in our society view suicide in those who face the distress of a fatal illness as "rational" and a means to regain control and maintain a dignified death (1–3). An internal debate thus often takes place in the cancer care professional that is not dissimilar from the public debate that surrounds celebrated legal cases in which the right to die is at issue (4,5). Information that can shed light on our understanding of the factors that contribute to suicidal ideation, requests for hastened death, or suicide in cancer patients will contribute greatly not only to the societal debate over these issues, but directly to humane patient care. What follows is a review of the current research data on suicide, suicidal ideation, and suicide risk factors in cancer patients, with particular focus on the roles of pain and psychiatric comorbidity.

The information presented in this chapter suggests that danger lies in the premature assumption that suicidal ideation or a request to hasten death in a cancer patient represents a "rational act," unencumbered by physical symptom distress or psychiatric comorbidity. Clearly there are suicides that occur in this population that many would view as rational expressions of personal autonomy; however, they represent only a small minority of suicides in cancer patients. The vast majority of cancer patients, particularly those with advanced disease, who express suicidal ideation or request a hastened death do so while suffering with unrecognized and untreated psychiatric disturbances (depression, confusional states), and poorly controlled physical symptoms (pain).

INCIDENCE

Studies show that, while relatively few cancer patients commit suicide (Table 46.1), the risk of suicide in cancer patients is twice that of the general population (6–14). The frequency of passive suicide and the degree to which noncompliance and treatment refusal represents a deliberate decision to end life is unknown, suggesting that the true incidence of suicide in cancer patients is underestimated. It has been our experience in working with cancer patients that, once a trusting and safe relationship develops, patients almost universally reveal that they have had occasional persistent thoughts of suicide as a means of escaping the threat of being overwhelmed by cancer. Suicidal ideation is discussed in more detail later in this chapter.

DEMOGRAPHICS

Men with cancer are clearly at an increased risk of suicide relative to the general population, with a relative risk as high as 2.3 times that of the general population (7,8,12,15). Studies indicate mixed results as far as women's risk of suicide in the cancer setting (7,8,12,15). In a group of 60 cancer suicides the male to female ratio was 4.5, compared to 3.4 for all suicides (16). In adolescent populations, cancer was associated with substantive suicidal ideation in females but not in males. Yet, females did not seek mental health services more often than males. This suggests that in adolescents, females with cancer are more at risk of suicide than their male counterparts (17). Several studies have concluded that older patients with cancer, in the sixth and seventh decades of life, are particularly vulnerable to suicide (7,8,12,16). Studies in Scandinavia show that suicide in men with cancer peaked at around age 70 years (7,8,12). In a recent study, the mean age of cancer suicides was 63 years compared to 45 years in a sex-matched noncancer suicide population (16). The same

TABLE 46.1. *Studies on Incidence of Suicide Among Cancer Patients*

Studies	Reference	Total Suicides	Total Cancer Deaths	Relative Risk	
				Men	Women
Finland	Louhivuori and Hakama (12)	63	28,857	1.3	1.9
United States	Fox et al. (15)	192	144,530	2.3	0.9
Sweden	Bolund (7,8)	22	19,000		

study also found that marital status did not differ between cancer and noncancer suicides, suggesting that marital status is no more a vulnerability variable in cancer suicide than in noncancer suicide (16).

SITE OF CANCER

Individuals with oral, pharyngeal, and lung cancers are at an increased risk of suicide compared to those with cancer of different types (Table 46.2). Cancer of these sites is often associated with heavy and prolonged use of alcohol and tobacco, and has profound impact due to facial disfigurement and impaired function (18). Gastrointestinal, urogenital, and breast cancers have been reported to increase the risk of suicide as well (7,8,12,19). There has long been speculation on the existence of a linkage between physiologic dysfunction of the pancreas and the generation of depressive and suicidal states (20). Numerous reports demonstrate mood changes in patients with pancreatic cancer who did not have knowledge of their diagnosis (9). In light of these reports, abnormalities of adrenocorticotrophic

hormone, parathyroid hormone, thyrotropin-releasing hormone, glucagon, serotonin, and insulin have been thought to cause depression in these patients (21).

CANCER SUICIDE AND VULNERABILITY VARIABLES

Identifying the cancer patient at risk for suicide is the first step in prevention and allows for appropriate psychosocial interventions to be initiated. Factors associated with increased risk of suicide in patients with cancer are listed in Table 46.3. These characteristics should be incorporated into the assessment of suicide potential in cancer patients and utilized as a framework for intervention in order to provide alternatives to suicide.

ADVANCED ILLNESS AND POOR PROGNOSIS

Cancer patients commit suicide most frequently in the advanced stages of disease (6–8,12,15,18). Eighty-six percent of suicides studies by Farberow et. al. occurred in the preterminal or terminal stages of illness, despite greatly reduced physical capacity (22). In a Finnish study of 60 cancer suicides, Hietanen et al. found that, for 62% of patients with cancer (of any stage) who committed suicide, cancer was the fundamental reason for the suicide, yet for 100% of those who committed suicide in the advanced stages of the

TABLE 46.2. *Sites of Cancer Associated with Suicide*

Studies	Primary Sites
UNITED STATES	
Weisman (46)	Oral, urogenital
Farberow et al. (22)	Tongue, larynx, lung
Farberow et al. (18)	Lymphoma, leukemia (<45 years)
Breitbart (27)	Lung, bronchus, trachea, intestine (45–65 years), pharynx, larynx (>65 years)
SCANDINAVIA	
Finland	
Louhivuori and Hakama (12)	Gastrointestinal, urogenital, breast
Hientanen et al. (16)	Gastrointestinal tract, head and neck
Norway	
Olafssen (47)	Breast, prostate
Sweden	
Bolund (7,8)	Oral, pharyngeal, stomach, renal (men), ovarian, breast (women), gastrointestinal (men and women)

TABLE 46.3. *Cancer Suicide Vulnerability Variables*

Advanced illness and poor prognosis
Depression and hopelessness
Delirium
Control and helplessness
Exhaustion and fatigue
Pain
Preexisting psychopathology
Prior suicide history, personal or family

disease, cancer was the fundamental reason for the suicide (16).

Poor prognosis and advanced illness usually coincide, so it is not surprising that, in Sweden, those who were expected to die within a matter of months were the most likely to commit suicide. Of 88 cancer suicides, 14 had uncertain prognoses, and 45 had poor prognoses (7,8). Patients with advanced illness are most likely to have cancer complications such as pain, depression, delirium, and deficit symptoms. These complications help to explain the high risk of suicide at this late stage.

DEPRESSION AND HOPELESSNESS

Depression is a factor in 50% of suicides, with or without terminal illness. People suffering from depression are at 25 times greater risk of suicide than the general population (23,24). The role depression plays in cancer suicide is equally significant. Approximately 25% of all cancer patients experience severe depressive symptoms (23–26), with about 6% fulfilling DSM-IV criteria for the diagnosis of major depression (24–26). Among those with advanced illness and progressively impaired physical function, symptoms of severe depression rise to 77% (25). At Memorial Sloan-Kettering Cancer Center, 31% of patients consulted by the psychiatry service had major depression and half of the patients had adjustment disorder with depressed mood (27).

Hopelessness is the key variable that links depression and suicide in the general population. Hopelessness is a significantly better predictor of completed suicide than is depression alone (28,29). With the typical cancer suicide being characterized by advanced illness and poor prognosis, hopelessness is an all too common experience (6). In Scandinavia, the highest incidence of suicide was found in cancer patients who were offered no further treatment and no further contact with the health care system (7,8,12). Being left to face illness alone creates a sense of isolation and abandonment that is critical to the development of hopelessness.

DELIRIUM

The prevalence of organic mental disorders, primarily delirium, among cancer patients requiring psychiatric consultation has been found to range from 25% to 40% (30,31), and as high as 85% during the terminal stages of illness (32). While earlier work (18) suggested that delirium was a protective factor with regard to cancer suicide, our clinical experience has found these confusional states to be a major contributing factor in impulsive suicide attempts, especially in the hospital setting.

CONTROL AND HELPLESSNESS

Loss of control and a sense of helplessness in the face of cancer are important factors in suicide vulnerability. Control refers to both the helplessness induced by symptoms or deficits due to cancer or its treatments, as well as the excessive need on the part of some patients to be in control of all aspects of living or dying. Farberow et al. noted that patients who were accepting and adaptable were much less likely to commit suicide than cancer patients who exhibited a need to be in control of even the most minute details of their care (18). This controlling trait may be prominent in some patients and cause distress with little provocation. However, it is not uncommon for cancer-related events to induce a great sense of helplessness even in those who are not typically controlling individuals. Impairments or deficits induced by cancer or cancer treatments include loss of mobility, paraplegia, loss of bowel and bladder function, amputation, aphonia, sensory loss, and inability to eat or swallow. Most distressing to patients is the sense that they are losing control of their minds, especially when they are confused or sedated by medications. The risk of suicide is increased in cancer patients with such physical impairments, particularly when accompanied by psychological distress and disturbed interpersonal relationships due to these deficit factors (16,18).

FATIGUE

Fatigue, in the form of exhaustion of physical, emotional, spiritual, financial, familial, communal, and other resources, increases risk of suicide in the cancer patient (27,33). Cancer is now often a chronic illness. Increased survival is accompanied by increased numbers of hospitalizations, complications, and expenses. Symptom control thus becomes a prolonged process with frequent advances and setbacks. Also, the dying process can become extremely long and arduous for all concerned. It is not uncommon for both family members and health care providers to withdraw prematurely from the cancer patient under these circumstances. A suicidal patient can thus feel even more isolated and abandoned. The presence of a strong support system for the patient which may act as an external control of suicidal behavior reduces the risk of cancer suicide significantly.

PAIN

Uncontrolled pain is a major risk factor for suicide and suicidal ideation in cancer patients (7,8,18,27,33). Pain is a leading cause of morbidity in the cancer patient. Fifteen percent of patients with nonmetastatic cancer have significant pain, whereas 60%–90% of patients with advanced cancer report debilitating pain, and up to 25% of all patients with cancer die in pain (34–36). The public perceives cancer as an extremely painful disease relative to other medical conditions. Sixty-nine percent indicated in a public opinion survey that cancer pain can get so bad that a person might consider suicide (37). Physicians who work with cancer patients report that persistent or uncontrolled pain accounts for the majority of requests they receive for physician-assisted suicide or euthanasia. The vast majority of cancer suicides, in several studies, occur in patients with severe pain that was inadequately controlled or poorly tolerated (16,18). Pain plays an important role in vulnerability to suicide; however, associated psychological distress and mood disturbance seem to be essential cofactors in raising the risk of cancer suicide. Cancer patients with pain are twice as likely to suffer from a psychiatric complication (anxiety or depressive disorder) as those without pain (38). Pain has adverse effects on a cancer patient's quality of life and sense of control. Pain interferes with a patient's ability to receive support from family and others. Cancer patients with advanced cancer and pain are especially vulnerable to suicide due to the increased likelihood of the presence of multiple risk factors such as depression, delirium, loss of control, and hopelessness.

The role of cancer pain in suicidal ideation is complex. There is evidence to suggest that it is not merely the extent or degree of pain that plays a role in cancer related suicidal ideation, but rather the suffering experienced as part of one's psychological reactions to cancer pain, such as depression and hopelessness. Studies at Memorial Sloan-Kettering Cancer Center examined the relationship of cancer pain to suicidal ideation (27,33). In a series of 71 cancer patients who had suicidal ideation with serious intent, significant pain was a factor in only 30% of cases. In striking contrast, virtually all 71 suicidal cancer patients had a psychiatric disorder (mood disturbance or organic mental disorder) at the time of evaluation (27). In a second study, we examined 196 cancer pain patients involved in ongoing research protocols of the Memorial Sloan-Kettering Cancer Center Pain and Psychiatry Service (33). Suicidal ideation occurred in 17% of the study population, with the majority reporting suicidal ideation without intent to act. Interestingly, in this population of cancer patients who all had significant pain (Visual Analog Scale Pain Intensity mean score of 5.4), suicidal ideation was not directly related to pain intensity, but rather was strongly related to the degree of depression and mood disturbance (as measured by the Beck Depression Inventory and the Memorial Pain Assessment Card–Visual Analog Scale Mood Scale). Duration of pain also did not predict suicidal ideation. Pain was related to suicidal ideation indirectly in that patients' perception of poor pain relief was associated with suicidal ideation. Perceptions of pain relief may have more to do with aspects of hopelessness than pain itself.

PREEXISTING PSYCHOPATHOLOGY

Holland (39) advises that it is extremely rare for cancer patients to commit suicide without some degree of premorbid psychopathology that places them at increased risk. Farberow et al. (18) described a large group of cancer suicides as the "dependent dissatisfied." These patients were immature, demanding, complaining, irritable, hostile, and difficult ward management problems. Staff often felt manipulated by these patients and became irritated by what they saw as excessive demands for attention. Suicide attempts or threats were often seen as "hysterical" or manipulative. Our consultation data on suicidal cancer patients showed that half had a diagnosable personality disorder (27,33).

PRIOR SUICIDE HISTORY AND FAMILY HISTORY

The frequency of suicide attempts in cancer patients has not been well studied. While the frequency of suicidal thinking in the cancer setting may be in question, its relationship to suicide attempts or completions is clearer. Bolund (7,8) reports that fully half of all Swedish cancer suicides had previously conveyed suicidal thoughts or plans to their relatives. In addition, many of the completed cancer suicides had been preceded by an attempted suicide. This is consistent with the statistics of suicide in general, which show that a previous suicide attempt greatly increases the risk of completed suicide (40,41). A family history of suicide is of increasing relevance in assessing suicide risk.

SUICIDAL IDEATION

Thoughts of suicide occur frequently in the setting of advanced cancer These thoughts serve to act as a steam valve for feelings, often expressed by patients as "If it gets too bad, I always have a way out." It has been our experience in working with cancer patients that, once a trusting and safe relationship develops, patients almost universally reveal that they have had occasionally persistent thoughts of suicide as a means of escaping the threat of being overwhelmed by cancer. Recent published reports, however, suggest that suicidal ideation is relatively infrequent in cancer, and is limited to those with more advanced disease, those who are hospitalized or in palliative care settings, or those who have pain or are significantly depressed (see Table 46.4). Any discrepancy between clinical impression and research conclusions may be due to the limitations of the research interview in eliciting report of suicidal ideation. Silberfarb et al. (42) found that only three of 146 breast cancer patients with local disease receiving ambulatory care reported suicidal thoughts to a research interviewer, while none of the 100 cancer patients interviewed in a Finnish study expressed suicidal thoughts (19). At Memorial Hospital, suicide risk evaluation accounted for 8.6% of psychiatric consultations in 1986, usually requested by staff in response to a patient verbalizing suicidal wishes (27,33). Three-quarters of those evaluated for suicide wishes ($n = 71$) in fact were found to be actively suicidal, requiring that steps be taken to assure their safety. The vast majority of those hospitalized cancer patients with suicidal ideation had serious psychiatric disorders that had not been recognized or treated. One-half of the group had an adjustment disorder, 30% had a major depression, and approximately 20% had a delirium at the time of their psychiatric evaluation. With appropriate psychiatric interventions, suicidal ideation disappeared or diminished significantly in this group of patients. Pasacreta and Massie (43) distributed a psychosocial survey to the entire nursing staff at Memorial Hospital in October 1987. Nurses were asked a number of questions including "Has your patient expressed suicidal ideas or wishes to you in the past week?" Eleven percent of the 550 hospitalized cancer patients at Memorial Hospital had expressed suicidal ideation to their nurse. We recently studied 196 cancer patients with pain at Memorial Hospital and found that suicidal ideation occurred in 17% of the study population (33). A study conducted in the Palliative Care Unit at St Boniface Hospice in Winnipeg, Canada, demonstrated that ten of 44 terminally ill cancer patients were suicidal or desired an early death, and that all ten were suffering from clinical depression (44).

THE AFTERMATH OF SUICIDE: IMPACT ON FAMILY AND HEALTH CARE PROVIDERS

When suicide complicates bereavement, the loss can be especially difficult for the survivors left behind. When cancer has played a role in suicide, the loss is often difficult and elicits complex emotions. The intensity and nature of the survivors' reactions will depend on such variables as the age and physical condition of the deceased, the nature of the suicide, the relationship with the deceased, and the survivor's individual personality and cultural background. A pattern of reactions that include feelings of rejection, abandonment, anger, relief, guilt, responsibility, denial, identification, and shame is often seen in those left behind. Assisting survivors of suicide through the bereavement period is often necessary and rewarding. Mutual support groups have been developed to reduce isolation, provide opportunities for ventilating feelings, and find ways to deal with the aftermath of suicide.

Reactions to the suicide of a cancer patient in the staff are similar to those seen in family members, especially feelings of responsibility, guilt, shame, relief, and questioning of professional judgment. It is helpful for the team that cared for a patient who committed suicide to review the case by carrying out a psychological autopsy, in an attempt to understand why and how it happened, the signs and signals or risk, and how routines might be altered to manage similar problems in the future. This type of meeting leads to discussion of personal feelings and allows for a sense of mutual

TABLE 46.4. *Suicidal Ideation and Cancer: Prevalence Studies*

Study	Prevalence (%)	Setting
Achte and Vaukonnen (19)	< 1	Ambulatory breast cancer
Silberfarb et al. (42)	< 1	Ambulatory mixed cancer types
Breitbart (27)	8.6	Psychiatric consultations, hospitalized cancer patients
Pasacreta and Massie (43)	11	Nurse reports, hospitalized cancer patients
Breitbart et al. (48)	16.3	Ambulatory and hospitalized patients with cancer pain
Brown et al. (44)	20	Palliative care unit

support. Psychiatric colleagues can often be of help as participants in such a review, or to assist on an individual level.

MANAGEMENT PRINCIPLES

Assessment of suicide risk and appropriate intervention are critical. Early and comprehensive psychiatric involvement with high-risk individuals can often avert suicide in the cancer setting (40). A careful evaluation (Table 46.5) includes a search for the meaning of suicidal thoughts, as well as an exploration of the seriousness of the risk. The clinician's ability to establish rapport and elicit a patient's thoughts are essential as he or she assesses history, degree of intent, and quality of internal and external controls. One must listen sympathetically, not appearing critical or stating that such thoughts are inappropriate. Allowing the patient to discuss suicidal thoughts often decreases the risk of suicide. The myth that asking about suicidal thoughts puts the idea in their head is one that should be dispelled, especially when dealing with cancer (45). Patients often reconsider the idea of suicide when the physician acknowledges the legitimacy of their option and the need to retain a sense of control over aspects of their death.

Table 46.3 outlines cancer vulnerability variables that can be utilized as a guide to evaluation and management. Once the setting has been made secure, the assessment of the mental status and the management of pain control can begin. Analgesics, neuroleptics, or antidepressant drugs should be utilized when appropriate to treat agitation, psychosis, major depression, or pain. Underlying causes of delirium or pain should be addressed specifically when possible. It is important to

initiate a crisis intervention–oriented psychotherapeutic approach that mobilizes as much of the patient's support system as possible. A close family member or friend should be involved in order to support the patient, provide information, and assist in treatment planning. Psychiatric hospitalization can sometimes be helpful when there is a clear indication and the patient's medical illness is stable. Most frequently, however, the medical hospital or home is the setting in which management takes place. Although it is appropriate to intervene when medical or psychiatric reasons are clearly the driving force in a cancer suicide, there are circumstances when usurping control from the patient and family with overly aggressive intervention may be less helpful. This is most evident in those with advanced illness with whom comfort and symptom control are the primary concerns.

The goal of intervention should not be to prevent suicide at all costs, but to prevent suicide that is driven by desperation. Prolonged suffering due to poorly controlled symptoms lead to such desperation, and it is our role to provide effective management of such problems as an alternative to suicide in the cancer patient.

TABLE 46.5. *Evaluation of Suicidal Patient*

Establish rapport — empathic approach

Obtain patient's understanding of illness and present symptoms

Assess relevant mental status — delirium (internal control)

Assess vulnerability variables

Assess support system (external control)

Obtain history of prior emotional problems, or psychiatric disorders

Obtain family history

Record prior suicide threats, attempts

Assess suicidal thinking, intent, plans

Evaluate need for one-to-one nurse in hospital or companion at home

Formulate immediate and long-term treatment plan

REFERENCES

1. Kastenbaum R. Suicide as the preferred way to death. In: Schneidman ES, ed. *Suicidology: Contemporary Developments*. New York: Grune and Stratton; 1976.
2. Roman J. *Exit House*. New York: Seaview Books; 1980.
3. Siegel K, Tuckel P. Rational suicide and the terminally ill cancer patient. *Omega*. 1984; 15: 263–69.
4. Annas GJ. When suicide prevention becomes brutality: the case of Elizabeth Bouvia. *Hastings Center Rep*. 1985; 114:20–21.
5. Kane FI. Keeping Elizabeth Bouvia alive for the public good. *Hastings Center Rep*. 1985; 15:5–9.
6. Holland JC. Psychological aspects of cancer. In: Holland JF, Frei E, eds, *Cancer Medicine*, 2nd ed. Philadelphia: Lea and Febiger; 1982.
7. Bolund C. Suicide and cancer I. Demographic and social characteristics of cancer patients who committed suicide in Sweden, 1973–1976. *J. Psychosoc Oncol*. 1985; 3:17–30.
8. Bolund C. Suicide and cancer II. Medical and care factors in suicides by cancer patients in Sweden, 1973–1976. *J. Psychosoc Oncol*. 1985; 3:31–52.
9. Forman B. Cancer and suicide. *Gen Hosp Psychiatry*. 1979; 1:108–114.
10. Campbell PC. Suicides among cancer patients. *Conn Health Bull*. 1996; 80:207–212.
11. Dorpat TL, Anderssen WE, Ripley HS. The relationship of physical illness to suicide. In: Resnik HLP, ed. *Suicidal Behaviors*. London: Churchill Livingstone; 1968.
12. Louhivuori KA, Hakama M. Risk of suicide among cancer patients. *Am J Epidemiol*. 1979; 109:59–65.
13. Sainsbury P. Suicide in London: an ecological study. *Mandsley Monograph* No. 1. London: Chapman and Hall; 1975.

14. Whitlock FA Suicide, cancer and depression. *Br J Psychiatry*. 1978; 132:269–274.

15. Fox BH, Stanek EJ, Boyd SC, and Flannery JT. Suicide rates among cancer patients in Connecticut. *J Chron Dis*. 1982; 35:85–100.

16. Hietanen P, Lonnqvist J, Henriksson M and Jallonoja P. Do cancer suicides differ from others? *Psycho-oncology*. 1994; 3:189–195.

17. Suris JC, Parera N, Puig C. Chronic illness and emotional distress in adolescence. *J Adolesc Health*. 1996; 19:153–156.

18. Farberow NL, Schneidman ES, Leonard CV. Suicides among general medical and surgical hospital patients with malignant neoplasms. *Med Bull*. 1963; 9. Washington DC: U.S. Veterans Administration.

19. Achte KA, and Vaukonnen ML. Suicides committed in general hospitals. *Psychiatr Fenn Yearbook Psychiatr Clin Helsinki Univ Gen Hosp*. 1971; 221–28.

20. Passik SD, Breitbart W, Depression in patients with pancreatic carcinoma: diagnostic and treatment issues. *Cancer*. 1996; 78:615–623.

21. Green A, Austin C. Psychopathology of pancreatic cancer: a psychobiologic probe. *Psychosomatics* 1993; 34:208–21.

22. Farberow NL, Ganzler S, Cutter F, Reynolds D. An eight year survey of hospital suicides. *Suicide Life Threat Behav*. 1971; 1:184–201.

23. Guze S, Robins E. Suicide and primary affective disorders. *Br J Psychiatry*. 1970; 117:437–438.

24. Robins E, Murphy G, Wilkenson RH Jr, et al. Some clinical considerations in the prevention of suicide based on 134 successful suicides. *Am J Public Health*. 1959; 49:888–899.

25. Bukberg J, Penman D, Holland H. Depression in hospitalized cancer patients. *Psychosom Med*. 1984; 46: 199–212.

26. Plumb MM, Holland JC. Comparative studies of psychological function in patients with advanced cancer. *Psychosom Med*. 1977; 39:264–276.

27. Breitbart W. Suicide in cancer patients. *Oncology*. 1987; 1:49–53.

28. Beck AT, Kovacs M. Weissman A. Hopelessness and suicidal behavior: an overview. *JAMA*. 1975; 234:1146–1149.

29. Kovacs M, Beck AT, Weissman A. Hopelessness: an indication of suicide risk. *Suicide*. 1975; 5:98–103.

30. Massie MJ, Gorzynski JG, Mastrovito RC, et al., The diagnosis of depression in hospitalized patients with cancer. *Proc Am Assoc Cancer Res Am Soc Clin Oncol*. 1979; 20:432–440.

31. Levine PM, Silberfarb PM, Lipowsky ZJ. Mental disorders in cancer patients. *Cancer*, 1978; 42:1385–1390.

32. Massie MJ, Holland JC, Glass E. Delerium in terminally ill cancer patients. *Am J Psychiatry*. 1983; 140:1048–1050.

33. Breitbart W. Cancer pain and suicide. In: Foley K, Bonica JJ, Ventrafridda V, eds. *Advances in Pain Research and Therapy*, vol. 16. New York: Raven Press; 1990: 399–412.

34. Cleeland CS. The impact of pain on patients with cancer. *Cancer*. 1984; 54:263–267.

35. Daut RI, Cleeland CS. The prevalence and severity of pain in cancer. *Cancer*. 1982; 50:1913–1918.

36. Twycross RG, Lack SA. Symptom control in far advanced cancer. In: Twycross RG, Lack SA, eds. *Pain Relief*. London: Pitman; 1984.

37. Levin DN, Cleeland CS, Dar R. Public attitudes toward cancer pain. *Cancer*. 1985; 56:2337–2339.

38. Derogatis LR, Marrow GR, Fetting J, et al. The prevalence of psychiatric disorders among cancer patients. *JAMA*. 1983; 249:751–757.

39. Holland JC. Psychological aspects of cancer. In: Holland JF, Frie E, eds. *Cancer Medicine*, 2nd ed. Philadelphia: Lea and Febiger; 1982.

40. Dubovsky SL. Averting suicide in terminally ill patients. *Psychosomatics*. 1978; 19:113–115.

41. Murphy GE. Suicide and attempted suicide. *Hosp Pract*. 1977; 12:78–81.

42. Silberfarb PM, Maurer LH, Cronthamel CS. Psychosocial aspects of breast cancer aptients during different treatment regimens. *Am J Psychiatry*. 1980; 137:450–455.

43. Pasacreta JV, Massie MJ. Nurses report of psychiatric complications in patients with cancer. *Oncol Nurs Forum*. 1990; 17:347–353.

44. Brown JH, Henteleff P, Baraket S, Rowe JR. Is it normal for terminally ill patients to desire death? *Am J Psychiatry*. 1986; 143:208–211.

45. McKegney PP, Lange P. The decision to no longer live on chronic hemodialysis. *Am J. Psychiatry*. 1971; 128:47–55.

46. Weisman AD. Coping behavior and suicide in cancer. In: Cullen JW, Fox BH, Ison RN, eds. *Cancer: The Behavioral Dimensions*. New York: Raven Press; 1976.

47. Olafssen D. Cancer and suicide. Report presented at the International Conference on Suicide, 1982, Paris.

48. Breitbart W, Passik SD, Eller K, Sison A. Suicidal ideation in AIDS: the role of pain and mood [abstract]. 145th Annual Meeting, American Psychiatric Association, 2–7 May 1992, Washington DC. New Research Program and Abstracts; 113.

47

Anxiety Disorders

RUSSELL NOYES JR., CRAIG S. HOLT, AND MARY JANE MASSIE

For many patients, cancer is an emotionally stressful, even traumatic event. In addition to physical discomforts, patients with cancer often are troubled by bodily dysfunction and alterations in appearance. The treatment they receive often adds, in various ways, to the distress related to their illness. Malignant disease also may force changes in social roles and may disrupt interpersonal relationships. Of course, serious illness such as cancer may be accompanied by the threat of death, a threat that can challenge the view patients have of themselves and their world (1,2). While anxiety is a normal reaction to such threats (3), some patients show an exaggerated response with symptoms that overwhelm them and impair their functioning. Such pathological anxiety is the focus of this chapter.

Anxiety appears at crisis or transition points such as the time of diagnosis or recurrence, awaiting new treatment or surgery, completion of lengthy treatment, and advanced or terminal stages (4,5). Such points represent threatening events of a kind often associated with anxiety disorders (6). According to Weisman (7), patients who receive a diagnosis of cancer, learn of a recurrence, or hear that treatment has failed react in a characteristic fashion. They experience initial shock and disbelief followed by emotional turmoil. The latter is accompanied by anxiety and depressive symptoms, together with irritability, loss of appetite, and difficulty sleeping. Patients often experience intrusive thoughts about their diagnosis and its impact upon their future. Their ability to concentrate and carry out their usual activities is temporarily impaired. However, these symptoms decline gradually and usually resolve over a 7–10 day period (8,9).

The literature dealing with anxiety in cancer patients is limited. Few studies have measured anxiety apart from overall psychological distress, and fewer still have identified pathological anxiety. Still, the subject is important for several reasons. One is that anxiety disorders are prevalent in cancer patients. Another is

that these disorders significantly undermine the quality of these patients' lives. Still another reason is that anxiety interferes with the ability of cancer patients to tolerate, even continue with, treatment. Finally, anxiety disorders in these patients are in some cases preventable but, in most cases, are responsive to treatment.

PATHOLOGICAL ANXIETY AND ITS ASSESSMENT

Pathological Anxiety

Anxiety that persists and causes impairment is considered pathological. It is characterized by moderate to severe apprehension or worry and associated anxiety symptoms (see Table 47.1). It must have persisted for 2 weeks or more and been present at least half the time (10). Patients report that such anxiety dominates their awareness and is uncontrollable. Severe anxiety reduces their threshold for physical distress, especially pain, and causes impairment in functioning. Because of poor concentration, patients may not comprehend what they are told about their disease and may find treatment decisions difficult (11). They may become disorganized and are further undermined by lack of sleep. Patients with such anxiety may be unable to cooperate with treatment and seek to avoid fear-provoking procedures.

The diagnosis of anxiety disorders in medically ill patients is problematic (2,12). Somatic symptoms involve many organ systems, especially the cardiovascular and gastrointestinal, and these overlap with the symptoms of cancer and side effects of treatment. For example, symptoms such as poor concentration, fatigue, and trouble sleeping may be due to advanced disease, especially when pain is present. Consequently, somatic symptoms are of less value in making an anxiety disorder diagnosis and greater reliance must be placed upon psychological symptoms, those falling

TABLE 47.1. *Anxiety Symptoms Contained in the DSM-III-R and DSM-IV Criteria for Generalized Anxiety Disorder*

Apprehensive expectation
   Excessive anxiety*
   Uncontrolled worry*

Motor tension
   Trembling, twitching, or feeling shaky
   Muscle tension, aches, or soreness*
   Restlessness*
   Easy fatigability*

Autonomic hyperactivity
   Shortness of breath or smothering sensations
   Palpitations or accelerated heart rate (tachycardia)
   Sweating, or cold clammy hands
   Dry mouth
   Dizziness or lightheadedness
   Nausea, diarrhea, or other abdominal distress
   Flushes (hot flashes) or chills
   Frequent urination
   Trouble swallowing or lump in throat

Vigilance and scanning
   Feeling keyed up or on edge*
   Exaggerated startle response
   Difficulty concentrating or mind going blank because of anxiety*
   Trouble falling or staying asleep*
   Irritability*

*DSM-IV criteria.

under the headings of apprehensive expectation and vigilance and scanning in Table 47.1.

It is also unclear how suitable the DSM-IV criteria are for the medically ill (13,14). Most cancer patients have adjustment disorders, but symptom criteria have not been developed for them. The criteria for generalized anxiety disorder (DSM-IV) were refined to make them more discriminatory, but they now include the overlapping symptoms referred to above (Table 47.1). Also, the anxiety seen in cancer patients is accompanied by greater autonomic hyperactivity than in patients with chronic anxiety (e.g., generalized anxiety disorder). Finally, anxiety and depressive symptoms commonly coexist and mixed states may be important in the medically ill (15,16). Empirical investigation of cancer patients is needed so that criteria for this and other medically ill populations may be developed (17).

The diagnostic recognition of anxiety disorders in cancer patients faces clinical obstacles as well. One is that patients often interpret their distress as a normal reaction to their disease and, therefore, do not seek relief from what they feel they must deal with on their own. Others, for example persons with phobias, may regard their anxiety as abnormal but be ashamed to reveal it. Also, physicians may fail to recognize patients' anxiety and, for this reason, not respond to it (18). Finally, physicians, like their patients, may interpret anxiety as a normal reaction to illness and not a problem needing treatment.

Measurement

The measurement of psychological distress in cancer patients has received increasing attention and, in the past decade, two instruments have been developed for this purpose. These are the Hospital Anxiety and Depression Scale (HADS) and the Rotterdam Symptom Checklist (RSCL). Prior to their introduction, several scales had been used to assess psychological distress and anxiety in particular. These included the Symptom Checklist-90 (19), which has an anxiety subscale, and the Profile of Mood States (20), which contains an anxiety (tension) subscale. Cella et al. (21) developed an abbreviated version of the Profile of Mood States for use in cancer patients. Also, the State-Trait Anxiety Inventory has frequently been administered to cancer patients (22). This scale is widely used in psychological research and a shortened version has been developed for these patients (23).

The Hospital Anxiety and Depression Scale is a brief, self-assessment scale developed for use in medically ill populations (24). Both the anxiety and depression subscales contain seven items that are rated on 4-point linear scales (0–3). The authors used only psychological items likely to distinguish anxiety and depression. Zigmond and Snaith (24) demonstrated that the scale is useful for screening (a score of 8–10 for doubtful cases, and 11 or more for definite cases on either scale) and is a valid measure of severity. Their findings have been confirmed in subsequent studies (25–30). A factor analysis identified two factors corresponding to the questionnaire's anxiety and depression subscales (31).

Studies examining the HADS as a screening instrument have tended to combine the subscales. Optimal scores have ranged from ≥ 10 or ≥ 19, depending upon the severity of illness in populations surveyed and the level of psychopathology identified (26,30,32). However, the anxiety subscale performed well when examined separately; Hopwood et al. (32) reported a sensitivity of 75%, a specificity of 90%, and a misclassification rate of 12% at a score of 11.

The Rotterdam Symptom Checklist was developed to measure psychological and physical distress in cancer patients (33,34). It is a self-administered 27-item scale calling for responses on 4-point linear scales. Although the psychological subscale includes anxiety items, the performance of these items has not been examined separately. The RSCL has shown predictive value equal to that of the HADS (32).

PREVALENCE OF ANXIETY DISORDERS

The prevalence of anxiety disorders among cancer patients remains uncertain because of limitations in research methodology. Studies over the past 25 years have used varying criteria for caseness and have examined widely differing populations. As shown in Table 47.2 (18,19,22,27,29,30,35–50), most studies used scale scores to identify patients with pathological anxiety and few used structured interviews or diagnostic criteria. Also, as may be seen in

TABLE 47.2. *Studies Examining the Prevalence of Pathological Anxiety in Cancer Patients*

Study	N	Sample	Stage	Criteria	Anxious	Comment
Maguire et al. (35)	75	Breast	Early	Clinical assessment, pre-DSM-III	27%	14% of benign breast disease controls had anxiety
Hughes (36)	44	Breast	Early	Clinical assessment	18%	Preoperative scores predicted postoperative anxiety
Dean (37)	125	Breast	Early	Clinical assessment, RDC criteria	1%	5% hospital control sample had anxiety disorders
Lee et al. (38)	197	Breast	Early	Present State Examination	18%	Anxiety declined after surgery
Fallowfield et al. (22)	269	Breast	Early	Modified Present State Examination	39%	Premorbid trait anxiety associated with posttreatment anxiety
Hopwood et al. (27)	222	Breast	Advanced	HADS ≥ 11	9%	9% with mixed anxiety–depression
Watson et al. (39)	380	Breast	Early	HADS ≥ 10	16%	Anxiety correlated with mental adjustment to cancer
Pinder et al. (40)	139	Breast	Advanced	HADS ≥ 11	19%	Anxiety unrelated to demographic or illness variables
Peck (41)	50	Mixed	Early	Clinical assessment, pre-DSM-III	44%	8% had preexisting anxiety disorders
Peck and Boland (42)	50	Mixed	Early	Clinical assessment, pre-DSM-III	6–16%	
Derogatis et al. (3)	215	Mixed	Mixed, Nonterminal	Clinical assessment	7%	13% adjustment disorder with mixed features
Ibbotson et al. (30)	513	Mixed	Mixed	Psychiatric Assessment Schedule, DSM-III criteria	17%	Excludes adjustment disorders
Sensky et al. (18)	149	Mixed	Mixed	HADS ≥ 11	15%	No relation between stage of disease and anxiety
Moorey et al. (31)	568	Mixed	Early	HADS ≥ 8	28%	
Carroll et al. (44)	930	Mixed	Mixed	HADS ≥ 11	18%	HADS ≥ 8 identified 41% as anxious
Craig and Abeloff (19)	30	Mixed	Mixed	Symptom Checklist-90, Anxiety Scale ≥2 SD	10%	SCL-90 ≥ 1 SD identified 30% as anxious
Plumb and Holland (45)	80	Mixed	Advanced	Current Past Psychopathology Scale ≥ severe symptoms	14%	33% had moderate symptoms
Farber et al. (46)	141	Mixed	Mixed	Symptom Checklist-90, Anxiety Scale ≥ 2 SD	13%	14% had moderate anxiety
Stefanek et al. (47)	126	Mixed	Mixed, Nonterminal	Brief Symptom Inventory, Anxiety Scale ≥ 2 SD	10%	BSI anxiety ≥ 1 SD identified 36% as anxious
Kaasa et al. (48)	247	Mixed	Advanced	Impact of Events Scale ≥ 20	33%	PTSD symptoms
Davies et al. (49)	75	Head/neck	Early	Leeds Self-Assessment of Anxiety Scale ≥ 7	40%	High rate reflects use as screening
Bergman et al. (50)	65	Lung	Early	HADS ≥ 11	9%	4% with mixed anxiety–depression
Brandenberg et al. (29)	93	Melanoma	Screening	HADS ≥ 8	15%	High risk control group
	123	Melanoma	Early	HADS ≥ 8	18%	Patients following first surgery
	57	Melanoma	Advanced	HADS ≥ 8	28%	

RDC, Research Diagnostic Criteria; HADS, Hospital Anxiety and Depression Scale; SCL-90, Symptom Checklist-90; BSI, Brief Symptom Inventory; PSTD, Posttraumatic Stress Disorder.

Table 47.2, samples have been quite diverse, including patients with early versus advanced disease, outpatients versus inpatients, single tumor type versus many types, and a particular treatment vs. many or different stages of treatment. A number of studies, not shown in the table, focused exclusively on depression or failed to separate anxiety and depression.

The most widely quoted study of the prevalence of psychiatric disorders by Derogatis et al. (43) used DSM-III criteria in a large sample of cancer patients. Based on clinical assessment, 44% of patients were diagnosed as having current, Axis I disorders. Approximately two-thirds of these were adjustment disorders. Twenty-one percent had prominent anxiety symptoms, including 2% anxiety disorders, 6% adjustment disorder with anxious mood, and 13% adjustment disorder with mixed emotional features. Most studies shown in Table 47.2 estimated the current prevalence of any anxiety disorders within a range of 15%–28%. Using a conservative cutoff on the HADS (i.e., ≥ 11 anxiety scale), five studies identified between 9% and 19% of cancer patients as having anxiety disorders (18,27,40,44,50). These studies tell us that anxiety disorders are prevalent and that adjustment disorder with anxious mood is the most common.

Table 47.2 is organized according to tumor site, and shows that the psychiatric morbidity of breast cancer has been the most widely researched. However, within studies of breast cancer patients, estimates of prevalence fall within the range for all studies. For the present then, there is no evidence of differing rates according to site. Also, there is no pattern across studies related to stage of disease. Beyond this, studies relying on clinical assessment and, in some cases, diagnostic criteria report rates that are similar to those employing scores derived from self-report measures. Yet, because the studies of prevalence shown in Table 47.2 are methodologically diverse, it is difficult to draw any very definite conclusions.

Anxiety disorders appear to be more common in persons with cancer than in persons without cancer or other chronic illnesses in the general population. Based on Epidemiologic Catchment Area Program data, Wells et al. (51) reported that nearly 12% of persons with chronic medical conditions had anxiety disorders compared to 6% of those without. Cancer was one of the conditions that showed an especially strong association with anxiety and other psychiatric disorders. These data support earlier studies showing a higher prevalence of anxiety among cancer patients than controls. For instance, Maguire et al. (35), found moderate to severe anxiety in 27% of breast cancer patients compared to 14% of controls, and Brandenberg et al. (29) identified 28% of advanced melanoma patients as having anxiety compared to 15% of familial melanoma patients with no disease. A third study found no difference (37). According to the National Comorbidity Survey the current (i.e. 12 months) prevalence of anxiety disorders in the general population is 17% (52).

Although most anxiety disorders develop after the onset of neoplastic disease, a smaller proportion represent preexisting conditions. The literature says little about this subgroup, but it is important because the outcome of preexisting disorders is likely to differ from that of adjustment disorders. In an early study, Peck and Boland (42) reported that a majority of anxiety disorders had been present before their patients developed cancer. Later, Wald et al. (53) reported that 40% of the anxious cancer patients they treated had preexisting anxiety disorders. In addition, not all reactive disorders are due to cancer (54). For instance, Robinson et al. (55) found that 29% with anxiety or depression had disorders related to circumstances other than cancer.

It is not clear from the literature whether anxiety disorders are more or less prevalent in patients with cancer than in patients with other medical illnesses. This comparison addresses the question of what it is about cancer that gives rise to anxiety. According to Cassileth et al. (56), the distress associated with chronic disease is similar for major illness groups including cancer. Existing studies indicate that anxiety disorders are also prevalent in medically ill patients in general. Rates of anxiety disorders among primary care outpatients have ranged from 7% to 15% (57–59), and among general medical inpatients rates of 20% have been reported (60). Of course, the populations studied have varied widely in severity and prognosis. Factors such as these are important and difficult to control across groups.

In cancer patients symptoms of anxiety often coexist with depression and mixed states are, perhaps, more common than anxiety alone. Cassileth et al. (61) noted a high correlation ($r = 0.81$) between scores on the State-Trait Anxiety Inventory and Beck Depression Inventory in patients with malignant disease. Also, studies using the HADS have reported high correlations between the subscales—e.g., Moorey et al. (31). Most studies have reported higher prevalences of adjustment disorders with mixed features than of anxiety features alone—e.g., Derogatis et al. (43). Measurement difficulties and negative affectivity may contribute to this apparent overlap, but mixed states are receiving increasing attention (15).

Anxiety is a frequent reason for psychiatric consultation among cancer patients. Massie and Holland (62) reported that it was the third most common reason (after depression and organic mental disorder), accounting for 16% of requests among mostly inpatients. Likewise, Hinton (63) identified anxiety as the reason for referral in 18% of terminally ill patients, but Levine et al. (64) were not asked to see anxious patients. In Massie and Holland's series the majority were found to have adjustment disorders; specifically, 4% had anxiety disorders and 21% had adjustment disorder with anxious mood. By way of comparison, 9% had major depression and 48% had adjustment disorder with depressed mood. Thus, patients with anxiety disorders were seen frequently, though less often, than patients with depression.

CLINICAL PRESENTATION

Acute Anxiety Symptoms

Although most anxiety disorders represent acute reactions to cancer or its treatment, some patients have long-standing disturbances that are exacerbated by their illness or challenged by the treatment setting (65). Regardless of cause, the symptoms experienced by most patients are similar. Their mood is anxious and they are troubled by uneasiness, anxious foreboding or, in more severe cases, a sense of impending doom. This mood is accompanied by an unpleasant feeling of arousal; patients feel keyed up, are irritable, and have a tendency to startle. They are unable to relax and have difficulty falling asleep.

Patients with anxiety find their minds filled with recurring, intrusive thoughts and images of cancer (48). They are beset by fears of bodily destruction or death and dwell upon obtaining urgently needed help or avoiding an overwhelming threat (66). The thinking of anxious patients is often catastrophic and overgeneralized; they see unlikely dangers as probable and unfortunate consequences as devastating. Typically, they view their situation as uncontrollable and see themselves as helpless victims.

Symptoms of autonomic arousal include rapid or forceful heartbeat, sweating, and a sinking sensation in the stomach. Many patients experience cardiovascular and respiratory symptoms; they report tightness in the chest, shortness of breath, feelings of dizziness, and paresthesias. Such sympathetically mediated symptoms often accompany anxiety attacks. With attacks, anxiety rapidly rises to panic proportions, leaving patients emotionally drained and fearful of future attacks.

Parasympathetically-mediated symptoms such as abdominal distress, nausea, and diarrhea are common. Vegetative disturbances are often part of the clinical picture and may include loss of appetite and sexual interest.

Acutely anxious patients show physiologic signs and behavioral manifestations. They appear worried and drawn. Many are distractible, perplexed, and emotionally labile. Others are fidgety, restless, and have trouble sitting still. They are often tremulous or diaphoretic. Trouble sleeping contributes to fatigue and low tolerance for frustration. In response to anxious preoccupation about cancer, many repeatedly check their bodies for signs of recurrence or progression. Acutely anxious patients feel an urge to avoid or escape from surroundings they see as threatening, prompting them to refuse treatment or to sign out of the hospital (67). Anxiety symptoms may contribute to physical disability as well. Loss of appetite, poor sleep, shortness of breath, fatigue, and pain are all cancer symptoms that may worsen with anxiety.

Chronic, Preexisting Anxiety Disorders

Many with chronic disturbances, such as generalized anxiety disorder and panic disorder, experience reemergence or intensification of symptoms with the development of cancer. Persons whose panic attacks have been controlled may experience them again upon learning the diagnosis or being exposed to painful procedures, toxic medications, or crowded treatment facilities. Panic attacks are characterized by sudden, extreme anxiety that is accompanied by sympathetic nervous system arousal and an overwhelming urge to escape. Attacks are not only painful but may prompt patients to abruptly terminate procedures or treatments. Posttraumatic stress disorder may also be reactivated by the stress of cancer (68).

Specific phobias, especially needle/blood phobia and claustrophobia (fear of closed places), may interfere with cancer treatment. These fears usually develop in childhood and are characterized by extreme anxiety on exposure to the feared objects and avoidance of them. Patients with blood/needle phobia may be unable to tolerate injections, blood draws, treatment procedures, etc., and experience persistent anxiety in anticipation of such procedures. These patients show a characteristic vasovagal response to the feared object (i.e., bradycardia and fall in blood pressure). Claustrophobic patients are unable to tolerate procedures that require confinement in small spaces. This may include imaging studies, radiotherapy, administration of anesthetic agents, etc. For example, Brennan et al. (69) observed extreme anxiety in 13% of patients undergoing magnetic resonance imaging scans.

ETIOLOGIC FACTORS FOR ANXIETY

Demographic Variables

In the general population, anxiety disorders are associated with female gender, younger age, and lower socioeconomic status (52). In cancer populations these demographic variables appear less important (70). In studies that examined the relationship to gender, four found greater anxiety in women (20,29,44, 50) and five found no difference (43,45,47,49,71). Concerning age, three studies found greater anxiety in younger patients (38,39,44), and five found no difference (40,43,45,49,71). Three studies found no relationship to marital status (40,43,47), and three found no relationship to social class or education (40,43,45). These differences suggest that, as illness variables become more important, demographic factors become less so.

Premorbid Adjustment

In his study of terminally ill patients, Hinton (63) noted that mood changes, including anxiety, were usually consistent with previous patterns of reaction. Among patients who became anxious and insecure in the face of advanced disease, he identified premorbid anxious tendencies and obsessional personality traits. Prospective studies of patients receiving treatment have tended to confirm these observations. For example, Fallowfield et al. (22) reported that breast cancer patients undergoing mastectomy who had high trait anxiety were more likely to have clinically significant anxiety over the next 12 months. Likewise, high neuroticism, as measured by the Eysenck Personality Inventory, predicted psychological morbidity after mastectomy (72). Such findings are in accord with evidence from epidemiologic studies of premorbid neurotic traits in persons who develop anxiety disorders (73).

Other factors that may contribute to anxiety include coping style, sense of control, and social support. In his review, Greer (74) noted that these factors had been identified by researchers as influencing the psychosocial adjustment of cancer patients. Most of the research deals with distress without looking specifically at anxiety. For example, emotional support reduced the psychological distress of women with breast cancer and improved their self-esteem and sense of control (75). Also, a large study of women with breast cancer showed that anxiety was positively correlated with helplessness, fatalism, and anxious preoccupation but negatively correlated with fighting spirit (39). Positive correlations between sense of control and subsequent psychological adjustment to breast, lung, and colorectal cancer were also observed (76).

Stage of Neoplastic Disease

Anxiety appears to increase as cancer progresses toward its terminal stage (77). In general, research has shown that mental health declines along with physical status (56,78). In studies that examined stage of cancer, six found greater anxiety among patients with more advanced disease (20,27,29,43,49,71), and four found no difference (18,40,44,47). In cancer outpatients, Cassileth et al. (79) observed that anxiety and overall mental health were associated with treatment status. State anxiety rose sequentially in patients receiving follow-up care, active treatment, and palliative treatment. The authors noted that patients receiving active treatment faced inconvenience, toxicity, and uncertainty, but that those receiving follow-up care had been freed from such stress. In a large sample, Cella et al. (20) observed a relationship between mood disturbance, including anxiety, and both the extent of disease and physical impairment. However, these risk factors only explained 10%–15% of the variability in distress.

Treatment of Cancer

Treatments of cancer, including surgery, chemotherapy, and radiotherapy are anxiety-provoking and may contribute to psychological morbidity (80). The psychological reaction to mastectomy has received considerable attention and high levels of anxiety as well as depression have consistently been reported (72). These symptoms are not only a response to the loss of a breast but also to cancer, factors that are difficult to separate. Studies indicate that anxiety increases with discovery of the tumor, peaks prior to surgery, remains high immediately afterwards, then declines in the first postoperative year (see Table 47.3) (35). The early literature contains accounts of mounting anxiety following hospitalization for surgery. According to Bard and Sutherland (81), hospital admission caused some patients to feel "trapped and helpless in the face of imminent disaster" and prompted some to leave the hospital.

Anxiety states in mastectomy patients have been viewed as the response to an emotionally traumatic event (72). Consistent with this view, the type of treatment and the tumor's response to that treatment have appeared to influence the level of anxiety (22,37,38,82). Recent studies comparing patients receiving alternative therapies, including lumpectomy versus mastectomy, have not consistently shown less anxiety with the lesser

TABLE 47.3. *Percent of Patients with Clinically Significant Anxiety from Before Diagnosis to 1 yr after Surgery in Breast Cancer Patients and Controls*

Time of Assessment	Mastectomy (%)	Controls (%)	χ^2
Before discovery	10	10	NS
After discovery	23	26	NS
Before surgery	27	14	0.05
After surgery (4 mo)	23	8	0.01
After surgery (1 yr)	18	8	0.01

NS, not significant.
Source: Adapted from Maguire et al. (35).

procedure (83). However, design limitations make studies difficult to interpret and the approach to treatment decisions may be important (22).

Chemotherapy is a major cause of emotional distress, including anxiety (84). Awareness of toxicity may cause anxiety before treatment begins, but repeated postinfusion nausea and vomiting often produces subsequent preinfusion distress (5,8). Anticipatory nausea and vomiting, that affect a quarter to a half of patients, is a classically conditional response to chemotherapy (85). It often generalizes beyond the treatment setting and may persist, sometimes for years (86). It adds to the overall distress of treatment and may lead to nonadherence or termination. However, recent studies indicate that anticipatory anxiety, which may be similarly conditioned, develops in many patients and interacts with anticipatory nausea, each increasing the other (87,88).

Research has shown that preexisting trait anxiety is predictive of high state anxiety before the first and subsequent infusions (86,87). It has also shown that state anxiety is correlated with infusion-related nausea and vomiting (88). Based on his review of the literature, Andrykowski (89) concluded that state anxiety plays a causal role in the development of anticipatory nausea and vomiting. Regardless of how these relationships are explained, it seems clear that anxiety contributes to the distress associated with chemotherapy, and that efforts to identify anxious patients and reduce their anxiety may improve the tolerability of this therapy (67).

Patients undergoing radiotherapy experience significant psychological distress including apprehension, anxiety, restlessness, feelings of helplessness, nightmares, and insomnia (90). Peck and Boland (42), who observed moderately severe anxiety in 26% of their patients, noted that many believed radiation might damage their bodies. This anxiety and associated psychological distress may even exceed the physical distress caused by radiation (91), and, unlike the anxiety associated with some forms of treatment, it may not decline as therapy progresses (92). This may be because of accumulating side effects and the anticipation of treatment's end (93).

Organic Factors

A variety of organic factors may also give rise to anxiety disorders in cancer patients (8). As with psychological factors, these may involve the neoplastic disease, treatment of the disease, or factors unrelated to the cancer or its treatment. Most disturbances fall under the DSM-IV category of anxiety disorders due to general medical conditions or substance-induced anxiety disorders (14). To make one of these diagnoses there should be: (*1*) a temporal association between the onset and course of the medical condition or substance use and anxiety symptoms; (*2*) features that are not typical of primary anxiety disorders; (*3*) evidence from the literature that the medical condition or substance may be associated with anxiety symptoms.

Poorly controlled pain is the most common cause of anxiety related to neoplastic disease (8). An association between psychiatric disorders and pain in cancer patients was demonstrated by Derogatis et al. (43). Among patients who received a psychiatric diagnosis, 39% had significant pain, whereas among those who did not receive a diagnosis only 19% had pain. Also, Ahles et al. (94) found high anxiety and depression in cancer patients with pain compared to those without pain. This anxiety may be a consequence of or a contributor to acute pain (95). Many patients believe that pain is indicative of disease progression and this not only increases their pain but their apprehension (94). There is often a disparity between a patient's interpretation and his or her actual condition because, although pain may be a symptom of cancer, there is no established link between its severity and progression of disease.

Patients who are experiencing acute uncontrollable pain appear drawn, diaphoretic, restless, and plead for help. If help is not forthcoming, they may become agitated and express suicidal thoughts (8). In the hospital, anxiety is heightened when pain medication is inadequate and the staff unresponsive. The ordering of analgesics on an as necessary basis usually fails to establish control and increases the patient's anxiety about being able to obtain relief. The patient's insistent demands or anger may trigger a request for psychiatric evaluation. According to Massie and Holland (96), it is not possible to evaluate anxiety until pain has been controlled. Anxiety must, in other words, be considered a consequence of pain initially. Usually the patient's anxiety is reduced when pain is relieved.

Altered metabolic states are often a cause of anxiety in cancer patients (97). And, because unexplained anxiety may signal serious or catastrophic events, it should prompt a review of the patient's medical status. The most common metabolic cause of anxiety in cancer patients is hypoxia (8). Hypoxic patients sense that something is wrong with their breathing and become fearful. Sudden anxiety with chest pain may be the result of a pulmonary embolus (98). Anxiety often contributes to respiratory distress but, once the cause is established, may be relieved by anxiety-reducing medication. Short-acting benzodiazepines have a dose-related effect upon the respiratory center but, when their use is carefully monitored, may reduce anxiety and improve respiratory function. Alternatively, an antihistamine may be used.

Sepsis that is accompanied by chills and fever is often associated with anxiety. Also, anxiety and restlessness may be early signs of delirium, regardless of the cause (99). As the disturbance progresses, anxiety may give way to agitation. A variety of endocrine abnormalities that are associated with anxiety may also occur in cancer patients (98). One of these is hypoglycemia. In this case, anxiety and restlessness may be early signs of a potentially life-threatening complication. Also, hypocalcemia may be associated with anxiety as well. Table 47.4 shows a list of medical conditions that are often accompanied by anxiety (100).

Hormone-secreting tumors may also give rise to anxiety disorders or to symptoms that resemble anxiety. Thyroid tumors often create a hyperthyroid state that resembles generalized anxiety disorder (101). Pheochromocytomas are also associated with anxiety or panic symptoms, although a recent study found them infrequent (102). Parathyroid tumors are another cause of anxiety (103). Certain tumors (e.g., pancreatic and lung cancer) produce paraneoplastic syndromes that may cause psychiatric disturbances including anxiety. Pancreatic cancer has frequently been associated

TABLE 47.4. *Medical Conditions Associated with Anxiety*

Cardiovascular conditions
  Angina pectoris
  Arrhythmia
  Congestive heart failure
  Hypovolemia
  Myocardial infarction
  Valvular disease

Endocrine conditions
  Carcinoid
  Hyperadrenalism
  Hypercalcemia
  Hyperthyroidism
  Hypocalcemia
  Hypothyroidism
  Pheochromocytoma

Metabolic conditions
  Hyperkalemia
  Hyperthermia
  Hypoglycemia
  Hyponatremia
  Hypoxia
  Porphyria

Neurological conditions
  Akathisia
  Encephalopathy
  Mass lesion
  Postconcussion syndrome
  Seizure disorder
  Vertigo

Peptic ulcer disease

Respiratory conditions
  Asthma
  Chronic obstructive pulmonary disease
  Pneumothorax
  Pulmonary edema
  Pulmonary embolism

Immunologic conditions
  Anaphylaxis
  Systemic lupus erythematosus

Source: From Goldberg and Posner (100).

with anxiety as well as depression. Holland et al. (104) demonstrated greater anxiety and depression in pancreatic cancer patients than in gastric cancer patients who had been matched for severity of illness. Tumors of the central nervous systems, especially those affecting the temporal lobes and limbic structures, may also give rise to anxiety (105).

Substance-induced anxiety disorders are commonly seen in cancer patients. The psychiatric effects of corticosteroids, which are widely administered to these patients, are well known; the incidence of major psychiatric disturbances is between 5% and 10% in patients receiving high doses (106). However, minor mood disturbances, including anxiety symptoms, are very common (106). These include anxiety, restlessness, emotional lability, insomnia, and agitation.

Dexamethasone, when given in high doses (e.g., for spinal cord compression), may cause this kind of disturbance. Prednisone does not usually produce anxiety but, in high doses or during a rapid taper, may do so (8). Steroid-induced anxiety may be difficult to distinguish from an adjustment disorder with anxious mood; however, during steroid treatment the sudden onset of symptoms in a previously stable patient suggests that the steroid is responsible.

Antiemetic drugs such as metoclopramide and prochlorperazine are an increasingly common cause of anxiety-like symptoms. These neuroleptic drugs are given in high doses to control chemotherapy-related nausea and vomiting. Akathisia or motor restlessness typically develops several hours to days after treatment. Uncontrollable movements involving the legs, hands and jaws are accompanied by anxiety that patients find hard to explain. According to Fleishman et al. (107), 50% of cancer patients receiving one of these drugs experience this side effect. Akathisia may be rapidly controlled by a benzodiazepine or β-blocking drug (108). Reduction in dose or substitution of another antiemetic drug (ondansetron) may also be helpful. Patients should be told that this side effect can occur but that the means to control it is available.

A variety of other drugs are capable of producing anxiety symptoms especially in high doses. Thyroid replacement, when excessive, may produce a hyperthyroid state associated with anxiety symptoms (109). Also, bronchodilators and β-adrenergic agonists used for treatment respiratory complications of neoplastic disease may cause anxiety symptoms (110). Stimulant drugs, such as pemoline, methylphenidate, and dextroamphetamine which are used to treat depression and stimulate appetite in cancer patients, may cause anxiety and insomnia if the dose is too high. Antidepressants, such as fluoxetine, may also give rise to anxiety. Likewise, caffeine, which some patients use to counteract fatigue and which is contained in some analgesic preparations, may produce typical anxiety symptoms.

Discontinuation of certain drugs is associated with withdrawal syndromes that have prominent anxiety symptoms. If alcohol is abruptly stopped as a result of illness or hospitalization, withdrawal symptoms, including severe anxiety, may appear within the first day (111). Patients with certain neoplasms (e.g., head and neck cancer) have an increased prevalence of alcohol disorders, and among them withdrawal states are common. Some patients develop delirium tremens under these circumstances. Patients dependent upon narcotics, such as heroin, may also experience anxiety

as part of a withdrawal syndrome. Also, benzodiazepines are an increasing cause of withdrawal symptoms. Shorter acting drugs, such as alprazolam and lorazepam, may cause severe anxiety if abruptly discontinued (112). Under these circumstances, withdrawal symptoms may develop within 24 h. Similarly, discontinuation of sedative-hypnotics and narcotic analgesics — often on admission or discharge from hospital — may precipitate withdrawal syndromes.

COURSE AND OUTCOME

Anxiety disorders that develop in cancer patients sometime disappear with resolution of the crisis that precipitated them. However, they tend to follow the course of the underlying disease. In a study of adjustment disorders among inpatients referred for psychiatric consultation, Popkin et al. (54) observed that two-thirds resolved, usually within 30 days. Also, Kathol and Wenzel (113) reported that most anxiety and depressive disorders in newly admitted medical patients resolve during hospitalization. Similarly, longitudinal studies of cancer patients, beginning at the time of diagnosis or initiation of treatment, show a gradual decline in the level of anxiety symptoms and number of patients with anxiety disorders (22,27,38,50). For instance, Maguire et al. (35) reported that, of patients who suffered moderate to severe anxiety before surgery, 12% lasted 2–8 months, 17% lasted more than 8 months, and 4% that had an onset after 4 months still persisted at 1 year. Others have observed a decline in anxiety disorders over 6 months to 1 year (114–116).

These same studies show that the progression of disease and/or treatment influences psychological morbidity and that new cases of anxiety develop along the way. For instance, Bergman et al. (50) reported that anxiety declined in lung cancer patients who completed chemotherapy and that this anxiety covaried with the tumor's response to therapy. In a study of advanced breast cancer patients, Hopwood et al. (27) observed considerable fluctuation in psychological well-being; 13 of 24 patients who were cases of anxiety initially were borderline or well 1–3 months later, but 11 more had become cases. Similarly, Devlen et al. (115) found anxiety in lymphoma patients highest before treatment, but new episodes of anxiety and depression developed throughout the year which were associated, in many instances, with toxicity of treatment.

Anxiety may also increase with the termination of prolonged treatment. In their study of women undergoing mastectomy and radiotherapy, Holland et al.

(93) observed a seemingly paradoxical increase in anxiety after the completion of treatment. This increase appeared to be related to patient fears that, without close surveillance and protective treatment, their cancer might recur. It was also related to the loss of emotional support provided by daily contact with the radiotherapy staff.

TREATMENT

Management

Awareness of successful management techniques is critical in bettering the care of the cancer patient and reducing anxiety. These techniques are often underappreciated for the simple power they possess. Management skills are often neither time-consuming nor training-intensive. For example, anxiety is best managed initially by providing emotional support and adequate information (117). The patient's physician should attempt to elicit and deal with thoughts and feelings that are causing distress. Anxiety about procedures or treatments may be reduced by adequate preparation so that patients will know what to expect. Although the value of such simple measures is well documented, they are too often neglected (118). Causes of anxiety to be explored include worry about practical matters such as finances, physical suffering, uncertainty about the future, loss of independence, loss of social role, fear of becoming a burden, fear of the manner of death, and spiritual concerns (10,19). Many patients with moderate levels of anxiety will be helped by this kind of opportunity to share their concerns and to feel understood (119).

Patients may also be helped by simple anxiety management techniques such as relaxation, distraction, and cognitive reframing. Progressive muscle relaxation is commonly used, and a number of studies have shown it to be effective in reducing anxiety and other symptoms in cancer patients (120). Cognitive reframing addresses many patients' anxiety that is generated or reinforced by excessively worrisome thoughts. Their anxiety may be reduced by replacing such thoughts with more realistic ones. For example, a patient might think, "This chemotherapy is poisoning my body." Such a thought might be replaced with, "This chemotherapy is helping to rid my body of cancer cells." With such measures anxiety often resolves quickly and easily, but patients should be monitored to be sure they do not develop an anxiety disorder.

The anxiety and anxiety disorders that occur in cancer patients often respond favorably to a variety of pharmacological and psychosocial approaches. Evidence for the efficacy of specific treatments is detailed elsewhere in this volume; here we briefly mention a range of options.

Pharmacological Treatment

Antianxiety drugs are widely prescribed for cancer patients and probably deserve even wider application. Surveys of advanced cancer patients have found that between a quarter and a third receive antianxiety agents during hospitalization (121,122). Benzodiazepines are the agents most often used. They are used not only for reducing anxiety but also insomnia, and the nausea and vomiting of chemotherapy. In addition to their anxiolytic effects, their sedative, muscle-relaxant, and amnestic properties make them valuable in these patients. There are few controlled trials, so that efficacy in cancer populations has not been established for some indications. In one randomized, nonblind trial of alprazolam versus progressive muscle relaxation, Holland et al. (123) found that both treatments resulted in a significant reduction in anxiety and depressive symptoms. However, patients receiving alprazolam (0.5 mg three times a day) showed a more rapid decrease in anxiety and a slightly greater reduction in depressive symptoms.

Benzodiazepines have been shown in controlled trials to significantly reduce the nausea and vomiting of chemotherapy and the anticipatory nausea, vomiting, and phobic anxiety that may accompany this form of treatment. Studies in this area have been reviewed by Triozzi et al. (124) and Greenberg (67). Lorazepam is commonly added to antiemetic regimens, but the mechanism of its action remains unclear. Regardless, patients who receive the drug experience less anxiety, more sedation, and less recall of the treatment in addition to less nausea and vomiting. When 2–4 mg of lorazepam is given intravenously before chemotherapy, many patients do not remember the treatment. Patients receiving benzodiazepines have been pleased with the effects and, in some instances, have been willing to continue an otherwise intolerable treatment (124).

Lorazepam, alprazolam, and clonazepam are the benzodiazepines most frequently prescribed for cancer patients (125). Lorazepam has no active metabolites and is unlikely to accumulate. It is, therefore, preferred for patients with hepatic disease. This drug, unlike most other benzodiazepines, may be administered by the oral, intramuscular, and intravenous (even sublingual) routes, making it versatile. Also, it is believed to have superior amnestic properties. Control of anxiety is rapid, often occurring within a few days. Drowsiness and fatigue, the most common side effects, usually respond to downward dose adjustment or the passage of time. Impaired coordination, imbalance, memory difficulty, sexual dysfunction, incontinence, and depressed mood are notable but infrequent. Elderly patients, those with advanced disease, those with impaired liver function, and those taking other psychotropic medication are more apt to experience these side effects. Alprazolam has been shown to have antidepressant properties and may be used where depressive symptoms coexist.

Procedure-related anxiety may be reduced by the use of a benzodiazepine, making the patient more comfortable and lessening the chance that conditioned aversion, including phobic anxiety, will develop (126). Treatment should begin with the earliest sign of anxiety hours or days before the next procedure or treatment. Low doses (e.g., lorazepam 0.5 mg three times a day) may be sufficient but on the day of treatment may be increased to a level that causes mild sedation (e.g., 2 mg three times a day). An intravenous dose of lorazepam that is sufficient to produce somnolence (e.g., 2–4 mg) may be given 15 min before the procedure and, in the case of chemotherapy, may be repeated afterwards if necessary. By reducing anxiety, benzodiazepines may facilitate the use of behavioral techniques.

Benzodiazepines are also useful for the rapid control of panic attacks and agoraphobia. Although preexisting anxiety disorders tend to be chronic, treatment usually substantially reduces symptoms and should be pursued as aggressively in cancer patients as in others. Patients with preexisting panic and other anxiety disorders often require higher doses (e.g., 4–6 mg alprazolam). Also, other drugs, especially the antidepressants, are used for the treatment of these conditions. Tricyclic antidepressants (e.g., imipramine) effectively control panic attacks and reduce phobic avoidance in the usual antidepressant doses. However, the response is slow to develop and, because many anxious patients are sensitive to side effects of these drugs, they must be started at a low dose and gradually increased. Serotonin reuptake inhibitors (e.g., paroxetine) appear to be effective and are well-tolerated by many patients. Monoamine oxidase inhibitors (e.g., phenelzine) are also effective but require a tryramine-free diet and carry the risk of hypertensive crises.

Psychological Treatment

Cancer patients appear to benefit from a wide variety of psychosocial interventions that have been used to reduce general distress, procedure-related discomfort, and acute anxiety. A number of controlled trials have been carried out that, on the whole, show improvements in psychological function following relatively brief interventions. In their recent review, Fawzy et al. (127) notes that four types of intervention have most commonly been examined. These are education, behavioral training, individual psychotherapy, and group interventions. Few of the studies reviewed examined change in anxiety specifically. Most measured psychological distress, using instruments such as the Profile of Mood States, from which inferences must be drawn about the treatment of anxiety disorders. In addition, most interventions were compared to ineffective procedures. This may show that a given treatment is better than no treatment but tells little about how it compares with other approaches.

Educational interventions that focused on cancer and its treatment have aimed at replacing the sense of helplessness with a sense of mastery, and, in the process, reducing psychological distress. In one study, Hodgkin's disease patients who received a booklet with disease-related information, showed less anxiety 3 months later than patients who did not receive the booklet (128). Also, patients with bladder cancer, who were encouraged to express their fears, had less anxiety postoperatively (129). However, in two other studies, no change in anxiety was observed (130,131). In fact, the authors of one attributed failure of patients to increase their knowledge to their high level of anxiety.

Behavioral training methods have been used along with many cancer interventions to reduce physical as well as psychological distress, and these methods have, in general, yielded more robust responses than education. Techniques have included progressive muscle relaxation, hypnosis, deep breathing, meditation, biofeedback, and guided imagery (127). With respect to anxiety, Davies (49) reported significant improvement in anxiety among breast cancer patients receiving biofeedback and cognitive therapy. Also, Gruber et al. (132) observed reduced anxiety levels among breast cancer patients who received progressive muscle relaxation and guided imagery. Similarly, Baider et al. (133) reported reductions in anxiety, as measured by the Brief Symptom Inventory and Impact of Events Scale, in a large group of patients receiving muscle relaxation and guided imagery.

Behavioral training has proven useful for managing chemotherapy-related nausea, vomiting, and anxiety (134–137). To control anticipatory nausea patients may be taught muscle relaxation together with pleasant, relaxing imagery (138). Systematic desensitization, a technique originally designed for the treatment of phobias, may also be helpful for reducing anticipatory anxiety. Also, distraction, by itself, is a technique that may block the perception of anxiety. For example, older children may use video games to reduce anxiety and nausea (136).

Behavioral techniques may also be useful for managing anxiety related to investigations or procedures (139). Relaxation training, systematic desensitization, and positive reinforcement have been used to reduce anxiety and phobic reactions to medical treatments and any, or a combination, may be useful for cancer patients (140). Behavioral approaches, especially those for children undergoing painful procedures, usually involve a combination of positive motivation, emotive imagery, and hypnosis. To enhance motivation, special treats or privileges are promised to those about to undergo procedures. Emotive imagery involves telling the child a story that distracts his or her attention from the procedure. Hypnosis helps patients to focus their attention away from pain.

Patients with claustrophobia or needle/blood phobia may be successfully treated with behavioral methods (141). Most behavioral treatments involve exposing the patient to the feared stimulus either in vivo or in imagination. With systematic desensitization, for example, the therapist guides the patient through a hierarchy of increasingly anxiety-provoking situations. For needle/blood phobia, Ost et al. (142) have developed a technique called applied tension that is effective in half the time required for other techniques. Patients are taught to recognize early signs of a drop in blood pressure and to apply a muscle-tensing procedure to reverse that drop. They are then exposed to an array of phobic situations in order to practice this coping skill.

Individual psychotherapy has, in most controlled trials, resulted in reduced psychological distress and better coping in cancer patients (127). In a study that attempted to reduce psychological morbidity including anxiety, Greer et al. (143) examined the effect of an adjuvant psychological therapy. At 4 months and again at 12 months, patients who had received the therapy had significantly lower scores on anxiety and psychological distress than did controls (144). Also, fewer therapy patients fell in the clinical range for anxiety (i.e., Hospital Anxiety and Depression Scale ≥10) than did controls. The study — one of the few to address anxiety specifically — demonstrated that a brief psychological intervention can not only reduce distress but also the rate of disorders a year afterward.

Controlled group intervention studies have likewise shown overall benefit in cancer patients (127). Group techniques have included education, emotional support, stress management, coping strategies, behavioral training, and others. In an important study by Spiegel et al. (145), patients who participated in psychological support groups for a year reported less tension and fewer phobias (trend) than did controls.

CONCLUSION

Anxiety disorders are frequently encountered among cancer patients. They contribute substantially to the psychological morbidity and interfere with the treatment of neoplastic disease. Most are reactions to the threat posed by the disease that respond to relatively simple measures. But, some have an organic cause and correction of that cause may be medically important. Research is needed to achieve better recognition of anxiety disorders and of patients likely to develop them.

REFERENCES

1. Maguire P. The psychological impact of cancer. *Br J Hosp Med.* 1985; 34:100–103.
2. Derogatis LR, Wise TN. *Anxiety and Depressive Disorders in the Medical Patient.* Washington, DC: American Psychiatric Press; 1989.
3. Viney L, Westbrook M. Patterns of anxiety in the chronically ill. *Br J Med Psychol.* 1982; 55:87–95.
4. Welch-McCaffrey D. Cancer, anxiety, and quality of life. *Cancer Nurs.* 1985; 8:151–158.
5. Holland JC. Anxiety and cancer: The patient and the family. *J Clin Psychiatry.* 1989; 50:20–25.
6. Finlay-Jones R, Brown GW. Types of stressful events and the onset of anxiety and depressive disorders. *Psychol Med.* 1981; 11:803–815.
7. Weisman A. *Coping with Cancer.* New York: McGraw-Hill; 1979.
8. Massie MJ. Anxiety, panic, and phobias. In: Holland JC, Rowland JH, eds. *Handbook of Psychooncology: Psychological Care of the Patient with Cancer.* New York: Oxford University Press; 1989; 300–309.
9. Massie MJ, Holland JC. Overview of normal reactions and prevalence of psychiatric disorders. In: Holland JC, Rowland JH, eds. *Handbook of Psychooncology: Psychological Care of the Patient with Cancer.* New York: Oxford University Press; 1989; 273–282.
10. Maguire P, Faulkner A, Regnard C. Managing the anxious patient with advancing disease — a flow diagram. *Palliative Med.* 1993; 7:239–244.
11. Scott DW. Anxiety: critical thinking and information processing during and after breast biopsy. *Nurs Res.* 1983; 32:24–28.
12. Strain JJ, Liebowitz MR, Klein DR. Anxiety and panic attacks in the medically ill. *Psychiatr Clin North Am.* 1981; 4:333–346.
13. Stoudemire GA, Strain JJ, Hales RE. DSM-IV issues for consultation psychiatry. *Psychosomatics.* 1989; 30:239–244.
14. American Psychiatric Association. *Diagnostic and Statistical Manual of Mental Disorders,* 4th ed. Washington, DC: American Psychiatric Association, 1994.

15. Zinberg RE, Barlow DH. Mixed anxiety-depression: a new diagnostic cateogry. In: Rapee RM, Barlow DH, eds. *Chronic Anxiety: Generalized Anxiety Disorder and Mixed Anxiety–Depression.* New York: Guilford Press; 1991; 136–152.

16. Liebowitz MR. Mixed anxiety and depression: Should it be included in DSM IV? *J Clin Psychiatry.* 1993; 54(suppl. 5):4–7.

17. Rosenbaum JF, Pollack MH. Anxiety. In: Cassem NH, ed. *Massachusetts General Hospital Handbook of General Hospital Psychiatry.* Boston: Mosby Year Book; 1991; 159–190.

18. Sensky T, Dennehy M, Gilbert A, et al. Physician's perceptions of anxiety and depression among their outpatients: Relationships with patients and doctors' satisfaction with their interviews. *J R Coll Phys Lond.* 1989; 23:33–38.

19. Craig TJ, Abeloff MD. Psychiatric symptomatology among hospitalized cancer patients. *Am J Psychiatry.* 1974; 131:1323–1327.

20. Cella D, Orofiamma B, Holland J, et al. The relationship of psychological distress, extent of disease and performance status in patients with lung cancer. *Cancer.* 1987; 60:1661–1667.

21. Cella DR, Jacobson PB, Orav EJ, et al. A brief POMS measure of distress in cancer patients. *J Chron Dis.* 1987; 40:939–942.

22. Fallowfield LJ, Hall A, Maguire GP, Baun M. Psychological outcomes of different treatment policies in women with early breast cancer outside a clinical trial. *Br Med J.* 1990; 301:575–580.

23. Van Knippenberg FCE, Duivenvoorden HJ, Bouke B, Passchier J. Shortening the State-Trait Anxiety Inventory. *J Clin Epidemiol.* 1990; 43:995–1000.

24. Zigmond AS, Snaith RP. The Hospital Anxiety and Depression Scale. *Acta Psychiatr Scand.* 1983; 67:361–370.

25. Aylard PR, Gooding JH, McKenna PJ, Snaith RP. A validation study of three anxiety and depression self-assessment scales. *J Psychosom Res.* 1987; 31:261–268.

26. Razavi D, Delvaux N, Farvaeques C, Robaye E. Screening for adjustment disorders and major depressive disorders in cancer inpatients. *Br J Psychiatry.* 1990; 156:79–83.

27. Hopwood P, Howell A, Maguire P. Psychiatric morbidity in patients with advanced cancer of the breast: prevalence measured by two self-rating questionnaires. *Br J Cancer.* 1991; 64:349–352.

28. Razavi D, Delvaux N, Bredart A, et al. Screening for psychiatric disorders in a lymphoma outpatient population. *Eur J Cancer.* 1992; 28A:1869–1872.

29. Brandenberg Y, Bolund C, Sigurdardottir V. Anxiety and depressive symptoms at different stages of malignant melanoma. *Psycho-oncology.* 1992; 1:71–78.

30. Ibbotson T, Maguire P, Selby T, et al. Screening for anxiety and depression in cancer patients: the effects of disease and treatment. *Eur J Cancer.* 1994; 30A:37–40.

31. Moorey S, Greer S, Watson M, et al. The factor structure and factor stability of the Hospital Anxiety and Depression Scale in patients with cancer. *Br J Psychiatry.* 1991; 158:255–259.

32. Hopwood P, Howell A, Maguire P. Screening for psychiatric morbidity in patients with advanced breast cancer: validation of two self-report questionnaires. *Br J Cancer.* 1991; 64:353–356.

33. De Haes JCJM, Pruyn JFA, van Knippenberg FCE. Klachtenlijst voor kankerpatienten, eerste ervaringen. *Ned Tijdschr Psychol.* 1983; 38:403–408.

34. De Haes JCJM, van Knippenberg FCE, Neijut JP. Measuring psychological and physical distress in cancer patients: structure and application of the Rotterdam Symptom Checklist. *Br J Cancer.* 1990; 62:1034–1038.

35. Maguire GP, Lee EG, Bevington DJ, et al. Psychiatric problems in the first year after mastectomy. *Br Med J.* 1978; 1:963–965.

36. Hughes J. Emotional reactions to the diagnosis and treatment of early breast cancer. *J Psychosom Res.* 1982; 26:277–283.

37. Dean C. Psychiatric morbidity following mastectomy: preoperative predictors and type of illness. *J Psychosom Res.* 1987; 31:385–392.

38. Lee MS, Love SB, Mitchel JB, et al. Mastectomy or conservation for early breast cancer: psychological morbidity. *Eur J Cancer.* 1992; 28A:1340–1344.

39. Watson M, Greer S, Rowden L, et al. Relationships between emotional control, adjustment to cancer and depression and anxiety in breast cancer patients. *Psychol Med.* 1991; 21:51–57.

40. Pinder KL, Ramirez AJ, Black E, et al. Psychiatric disorders in patients with advanced breast cancer: Prevalence and associated factors. *Eur J Cancer.* 1993; 29A:524–527.

41. Peck A. Emotional reactions to having cancer. *Am J Roentgenol Radiat Ther Nucl Med.* 1972; 114:591–599.

42. Peck A, Boland J. Emotional reactions to radiation treatment. *Cancer.* 1977; 40:180–184.

43. Derogatis L, Morrow G, Fetting J, et al. The prevalence of psychiatric disorders among cancer patients. *JAMA.* 1983; 249:751–757.

44. Carroll BT, Kathol, RG, Noyes R, et al. Screening for depression and anxiety in cancer ptients using the hospital Anxiety and Depression Scale. *Gen Hosp Psychiatry.* 1993; 15:69–74.

45. Plumb MM, Holland J. Comparative studies of psychological function in patients with advanced cancer. II. Interview rated current and past psychiatric symptoms. *Psychosom Med.* 1981; 43:243–254.

46. Farber JM, Weinerman BH, Kuypers JA. Psychosocial distress in oncology outpatients. *J Psychosoc Oncol.* 1984; 2:109–118.

47. Stefanek ME, Derogatis LR, Shaw A. Psychological distress among oncology outpatients: prevalence and severity. *Psychosomatics.* 1987; 28:530–539.

48. Kaasa S, Malt U, Jagen S, et al. Psychological distress in cancer patients with advanced disease. *Radiother Oncol.* 1993; 27:193–197.

49. Davies ADM, Davies C, Delpo MC. Depression and anxiety in patients undergoing diagnostic investigations for head and neck cancers. *Br J Psychiatry.* 1986; 149:491–493.

50. Bergman B, Sullivan M, Sorenson S. Quality of life during chemotherapy for small cell lung cancer. I. An evaluation of generic health measures. *Acta Oncol.* 1991; 30:947–957.

51. Wells KB, Golding JM, Burnam A. Psychiatric disorders in a sample of the general population with and without chronic medical conditions. *Am J Psychiatry.* 1988; 145:976–981.

52. Kessler RC, McGonagle KA, Zhao S et al. Lifetime and 12-month prevalence of DSM-III-R psychiatric disorders in the United States. *Arch Gen Psychiatry.* 1994; 51:8–19.

53. Wald TG, Kathol RG, Noyes R, et al. Rapid relief of anxiety in cancer patients with both alprazolam and placebo. *Psychosomatics.* 1993; 34:324–332.

54. Popkin MK, Callies AL, Colon EA, Stiebel J. Adjustment disorders in medically ill inpatients referred for consultation in a university hospital. *Psychosomatics.* 1990; 31:410–414.

55. Robinson JK, Bosher ML, Danak DA, Peterson KJ. Depression and anxiety in cancer patients: evidence for different causes. *J Psychosom Res.* 1985; 29:133–138.

56. Cassileth BR, Lusk EJ, Strouse TB, et al. Psychosocial status in chronic illness: A comparative analysis of six diagnostic groups. *N Engl J Med.* 1984; 311:506–511.

57. Hoeper EW, Nycz GR, Cleary PD, et al. Estimated prevalence of RDC mental disorder in primary medical care. *Int J Ment Health.* 1979; 8:6–15.

58. Schulberg HC, Saul M, McCelland M, et al. Assessing depression in primary medical and psychiatric practices. *Arch Gen Psychiatry.* 1985; 42:1164–1170.

59. Von Korff M, Shapiro S, Burke JD, et al. Anxiety and depression in a primary care clinic. *Arch Gen Psychiatry.* 1987; 44:152–156.

60. Schwab JJ, McGinness NH, Marder L et al. Evaluation of anxiety in medical patients. *J Chron Dis.* 1966; 19:1049–1057.

61. Cassileth BR, Lusk EJ, Hutter R, et al. Concordance of depression and anxiety in patients with cancer. *Psychol Rep.* 1984; 54:588–590.

62. Massie MJ, Holland JC. Consultation and liaison issues in cancer care. *Psychiatr Med.* 1987; 5:343–359.

63. Hinton J. Psychiatric consultation in fatal illness. *Proc R Soc Med.* 1972; 65:1035–1038.

64. Levine PM, Silverfarb PM, Lipowski ZJ. Mental disorders in cancer patients: a study of 100 psychiatric referrals. *Cancer.* 1978; 42:1385–1391.

65. Sharer AU, Schreiber S, Galai T, McLoud RN. Posttraumatic stress disorder following medical events. *Br J Clin Psychol.* 1993; 32:247–253.

66. Stefanek ME, Shaw A, DeGeorge D, Tsottles N. Illness-related worry among cancer patients: prevalence, severity, and content. *Cancer Invest.* 1989; 7:365–371.

67. Greenberg DB. Strategic use of benzodiazepines in cancer patients. *Oncology.* 1991; 5:83–95.

68. Hamner MB. Exacerbation of posttraumatic stress disorder symptoms with medical illness. *Gen Hosp Psychiatry.* 1994; 16:135–137.

69. Brennan SC, Redd WH, Jacobsen PB, et al. Anxiety and panic during magnetic resonance scans. *Lancet.* 1988; 2:512.

70. Goldberg RJ, Cullen LO. Factors important to psychosocial adjustment to cancer: a review of the evidence. *Soc Sci Med.* 1985; 20:803–807.

71. Cassileth BR, Lusk EJ, Strouse TB, et al. A psychological analysis of cancer patients and their next-of-kin. *Cancer.* 1985; 55:72–76.

72. Morris T. Psychological adjustment to mastectomy. *Cancer Treatment Rev.* 1979; 6:41–61.

73. Angst J, Vollrath M. The natural history of anxiety disorders. *Acta Psychiatr Scand.* 1991; 84:446–452.

74. Greer S. Psycho-oncology: its aims, achievements, and future tasks. *Psycho-oncology.* 1994; 3:87–101.

75. Bloom JR. Social support and adjustment to breast cancer. In: Anderson B, ed. *Women and Cancer.* New York: Springer; 1986; 204–229.

76. Ell KO, Mantell JE, Hamovitch MB, Nishimoto RH. Social support, sense of control, and coping among patients with breast, lung or colorectal cancer. *J Psychosoc Oncol.* 1989; 7:63-89.

77. Weisman AD, Worden JW. Coping and vulnerability in cancer patients. Boston, MA: Privately printed; 1977.

78. Noyes R, Kathol RG, Debelius-Enemark P, et al. Distress associated with cancer as measured by the Illness Distress Scale. *Psychosomatics.* 1990; 31:321–330.

79. Cassileth BR, Lusk EJ, Walsh WP. Anxiety levels in patients with malignant disease. *Hosp J.* 1986; 2:57–69.

80. Schag CAC, Heinrich RL. Anxiety in medical situations: adult cancer patients. *J Clin Psychol.* 1989; 45:20–27.

81. Bard M, Sutherland AM. Psychological impact of cancer and its treatment: IV Adaptation to radical mastectomy. *Cancer.* 1955; 8:656.

82. McArdle J, Hughson AJM, McArdle CS. Reduced psychological morbidity after breast conservation. *Br J Surg.* 1990; 77:1221–1223.

83. Cassileth BR, Knuiman MW, Abeloff G, et al. Anxiety levels in patients randomized to adjuvant therapy versus observation for early breast cancer. *J Clin Oncol.* 1986; 4:972-974.

84. Cella DF, Pratt A, Holland JC. Persistent anticipatory nausea, vomiting, and anxiety in cured Hodgkin's disease patients after completion of chemotherapy. *Am J Psychiatry.* 1986; 43:641–643.

85. Olafsdottir M, Sjoder P-O, Westling B. Prevalence and prediction of chemotherapy-related anxiety, nausea and vomiting in cancer patients. *Behav Res Ther.* 1986; 24:59–66.

86. Kvale G, Glimelius B, Hoffman K, Sjoden P. Pre-chemotherapy nervousness as a marker for anticipatory nausea: a case of a non-causal predictor. *Psycho-oncology.* 1993; 2:33–41.

87. Jacobsen PB, Bovberg DH, Redd WH. Anticipatory anxiety in women receiving chemotherapy for breast cancer. *Health Psychol.* 1993; 12:469–475.

88. Andrykowski MA, Gregg ME. The role of psychological variables in post chemotherapy nausea: anxiety and expectation. *Psychosom Med.* 1992; 54:48–58.

89. Andrykowski MA. The role of anxiety in the development of anticipatory nausea in cancer chemotherapy: a review and synthesis. *Psychosom Med.* 1990; 52:458–475.

90. Forester BM, Kornfeld DS, Fleiss J. Psychiatric aspects of radiotherapy. *Am J Psychiatry.* 1978; 135:960–963.

91. Munro AJ, Biruls R, Griffin AJ, et al. Distress associated with radiotherapy for malignant disease: A quantitative analysis based on patients perceptions. *Br J Cancer.* 1989; 60:370–374.

92. Andersen BL, Karlson JA, Anderson B, Tewfik HH. Anxiety and cancer treatment: Response to stressful radiotherapy. *Health Psychol.* 1984; 3:535–551.

93. Holland JC, Rowland J, Lebovits A, et al. Reactions to cancer treatment: Assessment of emotional response to adjuvant radiotherapy as a guide to planned intervention. *Psychiatr Clin North Am.* 1979; 2:347–358.

94. Ahles TA, Blanchard EB, Ruckdeschel JC. The multidimensional nature of cancer-related pain. *Pain.* 1983; 17:277–288.

95. Sternbach RA. *Pain Patients: Traits and Treatment.* New York: Academic Press; 1974.

96. Massie MJ, Holland JC. The cancer patient with pain: psychiatric complications and their management. *Med Clin North Am.* 1987; 71:243–258.

97. Lishman W. *Organic Psychiatry.* London: Blackwell; 1987: 428–485.

98. Dietch JT. Diagnosis of organic anxiety disorders. *Psychosomatics.* 21981; 2:661–669.

99. Massie MJ, Holland JC, Glass E. Delirium in terminally ill cancer patients. *Am J Psychiatry.* 1983; 140:1048–1050.

100. Goldberg RJ, Posner DA. Anxiety in the medically ill. In: Stoudemire A, Fogel BS, eds. *Psychiatric Care of the Medical Patient.* Oxford: Oxford University Press; 1993: 87–104.

101. Kathol RG, Dalahunt JW. The relationship of anxiety and depression to symptoms of hyperthyroidism using operational criteria. *Gen Hosp Psychiatry.* 1986; 8:23–28.

102. Starkman MN, Zelnik TC, Nesse RM, et al. Anxiety in patients with pheochromocytomas. *Arch Intern Med.* 1985; 145:248–252.

103. Lawlor BA. Hypocalcemia, hypoparathyroidsim, and organic anxiety syndrome. *J Clin Psychiatry.* 1988; 49:317–318.

104. Holland JC, Hughes A, Korzan AH, Tross S, et al. Comparative psychological disturbance in patients with pancreatic and gastric cancer. *Am J Psychiatry.* 1986; 143:982–986.

105. Strain F, Ploog D. Anxiety related to nervous system dysfunction. In: Noyes R, Roth M, Burrows GD, eds. *Handook of Anxiety,* vol. 2. Amsterdam: Elsevier; 1988: 431–475.

106. Stiefel FC, Breitbart WS, Holland JC. Cortiscosteroids in cancer: neuropsychiatric complications. *Cancer Invest.* 1989; 7:479–491.

107. Fleishman SB, Lavin MR, Sattler M, Szarka H. Antiemetic-induced akathisia in cancer patients. *Am J Psychiatry.* 1994; 151:763–765.

108. Fleischhacker WW, Roth SD, Kane JM. The pharmacologic treatment of neuroleptic-induced akathisia. *J Clin Psychopharmacol.* 1990; 10:12–21.

109. Hall RCW. Psychiatric effects of thyroid hormone disturbance. *Psychosomatics.* 1983; 24:7–18.

110. Weiner N. Norephedrine, ephedrine, and sympathomimetic amines. In: Goodman AG, Goodman LS, Gilman A, eds. *Pharmacological Basis of Therapeutics.* New York: Macmillan; 1980: 163.

111. Lerner WD, Fallon HJ. The alcohol withdrawal syndrome. *N Engl J Med.* 1985; 313:951–952.

112. Noyes R, Garvey M, Cook B, Perry PJ. Benzodiazepine withdrawal: a review of the evidence. *J Clin Psychiatry.* 1988; 49:382–389.

113. Kathol RG, Wenzel RP. Natural history of symptoms of depression and anxiety during inpatient treatment on general medicine wards. *J Gen Intern Med.* 1992; 7:287–293.

114. Lloyd GG, Parker AC, Ludlam CA, McGuire RJ. Emotional impact of diagnosis and early treatment of lymphomas. *J Psychosom Res.* 1984; 28:157–162.

115. Devlen J, Maguire P, Phillips P, et al. Psychological problems associated with diagnosis and treatment of lymphomas. II. Prospective Study. *Br Med J Clin Res Ed.* 1987; 295:955–957.

116. Grandi S, Fava GA, Cunsolo A, et al. Rating depression and anxiety after mastectomy: observer versus self-rating scales. *Int J Psychiatry Med.* 1990; 20:163–171.

117. Massie MJ, Shakin EJ. Management of depression and anxiety in cancer patients. In: Breitbart W, Holland JC, eds. *Psychiatric Aspects of Symptom Management in Cancer Patients.* Washington, DC: American Psychiatric Press; 1993: 1–21.

118. Egbert LD, Battit GE, Welch CE, Bartlett MK. Reduction of postoperative pain by encouragement and instruction of patients. *N Engl J Med.* 1964; 270:825–827.

119. Maguire P, Faulkner A, Regnard C. Eliciting the current problems of the patient with cancer. *Palliative Med.* 1993; 7:63-68.

120. Fleming U. Relaxation therapy for far-advanced cancer. *Practitioner.* 1985; 229:471–475.

121. Jaeger H, Morrow GR, Brescia F: A survey of psychotropic drug utilization by patients with advanced neoplastic disease. *Gen Hosp Psychiatry.* 1985; 7:353–360.

122. Stiefel FC, Kornblith AB, Holland JC. Changes in the prescription patterns of psychotropic drugs for cancer patients during a 10-year period. *Cancer.* 1990; 65:1048–1053.

123. Holland JC, Morrow G, Schmale A, et al. A randomized clinical trial of alprazolam versus progressive muscle relaxation in cancer patients with anxiety and depressive symptoms. *J Clin Oncol.* 1991; 9:1004–1011.

124. Triozzi PL, Goldstein D, Laszlo J. Contributions of benzodiazepines to cancer therapy. *Cancer Invest.* 1988; 6:103–111.

125. Massie MJ, Lesko L. Psychopharmacological management. In: Holland JC, Rowland JH, eds. *Handbook of Psychooncology: Psychological Care of the Patient with Cancer.* New York: Oxford University Press; 1989: 470–491.

126. Klein DS. Prevention of claustrophobia induced by MR imaging: use of alprazolam. *Am J Roentgenol.* 1991; 156:633.

127. Fawzy FI, Fawzy WW, Arndt LA, Pasnau RO. Critical review of psychosocial interventions in cancer care. *Arch Gen Psychiatry.* 1995; 52:100–113.

128. Jacobs C, Ross RD, Walker IM, Stockdale FE. Behavior of cancer patients: a randomized study of the effects of education and peer support groups. *Am J Clin Oncol.* 1983; 6:347–353.

129. Ali NS, Khalil HZ. Effect of psychoeducational intervention on anxiety among Egyptian bladder cancer patients. *Cancer Nurs.* 1989; 12:236–242.

130. Rainey LC. Effects of psychoeducational intervention on anxiety among Egyptian bladder cancer patients. *Cancer Nurs*. 1989; 12:236–242.

131. Richardson JL, Shelton DR, Krailom M, Levine AM. The effect of compliance with treatment on survival among patients with hematologic malignancies. *J Clin Oncol*. 1990; 8:356–364.

132. Gruber BL, Hersh SP, Hall NRS, et al. Immunological responses of breast cancer patients to behavioral interventions. *Biofeedback Self Regul*. 1993; 18:1–21.

133. Baider L, Uziely B, De-Nour AK. Progressive muscle relaxation and guided imagery in cancer patients. *Gen Hosp Psychiatry*. 1994; 16:340–347.

134. Contanch PH. Relaxation training for control of nausea and vomiting in patients receiving chemotherapy. *Cancer Nurs*. 1983; 6:277–283.

135. Sims SER: Relaxation training as a technique for helping patients cope with the experience of cancer: a selective review of the literature. *J Adv Nurs*. 1987; 12:583–591.

136. Redd WH. Behavioral approaches to treatment-related distress. *Cancer*. 1988; 38:138–145.

137. Jacobsen PB, Redd WH. Behavioral aspects of oncology. In: Byrne DG, Caddy GR, eds. *Behavioral Medicine: International Perspectives*. Norwood, NJ: Ablex Pub. Corp.; 1992; 293–315.

138. Redd WH. Use of behavioral methods to control the aversive effects of chemotherapy. *J Psychosoc Oncol*. 1986; 3:17–22.

139. Wilson-Barnett J. Psychological reaction to medical procedures. *Psychotherapy Psychosom*. 1992; 57:118–127.

140. Melamed BG, Seigal LJ. *Behavioral Medicine*. New York: Spring Publishing Co.; 1980.

141. Ost LG, Lindahl IL, Sterner U et al. Exposure in vivo vs. applied relaxation in the treatment of blood phobia. *Behav Res Ther*. 1984; 22:205–216.

142. Ost LG, Sterner U, Fellenius J. Applied tension, applied relaxation and the combination in treatment of blood phobia. *Behav Res Ther*. 1989; 27:109–121.

143. Greer S, Moorey S, Baruch J, et al. Adjuvant psychological therapy for patients with cancer: a prospective randomized trial. *Br Med J*. 1992; 304:675–680.

144. Moorey S, Greer S, Watson M, et al. Adjuvant psychological therapy for patients with cancer: Outcome at one year. *Psycho-oncology*. 1994; 3:39–46.

145. Spiegel D, Bloom JR, Yalom I. Group support for patients with metastatic cancer. *Arch Gen Psychiatry*. 1981; 38:527–533.

48

Delirium

WILLIAM BREITBART AND KENNETH R. COHEN

Delirium is an ancient disorder first described almost 2500 years ago (1). Delirium is derived etymologically from the Latin—*de* meaning down or away from, and *lira* meaning a furrow or track in the fields. Delirium thus means to "be off the track." More than 25 different terms have been commonly used to denote delirium over the last years, including confusion, acute confusional states, acute brain failure, acute dementia, acute organic syndrome, cerebral insufficiency, metabolic encephalopathy, organic brain syndrome, reversible toxic psychosis, and intensive care unit psychosis (2). Delirium is a common and often serious medical complication in the management of the patient with cancer. Behavioral dysregulation, cognitive disturbance, and lack of appropriate judgment can impede the delivery of good medical care. In addition, delirium is usually a sign of significant disturbance of multiple medical etiologies. Delirium in cancer is associated with significant morbidity for patients and families, and increased mortality. The signs and symptoms of delirium can be diverse and are sometimes mistaken for other psychiatric disorders such as mood or anxiety disorders. Practitioners in the psycho-oncology setting must be able to diagnose delirium accurately, recommend appropriate assessment, and be knowledgeable of complications of delirium and of the pharmacologic and nonpharmacologic interventions currently available.

PREVALENCE

Delirium is one of the most common mental disorders encountered in general hospital practice. Knight and Folstein (3) estimated that 33% of hospitalized medically ill patients have serious cognitive impairments. Massie and et al. found delirium in 25% of 334 hospitalized cancer patients seen in psychiatric consultation (4) and in 85% (11 of 13) of terminal cancer patients (5), Pereira et al. found the prevalence of cogivitive impairment in cancer inpatients to be 44%, and just

prior to death, the prevalence rose to 62.1% (6). Delirium also occurs in up to 51% of postoperative patients (1,7). The incidence of delirium is currently increasing, which reflects the growing numbers of elderly, who are particularly susceptible (8). Studies of elderly patients admitted to medical wards estimate that between 30% and 50% of patients age 70 years or older showed symptoms of delirium at some point during hospitalization (9,10). In two separate studies, the incidence of delirium in elderly patients admitted to general hospital wards was 16% (11,12). In a British geriatric multicenter study, 35% of patients age 65 years or older were found to be delirious upon admission or to develop delirium during the index hospitalization (13). This study also found that 25% of the elderly patients evaluated as cognitively intact on admission could be expected to develop delirium during the first month of hospitalization. In addition, those patients with dementia are at even greater risk, and thus as the prevalence of dementia increases with the aging of the population, so the incidence of delirium may also be expected to rise (Table 48.1).

CLINICAL FEATURES

The clinical features of delirium are quite numerous and include a variety of neuropsychiatric symptoms that are also common to other psychiatric disorders such as depression, dementia, and psychosis (2). Clinical features of delirium include: prodromal symptoms (restlessness, anxiety, sleep disturbance, irritability); rapidly fluctuating course; reduced attention (easily distractible); altered arousal; increased or decreased psychomotor activity; disturbance of sleep–wake cycle; affective symptoms (emotional lability, sadness, anger, euphoria); altered perceptions (misperceptions, illusions, delusions (poorly formed), hallucinations); disorganized thinking and incoherent speech; disorientation to time, place, or person; memory

TABLE 48.1. *DSM-IV Cognitive Disorders*

A. General cognitive impairment
  1. Delirium
    a. Delirium due to a general medical condition
    b. Substance-induced delirium
    c. Delirium due to multiple etiologies
    d. Delirium not otherwise specified
  2. Dementia
    a. Dementia of the Alzheimer's type
    b. Vascular dementia
    c. Dementia due to other medical conditions
    d. Substance-induced persisting dementia
    e. Dementia due to multiple etiologies
    f. Dementia not otherwise specified
B. Specific cognitive impairment
  1. Amnestic disorders
    a. Amnestic disorders due to a general medical condition
    b. Substance-induced persisting amnestic disorder
    c. Amnestic disorder not otherwise specified
C. Cognitive disorder not otherwise specified

Source: Adapted from Tucker (76).

impairment (cannot register new material). Neurologic abnormalities can also be present during delirium, including cortical abnormalities (dysgraphia, constructional apraxia, dysnomic aphasia), motor abnormalities (tremor, asterixis, myoclonus, reflex and tone changes), and electroencephalogram (EEG) abnormalities (usually global slowing). It is this protean nature of delirious symptoms, the variability and fluctuation of clinical findings and the unclear and often contradictory definitions of the syndrome that has made delirium so difficult to diagnose and treat.

The definitions and descriptions (including diagnostic criteria) of delirium over the years have reflected the evolution of our understanding of delirium, from first purely descriptive symptomatology towards pathophysiologic concepts. From the wide array of neuropsychiatric symptoms, certain clinical criteria have been recognized as being essential to and most specific to delirium diagnosis: (*1*) chronological features — i.e., acute or subacute onset, as well as the transient and reversible nature of the disorder, (*2*) pathognomonic clinical features. Lipowski (14) emphasized certain clinical symptoms as pathognomonic of delirium: disordered attention and cognition, accompanied by disturbances of psychomotor behavior and the sleep–wake cycle. The essential clinical features of delirium as described in the American Psychiatric Association's (APA) *Diagnostic and Statistical Manual of Mental Disorders*, DSM-III, in 1980 (15) were (*1*) clouding of consciousness and impaired attention, (*2*) impaired cognition (disorientation and memory disorders), and two of the following: (*3*) psychomotor behavior distur-

bance, (*4*) sleep-wake cycle (arousal systems?) anomalies, (*5*) perceptual disturbances, and (*6*) incoherent speech, in the context of acute onset and transitory duration. DSM-III-R (16) further added disorganized thinking. The DSM-IV diagnostic criteria are described in a following section.

PATHOPHYSIOLOGY

In spite of very little being known about the neuropathogenesis of delirium, its symptoms suggest that it is a dysfunction of multiple regions of the brain. Delirium has been characterized as an etiologically nonspecific, global, cerebral dysfunction characterized by concurrent disturbances of level of consciousness, attention, thinking, perception, memory, psychomotor behavior, emotion, and the sleep–wake cycle. Disorientation, fluctuation, or waxing and waning of these symptoms, as well as acute or abrupt onset of such disturbances, are other critical features of delirium. Delirium, in contrast to dementia, is conceptualized as a *reversible* process. Reversibility of the process of delirium is often possible even in the patient with advanced illness; however it may *not* be reversible in the last 24–48 h of life.

Our current understanding of delirium is that it involves a reversible disruption of cerebral attentional processes due to metabolic anomalies affecting certain neurotransmitters. Wise and Brandt (2) describe delirium as "a transient, essentially reversible dysfunction in cerebral metabolism that has an acute or subacute onset and is manifest clinically by a wide array of neuropsychiatric abnormalities." Although delirium involves widespread metabolic cerebral dysfunction, recent work in the pathophysiology of delirium has suggested several discrete etiologic models for this dysfunction.

Another view of delirium focuses on the extent of brain dysfunction: "Delirium is often considered a global and nonspecific disorder of brain function. This characterization may be appropriate for delirium caused by such widespread systemic processes as hypoxia, hypothermia, and acid-base disorders. However, several important etiologies of delirium may be associated with more limited and specific brain pathophysiology" (17). In other words, delirium can be seen either as (*1*) a global and nonspecific disorder for brain function implying a generalized dysfunction in cerebral metabolism or as (*2*) a more limited and specific brain pathology initially caused by the derangement of a specific neurotransmitter or set of neurotransmitters. Evidence is growing to support the contention that delirium is a heterogeneous group of different disorders with different symptomatologies. As examples, perturbations of certain neurotransmitters produce specific pathophysiologic changes resulting in delirious symptoms [adapted from Ross (17)]: (1) Anticholinergic drugs produce delirium through suppression of cholinergic systems; (2) some hallucinatory drugs such as lysergic acid diethylamide (LSD) involve antagonism of the serotonin system; (3) phencyclidine produces delirium by blocking glutamate-sensitive N-methyl-D-aspartate receptors in the central nervous system (CNS); (4) hepatic encephalopathy and benzodiazepine intoxication both produce delirium through overstimulation of γ-aminobutyric acid (GABA) systems; (5) benzodiazepine withdrawal states, as well as alcoholic withdrawal, produce delirium through acute understimulation of GABA systems; (6) in a variety of etiologies, such as the anticholinergic-induced type, delirium symptoms such as hallucinations seem to involve a further perturbation — a relative overactivation of the dopaminergic mesocortical system responsible for many of the features of hyperactive delirium.

The global dysfunction model, however, seems to apply more readily to deliria where multiple neurotransmitter systems or a cascade of interacting neurotransmitter systems are involved, such as in infection or hypoxia. This global model may also be interpreted as a final end pathway common to the different specific etiologies of delirium. The metabolic basis of the final common pathway, however, is open to question. Based on studies in Alzheimer's disease, perturbations in second messenger systems have been suggested: "The diversity of the changes in neurotransmitters suggests that alterations in second-messenger systems may be the more fundamental change. Results clearly implicate second messenger systems such as calcium, cyclic GMP, and the phosphatidylinositol cascade" (18).

SUBTYPES OF DELIRIUM

Lipowski (14) clinically described two subtypes of delirium, based on psychomotor behavior and arousal levels. The subtypes included the hyperactive (or agitated, or hyperalert) subtype and the hypoactive (or lethargic, or hypoalert) subtype (Table 48.2). Others have included a "mixed" subtype (2) with alternating features of each. Ross (17) suggests that the hyperactive form is most often characterized by hallucinations, delusions, agitation, and disorientation, while the hypoactive form is characterized by confusion and sedation, but is rarely accompanied by hallucinations, delusions, or illusions. Ross further suggests that specific delirium subtypes are related to specific etiologies of delirium and have unique pathophysiologies; i.e., hyperactive forms being typical of withdrawal syndromes and anticholinergic-induced delirium, while the hypoactive forms are typical of hepatic or metabolic encephalopathies, acute intoxications from sedatives, or hypoxia. The pathophysiology of a hyperactive delirium due to benzodiazepine withdrawal is characterized by elevated or normal cerebral metabolism, fast or normal EEG, and reduced activity in GABA systems, while the pathophysiology of a hypoactive delirium due to benzodiazepine intoxication is characterized by decreased global cerebral metabolism, diffuse slowing of the EEG, and overstimulation of GABA systems.

DIAGNOSTIC CRITERIA [FROM DSM-IV (19)]

The essential feature of a delirium is a disturbance of consciousness that is accompanied by a change in cognition that cannot be better accounted for by a preexisting or evolving dementia. The disturbance develops over a short period of time, usually hours to days, and tends to fluctuate during the course of

TABLE 48.2. *Contrasting Features of Subtypes of Delirium*

	Hyperactive	Hypoactive
Type	Hyperalert Agitated	Hypoalert Lethargic
Symptoms	Hallucinations Delusions Hyperarousal	Sleepy Withdrawn Slowed
Examples	Withdrawal syndromes (benziodiazepines, alcohol)	Encephalopathies (hepatic, metabolic) Benzodiazepine intoxication
Pathophysiology	Elevated or normal cerebral metabolism EEG: fat or normal Reduced activity in GABA systems	Decreased global cerebral metabolism EEG: diffuse slowing Overstimulation of GABA systems

the day. There is evidence from the history, physical examination, or laboratory tests that the delirium is a direct physiological consequence of a general medical condition, substance intoxication or withdrawal, use of a medication, or toxin exposure, or a combination of these factors (Table 48.3).

The disturbance in consciousness is manifested by a reduced clarity of awareness of the environment. The ability to focus, sustain, or shift attention is impaired (Criterion A). Questions must be repeated because the individual's attention wanders, or the individual may persevere with an answer to a previous question rather than appropriately shift attention. The person is easily distracted by irrelevant stimuli. Because of these problems, it may be difficult (or impossible) to engage the person in conversation.

There is an accompanying change in cognition (which may include memory impairment, disorientation, or language disturbance) or development of a perceptual disturbance (Criterion B). Memory impairment is most commonly evident in recent memory and can be tested by asking the person to remember several unrelated objects or a brief sentence, and then to repeat them after a few minutes of distraction. Disorien- tation is usually manifested by the individual being disoriented to time (e.g., thinking it is morning in the middle of the night), or being disoriented to place (e.g., thinking he or she is at home rather than in a hospital). In mild delirium, disorientation to time may be the first symptom to appear. Disorientation to self is less common. Language disturbance may be evident as dysnomia (i.e., the impaired ability to name objects), or dysgraphia (i.e., the impaired ability to write). In some cases, speech is rambling and irrelevant, in others pressured and incoherent, with unpredictable switching from subject to subject. It may be difficult for the clinician to assess for changes in cognitive function because the individual may be inattentive and incoherent. Under these circumstances, it is helpful to review carefully the individual's history and to obtain information from other informants, particularly family members.

Perceptual disturbances may include misinterpretations, illusions, or hallucinations. For example, the banging of a door may be mistaken for a gunshot (misinterpretation); the folds of the bedclothes may appear to be animate objects (illusion); or the person may "see" a group of people hovering over the bed when no-one is actually there (hallucination). Although sensory misperceptions are most commonly visual, they may occur in other sensory modalities as well. Misperceptions range from simple and uniform to highly complex. The individual may have a delusional conviction of the reality of the hallucinations and exhibit emotional and behavioral responses in keeping with their content.

The disturbance develops over a short period of time and tends to fluctuate during the course of the day (Criterion C). For example, during the morning hospital rounds, the person may be coherent and cooperative, but at night insist on pulling out intravenous lines and going home to parents who died years ago.

Thus, less diagnostic significance has now been placed on incoherent speech, disturbance of sleep–wake cycle, and increased or decreased psychomotor activity. These progressive changes in DSM criteria for delirium have resulted in varying sensitivity in the detection of delirium for the different versions (20).

AROUSAL AND COGNITION

The emphasis in defining delirium in recent years has thus shifted from an extensive list of symptoms to the two essential concepts of disordered attention (arousal) and cognition, while continuing to recognize the importance of acute onset and organic etiology. Ross (17) now defines delirium simply as "a disorder of cognition and alteration in arousal and attention", in contrast to dementia, which is a disorder primarily of cognition. Because the disorder of arousal/attention is pathognomonic to delirium, the pathophysiology of alterations in CNS arousal/attention has become paramount in delirium research. New models using

TABLE 48.3. *DSM-IV Criteria for Delirium due to a General Medical Condition*

Criterion A	Disturbance of consciousness (i.e., reduced clarity of awareness of the environment) with reduced ability to focus, sustain, or shift attention
Criterion B	Change in cognition (such as memory deficit, disorientation, language disturbance, or perceptual disturbance) that is not better accounted for by a preexisting, established, or evolving dementia
Criterion C	The disturbance develops over a short period of time (usually hours to days) and tends to fluctuate during the course of the day
Criterion D	There is evidence from the history, physical examination, or laboratory findings of a general medical condition judged to be etiologically related to the disturbance.

Source: Adapted from Tucker (76).

neural network theory have suggested that selective attention involves modulation of different neural systems so that competing perceptions of internal and external origin are held in relative abeyance, thereby allowing one to be selectively analyzed. In this view, delirium could involve an absence of modulation of competing perceptions so that the subject is uncontrollably and randomly dominated by them, probably with relative predominance of internal compared to external perceptions, especially for patients with hallucinations (21).

ASSESSMENT OF DELIRIUM

Historically, the major objective of clinical evaluation in the area of delirium has been to identification of delirious patients through the use of screening questionnaires; that is, instruments that are rapid and are easy to administer by minimally trained raters. More recently, with the development of standardized diagnostic classifications criteria of the DSM and International Classification of Diseases (ICD) systems, formally confirming the diagnosis of delirium for research purposes has become important. Emphasis has shifted to more sophisticated diagnostic instruments that maximize diagnostic precision and can be used by trained clinician and nonclinician raters. Measuring the severity of delirium once it has been diagnosed, differentiating subtypes, describing delirium in children, and identifying new specific etiologic subtypes (e.g., opioid-induced delirium) are some of the new challenges in this field (22).

Instruments for the evaluation of delirium have been grouped into four categories: (1) tests that measure cognitive impairment, which are usually used to screen for delirium, such as the Mini-Mental-Status Exam (MMSE); (2) delirium diagnostic instruments based on DSM or ICD criteria, which are used to make a yes/no judgment of the presence or absence of delirium (such as the confusion-assessment method); (3) delirium-specific numerical rating scales, whose scores can be used for likelihood of diagnosis or estimating severity, such as the Delirium Rating Scale (DRS); and (4) physiologic correlates of delirium using laboratory and paraclinical exams, whose precise role in screening, diagnosis, and severity evaluation has yet to be fully determined (see Table 48.4).

The MMSE, while not a screening tool specific for delirium, has become one of the most frequently used neuropsychological tests in clinical evaluation of delirium, and thus has become a de facto reference against which other instruments are judged (23). It was originally conceived as a brief (5–10 min) practical clinical instruments for distinguishing functional from organic mental status impairment. It includes 11 simple questions, including two with written answers, and yields a score that is a weighted sum of the items, with a maximum of 30 and a cutoff for cognitive impairment of 24. It assesses the subject's orientation to time and place, instantaneous recall, short-term memory, serial subtractions or reverse spelling, constructional capacities, and use of language. Although a score of 23 or less has generally been considered the cutoff for cognitive impairment, a three-tiered system is now becoming popular based on the results of new epidemiologic data: 24–30, no impairment; 18–23, mild impairment; 0–17, severe impairment (23). The MMSE has the advantage of being able to be administered by lay interviewers (24–27). Precise instructions for administering and scoring the exam have been provided (28), and useful suggestions such as using the three words "apple, penny, table" for the memory task as well as commonly used variations in administration have been published (23).

The DRS is a numerical rating scale that specifically integrates DSM-III criteria. It is a 10-item scale with items scored from 0 to 3 or 0 to 4 in the following domains: (1) temporal onset, (2) perceptual disturbance, (3) hallucinations, (4) delusions, (5) psychomotor behavior, (6) cognitive status, (7) physical disorder, (8) sleep–wake cycle disturbance, (9) lability of mood, and (10) variability of symptoms (29). A single validation study on a rather small clinical sample (20 delirious patients, nine schizophrenic patients, nine demented patients, and nine medical patients used as controls) offered some evidence of validation, but with certain methodologic shortcomings. A limitation of the DRS is that it was actually created and then validated using items more pertinent for diagnosing delirium than for rating its severity. Thus, although proposed as a severity-rating scale, it actually measures diagnostic certainty.

Because of the shortcomings with existing delirium assessment instruments, we developed a measure specifically designed to quantify the severity of delirium symptoms for use in clinical intervention trials. The Memorial Delirium Assessment Scale (MDAS) was designed with the intent that the instrument could be administered repeatedly within the same day, in order to allow for objective measurement of changes in delirium severity in response to medical changes or clinical interventions. Potential items were developed by the principal investigators (W.B., M.S.) and were reviewed with regard to content validity by a group of experienced consultation-liaison psychiatrists. The resulting instrument, the MDAS, is described below.

Memorial Delirium Assessment Scale (MDAS)

The MDAS is a 10-item, 4-point clinician-rated scale (possible range, 0–30) designed to quantify the severity of delirium in medically ill patients (30). Items included in the MDAS reflect the diagnostic criteria for delirium in the DSM-IV (19), as well as symptoms of delirium from earlier or alternative classification systems (e.g., DSM-III, DSM-III-R, ICD-9). Scale items assess disturbances in arousal and level of consciousness, as well as several areas of cognitive functioning (memory, attention, orientation, disturbances in thinking) and psychomotor activity. Items were anchored with statements reflecting the severity or intensity of the symptom, and were reviewed by experienced clinicians to ensure ease of administration and ability to generate accurate (reliable) ratings. The resulting scale, which requires approximately 10 min to administer (not including additional time necessary to establish rapport, review chart records, and speak to staff/family members), integrates behavioral observations and objective cognitive testing. When items cannot be administered, scores can be prorated from the remaining items to an equivalent 10-item score, however, this process was never necessary in the studies reported below (Table 48.4).[1]

ETIOLOGIES/DIFFERENTIAL DIAGNOSIS

Studies in patients with advanced cancer have demonstrated the potential utility of a thorough diagnostic assessment (31,32) When diagnostic information is available, specific therapy may be able to reverse delirium. One study found that 68% of delirious cancer patients could be improved, despite a 30 day mortality of 31% (32). Another found that one-third of the episodes of cognitive failure improved following evaluation that yielded a cause for these episodes in 43% (31).

The diagnostic work-up should include an assessment of potentially reversible causes of delirium. A full physical examination should assess for evidence of sepsis, dehydration or major organic failure. Medications that could contribute to delirium should be reviewed. A screen of laboratory parameters will allow assessment of the possible role of metabolic abnormalities, such as hypercalcemia, and other problems, such as hypoxia or disseminated intravascular coagulation. Imaging studies of the brain and assessment of the cerebrospinal fluid may be appropriate in some instances.

Delirium can be due either to the direct effects of cancer on the central nervous system CNS, or to indirect CNS effects of the disease or treatments (medications, electrolyte imbalance, failure of a vital organ or system, infection, vascular complications and preexisting cognitive impairment or dementia) (Table 48.5). Early symptoms of delirium can be misdiagnosed as anxiety, anger, depression, or psychosis. In any patient showing acute onset of agitation, impaired cognitive function, altered attention span, or a fluctuating level of consciousness, a diagnosis of delirium should be considered (33). A common error among medical and nursing staff is to conclude that a new psychological symptom is functional without completely ruling out all possible organic etiologies. Given the large numbers

TABLE 48.4. *Assessment Methods for Delirium in Cancer Patients*

Diagnostic classification systems
    DSM-IV
    ICD-9
    ICD-10

Diagnostic interviews/instruments
    Delirium Symptom Interview (DSI) (77)
    Confusion Assessment Method (CAM) (78)

Delirium rating scales
    Delirium Rating Scale (DRS) (29)
    Confusion Rating Scale (CRS) (79)
    Saskatoon Delirium Checklist (SDC) (80)
    Memorial Delirium Assessment Scale (MDAS) (30)

Cognitive impairment screening instruments
    Mini-Mental State Exam (MMSE) (81)
    Short Portable Mental Status Questionnaire (SPMSQ) (82)
    Cognitive Capacity Screening Examination (CCSE) (83)
    Blessed Orientation Memory Concentration Test (BOMC) (84)

1. Prorated scores are calculated by averaging the items completed and multiplying by 10. No data exist at present regarding the reliability of validity of prorated scores or the minimum number of items needed for accurate prorating. Whenever possible, the entire scale should be administered.

TABLE 48.5. *Causes of Delirium in Cancer Patients*

DIRECT
Primary brain tumor
Metastatic spread

INDIRECT
Metabolic encephalopathy due to organ failure
Electrolyte imbalance
Treatment side effects from
    Chemotherapeutic agents, steroids, and biological response modifiers
    Radiation
    Narcotics
    Anticholinergics
    Antiemetics
Infection
Hematologic abnormalities
Nutrition
Paraneoplastic syndromes

of drugs cancer patients require, and the fragile state of their physiologic functioning, even routinely ordered hypnotics are enough to tip patients over into a delirium. Narcotic analgesics such as levorphanol, morphine sulfate, and meperidine, are common causes of confusional states, particularly in the elderly and terminally ill (34). Chemotherapeutic agents known to cause delirium include methotrexate, fluorouracil, vincristine, vinblastine, bleomycin, BCNU (carmustine), cisplatin, asparaginase, procarbazine, and the glucocorticosteroids (Table 48.6) (35–40). Except for steroids, most patients receiving these agents will not develop prominent CNS effects. The spectrum of mental disturbances related to steroids includes minor mood lability, affective disorders (mania or depression), cognitive impairment (reversible dementia), and delirium (steroid psychosis). The incidence of these disorders range from 3% to 57% in noncancer populations, and they occur most commonly on higher doses. Symptoms usually develop within the first 2 weeks on steroids, but in fact can occur at any time, on any dose, even during the tapering phase (35). Prior psychiatric illness, or prior disturbance on steroids, is not a good predictor of susceptibility to, or the nature of, mental disturbance with steroids. These disorders are often rapidly reversible upon dose reduction or discontinuation (35).

When confronted with a delirium in the terminally ill or dying cancer patient, a differential diagnosis should always be formulated; however, studies should be pursued only when a suspected factor can be identified easily and treated effectively. Interestingly, Bruera et al. (41) reported that an etiology was discovered in less than 50% of terminally ill patients with cognitive failure.

MANAGEMENT

A standard approach for managing delirium in the cancer patient includes a search for underlying causes, correction of those factors and management of the symptoms of delirium. The treatment of delirium in the dying cancer patient is unique, however, because: (1) most often, the etiology of terminal delirium is often multifactorial or may not be found; (2) when a distinct cause is found, it is often irreversible (such as hepatic failure or brain metastases); (3) work-up may be limited by the setting (home, hospice); (4) the consultant's focus is usually on the patient's comfort, and ordinarily helpful diagnostic procedures that are unpleasant or painful (e.g., CT (computed tomography) scan, lumbar puncture) may be avoided.

In addition to seeking out and correcting the underlying cause for delirium, the first priority in managing a delirious patient is to ensure his or her safety. Symptomatic and supportive therapies are important (33). In fact, in the dying patient they may be the only steps taken. Fluid and electrolyte balance, nutrition and vitamins may be helpful. Measures to help reduce anxiety and disorientation (structure and familiarity) may include a quiet, well-lit room with familiar objects, a visible clock or calendar, and the presence of family. Judicious use of physical restraints, along with one-to-one nursing observation, may also be necessary and useful. Often, these supportive techniques alone are not effective, and symptomatic treatment with neuroleptic or sedative medications is necessary (Table 48.7). Sedation may be necessary to relieve severe agitation or insomnia (33).

TABLE 48.6. *Chemotherapies That Can Cause Delirium*

L-Asparaginase
Bleomycin
Carmustine (BCNU)
Cisplatin
Cytosine arabinoside (ara-C)
Fludarabine
Fluorouracil
Interferon
Interleukin
Isophosphamide
Methotrexate
Prednisone
Procarbazine
Vinblastine
Vincristine

TABLE 48.7. *Medications for Managing Delirium in Cancer Patients*

Generic Name	Approximate Daily Dosage
NEUROLEPTICS	
Haloperidol	0.5–5 mg every 2–12 h, PO, IV, SC, IM
Thiorodazine	10–75 mg every 4–8 h, PO
Chlorpromazine	12.5–50 mg every 4–12 h, PO, IV, IM
Molindone	10–50 mg every 8–12 h, PO
Risperidone	1–3 mg every 12 h, PO
Methotrimeprazine	12.5–50 mg every 4–8 h, IV, SC, PO
BENZODIAZEPINES	
Lorazepam	0.5–2.0 mg every 1–4 h, PO, IV, IM
Midazolam	30–100 mg every 24 h, IV, SC
ANESTHETICS	
Propofol	10–50 mg every h, IV

One hypothesis is postulated that an imbalance of central cholinergic and adrenergic mechanisms underlies delirium, and so a dopamine-blocking drug may initiate a rebalancing of these systems (42). Haloperidol, a neuroleptic agent that is a potent dopamine blocker, is the drug of choice in the treatment of delirium in the medically ill (33,43–45). Haloperidol in low doses (1–3 mg) is usually effective in targeting agitation, paranoia, and fear. Typically 0.5–1.0 mg haloperidol (PO, IV, IM, SC) is administered, with repeat doses every 45–60 min titrated against target symptoms (5,46,47). An intravenous route can facilitate rapid onset of medication effects. If intravenous access is unavailable, one can start with intramuscular or subcutaneous administration and switch to the oral route when possible. The majority of delirious patients can be managed with oral haloperidol. Parenteral doses are approximately twice as potent as oral doses. Delivery of haloperidol by the subcutaneous route is utilized by many palliative care practitioners (48,49). In general, doses need not exceed 20 mg of haloperidol in a 24 h period; however, there are those that advocate high doses (up to 250 mg per 24 h usually intravenously) in selected cases (43,44,50). A common strategy in the management of symptoms related to delirium is to add parenteral lorazepam to a regimen of haloperidol (43,44,50). Lorazepam (0.5–1.0 mg every 1–2 h, PO or IV), along with haloperidol, may be more effective in rapidly sedating the agitated delirious patient. In a double-blind, randomized comparison trial of haloperidol versus chlorpromazine versus lorazepam, Breitbart et al. demonstrated that lorazepam alone, in doses up to 8 mg in a 12 h period, was ineffective in the treatment of delirium, and in fact contributed to worsening delirium and cognitive impairment (51). Both neuroleptic drugs, however, in low doses (approximately 2 mg of haloperidol equivalent per 24 h) were highly effective in controlling the symptoms of delirium (dramatic improvement in DRS scores) and improving cognitive function (dramatic improvement in MMSE scores). In addition, halperidol has been found effective in improving cognitive deficits in both hypoactive and hyperactive delirium.

Methotrimeprazine (IV or SC) is often utilized to control confusion and agitation in terminal delirium (52). Dosages range from 12.5 mg to 50 mg every 4–8 h up to 300 mg per 24 h for most patients. Hypotension and excessive sedation are problematic limitations of this drug. Midazolam, given by subcutaneous or intravenous infusion in doses ranging from 30 to 100 mg per 24 h are also used to control agitation related to delirium in the terminal stages (53,54). The goal of treatment with midazolam, and to some extent with methotrimeprazine, is quiet sedation only. As opposed to neuroleptic drugs like haloperidol, a midazolam infusion does not clear a delirious patient's sensorium or improve cognition. Propofol, a short-acting anesthetic agent, carries the advantage over midazolam in that the level of sedation is more easily controlled and recovery is rapid upon decreasing the rate of infusion (55). While neuroleptic drugs such as haloperidol are most effective in diminishing agitation, clearing the sensorium and improving cognition in the delirious patient, this is not always possible in the last days of life. Processes causing delirium may be ongoing and irreversible during the active dying phase. Ventafridda et al. (56) and Fainsinger et al. (57) have reported that a significant group (10–20%) of terminally ill patients experience delirium that can only be controlled by sedation to the point of a significantly decreased level of consciousness.

The use of neuroleptics in the management of delirium in the dying patient remains controversial in some circles. Some have argued that pharmacologic interventions with neuroleptics or benzodiazepines are inappropriate in the dying patient. Delirium is viewed as a natural part of the dying process that should not be altered. Another rationale that is often raised is that these patients are so close to death that aggressive treatment is unnecessary. Parenteral neuroleptics or sedatives may be mistakenly avoided because of exaggerated fears that they might hasten death through hypotension or respiratory depression. Many are unnecessarily pessimistic about the possible results of neuroleptic treatment for delirium. They argue that, since the underlying pathophysiologic process often continues unabated (such as hepatic or renal failure), no improvement can be expected in the patient's mental status. There is concern that neuroleptics or sedatives may worsen a delirium by making the patient more confused or sedated. Clinical experience in managing delirium in dying cancer patients suggests that the use of neuroleptics in the management of agitation, paranoia, hallucinations, and altered sensorium is safe, effective, and quite appropriate. Management of delirium on a case by case basis seems wisest. The agitated, delirious dying patient should probably be given neuroleptics to help restore calm. A "wait and see" approach, prior to using neuroleptics, may be most appropriate with patients who have a lethargic or somnolent presentation of delirium. The consultant must educate staff and patients and weigh each of these issues in making the decision of whether to use pharmacologic interventions for the dying patient who presents with delirium.

Several interesting clinical questions in this area exist, and more research could helpfully inform clinical management. Must we always treat delirium in the terminally ill or dying patient? What are appropriate goals for treatment? What is the impact of delirium on patients, family, staff? What are effective pharmacologic and nonpharmacologic interventions? An interesting, currently important, topic is that of differential therapeutics. Hypoactive and hyperactive subtypes of delirium have been described and seem to have distinct phenomenologies and etiologies (58). Therefore, hypoactive and hyperactive deliria may require different treatment strategies. While some investigators suggest that neuroleptics may be equally effective for both subtypes of delirium (59), others suggest that hypoactive delirium may best respond to psychostimulations or combinations of neuroleptics and stimulant (60). Stimulants may also play a role in the experienced by patients on opioid infusions (61). Newer antipsychotic agents have fewer neurological side effects (e.g., extrapyramidal effects or tardive dyskinesia), such as clozaril, risperidone, olanzapine, or sulpiride (62). Risperidone has been useful in the treatment of dementia and psychosis in AIDS patients at doses of 1–6 mg per day, suggesting safe use in patients with delirium (63,64). These new agents and newer antipsychotics that will be become available in the near future may have important roles in managing delirium in the terminally ill.

PAIN ASSESSMENT AND DELIRIUM

Delirium often impacts on the assessment of other symptomatology in medically ill patients. For example, assessment of pain intensity in patients during an episode of cognitive failure was significantly higher than before and after the episode, when similar intensities suggested a stable pain syndrome. It is recognized that success in the treatment of cancer pain is highly dependent on proper assessment (65,66). Unfortunately, the assessment of pain intensity becomes very difficult in patients with cognitive failure. Fainsinger et al. (67) report that 40% of patients required treatment for delirium in the last week of life, and they and Ventafridda et al. (56) report that about 10% of terminally ill patients were sedated to control this symptom. Assessing the intensity of pain when patients develop agitated cognitive failure is, therefore, a frequent problem. It may be speculated that delirium can increase pain through associated emotional lability and affective disinhibition (i.e., increased anxiety, distress, or through distortion of the patient's ability to report pain accurately. Accurate pain reporting depends on

the ability to perceive the pain normally and to communicate the experience appropriately. Delirium could both impair the ability to perceive and report pain accurately.

MORPHINE AND ALTERNATIVE OPIOIDS

Delirium is a well-recognized side effect of opioid administration (68–70). Much of the literature that discusses this problem suggests that the effect usually is short-lived. Ellison (71) notes that euphoria and dysphoria are acute and usually evanescent problems, and that tolerance usually develops rapidly. Bruera et al. (72) suggest that it is escalation of the morphine dosage that leads to confusion, and this resolves quite quickly. The specific causes of acute confusional states in patients with advanced cancer are not determined in up to 75% of cases, and management usually focuses on the appropriate use of psychotropic agents (14, 48).

Rotation of opioid has been shown previously to improve delirium (73), and in one study 73% of patients in whom confusion was regarded as troublesome experienced improvement after a change in opioid (74). Experience in Finland (75) has previously suggested that oxycodone is less likely to cause delirium than morphine, but this has not previously been confirmed in prolonged use or in palliative care patients. Fentanyl, the opioid that is often used as an alternative, has a short duration of action. Consequently, it is suitable only for transcutaneous, continuous infusion or epidural use. Oxycodone, an opioid equipotent to morphine in the oral form, has been shown to be far less likely to cause delirium in an unpublished study by Maddocks et al. The improvement was progressive over the course of several days following a change from morphine, suggesting that a long-acting metabolite of morphine may be responsible for causing delirium. This study suggests that the ready availability of oxycodone in a wider range of formulations and administration routes would provide a major benefit for the great majority of patients requiring palliative care, particularly those who are unable to tolerate parenteral morphine.

SUMMARY

The mental health practitioner in the oncology setting is likely to encounter delirium as a common major psychiatric complication of cancer, particularly in hospitalized cancer patients where between 15% and 30% develop delirium. Proper assessment, diagnosis and management are important in minimizing morbidity and improving quality of life. For further information on delirium and cognitive disorder screening, the reader is referred to the *Handbook of Measures for Psychological, Social and Physical Function in Cancer*, vol. III: Cognitive Impairment Disorders, available through Memorial Sloan-Kettering Cancer Center.

REFERENCES

1. Lipowski ZJ. *Delirium: Acute Confusional States.* New York: Oxford University Press; 1990.
2. Wise MG, Brandt GT. Delirium. In: Yudofsky SC, Hales RE, eds. *Textbook of Neuropsychiatry*, 2nd ed. Washington, DC. American Psychiatric Association; 1992.
3. Knight EB, Folstein MF. Unsuspected emotional and cognitive disturbance in medical patients. *Ann Intern Med.* 1977; 87:723–724.
4. Massie MJ, Gorzynski JG, Mastrovito R, et al. The diagnosis of depression in hospitalized patients with cancer [abstract]. *Proc Am Assoc Cancer Res Am Soc Clin Oncol.* 1979; 20:432.
5. Massie MJ, Holland J, Glass E. Delirium in terminally ill cancer patients. *Am J Psychiatry.* 1983; 140:1048–1050.
6. Pereira J, Hanson J, Bruera E. The frequency and clinical course of cognitive impairment in patients with terminal cancer. *Cancer.* 1997; 69:835–841.
7. Tune LE. Post-operative delirium. *Int Psychogeriatr.* 1991; 3:325–332.
8. Lipowski ZJ. Transient cognitive disorders (delirium, acute confusional states) in the elderly. *Am J Psychiatry.* 1983; 140:1426–1436.
9. Gillick MR, Serrel NA, Gillick LS. Adverse consequences of hospitalization in the elderly. *Soc Sci Med.* 1982; 16:1033–1038.
10. Warsaw GA, Moore J., Friedman SW, et al. Functional disability in the hospitalized elderly. *JAMA.* 1982; 248:847–850.
11. Berman K, Eastham EJ. Psychogeriatric ascertainment and assessment for treatment in an acute medical ward setting. *Age Ageing.* 1974; 3:174–188.
12. Seymour DJ, Henschke PJ, Cape RDT, et al. Acute confusional states and dementia in the elderly: the role of dehydration/volume depletion, physical illness and age. *Age Ageing.* 1980; 9:137–146.
13. Hodkinson HM. Mental impairment in the elderly. *J R Coll Phys Lond.* 1973; 7:305–317.
14. Lipowski, ZJ. *Delirium: Acute Brain Failure in Man.* Springfield, IL. Charles C. Thomas; 1980.
15. American Psychiatric Association (APA). *Diagnostic and Statistical Manual of Mental Disorders*, 3rd ed. Washington, DC: APA; 1980.
16. American Psychiatric Association (APA). *Diagnostic and Statistical Manual of Mental Disorders*, 3rd ed. Washington, DC: APA; 1987.
17. Ross CA. CNS arousal systems: possible role in delirium. *Int Psychogeriatr.* 1991; 3:353–371.
18. Gibson GE, Blass JP, Huang H-M, Freemen GB. The cellular basis of delirium and its relevance to age-related disorders including Alzheimer's disease. *Int Psychogeriatr.* 1991; 3:373–395.
19. American Psychiatric Association (APA). *Diagnostic and Statistical Manual of Mental Disorders*, 4th ed. Washington, DC: APA; 1994.
20. Liptzin B, Levkoff S, Cleary P, et al. An empirical study of diagnostic criteria for delirium. *Am J Psychiatry.* 1991; 148:454–457.
21. Gray JA, Feldon J, Rawlins JNP, et al. The neuropsychology of schizophrenia. *Behav Brain Sci.* 1991; 4:1–84.
22. Smith M, Breitbart W, Platt M. A critique of instruments and methods to detect, diagnose, and rate delirium. *J Pain Symptom Manage.* 1995; 10:35–77.
23. Tombaugh TN, McIntyre NJ. The mini-mental state examination: a comprehensive review. *J Am Geriatr Soc.* 1992; 40:922–935.
24. Anthony JC, Leresche LA, Niaz U, et al. Limits of the "mini mental state" as a screening test for dementia and delirium among hospital patients. *Psychol Med.* 1982; 12:397–408.
25. Folstein MF, Folstein SE, McHugh PR. "Mini mental state:" a practical method of grading the cognitive state of patients for the clinician. *J Psychiatr Res.* 1975; 12:189–198.
26. Folstein MF, McHugh PR. Psychopathology of dementia: implications for neuropathology. In: Katzman R, ed. *Congenital and Acquired Cognitive Disorders.* New York. Raven Press; 1979:17–30.
27. Dick JPR, Guiloff RJ, Stewart A, et al. Mini mental state examination in neurological patients. *J Neurol Neurosurg Psychiatry.* 1984; 47:496–499.
28. Spencer MP, Folstein MF. The mini mental state examination. In: Keller PA, Ritt LG, eds. *Innovations in Clinical Practice: A Source Book.* Sarasota, FL: Professional Resource Exchange; 1985:305–310.
29. Trzepacz PT, Baker RW, Greenhouse J. A symptom rating scale for delirium. *Psychiatry Res.* 1988; 23:89–97.
30. Breitbart W, Rosenfeld B, Roth A, et al. The Memorial Delirium Assessment Scale. *J Pain Symptom Manage.* 1997; 13:128–137.
31. Bruera E, Miller L, McCallion J, et al. Cognitive failure in patients with terminal cancer: a prospective study. *J Pain Symptom Manage.* 1992; 7(4):192–195.
32. Tuma R, DeAngelis L. Acute encephalopathy in patients with systemic cancer. *Ann Neurol.* 1992; 32:288.
33. Lipowski ZJ. Delirium (acute confusional states). *JAMA.* 1987; 285:1789–1792.
34. Bruera E, MacMillan K, Kuehn N, et al. The cognitive effects of the administration of narcotics. *Pain.* 1989; 39:13–16.
35. Stiefel FC, Breitbart W, Holland JC. Corticosteroids in cancer: neuropsychiatric complications. *Cancer Invest.* 1989; 7:479–491.
36. Young DF. Neurological complications of cancer chemotherapy. In: Silverstein A, ed. *Neurological Complications of Therapy: Selected Topics.* New York: Futura Publishing; 1982; 57–113.
37. Holland JC, Fassanellows, Ohnuma T. Psychiatric symptoms associated with L-asparaginase administration. *J Psychiatr Res.* 1974; 10:165.
38. Adams F, Wuesada JR, Gutterman JU. Neuropsychiatric manifestations of human leukocyte interferon therapy in patients with cancer. *JAMA.* 1984; 252:938–941.

39. Denicoff KD, Rubinow DR, Papa MZ, et al. The neuropsychiatric effects of treatment with interleukin-1 and lymphokine-activated killer cells. *Ann Intern Med.* 1987; 107(3):293–300.

40. Weddington WW. Delirium and depression associated with amphotericin B. *Psychosomatics.* 1982; 23: 1076–1078.

41. Bruera E, Miller L, McCallion S. Cognitive failure in patients with terminal cancer: A prospective longitudinal study. *Psychosoc Aspects Cancer.* 1990; 9:308–310.

42. Itil T, Fink M. Anticholinergic drug-induced delirium: experimental modification, quantitative EEG and behavioral correlations. *J Nerv Ment Dis.* 1966; 143:492–507.

43. Adams F, Fernandez F, Andersson BS. Emergency pharmacotherapy of delirium in the critically ill cancer patient. *Psychosomatics.* 1986; 27:33–37.

44. Murray GB. Confusion, delirium, and dementia. In: Hackett TP, Cassem, NH, eds. *Massachusetts General Hospital Handbook of General Hospital Psychiatry*, 2nd ed. Littleton, MA: PSG Publishing; 1987; 84–115.

45. Fernandez F, Holmes VF, Adams F, Kavanaugh JJ. Treatment of severe refractory agitation with a haloperidol drip. *J Clin Psychiatry.* 1988; 49:239–241.

46. Breitbart W. Psychiatric management of cancer pain. *Cancer.* 1989; 63:2336–2342.

47. Breitbart W. Psychiatric complications of cancer. In: Brain MC, Carbone PP, eds *Current Therapy in Hematology Oncology—3.* Toronto: B.C. Decker; 1988; 268–274.

48. Fainsinger R, Bruera E. Treatment of delirium in a terminally ill patient. *J Pain Symptom Manage.* 1992; 7:54–56.

49. Twycross RG, Lack SA. *Symptom Control in Far Advanced Cancer: Pain Relief.* London, Pitman Brooks, 1983.

50. Fernandez F, Levy JK, Mansell PWA. Management of delirium in terminally ill AIDS patients. *Int J Psychiatry Med.* 1989; 19:165–172.

51. Breitbart W, Marotta R, Platt M, et al. A double-blind trial of halperidol, chlropormazine, and lorazepan in the treatment of delirium in hospitalized AIDS patients. *Am J Psychiatry.* 1996; 153:231–237.

52. Oliver DJ. The use of methotrimeprazine in terminal care. *Br J Clin Pract.* 1985;39:339-340.

53. Bottomley DM, Hanks GW. Subcutaneous midazolam infusion in palliative care. *J Pain Symptom Manage.* 1990; 5:259–261.

54. De Sousa E, Jepson A. Midazolam in terminal care. *Lancet.* 1988; 1:67–68.

55. Moyle J. The use of propofol in palliative medicine. *J Pain Symptom Manage.* 1995; 10:643–646.

56. Ventafridda V, Ripamonti C, DeConno F, et al. Symptom prevalence and control during cancer patients' last days of life. *J Palliat Care.* 1990; 6:7–11.

57. Fainsinger R, MacEachern T, Hanson J, et al. Symptom control during the last week of life in a palliative care unit. *J Palliat Care.* 1991; 7:5–11.

58. Ross CA, Peyser CE, Shapiro I, Folstein MF. Delirium: phenomenologic and etiologic subtypes. *Int Psychogeriatr.* 1991; 3:135–147.

59. Platt M, Breitbart W, Smith M, et al. Efficacy of neuroleptics for hypoactive delirium [letter]. *J Neuropsychiatry Clin Neurosci.* 1994; 6:66–67.

60. Stiefel F, Bruera E. Psychostimulants for hypoactive hypoalert delirium? *J Palliat Care.* 1991; 3:25–26.

61. Bruera E, Miller MJ, Macmillan K, Kuehn N. Neuropsychological effects of methylphenidate in patients receiving a continuous infusion of narcotics for cancer pain. *Pain.* 1992; 48:163–166.

62. Baldessarini R, Frankenburg F. Clozapine: a novel antipsychotic agent. *N Engl J Med.* 1991; 324:746–752.

63. Singh A. Safety of risperidone in patients with HIV and AIDS [Abstract]. Proceedings of the 149th Annual Meeting, American Psychiatric Association, May 1996; 4–9: 1–126.

64. Belzie L. Risperidone for AIDS—associated dementia: a case series [abstract]. Proceedings of the 149th Annual Meeting, American Psychiatric Association, May 1996.

65. Foley K. The treatment of cancer pain. *N Engl J Med.* 1984; 313:84–95.

66. Foley K. Pain syndromes in patients with cancer. *Med Clin North Am.* 1987; 71:169–184.

67. Fainsinger R, Bruera E, Miller MJ, et al. Symptom control during the last week of life on a palliative care unit. *J Palliat Care.* 1991; 1:5–11.

68. Kalso E. Vainio A. Hallucinations during morphine but not during oxycodone treatment [letter]. *Lancet.* 1988; 56:912.

69. Stiefel F, Fainsinger R, Bruera E. Acute confusional states in patients with advanced cancer. *J Pain Symptom Manage.* 1992; 7:94–98.

70. Caraceni A, Martini C, DeConno F, Ventafridda V. Organic brain syndromes and opioid analgesia for cancer pain. *J Pain Symptom Manage.* 1994; 9:527–533.

71. Ellison NM. Opioid analgesics for cancer pain: toxicities and their treatment. In: Patt R, ed. *Cancer Pain.* Philadelphia: JB Lippincott; 1993: 185–194.

72. Bruera E, Macmillan K, Hanson J, MacDonald RN. The cognitive effects of the administration of narcotic analgesics in patients with cancer pain. *Pain.* 1989, 39:13–16.

73. McDonald N, Der L, Allen S, Champion F. Opioid hyperexcitability: the application of an alternate opioid therapy. *Pain.* 1993; 53:353–355.

74. DeStoutz, Bruera E, Suarez-Almazor M. Opiate rotation (OR) for toxicity reduction in terminal cancer patients [abstract]. In: *Abstracts of the Seventh World Congress on Pain.* Paris: IASP; 1993:331.

75. Kalso E, Vainio A, Manri J, et al. Morphine and oxycodone in the management of cancer pain: plasma levels determined by chemical and radioreceptor assays. *Pharmacol Toxicol.* 1990; 67:322–328.

76. Tucker GJ. DSM-IV Organic Disorders Work Group. DSM-IV: proposals for revision of diagnostic criteria for delirium. *Int Psychogeriatr.* 1991; 3:197–208.

77. Albert MS, Levkoff SE, Reilly C, et al. The delirium symptom interview: an interview for the detection of delirium symptom in hospitalized patients. *J Geriatr Psychiatry Neurol.* 1991; 5:14–21.

78. Inouye SK, Vandyck CH, Alessi CA, et al. Clarifying confusion: the confusion assessment method, a new method for detection of delirium. *Ann Intern Med.* 1990; 113:941–948.

79. Williams MA. Delirium and acute confusional states: evaluation devices in nursing. *Int Psychogeriatr.* 1991; 3:301–308.

80. Miller PS, Richardson JS, Jyn IA. Association of low serum anticholinergic levels and cognitive impairment in elderly presurgical patients. *Am J Psychiatr.* 1988; 145:342–345.

81. Folstein MF, Folstein SE, McHugh PR. "Minimental status": a practical method for grading the cognitive state of patients for clinicians. *J Psychiatr Res.* 1975; 12:189–198.

82. Wolber G, Romaniuk M, Eastman E, Robinson C. Validity of the short Portable Mental Status Questionnaire with elderly psychiatric patients. *J Consult Clin Psychol.* 1984; 52:712–713.

83. Jacobs JC, Bernhard MR, Delgado A, Strain JJ. Screening for organic mental syndromes in the medically ill. *Ann Intern Med.* 1977; 86:40–46.

84. Katzman R, Brown T, Fuld P, et al. Validation of a short orientation-memory- concentration test of cognitive impairment. *Am J Psychiatry.* 1983; 140:734–739.

49

Substance Abuse Disorders

STEVEN D. PASSIK AND RUSSELL K. PORTENOY

Use of illicit substances and alcohol is highly prevalent in the United States. We live in a highly drug oriented society (1) and the specter of drug abuse and the fear of addiction colors how we view the treatment of pain and other forms of distress. Indeed, nearly 33% of the population of the United States reports having sampled illicit drugs, (2) and an estimated 6%–15% have a substance use disorder of some type (3). Substance abuse may result in serious morbidity or predispose to the development of chronic and life-threatening medical illnesses such as cancer (4).

Patients who have used illicit drugs are being encountered more frequently in medical settings. The management of substance use is crucial to adherence to medical therapy and safety during treatment. Strategies for management of substance use aid health care practitioners to treat patients respectfully and compassionately and to offer aggressive therapy for pain and other distressing symptoms without reservation or prejudice.

The use of drugs to manage psychiatric symptoms, pain and other distressing physical symptoms in patients with histories of extensive drug use is complex, labor intensive and multidimensional. The psycho-oncologist involved in this treatment must be able to: (1) diagnose and manage the spectrum of illicit drug use and abuse and its complicated emotional and psychiatric comorbidities; (2) set guidelines for the patient so that safe and compassionate treatment is possible; (3) interact with staff members who often have intense and ambivalent feelings about caring for these patients; (4) provide an aftercare or outpatient program that involves working with members of patients' families or their friends, who sometimes also have problems of drug abuse.

Concerns about drug abuse complicate every aspect of oncology treatment, including symptom manage-ment, because it disrupts a crucial aspect of the doctor–patient relationship—trust. Doctors may not trust the self-report of drug-abusing patients, and patients with histories of extensive drug abuse, who often come from backgrounds characterized by exploitation and neglect, may not have faith that those in authority will display adequate care and concern. These expectations often become self-fulfilling prophesies. Without mutual trust, the assessment, treatment, and follow-up of these patients can be disrupted. Cancer patients with histories of drug abuse who experience unrelieved emotional or physical distress may rely upon previously successful modes of coping such as use of illicit drugs and manipulative behaviors, and create a vicious cycle of undertreatment, drug abuse, and diminished trust.

Illicit drug use, actual or suspected misuse of prescribed medications, or actual substance use disorders are among the most serious of psychiatric complications in the psycho-oncology setting. In the treatment of potentially curable malignancies, the threat to treatment adeherence posed by unchecked substance use may be life-threatening. Untoward interactions between illicit drugs and medications prescribed as part of the patient's treatment can be dangerous. Ongoing substance abuse may alienate or weaken an already fragile social support network that is crucial for mitigating the chronic stressors associated with cancer and cancer treatment. The potential for morbidity and even mortality among cancer patients with active illicit drug abuse, those with a substance abuse history in drug-free recovery, and those on methadone maintenance can only be mitigated by a therapeutic strategy that addresses drug-taking behavior while facilitating the treatment of malignancy and distressing symptoms, as well as addiction.

PREVALENCE OF SUBSTANCE USE DISORDERS IN THE ONCOLOGY POPULATION

One of the authors (S.D.P.) noted in a review that only 3% of consultations performed by the Psychiatry Service at Memorial Sloan-Kettering Cancer Center were requested for management of issues related to drug abuse. The results of the Psychiatric Collaborative Oncology Group study (5) were similar: following structured clinical interviews, less than 5% of 215 ambulatory cancer patients qualified for a diagnosis of substance use disorders (SUD) using the DSM-III criteria (6). This low prevalence of SUD in the tertiary care oncology hospital population contrasts with that seen in the general medical setting. For example, a review of statistics from the consultation-liaison service in a large Midwestern hospital (7) observed that 30%–40% of consults involved SUD. These differences may reflect underreporting in the cancer population. Social forces may inhibit the reporting of drug use behaviors by patients. Many drug absuers are poor, feel alienated from the medical system, and/or self-treat a range of medical problems. They may not be able to afford cancer treatment or may not present to physicians until they are seriously or even terminally ill. The low recorded prevalence of drug abuse in cancer centers is likely not representative of the true prevalence of drug abuse in cancer patients treated in local and public hospitals.

PROBLEMS OF DEFINITION IN THE MEDICALLY ILL

Although the identification of patients who are actively abusing illicit drugs can be straightforward, the diagnosis of SUD in those who are receiving potentially abusable licit drugs for an appropriate medical indication (e.g., opioids for pain) can be challenging. The difficulties inherent in this process are both conceptual and related to nomenclature.

The DSM-IV criteria differentiate two types of substance use disorders: substance dependence (the more serious of the two) and substance abuse (Table 49.1).

TABLE 49.1. *DSM-IV Criteria for Substance Abuse Disorders*

Substance Dependence	Substance Abuse
A maladaptive pattern of substance abuse, leading to clinically significant impairment or distress, as manifested by three of more of the following occurring at any time in the same 12-month period:	A madadaptive pattern of substance abuse leading to clinically significant impairment or distress, as manifested by one (or more) of the following, occurring within a 12-month period:
A. Tolerance, as defined by either of the following: 　1. As need for markedly increased amounts of substance to achieve intoxication or desired effect 　2. Markedly diminished effect with continued use of the same amount of the substance	1. Recurrent substance use resulting in a failure to fulfill major role obligations at work, school, or home (e.g., repeated absences or poor work performance related to substance use; substance related absences, suspensions, or expulsions from school; neglect or children or household)
B. Withdrawal, as manifested by either of the following: 　1. The characteristic withdrawal syndrome for the substance 　2. The same (or closely related) substance is taken to relieve or avoid withdrawal symptoms	2. Recurrent substance use in situations in which it is physically hazardous (e.g., driving an automobile or operating a machine when impaired by substance use)
C. The substance is often taken in larger amounts or over a longer period than was intended	3. Recurrent substance-related legal problems (e.g., arrests for substance-related disorderly conduct)
D. There is a persistent desire or unsuccessful efforts to cut down or control substance use	4. Continued substance use despite having persistent or recurrent social or interpersonal problems caused or exacerbated by the effects of the substance (e.g., arguments with spouse about consequences of intoxication, physical fights)
E. A great deal of time spent in activities necessary to obtain the substance (e.g., visiting multiple doctors or driving long distances), use the substance, (e.g., chain-smoking), or recover from its effects	H. The symptoms have never met the criteria for Substance Dependence for this class of substance.
F. Important social, occasional, or recreational activities are gi en up or reduced because of substance use	
G. The substance use is continued despite knowledge of having a persistent or recurrent physical or psychological problem that is likely ot have been caused or exacerbaed by the substance (e.g., current cocaine use despite recognition of cocaine induced depression, or continued drinking despite recognition that an ulcer was made worse by alcohol consumption)	

While their application can be problematic to pain patients (see below), the adaptation of these criteria is helpful in standardizing the language that we use to describe substance use problems.

However, SUD and drug abuse must be distinguished from both tolerance and physical dependence in the setting of pain and symptom management. The latter are pharmacologic properties that develop with prolonged use of specific drugs – not limited to controlled substances – and are neither necessary nor sufficient for a diagnosis of SUD (yet they are included in the DSM-IV criteria and can thus be problematic). Tolerance reflects the need for higher doses of a drug to maintain an effect. Physical dependence is defined solely by the occurrence of an abstinence syndrome on abrupt dose reduction or administration of an antagonist drug.

Both clinicians and patients misinterpret tolerance and physical dependence as evidence of SUD or addiction. Waning effect or the request for a higher dose to maintain an effect requires making "differential diagnosis" in the medical setting (Table 49.2). The differential diagnosis includes: increased activity in nociceptive pathways (such as mechanical factors related to tumor growth), psychologic processes that worsen or alter the pain experience (such as increasing distress from anxiety or depression), and tolerance (due to pharmacologic, pharmacokinetic or psychologic processes) (8). In the cancer setting, progressive or recurrent disease is the most common cause; tolerance probably contributes only after progression of disease is taken into account.

The vast majority of cancer patients who receive chronic opioid therapy are physically dependent without evidence of SUD. Physical dependence may be associated with some morbidity, which, in the clinical setting, seems unrelated to SUD. Patients who are taking drugs that can cause physical dependence may express concern about the potential for withdrawal. This concern may reflect patients' more general fear of loss of control of aspects of their lives to illness. In this context, the inability to stop taking a drug promptly can be viewed as quite threatening.

Conceptual Problems
The diagnosis of SUD or aberrant drug taking in the cancer patient remains difficult even if tolerance and physical dependence are appropriately disregarded. There are three main conceptual problems related to this difficulty: (1) undertreatment of pain and other distressing physical symptoms; (2) difficulty in extrapolating the definition of addiction derived from physically healthy addicts to cancer patients; (3) the inappropriate focus on specific drugs or routes of drug administration as indicators of "addiction" or "addiction liability."

Any assessment of "addiction" in a cancer patient, especially those without a prior history of significant drug use, must begin with an assessment of the adequacy of pain and symptom control. There is compelling evidence that pain is undertreated in populations of medically ill patients, including cancer and AIDS (9, 10). Undertreatment may be associated with aberrant behaviors driven by the desparation associated with

TABLE 49.2. *A Differential Diagnosis for Declining Analgesic Effects in the Clinical Setting*

INCREASED ACTIVITY IN NOCICEPTIVE PATHWAYS
Increased activation of nociceptors in the periphery:
> Due to mechanical factors (e.g., tumor growth)
> Due to biochemical factors (e.g., inflammation)
> Due to peripheral neuropathic processes (e.g., neuroma formation)
Increased activity in central nociceptive pathways:
> Due to central neuropathic processes (e.g., sensitization, shift in receptive fields, change in modulatory processes)

PSYCHOLOGIC PROCESSES*
Increasing psychologic distress (e.g., anxiety or depression)
Change in cognitive state leading to altered pain perception or reporting (e.g., delirium)
Conditioned pain behavior independent of the drug

TOLERANCE
Due to pharmacodynamic processes
Due to pharmacokinetic processes
Dut to psychologic processes

*Other than conditioned responses to the drug.

unrelieved pain. Weissman and Haddox (11) coined the term "pseudo-addiction" to describe these effects. They note that these aberrant behaviors cease when adequate analgesia is restored.

Less dramatic behaviors, such as dose escalation by the patient or seeking out more than one prescriber when pain is unrelieved, are more common. Additionally, cancer patients with prior histories of drug abuse, including those who have been abstinent for long periods, can display even more dramatic examples of pseudo-addiction when undermedicated for pain. Such patients have greater experience with and access to sources of illicit drugs than do those who have no such history.

USE DESPITE HARM APPLIED TO THE ONCOLOGY SETTING

The second reason for confusion is that the core concepts used to define addiction—which have been derived from physically healthy drug abusers—do not readily apply to cancer patients. For example, one of the most widely accepted concepts in the definition of SUD, use despite harm (12), may be difficult to interpret in the setting of progressive disease. Commonly, cancer patients suffer gradual diminution of psychosocial functioning as disease- and treatment-related limitations mount. The harm done to psychosocial functioning that stems from illness and treatment is difficult to separate from the harm due to drug-taking behaviors. Those who harm their treatment (i.e., noncompliance), or jeopardize relationships with physicians, other health care providers and family members in the pursuit of continued use of substances, may be signaling a burgeoning addiction problem.

Another commonly used indicator of psychological dependence or addiction in the physically healthy drug abuser is obsessive use or the loss of control of the drug taking. This criterion, too, *can* have less clear application to cancer patients. Those with unrelieved pain can appear to be obsessed and driven in their attempts to procure various medications. They may hoard analgesic during periods when pain intensity is decreased and/or visit more than one physician to obtain prescriptions. All of these traditional "red flags" may be of little value in the setting of unrelieved symptoms.

Another core concept used in defining addiction, though not directly reflected in the DSM-IV nomenclature, is drug-taking behavior that is a deviation from societal norms (13). This criterion may be difficult to apply because there are ill-defined norms for cancer patients and most other medically ill populations. If a large percentage of patients engage in a given behavior, it may be normative and judgments about deviance may be influenced accordingly. For example, Passik et al. (14) noted that 26% of inpatients with cancer reported borrowing an anxiolytic from a family member at some time. Thus, the anxious patient who manifests this behavior is not necessarily fulfilling a criterion for SUD. Clearly there are behaviors that, based on their illegality alone, should be considered universally unacceptable, such as prescription forgery. However, there are many less extreme behaviors, such as borrowing a spouse's medication, that have less universal meaning. Nonetheless, clinicians would be more secure in making judgments about individual behaviors if there were empirical data examining the prevalence of various drug-taking attitudes and behaviors in different pain populations (such as cancer, AIDS, chronic nonmalignant pain, sickle cell, etc.).

The undue emphasis upon the addiction liability of certain drugs or routes of drug administration has stalled the development of a more complex and accurate psychological, social, and biological understanding of addiction in the cancer or medically ill patient. This emphasis has led to the faulty assumption by many health care professionals that the avoidance of certain drugs or certain routes of administration can effectively prevent problems of addiction in their patients. The clinical lore is that opioids, benzodiazepines and psychostimulants are highly addictive due to their rewarding properties (euphoria, avoidance of withdrawal). Similarly, there is a common perception that the parenteral route must be avoided because of its ability to deliver a drug in a rapid fashion. These perceptions derive from observations in the healthy addict population. It is clearly wrong to assume that large numbers of individuals with no personal or family history of SUD, no affiliation with a substance abusing subculture or premorbid psychopathology, will develop SUD de novo when administered these drugs or these routes for appropriate medical indications. These views persist despite contrary empirical data and clinical experience with cancer pain patients and patients with chronic nonmalignant pain (15,16).

In the Boston Collaborative Drug Surveillance Study (15), only four of 11,882 patients in Boston hospitals who had no history of SUD and were treated with opioids for pain during their hospital stays developed SUD upon follow-up. Perry and Heidrich (16) performed a national survey of burns centers, and could document no cases of SUD among 10,000 patients who had no history of SUD and were treated with opioids for burn pain.

The hypothesis that addiction liability resides solely in the pharmacology of a drug may be questioned on many grounds. As noted, drugs believed to have "high addiction potential," such as opioids, are not abused by a large majority of chronic pain patients. In contrast, many drugs that are thought to have "low addiction potential" are actually bought and sold on the streets of major metropolitan areas. For example, neuroleptics are commonly disliked by those who require them, possibly due to the fact that they diminish hedonic capacity. Nonetheless, neuroleptics are abused and fairly widely sold on the streets (for self-medication of insomnia, psychotic or anxiety symptoms, to get "high" on anticholinergic effects, or to diminish unpleasant withdrawal symptoms). Other drugs, such as anticholinergic agents and a range of antidepressants, thought to be low in addiction potential, are also abused.

Clinical experience suggests that the use of the parenteral route to deliver opioids and other medications for medical indications does not lead to the development of SUD in patients without a prior history of drug abuse. However, virtually all routes of drug administration can be abused. It should be kept in mind that those who abuse drugs generally seek a change in mental status, though not necessarily a pleasant one. The more rapidly this change can be effected the better. Moreover, many drug abusers want to return to normal as quickly as possible, so that they can continue to maintain their functioning (i.e., those who get high during their lunch hour but do not want to return to work intoxicated; the adolescent cancer patient who smokes pot while his parents are away but wants to be "straight" when they return from work).

Although it is true that selected drugs or routes that produce a rapid onset and rapid "offset" are more prone to abuse by those with SUD, these properties do not appear to associate with an increased risk of iatrogenic addiction. The simple avoidance of prescribing certain drugs or the use of certain routes of drug administration is not an effective way to avoid the issue of addiction. The effective management of the cancer patient with a substance abuse history necessitates far more multidimensional and sophisticated approaches. These approaches must take into account the biological, chemical, social and psychiatric aspects of patients with SUD and not solely focus on the chemical aspect.

THE SPECTRUM OF ABERRANT DRUG-TAKING ATTITUDES AND BEHAVIORS

To address the conceptual problems inherent in the assessment and diagnosis of SUD in the cancer pain patient, it is helpful to posit a construct that may be termed "aberrant drug-related behaviors" that defines the broad range of problematic behaviors that patients may exhibit during long-term therapy with a potentially abusable drug. These behaviors lie along a continuum from less to more aberrant (Table 49.3). Behaviors on the more prevalent, less aberrant, end of the spectrum (i.e., aggressively complaining about the need for medications) are more likely to reflect untreated distress of some type, rather than addiction-related concerns. Conversely, the less prevalent, more aberrant, end of the continuum includes behaviors that are more likely to reflect true addiction.

TABLE 49.3. *An Example of the Spectrum of Aberrant Drug-Taking Behaviors*

Aberrant Drug-Related Behaviors More Suggestive of Addiction	Aberrant Drug-Related Behaviors Less Suggestive of Addiction
Selling prescription drugs	Aggressive complaining about the need for more drugs
Prescription forgery	Drug hoarding during periods of reduced symptoms
Stealing or borrowing drugs from others	Requesting specific drugs
Injecting oral formulations	Openly acquiring similar drugs from other medical sources
Obtaining prescription drugs from nonmedical sources	Unsanctioned dose escalation or other noncompliance with therapy on one or two occasions
Concurrent abuse of alcohol or illicit drugs	
Multiple dose escalations or other noncompliance with therapy despite warning	Unapproved use of the drug to treat another symptom
	Reporting psychic effects not intended by the clinician
Repeatedly seeking prescriptions from other clinicians or from emergency rooms without informing prescriber	Resistance to a change in therapy associated with tolerable adverse effects with expressions of anxiety related to the return of severe symptoms
Evidence of deterioration in the ability to function at work, in the family, or socially that appear to be related to drug use	
Repeated resistance to changes in therapy despite clear evidence of adverse physical or psychological effects from the drugs	

The important implication of this behavioral categorization is that aberrant behaviors have a "differential diagnosis" (Table 49.4).

These behaviors can reflect addiction, pseudo-addiction, or criminal intent (i.e., the patient who is drug-seeking in attempt to sell or divert). On a more challenging level, they can indicate any of a diverse set of psychiatric disorders. The patient might be self-medicating symptoms of anxiety or depression, insomnia, or even problems of adjustment (such as boredom due to diminished ability to engage in usual activities and hobbies). Patients with borderline personality disorder will often manifest chaotic and impulsive medication use in attempts to regulate inner tension, anger at doctors, friends or family, or to medicate chronic emptiness or boredom. Their use of drugs is not unlike their use of food, exercise, sex, or other means to achieve the same goals.

After the clinician has considered the differential diagnosis of aberrant behaviors that have emerged, a response can be formulated. The response to less aberrant behaviors will generally be more vigorous efforts to manage pain and psychological distress. The response to the emergence of behaviors on the more aberrant end of the continuum is more problematic and complex. Even if these behaviors are understood to be due to an etiology other than true addiction (i.e., borderline personality disorders), they should trigger a change in management along the lines of tightening restrictions or consideration of discharging the patient if he/she is refractory to attempts to set limits. Discharge from the hospital or clinic should be reserved for truly intractable situations. While there is no set number of transgressions that should be tolerated, one must bear in mind that SUD is a chronic relapsing illness and clinicians should attempt to avoid punishing the patient for a manifestation of his/her psychiatric disorder. Good pain and symptom man-

agement may lower the likelihood of a relapse but does not exclude the possibility. Thus, in the management section below, we offer a range of interventions that can be employed to help set the stage for management of the patient with SUD.

CLINICAL MANAGEMENT OF SUD

Patients with SUD are heterogeneous. The broad categories comprise patients who are actively abusing drugs or alcohol, those in drug-free recovery, and those enrolled in methadone maintenance programs. The following sections focus mainly on the patient who is actively drinking or using drugs. The guidelines can also be useful in helping patients in drug-free recovery to accept the pain and symptom management they require and calm their fears of re-addiction (see below).

General Guidelines

Based on clinical experience, some general guidelines can be developed to facilitate the management of the patient with SUD (Table 49.5).

Involve a Multidisciplinary Team. The treatment of patients with cancer and SUD often must contend with multiple social, psychiatric, medical, and administrative problems. While staffing will no doubt vary at different hospitals and settings, a team approach minimally involving the oncologist, nurse, social worker, and psycho-oncologist can be very useful. Consultations from addiction medicine specialists may be helpful in some instances.

TABLE 49.4. *Differential Diagnosis of Aberrant Drug-Taking Behavior*

Pseudo-addiction (unrelieved pain)

Addiction (substance use disorder)

Other psychiatric diagnosis

    Depression

    Anxiety

    Borderline personality disorder

    Organic mental syndrome

Criminal intent

TABLE 49.5. *General Guidelines for the Management of Patients with Substance Abuse Disorders*

Involve a multidisciplinary team

Set realistic goals for therapy

Evaluate and treat comorbid psychiatric disorders

Prevent or minimize withdrawal symptoms

Consider tolerance when prescribing medications for pain and symptom control

Use accepted guidelines, such as those of WHO or AHCPR

Accept the patient's self-report of distress

Frequently reassess the adequacy of pain and symptom control

Use sound pharmacology

Recognize specific drug-abuse behaviors

Use nonopioids and psychological techniques as indicated but not as substitutes

---

Set Realistic Goals for Therapy. SUD is a chronic and relapsing condition, and good pain management does not preclude relapse. Therefore, total abstinence from illicit drug use is not a workable goal of pain therapy. Not all patients will receive optimum cancer therapy or pain management because of poor compliance or a pattern of binge use. Due to the heightened stress of life-threatening disease, preventing relapses of substance use may sometimes be impossible. In such cases, the goal of treatment might be changed to gathering enough social and emotional support and setting sufficient limits for the patient to contain the harm done by occasional relapses. Such patients may be able to comply with and complete simpler regimens. A small subgroup may never be able to make themselves available enough for cancer treatment due to intractable drug use and poor social support. The psycho-oncologist must be flexible and may need to restart treatment and reestablish limits on multiple occasions. The success rate for the psycho-oncologic management of such is unknown.

Evaluate and Treat Comorbid Psychiatric Disorders. The comorbidity of personality disorder, depression, and anxiety disorders in alcoholics and other patients with SUD is extremely high, ranging from 17%–75% (17). The treatment of anxiety and depression can increase patient comfort and possibly diminish the likelihood of relapse of SUD.

Prevent or Minimize Withdrawal Symptoms. Treatment guidelines for the management of withdrawal states for various substances are widely available (18). Psycho-oncologists need to be familiar with the signs, symptoms, and treatments of withdrawal states, as many constitute medical emergencies. Treatment of pain, anxiety, and depression cannot begin until the patient is stabilized, comfortable, and out of danger of withdrawing.

Consider Tolerance When Prescribing Medications for Pain and Symptom Control. Patients who are actively abusing drugs may be tolerant to the drugs administered for therapy. The extent of this tolerance is never known and it is best to start with a conservative estimate of the patient's requirement and then rapidly titrate the dose while reassessing frequently until the patient is comfortable. There are no standard transformations for converting the amount of street drugs and alcohol used to the amount of analgesic and other medications that will be required.

Use Accepted Cancer Pain Guidelines for Symptom Management. Well-established guidelines for pain management provide a useful framework for analgesic pharmacotherapy. These guidelines advocate accepting the patient's self-report of distress as a key to assessment and intervention, a strategy all too often discarded when patients with SUD are encountered. Additionally, virtually all accepted cancer pain guidelines discuss the need to frequently reassess the adequacy of pain and symptom control to facilitate communication and diminish pseudo-addiction.

Follow Sound Pharmacological Principles. A common error when prescribing analgesia to patients with a history of SUD is that clinicians commonly fail to follow pharmacologic principles and then erroneously conclude the patient is drug-seeking or problematic. For example, if intervals between doses of analgesics or anxiolytics are too long, the patient can appear to be drug-seeking or "clock-watching." Another common misconception involves methadone. Methadone blocks withdrawal for significantly longer periods than it relieves pain. It is usually required every 6 h for continuous analgesia; patients in methadone maintanence require additional doses or additional medications to achieve pain relief around the clock. The AHCPR guidelines contain suggestions for the dosing and scheduling of analgesics and psychotropic adjuvants for pain and symptom management. Unfortunately no such guidleines have yet been compiled for the treatment of psychiatric complications in cancer and in particular the cancer patient with SUD.

Select Appropriate Drugs and Routes of Administration for the Symptom and Setting. Given the possible difficulty of using short-acting formulations in patients with histories of SUD, the use of long-acting preparations in adequate amounts may help minimize the number of rescue doses required, diminish cravings, and lower the likelihood of abuse of prescribed medications. As was mentioned above, the prescribing of opioids and other potentially abusable drugs should be carried out in a setting of limits and guidelines rather than overly focusing on the choice of drug or route. The use (or avoidance) of any specific drug or route neither predicts abuse nor protects against it.

Recognize Specific Drug Abuse Behaviors. Rather than discussing drug addiction and alcohol use in generalities, the clinician and patient need to have a constant discourse guided by specific drug-taking behaviors. This may lead to early detection of drug-taking problems. The clinician must assess the full spectrum of aberrant drug-taking.

Utilize Nondrug Approaches and Psychological Techniques in Addition to, but not as, Substitutes. In helping patients with SUD cope with the rigors of cancer treatment, the psycho-oncologist can teach a range of helpful and highly specific techniques. They may include include relaxation techniques, ways of thinking about and describing the experience of pain, and methods of communicating physical and emotional distress to hospital staff members. Patients can be encouraged to experiment with different nondrug approaches to their pain and other symptoms. These are all helpful adjuvants to management but should not be seen as substitutes for potent analgesic drugs or medications for depression, anxiety, and other psychological symptoms.

Taking a Substance Use History

Clinicians often avoid asking patients about drug abuse (and other socially undesirable behaviors) for fear that patients will be offended, or become angry or threatened. Often there is the fatalistic expectation that the patient will not respond truthfully. Questions such as, "You don't use drugs or alcohol do you?" send a strong message about behaviors that the clinician believes are unacceptable. If the patient is not abusing drugs at the time of the initial meeting with the doctor but experiences a relapse at some future point, this type of history-taking may reduce the likelihood of truthful communication.

The clinician should be nonjudgmental when taking the patient's history of substance abuse. Adopting a professional and caring demeanor often necessitates some degree of self-observation and exploration of one's prejudices toward or feelings about members of subcultures who hold different values.

The clinician should anticipate defensiveness on the part of the patient. It can be helpful to mention that patients often misrepresent their drug use for valid reasons: stigmatization, mistrust of the interviewer, or concern about fears of undermedication. Clinicians must tell the patient that they need accurate information about drug use to help keep the patient as comfortable as possible by avoiding withdrawal states and prescribing adequate medication for pain and symptom control.

Polysubstance Use, History-Taking, and the Prevention of Withdrawal

In addition to gathering the history and mentioning the reasons for lying, the clinician must be inquisitive and knowledgeable about drug abuse. The use of street names for drugs should be avoided unless the clinician has current knowledge of the names in use. The use of terms that are out of date does not suggest to the patient that the clinician is current in his or her knowledge. However, the use of street names is secondary to the manner in which the history is taken. The interview should be conducted in a very methodical and curious manner, with a review of all drugs, the frequency of and triggers to their use, and a history of periods of sobriety and drug treatments if any. The so-called "pyramid" interview can be a useful way to slowly introduce the subject of drug use. This style of interviewing begins with broad and general questions about the role of substances in one's life (beginning with licit ones such as caffiene and nicotine). It then proceeds to more specific questions about illicit substances, and the frequency and quanitity used. Allowing the patient to describe his personal experiences with various substances may be *enjoyed* by the patient if the environment is right (it is, after all, an area in which they have tremendous expertise).

Desired Effects of Drugs of Abuse and the Treatment of Comorbid Psychiatric Disorders

In the cancer setting an additional question is very important and yet often omitted: the patient should be asked about the desired effects of all drugs used. This question can often lead to very valuable information about comorbid mood, anxiety, or pain problems that require treatment. The answer provides a key to helping patients with control of symptoms they find particularly noxious, and to diminish the need for drugs of abuse.

In follow-up assessments it is helpful to keep the continuum of aberrant drug-taking in mind as a guide. This effort helps to focus on specific aspects of drug-taking and compliance rather than deal in more general and ambiguous terms (such as speculating upon whether their use of pain medication constitutes "addiction" or "relapse"). Patients can also be asked to keep a drug-taking journal that describes how they are taking their medications. By assessing the patient's specific drug-taking behaviors the clinician can document an understanding of how well management is proceeding with regard to both pain control and addiction.

Inpatient Treatment of Acute Pain

Psycho-oncologists often utilize structured treatment guidelines in planning the inpatient treatment of the active substance abusing cancer patient (Table 49.6). Although the applicability and feasibility of these guidelines may vary from setting to setting, they allow for the surveillance of illicit drug use, control of manipulation by patients, and the safety of the staff and patient.

The clinician may employ various suggestions from among these guidelines according to the individual patient's requirements. Structured treatment guidelines set clear limits, help avoid conflicts surrounding the use of medications appropriately used for pain and symptom control, and communicate knowledge of pain and substance abuse management. In return for compliance with the treatment plan, the patient is offered a consistent approach to *all* aspects of care, including pain and symptom control. In extreme cases, patients may have to be informed that they will receive cancer treatment only if they comply with the guidelines.

When feasible, the patient with SUD should be seen as an outpatient by the psycho-oncologist or other member of the team prior to admission. This visit allows the clinician to anticipate withdrawal and when appropriate provide preadmission referral for detoxification. During this first outpatient meeting the management plan and the team's policies for violations of the plan are discussed with the patient.

Patients scheduled for a surgical procedure should be admitted to the hospital several days to a week early to allow for stabilization of drug regimens and to avoid the development of withdrawal syndromes (if this is possible within the context of the patient's insurance coverage). If possible the patient should have a private room close to the nursing station to allow for monitoring. Hospital staff members (security guards or nurses) conduct a search of the patient's possessions, during which illicit drugs, previously prescribed medications, or alcohol are to be removed from the patient's room. The search is conducted in the patient's presence with another member of the hospital staff present. Illegal substances are discarded per hospital protocol.

TABLE 49.6. *Structured Inpatient Management Plan*

Private room close to nursing station
Search patient's possessions and packages brought by visitors
Restrict patient's mobility (to room, floor, etc.)
Collect urine for toxicology screens daily
Involve hospital administration
Review plan with all involved hospital staff

The patient may be restricted to his room or floor until the danger of withdrawal or illicit drug use is judged to be diminished. The patient may be required to wear hospital pyjamas to reduce the risk of departure from the hospital to buy drugs. The team interviews those individuals whom the patient would like to have visit. The patient's visitors are then subsequently limited to family and friends that are known to be drug free. Packages brought to the hospital by family members and friends are searched by responsible staff to assure that they do not contain illicit drugs or alcohol.

Patients are instructed to produce periodic urine specimens. These specimens are sent for urine toxicology on admission and subsequently whenever the patient's physician believes a urine toxicology screen is needed. The physician may decide to discard some specimens after collection, but specimens should be obtained on a regular basis so that the patient is aware that surveillance is ongoing. Many laboratories cannot return results of urine toxicology screens in a timely fashion. Thus, a good strategy for suveillance is to collect daily specimens, but to send them to the laboratory only when clinically indicated.

Patients who are actively abusing substances and who are unwilling to abide by hospital policy may need to be discharged from the hospital and referred to drug rehabilitation programs before they are treated for cancer. The response to each patient must be individualized depending on the severity of the patient's medical condition and the safety of surgery or chemotherapy administration when the drug use is not under control. Ethical and legal considerations should be discussed in detail among members of hospital administration, the ethics committee, and senior clinicians depending upon the setting. Importantly, HIV infection should be considered in patients with a history of intravenous drug use.

Once a structure is established to control drug use, the medical management of the active abuser must proceed attentively. Frequent visits are usually needed to to assess and manage symptoms. The patient should be prescribed medications to prevent withdrawal and reduce distressing symptoms. Relatively high doses of medications may be needed and are completely acceptable if the therapy is systematic and monitored. It is usually better to treat symptoms, if possible, with a regularly scheduled drug regimen, thus avoiding frequent encounters with hospital staff members that center upon obtaining drugs. When approaching discharge, the patient may be able to undergo some tapering of opioids and other medications. Many must return home receiving drugs that will require close monitoring and a structured outpatient treatment plan.

Inpatient Management and Staff Issues

The already labor-intensive management of substance-abusing cancer patients is intensified by the need for constant team meetings and communication. Such meetings are beneficial in that they maintain consistency across shifts, allow staff members' expression of feelings and concerns, plan staff rotation in the care of such patients, and discuss ethical and legal issues. Having hospital administrators present at these meetings can be particularly useful in alleviating concerns about the legality of restrictive measures.

Outpatient Management

Other guidelines may apply to the management of the actively abusing outpatient who is undergoing treatment for cancer (Table 49.7). After discharge, referral to drug rehabilitation settings may be necessary. Patients who are undergoing cancer treatment may encounter difficulty in gaining entrance or adhering to such programs given the demands of their cancer treatment. The following approaches may be useful in managing this complex and less easily controllable aspect of care.

Use Written Contracts. The use of written contracts to state clearly the roles of the team members and the rules and expectations for the patient can be helpful in structuring outpatient treatment. The contract should explicitly state the consequences of aberrant drug use. A series of graded contracts in which the patient's behavior determines the level of restrictions can be a useful strategy.

Frequent Outpatient Visits, Limited Quantities of Medications per Prescription, Renewals Contingent on Outpatient Attendance. Patients with SUD should be seen as outpatients frequently. This helps to establish close ties with staff and allows re-evaluation of both symptom control and addiction-related concerns. Patients should be given limited quantities of medications to diminish the temptation

TABLE 49.7. *A Structured Outpatient Management Plan*

Use written contracts
Frequent clinic visits
Limited quantities of medications per prescription
Reschedules contingent on clinic attendance
Use 12-step programs where possible
Spot urine toxicology screens
Involve family in treatment planning

to divert drugs and to provide an incentive for keeping appointments. Policies for prescription loss or replacement should be explicitly stated and no prescription renewals should be given if sessions are missed. The need for communication before any changes in dose should be emphasized. Covering staff members should be told which patients should not have prescriptions replaced or called in to pharmacies. These restrictions should be made more or less stringent depending upon the patient's behavior and medical condition.

Use 12-Step Programs Where Possible. As an alternative to extensive, inpatient drug rehabilitation, some patients can document their attendance at 12-step groups. Contacting patients' sponsors can be useful in helping patients adhere to treatment and avoid ostracism when they return to their program while receiving controlled prescription drugs.

Spot Urine Toxicology Screens. To promote compliance and detect the concurrent use of illicit substances, patients should be periodically asked to supply urine specimens for toxicology screens. The team should have a predetermined response which the patient should be aware of should the screen be positive for illicit drugs.

Family Sessions and Meetings. Many drug-abusing patients come from dysfunctional and unsupportive families. Family meetings may identify family members who are using illicit drugs. Referral of family members to drug treatment can be offered and portrayed as a way of marshalling support for the patient. The patient should be prepared to cope with friends or family members who may try to buy or steal his/her medications. Identifying reliable individuals who can be sources of strength and support can help the patient through cancer treatment.

The Special Problem of the Patient in Drug-Free Recovery

The patient that has attained a period of extended sobriety and is in drug-free recovery is often fearful of taking pain and psychiatric medications. Many such patients are rightfully proud of having become sober. Their reluctance to take opioids or other medications may hinge on fears that they will become "re-addicted" (i.e., develop cravings for illicit or licit drugs, lose control of their medications), or jeopardize their social support networks if they are viewed as abusing by family or friends. Some may be afraid that friends or others who are actively using drugs will attempt to gain access to these medications. The clinician can be helpful to such patients by reassuring them that such syndromes appear to be rare in the context of pain treatment. The social context of pain treatment in the setting of life-threatening illness is tremendously different from that which surrounds recreational or even more serious drug abuse at times in the patient's life when he or she was physically healthy. It is perhaps social forces, amongst others, that leads to the not uncommon anecdotal experience that former addicts do not commonly experience euphoria when treated with opioids for pain (19). In setting the "social context" for pain control it can be helpful to negotiate with the patient that they forego opioid treatment until they feel it is necessary and safe for them. Presenting opioid treatment as an option can enhance a sense of control. It is also important to have the patient consider the risk of re-addiction that might be associated with being in uncontrolled pain for a length of time. Meetings with friends and family can be reassuring. Once opioid therapy is deemed necessary and acceptable to the patient, family and medical team, the voluntary use of some of the guidelines mentioned above can help such patients feel safe during treatment and as if there are controls in place to prevent drug-taking problems. Counseling can help them to identify possible triggers to drug and alcohol abuse that they might encounter during their cancer treatment (i.e., fatigue, fear, boredom) and develop strategies for avoiding illict drug use or uncontrolled use of prescribed medications at those times.

CONCLUSION

The diagnosis and management of patients with SUD is challenging, both conceptually and clinically, for the psycho-oncologist. The experience of working with such patients is very labor intensive and often frustrating and difficult. This work also offers a unique opportunity to be involved in a team approach that can accomplish extraordinary good for the patient and staff. A skilled approach implemented with consistency and sensitivity can result in humane and compassionate care for patients and enhanced support for the staff responsible for these challenging patients.

REFERENCES

1. Hills CS, Fields (eds). Drug treatment of cancer pain in a drug oriented society. Preface. *Advances in Pain Research and Therapy*. New York: Raven Press; 1989.
2. Groer J, Brodsky M. The incidence of illicit drug use in the United States 1962–1989. *Br J Addict*. 1992; 87:1345.
3. Regier DA, Meyers JK, Dramer, et al. The NIMH epidemiologic catchment area program. *Arch Gen Psychiatry*. 1984; 41:934–958.
4. Wells KB, Golding JM, Burnam MA. Chronic medical conditions in a sample of the general population with anxiety, affective, and substance use disorders. *Am J Psychiatry*. 1989; 146:1440.
5. Derogatis LR, Morrow GR, Fetting J, et al. The prevalence of psychiatric disorders among cancer patients. *J Am Med Assoc*. 1983; 249:751.
6. American Psychiatric Association. *Diagnostic and Statistical Manual for Mental Disorders*, 3rd ed. Washington, DC: American Psychiatric Association; 1983.
7. Burton RW, Lyons JS, Devens M, Larson DB. Psychiatric consults for psychoactive substance disorders in the general hospital. *Gen Hosp Psychiatry*. 1991; 13:83.
8. Portenoy RK, Foley KM. Chronic use of opioid analgesics in non-malignant pain: report of 38 cases. *Pain*. 1986; 25:171.
9. Cleeland C, Gonin R, Hatfield A, et al. Pain and its treatment in outpatients with metastatic cancer. *N Engl J Med*. 1994; 330:592.
10. Breitbart W, Rosenfeld BD, Passik SD, et al. The undertreatment of pain in ambulatory AIDS patients. *Pain*. 1996; 65:239.
11. Weissman DE, Haddox, JD. Opioid pseudoaddiction—an iatrogenic syndrome. *Pain*. 1989; 36:363.
12. Rinaldi RC, Steindler EM, Wilford BB, Goodwin D. Clarification and standardization of substance abuse terminology. *J Am Med Assoc*. 1988; 259:555.
13. Jaffe JH. Current concepts of addiction. *Res Publ Assoc Res Nerv Ment Dis*. 1992; 70:1–21.
14. Passik S, Breitbart W, Lowinson J, et al. Use and abuse of opioids and other licit and illicit drugs: Attitudes and behavior in cancer patients. Proceedings of American Pain Society 12th Annual Scientifc Meeting, Orlando, FL, 4–7 November 1993. Abstract 93650, A108.
15. Porter J, Jick H. Addiction rate in patients treated with narcotics. *N Engl J Med*. 1980; 302:123.
16. Perry S, Heidrich G. Management of pain during debridement: a survey of US burn units. *Pain*. 1982; 13:267.
17. Khantzian EJ, Treece C. DSM-III psychiatric diagnosis of narcotic addicts. *Arch Gen Psychiatry*. 1985; 42:1067.
18. Wise MG, Rundell JR. *Consultation Psychiatry*. Washington, DC: American Psychiatric Press; 1988: 84–93.
19. Gonzales GR, Coyle N. Treatment of cancer pain in a former opioid abuser: fears of the patient and staff and their influence on care. *J Pain Symptom Manage*. 1992; 7:246.

50

Alcoholism and Cancer

JEREMY C. LUNDBERG AND STEVEN D. PASSIK

According to the American Cancer Society, an estimated 1,252,000 individuals will be diagnosed with cancer in 1996 (1). Researchers have documented a relationship between the consumption of alcohol and neoplasms of the head and neck, breast, liver, colon, rectum, and it has been suspected to be related to cancer of the pancreas. According to Maxmen and Ward, an estimated 5% of the US population are alcoholic (with a male to female ratio of at least 3:1) (2). The peak prevalence of alcoholism is between 40 and 55 years of life, with studies suggesting a second peak at 65–74 years of age (3,4). The mean age of incidence for the cancers mentioned above corresponds with these peaks. Interestingly, alcoholism is more frequently encountered in the oncology setting than other forms of substance abuse. However, the abuse of illicit drugs (e.g., cocaine, heroin) receive greater attention from clinicians. This phenomenon is due to problems in pain management that arise as a result of drug interactions and abuse (see Chapter 49).

The role of the psycho-oncologist in the assessment and management of alcoholism and comorbid psychiatric disorders is crucial to improving both treatment adherence and the quality of life of the patient. Addiction medicine is not an area of expertise for many psycho-oncologists, and many feel inadequately prepared for the treatment of these challenging patients. This chapter reviews: (*1*) psychiatric syndromes frequently encountered in alcoholics; (*2*) the goals and strategies of management of patients with cancer who have comorbid alcohol abuse.

HISTORICAL PERSPECTIVE ON ALCOHOLISM

Alcoholism is a major health and clinical problem in the United States. Despite being defined as a disease by the American Medical Association in 1956, alcoholism has often been considered a form of deviance and moral weakness (5). The medical and mental health communities traditionally viewed the alcoholic as hopeless, while society has labeled them as useless. The prevailing societal stigma towards alcoholism is poignantly illustrated by the name chosen for the first 12-step recovery program in the 1930s, "Alcoholics Anonymous." Although a number of alcoholics were successfully recovering from their addiction and returning to productive lives, these individuals were considered "miracles" by both the general public and medical professionals. By the 1970s, alcoholism represented between 15% and 50% of medical/surgical admissions to general hospitals and was the most frequent discharge diagnosis for Medicare and Medicaid recipients in New York County (6,7). Given the enormous impact on society and the health care system, a movement was begun by medical and mental health professionals to take a comprehensive treatment approach to the socioeconomic, psychological and physical aspects of alcoholism.

Today, alcoholism is defined as a "chronic, progressive often fatal disease" and represents America's most serious drug problem (2,8). Alcoholics commonly experience serious socioeconomic (i.e., unemployment), legal, marital and family problems, psychological/psychiatric (i.e., depression, anxiety, dementia, and other co-existing psychiatric disorders) and physical (i.e., seizures, heart disease, cancer, liver disorders) problems resulting from their disease. An estimated 1 million Americans seek treatment for alcoholism each year and approximately 50% relapse within the first few months of treatment (9). The chronic, progressive nature of this disease is clearly illustrated by the fact that only 5% of alcoholics achieve treatment success (i.e., abstinence). Zimberg suggests that only 7–15% of alcoholics are able to return safely to normal drinking (3). Given these realities, modern substance abuse theorists have recognized harm reduction as a legitimate treatment goal (10,11). Harm reduction and crisis intervention therapies focus upon minimizing alcohol consumption and the subsequent negative consequences, rather than total abstinence. These goals characterize the approach commonly taken to help alcoholic cancer patients. The practical management of alcoholism in the oncology setting uses a range of approaches that constitute and emphasize harm reduction rather than abstinence in recognizing the unique stresses encountered by these patients during the course of a life-threatening illness.

In the following sections, we address the clinical aspects of alcoholism and cancer, beginning with an overview of comorbid disorders frequently found in the alcoholic.

ALCOHOLISM AND COMORBID PSYCHIATRIC DISORDERS

Introduced by Feinstein in 1970, comorbidity is defined as "any distinct additional clinical entity that has existed or that may occur during the clinical course of a patient who has the index disease under study" (12). Davidson and Ritson add that comorbidity should be restricted to diseases or disorders and, in the strict sense, does not apply to symptoms (13).

Alcoholic individuals have been found to be at higher risk for other psychiatric disorders (14). According to the Epidemiologic Catchment Areas Study, of 20,291 individuals in the USA, an estimated 33% have had a lifetime occurrence of at least one mental disorder. Alcohol dependence and abuse accounted for 13.5% of the total disorders. Among those with an alcohol disorder, 37% had a comorbid mental disorder. Most common comorbid mental disorders associated with alcoholism were: anxiety disorders (19.4%), antisocial personality disorder (14.3%), affective disorder (13.4%), and schizophrenia (3.8%) (15). Christie et al. estimate that 78% of people with drug and alcohol problems have had a psychiatric disorder in their lifetime (16). In the study of Penick et al., of 928 patients undergoing treatment for alcoholism at Veterans Administration Hospitals 38% met the criteria for alcoholism only (i.e., monosyndromatic alcoholics). The remaining 575 (62%) patients met the diagnostic criteria for one or more additional lifetime psychiatric disorders (i.e., polysyndromatic alcoholics). Thirty percent met the criteria for one additional syndrome, 16% for two additional syndromes, 12% for three, and 4% for four or more disorders in addition to alcoholism. In order of prevalence, depression was most common comorbid psychiatric disorder (36%), followed by antisocial personality disorder (24%), drug abuse and mania (17% each). Those patients studied were found to endorse symptoms that correspond to those used to define psychiatric disorders in nonsubstance-abusing populations (17). Thus, the psycho-oncologist assessing the alcoholic cancer patient must identify and treat any comorbid disorders present.

The occurrence of comorbid organic mental disorders in alcoholics may contribute to poor treatment compliance and success due to cognitive limitations and premorbid (in relation to the diagnosis of cancer) pain and neurologic deficits. In patients with a history of severe alcoholism and metabolic or nutritional problems, Maxmen and Ward estimate that 65% and 53% may develop Wernicke's encephalopathy or Korsakoff's psychosis, respectively. Interestingly, in terms of pain control issues, 70% develop alcoholic polyneuropathy. Delirium tremens (DTs) occurs in approximately 5% of alcoholic individuals during withdrawal, of which 5%–15% of cases are fatal (2).

Alcoholism: Primary or Secondary?

There has been some debate as to whether alcoholism is the primary or secondary disorder (occurring after the onset of the primary disorder) in relationship to other psychiatric disorders. Brown et al. caution that, since transient psychiatric symptoms (i.e., depression and anxiety) frequently manifest during intoxication and withdrawal from psychoactive drugs, a diagnosis based upon current symptoms of anxiety and depression should not, if possible, be made prior to 4 weeks of abstinence from alcohol (18). When attempting to tease out primary or secondary alcoholism, Schuckit reported that 43% of males alcoholics had primary alcoholism (19). A study by Winokur et al. found that individuals with a manic-depressive disorder (primary) may attempt to self-medicate through the abuse-dependence of alcohol (secondary) (20). Kushner et al. found the relationship between alcohol problems and anxiety disorders to be variable within the category of anxiety disorders. In individuals with agoraphobia and social phobia, alcohol problems appeared to represent attempts to self-medicate (secondary) the symptoms of anxiety. In contrast, symptoms of panic disorder and generalized anxiety disorder were likely to follow pathological alcohol consumption (primary). Simple phobia was not found to be related to alcohol problems in any significant way (21). Zimberg contends that, when appropriate treatment for the primary psychiatric disorder is effective, the secondary psychiatric disorder often lessens or remits completely (3). Other researchers feel that coexisting psychiatric disorders must be given equal attention because of issues regarding treatment compliance and other mitigating factors (22). In the oncology setting, comorbid psychiatric disorders may be easier to treat than alcoholism itself.

The symptomatic control of depression and anxiety can greatly enhance the patient's quality of life, possibly diminish the likelihood of drinking and enhance treatment compliance.

Prevalence of Alcoholism and Comorbid Psychiatric Disorders in the Medical and Oncology Settings

Alcoholism complicates medical care in many ways. Alcoholic individuals generally display poor, sporadic treatment compliance, have limited social support, and/or present with a comorbid psychiatric disorder(s). In 1976, Shevitz et al. studied 1000 medical and surgical inpatients referred to the Psychiatric Consultation Service at the Dartmouth-Hitchcock Medical Center. Sixty-eight percent of the patients referred presented with concurrent physical and psychiatric disorder. Alcoholism was a primary diagnosis in 3% of referrals, but was identified as a major problem in 9% of patients (23).

The diagnosis of cancer is a catastrophic stress. Individuals with cancer endure financial and lifestyle disruptions. Social isolation, stress and anxiety associated with fears of mortality and dependency take a psychological toll on the cancer patient, often resulting in the development of a psychiatric disorder. There have been relatively few studies that examine the prevalence of psychiatric disorders, and even fewer of alcoholism, specifically in an oncology population. A large institutional study carried out at three cancer centers in the United States found that 47% of cancer patients randomly assessed met the criteria for a diagnosis of a psychiatric illness, of which alcohol abuse and personality disorders constituted 3% (24). In 1986, Weddington et al. examined the prevalence of current and lifetime psychiatric disorders in patients with extremity sarcoma. Of the 35 patients assessed, two patients were excluded (one patient was intoxicated with alcohol at time of assessment). Alcoholism was reported in 12% of the 33 remaining patients (25). As previously discussed, the prevalence of alcoholism likely varies widely from one site-specific neoplasm to another with the highest rate found in the head and neck cancer population.

A history of alcohol abuse may contribute to poor adjustment to illness (26). Patients with a history of alcoholism appear to be at a higher risk for the development of major depression or adjustment disorder with depressed mood (27). A history of alcohol abuse is a risk factor for the development of suicidal thinking in the presence of illness. Cornelius et al. found that depressed alcoholics express suicidal thinking at a 59% higher rate than nondepressed alcoholics and is more predominant during times when questions regarding

treatment are pressing (28). In 1990, Breitbart reported that 4% of patients referred for psychiatric consultation for suicidal risk were given a diagnosis of alcoholism (29). In addition, an 8-year study of suicide rate in Veterans Administration Hospitals revealed that 50% of patients who committed suicide had neoplasms of head, neck, and lung, sites of cancer which are associated with heavy drinking and smoking and psychiatric comorbidity (30). Finally, ineffective pain management contributes to increased disease-related stress. Patients with a history of drug addiction or alcoholism are at substantial risk for poor control of cancer-related pain (31,32).

The prevalence of alcoholism in major cancer centers is most likely underestimated. Socioeconomic barriers such as low income or unemployment, lack of health insurance, ignorance of and possibly even attempts to self-medicate early signs of malignancies, may preclude patients with alcoholism from seeking care at tertiary care centers. In addition, alcoholism appears to be underreported and frequently misdiagnosed. A study by Bruera et al. of 100 terminally ill alcoholic cancer patients found that, despite multiple hospital admissions and screenings, only one-third had documentation of alcoholism in their medical records (33).

PSYCHOTHERAPEUTIC MANAGEMENT OF THE ALCOHOLIC CANCER PATIENT

This section provides an overview for planning an effective, multidisciplinary approach to the management of alcoholism in the oncology setting. Team care of the alcoholic cancer patient requires: (1) the collaborative effort of a multiple disciplines; (2) a plan for the management of acute alcohol withdrawal symptoms and delirium tremens; (3) a supportive psychotherapeutic approach emphasizing crisis intervention and harm reduction; (4) the development of an appropriate aftercare or outpatient program.

Assessment

The first member of the medical team (often the nurse) to suspect alcohol dependence/abuse should alert the team to the possibility of an alcohol problem. At this point, the process of multidisciplinary assessment and management should be set in motion. Too often, the fear of offending or stigmatizing the patient leaves obvious signs of alcohol dependence/abuse neglected (i.e., smell of alcohol on breath or intoxication during visits to clinic). A physician should obtain a history and evaluate the possibility of alcohol withdrawal or other emergent problems. In the wake of current pressures to treat the majority of patients in ambulatory setting, and to admit patients on the morning of major surgery, the swift identification of alcoholism and initiation of plans for social, medical and psychological needs of the patient must begin upon initial contact. Social work and/or psychiatric consultation/liaison service should be utilized early, to begin team management and planning.

Taking an accurate, detailed history from the patient is essential for the proper assessment and treatment of alcoholism and comorbid psychiatric disorders. Alcoholic individuals typically underreport the frequency, quantity and duration of their alcohol consumption when providing their medical history because of embarrassment, fear of being stigmatized by the medical staff, and/or strong defense mechanisms, primarily denial. Therefore, the empathetic and skillful taking of an indepth history is the first priority. Interviewer's should inquire in a nonjudgmental, empathetic manner about the duration, quantity and, importantly, the desired effect of the patient's alcohol consumption. The use of the CAGE Questionnaire, a four question screening instrument (Table 50.1), accurately detects alcoholism at a rate of 85% (34,35). Maxmen and Ward caution, however, that the CAGE misses more cases of alcohol dependence in women than it does in men (2). Clinicians should also inquire about past episodes of withdrawal, seizures, head trauma, medical and psychiatric hospitalizations and drug use, both licit and illicit. Because 17% alcoholics abuse other drugs, a clinician needs to be aware of possible polysubstance abuse/dependence on the part of the patient (17). Consultation with family members or close friends may be helpful in verifying the accuracy of the patient's report and level of denial. However, the presence of codependent behavior (i.e., denial or enabling) should also be considered when interviewing family or friends of an alcoholic cancer patient. In the actively drinking alcoholic, time of last consumption should be noted and the prevention of withdrawal should become first priority.

Alcohol Withdrawal Syndrome

All too frequently, alcoholism is not identified until the manifestations of alcohol withdrawal syndrome are present. According to the *Diagnostic Statistical Manual* (4th Edition) the alcoholic in withdrawal has decreased or stopped his or her prolonged ingestion of alcohol (see Table 50.2 for criteria) (36).

Alcohol withdrawal is dangerous and can seriously complicate cancer treatment. In some instances, it is fatal. The first symptoms of withdrawal typically appear in the first few hours following the cessation of alcohol consumption and may consist of tremors, agitation and insomnia. In cases of mild to moderate withdrawal, these symptoms tend to dissipate within 1–2 days without recurrence. However, in cases of severe withdrawal, autonomic hyperactivity, hallucinations and disorientation may follow. The onset of delirium tremens marks the individual's progression from the withdrawal state to a state of delirium that represents a serious medical emergency. Delirium tremens occurs in approximately 5–15% of patients in alcohol withdrawal, typically within the first 72–96 h of withdrawal, and is characterized by agitation, hallucination, delusions, incoherence and disorientation (2). Delirium tremens is self-limiting and usually ends in 72–96 h with the patient entering a deep sleep with amnesia for most of what had occurred. However, in the medically ill patients, the risk of further complications is high and the disorder must be treated.

Wernicke–Korsakoff's syndrome is indicative of a thiamine deficiency and represents a frequently underdiagnosed, debilitating disorder that causes permanent cognitive impairment. Although not a result of the development of delirium tremens, the level of alcohol consumption required for the development of delirium tremens is sufficient to cause thiamine depletion. Symptoms of Wernicke–Korsakoff syndrome may include a fixed upward gaze, alcoholic neuropathy, "stocking-glove" paresthesia, autonomic instability, and delirium encephalopathy.

TABLE 50.1. *CAGE Questionnaire*

C	Thought you should CUT back on your drinking?
A	Felt ANNOYED by people criticizing your drinking?
G	Felt GUILTY or bad about your drinking?
E	Had morning EYE-OPENER to relieve hangover or nerves?

Source: Ewing (34).

TABLE 50.2. *Alcohol Withdrawal*

The individual in withdrawal has decreased or stopped his or her prolonged ingestion of alcohol (generally >1 month) and presents with at least two of the following symptoms:

Autonomic hyperactivity (e.g., sweating or a pulse rate >100 beats/min)
Increased hand tremor
Insomnia
Nausea or vomiting
Transient visual, tactile, or auditory hallucinations or illusions
Psychomotor agitation
Anxiety
Grand mal seizures

Medical Treatment of Withdrawal. While a full discussion of the pharmacological approach to alcohol withdrawal is beyond the scope of this chapter, a basic approach to the treatment of this syndrome is given.

The use of hydration, benzodiazepines, and, in some cases, neuroleptics, is appropriate for the management of alcohol withdrawal syndrome (see Table 50.3). The administration of a vitamin–mineral solution is indicated to counteract the effects of malnutrition that results from the alcohol itself and poor eating habits. Thiamine 100 mg administered intramuscularly or intravenously for 3 days before switching to oral administration for the duration of treatment prevents the development of Korsakoff's syndrome and alcoholic dementia. A daily oral dose of folate 1 mg should also be given throughout the course of treatment. In cases of mild withdrawal, hydration alone may sufficient. Benzodiazepines (lorazepam, midazolam, diazepam, and chlordiazepoxide) are the drugs of choice for the management of alcohol withdrawal because of their sedative effects (see Table 4) (37,38). Careful consideration must be given to route, absorption, potency and dose of benzodiazepine prescribed. Dose should be based upon estimated alcohol consumption and the type of setting of detoxification (see below). Insufficient administration of benzodiazepines (too low dose, or too rapid taper) may allow the progression of withdrawal to a state of delirium tremens. The development of seizures is life-threatening and they may repeatedly recur in the patient while unconscious. The nonbenzodiazepine anticonvulsants are not prescribed prophylactically. In cases of severe withdrawal and confusion, neuroleptics (e.g., haloperidol 0.5–5.0 mg IV every 8 h) are added to the treatment regimen. Commonly, alcoholic patients report to the hospital either intoxicated or in the early stages of withdrawal. From a surgical perspective, serious complications can arise from the presence of alcohol withdrawal and its acute management is the primary treatment goal. Unfortunately, clinicians are frequently provided insufficient lead time to properly detoxify the patient prior to surgery (typically less than 24 h) and the patient stands at an increased the risk for the postoperative development of organic mental disorders, seizure, and delirium tremens. Since alcoholic cancer patients are already at high risk for delirium postoperatively due to poor nutrition, prior head trauma, brain injury from excessive alcohol consumption, the development of seizures and delirium tremens adds to the risk of fatality. It is important to note that, since it desirable for the patient to be alert postoperatively for ambulation and use of pulmonary toilet, the amount of sedation required for detoxification is much lower than the desired level of sedation in a nonsurgical alcoholic patient.

Treatment Modalities

Abstinence, though optimal, is not necessarily a treatment goal for the alcoholic in an oncology setting. Instead, a management plan that facilitates the effective implementation and continuation of cancer treatment is given priority. The most common approaches to the management of alcoholism are psychotherapeutic and pharmacological interventions.

Psychotherapeutic Approach. A psychotherapeutic treatment approach that focuses on crisis intervention, the development of effective coping skills, relapse prevention, and, most importantly, treatment compliance, appears to be most effective with medically ill individuals. The improvement of coping skills in the alcoholic individual is critical. Alcohol represents one of the dependent patient's

TABLE 50.3. *Guidelines for the Treatment of Alcohol Withdrawal*

Continual close monitoring of withdrawal status

Utilization of benzodiazepines

Taper dose slowly (generally not by more than 25% per 24 h period)

Administration of thiamine 100 mg IM or IV four times a day

Administration of folate 1 mg PO four times a day

Monitor for signs of the potential onset of delirium tremens

Consideration should be given to a loading dose of phenytoin for patients with a history of withdrawal seizures or for patients in whom seizures are likely (e.g., patients with brain metastases)

TABLE 50.4. *Types and Characteristics of Benzodiazepines for Treatment of Alcohol Withdrawal*

Drug	Dose	Duration of Action	Half-Life (h)
Chlordiazepoxide	25–100 mg IV every 3 h	Short	5–30
Diazepam	10–20 mg IV every 1–4 h	Short	20–100
Lorazepam	1–2 mg IV every 1–4 h	Intermediate	10–20
Midazolam	1–5 mg IV every 1–2 h	Very short	1–4

primary, though maladaptive, coping tools. When compounded with the stress associated with having cancer, the cessation of alcohol consumption can be overwhelming and contribute to noncompliance and discontinuation of treatment. Teaching specific, illness-related coping methods with an emphasis upon containing episodes of consumption is essential. The treatment of anxiety and depression may decrease the patients need and desire for alcohol.

Harm reduction and crisis intervention are central components of the treatment of alcohol dependence/abuse in the cancer patient. The goals of treatment are to minimize the frequency and intensity of the patient's alcohol consumption and, thereby, to reduce further damage to the patient and to facilitate treatment compliance. Should the patient relapses, treatment should be re-started and the emphasis upon treatment compliance re-established. The clinician should be aware of possible issues of countertransference (e.g., frustration and anger) towards the patient and take the necessary steps to remedy this situation in a professional manner. Staff should be reminded that alcoholism is a chronic, relapsing illness. Kranzler et al. described two patients with head and neck cancers who, despite being told of the negative medical consequences, continued to inject alcohol via their feeding tubes (39). This report represents the essence of alcohol addiction, even in the face of a disfiguring, life-threatening illness.

Despite the staff's best efforts at therapy and support, the patient may return to drinking. Relapse should be expected and tolerated; patients should not be "penalized" for their psychiatric disorder. The goal of crisis intervention is to restore the patient to baseline behavior through symptom management. By strengthening coping and problem-solving, the clinician can help the alcoholic patient to consider different methods of coping with disease-related stress and attempt to minimize the patient's reliance upon alcohol as a coping mechanism.

Pharmacological Approach. To date, there are no long-term, effective pharmacological treatments for alcoholism per se. However, pharmacological interventions directed towards the treatment of comorbid psychiatric disorders and the reduction of "cravings" in alcoholics have been found to be beneficial in reducing alcohol consumption. When selecting a medication for patients with alcoholism, consideration must be given to issues of drug efficacy, potential for the development of addiction and side effects, and possible negative interactions with other medical interventions. The following section addresses the use of antidepressants,

antianxiety medications and opioid receptor blocker (naltrexone) in alcoholic cancer patients.

Researchers hypothesized that the treatment of comorbid depression in alcoholics would significantly contribute to better treatment outcomes. Because of the neurophysiological changes that result from prolonged alcohol consumption, the efficacy of antidepressants for alcoholism has been difficult to establish. However, preliminary research has found the use of fluoxetine among alcoholic individuals with major depression beneficial in reducing levels of depression (40). Similarly, Mason and colleagues reported good results in the use of desipramine in the treatment of secondary depression in abstinent alcoholics. The treatment of depression secondary to alcoholism may reduce the risk for drinking relapse in some patients (41,42). A recent study by McGrath et al. reported the effectiveness of imipramine for primary depression in alcoholics. Although subjects were not physically dependent upon alcohol, this study found decreased levels of alcohol consumption in those individuals whose depression responded to treatment. These researchers concluded that imipramine contributes to harm reduction and may be beneficial to patients seeking treatment in acute care facilities for disorders other than alcoholism (43). Because of problems with treatment compliance in alcoholics, dietary restrictions and the potential for negative interactions of continued substance abuse should be taken into serious consideration when prescribing monoamine oxidase inhibitors for comorbid depression. It is important to note that research does not support a solely pharmacological approach to the treatment of comorbid depression in alcoholics. Therefore, brief psychotherapy should be implemented in conjunction with the use of antidepressants.

The presence of a comorbid anxiety-related disorder can contribute to poor treatment compliance and negatively impact the quality of life of the alcoholic cancer patient. The most widely used type of anxiolytic drugs are benzodiazepines. Although controversial, the long-term use of benzodiazepines has been found effective in reducing cravings and anxiety in recovering alcoholics. However, the sudden discontinuation of long-term benzodiazepine therapy (i.e., in favor of drinking) in dependent patients can result in seizures and death (44). Frances and Borg suggest that the potential for self-medication, dose escalation and the potential for abuse should be taken into consideration with benzodiazepines. They recommend oxazepam in the treatment of anxiety and alcohol disorders because it is not metabolized by the liver, has a slow onset of action, and is less reinforcing. However, Nunes et al.

recommend the use of benzodiazepines in alcoholics only in cases of acute alcohol withdrawal, because benzodiazepines may act as "triggers" to alcoholic relapse. Antidepressants have been shown to be useful in the treatment of anxiety disorders in alcoholic patients. Researchers suggest the use of tricyclic antidepressants and the serotonergic drugs imipramine or fluoxetine in the treatment of panic disorder and generalized social phobia. For generalized anxiety disorders, imipramine or busprone may be beneficial (45,46). As with depression, consideration of the side effects, potential for abuse and interactions with other medical interventions needs to be made when implementing any pharmacological approaches to the treatment of comorbid anxiety.

The introduction of naltrexone, an opioid receptor blocker, has been found useful in diminishing cravings for alcohol (47). O'Malley et al. found that alcoholics receiving naltrexone reported diminished rates of alcohol consumption. However, the effects of naltrexone therapy on rates of abstinence was only sustained through 1 mo of follow-up (48). It is important to note that naltrexone, has not yet been tested in medically ill populations. An opioid inhibitor, naltrexone, negates the effects of pain medications commonly used in an oncology setting. Thus, it cannot be prescribed for patients with pain who are taking opioids. Similarly, the safety of long-term use of naltrexone is presently unclear. Further research is necessary to document the efficacy of naltrexone on both a long-term basis and in medically ill populations.

Aftercare

The implementation of an appropriate aftercare program is necessary upon the patient's discharge from inpatient treatment. The aftercare program, developed in consultation with the patient, should promote continuous support and the treatment of comorbid psychiatric disorders. Consistent monitoring of medications and assessment of treatment compliance is indicated. Medications should be prescribed in small amounts (i.e., 1–2 week supply) to minimize possible drug-hoarding behaviors and to facilitate regular attendance at follow-up appointments.

The clinician and patient should develop a therapeutic contract that establishes firm guidelines for treatment compliance. Under the therapeutic contract, clinicians may require the patient to attend self-help programs such as Alcoholics Anonymous and to provide documentation verifying regular attendance. Most 12-step programs do not endorse the use of psychotrophic medications (chlordiazepoxide, diazepam, etc.) during recovery. Therefore, the clinician may want to contact the patient's Alcoholics Anonymous sponsor (with the patient's consent) and indicate the patient's medication requirements. The sponsor can assist the patient at meetings, helping to ensure that social support is not jeopardized because of medication use. Should the patient desire, a referral can be made to an alcohol treatment program. Similarly, the use of blood and urine analysis may be useful in encouraging abstinence. Because alcoholism is a chronic, relapsing illness, the clinician should expect the patient to violate the therapeutic contract at some point. The clinician should attempt to schedule follow-up appointments that coincide with medical follow-up visits.

Close interprofessional collaboration is required for the effective management of alcohol abuse, dependence and subsequent withdrawal. Fragmented communication among staff can lead to serious management problems. Meetings that involve all staff involved in the care of the alcoholic patient can greatly improve the development and implementation of an effective management plan.

CONCLUSION

Alcohol has been linked to cancer and the management of alcoholic cancer patient represents a serious and complicated challenge to the psycho-oncologist.

REFERENCES

1. American Cancer Society. *Cancer Facts and Figures–1995.* American Cancer Society; 1995.
2. Maxmen JS, Ward NG. Substance-related disorders. In: Maxmen JS, Ward NG, eds. *Essential Psychopathology and Its Treatment*, 2nd ed. New York: W.W. Norton & Co.; 1995: 132–172.
3. Zimberg S *The Clinical Management of Alcoholism.* New York: Brunner/Mazel; 1982.
4. Bailey MB, Harberman PW, Alksne H. The epidemiology of alcoholism in an urban residential area. *Q J Stud Alcohol.* 1965; 26:19–40.
5. Bickerton R. Employee assistance: a history in progress. *EAP Dig.* 1990; 91:34–42.
6. McCrusker J, Cherubin CE, Zimberg S. Prevalence of alcoholism in general municipal hospital population. *NY State J Med.* 1971; 71:751–754.
7. Zimber S. Alcoholism: prevalence of general hospital emergency room and walk-in clinic. *NY State J Med.* 1979; 79:1533–1536.
8. Wrona S, Tankanow R. Corticosteriods in the management of alcoholic hepatitis. *Am J Hosp Pharm.* 1994; 51:347–353.
9. Gordis E. Personal statement regarding naltrexone as a treatment for alcoholism. Letter on the Internet; 1995.
10. Gilman C. Smack in the eye. In: O'Hare P, ed. *The Reduction of Drug-Related Harm.* London: Routledge; 1992.

11. Saunders B. Illicit drugs and harm reduction education [editorial]. *Addict Res.* 1995; 2:i–iii.

12. Feinstein AR. The pre-therapeutic classification of comorbidity in chronic disease. *J Chron Dis.* 1970; 23:455–468.

13. Davidson KM, Ritson EB. The relationship between alcohol dependence and depression. *Alcohol Alcoholism.* 1993; 28(2):147–155.

14. Helzer JE, Pryzbeck TM. The co-occurrence of alcoholism with other psychiatric disorders in the general population and its impact on treatment. *J Stud Alcohol.* 1998; 49:219–224.

15. Reiger DA, Farmer ME, Rae DS, et al. Comorbidity of mental disorders with alcohol and other drug abuse. *J Am Med Assoc.* 1990; 264:2511–2518.

16. Christie KA, Burke JD, Reiger DA, et al. Epidemiological evidence for onset of mental disorders and higher risk of drug abuse in young adults. *Am J Psychiatry.* 1988; 145:971–975.

17. Penick E, Powell B, Nickel E, et al. Co-morbidity of life-time psychiatric disorders among male alcoholic patients. *Alcoholism: Clin Exp Res.* 1994; 18:1289–1293.

18. Brown SA, Inaba RK, Gillin C, et al. Alcoholism and affective disorder: clinical course of depressive symptoms. *Am J Psychiatry.* 1995; 152:45–52.

19. Schuckit M. Alcoholic patients with secondary depression. *Am J Psychiatry.* 1983; 140:711–714.

20. Winokur G, Coryell W, Akiskal HS, et al. Alcoholism in manic-depressive (bi-polar) illness: familial illness, course of illness, and the primary-secondary distinction. *Am J Psychiatry.* 1995; 152:365–371.

21. Kushner MG, Sher KJ, Beitman BD. The relationship between alcohol problems and the anxiety disorders. *Am J Psychiatry.* 1990; 147:685–695.

22. Oldham JM, Shodol AE, Kellman HD, et al. Comorbidity of axis I and axis II disorders. *Am J Psychiatry.* 1995; 152:571–578.

23. Shevitz S, Silberfarb P, Lipowski ZJ. Psychiatric consultations in a general hospital: a report on 1,000 referrals. *Dis Nerv Syst.* 1976; 37:295–300.

24. Derogatis LR, Morrow GR, Fetting J, et al. The prevalence of psychiatric disorders among cancer patients. *J Am Med Assoc.* 1983; 249:715–757.

25. Weddington WW, Segraves KB, Simon MA. Current and lifetime incidence of psychiatric disorders among a group of extremity sarcoma survivors. *J Psychosom Res.* 1986; 30:121–125.

26. Weisman D. Early diagnosis of vulnerability in cancer patients. *Am J Med Sci.* 1976; 271:187–196.

27. Massie MJ, Holland JC. Depression and cancer. *J Clin Psychiatry.* 1990; 51:12–17.

28. Cornelius JR, Salloum IM, Mezzich J, et al. Disproportionate suicidality in patients with comorbid major depression and alcoholism. *Am J Psychiatry.* 1995; 152:358–364.

29. Breitbart W. Suicide. In: Holland JC, Rowland JH, eds. *Handbook of Psychooncology: Psychological Care of the Patient with Cancer.* New York: Oxford University Press; 1990:291–299.

30. Farberow NL, Ganzler S, Cutter F, Reynolds D. An eight-year survey of hospital suicides. *Life-Threat Behav.* 1971; 1:184–201.

31. Foley KM. Pain syndromes in patients with cancer. In: Bonica JJ, Ventafridda V, eds. *Advances in Pain Research and Therapy.* New York: Raven Press; 1979:59–75.

32. Bruera E, MacMillan K, Hanson J, MacDonald RN. The Edmonton staging system for cancer pain: preliminary report. *Pain.* 1989; 37:203–209.

33. Bruera E, Moyano J, Sifert L, et al. The frequency of alcoholism among patients with pain due to terminal cancer. *J Pain Sympt Manage.* 1995; 10:599–603.

34. Ewing JA. Detecting alcoholism, the CAGE questionnaire. *J Am Med Assoc.* 1984; 252:1905–1907.

35. Beresford TP, Blow FC, Hill E, et al. Clinical practice: comparison of Cage questionnaire and computer-assisted laboratory profiles in screening for covert alcoholism. *Lancet.* 1990; 336:482–485.

36. American Psychiatric Association. *Diagnostic Statistical Manual of Mental Disorders*, 4th ed. Washington, DC: American Psychiatric Association; 1994.

37. Erstad B, Cotugno C. Management of alcohol withdrawal. *Am J Health-Syst Pharm.* 1995; 52:697–709.

38. Newman J, Terris D, Moore M. Trends in the management of alcohol withdrawal syndrome. *Laryngoscope.* 1995; 105:1–7.

39. Kranzler HR, Ginther L, Ttofi C. The intragastric infusion of ethanol by alcoholics after surgery for head and neck cancer. *Am J Addict.* 1992; 1:83–85.

40. Kranzler HR, Burleson JA, Korner P, et al. Placebo-controlled trial of flouxetine as an adjunct to relapse prevention in alcoholics. *Am J Psychiatry.* 1995; 152:391–397.

41. Mason BJ, Kocsis JH. Desipramine treatment of alcoholism. *Psychopharmacol Bull.* 1991; 27:155–161.

42. Mason BJ, Kocsis JH, Ritvo EC, Cutler RB. A double-blind, placebo-controlled trial of desipramine for primary lcohol dependence stratified on the presence or absence of major depression. *J Am Med Assoc.* 1996; 275:761–767.

43. McGrath PJ, Nunes EV, Stewart JW, et al. Imipramine treatment of alcoholics with primary depression. *Arch Gen Psychiatry.* 1996; 53; 232–240.

44. Krenzelok EP. Judicious use of flumazenil. *Clin Pharmacol.* 1993; 12:691–692.

45. Nunes E, McGrath PJ, Quitkin FM. Treating anxiety in patients with alcoholism. *J Clin Psychiatry.* 1995; 56:3–9.

46. Frances RJ, Borg L. The treatment of anxiety in patients with alcoholism. *J Clin Psychiatry.* 1993; 54:37–43.

47. Swift RM, Whelihan W, Kuznetsov O, et al. Naltrexone-induced alterations in human ethanol intoxication. *Am J Psychiatry.* 1994; 151:1463–1467.

48. O'Malley SS, Jaffe AJ, Chang G, et al. Six-month follow-up of naltrexone and psychotherapy for alcohol dependence. *Arch Gen Psychiatry.* 1996; 53:217–224.

51

Posttraumatic Stress Disorder

STEVEN D. PASSIK AND KATHY L. GRUMMON

Advancement in the treatment of many cancers has resulted in growing numbers of patients experiencing longer periods of disease-free survival. Paralleling this fortunate development, however, has been evidence that the experience of being diagnosed with, treated for, and surviving cancer can be accompanied by substantial problems in psychological well-being for a subset of individuals (1–3). Researchers have not reliably documented an increased prevalence of formal psychiatric disorders or major psychopathology in survivors as compared to normal controls or community samples (3–8). However, studies examining adult and child survivors of cancer have described heightened psychological distress (7,9,10), disturbances in self-esteem, body image, intimacy and sexuality, as well as subsyndromal symptoms of anxiety and depression related to fears of recurrence and the confrontation with one's mortality (3,4,6).

For some time, psycho-oncologists have been documenting an additional dimension to the cancer experience—discrete symptoms that are regarded as "conditioned" responses. Anticipatory nausea and vomiting, anxiety and other emotions that accompany these physiologic phenomena have been well studied as learned responses to repetitive, aversive treatments (11–13). A number of investigators have also reported the presence of stress- or trauma-related symptoms such as avoidance behaviors, intrusive thoughts, and heightened arousability in cancer survivors (4,6,9,10). These symptoms resemble those seen in individuals who have experienced extreme stressors, such as combat, natural disaster, rape or other life threats. Collectively, these symptoms are referred to as posttraumatic stress disorder or PTSD (14–20).

These observations in cancer patients and survivors parallel a recent change in thinking about the PTSD diagnosis. In the diagnostic nomenclature of the DSM-III-R (21), people with medical illnesses, including life-threatening ones, were specifically excluded from consideration for the diagnosis of PTSD. Illness as a stressor was not considered to be unusual enough or of high enough magnitude to induce the psychological aftermath of a traumatic experience. Thus, even those patients who fulfilled all of the other criteria for PTSD were not eligible for the diagnosis simply because having cancer did not meet the required definition of a high magnitude stressful event (21,22). Patients with symptoms of re-experience, arousal and avoidance were most likely diagnosed with an adjustment disorder or other anxiety or mood disorder, especially given the high comorbidity of PTSD with anxiety, mood and substance abuse disorders (14). Practicing psycho-oncology clinicians, who have always recognized the signs of trauma in their patients, may regard recent changes in the application of the PTSD diagnosis to cancer as mere nosologic hair-splitting. It is unlikely that these practitioners treated their patients differently or minimized the emotional impact of their experience simply because of the exclusive DSM diagnostic criteria. The diagnostic criteria for PTSD contained in the DSM-IV (14) represent a shift in emphasis away from the traumatic event itself and toward the psychological experience of the person who takes part in, undergoes or witnesses that event. In this regard, the philosophy behind the DSM criteria may have moved closer to the wisdom of practicing psycho-oncologists. However, perhaps in some instances, past philosophical biases may have led to a failure to assess for the specific symptom clusters that constitute the PTSD diagnosis, in clinical and empirical work alike. That is, researchers and clinicians may have potentially missed an opportunity to identify symptoms that cause significant distress, detract from quality of life, and require attention and treatment.

The physical and psychological impact of cancer and cancer treatment clearly constitute traumatic experiences for a subset of patients. The diagnosis of a potentially life-threatening disease and the recurring threats to bodily integrity and autonomy often have profound psychological effects (23). Patients commonly experience pain, fatigue, weakness, nausea, and vomiting and often undergo painful, toxic and intrusive procedures. Patients also endure repeated, sometimes lengthy, hospitalizations in an environment that can seem foreign and engender a sense of loss of control. Taken together, these aspects of the cancer experience often lead to a sense of helplessness that can be "traumatic." The impact may be greatest on those who have other risk factors that render them particularly vulnerable. Such risk factors have not been empirically linked to PTSD in cancer patients, but clinical experience and research on PTSD in other populations (17,18,24) suggest that they are likely to include poor social support, prior history of traumatization or victimization, or a history of psychiatric disorder. For example, vulnerable patients with Axis II disorders, such as a history of borderline and/or narcissistic personality disorder, would likely manifest problems during cancer treatment when they are asked to surrender a degree of their autonomy to insure effective treatment and maintain safety (25).

APPLYING PTSD TO CANCER: PITFALLS AND POTENTIAL

With the aforementioned changes in the philosophy of PTSD and the DSM criteria, there has been a rapid adoption of the PTSD diagnosis by many psycho-oncology researchers and clinicians. While some obvious benefits accompany this new perspective, there are also conceptual and practical problems that arise in the application of PTSD to cancer that threaten to dilute its theoretical and diagnostic specificity. One major problem in applying PTSD to cancer has been the lack of agreement as to when cancer survivors, who live with the threat of recurrence, can be defined as "post" the entirety of the cancer experience and, therefore, eligible for a diagnosis of PTSD. Also, the timing of PTSD assessment becomes a crucial issue for both diagnostic specificity and the clinical meaningfulness of the symptomatology. If patients are not afforded the appropriate time to proceed through the normal process of adjusting to a health threat(s), the percentage of patients "qualifying" for a psychiatric diagnosis will be inflated to the point that the diagnosis is of little value. The DSM-IV criteria try to guard against this by proposing a time frame (symptoms present for at least 1 month) and insisting that the symptoms have a discernable impact upon psychosocial functioning (14).

A related problem is the difficulty of defining the traumatic stressor for individual cancer patients. Within the multiple crises that constitute the totality of the cancer experience, it is much more difficult to identify a discrete stressor than with other traumas such as natural disaster or rape. In the cancer experience, the stressor may be the initial diagnosis, the perception that the disease could be fatal, an unrelieved period of pain, a symptom that signals recurrence, an aversive procedure, or an unexpected, even chance, occurrence (e.g., being present when a roommate in a shared hospital room is resuscitated or dies). In ideal situations, the timing of the PTSD assessment would be measured in relation to the stressor as viewed from the perspective of the patient. However, this may be difficult to implement, especially in large research designs. Often, the problem is only partially (and sometimes arbitrarily) addressed by waiting a uniform period of time since the discontinuation of cancer treatment (a common research strategy to date). The following cases illustrate how different and subtle the traumatic aspect of the stressor can be for individual patients.

Case Examples: What is the Stressor?

A young mother meeting full PTSD criteria following surgical resection of node-negative renal cancer was referred for psychiatric evaluation of anxiety symptoms 6 months after her cancer treatment ended. The patient reported that she was involved in a dispute with the oncologist about obtaining follow-up diagnostic imaging. At the time of the initial assessment she was hoping to obtain a CT scan of her chest after respiratory difficulties (likely representing panic/hyperarousal symptoms triggered by worry about metastatic disease). These symptoms led her to believe that she might have lung metastases. Her initial tumor was diagnosed somewhat serendipitously when she changed internists and received a work-up for blood in her urine by the new physician. Formerly an avid exerciser and self-described "diet and health nut," she was devastated by the diagnosis and had chronic troublesome thoughts that she could "do nothing to insure health." The patient and her therapist recognized that for her the traumatic event was the chance nature of the diagnosis and the undermining of her sense of control of her health via diet and exercise. In the initial stages of therapy, she was given "permission" to obtain imaging tests as frequently as she could afford, but was advised to assess their value in terms of whether or not they provided lasting reassurance. Subsequent CT of the chest was negative.

A 54-year-old man with laryngeal cancer, who was initially believed to have localized, node-negative disease, was referred for evaluation of symptoms of depression. He had undergone surgical resection and was in the process of obtaining a consultation regarding the use of brachytherapy versus external beam radiation when an enlarged lymph node in his neck was noted and a biopsy revealed more malignancy. Almost immediately following this development, he became reclusive, would not go to work or interact with his wife and child. When he did not improve over the course of a month, his wife insisted that he seek counseling. Initially the therapist anticipated that the patient was reacting to the increased threat to his life posed by the discovery. More specifically, the patient disclosed that it was the presence of a lymph node "in his neck" that had undermined him. His father had died of Hodgkin's disease when the patient was a young man. The father's disease began with discovery of a lymph node in his neck and he "wasted away" rapidly thereafter. The patient was filled with dread upon hearing this diagnosis and had been experiencing nearly constant visions of himself wasting away as his father did, as the disease spread from his neck throughout his body. He also reported nightmares in which he saw himself back at his dying father's bedside. When he looked down at his father in the dream, his own face would appear on his father's body. He reported that he had been avoiding his family because interacting with them triggered thoughts about his death and because he feared that his child would watch him waste away and would become as traumatized as he had been.

A male musician, 6 years post cancer treatment, was referred for socialization problems. He had a history of glioblastoma multiforme and awoke after resection in a neurology intensive care unit. On high dose steroids "his mind was a blur," with racing thoughts. He was terrified. Not long thereafter, the neurology team making rounds stopped by to assess him. They began asking him mental status questions that he could not answer. He felt tremendously humiliated and fearful that he was losing his mind. Years after treatment ended he was unable to erase this experience from his memory. Headaches served as a trigger to intrusive thoughts of the event.

Overextension of the PTSD diagnosis and uncertainty about the nature and timing of the target stressor continue to represent significant problems in the adoption of PTSD by psycho-oncologists. For researchers especially, these conceptual issues present some obviously troubling problems. How are researchers to capture the diagnostic subtleties? Such variables are simply "noise" in large between group designs.

In clinical practice, however, the diagnostic "details" may be less critical. The pragmatic, crisis intervention approach employed by most practicing psycho-oncologists dictates that distressing symptoms are always regarded as legitimate targets for intervention. For instance, the young woman with renal cancer clearly needed strategies to diminish panic (hyperarousal) symptoms so that they did not trigger intrusive thoughts about lung metastases. Such strategies also empowered her to take an active role in restoring a sense of personal safety. The man with laryngeal cancer needed help with diminishing intrusive thoughts and nightmares while reducing avoidance of work and family. The musician benefited from retelling and reframing his target experience and from learning strategies for stopping intrusive thoughts.

While the first patient discussed above met full DSM-IV criteria for PTSD, the second and third did not. These cases highlight the point that whether patients have a full-blown syndrome (PTSD) or only a subset of distressing symptoms, they should be afforded consideration of a range of interventions, from psychopharmacologic to psychotherapeutic, in an effort to enhance their quality of life and reduce their distress (see treatment section below). These cases also demonstrate that patients can be "posttraumatic" long before they are posttreatment. In such instances, PTSD serves less as a specific diagnosis and more as a heuristic for planning ways to intervene.

Despite these pitfalls, there is potential utility in applying PTSD to certain psychological aspects of the cancer experience. The diagnosis has been the subject of a high level of theoretical and clinical discourse and a large number of research studies. Collaboration with colleagues in the PTSD field will likely lead to the specification of new research hypotheses and possible importation of empirically-based, manualized psychotherapeutic approaches to psycho-oncology.

EVOLUTION OF THE PTSD DIAGNOSIS

PTSD is a diagnosis that has had a long, sometimes difficult, history within psychiatry (22,26). Its place among other mental disorders has been uncertain. Initially gaining entrance into the nomenclature in the post-Vietnam period, the initial philosophy was that PTSD resulted from mere exposure to a highly traumatic experience and could, therefore, happen to anyone—it was a "normal," or expected, mental disorder (20). More recent biological data have not supported this contention. Instead, there now appear to be distinct differences in the biology of those individuals who experience a trauma and develop PTSD and those who do not (27–29). Additional observations from research on personality and social factors in PTSD have led to a shift in focus from the traumatic event itself to the individual's experience of that event (30). Thus, as researchers and clinicians have refined their understanding of PTSD, they have begun to establish what is now an extensive knowledge base on the nature and etiology of this disorder. Additionally, some have begun to design and test psychotherapeutic interventions for traumatized individuals (15). For example, the trauma recovery approach to rape survivors is a highly structured psycho-educational and support group intervention that might be translated for work with cancer survivors.

DIAGNOSTIC CRITERIA AND CHARACTERISTICS OF PTSD

In 1994, the application of PTSD to cancer patients began with the redefinition of the trauma criterion in DSM-IV to include life-threatening illness (14) (see Table 51.1).

PTSD was initially characterized as an anxiety disorder that developed in response to severe trauma in which an individual experienced, witnessed or was confronted by actual or threatened death, injury or loss of physical integrity of self or others. DSM-IV stipulated, for the first time, that being "diagnosed with a life-threatening illness" or "learning that one's child" had such an illness were qualifying stressful events (14, p. 424). These events elicit responses of intense fear, helplessness or horror, and trigger three clusters of PTSD symptoms: reexperience of the trauma (nightmares, flashbacks, and intrusive thoughts), persistent avoidance of reminders of the trauma (avoidance of situations, numbing of general responsiveness, and restricted range of affect), and persistent increased arousal (sleep difficulties, hypervigilance, irritability). Other common emotional responses associated with such traumas are despair, helplessness, guilt over actions taken or avoided, and consuming loss (14). (see Table 51.2).

PREVALENCE OF PTSD IN CANCER PATIENTS AND SURVIVORS

Research on PTSD in cancer survivors has concentrated on defining the prevalence and characteristics of the disorder in patients undergoing treatment, adult and child survivors, and their family members. A wide variety of cancer types have been studied including, but not limited to, leukemia (31), breast cancer (32), and head and neck cancers (33). Using a model of stress and coping, researchers studying adult populations have identified that, in cancer, as in other major life stresses, increased arousal, avoidant and intrusive thinking are often seen (13). To date, the majority of these studies have focused on the symptoms rather than the diagnosis of PTSD syndromes per se (see Table 51.3).

Much of the recent research has focused on adult survivors of Hodgkin's disease, possibly due to the high rates of survival from this cancer (13). In a study of 273 disease-free survivors of advanced Hodgkin's disease, Kornblith et al. (2,4,9) found a high prevalence of both intrusive and avoidant symptoms even though their subjects were an average of 6.3 years from their last treatment. The researchers also noted that subjects with these symptoms tended to have high levels of psychological distress and sexual problems. Cella and Tross (3) also found higher levels of avoidant thinking in former Hodgkin's patients than in age-matched, physically healthy controls. These authors also noted lower levels of motivation for seeking intimate relationships in the post-Hodgkin's population, a symptom which is included in the DSM-IV diagnosis of PTSD.

In a sample of leukemia survivors treated with conventional chemotherapy and/or bone marrow transplant (BMT), Lesko and colleagues (31) found significant rates of intrusive and avoidant thoughts that were associated with reduced quality of life and other social sequelae. Similar results were obtained by Ostroff et al. (34) in an investigation of acute and chronic leukemia patients who were at least 1 year post-BMT. Finally, a recent study by Greenberg et al. (7) found that 23% of a sample of adult survivors of osteogenic sarcoma reported high rates of intrusive thoughts of cancer; 6% rated their symptoms as severe. Again, levels of intrusive symptoms were significantly correlated with psychological distress.

In some studies, the authors inferred a diagnosis of PTSD despite the fact that their research predated the DSM-IV redefinition (see Table 51.4). For example, Schwartz et al. (32) found that over half of a sample of women with a history of breast cancer had intrusive thoughts and sleep disturbances that they linked to their cancer treatment. Fifteen percent of these women were estimated to be eligible for a diagnosis of PTSD. Bobertz (35), in her assessment of gynecolo-

---

TABLE 51.1. *Differences in Criterion Event Definition (Criteria A) Between DSM-III-R and DSM-IV*

The essential feature of this disorder is the development of characteristic symptoms following exposure to a psychologically distressing event . . .

DSM-III-R	DSM-IV
. . . that is *outside the range of usual human experience* (i.e., *excluding* some common experiences such as simple bereavement, marital conflict, and *chronic illness*) and that would be markedly distressing to almost anyone.	. . . that involved actual or threatened death, serious injury, or threat to physical integrity of self or others. Such events include being *diagnosed with a life-threatening illness* or *learning that one's child has a life-threatening illness.*

Source: Adapted from Refs. 14 and 21.

TABLE 51.2. *Diagnostic Criteria for Posttraumatic Stress Disorder (Criteria B,C,D,E,F)*

Description	Examples of Symptoms
CRITERION B Persistent reexperiencing of the traumatic event	Recurrent, intrusive, and distressing images, thoughts, or perceptions Recurrent distressing dreams of the event Reliving the event through illusions, hallucinations, and dissociative flashbacks Intense distress when exposed to cues/symbols of the event Physiological reactivity when exposed to cues/symbols of the event
CRITERION C Persistent avoidance of stimuli associated with the trauma and Numbing of general responsiveness	Efforts to avoid thoughts, feelings, or conversations associated with the trauma Efforts to avoid activities, places, people that arouse recollections of the event Inability to recall aspecs of the event Diminished interest in usual activities Feelings of estrangement/detachment from others Restricted range of effect Sense of foreshortened future
CRITERION D Symptoms of increased arousal	Difficulty sleeping Irritability or angry outbursts Difficulty concentrating Hypervigilance Exaggerated startle response
CRITERION E Duration of the disturbance (symptoms in Criteria B, C, and D) is more than 1 month	
CRITERION F The disturbance causes clinically significant distress or impairment in social, occupations, or other important areas of functioning	

Source: Adapted from Ref. 14.

gic cancer patients, observed intrusive symptoms in 62% of her sample and estimated that over one-third of these women had symptoms severe enough to qualify for a PTSD diagnosis. Disease-related distress and treatment-related symptoms predicted which patients met criteria for PTSD. The higher prevalence of symptoms in the Bobertz study may be related to the timing of the assessment as these patients *were undergoing treatment* at the time of the assessment. Nevertheless, the results of the Bobertz survey should not be wholly discounted simply because the patients were not posttreatment. As mentioned above, there may well have been patients in the study who were reacting to a trauma that had occurred earlier in the course of their illness—patients who were "posttraumatic" before they were posttreatment.

In an early longitudinal investigation of patients with head and neck cancers, Manuel et al. (33) again demonstrated this notion that PTSD-related symptoms may be manifested at various times throughout the cancer experience. Specifically, subjects endorsed intrusive and avoidant symptoms shortly after diagnosis as well as during and after treatment. The authors also noted that, while the symptoms persisted, they were most notable at the time of diagnosis and receded as treatment progressed. These observations are consistent with the view of cancer as a series of sequential traumas rather than a single event and, again, indicate that PTSD may be a valid diagnosis in patients during treatment as well as former patients or survivors. This view is further supported by additional findings of PTSD-related symptoms in both men with prostate cancer (36) and patients with newly diagnosed recurrence of disease (37).

In 1992, Alter et al. (6) described a DSM-IV field trial that contributed to the redefinition of PTSD. Using a diagnostic clinical interview method, these authors compared cancer survivors who had

TABLE 51.3. *PTSD in Cancer: Review of Research PTSD Symptoms Assessed*

Author/Date	Sample	Time of Assessment	PTSD Assessment Tool	Results
Kornblith et al. (1990)	273 adult Hodgkin's disease survivors	At least 1 yr post-treatment (mean 6.3 yr)	Impact of Events Scale (IES)	Significant prevalence of intrusive and avoidant symptoms. Symptoms correlated with psychological distress and occurrence of sexual problems
Cella & Tross (1986)	60 adult, male Hodgkin's disease survivors compared to 20 age-matched healthy men	At least 6 mo post-treatment (median 2 yr)	IES	Patients had higher levels of avoidant thinking and lower intimacy motivation than controls
Lesko et al. (1992)	70 mixed leukemia survivors	At least 1 yr post-treatment (mean 61 mo)	IES	High rates of intrusive and avoidant symptoms which were associated with psychological distress/maladjustment
Ostroff et al. (1989)	44 acute and chronic leukemia patients compared to normative samples of physically healthy individuals	At least 1 yr post-BMT (mean 2.25 yr)	IES	Survivors had significantly higher levels of intrusive and avoidant symptoms than normative samples. Symptoms correlated with psychological distress
Greenberg et al. (1994)	89 adult survivors of osteogenic sarcoma	At least 1 yr post-treatment (mean 12 yr)	IES	23% reported high rates of avoidance and intrusive thoughts; 6% had more severe symptoms. Symptoms correlated with psychological distress
Kornblith et al. (1994)	172 men with prostate cancer and 83 spouses/partners	Not indicated; most undergoing treatment	Intrusion subscale of the IES	Both patients and spouses reported frequent intrusive thoughts and images. Spouses symptom levels were higher than patients
Cella et al. (1990)	40 patients with recurrent malignancies of mixed sites	Diagnosis of recurrence within 30 days	IES	High prevalence of avoidant and intrusive symptoms; those with first recurrence or "surprise" recurrence most symptomatic
Stuber et al. (1991)	6 children with AML or neuroblastoma	Immediately pre-transplant, 3-, 6-, and 12-mo post- BMT	Child interview and PTSD Reaction Index	Mild to moderate levels of intrusive/avoidant symptoms and emotional constriction at 3-, 6-, and 12-mo post-BMT
Stuber et al. (1994)	30 childhood cancer survivors (8–19 yr old)	At least 22 months post-treatment (mean 61.53 mo)	Posttraumatic Stress Reaction Index (adapted for use with children with cancer)	30% had mild post-traumatic symptoms; 17% had more severe PTSD-like experiences
Stuber et al. (1994)	Parents of 30 childhood cancer survivors	At least 22 mo post-treatment (mean 61.53 mo)	Posttraumatic Stress Reaction Index (adult version)	25% of fathers and 25% of mothers indicated moderate levels of post-traumatic symptoms. 7% of mothers endorsed severe symptom levels

completed their treatment an average of 4.6 years earlier to a community-based, healthy control group. They concluded that survivors have a higher rate of PTSD than that found in the community (see Table 51.5). Specifically, 4% of the subjects interviewed met criteria for current PTSD and 22% met lifetime criteria (incidence of symptoms at any time prior to 6 months before the interview). The latter group was also noted to have higher levels of general psychological distress suggesting that individuals with a history of PTSD may be at significant risk for continued emotional difficulties.

TABLE 51.4. *PTSD in Cancer: Review of Research with PTSD Diagnosis Inferred*

Author/Date	Sample	Time of Assessment	PTSD Assessment Tool	Results
Schwartz et al. (1995)	94 breast cancer survivors	At least 2 mo post-treatment; 67% 12 mo posttreatment; 33% less than 12 mo posttreatment	IES Intrusion Subscale	Over half of sample had intrusive thoughts and sleep disturbance related to treatment; 15% estimated eligible for PTSD diagnosis
Bobertz et al. (1992)	16 women undergoing treatment for gynecologic cancers	Not indicated	Trauma Exposure Questionnaire (developed specifically for this study)	62% had intrusive symptoms; 33% had symptoms severe enough for PTSD diagnosis
Manuel et al. (1987)	35 newly diagnosed head and neck cancer patients	At time of diagnosis and twice during treatment at 4–6 wk intervals	IES	Intrusive/avoidant symptoms prevalent both at diagnosis and during treatment. Symptoms most prevalent at time of diagnosis

Early research in children who had survived cancer also pointed to the presence of PTSD symptoms and the appropriateness of this diagnosis in this population. Stuber et al. (38) investigated stress responses after pediatric bone marrow transplantation and found that posttraumatic symptoms persisted for at least 1 year following treatment. A later and larger study also documented such symptoms in childhood cancer survivors with 30% reporting mild levels of symptoms and 17% demonstrating more severe PTSD-like experiences (23). Lastly, Pelcovic et al. (39) showed that 17.4% of adolescent survivors of pediatric cancer met full criteria for a diagnosis of current PTSD and 34% fulfilled criteria for PTSD some time since treatment (see Table 51.5).

The prevalence of symptoms typical of PTSD has also been noted in family members of cancer patients and survivors, leading to the inclusion of this group in the expanded DSM-IV definition of PTSD (14). It is thought that posttraumatic symptoms in this population may be due to the family member's confrontation with the potential life threat to the patient as well as the repeated witnessing of treatments and side effects. For instance, in an investigation of parents of childhood cancer survivors (40), roughly one-quarter of fathers described moderate levels of posttraumatic stress symptoms. A similar proportion of mothers endorsed moderate experiences and an additional 7% reported severe levels, suggesting that mothers may be particularly vulnerable to these reactions. Further,

TABLE 51.5. *PTSD in Cancer: Review of Research Studies which Assessed PTSD Diagnosis*

Author/Date	Sample	Time of Assessment	PTSD Assessment Tool	Results
Alter et al. (1996)	27 cancer survivors (mixed tumors; most with a history of breast cancer) compared to community-based control group	At least 3 yr from time of diagnosis (mean 5.4 yr); average of 4.6 yr from last treatment	Structured Clinical Interview for DSM-III-R (SCID)—PTSD portion	4% of survivors met criteria for current PTSD; 22% met criteria for lifetime diagnosis of PTSD. Higher rates of diagnoses than in community sample
Pelcovic et al. (submitted)	23 adolescent survivors of pediatric cancer compared with 27 adolescents with a history of physical abuse and 23 normal controls	Most off active treatment (time not indicated); some on maintenance treatment	SCID-PTSD module	17.4% of survivors met criteria for diagnosis of current PTSD; 34% met criteria for lifetime PTSD
Pelcovic et al. (1996)	24 mothers of adolescent survivors of pediatric cancer compared with a 23-member community control sample	Average of 3.28 yr post-treatment (range 0–11 yr)	Potential Stressful Life Events Interview; SCID-PTSD module; Modified Diagnostic Interview Schedule (DIS)—PTSD module	54% of mothers met full criteria for diagnosis of lifetime PTSD; 25 % met criteria for current PTSD

both mothers and fathers tended to report more severe posttraumatic symptoms than the child patients themselves and these symptoms did not appear to diminish over time. Additionally, Pelcovic et al. (41) found that 25% of mothers of adolescent survivors met the DSM-IV criteria for current PTSD (see Table 51.5). Finally, Kornblith et al. (36) found that the wives and partners of prostate cancer patients endorsed frequent intrusive thoughts and images regarding the disease. In fact, they reported significantly more of these symptoms than the patients themselves. Several explanations were posited for this finding including gender differences in stress adaptation styles and in willingness to report distress symptoms in general.

MECHANISMS, ETIOLOGY, AND RISK FACTORS FOR PTSD IN CANCER: THE CONVERGENCE OF CONDITIONING, STRESS, AND BIOLOGY

PTSD is, by definition, precipitated by an intensely distressing event. However, this factor alone is not sufficient to explain the phenomenon. Not everyone exposed to a traumatic stressor develops the full-blown syndrome or even subsets of PTSD symptoms. Attempts to explain these differences and to predict who is vulnerable (and who may be resilient) have focused upon psychological (i.e., learning theory), biological (i.e., neurological and endocrine), and social (i.e., social support) factors. Early studies of Vietnam veterans suggested a two factor learning theory to account for the trauma-related pathology (42,43). The same theory has more recently been applied to PTSD development in cancer (11–13). Specifically, PTSD symptoms are seen to develop as a function of both classical conditioning and instrumental learning. The former accounts for the fear responses elicited by various stimuli originally associated with the traumatic event. Neutral stimuli (e.g., smells, sounds, visual images) previously paired with the aversive stimuli (chemotherapy, painful procedures) eventually evoke anxiety, arousal and fear when presented alone even after the trauma has ended. Higher-order conditioning and stimulus generalization account for the exacerbation and extension of symptoms to additional stimuli. Once established, PTSD symptoms are maintained through instrumental learning. That is, avoidant responses are reinforced since avoidance of the stimuli prevents unpleasant feelings and thoughts.

Estimates from epidemiologic studies suggest that, on average, approximately 25%–33% of individuals exposed to traumatic events, including cancer, develop PTSD (28,44). While the disorder appears to be a result of the above-mentioned learning processes,

many factors have been suggested to explain why one person may develop PTSD and another may not.

According to DSM-IV, the severity, duration and proximity of an individual's exposure to the traumatic event are the most important factors affecting the likelihood of developing PTSD (14). In a review of studies encompassing a range of stresses and victim groups, Davidson and Foa (22) reported that stressor magnitude was directly proportional to the risk of PTSD. In addition, the suddenness of the event and the threat to life or physical integrity have been shown to be important predictors in various populations (30), including Vietnam veterans (24,45), disaster victims (46) and burn patients (18).

While the nature of the stressor may be a primary determinant in the response to traumatic events, other individual and social factors may also affect the outcome (30). Among the former, premorbid psychopathology (24,46), prior history of trauma (17,22), high levels of general psychological distress (18), and dysfunctional coping and attributional styles (22,30, 47) have been linked to a risk for PTSD in war veterans, holocaust survivors and other victims. In addition, several authors have posited predisposing genetic factors (27) as well as overly reactive hormonal systems and reduced hippocampal volume (28,29,48). Among social factors, the quality of the recovery environment, often measured in terms of social support, has been shown to reduce the likelihood of PTSD following combat exposure (24,45) and burn injury (18).

Research into the identification of moderating variables in oncology populations has been limited, is almost exclusively retrospective, and, to date, has been equivocal. With regard to the quality of the stressor, the effect of the threat to life and bodily integrity has been documented in both adult and family samples (e.g., 3,6,40), though not in children (23). In addition, the presence of pain and other physical symptoms has been shown to correlate with levels of intrusive thoughts (36). Cancer recurrence has also been shown to increase the likelihood of stress symptoms in patients (37). While severity or intensity of treatment were not related to intrusive or avoidant symptoms in adult survivors of Hodgkin's disease (2) or breast cancer (6), or in prostate cancer patients (36), these qualities were found to predict symptoms in survivors of childhood cancer (23).

Time elapsed since diagnosis and time elapsed since treatment completion have been shown to correlate with and predict posttraumatic symptoms in survivors of osteogenic sarcoma (7) and Hodgkin's disease (3,9). Specifically, those subjects who were farther from diagnosis and treatment tended to exhibit fewer symptoms.

However, this effect has not been found in studies of patients with recent recurrences (37), survivors of breast cancer (6) or childhood cancers (23). In fact, one intriguing finding involving a very small number of patients suggested that breast cancer survivors receiving tamoxifen chemotherapy exhibited a decreased risk of PTSD (6). This result was attributed to the perceived sense of protection and control over recurrence afforded by long-term therapy. Lastly, duration of treatment, rather than time since treatment, has been shown to predict stress symptoms in childhood cancer survivors (23).

Few patient characteristics have been shown to predict the occurrence of PTSD. High levels of psychological distress have been correlated with both stress symptoms (4,6,7) and actual PTSD diagnosis in adult survivors (6). In addition, trait anxiety was found to predict posttraumatic symptoms in the parents of childhood cancer survivors (40). Finally, women survivors with a diagnosis of lifetime PTSD tended to have a history of exposure to previous trauma (6).

Demographic characteristics such as age, gender and education at time of diagnosis, have not proven to be reliable predictors of stress symptoms (2,6,9). The effects of other powerful moderators in noncancer samples, such as premorbid psychological health and social support, have yet to be addressed prospectively in the cancer population. Indeed, most risk factors for PTSD have yet to be thoroughly evaluated in prospective studies of oncology populations although several such studies are presently underway.

ASSESSMENT OF PTSD IN THE CANCER SETTING

The review of early research clearly indicates that a significant percentage of cancer patients and survivors manifest symptoms of PTSD. However, research has yet to specifically address how these symptoms are to be differentiated from normal, cyclical adjustment processes nor has it extensively evaluated the impact of the symptoms upon quality of life and psychosocial functioning defined more broadly. A careful assessment of patients is critical to the identification of the symptoms and their deleterious impact upon functioning and to the planning of interventions targeted at the most distressing symptoms.

Perhaps the most difficult aspect of PTSD assessment in the cancer setting is the determination of precisely when to evaluate. Diagnosis is complicated by the fact that cancer is not an acute or discrete event, but rather an experience marked by repeated traumas and indeterminate length. Thus, an individual may exhibit the symptoms of PTSD at any point along a

continuum from diagnosis through treatment to treatment completion and, possibly, to recurrence (44). Patients with a history of past victimization, such as holocaust survivors (17), who have PTSD or its symptoms, can have symptoms activated by any number of stimuli (e.g., procedures such as magnetic resonance imaging and CT scans) encountered during their treatment. While such patients may have more difficulty adjusting to cancer and cancer treatment, in general, their PTSD symptoms are likely to vary depending upon circumstantial factors. Indeed, it has been reported that the relative predominance of specific PTSD symptoms may wax and wane throughout the cancer experience and beyond (14).

Case Example: When to Assess?

A 52-year-old woman learned that she was going to require a laryngectomy when it was found that her tumor progressed through chemotherapy and radiation on a "laryngeal preservation" protocol. She was referred for psychiatric consultation when she was unable to go forward with the surgery. The patient described that when she learned of the possible loss of her voice she began having obsessive and intrusive thoughts and "flash-forwards." In these episodes she envisioned herself in her home while it was burning down and she was unable to cry out for help or warn her husband (who was partially deaf but unwilling to consider a hearing aid). The patient had a history of being rescued from a fire while a young child. She had become withdrawn and startled easily and noted that she had become compulsive about checking the burners on the stove in her home before she could leave or go to sleep. She noted multiple comorbid depressive symptoms. Recognizing her symptoms as a case of "pre-TSD," the patient was started on multidimensional therapy including fluoxetine 20 mg daily, individual and family psychotherapy. She was encouraged to meet with a laryngectomy survivor who was skilled in esophageal speech. The patient had a complete response to this treatment, had an uncomplicated resection, and in her recovery became a patient-to-patient volunteer assisting other laryngectomy patients. Years later she noted that the visions and intrusive thoughts only seem to recur when she had to attend her annual check-ups.

These observations suggest the need for repeated evaluations beginning with initial diagnosis and extending throughout the life of the patient. The DSM-IV definition indicates that while PTSD symptoms usually begin within the first 3 months after trauma, there may be a delay of months, or even years, before symptoms appear (14). This has been demonstrated by research with noncancer populations that has shown that the onset of PTSD symptoms may be delayed. In fact, they may not be manifested until years following the traumatic event (16). These findings support the necessity for long-term monitoring of cancer survivors and family members. Delayed symptoms such as pathological grief reactions in surviving family members bear some resemblance to PTSD and may require similar treatment strategies (49). Such reactions often have elements of reexperiencing (intrusive replaying of events during the illness, nightmares and flashbacks about the deceased), avoidance (failure to resume normal activities, inability to approach the deceased person's possessions or maintaining them as a type of shrine), and hyperarousal (hypervigilance about the protection of the deceased's possessions, grave site or memory, irritability, poor sleep and concentration).

Finally, at least one study has shown that individuals who experienced a traumatic event may exhibit early symptoms without meeting the full criteria for a diagnosis of PTSD (18). Nonetheless, the appearance of these early symptoms was found to predict later development of a full PTSD syndrome. These results lend further credence to the need for both repeated and long-term follow-up of individuals exposed to the trauma of cancer.

The difficulty in proper diagnosis of PTSD may also be compounded by the overlap of PTSD symptoms with those of other psychiatric disorders and time-limited aspects of normal adjustment. For example, irritability, poor concentration, hypervigilance, exaggerated startle, and disturbed sleep are also symptoms of generalized anxiety disorder. Other arousal and avoidance symptoms are common to PTSD, phobias and panic disorder. Loss of interest, diminished motivation, sense of a foreshortened future, avoidance of other people, and sleep impairment might suggest both PTSD and depressive disorders. Furthermore, even the normal reactions to the diagnosis and treatment of life-threatening disease can consist of responses such as intrusive thoughts, dissociation and depersonalization, sleep disturbances and heightened arousal. Therefore, clinicians and researchers must be particularly attuned to the causes, duration and severity of PTSD-like symptoms when considering PTSD among several differential diagnoses.

Accurate diagnosis of PTSD also requires the use of reliable and valid instruments. To date, no measures have been developed specifically for use with cancer patients and survivors. However, of the many instruments designed during the post-Vietnam period, several have been used in cancer-related research and been proven applicable to this population. The Clinician-Administered PTSD Scale (50) provides both diagnostic and descriptive information. It measures the frequency as well as the severity of each PTSD symptom as required by DSM-IV. This instrument can be used to assess both current and lifetime diagnoses of PTSD as well as the impact of symptoms on

functioning. The Structured Clinical Interview for DSM-III-R (SCID) PTSD Subscale (51) systematically assesses the presence of reexperience, arousal and avoidance symptoms and provides the researcher or clinician with a reliable diagnosis of current or lifetime PTSD.

While not providing a comprehensive diagnosis, other instruments have proven useful in the measurement of certain symptoms of PTSD. For example, the Impact of Events Scale (52) is a widely used measure designed to assess the presence of intrusive thoughts or the blocking of thoughts and images related to a major stressor. This self-report instrument provides both "intrusion" and "avoidance" scores which have been shown to be elevated in many cancer populations (e.g., 7,9,33) and to predict later PTSD diagnosis in other trauma victims (18). The Post-Traumatic Stress Reaction Index, another self-report instrument, has been adapted for use with children and used in a study of childhood cancer survivors (23). This instrument rates 20 posttraumatic stress symptoms and provides an overall intensity, or summary, score. Although this measure does not allow for the diagnosis of PTSD itself, severe scores have been shown to correlate with DSM-based diagnoses of PTSD by clinical interview.

In attempting to make a diagnosis of PTSD, it is also important to be aware that the disorder is often marked by comorbid psychopathology. Although the percentages vary somewhat from study to study, substance abuse, affective disorders, and other anxiety disorders are consistently encountered in samples of subjects with PTSD (15,20,22,30). One study found that those Vietnam veterans with PTSD had, on average, one to two additional major psychiatric disorders (53), while another study estimated that patients averaged a total of 3.8 diagnoses (54). In their review of research, Keane and Wolfe (54) reported that combat veterans with PTSD exhibited significant comorbid pathology, including major depression (32%–72%), alcohol dependence (65%), drug dependence (40%), social phobia (50%) and obsessive-compulsive disorder (10%). High rates of concurrent disorders have also been documented in other trauma victims. For example, 40%–42% of disaster survivors with PTSD also qualified for a diagnosis of major depression and 20%–42% met criteria for concurrent generalized anxiety disorder (46,54). While not yet studied in cancer patients or survivors, the presence of co-occurring psychiatric disorders in post-Vietnam war veterans and other trauma victims would indicate that cancer clinicians should be alert to the need to identify and treat such related syndromes in their patients.

TREATMENT OF PTSD

The chronic and sometimes devastating psychological and interpersonal sequelae of PTSD (6,22) necessitate timely and effective treatment for people with this syndrome. Unfortunately, the avoidant responses associated with PTSD often prevent or delay these individuals from seeking professional assistance. While no specific, manualized therapies have been developed for PTSD in the cancer setting, treatment modalities used with other PTSD victims can be useful in alleviating distress in cancer patients and survivors. Most clinicians recommend using a multimodal approach, choosing various components to meet the specific needs of each patient and taking into account any concurrent psychiatric disorders such as depression or substance abuse. This is clearly the favored approach amongst psycho-oncologists, who frequently combine multiple modalities in their crisis intervention approach to facilitating adjustment.

The crisis intervention model comprises a broad range of therapies which can be helpful in the treatment of PTSD. The goals of this model are to reduce symptoms and restore patients to their usual level of functioning. The therapist often takes an active, directive stance with the patient, focusing on resolving concrete problems, teaching specific coping skills (15), and providing a safe and supportive environment for the patient (18).

Cognitive-behavioral techniques have proven especially helpful within the crisis intervention setting. Some of these methods include helping the patient to understand symptoms, teaching effective coping strategies and stress management techniques such as relaxation training, restructuring cognitions, and providing exposure to opportunities for systematic desensitization of symptoms (15,47). Behaviorally oriented approaches to sexual therapy may also be useful when the avoidance manifested by patients is most prominent in decreased frequency of sexual behavior and avoidance of intimate situations.

Support groups also appear to be beneficial for people experiencing posttraumatic symptoms. In the group setting, such patients can receive emotional support, encounter individuals with similar experiences and symptoms thereby validating their own, and learn a variety of coping and management strategies (15).

For those patients with particularly distressing or severe symptoms, psychopharmacology may provide an additional means of treatment. Several classes of medications have been used in the treatment of individuals with PTSD. For example, tricyclic and monoa-mine oxidase inhibitor antidepressants are commonly used, particularly when the symptoms of PTSD are accompanied by depression (15). Serotonin reuptake inhibitors, such as fluoxetine, are effective in reducing the hyperarousal and intrusive symptoms of PTSD (15, 22). Antianxiety medications may help to reduce overall arousal and anxiety symptoms. Finally, although used infrequently, antipsychotic medications may reduce severe, intrusive flashbacks (15).

FUTURE DIRECTIONS

Given the relatively recent inclusion of the cancer experience in the diagnostic definition of PTSD, it is not surprising that much remains to be learned about the nature, assessment and treatment of PTSD in cancer. Studies are needed to establish the epidemiology of PTSD and to determine how PTSD is associated with other comorbid disorders in cancer patients. Prospective research is needed to determine why certain individuals develop PTSD while others do not.

Prospective, longitudinal studies are also needed to better describe the nature and course of PTSD in the cancer setting. Such data will help to identify the ideal timing for both assessment and intervention. Assessment tools tailored to the specific experiences of cancer patients and survivors must be designed. Similarly, cancer-specific interventions are needed. While existing therapies have proven useful with cancer-related PTSD, additional treatments created to meet the particular needs of this population (such as pain interventions, physical therapy, and sexual and vocational counseling) might prove even more successful. Further, once specific risk factors for postcancer PTSD are identified, efforts should be directed toward developing prophylactic interventions thereby decreasing the incidence of this disorder in the cancer setting. Finally, since PTSD may develop at any time in the cancer experience, including years into survivorship, cancer care facilities should develop mechanisms to identify and treat PTSD within the context of long-term, comprehensive follow-up care.

REFERENCES

1. Zampini K, Ostroff JS. The post-treatment resource program: portrait of a program for cancer survivors. *Psychooncology*. 1993; 2:1–9.
2. Kornblith AB, Andersen J, Cella DF, et al. Comparison of psychosocial adaptation and sexual function of survivors of advanced Hodgkin Disease treated by MOPP, ABVD, or MOPP alternating with ABVD. *Cancer*. 1992; 70:2508–2516.

3. Cella DF, Tross, S. Psychological adjustment to survival from Hodgkin's Disease. *J Consult Clin Psychol.* 1986; 54:616–622.

4. Kornblith AB, Anderson J, Cella DF, et al. Quality of life assessment of Hodgkin's Disease survivors: a model for cooperative clinical trial. *Oncology.* 1990; 4:93–101.

5. Cella DF. Cancer survival: psychosocial and public issues. *Cancer Invest.* 1987; 5:59–67.

6. Alter CL, Pelcovitz D, Axelrod A, et al. Identification of PTSD in cancer survivors. *Psychosomatics.* 1996; 37:137–143.

7. Greenberg DB, Goorin A, Gebhardt MC, et al. Quality of life in osteosarcoma survivors. *Oncology.* 1994; 8:19–25.

8. Tross S, Holland J. Psychological sequelae in cancer survivors. In: Holland J, Breitbart W, eds. *The Handbook of Psycho-oncology.* New York: Oxford University Press; 1990:101–117.

9. Kornblith AB, Anderson J, Cella DF, et al. Hodgkin Disease survivors at increased risk for problems in psychosocial adaptation. *Cancer.* 1992; 70:2214–2224.

10. Koocher G, O'Malley J. *The Damocles Syndrome: Psychosocial Consequences of Surviving Childhood Cancer.* New York: McGraw-Hill; 1981.

11. Redd WH, Dadds MR, Futterman AD, et al. Nausea induced by mental images of chemotherapy. *Cancer.* 1993; 72:629–636.

12. Jacobsen PB, Bovbjerg DH, Redd WH. Anticipatory anxiety in women receiving chemotherapy for breast cancer. *Health Psychol.* 1995; 12:469–475.

13. Cella DF, Pratt A, Holland JC. Persistent anticipatory nausea, vomiting, and anxiety in cured Hodgkin's disease patients after completion of chemotherapy. *Am J Psychiatry.* 1986; 143:641–643.

14. American Psychiatric Association. *Diagnostic and Statistical Manual of Mental Disorders,* 4th ed. Washington, DC: American Psychiatric Association; 1994.

15. Keane, TM, Fisher LM, Krinsley KE. Post-traumatic stress disorder. In: Ammerman RT, Hersen M, eds. *Handbook of Prescriptive Treatments for Adults.* New York: Plenum Press; 1994.

16. Solomon Z, Garb R, Bleich A, Grupper D. Reactivation of combat-related posttraumatic stress disorder. *Am J Psychiatry.* 1987; 144:51–55.

17. Baider L, Sarell M. Coping with cancer among holocaust survivors in Israel: an exploratory study. *J Human Stress.* 1984; 10:121–127.

18. Perry S, Difede J, Musngi G, et al. Predictors of posttraumatic stress disorder after burn injury. *Am J Psychiatry.* 1992; 149:931–935.

19. Green BL, Lindy JD, Grace MC, Leonard AC. Chronic posttraumatic stress disorder and diagnostic comorbidity in a disaster sample. *J Nerv Ment Dis.* 1992; 180:760–766.

20. Rundell JR, Ursano RJ, Holloway HC, Silberman EK. Psychiatric responses to trauma. *Hosp Commun Psychiatry.* 1989; 40:68–74.

21. American Psychiatric Association. *Diagnostic and Statistical Manual of Mental Disorders,* 3rd ed. revised. Washington, DC: American Psychiatric Association; 1993.

22. Davidson JRT, Foa EB. Diagnostic issues in posttraumatic stress disorder: considerations for the DSM-IV. *J Abnormal Psychol.* 1991; 100:346–355

23. Stuber ML, Meeske K, Gonzalez S, et al. Post-traumatic stress after childhood cancer I: The role of appraisal. *Psycho-oncology.* 1994; 3:305–312.

24. Green BL, Grace MC, Lindy JD, et al. Risk factors for PTSD and other diagnoses in a general sample of Vietnam veterans. *Am J Psychiatry.* 1990; 147:729–733.

25. Passik SD, Hay, JL. Symptom control in patients with severe character pathology. In: Portenoy RK, Eduardo, EB, eds. *Supportive Care Medicine,* vol. 3. New York: Oxford University Press. [In press].

26. Yehuda R, McFarlane AC. Conflict between current knowledge about posttraumatic stress disorder and its original conceptual basis. *Am J Psychiatry.* 1995; 152:1705–1713.

27. True WR, Rice J, Eisen SA, et al. A twin study of genetic and environmental contributions to liability for posttraumatic stress symptoms. *Arch Gen Psychiatry.* 1993; 50:257–264.

28. Yehuda R, Resnick H, Kahana B, Giller EL. Long-lasting hormonal alterations to extreme stress in humans: normative or maladaptive? *Psychosom Med.* 1993; 55:287–297.

29. Yehuda R, Boisoneau D, Lowy MT, Giller EL. Dose-response changes in plasma cortisol and lymphocyte glucocorticoid receptors following dexamethasone administration in combat veterans with and without posttraumatic stress disorder. *Arch Gen Psychiatry.* 1995; 52:583–592.

30. Green BL, Lindy JD, Grace MC. Posttraumatic stress disorder: toward DSM-IV. *J Nerv Ment Dis.* 1985; 173:406–411.

31. Lesko LM, Ostroff JS, Mumma GH, et al. Long-term psychological adjustment of acute leukemia survivors: impact of bone marrow transplantation versus conventional chemotherapy. *Psychosom Med.* 1992; 54:30–47.

32. Schwartz M, Redd W, Bovbjerg D, et al. Predictors of intrusive symptomatology in breast cancer survivors. Paper presented at the annual meeting of the Society for Behavioral Medicine. San Diego: 1995.

33. Manuel GM, Roth S, Keefe FJ, Brantley BA. Coping with cancer. *J Human Stress.* 1987; 13:149–158.

34. Ostroff J, Mashberg D, Lesko L. Stress responses among bone marrow transplantation survivors [abstract]. *Psychosom Med.* 1989; 51:259.

35. Bobertz J, Hilliard C, Foy D. Trauma reactions among gynecologic oncology patients. Proceedings of Psychosocial Oncology, Enhancing Patient and Family Care; 1992 Sept 11–12; Los Angeles.

36. Kornblith AB, Herr HW, Ofman US, et al. Quality of life in patients with prostate cancer and their spouses. *Cancer.* 1994; 73:2791–2802.

37. Cella DF, Mahon SM, Donovan MI. Cancer recurrence as a traumatic event. *Behav Med.* 1990; 13: 15–22.

38. Stuber ML, Nader K, Yasuda P, et al. Stress responses after pediatric bone marrow transplantation: preliminary results of a prospective, longitudinal study. *J Am Acad Child Adolesc Psychiatry.* 1991; 50:407–414.

39. Pelcovic D, Goldenberg B, Mandel S, et al. PTSD and family functioning in adolescent cancer survivors. Submitted manuscript.

40. Stuber ML, Gonzalez S, Meeske K, et al. Posttraumatic stress after childhood cancer II: A family model. *Psycho-oncology*. 1994; 3:313–319.
41. Pelcovic D, Goldenberg B, Kaplan S, et al. Posttraumatic stress disorder in mothers of pediatric cancer survivors. *Psychosomatics*. 1996; 37:116–126.
42. Keane TM, Zimering RT, Caddell JM. A behavioral formulation of posttraumatic stress disorder in Vietnam veterans. *Behav Therapist*. 1985; 8:9–12.
43. Charney DS, Deutch AY, Krystal JH, et al. Psychobiologic mechanisms of posttraumatic stress disorder. *Arch Gen Psychiatry*. 1993; 50:294–305.
44. Passik, SD. The Greenberg et al. article reviewed [comment]. *Oncology*. 1994; 8:25–26.
45. Foy DW, Resnick HS, Sipprelle RC, Carroll EM. Premilitary, military, and postmilitary factors in the development of combat-related posttraumatic stress disorder. *Behav Therapist*. 1987; 10:3–9.
46. Smith EM, North CS, McCool RE, Shea JM. Acute postdisaster psychiatric disorders: Identification of persons at risk. *Am J Psychiatry*. 1990; 147:202–206.
47. Mikulincer M, Solomon Z. Attributional style and combat-related posttraumatic stress disorder. *J Abnormal Psychol*. 1988; 97:308–313.
48. Bremner JD, Randall P, Scott TM, et al. MRI-based measurement of hippocampal volume in patients with combat-related posttraumatic stress disorder. *Am J Psychiatry*. 1995; 152:973–981.
49. Rando TA. *Treatment of Complicated Mourning*. Champaign, IL: Research Press; 1993.
50. Blake DD, Weathers FW, Nagy LN, et al. A clinician rating scale for assessing current and lifetime PTSD: the CAPS-1. *Behav Therapist*. 1990; 18:187–188.
51. Spitzer RL, Williams JB, Gibbon M, First MB. The structured clinical interview for DSM-III-R (SCID). I: History, rationale, and description. *Arch Gen Psychiatry*. 1992; 49:624–629.
52. Horowitz M, Wilner N, Alvarez W. Impact of Events Scale: a measure of subjective stress. *Psychosom Med*. 1979; 41:209–218.
53. Roszell DK, McFall ME, Malas KL. Frequency of symptoms and concurrent psychiatric disorder in Vietnam veterans with chronic PTSD. *Hosp Commun Psychiatry*. 1991; 42:293–296.
54. Keane TM, Wolfe J. Comorbidity in post-traumatic stress disorder: an analysis of community and clinical samples. *J Appl Soc Psychol*. 1990; 20:1776–1788.

52

Somatoform and Factitious Disorders and Cancer

CHARLES V. FORD

The somatoform disorders are a group of syndromes, originally grouped together in the *Diagnostic and Statistical Manual of Mental Disorders* (3rd edition) in which a patient presents for medical care with symptoms and/or concerns that reflect a physical disease but for which the symptoms have a psychogenic etiology (1). The DSM-IV provides specific criteria for each of several somatoform disorders but most patients who somatize display atypical symptom presentations (2). Somatizing disorders tend to have a dimensional quality in that they represent a continuum from normal behaviors to clinical syndromes and, further, there tends to be a phenomenologic fluidity in that the disorders often merge into each other (3). The clinician must keep in mind in reading the following descriptions that the textbook clarity of symptomatic presentations is more for didactic purposes than a reflection of clinical reality.

Somatization has been described by Katon et al. as a culturally sanctioned idiom of psychosocial distress (4). It is a remarkably common phenomenon and it has been estimated that approximately 25% of primary care patients demonstrate some degree of somatization. (5) It is not an all-or-none phenomenon — rather, some degree of somatization in the form of excessive worry or elaboration of symptoms often occurs in conjunction with physical disease. Patients with concurrent depression and/or anxiety perceive themselves as being more sick and disabled than do nonanxious/depressed patients with comparable physical disease. Comorbid depression increases medical utilization by a factor of two to three times (6).

The process of somatization is caused or facilitated by a variety of different issues (7). Among these are: (*1*) decreased social support; (*2*) difficulties in communicating one's psychological distress (e.g., underlying cerebral dysfunction, lower intelligence, poor educa-

tion, or alexithymia); (*3*) cultural factors that discourage the overt display and/or communication of emotional states; (*4*) childhood environments that placed an emphasis upon somatic complaints; (*5*) stigmatization in that psychological disorders have often been regarded as a sign of weakness or poor character; (*6*) economic factors, because treatment of psychological disorders is often reimbursed more poorly than treatment of somatic diseases; (*7*) misattribution of the physiological signs and symptoms of anxiety or depression to physical illness.

The misattribution and/or psychological amplification of the severity of physical symptoms due to depression/anxiety is one of the most common forms of somatization. It is particularly referable to cancer in that cancer patients who have concurrent anxiety/depression are often preoccupied with physical symptoms and may misinterpret symptoms, including those of anxiety/depression, as evidence of a recurrence or worsening of their underlying disease. Patients may differentially focus upon these symptoms and seek treatment for them rather than recognize their psychological discomfort. Depression and anxiety disorders, including obsessive-compulsive disorder, are frequently associated with or underlie all of the somatoform disorders. A primary task of the clinician is to carefully evaluate each patient for the possibility of psychiatric comorbidity even when the patient presents with an apparently "classic" somatoform disorder. The prognosis for the somatizing cancer patient, as a general rule of thumb, is better when the somatization is associated with depression or anxiety (8).

THE SOMATOFORM DISORDERS

The somatoform disorders and cancer may be related one to another in several different ways. (*1*) The symptom and/or concern of the person with the somatoform disorder may mimic cancer; therefore, the diagnostic work-up for such an individual must take malignancy into account. (2) The person with a somatoform disorder may develop cancer. (3) A patient with cancer may develop a somatoform disorder as a means of coping with the cancer and/or concurrent psychosocial stressors; the new symptom may be mistakenly regarded as an extension and/or reoccurrence of the original disease. Each of these three possibilities will be discussed in reference to the individual somatoform disorders.

Hypochondriasis

The DSM-IV diagnostic criteria for hypochondriasis specify that the person be preoccupied with the fear or the conviction that one has a serious disease. This preoccupation persists despite adequate medical evaluation and reassurance.

Hypochondriasis is a relatively common disorder and in one study 4%–6% of the patients in an internal medicine clinic met specified criteria for hypochondriasis (9). The usual age of onset for hypochondriasis is young adulthood and it frequently persists through middle age into later life. Cancer is one of the most common fears of the hypochondriacal patient. In fact, the term "cancerphobia" is applicable to many hypochondriacal patients (10). Normal body sensations may be misinterpreted as due to disease with resultant preoccupation and fear that one suffers from cancer. A negative diagnostic evaluation, and reassurance, provides only transient relief and the patient soon returns with a new symptom and/or the obsessive fear that cancer is present but was not diagnosed. The patient's insistence upon continuing diagnostic tests may become irrational and a management problem. The following brief clinical vignette illustrates this phenomenon.

A 35-year-old married woman with mild fibrocystic breast disease became preoccupied with the idea that she might have breast cancer. She repetitively returned to her physician requesting manual examinations, mammograms and periodic biopsies, all of which were benign. She then became obsessed with the idea that she should have bilateral prophylactic mastectomies, despite the fact that she did not have a family history for breast cancer. Her physician recognized her behavior as a form of hypochondriasis and refused to perform the mastectomies. The patient then "doctor-shopped" until she found a surgeon who would operate.

The patient who has preexisting hypochondriasis may at some point in life develop malignancy. It is an interesting phenomenon that, given a genuine severe stressor about which to become concerned, the patient's worries and behaviors may become appropriate and realistic. Faced with a real threat, the prior obsessions often "melt away." Other hypochondriacal patients may incorporate their prior preoccupation with bodily symptoms, and conviction of disease, into illness behavior referable to their cancer treatment. Such patients who have both serious disease, and hypochondriacal behavior, are very difficult to manage (11).

Transient hypochondriasis is a common, and normal, response in any patient who has developed serious disease such as cardiac disorders and/or cancer. Following diagnosis and treatment, the cancer patient frequently becomes hypervigilant as to any new bodily sensations and may overinterpret them as evidence that the disease is spreading and/or recurring (12). These patients often respond to reassurance and, with time, the anxiety and hypervigilance decreases in many patients (13).

The management of hypochondriasis consists first of the identification of any underlying comorbid psychiatric disorders such as depression, panic disorder or obsessive-compulsive disorder. When the symptom (e.g., "cancerphobia") is a symptom of anxiety, depression, or obsessive-compulsive disorder it may respond to the appropriate treatment (14). Hypochondriacal patients require frequent office visits, evaluation including a physical examination of any new complaint, and limitation of invasive diagnostic procedures to those situations where there is evidence of objective findings. Education and reassurance, often repetitive, is the cornerstone of the effective management of these patients.

Somatization Disorder and Undifferentiated Somatization Disorder

Somatization disorder is a syndrome of multiple unexplained physical symptoms beginning before age 30 years. The DSM-IV diagnostic criteria specify that the patient have at least eight unexplained symptoms that include four pain symptoms from different sites, two gastrointestinal symptoms, one sexual symptom and at least one pseudoneurologic symptom (conversion symptom). Phenomenologic studies suggest that somatization disorder has a dimensional, rather than categorical, quality and that subsyndromal forms of the disorder (undifferentiated somatization disorder) differ only in the degree of the various findings associated with the disorder (15).

Patients with somatization disorder are usually women, often of lower socioeconomic status, who typically experience high stress in association with relatively low social support. Their illness behavior can be interpreted as the use of the sick role as a means of coping with life stressors. Somatization disorder patients are almost always comorbid for one or more psychiatric disorders such as depressive and anxiety disorders, substance abuse, and/or personality disorders. They often have a history of psychiatric hospitalizations and/or suicidal gestures. The somatization disorder patient frequently concurrently sees multiple physicians and may receive medications, including habituating agents, unknown to other physicians. "Doctor-shopping" behavior is a major problem in management of these patients who are also frequently inaccurate, dramatic historians who exaggerate details of their past medical histories. They may report a past history of cancer (e.g., as a reason for a hysterectomy) that cannot be verified from the medical records. Malignancy, because of these patients' dramatic symptomatic presentations and complicated medical history, is frequently a part of the differential diagnosis.

A 38-year-old divorced mother of three children was admitted via the emergency department because of severe recurrent pelvic pain. She gave a history of having had a hysterectomy for "cancer" 10 years previously and she thought that "they got it all." A review of medical records from another institution revealed that chronic pain had been the reason for the hysterectomy and the pathology report indicated only mild endometriosis.

The patient with somatization disorder is not immune from developing cancer. When this occurs, these patients often persist in their abnormal illness behavior and may exaggerate and/or dramatize symptoms, as needed, to obtain more attention and/or to cope with concurrent psychosocial stressors in their chaotic lives. The physician must be careful not to overreact and must proceed with further diagnostic/therapeutic procedures based upon objective evidence rather than subjective complaints. Comorbid psychiatric disorders should be appropriately treated. It must be kept in mind that these patients are often prone to habituation and/or suicidal gestures and there must be judicious prescription of potentially addictive drugs and/or potentially lethal medications.

Conversion Disorder

Conversion disorder, by definition, involves one or more symptoms of the voluntary motor or sensory functions that suggest neurologic or medical disease. Psychological issues are judged to be associated with initiating and/or perpetuating the symptom. Symptoms may be associated with secondary gains, but the symptom is not regarded to be initiated by conscious motivation. Symptoms, because they involve voluntary or sensory functions, may, at times, reflect

the possibility of a tumor of the nervous system. Common symptoms include pseudoseizures, paralyses, anesthesia/paresthesias, hysterical blindness/deafness, or vocal chord dysfunction. The most common differential diagnosis is often that of multiple sclerosis or other degenerative central nervous diseases, vascular disease such as stroke, and/or the possibility of a brain or spinal tumor. The diagnosis is usually established by determining that the symptom is nonphysiological, that there is an acute emotional stressor that precipitated and/or is associated with symptom perpetuation and that the patient has had a model for the symptom in the past.

Conversion is also frequently associated with concurrent underlying psychiatric disorders such as depression. Current etiologic concepts of conversion suggest that it is an attempt to use somatic mechanisms to communicate psychosocial distress when there is some neurological, cultural or environmental impairment to verbally communicate. Contrary to previous psychoanalytic views, it is usually impossible to determine the symbolic meaning, if any, of a specific symptom. Persons with cancer who are impaired, for any reason, in their ability to express ideas and feelings may develop conversion symptoms. The following case was reported by Massie (11).

A 45-year-old woman with terminal chronic myelogenous leukemia developed a severe gait disturbance that did not appear to have a neurologic cause. On psychiatric evaluation it was apparent that her symptoms were in response to a comment made by her husband that indicated his recognition of her terminal state. The woman was both terrified and angry at his comments but unable to express herself. With psychotherapy she recognized that she was terrified of dying but had never been able to admit her fears and that she felt guilty in leaving household responsibilities to her husband.

The evaluation of conversion disorder consists of: (1) recognition of any predisposition such as underlying neurologic dysfunction or psychiatric illness; (2) the identification of precipitating stress; (3) determination of factors that tend to reinforce or perpetuate the symptom. Treatment involves careful consideration of all these issues (3).

Amytal (or lorazepam) interviews, or hypnosis, which are techniques that create an altered state of consciousness, may provide immediate symptom resolution and/or sufficient psychological information to understand the psychological meaning of the symptom to the patient. At times, when the patient may be defending against psychosis and/or suicide, it may be prudent to allow the patient to maintain the symptom. It must be emphasized that patients may demonstrate considerable psychogenic symptomatic elaboration of genuine physical disease (16–18). Treatment by an amytal interview may *appear* to relieve the symptom when, in fact, there may be an underlying neurologic disease.

Comorbid psychiatric disease underlying conversion symptoms should be treated. Behavioral therapy techniques are often very useful, particularly with chronic symptoms. These may allow the patient face-saving ways to discard the symptom. When the symptom has resulted from overwhelming environmental stressors it may be necessary to make environmental changes in order to reduce the stress upon the patient.

Most conversion symptoms are short-lived and remit spontaneously or in response to the techniques mentioned above. When conversion is long-standing it has generally been reinforced by massive secondary gains. A comprehensive treatment plan is needed to address such factors.

Body Dysmorphic Disorder

Body dysmorphic disorder (BDD) is a diagnostic term first introduced in DSM-III-R. It has been called the "pain of imagined ugliness" and it is a syndrome manifested by the belief or preoccupation that one has a disfiguring deformity that causes humiliation (19). The person with BDD may spend much of the day repetitively reexamining him/herself and/or looking in the mirror or other reflective surfaces. Generally the deformity, if present at all, is so minor as to be essentially imperceptible to others. Fear of humiliation leads to concurrent symptoms of social phobia and the person with BDD may become housebound.

Persons with BDD are almost always comorbid for at least one additional psychiatric disorder, most frequently major depression and/or obsessive-compulsive disorder. Their preoccupation with their symptoms is so intense as to suggest that this is a somatic preoccupation of an obsessive-compulsive disorder. In fact, some authors believe that BDD is merely a subtype of obsessive-compulsive disorder. Lending credence to this theory are reports that most patients with BDD respond to treatments for obsessive-compulsive disorder (e.g., with specific, serotonin reuptake inhibitors (20)).

BDD, although a modern redefinition of "dysmorphophobia," is a relatively new diagnosis. There are no reports in the medical literature linking BDD with cancer, but it would not be surprising to find that some patients who have bodily changes secondary to their malignancies, and/or their treatment, may become obsessively preoccupied with these changes.

Pain Disorder

Pain disorder is the latest incarnation of a variety of previously unsatisfactory diagnostic terms such as psychogenic pain disorder or somatoform pain disorder (21). The current DSM-IV criteria state that the patient's pain appears in excess of physiologic findings and that psychological factors appear to be important in the initiation or the perpetuation of the pain. Pain disorder can be classified as occurring in association with a known physical disease. Pain disorder is further classified as being either acute or chronic (lasting longer than 6 months). As a general rule, acute pain is associated with concurrent anxiety and chronic pain is associated with depression.

Pain disorder is a very heterogeneous disorder both symptomatically and in terms of its psychological roots (22). Pain has been interpreted as an unconscious mechanism by which one seeks expiation from guilt. Persons with chronic pain syndromes frequently report histories that suggest self-defeating masochistic behaviors and/or a history of physical or sexual abuse. Pain can also be a learned behavior and the expression of pain can be used to manipulate other persons.

Irrespective of the etiologic importance for any one individual, chronic pain patients tend to be nonpsychologically minded and to resent any implication that their emotional distress is due to anything other than the pain that they experience. The treatment of pain syndromes includes treatment of concurrent psychiatric disorders, particularly depression; behavioral modification, particularly relaxation techniques; and operate conditioning in which the patient's pain behaviors are ignored and the patient is praised for efforts at self-care and increased activity. Pharmacologic strategies must be cautious in that these patients have a tendency to become habituated to medications, both analgesics and benzodiazepines. When medications are deemed necessary, it is important to place the patient on a fixed dosage schedule rather than on an as-needed basis. The latter encourages the patient to engage in more pain behaviors to communicate a need for medication while the former allows the patient to know that medication will be forthcoming at predictable times (21).

Cancer patients are at risk to develop pain syndromes. Malignancies and metastasis to the bones, particularly the spine, often result in pain (23). Notwithstanding the fact that cancer often involves pain, it is remarkable how many cancer patients are able to tolerate their pain and, despite every objective reason to be disabled, continue to demonstrate remarkable occupational and social function. Thus, the perception of pain is an amalgam of a number of complex factors, including personality type, organic physical issues, and concurrent emotional states.

FACTITIOUS DISORDERS AND MALINGERING

Factitious disorders and malingering represent the deliberate and conscious exaggeration, misrepresentation, simulation or production of a disease process. Both factitious disorders and malingering are consciously produced but the motivation for factitious disorders is, by definition, unconscious and presumably consists of a wish to attain the sick role. In contrast, malingering is consciously motivated with a determined incentive such as avoidance of military duty, disability payments, or a lawsuit.

Although malingering is defined by its motivation, the causes for factitious disorder are more complex. It has been proposed that persons engage in factitious behaviors to obtain nurturance from others, to achieve a sense of power and superiority by the capacity to fool and manipulate others, and/or as a defense against severe separation anxiety and incipient psychosis (13). Cancer is a highly emotionally charged disease and it is not surprising that there have been a number of reports in the literature of persons either misrepresenting themselves as having cancer and/or simulating symptoms to suggest malignant disease (24–28). The patient described below is illustrative of this syndrome (25).

Jenny, a 35-year-old reserved, quiet, but hardworking secretary experienced the unexpected breakup of her 1 year engagement. Her fiancé informed her that she would have to move out of his apartment. Emotionally distraught from this unexpected psychologic blow, Jenny announced one day at work that she had been recently diagnosed as having breast cancer. In response to this announcement, coworkers rallied about her and even helped share her workload. She suddenly felt that she was "someone" as people went out of their way to be helpful. Jenny maintained the charade by shaving her head, announcing that she had lost her hair through chemotherapy, and she started to attend cancer support groups. Her ruse was eventually discovered by group members who became aware of inconsistencies in her story. Discovery of her deception enraged her coworkers and, as a result, Jenny entered psychotherapy. It was clear to the therapist that she was both depressed (antidepressant medication was prescribed) and that she had an intense longing for nurturance.

Another patient, who had declared that she was terminal from cancer, permitted herself to be interviewed in front of a medical school class. She tearfully told the class that one of her dying wishes was to ride in a hot air balloon. The class then collected money in order that the wish could be fulfilled. It was later discovered that her entire story had been a fabrication (27).

Although rare, physicians must be alert to the possibility of factitious disorders. Some patients who have provided histories of cancer subsequently received both invasive and dangerous treatment for their nonexistent malignancies. One patient later sued her physician for failure to recognize that her illness was indeed factitious. The case was settled out of court with a substantial payment to the woman (29). This case raises a very interesting situation in that the physician, who had no reason not to be trusting, was punished for failure to detect his patient's lies.

SUMMARY

The most common form of somatization in the cancer patient is overinterpretation of bodily symptoms by depressed/anxious patients. Some patients with chronic somatoform disorders who develop cancer may incorporate their prior illness behaviors into their treatment for cancer. A few patients, overwhelmed with the stress of their malignancies, may use somatoform disorders, such as a conversion symptom, as a means to cope with their psychological stress. A few patients may go to the extreme of simulating cancer in an effort to obtain attention and nurturance.

REFERENCES
1. American Psychiatric Association. *Diagnostic and Statistical Manual of Mental Disorders*, 3rd ed. Washington, DC, American Psychiatric Press; 1980.
2. American Psychiatric Association. *Diagnostic and Statistical Manual of Mental Disorders*, 4th ed. Washington DC, American Psychiatric Press; 1994.
3. Ford CV. Dimensions of somatization and hypochondriasis. *Neurol Clin North Am.* 1995; 13:241-253..
4. Katon W, Ries RK, Kleinman AA. A prospective DSM-III study of 100 consecutive somatization patients. *Compr Psychiatry.* 1985; 25:305-314.
5. Bridges KW, Goldberg DP. Somatic presentations of DSMIII psychiatric disorders in primary care. *J Psychiatry Res.* 1985; 29:563-569.
6. Wells KB, Stewart A, Hays RD, et al. The functioning and well-being of depressed patients and results from the medical outcomes study. *JAMA.* 1989; 262:914-919.
7. Ford CV. Conversion disorder and somatoform disorder not otherwise specified. In: Gabbard GO, ed. *Treatments of Psychiatric Disorders*, vol II, 2nd ed. Washington, DC: American Psychiatric Press; 1995: 1735–1753.
8. Chaturvedi SK, Hopwood P, Maguire P. Non-organic somatic symptoms in cancer. *Eur J Cancer.* 1991; 27A:1006–1008.
9. Barsky AJ, Wyshak G, Klerman GL, et al. The prevalence of hypochondriasis in medical outpatients. *Soc Psychiatry Psychiatr Epidemiol.* 1990; 25:89–94.
10. Brown RS, Lees-Haley PR. Fear of future illness, chemical AIDS, and cancer phobia: a review. *Psychol Rep.* 1992; 71:187–207.

11. Massie MJ. Somatoform disorders and cancer. In: Holland JC, Rowland JH, eds. *Handbook of Psychooncology: Psychological Care of the Patient with Cancer.* New York: Oxford University Press; 1990: 317–319.

12. Grassi L, Rosti G, Albien G, Marangolo M. Depression and abnormal illness behavior in cancer patients. *Gen Hosp Psychiatry.* 1989; 11:404–411.

13. Ford CV. *The Somatizing Disorders: Illness as a Way of Life.* New York: Elsevier; 1983.

14. Viswanathan R, Paradis C. Treatment of cancer phobia with fluoxetine [letter]. *Am J Psychiatry.* 1991; 148:1090.

15. Escobar JI, Swatz M, Rubio-Stipee M, et al. Medically unexplained symptoms: distribution risk factors and comorbidity. In: Kirmayer LJ, Robbins JM, eds. *Current Concepts of Somatization: Research and Clinical Perspectives.* Washington, DC: American Psychiatric Press; 1991: 63–78.

16. Burch EA, Hutchison CF, Still CN. Hysterical symptoms masking brain stem glioma. *J Clin Psychol.* 1978: 39:75–78.

17. Epstein BS, Epstein JA, Postel DM. Tumors of spinal cord simulating psychiatric disorders. *Dis Nerv Syst.* 1971; 32:741–743.

18. Peterson LG, Popkin MK, Hall RCW. Psychiatric presentations of cancer and sequelae of treatment. *Psychiatr Med.* 1983; 1:79–92.

19. Phillips KA, McElroy SL, Keck PE, et al. Body dysmorphic disorder: 30 cases of imagined ugliness. *Am J Psychiatry.* 1991; 148:1138–1149.

20. Brady KT, Austin L, Lydiard RB. Body dysmorphic disorder: The relationship to obsessive compulsive disorder. *J Nerv Ment Dis.* 1990; 178:538–540.

21. King SA, Stoudemire A. Pain disorders. In: Gabbard GO, ed. *Treatments of Psychiatric Disorders,* vol II, 2nd ed. Washington, DC: American Psychiatric Press; 1995: 1755–1782.

22. Adler RH, Hurny C. Differential diagnosis of pain in cancer patients. *Recent Results Cancer Res.* 1988; 108:1–8.

23. Benjamin S. Psychological treatment of chronic pain: a selective review. *J Psychosom Res.* 1989; 33:121–131.

24. Bruns AD, Fishlein PA, Johnson EA, Lee YT. Munchausen's syndrome and cancer. *J Surg Oncol.* 1994; 56:136–138.

25. Feldman MD, Escalona R. The longing for nurturance: a case of factitious cancer. *Psychosomatics.* 1991; 32:226–228.

26. Feldman MD, Ford CV. *Patient or Pretender: The Strange World of Factitious Disorders.* New York: Wiley; 1994.

27. Baile WF Jr, Kuehn CV, Straker D. Factitious cancer. *Psychosomatics.* 1992; 33:100–105.

28. Broad JA, Hammond CB. Factitious trophoblastic disease, Munchausen's mole. *South Med J.* 1980; 73:831–832.

29. Lipsitt DR. The factitious patient who sues [letter]. *Am J Psychiatry.* 1986; 143:1482.

53

Schizophrenia

JOHN L. SHUSTER

Schizophrenia is probably the most dreaded and devastating of the mental disorders. With a lifetime prevalence of less than 1% schizophrenia infrequently complicates cancer (1). In one survey, only 4% of psychiatric consultations performed at Memorial Sloan-Kettering Cancer Center concerned cases of schizophrenia (2). However, when these two conditions do occur together, they present an imposing set of clinical challenges.

Schizophrenia is a psychotic disorder characterized by delusions, hallucinations, disturbances in interaction, and disorganization of thought, speech, and behavior (1). It may resolve completely after a severe symptomatic episode. Unfortunately, a chronic, deteriorating course is more common. Schizophrenia causes dramatic disturbances in social, occupational, and interpersonal functioning. The active psychotic (positive) symptoms of schizophrenia cause obvious impairment. The residual (negative) symptoms of the disorder (e.g., affective flattening, social withdrawal, alogia, avolition) are more subtle, but often cause as much or more impairment as the psychotic symptoms and are even more resistant to treatment. This chapter summarizes information about the epidemiology, evaluation, and management of schizophrenia in the setting of cancer.

EPIDEMIOLOGY OF CANCER IN THE SETTING OF SCHIZOPHRENIA

Cancer Rates Among Schizophrenic Patients

Studies of the risk of cancer in schizophrenia constitute the vast majority of articles in the medical literature pertinent to this chapter. Reports began to appear in the early part of this century (3). Many of the early studies found significantly reduced risks of all cancers and cancer death in patients with mental disorders, including schizophrenia (4–6). Consequently, it was believed for many years that schizophrenia conferred some protection from the development of some or all types of cancer.

Some recent reports have supported this association, as well. Modrzewska and Bøøk reported lower than expected cancer death rates among a population in Northern Sweden with a high incidence of schizophrenic psychoses (7). Mortensen found reduced incidence of cancers of all types in male schizophrenic patients as compared to the general population — an association strengthened after statistical correction for smoking (8, 9). The author found no similar difference in cancer incidence for female patients overall, though the incidence of some individual types of cancer were elevated or reduced in those women with schizophrenia.

Most of the more recent studies, however, have failed to find a consistent association between schizophrenia and cancer risk or cancer mortality (5,6,10–15). Furthermore, the studies of cancer mortality which found schizophrenia to have a protective effect have been criticized for methodologic flaws. For example, most of these studies measure proportionate mortality, not absolute mortality. Measurement of proportionate mortality can artificially lower the measured death rate in this setting, since schizophrenic patients are more likely to die of other causes (5,15). Measures of absolute, age-adjusted cancer mortality have found no difference or slight increases in schizophrenic patients compared to controls (5,14,16). Some authors have attributed any protective effect a schizophrenia diagnosis might have genuinely conferred in some of the older studies to the effects of long-term hospitalization (e.g., better diet, relative protection from environmental carcinogens). This is consistent with the common finding that the protective effects of a schizophrenia diagnosis were concentrated in those patients who had been chronically hospitalized (5,6,17).

Most of the evidence available today supports the notion that the presence of schizophrenia itself has little or no effect on the overall risk of developing or dying from malignancy. This does not, however, eliminate the possibility that there may be important associations between schizophrenia and the risk of specific types of cancer (8,9,11–13,17).

Schizophrenia and Cancer Risk Factors

Schizophrenia clearly does have an effect on some of the common risk factors for cancer (18). Dietary factors are estimated to account for as many of one-third of cancers in the United States. Persons with chronic schizophrenia may be exposed to an unbalanced diet (e.g., high in processed foods, deficient in fresh fruits and vegetables) due to limited finances and decreased attention to self-care. The possible risk-enhancing effects of chronic stress, which may be present in schizophrenia, are controversial (19,20). Comobid alcohol use (a risk factor for oral and esophageal cancer) may also increase cancer risk in schizophrenia.

Tobacco exposure is the clearest risk factor for cancer. Schizophrenia is associated with a marked increase in rate of cigarette use, number of cigarettes used daily, and use of high-tar cigarettes (21,22). Rates of cigarette use are substantially higher in schizophrenia than in other mental disorders (21). Numbers of cigarettes smoked by patients with schizophrenia appear to increase after neuroleptic exposure (23). Conversely, smokers with schizophrenia receive higher doses of neuroleptics than nonsmokers, partly due to increased metabolism of neuroleptics in the setting of tobacco use (24). The high rates of cigarette use by those who suffer from schizophrenia may also be partly related to improvements in cognitive impairment, drug-induced parkinsonism, or auditory sensory gating associated with smoking (24–26).

Other Hypotheses About the Possible Association Between Schizophrenia and Cancer Risk

In addition to modifications in risk factors (e.g., diet, tobacco, alcohol), a number of other interesting hypotheses have been proposed to explain alterations in the risk for certain cancers as a result of having schizophrenia. Environmental pollutants, exposure to psychotropic medications, reduced parity, nonspecific constitutional factors, and alterations in ability to somatize distress have all been proposed as possible mediators of these possible associations (11,13). Levi and Waxman proposed that a deficiency in methionine adenosyltransferase might contribute to symptoms of schizophrenia while conferring some degree of protection from cancer (27). McDaniel proposed that altera-

tions in natural killer cell activity, which may be increased in schizophrenia but decreased by exposure to neuroleptics, might also explain some of the variations in cancer risk among patients with schizophrenia (28).

CANCER AND SCHIZOPHRENIA: DIAGNOSTIC CONSIDERATIONS

Impediments to Diagnosing Cancer in the Setting of Schizophrenia

Clinical features of schizophrenia may interfere with cancer detection. Paranoia or avolition may prevent the patient from seeking ongoing preventive care or evaluation when symptoms emerge. Bizarre or nonspecific physical complaints may be minimized by family and physicians. Disorganization or psychotic symptoms may hinder evaluation of the schizophrenic patient, making underrecognition of subtle signs of cancer more likely. These and other factors which limit access to good medical care, or the effectiveness of that care, may increase the risk of cancer in the patient with schizophrenia. Since schizophrenia usually has its onset in young adulthood and commonly has a chronic course, patients who suffer from this disorder will likely be symptomatic at times in the lifespan when cancer is an important diagnostic consideration.

Differential Diagnosis of Schizophreniform Symptoms in the Cancer Patient

Since schizophrenia is a relatively rare disorder with a high degree of stigmatization and serious prognostic implications, it should be considered a diagnosis of exclusion. Additionally, the new onset of psychotic symptoms, hallucinations, or disorganized or bizarre behavior in a cancer patient is likely due to a cause other than schizophrenia. Assessment of schizophreniform symptoms should include evaluation of any previous history of similar symptoms, questioning about the possibility of a prodromal phase of the illness, inquiry regarding any family history of psychotic illness, and thorough mental status examination including application of the DSM-IV diagnostic criteria (1).

Differential diagnostic evaluation should include evaluation for primary or comorbid substance use disorders or withdrawal states (e.g., alcohol, benzodiazepines, cocaine, amphetamine, hallucinogens, phencyclidine), bipolar and other mood disorders (e.g., major depression with psychotic features), schizoaffective disorder, delusional disorders, severe anxiety disorders, dissociative disorders, and personality disorders. Mental disorders due to a general medical condition (e.g., steroid psychosis, symptoms induced by central nervous system metastases, neuropsychiatric symptoms as a consequence of partial complex seizures) should always be considered in the cancer patient exhibiting psychiatric symptoms.

Probably the most important diagnostic consideration in schizophreniform symptoms of new or sudden onset in the cancer patient is delirium. This disorder usually emerges in the oncology patient as a complication of the cancer or its treatment. Medical complications (e.g., metabolic imbalances, infections) and paraneoplastic syndromes can precipitate delirium. Many medications used in the treatment of cancer can lead to delirium. Chemotherapy drugs (e.g., methotrexate, vincristine, L-asparaginase), narcotics, and drugs with substantial anticholinergic effects should be considered as causative agents in the delirious cancer patient. See Chapter 48 for a more thorough discussion of delirium.

MANAGEMENT OF COMORBID CANCER AND SCHIZOPHRENIA

When cancer and schizophrenia occur together, some patients tolerate treatment well (29). However, the clinical management challenges facing the physician in this situation can be daunting. Generally, the elements of schizophrenia treatment are the same as in medically healthy patients with this disorder. Antipsychotic medications are the mainstay of treatment for schizophrenia, and are especially useful for controlling active psychotic symptoms and preventing their recurrence. Supportive individual and group psychotherapy or family psychotherapy aimed at education about schizophrenia and modulating expressed emotion are often helpful adjuncts. Psychosocial treatments may be especially beneficial in helping the patient tolerate and adhere to complex treatment recommendations. Patients should be closely monitored for compliance with recommended pharmacologic treatments, exacerbation of psychiatric symptoms, and development of substance abuse in the stressful setting of cancer treatment.

Massie has outlined a set of issues pertinent to the management of cancer in schizophrenic patients (30). She points out that most schizophrenic patients do not tolerate large teams of caregivers well and cooperate best when they are consistently cared for by the same doctor and nurse. Psychiatric consultation ordered early in the course of treatment can be helpful to assess the patient's mental condition, make treatment recommendations specific to that patient, and help the members of the oncology team optimize the patient's

cooperation with treatment. Family intervention, including education about schizophrenia, cancer, and their treatment, is very important to facilitate management of the patient at home. She advises physicians to pay particular attention to issues of informed consent, since patients often have difficulty understanding the nature of their illness and the proposed treatment. She also advises close monitoring for emergence of physical symptoms, especially pain, since patients with schizophrenia complain little of pain and discomfort (when others would suffer substantial distress) and are commonly inattentive to physical symptoms which might be important signals of advancing disease or treatment complications. Finally, though she points out that some patients with schizophrenia and cancer require little or no neuroleptic medication to tolerate cancer treatment, Massie recommends that a psychiatrist monitor psychotropic medications.

SPECIAL ISSUES IN THE PSYCHOPHARMACOLOGY OF SCHIZOPHRENIA IN THE CANCER PATIENT

Possible Indirect Benefits of Neuroleptic Medications in the Setting of Cancer

Antipsychotic drugs, particularly chlorpromazine, have been reported to have antitumor effects (31). Csatary comments on these observations in the literature and reports the case of a patient whose squamous cell carcinoma of the larynx regressed after treatment with chlorpromazine for psychiatric indications (32). This observation led to treatment with injections of chlorpromazine directly into the tumor, with further regression. Csatary reports that the patient committed suicide while his cancer was in remission. He cites several findings in the literature which might mediate an antineoplastic effect of chlorpromazine.

Mortensen reported the results of a study of 6168 schizophrenic patients followed over a 23-year period for risk of developing one of four cancers (lung, bladder, breast, cervix) (33). Each patient was compared to two controls (schizophrenic patients who did not develop cancer), matched for sex and age. Neuroleptic treatment was associated with reduced risk for all four tumor types studied. Ravn responded to this report with supportive anecdotal evidence (34). If the apparent protective effect of neuroleptics is real, it might be indirect (i.e., a result of better self care and risk factor reduction related to better symptom control).

Safety of Psychotropic Medications in the Setting of Cancer

In stark contrast to these reports, other recent evidence suggests that psychopharmacologic agents, especially some antidepressants, might act as tumor growth promoters (35–37). The authors proposed that interaction with an intracellular histamine receptor is the mechanism of the tumor promoting effect they reported for fluoxetine and amitriptyline. Antidepressants are often used in the comprehensive treatment of schizophrenia. Additionally, though neuroleptics have yet to be implicated in any of these studies, some neuroleptic drugs have significant antihistaminic activity. The results of these studies have been questioned since they were obtained in a rodent model with experimentally induced tumors and a small sample size. Additionally, two human epidemiologic studies, one a prospective study including more than 2200 cancer patients taking tricyclic antidepressants, failed to find a similar effect (38,39). Other reports have described cytostatic effects of fluoxetine, citalopram, and tricyclic antidepressants which might suppress tumor growth (40,41). Brandes and Friesen have recently reported two cases of patients with possible tumor growth promotion associated with lithium and an antihistamine decongestant (42). Miller (43) and Brandes (42) suggest that these apparently conflicting reports might be consistent with a tumor promoting effect of these drugs at lower doses and an antineoplastic effect at higher doses.

As pointed out in a series of editorial comments regarding these reports more investigation is needed to make clinical sense of these findings (43–45). In the meantime, all commentators agree that these studies do not provide enough evidence to justify any change in the careful and appropriate use of psychotropic agents in cancer patients. Unfortunately, media coverage of these preliminary reports might not be so careful with the facts. As similar studies are reported in the mass media, physicians should be prepared to discuss them with ambivalent patients who are appropriately treated with these drugs.

Antipsychotic drugs do not appear (so far) to increase the risk of cancer or accelerate tumor growth. This statement is supported by the fact that cancer incidence in schizophrenic patients did not appear to increase in the years following the development of neuroleptics (13). Studies aimed at assessing the effect of prolactin elevation commonly seen with neuroleptic administration on subsequent risk of developing breast cancer have found no effect (9,46). Benzodiazepines, often used adjunctively in schizophrenia, do not appear to influence the risk of cancer (47).

SUMMARY

When cancer and schizophrenia occur together, they can present an imposing set of clinical challenges. Most of the evidence available today supports the notion that the presence of schizophrenia itself has little or no effect on the overall risk of developing or dying from malignancy. However, schizophrenia clearly does have an effect on some of the common risk factors for cancer (especially smoking). Clinical features of schizophrenia may interfere with cancer detection and management. Since schizophrenia is a relatively rare disorder with a high degree of stigmatization and serious prognostic implications, it should be considered a diagnosis of exclusion. The new onset of psychotic symptoms, hallucinations, or disorganized or bizarre behavior in a cancer patient is likely due to a cause other than schizophrenia, with delirium deserving special diagnostic consideration. When cancer and schizophrenia occur together, some patients tolerate treatment well and easily. However, the clinical management challenges facing the physician in this situation can be daunting.

REFERENCES

1. American Psychiatric Association. *Diagnostic and Statistical Manual of Mental Disorders*, 4th ed. Washington, DC: American Psychiatric Press; 1994.
2. Massie MJ, Holland JC. The cancer patient with pain: psychiatric complications and their management. *Med Clin North Am.* 1987; 71:243–258.
3. Commissioners on Lunacy for England and Wales. *Annual Report.* HMSO: London; 1909.
4. Baldwin JA. Schizophrenia and physical disease. *Psychol Med.* 1979; 9:611–618.
5. Craig TJ, Lin SP. Cancer and mental illness. *Compr Psychiatry.* 1981; 22:404–410.
6. Fox BH, Howell MA. Cancer risk among psychiatric patients: a hypothesis. *Int J Edpidemiol.* 1974; 3: 207–208.
7. Modrzewska K, Bøøk JA. Schizophrenia and malignant neoplasms in a northern Swedish population. *Lancet.* 1979; 1:275–276.
8. Mortensen PB. The incidence of cancer in schizophrenic patients. *J Epidemiol Commun Health.* 1989; 43:43–47.
9. Mortensen PB. The occurrence of cancer in first admitted schizophrenic patients. *Schizophr Res.* 1994; 12:185–194.
10. Black DW, Winokur G. Cancer mortality in psychiatric patients: the Iowa record-linkage study. *Int J Psychiatry Med.* 1986–1987; 16:189–197.
11. Gulbinat W, DuPont A, Jablensky A, et al. Cancer incidence in schizophrenic patients: results of record linkage studies in three countries. *Br J Psychiatry.* 1992; 161 (suppl 18): 75–85.
12. Saku M, Tokudome S, Ikeda M, et al. Mortality in psychiatric patients with a specific focus on cancer mortality associated with schizophrenia. *Int J Edpidemiol.* 1995; 24:366–372.

13. Soni SD, Gill J. Malignancies in schizophrenic patients. *Br J Psychiatry*. 1979; 134: 447–448.
14. Tsuang MT, Woolson RF, Fleming JA. Schizophrenia and cancer death. *Lancet*. 1980; 1:480–481.
15. Tsuang, MT, Perkins K, Simpson JC. Physical diseases in schizophrenia and affective disorder. *J Clin Psychiatry*. 1983; 44:42–46.
16. Perrin GM, Pierce IR. Psychosomatic aspects of cancer. *Psychosom Med*. 1959; 21:397–421.
17. Katz J, Kunofsky S, Patton R, Allaway N. Cancer mortality among patients in New York mental hospitals. *Cancer*. 1967; 20:2194–2199.
18. Ames BN, Gold LS, Willett WC. The causes and prevention of cancer. *Proc Natl Acad Sci USA*. 1995; 92:5258–5265.
19. Dorian B, Garfinkel PE. Stress, immunity and illness: a review. *Psychol Med*. 1987; 17:393–407.
20. Schindler BA. Stress, affective disorders, and immune function. *Med Clin North Am*. 1985; 69:585–597.
21. Lohr LB, Flyn K. Smoking and schizophrenia. *Schizophr Res*. 1992; 8: 93–102.
22. Masterson E, O'Shea B. Smoking and malignancy in schizophrenia. *Br J Psychiatry*. 1984; 145:429–432.
23. McEvoy JP, Freudenrich O, Levin ED, Rose JE. Haloperidol increases smoking in patients with schizophrenia. *Psychopharmacology*. 1995; 119:124–126.
24. Goff DC, Henderson DC, Amico E. Cigarette smoking in schizophrenia: relationship to psychopathology and medication side-effects. *Psychopharmacology*. 1992; 149:1189–1194.
25. Adler LE, Hoffer LD, Wiser A, Freedman R. Normalization of auditory physiology by cigarette smoking in schizophrenic patients. *Am J Psychiatry*. 1993; 150:1856–1861.
26. Sandyk R. Cigarette smoking: effects on cognitive functions and drug-induced Parkinsonism in chronic schizophrenia. *Int J Neurosci*. 1993; 70:193–197.
27. Levi RN, Waxman S. Schizophrenia, epilepsy, cancer, methionine, and folate metabolism. *Lancet*. 1975; 2:11–13.
28. McDaniel, JS. Could natural killer cell activity be linked to the reduced incidence of cancer in schizophrenic patients? *J Epidemiol Commun Health*. 1990; 44:174.
29. Solomon S, McCartney JR, Saravay SM, Katz E. Postoperative hospital course of patients with history of severe psychiatric illness. *Gen Hosp Psychiatry*. 1987; 9:376–382.
30. Massie MJ. Schizophrenia. In: Holland JC, Rowland JH, eds. *Handbook of Psychooncology: Psychological Care of the Patient with Cancer*. New York: Oxford University Press; 1989: 320–323.
31. Driscoll JS, Melnick NR, Quinn FR, et al. Psychotropic drugs as potential antitumor agents: a selective screening study. *Cancer Treat Rep*. 1978; 62:45.
32. Csatary LK. Chlorpromazines and cancer. *Lancet*. 1972; 2:338–339.
33. Mortensen PB. Neuroleptic treatment and other factors modifying cancer risk in schizophrenic patients. *Acta Psychiatr Scand*. 1987; 75:585–590.
34. Ravn J. Neuroleptic treatment and other factors modifying cancer risk in schizophrenic patients. *Acta Psychiatr Scand*. 1988; 76:605.
35. Brandes LJ, Arron RJ, Bogdanovic RP, et al. Stimulation of malignant growth in rodents by antidepressant drugs at clinically relevant doses. *Cancer Res*. 1992; 52:3796–3800.
36. Brandes LJ, Warrington RC, Arron RJ, et al. Enhanced cancer growth in mice administered daily human-equivalent doses of some H1-antihistamines: predictive in vitro correlates. *J Natl Cancer Inst*. 1994; 86:770–775.
37. Brandes LJ. Letter regarding "Response to antidepressants and cancer: Cause for concern?" *J Clin Psychopharmacol*. 1995; 15:84–85.
38. Friedman GD. An editor comments. *Am J Epidemiol*. 1992; 136:1415–1416.
39. Linkins RW, Comstock GN. Two authors comment. *Am J Epidemiol*. 1992; 136:1416–1417.
40. Tutton PJM, Barkla DH. Influence of inhibitors of serotonin uptake on intestinal epithelium and colorectal carcinomas. *Br J Cancer*. 1982; 46:260–265.
41. Sauter C. Cytostatic activity of commonly used tricyclic antidepressants. *Oncology*. 1989; 46:155–157.
42. Brandes LJ, Friesen LA. Can the clinical course of cancer be influenced by non-antineoplastic drugs? *Can Med Assoc J*. 1995; 153:561–566.
43. Miller, LG. Psychopharmacologic agents and cancer: a progress report. *J Clin Psychopharmacol*. 1995; 15: 160–161.
44. Miller LG. Antidepressants and cancer: cause for concern? *J Clin Psychopharmacol*. 1993; 13:1–2.
45. Roy DJ, MacDonald N. The Brandes–Friesen case reports: how should we interpret the news? *Can Med Assoc J*. 1995; 153:569–571.
46. Hoover J. Breast cancer: epidemiologic considerations. Reserpine and Breast Cancer Task Force, Department of Health, Education, and Welfare Publication; 1977.
47. Rosenberg L, Palmer JR, Zauber AG, et al. Relation of benzodiazepine use to the risk of selected cancers: breast, large bowel, malignant melanoma, lung, endometrium, ovary, non-Hodgkin's lymphoma, testis, Hodgkin's disease, thyroid, and liver. *Am J Epidemiol*. 1995; 141:1153–1160.

54

Personality Disorders

PHILIP R. MUSKIN

We all have a personality—i.e., a style with which we relate to the world and to other people. Like ice cream, which takes on the taste of whatever is added to the basic ingredients, personality traits give each of us our flavor. Even people who we joke have "no personality" exhibit certain traits, characteristic ways of doing things, or predictable responses to certain situations or emotional stimuli. For most people personality style is a relatively invisible part of their make-up, while simultaneously it is one of a person's most distinguishing characteristics. The general public does not use the diagnostic labels of DSM-IV, but uses descriptors which relate more to the interpersonal problems that certain personality styles generate. Terms like "obnoxious," "hostile," "lay-back," "self-centered," "weird," and "bossy" are just a few of the ways a variety of different diagnostic categories might be described by people interacting with the person in question.

What is perhaps the most important part of personality is how it shapes the way a person will cope with life events. This aspect of personality is so important that an understanding of different personality types is crucial for those working with patients with serious medical illness (1). People who function well in everyday life may do very poorly under the stress imposed by a serious medical illness such as cancer. A major component of the disturbance in the person's ability to function can be attributed to the limitations imposed by his or her personality. In contrast, people with more severe personality disorders may experience regular problems in everyday life, stemming from their psychiatric disorder. When people with personality disorders become seriously medically ill they are likely to experience problems resultant from their habitual ways of handling life events (2–5). The ability to work with the patient may depend upon whether the physician recognizes the impact of personality or

personality disorder on the patient's manner of coping with the stress of the illness itself, as well as the stresses concomitant with hospitalization and treatment (1). This chapter will address several points regarding the interaction of personality with serious medical illness such as cancer.

NATURE VERSUS NURTURE

Are we born a certain way, or are we fashioned into a particular personality by the experiences of childhood? Parents recognize traits in their children that remain consistent from the earliest moments in childhood through the life of the individual. Several studies suggest that inborn aspects of character are present (6–9). However, it is also clear that experiences in childhood shape the individual in a powerful way (10). Our inherited genetic substrate is not an all-or-nothing phenomenon. Genes may turn on or turn off at different points in development, rendering the person more (or less) vulnerable to environmental influences. Certain traumatic experiences such as physical and/or sexual abuse have an effect on the person, but these experiences do not have a predictable effect resulting in a particular personality or personality disorder 100% of the time. Studies have demonstrated the negative effect of physical and sexual abuse on children resulting in an increase in psychopathology, particularly Axis II disorders (11–13). However, not all patients with personality disorders have a history of childhood abuse and not all children who are abused have personality disorders (11–13). Rather than a nature *versus* nurture relationship, there is a consensus that personality and personality disorders are the result of an interaction between both inherited characteristics and the influence of the environment (14).

PERSONALITY DISORDERS IN DSM-IV

Whereas a personality is a stable attitude towards life, love and the pursuit of happiness, a personality disorder is a diagnostic entity in DSM-IV (15). See Table 54.1 for the diagnostic criteria of a personality disorder.

DSM-IV has taken the approach that personality disorders represent qualitatively distinct clinical syndromes (the categorical perspective). An alternative to the categorical approach is the dimensional perspective—i.e., that personality disorders represent maladaptive variants of personality traits that merge imperceptibly into normality and into one another. It can be quite a challenge to determine the point where an experience moves from the normal to the abnormal. How much of an increase in "organic" findings such as blood pressure or heart rate are "within normal limits"? How sad can one be during bereavement before the sadness is diagnosed as a major depressive disorder? How much good feeling about oneself is normal before a diagnosis of narcissistic pathology or narcissistic personality disorder is appropriate? At what point does the person who pays close attention to detail deserve classification as having an obsessive-compulsive personality disorder? There is a point past which a medical finding is generally accepted as abnormal, a midrange where the finding may or may not be abnormal, and "nonnormal" findings which are not considered abnormal.

Certain personality disorders seem to have some overlap with Axis I conditions in DSM-IV, such as paranoid, schizoid and schizotypal (16–18). Since no diagnostic system is perfect, continued research will demonstrate whether alterations will be necessary in the separation between Axis I and Axis II. It may turn out that certain personality disorders are prodromes of Axis I disorders or subthreshold conditions of Axis I disorders. DSM-IV recognizes that genetic and biologic similarities may exist between some of the personality disorders and certain Axis I disorders. However, the rationale for the separation is to encourage clinicians to attempt to make appropriate personality disorder diagnoses even when the patient offers no complaint. Individuals with personality disorders, not just personality traits, may experience no discomfort from their behavior, in spite of observable dysfunction at work or in relationships (i.e., the symptoms are egosyntonic). On the other hand, it is important for the psychiatric consultant to not overemphasize diagnosis and recognize that the impact of severe medical illness may exacerbate the personality traits of an individual such that he or she appears to have dysfunction adequate to diagnose a personality disorder (19).

DSM-IV clusters the ten personality disorders into three groups based on common characteristics. See Table 54.2 for the DSM-IV personality disorder clusters.

MEDICAL ILLNESS AND PERSONALITY

This theoretical discussion takes on a real meaning when a patient with a medical problem presents difficulties related to constraints imposed by personality or by a personality disorder. Personality occurs in everyone, as noted above, but personality disorders are not uncommon, and are found in approximately 10% of the population (20). Patients with personality disorders may be more likely to be hospitalized medically than other people (21). Knowing how personality might shape the experience of medical illness becomes mandatory for the physician in order to work with the patient successfully.

TABLE 54.1. *Diagnostic Criteria for Personality Disorders*

A. An enduring pattern of inner experience and behavior that deviates markedly from the expectations of the individual's culture. This pattern is manifested in two (or more) of the following areas:

  1. *Cognition* or how the person perceives and interprets himself/herself, other people, and events

  2. *Affectivity* or how the persons reacts emotionally in terms of the range, intensity, lability and appropriateness of the response

  3. *Interpersonal functioning* or how the person relates with others

  4. *Impulse control*

B. The pattern is enduring, inflexible and is pervasive across a broad range of social and personal situations

C. The pattern leads to clinically significant distress and/or impairment in social, occupational or other important areas of function

D. The pattern is stable, of long duration and the onset of the pattern can be traced back at least to the person's adolescence or early adulthood

E. There is no other mental disorder, or consequence of a mental disorder that would better account for this enduring pattern of behavior

F. No general medical condition nor the direct physiological effects of a substance could account for this enduring pattern of behavior

TABLE 54.2 *Personality Disorders*

A. Odd/eccentric cluster

Paranoid personality disorder is a pattern of distrust and suspiciousness such that others' motives are interpreted as malevolent

Schizoid personality disorder is a pattern of detachment from social relationships and a restricted range of emotional expression

Schizotypal personality disorder is a pattern of acute discomfort in close relationships, cognitive or perceptual distortions, and eccentricities of behavior

B. Dramatic/emotional/erratic cluster

Antisocial personality disorder is a pattern of disregard for, and violation of, the rights of others

Borderline personality disorder is a pattern of instability in interpersonal relationships, self-image, and affects, and marked impulsivity

Histrionic personality disorder is a pattern of excessive emotionality and attention seeking

Narcissistic personality disorder is a pattern of grandiosity, need for admiration, and lack of empathy

C. Anxious/fearful cluster

Avoidant personality disorder is a pattern of social inhibition, feelings of inadequacy, and hypersensitivity to negative evaluation

Dependent personality disorder is a pattern of submissive and clinging behavior related to an excessive need to be taken care of by others

Obsessive-compulsive personality disorder is a pattern of preoccupation with orderliness, perfectionism, and control

Tentative diagnoses, dependent on the outcome of further study:

Passive-aggressive personality disorder is a pervasive pattern of negativistic attitudes and passive resistance to demands for adequate performance in social and occupational situations

Depressive personality disorder is a pervasive pattern of depressive cognitions and behaviors (including a persistent and pervasive feeling of dejection, gloominess, cheerlessness, joylessness, and unhappiness) that occur in a variety of contexts.

To understand how personality shapes the experience of illness it is necessary to understand the stress that illness and hospitalization impose upon the psychology of the individual. Serious illness, and many other expected and unexpected occurrences, all cause distress for patients and their families. Psychological stress is a situation that destabilizes a person's life. People vary in their vulnerability to stress and vary in their ability to adapt to the particular situation. How a patient adapts to the stress will depend upon prior experiences with illness and doctors, the person's characteristic manner of coping with stress, and the particular type and severity of stress that the patient is experiencing. The genetic endowment of the individual, the specific character style, and the external resources of the family will also play a powerful role. The experience of an illness severe enough to require hospitalization will be modulated by the individual's early experiences as a young child. The vestiges of the past, no matter how distant, will be reflected in this current life crisis; however, "The vast majority of patients are able to cope and to assume the role of patient without difficulty, and this is extraordinary in itself when one considers the magnitude of these stresses" (22). Strain and Grossman outline seven broad categories of psychological stress which affect the patient who is hospitalized (22). These categories are worth a brief review:

1. *The basic threat to narcissistic integrity.* Many people feel relatively indestructible and assume they will always be capable, independent and self-sufficient. Most of us believe, in spite of evidence to the contrary, that we are always in complete control of what happens to our bodies. Illness, particularly severe illness which requires hospitalization and may threaten a person's very existence, undermines these important, typically unconscious fantasies. The child's fantasy of all-powerful parents who guarantee his or her pleasurable existence is challenged by the experience of illness, pain, and suffering. When the infantile fantasy of parental omnipotence is transferred onto the patient's doctor, there exists a potential for rage targeted at the doctor who is perceived as having failed to protect the patient from the illness. Patients who handle stress in this way may generate reactive negative feelings in their physicians, which could result in a disruption of the patient–physician relationship.

2. *Fear of strangers.* Upon entering the hospital, patients put themselves, and even their lives, in the hands of complete strangers. This can reawaken early fears about the dangerousness of strangers. This fear can disrupt the routine of medical care by restricting access to one's body, bodily fluids, or by inhibiting the patient from revealing important information.

3. *Separation anxiety.* Hospitalized patients are separated from both important people and objects by which their world is defined, and sometimes by which the patients define themselves, resulting in intense anxiety. Hospitalization may be a special problem for those individuals whose capacity to adapt to new situations is limited by their cognitive abilities (patients with

moderate to severe dementia), or limited by their psychological abilities (patients with severe personality disorders).

4. *Fear of the loss of love and approval.* For some patients the very circumstance of being ill reactivates dependency conflicts from childhood and generates tremendous distress in the current situation that is both inappropriate and maladaptive. This stress may be overt in its manifestation, as with a patient who believes his illness will render him unlovable. For some women having a mastectomy or hysterectomy may stimulate a fear that she will no longer be loved by her partner. Some patients fear their need for nursing care and convalescence will result in disapproval from family or friends. Patients also fear loss of love and approval from their physicians because they have become ill, because they are not recovering at a rapid enough rate, because their pain continues despite treatment, or even because they are terminally ill.

5. *Fear of the loss of control of developmentally achieved functions.* Physical illness, and often the therapeutic measures to address the illness, may cause suspension of physical and mental functions that were previously under the patient's control. Patients frequently feel fatigued, occasionally lose control of bowel and/or bladder function, or experience physical incoordination and/or the inability to speak articulately. Such losses are painful and result in patients' anguish.

6. *Fear of loss of or injury to body parts.* As we know, both men and women experience castration anxiety, the fear of the loss of a part of one's body, or the loss of function, alteration or temporary dysfunction of a body part. This broader view of castration fears does not mean that for some patients an injury, illness, diagnostic procedure, or treatment may take on a sexual meaning. These patients experience such events as real threats to their genital integrity or sexual potency. Appropriate, compassionate, empathic and practical interpretation of all the forms of castration fears are often powerfully therapeutic.

7. *Reactivation of feelings of guilt and shame with accompanying fears of retaliation for previous transgressions.* Physical illness may be perceived as a punishment for prior crimes, real or imagined. When illness serves as a metaphor of guilt for the patient, the illness signifies that the person is bad or has done bad things.

REGRESSION AND MEDICAL ILLNESS

The stresses of illness and of hospitalization mimic the developmental stresses of childhood. The individual is placed in a situation of dependency which replicates the experience of childhood. Behavior, coping skills, experience of emotion and expression of emotion all take on qualities from previous stages of the person's development. The experience of being ill is thus a *regressive* one for the person. Regression may range from the temporary loss of recent gains in the patient's psychological make-up, to behavior of a fashion more appropriate for a young child. Physical illness commonly induces regression, and this phenomenon is most easily observed in children. For instance, a 5- or 6-year-old child with a high fever may suck her thumb, insist on her mother being present to go to sleep, or act in a clingy manner—behaviors the child abandoned some months or years previously. While regression may evoke a negative image for some, this is not necessarily the case. Regression is a dedifferentiation of the individual such that the person is in a more plastic state. This is a state that is simultaneously more primitive than the person's typical behavioral and emotional level of function. Regression implies that the person is using defenses that are less reality-oriented, based more upon unresolved conflicts from childhood, less stable and less adaptive to the demands of the environment (23). The experience of regression potentially offers the person more flexibility to adapt to the environment and creates the potential for positive change. However, while in this state, the person may function in a manner somewhat or totally different from his or her usual way of dealing with the world. This alteration exerts a stress upon friends, family *and* care givers. The regressed adult is operating with a defensive structure more appropriate for someone who typically functions at a lower level of psychiatric health. The adequacy with which the individual negotiated the stresses and conflicts of development, and the strengths and/or deficiencies of parental relationships, will play a crucial role in how this adult will cope with illness and hospitalization. The typical level of function is the starting point for the patient. The lower the level of function, the more primitive the defensive structure to which the patient will regress. Simultaneous with this process are patients' reactions to their regression and their attempts to return to their usual level of function and control. The attempts at regaining control over the regression are occasionally what generates the request for a psychiatric consultation, rather than the behavior induced by the regression itself.

It is worth noting the influence of the medical setting itself on the distress generated by hospitalization. Major medical centers are complex, vibrant and ever-evolving organizations which are often disorienting, bewildering and frightening to patients, families, and visitors. Thus the physical structure of the hospital can provide additional stress for the patient. The tertiary care medical center, where the majority of patients with malignancies go for evaluation and treatment, are usually a series of structures connected in a heterogeneity of logical and often remarkably illogical ways. Negotiating the physical characteristics of the hospital can be a daunting undertaking. There is an increase in anxiety in patients as the size of the health care setting increases (24). This anxiety is separate from, but in addition to, the anxieties concerning their health. People come to hospitals because they experience themselves as being sick, in pain, suffering, needing information, care or help. Sometimes the experience of negotiating transportation to the hospital, the experience of the emergency room or the time spent in the admitting office, will all contribute to the stress of hospitalization for a patient.

Hospitals also have unique smells. In addition to the many different types of disinfectants, all of which have odors, there are other scents which we associate with pain, suffering and death, or with feelings connected to sexuality, loss of impulse control and shame. Doctors and nurses usually habituate to these olfactory stimuli, but patients experience this primitive sensory stimulation, even if the experience is not conscious. Various parts of the hospital may even have distinct scents. In the patient's room intimate bodily functions are exposed. There are few circumstances of life, with the exception of the earliest years of childhood, where this occurs without resultant shame and humiliation for the patient. These olfactory experiences also contribute to the regressive effect of illness and hospitalization.

Admission to the hospital also signifies relinquishing the comfort of and the control over one's personal environment. Not only does the patient leave home, he or she is asked to give up personal belongings. Most importantly, patients are asked to relinquish their clothing. In giving up their clothes, their belongings and their home, individuals attain a new status, that of "patient." The individual must adapt to the patient role instantaneously and accept that all patients are viewed as the same in the health care setting. The typical trappings of power, wealth and position are often unavailable for the "patient." The patient is expected to follow a rather rigid set of rules, though the rules are often vaguely defined. When and often *what* a patient eats may no longer be under the person's control. Access to family and friends is restricted and typically privacy not possible. As the severity of the medical illness increases, the patient suffers ever increasing loss of control, sometimes to the point of the loss of bodily functions, respiration, even cardiac function. It is this set of cir-

cumstances that each patient must negotiate and it is the patient's personality or personality disorder that will shape the adequacy of the journey. How the individual copes with the inescapable stress of hospitalization will emerge as the central focus of the psychiatrist asked to consult for this "difficult patient." In addition, how the hospital structure, the personnel, the resources of the patient (financial, social, cognitive) limit the ability of the patient to cope with the stress of hospitalization may determine whether a particular patient successfully copes with illness and with the hospitalization.

PERSONALITY TYPES AND MEDICAL ILLNESS

The assessment and the management of patients with various personality types has been the focus of literature directed towards both psychiatrists and physicians with primary medical responsibility towards patients (1,19). Recently, Oldham recommended an updated version of the original Kahana and Bibring terminology that reflects DSM-IV (25). A useful general principle in management is to use medication at times when the severity of the patient's symptoms prevents any other approach. For the most part, however, the management will be psychotherapy, which may be a modality of treatment offered by the psychiatrist or the primary care physician. Much excellent psychotherapy can be delivered by the patient's personal physician. At times the regular doctor is the only professional with whom the patient can interact. Occasionally the psychiatrist is utilized as a supervisor, even when the patient's personal physician is more senior than the consultant. Using Oldham's terminology (25), the following sections focus on an illustrative case description of a patient with a serious medical illness from each of the eight personality types. Some of these individuals have psychopathology in more than one area. Human beings are rarely "pure cultures"—mixtures of personality traits occur within each of us, and within people who have personality disorders.

Dependency and Overdemandingness (DSM-IV Dependent PD, Borderline PD)

The consultation request for Ms. S came from the chief of the OB/GYN service after numerous telephone calls from the president of the hospital. Ms. S called the president if anything bothered her about the hospital, the nurses, the food, etc. She had grown up in a middle class neighborhood in modest circumstances, but claimed a relation to an extremely important national figure, whom she threatened to call upon if disappointed. Admitted for evaluation of vaginal bleeding, her surgeon could hardly manage the patient and insisted on a psychiatrist being involved in the case if she was to continue with the work-up. Ms. S "held court" daily, dressed provocatively, insisting upon special treatment from nurses. She did not appear as if she was ill, nor did she accept that she might have a serious medical condition. Many of the nursing staff admitted to "hating" the patient, but there were several staff members who, following "private" conversations with Ms. S, defended her and blamed the other staff for not being understanding. Ms. S insisted only a certain resident could draw her blood because he was "the best" and she refused phlebotomy if he was not available.

The psychiatrist entered this situation with the belief this was a woman with a borderline personality disorder because of the impulsivity, use of splitting, lability of emotion, narcissism and manipulativeness of the patient. She also recognized that much of the behavior defended against the tremendous fear Ms. S had that the work-up would reveal uterine cancer and that she would require a hysterectomy. Ms. S directed many of her attacks at the consultant, whom she criticized for being "too young and too skinny." At other times the psychiatrist was "the golden girl" of the institution. The psychotherapeutic approach the consultant chose was to set limits on the disruptive behaviors, the telephone calls and the private meetings with staff members, while empathizing with Ms. S for having a condition that might so affect her image of herself as woman. A considerable amount of time was spent "chatting" with the nursing staff daily. The psychiatrist and the gynecologist spoke daily about the care of Ms. S. The therapy, which lasted over a period of 2 weeks, gave Ms. S a chance to talk about her terror of being "mutilated" and losing her "sexual appeal." When a diagnosis of cancer was made, and a hysterectomy recommended, the psychiatrist helped Ms. S negotiate the placement of the incision so that she could still wear a bikini bathing suit. When Ms. S decided to have her follow-up treatment in her home state, the psychiatrist arranged a consultation with a psychiatrist she knew from her residency to continue to "talk things over" during the chemotherapy.

Ten years later the consultant was sitting in nursing station on the private medical unit. She noticed a patient who looked vaguely familiar walking by and heard a nurse's comment, "can't wait until she leaves." Several nurses laughed at that point and mentioned the patient's name. The consultant was shocked to hear that this was the same patient, hospitalized for a "chronic pain syndrome" but thought to be narcotic-seeking by the staff. Speaking with the psychiatric consultant on the case she discovered that the patient had been in and out of the hospital several times, all related to narcotic abuse. The old chart had been "lost," with a question of whether or not the patient had stolen her old chart. The major difference was the absence of the connection to the national figure. Otherwise, the description of the patient and her behavior was unchanged from the initial consultation a decade earlier.

Orderliness and Compulsiveness (DSM-IV Obsessive-Compulsive PD)

Dr. F was referred for outpatient psychotherapy from a psychopharmacologist who had recently tried a course of electroconvulsive therapy for her refractory depression and obsessions. A survivor of the Holocaust she was the first person in her family to go to college and was a full professor at a major university. She dated her obsessions from childhood, including the thought that someone she knew would get cancer. For a period of 20 years or more she had compulsively examined her breasts for signs of a mass, particularly when under stress or when a family member or friend was ill. At these times she had the conviction that she would develop breast cancer and die. Her self-examinations would cause her breasts to swell from the harsh manipulation. She believed that she would not get cancer if she carried out the ritual examination, but felt tremendous guilt that others were ill. Simultaneous with her obsession about cancer she took very poor care of herself physically. When she developed vaginal bleeding she ignored the symptom, assuming it was a "long period." While on a trip abroad she required hospitalization following a syncopal episode and was discovered to have a very low hematocrit. She refused any treatment for her gynecologic disorder but returned to the USA where she had a hysterectomy. Her academic career continued successfully but she had few intimate relationships with the exception of her mother and her sister.

When she first discovered a mass in her breast Dr. F ignored the finding, believing this was "nothing important." She did not contact her gynecologist or internist. Her belief that she would be immune from cancer by continued self-examination was not shaken by the discovery of the mass. Almost a year after Dr. F first discovered the mass, she went to her physician for a yearly physical. A diagnosis of breast cancer was made and she had a radical mastectomy with several positive lymph nodes. Following her surgery and radiotherapy Dr. F experienced no anxiety about recurrence of the cancer. Approximately a year later she developed back pain which she ignored until the pain became excruciating and she had trouble walking. Metastatic cancer was discovered in her spine which was treated with radiation. She suffered a collapse of a vertebrae leading to a stooped posture. At this point her obsessions about cancer increased markedly and she was reluctant to see her doctor for fear he would give her "bad news." Her anxiety was so intense around the time of an appointment that she could not function. An arrangement was made that her doctor only call her if the results of her tests were significant, as "no news is good news." She was chronically depressed, unable to do her academic work, and constantly obsessed about having cancer. The electroconvulsive therapy had little effect on her symptoms.

After the referral Dr. F was started on chloripramine and clonazepam. After 8 weeks on both medications Dr. F experienced a reduction in her depression and a lessening of her obsessions. She was able to sleep through the night for the first time in years. Over a period of 3 years in psychotherapy she explored her dependent relationship with her mother and her gender conflicts. Her academic work improved to the point that she could enjoy the fruits of her labors. She was able to appear for doctors appointments without a companion and she could now call the doctor to check on her laboratory results. At times of stress she would become concerned that a minor ache signified another metastasis, but she was reassured when the evaluation was negative. After 3 years she felt comfortable discontinuing psychotherapy, remaining on the two medications and having psychiatric follow-up every 6 months.

Dramatization (DSM-IV Histrionic PD)

Mrs. D was referred for inpatient treatment of major depressive disorder and concomitant cardiac disease. At the time of her referral selective serotonin reuptake inhibitory were not available and a tricyclic antidepressant was being considered. Mrs. D was an uncommonly attractive woman who looked considerably younger than her actual age (65 years). When the medical intern asked her to take off her clothes so he could examine her, she disrobed completely and stood in front of him revealing her body, and her mastectomy scar. A psychiatric consultation was requested immediately for "patient out of control." The consultant arrived to find Mrs. D dressed in a lacy and revealing nightgown she had brought from home. The gown was notable in his mind for being see-through and cut very high, but that he would not have known Mrs. D had had a mastectomy. Mrs. D gave a history of having a "wonderful life" until her husband discovered a mass in her right breast during sex. She was aware of the pride she took in her figure and in her beauty as a

woman. During the surgery that was to have been a biopsy, the surgeon sought permission from her husband to perform a radical mastectomy because the mass was clearly malignant on frozen section. "They decided not to wake me up," she related with unconcealed rage. Her anger at her husband and her doctor was maximal. She felt mutilated by these two men. When she developed a recurrence she welcomed the opportunity to die from the cancer, but the recurrence responded well to treatment. Following her recovery she prohibited her husband from seeing her without her clothes on and sex was permitted only in pitch-black darkness. In her everyday life she took tremendous care that no-one be aware of her "disability." She often thought of suicide. About 8 years after her breast surgery she developed crushing chest pain while rushing to catch a bus. As she collapsed, Mrs. D thought to herself that she was finally going to be released from her misery.

The consultant started Mrs. D on an antidepressant and her cardiologist monitored her ECG. After about 3 weeks she felt like a "changed person" including a decrease in the chronic pain in her right arm. The consultant decided to propose to Mrs. D a psychodynamic life narrative formulation about her response to the mastectomy (26). Mrs. D listened to the consultant's formulation that her appearance had always been central to her feelings about herself and that her husband and surgeon had not understood what it would mean to lose a breast for her. Her anger at her husband was genuine but she was also terrified that she was no longer an attractive, desirable woman. The loss had been so tremendous that life wasn't worth living for Mrs. D. The consultant suggested that Mrs. D had ignored reality, that she was an attractive woman, desired by her husband, and no less of a woman to the world. He recommended that she consider talking with other women who had had mastectomies, which she had never done. Mrs. D was not sure she could forgive her husband for making the decision for her about the mastectomy. She admitted that she was often puzzled when men found her attractive because she felt "damaged," but she accepted the consultant's idea that this was her fear, not reality. Several months after the consultation Mrs. D called to ask the consultant for a referral for a "marriage counselor" because she believed she and her husband could not work out their problems without a "referee."

Self-Sacrifice (DSM-IV Dependent PD, Passive-Aggressive PD, Depressive PD)

A consultation was requested for Ms. B after she told a nurse she would kill herself if she had cancer. Ms. B had been admitted for evaluation of a painful mass in her thigh. She worked as a secretary in the hospital where she was well known for her efficiency. The chart note stated that she noticed the mass several days prior to the office visit. Ms. B started by asking the consultant if what she said was confidential and whether the information would go into her chart. She was assured that all the information was confidential and that little of what she said belonged in the chart. Ms. B related a story detailing many years of physical abuse by her ex-husband. The mother of three children by the time she was 21, she did everything she could to protect them from his "drunken attacks," while trying to keep the family together so the children would not come from a broken home, as had Ms. B. She was physically abused often during the 10-year marriage but felt this was her "portion." With great shame she revealed that her husband would beat her on her thigh during sex to get her to respond, exactly at the spot where she had the mass. She had always feared that her compliance with his abuse would come back to haunt her. The mass had been present for years but had become painful after a minor car accident a few days prior to her seeing her doctor. She was convinced she had cancer of the bone which was her "punishment for bad things." She had also convinced herself that she would require an amputation of her leg, lose her job and lose her current partner. The consultant obtained a promise from Ms. B not to kill herself until a diagnosis was made and the two of them had a chance to review the situation together. She suggested that Ms. B's whole life had been focused on her children and a suicide would harm them forever. The psychiatrist commented on Ms. B's great courage to have suffered so greatly in order to protect her children and what a great burden she must have carried waiting for something bad to happen.

A bone scan and biopsy revealed a large calcified hematoma in her thigh. There was no indication that the mass was malignant. When the consultant and Ms. B met the day of her discharge the consultant found her to be cheerful, almost euphoric in her mood. "I feel free," Ms. B told her, "for the first time." The consultant discussed with Ms. B how she might tell her children something about the abuse she had suffered so they could understand what she had been through. This idea had never occurred to Ms. B because she believed "people don't talk about such things." However, she believed that the consultant would not "steer me astray" and planned to communicate her feelings and some of the facts about herself to her children when she left the hospital.

Self-Importance (DSM-IV Narcissistic PD)

Mr. G was admitted to the most exclusive part of the hospital at an additional out-of-pocket cost of $375 per day. The brother of a famous film star, he made sure everyone knew his connections. Every note in his chart mentioned his famous relative in the history, though there was no importance of that fact to his medical condition. He was a poor historian because he would not cooperate with the routine of admission history and physical. Mr. G lived in another city and his regular physician was not available. His admission for excision of a basal cell carcinoma seemed secondary to his loudly stated concerns that the "plastics guy" leave him without a scar. From the moment he was admitted his famous relative was involved, calling doctors' offices but not being available to be called back until late in the evening.

As the hospitalization progressed, Mr. G became more agitated, more difficult, and more confused. A psychiatric consultation was requested by the attending plastic surgeon for "noncompliance." A senior resident in psychiatry saw Mr. G, who, though confused and agitated, was "upset" that a resident was the consultant. After speaking with Mr. G and his famous sibling, the resident discovered that Mr. G was under psychiatric care and tried to contact the psychiatrist. Mr. G's sibling asked the surgeon to get the "head of psychiatry" to consult on the case. Several telephone calls were made to the C.-L. Service by various physicians involved with Mr. G and the chief of the service reviewed the case with the resident. He found Mr. G to be delirious and raised the issue of withdrawal from alcohol, which was denied by Mr. G, his sibling, and the surgeon. While reading the chart the attending found one of the pieces of paper stuck to the front of the chart. On that page was a note from a resident who had seen Mr. G on the day of admission noting that he took ethchlorvynol (Placidyl) nightly. The psychiatrist placed a call to Mr. G's regular psychiatrist as an emergency. He obtained a history that Mr. G had taken sleeping medication for many years but that he "only takes one." Confronting Mr. G with this history the psychiatrist learned that he took "a few" every night. The plastic surgeon was called who refused to believe this "type of man" could be addicted and withdrawing. He insisted on a neurological consultation and called a neurologist who was also one of the deans of the medical school. The psychiatrist related his findings to the neurologist and his impression that Mr. G was at risk for seizures and other complications from untreated withdrawal. The neurologist came to the floor and personally started an infusion of intravenous phenobarbital. Mr. G's delirium cleared over the next 24 h and he was detoxified from ethchlorvynol with phenobarbital over a period of 3 weeks. A recommendation was made by the psychiatrist that Mr. G have treatment directed towards his long-standing substance abuse, with inpatient treatment following discharge from the current admission. Mr. G immediately discharged the psychiatrist in order to find a "top expert" in substance abuse treatment.

Detachment (DSM-IV Schizoid PD, Schizotypal PD, Avoidant PD)

The consultation requested for Mr. Q was to "evaluate capacity for discharge planning." A 50-year-old man admitted for shoulder pain following an accident, Mr. Q was discovered to have a large thyroid mass causing a 40% occlusion of his trachea. It was not clear if the mass was a thyroid nodule or a malignancy but Mr. Q declined to pursue further work-up or surgery because he "did not like to be cut." He seemed unconcerned about the possibility of increasing occlusion of his trachea and did not want to discuss the matter. His aunt, the only family member that could be found, told the psychiatrist that Mr. Q always "kept to himself." Over the next few days the consultant learned that Mr. Q had been married but had been divorced more than 25 years ago. He had no friends and worked as a filing clerk with a good work history. There was no drug or alcohol use and, besides his aunt, no relationships. The psychiatrist could not elicit a prior history of hallucinations or delusions or any prior psychiatric contact. Mr. Q had "idiosyncratic" ideas about surgery and doctors, which, while not delusional, prevented him from permitting the evaluation to proceed. The surgical staff were ready to discharge Mr. Q as he was not in acute distress.

Exploration with Mr. Q revealed that he kept to himself and wrote horror stories in which he identified with the detective who solved the mystery. He believed that surgery of any sort would be too painful and might change him. As he was in no discomfort he could not believe that the thyroid mass was placing him at risk. The psychiatrist did not feel Mr. Q lacked capacity and used the time to discuss the horror stories rather than confront the denial of illness. Mr. Q became increasingly uncomfortable in the hospital and wanted to return home to his cats. He had a good relationship with his personal physician with whom he agreed to discuss the need for further evaluation. The psychiatrist found that his aunt had been treated surgically for a similar condition, discovered to be a benign thyroid nodule. She agreed to meet with Mr. Q and his physician after discharge to describe her experience to Mr. Q. Without evidence

to hold Mr. Q against his will, he was discharged by the surgical team. The psychiatrist attempted to reach Mr. Q several times over the next 2 weeks, without success.

Suspiciousness (DSM-IV Paranoid PD)

An urgent consultation request came from the cardiac care unit about a 45-year-old man, admitted with crescendo angina, who had touched a nurse on the buttocks and was "threatening to the other staff." The psychiatrist, who rounded regularly with the CCU staff, decided to see this patient along with the team on morning rounds. Mr. C was sitting up in bed when the team came to his room. He was not wearing a hospital gown and the sheets were carefully tucked in, sharply outlining his legs and groin. The consultant was aware of his anxiety that Mr. C was naked under the sheet which would be revealed when the attending examined his legs. He also realized that Mr. C's intern, resident and attending were all women. Mr. C was anxious and hostile during the brief examination, asking numerous questions about what was being done to him. He frequently brought up his concerns that he would be harmed by the tests and was particularly focused on the angiogram planned for later that day. Talking with Mr. C after rounds, the consultant found him to be overtly paranoid, though not delusional. In the middle of a divorce, Mr. C believed his wife would "relish the thought" that he was "weakened." He described a lifelong fear of women, starting with a mother who was intrusive, controlling and suspicious. Mr. C felt "less of a man" since his admission. He found the numerous tests and discussion of procedures confusing and he was angry that his requests for detailed information were met with annoyance by the doctors and nurses. Mr. C also revealed that he was afraid to go to sleep lest someone come into his room and "do something" to him, but he would not reveal the details of his fear.

The consultant recommended that Mr. C receive a small dose of a neuroleptic at night to help with sleep. Mr. C accepted the recommendation and was pleased that he was not being given a drug to which he could become dependent. In discussion with the intern and resident the consultant suggested that the resident set aside time to literally sit down with Mr. C and discuss her impression of his medical condition. The resident was reluctant to undertake this task, admitting Mr. C frightened her and she feared he would assault her. Using the resident's experience the consultant proposed that was exactly the situation Mr. C was trying to create, he wanted the women upon whom he was dependent to fear him. This made him feel stronger at a time when he felt weak. At the same time, the consultant noted, the fear made him anxious that he would be harmed by the people who he knew could help him. The consultant suggested the way to resolve this conflict was for the resident to openly discuss all the facts of Mr. C's case and to tell him, overtly, that he would completely recover and be "as strong as ever." The resident agreed under the condition that the consultant be physically present in the intensive care unit during her discussion with Mr. C.

Mr. C was initially hostile but, to the medical resident's amazement, he responded warmly to her as the conversation progressed. He confided that he had never felt he could trust any woman in his life. His wife's betrayal (he revealed that his wife had left him for another man), and his subsequent chest pain, left him feeling intolerably helpless and weak. At this point the resident told Mr. C her version of the statement that the consultant had suggested. Mr. C started to cry. He took the resident's hand, telling her he "knew" she would not lie, but he had been expecting her to tell him the opposite—i.e., that he would become an invalid. When the resident outlined a program of physical rehabilitation, diet and medication which Mr. C would have to follow religiously, Mr. C expressed overt joy at having a plan to return him to health. While the nursing staff remained anxious about Mr. C until his discharge, there were no further problems. The neuroleptic was discontinued after 3 days without a return of the previous inappropriate behavior. After his discharge Mr. C sent a bouquet of flowers to the unit in thanks for "extraordinary care in my time of need."

Manipulativeness (DSM-IV Antisocial PD)

An emergency consultation was called in for a 34-year-old man admitted with fevers, coughing and weight loss. He was in isolation while a diagnosis of TB was being ruled out. The consultation request came after he told a nurse that he would kill her if she didn't do what he wanted and that there was nothing that could be done to him as he was going to die of AIDS anyway. He was alleged to have also threatened several nurses that he would "infect them with AIDS." When the psychiatric consultant came into Mr. H's room she noticed that an elderly woman was sitting in the corner. Though the consultant, and everyone else who entered the room wore a protective mask, this woman did not. Mr. H was a large Hispanic man, lying in bed, propped up and eating a sandwich. He had several tattoos on his arms and a long, angry-looking scar across his neck. The consultant asked Mr. H to tell her what had happened and listened to his series of complaints about the nurses and doctors.

He repeatedly said "nothing mattered" as he was going to die anyway, and that his threats were real. As Mr. H started his complaints she asked him who the woman was sitting in the corner. He introduced the psychiatrist to his mother, who spoke no English. When the consultant asked Mr. H to tell his mother she needed to wear a mask as he might have TB, he translated for her and asked if the psychiatrist would show his mother how to use the mask. After about 30 minutes the psychiatrist gave Mr. H a tranquilizer to "take the edge off," and started chlorpromazine 100 mg three times a day. She promised to return later that day to see how the drug was working. Later that day Mr. H was sleepy but awake. He protested that the drug was "too strong" but he agreed it had calmed him down considerably.

Over the next few days Mr. H told the psychiatrist about his life on the streets, his drug use, his many fights including the knife fight that left him with the scar on his neck. He continued to make occasional threats to the nurses when they did not answer his call bell quickly enough. The psychiatrist told Mr. H that he was scaring everyone with his threats resulting in the staff staying away from him. She suggested he could get more of what he felt he deserved if he stopped threatening to kill people. When he maintained that there was "nothing that could be done to me" because of his AIDS, she confronted him with the fact that people with AIDS still went to jail for their crimes. She brought in a translator who told his mother that he was threatening people and, if he hurt someone, he would go to jail. His mother scolded him and told the psychiatrist through the translator that her son would "behave himself." His sputum was repeatedly negative for acid-fast bacilli and he was taken off isolation. At the psychiatrist's suggestion, he was left in a single room, with his mother in almost constant attendance. He remained on chlorpromazine for the entire 2 weeks that he was hospitalized, during which time he made no further threats to the staff. He was discharged home, in the care of his mother, with follow-up at the hospital's HIV clinic.

CONCLUSION

Recognizing the style with which a patient functions in the world provides a basis for understanding how that person will cope with the stress of a serious medical illness. Using this understanding the physician can form a foundation upon which he or she can build a strategy for communication with the patient. Most, but not all of the time, the obstacles created by the patient's personality can be negotiated using this foundation of understanding to enable the patient to receive the best possible medical care. When the physician approaches each interaction as a therapeutic encounter with the patient, the role of personality becomes even more important. The case histories illustrate how personality and personality disorders limit patients in the way they handle medical illness. The success of the psychiatric consultant came from his or her ability to comprehend what it was about the person that was causing the maladaptive response. Rather than requiring a large factual knowledge base, the majority of therapeutic interactions rely upon the ability of the physician to experience and then to appropriately respond to emotional currents in the patient. These skills are cardinal ingredients in the art of being a physician.

REFERENCES

1. Kahana RJ, Bibring GL. Personality types in medical management. In: Zinberg N, ed. *Psychiatry and Medical Practice in a General Hospital.* New York: International Universities Press; 1964:98–123.
2. Groves JE. Management of the borderline patient on a medical or surgical ward: the psychiatric consultant's role. *Int J Psychiatry Med.* 1975; 6(3):337–348.
3. Groves JE. Taking care of the hateful patient. *N Engl J Med.* 1978; 298:883–887.
4. Groves JE. Current concepts in psychiatry, borderline personality disorder. *N Engl J Med.* 1981; 305:259–262.
5. Bindwell BG, Herbers JE, Kroenke K. Evaluating chest pain. The patient's presentation style alters the physician's diagnostic approach. *Arch Intern Med.* 1993; 153:1991–1995.
6. Kagan J. *Change and Continuity in Infancy.* New York: Wiley; 1971.
7. Thomas A, Chess S. *Temperament and Development.* New York: Bruner/Mazel; 1977
8. Torgerson AM. Temperamental differences in infants and 6-year old children: a follow-up study of twins. In: Strelau J, Farley FH, Gale A, eds. *The Biological Basis of Personality and Behavior: Theories, Measurement, Techniques and Development.* Washington, DC: Hemisphere; 1985.
9. Kagan J, Reznick JS, Snidman N. Biological bases of childhood shyness. *Science.* 1988; 240:167–171.
10. Freud S. *The Standard Edition of the Complete Psychological Works of Sigmund Freud.* London: Hogarth Press; 1966.
11. Brown GR, Anderson B. Psychiatric morbidity in adult inpatients with childhood histories of sexual and physical abuse. *Am J Psychiatry.* 1991; 148:55–61.
12. Nigg JT, Silk KR, Westen D et al. Object representations in the early memories of sexually abused borderline patients. *Am J Psychiatry.* 1991; 148(7):864–869.
13. Goldman SJ, D'Angelo EJ, DeMaso DR. Physical and sexual abuse histories among children with borderline personality disorder. *Am J Psychiatry.* 1992; 149(12):1723–1726.
14. Livesley WJ, Jang KL, Jackson DN, Vernon PA. Genetic and environmental contributions to dimensions of personality disorder. *Am J Psychiatry.* 1993; 150:1826–1831.
15. American Psychiatric Association. *Diagnostic and Statistical Manual of Mental Disorders*, 4th ed. Washington, DC: American Psychiatry Press; 1994.
16. Kendler KS, Gruenberg AM. An independent analysis of the Danish adoption study of schizophrenia, VI: The relationship between schizotypal personality disorder and schizophrenia. *Arch Gen Psychiatry.* 1981; 38:982–984.
17. Kendler KS, Gruenberg AM. Genetic relationship between paranoid personality disorder and the "schizophrenic spectrum" disorders. *Am J Psychiatry.* 1982; 139:1185–1186.
18. Siever LJ, Silverman JM, Horvath TB, et al. Increased morbid risk for schizophrenia-related disorders in relatives of schizotypal personality disordered patients. *Arch Gen Psychiatry.* 1990; 47:634–640.
19. Geringer ES, Stern TA. Coping with medical illness: the impact of personality types. *Psychosomatics.* 1986; 27:251–261.
20. Weissman MM. The epidemiology of personality disorders: a 1990 update. *J Pers Disord.* 1993; 7:44–62.
21. Reich J, Boerstler H, Yates W, Nduaguba M. Utilization of medical resources in persons with DSM-III personality disorders in a community sample. *Int J Psychiatry Med.* 1989;19:1–9.
22. Strain JJ, Grossman S. *Psychological Care of the Medically Ill.* New York: Appleton-Century-Croft; 1975.
23. Field HL. Defense mechanisms in psychosomatic medicine. *Psychosomatics.* 1979; 20:690–700.
24. Lucente FE, Fleck S. A study of hospitalization anxiety in 408 medical and surgical patients, *Psychosom Med.* 1972; 34:304–312.
25. Oldham JM. Personality disorders. *JAMA.* 1994; 272(22):1770–1776.
26. Viederman M, Perry, SW. Use of a psychodynamic life narrative in the treatment of depression in the physically ill. *Gen Hosp Psychiatry.* 1980; 3:177–185.

55

Chemotherapeutic Agents and Neuropsychiatric Side Effects

STEWART B. FLEISHMAN AND GLENN R. KALASH

One must approach the attribution of psychiatric side effects to drugs used in cancer treatment cautiously. More interest has developed in this area as patients are diagnosed with cancer earlier, undergo more complex treatment, and live with cancer longer than ever before.

We know less than we should about these effects for a variety of reasons. One main reason stems from the coding of side effects or "toxicity grading." As clinical trials replaced the anecdotal report as the basis for judging clinical worthiness of a treatment, standardized toxicity ratings have specified "neurological," with subheadings "cortical" or "other neurologic-behavioral," specifying agitation, somnolence or psychosis. Secondly, less dramatic untoward effects of newer agents are often discovered well after completion of a clinical trial, after a drug is licensed and more widely used. Use of therapies in tandem or in a new sequence may also produce a spectrum of drug–drug interactions not measured in the original testing. Lastly, only recently has newer technology such as better imaging techniques, improved encephalography, and more exacting neuropsychological testing allowed finer quantification of subthreshold signs and symptoms as well as distress. Yet, access to confirmatory tissue sample for biopsy or assay and the reluctance to order imaging studies without clear-cut deficits further limits the corroboration of subtle findings. In the central nervous system (CNS), a brain biopsy or lumbar puncture is limited to times when test results would change a treatment plan, not merely to verify subtle side effects.

By listening to patients carefully, and giving credence to their reports, we find that many experience subtle CNS effects of cancer treatment, such as transient confusional states or a period of cognitive impairment. Some attribute these changes to the treatments themselves, assume them to be temporary, and wait for them to pass. Others become quite concerned but are loathe to mention them to a caregiver, afraid that they are "going crazy" or becoming senile in addition to having cancer. Out of the need to be considerate and thought of as "good patients," others neglect to mention these effects as they perceive the oncologists and nurses as "too busy" (1). Perhaps the reticence to probe further into these areas is promoted by lack of familiarity and skills to measure mood, cognition or attention span, or a lack of confidence in successful corrective intervention.

Review of the literature concerning this area reveals a paucity of documentation of the subthreshold morbidity of cancer treatment on the brain, mind, and emotions. Landmark work by Posner and colleagues at Memorial Sloan-Kettering began to quantify the CNS toxicity of drugs used to treat primary brain tumors or brain metastases. Such an effort necessitates differentiating these toxicities from the systemic metabolic and physiologic changes that lead to secondary CNS effects, ranging from commonly encountered hypoxic and hypoglycemic states to more esoteric paraneoplastic phenomena. Evidence of the loss of integrity of the blood–brain barrier itself with cancer (2,3), lends potential pathophysiologic explanation to the occurrence of subthreshold phenomena (4). Others have delved into the acute, early delayed, and late delayed effects of radiation to the brain (5).

Summarized here are the side effects of those drugs commonly used in cancer treatment, both those whose activity is primarily in the CNS, and those that have collateral effects there. Two classes of drugs that are mainstays of cancer treatment—opiate analgesics and antiemetics—primarily act on the brain, so their effects on attention, cognition and even emotional states are expected. Other classes of medications (antineoplastic agents themselves, antibiotics, antifungals, antivirals and anti-inflammatory drugs) have some incidental CNS effects. Familiarity with usual side effects can help differentiate motor, sensory, cognitive, or mood changes that result from primary or metastatic disease in the CNS from transient or more easily reversible changes resulting from drug administration.

INTERPRETING REPORTS OF SIDE EFFECTS

When considering reports of side effects, the context and circumstances of the report should be considered. Seminal questions include:

- Is it an isolated or commonly seen side effect?
- Is it reported as the result of a trial, a collection of reports or a single patient encounter?
- Has a drug–drug or drug–food interaction been considered?
- Was the cancer treatment multimodal (chemotherapy accompanied by radiation therapy or a postoperative course)?
- Was the patient rechallenged with the implicated agent to see if the effect recurred, providing additional evidence that the side effect was indeed caused by the drug in question?
- Was it reported for a child or an adult?

- Can the underlying illness, rather than its treatment, cause the implicated side effect (e.g., delirium from antivirals caused by drug effect or encephalitis)?
- Is there a comorbid medical or psychiatric problem? (e.g., hepatic or renal dysfunction, or preexisting dementia).
- What nomenclature was used? Descriptions vary; words used are those most familiar to the type of specialist submitting the finding. How specific is the language used?

DRUGS WHOSE PRIMARY ACTION IS THROUGH THE CNS

Two types of drugs—antiemetics and analgesics—commonly used in cancer treatment act primarily through the CNS. It is not surprising, but expectable, that the side effects of these drugs would likewise be manifest through the CNS.

Antiemetics (6)

With the exception of glucocorticoids, all drugs commonly used as antiemetics work through the CNS. These are: dopamine-blockers (neuroleptics and benzamides), antihistamines (anti-H1), benzodiazepines, and cannaboids. Their mechanisms of action and side effects are listed in Table 55.1. The mechanisms under-

TABLE 55.1. *Antiemetic Drugs Which Act Primarily Through the CNS*

Drugs and Mechanisms	Side Effects
NEUROLEPTICS Block chemoreceptor trigger zone effect on vomiting center in area postrema	Extrapyramidal side effects, dystonias
	Akathisia (reversible) and tardive dyskinesias
Chlorpromazine (Thorazine) Prochlorperazine (Compazine) Haloperidol (Haldol) Promethazine (Phenergan)	Anticholinergic: dry mouth, blurred vision, tachycardia, constipation, sedation, hallucinations, delirium, catatonia
	Galactorrhea, breast tenderness, irregular menses (85)
BENZAMIDES Same as neuroleptics but are prokinetic (cholinergic) drugs which enhance motility	Extrapyramidal side effects (as above)
	Flatulence, diarrhea
Metoclopramide (Reglan) Trimethobenzamide (Tigan)	Decreased bioavailability of foods (rapid transit to intestines)
ANTIHISTAMINES Block H1 stimuli in gastrointestinal tract and vestibular apparatus	Anticholinergic side effects (as above)
Diphenhydramine (Benadryl)	Weakness, irritability, depression (86,87)
BENZODIAZEPINES Enhance other antiemetics, dull cognition and memory to cause anterograde amnesia and prevent anticipatory nausea and vomiting; reduces akathisia from neuroleptics and benzamides	Sedation
	Cognitive and memory dysfunction (88)
	Psychomotor impairment
Lorazepam and others (Ativan)	Disorientation, delirium (89)
	Amensia, rebound insomnia
CANNABOIDS Euphoria	Sedation
Dronabinol (Marinol)	"Disinhibition"—reduces conscious control of behavior

Source: Ref. 6.

lying the effects of dexamethasone and other corticoids is poorly understood.

Opiate Analgesics (7)

Working at multiple sites within the CNS, morphine and its congeners—hydromorphone (Dilaudid), levorphanol (Levodromoran), codeine, hydrocodeine, oxycodone (Percocet), meperidine (Demerol)—inhibit the release of neurotransmitters, such as substance P, at the terminals of primary afferent nerves. They also inhibit the spinothalamic transmission of the nociceptive message to higher centers, where they most often produce euphoria, a sense of tranquility and mental "clouding" (changes in orientation, cognition and memory). Patients and caregivers most dislike the loss of clear thinking and accurate recall, perhaps associated with prelude to disease progression and death. Less often, these effects may be accompanied by a sense of alarm, panic, fear, anxiety, and dysphoria. These excitatory effects may lead to seizures, but only at the highest doses. Miotic (pinpoint) pupils and muscle rigidity are more common, as is constipation. Respiratory depression results more from dose escalation, especially from parenteral administration, and less from slow-release oral or transdermal preparations.

Amphetamines

Though less often used, stimulants such as dextroamphetamine (Dexedrine), methylphenidate (Ritalin), and pemoline (Cylert) can counteract the sedative effects of analgesics or antiemetics. Their use to offset the fatigue brought on by cancer itself is innovative, and currently under investigation.

As a group, stimulants may cause restlessness, insomnia, euphoria or overstimulation (8). They may elicit psychotic thinking when it may otherwise be suppressed, as well as seizures, extrapyramidal symptoms, and even Tourette's syndrome (9–11). Their appetite suppressant effects are usually overshadowed by an improvement in energy and activity, which then has salutary effects on appetite.

INCIDENTAL EFFECTS ON CNS

Antineoplastic Agents

Most cancer chemotherapeutic drugs do not cross the blood–brain barrier to any great extent, limiting the effectiveness of the treatment of CNS tumors, whether primary or metastatic. With more widespread use in the last 40 years, innovative drug delivery (higher cumulative effects of frequent dosing, intrathecal administration) and concurrent radiation therapy

there have been an increasing number of reports of chemotherapy-related morbidity to the CNS. Considered here are reports collected about the most commonly used agents with CNS effects. Subthreshold effects on mood, cognition, and memory from chemotherapy remains an insufficiently understood area.

Methotrexate. Given intrathecally or intravenously on a weekly schedule, acute meningeal irritation with headache, nausea, stiff neck, lethargy, fever, and occasional encephalopathy may be seen. A transverse myelopathy with paraplegia or parapareses may also occur. A delayed leukoencephalopathy may develop months to years afterwards, characterized by personality change, confusion, forgetfulness, dysarthria, dysphagia, dementia, ataxia, tremor, spasticity or seizures, and lead to coma or death.

It has been postulated that these effects may result from the diluent used in preparation or a metabolic result of methotrexate's effect on folic acid metabolism in the brain, since its primary systemic mechanism of action is folic acid antagonism. Although severe encephalopathy is uncommon, milder forms of encephalopathy undoubtedly occur (12–15).

5-Fluorouracil (5-FU). A pyrimidine analogue that interferes with DNA synthesis, 5-FU has been found to cross the blood–brain barrier and concentrate most in the cerebellum. A transient reversible cerebellar ataxia has been identified in less than 7% of patients receiving 5-FU. The symptoms include difficulty walking and performing fine tasks, ataxia of the extremities and trunk, titubation, intention tremor, dysmetria, scanning speech, nystagmus and a positive Romberg's sign (12,13,16). Memory loss has been reported with the preservation of other cognitive functions (17–19). Episodes of confusion and disorientation have also been reported as an "organic brain syndrome" (15,20).

Cisplatin (Platinol). An inorganic platinum-containing agent, cisplatin is associated with significant morbidity of the special sensory systems, and peripheral neuropathy. Autonomic effects and encephalopathy are known and are less common. Being a heavy metal, its neurotoxic effects are expectable.

A sensory peripheral neuropathy, evidenced by numbness, tingling and decreased vibratory sense, often begins in the hands and feet. It can occur within the first few days of treatment, then stabilize or improve after cisplatin is discontinued. Symptoms may also begin and progress after cisplatin is

TABLE 55.2. *Less Often Used Antineoplastic Drugs with Neurotoxicity*

Drug	Neurotoxic Effects
Hexylmethylmelamine (Hexalen, Altretamine)	Confusion, anxiety, hallucinations, "depression", dizziness, ataxia, tremos, parkinsonian-like effects (16,90–93)
L-Asparaginase	Mild to severe encephalopathy, usually reversible, somnolence, agitation, fatigue due to ?depletion in CNS glutamine and (Elspar) asparaginase levels or ?hepatic encephalopathy (13,94)
Hydroxyurea (Hydrea)	Drowsiness (high dose) (12)
N-Phosphonoacetyl-L-aspartate (PALA)	Severe encephalopathy with or without seizures; may be delayed (animal studies) (12)
Mitotane (Lysodren)	Somnolence, lethargy, confusion, mood change, depression, headache, vertigo, blurred vision (12), decreased memory (95)
5-Azacytidine (AZQ)	Weakness, lethargy, myositis, irritability, confusion, somnolence
Bleomycin (Blenoxane)	Encephalopathy (23)
Aminoglutethimide (Cytadren)	Drowsiness, lethargy (96,97)
Dacarbazine (DTIC)	Dementia, hemiparesis, jaw pain, facial burning (98,99)
Suramin	Cognitive and memory losses, polyneuropathy (loss of Schwann cell substrate) (100)
Fludarabine (Fludara)	Confusion, somnolence, fatigue, optic nerve demyelination, necrotizing leukoencephalopathy (101–105)
Chlorambucil (Leukeran)	Confusion, agitation, hallucination (106)
Levamisole (Ergamisol)	Excitation, insomnia, fatigue, weakness, anxiety, irritability, confusion, depression (107)

discontinued and rarely, fail to improve (15). No correlation has been found to smoking history, alcohol ingestion or familial diabetes (21). Motor function remains unaffected.

Ototoxicity is a well-known and common toxicity. Most often it is bilateral, irreversible, and of moderate severity. Hearing impairment is more likely in older patients with preexisting hearing loss. It is generally dose dependent (12,15). Loss of high frequency preserves most patients' ability to hear the spoken voice (22).

Other neurotoxic effects include autonomic parasympathetic effects, including impotence. Lhermitte's sign, a sudden electric shock-like feeling traveling through the spine to the legs upon flexion, highlights the spinal cord effects of cisplatin. Neuro-ophthalmologic effects, such as retrobulbar neuritis, transient blindness and altered color perception, have also been noted. Ptosis or strabismus may be manifestations of heavy metal intoxication. Encephalopathy with visual disturbance has also been reported (23).

Ifosfamide (Ifex). Unlike cyclophosphamide, which has a closely related chemical structure, ifosfamide causes effects toxic to the CNS in 10%–50% of

patients. Episodes of confusion, somnolence, hallucinations, incontinence, seizures, weakness, mutism, cranial nerve, cerebellar and extrapyramidal signs have been reported (15,24,25). These effects may be related to the accumulation of chloracetaldehyde (26). Ifosfamide encephalopathy has been successfully reversed with intravenous methylene blue (27).

Vinca Alkaloids—Vincristine, Vinblastine, Vindesine, Vinorelbine (Oncovin, Velban, Navelbine). The vinca alkaloids cause sensory and motor changes in peripheral nerves in almost all patients. Beginning with a weak or absent ankle jerk (Achilles tendon) reflex, other effects, such as paresthesias, weakness in the hands and feet, a broad-based "slapping" gait, and foot drop, may also occur. Cranial nerves may also be affected, with resulting ptosis, pupillary, or vocal cord dysfunction. Autonomic toxicity may show as constipation, impotence, bladder atony or orthostatic hypotension. Seizures, paraplegia or quadriplegia have also been reported (12,28).

The peripheral nerve dysfunction is often the dose-limiting side effect of vincristine. Vinblastine causes myelosuppression and was often discontinued before the neurotoxicity developed. With the use of marrow stimulating growth factors allowing higher doses of vincas to be prescribed, the neurologic effects of vinblastine may increase. Major depression has been reported with vinblastine (29,30). Recently marketed, vinorelbine is a new agent which appears less neurotoxic thus far.

Cytosine Arabinoside (Ara-C, Cytosar-U). Used both intravenously and intrathecally, Ara-C can cause transient irritative symptoms of weakness, paraplegia, blindness or peripheral neuropathy, with a profile similar to methotrexate, but seen less often. Cerebellar degeneration with severe ataxia dysarthria and nystagmus have also been related to Ara-C (31–34). Personality change, somnolence and coma have also been reported (35).

Procarbazine (Matulane). A weaker monoamine oxidase inhibitor (MAOI) than those used to treat major depression, procarbazine crosses the blood–brain barrier easily. It commonly causes sedation, lethargy, somnolence, or disorientation which is dose dependent. Review of reports that it causes "depression" (36–41) reveals an unfortunate clash of nomenclature. With a chemical structure very similar to MAOIs used to treat major depression, it would be unlikely for a drug of this category to cause major depression. Description of its soporific side effects, described as "CNS depression," is responsible for this point of confusion. Procarbazine has the opposite effect on mood, implicated in causing a euphoric or manic mood change, consistent with its antidepressant effect. Like antidepressant MAOIs, it causes hypotension, secondary orthostatic changes, and, rarely, hypertension when mixed with foods containing tyramine. Avoidance of using procarbazine with sympathomimetic drugs is also prudent. Dermatitis and a mild peripheral neuropathy have also been reported (12,28).

Less often used antineoplastic agents with neurotoxic effects are listed in Table 55.2. Of historical note are the side effects of L-asparaginase (Elspar),

TABLE 55.3. *Antineoplastic Agents without Significant Neurotoxicity**

Mechlorethamine (Mustargen)
Cyclophosphamide (Cytoxan)
Doxorubicin (Adriamycin)
Busulfan (Myeleran)
L-Phenylalanine mustard (Melphalan)
6-Mercaptopurine (Purinethol)
Etoposide (VP-16, VePesid)
BCNU (BiCNU)
CCNU (lomustine, CeeNU)
Thiotepa

* At usual doses and via usual routes of administration.

which has been associated with disorientation, convulsions, and/or coma, somnolence, fatigue, agitation of hallucinations. This constellation of higher CNS dysfunction has been reported to occur in up to 25% of those patients treated with L-asparaginase (13,42). Table 55.3 lists those agents devoid of significant neurotoxicity. Hormonal agents used in cancer are listed in Table 55.4, and biologic modifiers in Table 55.5.

Antibiotics, Antifungals, and Antivirals

Consideration of the effects of antibiotics is important as a significant proportion of patients with cancer require them as a result of becoming immunosuppressed from the underlying disease process, postoperatively or from chemotherapy and radiation therapy. As a group, antibiotics of the penicillin family have been reported to cause encephalopathy and seizures (43,44). Cephalosporin derivatives such as cephalexin (Keflex) and cephazolin (Ancef) have been implicated in similar reactions (45–47), along with lethargy, disorientation, memory loss, and psychosis. Cefaclor has been associated with hyperactivity as well as somnolence, nervousness, insomnia, and confusion (48,49). Ticarcillin (Ticar, Timentin) (50,51) has been reported to cause hallucinations, giddiness, and seizures.

TABLE 55.4. *Hormonal Agents with CNS Effects*

Flutamide (Eulexin)	Drowsiness, confusion, depression (108), anxiety, nervousness, insomnia, mania (109)
Tamoxifen (Nolvadex)	Depression, lassitude confusion (110–112), emotional liability, delusions
	Reduction in plasma doxepin and desmethyldoxepin levels (through cytochrome P450 enzyme induction) (113)
Megesterol acetate (Megace)	"Mild" depression (114)

TABLE 55.5. *Biologic Modifiers*

Interferon alpha (Intron A, Roferon A)	Lethargy, fatigue, somnolence, agitation, malaise, confusion, emotional lability, depersonalization, suicide attempts, dementia, personality change (115–117), metabolic encephalopathy (120)
Sargramostim (GM-CSF, Leukine)	Lethargy, malaise, fatigue (118–120)
Erythropoietin (EPO, Epoetin)	Visual hallucinations (121)
Interleukin (Aldesleukin)	Insomnia, agitation, delirium, somnolence (122,123)

Gentamicin and tobramycin have caused delirium and seizures (52,53). The fluoroquinolones—ciprofloxacin (Cipro), norfloxacin (Noroxin) and ofloxacin (Floxin)—may cause insomnia, drowsiness, delirium, hallucinations, mania or depression, phobic reactions, irritability, or depersonalization (54–57). Even the newest agents such as imipenem/cilastin (Primaxin) are implicated in causing encephalopathy, tremor, parathesia, vertigo, headache, and seizures (58).

Antifungal agents—ketoconazole (Nizoral), fluconazole (Diflucan), clotrimazole (Mycelex), and griseofulvin (Fulvicin, Grisactin)—have been reported to cause delirium, depression, seizures, memory impairment, somnolence, apathy, and headache (59–63). Amphotericin B (Fungizone) has been reported to cause parkinsonian symptoms, a reversible encephalopathy, and an irreversible leukoencephalopathy (64–66). Metronidazole (Flagyl) has been implicated in causing depression, disorientation, seizures, and headache (67,68). Pentamidine (Pentam 300, Pentacarinat) when used intravenously has been reported to cause hallucinations, seizures, delirium, vertigo, ataxia, anxiety, and memory impairment (69,70).

Antiviral agents, such as acyclovir (Zovirax), ganciclovir (Cytovene), and foscarnet (Foscavir), may cause encephalopathic, cognitive, perceptual and mood changes, lethargy, agitation, and seizures (71–73). Zidovudine, or azidothymidine, AZT (Retrovir), has been noted to cause insomnia, somnolence, seizures, and mania (74–76).

Anti-inflammatory Drugs

Anti-inflammatory agents are used as adjuvant analgesics in patients who have finished platelet-reducing chemotherapy or radiation. Aspirin has been reported to cause delirium, combativeness, and agitation (77). Ibuprofen (Motrin, etc.) has been implicated in causing anxiety, depression, drowsiness, insomnia, giddiness, extrapyramidal symptoms, and cognitive dysfunction (78–81). Reports of depression, hallucinations, delusions, depersonalization, and extrapyramidal symptoms have been associated with indomethacin

(Indocin) used to treat tumor-induced fever and as an anti-inflammatory (82–84).

The wide range of effects of the glucocorticoids on mood, anxiety, perception, and cognition has been addressed elsewhere.

CLINICAL SCREENING OF NEW DRUGS FOR NEUROTOXICITY

Tuxen and Hansen (15) advise careful neurological examination and history-taking with regard to central peripheral and autonomic symptoms. If the screening procedure suggests neurotoxicity, referral for electrophysiologic, imaging and neuropsychological studies may be indicated.

Extending the examination to include items about cognition, memory and mood will sensitize caregivers and patients to these less understood effects. Documentation and understanding of these collateral effects can then encourage prevention and intervention.

REFERENCES

1. Fleishman SB, Lavin MR, Sattler M, Szarka H. Antiemetic-induced akathisia in cancer patients receiving chemotherapy. *Am J Psychiatry.* 1994; 151(5): 763–765.
2. Donelli MG, Zucchetti M, D'Incalci M. Do anticancer agents reach the tumor target in the human brain? *Cancer Chemother Pharmacol.* 1992; 30:251–260.
3. Stewart DJ. A critique of the role of the blood–brain barrier in the chemotherapy of human brain tumors. *J Neuro-Oncol.* 1994; 20:121–139.
4. Posner J. Neoplastic disorders. *Sci Am Med.* 1994; 11(VI):1–16.
5. Berger PS. Neurological complications of radiotherapy. In: Silverstein A, ed. *Neurological Complications of Radiotherapy.* Mt Kisco: Futura Publishing; 1992: 137–185.
6. Brunton LL. Agents affecting gastrointestinal water flux, motility, digestants and bile acids. In: Goodman-Gilman A, Rall TW, et al, eds. *The Pharmacological Basis of Therapeutics.* New York: Pergamon Press; 1990.
7. Jaffee JH, Martin WR. Opiate analgesics and antagonists. In: Goodman-Gilman A, Rall TW, et al, eds. *The*

Pharmacological Basis of Therapeutics. New York: Pergamon Press; 1990.

8. Product Information. Dexedrine (R), dextroamphetamine sulphate. Pittsburgh, PA: Smith, Kline & French; 1982.

9. Lowe TL, Cohen DJ, Detlor J, et al. Stimulant medications precipitate Tourette's syndrome. *JAMA.* 1982; 247:1729–1731.

10. Lundh H, Tunving K. An extrapyramidal choreiform syndrome caused by amphetamine addiction. *J Neurol Neurosurg Psychiatry.* 1981; 44:728–730.

11. Chadwick D. Drug-induced convulsions. In: Rose FC, ed. *Research Progress in Epilepsy.* London: Pitman Press; 1983: 151–160.

12. Young DF, Posner JB. Nervous system toxicity of the chemotherapeutic agents. In: Viken PJ, Bruyn GW, eds. *Handbook of Clinical Neurology*, vol 39, *Neurological Manifestations of Systemic Diseases*, Part II. New York: Elsevier; 1980: 91–129.

13. Weiss HD, Walker MD, Wiernik PH. Neurotoxicity of commonly used neoplastic agents. *New Engl J Med.* 1974; 291:75–81.

14. Pizzo PA, Poplack DG, Bleyer WA. Neurotoxicities of current leukemia therapy. *J Pediatr Hematol Oncol.* 1979; 1(2):127–140.

15. Tuxen MK, Hansen SW. Complications of treatment: neurotoxicity secondary to antineoplastic drugs. *Cancer Treat Rev.* 1994; 20:191–214.

16. Goldberg ID, Bloomer WD, Dawson DM. Nervous system toxic effects of cancer therapy. *JAMA.* 1982; 247:1437–1441.

17. Moertel CG, Rettemeier RJ, Bolton CF, Shorter RG. Cerebellar ataxia associated with fluorinated pyrimidine therapy. *Cancer Chemother Rep.* 1964; 41:15–18.

18. Nichols M, Bergevin PR, Vyas AC, et al. Neurotoxicity from 5FU (NSC-19893) administration reproduced by mitomycin C (NSC-26980). *Cancer Treat Rep.* 1976; 60:293–294.

19. Bergevin PR, Pawardhan VC, Weismann J, et al. Neurotoxicity of 5-fluorouracil. *Lancet.* 1975; 1:410.

20. Lynch HT, Droszcz CP, Albano WA, Lynch JF. "Organic brain syndrome" secondary to 5-fluorouracil toxicity. *Dis Colon Rectum.* 1981; 24:130–131.

21. Mollman JE, Glover DJ, Hogan WM, Furman RE. Cisplatin neuropathy: risk factors, prognosis, and protection by WR-2721. *Cancer.* 1988; 61:2192–2195.

22. Piel IJ, Meyer D, Perlia CP, et al. Effects of cis-diamminedichloroplatinum (NSC-119,875) on hearing function in man. *Cancer Chemother Rep.* 1974; 58:871–875.

23. Hitchkins RN, Thomson DB. Encephalopathy following cisplatin, bleomycin and vinblastine therapy for non-seminomatous germ cell tumor of testis. *Aust NZ J Med.* 1988; 18:67–68.

24. Heim ME, Fein R, Schick E et al. Central nervous side effects following ifosfamide monotherapy of advanced renal carcinoma. *J Cancer Res Clin Oncol.* 1981; 100:113–116.

25. Anderson NR, Tandon OS. Ifosfamide extrapyramidal neurotoxicity. *Cancer.* 1991; 68:72–75.

26. Goren MP, Wright RK, Pratt CB, Pell FE. Dechlorethylation of ifosfamide and neurotoxicity (letter). *Lancet.* 1986; 2:1219–1220.

27. Zulian GB, Tullen E, Maton B. Methylene blue for ifosfamide-associated encephalopathy. *N Engl J Med.* 1995; 332:1239–1240.

28. Weiss HD, Walker MD, Wiernik PH. Neurotoxicity of commonly used antineoplastic agents. *N Engl J Med.* 1974; 291:127–133.

29. Product Information. Velban(R), vinblastine sulfate. Indianapolis, IN: Eli Lilly and Company; 1990.

30. Olin B, ed. *Facts and Comparisons.* St. Louis, MO: JB Lippincott Co; 1988.

31. Cerosimo RJ, Carter RT, Matthews SJ, Coderre M, Karp DD. Acute cerebellar syndrome, conjunctivitis, and hearing loss associated with low-dose cytarabine administration. *Drug Intell Clin Pharm.* 1987; 21:798–803.

32. Sylvester RK, Fisher AJ, Lobell M. Cytarabine-induced cerebellar syndrome case report and literature review. *Drug Intell Clin Pharm.* 1987; 21:177–180.

33. Watson PR, Brubaker LH, Yaghmai F. Severe central nervous system toxicity from high-dose cytarabine expressive aphasia occurring after the second day of treatment. *Cancer Treat Rep.* 1985; 69:313–314.

34. Baker WJ, Royer GL, Jr., Weiss RB. Cytarabine and neurologic toxicity. *J Clin Oncol.* 1991; 9:67–93.

35. Product Information. Cytosar-U(R), cytarabine. Kalamazoo, MI: Upjohn; 1994.

36. DeConti RC. Procarbazine in the management of late Hodgkin's disease. *J Am Med Assoc.* 1971; 215:927–930.

37. Greenwald ES. Cancer chemotherapy. Part II. *NY State J Med.* 1966; 66(20):2670–2681.

38. Mann AM, Hutchinson JL. Manic reaction associated with procarbazine by hydrochloride therapy of Hodgkin's disease. *Can Med Assoc J.* 1967; 97:1350–1353.

39. Samuels ML, Leary WB, Alexanian R, et al. Clinical trials with *N*-isopropyl-α-(2-methylhydrazino)-*p*-toluamide hydrochloride in malignant lymphoma and other disseminated neoplasia. *Cancer.* 1967; 20:1187–1194.

40. Product Information. Matulane (R), procarbazine. Nutley, NJ: Roche Laboratories; 1994.

41. Chabner BA, Spanzo R, Hubbard SS. High dose intermittent intravenous infusion of procarbazine (NSC-77213). *Cancer Chemother Rep.* 1973; 57:361–363.

42. DeVita VT, Hellman S, Rosenberg SA, eds. *Cancer: Principles and Practice in Oncology*, 4th ed. Philadelphia, PA: Lippincott; 1974: 388.

43. Conway N, Beck E, Sommerville J. Penicillin encephalopathy. *Postgrad Med J.* 1968; 44:891.

44. Nicholl PJ. Neurotoxicity of penicillin. *J Antimicrob Chemother.* 1980; 6:161–172.

45. Weber DJ, Tolkoff-Rubin NE, Rubin RH. Amoxicillin and potassium clavulanate: an antibiotic combination mechanism of action, pharmacokinetics, antimicrobial spectrum, clinical efficacy and adverse effects. *Pharmacotherapy.* 1984; 4:122–136.

46. Herd AM, Ross CA, Bhattacharya SK. Acute confusional state with post-operative intravenous cefazolin [letter]. *Br Med J.* 1989; 199:393–394.

47. Schwankhaus JD, Masucci EF, Kurtzke JF. Cefazolin-induced encephalopathy in a uremic patient [letter]. *Am Neurol.* 1985; 17:211.

48. Gardner ME, Fritz WL, Hyland RN. Antibiotic-induced seizures. A case attributed to cefazolin and a

review of the literature. *Drug Intell Clin Pharm.* 1978; 12:268–271.

49. Product Information. Ceclor (R), cefaclor. Indianapolis, IN: Eli Liley; 1988.

50. Glynne A, Goulbourn, RA, Ryden R. A human pharmacology study of cefaclor. *J Antimicrob Chemother.* 1978; 4:343–348.

51. File TM, Tan JS, Salstrom SJ, et al. Timentin versus piperacillin or moxalactam in the therapy of acute bacterial infections. *Antimicrob Agents Chemother.* 1984; 26:310–313.

52. Product Information. Timentin(R), ticarcillin/clavulanic acid. Philadelphia, PA: Smith Kline Beecham Pharmaceuticals; 1992.

53. McCartney CF, Hatley LH, Kessler JM. Possible tobramycin delirium. *JAMA.* 1982; 247:1319.

54. Byrd GJ. Report of gentamycin-associated organic brain syndrome. *Drug Ther.* 1976; 6:11.

55. Scully BE, Parry MF, Neu HC, et al. Oral ciprofloxacin therapy of infections due to *Pseudomonas aeruginosa. Lancet.* 1986; 1:819–822.

56. Product Information. Ciloxan (R), ciprofloxacin ophthalmic solution. Fort Worth, TX: Alcon Ophthalmic; 1995.

57. Deany NB, Vogel R, Vandenburg MJ, et al. Norfloxacin in acute urinary tract infections. *Practitioner.* 1984; 228:111.

58. Blomer R, Bruch K, Krauss H, et al. Safety of ofloxacin: adverse drug reactions reported during phase II studies in Europe and in Japan. *Infection.* 1986; 14:S332–S334.

59. Brotherton TJ, Kelber RL. Seizure-like activity associated with imipenem. *Clin Pharm.* 1984; 3:536–540.

60. Sawyer PR, Brogden RN, Pinde RM, et al. Clotrimazole: a review of its antifungal activity and therapeutic efficacy. *Drugs.* 1975; 9:424.

61. Ross JB, Levine B, Catanzaro A, et al. Ketoconazole for treatment of chronic pulmonary coccidiomycosis. *Ann Intern Med.* 1982; 96:440–443.

62. Lastnick G. Psychotic symptoms with griseofulvin. *JAMA.* 1974; 229:1420.

63. Hanash KA. Neurologic complications of ketoconazole therapy for advanced prostatic cancer. *Urology.* 1989; 33:466–467.

64. Stern JJ, Hartman BJ, Sharkey P, et al. Oral fluconazole therapy for patients with acquired immunodeficiency syndrome and cryptococcosis: experience with 22 patients. *Am J Med.* 1988; 85:477–480.

65. Walker RW, Rosbenblum MK. Amphotericin B-associated leukoencephalopathy. *Neurology.* 1992; 42:2005–2010.

66. Balmaceda CM, Walker RW, Castro-Malaspina H, et al. Revisal of amphotericin-B related encephalopathy. *Neurology.* 1994; 44:1183–1184.

67. Fisher JF, DeWald J. Parkinsonism associated with intra-ventricular amphotericin B. *J Antimicrob Chemother.* 1983; 12:97–99.

68. Giannini AJ. Side effects of metronidazole. *Am J Psychiatry.* 1977; 134:324–330.

69. Frytak S, Moertel CH, Childs DS, et al. Neurologic toxicity associated with high dose metronidazole therapy. *Ann Intern Med.* 1978; 88:361.

70. Western KA, Penera DR, Schultz MD. Pentamidine isothionate in the treatment of *Pneumocystis carinii* pneumonia. *Ann Intern Med.* 1970; 73:695–702.

71. Walzer PD, Perl DP, Krogstad DJ, et al. *Pneumocystis carinii* pneumonia in the United States. Epidemiologic diagnostic, and clinical features. *Ann Intern Med.* 1974; 80:83–93.

72. Arndt KA. Adverse effects to acyclovir: topical, oral and intravenous. *J Am Acad Dermatol.* 1988; 18:188–190.

73. Product Information. Foscavir (R), foscarnet sodium. Westborough, MA: Astra Pharmaceutical Products; 1994.

74. Product Information: Cytovene(R), ganciclovir. Palo Alto, CA: Syntex Laboratories; 1994.

75. Product Information. Retrovir(R), Research Triangle Park, NC: Glaxo Wellcome; 1994.

76. Saracchini S, Vaccher E, Covezzi E, et al. Lethal neurotoxicity associated to azidothymidine therapy. *J Neurol Neurosurg Psychiatry.* 1989; 52:544–545.

77. O'Dowd MA, McKegney FP. Manic syndrome associated with zidovudine [letter]. *JAMA.* 1988; 260:3587.

78. Steele TE, Morton WA Jr. Salicylate-induced delirium. *Psychosomatics.* 1986; 27:455–456.

79. Blechman WJ, Schmid FR, April PA, et al. Ibuprofen or aspirin in rheumatoid arthritis therapy. *JAMA.* 1975; 233:336–340.

80. Jasani HK, Downie WW, Samuels BM, et al. Ibuprofen in rheumatoid arthritis: Clinical study of analgesic and anti-inflammatory activity. *Ann Rheum Dis.* 1968; 27:457.

81. Wood N, Pall HS, Williams AC, et al. Extrapyramidal reactions to anti-inflammatory drugs. *J Neurol Neurosurg Psychiatry.* 1988; 51:731–732.

82. Goodwin JS, Regan M. Cognitive dysfunction associated with naproxen and ibuprofen in the elderly. *Arthritis Rheum.* 1982; 25:1013–1015.

83. Carney MWP. Paranoid psychosis with indomethacin. *Br Med J.* 1977; 2:994.

84. Wood N, Pall HS, Williams AC, et al. Extrapyradmidal reactions to anti-inflammatory drugs. *J Neurol Neurosurg Psychiatry.* 1988; 51:731–732.

85. Schwartz JI, Moura RJ. Severe depersonalization and anxiety associated with indomethacin. *South Med J.* 1983; 76:679–680.

86. Ananth JV, Ban TA, Lehmann HE, et al. Toxic psychosis syndrome associated with chlorpromazine administration. *Can Med Assoc J.* 1970; 102:642.

87. Murray WJ, Bechtoldt AA, Berman L, et al. Efficacy of oral psychosedative drugs for preanesthetic medication. *JAMA.* 1968; 203:327.

88. Filoux F. Toxic encephalopathy caused by topically applied diphenhydramine. *J Pediatr.* 1986; 108:1018–1020.

89. Ghoneim MM, Mewaldt SB, Berie JL, et al. Memory and performance effects of single and 3-week administration of diazepam. *Psychopharmacology.* 1981; 73:147–151.

90. Scharf MB, Khosla N, Lysaght R, et al. Anterograde amnesia with oral lorazepam. *J Clin Psychiatry.* 1983; 44:362–364.

91. Louis J, Louis NB, Linman JW, et al. The clinical pharmacology of hexamethylmelamine: phase I study. *Clin Pharmacol Ther*. 1967; 8:55–64.

92. Wilson WL, Bisel HF, Cole D, et al. Prolonged low-dosage administration of hexamethylmelamine (NSC-13875). *Cancer*. 1970; 25:567–570.

93. Stolinsky DC, Bodgon DL, Solomon J, et al. Hexamethyl-melamine (NSC-18375) alone and in combination with 5-(3,3-dimethyltriazeno)imidazole-4-carboxamide (NSC-45388) in the treatment of advanced cancer. *Cancer*. 1972; 30:654–659.

94. Stolinsky DC, Bateman JR. Further experience with hexamethylmelamine (NSC-13875) in the treatment of carcinoma of the cervix. *Cancer Chemother Rep*. 1973; 57:497–499.

95. Oettgen HF, Stephenson PA, Schwartz MK, et al. Toxicity of *E. coli* L-asparaginase in man. *Cancer*. 1970; 25:253–278.

96. Schteingart DE, Tsao HS, Taylor CI. Sustained remission of Cushing's disease with mitotane and pituitary irradiation. *Ann Intern Med*. 1980; 92:613–619.

97. Santen RJ, Misbin RI. Aminoglutethimide: review of pharmacology and clinical use. *Pharmacotherapy*. 1981; 1:95–120.

98. Santen RJ, Samojilik E, Lipton A, et al. Kinetic, hormonal and clinical studies with aminoglutethimide in breast cancer. *Cancer*. 1977; 39 (suppl): 2948–2958.

99. Moertel CG, Rettemeier RJ, Hahn RG, et al. Study of 5-(3,3-dimethy-1,1-triazeno)imidazole-4-carboxamide (NSC-45388) in patients with gastrointestinal carcinoma. *Cancer Chemother Rep*. 1970; 54:471–473.

100. Samson MK, Baker LH, Izbicki RM, et al. Phase I–II study of DTIC and cyclocytidine in disseminated malignant melanoma. *Cancer Treat Rep*. 1976; 60:1369–1371.

101. LaRocca R, Stein C, Myers C, et al. Suramin induced acute polyneuropathy. *Proc ASCO Abstr*. 1989; 277.

102. Cohen RB, Abdallah JM, Gray JR, Foss F. Reversible neurologic toxicity in patients treated with standard-dose fludarabine phosphate for mycosis fungoides and chronic lymphocytic leukemia. *Ann Intern Med*. 1993; 118:114–116.

103. Spriggs DR, Stopa E, Mayer RJ, et al. Fludarabine phosphate (NSC 312878) infusions for the treatment of acute leukemia: phase I and neuropathological study. *Cancer Res*. 1986; 46:5953–5958.

104. Warrell RP, Berman E. Phase I and II study of fludarabine phosphate in leukemia: therapeutic efficacy with delayed central nervous system toxicity. *J Clin Oncol*. 1986; 4:74–79.

105. Harvey WH, Fleming TR, Beltram G, et al. Phase II study of fludarabine phosphate in previously untreated patients with hepatoma: a Southwest Oncology Group Study. *Cancer Treat Rep*. 1987; 71:1111–1112.

106. Harvey WH, Fleming TR, Von Hoff DD, et al. Phase II study of fludarabine phosphate in previously untreated patients with colorectal carcinoma: a Southwest Oncology Group Study. *Cancer Treat Rep*. 1987; 71:1319–1320.

107. Product Information. Leukeran (R), chlorambucil. Research Triangle Park, NC: Burroughs-Wellcome; 1993.

108. Colizza S, Bagolan P, DiPaola M. Side effects of levamisole given to neoplastic patients as adjuvant to surgery. *J Surg Oncol*. 1984; 16:259–543.

109. Technical Information. Euflex (R), flutamide. Kennilworth, NJ: Schering; 1986.

110. Lajeunesse C, Parent R, Villaneuve A. Manic-like episode following flutamide treatment. *Am J Psychiatry*. 1986; 143:1498–1499.

111. Pluss JL, DiBella NJ. Reversible central nervous system dysfunction due to tamoxifen in a patient with breast cancer. *Ann Intern Med*. 1984; 101:652.

112. Ron IG, Inbar MJ, Barak Y, et al. Organic delusional syndrome associated with tamoxifen treatment. *Cancer*. 1992; 69:1415–1417.

113. Heel RC, Brogden RN, Speight TM, et al. Tamoxifen: a review of its pharmacological properties and therapeutic use in the treatment of breast cancer. *Drugs*. 1978; 16: 1–24.

114. Jefferson JW. Tamoxifen-associated reduction in tricyclic antidepressant levels in blood. *J Clin Psychopharmacol*. 1995; 15:223–224.

115. Gal D, Edman CD, Vellios F, et al. Long-term effect of megestrol acetate in the treatment of endometrial hyperplasia. *Am J Obstet Gynecol*. 1983; 146:316–322.

116. Yung WKA, Prados M, Levin VA, et al. Intravenous recombinant interferon beta in patients with recurrent malignant gliomas: a phase I/II study. *J Clin Oncol*. 1991; 9:1945–1949.

117. Quesada JR, Talpaz M, Rios A, et al. Clinical toxicity of interferon in cancer patients: a review. *J Clin Oncol*. 1986; 4:234–243.

118. Renault PF, Hoofnagle JH, Park Y, et al. Psychiatric complications of long term interferon therapy. *Arch Intern Med*. 1987; 147:577–580.

119. Antin JH, Smith BR, Holmes W, et al. Phase I/II study of recombinant human granulocyte-macrophage colony stimulating factor in aplastic anemia and myelodysplastic syndrome. *Blood*. 1988; 72:705–713.

120. Lieschke GJ, Cebon J, Morstyn G. Characterization of the clinical effects after the first dose of bacterially synthesized recombinant human granulocyte-macrophage colony-stimulating factor. *Blood*. 1989; 74:2634–2643.

121. Trudeau M, Zukiwski A, Langleben A, et al. A phase I study of recombinant human interferon alpha-2b combined with 5-fluorouracil and cisplatin in patients with advanced cancer. *Cancer Chemother Pharmacol*. 1995; 35(6):496–500.

122. Steinberg H. Erythropoietin and visual hallucinations [letter]. *N Engl J Med*. 1991; 325(4):285.

123. Denicoff KD, Burinow DR, Papa MZ, et al. The neuropsychiatric effects of treatment with interleukin-2 and lymphokine-activated killer cells. *Ann Intern Med*. 1987; 107:293–300.

56

Metabolic Disorders and Neuropsychiatric Symptoms

WILLIAM BREITBART AND SIMON E. WEIN

Neuropsychiatric signs and symptoms caused by cancer-related metabolic, endocrine, and paraneoplastic disorders are diagnostically and therapeutically challenging clinical problems. This chapter reviews the neuropsychiatric disorders due to metabolic disorders and endocrine and paraneoplastic manifestations of cancer (Table 56.1), emphasizing the range of clinical presentations, differential diagnoses and treatment options. Disorders of endocrine and metabolic function are caused by primary endocrine gland tumors, by paraneoplastic syndromes, and by various cancer therapies (1). Endocrine tumors are uncommon and present with a spectrum of problems reflecting the sites of origin and the hormones produced. Many neoplasms, endocrine and nonendocrine, produce a range of hormones and other proteins that act at a distance from the original tumor (Table 56.2). Neurological paraneoplastic syndromes, however, such as limbic and bulbar encephalitidies (Table 56.3), are caused by cancer inducing an antibody that cross-reacts with antigens in normal tissue to produce the clinical picture. Endocrine and paraneoplastic complications in the cancer patient have such diverse etiologies that a review of the neuropsychiatric manifestations is best approached from the perspective of their physiologic disturbances. The cancer-related disorders of cortisol, thyroxine, calcium, glucose, sodium, magnesium, and phosphate are reviewed with emphasis on their neuropsychiatric features. Carcinoid syndromes and pheochromocytoma (as part of multiple endocrine neoplasia) are also discussed.

CORTISOL

Hypercortisolism (Cushing's Syndrome)

Cushing's syndrome (adrenocortical hypersecretion of cortisol) in cancer is caused by pituitary adenoma (Cushing's disease), hypothalamic tumors, adrenal neoplasm, ectopic adrenocorticotropin (ACTH) production, or exogenous corticosteroids. Among adrenal neoplasms, only about 20% produce Cushing's syndrome (2). Ectopic ACTH production is associated with many tumors, although only a small percent actually develop Cushing's syndrome (Table 56.4). In a study of small cell lung cancer, 3%–7% had Cushing's syndrome with a much higher percent having a subclinical picture and an even greater number (up to 50%) with elevated levels of serum ACTH (3). Cushing's syndrome, irrespective of its etiology, has the highest incidence of neuropsychiatric symptoms of any endocrine disorder.

Studies have confirmed no difference in incidence with respect to depression between the differing forms of Cushing's syndrome (4,5). Clinical experience has shown that neither the dose of corticosteroids nor the duration of treatment consistently predicts the type, timing or severity of neuropsychiatric disturbance. Further, for a given patient there is no predictable, consistent pattern of neuropsychiatric symptoms. Neither a past psychiatric history nor a current psychiatric illness is a contraindication to using steroids in the cancer patient. Personality disorders and traits may influence the content but not the incidence or nature of steroid-induced psychosis. Psychiatric symptoms most often start within the first 2 weeks of corticosteroid treatment although the onset can range from as early as day one, to as late as 3 months. Conversely, tapering the dose of steroid can precipitate withdrawal symptoms which usually present as depression, although agitation, anxiety and even psychosis may result. Reintroduction of steroids with a slower taper generally controls the problems. A number of studies have shown that euphoria and increased motor activity are likely to occur earlier in the course of hypercortisolism,

TABLE 56.1. *Neuropsychiatric Manifestations of Metabolic Complication in Cancer Patients*

	Depression	Mania	Delirium	Cognitive Impairment	Psychoses	Anxiety and/or Panic Attacks	Personality Change
Hypercortisolism	+ + +	+ +	+ +	+	+ + +		
Hypocortisolism	+ +		+	+	+		+
Hyperthyroidism	+	+	+ +	+	+ +		
Hypercalcemia	+ +		+ +	+ +	+ +		+ +
Hypocalcemia	+	+	+ + +	+ +	+	+ + +	
Hyperglycemia			+	+ +			
Hypoglycemia	+ +	+	+ + +	+ +	+ +	+ + +	+
Hyponatremia (SIADH)	+ +		+ +	+ +	+		
Hypomagnesemia	+ +		+				
Hypophosphatemia	+		+				
Carcinoid	+		+				
Pheochromocytoma						+ + +	+ +

SIADH, syndrome of appropriate antidiuretic hormone secretion.

whereas depression, emotional lability, insomnia, fatigue, loss of libido and cognitive defects are more common later. Psychologic dependence is rare; however, not infrequently corticosteroids are abused by patients for their euphoric or pain-relieving benefits (6,7). Steroid-related psychiatric symptoms are largely reversible by reducing or discontinuing medication, and suicidal acts, though rare, do occur. The Boston Collaborative Drug Surveillance Program (8), in a prospective study of steroid side effects, showed that

TABLE 56.2. *Protein and Hormone Precursors Produced by Neoplasms*

Proopiomelanocortin and related peptides

Corticotropin-releasing hormone

Chorionic gonadotropin and its subunits (α and β)

Vasopressin

Cytokine growth factors (e.g., transforming growth factor-beta, epidermal growth factor, insulin-like growth factor II)

Parathyroid hormone-related protein

Parathormone

Erythropoietin

Eosinophilopoietin

Growth hormone

Growth hormone releasing hormone

Prolactin

Gastrin

Gastrin-releasing peptide (and bombesin)

Secretin

Glucagon

Calcitonin

Renin, prorenin

Vasoactive intestinal peptide

Somatostatin

Hypophosphatemia-producing factor

Endothelin-1

higher doses correlated with increased psychiatric complications. The mean daily dose for patients with neuropsychiatric reactions was 59.5 mg. compared with 31.1 mg. per day for those with no reaction.

Breitbart et al., at Memorial Sloan-Kettering Cancer Center, studied 50 patients with malignant spinal cord compression who were treated with a tapering dose of 100 mg of dexamethasone. They were compared with 50 equally ill patients without cord compression (9). They found the corticosteroid group had a significantly greater incidence of major depression syndromes ($p < 0.05$) and a tendency to a higher incidence of delirium. Other studies have shown no correlation between duration of corticosteroid treatment and incidence of mental disturbances. Even a single dose can produce psychiatric symptoms. The neuropsychiatric spectrum of Cushing's syndrome includes affective disorders, delirium, cognitive impairment, and minor disturbances such as sleep, tremor, nervousness, hyperkinesia and subtle alteration in sensation and perceptional (10–12). Affective disorders run the gamut between mania, major depression and mild alterations in mood. Euphoria is quite common, in up to 30% in one study, with an additional 11% developing frank mania (6). This mood-elevating effect is used in the palliative care of patients with advanced cancer in order to improve their appetite and enhance their sense of well-being. The incidence reported in the literature of depressive symptoms in cancer patients on steroids varies widely from 6% to 17% (13). In cancer patients on steroids, delirium, often inappropriately called "steroid psychosis," is common, though often in a mild form (14). The incidence of delirium and cognitive impairment in cancer is likely increased by the frequency of comorbid medical illnesses and the common use of narcotic analgesics. Nonetheless, clinically at least, steroid use appears to be the critical and

TABLE 56.3. *Paraneoplastic Neurological Syndromes*

Syndrome	Associated Cancer*	Clinical Features
Limbic encephalopathy†	SCLC	Depression, memory loss, confusion, abnormal CSF
CSF/brain-stem encephalopathy†	SCLC	Ataxia, cranial nerve dysfunction, corticospinal dysfunction, abnormal CSF
Subacute cerebellar degeneration	Breast, ovary, SCLC, Hodgkin's	Ataxia, dysarthria, nystagmus, normal CSF, dementia
Opsoclonus, myoclonus	Lung	Jerky, irregular movements of eyes and skeletal muscles, anxiety
Optic neuritis, retinal degeneration	SCLC	Painless loss of vision, transient visual obscurations, anxiety

*Only the most commonly associated tumors are listed.
†Often occur in association with each other.
  SCLC, small cell lung cancer.

frequently reversible factor (15). Some clinicians feel that patients with steroid-induced delirium have hallucinations or delusions that are more often paranoid in nature. For example, a 65-year-old woman who received high dose dexamethasone suddenly became mute and catatonic, and later during an Amytal interview she described her paranoid fear that if she spoke or moved she would be thrown into a pit full of snakes next to her bed.

Cognitive impairment, or reversible dementia, can also be caused by steroids and presents with deficits in memory, concentration, laryngeal and slowed higher cortical mentation (16,17). It is important to note that most patients experience only mild neuropsychiatric symptoms and that long-term or chronic sequelae in general do not occur (18). Cushing's syndrome is palliated by giving drugs that inhibit steroid synthesis such as aminoglutethimide, metapyrone, mitotane, ketoconazole, and octreotide. Rarely bilateral adrenalectomy is required.

Hypocortisolism (Adrenal Insufficiency)

Adrenal insufficiency in cancer can be due to anatomic destruction of the adrenal glands by tumor invasion or surgical removal, by suppression of the hypothalamic-pituitary axis via ectopic ACTH secretion (paraneoplastic) or exogenous steroid administration, by tumor or cancer-related hypopituitarism, and, rarely, to metabolic failure in hormone production secondary to cytotoxics such as 5-fluouracil (19).

Adrenal insufficiency can present acutely (as in an addisonian crisis) or chronically (15). The clinical pictures differ somewhat. In an acute presentation there is no definite set of psychiatric symptoms, although cognitive impairment, delirium, clouding of consciousness, and even coma have been documented. In the chronic picture classical features include lethargy, weakness, fatigue, anorexia, hypotension, cutaneous pigmentation, and severe electrolyte disturbances. Psychiatric manifestations include irritability, negativism, poor concentration, withdrawal, and depression (20). Because primary muscle weakness is a prominent symptom of hypocortisolism, most authors do not include it as a depressive symptom. Occasionally, especially early in the disease when symptoms are vague, patients can be misdiagnosed with a somatoform illness such as a conversion disorder or hypochondriasis. Also described, though uncommonly, are profound perceptual disturbances, including lowering the threshold of sensitivity to smell, taste, touch, and hearing

TABLE 56.4. *Neoplasms Associated with "Ectopic" Cushing's Syndrome*

Neoplasms	Approximate Percentage of Reported Patients
Carcinoma of the lung (predominantly small or oat cell)	50
Carcinoma of the thymus	10
Carcinoma of the pancreas (including carcinoid and islet cell	10
Pheochromoytoma, neuroblastoma, ganglioma and paraganglioma	5
Medullary carcinoma of the thyroid	5
Bronchial adenoma and carcinoid	2
Miscellaneous carcinomas or hematologic malignancies*	18

*For example, carcinoma of the ovary, prostate, breast, thyroid, kidney, salivary glands, testes, stomach, colon, gallbladder, esophagus, appendix and acute myeloblastic leukemia.

(21). The neuropsychiatric symptoms are likely due to adrenal hormone deficiency per se or to compensatory increases in the levels of ACTH and corticotropin releasing hormone. Therefore, correction of electrolyte imbalances alone will not reverse the symptom.

THYROID HORMONE (THYROXINE)

Hyperthyroidism (Thyrotoxicosis)

Thyroid cancer is quite rare, with a prevalence of 0.2%–0.8%. Radiation and prolonged high levels of thyroid-stimulating hormone (TSH) (e.g., chronic iodine deficiency states) contribute to the incidence of thyroid neoplasms. Exposure to low dose radiation by nuclear power-plant accidents, atomic bomb fallout, and, historically, treatment of thymic hyperplasia and acne by radiation therapy all produce papillary cell thyroid cancer (15). Patients with thyroid cancer are virtually always euthryroid. Only a few cases of hyperthyroidism have been reported in association with follicular carcinomas. Usually patients present in a hyperthyroid state due to inappropriate thyroxine replacement following surgical or ^{131}I thyroid gland ablation. In the oncology setting hyperthyroidism can also be seen following excessive exposure to the iodide in contrast given for radiological studies. Choriocarcinomas and embryonal carcinoma of the testis can uncommonly be ectopic sources of TSH.

Hyperthyroidism is almost always associated with neuropsychiatric symptoms (22) of mild to severe anxiety, depression, cognitive or intellectual impairment, psychosis and delirium (Table 56.1) . Anxiety and nervousness are common, occurring in up to 53%–69% of patients in prospective studies (23). Motor restlessness, irritability, emotional lability and sleep disturbance are typical, while panic attacks are rare. Depression occurs in 30%–70% of patients with hyperthyroidism, though less frequently than in hypothyroidism (24). More commonly, hyperthyroidism presents with apathy, fatigue and cardiac complications in the elderly. Cognitive symptoms of guilt and hopelessness are less common in the elderly subgroup. Delirium, mania, psychosis and even coma are rare and occur only in the severely neglected hyperthyroid (25). The degree of anxiety tends to correlate with thyroid hormone levels, which is not true for depression.

Hypothyroidism

Surgery, ablative doses of ^{131}I, radiation therapy, some chemotherapy agents and lithium treatment can impair thyroid function and cause frank hypothyroidism, while severe infection, prolonged exposure to cold or alcohol abuse can precipitate a hypothyroid state. Patients receiving radiation therapy to the neck after hemithyroidectomy have a high incidence of hypothyroidism (26). Patients with Hodgkin's and non-Hodgkin's lymphomas have a higher incidence of hypothyroidism than head and neck cancer patients, even though the latter receive higher doses of neck radiation. This may be related to the use of iodide contrast in the lymphangiogram for the lymphoma patient (27). L-Asparaginase has been associated with low levels of thyroxine (T_4) (28), and aminoglutethimide, which is used to treat adrenal, breast and occasionally prostate cancer, can cause hypothyroidism (29). The diagnosis of hypothyroidism is frequently delayed because fatigue, cold intolerance, weight gain and constipation can be subtle and easily missed.

Cognitive impairment in the form of a subcortical dementia occurred in up to 30% of patients in one study (30). Typical features include difficulty in concentration, slowed responses to questions, impaired short-term memory and a facetious demeanor. In severe cases the cognitive deficits, in particular memory, can persist for years even following treatment of the hypothyroidism. Major depression occurs in 33%–43% of cases with vegetative symptoms more commonly than cognitive symptoms (hopelessness, guilt, low self-esteem) (15). "Myxedema madness," a severe presentation of hypothyroidism, accounts for a small number of patients (5%) who present with psychosis and delirium. Anxiety can also be a part of the presenting syndrome. In view of the association of depression with hypothyroidism and the considerable overlap of clinical features (up to 14% of psychiatric patients with depression have evidence of hypothyroidism) it is essential to do thyroid function tests, including TSH, when evaluating depressive symptomatology (25).

CALCIUM

Hypercalcemia

Hypercalcemia is one of the most common metabolic complications of cancer. The diagnosis can often be missed, as many of its clinical features (see Table 56.5), such as lethargy, constipation, confusion, drowsiness, nausea and vomiting are nonspecific and may be attributed to side effects of chemotherapy and radiation therapy, or to progression of the tumor itself. Nonetheless, it is important to diagnose, as effective treatment is available to prevent progression to severe hypercalcemia. It is worth noting that most patients with hypercalcemia have metastatic disease and 80% will die within 12 months (31). Table 56.6 lists the types

TABLE 56.5. *Clinical Features of Hypercalcemia of Malignancy*

GENERAL
Dehydration
Anorexia
Polydipsia
Poluria
Pruritus

GASTROINTESTINAL
Anorexia
Nausea
Vomiting
Constipation
Ileus

NEUROPSYCHIATRIC
Fatigue
Lethargy
Myopathy
Hyporeflexia
Psychosis
Depression
Delirium
Seizures
Coma

CARDIOLOGIC
Bradycardia
Atrial arrhythmias
Ventricular arrhythmias
PR interval prolonged
QT interval reduced
Wide T waves

of cancer associated with, and the mechanisms of hypercalcemia. Overall, 10% of cancer patients develop hypercalcemia. Cancers of the breast and lung (specifically squamous cell) account for over 50% of all case cases.

TABLE 56.6. *Neoplasms Associated with Hypercalcemia*

Neoplasms	Approximate Percentage of Reported Patients
CARCINOMA	
Lung	35
Kidney	24
Ovary	8
Miscellaneous*	< 2
HEMATOLOGIC MALIGNANT NEOPLASMS	
Multiple myeloma	7
T-cell lymphoma	2
Other	1
TUMORS WITH BONY METASTASES	
Breast carcinoma	50
Others not include in frequency estimates	5

*This includes almost every type of carcinoma (e.g., pancreas, urinary bladder, colon, prostate, penis, eosphagus, parotid glands, testes, liver, and stomach).

There are three commonly proposed mechanisms to explain hypercalcemia of malignancy (32,33). The hematologic malignancies, namely multiple myeloma and certain lymphomas (T-cell and Burkitt's), secrete cytokines with osteoclast-activating activity, including tumor necrosis factor-beta (lymphotoxin), tumor necrosis factor-alpha (cachectin) and interleukin 1, all of which cause osteoclasts to resorb bone, thereby releasing calcium. The second mechanism, humoral hypercalcemia of malignancy, is typified by solid tumors without bone metastases, especially renal and various squamous cell cancers. In these cancers hypercalcemia is caused by the secretion of proteins which bind to the parathyroid receptor, mimicking the parathyroid hormone. If no metastases are present, removal of the primary lesion will lead to resolution of hypercalcemia. The parathyroid hormone-related protein (PTHrP), an ectopic tumor protein, has been identified as causing hypercalcemia by this mechanism. Thirdly, solid tumors with bone metastases, typically breast and lung, directly erode bone, and, in conjunction with locally produced proteins such as prostaglandins and cytokine, release calcium into the circulation. Nonetheless there is poor correlation between extent of metastases and level of serum calcium, suggesting that other mechanisms, namely humoral, are also involved. Other mechanisms causing hypercalcemia in cancer patients, all uncommon, should be considered. Rarely a tumor can produce ectopic parathyroid hormone (PTH), itself resulting in hyperparathyroidism (34).

Another scenario is the coincidental association of benign primary hyperparathyroidism and cancer. Ectopic production of vitamin D_3 has resulted in release of calcium from bone via vitamin D receptors. And lithium, a mood stabilizer, as been reported to cause hyperparathyroidism and hypercalcemia. Nonmalignant parathyroid adenoma (and hyperplasia) can cause severe hypercalcemia due to secretion of PTH; 40% of these cases have neuropsychiatric symptoms, and in 12% of cases they are the presenting feature. Parathyroid adenoma and hyperplasia are part of multiple endocrine neoplasia (MEN) syndrome. This syndrome is transmitted as an autosomal dominant trait with high penetrance but variable clinical expressivity (Table 56.7).

Calcium is necessary for normal neural membrane function and synaptic transmission. Thus it is not surprising that loss of calcium homeostasis results in neuropsychiatric complications (see Table 56.5). In general, the psychiatric symptoms vary directly with the level of serum calcium. However, some authors (3) observed that the rate of rise of calcium and the patient's general performance status, including age,

TABLE 56.7. *Multiple Endocrine Neoplasia Syndromes*

MEN-I	Parathyroid hyperplasia
	Pancreatic endocrine tumor
	PPomas (80%–100%)
	Gastrinoma (54%)
	Inslinoma (21%)
	Glucagonoma (3%)
	GRFoma (rare)
	VIPoma (rare)
MEN-IIa	Medullary thyroid carcinoma, bilateral
	Phaeochromocytoma, bilateral (70%)
	Parathyroid hyperplasia
MEN-IIb	Medullary thyroid carcinoma, bilateral
	Phaeochromocytoma, bilateral (70%)
	Specific body phenotype: multiple mucosal neuromas, marfanoid habitus, bony abnormalities, bumpy lips

MEN, multiple endocrine neoplasia; MTC, medullary thyroid carcinoma; PPoma, pancreatic endocrine tumor releasing pancreatic polypeptide; VIPoma, vasoactive intestinal peptide tumor; GRFoma, growth hormone releasing factor tumor.

renal and liver function, influence the presentation. When calcium is elevated to between 12 and 16 mg/100 ml, typically depression, apathy, weakness (myopathy) and slowed mentation are present. As levels rise to 19 mg/100 ml delirium becomes more likely, with confusion, paranoia, disorientation and hallucinations. With calcium levels of 20 mg/100 ml and above, somnolence, seizures and eventually coma manifest. Coincident with these neuropsychiatric features, gastrointestinal and cardiologic problems will be present.

Hypercalcemia in metastatic breast cancer is not always reversible, but the biochemical and clinical features are often able to be ameliorated. Hypercalcemia of whatever cause is treated with saline hydration (with or without furosemide) and bisphosphonates, with mithramycin, gallium nitrate and calcitonin as backup treatments. Corticosteroids are added if a hematologic malignancy is driving the hypercalcemia.

Hypocalcemia

Hypocalcemia is comparatively uncommon in patients with cancer unless related to surgical ablation of parathyroids, renal insufficiency, malabsorption due to drug or other cancer-related complications, or as a result of drugs given to lower calcium levels, such as mithramycin, bisphosphonates and calcitonin and L-asparaginase. Calcitonin, which is normally produced by parafollicular cells of the thyroid, is secreted by some medullary carcinomas of the thyroid as well as breast, pancreas, colon, and lung cancer (35). However, hypersecretion of calcitonin by these or

any tumors does not produce symptoms of hypocalcemia.

In hypocalcemic states, the tetany and neuromuscular twitching can manifest as anxiety. However, the most common mental changes are cognitive impairment and delirium, which occur in 33% of patients (36). Cases of hypomania and depression have been described, as well as a diverse range of psychiatric disorders (36) (Table 56.1). It is vital, therefore, to measure serum calcium when evaluating mental disturbances in cancer patients, remembering that these symptoms generally resolve with calcium replacement.

GLUCOSE

Hypoglycemia

Hypoglycemia in cancer patients is caused by either nonmalignant metabolic disorders or the cancer itself. Metabolic etiologies vary widely: hepatic insufficiency, adrenocortical failure, hypopituitarism and improper use of exogenous insulin or oral hypoglycemic agents. Rarely fluoxetine (Prozac) causes hypoglycemia and should be monitored in diabetics. Cancer-related hypoglycemia is found with beta-islet cell tumors of the pancreas (insulinomas, which secrete insulin) and in other nonislet tumors. The latter group produce hypoglycemia by increased tumor use of glucose, by production of insulin-like growth factors (IGF-I and IGF-II) and by failure of normal homeostatic mechanisms (37).

Insulinomas are diagnosed by high plasma levels of insulin in the presence of hypoglycemia. Rarely malignant bronchial carcinoids and liposarcomas produce ectopic insulin (38). The tumors that do not produce insulin tend to be large (average 2.4 kg), intrathoracic or retroperitoneal, with liver metastases (39). Most of these tumors are mesenchymal in origin (Table 56.8). Of interest, lung cancer, which is a common cause of other endocrine complications is rarely, if ever, asso-

TABLE 56.8. *Neoplasms Associated with Hypoglycemia*

Tumor	Approximate Percentage of Cases
Mesenchymal*	45
Hepatic carcinoma	23
Adrenal carcinoma	10
Gastrointestinal carcinoma†	8
Hematologic neoplasms	6
Miscellaneous	8

*Includes fibrosarcomas, mesotheliomas, neurofibromas, neurofibrosarcomas, spindle cell carcinomas, rhabdomyosarcomas, and leiomyosarcomas.

†Includes cholangiomas, gastric carcinomas, colon carcinomas, pancreatic carcinomas, and carcinoid tumors.

ciated with hypoglycemia. The clinical presentation of hypoglycemia depends upon the rate of fall of plasma glucose as well as the absolute level. Clinical manifestations relate to cerebral hypoglycemia and secondary secretion of catecholamines. Chronic neuroglycopenia can present as depression, dementia, or as a schizophreniform syndrome. Acute hypoglycemia may present initially with tachycardia, sweating, pallor and light-headedness. Neuropsychiatric symptoms vary with the level of glucose: down to 70 mg/100 ml, anxiety is prominent; as the glucose level falls further, agitation, delirium, stupor, seizures and coma (at levels near 10 mg/100 ml) ensue. Focal neurological signs and symptoms, resembling a stroke, may be irreversible if rapid treatment is not initiated (40,41).

Hyperglycemia

Hyperglycemia is generally not a problem specific to the cancer setting. Very high levels of glucose can be seen in untreated or uncontrolled diabetics, particularly under the stress of infection, treatment with exogenous corticosteroids, or with renal impairment. Patients who have had surgical pancreatectomy require careful attention to blood glucose levels with appropriate insulin replacement therapy. Several chemotherapeutic agents can impair glucose regulation through effects on beta-cells of the pancreas. Streptozotocin has a cytotoxic effect on beta-cells (42), vincristine may impair glucose-induced insulin release (43), and L-asparaginase interferes with insulin synthesis (44,45). Excessive secretion of glucagon by a glucagonoma can cause a modest hyperglycemia that is rarely clinically significant. Hyperosmolar states caused by hyperglycemia may result in an encephalopathy, even coma, that may be fatal. Recovery of intellectual function after this insult may be incomplete (6).

PHEOCHROMOCYTOMA

Malignant or benign functional pheochromocytomas have the capacity to secrete excessive amounts of epinephrine and norepinephrine. Among these tumors of the adrenal medulla, 10%–15% are malignant. Pheochromocytomas are derived from the amine precursor uptake and decarboxylase system, and familial pheochromocytoma is a component of type II multiple endocrine neoplasia (MEN) (Table 56.7). Diagnosis of functional pheochromocytoma is aided by measuring urinary metanephrine and plasma catecholamines. Excessive secretion of catecholamines is responsible for the physical and psychiatric manifestations of pheochromocytoma. Paroxysmal episodes of hypertension, palpitations, headache, sweating, weight loss, tachycardia, and postural hypotension are only a few of the manifestations of pheochromocytoma. Often there is a family history of pheochromocytoma or a hypertensive response to anesthesia. Pheochromocytoma is best managed by reducing the tumor bulk and initiating alpha- and beta-adrenergic blockade to relieve symptoms. Psychiatric symptoms seen with pheochromocytoma are personality changes, anxiety, and panic disorders; their prominence may lead to primary psychiatric disorder.

CARCINOID TUMOR

Carcinoid tumors are relatively common but the symptomatic carcinoid syndrome is rare (46). The tumor arises from enterochromaffin cells located mainly in the gastrointestinal mucosa. Most carcinoid tumors are found in the appendix or rectum but rarely produce enough biologically active amines and peptides to be symptomatic. Carcinoid tumors from the ileum typically produce the syndrome, although the carcinoid syndrome can also arise from tumors of the stomach, bile duct, duodenum, pancreas, lung and ovary. Many active substances are produced by the enterochromaffin cell, including serotonin, bradykinin, prostaglandins, histamine and vasoactive intestinal peptide. However, serotonin is the likely common biochemical denominator of the carcinoid syndrome. Most ileal tumors that produce the carcinoid syndrome have overt liver metastases. Presumably the liver (and lung in the case of bronchial carcinoids) removes biologically active mediators from the circulation, but when liver metastases are present clearance is impaired.

Typical features of the carcinoid syndrome are cutaneous flushing (in over 90% of patients) with vasomotor instability. The flushing, which can be intense, usually lasts for minutes and can be mistaken for anxiety or panic attacks, but may continue for hours. Diarrhea (75%), right-sided endocardial fibrosis (35%), bronchoconstriction and dyspnoea (20%) are the other main features. Pellagra (niacin deficiency) is sometimes seen as a result of the body's store of tryptophan being diverted to the production of serotonin instead of niacin (9). The psychiatric manifestations associated with carcinoid tumors (and serotonin metabolism) are depression and encephalopathy. This is of interest because a low level of central nervous system serotonin is thought to be the neurotransmitter abnormality in depression. In carcinoid syndrome, it is possible that the tumor may consume all available tryptophan in the periphery. A paradoxical situation occurs in which there is an excess of serotonin in the serum but a profound deficiency of serotonin in the brain. A retrospective chart review of 22 patients with carcinoid reported that 50% had depression and 35% had signs of delirium (47). Patchell and Posner (48) reviewed the neurological complications of 219 patients with carcinoid seen at Memorial Sloan-Kettering Cancer Center. In their study, only 1% of all patients had depression, whereas 11% of patients with evidence of hypersecretion of serotonin had depression. They felt that there was a suggestion of increased incidence of depression in patients with carcinoid tumors.

Encephalopathy has been reported with carcinoid tumors which has improved after tryptophan and niacin were replaced in the diet (49). Pharmacologic control of the carcinoid syndrome is aimed at inhibiting hydroxtryptamine, especially its receptors; therefore, cyprohepatidine, ketanserin, and ondansetron are used, and, more recently, octreotide.

PHOSPHATE

Hypophosphatemia

Phosphate is an element crucial to widespread biochemical processes. In cancer, low levels are found associated with mesenchymal, prostate, and endodermal tumors. Mostly the mechanism is not known, although occasionally renal phosphate wasting with low vitamin D is the cause. Hypophosphatemia is also found in the very sick patient with multiple medical problems. Acute hypophosphatemia (less than 0.8 mg/dl) presents with muscle weakness, hyporeflexia, parasthesia, and nonspecific encephalopathy including cranial nerve palsies with delirium. In chronic hypophosphatemia (less than 1.5 mg/dl), weakness, debility, and anorexia prevail with later progression to neuropathy, paralysis, and rarely seizures (Table 56.1).

MAGNESIUM

Hypomagnesemia

Magnesium is involved in the homeostasis of cell membrane activity. Prolonged hypomagnesemia can cause secondary hypocalcemia and hypokalemia. At plasma magnesium levels of less than 1.2 mg/dl, anorexia and nausea followed by apathy, depression, anxiety, agitation, and confusion are prone to occur (Table 56.1). In cancer patients, causes are parathyroidectomy, impaired gastrointestinal absorption (including naso-

gastric suctioning and renal losses due to cisplatin, diuretics, hypercalcemia, and aminoglycosides.

HYPONATREMIA

Syndrome of Inappropriate Antidiuretic Hormone (SIADH)

Ectopic secretion of antidiuretic hormone (ADH) by tumors is a common paraneoplastic syndrome. It was first described in 1957 as the Schwartz–Bartter syndrome (50). The key to diagnosis is demonstrating hyponatremia and hypo-osmolality in the presence of an inappropriately concentrated urine and normal extracellular fluid volume (49). There are many causes of SIADH in cancer (Table 56.9), some directly related

TABLE 56.9. *Differential Diagnosis of SIADH in Cancer Patients*

Cause	Examples
Ectopic ADH secretion	Lung cancer (small cell)
	Prostate cancer
	Adrenocortical cancer
	Hodgkin's disease, lymphosarcoma
	Thymoma
	Carcinoma of duodenum
	Pancreatic cancer
Drug-induced SIADH	Chemotherapy
	Vincristine
	Cyclophosphamide
	Psychotropics
	Fluoexentine
	Amitriptyline
	Nortriptyline
	Haloperidol
	Thioridazine
	Thiothixene
	Fluphenazine
	Other drugs
	Ethanol
	NSAIDs
	Chloropropamide
	Carbarnazepine
	Narcotics
	Barbiturates
	Thiazide diuretics
	General anesthesia
Pulmonary disease	Pneumonia
	Tuberculosis
	Lung abscess
CNS disorders	Metastases
	Tumor
	Trauma
	Cerebrovascular accidents
	Encephalitis
	Meningitis
	Pain
Idiopathic	

to tumor, while others are associated indirectly. The commonest tumor associated with ectopic secretion of ADH is small-cell lung cancer. Estimates vary, but some studies found 32% of small cell lung cancers having biochemical evidence of SIADH with a lower incidence of clinically apparent hyponatremia (3). SIADH can present up to a year before radiological evidence of a lung cancer (25). Cerebral metastases of any origin can cause SIADH. Medications implicated include morphine, phenothiazines, tricyclic antidepressants, and fluoxetine (Prozac), all frequently used in palliative care (51). Vincristine and cyclophosphamide, also known causes, are both commonly used in the treatment of lung cancer which can prove diagnostically challenging. Hyponatremia causes a range of symptoms at serum levels below 125 mmol/l. Clinical features depend on both the level and the rate of fall. With a rapid drop of sodium, cerebral edema develops, and nausea, vomiting, and anorexia occur early progressing to lethargy, stupor, delirium, cognitive impairment, agitation, seizures, focal neurological deficits, and coma. The latter occur at serum sodium levels below 110 mmol/l. When hyponatremia evolves slowly, the brain protects itself against edema and presenting features are depression, and minor behavioral and cognitive changes.

SIADH, which is not due to low total body sodium, must have the underlying cause, where possible, reversed and the concentration of sodium in the blood carefully raised. If sodium is raised too quickly central pontine myelinosis can occur with fatal consequences. The key to treatment is water restriction, even down to 500 ml daily, supplemented by demeclocyline and at times oral urea. Occasionally in emergency situations hypertonic (twice-normal) saline can be given intravenously and very cautiously. Medical and psychiatric interventions need to be coordinated. Improvement of neuropsychiatric symptoms may lag behind biochemical normalization.

CASE REPORT

A 63-year-old white male with small cell lung cancer developed hyponatremia secondary to SIADH. As the serum sodium fell to levels as low as 113 mEq/l, he became quite lethargic and listless with disorientation, severe confusion and difficulty in motor coordination. Efforts to raise sodium levels were quickly successful, but at serum sodium levels of 120–125 mEq/l the patient's behavior became bizarre. His speech and thinking were quite slow with associated difficulties in concentration, attention, orientation, and short-term memory. The patient experienced episodes of depersonalization and dissociation accompanied by visual hallucinations. In addition, he developed a delusional belief that he was locked in a bare prison cell and was a prisoner of God. Without any psychiatric intervention, the patient's mental status cleared completely as the serum sodium returned to 132–136 mEq/l level. An EEG done during the period of abnormal behavior demonstrated diffuse slowing. CT and MRI scans of the brain, as well as repeated CSF examinations, were all normal. Similarly, a repeat EEG had normalized.

CENTRAL NERVOUS SYSTEM PARANEOPLASTIC DISORDERS

Nonmetastatic or paraneoplastic neurological complications of cancer are uncommon. A small subset of this group presents with neuropsychiatric symptoms and signs affecting the cortex, brain-stem and cerebellum. (Table 56.3) . These syndromes can precede the diagnosis of cancer and usually run a course independent to that of the tumor because the mechanism is probably due to the abnormal cancer cell inducing an antibody which cross-reacts with antigens in normal tissue (1). Dementia is a well-documented paraneoplastic disorder. If the onset is acute, metabolic and infectious etiologies need to be excluded also. Similar principles apply to cerebellar dysfunction. Clinically, subacute cerebellar degeneration presents with dysarthria and limb incoordination without nystagmus. It is classically associated with lung and ovarian tumors and is inexorably progressive. Metastatic cerebellar disease is usually unilateral and has no speech involvement. The final important clinical point is that paraneoplastic dementia, cerebellar, and brain-stem lesions often coexist. Unfortunately there is no specific treatment available.

SUMMARY

This chapter has outlined the neuropsychiatric complications of metabolic, endocrine, and paraneoplastic syndromes in malignancy. The clinical appearance, diagnostic difficulties and management principles have been emphasized. Review of the literature showed that there is a need for prospective studies utilizing modern investigative techniques such as single photon emission computerized tomography and functional magnetic resonance imaging scans. Both of these modalities study neurophysiologic abnormalities providing a window to the study of pathogenesis and therapy. In reviewing the psychiatric symptoms of metabolic, endocrine, and paraneoplastic disorders, distinguishing physiological from psychological mechanisms is diifficult (52). This problem is best illustrated in idiopathic depression, where neurophysiological abnormalities are similar to those of Cushing's syndrome. A review by Fava et al. (53). Emphasized the value of studying "the interaction between affective disorders and endocrine disease in order to find a common etiological mechanism." Hence, more information is needed to assess the best psychopharmacologic interventions in neuropsychiatric syndromes due to medical disorders.

REFERENCES

1. Posner JB. *Neurologic Complications of Cancer.* Philadelphia: Davis; 1995.
2. Soffer LJ, Lannaccone A, Gabrilove JL. Cushing's syndrome. *Am J Med.* 1961; 39:129–146.
3. Warrell RP, Bockman RS. Metabolic emergencies. In: DeVita VT, Heilman S, Rosenberg SA, eds. *Cancer,* 3rd ed. Philadelphia: JB Lippincott; 1989: 1986–2002.
4. Haskett RF. Diagnostic categorization of psychiatric disturbance in Cushing's syndrome. *Am J Psychiatry.* 1985; 142:911–916.
5. Haskett RF, Rose RM. Neuroendocrine disorders and psychopathology. *Psychiatr Clin North Am.* 1981; 4:239–252.
6. Wyszynski AA, Wyszynski B. The patient on steroids. In: *A Case Approach to Medical-Psychiatric Practice.* Washington, DC: American Psychiatric Press; 1996:193–212.
7. Morgan HG, J Boulnois, Burns-Cox C. Addiction to prednisone. *Br J Med Psychol.* 1973; 2:93.
8. Boston Collaborative Drug Surveillance Program (BCDSP). Acute adverse reactions to prednisone in relation to dosage. *Clin Pharmacol Ther.* 1972; 1 3:694–698.
9. Breitbart WS, Stiefel F, Kornblith AB, Pannullo S. Neuropsychiatric disturbance in cancer patients with epidural spinal cord compression receiving high dose corticosteroids: prospective comparison study. *Psycho-Oncology.* 1993; 2:239-245.
10. Cohen SI. Cushing's syndrome in psychiatric study of 29 patients. *Br J Psychiatry. 1980; 136:120-4.*
11. Lewis DA, Smith RE. Steroid-induced psychiatric syndromes: a report of 14 cases and a review of the literature. *J Affect Dis.* 1983; 5:31 9–332.
12. Ling MHM, Perry PJ, Tsung MT. Side effects of corticosteroid therapy. *Arch Gen Psychiatry.* 1981; 38: 471–477.
13. Starkman MN, Schteingart DE, Schork MA. Depressed mood and other psychiatric manifestations of Cushing's syndrome: relationship to hormone levels. *Psychosom Med.* 1981; 43:3–18.
14. Hall RCW, Popkin MK, Stickney SK, Gardner ER. Presentation of the steriod psychoses. *J Nerv Ment Dis.* 1979; 167:229–236.
15. Gadde KM, Krishnan KRR. Depression in endocrine disorders. *Dir Psychiatry.* 1996; 1:60–65.
16. Vincent FM. The neuropsychiatric complications of corticosteroid therapy. *Compr Ther.* 1995; 21:524–528.
17. Whelan TB, Schteingart DE, Starkman MN. Neuropsychological deficits in Cushing's syndrome. *J Nerv Ment Dis.* 1980; 168:753–757.
18. Varney NR, Alexander B, Macindoc JH. Reversible steroid dementia in patients without steroid psychosis. *Am J Psychiatry.* 1984; 141:369–372.
19. Bajorunas DR. Disorders of endocrine function following cancer therapies. *Clin Endocrinol Metab.* 1980; 9: 405–430.
20. Whybrow PC, Hurwitz T. Psychological disturbance associated with endocrine disease and hormone therapy. In: Sachar EJ, ed. *Hormones, Behavior and Psychopathology.* New York: Raven Press; 1976: 11–25.
21. Henkin RI. The neuroendocrine control of perception. In: Hamburg D, ed. *Perception and Its Disorders.* Baltimore: Williams & Wilkins; 1970:62–73.
22. Taylor JW. Depression in thyrotoxicosis. *Am J Psychiatry.* 1973; 132:552–553.
23. Kathol R. Endocrine disorders. In: Rundell JR, Wise MG, eds. *Textbook of Consultation-Liaison Psychiatry.* Washington DC: American Psychiatric Press; 1996: 579–584.
24. Whybrow P, Ferrell R. Thyroid state and human behavior: contributions from a clinical perspective. In: Prange AJ Jr, ed. *The Thyroid Axis, Drugs and Behavior.* New York Raven Press; 1974: 5–21.
25. Corn TH, Checkley SA. A case of recurrent mania with recurrent hyperthyroidism. *Br J Psychiatry.* 1983; 143:74–76.
26. Murken RE, Duvan AJ. Hypothyroidism following combined therapy in carcinoma of the laryngopharynx. *Laryngoscope.* 1972; 82:1306–1314.
27. Fuks Z, Glatstein E, Marsa GW, et al. Long-term effects of external radiation on the pituitary and thyroid glands. *Cancer.* 1976; 37:1152-11-61.
28. Garrick MB, Larsen PR. Acute deficiency of thyroxine-binding globulin during L-asparaginase therapy. *N Engl J Med.* 1979; 301:252–253.
29. Fishman LM, Liddle GW, Island DP, et al. Effects of aminoglutethimide on adrenal function in man. *J Clin Endocrinol Metab.* 1967; 27:481–490.
30. Touks CM. Mental illness in hypothyroid patients. *Br J Psychiatry.* 1974; 110:706–710.
31. Odell WD. Paraneoplastic syndromes. In: Holland JF, et al., eds. *Cancer Medicine,* 4th ed. Baltimore: Williams & Wilkins; 1997: 1149–1165.
32. Grill V, Martin TJ. Parathyroid hormone-related protein as a cause of hypercalcemia in malignancy. In: Bitezikian JP, Levine MA, Marcus R, eds. *The Parathyroids.* New York: Raven Press; 1994: 295–309.
33. Denko JD, Kaebbing R. The psychiatric aspects of hypoparathyroidism. *Acta Psychiatr Scand.* 1960; 38: 1–70.
34. Karpati G, Frame B. Neuropsychiatric disorders in primary hyperparathyroidism. *Arch Neurol.* 1964; 10: 387–397.
35. Schwartz KE, Wolfsen AR, Forste B, Odell WD. Calcitonin in non-throidal cancer. *J Clin Endocrinol Metab.* 1979; 49:438–444.
36. Smith KC, Barish J, Corren J, Williams RH. Psychiatric disturbance in endocrinologic disease. *Psychosom Med.* 1972; 34:69–86.
37. Gorden P, Hendricks CM, Kahn CR, et al. Hypoglycemia associated with non- islet cell tumor and insulin-like growth factors. *N Engl J Med.* 1981; 305:1452–1455.
38. Shames JM, Dhurandha NR, Blackard WG. Insulin-secreting bronchial carcinoid tumor with widespread metastasis. *Am J Med.* 1968; 44:632.

39. Carey RW, Pretlow TG, Ezdinli EZ, Holland JF. Studies on the mechanism of hypoglycemia in a patient with massive intraperitoneal leiomyosarcoma. *Am J Med.* 1966; 40:458.

40. Roth AJ, Breitbart WS. Psychiatric complications of cancer. In: Cherny NI, Foley KM eds. *Hematol/Oncol Clin N Am.* 1996; 10:235–260.

41. Sachs W. Disorders of glucose metabolism in brain dysfunction. In: Guall EG, ed. *Biology of Brain Dysfunction.* New York: Plenum; 1973:143.

42. Junod A, Lambert AE, Orci L, et al. Studies of the diabetogenic action of streptozotocin. *Proc Soc Exp Biol Med.* 1967; 126:201–205.

43. Shah J, Stevens B, Sorensen B, et al. Dissociated effect of vincristine on insulin release and Beta cell microtubular content in the intact rat. *Diabetes.* 1979; 28:372A.

44. Oettgen RIF, Stephenson PA, Schwartz MK, et al. Toxicity of *E. coli* L-asparaginase in man. *Cancer.* 1970; 25:253–278.

45. Whitecar JP Jr., Bodey GP, Hill CS Jr., Samaan NA. Effect of L-asparaginase on carbohydrate metabolism. *Metabolism.* 1970; 19:581–586.

46. Bower M, Coombes RC. Endocrine and metabolic complications of advanced Cancer. In: Doyle D, Hanks GWC, MacDonald N, eds. *Oxford Textbook of Palliative Medicine.* Oxford, England: Oxford University Press; 1993: 447–460.

47. Major LF, Brown GL, Wilson WP. Carcinoid and psychiatric symptoms. *South Med J.* 1973; 66:787–789.

48. Patchell RA, Posner JB. Neurologic complications of carcinoid. *Neurology.* 1986; 36:745–749.

49. Trivedi S. Psychiatric symptoms in carcinoid syndrome. *J Indian Med Assoc.* 1984; 82:292–294.

50. Schwartz WB, Bennett W, Curelops S, Banter FC. A syndrome of renal sodium loss and hyponatremia probably resulting from inappropriate secretion of antidiuretic hormone. *Am J Med.* 1957; 23:529–543.

51. Sandifer MG. Hyponatremia due to psychotropic drugs. *J Clin Psychiatry.* 1983; 44:301–303.

52. Stiefel FC, Brietbart WS, Holland JC. Corticosteroid in cancer: neuropsychiatric complications. *Cancer Invest.* 1989; 7:479–491.

53. Fava GA. Affective disorders and endocrine disease. *Psychosomatics.* 1994; 35:341–353.

X

INTERVENTIONS

EDITOR: MATTHEW LOSCALZO

57

Screening Procedures for Psychosocial Distress

JAMES R. ZABORA

Cancer disrupts all aspects of patients' and families' lives. Cancer engenders fear, produces uncertainty and creates significant demands for any patient or family. At the time of diagnosis, cancer generates distress for virtually every patient (1). However, in spite of this early trauma, significant evidence indicates that the majority of newly diagnosed cancer patients gradually adapt to the crisis, their diagnosis and its related treatments (2). Patients, who fail to adapt challenge the health care team to respond to a multitude of psychological and social problems. Often, the distress associated with these problems may not become manifest to the health care team until the patient reaches an observable crisis event (3). Frequently, referrals to psychosocial providers occur when the patient is severely depressed or anxious, experiencing significant conflicts within the family, or is suicidal (4). Psychosocial interventions at these acute points in time have been shown to be effective, but the major question is whether an early screening program would enable health care providers to identify patients who are at a higher risk in order to initiate clinical interventions and consequently prevent a crisis event. Since psychological distress may actually increase health care costs and prolong medical treatments, early identification and intervention may also produce a significant financial impact (5). Costs associated with early identification and intervention may be significantly less than the costs related to elevated distress, which may contribute to adverse medical events and rehospitalizations.

Weisman et al. described the high distress profile among newly diagnosed patients (2). Table 57.1 details the critical psychosocial variables associated with elevated psychological distress. It is clear that there is not one predominant factor, but rather, a series of variables which may contribute to elevated levels of psychological distress. In other words, any profile of a high distress patient might contain variables from each of the four categories in Table 57.1.

Weisman et al.'s Omega instruments must be considered as the standard against which new instruments or methods for psychosocial screening should be compared. However, one disadvantage to the Omega structured interview is simply time. Completion of the interview and one self-report measure (with scoring) may require 20–25 min. While this time period seems reasonable, it becomes unmanageable in any institution or clinic with a large volume of cancer patients. For example, in a cancer center which sees 4000 new patients annually, the Omega instruments could require 1.5 employees simply to screen every patient. This approach may not be cost-effective since the majority of patients do not require clinical interventions (6). Consequently, in relation to any psychosocial screening and intervention program, a critical issue is the exact prevalence of elevated psychological distress among cancer patients. Numerous prevalence studies (7–9) suggest that one of every three newly diagnosed cancer patients will experience significantly higher levels of distress and may benefit from social work, psychological or psychiatric intervention. Table 57.2 details these prevalence studies, their measures of distress, and rates of psychological distress.

Given a relatively consistent prevalence rate of approximately 30%, use of the Omega instruments in large volume clinics may require a significant amount of staff time with a low positive case yield. Self-report measures offer a valuable alternative for cancer centers that see a high number of cancer patients per year and wish to screen for psychological distress (6).

Since screening attempts to identify distress through measurement, the concepts of sensitivity and specificity must also be considered and demonstrated. Sensitivity is the ability to predict the number of patients as high

TABLE 57.1. *Variables Associated with Psychosocial Adaptation*

Social Support	Past History	Current Concerns	Other
Marital status	Substance abuse	Health	Education
Living arrangements	Depression	Religion	Employment
Number of family members and relatives in vicinity	Mental health	Work/finance	Physical symptoms
	Major illness	Family	Anatomical staging
Church attendance	Optimism versus pessimism	Existential	
		Self-appraisal	

distress divided by the actual number of patients who are highly distressed. On the other hand, specificity is the number of patients who are predicted to be low distress divided by the actual number of low distress patients (10). Therefore, if the specificity of a screening measure were .50, the false negative rate may be unacceptable. In other words, too many positive cases may be missed, which diminishes the effectiveness of any screening program.

Given these initial issues, screening must also be differentiated from assessment. Screening is a rapid method to prospectively identify potential patients who may experience significant difficulty in their attempts to cope and adapt to their diagnoses and treatments. Screening is a predictive model. Assessment seeks to accomplish a series of tasks in the early phases of a relationship with a patient. These tasks include an estimate of the severity of the patient's distress, definition of the initial course of action, development of a dynamic understanding of the patient, the establishment of a diagnosis and the first step in the development of a therapeutic relationship (11).

Finally, methods for psychosocial screening must be brief and pragmatic. Although improvements in screening techniques continue to be developed, further research is necessary to identify brief, simple and accurate tools to accomplish this vital task. Through screening, the early incorporation of psychosocial and behavioral interventions in cancer treatment may be more readily accepted by patients and less stigmatizing (12). In addition, these interventions complement cancer therapies and may enhance medical outcomes while reducing the overall costs of health care (5).

RATIONALE FOR PSYCHOSOCIAL SCREENING

Given the prevalence rate of psychological distress among cancer patients, it is clear that the current system of referrals to psychosocial providers is inadequate. Referrals are reactions to elevated and observable levels of distress which may have been gradually increasing over time (4). A number of studies have documented the unmet psychosocial needs of cancer patients (13,14).

Another challenge for the health care team is a patients' inability or unwillingness to share his/her distress. Quite often, patients intentionally conceal their distress and suppress their emotional concerns. Their motivation to do so is understandable. Any revelation concerning their distress may divert the health care team's attention from the tumor, its treatment, and achieving the best outcome. Patients fear being considered as weak and unable to cope. Furthermore, factors such as social stigma, denial, distancing, disapproval, and fear of rejection also play a role in patients' reluctance to reveal their distress.

In response to these issues, a screening questionnaire enables the health care team to examine critical issues

TABLE 57.2. *Prevalance Studies of Psychological Distress Among Cancer Patients*

Authors	Year	Measures	n	Rates of Distress
Derogatis et al. (7)	1983	SCL 90-R and psychiatric interview	215	47% received a DSM-III diagnosis; 68% of these were adjustment disorders
Farber et al. (8)	1984	SCL-90	141	34.4% had elevated scores
Stefanek et al. (9)	1987	BSI	126	28% demonstrated moderate to high distress

in an apparently anonymous manner. Patients complete questionnaires with the full understanding that someone will review their responses. However, because they are responding to a questionnaire, they may respond more readily to sensitive questions than they would in a face-to-face encounter. Early identification of distressed patients creates the potential to avert crisis events, yields pertinent psychological data (which may not be available from other sources) and maximizes the effective utilization of psychosocial services. In addition, screening and early interventions significantly contribute to the total and comprehensive medical care of patients and their families. Successful interventions can decrease distress, enhance quality of life and increase patient satisfaction (15). As managed care continues to evolve, patient satisfaction and quality of life are two critical outcomes to be closely considered immediately after cancer survival data in the development of global contracts. Managed care payers demand quality care that is comprehensive and meets the diverse and complex needs of cancer patients and their families.

METHODS OF PSYCHOSOCIAL SCREENING

Structured Interview

Weisman et al. (2) offer the only true structured interview which combines with a self-report measure to form the Omega Screening Instruments. Essentially, the interviewer seeks to acquire objective data in order to form an overall patient profile. As seen in Table 57.1, the majority of the items fall into two major categories: past history and social support. Additional items such as socioeconomic status indicators, perception of physical symptoms and tumor staging are also included. Some responses are weighted (e.g., being a widow or widower under marital status). Given the framework for each question, the interviewer can quickly construct a profile. When combined with the Inventory of Current Concerns (ICC), an objective score can be calculated. A score that totals or exceeds 7 should result in an offer of psychosocial intervention. Two case examples illustrate this process.

In one situation, a 60-year-old widow, who lives alone, has few family members in the immediate area, never attends religious services, has a history of depression, possesses significant past regrets and scores positive on three of seven domains of the ICC would yield an overall score of 9. Such a profile can be contrasted with a 65-year-old married women who has many family members in the immediate area, frequently attends religious services, is generally optimistic, but has experienced another major illness in her life, has received mental health counseling in the past, and scores positive on two domains on the ICC. This profile would yield a score of 4.

The Omega Screening Instruments are ideal for low volume areas such as a bone marrow transplant unit where staff can devote 20–25 min to each patient in order to gather preliminary data prior to a comprehensive psychosocial assessment. If the interviewer can be trained to maintain the focus on the individual items (rather than tangential discussions), the instruments can be completed with scoring in about 25 min. A key point to remember is that screening cannot be equated with assessment, which can easily require 90 min. The Omega Screening Instruments dramatically reduce time allocations; however, in high volume areas, a 25 min screening interview may not be feasible.

Self-Report Screening Measures

Any attempt to screen patients through self-report instruments must consider basic principles of measurement. Clinicians must decide what they seek to measure. If measurement of psychological distress is the goal, critical concepts such as reliability and validity must be incorporated into the selection of any standardized instrument. Reliability demonstrates the consistency of the measure over time, while validity establishes the ability of the instrument to truly measure its targeted domain (16). Needless to say, a number of psychological measures exist, but the Brief Symptom Inventory (BSI), the Profile of Mood States (POMS), the General Hospital Questionnaire (GHQ), the Hospital Anxiety and Depression Scale (HADS), and the Medical Outcomes Study Short Form (SF-36) offer potential as screening instruments for use with cancer patients. Table 57.3 provides the critical elements of each of the five scales that are described in this section.

Brief Symptom Inventory (BSI). The BSI is a 53 item measure of psychological distress which contains three global scales and nine subscales (17). The BSI is written on a sixth grade reading level and only requires 5–7 minutes to complete. Each item is on a 5 point Likert scale from 0 (not at all) to 4 (always). The patient is asked to respond to each item in terms of "how they have been feeling during the past 14 days." Positive cases can be identified by a Global Severity Index T score of ≥ 63 or any two subscales where the T score is ≥ 63 (18). Within a cancer setting, the somatization score should be eliminated from the equation since many patients report significant physical symptoms. The BSI has been utilized in prevalence studies related to psychological distress (9)

TABLE 57.3. *Critical Elements of the BSI, POMS, GHQ, HADS, and MOS-36*

Measure	No. of Items	Global Scales	Subscales	Psychometrics
BSI	53; 5 point Likert scale	Global Severity Index (GSI) Positive Symptom Distress Index Positive Symptom Total	Somatization Hostility Anxiety Depression Phobic anxiety Interpersonal Sensitivity Obsessive-compulsive Paranoid Ideation	Test–retest coefficient = .68–.91; α = .71–.85
POMS	65; 5 point Likert scale	Total Mood Disturbance	Tension-anxiety Depression-dejection Anger-hostility Vigor-activity Fatigue-inertia Confusion-bewilderment	Test–retest coefficient = .65–.74; α = .87–.95
GHQ	60, 30, 20 or 12; 4 point Likert scale	—	Anxiety Depression Hypochrondriasis Social impairment	Test–retest coefficient = .90; split-half coefficient = .95; α = .85 for 30 item version
HADS	14; 3 point Likert scale	—	Anxiety Depression	Test–retest coefficient = .74 for anxiety, .70 for depression; α = .41–.76 and .30–.60
MOS Short Form (SF-36)	36; varied response format	—	Physical Physical role limitations Pain Social Psychological Emotional role limitations Vitality Health perceptions	α = .78–.93

and has been tested for its efficacy as a screening instrument against the Omega instruments (6).

Profile of Mood States (POMS). In order to understand the psychology of emotional distress, subjective data such as affect and mood must also be considered as well as physiological and behavioral data. The POMS was developed to rapidly and economically identify transient and fluctuating affective states. The POMS measures six identifiable mood or affective states through the 65 item version, and can be completed in 10–16 min (19).

The POMS requires respondents to read each item carefully and select the response which describes how he/she has been feeling during the past week including today. Each item is an adjective which relates to one of the six mood or affective states. Each adjective can be rated on a 5 point Likert scale from 0 (not at all) to 4 (extremely). The 1-week time frame allows the opportunity to depict each patient's typical and persistent mood state. Raw scores on each mood state can be converted to T score norms in order to compare results to normative samples.

General Hospital Questionnaire (GHQ). The GHQ was originally constructed to screen for psychiatric illness in general populations, in primary health care settings, or among medical outpatients (20). The format for questions seek a response to a specific symptom (e.g., abnormal thoughts) or a type of behavior (e.g., managing to keep busy or occupied). Each item compares the patient's normal situation to his/her present perception of the problem or symptom. Response formats range from "less than usual" to "much more than usual." Scores can be calculated on a 0-1-2-3 Likert system or a 0-0-1-1 method. Scores can be interpreted as an indication of the severity of psychological distress. For the GHQ-60, 12 positive responses identify a probable case. For the 30, 20 and 12 item formats, 24, 15, and 9 positive responses require further evaluation (21). Given the variation in formats, patients can complete the GHQ in 5–20 min.

Hospital Anxiety and Depression Scale (HADS). Essentially, the HADS has two subscales: one for anxiety and the other for depression. Since anxiety and depression are the two most frequently encountered psychiatric symptoms in general hospitals and primary health care clinics, an instrument that specifically targets these domains could be of great benefit. The two subscales of the HADS each consist of seven items whose scores are divided into three categories according to severity which produces a maximum score of 21 on each subscale. Definitive cases for either subscales are indicated by a score of 11 or higher, doubtful cases in a range from 8 to 10, and non-cases by a score of 7 or less (22). The success of the HADS as a true screening instrument is mixed (23). Time for completion of the HADS is 5–7 min.

Medical Outcomes Study Short Form Health Survey (SF-36). The MOS SF-36 was designed to measure health status in the Medical Outcomes Study and has been utilized in clinical practice, health services research, policy evaluations, and general population surveys (24). The SF-36 is one multiitem scale which assesses eight health concepts; these are detailed in Table 57.3. This measure can be self-administered by patients age 14 years or older, or can be completed with the assistance of an interviewer in 7–10 min. Individual items can be rated on a 5 point Likert scale, although the descriptive choices on each item varies. Low scores indicate limitations in physical activities, emotional problems or high levels of pain. High scores demonstrate positive health beliefs and

performance, or little or no evidence of physical limitations. Within the SF-36, the general mental health subscale has been utilized as the Mental Health Inventory which has demonstrated the capability to discriminate psychiatric and medical patients (25).

PSYCHOSOCIAL SCREENING OF FAMILIES

Since virtually all patients enter their cancer experience as members of a family system, clinicians may wish to consider incorporation of a measure of family functioning into a psychosocial screening program. Given the dramatic shift in care from inpatient units to ambulatory care over the past 10 years, expectations concerning families as caregivers have significantly increased. Consequently, a family's level of adjustment to a cancer diagnosis and related treatments may parallel the patient's attempts to adjust to this significant threat in their lives. As with patients, families' level of adaptation may also be directly related to salient variables which actually precede the cancer diagnosis. Diverse family theories provide a range of explanations which detail how functioning is modified following crisis or stressful events. Family unity, intergenerational boundaries, and internal coalitions are concepts that describe aspects of family functioning. Utilization of specific family theoretical models guides clinicians and investigators in their selection of critical concepts that can be measured in an attempt to categorize the level of family functioning. As a result, family adaptation can be predicted along with potential problematic behaviors which a portion of families may exhibit (26). Families that are defined as problematic require attention and time from the health care team. When the focus of care shifts from the patient to the family, medical outcomes are jeopardized. Problematic families can be identified early in the treatment process and clinical interventions and management strategies can be offered prospectively rather than at the time of discharge from the hospital or at another critical point in the treatment process (27). Specific family measures and their psychometric properties that are suitable for screening are detailed in Table 57.4. Given the brevity of the Family APGAR and the Family Adaptability Cohesion Evaluation Scale, these hold the greatest likelihood as effective screening instruments.

SPECIAL ISSUES

Screening of Children
In pediatric settings, a child's health and response to treatment is often profoundly influenced by psychoso-

TABLE 57.4. *Potential Family Screening Instruments*

Measure	Author(s)	No. of Items	Response Format	Psychometrics
Family Environment Scale (28)	Moos et al. (1974)	90 or 40	True/false	Test–retest coefficient = .68–.86; α = .61–.78
Family APGAR (29)	Smilkstein (1978)	5	3 point Likert	Test-retest coefficient = .83; α = .80
Family Adaptability Cohesion Evaluation Scale (30)	Olson et al. (1979)	20	5 point Likert	Test-retest coefficient = .80 for adaptability and .83 for cohesion; α = .62 and .77

cial factors which are not routinely assessed. Clearly, routine screening for psychosocial problems will uncover more problems and greater needs than are detected in routine medical histories or are recorded in medical records. Psychosocial screening in pediatric settings can supplement the team's sense of the child's level of functioning, as well as alert the team concerning children who may be at a higher level of risk (31). In addition, screening results also enable the team to develop a specific treatment plan while providing important information to encourage parents to accept a referral for psychosocial services. To date, the most widely utilized instrument is the Pediatric Symptom Checklist (32). Given the predominant role played by parents, utilization of a psychological instrument in conjunction with a family measure may provide significant insight into how each parent may respond as care proceeds.

Screening for Alcoholism

In certain populations such as head and neck cancer patients, clinicians may wish to screen for alcoholism in an attempt to identify current problematic drinkers as well as the severity of the problem. Alcohol abuse in the context of chemotherapy or radiotherapy may significantly influence patients' decision making and their ability to adhere to complex medication schedules. Either the four item CAGE questionnaire (33), or the two item test developed by Cyr and Wartman (34) provide the clinician with the ability to quickly identify problem drinkers during the initial phase of care following their cancer diagnosis.

Screening for Home Care Needs

One of the most pragmatic ways to determine the need for home care services as the time of discharge draws closer is to examine whether the patient and family have utilized these services in the past. Consequently, incorporation of a single question, "Have you used home care services in the past year?" into the routine assessment at the time of admission will predict with

acceptable sensitivity and specificity which patients will require home care at discharge.

Screening for Physiological Symptoms

Cancer pain and fatigue are two problems that often are underdiagnosed and, consequently, are undertreated. Screening programs possess the potential for patients to identify specific problems such as fatigue, pain, nutritional deficits, sexual dysfunction, or shortness of breath in order to prospectively offer relief for these symptoms. Given the emphasis on patient satisfaction and quality of life by managed care companies, identification of the problems and symptoms by the Patient Needs Assessment Tool (35) can enhance and facilitate comprehensive patient care.

THE JOHNS HOPKINS PSYCHOSOCIAL SCREENING PROGRAM

For the past 5 years, numerous models have been tested in order to implement a psychosocial screening program in a cancer center which evaluates over 4000 new patients per year. Utilization of professional staff to distribute and collect screening questionnaires is not cost-effective. Distribution of screening instruments via mail prior to the first clinic visit produces a low compliance rate. Incorporation of family members to assist the patient with the completion of the questionnaire introduces a potential source of influence or bias. Consequently, the program detailed in Figure 57–1 describes the psychosocial screening program at Johns Hopkins.

This psychosocial screening program is automated and utilizes existing clerical and support staff to distribute and retrieve standardized questionnaires. Professional staff enter this sequence at the point of offer of interventions. Screening occurs during the first or second visit in medical oncology outpatient clinics after patients have decided to receive care in this setting. Within the radiation therapy department, screening is incorporated into the "simulation schedule"

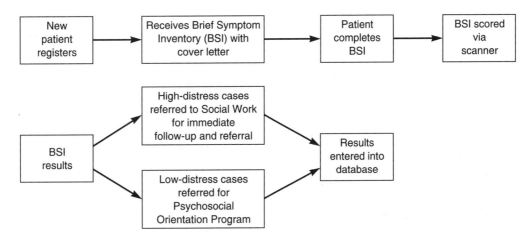

FIG. **57–1.** Psychosocial screening program at Johns Hopkins Hospital, Baltimore, MD.

since these patients will most likely receive care at Johns Hopkins. Ideally, screening should occur for all patients, including those who may only be seeking a medical consultation or "second opinion." In these cases, screening results can be communicated to referring physicians in order to alert them to potential psychosocial problems.

The Brief Symptom Inventory (BSI) was selected as the screening instrument due to its brevity, ease of understanding, and sixth grade reading level. Even though the BSI possesses a number of emotionally laden items, patients find it acceptable, with less than 10% of patients preferring not to complete it. Patient satisfaction surveys confirm the 5–7 min time frame to complete as well as a positive response that staff are concerned about patients' emotional concerns. High distress patients express more interest in the scores and results than do those with low distress. The BSI may increase their awareness concerning their level of psychological distress.

High distress pateints are identified based on a Global Severity Index (GSI) Score $\geq$ 63, or any two subscales $\geq$ 63, with the exclusion of the somatization subscale. Utilization of these "cut-off" scores yields a consistently high sensitivity of .87 and specificity of .89. In a recent analysis of the Hopkins database, 2388 newly diagnosed patients were examined for the overall prevalence of psychological distress by the site of the cancer diagnosis. Ten cancer diagnoses were represented in this sample with a minimum of 100 patients in each diagnostic category. Lung cancer patients exhibited a significantly higher level of distress than the other diagnoses with the exception of brain and

hepatoma. The overall prevalence of distress identified by the BSI was approximately one-third of the patients in this large sample (36). These results confirm the need for early psychosocial intervention and the potential utilization of instruments such as the BSI to implement psychosocial screening programs.

Costs associated with use of the BSI include the purchase of a scanner and the appropriate BSI scannable forms. Initial start-up costs are approximately $7500, with annual operating expenses of $4000. These figures do not include costs associated with staff time.

Critical to this program is the utilization of nonprofessional support staff to coordinate the screening program, and offer concrete assistance to patients who may experience difficulty in the completion of any instrument or questionnaire. Illiteracy, physical status, or anxiety may directly prevent a patient from reading the questionnaire and responding to each item. In our case, the resource coordinator (a nonprofessional position which requires positive interpersonal skills) responds to specific concerns or problems which patients or families may verbalize. Availability for timely problem-solving is a major function for support staff in order to enhance the potential for completion of questionnaires.

High distress patients receive an immediate follow-up contact with the focus being a referral to the Cancer Counseling Center (CCC). The CCC is a comprehensive mental health program staffed by masters prepared social workers who provide psychotherapy, psychiatric liaison nurses, and consulting psychiatrists. Low distress patients are referred to the psychosocial orientation program which is primarily staffed by volunteers. These specially trained volunteers possess strong interpersonal skills, and educate new patients and families concerning a range of psychosocial programs which are available. These programs are intended to enhance the adaptation of these patients and include disease-specific support groups, volunteer patient-to-patient counselors, psychoeducational programs related to survivorship concerns, and a program for children who have cancer in the family. The 20 min orientation program is provided to all new patients through the use of specially trained volunteers, and is scheduled during the first week of treatment.

CONCLUSIONS

Given the prevalence of psychological distress among cancer patients, psychosocial screening provides the opportunity to identify vulnerable patients during the first week of care. Early identification of high distress patients enables psychosocial providers to prospectively offer services and interventions which may provide the greatest benefit to specific patients. Educational programs may benefit patients with lower levels of distress, whereas support groups might be best suited for patients with moderate levels of distress. On the other hand, patients and families with high levels of distress should receive psychotherapy and/or family therapy. A match of intervention with level of distress maximizes the benefit of any psychosocial intervention, and the offer of interventions as early as possible in the treatment process lessens the stigma associated with mental health services. In addition, identification of psychological and social concerns can be incorporated into a definition of comprehensive care. Mental health services which address psychological distress can potentially improve medical outcomes, reduce health care costs and increase patient satisfaction as well as quality of life. In the evolving managed care environment, variables such as patient satisfaction and quality of life will continue to be strongly considered as salient outcomes in addition to survival data.

Psychosocial screening not only provides the opportunity to prospectively link patients to specific psychosocial services, but use of a standardized psychological instrument can also serve as a baseline measure. Consequently, if patients with a high level of distress are directly referred to a counseling service, a standardized measure such as the Brief Symptom Inventory can again be administered upon the completion of the intervention. In effect, the screening instrument serves as the pretest to the intervention as

well as a posttest measure in order to determine any change in psychological status. In order for psychosocial programs to survive in a managed care environment, psychosocial services must also position themselves to compete for mental health capitated contracts. Psychosocial screening creates the opportunity to establish a baseline measure in order to examine the effectiveness of mental health services within the overall program or for each individual psychosocial provider. A screening program also enables psychosocial providers to develop a clinical database in order to undertake specific analyses in large samples of cancer patients. For example, psychological distress can be examined in relationship to age, gender, socioeconomic status, race, ethnicity or cancer diagnosis. As a result, psychological interventions can be employed and tested for efficacy in relation to the resolution of psychological symptoms in specific populations at different points in time. Furthermore, the link between intreated psychological distress and increased health care costs requires investigation. A critical objective is to develop a brief screening instrument which is reliable, valid, easy to score. Such a tool enables psychosocial providers to identify high risk patients and offer early intervention, and to explore the relationship between psychological distress and health care costs.

REFERENCES

1. Weisman AD, Worden JW. The essentential plight in cancer: significance of the first 100 days. *Int J Psychiatry Med.* 1976; 7:1–15.
2. Weisman AD, Worden JW, Sobel HJ. Psychosical screening and intervention with cancer patients: research report. Boston: Harvard Medical School and Medical School and Massachusetts General Hospital; 1980.
3. Weisman AD. A model of psychosocial phasing in cancer. *Gen Hosp Psychiatry.* 1979; 1:187–195.
4. Rainey LC, Wellisch DK, Fawzy FI. Training health professionals in psychosocial aspects of cancer: a continuing education model. *J Psychosoc Oncol.* 1983; 1(2):41–60.
5. Allison TG, Williams DE, Miller TD, et al. Medical and economic costs of psychologic distress in patients with coronary artery disease. *Mayo Clin Proc.* 1995; 70: 734–742.
6. Zabora JR, Smith-Wilson R, Fetting JH, et al. An efficient method for the psychosoical screening of cancer patients. *Psychosomatics.* 1990; 31:192–196.
7. Derogatis LR, Morrow GR, Fetting J. The prevalence of psychiatric disorders among cancer patients. *JAMA.* 1983; 249:751–757.
8. Farber JM, Weinerman BH, Kuypers JA. Psychosocial distress in onocology outpatients. *J Psychosoc Oncol.* 1984; 2(3/4):109–118.

9. Stefanek M, Derogatis L, Shaw A. Psychological distress among oncology outpatients. *Psychosomatics*. 1987; 28:530–538.

10. Lilienfeld AM, Lilienfeld DE. *Foundations of Epidemiology*. New York: Oxford University Press; 1980.

11. Tomb DA. *Psychiatry for the House Officer*, 3rd ed. Baltimore: Williams & Wilkins; 1988.

12. Fawzy FI, Fawzy NW, Arndt LA, Pasnau, RO. Critical review of psychosocial interventions in cancer care. *Arch Gen Psychiatry*. 1995; 52:100–113.

13. Guadagnoli E, Rice C, Mor V. Cancer patients knowledge of and willingness to use agency-based services: Toward application of a model of behavioral change. *J Psychosoc Oncol*. 1991; 9(3):1–21.

14. Mor V, Guadagnoli E, Wool M. An examination of concrete service needs of advanced cancer patients. *J Psychosoc Oncol*. 1987; 5(1):1–17.

15. Andersen, BL. Psychological interventions for cancer patients to enhance the quality of life. *J Consult Clin Psychol*. 1992; 60(4):552–568.

16. Nunnally JC. *Psychometric Theory*, 2nd ed. New York: McGraw-Hill; 1978.

17. Derogatis LR, Melisaratos N. The brief symptom inventory (BSI): an introductory report. *Psychol Med*. 1983; 13:595–605.

18. Derogatis LR. *The Brief Symptom Inventory: Administration, Scoring, and Procedures Manual*. Minneapolis: National Computer Systems; 1993.

19. McNair DM, Lorr M, Droppleman, LF. *Profile of Mood States*. San Diego: Educational and Industrial Testing Service; 1971.

20. Goldberg D. *Manual of the General Hospital Questionnaire*. Windsor, UK: NFER Publishing; 1978.

21. Banks MH. Validation of the general hospital questionnaire in a young community sample. *Psychol Med*. 1983; 13:349–353.

22. Ford S, Lewis S, Fallowfield L. Psychological morbidity in newly referred cancer patients. *J Psychosom Res*. 1995; 39(2):193–202.

23. Johnson G, Burvill JG, Anderson CS, et al. Screening instruments for depression and anxiety following stroke: Experience in the Perth Community stroke study. *Acta Psychiatr Scand*. 1995; 91:252–257.

24. Ware JE, Sherbourne CD. The MOS 36-item short form health survey (SF-36): Conceptual framework and item selection. *Med Care*. 1992; 30(6):473–483.

25. McHorney CA, Ware JE, Raczek AE. The MOS 36-item short form health survey (SF-36): psychometric and clinical tests of validity in measuring physical and mental health constructs. *Med Care*. 1993; 31(3):247–263.

26. Zabora JR, Fetting JH, Shanley VB, et al. Predicting conflict with staff among families of cancer patients during prolonged hospitalizaitons. *J Psychosoc Oncol*. 1989; 7(3):103–111.

27. Zabora JR, Smith ED. Early assessment and intervention with dysfunctional family systems. *Onocology*. 1992; 5(2):31–35.

28. Moos RH, Moos BS. *The Family Environment Scale Manual*. Palo Alto: Consulting Psychologists Press; 1984.

29. Smilkstein G. The family APGAR: a proposal for a family function test and its use by physicians. *J Fam Pract*. 1978; 6:1231–1239.

30. Olson DH, Portner J, Lavee Y. *FACES III Manual*. Minneapolis: Family Social Science; 1985.

31. Kemper K. Self-administered questionnaire for structured psychosocial screening in pediatrics. *Pediatrics*. 1992; 89(3):433–436.

32. Bishop SJ, Murphy JM, Jellinek MS, Dusseault K. Psychosocial screening in pediatric practice: a survey of interested physicians. *Clin Pediatr*. 1991; 30(3):142–147.

33. Woodruff RA, Clayton PJ, Cloninger CR, Guze SB. A brief method of screening for alcoholism. *Dis Nerv Syst*. 1976; 37:434–435.

34. Cyr MG, Wartman MA. The effectiveness of routine screening questions in the detection of alcoholism. *JAMA*. 1988; 259(1):51–54.

35. Coyle N, Goldstein ML, Passik S, et al. Development and validation of a patient needs assessment tool for oncology clinicians. *Cancer Nurs*. 1996; 19(2):81–92.

36. Zabora JR, BrintzenhofeSzoc KM, Smith ED. Prevalence of psychological distress by cancer site. *Proc Am Soc Clin Oncol*. 1996; 15:507.

58

Brief Crisis Counseling

MATTHEW LOSCALZO AND KARLYNN BRINTZENHOFESZOC

Lindemann's seminal description of the acute grief reactions experienced by individuals involved in the tragic Coconut Grove fire in 1943 laid the groundwork for an objective appreciation of the impact of crisis on humans (1). Later, Caplan proffered the following definition of crisis: "A crisis occurs when a person faces an obstacle to important life goals that is, for a time, insurmountable through the utilization of his customary methods of problem-solving" (2). Caplan (3) developed a model of stress based on psychological and physiological arousal caused by the demands of the situation that exceed the individual's perceived resources. Within Caplan's model, reduced psychophysiological arousal results in a higher level of integration and functioning that leads to a sense of mastery. Lazarus then formulated a model of adaptation to stress within general principles of biology focusing on homeostatic response to disturbances of psychic equilibrium (4). These theorists contributed to an understanding of crisis which appreciates the significance of social, psychological and physiological manifestations of the crisis experience.

Crisis is unique in that it is the one biological, psychological, social, and, for some people, spiritual event, that virtually everyone will experience at least once in their lives. Despite the fact that a crisis involves individuals, families, or communities, the person in crisis always perceive themselves as being the focus of tension and isolation. If the individual or family fails to provide immediate attention to a crisis, negative consequences will certainly result. Crises are an inevitable and expected aspect of human growth and development and occur on a continuum from a minor event to a grave catastrophe.

Crisis is a temporary state, lasting about 6–8 weeks, accompanied by confusion, disorganization, and an inability to manage the event using traditional problem-solving skills (5). The crisis state is precipitated by an actual or threatened hazardous event, a loss or a challenge (6,7). In the case of people with cancer and their families, the crisis may be precipitated at any point along the disease continuum. The initial crisis precipitant is usually an alarming symptom, physical change or positive test result and eventual confirmation of a cancer diagnosis. However, the initial diagnosis of a malignancy is only the first point on the disease continuum that presents a series of crisis points, each fraught with significant challenges to coping and adaptation. The opportunity to intervene early in the illness, before maladaptive interactions become solidified, creates a therapeutic environment where future obstacles and setbacks can be anticipated and managed (8).

Crises may be developmental or situational. Developmental crises are the normal challenges that individuals confront. Erikson described life cycle tasks which are necessary to attain healthy maturity (9). Within this model, normal developmental crises represent problems to be overcome by the individual before the next step of psychological growth can occur. For example, a 53-year-old woman who at the height of her professional life perceives that she is simply not as physically attractive, active or capable as she once was. She may also be concerned about her child who is about to graduate from college and leave home.

A situational crisis, on the other hand, occurs with an event that is beyond the control of the individual. For example, for the woman described above, who is already facing a life cycle crisis, is diagnosed with breast cancer. The situational crisis is superimposed on the person within the context of that individual's life cycle phase.

Another level of crisis relevant to cancer is that of exhaustion. That is, the exhaustion of both patient and family in the face of a chronic, traumatic illness course. This occurs when the patient and family have lived with the demands of cancer for an extended period of time (6). Within the present health care environment, family caregivers are at particular risk for an exhaustion crisis.

The precipitating stressful event resulting in crisis can only be understood in the personal context of the individual, determined in part by personal meaning of the experience. Meaning and mastery are intertwined. Assigning cause in itself leads to a sense of control in the face of ambiguous and complex information (10). The nature and duration of the precipitating event influences the person's attempts to respond effectively to overwhelming demands: i.e., how the person reacts to and integrates the crisis experience is significantly influenced by how the event is interpreted. Lazarus defined cognitive appraisal as processes that "are complex and symbolic, permitting us to distinguish among actual harm-loss (future) threat, and challenge, and to make many other subtle cognitive distinctions that give our lives their highly rich and complex emotional qualities." (11). Thus, a person's cognitive appraisal of the event that precipitates the crisis will influence the emotional response, as well as associations, psychic maneuvers to ward off overwhelming anxiety, social demands, and behaviors aimed at restoring homeostasis. Maneuvers or coping methods that have worked in the past will be used again. When the person's attempts to ward off overwhelming distress are unsuccessful, signs and symptoms of confusion and disorganization appear. Insomnia, poor concentration, loss of daily patterns of behavior and preoccupation with thoughts of illness and death occur. The ability to accurately access and plan an action is impaired (12). While there is no psychiatric diagnosis for this crisis state, it is best described in the DSM-IV, in which an individual has experienced an event within the past 3 mo in which the distress is in excess of that which would be anticipated (13). This is called Adjustment Disorder with Depressed, Anxious or Mixed Mood.

Paradoxically, despite impaired psychic functioning, the anxiety and distress experienced by people in crisis often lead to a brief period of enhanced openness to outside counsel and motivation for relief. The universality of the crisis experience makes it an event that is communicated readily to others and for which emotional support is provided with minimal stigma and little loss of self-esteem. Social rituals exist for support of persons during crisis events. Fewer supportive rituals exist for people with chronic life-threatening diseases.

Crisis intervention counseling as a treatment modality is time-limited and is focused directly on overcoming problems of the here and now. Attention is not directed to unresolved problems of the past, personality problems, or intrapsychic problems which are the purview of traditional therapies (14–16). The goal is to rapidly restore the individual and family to their level of functioning that existed before the onset of the crisis (4,16,17).

This chapter offers a guide to interventions to deal with cancer-related crises. Brief crisis counseling seeks to enable patients and families to quickly regain a sense of equilibrium, maintain hope and focus on meaningful and effective activity. The chapter outlines the transitions or crisis points in cancer, how patients respond and how counseling may help them adjust.

CRISIS AND CANCER

Crisis counseling has been described most extensively during the period of diagnosis. Weisman and Worden (18) called the first 100 days after diagnosis a period of "existential plight." Specifically, patients experience a period of acute emotional distress (described earlier) that diminishes as the reality of the illness is integrated and as they return to their usual level of functioning. Weisman identified the medical, social, and psychological/psychiatric characteristics of people with cancer that predict poor psychosocial adjustment (19). They found that preventive psychosocial interventions lowered distress, enhanced coping skills and significantly increased the level of problem resolution (20). These psychosocial interventions have come to be called brief crisis counseling. This is an active problem-solving approach focusing on the rapid restoration of physical, psychological, social and spiritual coping abilities, achieved through psychosocial and behavioral interventions and referral. Effective for acute phases of disorganization, it cannot address issues related to deeper problems or dysfunctional family structures.

The cancer experience is comprised of a series of crises that occur over the course of the illness. Massie and Holland (21) stated, "The response to a crisis in cancer, either at the time of diagnosis or at some later transitional or crisis point, is characterized by an initial phase in which the person experiences either disbelief or temporary denial of the diagnosis." Each transitional or crisis event confronts the patient and family with new challenges to their ability to function in a directed, effective and meaningful way. Because of the nature of the disease and its multimodal treatments, the person with cancer is often confronted with an ongoing series of powerful assaults, without respite. Cohen described the emotional reactions associated with cancer as being disbelief, hope, anguish, terror, acquiescence, surrender, rage, envy, disinterest, ennui, and yearning for death (22). Many people report that the ongoing frustration and inherent struggles of cancer and its unpleasant treatments makes them feel like Sisyphus: continually challenged, exhausted, and frustrated.

In addition to the personal reactions to the demands of the illness, cancer maintains a firm hold on the dark side of the imagination, engendering terrifying glimpses of evil, deterioration, wasting, and uncontrolled loss of vitality (23,24). Patients and their families, confronted with the physical reality of illness, become acutely aware of a sense of vulnerability and uncertainty. This sense of exposure and sudden dependence on others assaults their sense of safety, control and confidence. Primitive emotional reactions occur and the impulse to flight is real, which may be poorly understood by medical staff (25).

Clinicians working in oncology must recognize and understand the acute distress exhibited by the patient and the family. Because hospital stays are shorter and more treatment is in ambulatory settings, services provided to patients and families must be tailored to these changes. Cancer, AIDS, Parkinson's disease or other chronic life-threatening medical conditions characterized by superimposed acute episodes create significant distress, with a high likelihood of psychosocial crises occurring at these points. The staff may minimize psychosocial concerns which they perceive as time consuming and less important. The psycho-oncologist must be a part of the treatment team and integrate brief counseling into the care. Introducing crisis counseling should be done in a way to minimize the stigma many people associate with psychological problems. Once the patient is incorporated as a team member, they can be assessed by the team's discussion of their problems, or by brief interview in clinic or hospital which they perceive as part of the overall services.

THE DISEASE CONTINUUM

The cancer experience is composed of predictable events which, as a whole, are described as the disease continuum (26,27). These events begin with the diagnosis, followed by treatment, remission, recurrence or progression, advanced disease, and the terminal stage. Cancer treatment, whether it is surgery, chemotherapy, or radiation therapy, is perceived as a crisis (28–30). The end of treatment and remission has its crisis aspects, as does survivorship (30,31). Recurrence or progression presents existential issues (28,29). Survivors face their own crisis (30); the time near the end of life and terminal stage is particularly poignant with spiritual and psychological issues (32–34). For the families of cancer patients, there is also distress at each stage of the disease continuum (35–37) as well as the bereavement phase following the patient's death (38).

IMPACT ON PATIENT AND FAMILY

The manner in which the patient and family react is variable for each individual and for each event along the disease continuum. Indeed, patients and families do not always share the same responses or attitudes or priorities. Studies have found significant dissonance between patients and their families as to how they experience, interpret and respond to cancer (39–42). Reactions associated with each of the cancer crises or transition points are described in Table 58.1 from the patient's perspective and from the family's in Table 58.2.

However, there are several psychosocial issues that are similar. A sense of being trapped and the dread that accompanies the treatment and illness process, and the confrontation of mortality are shared. The loss of aspirations and the loss of dreams for self and family can be overwhelming. Some perceptions of cancer, if not corrected or reframed early in the cancer experience, can affect the patient and the family long after the resolution of the disease. For example, the uncertainty about diagnosis and treatment initially may cause blaming of each other, leading to conflict and poor communication.

A lack of information and misbeliefs of family members about the cause of cancer can lead to beliefs that stress caused it, it is a punishment for a past deed, or that it was wished on the person by someone else (43). It is essential in the early stages that accurate information is shared among the patient, family and health care team. Important medical information is best delivered in the presence of the patient and a family member. This role-modeling of open communication in which key family members hear the same information simultaneously supports subsequent problem-solving.

The sections below outline responses at each stage.

Diagnosis

Fear, shock, and numbing are common manifestations of the crisis of diagnosis. This may include fear of the disease, of what the future holds (both in terms of the actual treatment and how to maintain a normal life), of the treatment outcome and death. Confrontation with mortality and existential issues results in distress, anxiety, depression and a search for meaning that may have spiritual aspects for many patients. However, the acute level of distress dissipates over 7–14 days as the reality of the illness is incorporated into daily living and a plan of action is developed (44).

TABLE 58.1. *Impact of Cancer Along the Disease Continuum for the Patient*

Crisis Event	Personal Meaning	Manifestation	Coping Tasks	Survivor Goals	Professional Interventions
Diagnosis	Why me? What did I do? I caused the cancer Someone wished this on me—who was it? Is this retribution? Am I going to die? Death sentence	Fear Anxiety/depression Denial Psychic numbing Confusion Confronting one's mortality Terror Anger Loss of trust in God, in self, in one's body, and in others	Integrate reality of diagnosis Tolerate emotional turmoil and stress Accept increased dependency Accept help Adjust to the mileu of the health care system Forestall regular daily routines to undergo treatment Make decisions about treatment options Communicate illness/diagnosis and its implications to others Search for meaning	Best care possible with the least disruption to life	Physical availability Information Support Education Cognitive-behavioral skills Training Resource provision/referral Advocacy
Treatment (Surgery, Chemotherapy, Radiation)	I have a chance to beat this thing. Will I survive this? How will I manage with (whatever organ) gone? Will they get it all? I have to take this poison to beat the cancer but it might kill me If I miss an appointment will I die? Will my hair fall out? What will I look like bald? Do they really know what they are doing? I have to believe in this for it to work Am I radioactive?	Fear Anxiety Depression Agitation Confusion Need to control Sense of purpose Confronting changes in one's body Fear of intimacy and sexual contact Relief Denial Nausea and vomiting Anticipatory nausea and vomiting. Avoidance Vulnerability Pain	Adapt to chronicity of disease and treatment Make decisions regarding course of treatment See treatment as "new job" to be learned, mastered and paid attention too Develop and maintain satisfactory relationship with health care professionals Correct faulty thinking and feeling Reorganize family to incorporate the demands of treatment Incorporate physical demands of treatment into daily life Cope with ambivalence about treatment Rebuild self-esteem following changes in body	Optimal independence and control Insurability, employment Strive to maintain normalcy Get through treatment	Crisis intervention Information Education Support Cognitive-behavioral skills Training Problem solving Physical availability Resource provision/referral

(continued)

TABLE 58.1. *Impact of Cancer Along the Disease Continuum for the Patient—continued*

Crisis Event	Personal Meaning	Manifestation	Coping Tasks	Survivor Goals	Professional Interventions
Remission	I have a second chance so I have to be good I have to keep a positive attitude Will I jinx myself if I question success of treatment? I made it through does this mean I can go back to normal? I'm on borrowed time I got a break now I have to stay on top of it Life is unpredictable—I am waiting for it to come back Do they really know? I don't know if I can ever truly trust my body again I am in control again. I can have a life again. I want to help others going through what I did. I knew all along I would win this battle	Gratitude Fear of recurrence Relief Fear of abandonment Hypervigilance over health Hypochondriacism Obsessive thoughts Loneliness Anger Exerting control Altruistic bargaining Search for meaning Fear Anxiety	Rejoice in the end of treatment Deal with the reality that life has changed forever Live with uncertainty Adjust to late effects of treatment Seek information regarding long-term adaptation and survival. Adjust to less medical surveillance Resum a "normal" life Fend off fear of recurrence Assume redefined role in family, community and work Establish or restablish goals and aspirations Learn to trust self and environment again Accept one's mortality without distress of immediacy	Rehabilitation—psychological and physical, cognitive difficulties, restoration of self-worth Return to work, role in family and community Redevelop intimacy	Education Information Support Cognitive-behavioral skills Training Supportive psychotherapy Resource provision/referral
Recurrence/new Primary	What did I do wrong? Was it my negative attitude? Was I foolish to hope this was over forever? God has failed me I beat this last time I will beat it again Nothing ever works out good for me They said I was okay but I'm not Do I have to start all over again?	Anger Fear Depression Anxiety Shock Loss of hope Denial Guilt Loss of trust Feelings of alienation Increased vulnerability Loss of control Confronting mortality Search for meaning	Re-establish hope Accept the uncertainty about the future Understand information about new situation Regain a life focus and time perspective appropriate to the changed prognosis Communicate new status to others Make decisions about the new treatment course Integrate reality of ongoing nature of disease to probable death from cancer Tolerate changes in routine and roles again Adjust to increased dependency again Reinvest in treatment	Integrate reality with family functioning Maintain self-worth	Information Support Education Cognitive-behavioral skills training Physical ability Supportive psychotherapy resource Provision/referral

Stage	Issues/questions	Emotional responses	Goals		Interventions
Advanced disease	I'm out of control Will they offer new treatment? What am I doing wrong? Will it be as bad as the last time? Will I go broke?	Depression Anxiety Demoralization Fear Denial Anger Fear of intimacy	Maintain hope and direction Tolerate medical care Enhance coping skills Maintain open communication with family, friends and health care professionals Assess treatment and care options Maintain relationships with medical team	Dignity Direction Role in work, family and community	Support Cognitive-behavioral skills training Supportive psychotherapy Physical availability resource Provision/referral Information Education
Terminal	When am I going to die? Does dying hurt? What happens after you die? Why me? Why now? What did I do to deserve this? What will happen to my family? Will I be remembered by my family and friends? What if I start to die and I'm all alone? Can't the doctors do something else, are they holding back on me, have they given up on me?	Depression Fear Anxiety Denial Demoralization Self-destructive behavior Loss of control Guilt Anger Fear of abandonment Fear of isolation Increased dependency Acceptance Withdrawal Search for meaning in past as well as present Pain/suffering Need to discuss afterlife	Maintain a meaningful quality of life Adjust to physical deterioration Plan for surviving family members Accept reality of prognosis Mourn actual losses Mourn the death of dreams Get things in order Maintain and end significant relationships Say good-bye to family and friends Accept impending death Confront the relevant existential and spiritual issues Talk about feelings Review one's life	Dignity Family support and bereavement	Physical availability Support Cognitive-behavioral skills training Therapeutic rituals Coordination of services Advocacy Information

TABLE 58.2. *Impact of Cancer on Family*

Crisis Event for Patient	Manifestation in Family Members	Family Survival Goals	Professional Interventions
Diagnosis	Survivor guilt Desire to rescue Vulnerability through identification Fear of contagion Blame the victim	Reassignment of family roles and tasks Potential shift in power structure Learn to communicate about diagnosis Deal with own sense of vulnerability	Information Support Education Physical availability Resource provision/referral Cognitive-behavioral skills training Develop a plan of action
Treatment (surgery, chemotherapy, radiation)	Balance competing needs of family members and patient Regulate hopefulness Adjust to patients physical changes Powerless to control the side effects of treatment	Accept financial constraints Learn to communicate about effects of treatment Integrate the experience into everyday life	Information Support Education Physical availability Resource provision/referral Cognitive/behavioral skills training Develop a plan of action
Remission	Restore family roles and tasks Reestablish power structure Learn to live with uncertain future Reintroduce family goals	Accept long-term financial issues Adjust to living with a changed person Tolerate the patient always wanting to talk about the cancer experience Learn to be a normal family again Integrate the experience into everyday life	Information Support Education Physical availability Resource provision/referral Cognitive/behavioral skills training Develop a plan of action
Recurrence/new primary	Adjust family roles and tasks again Address growing mistrust of the health care setting Desire to rescue Moderate sense of failure and betrayal	Cope with physical and psychological exhaustion Integrate the experience into everyday life	Information Support Education Physical availability Resource provision/referral Advocacy Cognitive/behavioral skills training Develop a plan of action
Advanced Disease	Disappointment. Sense of failure Acceptance of loss Financial concerns	Maintain sense of hope and meaning Maintain open communication Maintain financial solvency Anticipate life without patient	Information Support Physical Availability Resource provision/referral Cognitive/behavioral skills training Develop a plan of action
Terminal	Guilt Focus of resources on patient Delay or cancel life plans Emotional withdrawal from patient Having strangers in home Physical changes to home Time away from work, school, friends	Need to accept impending loss Determine caregiving roles Accept the death of dreams	Information Support Education Physical availability Resource provision/referral Advocacy Cognitive/behavioral skills training

(continued)

TABLE 58.2. *Impact on Cancer on Family—continued*

Bereavement	Anger	Develop a new relationship with the deceased	Information
	Intense acute grief		Support
	Heightened emotional arousal	Permanently reassign family roles, tasks and power structure	Education
	Fears about emotional and financial solvency	Revaluate financial solvency	Physical availability resource
	Confusion	Integrate the experience into everyday life	Provision/referral
	Insecurity		Cognitive-behavioral skills training
	Longing		Therapeutic rituals
	Sadness		

Each crisis that the patient experiences impacts upon the family (45). At time of diagnosis, the family members search for explanations, and they may have fears about genetic risk for themselves or communicability. Family members may express their fear and frustration by becoming angry at the patient and may blame the victim because they feel powerless to protect the loved one, as they are suddenly flooded with intense waves of conflicting feelings. They may also experience survivor guilt or become hypochondriacal with concern about minor symptoms. Overall, at times of crisis there is a weakening and blurring of ego boundaries as families "circle the wagons" to protect each other from this external threat.

The place the patient holds in the family hierarchy also influences reactions of the ill person and the family. One of the immediate and challenging needs is to reassign family roles and tasks, to fill in the gaps left by the patient, and to adjust the power structure. Concerns around disruption of family functioning (46) and the need to realign the power structure is a significant concern for the patient (47,48).

Treatment

During the treatment phase, crises are related to the painful procedures, noxious side-effects and an increasing awareness of the long-term negative physical and psychological effects which may continue for months. However, the ultimate question revolves around eradication of the disease, making the chronic stresses tolerable for long-term gain. Anxiety and confusion concerning the effectiveness and repercussions of treatment may lead to difficulty in decision making. Nausea and vomiting, alopecia, physical debilitation, and fatigue are common symptoms which result in acute distress and treatment avoidance. Side effects interfere with daily functioning, the ability to maintain roles in the family, work, and community, and threaten self-image and self-confidence. For both the person

with cancer and the family member, the focus is on the passage of time. Understandably, there is a great desire for time to move quickly. Distortion of time perception is to be expected during times of significant stress and when there is a sense of being trapped. The act of waiting (in the absence of focused activity) is difficult for people in crisis.

For the family, the need to balance the needs of the member with cancer with those of the other family members becomes a concern; it can result in guilt and shame. The practical requirements to assure that the patient gets the treatments supersedes the needs of other family members. This may lead to the family having to confront the dawning realization (for the first time) that they have limits. It is the hope for cure or extending life coupled with the need to do something meaningful to address the problem which enables patients and families to control their fear and maintain focus during the treatment phases. The financial impact and lost productivity become apparent during this phase of care. Financial concerns are often a source of worry throughout the treatment and beyond.

Remission

For those patients who experience remission as a crisis, there is an overwhelming sense of exposure, vulnerability to recurrence and fear. The Damocles syndrome is described as the person partaking in the fruits of life while the threat of death hangs above by a thin thread (49). During remission, hypochondriacal concerns are common (50). Heightened anxiety and hypervigilance occur before follow-up visits. As follow-up appointments are spaced further apart, fear of not being adequately checked and loss of contact with the doctor are common fears during remission (51).

Recurrence

According to Silberfarb et al., first recurrence is the most distressing point along the disease continuum

(52). Schmale reported that recurrence is similar to the initial diagnosis but with the significant difference being a shift in the goals to control of the disease over cure (53). The precipitant of crisis around recurrence concerns the sense of immediate vulnerability, viability of life, perception and reality of treatment options and the person's ability and willingness to become actively reinvested in the treatment process. Often the individual feels frustrated and betrayed, vacillating between wanting immediate medical intervention and verbalizing doubts over the utility of further efforts. These responses generally activate the patient and family to action, resulting in a commitment to identify the best course of action. If threat to life is imminent, the crisis response can be expected to be considerable, as the system has not had ample opportunity to integrate the implications of this harsh new reality. Recurrence is a confrontation to patient and family that the cancer may not be controllable and that death may be inevitable. Anger at the health care staff may communicate their distress and need for reassurance.

Advancing Disease

Awareness that the disease is not responding to treatment results in redoubled attempts to find new therapeutic modalities or the acceptance that further aggressive curative treatment is unrealistic (see Chapter 87). Either way, the crisis is focused around identifying unexplored treatment options or reframing the situation to one in which care, comfort and communication become the focus of activity. For those patients and families who continue to rigidly perceive cure as the only acceptable outcome, periods of ongoing crisis manifested by panic and anxiety are expected as their defense mechanisms periodically falter under such a psychic burden. For those patients and families who are unable to tolerate even the discussion concerning the possibility of loss, support of defensive maneuvers and coping skills within a hopeful therapeutic context is necessary. Many patients prefer to enter clinical trials of new agents at this point. It is also at this time that alternative treatments are sought by patients and family members who may feel that the traditional medical care has little to offer (see Chapter 70).

Psychosocial distress is more evident in those with poor functional status and advanced disease (54). Patients in deteriorating health find it especially difficult to maintain social relationships as the illness consumes increasing amounts of valuable physical and psychic energy. As the focus of social relationships become increasingly limited, depression and self-absorption are more likely to occur. This can lead to acute psychosocial distress as the patient and family sense the withdrawal of significant others (who were actively supportive and hopeful during the earlier phases) as disability increases and death becomes a likely possibility.

Terminal Stage

At this point, the control of distressing symptoms and attention to their psychological well-being predominate. The family has great need to stay informed of physical changes and to feel involved as much as possible in care (see Chapter 87). The spiritual needs must be considered as well, for patient and family. Crisis counseling is needed to assure that these physical, psychological, social and spiritual dimensions are being met.

Bereavement

Responses of the family following the death of the patient will be influenced by the quality and meaning given to the death event, the ongoing relationship with the deceased and the psychological health of the individuals involved. Pining, sadness, guilt, shame, confusion, and anger are to be expected immediately following the loss. Potential crises revolve around family conflicts, distribution of financial benefits and liabilities, resumption of the long-ignored demands of normal living and psychiatric reactions. Of particular relevance during this period is the quality of the patient's management prior to death. Family members have the potential to gain great satisfaction and emotional growth from maintaining an ill loved one at home if the outcome is perceived as positive. Inadequately managed noxious symptoms, especially pain, on the other hand, can leave a family member guilt-ridden, filled with shame and depressed. In the absence of counseling and support, ongoing rage at the health care team can manifest itself in a wide variety of destructive ways including dissatisfaction and litigation.

BRIEF CRISIS COUNSELING

Dunkel-Schetter et al. identified the primary aims of counseling to control distress about pain, frightening symptoms, ambiguity concerning prognosis, and changes in social relationships (55). They found in a study of 668 multisite and multistage cancers that, except for a small difference with breast cancer (where help was increasingly sought), the type of cancer and time since diagnosis did not influence coping patterns. Escape-avoidance led to more distress, while positive reinterpretation of the event resulted in less distress; seeking and using social support also decreased distress. Dunkel-Schetter also reported that, "psychosocial adjustment to cancer might focus less on biomedical and disease characteristics often presumed to be determinants of coping and more on subjective appraisals of stress from cancer and their effects. Nonetheless, medical factors seem to influence coping only as they are filtered through the person's cognitive appraisal system."

Given the nature of cancer, successful coping will not always lead to mastery over the illness. White has proposed that striving toward an acceptable compromise may represent the optimal adaptive response (56). According to Holland, the best way to help people with cancer is to support their usual ways of coping by helping them apply the strategies that have worked in the past (57).

Psychosocial and educational interventions make a significant difference in the lives of persons with cancer and their families. Emanating from Project Omega, in the late 1970s, Weisman et al. (58) developed a composite of those people with cancer who coped effectively with the demands of the illness. The individuals who were the best copers were flexible and resourceful, tended to revise, correct, and substitute strategies, and they anticipated change for the better. Their family members were more practical, they were able to develop specific plans, and allowed few regrets. Those who coped poorly were beleaguered by pessimism, a sense of futility and a poor sense of control. Their self-esteem was compromised by a combination of already existing problems and feelings of weakness, helplessness, and discouragement.

Capone et al. found that crisis intervention techniques led to better self-image, faster return to work and return to prior level of sexual functioning for 97 women with newly diagnosed gynecological cancer (59). Gordon et al., in a study of the efficacy of psychosocial interventions with 308 newly diagnosed cancer patients with mixed tumor sites, found that those who received intervention were more realistic about issues and moved on from the problems of the initial diagnosis (60). Worden and Weisman demonstrated lower distress and better problem resolution in newly diagnosed people with cancer following psychological intervention (61). Other studies have reported the usefulness of psychological interventions, focusing on enhancing coping skills, counseling, social and emotional support (62–64), and education (65). In their review of 22 controlled studies from 1976 to 1990, Trijsburg et al. found that 19 of the studies reported positive effects of psychological and somatic function-

ing of patients and that they were present one year after the intervention. Distress, self-concept, health locus of control, fatigue, sexual problems, depression, anxiety, pain, and nausea and vomiting were improved by the interventions (66).

In general, brief interventions focus on presenting problems which are described in clear and practical ways. Horowitz developed a stress response model relevant to the crisis of cancer, which divides response into three phases: initial, dysphoria, and adaptation (67). The initial response is marked by denial, despair, and disbelief. Psychophysiological responses consistent with the flight–fight response are expected (68). The second phase, dysphoria, is notable for the expression of emotional reactions, especially anxiety, depressed mood, cognitive impairment, and disruption in daily functioning. The third phase is adaptation. In cancer there is a process which begins after approximately 2 weeks, when distressing emotions are less intense and focus returns to the problems of living with cancer and its treatment. For, as the person affected by cancer is confronted with other significant challenges resulting from the illness, this unpleasant emotional rollercoaster-like experience may be repeated many times. For the patient with advancing disease, periods of respite between transitional phases are short, with increasing disability more likely after each episode. Brief crisis counseling is focused on emotional negotiation of this process.

The experience of cancer is an environment where tension and, motivation are high to achieve change and therefore, brief counseling is very effective. Corrective emotional experiences with significant others and supportive health care staff may lead to more meaningful emotional connections with others, and the acquisition of new coping skills. The experience can have implications for future functioning.

Camille was the 27-year-old Hispanic daughter of her 67-year-old father who was sent home to die of metastatic cancer. The relationship had always been one of distant respect and love. Camille felt increasingly excluded from her father as his disease progressed. She became depressed and withdrew from her family. The patient tried to protect his family from the reality of his progressing disease by maintaining a positive attitude and focusing on hope. Upon return home, he quietly complained of severe unrelenting pain. The attending physician was aware of the patient's pain and told the family that there was nothing else that he could do. Camille and her mother felt they could not insist on pain medicines, despite the patient's increased pain, with moaning, crying and begging to die. They were immobilized by the crisis. Through much encouragement and emotional support, and helping them to understand that pain control was possible, they were able to act. Camille was asked to role play and practice asking the doctor for more help. When the physician would not prescribe additional medications, she asked him for a referral to the local hospice. As a result, the patient's pain was quickly controlled and hospice care provided support for all three. Camille had been able to do something meaningful for her father. Communication in the family was improved. The patient died at home with his family at his side. Camille reported later that caring for her father changed her life forever; she felt stronger and better able to do things on her own.

People with cancer are generally in good psychological health relative to the general population (69). However, there is a subset of people who have significant psychiatric disturbances and disabling distress which requires psychiatric management. These individuals need to be recognized early (see Part IX for common psychiatric disorders and their management).

Patients and families accept psychological assistance with the expectation that the therapist is willing to listen and is capable of helping. Active listening, encouraging expression of opinions, joining the individual in approaching the problem and jointly developing a plan of action is effective (70). The first aim is to stabilize the situation by offering support and listening, and then offering guidance and direction (71). Although listening in itself may be helpful, it is inadequate to provide ample relief in the absence of a plan of action. Open communication and problem-solving, a realistic appraisal of the situation and a sense of confidence that appropriate joint and planned activities will lead to relief of the immediate distress are important. Hope is a by-product of directed and meaningful action.

Brief crisis counseling entails physical availability, emotional and practical support, expert and accurate information, insight into relevant past patterns and present functioning, and identification of resources. The application is different at each stage of the disease and is dependent on the needs of the individual.

Table 58.1 describes the normal and expected reactions of the crises of cancer, how they are manifested, coping tasks of the patient, survivor goals, and the appropriate interventions for patients. Table 58.2 addresses the manifestation of family members at the same crisis points, family survival goals and relevant interventions.

Physical availability and the presence of a counselor is comforting and in itself helps to focus at a time of overwhelming emotion and confusion. The counselor provides information and encourages thoughtful consideration of treatment options. Assessment of their cognitive appraisal is important (59,72). The sudden need to trust an unfamiliar medical team may be disconcerting to the patient and family. They may need reassurance about the situation and the care.

The provision of resources is especially important during a crisis. Timely referrals, understanding of medical insurance coverage, transportation, temporary housing, communication and advocacy with the social network (family, job, religious community, etc.) may demand immediate attention. The anxiety and frustration of the person with cancer and family members are readily communicated to medical staff. Interpretation to the medical team of the emotional reactions of the patient and family provides objectivity and a sense of control which minimizes potentially distancing behaviors by staff. The clinician must intercede as needed in the hospital system. Practical tasks are used therapeutically as part of crisis intervention. They help to focus on activities that contribute to resolution (4,5,16).

GUIDELINES FOR CRISIS COUNSELING

Weisman and Worden recommended that the counselor instill a sense of optimism, practicality, flexibility, and resourcefulness (20). The counselor, by attitude, can model the behaviors that are most helpful during times of acute stress. Part of the psycho-oncologist's role is also to support and inform the medical staff about patients' and families' responses.

Suggestions below are useful guidelines for managing patients during crises.

- *What you say really matters.* The crisis experience is particularly time-sensitive and cognitive integration malleable during times of such intense interaction. Communications during these emotionally difficult but opportunistic interactions can best be seen as powerful hypnotic suggestions. Statements may be taken quite literally and can have long-lasting affects (73).

- *Accepting your limitations helps patients to accept theirs.* Conveying an openness to the need for emotional and psychological support by role-modeling through an appropriate and timely referral to a mental health professional can minimize stigma and encourage adaptation. Telling the patient and family at the first session that it is normal to seek help during times of crisis can relieve anxiety and encourage problem solving early on in the illness process.

- *Promise only what you personally can insure will happen.* It is better to tell a person with cancer and their significant other that you do not have the time right now or that there is a person better suited to manage their specific concerns than to use behaviors which lead to the premature closure or minimization of legitimate concerns. Do not say you will be back later to address a concern if you are not certain that you will in fact return. This will lead to an erosion of confidence at a time when the helping relationship may represent all the patient and family may perceive as real.

- *Do not prematurely stop the expression of intense emotional feelings.* Expression of emotions may lead to a sense of physical relief, renewed energy and enhanced ability to problem solve. Not being allowed to work through these intense feelings can lead to ineffective coping on the part of the patient or family (74).
- *Saying "I know how you feel," may not be helpful.* To tell a patient that their internal personal experience is understood may limit communication at a time when repeated recounting of the concerns is necessary to maintain a sense of control.
- *Telling the patient and family that everything is going to be all right may not make anybody feel better.* Telling a patient or family that "everything will be all right" or "everything is for the best" minimizes their situation and the clinician loses credibility. Often, everything is not going to be all right. The patient or family in acute distress needs to be reassured rather that someone is there to share the experience and that they will not be abandoned. Patients and families need to believe that you will be there to assist them through this difficult and trying experience, regardless of the outcome.
- *Demanding a positive attitude can be an unrealistic burden.* Positive thinking may not be a beneficial way to deal with life threatening illness even though it is seen as helpful in dealing with other stressful situations. Positive thinking may actually be self-deception and result in decreased energy and increased psychological distress (9). For example, allowing the person to express the negative is important.

CONCLUSION

In summary, cancer creates a series of crises. The crises offer many opportunities for patients and families to unify as a cohesive and directed unit to reach out for additional social and emotional support. Brief crisis counseling, representing the mainstay of psychological interventions for cancer patients and their families, is a highly focused approach, potentially resulting in therapeutic gain well beyond the limits of the time-limited event. The physical presence and intervention of a supportive counselor who understands both the medical and psychosocial situation holds the greatest promise for

rapid resolution of the crisis situation. Brief crisis counseling attempts to restore a sense of control, direction, and hope, using a cost-effective model.

REFERENCES

1. Lindemann E. Symptomatology and management of acute grief. *Am J Psychiatry.* 1944; 101:141–148.
2. Caplan G. *An Approach to Community Mental Health.* New York: Grune and Stratton; 1961.
3. Caplan G. Mastery of stress: psychosocial aspects. *Am J Psychiatry.* 1981; 12:67–81.
4. Lazarus RS. Psychological stress and the coping process. New York: McGraw-Hill, 1966.
5. Roberts AR. *Crisis Intervention Handbook: Assessment, Treatment and Research.* Belmont, CA: Wadsworth Publishing; 1990.
6. Parad HJ, Parad LG. *Crisis Intervention: Book 2.* Milwaukee, WI: Family Service America; 1990.
7. Golan N. Crisis theory. In: Turner FJ, ed. *Social Work Treatment: Interlocking Theoretical Approaches.* New York: Free Press; 1986: 296–340.
8. Horwitz M. *Stress Response Syndromes.* New York: Jason Aronson; 1976.
9. Erikson EH. *Childhood and Society*, 2nd ed. New York: WW Norton; 1963.
10. Taylor SE. Adjustment to threatening events: a thoery of cognitive adaptation. *Am Psychol.* 1983; 38:1161–1173.
11. Lazarus, RS. Stress and coping as factors in health and illness. In: Cohen J et al., eds. *Psychosocial Aspects of Cancer.* New York: Raven Press; 1982: 163–190.
12. Janosik EH. Crisis *Counseling: A Contemporary Approach*, 2nd ed. Boston: Jones and Bartlett; 1994.
13. *Diagnostic and Statistical Manual of Mental Disorders*, 4th ed. Washington, DC: American Psychiatric Association; 1994.
14. Epstein L. *Brief Treatment and a New Look at the Task-Centered Approach*, 3rd ed. New York: Macmillan; 1992.
15. Hughes, JE. Psychological and social consequences of cancer. *Cancer Surv.* 1987; 66:455–475.
16. Weisman AD. Coping with illness. In: Hacket TP, et al., eds. *MGH Handbook of General Hospital Psychiatry.* Littleton, MA: PSG Publishing; 1987.
17. Payne M. *Modern Social Work Theory: A Critical Introduction.* Chicago: Lyceum; 1991.
18. Weisman AD, Worden JW. The existential plight in cancer: significance of the first 100 days. *Int J Psychiatr Med.* 1976; 7:1–15.
19. Weisman AD. Early diagnosis of vulnerability in cancer patients. *Am J Med Sci.* 1976; 271:187–196.
20. Worden JW, Weisman AD. Preventive psychosocial intervention with newly diagnosed cancer patients. *Gen Hosp Psychiatry.* 1984; 6:243–249.
21. Massie MJ, Holland JC. Overview of normal reactions and prevalence of psychiatric disorders. In: Holland JC, Rowland JH, eds. *Handbook of Psychooncology: Psychological Care of the Patient with Cancer.* New York: Oxford University Press; 1989: 273–282.
22. Cohen M. Psychosocial morbidity in cancer: a clinical perspective. In: Cohen J, et al., eds. *Psychosocial Aspects of Cancer.* New York: Raven Press; 1982: 117–128.

23. Sontag S. *Illness as Metaphor*. New York: Farrar, Strauss & Giroux; 1977.

24. Murray M, McMillan CL. Gender differences in perceptions of cancer. *J Cancer Educ*. 1993; 8:53–62.

25. Marteau TM, Riordan DC. Staff attitudes towards patients: the influence of causal attributions for illness. *Br J Clin Psychol*. 1992; 31:107–111.

26. Cella D, Mahon S, Donovan M. Psychosocial adjustment to recurrent cancer. *Oncol Nurs Forum*. 1990; 17(suppl 3):47–52.

27. Mor V. Cancer patients' quality of life over the disease course: lessons from the real world. *J Chron Dis*. 1987; 40:535–554.

28. Silberfarb PM, Philibert D, Levine PM. Psychosocial aspects of neoplastic disease: II. Affective and cognitive effects of chemotherapy in cancer patients. *Am J Psychiatry*. 1980; 137:597–601.

29. Cull, A. Psychological aspects of cancer and chemotherapy [invited review]. *J Psychosom Res*. 1990; 34: 129–140.

30. Fawzy FI, Fawzy NW. A structured psychoeducational intervention for cancer patients. *Gen Hosp Psychiatry*. 1994; 16:149–192.

31. Spiegel D. Health caring: psychosocial support for patients with cancer. *Cancer*. 1994; 74:1453–1457.

32. Stefanek M. Psychological distress among oncology patients. *Psychosomatics*. 1987; 28:530–539.

33. Worden JW. The experience of recurrent cancer. *CA Cancer J Clin*. 1989; 39:305–310.

34. Ganz PA, Rofessart J, Polinsky ML, et al. A comprehensive approach to cancer patients' needs assessment: the cancer inventory of problem situation and a companion interview. *J Psychosoc Oncol*. 1986; 4:27–42.

35. Wainstock JM. Breast cancer: psychosocial consequences for the patient. *Semin Oncol Nurs*. 1991; 7:207–215.

36. Cassidy S. Emotional distress in terminal care: discussion paper. *J R Soc Med*. 1986; 79:717–720.

37. Kinzel T. Relief of emotional symptoms in elderly patients with terminal cancer. *Geriatrics*. 1988; 43:61–68.

38. Stedeford A. Psychological aspects of the management of terminal cancer. *Compr Ther*. 1984; 10:35–40.

39. Ell K, Nishimoto R, Mantell J, Hamovitch M. Longitudinal analysis of psychological adaptation among family members of patients with cancer. *J Psychosom Res*. 1988; 32(4/5):429–438.

40. Sales E. Psychosocial impact of the phase of cancer on the family: an updated review. *J Psychosoc Oncol*. 1991; 9(4);1–18.

41. Sales E. Schulz R, Biergel D. Predictors of strain in families of cancer patients: a review of the literature. *J Psychosoc Oncol*. 1992; 10(2):1–26.

42. Kaplan DM. Intervention strategies for families. In: Cohen J, et al., eds. *Psychosocial Aspects of Cancer*. New York: Raven Press; 1982: 221–233.

43. Parkes CM. *Bevereavement: Studies of Grief in Adult Life*, 2nd ed. Madison, CN: International Universities Press; 1986.

44. Gotay CC. The experience of cancer during early and advanced stages: the views of patients and their mates. *Soc Sci Med*. 1984; 18:605–613.

45. Oberst MT, James RH. Going home: patient and spouse adjustments following cancer surgery. *Top Clin Nurs*. 1985; 7(1):46–57.

46. Grobe ME, Ahmann DL, Ilstrup DM. Needs assessment for advanced cancer patients and their families. *Oncol Nurs Forum*. 1982; 9(3):26–30.

47. Cohen J, Cullen JW, Martin LR. *Psychosocial Aspects of Cancer*. New York: Raven Press; 1982.

48. Holland JC. Clinical course of cancer. In: Holland JC, Rowland JH, eds. *Handbook of Psychooncology: Psychological Care of the Patient with Cancer*. New York: Oxford University Press; 1989; 75–100.

49. Casseleth Br, Hamilton JH. The family with cancer. In: Cassileth BR, ed. *The Cancer Patient: Social and Medical Aspects of Care*. Philadelpha: Lea & Febiger; 1979.

50. Levin DN, Cleeland CS, Dar R. Public attitudes toward cancer pain. *Cancer*. 1985; 56:2337–2339.

51. Liang LP, Dunn SM, Gorman A, Stuart-Harris R. Identifying priorities of psychosocial need in cancer patients. *Br J Cancer*. 1990; 62:1000–1003.

52. Silberfarb PM, Maurer LH, Crouthamel S. Psychosocial aspects of neoplastic disease: I. functional status of breast cancer patients during different treatment regimens. *Am J Psychiatry*. 1980; 137:450–455.

53. Schmale A. Psychological reactions to recurrent metastasis of dissemination cancer. *Int J Radiat Oncol Biol Phys*. 1976; 1:515–520.

54. Fitch MI, Osoba D, Iscoe NJ, Szalai JP. Prediction of psychosocial distress in patients with cancer: conceptual basis and reliability of a self-report questionnaire. *Anticancer Res*. 1995; 15(4):1533–1542.

55. Dunkel-Schetter C, Feinstein LG, Taylor SE, Folks RL. Patterns of coping with cancer. *Health Psychol*. 1992; 11(2):79–87.

56. White RW. Strategies of adaptation: An attempt at systematic description. In: Coehlho GV, Hamburg DA, Adams JE, eds. *Coping and Adaptation*. New York: Basic Books; 1974: 47–68.

57. Holland JC. *Psychologic Aspects of Cancer*. In: Holland J, Fei E, eds. *Cancer Medicine*. Philadelphia: Lea Febiger; 1973: 991–1021.

58. Weisman AD, Worden JW, Sobel HJ. Psychosocial screening and intervention with cancer patients—research report. Project Omega, Department of Psychiatry, Harvard Medical School, Massachusetts General Hospital, Boston, Mass.; 1980.

59. Capone MA, Good RS, Westie S, Jacobsen AF. Psychosocial rehabilitation in gynecologic oncology patients. *Arch Phys Med Rehabil*. 1980; 61:128–132.

60. Gordon WA, Freidenbergs I, Diller L, et al. Efficacy of psychosocial intervention with cancer patients. *J Consult Clinical Psychol*. 1980; 48:743–759.

61. Worden JW, Weisman AD. Preventive psychosocial intervention with newly diagnosed cancer patients. *Gen Hosp Psychiatry*. 1984; 6:243–249.

62. Fawzy FI, Fawzy NW, Hyun CS. Short-term psychiatric intervention for patients with malignant melanoma: effects of psychological state, coping, and the immune system. In: Lewis CE, O'Sullivan C, Barraclough J, eds. *The Psychoimmunology of Cancer*. Oxford University Press; 1994: 292–319.

63. Edgar L, Rosberger Z, Nowlis D. Coping with cancer during the first year after diagnosis. *Cancer*. 1992; 69(3):817–828.

64. Greer S, Moorey S, Baruch JDR, et al. Adjuvant psychological therapy for patients with cancer: a prospective randomised trial. *Br Med J.* 1992; 304:675–680.

65. Brandeburg Y, Bergenmar M, Bolund C, et al. Information to patients with malignant melanoma: a randomized group study. *Patient Ed Counsel.* 1994; 23:97–95.

66. Trijsburg RW, van Knuppenberg FCE, Rijma SE. Effects of psychological treatment of cancer patients: a critical review. *Psychosom Med.* 1992; 54:489–517.

67. Horowitz M. *Phase-oriented Treatment of Stress Response Syndromes.* New York: Jason Aronson; 1973.

68. Cannon WB. *The Wisdom of the Body.* New York: WW Norton; 1932.

69. Bond MR, Pearson IB. Psychological aspects of pain in women with advanced cancer of the cervix. *J Psychosom Res.* 1969; 13:13.

70. Novalis PN, Rojcewicz SJ, Peele R. *Clinical Management of Supportive Psychotherapy.* Washington, DC: American Psychiatric Press: 1993; 235–255.

71. Rusk TN, Gerner RH. A study of the process of emergency psychotherapy. *Am J Psychiatry.* 1972; 128:882–886.

72. Cade B, O'Hanlon WH. *A Brief Guide to Grief Therapy.* New York: WW Norton; 1993.

73. Bellak LB. Intense brief and emergency psychotherapy. In: Grinspoon L, ed. *Psychiatry Update* (The American Psychiatric Association Annual Review, vol. III). Washington, DC: American Psychiatric Press; 1984: 11–24.

74. Berglund G, Bolund C, Gustafsson U, Sjoden P. A randomized study of a rehabilitation program for cancer patients: the 'starting again' group. *Psycho-Oncology.* 1994; 3:109–120.

59

Psychoeducational Interventions

FAWZY I. FAWZY AND NANCY W. FAWZY

In the late 1970s there was a dawning awareness of a growing need to address the psychological issues faced by cancer survivors in contrast to the previous emphasis on death and dying (1,2). This chapter reviews the 31 psychoeducational interventions reported in the literature from 1978 to 1994. These interventions have taken many different forms for a variety of cancer diagnoses and disease stages. Among the interventions, four major content themes have emerged:

1. *Education.* The overall goal of education for cancer patients is to reduce the sense of helplessness and inadequacy due to uncertainty and lack of knowledge. Many patients have inadequate levels of information and desire more (3). Patient education not only offers diagnosis and treatment specific information to patients who may have misconceptions, no conceptions at all, and who may be hesitant to ask for such information, but may also enhance coping skills (4). Such intervention seeks to replace helplessness with a sense of mastery and control. Education for cancer patients may cover technical disease and treatment information, and it may also include information about coping, emotional issues, and much more.

2. *Coping.* The goal of coping-skills training is to teach patients how to deal effectively with their diagnosis, treatment, and life in general using cognitive and behavioral methods. Specific components of coping include cognitive restructuring, problem-solving, stress management, relaxation training, deep breathing, meditation, biofeedback, hypnosis, self-hypnosis, guided imagery, and visualization.

3. *Emotional support.* Emotional support includes allowing patients the opportunity to vent the many feelings and emotions which they may have about their disease and its treatment and providing them with a sense of personal validation.

4. *Psychotherapy.* Psychotherapy is a long-established method used to ease the distress and disruption that accompanies the diagnosis of cancer. Support,

compassion, and empathy from a therapist form the cornerstone of successful psychotherapy. A major problem, however, is that the exact form of the psychotherapy employed in many studies is not explained. Therapy, psychotherapy, and counseling are the terms most commonly used without any clear definition or attempt to differentiate between them. It appears from all the studies reviewed that the critical component of these interventions was the support and emotional engagement of the patient regardless of which term was used.

The formats employed have been fairly evenly divided between individual and group interventions. Psychological and behavioral outcomes include coping, affective state, quality of life, knowledge, and compliance. Physiological outcomes include physical functioning and immune parameters, as well as recurrence and survival.

According to Holland (5), the goals of these interventions are to decrease feelings of alienation by talking to others in a similar situation, to reduce anxiety about the treatments, to assist in clarifying misperception and misinformation, and to lessen feelings of isolation, helplessness, and being neglected by others. Interventions which are designed to help the person feel less helpless and hopeless have the added benefit of encouraging more responsibility to get well and comply with medical regimens. Aware of the benefits of these psychosocial therapeutic interventions, today's patients often specifically request such services.

The purpose of this chapter is to describe and contrast these interventions, addressing the type of patient population, the research design, the details of the interventions, and the outcomes. Because the majority of the studies use varying instruments and do not specifically measure the outcome categories delineated above, the authors have used reasonable judgment in determining into which category each outcome measure falls. For example, anxiety and depression both are included in affective state. However, Quality of Life is only used if the research actually indicates that this is measured.

The studies are presented chronologically in four time periods for ease of review.

1978–1980 (Table 59.1)

In the late 1970s, reports began appearing in the literature of group interventions for cancer patients. Wood et al. reported on a pilot study with 15 cancer patients of various diagnoses. Eight weekly $1\frac{1}{2}$ hour sessions were held (6). The groups were co-led by a psychiatrist, a registered nurse, and a social worker. The focus of the discussions was on issues of living and coping with cancer. A survey using a Likert scale and covering 20 areas of changed experience was used to evaluate effectiveness. The authors reported difficulty in keeping the group focused, though patients reported that the intervention was useful in helping them to talk about and face fears and anxieties, to get information, to feel less isolated, and to feel supported in general.

Ferlic et al. provided 30 newly diagnosed cancer patients with six $1\frac{1}{2}$ hour group counseling sessions over 2 weeks (7). The content consisted of: *(1)* patient education; *(2)* team presentations (nursing perspectives, medical and psychological aspects, religion, sexuality, and nutrition); *(3)* group support. A social worker (MSW) co-led the session each week with the help of one other team member (i.e., one of three nurses, two physicians, two chaplains, an occupational therapist, and a dietitian). Each group contained members at varying stages in their cancer treatment, although the emphasis of the groups was on the newly diagnosed patient with advanced cancer. Group members were compared to a similar group of patients who did not attend the sessions. It was not clear how patients were assigned to groups. The Patient Perception test and Self-Concept questionnaire were administered pre- and postintervention and 6 months later by mail. However, not enough tests were returned to provide valid 6 months data. The intervention proved useful in improving patients' scores in group aptitude, hospital adjustment, relationship strength, cancer knowledge, and perceptions about death. It also served to enhance self-concept.

The Omega Project concentrated primarily on patients' thought processes and cognitive skills training, by using a structured problem-solving intervention to address common questions and concerns of cancer patients, provide education, and teach relaxation techniques (8). The program employed four educational audio tapes, and the Cancer Problem Solving

Instrument (CPSI), which contained 20 illustrated "problem" cards used to focus discussions, and consisted of four sessions during a 6 week period. During session 1, counselors introduced the overall plan and rationale of the program, and introduced and demonstrated relaxation training. In session 2, which took place one week to 10 days following session 1, counselors reviewed session 1, lead a 20 minute relaxation exercise, and introduced the CPSI. Sessions 3 and 4 followed the same pattern as session 2, emphasizing application of the problem-solving techniques via discussion and role-playing. With mixed cancer sites, 59 subjects participated in the intervention while 58 were in the control condition. Screened for variables such as religion, socioeconomic status, race, and demographics, the assessment instruments, including the Profile of Mood States (POMS), the Index of Vulnerability, Therapist Rating Form, Patient Evaluation of Psychosocial Intervention, and the Inventory of Current Concerns, demonstrated the positive psychological impact of the intervention. This intervention increased communication and coping skills in subjects when compared to controls after 6 months. In 1982, Sobel and Worden published the practitioner's manual to guide other professionals in implementing their intervention program for cancer patients (9).

Capone et al. investigated the effectiveness of in-hospital, individual therapy for newly diagnosed patients with gynecologic malignancies (10). Ninety-seven subjects were randomly assigned, regardless of age, race or prognosis, to one of two conditions. The experimental condition of 56 subjects underwent a minimum of four psychological counseling sessions during their hospitalizations for initial gynecologic treatment. The counseling sessions focused on molding reality-based expectations, encouraging adaptive changes in behavior, and processing information. The early counseling sessions, including at least one session prior to initial treatment, concentrated on helping patients express their feelings and fears about their disease and its treatment. These early counseling sessions were also used to help patients better understand their disease and possible treatment outcomes. The middle counseling sessions focused on patients' self-esteem and femininity. The final sessions, including a session shortly prior to discharge from the hospital, dealt primarily with patients' interpersonal relationships. Patients were encouraged to return to their usual roles within their families and social networks. Throughout all of the sessions, discussions of sexuality and sexual concerns were initiated. The experimental group was assessed prior to initial medical treatment, and reassessed

TABLE 59.1. *Psychoeducation Studies, 1978–1980*

Study	Patient Population			Design (No. of Groups)			Time	Intervention	Follow-up end-point	Outcomes							
	Dx	N/M	M/F (n)	R/NR	Exp (n)	Contr. (n)		Content Format Individual or group		Coping	Affect	QOL	Know	Comp	Phys	Immune	R/S
Wood et al. (1978)	Mixed	N & M	M&F	NR	1 (15)	None	8 × 1.5 h over 8 wk	Ed, C (Common issues and concerns) Group	8 wk	+	+		+				
Ferlic et al. (1979)	Mixed	N	M = 30	NR	1 (30)	1 (30)	6 × 1.5 h over 2 wk	Ed, C, ES (Medical, psychological, religious, sexuality, and nutrition issues) Group	6 mo	+			+				
Weisman et al. (1980)	Mixed	NS	M = 41 F = 74	R	1 (59)	1 (58)	4 × ? h over 6 wk	Ed, C, SM, B (Audiotapes, illustrated cards) Group	6 mo	+	+						
Capone et al. (1980)	Gynecologic	N	F = 97	R	1 (56)	1 (41)	4 × ? h during initial hospitalization	Ed, Psy (Concerns about Tx outcome, self-esteem, sexuality, adaptive behavior/role changes molded) Individual	12 mo	+	+						
Gordon et al. (1980)	Breast, lung, MM	N	M = 70 F = 147	NR	1 (157)	1 (151)	≈ 24× 0.5 h × 6 mo	Ed, Psy, C (Medical info, emotional venting, consults and referrals) Individual	6–12 mo	+	+						
Maguire et al. (1980)	Breast	N	F = 153	R	1 (75)	1 (77)	4 × ? h × ? mo	Ed, Psy (Medical/prosthesis info) Individual	18 mo	NC	NC						

Dx, diagnosis; N/M, newly diagnosed versus metastatic recurrence; M/F, male and female; R/NR, randomized/nonrandomized; Exp., experiment; Ed, education; C, coping; SM, stress management; B, behavioral training; ES, emotional support; Psy, psychotherapy; QOL, quality of life; Know, knowledge; Comp, compliance; Phys, physical; R/S, recurrence/survival; MM, malignant melanoma; NC, no changes; blank spaces indicates areas not measured; +, an improvement in intervention group(s); –, a decrease in improvement group(s); X, change over time occured but no difference between groups at end-point; NS, not specified.

upon returning for their 3, 6, and 12 months post-treatment examinations using the Self-Rating Symptom Scale, the POMS, and the Tennessee Self-Concept Scale. Forty-one patient controls who did not receive any counseling were assessed at their 3, 6, and 12 months posttreatment gynecologic exams using the same set of instruments. All of the subjects had similar levels of psychological distress at the start of the study (pretreatment). However, at 3 months post-treatment, the counseled patients reported significantly less emotional upset, confusion, and social isolation than the control patients. Individual counseling interventions during the initial hospitalization had a significant effect in reducing sexual dysfunction specifically related to the diagnosis and treatment of genital cancer. Follow-up results suggested that intervention patients were more likely to return to normal vocational and sexual functions after the first year of treatment.

Gordon et al. collected five different types of data: medical, demographic, behavioral, psychosocial, and a personal interview, to determine the efficacy of counseling interventions for oncology patients (11). The experimental group of 138 patients underwent a systematic program of rehabilitation which included three types of interventions: an educational intervention, which provided patients with information about their disease, the medical system, and how to effectively live with their illness; a counseling intervention, which encouraged patients to express their feelings and reactions; and an environmental manipulation intervention, which included consultations with health care personnel and referral services. One hundred and thirty-one control subjects were evaluated but not offered any form of psychosocial intervention. The intervention patients had a more rapid decline of negative affect, a more active use of time, a higher proportion of vocational return, and a more realistic outlook on life than the control patients. Most importantly, the individual counseling, education, and personnel consultations provided to the experimental group appeared to help them deal more effectively with some of their psychosocial problems.

Maguire et al. conducted a study to determine if counseling by a specialist nurse would prevent the psychiatric morbidity associated with mastectomy in breast cancer patients (12). Seventy-five women were randomized to a counseling intervention condition during their stay on a surgical unit and 77 women to a control condition. The experimental condition consisted of individual sessions with a specialist nurse before and after surgery, as well as follow-up home and clinic visits to monitor progress. During initial contact with the patients in this group, the specialist nurse explored each patient's feelings about her illness, and assessed each patient's available social support. Prior to surgery, the specialist nurse met with each patient for about one hour to assess her ability to cope with daily functioning before and after the onset of disease. The nurse also explored patients' feelings about the disease, attitudes about their bodies, emotional states, and provided any needed information concerning their disease or impending medical procedures. Within a week of surgery, the nurse met with each patient to discuss her reaction to the surgery, and to explore the patient's feelings about her new scar. The patient was provided with information about the various prostheses available, and the nurse reassessed each patient's level of coping. The first home visit by the nurse followed the same format of the postsurgical assessment, as did subsequent follow-up visits. Results of this design failed to show any significant prevention in psychiatric morbidity. However, with regular individual assessment, the nurse was able to refer those patients who needed further psychiatric help. In the absence of close personal contact, only a few control subjects were recognized as being in need of referral. Thus, some individuals who might have benefited from psychiatric care did not receive it. On the other hand, distressed patients in the experimental condition were readily identified and referred for appropriate psychiatric treatment. As a result, the experimental patients showed a reduced level of morbidity 12–18 months after the mastectomy. Overall, this study indicated that the recognition and early detection of psychiatric morbidity and subsequent referral service is a successful way to reduce the high levels of distress and morbidity in breast cancer patients.

1981–1985 (Table 59.2)

Spiegel et al. (1981) performed a prospective intervention study of patients with metastatic breast cancer (13). Experimental patients met weekly in psychological support groups of seven to ten members each for a year. Groups were led by a psychiatrist or social worker and a counselor who had had breast cancer that was in remission. Meetings were informal and consisted of heuristic interpersonal exploration, as well as discussions of death and dying, family problems, treatment issues, communication problems, and living with a terminal illness. Members discussed their issues, concerns, and fears with one another, and taught each other what they had learned from their own personal experiences. At 12 months, experimental

TABLE 59.2. *Psychoeducation Studies, 1981–1985*

Study	Patient Population Dx	N/M	M/F (n)	Design (No. of Groups) R/NR	Exp (n)	Control (n)	Time	Intervention Content Format Individual or group	Follow-up endpoint	Coping	Affect	QOL	Know	Comp	Phys	Immune	R/S
Spiegel et al. (1981)	Breast	M	F = 58	R	1 (34)	1 (24)	52 × 1.5 h over 1 yr	Ed, C, B, ES (Mutual instruction and support based on personal experience) Group	1 yr	+	+						
Johnson (1982)	Mixed	N & M	NS	R	1 (26)	1 (26)	8 × 1.5 h over 4 wk	Ed, C, ES (Course and resource center) Group	4 wk	+	+		+				
Vachon et al. (1982)	Breast RTX	N	F = 168	NR	1 (64)	1 (104)	? × ? h over 3 wk	Ed, C, ES (Met with experienced patients) Group	3 wk		+						
Jacobs et al. (1983)	Hodgkin's	N	M = 32 F = 16	R	1 (21)	1 (26)	Pt. determined	Ed (Info booklet and newsletters) Individual	3 mo	+	+		+				

Study	Dx				n (control)	Duration	Intervention	Follow-up				
Worden and Weisman (1984)	Mixed	N	NS	R	1 (59)	1 (58)	4 × ?h × 1 mo	1: Ed, Psy (Emotional venting, problem-solving) 2: Ed, B (PMR, illustrations) Individual	12 mo	+	+	+	
Forester et al. (1985)	Mixed radiation	N & M	M=50 F=50	R	1 (48)	1 (52)	Weekly × 30 min × 10 wk	Ed, Psy, ES (Q/A, interpretation, catharsis) Individual	10 wk	+	+	+	+
Rainey (1985)	Mixed RTX	N & M	M=30 F=30	NR	1 (30)	1 (30)	12 min	Ed (Radiation therapy slide show) Individual	4–6 wk	+	+	+	+ X
Heinrich and Schag (1985)	Mixed	M	M=35 F=16	NR	1 (26)	1 (25)	6 × 12h over 6 wk	Ed, C, SM, B, ES (Discussions, lectures, handouts, tapes) Group	4 mo	+	+	+	NC

Dx, diagnosis; N/M, newly diagnosed versus metastatic recurrence; M/F, male and female; R/NR, randomized/nonrandomized; Exp., experiment; Ed, education; C, coping; SM, stress management; B, behavioral training; ES, emotional support; Psy, psychotherapy; PMR, progressive muscle relaxation; QOL, quality of life; Know, knowledge; Comp, compliance; Phys, physical; R/S, recurrence/survival; NC, no changes; RTX, radiotherapy; Q/A, questions and answers; blank spaces indicate areas not measured; +, an improvement in intervention group(s); −, a decrease in intervention group(s); X, change over time occured but no difference between groups at end-point; NS, not specified.

patients showed significantly less tension, less fatigue, less confusion, and more vigor than those in the control group. In addition, there was a significant reduction in levels of pain. A trend toward having less depression, fewer maladjusted coping responses, and fewer phobias was also apparent.

Johnson (1982) paired, then randomized, 52 newly diagnosed or recurrent cancer patients to an education group, who participated in eight 90 minute structured educational sessions over a period of 4 weeks, or to a control group (14). The patient education course, titled "I Can Cope," covered topics such as learning about the disease, coping with daily health problems, communicating with others, liking yourself, living with limits, and finding appropriate resources. A learning resource center was available for the group, containing books, tapes, films, and games related to each topic. The control group was exposed to neither the education group nor the learning resource center. Patients were measured pre- and postintervention for anxiety, knowledge about cancer, and perceived purpose and meaningfulness in life (i.e., cognitive coping). The structured intervention positively affected all three dependent variables.

Vachon et al. (1982) compared 64 women with breast cancer who resided at a Hospital Lodge while going through approximately 3 weeks of radiation therapy to 104 women who went through their therapy while living at home (15). Patients stayed in the Lodge because they lived too far from the hospital to commute for their radiation therapy treatments. The Lodge provided "Coping with Cancer" support groups. In these groups patients were given disease and treatment information, they discussed their concerns about survival, self-esteem, relationships, and role changes, and they met with patients who had completed therapy and were doing well. These experienced patients served as role models, and were able to provide patients with suggestions about maintaining autonomy, coping with others, and communicating with physicians. It was not clear how many group sessions were held during the 3 weeks. Affective state was assessed via the General Health Questionnaire. Residence in the Lodge with attendance in the groups was associated with a decreased chance of change for the worse in affective state and an increased chance of change for the better.

Jacobs et al. (1983) employed a purely educational intervention in a randomized study of patients with Hodgkin's disease (16). Twenty-one experimental patients received a 27 page booklet including information about the diagnosis, staging, treatment methods and problems, and prognosis. The experimental groups also received newsletters regarding current advances in Hodgkin's disease treatment and a question and answer section. Three months later the intervention group had increased their knowledge levels compared to the 26 control patients. On the Cancer Patient Behavior Scale, intervention patients also showed decreased anxiety and treatment problems. They showed a trend for decreased depression and life disruption but also, interestingly, a decrease in social competency. The authors suggested that increased knowledge led to more self-awareness and therefore more self-consciousness in social situations.

Examining a completely different oncology population, Worden and Weisman (1984) studied the effectiveness of preventive psychosocial interventions in 381 newly diagnosed cancer patients (17). Prescreened and approached if at a high risk for emotional distress and poor coping, subjects were randomly divided into either a 1 month or a 2 months intervention program or a control condition. Intervention A was based on a patient-centered, psychotherapeutic model which focused on clarifying personal problems, expressing appropriate affect, and encouraging the patient to explore methods of problem solving. Intervention B emphasized cognitive skill training and behavior therapy to help patients learn a specific approach to cope with common problems generally experienced by cancer patients. Patients in this intervention group were presented with illustrations depicting a problem followed by corresponding illustrations which showed the same problem solved. Patients in this group were also trained in progressive body relaxation. Each intervention consisted of individual sessions with a psychologist and a follow-up meeting with a social worker at 2, 4, 6, and 12 months after the therapist–patient relationship was terminated. Using the POMS, Index of Vulnerability, and Inventory of Current Concerns, they reported a significant lowering of emotional distress as well as an increase in coping skills in the intervention group. Although the number of problems experienced by both groups was similar, the patients receiving counseling had a significant increase in their level of problem resolution.

Forester and colleagues (1985) set out to determine the effects of ongoing individual psychotherapy for patients receiving radiotherapy treatment (18). Fifty-two randomly assigned subjects served as controls while 48 subjects received weekly counseling sessions for 10 weeks, 4 weeks beyond the period of radiotherapy. Counseling sessions combined supportive therapy with educational, interpretive, and cathartic components. The educational components included answering patients' questions and providing appropriate reassurances. Interpretive components involved therapist's interpretations of patients' issues and psychological coping mechanisms, and encouraging patients to develop more appropriate ways of dealing with their emotions. Cathartic components involved therapists encouraging patients to openly express their emotions. This component of the therapy was particularly useful among the men, who may have been less inhibited about spontaneous communication during the therapy sessions. A significant reduction in physical and emotional distress was found in the psychotherapy patients. Within the experimental group there were further differences. For example, even though men seemed to suffer more distress than women, they demonstrated a better therapeutic response to psychotherapy.

Rainey (1985) tested 30 sequential radiation therapy patients for knowledge and emotional status using the state component of the State-Trait Anxiety scale and the Profile of Mood States Total Mood Disturbance score (TMD) (19). The next 30 patients were provided with a 12 minute educational slide-show about radiation therapy prior to testing. The slide program included: an introduction of the radiation oncology professionals and their roles; types of radiation therapy equipment; an outline of the treatment procedures; an explanation of what the patient will experience during the treatment; information on how radiation therapy works; clarification of common misconceptions about radiation therapy; an explicit statement encouraging patients to seek further information about their treatment. Both groups were then retested at the end of radiation therapy approximately 4–6 weeks later. The intervention group scored higher on the initial knowledge test but there was no difference between groups for anxiety or TMD. By the follow-up point both groups demonstrated equally high levels of knowledge, but the intervention group had lower levels of state anxiety and TMD.

Heinrich and Schag (1985) studied 26 patients with various cancer diagnoses who participated in a Stress and Activity Management group (SAM) to 25 patients who were in a Current Available Care (CAC) control group (20). Patients were not randomized but recruited in sequential groups of about ten to whatever condition was open at the time they were recruited. Twelve spouses in the treatment group and 13 in the control group also participated. SAM was a comprehensive, structured 6 week group designed to educate patients and their spouses about cancer and its impact, and to teach skills for stress management and physical activity. Components of the treatment included cancer and stress education, relaxation exercise, problem solving,

and physical exercise. Groups lasted 2 hours, and information was presented through discussions, handouts, audio tapes, slides, lectures, and homework. Patients were assessed pretreatment, posttreatment, and 2 and 4 months later using the Karnofsky Performance Status Scale, Cancer Information test, the Psychosocial Adjustment to Illness Scale (PAIS) and the Depression, Anxiety, and Global Severity Index from the SCL-90-R, Quality of Life, and Daily Activity Diary. Patients and spouses in the SAM group all showed an increase in knowledge even though most of the patients had been dealing with their cancer for over 2 years. SAM patients and spouses reported being able to cope better and had a better attitude towards treatment. There was no difference between groups in psychosocial adjustment to illness. This may have been a function of the instrument used (PAIS), which may not have been sensitive enough to pick up differences in this population even though it is very useful in extremely ill patients.

1986–1990 (Table 59.3)

Houts et al. (1986) randomly assigned 32 newly diagnosed gynecological cancer patients to either extra counseling services or regular support services (21). They created four possible coping strategies within the experimental condition. These were to maintain normal relations with family and friends, to make positive plans for the future, to ask the medical staff any and all questions, and to keep up "normal" routines whenever possible. These four coping skills were presented to the experimental condition in two separate interventions: the first group was introduced to the coping skills by experienced social workers who had once had cancer themselves, the second group was simply given a notebook and audio cassette which explained the coping strategies. Measured with the POMS questionnaire at baseline, 6 weeks, and 12 weeks, this study found no statistically significant data to support the authors hypothesis that former cancer patients would serve as better counselors to newly diagnosed patients than other therapists.

Cain et al. (1986) randomly assigned 80 women with gynecological cancer to a thematic individual, thematic group, or standard counseling modes (22). Patients in the thematic individual or thematic group counseling modes participated in eight weekly sessions conducted by social workers. The themes of these counseling sessions included the nature of cancer, causes, impact of treatment particularly on body image and sexuality, relaxation, diet and exercise, relating to caregivers, talking with family and friends, and goal setting.

TABLE 59.3. *Psychoeducation Studies, 1986–1990*

Study	Patient Population Dx	N/M	M/F (n)	Design R/NR	Exp (n)	Control (n)	Time	Intervention Content Format Individual or group	Follow-up endpoint	Coping	Affect	QOL	Know	Comp	Phys	Immune	R/S
Houts et al. (1986)	Gynecologic	N	F=32	R	1 (14)	1 (18)	Three calls over 12 wks	Ed, Psy C 1: Instructor with cancer 2: Book and audiotape Individual	12 wk	NC	NC						
Cain et al. (1986)	Gynecologic	N	F=80	R	1 (21) 2 (28)	1 (31)	8 × 2 h over 8 wk	Ed, C, B, ES (Exercise, relaxation, goals) 1: Individual 2: Group	6 mo	+ +	+ +						
Telch and Telch (1986)	Mixed	N & M	M=14 F=27	R	1 (13) 2 (14)	1 (14)	6 × 1.5 h over 6 wk	1: Ed, C, SM, B (PMR, role-playing) 2: ES (venting) 3: Control Group	3 mo	+ NC —	+ NC —						
Eardly (1987)	Mixed	N	M=29 F=71	R	1 (200)	1 (215)	Booklet received prior to radiotherapy	Ed (Radiotherapy booklet) Individual	? days				+				

Author	Dx	N/M	M/F	R/NR	Group (n)	Duration	Intervention	Individual/Group	Follow-up	Outcomes
Ali and Khalil (1989)	Bladder	N	M=23 F=7	R	1 (15); 1 (15)	30–60 min	Ed (Preop information)	Individual	12 days	+
Cunningham and Tocco (1989)	Mixed	N & M	M=14 F=35	R, N, R	1 (28); 2 (25); 3 (39)	6 × 2h over 6 wk	1: Ed, C, ES; 2 & 3: Ed, C, ES, SM, B, PMR, GI, lifestyle management	Group	3 mo	+ +
Spiegel et al. (1989)*	Breast	M	F=58	R	1 (34)	52 × 1.5h over 1 yr	Ed, C, B, ES	Group	10 yr	+
Richardson et al. (1990)	Mixed hematology	N	M=59 F=35	R	1 (22); 2 (23); 3 (24)	1: 1h + home visit; 2: 1h + hospital; 3: 1h + hospital and home visit	1: Ed Cueing; 2: Ed Shaping; 3: Ed Cueing and Shaping	Individual	6 mo	+ +
Fawzy et al. (1990)	MM	N	M=47 F=53	R	1 (38); 1 (28)	6 × 1.5h over 6 wk	Ed, C, SM, B, ES (PMR, GI, illustrations)	Group	6 mo	+ + +

Dx, diagnosis; N/M, newly diagnosed versus metastatic recurrence; M/F, male and female; R/NR, randomixed/nonrandomized; Exp., experiment; Ed, education; C, coping; SM, stress management; B, behavioral training; ES, emotional support; Psy, psychotherapy; PMR, progressive muscle relaxation; GI, guided imagery; QOL, quality of life; Know, knowledge; Comp, compliance; Phys, physical; R/S, recurrence/survival; MM, malignant melanoma; NC, no changes; RTX, radiotherapy; Q/A, questions and answers; blank spaces indicates areas not measured; +, an improvement in intervention group(s); X, change over time occured but no difference between groups at end-point; NS, not specified.
*Follow-up of earlier study.

Patients in the individual mode were seen either in the hospital or at home, and also received information from an oncology nurse about cancer, treatment, and diet. The group mode included four to six women who participated in meetings held at the hospital, and received information from a dietitian and an oncology nurse, an oncologic fellow, or a radiologist. The patients in the standard counseling mode served as control subjects, and participated in the usual interactions between patients and their physicians, nurses, and social workers. Coping and adjustment was measured by the PAIS and affective state via the Hamilton Depression Rating Scale. It was concluded that either the individual or group counseling were equally effective in decreasing anxiety and depression and increasing adjustment to the illness up to 6 months later. The authors also claimed that the intervention patients were significantly more knowledgeable about their illness and treatment, but there was no objective measurement of knowledge included in the design.

Forty-one cancer patients with different diagnoses and stages of disease who were exhibiting marked levels of psychosocial distress were randomized by Telch and Telch (1986) to: *(1)* a coping skills instruction group; *(2)* an emotional support group; or *(3)* a no treatment control group (23). Groups were led by either a doctoral student in counseling psychology or a licensed clinical social worker. The two intervention groups met once a week for 6 weeks for about 90 minutes each session. The coping skills groups had a set agenda emphasizing the teaching and rehearsal of cognitive, behavioral, and affective coping strategies. One of five topics was presented each week, including relaxation and stress management, communication, problem-solving and constructive thinking, feelings management, and activity planning. Patients learned coping techniques through coaching, rehearsal and role-playing, homework assignments, and self-monitoring. The emotional support group was unstructured and geared towards encouraging patients to express feelings and emotions. The control group received no psychological intervention. Patients were assessed pregroup and immediately after the 6 week groups. The primary instruments were the POMS, to assess affective state and the Cancer Inventory of Problem Situations (CIPS). The coping skills group showed consistent improvement in affective state, satisfaction related to work, social activities, physical appearance, sexual intimacy, physical and social activities, cognitive distress, communications, and coping with medical procedures. Patients in the emotional support group showed little or no improvement while

the control patients actually had deterioration in their psychological functioning.

Eardly (1987) conducted a study of the impact of pretreatment education on levels of worry among patients scheduled for a course of radiotherapy (24). Along with a letter of admission to the radiotherapy center, patients in an experimental group received a booklet which provided a description of the treatment, side-effects, and follow-up care. A control group received only a letter of admission. Shortly after receiving the admission letters, patients in both groups received questionnaires designed to assess levels of worry about radiotherapy; 200 patients who had received education booklets and 215 who had not received booklets responded to the questionnaire. In terms of overall worry, there were no differences between those who had received the booklet and those who had not. However, there was a significantly smaller proportion of patients in the experimental group who expressed concerns about hair loss, and who had worries other than those listed on the questionnaire. A significantly greater proportion of patients who had received the booklet reported that they were satisfied with the amount of information that they had received about their treatment.

Ali and Khalil (1989) conducted a 30–60 minute preoperative intervention for 30 bladder cancer patients 1–2 days prior to urinary diversion (25). This consisted of providing information about the procedure, site, and appearance of the stoma, and external collection devices and a visit from a "well-functioning" ostomate patient. In addition, patients were encouraged to express their fears and anxieties. The outcome measure used was state anxiety, which they found to be decreased on the third and twelfth days postoperatively.

Cunningham and Tocco (1989), randomly assigned 60 cancer patients with mixed diagnoses to one of two treatments: *(1)* supportive discussion group with education in coping skills, or *(2)* a supportive discussion group alone (26). Both groups of seven to ten members each participated in six weekly, 2 hour sessions with one leader. In addition to supportive discussion, ventilation of feelings, general problem-solving, and information sharing, the psychoeducational intervention included the following components: two sessions of relaxation training, including progressive muscle relaxation and self-hypnosis, two sessions on the use of guided imagery, a session on goal setting and a session on general lifestyle management. The latter session specifically dealt with diet, exercise, work, recreation, and discussion of spiritual issues. The authors referred to the second group as the "control" intervention which consisted of just the supportive discussion, ventilation of feelings, general problem-solving, and information sharing. Another group of 18 patients who delayed starting the intervention for 6 weeks were also tested and served as a nonrandomized control group. These three groups were all tested pregroup, immediately postgroup, and 2–3 weeks later. Furthermore, a fourth group of 39 patients, who were also nonrandomized, participated in the psychoeducational intervention and were followed for 3 months. Assessments were done with the POMS and the SCL-90-R, both measures of affective state. Both intervention groups showed a significant improvement in affective state compared to the no treatment "control" group. The psychoeducational group showed a greater gain. The 39 patients in the fourth group demonstrated a sustained improvement to the 3 months follow-up period.

In 1989, Spiegel et al. performed a 10-year follow-up of their previous study (13). Of the original 86 subjects, only three patients were alive and death records were obtained for the remaining 83. Survival time was significantly different, with means of 36.3 months in the intervention' group compared with 18.9 months in the control group. Lower mood disturbance and higher ratings of vigor on the POMS at the end of the intervention period were significantly associated with greater longevity (27).

Richardson et al. randomly assigned 94 newly diagnosed hematology patients to either a control group or one of three educational intervention groups (28). The purpose of the intervention was to increase compliance in taking the medications allopurinol and prednisone. Each of the intervention groups consisted of a one-hour educational session using an interactive slide-tape presentation with a nurse who discussed the disease, its treatment, side effects, and patient's responsibility in compliance. In addition to this educational component, each of the three experimental groups also underwent one of the following intervention programs. One program was a four level pill-shaping component carried out in the hospital prior to discharge, in which patients increasingly took more responsibility for the administration of their medications. Patients began by learning the purpose, nature, side effects, and schedules of the drugs, then identified their pills by name and dosage to the nurse, then alerting the nurse when it was time to take their medication, and finally being given the responsibility of self-medication under the nurse's supervision. Another intervention program included a home visit from the nurse within one week of discharge from the hospital. During this visit, the nurse helped the patient to develop a system for pill

taking which was related to their daily routines. The final intervention program comprised a combination of the pill-shaping and home visit. Patients in the control group did not receive any of these interventions, but did receive standard explanations of their disease, treatment, and side effects. Compliance was measured using blood levels of two drugs and a record of whether or not the patients kept the monthly clinic appointment during 6 months. Survival was measured in days from enrollment in the study to death within the 6 months. Compliance was accomplished equally by all three of the educational interventions for allopurinol but not for prednisone. Appointment keeping was positively enhanced by all three interventions. Using regression analysis it was concluded that low severity of disease, assignment to an educational program (any one), plus high allopurinol compliance were predictive of increased survival in patients with newly diagnosed hematological malignancy.

Fawzy et al. (1990) recognized that a variety of therapies resulted in some positive effects but that the variance accounted for by each of these alone was small. Therefore, specific portions of those interventions that were found to be effective and appropriate were combined in a 6 week structured group intervention which was tailored to encompass health education, stress management, coping skills, and supportive group psychotherapy (29).

Health care information specific to the particular type of cancer was provided. The stress management component was divided into two main sections. First, the patients were taught about stress awareness which was defined as identifying the sources of stress and their personal reactions to it. The second component was the actual management of stress. Patients were taught simple relaxation exercises, including progressive muscle relaxation followed by guided imagery or self-hypnosis. In the coping skills component of the intervention, patients were first taught the components of problem-solving and were then introduced to the concept of coping methods. The final part of the coping skills component involved integrating the stress management and problem-solving techniques with the information on coping methods and applying these to specific situations. The method used was modeled after Project Omega (8,9). New pictures illustrating ten common problems/situations encountered by cancer patients were developed (30). Psychological support was inherent throughout the intervention. The interaction of patients within the group provided a significant source of emotional support.

This intervention was used for a group of newly diagnosed malignant melanoma patients who had undergone standard surgical treatment. Patients were randomly assigned to either a control group receiving routine medical care or to an experimental group receiving the same kind of routine medical care plus the intervention described above.

All the patients reported moderate to high levels of psychological distress at baseline comparable to other cancer patients. However, at the end of the 6 week structured group intervention, the experimental subjects exhibited significantly lower levels of distress than the control subjects. Six months following the intervention, the group differences were even more pronounced. The experimental group reported significantly lower levels of confusion, depression, fatigue, and total mood disturbance, and higher levels of vigor on the POMS.

Immediately following the 6 week structured intervention, the experimental subjects showed significantly greater use of active-behavioral coping methods than the control subjects. In addition, the experimental subjects used significantly more active-positive, active-expressive, active-reliance, cognitive-positive, and distraction coping strategies. Six months following the intervention, the experimental patients continued to use significantly more active-behavioral coping methods as well as more active-cognitive coping methods than the controls.

At the end of the 6 week intervention, there was a significant increase in the percentage of LGLs (defined as CD57 with Leu7). Six months following the intervention, there continued to be an increase in the percentage of LGLs (defined as CD57 with Leu7) as well as increases in NK cells (defined as CD16 with Leu11 and CD56 with Leu19) and interferon-α augmented NK cell cytotoxicity (31).

In both experimental and control subjects combined, quality of life was strongly negatively correlated with anxiety, depression, anger, confusion, and total mood disturbance at 6 months follow-up. As negative affective state decreased through lower levels of anxiety, depression, anger, confusion, and total mood disturbance, the quality of life of these patients increased.

1991–1994 (Table 59.4)

Edgar et al. evaluated the emotional coping skills of 205 newly diagnosed cancer patients throughout a one-year period using 4 month assessments (32). Two interventions were tested: *(1)* an early intervention condition which began immediately after diagnosis; and *(2)* a later intervention, which began after a 4 month delay. Both conditions included five individual one-hour sessions with a nurse, with each one addressing

a specific issue: goal setting, in which patients set gradual, realistic goals in order to accomplish tasks and increase their sense of personal control; cognitive reappraisal, in which patients were taught to recognize and control thought processes which may contribute to negative moods; problem-solving techniques, in which patients were taught specific steps for problem-solving; effective use of resources, a multidisciplinary workshop which provided basic information about the health care system, professionals, and resource groups; and relaxation training, including progressive muscle relaxation, passive relaxation, visualization, and autogenic imagery. At the 8 month assessment, the later intervention group was found to be less depressed, anxious and worried than the early intervention participants. During the course of the year-long study, the later intervention group continued to have less anxiety, though all subjects improved in emotional coping skills by the end of the year. The authors suggested that patients with low ego strength pose a higher risk for psychological complications and may benefit from a psychosocial intervention.

Pruitt et al. (1992) randomized 31 radiation therapy patients with mixed diagnoses to either a three session intervention (one hour each session) or to a standard control group (33). The first session usually occurred during the second week of radiotherapy, and was performed by a chaplain with expertise in oncology. This session, which focused on basic radiation therapy information, included a video-tape and a question/answer component. A week after the first session, the second session was performed by a clinical nurse-specialist. Following a review of session one, the second session focused on common problems and coping skills. A week after the second session, the third session was performed by a social worker. Following a review of session two, session three focused on the importance of communicating areas of concern, and included a communication skills assessment. Knowledge using an author constructed instrument, psychological distress using the Brief Symptom Inventory, and current concerns using the Inventory of Current Concerns were measured at baseline, 1 month and 3 months post-intervention. Knowledge levels were unchanged in both groups. This finding which was attributed to the older age of the patients and their high anxiety levels. Depression was the only measure of affective state found to improve. Health concerns, existential concerns and self-appraisal were the areas of concern that showed the greatest correlation with affective state measures. Although coping strategies and communication skills were taught, they were not directly measured.

TABLE 59.4. *Psychoeducation Studies, 1991–1994*

Study	Patient Population			Design (No. of Groups)			Time	Intervention Content Format Individual or group	Follow-up endpoint	Outcomes							
	Dx	N/M	M/F (n)	R/NR	Exp (n)	Control (n)				Coping	Affect	QOL	Know	Comp	Phys	Immune	R/S
Edgar et al. (1992)	Mixed	N & M	M = 52 F = 153	R	1 (103) 2 (102)	None	5 × 1 h	Ed, Psy, B (PMR, GI, goal-setting) 1: Early 2: Late Individual	1 yr	+ +	+						
Pruitt et al. (1992)	Mixed RTX	N	M = 22 F = 9	R	1 (15)	1 (16)	3 × 1 h	Ed, C, ES (Radiation therapy info, video, Q/A) Individual	3 mo		+	NC					
Greer et al. (1992)	Mixed	M	M = 32 F = 124	R	1 (72)	1 (84)	6 × 1 h × 8 wk	Ed, Psy, C, B (PMR, role-play, emotional venting) Individual	4 mo	+	+						
Cunning-ham et al. (1993)	Mixed	N & M	M = 95 F = 307	N R	1 (402)	None	7 × 2 h over 7 wk	Ed, C, B, ES Group	5 mo	+	+						
Cella et al. (1993)	Mixed	N & M	M = 14 F = 63	N R	1 (77)	None	8 × ?h over 8 wk	Ed, C, ES (Mutal exchange, support) Group	8 wk	+	+	+					

(continued)

TABLE 59.4. *Psychoeducation Studies, 1991–1994—Continued*

Study	Patient Population			Design (No. of Groups)				Intervention		Follow-up end-point	Outcomes							
	Dx	N/M	M/F (n)	R/NR	Exp (n)	Control (n)	Time	Content Format Individual or group			Coping	Affect	QOL	Know	Comp	Phys	Immune	R/S
Fawzy et al. (1993)	MM	N	M=33 F=35	R	1 (34)	1 (34)	6 × 1.5h over 6 wk	Ed, C, SM, B, ES	Group	6 yr								+
Moorey et al. (1993)*	Mixed	N & M	M=32 F=124	R	1 (72)	1 (84)	1 year follow-up	Ed, Psy, B, C	Individual	1 yr	+	+						
Berglund et al. (1994)	Mixed	N & M	M=7 F=192	R	1 (98)	11 (101)	11 × 2h over 7 wk	Ed, C, SM (Physical training, diet, medical info)	Group	12 wk	+		+	+		+		
Brandenberg et al. (1994)	MM		M=107 F=124	R	1 (77)	1 (72) Interested 1 (67) Not interested	1 × 1.5h	Ed (Brochure and meeting)	Group	3 mo	+	+		+		+		

Dx, diagnosis; N/M, newly diagnosed versus metastatic recurrence; M/F, male and female; R/NR, randomized/nonrandomized; Exp., experiment; Ed, education; C, coping; SM, stress management; B, behavioral training; ES, emotional support; Psy, psychotherapy; PMR, progressive muscle relaxation; GI, guided imagery; Know, knowledge; Comp, compliance; Phys, physical; R/S, recurrence/survival; MM, malignant melanoma; NC, no changes; blank spaces indicate areas not measured; +, an improvement in intervention group(s); –, a decrease in intervention group(s); X, change over time occured but no difference between groups at end-point; NS, not specified.
*Follow-up of earlier study.

Cancer patients with confirmed malignant disease were selected to participate in a randomized controlled trial to determine the effects of adjuvant psychological therapy. Greer et al. (1992), measured 174 patients using the Hospital Anxiety and Depression Scales, the Rotterdam Symptom Checklist, Mental Adjustment to Cancer Scale, and the Psychosocial Adjustment to Illness Scale (PAIS) over a period of 8 weeks (34). The experimental condition included a brief, problem focused, cognitive-behavioral program specifically designed to meet the needs of individual cancer patients. The six one-hour therapy sessions focused on the current problems experienced by the patient, and used cognitive and behavioral techniques to approach various coping strategies. Techniques included: identifying the patient's personal strengths to promote self-esteem and overcome feelings of helplessness; identifying and challenging negative thoughts; using role-playing to cope with impending stressful events; encouraging open expression and communication of emotions between patient and spouse; and teaching progressive muscle relaxation to reduce anxiety. The control condition received no therapy. At 8 weeks, the therapy group had statistically significant lower scores than control patients on helplessness, fatalism, anxiety, and psychological symptoms, and they had higher scores on fighting spirit. During a follow-up assessment 4 months later, therapy patients continued to have lower scores than control subjects on anxiety, psychological symptoms, and psychological distress. The authors concluded that the adjuvant psychological therapy approach, geared towards assisting cancer patients, produced significant improvement in dealing with their serious illnesses.

Cunningham et al. (1993) used the POMS, the Functional Living Index for Cancer, and the Stanford Inventory of Cancer Patient Adjustment to assess improvements in the quality of life among 400 cancer patients who completed a brief support group program intended to train patients in coping skills (35). Results showed that subgroups based on religious status, gender, education level, marital status, and previous experience with mental self-help techniques did not vary significantly, but the overall program increased coping skills and enhanced mood states for most subjects involved. The seven session intervention appeared to benefit younger patients somewhat more than older ones, and, at the 3 month follow-up, positive improvements remained. There was no random selection or a control group used in this study.

Cella et al. (1993) detailed an 8 week support group for 77 cancer patients in a local community (36). Groups were comprised of 8–12 persons with cancer and a professional facilitator. Facilitators encouraged open exchange and mutual support between group members. There was no random selection or a control group in this study. As expected, self-reported quality of life improved significantly by the final session, compared to reports completed at the start of the intervention. Community and peer support was noted by participants as the most helpful aspect of the program and the group evaluations showed high satisfaction levels in all areas.

In a follow-up of their previous study (30,31), Fawzy et al. (1993) measured recurrence and survival in patients with malignant melanoma who had participated in a 6 week structured psychiatric group intervention 5–6 years earlier. For the control group, there was a trend for recurrence (13/34) and statistically significant greater rate of death (10/34) than for the experimental patients (7/34 and 3/34, respectively).

Treatment effect remained significant even after adjusting for significant covariates. Moreover, results indicated that *higher levels* of baseline affective distress, baseline coping, and enhancement of active-behavioral coping were predictive of *lower rates* of recurrence and death. These results suggest that the psychiatric intervention may have enhanced effective coping, reduced affective distress, and ultimately had a beneficial effect on survival and recurrence at 6 year follow-up (37).

In 1993, Moorey et al. (1994) completed a one-year follow-up of their previous study (38). The experimental patients continued to exhibit less anxiety and depression than controls, justifying further investigation of the benefits and efficacy of brief, adjuvant psychological therapy interventions for newly diagnosed cancer patients.

Berglund et al. established a prospective randomized study with 98 cancer patients who took part in a rehabilitation program and 101 patients who served as controls (39). The intervention, which focused on "starting again," consisted of 11 structured, 2 hour sessions led by an oncology nurse during a period of 7 weeks. A physical trainer led four sessions to increase mobility, strength, and fitness, and taught relaxation techniques, including progressive muscle relaxation, and guided imagery. A psychologist led three sessions to teach coping skills, including how to handle returning to work, interacting with others, anxiety, and medical check-ups. Four information sessions were conducted by the following professionals: an oncologist, who provided information about cancer, radiation, chemotherapy, and hormonal treatments; a psychologist, who provided information about emotional reactions to different phases of the illness;

a dietitian, who provided information about health, diet, and food preparation; and an oncological nurse, who provided information about alternative treatments and health centers. Assessments were made using the Cancer Inventory of Problem Situations, the Quality of Life (two global items) scale, and the Mental Adjustment to Cancer Scale. Subjects in the experimental condition improved significantly in physical training, physical strength, fighting spirit, body image, sufficient information, and decreased sleeping problems, when compared to the control patients. All three goals of the intervention were met, and results indicated that the "Starting Again" program has many beneficial effects for cancer patients.

Brandenberg et al. (1994) randomly assigned 149 patients who had received surgical treatment for malignant melanoma to either a an experimental information group (I) or a control (C) group (40). A group of 67 patients not interested (NI) in participating in the intervention group served as a second control group. Prior to their first follow-up visit, patients in the I group received a brochure "Malignant Melanoma and Skin Cancer," and attended a $1\frac{1}{2}$ hour information meeting lead by a nurse with melanoma expertise. At the information meeting, patients were provided with further information about melanoma, risk factors, prevention, and medical procedures. The C and NI groups did not receive additional information prior to their first follow-up visit. Questionnaires were administered to each group at discharge following their surgery and again at their first follow-up visit. Both questionnaires included items concerning psychosomatic complaints, the HAD scale to measure depressive and anxiety symptoms, and knowledge of melanoma. The second questionnaire also included items measuring concern for nevi (a risk factor), emotional reactions, and satisfaction with information. Assessment after first follow-up indicated that higher proportion of patients was satisfied with the information and a higher level of knowledge was found in the I group as compared to the C group. No differences were noted in concern for nevi on any of the psychological or psychosomatic measures between the I and C groups.

CONCLUSION

The psychological and medical problems encountered by cancer patients are numerous and unique. Based on a review of the literature and the authors' clinical and research experience, cancer patients may benefit from a variety of psychological intervention programs. A structured, psychoeducational intervention consisting of health education, coping including problem-solving techniques, stress management, and/or behavioral training, and psychosocial group support offers the greatest potential benefit for patients newly diagnosed or in the early stages of their treatment. Patients are usually distressed, anxious, and unable to effectively utilize their normal coping styles. A structured intervention offered early on during the course of cancer diagnosis and treatment may be less stigmatizing and more readily accepted by both patients and staff and easily integrated into the comprehensive medical care of cancer patients. The advantages of such a program include easy implementation and replication, promotion of important illness-related problem-solving skills, and increased participation in decision making and active coping. A short-term, structured, psychoeducational group intervention is the model that the authors propose to be used for newly diagnosed and/or patients with good prognosis. The focus is on learning how to live with cancer. We also encourage the development of ongoing weekly group support programs for patients with advanced metastatic disease based on Spiegel's work (13,26) that focus on daily coping, pain management, and dealing with the existential issues related to death and dying. Psychoeducational interventions should be used as an integral part of competent, comprehensive medical care and not as an independent treatment modality for cancer.

REFERENCES

1. Cohen J, Cullen J, Martin L. *Psychosocial Aspects of Cancer.* New York: Raven Press; 1982.
2. Fawzy FI, Fawzy NW. Psychosocial aspects of cancer. *Diagnosis and Management of Cancer.* Menlo Park, CA: Addison-Wesley; 1982.
3. Cassileth B, Volckmar D, Goodman RL. The effect of experience on radiation therapy patients desire for information. *Int J Radiat Oncol Biol Phys.* 1980; 6: 493–496.
4. Massie MJ, Holland JC, Straker N. Psychotherapeutic interventions. *Handbook of Psychooncology.* New York: Oxford University Press; 1989: 455–469.
5. Holland J. The current concepts and challenges in psychosocial oncology. *Current Concepts in Psychosocial Oncology: Syllabus of Postgraduate Course.* New York: Memorial Sloan-Kettering Cancer Center; 1982.
6. Wood PE, Milligan M, Christ D, Liff D. Group counseling for cancer patients in a community hospital. *Psychosomatics.* 1978; 19(9):555–561.
7. Ferlic M, Goldman A, Kennedy BJ. Group counseling in adult patients with advanced cancer. *Cancer.* 1979; 43:760–766.
8. Weisman AD, Worden JW, Sobel HJ. *Psychosocial Screening and Intervention with Cancer Patients: Research Report.* Cambridge, MA: Shea; 1980.

9. Sobel HJ, Worden JW. *Practitioner's Manual: Helping Cancer Patients Cope.* New York: Guilford Publications; 1982: 1–32.

10. Capone MA, Good RS, Westie KS, Jacobson AF. Psychosocial rehabilitation of gynecologic oncology patients. *Arch Phys Med Rehabil.* 1980; 61:128–132.

11. Gordon WA, Freidenbergs I, Diller L, et al. Efficacy of psychosocial intervention with cancer patients. *J Consult Clin Psychol.* 1980; 48(6):743–759.

12. Maguire P, Tait A, Brooke M, et al. Effect of counseling on the psychiatric morbidity associated with mastectomy. *Br Med J.* 1980; 281:1454–1456.

13. Spiegel D, Bloom JR, Yalom I. Group support for patients with metastatic cancer. *Arch Gen Psychiatry.* 1981; 38:527–533.

14. Johnson J. The effects of a patient education course on persons with a chronic illness. *Cancer Nurs.* 1982; April:117–123.

15. Vachon MLS, Lyall WAL, Rogers J, et al. The effectiveness of psyhosocial support during post-surgical treatment of breast cancer. *Int J Psychiatry Med.* 1981/82; 11(4):365–372.

16. Jacobs C, Ross RD, Walker IM, Stockdale FE. Behavior of cancer patients: a randomized study of the effects of education and peer support groups. *Am J Clin Oncol.* 1983; 6:347–353.

17. Worden JW, Weisman AD. Preventive psychosocial intervention with newly diagnosed cancer patients. *Gen Hosp Psychiatry.* 1984; 6:243–249.

18. Forester B, Kornfeld DS, Fleiss JL. Psychotherapy during radiotherapy: effects on emotional and physical distress. *Am J Psychiatry.* 1985; 142:22–27.

19. Rainey LC. Effects of preparatory patient education for radiation oncology patients. *Cancer.* 1985; 56:1056–1061.

20. Heinreich RL, Schag CC. Stress and activity management: group treatment for cancer patients and spouses. *J Consult Clin Psychol.* 1982; 33(4):439–446.

21. Houts PS, Whitney CW, Mortel R, Bartholomew MJ. Former cancer patients as counselors of newly diagnosed cancer patients. *J Nat Cancer Inst.* 1986; 76(5):793–796.

22. Cain EN, Kohorn EI, Quinland DM, et al. Psychosocial benefits of a cancer support group. *Cancer.* 1986; 57: 183–189.

23. Telch CF, Telch MJ. Group coping skills instruction and supportive group therapy for cancer patients: a comparison of strategies. *J Consult Clin Psychol.* 1986; 54(6):802–808.

24. Eardley, A. Patient's worries about radiotherapy: evaluation of a preparatory booklet. *Psychol Health.* 1988; 2:79–89.

25. Ali NS, Khalil HZ. Effect of psychoeducational intervention on anxiety among Egyptian bladder cancer patients. *Cancer Nurs.* 1989; 12(4):236–242.

26. Cunningham AJ, Tocco EK. A randomized trial of group psychoeducational therapy for cancer patients. *Patient Educ Counsel.* 1989; 14:101–114.

27. Spiegel D, Bloom JR, Kraemer HC, Gottheil E. Effect of psychosocial treatment on survival of patients with metastatic breast cancer. *Lancet.* 1989; 2(8668):888–891.

28. Richardson JL, Shelton DR, Krailo M, Levine AM. The effect of compliance with treatment on survival among patients with hematologic malignancies. *J Clin Oncol.* 1990; 8(2):356–364.

29. Fawzy FI, Fawzy NW, Hyun CS. Short-term psychiatric intervention for patients with malignant melanoma: effects on psychological state, coping, and the immune system. *The Psychoimmunology of Cancer.* Oxford University Press; 1994: 292–319.

30. Fawzy FI, Cousins N, Fawzy N, et al. A structured psychiatric intervention for cancer patients: 1. Changes over times in methods of coping and affective disturbance. *Arch Gen Psychiatry.* 1990; 47:720–725.

31. Fawzy FI, Kemeny ME, Fawzy N, et al. A structured psychiatric intervention for cancer patients: 2. Changes over time in immunological measures. *Arch Gen Psychiatry.* 1990; 47:729–735.

32. Edgar L, Rosberger Z, Nowlis D. Coping with cancer during the first year after diagnosis. *Cancer.* 1992; 69(3):817–828.

33. Pruitt BT, Waligora-Serafin B, McMahon T, et al. An educational intervention for newly-diagnosed cancer patients undergoing radiotherapy. *Psycho-Oncology.* 1993; 2:55–62.

34. Greer S, Moorey S, Baruch JDR, et al. Adjuvant psychological therapy for patients with cancer: a prospective randomised trial. *Br Med J.* 1992; 304:675–680.

35. Cunningham AJ, Lockwood GA, Edmonds CVI. Which cancer patients benefit most from a brief, group, coping skills program? *Int J Psychiatry Med.* 1993; 23(4):383–398.

36. Cella DF, Sarafian B, Snider PR, et al. Evaluation of a community-based cancer support group. *Psycho-Oncology.* 1993; 2:123–132.

37. Fawzy FI, Fawzy NW, Hyun CS, et al. Malignant melanoma: effects of an early structured psychiatric intervention, coping, and affective state on recurrence and survival six years later. *Arch Gen Psychiatry.* 1993; 50:681–689.

38. Moorey S, Greer S, Watson M, et al. Adjuvant psychological therapy for patients with cancer: outcome at one year. *Psycho-Oncology.* 1994; 3:39–46.

39. Berglund G, Bolund C, Gustafsson U, Sjoden P. A randomized study of a rehabilitation program for cancer patients: the "starting again" group. *Psycho-Oncology.* 1994; 3:109–120.

40. Brandenburg Y, Bergenmar M, Bolund C, et al. Information to patients with malignant melanoma: a randomized group study. *Patient Educ Counsel.* 1994; 23: 97–105.

60

Psychotherapeutic Issues

BARBARA M. SOURKES, MARY JANE MASSIE, AND
JIMMIE C. HOLLAND

Although psychological interventions for patients with cancer were slow to develop, since the 1950s efforts to develop and test interventions have grown steadily because of greater emphasis on quality of life of patients with cancer. The types of interventions most commonly utilized by health professionals working with cancer patients are education, behavioral training, group interventions, and individual psychotherapy. This chapter provides an overview of psychotherapy with cancer patients, outlining its indications, goals, and clinical management issues which arise for the psycho-oncologist.

It has been assumed that psychotherapy is beneficial to cancer patients; personal and clinical accounts support this view (1–4). It has been difficult, however, to carry out studies that test in a standardized way because psychotherapy is usually individualized to some extent for each patient. Psychotherapy research in general, however, has become more sophisticated, and methods for testing efficacy in medically ill patients have been developed. Relevant work has been reviewed by several individuals in recent years (5–8). For a detailed critique of the studies of psychosocial interventions see Chapter 59. Crisis and brief therapy is reviewed in Chapter 58.

WHO SHOULD RECEIVE INTERVENTIONS?

As attention to psychological aspects of cancer has grown, and studies have shown the efficacy of psychosocial interventions, the issue has repeatedly been raised of which patients should receive psychosocial interventions. Some enthusiasts have advocated offering counseling to all patients on the assumption that they need help, and, of course, want it. In fact, however, Worden and Weisman found that many patients rejected the offer of help (9). Investigative efforts turned to attempts to assure early identification of

patients who were most distressed and for whom an intervention might prevent poor adaptation and more serious psychological problems.

Worden and Weisman used this approach with 372 patients with newly diagnosed cancer in the aforementioned study. Utilizing their Index of Vulnerability as a screen for risk of poor adjustment, they identified patients who were found to be at high risk (10). Only about two-thirds of the patients identified as at high risk accepted counseling. Those who refused had a positive outlook, minimized the implications of their diagnosis, and viewed the offer of therapy as a threat to their emotional equilibrium by opening the possibility of increasing their distress by unleashing suppressed emotions. Patients who accepted counseling were less able to deny the diagnosis and its implications; they were less hopeful and were more apt to experience their situation in religious or existential terms. Among those who accepted counseling, an improvement in their psychological state was seen, supporting the concept that early identification of those at risk allows for helpful intervention. One might speculate that, among those who refused counseling initially, some might have accepted it later, if their positive stance was seriously threatened. At any rate, those who were identified as vulnerable and accepted help did benefit from it.

In Canada, Stam et al. found that 20% of 449 ambulatory cancer patients seen in a single cancer center, which received most cancer patients within the geographic area, were referred and seen for psychosocial counseling over a 1 year period (11). This may be an underestimate of actual need for help. Family and personal problems were the most common reasons for seeking help. Interventions were either psychotherapeutic or educational in type. Clearly, a subset of patients in the range of a quarter to a third of them have greater distress and interventions would likely be quite beneficial.

DEFINITION, GOALS, AND PSYCHOTHERAPEUTIC METHODS

Psychotherapeutic intervention is a one-on-one interaction of a patient with cancer and a therapist with the goal of increasing morale, self-esteem, and coping, while simultaneously decreasing distress. It has the effect of enhancing the individual's sense of personal control during the struggle with illness and helps bring a better resolution of the practical problems being faced (12). The goal of providing insight is limited to recognition of relationships to the past that bear on adaptation to illness (e.g., the experience of having the same type of cancer as a parent). The therapy described here is an integration of crisis intervention, supportive psychotherapy, and is based on psychodynamic principles which must be modified somewhat for application in the medically ill.

Psychotherapy with a patient who has cancer has several goals that include maintaining a primary focus on the illness and its implications, while exploring those issues from the past and present that affect the adjustment to illness (6,13). Using a brief therapy crisis intervention model, focus is kept on the illness and present concerns. Feelings and fears about the illness and its outcome are foremost in the patient's mind; they are often considered to be too painful and too burdensome to reveal to family and friends. Hence, the therapist, by virtue of being outside the situation, plays a useful role by encouraging exploring feelings which otherwise are unexpressed. The patient rapidly sees that most of the fears are not unique to his or her situation; they are, in fact, universal.

WHO SHOULD PROVIDE PSYCHOTHERAPY?

Psychotherapy is best provided by mental health professionals, or by those who develop skills through added special training in psychotherapy. Both should be familiar, however, with the special issues involved in psychotherapy with a patient with medical illness and cancer in particular. Social workers, psychiatric nurse-clinicians, psychologists, and psychiatrists have a background and training that equips them to work effectively with medical patients, however; it is essential that the therapist from any of these backgrounds be generally familiar with types of neoplasms, stages of disease, and treatments available with each type of cancer since patients are struggling with medical decisions and clinical outcomes which the therapist must understand.

The term therapist is used to indicate such a mental health professional who, irrespective of background, undertakes the difficult psychotherapeutic task of working with individuals who have a life-threatening illness or cancer. It is important to keep in mind that some patients require that a therapist have some special skill to achieve the desired outcome, such as cognitive behavioral techniques. Each mental health professional should, therefore, be aware of his or her own strengths and limitations, and should be able to recognize when the special skills of another mental health discipline might be better applied. A willingness on the part of the professional to obtain consultation for specialized skills is important.

In many settings, however, a single mental health professional assumes all these responsibilities simultaneously and must function truly as a generalist without opportunity for consultation. In larger centers, where several mental health professionals may be present and where the role of each is new and evolving, the potential for nonproductive professional jealousies to develop is great. The issues arise because neither the staff nor the newly assigned mental health professionals have a clear picture of expected roles or functions in a setting in which these roles are new and ill-defined (see Chapter 90). Conflicts can be avoided by mutual respect for the contributions of each discipline, and by maintaining a constant review of the nature and quality of management of all psychosocial aspects of care given within a unit or center, making changes in staff members and disciplinary background as needed. The most effective model is to provide these services in a single integrated unit by a single multidisciplinary team. Such a model encourages full and constructive use of all resources.

PSYCHOTHERAPEUTIC FRAMEWORK

The diagnosis of cancer leads many individuals to enter psychotherapy. The primary focus is the emotional stress engendered by the illness, rather than more general intrapsychic and interpersonal concerns of the physically healthy person. Aspects of the psychotherapeutic framework to which a psycho-oncologist must give special attention are: *(1)* time; *(2)* space; *(3)* the identity of the patient; *(4)* the therapeutic content and process; and *(5)* the therapeutic relationship. How that framework is defined will vary with the exigencies of the illness. However, flexibility does not give the therapist license to ignore, reject or take lightly the basic ground rules. Rather, the utmost challenge lies in adapting a structure to the illness reality, even as the illness changes, without sacrificing the uniqueness of the therapeutic interaction.

Time

Awareness of the irreversible passage of time pervades any experience of potential or imminent loss. Thus a diagnosis of cancer acutely heightens the sense of time for the patient and family. Its subjective meaning is inextricably entwined with the reality of the clock and calendar (13). Time becomes the organizing pivot of the experience: "If one can eliminate time sense, one can also avoid the ultimate separation that time brings—death" (1:6). It is this omnipresent awareness of time that makes the threat of loss more critical than any other life stress.

The time commitment in psychotherapy is composed of these facets: frequency, duration and appointed time of sessions. In traditional psychotherapy, a consistent structure is critical to the containment of the process. Thus, there is both theoretical and practical adherence to the "50 minute hour". With increasing levels of illness or approaching death as the reality at hand, the scheduling of sessions will need to be flexible and may vary considerably. In cancer survivors or those in remission, the adherence to the traditional structure is more appropriate. Equally important is the therapist's availability to meet these time commitments, since the therapist's consistent and abiding presence is an aspect of the time component of psychotherapy with patients with cancer.

Not only is there an ebb and flow in the frequency of sessions, but also the patient must be given specific "permission" to participate in the regulation. The patient's request for more frequent contact during a stressful period often parallels the reality of the severity of illness or the toxicity and side effects of treatment. Conversely, one encounters phases when patients request diminished frequency, or cessation, of sessions. The reasons for such a request may be highly adaptive to the individual's functioning. The patient who is facing the enormity of loss may at times need to control his or her emotional "thermostat," and shut off confrontation and intensity. In exercising this option, the patient must be secure in the knowledge that contact with the therapist may be reinitiated without fear of reprisal. The understanding that the frequency of sessions may vary is a sine qua non of psychotherapy with patients with cancer. A therapist who responds to the patient's "self-regulation" as a narcissistic blow has not accepted this modification. A therapist's sense of relief at lapses in the process may reflect his or her own difficulty in handling the level of intensity on a sus-

tained basis; a patient's retreat may be in reaction to such cues. While the therapist must certainly be alert for manipulation or resistance on the part of the patient, such motivation should be inferred with caution in the patient with cancer.

The frequency of sessions also depends upon whether the patient is being treated in the hospital or in an outpatient clinic. Time assumes a different meaning in the hospital. Hours and days often stretch out so that more frequent meetings, even on a daily basis, may not feel different to the patient from weekly sessions. During brief or uneventful admissions, there may be no need for such an increase. Whether or not the therapist works at the treatment institution will place bounds on his or her availability. However, telephone contact can bridge time between sessions or, if necessary, serve as a temporary substitute for face-to-face encounters.

Duration

The duration of individual sessions depends on the patient's physical status, as well as the concerns at hand. On occasion, particularly during hospitalizations, the therapist must interpret the meaning of a patient's illness behavior. For example, the patient may claim to be too sick to see or talk at any length with the therapist. Is the patient really incapable of interaction, or is the illness being used as a means of avoidance? An error in interpretation in either direction can be damaging to the theraeputic alliance.

If the therapist implies that the patient is using the illness to avoid emotional issues, when the patient is in fact physically drained, a "blame-the-victim" cycle is set in motion. The patient experiences justifiable resentment at the accusation. At some later point he or she may confront the therapist. However, it is often too threatening for a patient to express anger toward a caregiver and thus the basic trust of the therapeutic alliance may be ruptured beyond repair. Another avenue is that taken by the patient who passively accepts being labeled an "avoider." the vulnerability and powerlessness in the face of physical illness are now further exacerbated for this individual.

The therapist must maintain caution in another direction: that of permitting a patient to disengage under the guise of the illness when, in fact, the patient is clinically depressed. While the patient gives messages of wanting only to be left alone, on a more basic level he or she may be overwhelmed by depression, yearn for contact, and yet be unable to take the initiative. The firm, persistent, and gentle efforts of the therapist are often a turning point in the patient's reengagement.

What cues are available for the therapist to make a differential interpretation of illness behavior? First, it is imperative that the therapist understand the patient's medical condition. There is no substitute for facts. Second, the therapist weighs the patient's self-report with his or her own observations. Third, and of utmost importance, the therapist must communicate with other members of the caregiving team. They can give a general index of the patient's physical and emotional status, which then serves as a baseline for the therapist's assessment.

Appointment Time

The structured and secure expectation of meeting at a regular time can do much for the patient's sense of stability within the therapeutic relationship and in coping more effectively with illness. During hospitalizations, an appointed time provides the patient with a critical pivot for the day. However, as much as is positive in the regularity, there are obvious drawbacks to the "office-hours" regimen:

It is in the middle of the night when I feel most depressed. The dark is associated with death; there is the feeling that you are going to die alone; and there are times when I really feel the need to talk to somebody. (2:177)

Although the patient is encouraged to discuss such night fears during regular therapy sessions, it is common knowledge that he or she may never mention them, even in response to the therapist's direct inquiry. What emerges is the necessity for a flexible "on-call" schedule among therapists working with these patients. A patient's night anxieties are often assuaged simply by knowing of the therapist's availability. Furthermore, night staff can be trained in focused listening skills and thus provide a measure of comfort and relief.

Space

Space—the physical setting—establishes concrete boundaries for the therapeutic process. As the therapy hour is a time apart, so the setting affords a private space from daily life. The office becomes an extension of the therapist, with some of the same projective attributes.

A woman had a regularly scheduled therapy session prior to each hospital admission. She often verbalized how the therapist's office was a "refuge" before the onslaught. Upon hearing that the therapist would be away at the time of her next admission, the patient asked whether she might sit in the office alone. She felt that just being in the setting would help to prepare her.

In oncology, a consistent setting cannot always be depended upon for structure and "protection." Whereas the therapist's office serves as the base, other locations which may need to be additional bases are the clinic, hospital, or the patient's home. Especially when the patient is seen in the hospital, the setting no longer stands protected and apart. Rather, the therapeutic process is enmeshed in the physical and emotional confrontation of the illness.

A hospital room affords little privacy. During hospitalizations, psychotherapy sessions may be constricted, interrupted, or abbreviated by the presence of other patients, staff or visitors. At other times, the hospitalized patient may experience the therapist's presence as engulfing because the framework is altered: the therapist comes to the patient. With curtailment of physical autonomy, the patient's anxiety may escalate dramatically. It is a rare patient who asks directly that the therapist leave or that a session is ended. In compensation for this sense of "captivity," the therapist must be acutely sensitive to the patient's cues concerning spatial boundaries.

Visits to the home for the patient who is no longer physically able to come to the therapist's office are important for the patient and the therapist, since it may become the setting for saying goodbye. The sense of such a patient that the therapist's commitment extends to making home visits can be extremely reassuring in the face of advancing illness (see Chapter 87).

Identity of the Patient

In traditional psychotherapy, the identity of the patient is strictly defined: as an individual, a couple, a parent-child dyad, or a family. When a therapist works with a patient with cancer, the contract regarding "who is seen" is more open from the start. Although psychotherapy may be initiated with the physically ill patient, or with a family member, this one individual becomes the therapist's point of entry into the family system. By no means does all individual therapy become family-based. However, in the face of life threatening illness, bridging maneuvers to involve the entire family can be critical (see Chapter 85). Because of this broader definition of the identity of the patient, the boundaries of confidentiality may be more permeable than is traditionally dictated. The therapist bears heightened responsibility for handling privileged communication within the emotionally intense family system.

The therapist plays a pivotal role in the integration of the patient's total care. With the ethic of confidentiality as a guide, and with the patient's consent, the therapist may share selective aspects of the therapeutic material with the care-giving team. The therapist communicates only essential content which bears directly on the care of the patient. For example, it may be important to make a statement about the patient's emotional or mental status in relation to a precipitating event, if relevant; discussion of the individual's ability to cope; and, recommendations for aspects of medical care by other team members that will affect coping. Information that does not contribute to these categories is generally best left unsaid. The intimate nuance and subtlety of the material belong exclusively within the therapeutic relationship.

Rumors abounded as to whether the mother of an adolescent patient died naturally, or had committed suicide. The girl confided to the therapist that the death had been a suicide, and talked at length about its impact on her. The therapist's communication to the staff outlined: the fact that the patient's mother had committed suicide after a long psychiatric history; the feelings of abandonment and guilt described by the girl; how the experience might affect her coping with the illness; and her need for reassurance despite a counter-dependent facade. When the therapist provided factual data, the "sensationalism" vanished, and the staff developed a new sensitivity toward this patient.

Therapeutic Content and Process

A hallmark of traditional psychotherapy is the unstructured flow of content and process. Past, present, and future interweave in the unfolding of themes. Letting a process emerge at its own pace and time is a luxury precluded by the very nature of life-threatening illness. Its immediacy demands a focus on the present, framed by the themes of separation and loss.

The patient's and family's previous experiences with loss will bear significantly on the present. Thus, an individual's "loss history" is a critical tool in highlighting areas of strength and vulnerability. The history encompasses loss in its broadest sense; for example, through illness and death, termination of relationships (such as divorce), geographical separation, and loss of employment. The history should include the person's earliest memory of loss from childhood, subsequent experiences up to the present, and a description of how he or she functioned in each context. What were the most stressful aspects of the experience? What type of support was positive, deleterious, or lacking altogether? It is of utmost importance to know the patient's and family's past "acquaintance" with the illness they are now facing. Have they known anyone with the disease, and if so, what was its trajectory and outcome? Was a parent, sibling, or grandparent treated for cancer? What was the outcome and how did it affect the person? The meaning of the same diagnosis can vary dramatically depending upon these factors.

Through this carefully focused assessment, the groundwork is laid for therapeutic intervention.

A man diagnosed with an early stage malignancy was given an excellent prognosis by his physician. Despite this reassurance, the patient maintained that he was sure to die within the year. It turned out that the one person he had known with the same disease had died, and thus he viewed his own diagnosis as an unequivocal death sentence.

For the individual with cancer, psychological defenses are coping mechanisms for the present, rather than barriers to the past. An individual's defensive structure has developed over a lifetime of negotiating reality. Faced with the ultimate reality—the threat of death—his or her defenses may be mobilized to the hilt. Defensive patterns which appear to be constructive for the patient are identified as "psychological tools." Those with deleterious impact become grist for the therapeutic process of change. The therapist thus serves as an advocate of the patient's defensive structure, in the service of optimal coping.

There is a future for both patient and family, albeit in markedly different ways. The family must focus on plans which go beyond the patient's illness and death. Fear and guilt often accompany the acknowledgment that despite the loss of one family member, life does continue. The patient, on the other hand, can consider the future only within the context of the present illness.

And as my diet and my tumor have restricted my movements in space, so the probability that I shall die soon has restricted me to the immediate present in time. It has erected around me an invisible barrier that I bump into a dozen times a day . . . I'm reasonably sure I'll be alive a month from now, and I sincerely hope I'll be alive three months from now; but beyond that I don't know . . . In short, I have no future any more. And that I think is the greatest change of all. (3:46)

The therapist must constantly maintain an acute awareness of both the "real" and affective facets of time. On a cognitive level, the therapist monitors the reality of temporal issues; for example, how long the patient is expected to live, when the family is available, how much time should be devoted to therapeutic intervention at different points in the illness. For the patient and family, however, cognitive time may be out of phase with its affective counterpart. Thus, a family may panic over separation when, in fact, the patient's condition is stable and death is not imminent. Or, in contrast, a denial of impending loss may occur when time is short. These seeming inconsistencies arise from the fact that the patient and family live within a dualistic realm of time. The clock and calendar, by their imposition of finite limits, bespeak the reality of adult time. Especially in confronting life-threatening illness, "the calendar is the ultimate materialization of separation anxiety." (13:190) The contrast is child time: the magical, omnipotent belief in endless time forever. While the context for psychotherapy is finite time, a shift into child time does not necessarily imply denial or blocking.

A man acknowledged that there were no further treatment options for his advanced disease. Within the same sessions, he talked about travel plans for the following summer. When the therapist confronted him with the juxtaposition, the man replied: "Of course I am aware of the reality of my illness and—I nonetheless hope for something better."

The patient may also be testing the therapist: "Which time framework will you buy? Or, can you tolerate the fluctuation which is the essence of my experience?" Adherence to child time, to the exclusion of impinging reality, may signify fear dysfunction. However, most families flow between the two sets of time, in a normal and adaptive process of maintaining hope. The therapist need only follow.

The Therapeutic Relationship

The therapist's role for the patient is highly specific: he or she is an anchoring presence in a life situation that otherwise feels unstable and vulnerable. The transference and countertransference come to mirror the themes of attachment and loss that the patient is confronting in every relationship. In the urgency of life-threatening illness, the luxury of operating exclusively with the transference simply does not exist. Rather, the therapist must constantly translate back to the patient's "outside" life, maintaining a close correspondence between the transference material and its implications for the patient's significant relationships. Ideally, the therapist strives to foster a transference whose depth and intensity can fuel the tasks of living so crucial for the patient with limited life expectancy.

An aspect of the countertransference that is aroused in therapists who work with seriously ill individuals is the "rescue fantasy." In wanting to protect the vulnerable patient, the therapist encounters the danger of overinvolvement, a loss of boundary and role. The patient may feel threatened by an inordinate closeness to the therapist, while at the same time welcoming and needing the relationship. Ultimately, the patient may feel trapped into "choosing" between family and therapist, with a simultaneous fear of alienating either. The therapist must prevent the patient from ever experiencing such a forced choice position. One safeguard is to be found in the interpretation of the transference material. If the patient understands that the intense feelings which develop toward the therapist also have meaning for his or her other relationships, the sense of threat is minimized.

The family could feel estranged and supplanted just at the time they are desperately trying to "keep" the patient. Their pain is only exacerbated if they feel that the therapist is "better" than they in achieving closeness. The therapist and other caregivers must be aware of their own feelings of competition: such rivalry often serves as a danger signal of inappropriate involvement, coupled with a family's difficulty in relating to the patient.

The discussion at a case conference focused on a man's inadequate support of his wife during her prolonged hospitalization. The staff noted the husband's infrequent visits, and his discomfort in his wife's presence. Both the therapist and the nurses described their closeness to the patient. It was at this point that the therapist realized the staff's error: all were vying for a "special relationship" with the woman to compensate for the apparent problems within her marriage. Furthermore, the husband's behavior was clearly an indication of his own difficulty in coping with his wife's illness. The therapist was able to highlight these issues in the conference, and subsequent work focused on the couple's relationship.

COUNTERTRANSFERENCE

Psychotherapy with patients with cancer does not allow the luxury of maintaining an objective stance as one would with a physically healthy patient. More interaction is necessary with the patient and hence the issues of countertransference become critically important in the psychotherapist. Knowing one's own "loss history" becomes important to help in understanding why a certain patient's illness or impending death is more painful than another. Understanding this is critical to "survival" as a psycho-oncologist. Equally important is the assurance that someone is available to review and discuss the patient who has raised significant distress in the therapist. It is sometimes wise to transfer such a patient to a colleague, if the therapist senses some deep-seated relationship from the past that may be confounding the care of a particular patient and resulting in countertransference that is interfering.

Although no psychotherapy is ever complete, this fact is strikingly evident in work with individuals with cancer. The therapeutic process and the illness reality are inextricably bound: interruption or termination may occur at any point. Thus, each encounter should be complete in and of itself. The therapist must possess a high tolerance for ambiguity in order to step into the lives of those whose existence is predicated on such uncertainty. In essence, the therapist must be committed to the individual's quality of life—for however long that life may last. Furthermore, in the absence created by the patient's death, he or she must acknowledge the loss with the family, provide a sense of continuity for them, and offer grief counseling, if appropriate, or refer them for treatment. There is often a strong bond felt by families for the therapist who took care of their relative, and a desire to continue because of the fact that the therapist knew the deceased and provides an intimate continuing link. Bereavement counseling with the family is sometimes a useful interaction for grieving members.

SUMMARY

Therapists who provide psychotherapy for patients with cancer should know both theory and techniques of individual psychotherapy, be familiar with oncological diagnosis, prognosis, and treatment, and be aware of their personal responses to patients who have a life-threatening illness. Finally, psychotherapeutic work with cancer patients is challenging and requires commitment to do it effectively; it is also highly personally rewarding.

REFERENCES

1. Bard M. Implications of analytic psychotherapy with the physically ill. *Am J Psychother*. 1959; 13:860–871.
2. Creech RH. The psychological support of the cancer patient: a medical oncologist viewpoint. *Sem Oncol*. 1975; 2:285–292.
3. Cunningham J, Strassberg D, Roback H. Group psychotherapy for medical patients. *Compr Psychiatry*. 1978; 19:135–140.
4. Cain E, Kohorn EI, Quinlan DM, et al. Psycholsocial benefits of a cancer support group. *Cancer*. 1986; 57:183–189.
5. Watson M. Psychosocial interventions with cancer patients: a review. *Psychol Med*. 1983; 13:839–846.
6. Massie M, Holland JC, Straker N. Psychotherapeutic interventions. In: Holland JC, Rowland JR, eds. *Handbook of Psychooncology: Psychological Care of the Patient With Cancer*. New York: Oxford University Press; 1990:455–469.
7. Edgar L, Remmer J, Rosberger Z, Rapkin B. On oncology volunteer support organization: the benefits and fit within the health care system. *Psycho-Oncology*. 1996; 5:331–343.
8. Moorey S, Greer S, Watson W, et al. Adjuvant psychological therapy for patients with cancer: outcome at one year. *Psycho-Oncology*. 1994; 3:39–46.
9. Worden JW, Weisman AD. Do cancer patients really want counseling? *Gen Hosp Psychiatry*. 1980; 2:100–103.
10. Worden JW, Weisman AD. Preventive psychosocial intervention with newly diagnosed cancer patients. *Gen Hosp Psychiatry*. 1984; 6:243–249.
11. Stan HJ, Bultz BP, Pittman CA. Psychosocial problems and interventions in a referred sample of cancer patients. *Psychosom Med*. 1986; 48:539–547.
12. Gordon WA, Freidenberg SI, Diller L, et al. Efficacy of psychosocial interventions with cancer patients. *J Consult Clin Psychol*. 1980; 48:743–759.
13. Sourkes BM. *The Deepening Shade: Psychological Aspects of Life-threatening Illness*. Pittsburgh: University of Pittsburgh Press; 1982.

61

Group Therapies

JAMES L. SPIRA

Group psychotherapy specifically designed for persons with cancer may very well be the most powerful psychosocial intervention available for the vast majority of patients. Beyond the scope of individual therapy, group therapy can address the major issues facing persons with cancer in a way that members can garner the emotional support of persons with similar experiences and use the experiences of others to buffer the fear of future unknowns. Yet beyond it's effectiveness, group therapy is also extremely time- and cost-efficient (1).

For decades, group psychotherapy has been utilized effectively with patients facing a variety of psychosocial issues (2,3). Several professional societies and journals have been founded specifically to advance the discipline of group psychotherapy (e.g., International Group Therapy Association (Guilford Press), American Psychological Association, Division of Group Psychology and Group Psychotherapy). However, groups specifically designed for cancer patients have been utilized, described, and researched far less frequently. This chapter is intended to help reduce that deficiency by providing a clinical framework for health professionals who wish to offer psychosocial support to cancer patients. Toward that end, this chapter describes the type of patients most likely to benefit from group intervention, the formats that best serve them, and therapeutic guidelines for successful intervention. Before addressing clinical implementation, however, psychosocial factors which impact on psychological and physical health in cancer patients, and therapeutic groups which have demonstrated improvement in patients' health will be discussed.

THE BENEFITS OF GROUP THERAPY FOR PERSONS WITH CANCER

Certainly, group formats are extremely cost-effective for the patient, and time-effective for the therapist. Efficacy of time is especially noticed where teaching specific information or skills is involved, as can be presented in psychoeducational classes or brief group formats. Yet, as is evident from the brief review of research discussed below, group therapy is also highly effective in terms of assisting with improving quality of life, and possibly even physical health.

Not surprisingly, persons diagnosed with cancer undergo substantial changes in mood, psychophysical functioning, and existential aspects of their lives. The way that patients cope with their illness influences their emotional state and ability to adjust to living with the illness (4,5). Moreover, it is also possible that psychosocial factors may be of influence in the course of the disease itself (6). Specifically noteworthy is research emphasizing the importance of social support versus isolation in survival (7,8), open expression of affect versus inhibition of expression (9) or uncontrolled hostility (10), honest expression of cognitive concerns versus denial/avoidance (11), and active coping versus passive compliance (12). In brief, avoidance of feelings, denial of concerns, feeling helpless or passive, compliance with other's demands, and social isolation are bound to result in poor quality of life, if not increased risk of disease incidence, progression, or survival. Higher quality of life may even be related to one's physical health (13). Fortunately, all these psychosocial factors can be improved through the group psychotherapy format. Improving these factors is the intent of most studies investigating the impact of group psychosocial support for cancer patients. Many descriptions of group therapy for cancer patients exist in the literature (14–17). However, while helpful descriptions of group therapy formats, relatively few of these descriptions have been prospective randomized designs attempting to demonstrate specific benefits with specific interventional styles. Although in-depth reviews of these intervention studies can be found elsewhere (18–21), it is valuable at least to note that empirical studies of group intervention have served to illustrate the benefit of group therapy for cancer patients.

Beginning in the late 1970s, research has demonstrated the benefits of group therapy for improving cancer patients' quality of life (such as mood, coping, psychophysical distress, and physical functioning) and increasing patients' familiarity about the disease and treatment. With one exception, all reported studies of group therapy have been short-term (fewer than 12 meetings), for the most part following a cognitive-behavioral format combining educational information, coping skills, and emotional/social support (22–26). The exception was a research group based on the seminal work of Yalom (27) which met weekly for the entire year, and emphasized more traditional interactive, emotionally supportive therapeutic style (28). This is not surprising, since briefer meetings require greater structure whereas the longer groups can afford to utilize more inductive methodology (29).

Although not strictly group psychotherapy in the "traditional" sense, psychoeducational groups are also of significant value, especially for recently diagnosed patients and those at risk for developing disease. For these patients, focusing on information and improving compliance with treatment and future prevention hold great promise for improving the effectiveness of medical treatment or preventing future disease (30–33).

Several studies have attempted to separate interventional styles to determine which methods might be most effective. When examining gynecologic cancer patients' psychological adjustment 6 months after treatment, Cain et al. (34), found that both individual and group therapies were equally beneficial compared to a control group. Telch and Telch (35) reported improved coping and self-efficacy for cancer patients attending a cognitive-behavior style group compared to an unstructured and nontherapeutically led support group. Cunningham and Tocco (36) also found that a short-term cognitive-behavioral group was superior to unstructured support groups where patients were encouraged to express emotions, although both groups benefited from their respective interventions. In contrast, Evans and Connis (37) found that while cognitive-behavioral and supportive group therapy were both beneficial for depressed cancer patients, supportive therapy was superior in the long run. Taken together with other research, these studies point to the benefits of therapeutically led groups versus unstructured support groups that are not therapeutically guided by a skilled facilitator, and appear to be at least as beneficial as individual therapy for cancer patients.

Two studies indicate that group therapy may also be effective for improving physical health. The year long group therapy based on Yalom's approach to group psychotherapy found in a retrospective follow-up that patients who had been randomly assigned to receive group therapy lived an average of 18 months longer from study entry than did control patients (38) (see Chapter 63). However, Fox (39) has pointed out that the treatment group lived only as long as the national and local average whereas the control group died at a faster than expected rate, suggesting that statistical sampling error accounted for the survival effect. Other evidence for the benefits of group therapy on reduction of disease recurrence and improved survival comes from a study of malignant melanoma patients conducted by Fawzy et al. A brief structured intervention was found to improve not only mood and coping, but immunity as well in treatment patients for up to 1 year following treatment (40). These authors' 6 year follow-up also showed improvement in recurrence and survival rates for treatment patients (41). A group based on the work of Siegel, however, failed to find survival benefits for treatment subjects (42). One major distinction between this study and the others showing positive survival outcomes lies in the style of therapy. The Siegel groups emphasized considering a more positive future without dwelling on the negative, whereas the Yalom-style and coping-skills group directly addressed negative feelings and thoughts, encouraged expression of distress, as well as considered active coping strategies (43). This difference parallels the literature which suggests that confronting distress in an open and honest manner rather than avoid feelings and thoughts may contribute to improved health outcomes (44).

Which group approach is best? A meta-analysis was performed for of all prospective randomized studies examining the effects of educational, behavioral, and counseling interventions for cancer patients (45). Not surprisingly, informational/educational approaches were most effective for improving medical knowledge and compliance as well as with functional adjustment, behavioral approaches were most effective with managing specific symptoms, and nonbehavioral counseling therapy was superior for assisting with emotional adjustment as well as in more global measures examined. Importantly, support groups that lacked psychotherapeutic interventions were not found to be of value for any outcomes examined. Clearly, therapists should select the style of intervention which will best facilitate the desired outcome.

GROUP THERAPY FOR THE MEDICALLY ILL COMPARED TO OTHER FORMATS

Understanding how group therapy for cancer patients differs from both individual therapy and group psychotherapy for persons with psychosocial disturbance will lay a foundation for understanding the power as well as the limits of this treatment.

Group versus Individual Treatment

Whereas group therapy has tremendous potential to assist most cancer patients, individual psychotherapy can be of incomparable value for certain persons with cancer, especially those with personality characteristics that interfere with adjusting to living with cancer and coping with treatment (see Chapter 60). Yet, whenever possible, group therapy can be considered the "treatment of choice" for most cancer patients. In contrast to the usual emphasis on examining and modifying personality patterns prevalent in individual therapy, group therapy for persons with cancer emphasizes living more fully in each moment, and garnering supportive experiences from others regarding ways to handle the stresses faced in coping with life as a cancer patient. Certainly individual therapy can assist patients with such adjustments, and group therapy can emphasize personality patterns. Still, each is better suited to different therapeutic processes due to their special contextual circumstances. An individual therapist can focus on the complex puzzle that comprises each person's life, whereas a group setting is better suited to utilize the invaluable experience of others in coping with and adjusting to issues common to most cancer patients. Nowhere can the power of the group be so beneficially utilized as with the medically ill.

Group Therapy for Persons with Psychosocial Disturbance versus Persons with Cancer

Typically, group psychotherapy is conducted for persons with various levels of psychosocial dysfunction, yet members are selected to participate on the basis of similar levels of ego functioning. Group therapy for the medically ill is very different, however. A serious illness can attack anyone at any time. Therefore, these groups typically comprise persons with a wide range of past experiences, personal and external resources, and personality styles. Nonetheless, they have much in common. Typical themes discussed in groups of cancer patients include communication with medical professionals; relationships with family, friends, and coworkers; coping with medical treatment and ill effects of the disease; adjusting to living with a cancer diagnosis; existential issues such as addressing the possibility of

dying, examining one's priorities, and shifting self-image (19,46). Although there is much in common among issues addressed by cancer patients, the range of personality types in these groups are as varied as those who can develop cancer—i.e., the general population. In this way, groups with a psychosocial focus differ from those comprising the medically ill (see Table 61.1).

Group therapy for persons with psychosocial dysfunction most typically follows an interpersonal format (27). Group therapy for cancer patients includes a variety of formats, including drop-in meetings with a cancer patient serving as coordinator, educational/didactic class format, teaching and practice of coping skills, allowing for emotional distress, interpersonal support, and improving coping styles that affect current functioning (47). Naturally, the style of facilitating groups depends upon group format, patient make-up, stated goals, and therapist training.

FACILITATING GROUP PSYCHOTHERAPY FOR CANCER PATIENTS

Clearly, psychosocial support is of great value for persons with cancer. Yet the type of support offered depends to a great extent upon the stage of illness and the goals of therapy. Styles of group therapy and structure of groups which optimally facilitate various populations in their psychosocial development are considered below. Nevertheless, there are commonalities which exist across most types of groups, such as basic group facilitation methods, choice of topics, and dealing with special problems which are bound to arise in group formats. These are considered first, and finally summarized in a description of a typical group.

Topics Discussed in Groups

The focus of the group needs to address the most relevant issues immediately facing the patients' quality of life and physical health. Patients' issues will, of course, vary depending upon their stage of illness, and this will be considered below. Independent of stage of illness,

TABLE 61.1. *Characteristics of Groups Presenting for Psychosocial versus Medical Concerns*

Group Interest	Group Characteristics	
	Presenting Problem	Ego Strength
Psychopathology	Heterogeneous	Homogeneous
Medical	Homogeneous	Heterogeneous

TABLE 61.2. *Examples of Deductive (Therapist-Driven) and Inductive (Patient-Driven) Topics of Discussion*

Scientifically Determined Topics	Patients' Personal Concerns
Social support/isolation	Psychophysical (pain, nausea, sleeplessness)
Confronting fears/avoidance	Psychological (negative mood; intrusive thoughts)
Emotional expression/suppresion	Functional changes (physical fatigue, disability)
Active coping/helplessness	Appearance (cosmetics, prosthesis, reconstruction)
	Communication (doctor, family, friends, coworkers)

however, two perspectives can be followed with regard to what is addressed in the groups: scientifically determined risk factors for worsening quality of life and physical health, and personal concerns as stated by the patient (Table 61.2). Whereas in many cases, these overlap, there are instances where they do not.

Topics most commonly discussed in groups are both those of concern to the patients, as well as those deemed of value by the therapists. Topics generated by the patients stem directly from patients' immediate needs and concerns, such as coping with pain, nausea, sleeplessness, negative mood, intrusive thoughts, physical fatigue, improving appearance, and improving communication with doctors, family, and friends (46). Addressing these issues early and often will go far in establishing rapport with the patients. And as Maslow described, one must take care of basic functional concerns before one is able to adequately address existential issues (48).

Topics chosen by the therapists are often emotionally difficult for the patients to pursue at the time, even though they may well feel better afterwards. These include issues of establishing meaningful social support, confronting fears, expressing negative emotions, and seeking control over what can be improved, while letting go of what cannot be controlled. Although patients may not choose to discuss or express negative emotions or issues of death and dying, it ends up being very beneficial and appreciated by the patients. It appears that, by discussing these difficult issues in the groups, patients are able to focus on living more fully in each moment without as much distraction the rest of the week. Moreover, directly addressing the difficult

issues of illness and dying assists patients to reexamine the way they live, with the result of choosing to spend more time in activities that are more meaningful and valuable to them. Rather than *what* is discussed, it is often the therapeutic style that leads patients to examine these aspects of their lives. When therapists lead patients into exploring difficult realms, they must do so gently, lest they meet resistance and lose the trust of the group. The best leader is usually one who can follow the patient, gently introducing new ideas within the context of the patient's relevant experience (49). Exactly what, how, and when topics are discussed will vary greatly, depending on the special issues faced by each population, as well as the therapeutic goals, methods, and structure. Certainly, some forms of group treatment are more inductive in nature while others are almost entirely deductive. The style will lead to differing results, and so should be selected with specific goals in mind.

Styles of Therapeutic Facilitation

Three fundamental styles of therapeutic intervention can be described: *deductive,* didactically directed by the therapist; a balanced *interaction* between therapist and patients; or, *inductive* facilitation, with patient generated topics subtly facilitated by therapists (see Table 61.3).

Deductive Process. There are situations, such as a health education series for prevention or information for the newly diagnosed, where the therapist serves as a health educator. The therapist presents topics to be learned, with a goal of patients obtaining

TABLE 61.3. *Styles of Therapeutic Facilitation*

Deductive	Interactive	Inductive
Lecture about set topics for education	Lecture about set topics Provide exercise to personalize Facilitate discussion for integration into patients' lives	Discussion of any topic of concern raised by patients is facilitated by the therapist to enable authentic expression, stimulate active coping, and provide group support

information helpful to them now or in the future. At its best, this approach utilizes sound educational principles, presenting information in the context of patients' lives, world view, and motivational concerns so that each patient can best integrate the information into their lives in a way that works for them.

Interactive Process. Therapist's facilitation may emphasize interaction with patients around certain topics, such as improving communication, dealing with stress. A structured approach is most commonly utilized to balance lecture, experience, and discussion, as per the following example:

1. Therapists present issues in general, lecturing for 5–10 minutes on subject.
2. Participants do an exercise (paper and pencil, diads, self-hypnosis) in order to personalize the exercise for their specific circumstances, lasting about 20–30 minutes.
3. Therapists facilitate a general discussion about how these strategies can be implemented in one's life, touching on successes and barriers to successful implementation. Or, therapists can ask leading questions about specific topics in order to structure a group discussion about a topic (e.g., "Let's go around the group and each person say what his biggest stressor is when going for treatment."). The discussion lasts the rest of the 1–2 hour meeting.

Inductive Process. Another, more traditional form of group therapy facilitation occurs when therapists facilitate discussion of any topic that patients' raise. Rather than presenting specific topics to be learned or practiced, the focus here is on facilitating the *process* of discussion, such that participants are speaking of issues in personal, specific, affective terms, interacting with others to find active coping strategies (50). In this approach, therapists rarely lecture or give advice. Nor do they give specific exercises to structure the interactions among patients. Instead, therapists facilitate discussion among participants by asking questions as needed to get patients "back on track." When the discussion is going well, there is no need for the therapists to speak at all. Since this approach can serve as a basis for all types of groups and styles of facilitation, it is presented in some detail, below.

Facilitating Group Discussion

Before asking a leading question, it is usually a good idea to make a rapport statement. Therapists who rephrase or summarize patients' feelings and topics make sure they themselves understand what has been said, and increase the patients' confidence that the therapist truly does understand their concerns. Patients are more likely to follow a therapist's lead if they believe the therapist has been following their feelings and thoughts (51). Asking a few simple open-ended questions to help patients express their concerns in more personal, specific, effective ways to others can assist in accessing more authentic intimate personal feelings and also to explore other ways of coping with a problem. Below are some examples of the types of leading questions which are useful in facilitating authentic expression and further exploration of concerns. They are organized by the subject and object of the patient's concern, their affect and approach to coping with a problem, and the style of interaction they engage in (see Table 61.4).

SUBJECT. When the subject of the patient's expression is externally focused on a subject other than him or herself, the therapist should ask the patient a question which will lead them to phrase their concerns in more personal terms. In general, when the patient is talking about someone or something else, the therapist should ask how the matter affects the patient personally. For example, if a patient says: "My doctor simply is not interested in listening to what options his patients might want. He's pretty sure of himself," the therapist can redirect: "How do you react when you are speaking with him and want him to listen to your concerns, but he doesn't?"

OBJECT. When the object of the patient's expression is in general or abstract terms, the therapist should ask a question which leads the patient to phrase their concerns in more specific and concrete terms. In general, when the patient is speaking abstractly or vaguely, without reference to specific time and place, the therapist should ask the patient to give a very specific example of how he or she has experienced this situation. For example, if a patient says: "Doctors are really not interested in listening to what options patients want. They are trained to tell, not to listen," the therapist can redirect: "Has this happened to you? Can you give us an example of an interaction with your doctor when he did not listen to your concerns?" If the patient has no such experiences, then they were simply engaging in speculative intellectualization and the therapist should simply ask the group about their personal experiences in this type of situation.

TABLE 61.4. *Facilitating Group Therapy Discussion*

Lead	Quality of Expression From inauthentic	Therapeutic Leads → To authentic	
Subject	Impersonal/external	———————————→ "How does that affect you personally?"	Personal/internal
Object	Abstract/general	———————————→ "Can you give a specific example of that problem?"	Concrete/specific
Affect	Intellectual/repressed	———————————→ "How does that make you feel?"	Emotional/expression
Relationship	Solipsistic/isolated	———————————→ "Has anyone else had that type of experience?"	Supportive/interactive
Coping	Passive/Helpless	———————————→ "What can you do to handle the situation in a way that works better for you?"	Active/appropriate control

When needed, therapists ask open-ended questions to elicit more authentic patient expression. For example, in response to: "Doctors never care what's going on with *you*, only what's going on with the *tumor!*" the therapist might ask one or several of the above questions, depending on patients' subsequent responses.

AFFECT. When the expression is personal and specific, and of obvious concern to the patient, but is stated intellectually or void of emotion, the therapist should probe their emotional state. In general, when a patient is talking about a difficult subject in emotionally neutral or even overly positive terms, the therapist should ask them what negative feelings that brings up for them. For example, if a patient says: "I know exactly how I am going to end my life, once it is clear that there is no more hope. I am going to fly to Paris, get a hotel room with a view of Sacre Coeur, and take an overdose of sleeping pills." If this is said in an intellectual fashion, void of emotion, as if in casual conversation, the therapist might respond: "This is a VERY major step you are considering. And you seem to be talking about it so lightly. But when you think about getting sicker, there being no hope, and taking your own life, doesn't that bring up a lot of feelings in you?"

It is important for the therapist not to push too hard when eliciting a patient's expression of feelings. Simply offer an opportunity to explore. Point to the door, even open it a crack, but don't drag the patients through. Overzealousness on the part of the therapist will usually result in either *(1)* a patient having a rush of feelings that they are unable to cognitively integrate, and thus becoming more distressed than relived, *(2)* a feeling that they are being unduly pressured by the therapist or group, or *(3)* both. Ultimately, it is up to the patient whether, and to what extent, to explore frightening emotions. Another, more emotionally expressive person in the group can serve as a good model for exploring negative emotions. Eventually,

the fear of the "flood gates opening and never closing again" will subside as it becomes clear from observing others in the group that crying which comes freely during one's expression of concern is usually a positive release, leaving one feeling better, not worse.

Also, note the tendency of the group as a whole to become "informational" when difficult issues and emotions arise, or following an especially emotional session. Appreciate the emotional threshold of each person, and the group as a whole. Part of not "pushing too hard" includes allowing some lightness, even humor to emerge, before returning to difficult topics.

COPING. When patients discuss problems in a way that implies helplessness and lack of control, it is helpful to ask a question which leads them to explore ways that they can cope actively, rather than merely give up in despair. Of course, there is in reality a great deal over which a cancer patient has no control. Yet there is always something in which a patient can actively participate with regard to their problem. They may learn to react in a better way to the crisis, improve communication with others involved in the situation, or, if possible, to seek ways to improve the situation itself other than those already attempted. In general, when a patient states that there is nothing they can do regarding their cancer in general, or some aspect of it, therapists can ask questions which will lead patients to explore areas over which they in fact *do* have some degree of participation. For instance, if a patient says: "The doctor says that I have to go back for more hyperthermia treatment. But it hurts so much that I just don't think I can take it again," the therapist might ask: "Have you tried discussing this with your radiologist or the technicians?" Or ask the group, truly a "panel of experts," if anyone has a suggestion.

Rather than offering ready-made solutions to patients, it is almost always better to find a way for the patient to actively seek solutions in the group. After all, if the goal is for patients to develop active coping skills, simply giving them advice makes for a poor learning experience. It is usually useful to follow a stepwise progression in leading patients to explore active solutions to their problems. Ask questions which have the patients find a solution to their own problems ("What can you do to improve the situation?"). If this proves too difficult, it can be helpful to ask questions which will bring principles of active coping to light: ("How would you rather react to this difficult situation, in a way that would leave you feeling better afterwards?"). If this still does not lead to active exploration on the part of the patient, the therapist can ask for suggestions from the group as a whole. Finally, as a last result, it may be useful to offer an interpretation of what seems to be happening with a patient, and then ask the patient or the group to comment on this interpretation ("Sometimes people become more distressed when they feel out of control. I wonder if you are experiencing so much distress because you feel out of control with the treatment?").

RELATIONSHIP. One of the benefits of group therapy is that it offers patients the ability both to express emotions about their condition, as well as to give and receive support within a community of persons whose experiences are somewhat close to their own. Therefore, while allowing personal expression is important, therapists should attempt to have the expression directed to another person, the group as a whole, or, if necessary, the therapist. Yet therapists should be wary of turning a group into a series of individual patient expressions or conversations with the therapist. In fact, the therapist is relatively silent in this type of group. When needed in order to get a patient or the group "back on track," therapists will typically ask one to three questions before turning the focus to another person or opening the discussion to the group as a whole in order to maintain an interactive discussion among members.

In general, when a patient is expressing, but not relating, the therapist has several methods to elicit interaction. The therapist can facilitate interaction with:

1. *The therapist*. It is useful for the therapist to establish a connection with the patient by asking questions (eliciting personal, specific, and affective statements about their distress and ability to cope with it). Following a patient's statement that is external, abstract, intellectual or is evidence of passive coping, the therapist should probe for more authentic types of expressions in two or three questions, then redirect the next question to the group or to another group member to commence a dialogue between patients (see 3 below).

2. *The group*. Therapists should limit their interaction with a group member to just a few questions and responses before asking the group as a whole to get involved. It is useful for the therapist to briefly summarize what the patient has been saying (e.g., It sounds as if you have been finding it difficult to get your concerns across to your doctor"), followed by statements such as: "Has anyone else had a similar difficulty?", or perhaps: "Does anyone who has faced these same difficulties have some advice for (patient)?"

3. *Another member*. Whenever possible, it is very useful to facilitate an interaction between two group members. This direct patient interaction is an ideal way to give and get support, and establish a more intimate relationship than can be established with the therapist alone, or with the group in general. Therefore, following a patient's statement, whether a second patient responds, a second patient responds to a general question addressed to the group as a whole, or the therapist happens to recall that another patient has had a similar experience, the therapist should attempt to establish a two-way conversation for a time, before redirecting to the group. For example: "Sarah, you told us last week that you were finding ways to tell your doctor your concerns about reconstructive surgery. Can you offer any suggestions to Jodie that might help her out in her current situation?" And then, after some discussion: "Jodie, do you think the way Sarah handled her situation could assist you in your situation?" This approach is especially effective if the therapist can have two patients taking roles that help both them as well as each other. Consider a group in which one member is very quiet and tends to ask for help and then reject it, while another member is very free in giving advice to others yet rarely discusses his own situation with the group. It would be an ideal situation if the therapist could facilitate a discussion where the "quiet" member is able to use his experience to offer advice to the "helper" member who would be encouraged to reflect upon this advice.

Typically, therapists will find it easier to facilitate interaction in the order presented above (1 → 2 → 3). However, these are presented in reverse order of value to the patients. Interaction with other members of the group are in many ways superior to interaction with the group leader. This is evident when group leaders find that they may give advice at some point, yet it is only when another group member offers similar advice that the patient becomes excited and decides to act on the suggestion.

Heuristic Concerns in Facilitating the Group Process. In addition to the specific methods of facilitation, some general guidelines are helpful to keep in mind. It is useful to have an existential and experiential focus in the group, and to remain a facilitator of process rather than a lecturer (see Table 61.5).

EXISTENTIAL FOCUS. The therapeutic process described above allows for authentic examination of existential concerns, without the impression of psychological "games" that are often experienced in deductive or interactive brief coping skills groups. Since issues are patient driven, discussion stays close to the concerns of the patients. Process facilitation by the therapist assures continued authenticity in patients' quality of expression. In addition, this process can facilitate patients' ability to be more fully "in the moment," rather than linger in the past or worry about the future.

GIVING ADVICE. When facilitating discussion, therapists must avoid the trap of answering questions with definitive information. Instead, they can draw upon the knowledge of the group, which is a superb source of expertise. In educational groups, therapists are teachers relaying information. But in group discussion, therapists' emphasis should be on facilitating the *process*, not providing *content*. Once the therapist becomes the "expert" it will be extremely difficult to return to facilitating the process—the patients simply will not permit the therapist to "shift gears." Avoiding giving advice may be difficult for a therapist with expertise, but it is also very important. The expert-therapist should find ways to diffuse the question, such as suggesting that the patient ask their oncologist, or that the subject could be discussed after the group. This approach focuses the patients on the group process rather than the group becoming an informational meeting (and correspondingly void of interaction with each other in personal, specific, and affective terms).

EXPERIENTIAL EMPHASIS. Therapists can look for situations where the patients can experience a problem and solution first-hand in the group, rather than to merely comment about it. Rather than attempting to point out habitual ways of thinking and then asking a patient to reflect about their beliefs which formed this way of thinking, therapists can offer the opportunity for the patient to directly experience healthy ways of dealing with a problem (52). If Alice is having difficulty with her husband understanding some of her needs, the therapist attempting to foster reflection and awareness of personality patterns might say: "I notice (or you've said) that you sometimes have difficulty expressing your needs and problems here in the group, as well. Is this a common pattern in your life? In what other situations does this pattern arise?" Certainly, this line of questioning might be useful in a cognitive-behavioral psychotherapy group which attempts to make unconscious patterns conscious. In groups facilitating emotional expression and support among cancer patients, however, it might be more useful to say: "Sometimes it's hard to let others know what you need. Is there a way you can let those of us in the

TABLE 61.5. *Comparing Educational, Cognitive-Behavioral, and Social/Emotional Supportive Group Therapy*

Type of Group	Therapeutic Emphasis		
	Advice	Focus	Experience
Education	Mostly given	Information	None
Cognitive-behavioral	Sometimes given	Skill-oriented	Reflection about problem occurring throughout one's life; practice specific skills in special exercises
Social/emotionally supportive	Rarely given	Existential	Directly experience alternative ways of active coping through interactions naturally arising in group

group know what you need, so that we can better understand what you're going through?". Or, "Julie, do you know what Alice needs?. Alice, can you let Julie know what your needs are?" Thus, rather than stimulating reflection about one's patterns, therapists should look for an opportunity for a patient to directly experience their restrictive way of coping in the group and try out a healthy alternative. A reflective remark *after* such an experience has far greater impact than when stated alone. And when the experience is strong enough, such reflective remarks may be totally unnecessary.

The above process guidelines for inductive facilitation should be followed whenever group discussion occurs, even if discussion follows a deductively presented informational lecture, or special exercises in a skills-building format. However, as has been noted, once deductive teaching has occurred, shifting to an inductive facilitative format is problemmatic. Yet whatever method of facilitation predominates should be guided by the structure and goals of the group.

DETERMINING THE FORMAT FOR THERAPEUTIC GROUPS

The therapeutic style utilized for helping cancer patients will depend upon the specific population and the structure employed to serve these patients' special needs. These factors are reviewed below.

Structure of the Group

Choices must be made in organizing a group for cancer patients, in terms of therapeutic intention, method of facilitation, populations comprising the group, and size and time course of the group. These are each considered below.

Therapeutic Intent. There are three basic structures of group therapy: informational education, training in coping skills, and those offering social and emotional support, as well as combinations of these. Each of these structured formats is best served by a different therapeutic style. In general, informational education is best delivered through a deductive presentation, cognitive-behavioral training in coping skills by an interactive therapeutic style, and social and emotional support in an inductive facilitory style. However, each of these formats may benefit at times from partial use of another therapeutic style (see Table 61.6).

INFORMATIONAL EDUCATION. Informational groups are useful for those concerned with preventing cancer, and may focus on smoking cessation, breast self-exam,

TABLE 61.6. *Therapeutic Style Differs by Group Structure and Goals*

Goals of Group	Therapeutic Style		
	Deductive	Interactive	Inductive
Informational knowledge	X	x	–
Coping skills	x	X	x
Social and emotional support	–	x	X

X, primary therapeutic emphasis; x, minor emphasis; –, negligible emphasis.

the need for regular screening, the benefits of low fat diets and exercise, and the like. An educational focus is also commonly offered for those recently diagnosed who wish to learn more information about their disease, what treatments are available, rehabilitative options following surgery (physical therapy, cosmetic surgery, prostheses, etc.), and what, if any, preventive measures they can take in the future (sun exposure, skin creams, and self-exams for melanoma patients). Typically brief (one to four meetings), these groups are either lecture-oriented, with patients merely asking questions of the professional (arguably *not* group therapy), or with more of an active educational focus (e.g. teaching prevention skills as in smoking cessation or self-exam). Such groups are frequently coordinated by social workers with clinical nurse specialists as guest speakers, and are usually offered as a free service by the institution (53).

COPING SKILLS. The most common type of groups for cancer patients teach active coping strategies focusing on specific and immediate concerns for the patient. These concerns include identifiable stressors and stress reactions, communication issues, practicing health behaviors such as diet and exercise, specific self-help techniques for reducing pain and nausea, etc. Such groups are usually short-term (six to ten meetings), run 90–120 minutes per session, and most commonly utilize a cognitive-behavioral orientation. Typically, a therapist will present a topic for the first few minutes of a group, followed by the patients engaging in a paper and pencil exercise or an interaction with a partner to practice a strategy. The rest of the group will be taken up with discussion on how one can implement these active coping strategies in one's life. Many times such groups will begin and end with a brief physical relaxation or cognitive meditation training. Most often run by psychologists, social workers, or mental health nurse specialists trained in behavioral medicine techniques, these groups are effective for patients who have specific concerns about a recently diagnosed cancer (54).

SOCIAL AND EMOTIONAL SUPPORT. Persons with more advanced disease, or who are having difficulty adjusting to having cancer, can benefit from longer-term therapy (3 months to 1 year or longer). Since longer groups have the opportunity to form intimate bonds of support, patients are able to discuss virtually any issue of personal concern related to their living with having cancer. Specific topics rarely need to be introduced by the therapists as all topics will eventually be raised by the patients. Such groups have the potential to address both immediate issues of coping with distress, as well as deeper existential considerations of changing priorities, self-image, and directly confronting issues of death and dying. In these groups, the patients are most active, with the therapists typically taking a back seat, only to emerge to keep the patients "on track" and to facilitate interactions. These types of groups are most similar to traditional group psychotherapy, with the modifications made for cancer patients rather than patients with strictly psychosocial dysfunction, as described above.

COMBINATIONS OF EDUCATIONAL, COPING SKILLS, AND SOCIAL-EMOTIONAL SUPPORT. Combinations of two or three of these major approaches are certainly not uncommon. Clearly, a health educator may provide mainly lecture, but then ask participants to practice a skill, and then facilitate discussion among the participants. A psychologist in a coping skills class may tend to focus on lecturing about and practice of specific skills, or else spend more time in facilitation of discussion, depending upon therapeutic orientation or persons in the group. Or, a typical 12-session group for new breast cancer patients may include *(1)* basic education of prosthesis or reconstructive surgery, *(2)* relaxation skills and pain management, and *(3)* discussion of how to communicate needs and desires to one's spouse, etc. When resources permit, a different therapist may present different aspects of such mixed orientation groups.

The Time Course of a Group

FIRST MEETINGS. Initial introductions are important as they set the tone for the rest of the meetings. Allow members to express their stories. Beyond discussing members names, and type of cancer, members can also tell their story about the diagnosis, treatment, and how they are coping with it. This method, used by mental health workers in debriefing participants of disasters (55), is useful to reduce the stress reaction and

possibly future posttraumatic stress reactions (56,57). It is also an excellent way to set the tone of the group as one of seriousness, openness, and support. In longer term inductive groups, these can take several sessions, and group discussions can spin-off from a patient's story. In shorter groups, the therapist may need to draw out silent or shy members and manage more verbose members. It is paramount to have each patient's expression met with understanding and compassion, which allows the other members to feel safer in addressing their own fears. It is important to remember that persons from all walks of life and ways of viewing the world come together in this (for them) unusual setting. They are looking for guidance as to how the group functions, both in terms of *what* is discussed as well as *how* topics are to be discussed. The initial meeting is critical in forming the "group style" that is to continue in future meetings.

MIDDLE MEETINGS. Opening each meeting with some ritual is helpful. When members arrive initially, there is going to be some light chatting. At some point, it is valuable for the therapist to get up and close the door as a signal that the meeting is going to formally begin. Checking-in with everyone (anyone missing?) and showing honest concern for them will help the group know that they are cared for, as well as insuring better compliance with attendance or at least being informed of planned absences. A brief (5 minute) meditation or relaxation (58) is useful to begin with. Such meditation can serve to settle and focus one's mind and the group as a whole. It also serves to teach stress and pain management and self-comforting. The *body* of the meetings will consist of either presenting information (didactic), discussing the topic to be addressed for the meeting (interactive), or asking if there are any important issues that need to be discussed (inductive), depending upon the format of the group. *Closing* each meeting can sometimes be difficult, especially when emotional issues are being discussed. Letting the group know that there are 15 minutes left can serve to focus the group on essentials and help members begin to summarize important points. It can also be a message that new "hot" topics should not be pursued in much detail at this time, and should be picked up again at the next meeting. Finishing on time is important, as it offers the security of a much needed structure to often unexpected feelings that arise. Consistent closure also serves to let the group know that whatever occurs in the group, there is someone in charge monitoring the group. Finishing with another 5–10 minutes of meditation/relaxation helps not to only reinforce the value of learning to calm the mind and relax the body, but also to settle down after an arousing session. If participants know that they will leave feeling relatively calm and relaxed, they can allow more openness of expression during the meeting itself. It is also possible to lead a "guided meditation" or self-hypnosis as part of the relaxation at the end of a meeting as a way of summarizing the main topic that has been discussed, perhaps helping patients to imagine positive ways of dealing with a negative issue (59).

FINAL MEETINGS. The last several meetings can be difficult for members. Bonds that have been formed will be coming to a close, with associated feelings of loss. In long-term groups of 6 months or longer, closure should be discussed for the final month, with emphasis on how members will continue to find social support in their lives, as well as what the group has meant to them. Grieving the loss of the group may well prepare them for grieving other aspects of their lives. Shorter groups should also address the ending of the group and what it means to each patient at a final meeting, although such issues may arise with less intensity. In all cases, it is useful to recommend follow-ups to other groups, activities, or therapy, as required by each individual member.

Open or Closed Groups. Closed groups are those which require all patients to join the group at the same time, and remain in the group for a committed duration (e.g., 16 weekly meetings), during which time no other patients can join. *Open groups*, in contrast are those which allow members to join at any time, for any length, as is common in American Cancer Society monthly drop-in support groups. Effective groups intending therapeutic improvement are either closed or semiclosed groups (60). *Semiclosed* groups allow members to join when there is an opening in the group (member leaves, dies, or completes their commitment), but the patient must make a commitment for a specified duration.

Advantages of closed groups are primarily in the consistency and ease of treatment. Disadvantages of closed groups are found in several areas. If a program has limited resources and has not been able to fill a group, beginning a group with six patients while requiring newly interested patients to wait for months until the present group ends may be impractical. Short-term groups which have a specific agenda to cover may be able to demand a closed group. Yet in a long-term group with recurrent cancer patients, illness and death will reduce the size of the group to a point where it is

difficult to continue effectively. Therefore, semiclosed groups are often utilized in longer-term formats.

Size of Groups. The number of participants in a group depends upon the type of the group and outcomes expected. Educational groups can number in the dozens while emotion-focused social-interactive groups do better with about 12 members. Skill-oriented groups lie somewhere in the middle. The more one seeks serious and emotion-based interaction between group members, the smaller the group size needs to be. About a dozen members provide a minimum synergy of diverse experiences and personality styles to keep a group going well. Still, groups as small as six or as large as 20 can often be very engaging and productive, assuming that therapists have the skills to handle such groups.

Choosing the Setting. It is not always possible to choose a pleasant location for group therapy. If psychosocial treatment must be held in a medical center, then having the meetings substantially away from the place patients receive oncological treatment can avoid problem associations (such as anticipatory nausea, etc.). However, if one can only offer the treatment in a medical setting, then learning to relax and receive psychosocial support in this setting can aid in relaxing and receiving medical support next time they come for treatment.

Applications to Specific Populations

In deciding which therapeutic structures and styles to employ, it is necessary to consider factors associated with the patients being served. These factors include stage of disease, disease type, and the personal characteristics of those who make up the groups.

Stage of Disease. Each stage of illness has it's own special issues, which psychotherapists must be sensitive to in order to determine the appropriate therapeutic goals and select optimal methods and group structures to achieve these goals. The various group structures and therapeutic methods discussed above can be appropriately utilized to assist various types of persons with cancer (see Table 61.7).

PREVENTION. Persons who are at increased risk for disease incidence or recurrence frequently have education about preventive measures as their goal, although some discussion of stress and its management might be included in such education. Method of education is didactic which most often occurs in a brief format (between one and six weekly meetings).

TABLE 61.7. *Therapeutic Goals, Methods, and Structures Useful for Addressing the Special Issues of Specific Cancer Populations*

Stage of Illness	Special Issues	Goals	Methods	Structure
Prevention	At increased risk for disease incidence or recurrence	Education	Deductive: Didactic information	Brief class (1–4 meetings)
Diagnosis	Distress over diagnosis Confusion about cancer	Education Coping in moment Emotional support	Interactive: Didactic information Experiential skills Inductive: Supportive discussion,	Brief group (1–6 weeks)
Treatment	Discomfort: nausea, mucus Membranes, fatigue, weight Reality of illness sets- in	Coping with treatment Adjusting one's life to having cancer Emotional support	Interactive: Experiential skills Inductive: Supportive discussion,	Brief to short-term (4–12 weeks)
Recovery	Aelf-image (cancer patient?) Questioning life activities Relationships Sense of control Possible recurrence or death Attitudes/behavior affecting health	Active coping Emotional/social support Ee-examining life values, beliefs, priorities Considering one's future Living a healthy lifestyle	Interactive: Cognitive therapy Experiential skills Inductive: Supportive discussion	Short-term (8–16 weeks)
Recurrence and Dying	Emotional distress Death and dying Coping with treatment Loss of control Family and friends Physical discomfort/fatigue	Active coping Pain and stress management Emotional/social support Existential issues Lving fully in the moment	Inductive: Supportive discussion Interactive: Experiential skills	Long-term (24 weeks to ongoing)
Family Members and Bereavement	Emotional distress Existential issues Guilt	Emotional support Work through distress Living more in the moment Planning for the future	Inductive: Supportive discussion Interactive: Experiential skills	As needed, Brief formats, support persons attend with patients Longer formats, support and bereaved members meet separately

DIAGNOSIS. Patients who have recently received a first diagnosis of cancer are naturally distressed over the diagnosis, and are no doubt confused about cancer, its etiology, treatment, and prognosis. Goals for this population should include basic education, initial stress management in order to attend more to the present and cope with immediate decisions regarding treatment, and emotional support. While some deductive intervention is useful for offering basic information, therapeutic facilitation is primarily interactive for developing active coping skills, with some inductive facilitation for supportive discussion. It is difficult to mix didactic and interactive formats, since, once they have been lectured to, patients find it difficult to engage in discussion or open emotionally. Therefore, many therapists find it most beneficial to separate the didactic education from the interactive

components. Different meetings, different parts of meetings separated by a break, or even different facilitators, can help patients to get the most out of each type of method.

TREATMENT. Special issues for persons undergoing treatment may include the need to deal with recovery from surgery and discomfort from chemotherapy and radiotherapy which often includes fatigue, nausea, dry or sore mucus membranes, weight changes, flu-like symptoms, etc. Changes in appearance (e.g., hair loss) and daily functioning are also common. With these changes occurring, the urgency of dealing with the initial diagnosis and treatment decisions passing, and the initial shock subsiding, the reality of the illness begins to set in. Patients at this stage are concerned with coping with treatment, adjusting to a lifestyle of being a cancer patient, and receiving emotional support. An interactive therapeutic style which offers emotional support and discussion along with experiential skills is therefore appropriate, and can be delivered effectively for most patients in a brief (4–12 week) group, at least initially.

RECOVERY. Once treatment is completed, a patient's concerns turn to changes in self-image ("Am I a cancer patient?"), changes in relationships, questioning and reprioritizing daily activities, wanting more control over one's health and course of disease, wondering whether personality or behavior affects their health, and considering the possibility of disease recurrence and death. Therapeutic goals for this stage include training in active coping strategies, offering emotional and social support, reexamining life values, beliefs, priorities, considering one's optimal future way of living, and learning to live a mentally and physically healthy lifestyle. Utilizing an interactive therapeutic style with a cognitive-behavioral therapy orientation, teaching experiential coping skills, and then switching to an inductive therapeutic style allowing for supportive discussion will help achieve these skills, usually in a short-term (8–16 week) group format.

RECURRENCE AND DYING. Patients who have disease recurrence face substantial emotional distress—quite likely reexperiencing distress from the initial diagnosis (61)—protracted and intensive treatment, greater loss of control, physical discomfort and fatigue, reduced daily functioning and decisions regarding retirement and disability, new ways of relating to family and friends, and also more directly confronting the likelihood of dying. Learning to cope more actively, managing pain and stress, receiving emotional support, addressing existential issues, and living more fully in each moment are goals that are extremely beneficial to patients at this stage of illness. An inductive approach allowing for supportive discussion and occasional interactive facilitation of experiential skills (relaxation, self-hypnosis) can facilitate these goals in a longer format (24 weeks to ongoing).

FAMILY MEMBERS AND BEREAVEMENT. Families of cancer patients should not be neglected. Assisting the family members to cope better themselves goes a long way in supporting the patient. Family members to some extent suffer all the same issues as does the patient. Therefore, a similar style of therapy is appropriate for them as for the patient. In early stages of treatment (for patients confronting prevention, diagnosis, and possibly brief groups for coping with treatment), it is

valuable to have family members present in the groups. However, for longer-term groups (greater than 4 weeks), patients and family members are better served in separate groups, so that they each can discuss their own concerns and not worry about distressing the other. Resources permitting, it can be convenient to have patients and family members meet at the same time, in adjacent rooms. Of course, not all patients have family members in the area, or who can attend such groups, and this lack of support should be addressed in the patient groups.

Family members of patients who have died face considerable emotional distress, existential considerations, and possibly guilt (see Chapter 88). Offering emotional support to work through distress and helping them to live more fully in the moment and plan for the future requires an inductive, interactive format, along with teaching some experiential skills (relaxation, self-hypnosis). Family members who have been involved in family groups while the patient was alive should be invited to stay on in the group for as long as they like.

Disease Type. In the same way that stages of disease can be broken down to address specific issues, type of cancer needs to be considered as well. Cancer patients, no matter what organ is affected, have many issues in common that should be addressed in groups. However, women with breast cancer have some very different concerns than do men with prostate cancer. Members of mixed-gender groups may find it difficult to discuss issues of prosthesis, reconstruction, or sexuality. Lung cancer patients may need to address feelings of guilt and acknowledge the severity of the disease, while Hodgkins' patients typically try and put the disease behind them and learn to move on.

Demographic Differences. Age, race, income, education, etc., all need to be considered in developing groups. Groups designed specifically to educate poor minority women about the need to receive regular Pap-smears and follow-up in case of cervical dysplasia need to address different coping strategies (62) than a group of women in a wealthy community who meet to discuss the implications of cervical dysplasia.

Choosing the Make-up of Groups. For the most part, therapists attempt to offer treatment to the most specific population possible. It is not infrequent, however, that multiple populations are combined to include any stage of illness, any type of cancer, and any type of individual. There are advantages and disadvantages to homogeneous or heterogeneous groups. Groups can be organized around disease type or staging, gender, depression, specific issues corresponding to specific organs (skin, gynecologic), etc., or any combination of these.

HOMOGENEOUS GROUPS. The more homogeneous the group, the more specific the goals, and the more focused the intervention. Towards this end, it is usually advisable to organize groups with similar disease site and stage, and with age and sex being a factor when possible. For instance, groups of breast cancer patients in treatment who are under 50 years of age would have a more common focus than mixed cancer groups. It is often difficult for patients with earlier stage disease to discuss issues such as wigs or dating when there are also patients with recurrent disease in the groups discussing their funeral arrangements. Homogeneous groups are certainly the easiest to facilitate.

HETEROGENEOUS GROUPS. Although more difficult to facilitate, finding sufficient numbers of patients to comprise a homogeneous group often proves difficult, especially with less common types of cancer. On the positive side, the value of early stage patients in seeing others at later stages of illness can be helpful in confronting their fears of death and dying, and to see how well these patients handle the later stages of disease. Also, the more varied a group in terms of personality, demographics, gender, and disease type, the more varied will be the experiences that members can bring to any given problem.

Often members feel isolated when others in a group don't share some specific factor that they identify with, such as their type of cancer. (Of course, even in a group of first occurrence breast cancer patients under 50 years of age there can be a patient who claims that there is no one who can really understand her since no-one else has her specific subtype of breast cancer.) One solution is to ask such patients to describe their special issues in order to help others understand their situation better. This assists the speaker to express and connect, and help others to better appreciate the speaker's concerns.

Assuming the therapists are sufficiently trained to handle the problems that arise from mixed groups, it is better to have a group of mixed cancer patients than no group at all. Some groups that offer an educational format or a coping skills format to large groups of persons with any type or stage of cancer as well as support persons are apparently quite popular and helpful. However, inductive intervention useful for eliciting emotion-focused and supportive interactions among patients are almost certainly sacrificed.

SUMMARY

Group therapy is a potent effective modality for giving psychological support to cancer patients. Studies have proven its efficacy repeatedly. This chapter provides a "nuts and bolts" approach for how to plan and conduct group psychotherapy sessions with cancer patients. The need for attention to stage of disease, homogeneity of the group members, and intervention method are reviewed. The development of group interventions is being more extensively researched using better methods which should begin to prove scientifically what has been observed by many patients.

REFERENCES

1. Hellman CJ, Budd M, Borysenko J, et al. A study of the effectiveness of two group behavioral medicine interventions for patients with psychosomatic complaints. *Behav Med.* 1990; 16(4):165–173.
2. Corsini RJ, Rosenberg B. Mechanisms of group psychotherapy processes and dynamics. *J Abnorm Soc Psychol.* 1955; 51:406–411.
3. Presberg BA, Levenson JL. A survey of cancer support groups provided by the National Cancer Institute. *Psycho-Oncology.* 1993; 2:215–219.
4. Dunkel-Schetter C, Feinstein LG, Taylor SE. Patterns of coping with cancer. *Health Psychol.* 1992; 11(2):79–87.
5. Goldstein DA, Antoni MH. The distribution of repressive coping styles among non-metastatic and metastatic breast cancer patients as compared to non-cancer patients. *Psychol Health.* 1989; 3:245–258.
6. Greer S. Psychological response to cancer and survival. *Psychol Med.* 1991; 21:43–49.
7. Hann D, Oxman T, Ahles T, et al. Social support adequacy and depression in older patients with metastatic cancer. *Psycho-Oncology.* 1994; 4:213–223.
8. Reifman A. Social relationships, recovery from illness, and survival: a literature review. *Ann Behav Med.* 1995; 17(2):124–131.
9. Temoshok I. Biopsychosocial studies on cutaneous malignant melanoma: psychosocial factors associated with prognostic indicators, progression, psychophysiology, and tumor-host response. *Soc Sci Med.* 1985; 20:833–840.
10. Shekelle RB, Gale M, Ostfeld AM, Paul O. Hostility, risk of coronary heart disease, and mortality. *Psychosom Med.* 1983; 45(2):109–114.
11. Dunkel-Schetter C, Feinstein LG, Taylor SE. Patterns of coping with cancer. *Health Psychol.* 1992; 11(2):79–87.
12. Fawzy FI, Kemeny ME, Fawzy N, et al. A structured psychiatric intervention for cancer patients. II: Changes over time in immunological measures. *Arch Gen Psychiatry.* 1990; 47:729–735.
13. Ruckdechel J, Peantadosi S. The lung cancer study group quality of life assessment in lung cancer for bronchogame carcinoma. *J Thor Surg.* 1991; 6:201–205.
14. Winick L, Robbins GF. Physical and psychologic readjustment after mastectomy: an evaluation of Memorial Hospitals' PMRG program. *Cancer.* 1977; 39(2):478–486.

15. Wood PE, Milligan M, Christ D, Liff D. Group counseling for cancer patients in a community hospital. *Psychosomatics.* 1978; 19:555–561.

16. Frenkel EM, Torem M. Management of a dying patient in group therapy. *Group.* 1981; 5(1):54–61.

17. Cella D, Sarafian B, Snider P, et al. Evaluation of a community-based cancer support group. *Psycho-Oncology.* 1993; 2:123–132.

18. Trijsburg RW, van Knippenberg FCI, Rijpma SE. Effects of psychological treatment on cancer patients: a critical review. *Psychosom Med.* 1992; 54:489–517.

19. Spira J, Spiegel D. Group psychotherapy of the medically ill. In: Stoudemire A, Fogel B, eds. *Psychiatric Care of the Medical Patient,* 2nd ed. New York: Oxford University Press; 1993: 31–50.

20. Fawzy FI, Fawzy NW, Arndt LA, Pasnau RO. Critical review of psychosocial interventions in cancer care. *Arch Gen Psychiatry.* 1995; 52:100–113.

21. Forester B, Kornfelf DS, Fleiss JL, Thompson S. Group psychotherapy during radiotherapy: effects on emotional and physical distress. *Am J Psychiatry.* 1993; 150(11):1700–1706.

22. Weisman A, Worden J, Sobel H. *Psychosocial Screening and Intervention With Cancer Patients: Research Report.* Cambridge, MA: Shea; 1980.

23. Vachon ML, Lyall WA, Rogers J, et al. The effectiveness of psychosocial support during post-surgical treatment of breast cancer. *Int J Psychiatr Med.* 1982; 11:365–372.

24. Heinrich R, Schag C. Stress and activity management: group treatment for cancer patients and spouses. *J Consult Clin Psychol.* 1985; 33:439–446.

25. Berglund G, Bolund C, Gustafsson U, Sjoden P. A randomized study of a rehabilitation program for cancer patients: the "starting again" group. *Psycho-Oncology.* 1994; 3:109–120.

26. Fawzy FI, Fawzy NW, Hyun CS. Short-term psychiatric intervention for patients with malignant melanoma: effects on psychological state, coping, and the immune system. *The Psychoimmunology of Cancer.* New York: Oxford University Press; 1994; 292–319.

27. Yalom I. *The Theory and Practice of Group Psychotherapy,* 3rd ed. New York: Basic Books; 1985.

28. Spiegel D, Bloom J, Yalom I. Group support for patients with metastatic cancer. *Arch Gen Psychiatry.* 1981; 38:527–533.

29. Spiegel D, Spira J. *Supportive-Expressive Group Therapy: A Treatment Manual of Psychosocial Intervention for Women with Recurrent Breast Cancer.* Stanford, CA: Stanford University School of Medicine Department of Psychiatry; 1991.

30. Richardson JL, Shelton D, Krailo M, Levine AM. The effect of compliance with treatment on survival among patients with hematologic malignancies. *J Clin Oncol.* 1990; 8:356–364.

31. Fawzy FI, Fawzy NW, Wheeler JG. A post hoc comparison of the efficiency of a psychoeducational intervention for melanoma patients delivered in groups vs individual format. *Psycho-Oncology.* 1996; 5:81–91.

32. Johnson J. The effects of a patient education course on persons with a chronic illness. *Cancer Nurs.* 1982; April:117–123.

33. Lerman C, Lustbader E, Rimer B, et al. Effects of individualized breast cancer risk counseling: a randomized trial. *J Natl Cancer Inst.* 1995; 87(4):286–292.

34. Cain EN, Kohorn EI, Quinlan DM, et al. Psychosocial benefits of a cancer support group. *Cancer.* 1986; 67:183–189.

35. Telch CF, Telch MJ. Group coping skills instruction and supportive group therapy for cancer patients: a comparison of strategies. *J Consult Clin Psychol.* 1986; 54:802–808.

36. Cunningham AJ, Tocco EK. A randomized trial of group psychoeducational therapy for cancer patients. *Patient Educ Couns.* 1989; 14:101–114.

37. Evans RL, Connis RT. Comparison of brief group therapies for depressed cancer patients receiving radiation treatment. *Public Health Rep.* 1995; 1110(3):306–311.

38. Spiegel D, Bloom JR, Kraemer HC, Gottheil E. Effect of psychosocial treatment on survival of patients with metastatic breast cancer. *Lancet.* 1987; 2(8668):888–891.

39. Fox B. The role or psychological factors in cancer. *Incidence Prognosis Oncol.* 1995; 9:245–252.

40. Fawzy FI, Kemeny ME, Fawzy N, et al. A structured psychiatric intervention for cancer patients. II: Changes over time in immunological measures. *Arch Gen Psychiatry.* 1990; 47:729–735.

41. Fawzy FI, Fawzy NW, Hyun CS, et al. Malignant melanoma: effects of an early structured psychiatric intervention, coping, and affective state on recurrence and survival 6 years later. *Arch Gen Psychiatry.* 1993; 50:681–689.

42. Gellert GA, Maxwell RM, Siegel BS. Survival of breast cancer patients receiving adjunctive psychosocial support therapy: a 10-year follow-up study. *J Clin Oncol.* 1993; 11(1):66–69.

43. Siegel B, Spira J, Ulmer D. Panel discussion: the effects of group therapy on medically ill patients. *Fourth Mind, Body, and Immunity Conference.* Hilton Head, SC: Institute for the Clinical Application of Behavioral Medicine; December 1992.

44. Mooney S, Greer S, Watson M, et al. Adjuvant psychotherapy for patients with cancer. *Psycho-Oncology.* 1994; 3:39–47.

45. Meyer J, Mark MM. Effects of psychosocial interventions with adult cancer patients: a meta-analysis of randomized experiments. *Health Psychol.* 1995; 14(2):101–108.

46. Spira J. Educational Therapy: Existential, Educational, and Counseling Approaches to Behavioral Medicine Intervention. Doctoral Dissertation, University of California, Berkeley, 1991.

47. Spira J, ed. *Group Therapy for the Medically Ill.* New York: Guilford Press; 1997.

48. Maslow A. *Toward a Psychology of Being,* 2nd ed. Princeton: Insight Books; 1968.

49. Roter DL, Hall JA, Kern DE, et al. Improving physicians' interviewing skills and reducing patients' emotional distress. *Arch Intern Med.* 1995; 155:1877–1884.

50. Spira J. Existential group psychotherapy for women with metastatic breast cancer and other advanced stage illnesses. In: Spira J, ed. *Group Therapy for the Medically Ill.* New York: Guilford Press; 1997.

51. Roberts CS, Cox CE, Reintgen DS, et al. Influence of physician communication on newly developed breast

patients' psychological adjustment and decision-making. *Cancer.* 1994; 74:336–341.

52. Spigel D, Spira J. *Supportive-Expressive Group Therapy: A Treatment Manual For Women with Recurrent Breast Cancer.* Palo Alto, CA: Department of Psychiatry, Stanford University Medical Center; 1991.

53. Lerman C, Lustbader E, Rimer B, et al. Effects of individualized breast cancer risk counseling: a randomized trial. *J Natl Cancer Inst.* 1995; 87(4):286–292.

54. Fawzy FI, Fawzy NW, Hyun CS. Short-term psychiatric intervention for patients with malignant melanoma: effects on psychological state, coping, and the immune system. In: Lewis CE, O'Sullivan C, Barraclough J, eds. *The Pyschoimmunology of Cancer.* New York: Oxford University Press; 1994:292–319.

55. Mitchell J, Everly G. *Critical Incident Stress Debriefing: CISD.* Ellicott City, MD: Chevron Publishing; 1993.

56. Spira J. Dissociation and PTSD in the Medically Ill [abstract]. Academy of Psychosomatic Medicine, New Orleans, LA; November, 1993.

57. Tremsland L, Soreide J, Malt U. Traumatic distress symptoms in early breast cancer. *Psycho-Oncology.* 1996; 5:1–9.

58. Spira J. *Tai Chi Chuan and Zen Meditation For the Medically Ill: Videotape and Manual.* Durham, NC: Duke University School of Medicine; 1994.

59. Spira J, Spiegel D. Hypnosis and related techniques in pain management for the terminally ill. *Hospice J.* 1992; 8(1/2):89–120.

60. Trijsburg RW, van Knippenberg FCI, Rijpma SE. Effects of psychological treatment on cancer patients: a critical review. *Psychosom Med.* 1992; 54:489–517.

61. Miller SM, Roussi P, Altman D, et al. The effects of coping style on psychological reactions to colposcopy among low-income minority women. *J Reprod Med.* 1994; 39:711–718.

62. Gawler I. *You Can Conquer Cancer.* Melbourne: Hill of Content; 1984.

62

Cognitive-Behavioral Interventions

PAUL B. JACOBSEN AND DANETTE M. HANN

A recent survey found that cognitive-behavioral interventions were among the most widely offered psychosocial services in comprehensive cancer centers (1). The widespread use of these interventions can be attributed to several factors. First, and perhaps most important, cognitive-behavioral interventions have been shown to be effective in reducing emotional distress and controlling physical symptoms in cancer patients (2). Second, the interventions can usually be administered in a brief period of time and thus are well suited for use in oncology where rapid control of aversive symptoms may be necessary. Third, the interventions can be easily tailored to deal with the unique symptom control problems and quality of life issues that cancer patients experience. And fourth, the interventions are readily accepted by patients because of the emphasis that is placed on increasing the patient's sense of personal control and self-efficacy.

The aim of this chapter is to provide readers with an overview of the use of cognitive-behavioral interventions with cancer patients. We begin by describing the cognitive-behavioral approach and the types of interventions that comprise this approach. We then focus on three areas in oncology where cognitive-behavioral interventions have had a major impact on patient care: *(1)* relief of pain related to cancer and its treatment; *(2)* control of aversive reactions to chemotherapy administration; and *(3)* enhancement of emotional well-being. The review concludes with an appraisal of the current and future status of the use of cognitive-behavioral interventions with cancer patients. It should be noted our review is limited to the use of cognitive-behavioral interventions with adult cancer patients. Information about the many uses of cognitive-behavioral interventions with pediatric cancer patients can be found in Chapter 84.

THE COGNITIVE-BEHAVIORAL PERSPECTIVE

The cognitive-behavioral perspective is based on the postulate that mental and physical symptoms are in part a function of underlying thoughts, feelings, and/or behaviors of a maladaptive nature (3). Consequently, a cognitive-behavioral approach to reducing or eliminating symptoms involves the identification and correction of thoughts, feelings, and behaviors that contribute to symptom development and symptom maintenance. As the name implies, the cognitive-behavioral perspective incorporates both behavioral and cognitive approaches to psychological change. Reflecting its behavioral origins, the cognitive-behavioral perspective uses techniques for behavior change derived from the principles of operant conditioning (4) and respondent conditioning (5). Examples of behavioral techniques are contingency management, systematic desensitization, biofeedback, and various methods of relaxation training including some forms of hypnosis. Reflecting its cognitive origins, the cognitive-behavioral perspective also uses techniques for changing cognitions derived from principles of information processing (6). Examples of cognitive techniques are distraction, thought monitoring, cognitive restructuring, coping self-statements, and mental imagery exercises. Descriptions of commonly used cognitive and behavioral techniques can be found in Table 62.1 and in several sources (7–10).

In order to maximize therapeutic effectiveness, developers of cognitive-behavioral interventions often combine several cognitive and behavioral change techniques into a "package." Standardized multicomponent intervention packages have been developed for a range of purposes including the management of stress reactions (13) and chronic pain (3) and the treatment of anxiety disorders (28).

As stated previously, this chapter will focus on the use of cognitive-behavioral interventions with adult

TABLE 62.1. *Commonly Used Cognitive and Behavioral Techniques*

Technique	Description	Source of Additional Information*
Cognitive restructuring	Critical examination and reevaluation of negative interpretations of events in order to reduce feelings of distress, helplessness and hopelessness	Beck et al. (1979) (7) Beck and Emery (1985) (11)
Contingency management	Use of positive or negative reinforcement to increase the frequency of desired behaviors or reduce frequency of undesired behaviors	Turner et al. (1993) (12) Wolpe (1990) (9)
Coping self-statements	Silent or spoken self-statements used to manage, master, or reinterpret noxious or threatening situations and experiences	Turk et al. (1983) (3) Meichenbaum (1985) (13)
Distraction	Redirection of attentional processes for purposes of reducing awareness of threatening events or aversive sensations	McCaul and Malott (1984) (14)
Biofeedback	Provision of relatively immediate information about a normally subliminal aspect of physiologic functioning in order to facilitate learning of voluntary control over this functioning	Basmajian (1989) (15) Stoyva and Budzynski (1993) (16)
Progressive muscle relaxation	Tensing and relaxing of specific muscle groups and controlled deep breathing for purposes of reducing autonomic activation and inducing subjective feelings of relaxation	Bernstein and Borkevec (1973) (17) Bernstein and Carlson (1993) (18)
Systematic desensitization	Presentation of a series of increasingly potent anxiety-arousing stimuli (either in vivo or in imagination) to a deeply relaxed individual resulting in reduction of phobic responses	Wolpe (1990) (9)
Hypnosis	Formal induction of a state characterized by sustained attention and concentration, reduced peripheral awareness, and openness to suggestion	Barber (1993) (19) Spiegel and Spiegel (1978) (20)
Autogenic training	Use of suggestion and deep breathing to reduce autonomic arousal and induce a sense of relaxation	Linden (1993) (21) Schultz and Luthe (1969) (22)
Problem-solving therapy	Package of cognitive and behavioral techniques used to promote identification and implementation of effective problem-solving strategies	D'Zurilla (1986) (23) D'Zurilla (1988) (24)
Stress inoculation training	Package of cognitive and behavioral techniques designed to foster more adaptive responses to potentially stressful situations and events	Meichenbaum (1985) (13) Meichenbaum (1993) (25)
Guided imagery	Use of mental imagery to promote relaxation, to enhance perceived control, or to rehearse coping responses	Edwards (1989) (26) Sheikh (1983) (27)

*Number in parentheses refers to reference list.

cancer patients to relieve disease- and treatment-related pain; to control aversive reactions to chemotherapy administration, and to improve emotional well-being. Controlled randomized trials that have examined these uses of cognitive-behavioral interventions are listed in Tables 62.2–62.4 and are described below.

PAIN

The application of cognitive-behavioral techniques to the management of cancer pain is based on the premise that pain is a subjective experience that is influenced by attitudes and beliefs, as well as emotional distress (29). For example, the meaning that patients ascribe to their pain can affect the perception of pain severity as well as the perceived ability to manage pain (30). Patients who interpret pain as a signal of disease progression are likely to experience their pain as more severe and less controllable than patients who interpret pain as a

temporary consequence of treatment (31). The basic goals when using cognitive-behavioral interventions in the management of cancer-related pain are: *(1)* to alleviate pain, *(2)* to increase patients' sense of self-efficacy and control, and *(3)* to reduce the impact of pain on daily functioning, mood, and interpersonal relationships (32). When incorporated into a comprehensive pain management program, cognitive-behavioral techniques can help to relieve the physical sensations of pain as well as its accompanying psychological distress (e.g., depression and anxiety), thereby improving the patient's quality of life (33).

It should be noted that there are some patients for whom a cognitive-behavioral approach to cancer pain management may not be appropriate. If the patient is rapidly deteriorating, is in severe pain that is not being adequately controlled by other means, or is delirious, psychotic, or clinically depressed, cognitive-behavioral treatment should probably not be attempted (34). The appropriateness of a cognitive-behavioral intervention for an individual patient should be determined by medical and psychosocial staff in collaboration with the patient and family members.

The first step in planning an intervention is to conduct a comprehensive assessment that takes into account the multidimensional nature of cancer pain (35). Pain may have physical, cognitive, social, emotional, and behavioral sources and/or manifestations, all of which may be targeted for treatment. Millard (36) suggests that a comprehensive pain assessment include administration of a semistructured interview as well as standard pain assessment tools. In addition to improving clinical care, the inclusion of standard, reliable, and valid assessment instruments yields a database that can be used for research purposes. As part of the initial assessment phase of treatment, patients should be instructed to keep a daily pain diary. Ideally, patients should record the intensity, severity, and duration of their pain (average ratings for an entire day or separate hourly ratings), behavioral, physical, and emotional triggers for pain, the impact of pain on daily functioning (e.g., work activity, social activity, and family relationships), and maneuvers that successfully relieve the pain (e.g., medication, a warm bath, mild exercise). This initial record is helpful for the clinician and the patient in developing a full understanding of the nature of the pain, its patterns, and its potential treatment. A principal goal of assessment is to identify targets for cognitive and behavioral interventions. Once target behaviors and cognitions have been identified, there are several skills that can be taught to the patient. Some of the more commonly used interventions which have been studied empirically are described below.

Relaxation training is often used, either alone or as an adjunct to pharmacotherapy, in the management of cancer pain (37). Despite considerable anecdotal evidence of the efficacy of relaxation training for cancer-related pain (31,36), an extensive literature search uncovered only one study that used a controlled randomized design to examine the effectiveness of this technique (38) (see Table 62.2). In this study, researchers examined the effects of an intervention that combined progressive muscle relaxation with "mental imagery" on patients' reports of pain and their use of analgesic medications. Hospitalized patients with cancer pain were randomly assigned to a no intervention condition or to conditions in which relaxation training was provided either by audiotape or by a nurse. Compared to the control group, patients who received either audiotaped instruction or live instruction reported significantly less pain and used fewer nonopioid analgesics. Although this study will require

replication, it provides the strongest evidence to date of the effectiveness of relaxation training in alleviating cancer-related pain.

Imagery is a technique that involves having patients develop a mental image associated with feelings of peacefulness and calmness. It is frequently used in conjunction with relaxation training, but can also be used alone. Guided visualizations, in which patients are instructed to focus on an image which symbolizes their disease or a specific symptom like pain, then modify their image in a therapeutic manner, can help patients experience a greater sense of control over their disease process (39). As with relaxation, anecdotal reports support the use of imagery (31,39). Unfortunately, there has been little systematic study of its effectiveness in relieving cancer pain. In one of the few randomized studies (40), cancer patients with pain were assigned to listen to audiotapes that featured either guided imagery or progressive muscle relaxation exercises. Both interventions were found to be effective in reducing cancer-related pain and distress. However, few conclusions can be drawn about the efficacy of imagery since this study did not include random assignment to a no treatment control group.

Hypnosis may offer cancer patients the advantages of pain relief without the risks of tolerance, unpleasant side effects, or disruptions of cognitive or physical functioning associated with the use of pain medications (41). However, as Millard (36) points out, some patients are not receptive to the idea of being hypnotized by another person and prefer to be taught a relaxation exercise which they can control. Clearly, patient preference should be taken into account when considering the use of hypnosis. Although there is some anecdotal evidence in support of the use of hypnosis to relieve cancer-related pain (42,43), empirical evidence is again limited. One of the only controlled investigations of the efficacy of hypnosis in relieving cancer-related pain was conducted by Spiegel and colleagues (44,45). In this study, women with metastatic breast cancer were randomly assigned to a no intervention condition or to group therapy. Patients assigned to the group therapy condition were then nonrandomly assigned to groups that either did or did not include instruction in hypnosis for pain control. Results indicated that, compared to patients in the control condition, patients who received group therapy reported less severe pain and less suffering over a 1 year period. Additional analyses indicated that patients who received group therapy and hypnosis experienced less pain than patients who received group therapy alone. Although these findings support the use of hypnosis for relief of pain related to meta-

TABLE 62.2. Summary of Controlled Randomized Studies of Cognitive-Behavioral Interventions to Relieve Cancer-Related Pain

Study	Participants Diagnosis	Females/ Males	Control groups (n)	Experimental groups (n)	Format	Intervention Number and length of sessions	C-B components Coping	Relax	Hypnosis	Guided Imagery	Outcomes Coping	Emot Well-Being	Phys Well-Being	Func-tioning	Phys Arousal
Sloman et al. (1994) (38)	Mixed	F = 19 M-48	No tx (20)	#1 (20)	Indiv	4 sessions (adm. by audiotape)		x		x			+		
				#2 (20)	Indiv	4 sessions (adm. by nurse)		x		x			+		
Speigel and Bloom (1983) (45)	Breast	F = 54	No tx (24)	#1 (30)	Group	52 sessions, 90 min			x				+		
Syrajala et al. (1992) (50)	Hematalogic malignancy or lyphoma	F = 19 M = 26	No tx (10) Attn (12)	#1 (11)	Indiv	2 sessions, 90 min	x	x	x	x		+	+		
				#2 (12)	Indiv	2 sessions, 90 min		x	x	x		0	0		

x = Component included in intervention.
+ = Significant improvement relative to controls.
0 = Nonsignificant improvement relative to controls.

static disease, they require replication for at least two reasons. First, the assignment to self-hypnosis in this study was not based on random assignment. Second, since many subjects died before the 1 year follow-up, the outcome analyses required extensive use of statistical corrections for missing data. Future studies could best deal with this issue by examining the efficacy of hypnosis over shorter time intervals.

Biofeedback is a technique designed to teach patients how to modify specific aspects of physiologic functioning. Patients are instructed in ways to modify their muscle tension, body temperature, respiration or skin conductance while receiving visual and/or auditory feedback of their current functioning on these dimensions. Clinical reports suggest that both electroencephalographic (EEG) and electromyographic (EMG) biofeedback may be of use in the treatment of cancer-related pain (46,47). However, a review of the literature failed to uncover any randomized controlled studies of the efficacy of this approach in treating cancer patients with pain.

Multicomponent cognitive-behavioral interventions are designed to help patients modify thoughts, beliefs, or behaviors that may exacerbate pain and its psychological sequelae (e.g., depression, anxiety) and to provide them with skills that can be used to cope with pain. Turk and Rennert (48) were among the first to describe a multicomponent cognitive-behavioral intervention designed to relieve cancer-related pain. Their approach involved education about the contribution of beliefs, attitudes, and emotions to the experience of pain as well as training in the use of both behavioral and cognitive techniques (e.g., relaxation, imagery, attention diversion, problem solving) for coping with pain. Clinical reports suggest that multicomponent cognitive-behavioral interventions are effective against cancer-related pain (34,49). However, the first controlled study to evaluate this approach yielded equivocal results. In this study (50), patients receiving chemotherapy before bone marrow transplantation were randomized to one of four conditions: *(1)* cognitive-behavioral coping skills training; *(2)* hypnosis training; *(3)* attentional control; or *(4)* no treatment control. Of principal interest was the impact of the interventions on the severity of chemotherapy-induced oral mucositis pain. Results indicated that patients who underwent hypnosis training, but not cognitive-behavioral training, experienced less pain than controls. The authors of this study caution, however, that the numerous components included in the two cognitive-behavioral training sessions (relaxation training, cognitive restructuring, development of coping self-statements, and psychoeducation about symp-

toms and side effects) may have exceeded what patients could learn in such a short time. A description of a subsequent study conducted by the same group of researchers (32) suggests that patients who received a simplified version of this cognitive-behavioral intervention experienced less pain than controls.

AVERSIVE REACTIONS TO CHEMOTHERAPY

The use of cognitive-behavioral interventions with chemotherapy patients initially focused on the clinical problem of anticipatory nausea and vomiting (ANV). In the early 1980s, a series of clinical reports described patients who had previously received emetogenic chemotherapy and who became nauseated and/or vomited in anticipation of subsequent treatments (51,52). In addition to describing this phenomenon, these clinical reports hypothesized that anticipatory reactions in chemotherapy patients were examples of classically conditioned responses. Similar to conditioned vomiting responses that could be experimentally induced in laboratory animals (4), cancer patients appeared to develop ANV when previously neutral stimuli (e.g., the sights, sounds, and smells of the treatment environment) acquired nausea/emesis eliciting properties due to repeated association with chemotherapy administration and its aversive aftereffects. Based on this respondent conditioning conceptualization, several researchers investigated the efficacy of cognitive-behavioral interventions for controlling ANV. Two interventions were found to be effective in the first round of controlled clinical trials: progressive muscle relaxation training combined with guided imagery (53,54) and systematic desensitization (55) (see Table 62.3). In both these studies, patients with ANV who were randomly assigned to a cognitive-behavioral intervention subsequently experienced less anticipatory nausea and/or vomiting than patients randomly assigned to either no treatment or attention control conditions.

In the studies cited above, the cognitive-behavioral interventions were delivered to chemotherapy patients by specially trained mental health professionals. At least one study has investigated whether the potential availability of these interventions could be increased by training oncology personnel in the use of cognitive-behavioral techniques. In this study (56), patients with ANV were randomly assigned to receive no treatment or to receive systematic desensitization from either a clinical psychologist, an oncologist, or an oncology nurse trained in the technique. Results indicated that patients in each intervention condition experienced significant declines in anticipatory nausea relative to patients who received no treatment.

TABLE 62.3. *Summary of Controlled Randomized Studies of Cognitive-Behavioral Interventions to Relieve Aversive Reactions to Chemotherapy*

Study	Diagnosis	Females/Males	Control groups (n)	Experimental groups (n)	Format	Number and length of sessions	Prep info	Coping	Relax	Distr	Coping	Emot Well-Being	Phys Well-Being	Functioning	Phys Arousal
Burish and Lyles (1981) (53)	Mixed	F = 14 M = 2	No tx (8)	#1 (8)	Indiv	5 sessions			x		+	+	+		−
Lyles et al (1982) (54)	Mixed	F = 31 M = 19	No tx (18) Attn (14)	#1 (18)	Indiv	5 sessions			x			+	+		−
Morrow and Morrell (1982) (55)	Mixed	F = 42 M = 18	No tx (20) Attn (20)	#1 (20)	Indiv	2 sessions, 1 hour			x				+		
Morrow et al (1992) (56)	Mixed	?	No tx (14)	#1 (29)	Indiv	2 session, 1 hour (adm. by oncology staff)			x				+		
				#2 (29)	Indiv	2 sessions, 1 hour (adm. by psychologist)			x				+		
Vasterling et al (1993) (54)	Mixed	F = 39 M = 21	No tx (20)	#1 (20)	Indiv	5 sessions			x			+	+		−
				#2 (2)	Indiv	5 sessions				x		+	+		−
Burish et al (1987) (60)	Mixed	?	No tx (12)	#1 (12)	Indiv	6–8 sessions			x			+	+		−
Lerman et al (1990) (61)	Mixed	F = 32 M = 16	No tx (23)	#1 (25)	Indiv	1 session, 30 mins			x			0	+		
Burish et al (1991) (62)	Mixed	F = 29 M = 31	Attn (15)	#1 (15)	Indiv	1 session, 90 min	x	x				+	+	+	
				#2 (15)	Indiv	4 sessions		x	x			+	0	0	
				#3 (15)	Indiv	5 sessions	x	x	x			0	+	0	

x = Component included in intervention.
+ = Significant improvement relative to controls.
0 = Nonsignificant improvement relative to controls.

Moreover, there were no differences in the magnitude of the therapeutic effects based on whether the intervention was delivered by a psychologist, a physician, or a nurse.

The means by which relaxation training and systematic desensitization reduce ANV have been the subject of considerable debate. Speculation among researchers (57,58) has centered around two possible mechanisms of action: physiological relaxation and cognitive distraction. The relaxing effects of these interventions may serve to inhibit the muscular contractions in the gastrointestinal tract involved in nausea and vomiting. Alternatively, the cognitive demands of these interventions could serve to direct attention away from sensations of nausea or from stimuli that have acquired nausea-eliciting properties. To isolate the possible role of distraction in ANV control, one study (59) evaluated an intervention that has both distraction and relaxation components (progressive muscle relaxation training) as well as an intervention that has a distraction component but no relaxation component (videogame playing). Compared to a no treatment control condition, patients in both intervention conditions experienced significantly less anticipatory nausea. Moreover, the two interventions did not differ in their effectiveness. Thus, results suggest that control of ANV can be achieved by distraction alone.

Other research has examined whether cognitive-behavioral interventions conducted before the start of chemotherapy are effective in preventing or postponing development of ANV. Two studies that examined this issue (60,61) yielded mixed results. In both studies, patients scheduled to begin chemotherapy were randomly assigned to receive either progressive muscle relaxation and guided imagery or no intervention before the start of treatment. One study (60) found that by the fourth infusion (i.e., after several "conditioning trials") patients in the no intervention condition were experiencing significantly more anticipatory nausea and anticipatory anxiety than patients in the intervention condition. The same study also found that patients in the intervention condition experienced significantly less nausea, vomiting, and anxiety after chemotherapy than patients in the no intervention condition. The other study (61) found no significant group differences in anticipatory nausea when it was assessed at the third infusion. However, patients in the intervention condition did experience significantly less nausea after chemotherapy than patients in the no intervention condition.

Although findings regarding ANV prevention are inconclusive, both studies suggest that cognitive-behavioral interventions conducted before the start of che-

motherapy may have other beneficial effects. Specifically, these interventions may serve to limit posttreatment nausea and vomiting and reduce treatment-related emotional distress. In one of the few controlled studies designed specifically to address this issue (62), patients about to begin chemotherapy were randomly assigned to one of four intervention conditions: relaxation training, coping preparation, relaxation training and coping preparation, or no treatment. Relaxation training consisted of instruction in progressive muscle relaxation immediately before the first infusion. Coping preparation consisted of four components: *(1)* a tour of the oncology clinic that provided patients with procedural information as well as concrete sensory information regarding chemotherapy administration; *(2)* a videotape presentation of a patient modeling successful coping with chemotherapy treatment; *(3)* a discussion and question and answer session that offered patients an opportunity to express feelings and concerns and to receive suggestions on how to cope with treatment and its side effects; and *(4)* a booklet that patients could use to review previously presented information. This 90 minute intervention was conducted on a day prior to the first chemotherapy administration. Findings indicated that the coping preparation yielded a number of beneficial effects. Compared to patients in the no treatment condition, patients who received coping preparation reported less anticipatory nausea, posttreatment vomiting, and depression. Moreover, among patients working outside the home, those who underwent the coping preparation reported less interference associated with cancer and its treatment on their ability to work. The benefits of relaxation training were less extensive, and the addition of relaxation training to coping preparation did not yield additional benefits. Findings from this study suggest that brief training in coping skills before the start of treatment may be an effective means of improving quality of life during chemotherapy.

EMOTIONAL WELL-BEING

The use of multicomponent cognitive-behavioral interventions to improve well-being in cancer patients has been the subject of considerable attention in recent years. This interest can be attributed, in part, to evidence suggesting that psychosocial interventions designed to improve emotional and physical well-being in cancer patients may also improve survival (63,64). Interest in this area has also been stimulated by the increased recognition of the importance of quality of life (a construct that includes both emotional and physical well-being) as an end-point in cancer treatment (65,66). Although there is considerable enthusiasm for the use of cognitive-behavioral interventions to improve emotional well-being, a review of the literature indicates that only a handful of studies have evaluated these interventions using controlled randomized designs (see Table 62.4).

Worden and Weisman were among the first to develop and evaluate cognitive-behavioral interventions to reduce distress and improve well-being in cancer patients. In a landmark study (67), these investigators evaluated two interventions designed to promote coping and adaptation among newly diagnosed patients. Both interventions focused on the development of problem-solving skills. In the first approach, the therapist focused on the specific problems the patient was currently facing. In the second approach, the therapist focused more on the development of general problem-solving skills and discussed the solution of common problems faced by cancer patients. The second approach also included training in progressive muscle relaxation. Participants in the study were newly diagnosed cancer patients who were identified as being at high risk for psychological distress using well-defined criteria. These individuals were randomized to one of the two intervention conditions and their responses were compared to those of a nonrandomized control group. Results indicated that patients in both intervention groups experienced less psychological distress at follow-up than controls. Despite its methodologic limitations (i.e., the lack of a nonrandomized control group), this study has had an enormous impact on the field of psychosocial oncology. Elements of this intervention have been incorporated into several other multicomponent interventions that have been clinically validated and are described below.

Building on the work of Worden and Weisman (67), Heinrich and Schag (68) evaluated a stress and activity management program designed for cancer patients and their spouses. In multicouple groups, participants were taught specific problem-solving skills, received training in relaxation and information about coping with cancer and its treatment, and were encouraged to engage in physical exercise and to increase positively valued activities. The responses of couples randomized to this program were compared with those of couples randomized to standard care. Contrary to predictions, patients who received stress and activity management training did not demonstrate better psychosocial adjustment or activity levels than patients who received standard care.

Other studies that have evaluated similar cognitive-behavioral interventions have obtained different results. Telch and Telch (69) examined the impact on quality of life of a group-administered program of coping skills training. The program consisted of five modules that covered: (1) relaxation and stress management; (2) communication and assertion; (3) problem solving and constructive thinking; (4) feelings management; and (5) pleasant activity planning. The effects of this intervention were tested by randomly assigning cancer patients to receive group coping skills instruction, supportive group therapy, or no treatment. Results indicated that, immediately following the 6 week intervention, patients who underwent coping skills training were less emotionally distressed and reported fewer problems than patients in the other two conditions.

A study by Fawzy et al. (64) provides additional evidence that cognitive-behavioral interventions are effective in promoting adaptive coping and reducing emotional distress. In this study, patients with early stage melanoma were randomly assigned to a no treatment control condition or to a group administered program that included: health education, problem-solving skills training modeled after the work of Worden and Weisman (67), stress management training, and psychological support. At a 6 month follow-up, the intervention group was found to be experiencing less emotional distress and to be using more active coping methods than the control group.

Greer et al. (70) tested an individually administered cognitive-behavioral intervention designed to improve emotional well-being. The intervention, referred to as "adjuvant psychological therapy," has multiple components, including coping skills training, cognitive restructuring, and progressive muscle relaxation training. In a controlled outcome study designed to evaluate the effectiveness of this intervention, cancer patients who met specific criteria for psychological morbidity were randomized to receive either adjuvant psychological therapy or no treatment. At a 4 month follow-up, patients who had received the cognitive-behavioral intervention were found to be experiencing less emotional distress than patients who received no treatment. These effects remained evident at a 12 month follow-up (71).

At least one study has directly compared individual versus group administered forms of cognitive-behavioral interventions to promote emotional well-being. In this study (72), women with gynecologic cancer were randomized to either individual or group forms of "thematic counseling" or no treatment. Both the individual and group interventions included the following

TABLE 62.4. *Summary of Controlled Randomized Studies of Cognitive-Behavioral Interventions to Improve Emotional Well-Being*

Study	Participants		Control groups (n)	Experimental groups (n)	Intervention		C-B components				Outcomes		
	Diagnosis	Females/Males			Format	Number and length of sessions	Info	Coping/Problem Solving	Relax	Activity Planning	Coping	Emot Well-Being	Functioning
Heinrich and Schag (1985) (68)	Mixed	?	No tx (25)	#1 (26)	Group	6 sessions, 2 hours	x	x	x	x		0	
Telch and Telch (1986) (69)	Mixed	F = 27 M = 14	No tx (14)	#1 (13) #2 (14)	Group Group	6 sessions, 90 min 6 sessions, 90 min		x	x	x	+ +	+ +	
Fawzy et al (1990) (64)	Melanoma	F = 35 M = 31	No tx (28)	#1 (38)	Group	6 sessions, 90 min	x	x	x		+	+	
Greer et al (1992) (70)	Mixed	F = 32 M-124	No tx (84)	#1 (72)	Indiv	6 sessions, 1 hour		x	x	x		+	
Cain et al (1986) (72)	Gynecologic	F = 80	Std Care (29)	#1 (21) #2 (22)	Indiv Group	8 sessions 8 sessions		x x	x x	x x		+ +	+ +

x = Component included in intervention.
+ = Significant improvement relative to controls.
0 = Nonsignificant improvement relative to controls.

components: psychoeducation about cancer and its treatment, relaxation training, development of problem-solving skills, and discussion of diet and exercise. Data collected at a 6 month follow-up indicated that women who received thematic counseling either as individuals or in groups were less emotionally distressed and had made a better adjustment to their illness than women in the control group. Women who received thematic counseling also report better sexual functioning and greater participation in leisure activities. Thus, there does not appear to be any difference in efficacy associated with the format (i.e., group versus individual) of cognitive-behavioral intervention.

SUMMARY AND FUTURE DIRECTIONS

The cognitive-behavioral perspective has had a major impact on the psychosocial care of cancer patients. Interventions have been developed and empirically validated for the relief of pain related to cancer and its treatment, for the relief of aversive reactions to chemotherapy administration, and for the promotion of emotional well-being.

With regard to cancer-related pain, controlled randomized studies indicate that relaxation training is an effective means (38) and that hypnosis may be an effective means (45) of providing pain relief. Several multicomponent cognitive-behavioral interventions that involve training in problem-solving skills have been developed for use against cancer-related pain (48) and anecdotal reports suggest that patients benefit from these approaches (49). However, there do not appear to be any controlled randomized trials that have investigated this issue. Conducting such trials should be considered a high priority in light of recent guidelines that recommend the use of psychological interventions as part of multidisciplinary treatment of cancer-related pain (73). In addition to investigating the effects on reported pain intensity, researchers may also wish to evaluate the impact of cognitive-behavioral interventions on other important clinical outcomes (e.g., analgesic medication use, emotional well-being, and level of functioning).

With regard to aversive reaction to chemotherapy treatment, controlled randomized studies indicate that both relaxation-based interventions and distraction-based interventions are effective in controlling ANV (53–59). In addition, relaxation-based interventions conducted before the start of treatment appear to be effective in reducing posttreatment nausea and vomiting (60,61). In light of these findings, future efforts in this area should focus on increasing patient access to empirically validated interventions.

Preliminary research along these lines shows that oncology personnel can be trained to deliver cognitive-behavioral interventions to chemotherapy patients as effectively as mental health professionals (56). A key issue that has yet to be addressed is the relative cost-effectiveness of different methods of delivering cognitive-behavioral interventions. It remains unclear whether training oncology personnel to provide relaxation training, rather than using mental health professionals, yields any cost savings. Another delivery method that has yet to be examined is patient self-administered interventions. Effective self-administered forms of relaxation training have been developed for other clinical populations (e.g., headache sufferers) (74) and could be adapted for use with chemotherapy patients. In addition to investigating different delivery methods, future research with chemotherapy patients should consider a broader range of quality of life outcomes. Preliminary work suggests that administration of cognitive-behavioral interventions prior to outpatient chemotherapy may relieve emotional distress and improve daily functioning (62).

With regard to emotional well-being, controlled randomized studies indicate that multicomponent cognitive-behavioral interventions are an effective means of improving psychological functioning. Interventions that have been found to be effective involve training in relaxation, problem-solving, and adaptive coping skills. Three issues can be identified as foci for future work in this area. First, current multicomponent interventions can be refined by testing the efficacy of their individual components. Research along these lines could lead to interventions that are briefer and more economical and could help to identify the mechanisms responsible for the therapeutic effects of cognitive-behavioral techniques. Second, as in the case of aversive reactions to chemotherapy, research in this area should assess a broader array of quality of life outcomes. In addition to improving emotional well-being, cognitive-behavioral techniques may also be effective in relieving common physical symptoms (e.g., pain and fatigue) and improving physical and psychosocial functioning. Third, the use of cognitive-behavioral interventions to improve the quality of life of long-term cancer survivors deserves greater attention. Training in problem-solving and adaptive coping skills may prove to be particularly effective in assisting former patients who are experiencing poor quality of life due to persistent emotional concerns (e.g., fears of disease recurrence) and/or physical sequelae of cancer treatment (e.g., changes in physical function or appearance).

In conclusion, the use of cognitive-behavioral interventions with cancer patients is supported by an impressive number of controlled randomized studies. However, there are important gaps in this empirical foundation that should be the focus of future research (e.g., efficacy of cognitive-behavioral interventions for cancer pain). Future work in this area should also focus on examining the impact that cognitive-behavioral interventions have on patients' social and occupational functioning, on evaluating the cost-effectiveness of providing cognitive-behavioral interventions in oncology settings, and on identifying the mechanisms by which cognitive-behavioral interventions improve quality of life during and after active treatment.

ACKNOWLEDGMENTS
Preparation of this manuscript was supported in part by an American Cancer Society Junior Faculty Research Award to Dr. Jacobsen.

REFERENCES

1. Coluzzi PH, Grant M, Doroshow JH, et al. Survey of the provision of supportive care services at National Cancer Institute-designated cancer centers. *J Clin Oncol.* 1995; 13:756–764.
2. Meyer TJ, Mark MM. Effects of psychosocial interventions with adult cancer patients: a meta-analysis of randomized experiments. *Health Psychol.* 1995; 14:101–108.
3. Turk DC, Meichenbaum D, Genest M. *Pain and Behavioral Medicine: A Cognitive-Behavioral Perspective.* New York: Guilford Press; 1983.
4. Skinner BF. *Science and Human Behavior.* New York: Macmillan; 1953.
5. Pavlov IP. *Conditioned Reflexes.* Oxford: Oxford University Press; 1927.
6. Hamilton V. Cognition and stress: an information processing model. In: Goldberger L, Breznitz S, eds. *Handbook of Stress: Theoretical and Clinical Aspects.* New York: Free Press; 1982: 105–120.
7. Beck AT, Rush AJ, Shaw BF, Emery G. *Cognitive Therapy of Depression.* New York: Guilford; 1979.
8. Hawton K, Salkovskis P, Kirk J, Clark DM. *Cognitive Behavior Therapy for Psychiatric Problems.* Oxford: Oxford University Press; 1989.
9. Wolpe J. *Practice of Behavior Therapy.* New York: Pergamon Press; 1990.
10. Barlow DH. *Clinical Handbook of Psychological Disorders.* New York: Guilford; 1994.
11. Beck AT, Emery G. *Anxiety and Phobias: A Cognitive Approach.* New York: Basic Books; 1985.
12. Turner SM, Calhoun KS, Adams HE, eds. *Handbook of Clinical Behavior Therapy,* 2nd ed. New York: Wiley; 1993.
13. Meichenbaum D. *Stress Inoculation Training.* Elmsford, NY: Pergamon Press; 1985.
14. McCaul KD, Malott JM. Distraction and coping with pain. *Psychol Bull.* 1984; 95:516–533.
15. Basmajian JV, ed. *Biofeedback: Principles and Practice for Clinicians,* 3rd ed. Baltimore: Williams & Wilkins; 1989.
16. Stoyva JM, Budzynski TH. Biofeedback methods in the treatment of anxiety and stress disorders. In: Lehrer PM, Woolfolk RL, eds. *Principles and Practice of Stress Management.* New York: Guilford; 1993:263-300.
17. Bernstein DA, Borkevec TD. *Progressive Relaxation Training: A Manual for the Helping Professions.* Champaign, IL: Research Press; 1973.
18. Bernstein DA, Carlson CR. Progressive relaxation: abbreviated methods. In: Lehrer PM, Woolfolk RL, eds. *Principles and Practice of Stress Management.* New York: Guilford; 1993:53–88.
19. Barber TX. Hypnosuggestive approaches to stress reduction: data, theory, and clinical applications. In: Lehrer PM, Woolfolk RL, eds. *Principles and Practice of Stress Management.* New York: Guilford; 1993:169-204.
20. Spiegel H, Spiegel D. *Trance and Treatment: Clinical Uses of Hypnosis.* New York: Basic Books; 1978.
21. Linden W. The autogenic training method of JH Schultz. In: Lehrer PM, Woolfolk RL, eds. *Principles and Practice of Stress Management.* New York: Guilford; 1993: 205–230.
22. Schultz JH, Luthe W. *Autogenic Therapy:* vol 1. *Autogenic Methods.* New York: Grune & Stratton; 1969.
23. D'Zurilla TJ. *Problem-solving Therapy: A Social Competence Approach to Clinical Intervention.* New York: Springer; 1986.
24. D'Zurilla TJ. Problem-solving therapies. In: Dobson KS, ed. *Handbook of Cognitive-Behavioral Therapies.* New York: Guilford; 1988: 85–135.
25. Meichenbaum D. Stress inoculation training: a 20-year update. In: Lehrer PM, Woolfolk RL, eds. *Principles and Practice of Stress Management.* New York: Guilford; 1993: 373–406.
26. Edwards DJA. Cognitive restructuring through guided imagery: Lessons learned from Gestalt Therapy. In: Freeman A, Simon KM, Beutler LE, Arkowitz H, eds. *Comprehensive Handbook of Cognitive Therapy.* New York: Plenum; 1989: 283–297.
27. Sheikh AA, ed. *Imagery: Current Theory, Research, and Application.* New York: Wiley; 1983.
28. Barlow DH, Cerny JA. *Psychological Treatment of Panic.* New York: Guilford Press; 1988.
29. Turk DC, Fernandez E. On the putative uniqueness of cancer pain: do psychological principles apply? *Behav Res Ther.* 1990; 28:1–13.
30. Barkwell DP. Ascribed meaning: a critical factor in coping and pain attenuation in patients with cancer-related pain. *J Palliat Care.* 1991; 7:5–14.
31. Ahles TA. Psychological techniques for the management of cancer-related pain. In: McGuire DB, Yarbro CH, eds. *Cancer Pain Management.* Orlando, FL: Grune Stratton; 1987: 245–258.
32. Syrjala KL. Integrating medical and psychological treatments for cancer pain. In: Chapman CR, Foley KM, eds. *Current and Emerging Issues in Cancer Pain: Research and Practice.* New York: Raven Press; 1993: 393–409.
33. Breitbart W. Psychiatric management of cancer pain. *Cancer.* 1989; 63:2336–2342.

34. Loscalzo M, Jacobsen PB. Practical behavioral approaches to the effective management of pain and distress. *J Psychosoc Oncol.* 1990; 8:139–169.

35. Ahles TA. Cancer pain: research from multidimensional and illness representation models. *Motiv Emotion.* 1993; 17:225–243.

36. Millard RW. Behavioral assessment of pain and behavioral pain management. In: Patt RB, ed. *Cancer Pain.* Philadelphia, PA: JB Lippincott; 1993: 85–97.

37. Cobb SC. Teaching relaxation techniques to cancer patients. *Cancer Nurs.* 1984; 7:157–162.

38. Sloman R, Brown P, Aldana E, Chee E. The use of relaxation for the promotion of comfort and pain relief in persons with advanced cancer. *Contemp Nurse.* 1994; 3:6–12.

39. Simonton OC, Matthews-Simonton S, Sparks TF. Psychological intervention in the treatment of cancer. *Psychosomatics.* 1980; 21:226–233.

40. Graffam S, Johnson, A. A comparison of two relaxation strategies for the relief of pain and its distress. *J Pain Symptom Manage.* 1987; 2:229–231.

41. Barber J, Gitelson J. Cancer pain: psychological management using hypnosis. *CA Cancer J Clin.* 1980; 30:130–136.

42. Hilgard ER. *Hypnosis in the Relief of Pain.* Los Altos, CA: William Kaufman; 1975.

43. Margolis CG. Hypnotic interventions for pain management. *Int J Psychosom.* 1985; 32:12–19.

44. Spiegel D, Bloom JR, Yalom I. Group support for patients with metastatic breast cancer. *Arch Gen Psychiatry.* 1981; 38:527–533.

45. Spiegel D, Bloom JR. Group therapy and hypnosis reduce metastatic breast carcinoma pain. *Psychosom Med.* 1983; 45:333–339.

46. Fotopoulos SS, Graham C, Cook MR. Psychophysiologic control of cancer pain. In: Bonica JJ, Ventifridda V, eds. *Advances in Pain Research and Therapy.* New York: Raven Press; 1979:231–243.

47. Fotopoulos SS, Cook MR, Graham C, et al. Cancer pain: evaluation of electromyographic and electrodermal feedback. *Prog Clin Biol Res.* 1983; 132D:33–53.

48. Turk DC, Rennert K. Pain and the terminally ill cancer patient: a cognitive-social learning perspective. In: Sobel HJ, ed. *Behavior Therapy in Terminal Care: A Humanistic Approach.* Cambridge, MA: Ballinger; 1981.

49. Fishman B, Loscalzo M. Cognitive-behavioral interventions in management of cancer pain: principles and applications. *Med Clin N Am.* 1987; 71:271–287.

50. Syrjala KL, Cummings C, Donaldson G. Hypnosis or cognitive-behavioral training for the reduction of pain and nausea during cancer treatment: a controlled clinical trial. *Pain.* 1992; 48:137–146.

51. Nesse RM, Carli T, Curtis GC, Kleinman PD. Pretreatment nausea in cancer chemotherapy: a conditioned response? *Psychosom Med.* 1980; 42:33–36.

52. Redd WH, Andresen GV. Conditioned aversion in cancer patients. *Behav Thera.* 1981; 4:3–4.

53. Burish TG, Lyles JM. Effectiveness of relaxation training in reducing adverse reactions to cancer chemotherapy. *J Behav Med.* 1981; 4:65–78.

54. Lyles JN, Burish TG, Krozely MG, Oldham RK. Efficacy of relaxation training and guided imagery in reducing the aversiveness of cancer chemotherapy. *J Consult Clin Psychol.* 1982; 50:509–524.

55. Morrow GR, Morrell C. Behavioral treatment for anticipatory nausea and vomiting induced by cancer chemotherapy. *N Engl J Med.* 1982; 307:1476–1480.

56. Morrow GR, Asbury R, Hammon S, et al. Comparing the effectiveness of behavioral treatment for chemotherapy-induced nausea and vomiting when administered by oncologists, oncology nurses, and clinical psychologists. *Health Psychol.* 1992; 11:250–256.

57. Carey MP, Burish TG. Etiology and treatment of the psychological side effects associated with cancer chemotherapy: a critical review and discussion. *Psychol Bull.* 1988; 104:307–325.

58. Jacobsen PB, Redd WH. The development and management of chemotherapy-related anticipatory nausea and vomiting. *Cancer Invest.* 1988; 6:329–336.

59. Vasterling J, Jenkins RA, Tope DM, Burish TG. Cognitive distraction and relaxation training for the control of side effects due to cancer chemotherapy. *J Behav Med.* 1993; 16:65–80.

60. Burish TG, Carey MP, Krozely MK, Greco FA. Conditioned side effects induced by cancer chemotherapy: prevention through behavioral treatment. *J Consult Clin Psychol.* 1987; 55:42–48.

61. Lerman C, Rimer B, Blumberg B, et al. Effects of coping style and relaxation on cancer chemotherapy side effects and emotional responses. *Cancer Nurs.* 1990; 13:308–15.

62. Burish TG, Snyder SL, Jenkins RA. Preparing patients for cancer chemotherapy: effect of coping preparation and relaxation interventions. *J Consult Clin Psychol.* 1991; 4:518–525.

63. Spiegel D, Bloom JR, Kraemer HC, Gottheil E. Effect of psychosocial treatment on survival of patients with metastatic breast cancer. *Lancet.* 1989; 2:888–891.

64. Fawzy FI, Cousings N, Fawzy W, et al. A structured psychiatric intervention for cancer patients: I. Changes over time in methods of coping and affective disturbance. *Arch Gen Psychiatry.* 1990; 47:720–725.

65. Osoba D. Lessons learned from measuring health-related quality of life in oncology. *J Clin Oncol.* 1994; 12:608–616.

66. Cella DF. Quality of life as an outcome of cancer treatment. In: Groenwald SL, Goodman M, Frogge MH, Yargro CH, eds. *Cancer Nursing: Principles and Practice.* Boston, MA: Jones and Bartlett; 1993.

67. Worden JW, Weisman, AD. Preventive psychosocial intervention with newly diagnosed cancer patients. *Gen Hosp Psychiatry.* 1984; 6:243–249.

68. Heinrich RL, Schag CC. Stress and activity management: group treatment for cancer patients and spouses. *J Consult Clin Psychol.* 1985; 53:439–446.

69. Telch CF, Telch MJ. Group coping skills instruction and supportive group therapy for cancer patients: a comparison of strategies. *J Consult Clin Psychol.* 1986; 54:802–808.

70. Greer S, Moorey S, Baruch JDR, et al. Adjuvant psychological therapy for patients with cancer: a prospective randomized trial. *Br Med J.* 1992; 204:675–680.

71. Moorey S, Greer S, Watson M, et al. Adjuvant psychological therapy for patients with cancer: outcome at one year. *Psycho-Oncology.* 1994; 3:39–46.

72. Cain EN, Kohorn EI, Quinlan DM, et al. Psychosocial benefits of a cancer support group. *Cancer*. 1986; 57:183–189.

73. Jaycox A, Carr D, Payne R, et al. *Managing Cancer Pain: Patient Guide. Clinical Practice Guideline Number 9* (Adult Version—English). Rockville, MD: US Department of Health and Human Services, Public Health Service, Agency for Health Care Policy and Research. AHCPR Publication No. 93-0595, 1994.

74. McGrath PJ, Humphreys P, Keene D, et al. The efficacy and efficiency of a self-administered treatment for adolescent migraine. *Pain*. 1992; 49:321–324.

63

Studies of Life-Extending Psychosocial Interventions

CATHERINE CLASSEN, SANDRA E. SEPHTON, SUSAN DIAMOND, AND
DAVID SPIEGEL

It should no longer be surprising that psychotherapeutic and social support interventions provide emotional and other psychological benefits to cancer patients. A growing number of studies attest to the effectiveness of various group, individual, and family interventions in reducing depression and anxiety, improving coping, and mobilizing social support (1). More unexpected are findings that such psychosocial interventions may affect the course of the disease as well as adjustment to it. This is still an exploratory area, but one which merits further investigation. If we are to pay more than lip service to the idea that mind and body interact, it makes sense that intervention in one domain might affect the other. We have little doubt that changes in physical status influence cognition and affect. Given the complex neural and endocrine outflow from the nervous system, a variety of means by which improved support and coping might influence somatic response to carcinoma are possible, including influences on health-related behaviors, utilization of medical care, endocrine, autonomic, and immune function. The progression of cancer reflects not merely the invasiveness of the malignantly transformed cells, but also the efficacy of the host's various mechanisms for resisting progression. These include the endocrine environment, angiogenesis, and various components of the immune system which play a role in cancer surveillance. The field to this point has been stymied from opposite directions, initially by a tendency in medicine to downplay psychosocial influences on disease. More recently resistance to scientific examination of the mind/body interaction in cancer has been fueled by the "alternative medicine" approach which often overemphasizes the power of the mind to directly influence the body, thereby inducing guilt when cancer progresses. This domain is ripe for systematic scientific investigation

of possible effects of psychosocial intervention on the quantity as well as the quality of life with cancer.

To date only a handful of studies have been published regarding the impact of psychosocial interventions on survival and, while some of the results are encouraging, they are not definitive. Fortunately, several more clinical trials are currently underway in the United States, Canada, Switzerland, Denmark, and Australia. The results of these studies will be critical for drawing conclusions regarding the survival benefits of psychosocial interventions and making recommendations for patient care.

Although the research examining the effect of psychosocial interventions on survival is in its infancy, there is a broad tradition of research that has preceded this work (2). This includes the research on the association between social relationships and health. Several prospective community studies have shown that the number of social relationships is inversely related to mortality for all causes of death (3–7). However, recent meta-analyses have suggested that the effect of social support on health is moderate at best (8,9) and complex (10).

The complexity of the relationship between social support and health is evident in the research on cancer. In general the research suggests that social support has a beneficial effect on survival. Based on a sample of 6848 adults, one study examined the association between social support and cancer survival and found that women who were socially isolated were at significantly higher risk of dying from cancer (11). Among the men in this study, those with fewer social connections had significantly poorer survival rates. Another study, based on a sample of 27,779 cancer patients, found that being unmarried was associated with decreased survival, diagnosis at a more advanced stage of the disease, and a greater likelihood of being untreated (12). Other studies of cancer patients have also found social support to be associated with survival (13–16), although some studies have not demonstrated this relationship (17,18). In these latter studies, however, the measures used to assess social support had substantial limitations.

A study by Ell et al. (19) exemplifies the complexity of the relationship between social support and cancer survival. They examined the relationship between social relationships (defined as marital status and access to more distant social ties), social support (defined as perceived emotional support from close relationships) and survival among patients diagnosed with breast, colorectal, or lung cancer. They found that perceived emotional support was a protective factor among women with breast cancer and in the early stages of disease. However, among colorectal and lung cancer patients or for patients with advanced stages of disease, there was no relationship of perceived emotional support with survival. They also found marital status among women with breast cancer to be negatively associated with survival. This contradicts the research showing marriage to be a protective factor and suggests that breast cancer places a unique strain on marital relationships.

Another way of viewing this literature is that it demonstrates how a nonphysiological factor, such as social support, may have physiological ramifications. The potential for physiological effects from nonphysiological interventions has been demonstrated in other ways and in other populations as well. Studies examining the risk of death after a myocardial infarction have shown that good adherence to a medical regimen, regardless of whether the treatment is an active or placebo therapy, is associated with decreased risk of death (20,21). This was true even when taking medical and demographic variables into account for both men and women and additionally taking psychosocial variables into account for men. (The psychosocial measures were not available for the women.) At this point we can only speculate as to what mediated the health benefit of adhering to a placebo therapy.

There is also evidence that a patient's coping style is related to the degree of disease progression and mortality. Derogatis et al. (22) found that breast cancer patients who survived more than 1 year were more likely to be rated as unpleasant and uncooperative by medical staff than those who died in the initial year, although the study is confounded by the fact that the long-term survivors had received substantially less radiotherapy, and therefore may have been more capable of "healthy" assertiveness. Greer et al (23–25)

found that an attitude of "fighting spirit" rather than denial or hopelessness/helplessness was associated with slower disease progression, and this finding has been confirmed by others (14,26). Similarly, passive coping and hopelessness/helplessness have been found to be associated with poorer outcome (27,28) as was a need for sympathy and being emotionally reserved (29). Temoshok (30) found that a self-effacing personality constellation (so-called "type C") predicted more rapid progression of malignant melanoma. It should be noted that some studies have found no relationship between psychological factors and disease outcome (17,31,32). While these findings may reflect inherent weakness in the relationship between psychological variables and disease course, the independent variables in these studies were standard measures of distress rather than the putative personality constructs of affect suppression versus expression, or passive versus active coping style. Thus they may not have been sensitive to the constructs measured in the studies cited above.

These bodies of research on social and psychological factors associated with the course of cancer progression and mortality lead naturally to the question of whether it is possible that a psychosocial intervention for cancer patients might have an effect on medical outcome. Below we examine the handful of studies that have addressed this question.

REVIEW OF STUDIES EXAMINING THE IMPACT OF A PSYCHOSOCIAL INTERVENTION ON SURVIVAL

Studies That Demonstrated a Beneficial Effect on Survival (Table 63.1)

In the 1970s Spiegel et al. conducted a study to examine the effects of weekly support groups for metastatic breast cancer patients (33). Eighty-six patients were recruited into the study with 50 women randomly assigned to the treatment group and 36 women to the control group. Subjects in the treatment condition participated in weekly 90 min support group meetings that were co-led by two mental health professionals. There were 7–10 patients in each group and the intervention lasted for a year. In addition, both the treatment and control groups continued to receive routine oncological care.

Although the meetings were relatively unstructured, they were designed primarily to be supportive and to encourage direct discussion about living with cancer. The goal was to provide an environment in which patients could talk about their fears and concerns regarding the disease and its progression and express the associated dysphoric affect. In the group, patients

TABLE 63.1. *Intervention Studies That Influenced Survival*

Author	Subjects	Intervention	Outcome
Spiegel et al. (1989) (36)	86 women with metastatic breast cancer Subjects assigned to either the control or treatment condition	Weekly 90 min support group	Women in the support groups lived significantly longer—an average of 18 months from time of randomization
Richardson et al. (1990) (37)	94 patients with hematologic malignancies Subjects assigned to either a control or one of three treatment conditions	Three treatment conditions: 1. Education and home visit 2. Education and shaping 3. Education, shaping and home visit	Assignment to any of the three treatment conditions predicted survival
Fawzy et al. (1993) (38)	68 malignant melanoma patients	6-week intervention consisting of education, stress management, building coping skills, and psychological support	Treatment group had significantly longer survival and a trend for longer time to recurrence compared to the control group

freely discussed the effect of the disease on their lives. Group members discussed issues concerning their doctors and medical treatment, the effect of the illness on their families, fears about dying and death, and how to live fully in the time that was left. Because they were all in a similar situation, it enabled them to discuss these issues without undue concern about the impact it might have on others. In addition, it gave them the opportunity to share what they had learned from living with a life-threatening illness and help others who struggled with the same issues, thereby enhancing their own sense of competence and value via the "helper-therapy" principle (34). The patients assigned to the support group condition were provided with an environment where they benefited from social support, a sense of belonging, and the opportunity to express their thoughts and feelings about living with cancer, thereby improving their coping abilities and enhancing social support, both within the group and outside it (33,35).

This study was originally conceived as a randomized prospective psychotherapy trial with reduced mood disturbance as the primary outcome variable. There was no expectation of prolonging survival. Over 10 years after the study was completed, Spiegel et al. (36) collected survival data on all subjects who had participated. They hypothesized that the group intervention improved patients' quality of life, but it would have no effect on survival. To their surprise, women who were assigned to the support groups lived an average of 36.6 months from time of randomization as compared to the control subjects who lived an average of 18.9 months, a difference which was both statistically and clinically significant. By 4 years after the

study had begun all of the control patients had died, but a third of the treatment sample were still alive. The limitations of this study are that it involves a sample of moderate size and it was not originally designed to answer the question of whether a psychosocial intervention would improve survival.

A report by Richardson et al. (37) provided outcome data on the effect of treatment compliance on survival among patients with newly diagnosed hematologic malignancies. The aim of this study was to examine the relationship between compliance with medical treatment and survival time among these patients. Ninety-four patients were assigned either to the control group or to one of three conditions designed to increase compliance with treatment: *(1)* education and home visit; *(2)* education and shaping; and *(3)* education, shaping, and home visit.

The educational component included a 1 hour session with a project nurse giving an interactive slide and tape presentation. The presentation described the disease, its treatment, the side effects of treatment, and the responsibility of patients to comply with treatment and to take care of themselves. After each section, the nurse stopped the tape for discussion and to answer questions. The home visit was conducted by the same project nurse shortly after discharge. The nurse assisted the patient in establishing a routine that would facilitate taking the required pills. She left the patient with a discharge poster and got a family member to agree in writing to help the patient remember to take his or her pills, to assist the patient in problem-solving and to help the patient keep his or her doctors' appointments. The shaping component was a four level pill-shaping procedure that occurred while the patient was still in the hospital. The procedure involved working with a nurse to gradually take over the responsibility for self-medication.

Two to 5 years after entering the study, subjects were evaluated for survival status. Richardson and colleagues found that the factors predicting survival were severity of the disease, compliance with taking allopurinol, and assignment to any of the three educational conditions. The improved survival for those assigned to intervention held even after differences in treatment compliance were controlled. They theorized that the benefit from the educational program included learning the importance of self-care such as monitoring side effects, keeping appointments, going to the hospital for fever and bleeding, drinking liquids, keeping active, talking openly with medical caregivers and families and thereby facilitating problem solving. In addition, patients learned responsibility for their own care, giving them an enhanced sense of control and decreased fear and anxiety.

Fawzy et al. (38) conducted a study examining the effects of a brief, structured intervention on recurrence and survival among malignant melanoma patients. Sixty-eight subjects were recruited shortly after diagnosis and initial surgical treatment and randomly assigned to either the control or treatment group. The treatment group received a 6-week intervention that consisted of: *(1)* education, *(2)* stress management, *(3)* building coping skills, and *(4)* psychological support. The intervention groups consisted of 7–10 patients, were professionally led, and met once a week for 90 minutes.

Fawzy and colleagues evaluated time from surgery to recurrence and time from surgery to death at 6 years. They found that the treatment group experienced significantly longer survival than the control subjects and there was a trend for longer time to recurrence compared to the control group. They speculated that the increased knowledge and support received in the intervention group may have facilitated better health habits, such as protecting the skin from sun exposure, and lifestyle. Coping strategies may have improved as a result of the intervention, leading to better doctor–patient relationships, improved mental attitude, and greater treatment compliance. Intervention patients may have learned to manage their stress better, as well as benefiting from increased social support along with the opportunity to express their feelings to a sympathetic and understanding audience. Similar to the Spiegel study, this study was not originally designed to examine the effect of the intervention on recurrence and survival. Another limitation is that it involved a small sample. Consequently, both the Spiegel and Fawzy studies require replication.

Psychosocial Interventions Without Effect on Survival (Table 63.2.)

Four studies with adequate controls have examined the effect of a psychosocial intervention on survival and found no difference in survival (39–41). Linn et al. (39)

TABLE 63.2. *Intervention Studies That Did Not Influence Survival*

Author	Subjects	Intervention	Outcome
Linn et al. (1982) (39)	120 males with tumours of various sites, although primarily lung (n = 65)	Individual supportive counseling	No effect on survival
Gellert et al. (1993) (40)	34 women with breast cancer who were self-selected for the intervention and three matched controls for each intervention subject Subjects matched for demographic and medical variables	Siegel's Exceptional Cancer Patients program; consists of weekly 90 min groups for individual counseling, peer support and family therapy	No effect on survival
Ilnyckyj et al. (1994) (41)	127 patients with cancer of all types and stages	Three intervention groups: 1. Professional led 2. Professionally led for 3 months and then peer led 3. Peer led Intervention consisted of weekly 90 min support groups	No effect on survival

conducted a randomized prospective trial of 120 men in a Veterans Administration hospital with a tumors of several sites, primarily lung ($n = 65$), but including colon and stomach, pancreas, prostrate, bladder, and other sites. Patients in the intervention group received intensive and supportive individual counseling, modeled on the work of Kubler–Ross. The aim was to develop a trusting relationship with the counselor to enable talking about concerns. The patients were encouraged to maintain hope yet be realistic about their illness, to exercise control over aspects of their environment, to complete unfinished business, and to try to find meaning in their lives despite illness. Significant reductions in depression and alienation and improvement in life satisfaction, self-esteem and locus of control were reported by the intervention group over a 1 year follow-up period. There was approximately 85% mortality during this period. The authors found no difference in survival time for treatment versus control patients, either in the sample as a whole or for the subsample with lung cancer. All patients had advanced metastatic disease with a prognosis of between 3 and 12 months. The authors speculated that the absence of survival differences could be attributable to the advanced nature of the disease.

The second study by Siegel and his colleagues (40) examined the effect of participating in Siegel's Exceptional Cancer Patients (ECaP) program (42,43). ECaP is a nationally available program that offers groups in which patients can receive individual counseling, peer support, and family therapy as well as instruction in relaxation, imagery, and meditation. The groups meet weekly for 90-minute unstructured sessions, and consist of 8–12 patients plus relatives and friends. The objectives of the program are to enhance patients' sense of control, instil hope, and encourage acceptance of the disease. This program also encourages the idea that psychological factors may have caused cancer and that patients can be in control of the course of the disease through their attitude about it.

Thirty-four women with breast cancer who entered the program over a 2 year period were each matched with three control patients chosen for demographic and medical variables from the tumor registry. Patients were compared at 10 years. There were no significant differences in survival between the intervention and control subjects. Limitations of the study include an absence of randomization to intervention and comparison to a tumor registry population.

The third study by Ilnyckyj et al. examined the survival of 127 cancer patients who were randomly assigned to one of three psychosocial intervention groups or to a control group (41). The intervention consisted of weekly 1 hour sessions that continued for a period of 6 months. There were approximately 15 members per group. One group was professionally led by a social worker. A second group was professionally led for 3 months and then continued to meet for another 3 months without a leader. A third group was solely peer-led. The group leaders were not instructed in any specific technique although they were instructed to be informative and supportive. The peer-led group was told to meet and talk or to do whatever they wanted. The patients consisted of all types of cancer patients at all stages, although most patients had stage I disease.

Eleven years later, survival data were examined. The intervention groups were combined and compared to the control group. No differences in survival were found. Despite adequate numbers, limitations to this study may be the variable intervention and lack of a protocol-derived replicable intervention model. Furthermore, the groups consisted of patients of all disease types and at all stages. This would further compound a lack of cohesion in the groups and would diffuse the focus.

COMPONENTS OF EFFECTIVE INTERVENTIONS

Supportive Environment

In the three studies that demonstrated a survival benefit from a psychosocial intervention (36–38), there were a few key components that the interventions had in common and which may have contributed significantly to their overall effectiveness. In all three studies the subjects were provided a supportive, stable, and consistent environment. Both the Spiegel and Fawzy studies (36,38) were explicitly designed to provide support to the patients. In the Spiegel study (36) the treatment intervention consisted of weekly 90 minute group meetings that met regularly for one year and were co-led by two leaders who were trained specifically in that therapeutic modality. The aim of the therapy was to provide a supportive environment where patients would feel free to talk about their cancer-related concerns. In the Fawzy trial (38) the treatment consisted of six 90-minute sessions held once a week, led by two professionals. The intervention was structured to include education, stress management, building coping skills and psychological support.

The Richardson study (37) was rather different in that it was designed as a treatment compliance intervention and involved an individual intervention rather than a group intervention. All treatment subjects received an educational intervention which consisted of a slide and tape presentation by a nurse facilitator who answered the patient's questions and facilitated a discussion. Two of the three treatment conditions received a shaping component to assist the patient with medication compliance and was provided by a nurse facilitator. Also, in two of the three treatment conditions there were home visits by a project nurse to help the subject establish a routine for taking his or her pills. Although having the nurse provide emotional support was not a stated goal of the intervention, the nurse gave the patient individual attention with the explicit purpose of being helpful to the patient.

In each of these studies, the intervention was clearly delineated and was implemented by trained professionals. Both of these factors are important for having the patient feel confident in the treatment and thereby willing to participate fully. In contrast, in the Ilnyckyj study (41) the group was either peer-led with no attempt made to provide any direction, or it was led by a leader who had not been trained in any particular treatment approach and, to make matters worse, one of the groups had their leader leave the group midway through treatment so that they were left to fend for themselves. It is therefore unlikely that Ilnyckyj's groups felt considerable confidence in the intervention.

Homogeneous Groups

Another factor that we believe contributes to the creation of a safe and supportive environment is when the groups are homogeneous to disease and stage. This was true for both group intervention studies that found an effect on survival (36,38), and it was not true for the group intervention studies that did not find a survival effect (39,40).

A common complaint among cancer patients is that people in their daily lives simply do not understand what they are going through. Consequently, being in a group with others who are in a similar situation can be extremely helpful. In our experience, a natural bonding occurs in groups where patients share a similar disease and prognosis. For many patients there is an immediate sense of kinship. Our breast cancer patients often comment that they feel an understanding amongst themselves that goes beyond words. In addition, content analysis of the metastatic breast cancer groups at Stanford indicates that a substantial proportion of time is devoted to discussing and reacting to the condition of group members (44). Thus, the feeling of commonality and kinship that comes from being in a group is important for undoing the sense of isolation so often reported.

There is ample evidence that it is possible to lead psychologically effective groups that are heterogeneous to disease and stage (1). Nevertheless, heterogeneous groups are challenging and require greater skill. The leaders cannot count on a natural understanding to exist among the group members but instead will need to facilitate it. To date, there is no evidence that such heterogeneous groups affect survival time.

Educational Component

Another factor that the three interventions had in common is that they included an educational component. Each of these studies provided education either formally or informally. Both Richardson's (37) and Fawzy's (38) interventions had an educational component and these authors speculated that this resulted in patients changing their health habits, coping styles, improving communication with their doctors and better adhering to treatment. The educational component in Spiegel's study (36) was more informal. In the support groups patients shared their experiences, often exchanging medically relevant information. In addition, group members in the Spiegel study also tended to encourage one another to seek medical attention whenever a new symptom emerged. The patients were thereby encouraged to attend to physical complaints or concerns sooner rather than later. They were also relieved of anxiety when learning about the experiences of others who underwent similar treatments. In all three studies, the education served to diminish uncertainty and bolstered a sense of mastery and control.

Teaching Stress Management and Coping Strategies

Each of the three studies also included in their respective designs either a formal or informal stress management and coping skills component. Patients in the Richardson study (37) were instructed to assume greater responsibility for and knowledge about their own care. This kept them focused on their immediate concerns, thereby helping them cope with fear and anxiety and enhancing their sense of control. Fawzy's intervention (38) specifically taught stress management and coping techniques. This tightly structured intervention taught patients to consider different coping strategies for different situations. Having a greater repertoire of coping strategies is likely to have enhanced their sense of control and mastery and altered the way they dealt with their disease along with their feelings about it. The Spiegel study (36) offered stress management and coping in two ways. Specific instruction in self-hypnosis was given for pain management and resulted in significantly reduced pain (45). Stress management and coping were also informal topics of discussion. Thus, coping was facilitated through the discharge of emotions which were otherwise experienced as virulent and potentially overwhelming. In addition, patients served as role models for one another, modeling a broad range of coping strategies.

In each of these intervention studies, learning how to manage the disease provided patients with the opportunity to enhance their sense of mastery and control and instill optimism about their ability to deal with their disease. They all involved realistic acceptance of the medical realities of the illness, but coupled this awareness with active means of controlling those aspects of the illness, its treatment, and the time available that were influenceable. Thus, these interventions helped cancer patients to prepare for the worst, but hope for the best. None had the goal of living longer—rather they assisted these individuals in living better despite the impact of the disease on their lives.

The three studies that have reported an impact of psychosocial interventions on survival are provocative. They have stimulated further research on the interaction between mind and body and efforts at replication are underway in several centers in the United States and internationally. It is critically important that replication studies involve adequate sample size to reach valid conclusions, that they control for medical and cancer treatment variables, and that the intervention be protocol-driven and given by trained individuals. An obvious extension to this work is to examine possible health benefits for illnesses other than cancer.

In addition, if psychosocial interventions are proven to increase cancer survival it will not only be important to identify the most effective psychosocial treatments, it will also be essential to understand the mechanisms of their effects on survival.

POSSIBLE MEDIATORS OF PSYCHOSOCIAL TREATMENT EFFECTS ON CANCER SURVIVAL

Three general methods by which psychosocial treatments may affect disease course are: *(1)* psychosocial treatments may improve patient self-care behavior; *(2)* they may increase patient compliance with medical treatment; and *(3)* they may influence activity in biological pathways of disease resistance.

Health-Related Behavior

Health practices such as diet, exercise, smoking and sleep habits have been associated with the incidence and progression of neoplastic disease (46–49), while obesity, alcohol consumption, and other dietary fac-

tors have been associated particularly with breast cancer risk (49–52).

There are several means by which psychosocial treatments may motivate improvement in patient self-care: first, treatments may formally or informally educate patients about healthier behavior (1); second, treatments can provide social support and encouragement from peers and health care professionals (53); and third, interventions have been shown to alleviate distress and pain (33,45), which aggravate sleep disturbance (54).

In addition to self-care habits, patients' inclination to seek treatment and ability to interact with the medical system influence the quality of care they receive. For example, patients who delay seeking treatment, or encounter delay in the medical system, are prone to poor cancer outcomes (55). Psychosocial interventions can help patients use the medical system to their best advantage. In our supportive/expressive therapy groups, for example, patients often discussed how to interact successfully with physicians in order to receive better care (33,36). Thus, improved survival may result from both better self-care and better medical care in patients receiving effective psychosocial treatments.

Compliance with Medical Treatment

The side effects, intensity, and complexity of various cancer treatments make adherence to medical regimens particularly difficult for cancer patients (56–58). In a survey of 246 randomly selected oncologists, 85% reported that patient noncompliance was a significant problem, and patients' psychological problems were cited as the primary reason for noncompliance (59). Fear, uncertainty, and loss of control are the most commonly cited reasons for non-adherence to cancer treatment regimens (60). Among patients with breast cancer and other carcinomas, withdrawal from all or part of recommended treatment is estimated to range from 16%–33% (58,61–64). Richardson et al. (37) have shown that compliance improves survival among patients with hematologic malignancies. The survival value of treatment adherence has also been demonstrated in breast cancer patients (65). In spite of such reports, compliance continues to be a serious problem for patients and physicians confronting breast cancer (59).

By educating patients about their disease, psychosocial interventions strengthen feelings of control and perceived predictability, and may thereby improve psychological adjustment (66). Compliance may be facilitated as patients' understanding increases, their mood improves, and social support is received to help them overcome the psychological obstacles to adherence

(56,67–70). Indeed, telephone counseling alone has been shown to increase adherence to treatment among low-income women at risk for cervical cancer (60); and in the Richardson study, better compliance and a related increase in survival was observed in patients involved in an education-based intervention (37). This match between the patient's behavior and health care advice may be life-saving (37,59,65).

In support of the potential of psychosocial factors to affect cancer outcomes, longer survival times observed with better compliance may not be entirely due to pharmacological effects: In a few studies, adherence to treatment with a placebo also increased survival time (71,72).

Biological Pathways

Receiving a diagnosis of cancer is a difficult experience which engenders feelings of anxiety, depression, and confusion (73). Cancer patients are faced with the threat imposed by the disease in addition to other life stressors they may be experiencing. A link between stress and the outcome of a cancer diagnosis has been proposed (74–76). Neuroendocrine correlates of stress, including glucocorticoid and catecholamine hormone elevations, have been associated with suppression of the body's defenses against disease (77,78). Some neuroendocrine factors have been shown to promote tumor growth (79,80), although the clinical relevance of these mechanisms has not yet been established. Psychosocial interventions may act conversely, reducing stress-induced suppression of immunity and improving cancer survival by buffering the biological effects of stress.

Stress may, in fact, play a mediating role in the endocrine and immune modulation of cancer progression. Having cancer can be considered a chronic stressor. Reminders of the illness are a daily occurrence, with arduous treatments providing additional sources of stress. Symptoms of stress such as anxiety and depression are elevated in cancer patients (23,73), as are plasma levels of glucocorticoids and catecholamines (81–84). Elevated cortisol, a classic physiological hallmark of stress (85), is particularly evident in depressed subjects (86,87) as well as in cancer patients (81,82). These findings suggest that hyperactivity of the hypothalamic–pituitary–adrenal (HPA) axis, a typical response to stress and depression (87,88), may be associated with poor adjustment to cancer. Chronic stress and hyperactivity of the HPA axis may, indeed, be a factor of disease progression (88,89).

Mechanisms by which glucocortiscoids may influence tumor growth include the possible indirect activation of oncogenes by HPA axis hormones. A molecular

mechanism has recently been proposed whereby corticotropin-releasing hormone, the hypothalamic regulator of cortisol production, may promote expression of breast cancer oncogenes (90). Thus, stress-induced activation of the cortisol system (85) may be related to more rapid tumor progression, an effect which has been demonstrated in animals (79,80,91).

Others have proposed that glucocorticoids may influence the rate of tumor growth more directly. Several studies have found an association between stress-related elevation of glucocorticoids and more rapid tumor growth in animals (79,80,91). These authors cite several theories about how tumor growth may be modulated, including possible action of glucocorticoids to suppress antitumor immunity (91,92), stimulate tumor angiogenesis (93), stimulate tumor growth factors (94), or create a hyperglycemic environment in which tumor cells with enhanced abilities to transport and utilize glucose (95) experience a metabolic advantage over normal cells.

Alternatively, neuroendocrine-immune pathways may mediate psychosocial effects upon cancer progression: (74–76). There is growing evidence that functions of the nervous, endocrine and immune systems are interactive (96,97). Indeed, studies have shown suppression of immune function with psychological factors such as bereavement (98–100), marital disruption (101,102), stress (e.g., difficult life events, examinations) (103,104), caring for a spouse with Alzheimer's disease (105), depression (103,106,107), and negative fluctuations of daily mood (108). Interestingly, some of these effects may be mitigated by active coping style (109,110) or social support (104,111). Since immune mechanisms which combat neoplastic disease have been documented (112), thus, it may reasonably be proposed that psychosocial interventions may enhance cancer survival by relieving stress-induced suppression of immune defenses to disease (74–76).

Evidence in support of this postulate shows that psychosocial treatments are capable of mitigating the effects of stress on both endocrine and immune function (38,113). Psychosocial interventions have been shown to buffer the psychological stress engendered by a cancer diagnosis. Improvements in adjustment to cancer, coping abilities, pain and other quality of life measures have been noted in intervention subjects (1,33,45). The potential held by psychosocial treatments to buffer the endocrine stress response is suggested by the results of an intervention study in which biofeedback and cognitive therapy were associated with reduced cortisol levels in newly diagnosed breast cancer patients (113). One recent study (114) reports that breast cancer patients randomized to 13 weeks of group psychotherapy showed decreased plasma cortisol levels relative to controls at the end of the treatment period (although measures of immunity also decreased).

There is some data suggesting the clinical relevance of glucocorticoid levels. Recovery of the HPA axis after surgical stress has been related to cancer survival: Among patients operated for breast and stomach carcinoma, the failure of morning cortisol levels to decrease within 2 weeks after admission was associated with shorter survival times (115). Thus, having potential to influence endocrine function, psychosocial treatments may mediate survival benefits via neuroendocrine factors.

Immune function may be an important link in the relationship between neuroendocrine function and the course of cancer. Psychosocial treatments have been associated with improvements in immune function and physical health in cancer patients (36,38,113). After a 6 week psychiatric intervention for newly diagnosed malignant melanoma patients conducted by Fawzy et al., functional activity of natural killer (NK) cells was elevated in the intervention subjects 6 months later, and a survival benefit was observed (38). Social support is one component of psychosocial treatments with noted physiological benefits. For example, a change in the social environment has been shown to alter profoundly the endocrine, immunological, and cardiovascular consequences of a stressor (104,111,116,117). In breast cancer patients, higher perceived social support and active seeking of social support have been related to increased NK cell activity (118). Although the importance of a single immune parameter should not be emphasized, and a causative association with tumor stasis cannot be made, NK cell activity, which has been implicated both in cancer progression and in response to psychosocial factors (74,119), has also been shown to predict disease recurrence in breast cancer patients (120).

Thus, there is good reason to believe that psychosocial stress and social isolation caused by the diagnosis of cancer may adversely affect the endocrine and immune systems, with clinically relevant consequences for the body's ability to resist disease progression. Conversely, enhanced social support, coping abilities, self-care and compliance resulting from participation in psychotherapeutic interventions may plausibly improve medical outcome by buffering the consequences of stress and thereby ameliorating immune and endocrine function.

In conclusion, the research investigating the life-extending potential of psychosocial interventions is promising, although more studies are required. The research to date provides some evidence that changing the psychosocial environment and coping abilities of cancer patients not only improves their quality of life, but may affect the quantity of life. This body of work points to the need for further replication, examination of crucial elements of intervention, and the study of mechanisms which mediate the relation between mind and body in disease. If we replicate these findings, and standardize the interventions so that they are transferable to the community, we have the potential to alter our standards of what constitutes good health care.

SUMMARY

The facility of psychosocial interventions to alleviate adjustment difficulties resulting from a cancer diagnosis has been established. The effects of such treatments on disease course, however, are currently under scrutiny. In this chapter we have reviewed the handful of controlled studies that examined the effect of a psychosocial intervention on cancer survival. Out of six studies, three have demonstrated that a psychosocial intervention can reduce mortality. Studies which have demonstrated positive survival effects of psychosocial intervention have certain treatment components in common: provision of a supportive environment, use of groups that are homogeneous to disease and stage, an educational component, and teaching of coping strategies. Nevertheless, a causal association between these aspects of psychosocial treatment and survival cannot easily be assumed. Further work is needed to examine how effective treatment modalities might exert effects on disease course. Several potential pathways of survival effects are explored, including treatment effects on patients' health-related behaviors, compliance with medical treatment, and effects on biological pathways of disease resistance.

REFERENCES

1. Fawzy FI, Fawzy NW, Arndt LA, Pasnau RO. Critical review of psychosocial interventions in cancer care. *Arch Gen Psychiatry*. 1995; 52:100–13.
2. Mulder CL, van der Pompe G, Spiegel D, Antoni MH, De Vries MJ. Do psychosocial factors influence the course of breast cancer? A review of recent literature, methodological problems and future directions. *Psycho-Oncology*. 1992; 1:155–67.
3. Berkman LF, Syme SL. Social networks, host resistance and mortality: A nine-year follow-up study of Alameda County residents. *Am J Epidemiol*. 1979; 109:186–204.
4. House JS, Robbins C, Metzner H. The association of social influences and activities with mortality: prospective evidence from the Tecumseh Community Health Study. *Am J Epidemiol*. 1982; 116:123–140.

5. Schoenback VJ, Kaplan BH, Fredman L, Kleinbaum DG. Social ties and mortality in Evans County, Georgia. *Am J Epidemiol.* 1986; 123:577–591.

6. Tibblin G, Svrdsudd K, Welin L, Larsson B. The theory of general susceptibility. In: Isacsson SO, Janzon L, eds. *Social Support—Health and Disease.* Stockholm: Almqvist & Wiksell International; 1986: 1–19.

7. Welin L, Tibbin G, Svardsudd K. et al. Prospective study of social influences on mortality: the study of men born in 1913 and 1923. *Lancet.* 1985; 1:915–918.

8. Smith CE, Fernengel K, Holcroft C, Gerald K. Meta-analysis of the associations between social support and health outcomes. *Ann Behav Med.* 1994; 16(4):352–362.

9. Schwarzer R, Leppin A. Social support and health: a meta-analysis. *Psychol Health.* 1989; 3(1):1–15.

10. Schwarzer R, Leppin A. Social support and health: a theoretical and empirical overview. *J Soc Pers Relat.* 1991; 8(1):99–127.

11. Reynolds P, Kaplan GA. Social connections and risk for cancer: prospective evidence from the Alameda County study. *Behav Med.* 1990; 16:101–110.

12. Goodwin JS, Hunt WC, Key CR, Samet JM. The effect of marital status on stage, treatment, and survival of cancer patients. *J Am Med Assoc.* 1987; 258:3125–3130.

13. Funch DP, Marshall J. The role of stress, social support and age in survival from breast cancer. *J Psychosom Res.* 1983; 27(1):77–83.

14. Hislop TG, Waxler NE, Coldman AJ, et al. The prognostic significance of psychosocial factors in women with breast cancer. *J Chron Dis.* 1987; 40(7):729–735.

15. Neale AV, Tilley BC, Vernon SW. Marital status, delay in seeking treatment and survival from cancer. *Soc Sci Med.* 1986; 32:305–312.

16. Waxler-Morrison N, Hislop TG, Mears B, Kan L. Effects of social relationships on survival for women with breast cancer: a prospective study. *Soc Sci Med.* 1991; 33:177–183.

17. Cassileth BR, Lusk EJ, Miller DS, et al. Psychosocial correlates of survival in advanced malignant disease: *N Engl J Med.* 1985; 312:1551–1555.

18. Neale AV. Racial and marital status influences on 10 year survival from breast cancer. *J Clin Epidemiol.* 1994; 47(5):475–483.

19. Ell K, Nishimoto R, Mediansky L, et al. Social relations, social support and survival among patients with cancer. *J Psychosom Res.* 1992, 36(6):531–541.

20. Horwitz RI, Viscoli CM, Berkman L, et al. Treatment adherence and risk of death after a myocardial infarction. *Lancet.* 1990; 336:542–545.

21. Gallagher EJ, Viscoli CM, Horwitz RI. The relationship of treatment adherence to the risk of death after myocardial infarction in women. *J Am Med Assoc.* 1993; 270:742–744.

22. Derogatis LR, Abeloff MD, Melisaratos N. Psychological coping mechanisms and survival time in metastatic breast cancer. *J Am Med Assoc.* 1979; 242(14):1504–1508.

23. Greer S, Morris T, Pettingale KW. Psychological response to breast cancer: effect on outcome. *Lancet.* 1979; 2(8146):785–787.

24. Greer S, Morris T, Pettingale KW, Haybittle JL. Psychological response to breast cancer and 15-year outcome [letter]. *Lancet.* 1990; 335(8680):49–50.

25. Greer S. Psycho-oncology: its aims, achievements and future tasks. *Psycho-Oncology.* 1994; 3:87–101.

26. Levy SM, Wise BD. Psychosocial risk factors and cancer progression. In: Cooper CL, ed. *Stress and Breast Cancer.* Chichester: Wiley; 1988: 77–96.

27. Schmale AH, Iker H. Hopelessness as a predictor of cervical cancer. *Soc Sci Med.* 1971; 5(2):95–100.

28. Goodkin K, Antoni MH, Blaney PH. Stress and hopelessness in the promotion of cervical intraepithelial neoplasia to invasive squamous cell carcinoma of the cervix [published erratum appears in *J Psychosom Res.* 1987;31(5):659]. *J Psychosom Res.* 1986; 30(1):67–76.

29. Stavraky KM, Donner AP, Kincade JE, Stewart MA. The effect of psychosocial factors on lung cancer mortality at one year. *J Clin Epidemiol.* 1988, 41(1):75–82.

30. Temoshok L. Biopsychosocial studies on cutaneous malignant melanoma: psychosocial factors associated with prognostic indicators, progression, psychophysiology, and tumor-host-response. *Soc Sci Med.* 1985; 20:833–840.

31. Jamison RN, Burish TG, Wallston KA. Psychogenic factors in predicting survival of breast cancer patients. *J Clin Oncol.* 1987; 5(5):768–772.

32. Buddeberg C, Wolf C, Sieber M et al. Coping strategies and course of disease of breast cancer patients. Results of a 3-year longitudinal study. *Psychother Psychosom.* 1991; 55(2-4):151–157.

33. Spiegel D Bloom JR, Yalom ID. Group support for patients with metastatic cancer: a randomized prospective outcome study. *Arch Gen Psychiatry.* 1981; 38(5):527–533.

34. Riessman F. The "helper therapy" principle. *Soc Work.* 1965; 10:27–32.

35. Spiegel D. *Living Beyond Limits.* New York: Times Books; 1993.

36. Spiegel D, Bloom JR, Kraemer HC, Gottheil E. Effect of psychosocial treatment on survival of patients with metastatic breast cancer. *Lancet.* 1989; 2:888–891

37. Richardson JL, Shelton DR, Krailo M, Levine AM. The effect of compliance with treatment on survival among patients with hematologic malignancies. *J Clin Oncol.* 1990; 8(2):356–364.

38. Fawzy FI, Fawzy NW, Hyun CS, et al. Malignant melanoma: effects of an early structured psychiatric intervention, coping, and affective state on recurrence and survival 6 years later. *Arch Gen Psychiatry.* 1993; 50:681–689.

39. Linn MW, Linn BS, Harris R. Effects of counseling for late stage cancer patients. *Cancer.* 1982; 49(5): 1048–1055

40. Gellert GA, Maxwell RM, Siegel BS. Survival of breast cancer patients receiving adjunctive psychosocial support therapy: a 10-year follow-up study. *J Clin Oncol.* 1993; 11(1):66–69.

41. Ilnyckyj A, Farber J, Cheang MC, Weinerman BF. A randomized controlled trial of psychotherapeutic intervention in cancer patients. *Ann R Coll Phys Surg Can.* 1994; 27:93–96.

42. Siegel B. *Love, Medicine and Miracles.* New York, NY: Harper & Row; 1986.

43. Siegel B. *Peace, Love and Healing.* New York, NY: Harper & Row; 1989.

44. Spiegel D, Glafkides MC. Effects of group confrontation with death and dying. *Int J Group Psychother*. 1983; 33:433–447.

45. Spiegel D, Bloom JR. Group therapy and hypnosis reduce metastatic breast carcinoma pain. *Psychosom Med*. 1983; 45(4):333–339.

46. Doll R, Peto R. The causes of cancer: quantitative estimates of avoidable risks of cancer in the United States today. *J Natl Cancer Inst*. 1981;66:1191–1308.

47. Albanes, D. Caloric intake, body weight, and cancer: a review. *Nutr Cancer*. 1987; 9(4):199–217.

48. Blot WJ. Alcohol and cancer. *Cancer Res*. 1992; 52:2119s–2123s.

49. Eberlein T, Simon R, Fisher S, Lippman ME. Height, weight, and risk of breast cancer relapse. *Breast Cancer Res Treat*. 1985; 5(1):81–86.

50. Zumoff B, Gorzynski JG, Katz JL, et al. Nonobesity at the time of mastectomy is highly predictive of 10-year disease-free survival in women with breast cancer. *Anticancer Res*. 1982; 2(1-2):59–62.

51. Schatzkin A, Longnecker MP. Alcohol and breast cancer. Where are we now and where do we go from here? *Cancer*. 1994; 74(3 suppl):1101–1110.

52. Garland M, Willett WC, Manson JE, Hunter DJ. Antioxidant micronutrients and breast cancer. *J Am Coll Nutr*. 1993; 12(4):400–411.

53. Spiegel D. Essentials of psychotherapeutic intervention for cancer patients. *Support Care Cancer*. 1995; 3(4):252–256

54. Strang P, Qvarner H. Cancer-related pain and its influence on quality of life. *Anticancer Res*. 1990; 10(1):109-112.

55. Facione NC. Delay versus help seeking for breast cancer symptoms: a critical review of the literature on patient and provider delay. *Soc Sci Med*. 1993; 36(12):1521–1534.

56. Given BA, Given CW. Compliance among patients with cancer. *Oncol Nurs Forum*. 1989; 16(1):97–103.

57. Laszlo J, Lucas V. Emesis as a critical problem in chemotherapy. *N Engl J Med*. 1981; 305(16):948–949.

58. Barofsky I. Therapeutic compliance and the cancer patient. *Health Educ Q*. 1984; 10(Suppl):43–56.

59. Hoagland AC, Morrow GR, Bennett JM, Carnrike C. Oncologists' views of cancer patient noncompliance. *Am J Clin Oncol*. 1983; 6(2):239–244.

60. Lerman C, Hanjani P, Caputo C, et al. Telephone counseling improves adherence to colposcopy among lower income minority women. *J Clin Oncol*. 1992; 10(2):330–333.

61. Glass A, Wieand HS, Fisher B, et al. Acute toxicity during adjuvant chemotherapy for breast cancer: the National Surgical Adjuvant Breast and Bowel Project (NSABP) experience from 1717 patients receiving single and multiple agents. *Cancer Treat Rep*. 1981; 65(5–6):363–376.

62. Lee YT. Adjuvant chemotherapy (CMF) for breast carcinoma. Patient's compliance and total dose achieved. *Am J Clin Oncol*. 1983; 6(1):25–30.

63. Wilcox PM, Fetting JH, Nettesheim KM, Abeloff MD. Anticipatory vomiting in women receiving cyclophosphamide, methotrexate, and 5-FU (CMF) adjuvant chemotherapy for breast carcinoma. *Cancer Treat Rep*. 1982; 66(8):1601–1604.

64. Itano J, Tanabe P, Lum JL, et al. (1983). Compliance of cancer patients to therapy. *West J Nurs Res*. 1983; 5(1):5–20.

65. Bonadonna G, Valagussa P. Dose-response effect of adjuvant chemotherapy in breast cancer. *N Engl J Med*. 1981; 304(1):10–15.

66. Taylor SE, Lichtman RR, Wood JV. Attributions, beliefs about control, and adjustment to breast cancer. *J Pers Soc Psychol*. 1984; 46(3):489–502.

67. Ferguson K, Bole GG. Family support, health beliefs, and therapeutic compliance in patients with rheumatoid arthritis. *Patient Couns Health Educ*. 1979; 1(3):101–105.

68. Ayres A, Hoon PW, Franzoni JB, et al. Influence of mood and adjustment to cancer on compliance with chemotherapy among breast cancer patients. *J Psychosom Res*. 1994; 38(5):393–402.

69. Wyszynski AA. Managing noncompliance in the "difficult" medical patient: the contributions of insight. A case report. *Psychother Psychosom*. 1990; 54(4):181–186.

70. Haynes B, Taylor D, Sackett D, eds. *Compliance in Health Care*. Baltimore, MD: Johns Hopkins University Press; 1979.

71. Pizzo PA, Robichaud KJ, Edwards BK, et al. Oral antibiotic prophylaxis in patients with cancer: a double-blind randomized placebo-controlled trial. *J Pediatr*. 1983; 102(1):125–133.

72. Epstein LH. The direct effects of compliance on health outcome. *Health Psychol*. 1984; 3(4):385–393.

73. Andersen BL, Anderson B, deProsse C. Controlled prospective longitudinal study of women with cancer: II. Psychological outcomes. *J Consult Clin Psychol*. 1989; 57(6):692–697.

74. Bovbjerg D. Psychoneuroimmunology and Cancer. In: Holland JC, Rowland JH, eds. *Handbook of Psychooncology: Psychological Care of the Patient with Cancer*. New York: Oxford University Press; 1989: 727–754.

75. Bergsma J. Illness, the mind, and the body: cancer and immunology: an introduction. *Theor Med*. 1994; 15(4):337–347.

76. Andersen BL, Kiecolt-Glaser JK, Glaser R. A biobehavioral model of cancer stress and disease course. *Am Psychol*. 1994; 49(5):389–404.

77. Callewaert DM, Moudgil VK, Radcliff G, Waite R. Hormone specific regulation of natural killer cells by cortisol. *Fed Eur Biochem Soc J*. 1991; 285(1):108–110.

78. Landmann RMA, Muller FB, Perini CH, et al. Changes of immunoregulatory cells induced by psychological and physical stress: relationship to plasma catecholamines. *Clin Exp Immunol*. 1984; 58:127–135.

79. Rowse GJ, Weinberg J, Bellward GD, Emerman JT. Endocrine mediation of psychosocial stressor effects on mouse mammary tumor growth. *Cancer Lett*. 1992; 65(1):85–93.

80. Sapolsky RM, Donnelly TM. Vulnerability to stress-induced tumor growth increases with age in rats: role of glucocorticoids. *Endocrinology*. 1985; 117(2):662–666.

81. Williams JW, Mutgi A, Noyes R, et al. Comparison of urinary-free cortisol in depressed and nondepressed patients with malignancy. *Biol Psychiatry*. 1990; 28:522–525.

82. Schaur RJ, Fellier H, Gleispach H, et al. Tumor host relations I. Increased plasma cortisol in tumor-bearing humans compared with patients with benign surgical diseases. *J Cancer Res Clinical Oncol.*1979; 93:281–285.

83. Schaur RJ, Semmelrock HJ, Schauenstein E, Kronberger L. Tumor host relations II. Influence of tumor extent and tumor site on plasma cortisol of patients with malignant diseases. *J Cancer Res Clin Oncol.* 1979; 93:287–292.

84. Russell McRD, Shike M, Marliss EB. Effects of total parenteral nutrition and chemotherapy on the metabolic derangements in small cell lung cancer. *Cancer Res.* 1984; 44:1706–1711.

85. Rose RM. Overview of endocrinology of stress. In: Brown GM, ed. *Neuroendocrinology and Psychiatric Disorder.* New York, NY: Raven Press; 1984: 95–122.

86. Yehuda R, Boisoneau D, Mason JW, Giller EL. Glucocorticoid receptor number and cortisol excretion in mood, anxiety, and psychotic disorders. *Biol Psychiatry.* 1993; 34(1–2):18–25.

87. Nemeroff CB, Widerlov E, Bissette G, et al. Elevated concentrations of CSF corticotropin-releasing factor-like immunoreactivity in depressed patients. *Science.* 1984; 226(4680):1342–1344.

88. Chrousos GP, Gold PW. The concepts of stress and stress system disorders. Overview of physical and behavioral homeostasis. *J Am Med Assoc.* 1992; 267(9): 1244–1252.

89. McEwen BS, Stellar E. Stress and the individual. Mechanisms leading to disease. *Arch Intern Med.* 1993; 153(18):2093–2101.

90. Licinio J, Gold PW, Wong ML. A molecular mechanism for stress-induced alterations in susceptibility to disease. *Lancet.* 1995; 346(8967):104–106.

91. Ben-Eliyahu S, Yirmiya R, Liebeskind JC, et al. Stress increases metastatic spread of a mammary tumor in rats: evidence for mediation by the immune system. *Brain Behav Immun.* 1991; 5(2):193–205.

92. Masera R, Gatti G, Sartori ML, et al. Involvement of Ca^{2+}-dependent pathways in the inhibition of human natural killer (NK) cell activity by cortisol. *Immunopharmacology.* 1989; 18(1):11–22.

93. Folkman J, Langer R, Linhardt RJ, et al. Angiogenesis inhibition and tumor regression caused by heparin or a heparin fragment in the presence of cortisone. *Science.* 1983; 221(4612):719–725.

94. DeLarco J, Todaro G. Growth factors from murine sarcoma virus-transformed cells. *Proc Natl Acad Sci.* 1978; 75:4001–4005.

95. White M, Bramwell M, Harris H. Kionetic parameters of hexose transport in hybrids between malignant and non-malignant cells. *J Cell Sci.* 1983; 62:49.

96. Ader R, Cohen N, Felten D, Psychoneuroimmunology: interactions between the nervous system and the immune system. *Lancet.* 1995; 345(8942): 99–103.

97. Ader R, Cohen N. Psychoneuroimmunology: conditioning and stress. *Ann Rev Psychol.* 1993; 44:53–85.

98. Bartrop RW, Luckhurst E, Lazarus L, et al. Depressed lymphocyte function after bereavement. *Lancet.* 1977; 1:834–836.

99. Schleifer SJ, Keller SE, Camerino M, et al. Suppression of lymphocyte stimulation following bereavement. *J Am Med Assoc.* 1983; 250(3):374–377.

100. Irwin M, Daniels M, Smith TL, et al. Impaired natural killer cell activity during bereavement. *Brain Behav Immun.* 1987; 1:98–104.

101. Kiecolt-Glaser JK, et al. Marital quality, marital disruption, and immune function. *Psychosom Med.* 1987; 49(1):13–34.

102. Kiecolt-Glaser JK, Kennedy S, Malkoff S, et al. Marital discord and immunity in males. *Psychosom Med.* 1988; 50(3):213–229.

103. Irwin M, Daniels M, Bloom E, et al. Life events, depressive symptoms, and immune function. *Am J Psychiatry.* 1987; 144:437–441.

104. Kiecolt-Glaser JK, Garner W, Speicher C, et al. Psychosocial modifiers of immunocompetence in medical students. *Psychosom Med.* 1984; 46(1):7–14.

105. Kiecolt-Glaser JK, Glaser R, Dyer C, et al. Chronic stress and immunity in family caregivers of Alzheimer's disease victims. *Psychosom Med.* 1987; 49:523–535.

106. Schleifer SJ, Keller SE, Sirus SG, et al. Depression and immunity. *Arch Gen Psychiatry.* 1985; 42:129–133.

107. Evans DL, Leserman J, Pedersen CA, et al. Immune correlates of stress and depression. *Psychopharmacol Bull.* 1989; 25(34):319–324.

108. Stone AA, Cox DS, Valdimarsdottir E, Jandorf L, Neale JM. Evidence that secretory IgA antibody is associated with daily mood. *J Pers Soc Psychol.* 1987; 52(5):988–993.

109. Goodkin K, Fuchs I, Feaster D, et al. Life stressors and coping style are associated with immune measures in HIV-1 infection, a preliminary report. *Int J Psychiatry Med.* 1992; 22(2):155–172.

110. Goodkin K, Blaney NT, Feaster D, et al. Active coping style is associated with natural killer cell cytotoxicity in asymptomatic HIV-1 seropositive homosexual men. *J Psychosom Res.* 1992; 36(7)635–650.

111. Kennedy S, Kiecolt-Glaser JK, Glaser R. Immunological consequences of acute and chronic stressors: mediating role of interpersonal relationships. *Br J Med Psychol.* 1988; 61(Pt 1):77–85.

112. Souberbielle B, Dalgleish A. Anti-tumor immune mechanisms. In: Lewis CE, O'Sullivan C, Barraclough J, eds. *The Psychoimmunology of Cancer: Mind and Body in the Fight for Survival.* Oxford: Oxford University Press; 1994: 267–290.

113. Davis H. Effects of biofeedback and cognitive therapy on stress in patients with breast cancer. *Psychol Rep.* 1986; 59(2, Pt 2):967–974.

114. van der Pompe G, Duivenvoorden HJ, Antoni MH, Visser A, Heijnen CJ. Effectiveness of a short-term group psychotherapy program on endocrine and immune function in breast cancer patients: an exploratory study. *J Psychosom Res.* 1997; 42(5):453–466.

115. Audier AG. Determination of a constitutional neuroendocrine factor probably influencing tumor development in man: prophylactic and therapeutic aspects. *Cancer Detect Prev.* 1988; 11:203–208.

116. Kirschbaum C, Klauer T, Filipp SH, Hellhammer DH. Sex-specific effects of social support on cortisol and subjective responses to acute psychological stress. *Psychosom Med.* 1995; 57(1):23–31.

117. Gerin W, Milner D, Chawla S, Pickering TG. Social support as a moderator of cardiovascular reactivity in

women: a test of the direct effects and buffering hypotheses. *Psychosom Med.* 1995; 57(1):16–22.

118. Levy SM, Herberman RB, Whiteside T, et al. Perceived social support and tumor estrogen/progesterone receptor status as predictors of natural killer cell activity in breast cancer patients. *Psychosom Med.* 1990; 52(1):73–85.

119. Herberman R. Natural killer cells: characteristics and possible role in resistance against tumor growth. In: Reif AE, Mitchell MS, eds. *Immunity to Cancer.* San Diego: Academic Press; 1985: 217–229.

120. Levy SM, Herberman RB, Lippman M, et al. Immunological and psychosocial predictors of disease recurrence in patients with early-stage breast cancer. *Behav Med.* 1991; 17(2):67–75.

64

Art Psychotherapy

PAOLA LUZZATTO AND BONNIE GABRIEL

ART THERAPY AS A FORM OF PSYCHOTHERAPY

The Historical Roots of Art Therapy

Art therapy as a form of psychotherapy (also called art psychotherapy) started in the 1940s and 1950s, in Europe and in the United States. Art therapy has its roots, on one hand, in art and art education, and on the other, in psychology and psychoanalysis, as it is based on the notion that visual image-making is an important part of mental functioning, and that individuals may project their internal world, both consciously and unconsciously, into visual forms (1). The first pioneers of art therapy were mainly artists who introduced image-making to traumatized soldiers, to long-term psychiatric patients, and to children with emotional difficulties, emphasizing the healing property of the creative process in itself. Also the connection with medically ill patients goes back to the first pioneers: the English artist Adrian Hill started to work with patients treated for tuberculosis in a sanatorium and coined the term "art therapy" to describe the role of art-making for patients in isolation (2). His goals were to provide release from boredom and frustration, and to give back a sense of life and hope to the depressed tuberculosis patients. The influence of psychoanalysts like Naumberg (3) in the United States and Winnicott (4) in the United Kingdom helped to develop art therapy in the direction of promoting insight, and of facilitating change in the patients' inner world and in dysfunctional behaviors. Formal training in art therapy, which started in the 1970s, added a psychodynamic orientation to art therapy practice, and emphasized the use of transference and countertransference, and the dynamic relationship between patient(s) and therapist. At present the field of art therapy is characterized by a stimulating tension between the two approaches: one more focused on the healing property of the intrapsychic personal creative process, the other more focused on the therapeutic use of the interpersonal relationship. In this chapter we present an integrative approach, which makes use of both aspects of art therapy as a form of psychotherapy (5).

The Use of Visual Imagery in Art Therapy

The therapeutic use of mental images is an integral part of many forms of psychotherapy. Ways of using mental images were developed by Freud through his use of dreams and free associations (6), by Jung through his technique of active imagination (7), and, more recently, by the schools of cognitive therapy (8), Gestalt therapy (9) and psychosynthesis (10). The specificity of art therapy, in comparison to other forms of psychotherapy using mental imagery, may be seen in the actual *externalization* of the mental content of the patient into *visual* images. This factor transforms the therapeutic setting from the bipolar field of verbal psychotherapies (11) to a tripolar field, where the three poles are: the patient, the therapist, and the image (Fig. 64–1). A range of communicative dimensions may then be activated, which are specific to the art therapy field and which are not mutually exclusive approaches. On the contrary, the therapeutic process in art therapy is a continuous movement involving the three dimensions: expressive-creative, cognitive-symbolic, interactive-analytic (Fig. 64–2).

1. The *expressive-creative dimension* is based on the relationship between the patient and the image, with the therapist in the role of facilitator of the image-making process. This dimension was emphasized by the pioneers of art therapy, who favoured a studio-based approach, where patients could work individually, in the presence of the therapist, and reach an in-depth experience of image-making. Patients vary in how much they need to be facilitated, and how capable they are to reach a symbolic level in their imagery.
2. The *cognitive-symbolic dimension* is based on the relationship between therapist and patient, through

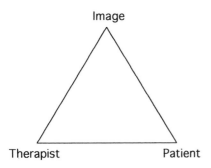

FIG. **64–1.** The tripolar field of art therapy: patient, image, therapist.

and about the image made by the patient. When patients are able to externalize and objectify their internal world into symbolic imagery, the therapist's role is that of a therapeutic ally, who can help them to own their pictures, to share and understand their meaning. This dimension is emphasized by the many art therapists who use a theme-oriented approach, or who employ Gestalt techniques, or who develop their own techniques to "work on the image." Working on the image may be done at many different levels: aesthetic, cognitive, symbolic. The symbolic work (helping patients to develop and understand their symbolic language and their system of personal meanings) may be regarded as the most specific tool of art therapy as a form of psychotherapy.

3. The *interactive-analytic dimension* combines the communication through the image, and the direct communication between therapist and patient. In this dimension the therapist offers himself/herself as an object of projection for the patient. This is the area of attention to transference and counter-transference issues, and it is emphasized by the art therapists who work psychoanalytically. The patient may use the image to express the transference to the therapist, or may project one aspect of himself/herself into the image, and another on to the therapist. Connections between these two aspects may further contribute to developments and transformations of the internal world of the patient.

These three dimensions are always present in the art therapy field, but they may be activated at different times. This gives a great flexibility to art therapy, which may be used as a supportive, as a cognitive, or as a psychoanalytic form of psychotherapy. Cancer patients do not constitute a homogeneous population: some of them may need to find a new form of relaxation; others may need to explore their way of coping with the traumatic experience of cancer diagnosis and treatment; others may need a psychodynamic approach to deal with unresolved conflicts and resentments which precede their illness.

The Three Types of Art Therapy Interventions
The structure of an art therapy intervention may activate different communicative dimensions, and stimulate different therapeutic factors.

Studio-Based Art Therapy. Studio-based art therapy is the ideal structure to facilitate self-expression and creativity. It is based on the provision of a safe and nonjudgmental environment, with a variety of art materials to experiment with, and combining silence and supportive verbal intervention to facilitate concentration and the development of personal imagery. Patients are encouraged to be in touch with their internal world of thoughts and feelings. Both

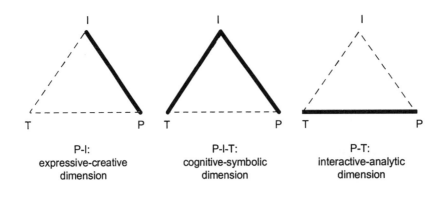

P-I:
expressive-creative
dimension

P-I-T:
cognitive-symbolic
dimension

P-T:
interactive-analytic
dimension

FIG. **64–2.** The three communicative dimensions in art therapy.

positive and negative feelings may be expressed symbolically, without disrupting the group, and without upsetting the relationship between the patient and the therapist.

Group Art Therapy. There are many forms of group art therapy—short-term and long-term—but in all of them the dynamics of the group interaction is used as a therapeutic tool. Some groups work around a common theme, selected by the therapist or by the patients; other groups evolve out of the expression of each patient's state of mind. Often the groups follow a simple structure, comprising three stages: *(1)* an introduction, which may or may not be verbal; *(2)* an image-making activity; *(3)* time for sharing about image-making and the meaning of the image, and time for feedback and group interactions.

Individual Art Therapy. Individual art therapy is a very flexible type of intervention. According to each patient's needs, the art therapist may decide to use mainly the expressive, or the cognitive, or the interactive approach. The movement from silent image-making to the use of words, or from words to image, becomes the individual style of each therapeutic encounter. Some patients always start a session by making an image, while others prefer to talk first. In the end, the image-making process becomes therapeutic when it leads to self-expression, containment, and transformation.

MEDICAL ART THERAPY: THE MAIN ISSUES

There are no distinct or predictable art therapy approaches which can be generalized as more suitable for one or the other patient population (12). The three communicative dimensions mentioned above (expressive, cognitive, interactive), and the three basic types of interventions (studio-based, group, individual) ought to be available all the time within any art therapy setting, and with any type of patient. There is so much variability among patients affected by cancer, that it would be inappropriate to label "cancer patients" as a population that needs to use only the creative dimension; or only group-work, or that needs stress management more than psychoanalysis, or free expression more than structured work. Nevertheless, it is useful to review clinical reports and case studies of art therapists working in this field in order to see the issues which have emerged, and how art therapists have perceived them. This can help in future planning and setting up of programs of art therapy in Cancer Centers,

and in defining the role of an art therapist within a psycho-oncology service.

The term "medical art therapy" has been applied to the use of art therapy with individuals who are physically ill, experiencing trauma to the body, undergoing aggressive or long-term medical treatments (13). Over the past 10 years a growing number of art therapists have been working with medically ill populations: in the United States at present they are almost 20% of the registered art therapists. In the United Kingdom a subset of art therapists from the British Association of Art Therapy, working with cancer and AIDS patients, has been called "The Creative Response." The general aim of medical art therapy is to improve the quality of life of medically ill patients, and the greatest challenge is the attempt to integrate somatic, psychological and existential themes such as pain, loss, and death.

Need for Innovative Interventions

When art therapists, who are primarily familiar with mental health or educational settings, start to work with medically ill patients, they feel challenged by the new situations (14). Time and Space factors of the sessions are different, and the combination of physical pain and psychological distress is new. There is need for more flexibility and for short-term "crisis interventions" (15). The therapeutic encounters may take place at the patient's bedside in the hospital room, or in waiting rooms (while the patients wait for chemotherapy, radiotherapy or check-ups) or at the patient's home. Issues of confidentiality must be confronted and sometimes adapted flexibly, as family and health aides often get included. Family work, bereavement groups and staff support groups become more relevant. Attention must be given to the whole range of human needs, from the most physical to the most spiritual: art therapists might have to focus on the expressions of bodily sensations, on images of pain, on different issues of loss and self-identity, on thoughts about death and dying, possibly including the terror of nothingness or the exploration of spiritual beliefs. Zeller (16) has stressed the need to teach art therapy students how to work with cancer patients.

The "Therapeutic Play" with Hospitalized Children

Early art therapy with severely ill children revealed the diagnostic and therapeutic value of their spontaneous drawings (17). Langarten (18) presents clinical art therapy as an important part of the treatment for medically hospitalized children on a pediatric unit. She focuses the individual treatment on a playful approach to hospital procedures and hospital authorities (encouraging drawings and role-playing about them), on bringing to the surface areas of concern (which often are not verbalized), and working-through process (using comic strip type drawings, and making up stories about people or animals who are in situations similar to their own). In a group of preadolescent boys and girls she helped them to visualize and explore positive and negative aspects of being in hospital, concerns and worries, fantasies and needs.

Rode (19) discussed the interface between the two professions of art therapist and child life specialist, as these two disciplines collaborate within a pediatric medical setting: they both use "therapeutic play" in order to reach the broadest range of patients and families. In some pediatric-oncology departments as many as 80% of the child life specialists are trained art therapists. Rode has directed pediatric patients (ages 9–20 years) with chronic illness into making their own "live with illness" videos, where children film each other painting and dancing; interview each other about their physical and emotional experience, from diagnosis to treatment; interview staff in the hospital and persons on the street; the filming itself was used as an innovative form of art therapy (20).

The concept of "therapeutic play" is illustrated also by Walker (21): children seem to be able to reveal their deepest anxieties while having fun with art material. On the whole, the use of images emerges as invaluable in the therapy with children and adolescents with cancer. Some art therapists emphasise the value of free expression, while others have devised special themes to help the children to draw what they cannot talk about.

In the attempt to facilitate the emotional expression of children with cancer, Sourkes (22) has created a structured intervention, based on three drawings: *(1)* the color-feeling wheel; *(2)* the change-in-family drawing; *(3)* the "scariest" drawing.

The need for flexibility is emphasized by Prager (23), who advocated the "single session" as a useful intervention for children with cancer, before or during medical procedures; at times the "session" may only last a few minutes. She also describes group art therapy in the dayroom, as an attempt to provide a kind of "sanctuary" for the children with cancer: no medical procedures are allowed in, and there is no right or wrong, no good or bad, the children can draw whatever they like.

Councill (24) pinpointed different art therapy interventions that may be useful during the three main stages: *(1)* diagnosis and treatment; *(2)* maintenance phase, *(3)* relapse or advanced stage. During the first stage it may be useful to focus on the use of art material as a safe tool for self-expression; during the middle

phase image-making can provide a special outlet for feelings of loss; during the third phase, art can give expression to the profound sense of isolation and fear of the unknown, and help in the communication between the child and the family when words are too difficult to say or to hear.

Hospitalized children have to cope with separation from parents, feelings of loss, and many fears. The inclusion of the art therapist as part of the pediatric treatment team has been seen as a unique humanizing influence during the child's hospitalization, which threatens the sense of self and trust in the world (25).

Working with Pain, Fatigue, and Stress

Art therapy, combining the physicality of the art material with the cognitive and emotional impact of image-making, has a special contribution to make in this area, where body and mind influence each other. Interventions focused on pain may range from a cathartic "drawing out the pain" (26) to an existential "integration" of the pain into the meaning of life (27). The literature shows that art therapists may establish meaningful communication with patients in physical pain. Some interventions used with patients who have been physically traumatized, like in a hospital burn unit, may be applied for cancer patients. Russell (28) described how art therapy may help the patients with physical pain to move through different stages: *(1)* express survival anxiety; *(2)* describe physical pain and provide relaxation; *(3)* offer search for meaning ("why me?"); *(4)* contribute towards recuperation through creation of tangible art products; *(5)* help patients to accept loss.

Langarten (29) described ways of working with adult patients with chronic pain: a woman who had one foot amputated, a man with chronic severe head pain, and long-term treatment with a couple in whom the husband had paralysis of right arm and leg and dysphasia from a stroke-affected speech. She worked toward the reintegration of the self, through various steps: eliminating the defense of denial; ventilation of fear; release of rage; and mourning. The art therapy approach provided means for recording conscious thoughts and emotions, as well as the unconscious mechanisms at work. In the marital therapy where the man could not speak, the art medium was invaluable to allow and facilitate genuine communication.

Long (30) listed four ways of utilizing art therapy in a pain management service: *(1)* focused work, to evaluate pain levels: using drawings of pain in the body; colored modeling clay to give shape to internal sensations; collage work to connect images of pain states with psychosocial stressors; *(2)* free drawing and painting to allow and deepen the expression of the pain experience and its transformation over time; *(3)* family art psychotherapy, when there is a pathological dynamics in the family system with an investment in psychosomatic symptoms; *(4)* drawing about pain 'before' and 'after' physiotherapy, to amplify and reinforce positive change.

The concept of "fatigue" is used more and more by patients who experience generalized weakness of their bodies. Fatigue is often associated with feelings of inadequacy and hopelessness. The use of imagery seems to enhance the individual's active participation in the healing process (31). Some art therapy techniques may be used with little physical effort to counteract fatigue through the production of meaningful images: pictures from magazine may be used for collages; simple marks on paper may stimulate free associations and creative patterns; symbolic images (e.g., a door, a wall, a flower, a tree, a path) may be offered as guided fantasies exercises (32).

Stress reduction is an important goal with cancer patients. The two basic aspects of stress reduction—*tension release* and *problem-solving*—find corresponding approaches in art therapy, through the relaxing and cathartic factors of image-making on one level, and through the more cognitive working-through process. Art therapy offers specific techniques for objectification of mental content and "distancing" (which is different from "avoidance").

Lusebrink and Scifres (33) investigated the imagery processes encountered in brief supportive therapy with mastectomy patients, using a sand tray. The "world" the patients built in the sandtray reflected the patients'' stressful situations, and their coping styles. Relaxation was enhanced by the tactile aspects of manipulating the sand. The use of the sand tray provided the opportunity for rearrangements of the metaphorical images, to explore alternative ways of coping. The authors also felt it was important to work with the patients on the externalization of dream images, which usually portray both emotional and bodily reactions to the illness.

Art Therapy with Patients in Isolation

The issue of isolation emerges as a multilevel issue. First of all it relates to hospitalization in general; then more specifically to some aspects of cancer treatment, like bone marrow transplantation. Furthermore, feelings of psychological and social isolation may follow the treatment.

Rosner-David, through her work with patients with tuberculosis, provided a significant contribution to the use of art therapy with patients in isolation (34). Isolation involves loss of control, loss of relationships,

anxiety and anger: participation in art therapy provides an opportunity for the patients to exercise control, choice and criticism, with a general decrease in anxiety.

Connell (35), working at the Royal Marsden Cancer Hospital in London, described one technique of overcoming the feeling of isolation of hospitalized cancer patients: she collects the individual patients'' drawings, poems, reflections into a big book which she keeps on the ward, and which the patients can look at and read at any time, especially when they feel lonely, or when they cannot sleep during the night. Patients who lie in their hospital bed and do not see each other may also communicate through writing or drawing on the same piece of paper, which the art therapist may take from one room to the next: this silent non-intrusive interaction may be comforting and stimulating.

Art therapy with a 11 year old girl within a bone marrow transplant unit is described by Gabriel (36). Although physically very weak and often unable to get up and talk, this patient was able to move from the pleasure of using art material, to the satisfaction of completing a project, to the sharing and unburdening herself about a guilty feeling in relationship to her mother.

Luzebrink and Scifres (33) felt that free expression was particularly useful in her work with mastectomy patients who had withdrawn from communicating with others, due to their anxieties and to their impaired self-worth. This is particularly so for laryngectomy patients, whose capacity to speak may be lost transiently or permanently. Art therapy was employed as an important diagnostic and therapeutic adjunct for laryngectomy patients at the University of Mississippi Medical Center (37). The German social insurance institutions extended coverage for creative therapies—including art therapy—to cancer patients, after their 3 year study on the effect of the individualized use of creative therapies demonstrated an improvement of the patients'' quality of life, overcoming the previous feeling of psychological and social isolation (38).

The Existential Issue of Death

Art images have historically served to express much of the emotion surrounding the issue of death and dying. Some art therapists have illustrated through their case studies how death and dying, bereavement and loss can be clearly communicated and worked through in art therapy, both in children (39) and in adults (40). Image-making may allow the expression of negative feelings, but it may also increase hope and understanding. The possibility of elaborating visual symbols of death and dying seems to be the specific contribution art therapy can make in this area (41): on one hand, the art therapist may help the dying and the grieving person to find their "personal symbols" to express something so powerful and so mysterious like the end of life; on the other side, there appear to be "universal symbols" (circles, energy, light, infinity, spirals, windows, tunnels) that may express the meaning of the cycle of death and rebirth. Art therapy may be particularly suitable to express the ambivalent nature of the death experience, based on loss and hope. Death may be seen as a mourning process, mourning a different loss from one stage to another of the illness, with different types of hope in each stage (42); in art therapy each stage may find a form and a symbol. Sourkes (43) emphasized the fluidity in the awareness of the dying child and the importance of working symbolically. Monsters and devouring animals predominate in the remembered nightmares: when the terror is brought to light, the intensity and frequency of the nightmares diminish. Children may project their feelings and thoughts on a favored stuffed animal, which may be described as ill, or sad, or peaceful, or happy. Sourkes gives a beautiful example of helping a child to integrate the complex experience with life-threatening illness with the use of symbolic imagery: a story, entitled "My Life is Feelings: starring Poly Polar Bear" was written by the child, with the help of the therapist, over a 3 month period, and it was illustrated with the photographs of the teddy bear in various sad and happy situations. Bjornsdottir (44) worked for 6 months with a depressed, dying 11-year-old boy who was concealing his distress. When, through his imagery, he started to communicate his concern about death, he became more secure and less depressed.

Other art therapists have focused on the family process. Art work made by children affected by cancer, during their hospitalization, may function as a bridge between the children and the staff in the hospital, or between the children and their family (45). Communication can be accomplished through artwork to say goodbye and subsequently serves as a legacy from the deceased. Junge (46) described the making of a book in which the whole family participates when one of its members dies: the book contains family memories, photographs, questions and answers about death; and all their feelings. Sourkes (22) has often worked with bereaved siblings, using the "letter-writing technique," to express unfinished business. Grief process is a time of rebuilding and reordering one's world (47); the goal is not to forget the deceased, but to complete the emotional relationship and to choose to reenter life.

Art Therapy and Cancer Patients with Psychiatric Symptoms

Cancer patients do experience a wide range of emotional distress and may present psychiatric symptoms of anxiety, depression, posttraumatic stress disorder, substance abuse, especially in the case of pathologic premorbid personalities. What is the role of the art therapist in these cases? Although art therapists function effectively in the treatment of psychiatric patients, in working with cancer patients they tend to channel their interventions more towards supportive art making and seem to be tentative about fully using the therapeutic process (48). But cancer patients deserve more than this: they deserve both support and confrontation. In fact, often patients interpret cancer in their body as a punishment, or an attack, or the sign of not being loved, or not being lovable: they may need to change the meaning they have given to their illness, or to change the response they have adopted to cope with that meaning. This is an important area for art therapists, as images are very suitable to communicate meanings, and to create new meanings (49). Art therapy has offered significant contributions with patients in psychotic states of mind (50,51), with borderline personalities (52), with eating disorders (53), substance abuse (54), and with symptoms of posttraumatic stress disorder (55,56). Art therapy has been effective as a form of family therapy, in working with troubled children and their families (57). The two stages of "mental visualization," followed by "giving shape to the internally perceived images," have been seen in psychiatry as good tools for strengthening a vulnerable ego (58), and the experience of the patient as "active creator" instead of "passive victim" may prevent or reduce depressive feelings (23). Art therapy may also be used to clarify cognitively the focal conflict in the patient's personality (59). If we consider that the major fears of psychiatric patients are either depressive (fears of separation and abandonment) or persecutory (fears of engulfment or persecution), "the image" as a transitional object may help in both cases. In fact, the patient may keep the "image" made in therapy as a bridge against the fear of separation; or the patient may use the space for image-making as a defence against the fear of intimacy and engulfment.

According to Skaife (48), there could be two main obstacles preventing the art therapist from providing in-depth psychotherapy to medically ill patients: on one hand, the medically ill patient may be threatened by the popular image of psychotherapy as connected with mental illness; on the other hand, the therapist may tend to provide diversional activities in order to be liked, and forgiven for being healthy, and to avoid envious feelings by the patient. The importance of being aware of one's countertransference, in working with cancer patients, has been stressed also by Dreifuss-Kattan (60), and by Kramer and Rosner (61): they both insist that special attention should be given to the therapist's own fears about illness and death.

Working with Staff, Caregivers, and Relatives

The need for support groups and professional supervision has been advocated by many art therapists working in this field. The same need arises for other professionals working with these patients; in fact art therapy can be used effectively to provide staff support groups. Rubin (12: 210) noted that the phenomenon of burnout is very real, but is probably less common among art therapists than among other mental health professionals. She believes it may be related to the tapping of strengths and creativity in people, which is often exciting to the art therapists as well as to the patients, and to the familiarity of the art therapist with primary process thinking, which may not be so familiar to other professionals.

Belfiore (62) provided an art therapy experience for nurses and doctors caring for terminally ill patients: through art therapy, a new language emerged, that enabled participants to express the deepest and hidden levels of their personal experience. A staff art therapy program with monthly art groups was led by an art therapist in Alabama (63), as an expressive outlet for highly stressed workers, in a clinic for terminally ill patients. Materials available were pastels, paints and clay. Group process was minimized. The participants attempted to focus on themselves, to nurture themselves, to free up their energy and rechannel it to attend again to the needs of others. Bertman (64) described an educational process for family members and health care professionals using visual images of illness and death from the art world, to elicit personal feelings and reactions to dying and grief. She used slide presentations, followed by discussions, as a teaching aid and also as an avenue for self-discovery, to medical students, graduate nurses, hospice volunteers.

At the Edge of Art Therapy: Art and Psychological Self-Healing

There is an overwhelming literature on the self-healing property of art making. Art therapy, as we defined it at the beginning of this chapter, implies the presence of three elements: the patient, the image-making, and the therapist. When the three elements are not all present, it is not art therapy. Nevertheless, this is an issue at the border between art and art therapy, and we wish to touch on a few points.

All art therapists know that there are categories of patients who do not benefit from being encouraged to draw or paint by themselves: some patients get very frustrated by what they perceive as their lack of imagination, or lack of artistic skill; other patients develop disturbing images (nightmares, flashbacks, obsessive thoughts, visual hallucinations, etc). When is the engagement into image-making, without the presence of the therapist, inherently therapeutic? We can identify three categories:

1. Some patients developed cancer when they were already familiar with the creative process, or with the introspective process (as artists, art therapists, or psychoanalysts, or just as creative and insightful patients), and they have been able to use their creativity as an individual therapeutic activity. Dreifuss-Kattan (60) analyzed first-person accounts of artists and writers with cancer, and she concluded that many of them can use their personal creativity to rediscover an internal "'good object'" and to connect with it, as a form of self-repair against loss. She found that the art work from cancer patients is often an account of having found a new identity: describing the fear and the pain of loss is itself a process of accepting and overcoming these emotions. Making images may be the beginning of a long therapeutic process. Nevertheless, the author also mentions the existence of a "'manic creativity,'" which is not a transformation of mourning so much as a defense against it. In this case, she believes that actual creativity can be attained only after the defense has subsided, and the patient has been helped to work through necessary mourning.

2. Other patients discovered their creativity as part of self-help groups, where the group provided the therapeutic support. This has happened more frequently in women's groups. In this spirit, a collective of women survivors of breast cancer worked for a 6 month period, allowing the meaning of the cancer experience to become visible through art (65). At UCLA Medical Center an organization called Art That Heals developed, through 7 years of operation, several programs which used arts interventions to reduce stress and facilitate coping with hospitalization (66)

3. Other patients find support in following the guidance offered in books, workbooks, visual journals, where they can move on, by themselves, step by step. If they feel bored, tense or uncomfortable, they may stop at any time. The workbook may become a

benign silent therapist, who can witness their process of self-expression and self-understanding. Capocchione (67) is the most well known representative of this approach. According to her, the method works only if it is private and confidential. The visual journal has limitations, and the readers may need to find outside support, to engage into other types of therapeutic interventions, and to select the activities which best suit their needs, and sometimes to develop their own exercises, developng their own self-help books. Sourkes has used the Mandala, based on drawing into a circle, following Jung's suggestion that the circle may be experienced as a symbol of the Self, and may be used to increased personal awareness. Sourkes' experience of this and other drawings in children with life-threatening illness has been highly positive (43)

The approach to art as self-healing leaves aside the silent crowd of patients who do not fall into those three categories, either because they are not "artistic," or because they dislike joining groups, or because they do not have the motivation to follow a workbook. This self-help approach places a strong emphasis on "positive imagery" because it is obvious that one cannot encourage a patient to delve into negative imagery and leave the patient alone with it. As a consequence, this field sometimes colludes with the defense of the patient in denying reality and not dealing with what would be initially disturbing, but more truly healing. On the whole, this area is not art therapy, but it borders on it. It becomes particularly important as a form of self-development for the patients who feel it is appropriate for them, and as a form of follow-up, after an art therapy intervention, so that the patients may continue to benefit from what they have learned.

ART THERAPY AND CANCER PATIENTS: ILLUSTRATION OF THE SIX THERAPEUTIC FACTORS

From the analysis of the literature and from our own clinical experience, six therapeutic factors of art therapy emerge, which we call the six "Cs" of art therapy: Catharsis; Creativity; Communication; Containment; Connections; Changing the image (Table 64.1). We have selected six pictures made by cancer patients during theme-oriented art therapy workshops, to illustrate these therapeutic factors (Figs. 64–3 to 64–8).

TABLE 64.1 *The Six Therapeutic Factors of Art Therapy*

1. *Catharsis*
It has a physical element
It does not threaten the therapeutic relationship
The experience is objectified
It can be discarded and/or transformed

2. *Creativity*
Perceiving oneself as agent
Allowing preconscious/unconscious material to emerge
Giving form to formless mental content
Giving meaning to meaningless material

3. *Communications*
Silent listening
Verbal sharing
Receiving feedback
Giving feedback

4. *Containment*
It offers a spacial metaphor for the inner space
It offers a double containment (= image and therapist)
It may contain opposite feelings which need to be integrated
It may contain fragmented feelings that need to find unity

5. *Connections*
Between images and affects
Between images and memories
Between present and past images
Between aspects of self

6. *Changing the Image*
Adding something
Removing something
Developing something
Finding alternative images

Catharsis: To Offer a Safe Place for Self-Expression
I was relieved of my pent-up anger, and I was made more calm. (Picture 1; Fig. 64–3)
During one workshop we encouraged patients to feel free to "make a mess" on paper. Cancer patients often feel under pressure to show that they can cope; being allowed to make a mess was reassuring for this patient, who could express confusion and anger having fun, in a liberating way, without crying, or shouting, that would have been embarrassing for this patient in front of the group. The free and playful use of art material was cathartic. The patient could look at "the mess" afterward, think about it, talk about it.

The cathartic factor, which is important in any form of psychotherapy, has some special features in art therapy: its kinesthetic quality offers a special kind of release and relief; the objectification of intense affects into the art work does not threaten the therapeutic

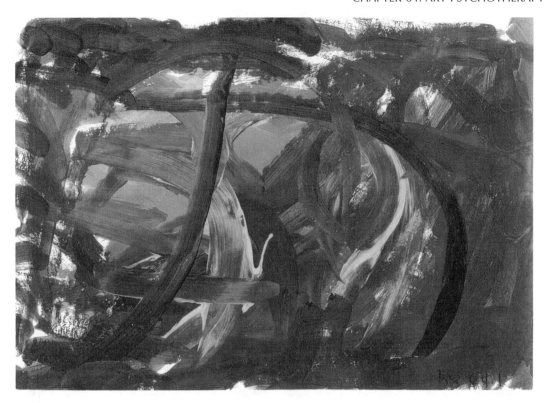

FIG. **64–3.** Catharsis.

relationship; the expression of negative feelings does not generate shame in the patient, nor remorse, nor fear of retribution. The space for image-making may be used by the patient to get rid of a painful feeling, and the drawing may be discarded, but it may also be looked at later on, and transformed (see below).

Creativity: To Increase Self-Esteem and Feelings of Autonomy

I felt things did not come directly from me, they just happened, then I saw something in them. (Picture 2; Fig. 64–4)

During another art therapy workshop the patients were told to focus their attention on an object placed on the table (in this case it was a candle), then to use visual free association, to see what would come to their mind, and to choose what to paint. Free association in art therapy is different from the verbal free association of psychoanalysis: through the combination of unconscious and conscious elements, an image may lead to another one, without the bridge of verbal connection. It gives a feeling of personal choice and autonomy.

This patient associated the image of the candle with a tree and with a face ("It just happened"); the external imagery was combined creatively with an internal imagery, and the picture came to embody a special meaning for the patient.

In the history of philosophy the concept of creativity has been identified with some special factors like the feeling of freedom and autonomy connected with the use of imagination (68), and the capacity to give form and meaning to formless and meaningless material (69). These factors may be used therapeutically with patients who do not wish to move into self-revelation, and who therefore have difficulty in engaging in formal therapy. The capacity to "'give meaning'" is particularly important to cancer patients, as illness and death may be threatening to deprive their life of meaning.

Communication: To Reduce Feelings of Isolation and Depression

I became more aware of genuine feelings, of stress and love, in my own life and in the life of others. (Picture 3; Fig. 64–5)

In this workshop patients were asked to choose pictures and words from the magazines which were placed on the table, and to use them to express "something about themselves." This patient expressed the pleasure of being able to communicate her true self, instead of hiding it.

Through the simple act of making an image, the patient's capacity to communicate is facilitated at various levels—intra-psychic and interpersonal—through both conscious and unconscious processes. Sometimes

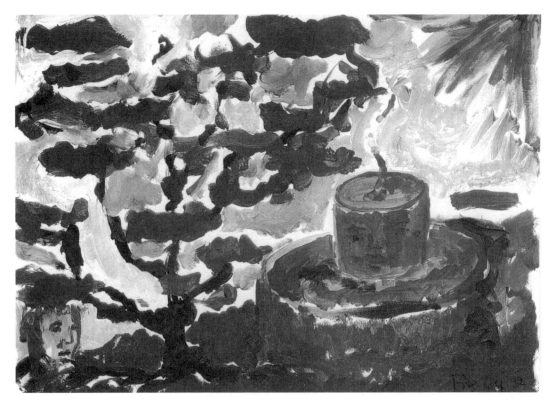

FIG. **64–4.** Creativity.

a patient wants to share an experience without talking about it, and may be happy to offer the image just to be looked at. This is particularly important for cancer patients who may feel ashamed about sharing "negative" feelings of fear or confusion, or may not like to listen to the stories of painful treatment or relapse of the illness in other patients. This ambivalence often prevents cancer patients from attending verbal support groups. The emerging of symbolic visual imagery in art therapy is often intriguing, and sometimes funny, and this triggers feelings of surprise in the patients, which facilitates a special kind of sharing that is not intrusive. The interplay of nonverbal and verbal communication becomes a precious tool that makes the therapeutic process unfold.

Containment: To Express Difficult Feelings and Prevent Anxiety

I was able to draw my pain, make it a thing, and distance from it. (Picture 4; Fig. 64–6)

One workshop was devoted to the concept and visualization of the experience of "stress." This patient decided to give a visual form to her traumatic experience of mastectomy. She had never expressed this fear of fragmentation before, as she always appeared strong and coping very well. Other patients, after looking at

her picture, shared in the group the same indescribable fear of bodily disintegration, following a surgical intervention, and thanked her for giving a form to their own feeling. Making and sharing her picture helped this patient to unburden herself of a "secret," and to feel accepted in her vulnerability.

During the therapeutic process patients may encounter feelings that are difficult to contain: opposite feelings that need to be reconciled; fragmented feelings that need to be integrated; hidden fears and old resentments; positive feelings that the patient was not able to develop. Art therapy offers a special form of multiple containment: the experience of the patient may be contained in the space of the picture *and* in the mind of the therapist (*and* in the group, if it is group therapy). An extra containment is the offer of an individual session, if a patient needs to talk more about the image that has emerged.

Connections: To Provide Self-Understanding and Improve Coping

The workshop made me think more about myself, and made me see myself clearer. (Picture 5; Fig. 64–7)

Here the patient described visually her own way of reacting to a traumatic situation: feeling powerless, feeling "like going down into a vortex," from where

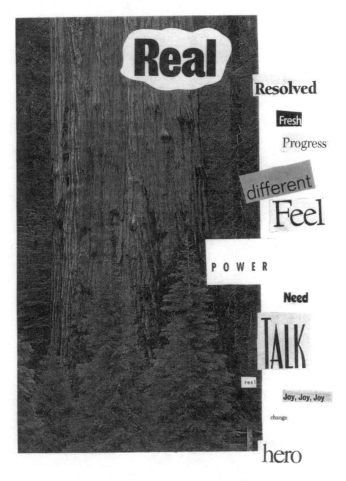

FIG. **64–5.** Communication.

there is no exit, and no hope. Recognizing this pattern helped this patient towards thinking about this feeling, instead of just "feeling it." Some patients are ready to connect their pictures to recurrent feelings and behaviours in their life, or even to early traumatic experiences, and this may increase their insight.

Once a mental content is externalized into a visual image, and the image is shared, it is easier for the patient to create a distance from it, and to think about it. The patient's observing ego may become more capable of making connections, which is the basis of the therapeutic "working through." An image may become connected to a state of mind, a memory, a repressed thought, a denied emotion. An image may be compared with others that the patient has made previously, and the therapist may help the patient to uncover recurrent patterns of behaviour, which may now be questioned: a new perspective may emerge.

Changing the Image: To Facilitate New Meanings and Acquisition of Hope

I have experienced how I can transform or trasmute my pain. (Picture 6; Fig. 64–8)

During this workshop the patients were encouraged to paint a landscape where there was "no life," and then to slowly transform it into a landscape where a seed might actually grow ("how will it grow?"). For this patient the first image was a dark brown mountain without any vegetation, and for her it was symbolic

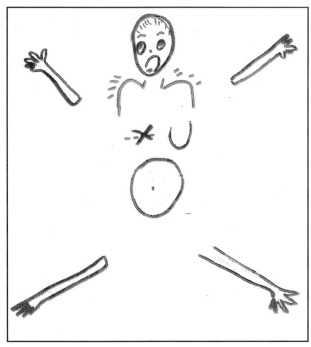

FIG. 64–6. Containment.

of death. After contemplating the possibility of a seed in the ground, she developed the image of a huge tree, which was as large as she could make it. She called this picture "The Embrace," and she gave to the image a deep existential and spiritual meaning, about the relationship between death and life.

It is a common experience of both therapists and patients that visual images made in the therapeutic setting develop and change. The visual distance between the patient and the image allows space for reframing. The playful attitude which often accompanies image-making also stimulates change. The patient may remove or add something, or develop another picture. The issue of whether and how the change in visual images "reflects" or "affects" the actual change in the mental attitude of the patient is a complex one. However, it is certain that, through the dynamic transformation of symbolic images, cancer patients may experience their potential to transform feelings of despair and gain hope. Developing alternative images may have a strong therapeutic impact on the psychic reality of the patient.

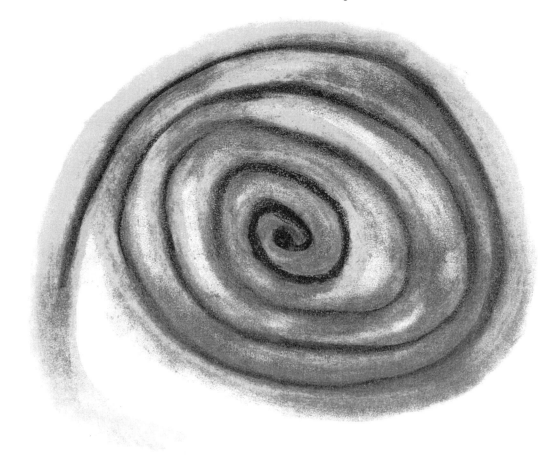

FIG. 64–7. Connections.

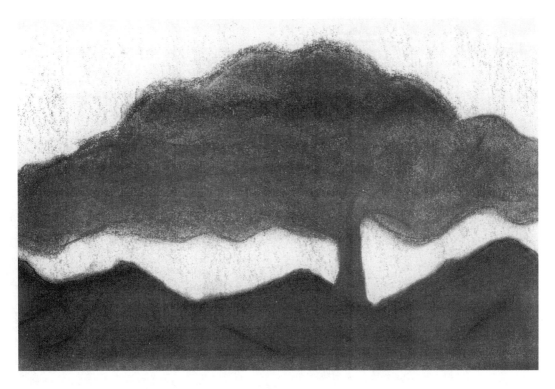

FIG. **64–8.** Changing the image.

FUTURE DIRECTIONS AND LINES OF RESEARCH

Therapeutic issues for cancer patients may vary from having to cope with the pain and the stress of cancer diagnosis and treatment, to psychiatric symptoms (anxiety, depression, substance abuse, posttraumatic stress disorder), from the wish to improve the quality of life of the posttreatment stage, to the search for new identity (following physical and social changes), and to existential issues about pain, death and life meaning.

Art therapy may offer useful clinical interventions with cancer patients, as it may be adapted to their different needs: *(1)* some cancer patients seem to benefit from the silent creative endeavor, as a form of self-repair against an internal feeling of damage and loss; *(2)* other patients may use their image-making to come out of their isolation, to communicate and interact with other patients, their family, the therapist; *(3)* other patients, who have become psychologically distressed, or disturbed, may use the verbal and nonverbal process of art therapy as a form of psychotherapy, for personal development and psychic change.

We propose a model of an integrated art therapy service, which could be appropriate to any large cancer center, and we suggest a few lines of research into the effectiveness of art therapy with cancer patients.

Art therapy could be provided by a team of art therapists working in five separate areas, but working together closely: *(1)* pediatric oncology; *(2)* adult in-patients; *(3)* ambulatory cancer patients; *(4)* home-based patients; *(5)* supportive service for caregivers and relatives. In this way a cancer patient may be offered art therapy at the time of admission on the ward, and then the same patient could continue to use it through a choice of ongoing or recurrent individual or group interventions.

Some interventions which appear to have been particularly appreciated by cancer patients merit listing: *(1)* an active and playful approach to help children describe their experience through pictures, photos, videos; *(2)* an art therapy book on the ward, where hospitalized adult patients can contribute images, words, reflections; *(3)* a program of art therapy workshops for ambulatory cancer patients, to stimulate the activation of the six therapeutic factors—catharsis, creativity, communication, containment, connections, change; *(4)* the provision of home visits from an art therapist, who helps the terminally ill patient to leave a visual legacy; *(5)* the availability of art therapists for psychotherapeutic interventions when cancer patients develop psychiatric symptoms, especially panic states, depression, suicidal ideations, posttraumatic stress syndrome, substance abuse; *(6)* support groups and bereavement groups for caregivers and relatives.

Some promising lines of research are apparent: *(1)* effectiveness of relief from pain, fatigue, and psychological distress after engagement into a series of art therapy workshop; *(2)* research into possible changes in brain imaging during involvment into creativity workshops; *(3)* a comparison on the effectiveness of short-term art psychotherapy versus verbal psychotherapy, or versus a combination of verbal psychotherapy plus art therapy; *(4)* a comparative study on the images about death and dying in suicidal, or non-suicidal terminally ill patients.

REFERENCES

1. Waller D. *Becoming a Profession*. London: Tavistock; 1991.
2. Hill A. *Art Versus Illness*. London: George Allen & Unwin; 1945.
3. Naumberg M. *An Introduction to Art Therapy*. New York: Teachers College; 1973.
4. Winnicott DW. *Therapeutic Consultations in Child Psychiatry*. London: Hogarth Press; 1971.
5. Luzzatto P. Letter to Editor. *Inscape: J Br Assoc Art Ther*. 1989; 5(autumn):31–35.
6. Breuer J, Freud S. *Studies on Hysteria*, standard ed. 2; 1955.
7. Jung CG. *The Archetypes and the Collective Unconscious*. New York: Pantheon; 1959.
8. Beck AT. Role of fantasies in psychotherapy and psychopathology. *J Nerv Ment Dis*. 1970; 150:3.
9. Perls FS. Dream seminars. In: Fagan J, Sheperd IL, eds. *Gestalt Therapy Now*. Palo Alto, CA: Science and Behavior; 1970.
10. Assagioli R. *Psychosynthesis: A Manual of Principles and Techniques*. New York: Hobbs and Dorman; 1965.
11. Langs R. Some communicative properties of the bipersonal field. In: Grotstein J, ed. *Do I Dare Disturb the Universe?* London: Karnac; 1981.
12. Rubin J. *The Art of Art Therapy*. New York: Brunner and Mazel; 1984.
13. Malchiodi CA. Introduction to special issue: Art and Medicine. *Art Ther*. 1993; 10(2):66–69.
14. Long J, et al. Innovations in medical art therapy: defining the field. *Proceedings of the 20th Annual American Art Therapy Association Conference*. Mundelein, IL: AATA; 1989.
15. Appleton V. An art therapy protocol for the medical trauma setting. *Art Ther*. 1993; 10(2):71–77.
16. Zeller J. The art of cancer care. *Proceedings of the 27th Annual American Art Therapy Association Conference*. Philadelphia, PA: AATA; 1996.
17. Luzzatto P. Anorexia nervosa and art therapy. *Arts Psychother*. 1994; 21:139–143.
18. Landgarten H. *Clinical Art Therapy*. New York: Brunner/Mazel; 1981; 121–135.
19. Rode D. Building bridges within the culture of pediatric medicine: the interface of art therapy and child life programming. *Art Ther*. 1995; 12(2):104–110.
20. Rode D. *Information Accompanying Videos*. The Mt. Sinai Child Life Program, New York: Through Our Eyes Productions; 1994.
21. Walker C. Use of art and play therapy in pediatric oncology. *J Pediatr Oncol Nurs*. 1989; 6:121–126.
22. Sourkes BM. Truth to life: art therapy with pediatric oncology patients and their siblings. *J Pyschol Oncol*. 1991; 9(2):81–96.
23. Prager A. Pediatric art therapy: strategies and applications. *Art Ther*. 1995; 12(1):32–38.
24. Councill T. Art therapy with pediatric cancer patients: helping normal children cope with abnormal circumstances. *Art Ther*. 1993; 10(2):78–87.
25. Rollins J. Helping children cope with hospitalization. *Imprint*. 1990; 37(4):79–83.
26. Berstein J. Art and endometriosis from an artist's sketchbook. *Art Ther*. 1995; 12(1):14–20.
27. Halliday D. My art healed me. *Inscape*. 1987; 3 (Summer):18–22.
28. Russell J. Art therapy on a hospital burn unit: a step towards healing and recovery. *Art Ther*. 1995; 12(1):39–45.
29. Langarten H. *Clinical Art Therapy. A Comprehensive Guide*. New York: Brunnel/Mazel; 1981: 335–372.
30. Long J. Establishing medical art therapy in a new out-patient pediatric pain management service. *Proceedings of the 26th Annual American Art Therapy Association Conference*. San Diego, CA: AATA; 1995.
31. Achterberg J, Lawlis G. *Bridges of the Bodymind, Behavioural Approaches to Healthcare*. Champaign, IL: Institute for Personality and Ability Testing; 1980.
32. Engelen H. Using the wall symbol in art therapy with cancer patients. *Proceedings 26th AATA Conference*. AATA; 1995.
33. Lusebrink V, Scifres K. Visual and tactile interventions in healings: sandtray with mastectomy patients. *Proceedings 26th AATA Conference*. AATA; 1995.
34. Rosner-David I, Illusorio S. Tuberculosis: art therapy with patients in isolation. *Art Ther*. 1995; 12(1):24–31.
35. Connell C. Art therapy as part of a palliative care programme. *Palliat Med*. 1992; 6:18–25.
36. Gabriel B. Art therapy in the bone marrow unit (personal communication).
37. Anand S, Anand V. Art therapy with laryngectomy patients. *Proceedings 26th AATA Conference*. AATA; 1995.
38. Heyde W, von Langsdorff P. Rehabilitation of cancer patients including creative therapies. *Rehabilitation (Stuttg)*. 1983; 22:25–27.
39. Cotton MA. Creative art expression from a leukemic child. *Art Ther*. 1985; 2(2):55–65.
40. Miller B. Art therapy with the elderly and the terminally ill. In: Dalley T, ed. *Art as Therapy*. London: Tavistock Publications; 1984.
41. Tate F. Symbols in the graphic art of the dying. *Arts Psychother*. 1989; 16:115–120.
42. Bluelbond-Langner M. *The Private Worlds of Dying Children*. Princeton, NJ: Princeton University Press; 1978.
43. Sourkes B. *Armfuls of Time (The Psychological Experience of the Child with a Life-threatening Illness)*. Pittsburgh, PA: University of Pittsburgh Press; 1995.

44. Bjornsdottir S. Art therapy for children with longstanding disorders. *Proceedings VI Nordic Seminar in Art Therapy*. Iceland; 1985.

45. Scudder Teufel E. Terminal stage leukemia: integrating art therapy and family process. *Art Ther*. 1995; 12(1):51–55.

46. Junge M. The book about daddy dying: a preventive art therapy technique to help family to deal with the death of a family member. *Art Ther*. 1985; March:4–10.

47. Raymer M, Betker McIntyre B. An art therapy support group for bereaved children and adolescents. *Art Ther*. 1987; March:27–35.

48. Skaife S. Sickness, health and the therapeutic relationship: thoughts arising from the literature on art therapy and physical illness. *Inscape*. 1993; Summer:24–29.

49. Horowitz MJ. *Image Formation and Psychotherapy*. New York: Jason Aronson; 1983.

50. Killick K. Working with psychotic processes in art therapy. *Psychoanal Psychother*. 1993; 7(1):38–49.

51. Wadeson H. *The Dynamics of Art Psychotherapy*. New York: Wiley; 1987.

52. Silverman D. Art psychotherapy: an approach to borderline adults. In: Landgarten H, Lubbers D, eds. *Adult Art Psychotherapy*. New York: Brunner/Mazel; 1991.

53. Wood M. Art therapy and eating disorders: theory and practice in Britain. *Inscape*. 1996; 1(1):13–19.

54. Luzzatto P. Drinking problems and short-term art therapy: working with images of withdrawal and clinging. In: Gilroy A, Dalley T, eds. *Pictures at an Exhibition*. London: Routledge; 1989: 207–219.

55. Golub D. Symbolic expression in PTSD: Vietnam combat veterans in art therapy. *Arts Pyschother*. 1985; 12:285–296.

56. Stern-Buck A. The use of art therapy in the treatment of PTSD. *Proceedings of the 27th AATA Conference*. Philadelpha, PA: AATA; 1994.

57. Riley S. *Integrative Approaches to Family Art Therapy*. Chicago: Magnolia Street Publishers; 1994.

58. Wellendorf E. Art therapy in psychiatry. *Psychiatr Prax*. 1980; 7:26–33.

59. Jadi F, Trixler M. The use of focal conflict model in art therapy. *Confin Psychiatr*. 1980; 23:93–102.

60. Dreifuss-Kattan E. *Cancer Stories: Creativity and Self-Repair*. Hillsdale, NJ: The Analytic Press; 1990.

61. Kramer E, Rosner I. Art therapy: a bridge between worlds. *Proceedings of the Twelfth Annual Conference of the AATA*. Liberty, NY, 22–25 October, 1981.

62. Belfiore M. The group takes care of itself: art therapy to prevent burn out. *Arts Psychother*. 1994; 21(3):119–126.

63. Elkinson-Griff A. Let me wipe my tears so I can help with yours. *Art Ther*. 1995; 12(1):67–69.

64. Bertman S. *Facing Death: Images, Insights and Interventions (A Handbook for Educators, Healthcare Professionals and Counselors)*. Bristol, PA: Taylor & Francis; 1991.

65. Predeger E. Womanspirit: a journey into healing through art in breast cancer. *Adv Nurs Sci*. 1996; 18:48–58.

66. Breslow DM. Creative arts for hospitals: the UCLA experiment. *Patient Educ Couns*. 1993; 21:101–110.

67. Capocchione L. *The Picture of Health: Healing Your Life with Art*. Carson, CA: Hay House; 1990.

68. Sartre JP. *The Psychology of Imagination*. London: Methuen; 1983.

69. Langer S. *Philosophy in a New Key*. Cambridge, MA: Harvard University Press; 1951.

65

Telephone Counseling

JULIA A. BUCHER, PETER S. HOUTS, MYRA GLAJCHEN, AND
DIANE BLUM

The need for information, guidance, and support among persons with cancer and their family caregivers has been well documented and continues to grow as a result of shortened hospital stays and greater reliance on outpatient care (1–3). Despite the development of a number of excellent and comprehensive psychosocial support programs (4,5), important barriers to these services still exist. Persons with cancer remember little of what they are told in medical care settings; communicating medical information in written form to persons with low reading skills remains a serious problem; and recruitment to educational programs or support groups remains a consistent challenge. For example, attendance at I Can Cope, a nationwide educational program, continues to be low; an estimated 7000 are reached yearly out of 1 million newly diagnosed cases (6). This low attendance is matched by low attendance at other support groups (7). As a result, we need to devise new ways to reach out to persons with cancer and families and provide them with the information and support that they need.

As a communication tool, the telephone has the potential to overcome many barriers to learning and gaining support. It reaches out to families at home where they are less anxious, able to integrate information, and can think through plans for purposive action. Information delivered over the telephone also bypasses problems with reading skills and bypasses the need to leave the home to receive information and support. The principal disadvantage of using the telephone is the lack of face-to-face contact, thus limiting the range of stimuli. On the other hand, many people are accustomed to using the phone for very personal commuxication and, for some, the lack of face-to-face contact may facilitate open communcation and exchanges about sensitive issues. Providing psychoeducational interventions over the telephone presents a cost-effec-

tive way to reduce barriers to support and help persons with cancer and their families cope.

This chapter will review four types of telephone interventions that have been used with persons with cancer and their families or that have promise for contributing to their care. We will discuss: using one-on-one telephone contacts for information, referral, and counseling; telephone groups for health education; and telephone groups for support. In addition, a new approach will be described: a voicemail bulletin board for education and group support with implications for case management and counseling.

USING ONE-ON-ONE TELEPHONE CONTACTS FOR INFORMATION, REFERRAL, AND COUNSELING

Literature abounds on the use of telephones for one-on-one interventions. These will be discussed first among findings for persons with cancer and then among those with other illnesses.

The Efficacy of One-on-One Telephone Interventions for Individuals with Cancer and Their Families

The usefulness of the telephone helpline as a source of information is well documented. An early cancer helpline, Can-Dial, was prerecorded and provided information about cancer treatments as well as preventive advice. Users dialed a toll-free number that was open 16 hours a day, 7 days a week and requested a prerecorded tape listed on a menu of up to 36 selections. Lectures by physicians were from 1 to 7 minutes in length. Early evaluation revealed that the most frequently requested tapes pertained to smoking (8). Later data revealed significant increases in service use, increases in cancer knowledge, and self-reports of adoption of healthy behaviors (9,10). Demographic analysis showed greatest use by younger urban females of higher socioeconomic status when compared to nonusers (11).

Other cancer helplines are interactive. Two are most prominent: the 1-800 Cancer Response System sponsored by the American Cancer Society and the 1-800 telephone line offered by the Counseling and Information Service (CIS), a nationwide network of 19 regional offices funded by the National Cancer Institute (12). Originally designed as a health education service for the general public and for cancer patients, callers to the CIS can order free printed materials, locate certified mammography centers, learn about clinical trials, request searches from the Physician Data Query (PDQ), or talk with information specialists who provide information, support, and referral information. Available 5 days per week during business hours, recent reports chronicle a steady increase in numbers of calls for personalized counseling offered since 1976 with 506,000 calls registered in 1990 (13). The most frequent requests are placed to the prerecorded Publication Ordering Service for written materials and national user profiles match one published statewide report (13,14). Callers tend to be younger white females with at least a high school education. Examination of both databases confirms the finding that persons with cancer call half as often as family members or friends who express a wide variety of needs for information (13,14).

Very few cancer helplines specialize in psychological and interpersonal counseling. In 1978 such a service was designed as part of the National Cancer Institute's Cancer Communications Network—the UCLA Psychosocial Cancer Counseling Line, which provides telephone counseling and referral services to persons with cancer and their families and also consultation to health professionals. After intensive educational sessions, volunteers staff the service, which is available 5 days per week during business hours. Calls average 20–25 minutes with 80% of users calling once. User profiles matched those of other helplines; a high percentage had college degrees. Twice as many family members and friends called as compared to the number of persons with cancer who called and the most frequent request was a referral to support groups (15,16).

The largest counseling helpline service, Cancer Care, Inc., has been in operation since 1944 offering a Counseling Line as well as taking calls at its offices in New York, New Jersey, and Connecticutt. Toll-free calls are made from all 50 states, and calls for counseling have increased dramatically in the past year providing practical assistance to nearly 7500 persons with cancer (17). The average length of these calls is between 20 and 50 minutes, and families initiate this option more often than persons with cancer. Patients request help with adjustment as do relatives who also want help with financial problems, anxiety, family problems, doctor–patient communications, and other psychosocial needs. Evaluation data reveal that nearly 80% of callers telephoned the Counseling Line within 1 day after learning about the service and were very satisfied (17).

More intensive interpersonal intervention is provided outside of helplines; however, few studies have demonstrated their psychological efficacy for persons with cancer. Nail et al. outlined reasons for calls made between nurses and users of an ambulatory oncology clinic. Although the program was not systematic, the majority of calls addressed more than one purpose and were for information, comfort, and coping. The authors concluded that telephone contact is helpful for more than filling prescriptions or scheduling appointments (18).

Siegel et al. (19) designed an automated telephone needs assessment followed by a social work telephone call to reduce the prevalence of unmet concrete needs among chemotherapy outpatients. Systematic outreach over 6 months resulted in early identification of problems, such as handling medical bills, transportation, or household needs, and social work follow-up for information and referral.

Similarly Polinsky et al. (20) followed 69 newly diagnosed women with breast cancer by telephone for 1 year who enrolled in a case management intervention study. Participants received a package of written material and assessments were conducted between 3 and 5 weeks after cancer surgery. Follow-up contacts were made at least once every 6 weeks by social workers who gave reassurance, information, and referral averaging less than 0.5 hour per contact. The most intense period of contact occurred during the first 3 months when physical problems were discussed. Psychological and treatment-related issues became more prominent over time and total contacts averaged 5.4 hours per person per year. Persons with cancer were more than willing to discuss psychosocial concerns over the telephone, supporting findings from other feasibility studies in which persons with cancer openly accepted calls made to them that they did not initiate (21,22).

The telephone's role in psychotherapy has been reported in only one study. In a description of two case studies, Mermelstein and Holland (23) included an overview of the advantages and disadvantages of this mode of delivery for long-term psychotherapy with adults with cancer. The same therapeutic processes occurred and its anonymity was particularly effective.

The Efficacy of One-on-One Telephone Interventions for Noncancer Populations

Most studies measuring effects of telephone interventions were conducted on noncancer populations. A general outcome of these studies was earlier detection of problems, multidisciplinary follow-up, and continuation in treatment programs (24,25). Unlike calls made to helplines, the majority of other one-on-one telephone interventions are initiated by health professionals and offer a combination of services. The conduct of these interventions differs very little from in-person case management type meetings and can be made by appointment or not scheduled.

The early literature on telephone interventions with other populations was confined to crisis intervention and suicide hotlines (26–28). Now telephone technology is used in primary health care (29,30), reminders about screenings and appointments (31), routine clinic follow-up (32,33), general clinical assessment and triage (34), and management of acute illnesses (35,36). Evaluation data confirm that it is an efficient mode of contact for health care delivery; patients and families find it acceptable; and they appreciate its ease.

Most studies of one-on-one telephone interventions dealt with reports of physical health outcomes. Effects on functional status have been documented, mostly among patients with osteoarthritis. Three randomly assigned intervention groups of 439 patients with primary or secondary osteoarthritis received the same intervention either in person, on the telephone, or by both methods. Those contacted by phone reported a significant improvement in physical health and reduction in pain compared to those not contacted by phone (37). Similarly, 79% of users of an interactive arthritis information helpline reported taking at least one positive action because of service usage, such as asking more questions of doctors, while 50% felt more in control of their arthritis after receiving helpline services, such as information, printed material, and, when necessary, physician consultation (38).

In another study, researchers added a telephone contact to face-to-face personal interventions with an experimental group of persons with chronic lung disease to review individual progress and reinforce individualized teaching plans to manage stress (39). The researchers concluded that an in-person and telephone follow-up intervention had a modest effect on functional status and that comprehensive management of these patients must include multiple strategies, such as periodic reinforcement of coping strategies at home

through telephone calls. In addition, Beckie (40) documented greater levels of knowledge and lower anxiety among patients who received 4–6 supportive and informational calls from a rehabilitation nurse after coronary artery bypass surgery compared to a control group. These studies attest to the usefulness of telephone services to improve knowledge, coping, and health.

Unfortunately, studies of the behavioral effects of telephone information and counseling are few . One randomized design compared the effects of four different self-help quit smoking interventions: no intervention; a self-quitting guide; this guide with an additonal one for the family; and the two guides with four brief counseling calls. They found that telephone counseling in either group increased adherence to the quitting protocol and increased quit rates (41). In another study, rates of smoking cessation also were affected significantly by follow-up telephone calls from cardiac rehabilitation nurses to patients discharged after a myocardial infarct. A randomly assigned group received information on the risks of smoking, reviewed printed and taped materials, and then received weekly calls for 2–3 weeks and then monthly calls for 4 months. This telephone group revealed a cessation rate that was almost 30% higher compared to a control group who received regular inpatient care (42). However, another randomized clinical trial showed no effect on smoking behavior delivered by behavioral counselors compared to effects derived from face-to-face counseling by physicians (43). Other behavioral studies clearly indicated that telephone case management worked well when combined with other strategies. For example, one home visit and four telephone calls over a 3 month time period improved compliance to self-monitoring of blood glucose when compared to a control group (44), and follow-up calls 2–4 days after emergency room visits increased patient compliance with scheduling and keeping appointments after treatment for urinary tract infections (45).

Recently, research indicates that telephone communication affects health care utilization. One randomized controlled trial found that regular calls from a public health nurse to nonacutely ill elderly were associated with one less physician visit per year (46). A more recent randomized trial substituted telephone care for clinic visits among a population of men receiving primary care (47). Three telephone contacts were made while the reguarly scheduled appointment was extended to twice as long as ususal. Telephone-care patients fared better on a variety of outcomes: fewer unscheduled clinic visits, less medication use, fewer admissions, shorter stays in hospitals, and lower estimated total expenditures. These findings among non-psychiatric populations challenge earlier conclusions made by mental health specialists that telephone counseling did not produce behavioral change (48).

USING THE TELEPHONE FOR GROUP EDUCATION

Teleconferences are used now to educate groups of patients or family caregivers. This technology allows small groups of callers to be united on the telephone, listening and speaking to one another as though they were in one room. Commonly presented by doctors, nurses, social workers, or cancer survivors, typical topics range from coping at home to dealing with the health care system. Programs are usually targeted for groups sharing a specific diseases, such as "Coping With Lung Cancer" and "Managing Advanced Prostate Cancer and Pain" (17,49).

The planning and organization of teleconference education is similar to traditional educational programs. After experiences with this method, Cancer Care, Inc. staff recommend that recruitment takes place 1 or 2 months in advance. Participants register in person, by telephone, or by mail. It is advisable to orient participants ahead of time with either a video or written instruction packet on how to prepare for the session, join the group, participate, and observe basic group rules. They also recommended including an evaluation survey in preconference packets.

Members of smaller telephone groups can ask questions throughout a presentation under a moderator's direction. However, participants in larger groups, such as those of 40 or more, are placed on a listen-only mode during the didactic portion of the presentation. Feedback from recent field testing (17) indicate that the suggested length of "lectures" is 1 hour, although information has been delivered from 45 minutes to as long as 90 minutes. After the formal delivery, the telephone line is switched to an interactive mode for a question and answer session lasting a recommended 20 minutes.

Educational teleconferences can be costly, particularly if large numbers of people participate. Most phone systems allow a maximim of 6–8 participants on a call initiated through a conventional phone system. Once group numbers increase beyond eight, outside conference operators are needed and costs quickly escalate. At the time of this writing, most conference calls cost 25 cents per minute no matter what the distance; therefore, a 1 hour call costs an average of $15 for each participant phone line. Just as with other presentations, these sessions can be taped and distributed to participants and to wider audiences.

Only one study has reported the effects of teleconference education. Glajchen and Moul (49) offered a teleconference on advanced prostate cancer and pain to 107 men who participated in two 1 hour presentations. The majority of listeners were patients. Fifty-two (63%) participants were interviewed 4 weeks later and their comprehension and recall of educational material were found to be high. The most correct answers were about treatment options for prostate cancer and availability of pain medication. The poorest recall included information on noncancerous causes of pain, hormonal therapy, and the use of strontium for pain. A majority reported that they found the information useful and felt more encouraged about their prognosis. The men were more likely to recommend a longer question and answer session than the allotted 10 minutes and requested audiocassette recordings of the teleconference. They also requested that depressing statistics about morbidity and mortality be eliminated.

USING THE TELEPHONE FOR SUPPORT GROUPS

Like telephone education, telesupport groups reach people who are unable or unwilling to participate in face-to-face groups. Mental health professionals focus on group discussion and emotional support. Education about stress management and coping skills also occurs. Similar to other support groups, telephone support groups can take many forms. They can be closed to a set number of participants or open to participants entering at any time. They can be time limited, such as 1 hour weekly sessions, or they can be ongoing with members joining in at any tine. Options also can be built in for participants to call one another outside of the set group time to talk informally or to initiate conference calls among members.

Outcomes of telephone support groups have been reported with other populations, such as Alzheimer's family caregivers and persons with HIV/AIDS. One method is to establish a network where participants call each other according to previously arranged call schedules. This method was piloted among two groups of Alzheimer's family caregivers. One group of five spouse caregivers called each other weekly over 12 weeks, as did a second group of adult children caregivers. Thus, group members made and received one call per week after listening to a selected topical audiotape before the calls to guide their discussion. The network of spouses was more cohesive than the group of adult children but both groups reported benefits, such as feelings of shared struggle and greater self-awareness (50).

Other telephone support groups use a more traditional teleconference format. Cancer Care, Inc. reports that their most common telephone support group for persons with cancer and their caregivers meets weekly for 1 hour for 8 weeks. Conference calls are limited to 12–14 participants although smaller groups can be justified. Groups larger than 14 require coordination by a telephone operator. In either case, each participant is called and placed on hold until the group leader joins the call. It is advisable at the start of the call to give clear instructions on how to contact the conference operator should any technical difficulties arise. Then, after a roll call, the leader begins the session and leads discussion. Participants should be asked to follow these procedures, which apply to time-limited (shorter term) groups and to ongoing groups (who meet indefinitely):

- Leave their phone lines open for 15 minutes prior to the start of the group.
- State their names each time before speaking until group members know each other.
- Keep background noise to a minimum wherever they receive the call.
- Ignore call-waiting, doorbells, beepers, or other deployments.
- Speak one at a time.
- Let the group leader know if they will be late or absent from the meeting.

Telephone support groups can be organized in a number of different formats. Open-ended telephone groups allow people to drop-in as needed, thus participants join and leave the group at different times. Open-ended groups for persons with cancer are more flexible, can accommodate arduous treatment schedules, and are appropriate for those who do not want to make a commitment to a series of sessions. Because they are longer term, with a fluid membership, open-ended groups risk becoming unfocused. Whereas closed-ended telephone groups, whose membership is "closed" to a select set of participants, develop more cohesion and intimacy and participants can tackle more in-depth topics. In general, these groups follow a more intense pace and are guided more closely by group facilitators.

According to the Cancer Care Inc. experience, the recommended size for any type of group is 12 participants. No matter what form telesupport groups take, they challenge health care professionals to listen very closely, deal with monopolizers, include more reticient members, and concentrate on both verbal cues and silences, all without visual feedback. Neophyte group leaders should not lead groups until they have first participated in groups and have listened to skilled facilitators.

Although no experimental–control group comparison research has been conducted to date, Glajchen and Magen (51) reported follow-up results of three different types of cancer telephone groups: patient, family, and bereaved. After finishing their 1 hour 8 week series, 392 participants (representing 63 groups) completed questionnaires about group processes and satisfaction. Participants in all groups reported very high levels of satisfaction with group experience; those in bereavement groups reported the highest overall satisfaction, and patient groups the lowest. Many members stated that they liked the opportunity to ventilate, experienced a sense of not being alone, and liked the support. A number of patients, however, reported that they did not like ending the sessions.

Colon (52) described the outcomes of one group of persons with cancer who have met weekly over the phone for 1 hour. Described as an ongoing format, such groups are not limited to 6 or 8 week sessions but meet indefinitely. In this instance, group size was limited to 12 and participants understood that the weekly group would not be terminated. Thus far, 30 people have participated since the group began 5 years ago. One result was unanticipated. Some members have become activists for cancer care, research and support; they advocated for change about cancer rehabilitation and even educated legislators about their needs.

Efficacy of Telephone Groups in Noncancer Populations

Studies of the usefulness of telephone groups in noncancer populations indicate that facilitator-led, cognitive-behavioral interventions are effective. Grouping participants by similar characteristics is reported to be helpful according to Evans et al. (53). For example, two groups of physically disabled adults and a professional group leader participated in 1 hour calls over 8 weeks to share information, solve problems, and build relationships. Counselors adopted a cognitive therapy approach that focused on goal achievement and used various "shaping techniques" to help members rehearse new behavior in coping with the attitudes of outsiders. Participants expressed satisfaction with phone conferencing and with attainment of their goals (53). The intervention was repeated with a larger group of disabled elderly and 86% reported goal achievement (54). The intervention was tested again on disabled adults using an experimental–control group design, and the treatment group reported less loneliness while their families reported observing more social role skills (55). Investigators emphasized that benefits may have been enhanced by group homogeneity, which contributed to developing a sense of cohesion and intimacy.

A study of telephone groups with blind elders also reported results (56). Participants were randomly selected and placed into experimental and control groups. The experimental group met with a counselor and other selected blind elders for 8 weekly 1 hour telephone conferences. Counselors used a cognitive-behavioral approach. The experimental group showed greater task-centered goal attainment along with decreased feelings of hopelessness and increased socialization. Telephone group work also has been piloted with persons with HIV/AIDS. Interventions with participants showed that they definitely would refer others to this telephone service (57) and that they felt others would benefit from small group exchange even near the end of life (58).

THE VOICEMAIL BULLETIN BOARD: A NEW APPROACH FOR EDUCATION AND SUPPORT

The recent development of telephone bulletin board helplines was based on innovations in computer screen programs that provided information and support. For example, the CHESS program used an at-home computer screen program to enable participants to locate facts and advice about breast cancer and its treatment (59). Interestingly, users of this at-home computer screen option for education and support selected the 'discussion section' or support group option more frequently than other options, such as dictionaries or question and answer exchanges with health professionals. Another study also showed that HIV/AIDS patients who received psychosocial support through at-home computer screen bulletin boards demonstrated that the social support feature was the one option most frequently accessed (60). Patients with access to the system were more likely to modify risk-taking behavior than those without access, suggesting the importance of social support provided by electronic groups in bringing about behavioral change.

Computer screen programs require access to a modem whereas computer-driven telephones do not. All that is needed to use the system is a touch-tone phone. Thus, potential for telephone systems to reach more users is higher. In addition, the telephone version of an Internet bulletin board allows messages to be voiced instead of typed. Users find this more personal. Messages are posted and callers can browse the list, communicate by telephone with health professionals

and other callers, ask questions, and support each other. It can be accessed through a 1-800 number at any time of the day or night and is managed by a computer that stores and plays messages as directed from telephone signals. The voicemail system is centrally located and run by a small staff who can access the system from any location. Health professionals monitor the content of discussions and remove statements whenever necessary to insure that accurate information is given in a supportive way. They also monitor problem-solving and coping strategies and can provide support and information to an asynchronous sample in an ongoing manner. Thus voicemail bulletin board contacts are more efficient than those made through teleconference support groups, which are time consuming to organize and limited to shorter weekly interactions.

Results of field tests suggest that 'talking computers' encourage users to participate in self-care and users report high levels of participation and satisfaction (61,62). The telepractice system has been used successfully to help different types of groups, including those of low socioeconomic status, obtain help and support. In a random assignment of 179 pregnant women who had used cocaine during or 1 month before pregnancy, the experimental group had access to the telecommunications system. Compared to the control group, the use of the system was associated with increased participation in formal drug treatment, which leads to reductions in drug use by implication (62). In a follow-up study, 53 of these women agreed to either participate in the voice bulletin board or attend biweekly face-to-face meetings. Clients were more likely to participate in the voice bulletin board and they reported significantly lower rates of health service utilization. Interestingly, the majority of comments left on the bulletin board were for emotional support. Follow-up has revealed increased participation in formal drug treatment and reduced rates of inappropriate health service utilization (63).

This technology recently has been adapted for use with cancer family caregivers who completed the Prepared Family Caregiver Program, which focuses on teaching basic problem-solving steps to improve coping (64). Participants receive video-led instruction about solving common problems related to cancer and guidance on how to use a written reference text, the Home Care Guide for Cancer (65). The follow-up voicemail system reinforces problem-solving strategies by allowing users to hear other caregivers talk about their caregiving problems, plan solutions to tackle those problems, and receive emotional support. Professionals also contribute to discussions thereby guiding users in positive directions and reinforcing problem-solving learning.

Future applications of voicemail systems for persons with cancer and their caregivers offer a promising combination of all the other types of telecommunication interventions: *(1)* health education from peers and health professionals, *(2)* explanations about cancer treatments, symptom management, and diagnosis, *(3)* problem-solving, and *(4)* group support. The technology allows small groups of caregivers in similar circumstances to form. In addition, health professionals can monitor how individudals are coping and intervene with personal messages and case management.

CONCLUSION

Continued use of the telephone to provide information and support is an appropriate practice in psycho-oncology, given a future in which efficiency and outpatient treatments are the norm and as delivery systems change (66,67). The telephone offers a strategic combination of intimacy and safety, mutual support systems for people isolated by illness or circumstances, and enhanced capacity for independent functioning. As with all interventions, its fit for individuals with cancer and their families must be assessed according to specific needs and evaluated regularly for valid outcomes and actions. Most importantly, its use must be integrated into comprehensive psychoeducational programs and research suggests that it fits into the complex process of cancer care.

REFERENCES

1. Houts PS, Yasko JM, Kahn SB, et al. Unmet psychological, social, and economic needs of persons with cancer in PA. *Cancer.* 1986; 58:2355–2361.
2. Farber JM, Weinerman BH, Kuypers JA. Psychosocial distress in oncology outpatients. *J Psychosoc Oncol.* 1984; 2:(3/4):109–118.
3. Derogatis LR. Psychology in cancer medicine: a perspective and overview. *J Consult Clin Psychol.* 1986; 54: 632–638.
4. Ganz PA. Patient education as a moderator of psychological distress. *J Psychol Oncol.* 1988; 6:(1/2):181–197.
5. Zabora J, Loscalzo, M. Comprehensive psychosocial programs: a prospective model of care. *Oncol Issues.* 1996; 11:(1):14–18.
6. McMillan SC, Tittle MB, Hill D. A systematic evaluation of the "I Can Cope" program using a national sample. *Oncol Nurs Forum.* 1993; 20:(3):455–461.
7. Bocanegra T. Cancer patients' interest in group support program. *Cancer Nursing.* 1992; 15:(5):347–352.
8. Wilkinson GS, Mirand EA, Graham S. CAN-DIAL—an experiment in health education and cancer control. *Public Health Rep.* 1976; 91:(3):218–222.
9. Wilkinson GS, Mirand EA, Graham S. Cancer intervention by telephone: a two-year evaluation. *Health Educ Monogr.* 1977; 5:(3):251–264.
10. Wilkinson GS, Mirand EA, Graham S. Measuring response to a cancer information telephone facility: Can-Dial. *Am J Public Health.* 1978; 66:367–371.
11. Wilkinson GS, Wilson J. An evaluation of demographic differences in the utilization of a cancer information service. *Soc Sci Med.* 1983; 17:(3):169–175.
12. Poe MR, DeVore LM. Using the telephone for cancer information. *Cancer Pract.* 1996; 4:(1):47-49.
13. Anderson DM, Duffy K, Hallett CD, Marcus AC. Cancer prevention counseling on telephone helplines. *Public Health Rep.* 1992; 107: 278–283.
14. Reiches NA, Brandt NK. The Ohio cancer information service: callers, inquiries, and responses. *Public Health Rep.* 1982; 97;(2):150–155.
15. Rainey LC. Cancer counseling by telephone help-line: the UCLA psychosocial cancer counseling line. *Public Health Rep.* 1985; 100:(3):308–315.
16. Meissner HI, Anderson DM, Odenkirchen JO. Meeting information needs of signfiicant others: use of the Cancer Information Service. *J Patient Educ Counsel.* 1990; 15:171–179.
17. Glajchen M. Personal communication. Cancer Care, Inc; 1996.
18. Nail LM, Greene D, Jones LS, Flannery M. Nursing care by telephone: describing practice in an ambulatory oncology center. *Oncol Nurs Forum.* 1989:16:(3): 387–395.
19. Siegel KS, Mesagno FP, Karus DG, Christ G. Reducing the prevalence of unmet needs for concrete services of catients with cancer: evaluation of a computerized telephone outreach system. *Cancer.* 1992;69:1873–1883.
20. Polinsky ML, Fred C, Ganz PA. Quantitative and qualitative assessment of a case management program for cancer patients. *Health Soc Work.* 1991; 16:176–183.
21. Marcus AC, Cella D, Sedlacek S, et al. Psychosocial counseling of cancer patients by telephone: A brief note on patient acceptance of an outcall strategy. *Psycho-Oncology.* 1993; 2:209–214.
22. Hagopian GA, Rubenstein JH. Effects of telephone call interventions on patients' well-being in a radiation therapy department. *Cancer Nurs.* 1990; 13;(6):339–344.
23. Mermelstein HT, Holland JC. Psychotherapy by telephone: a therapeutic tool for cancer patients. *Psychosomatics.* 1991; 32: 407–412.
24. McCullough MA, Day S, Herlihy E, Rapp, P. Use of a multidisciplinary follow-up program to assist patient adjustment following temporal lobectomy. *J Neurosci Nurs.* 1989; 21:(5):295–304.
25. Intagliata J. A telephone follow-up procedure for increasing the effectiveness of a treatment program for alcoholics. *J Stud Alcohol.* 1976: 37:(9):1330–1335.
26. Bleach G, Claiborn WL. Initial evaluation of hotline telephone crisis centers. *Commun Ment Health J.* 1974; 10:387–394.
27. Stein DM, Lambert MJ. Telephone counseling and crisis intervention: a review. *Am J Commun Psychol.* 1984; 12:101–126.

28. Slaikeu KA, Leff-Simon SI. Crisis intervention by telephone. In: Slaikeu KA, ed. *Crisis Intervention: A Handbook for Practice and Research*, 2nd ed. Boston: Allyn & Bacon; 1990: 319–328..

29. Curtis P, Talbot A. The telephone in primary care. *J Commun Health*. 1981; 6(3):194–203.

30. Radecki SE, Nelelle MA, Girard RA. Telephone patient management by primary care physicians. *Med Care*. 1989; 27:817–822.

31. Burgoyne RW, Acosta FX, Yamamoto J. Telephone prompting to increase attendance at a psychiatric outpatient clinic. *Am J Psychiatry*. 1983; 140: 345–347.

32. Wasson J, Gaudette C, Whaley F, et al. Telephone care as a substitute for routine follow-up. *J Am Med Assoc*. 1992; 267:1788–1793.

33. Nelson EW, Van Cleeve S, Swartz, MK, et al. Improving the use of early follow-up care after emergency department visits. *Am J Dis Child*. 1991; 145:440–444.

34. Murphy D, Dineen E. Nursing by telephone. *Am J Nurs*. 1975; 75(7):1137–1139.

35. Perrin EC, Goodman HC. Telephone management of acute pediatric illnesses. *N Engl J Med*. 1978; 298: 130–135.

36. Nicklin WM. Postdischarge concerns of cardiac patients as presented via a telephone callback system. *Heart Lung*. 1986; 5(3):268–272.

37. Weinberger M, Tierney WM, Booher P, Katz, BP. Can the provision of information to patients with osteoarthritis improve functional status? A randomized controlled trial. *Arthritis Rheum*. 1989; 32(12):1577–1583.

38. Maisiak R, Koplan S, Heck LW . Subsequent behavior of users of an arthritis information telephone service. *Arthritis Rheum*. 1990; 33(2):212–218.

39. Blake RL, Vandiver TA, Braun S, et al. A randomized controlled evaluation of a psychosocial intervention in adults with chronic lung disease. *Family Med*. 1990; 22(5):365–370.

40. Beckie T. A supportive-educative telephone program: impact on knowledge and anxiety after coronary artery bypass graft surgery. *Heart Lung*. 1989; 18(1):46–55.

41. Orleans C T, Shoenbach VJ, Wagner EH, et al. Self-help quit smoking interventions: effects of self-help materials, social support instructions, and telephone counseling. *J Consult Clin Psychol*. 1991; 59(3):439–448.

42. Taylor CB, Houston-Miller N, Killen JD, DeBusk RF. Smoking cessation after acute myocardial infarction: effects of a nurse-managed intervention. *Ann Intern Med*. 1990; 113(2):118–123.

43. Ockene JK, Kristellar J, Goldberg R, et al. Increasing the efficacy of physician-delivered smoking interventions: a randomized clinical trial. *J Gen Int Med*. 1991; 6(1):1–8.

44. Estey A L, Tan MH, Mann K. Follow-up intervention: its effect on compliance behavior to a diabetes regimen. *Diabetes Educ*. 1990; 16(4):291–295.

45. Jones PK, Jones SL, Katz J. A randomized trial to improve compliance in urinary tract infection patients in the emergency department. *Ann Emerg Med*. 1990; 19:16–20.

46. Infante-Rivard C, Krieger M, Petitcierc M, Baumgarten M. A telephone support service to reduce medical care use among the elderly. *Am Geriatr Soc*. 1988; 36:306–311.

47. Wasson J, Gaudette C, Whaley F, et al. Telephone care as a substitute for routine follow-up. *J Am Med Assoc.*. 1992; 267:1788–1793.

48. Hornblow AR. The evolution and effectiveness of telephone counseling services. *Hosp Commun Psychiatry*. 1986; 37(7):731–733.

49. Glajchen MG, Moul JW. Teleconferencing as a method of educating men about managing advanced prostate cancer and pain. *J Psychosoc Oncol*. 1996; 14(2):73–87.

50. Goodman CC, Pynoos J. Telephone networks connect caregiving families of Alzheimer's victims. *Gerontologist*. 1988; 28(5):602–605.

51. Glajchen M, Magen R. Evaluating process, outcome, and satisfaction in community-based cancer support groups. In: Galinsky MJ, Schopler JH, eds. *Support Groups: Current Perspectives on Theory and Practice*. New York: Haworth Press; 1995: 27–40.

52. Colon Y. Telephone support groups—a nontraditional approach to reaching underserved cancer patients. *Cancer Pract*. 1996; 4(3):156–159.

53. Evans RL, Fox HR, Pritzl DO, Halar EM. Group treatment of disabled adults by telephone. *Soc Work Health Care*. 1984; 9(3):77–84.

54. Evans RL, Smith KM, Werkhoven WS, et al. Cognitive telephone group therapy with physically disabled elderly persons. *Gerontologist*. 1986; 26(1):8–11.

55. Evans RL, Huller EM, Smith KM. Cognitive therapy to achieve personal goals: results of telephone group counseling with disabled adults. *Arch Phys Med Rehabil*. 1985; 66(10):693–696.

56. Evans RL, Jaureguy BM. Phone therapy outreach for blind elderly. *Gerontologist*. 1982; 22(1):32–35.

57. Ritter B, Hammons K. Telephone group work with people with end stage AIDS. *Soc Work Groups*. 1992; 15(4):59–72.

58. Rounds KA, Gallinsky MJ, Stevens LS. Uniting people with AIDS in rural communities: the telephone group. *Soc Work*. 1991; 36(1):13–18.

59. Gustafson D, Wise M, McTavish F, et al. Development and pilot evaluation of a computer-based support system for women with breast cancer. *J Psychosoc Oncol*. 1993; 11(4):69–93.

60. Gustafson DH, Hawkins RP, Boberg EW, et al. The use and impact of a computer-based support system for people living with AIDS and HIV infection. *JAMIA Symposium Supplement, SCAMC Proceedings*, American Medical Informatics Association. Philadelphia, PA: Hanley & Belfus; 1994.

61. Alemi F, Stephens RC, Muise K, et al. Educating patients at home: community health Rap. *Med Care Suppl*. Computer Services to Patients' Homes Through Their Telephones 1996; 34:(10):0521-0531.

62. Alemi F, Stephens RC, Javalghi RG, Dyches H, Butts J, Ghardiri A. A randomized trial of a telecommunications network for cocaine using pregnant women. *Med Care Suppl*. 1996; 34(10):510–520.

63. Alemi F, Mosavel M, Stephens RC, et al. Electronic help and support groups. *Med Care Suppl*. 1996; 34(10):532–544.

64. Houts PS, Nezu AM, Maguth Nezu C, Bucher JA. The prepared family caregiver: a problem-solving approach to family caregiver education. *Patient Educ Counsel*. 1996; 27:63–73.

65. Houts PS, Nezu AM, Nezu C, et al. *The American College of Physicians Home Care Guide for Cancer.* Philadelphia, PA: American College of Physicians; 1995.

66. Schoech D, Cavalier AR, Hoover R. Using technology to change the human services delivery system. *Admin Soc Work.* 1993; 17(2):31–52.

67. Curry SJ, Ludman E, Wagner EH. A model for health behavior change in managed care. *Outlook.* 1996; 3:5–6.

66

Meditation

JON KABAT-ZINN, ANN OHM MASSION, JAMES R. HEBERT, AND
ELANA ROSENBAUM

Medicine: the restoration of right inward measure when it is disturbed
Meditation: the direct perception of right inward measure—modified
from Bohm (1)

An illness such as cancer can create an immediate and
enduring crisis of being. It may challenge the integrity
of one's ideas about oneself, and long-held concepts
about one's life trajectory, one's body past and future,
and one's relationships. A personal world which was
felt to be relatively stable can be quickly disrupted as a
person is plunged into the role of patient in a universe
of doctors, tests, hospitals, and uncertain but critically
important choices. If, as often happens, there is a
strong focus on aggressively treating the disease, without adequately attending to the person with the disease, the person may be unwittingly disempowered by
the health care system at just that time when he or she
most needs to be able to marshal personal resources.
Lerner (2) has described receiving a cancer diagnosis as
akin to a soldier dropped unexpectedly into a jungle
war zone without map, compass, or training of any
kind. Shock, isolation, depression, fear, bewilderment,
self-pity, anger, bitterness, and feelings of helplessness
are not uncommon sequelae to a cancer diagnosis and
its immediate aftermath. In and around such times, an
inward orientation toward one's experience can be
extremely valuable in making sense of it and charting
a course of action. Meditation practice can be extremely useful in this regard, as a complement to medical
care, psychotherapy (if warranted), and social support
from family and friends.

Meditation can provide a powerful psychological
framework as well as specific methods for coming to
terms with one's personal situation in ways that can
provide deep comfort, meaning, and direction in times
of high stress and uncertainty. This includes specific
approaches for facing and working with emotional turmoil, pain, and suffering. In the process, meditation
can help individuals connect with what is deepest and
most nourishing in themselves, and to mobilize the full
range of inner and outer resources available to them.
However, meditation needs to be thought of as a "way
of being" rather than as a technique or set of techniques. Its practice requires disciplined and consistent
inner work. If possible, it is best learned within the
context of a class or group so that one has ongoing
support and opportunities for clarification and refinement in the early stages of practice.

In the past two decades, meditation has expanded
beyond the religious and spiritual contexts with which
it traditionally had been associated, to become the
foundation of some medically based group interventions (3), and an important element in others (4,5).
In most cases, these interventions make use of the
basic and universal characteristics of meditation, without its particular cultural and religious overtones and
elements, as methods to deepen awareness, self-understanding, self-acceptance, self-efficacy, and to increase
one's capacity for effective decision-making and
action.

The use of meditation in cancer therapy has yet to be
tested scientifically through clinical trials. However, its
generic value as a form of stress reduction and as a
long-practiced method of calming the mind and body
and developing clarity, insight, acceptance, and equanimity recommend it as an adjunct to other forms of
treatment for cancer patients, and it is generally used
in this context. Meditation can have a profound influence on quality of life in medical patients (3), and can
be instrumental in evoking a greater commitment and
sense of partnership when undergoing medical procedures and treatments, and in fostering a greater sense
of agency and engagement in life.

In this chapter, we outline the ways in which meditation in general, and meditative awareness, or *mindfulness* in particular, as used in the Stress Reduction

Clinic at the University of Massachusetts Medical Center, can be used to face and grapple with the physical, psychological, and spiritual dimensions of cancer and its aftermath. We also briefly discuss meditation-based interventions in relation to psychosocial interventions, the state of current research findings, and potential implications for health attitude and health behavior change in cancer prevention.

WHAT IS MEDITATION?

Meditation is the intentional self-regulation of attention (6,7). It enhances concentration and awareness as an individual focuses systematically and intentionally on particular aspects of his inner or outer experience. It is a refined and systematic way to pay attention on purpose, in the present moment, and nonjudgmentally.

There are two large generic categories of meditation practices: those emphasizing *concentration* and those emphasizing *mindfulness* (8). Concentrative methods cultivate one-pointedness of attention. Mindfulness practices start from a degree of one-pointedness and then expand the field of awareness to include a range of objects of attention as they change from moment to moment in the field of awareness.

Examples of concentrative practices include the use of mantras (sounds or phrases used repetitively to concentrate attention; transcendental meditation (TM) is an example), koans (phrases or questions in the Zen tradition that are aimed at cutting through discursive thinking), and the breath, when these objects serve as the singular, invariant focus attention. Concentration practices can bring about profound states of calmness, inner stillness, and nonreactivity of mind.

Mindfulness practices, exemplified in the *vipassana* (9–13) and *Soto Zen* (14–16) traditions, cultivate an intentionally nonreactive, nonjudgmental moment-to-moment awareness of a changing field of objects. Rather than becoming absorbed, as in concentrative practices, which to a degree shuts out the world, the practitioner attends to the full range of whatever is present in the field of his unfolding experience, no matter what it is. This makes mindfulness a highly practical inner orientation for people with busy, engaged lives, especially if they are faced with a life-threatening illness and all its accompanying emotional turbulence in addition to other life stressors. Mindful attention helps in facing and embracing all aspects of life, however painful or frightening, with increasing degrees of equanimity and wisdom. These qualities develop as the practitioner spends time each day in periods of silence and nondoing (formal meditation practice), with the focus on present-moment experience

as it unfolds, and then, as the practitioner carries that moment-to-moment awareness into various aspects of daily living (informal meditation practice).

All cultures acknowledge and, to varying degrees, value the human capacity to relate consciously to the present moment, and its potentially transformative power for seeing more clearly and conducting one's life with greater authenticity. Sir William Osler (17), one of the founders of modern medicine, extolled "the practice of living for the day only, and for the day's work" rather than becoming distracted by preoccupations with future and past concerns, however enticing or overwhelming. He seems to have discovered, in the conduct of his own life as a physician, the discipline of mindfulness practice in daily living, and the value of cultivating equanimity, and urged his students to follow it as a way of life (17,18). Thoreau extolled the virtues of what he called "the bloom of the present moment" as the major theme of *Walden* (19). Many great western poets, including TS Eliot ("A condition of complete simplicity/Costing not less than everything") (20) and Ranier Maria Rilke ("I am the rest between two notes") (21) captured the power of inner stillness and silence characteristic of present moment awareness.

A NONDOING ORIENTATION

Health care providers should keep in mind that meditation is fundamentally different from relaxation techniques in both its methods and objectives. Meditation is commonly but erroneously thought of as a technique that aims at achieving a specific, highly pleasant "meditative state" akin to deep relaxation. However, there exists no single "meditative state" that the meditator is trying to achieve. The overall orientation is one of nonstriving and nondoing, as noted above (14,22). In mindfulness meditation, there is no attempt to achieve any objective other than awareness, attained through the systematic deployment of moment-to-moment attention. Pleasant, unpleasant, and neutral feeling states, including deep states of relaxation, arise during meditation. The meditation instructions call for all to be observed nonjudgmentally moment by moment. Other states or qualities, such as patience, generosity, openness, compassion, can be invoked through specific meditation practices. However, no state can be said to be the goal of practice. The goal is simply awareness of whatever is happening in any moment. Any goals that are formulated in association with meditation practice, such as wanting to feel better, different, more relaxed, or less reactive, are intentionally observed as part of the practice itself, and thus, as best one can, held lightly in awareness, with an overall sense of non-attachment.

Thus, meditation teaching and practice contain a paradoxical element. In the medical setting, people are typically referred by health professionals for specific reasons and to achieve specific personal goals. The most common reasons patients give for pursuing meditation practice are stress and anxiety reduction, pain reduction, greater clarity in decision making, relaxation, inner peace, and improved coping. Yet, paradoxically, patients are told early on that the best way to "get somewhere" is to not try to get anywhere at all but simply to be where they are already, with awareness. Goals or specific objectives that the individual hopes to achieve through practice, aside from their motivating function to practice the meditation itself, are seen as thought formations, something like clouds in the sky, beyond their personal meaning and content, just like all other thoughts in the field of awareness.

This does not mean that people do not achieve their targeted goals as a result of attending such a program. They frequently do. Rather, it suggests that "progress" in meditation practice is best measured by an accepting of *the process itself* (reflected in continued regular practice, and in the feeling that the practice continues to be meaningful), and by whether the patient begins to have experiences of enhanced self-efficacy, well-being, and a sense of greater agency and coherence in facing life experience.

INSIGHT

During mindfulness practice, there may be moments in which the practitioner realizes that the observer, commonly associated with the pronoun, "I," is different from what is being observed, whether it is an experience of pain or grief or of any thought, feeling, impulse or sensation. In other moments, any sense of separation may dissolve, and there is simply *observing*. Emotional reactivity, self-absorption, and self-preoccupation can dissipate to a significant degree (23), resulting in profound feelings of unity, connectedness, and well-being.

Sustained self-reflective awareness (24), frequently described as "bare attention," (9) or simply "wakefulness," can give rise to varying degrees of insight into interconnectedness and into the limits of our conventional personal descriptions of who we are, the nature of what we commonly call the "self," and of how we find ourselves in relationship to others and to the world (self-in-relationship). Pain and suffering can be held in awareness and seen with greater patience, clarity, and intimacy, possibly over time giving rise

to useful insights and to new ways of understanding and coping with pain and suffering (23). The element of constant inquiry characteristic of mindfulness practice (22), promoted not through thinking but through bare attending and a continual nondiscursive examination of what one is actually experiencing, lays the foundation for such insights and for their potentially liberating effects. Such experiences of insight and growth, when they arise, also are held with the same quality of awareness and nonattachment that is brought to all other aspects of experience during meditation practice.

In spite of its nonstriving orientation, the effects of meditation are directly verifiable in a number of ways. Reports from the personal experiences of meditators and from clinical studies show that regular practice over extended periods of time can lead to an enhanced capacity to perceive oneself and oneself in relationship to the world with acuity, precision, and acceptance (3). Greater awareness and familiarity with the entire field of one's own experience, and particularly an ability to recognize thoughts as thoughts and feelings as feelings, can be accompanied by increasing degrees of equanimity, inner stillness, a personal sense of agency and authority, and, paradoxically, greater nonattachment and selflessness. This range of psychological attributes can support effective coping with high levels of stress and uncertainty. At the same time, it cultivates wisdom, the capacity to see and act based on the direct experience of interconnectedness and compassion, beyond the confines of narrowly defined self-interest.

APPLICATIONS TO PAIN AND SUFFERING

The practice of mindfulness encourages a willingness to look deeply into any and all emotional states and life circumstances that arise, even highly aversive and frightening ones, simply because they are already present and a part of one's experience. It suggests that whatever one's circumstances, it is possible to "work with" a situation by holding it in awareness. Mindfulness practice encourages creativity, self-reliance, imagination, and a willingness to be doggedly true to one's own history, experience, and intuition (25). Ultimately, the practitioner sets the agenda and pursues it based on his or her motivation, commitment, and constraints, especially after leaving the context in which the meditation practice is learned.

Although the terms are frequently used interchangeably, from the perspective of mindfulness, pain and suffering describe different domains of experience. The word "pain" describes basic perceptual and sensory inputs, whether physical or emotional, that are interpreted as dysphoric, hurtful. The term "suffering" describes one's emotional relationship to the bare actuality of the input—namely, how it is interpreted. There are many interpretive responses possible to any particular level of perceived pain or threat, from extreme suffering with very little stimulus, to minimal suffering even in the face of severely traumatic events or noxious stimuli. Suffering has been described as the state of severe distress associated with events that threaten the intactness of the person (26).

Meditation offers a life-affirming approach to the experience of both pain and suffering (3,9). It can sometimes be used to complement the use of medication when needed for the control of pain in cancer. The meditation instructions call on the patient to attempt to look deeply and nonjudgmentally into the experience of pain as bare sensation, if only for a few moments at a time at first. Slowly one attempts to observe sensation with nonattachment over more extended periods of time. For someone in pain, this might involve directing attention to the sensations in a particular region of the body and coupling that attention to a sense of the breath moving in *to* and out *from* that region, observing any changes in the sensations themselves from moment to moment. Frequently, this approach leads the person to perceive that thoughts and feeling about the pain, such as "this is killing me," and "I don't know if I can stand this" are different from the actual sensations of discomfort, such as burning, shooting, squeezing, tearing, aching. If one asks "Is this killing me *right now*?" the answer is frequently and surprisingly "No." For it is the thought about its duration or its meaning or intensity that often produces heightened suffering. This observation can result in reductions in emotional arousal and suffering from physical pain that is poorly controlled through medication, and from emotional pain related to the threat to one's well-being. It can also lead to questioning one's doctor about the meaning of the pain in terms of the disease, and what it might or might not indicate, thus reducing unwarranted interpretations and fears.

WHY RECOMMEND MEDITATION PRACTICE FOR PEOPLE WITH CANCER?

Meditation can play a useful role for people coping with cancer precisely because it is fundamentally concerned with present-moment reality, with what is here now (22). In addition to meditation's usefulness in dealing with the stress and the physical and emotional pain sometimes associated with cancer, dwelling in the present moment can slow perception of the passage of time and enhance an appreciation of each moment of living. At times of profound doubt, fear, and confusion, when a person may not know what path to take, knowing how to be still without having to make anything happen, go away, or change, can be an extremely valuable inward stance to adopt.

The disciplined practice of residing in stillness can lead, in time, to new ways of seeing, new pathways for knowing, and new choices for action that might not have been seen but for the stillness itself. From the meditative perspective, any situation, however painful, even cancer, can becomes one's teacher. In illness, a willingness to look and listen to the actuality of one's "lived experience" can significantly transform its meaning (27). One of us (ER), a senior Mindfulness-based Stress Reduction Instructor diagnosed with non-Hodgkin's lymphoma, recently wrote:

I am tired. I tire easily. Yet I am committed to fanning the flame of my spirit and I find that this requires true wisdom, *sachel* (common sense in Hebrew) my mother would say. It means that tonight I can't go out to be with my friends, even to meditate. Instead, I must rest to recover from the emotions of the day so I can rise tomorrow and be refreshed. I do not like making this decision to stay home even though it is "wise." But I know that I must listen to my body, not to necessarily live longer but because my fatigue doesn't allow me to be fully present with anyone or anything except the feelings of heavy eyelids and the effort to stay awake. I have learned that, to maintain my equilibrium, I must be ruthlessly honest with myself and admit when I have to "stop." This is new to me and confronts any shred of omnipotence I might once have held. I may not be my body but my body does certainly affect my mental and emotional state and I MUST pay attention.

I find that my meditation practice colors my belief system. I am consciously aware now that every moment is a precious moment. This means I walk the tightrope between wanting every moment to be "special" and simply dropping into a space where every moment, be it going to the bathroom or paying a bill, *is* special. To be fully in the moment, here, not lost in the thought of a wish or a "should," is my challenge and I find it necessary to be a warrior through the jungle of my self . . .

And as I open to these thoughts, these fears, these illusions of control, these wishes for things to be different, I also open to a deep sense of peace and appreciation of life itself. I receive succor from nature. I have celebrated snowfall and rain. I feel the wind on my cheek and appreciate my warm coat, the solace of my home and my husband, friends and colleagues. I feel more deeply connected not only to my selves but to others and the universe around.

As I teach my classes, my eyes frequently tear up as I am awed by the simple acts of courage I hear and observe again and again in people who are in pain, who struggle to eat or walk, or brush their hair. We practice meditation together and share and laugh, crying and questioning together, "Why me?" And in response, it is easier to tolerate and understand, "Why *not* me?" We sit quietly together in deep appreciation of each other and our daily bravery as we come to class and go about the routines of the day, choosing to live and face our suffering, our enemy, my enemy, our selves as we are, human, and imperfect. And in confronting the truth of ourselves/myself, pain and imperfections become acceptable, even beautiful, for to allow my humanness is to be free, and to be naked in my imperfections allows for a perfection that is life affirming. I can feel whole regardless of what the CT scan shows or the statistics say, and I can begin to truly believe that I am perfect and the pain, the anger, the negative mind states are as transitory as the bloom of the violet or the weather in New England. This allows me to go on and to be able to open up to receive light and love, bringing with it caring and compassion to myself and all others.

These personal reflections highlight the importance of keeping in mind that meditation involves facing and accepting the totality of one's experience as it is, rather than forced or mechanical attempts to achieve particular ends, even relaxation, insight, or greater well-being. It is out of that kind of embrace and acceptance than relaxation, insight, and well-being are most likely to come by themselves. With a simultaneously gentle yet very firm touch, meditation practice works on three interrelated and universal aspects of our experience as human beings:

1. A direct, moment-to-moment sense of connection between one's own body and sense of self. Here meditation serves as a way of being that involves varying degrees of mindfulness, wisdom, self-compassion, and self-acceptance. For someone with cancer, this dimension of meditation might include the painful realization that one's own health and well-being and the state of one's body can no longer be taken for granted, and then making the commitment to work with that situation mindfully and intentionally, however turbulent and tumultuous the mind states one encounters may be at times.

2. An understanding, through self-observation, of the ways in which sensations, impulses, thoughts, feelings, and meaning emerge in coherent patterns that can be seen and held in awareness. For a person with cancer, this might involve admitting that the disease may have shattered all personal sense of predictability and control, but recognizing that it does not represent a total loss or shattering of being. A range of options open up out of meditation for perceiving, understanding, and responding to situations in new ways. As a consequence, a new degree of mastery and wisdom may be reached in facing and comprehending one's own situation.

3. A sense of belonging, of being in community in the largest sense, of connectedness. Meditation often is thought of as something one "does" alone, isolated from the rest of the world. Actually, it is a way of being *in* the world in two interpenetrating contexts: as an individual self, and, simultaneously, as an integral part of a larger whole. The value of perceiving interconnectedness within the domain of community for a person facing cancer may be gleaned from the following anecdote:

A professor at a prestigious university who had struggled mightily with his doctors and insurer to develop and pay for the meditation-based treatment plan he felt he needed, commented one day in a stress reduction class in our clinic that his leukemia and the impending bone marrow transplant he faced had brought him into what he called "this community of the afflicted" where he felt more at home, in a funny way, than with his colleagues at work. One day, while riding on the subway, an insight came to him that the people sitting on either side of him might very well be suffering every bit as deeply as he was or as the other people in the class were. He saw that the community of the afflicted potentially extends to everybody. What started as a feeling of separation blossomed into a deeper feeling of inclusion and unity, one from which he took considerable satisfaction since it was in resonance with his deepest values (28).

This insight into interconnectedness came directly out of his meditation practice. In fact, spontaneous experiences of mindfulness and insight signal a maturation in one's practice of meditation, as mindfulness emerges from efforts at formal practice and becomes an attentional stance that can affect every moment of one's waking life.

APPLICATIONS OF MEDITATION IN CANCER

Meditation practice is a rigorous and demanding discipline, calling on the practitioner to devote some time on a daily basis to its formal practice, as well as to the equally challenging task of then bringing it into everyday life. Learning meditation under crisis conditions, such as immediately following a diagnosis of cancer, may be difficult and is not always advisable. Considerable discretion and sensitivity at the time of referral by the health care provider need to be exercised so that the recommendation is not misunderstood or rejected as inappropriate. The timing and the context in which meditation is offered are extremely important to maximize the receptivity of people in crisis who might benefit from its practice. The suggestion that one learn stress reduction methods or start practicing meditation close to the time that one learns one may be fighting for one's life may make no sense to the patient, may be seen as insulting or undermining of self-esteem, or may be too difficult to combine with the demands of radiation, chemotherapy, or other medical appointments. A high degree of sensitivity to timing and manner of presentation is required. Provider and patient need to explore together the appropriateness of such a suggestion, the degree of involvement it might require, and the potential benefits and costs associated with such an approach.

For people with cancer, it is sometimes wise to delay a recommendation or referral to a meditation-based program until after the immediate period of diagnosis. One approach is to raise the option of a meditation-based program at the second or third appointment after diagnosis and have the patient determine whether and when to enroll. Alternatively, provider and patient can decide to re-visit the subject at a later time chosen by the patient. Meditation can be helpful to some people in dealing with the side effects of treatment and in overcoming the sense of loss of control and mastery over their lives. It may be most helpful when treatments have ended and the person is attempting to return to normal activities as a "survivor" (4) and to change lifestyle to promote health and reduce risk of recurrence.

Meditation has also been used to great advantage in caring for terminally ill and dying patients in hospice settings and at home (29,30). This involves the use of meditation to help with the relief of physical pain and with the emotional pain and suffering due to the disease. It is used to best advantage when integrated into a comprehensive palliative care approach, which includes, if desired, discussing death and dying and feelings of loss within the context of mindfulness practice and the feeling states and thoughts that arise during meditation and at other times. Many dying patients also find that the calmness and silence of meditation bring profound feelings of acceptance, well-being, and inner peace.

Healthy persons at higher genetic risk of cancer also may be drawn to meditation to reduce environmental and lifestyle risk and to control anxiety, and may derive comfort and benefit from meditation-based stress reduction programs.

MINDFULNESS-BASED STRESS REDUCTION (MBSR)

This section briefly describes mindfulness-based stress reduction (MBSR), which originated with the Stress Reduction Clinic, an outpatient service within the Department of Medicine at the University of Massachusetts Medical Center. The intervention is structured as an 8 week course. The core curriculum is intensive training in mindfulness meditation and its applications in daily living (3,7). MBSR programs are currently in use in over 80 clinics, hospitals, and HMOs nationwide and abroad.

Medical patients with a wide range of diagnoses, including cancer, are referred to the program by their physicians. Patients meet with an instructor in classes of approximately 30 people for 2.5 hours once a week for 8 weeks. In the sixth week, there is a day-long silent meditation retreat on the weekend. The classes are composed of people with a wide range of chronic conditions and levels of disability, from cancer to cardiac disease, hypertension, gastrointestinal problems, and chronic pain. The mix of patients with different diagnoses allows for a generic approach, focusing on commonalities across diagnoses (stress, anxiety, suffering), on "what is right with a person rather than exclusively on what is wrong," on shared experiences such as breathing, proprioception, thoughts and emotions, work and family life, health and illness, and on seeing oneself as a whole person, rather than solely as a patient with a particular disease.

Other interventions that make use of meditation are designed specifically for cancer patients (2,5,31,32). The MBSR intervention has been modified to make it more disease-specific by the addition of "wraparound" sessions (one before and five after the 8 week course) which are attended by women with breast cancer participating in a current research trial. These sessions extend and deepen the MBSR experience and provide additional social support and community. MBSR is not meant to substitute for a cancer support group, and many cancer patients enrolled in MBSR programs make use of such groups. However, there is no reason why the MBSR format cannot be adopted for groups of patients with a single diagnosis.

Prior to enrolling in the MBSR program, a prospective candidate attends an individual meeting with a clinic staff member (preintervention interview) in which the individual's history, reasons for the referral, and motivation for taking the program are explored together. The patient is given a brief description of the 8 week format and requirements of the program for class attendance and meditation practice. Data are obtained on a battery of measures for individual and group assessments of clinical outcomes. Following completion of the program, all participants meet individually with their class instructors in hour-long interviews to review and discuss their experiences. Together they develop strategies for maintaining continuity in the meditation practice and for continuing community support, if appropriate. The interviews are conducted with a high degree of intentional mindfulness on the part of the interviewer, in both listening and in speaking with the patient (33). Participants can request additional individual time with instructors during the course as well so that private matters can be discussed outside of the class and large group format.

During the program itself, participants are exposed to three formal meditation techniques: *(1)* a *body scan meditation*, practiced lying down (supine if possible); *(2) sitting meditation,* practiced on straight-backed chairs or on the floor; and *(3) mindful hatha yoga*, which involves a range of body postures (see Appendices 1 and 2). These techniques and the rationale for their use are described in detail elsewhere (3,22). Offering a mix of practices with varying degrees of movement and stillness, and different primary foci for attention, is instrumental in reaching a broad range of individuals with different dispositions and degrees of mobility and receptivity.

As "homework," patients are required to practice a mix of these methods a minimum of 6 days per week for 45 minutes at a time, using audiotapes for guidance. In addition, informal mindfulness practices are assigned each week, and participants are encouraged to create their own to sustain mindfulness throughout the day. Informal practices include awareness of different aspects of daily life experience such as breathing, walking, driving, cooking, eating, cleaning, ironing, showering, talking, listening, working, parenting, and playing. Informal mindfulness practices also include awareness of emotional states, thoughts, and perceptions during daily activities, as well as bringing awareness to particularly stressful situations, to options for responding to them mindfully, and to the tendency to react automatically and unconsciously, especially when under stress.

In addition to formal meditation practice in the classes, participants and instructors spend considerable class time discussing various aspects of the meditation practice as experienced by the patients in the preceding week, and its potential relevance to what is happening in their lives.

PROFESSIONAL INSTRUCTOR QUALIFICATIONS

The clinical use of meditation training for patients within the context of medicine and health care is an emerging area of specialization. Significant professional training is required to develop a high degree of effectiveness in instructing and guiding an individual or large groups of people in its use. This is particularly so if those who wish to learn it are suffering from a life-threatening illness. The cardinal principle, necessary but not in itself sufficient, in using meditation with medical patients is that the instructor must be personally grounded in the practice of meditation. Years of experience through daily personal practice are necessary before a person might be competent to instruct others in its practice and its applications to stress, pain, and chronic illness. In addition, a MBSR instructor must have experience in teaching, in group process, and in dealing sensitively with medically ill individuals. A number of training opportunities are available for learning the clinical uses of meditation through the MBSR model. These are listed at the back of this chapter.

Since the field is an emerging one, formal certification of meditation teachers for mindfulness-based stress reduction is not yet available. Nor is there any formal certification for medically oriented meditation instructors using any other meditative approach. As the field develops further, certification will no doubt follow.

As with any new field, there is always a potential risk that incompetent and/or unethical practitioners will capitalize on patient interest and institutional demand for such programs. In the absence of certification procedures, the patient and referring health care providers must rely on their own perception of instructors and their appropriateness, sincerity, and competency, and on the reports of others with first hand knowledge.

TEACHING APPROACHES IN THE MEDICAL APPLICATIONS OF MINDFULNESS MEDITATION

As noted above, effective teaching of meditation can only be done by people who are themselves deeply committed to their own personal meditation practice, so that the instructor is not asking the patient to do something that the instructor him or herself does not actually do and understand through direct experience. Appendix 1 provides an example of basic instructions for cultivating mindfulness through awareness of breathing. As an alternative to guiding a person through an extensive session which might last from 5 to 45 minutes, guided mindfulness meditation practice tapes of a number of different techniques are available (see back of chapter) that can be used for this purpose. If the health care practitioner uses them personally on a regular basis, as well as prescribing them for the patient, their shared experience of meditation practice can form the basis for useful periodic discussions than can be profoundly beneficial to the patient as his or her meditation practice develops and is applied in coping with illness and its treatment. Typically, guided meditation instructions such as those in Appendix 1 could be given over a period of from 10–45 minutes. Extended periods of silence are interspersed between short periods of guidance, during which the person or group of people is actually practicing according to the instructions, which serve as intermittent reminders to stay focused on the breath or return to it if the mind has wandered away.

All other mindfulness meditation techniques can be seen as extensions or variations of the basic practice of awareness of breathing described above. The practitioner can intentionally expand the field of awareness around the breath to include sensations in specific parts of the body, a sense of the body as a whole, perceptions of all kinds, including sounds and sights, mood states and emotions, and thoughts, or practice "choiceless awareness" (34,35), in which there is no specific focus (3).

In clinical work using MBSR in a classroom setting, there is a graduated introduction of different formal meditation techniques over a period of 8 weeks (see Appendix 2). These include, as noted above, *a body scan meditation, sitting meditation,* and *mindful hatha yoga.* In addition, *walking meditation* is also frequently taught as a formal practice. The formal meditation practices are introduced and nested within a context of informal practices, some of which are done together as a group in class and then discussed, while others are assigned for homework. In the MBSR format, meditation and mindfulness are often introduced through an "eating meditation" exercise. One raisin is eaten very slowly, with an emphasis on seeing, feeling, tasting, chewing, and swallowing. The message is that attention can be focused on an "ordinary" everyday experience to such a degree that it becomes a universe of novel experience, previously unattended to. People frequently report changes in behavior related to eating on the basis of this one exercise. Other informal meditation exercises, including figure/ground drawings, puzzles, communications exercises based on the martial art of Aikido, observing the weather and activity in the street from the window of the classroom, theater

exercises with larger numbers of people during the all day session, involving fast, slow, and chaotic walking, and slow backwards walking with eyes closed, are used in the MBSR intervention to produce multisensory "in vivo" experiences in which mindfulness can be used to illustrate, identify, and break out of a broad range of conditioned patterns of perception and behavior (3).

A COMPARISON OF MEDITATION WITH OTHER INTERVENTIONS

There are commonalities and significant differences in structure, approach, and philosophy between clinically based uses of meditation, other self-regulatory or relaxation-based strategies and other psychosocial interventions such as supportive-expressive therapy (36), and cognitive-behavioral therapy (37,38). These are outlined in Tables 66.1 and 66.2.

RESEARCH ON MINDFULNESS-BASED STRESS REDUCTION

To our knowledge, to date there have been no randomized controlled trials conducted in which meditation was used as the core or single component of a psychosocial intervention for patients with cancer. At least two studies are currently under way: *(1)* a controlled randomized study by James Spira (personal communication) of patients with recurrent, breast, prostate or colon cancer, comparing Zen meditation plus Tai chi, walking plus progressive muscle relaxation, and lecture only; *(2)* a randomized study of women with stage I and II breast cancer comparing MBSR training, a nutrition education intervention, and a usual-treatment control at the University of Massachusetts Medical Center.

Although there are no published studies on MBSR and cancer, the intervention has been shown to lead to

TABLE 66.1. *Meditation vs Other Self-regulatory or Relaxation Strategies: Major Differences*

Meditation	Other Self-Regulatory/Relaxation Strategies
Nonstriving and nondoing orientation; nonattachment to goals	Relaxation or coping with some specific condition (e.g., anxiety or overcoming cancer cells) is targeted as the goal
Experiencing whatever is present in the moment, allowing present sensations, thoughts and feelings to be as they are, without having to hold on to them or push them away	Attempting to create a change in the present and future (e.g., creating relaxation, anxiety or pain reduction)
Presented as a way of being rather than a technique, a way to live fully and attend to all experience, pleasant, unpleasant, and neutral	Usually presented as a technique for solving or coping with a condition
Practiced daily, for its own sake, to be awake, not based on an attempt to induce a change in state	Often practiced as needed, a maneuver to relieve or cope with a particular condition or mood state (e.g., tension, anxiety or pain)

TABLE 66.2. *A Comparison of Meditation with Other Psychosocial Interventions*

Meditation	Cognitive-Behavioral Therapy*	Supportive-Expressive Therapy†
GOAL		
Presented as a way of being or general lifestyle approach	Generally presented as a way to cope with a particular mood, feeling state or illness (e.g., depression, anxiety, or cancer)	Goals are to: *(1)* facilitate full expression of emotions and thoughts about the illness, based on the therapeutic; *(2)* provide a support system as alleviating social isolation; and *(3)* live life as fully as possible
Group support is present but is not a stated goal or predominant focus	Group support usually occurs spontaneously, and may or may not be a stated goal	
Emphasis is on living life fully and being in touch with the full range of emotions		
INDIVIDUAL/GROUP FORMAT		
Can be taught in large or small groups of people with either homogeneous or diverse problems and concerns	Usually presented to individuals or groups with one overall concern (e.g., depression or anxiety)	Usually provided in small intimate groups which are homogeneous for a particular illness or common concern
Taught as a class to large or small groups (up to 40 people)	Provided as individual or small-group therapy (6–10 people)	Provided as group therapy, usually with smaller groups (8–10 people)
SKILLS/PRACTICES PRESENTED		
Coping skills are presented in the larger framework of everyday life, as a practice for living, using formal and informal practices and demonstrating how these are mirrored in everyday life	Coping skills are presented largely in relation to the mood or feeling state to be dealt with, and may be secondarily related to a more general lifestyle change	Coping strategies specific to the common illness or concern are learned by hearing what other group members have found helpful, through suggestions by the group leaders, or both
The practices are used for the purpose of cultivating greater present-moment awareness and self-acceptance, rather than as technique-based coping strategies		Uses a breathing technique based on self-hypnosis which shares some features with sitting meditation practice in having the primary focus on the breath
No attempt is made to either monitor or reframe particular thoughts or feeling states	Thoughts and reactions to physical sensations are monitored and reframed, sometimes induced (e.g., symptoms of panic attacks)	A forum for expressing feelings and concerns is presented, usually oriented around a specific illness; thoughts and feelings are not specifically induced or systematically monitored and reframed
Whatever appears in awareness is simply held as the salient aspect of the present moment experience	Through systematically looking at thought patterns or attributions to sensations, a change in perception is facilitated which may be associated with improvement (e.g., less anxiety or depression, greater ability to cope with the illness) and may secondarily include greater self-acceptance	Changes in lifestyle or perception usually are related to coping with the illness
If there is a change in perception, it emerges spontaneously		

*References: 37, 38, 42, 53–58 (discusses the differences between meditation-based stress reduction and cognitive-behavioral therapy for anxiety disorders).

†References: 36, 59, 60.

clinically significant short- and long-term reductions in physical and psychological symptoms as well as enhanced psychological well-being in patients with a broad range of chronic medical conditions (3), including chronic pain (7,39–41) and anxiety disorders (42,43). Other studies, using measures of *psychological hardiness* (44) and *sense of coherence* (45), trait-related personality factors normally conceived of as invariant in adulthood, showed significant increases in both measures over the course of MBSR training in large numbers of participants, and maintenance of these changes over 3 year follow-up in an unpublished study by Kabat-Zinn et al. This finding suggests that the intervention has the potential to transform outlook

and coping capacity in patients with serious medical conditions, including cancer.

A clinical trial of patients with moderate to severe psoriasis undergoing phototherapy or photochemotherapy, testing the use of guided mindfulness meditation audiotapes, which included a disease-specific visualization exercise, during their ultraviolet treatment sessions showed that meditators had an increased rate of skin clearing over patients undergoing phototherapy alone (46). This finding may have implications for skin cancer as well. Psoriasis and basal cell carcinomas have been characterized as showing overexpression of similar genes which may play a role in the loss of control over apoptosis (47).

POTENTIAL ADVERSE EFFECTS OF MEDITATION

Some case reports in the literature and several descriptive studies have reported adverse effects of meditation, ranging from increased episodes of anxiety, depression, and confusion in some people, to more pronounced disorientation and psychiatric crises in others (48). One study followed participants after an intensive silent mindfulness meditation retreat that some subjects undertook for 2 weeks and others for 3 months. Results showed that between one-third and one-half of a small sample of the retreat participants reported increased tension, anxiety, depression, and confusion. However, almost all subjects also reported strong positive effects (49). A study of people who practiced transcendental meditation found similar results (50). Both studies are important in documenting that not everyone responds positively to meditation. However, the studies suffer from methodological problems which make it difficult to differentiate the frequency of serious psychiatric disturbance from normal emotional turbulence. Many of the problems reported by the study subjects may have stemmed as much from the context, setting, and the cultural and ideological slant given to the meditation practice and a possible mismatch between subject and practice, as from the practice itself. In addition, many of the effects reported in the mindfulness study may have been related to adjustment difficulties following an extended silent meditation retreat. These observations do suggest the need for concurrent individual psychotherapy along with meditation training for certain individuals at high risk for flooding or uncovering repressed material, such as those with past or present suicidal ideation, reality testing disturbances such as psychotic disorders, or posttraumatic stress disorder. They also suggest that modification of the meditation approach used may be helpful in certain cases, such as emphasizing movement meditation such yoga or Tai chi, and/or shorter periods of sitting meditation with people experiencing difficulty with the body scan or with intensive sitting practice.

To date, we have not systematically studied negative reactions to the MBSR intervention. Anecdotally, serious psychiatric disturbance appears to occur at a very low frequency. Experience with over 8000 medical patients who completed the intervention suggests, however, that certain individuals may be at higher risk for experiencing increased anxiety due to practicing meditation (51). For example, people with a diagnosis of hyperventilation syndrome or panic disorder can become anxious in focusing on their breathing in the early weeks of practice. However, this anxiety rapidly disappears in the large majority of cases within a few weeks, and alternatives to attending to the breath can be implemented if such anxiety persists. People suffering from posttraumatic stress disorder can experience anxiety, dissociative symptoms, and flashbacks simply from being still. However, with adequate support, which mostly takes the form of concurrent psychotherapy in addition to instructor support, medical patients in MBSR are for the most part able and motivated to continue the meditation practice in one form or another and are able to use it to move toward greater psychological stability. They may, however, change the specific balance of elements comprising their meditation practice, such as less body scanning and more yoga. In rare instances, an instructor may advise a participant to discontinue all forms of formal practice at home for a period of time and just attend the classes, if the person is motivated to continue in the program but is experiencing life circumstances that makes it painful or frightening to practice on his or her own.

IMPLICATIONS FOR CHANGE IN LIFESTYLE AND HEALTH BEHAVIORS

Regular meditation practice constitutes a major lifestyle change for most individuals. Because of the disciplined commitment of time and the profound reorientation to present moment experience characteristic of mindfulness practices, meditation might play an important role in increasing self-efficacy (52) through awareness-based mastery experiences (i.e., regarding pain, anxiety, anger, tension, musculoskeletal flexibility and balance experienced during practice of the various MBSR methods). Self-efficacy is intimately intertwined with self-esteem and quality of life. While improvements in behaviors such as smoking, drinking, and diet due to MBSR-mediated increases in self-efficacy may or may not affect the course of cancer in an one individual, they would have an important and predictable effect on the primary prevention of many types of cancer. Because MBSR programs are designed to teach large numbers of people the rudiments of taking better care of themselves as a complement to what the health care system can do for them, such programs might serve a significant public health function, in addition to their clinical role.

CONCLUSION

Meditation practice may be of profound value to people who are living with cancer. The growing presence of mindfulness-based stress reduction programs in the clinical setting attests to the practical benefits of meditation training as an adjunctive intervention for cancer patients and an increasingly practical referral option for health providers. There are to date, however, no studies of meditation as a primary intervention modality in any psychoeducational program oriented toward cancer patients, although studies are underway in at least two centers. There is an important need for longitudinal randomized controlled studies in this area that take problematic design issues into account and simultaneously monitor biological, psychological, compliance, and lifestyle change variables. Limiting design issues also need to be considered in interpreting the medical literature reporting on all psychosocial interventions for health enhancement and behavior change, including our own work.

Most clinical interventions cited in the literature use self-regulatory practices such as progressive muscle relaxation, autogenic training, guided imagery, or self-hypnosis rather than meditation. These are commonly elements of a multimodal approach. Some programs use meditation-like exercises as one program component. These are employed primarily for relaxation rather than for systematic cultivation of awareness and ongoing human development. In contrast, mindfulness-based stress reduction programs use meditation as the unifying principle and practice that informs all other aspects of the intervention. Meditation in this framework is practiced as a "way of being" rather than as a technique. It emphasizes bringing mindfulness to all aspects of one's life experience, including physical illness, emotional turbulence, and the activities of everyday living.

TRAINING OPPORTUNITIES IN MBSR

There are a number of different formats in which health professionals can receive training in MBSR. These range from 5 and 7 day intensives in the form of retreats held at various sites around the United States, to a multi-phase internship in MBSR at the Center for Mindfulness in Medicine, Health Care, and Society, University of Massachusetts Medical Center. Information on programs can be obtained from: The Center for Mindfulness, Profession Training Office, UMass Medical Center, Worcester, MA 01566-0267, U.S.A. Tel: 508-856-1616; Fax: 508-856-197. Ordering information for guided mindfulness meditation audiotapes can be obtained from the same address.

REFERENCES

1. Bohm D. *Wholeness and the Implicate Order.* London: Routledge & Kegan Paul; 1980.
2. Lerner M. *Choice in Cancer Integrating the Best of Conventional and Alternative Approaches to Cancer.* Cambridge, MA: MIT Press; 1994.
3. Kabat-Zinn J. *Full Catastrophe Living.* New York: Delacorte; 1990.
4. Cunningham A, Edmonds C. Group psychological therapy for cancer patients: a point of view, and discussion of the hierachy of options. *Int J Psychiatry Med.* 1996; 261:51–82.
5. Lerner M, Remen R. Trade craft of the commonwealth cancer help program. *Advances.* 1987; 4(3):11–25.
6. Goleman D, Schwartz G. Meditation as an intervention in stress reactivity. *J Consult Clin Psychol.* 1976; 44:456–466.
7. Kabat-Zinn J. An out-patient program in behavioral medicine for chronic pain patients based on the practice of mindfulness meditation: theoretical considerations and preliminary results. *Gen Hosp Psychiatry.* 1982; 4:33–47.
8. Goleman D. *The Varieties of Meditative Experience.* New York: Dutton; 1977.
9. Thera N. *The Heart of Buddhist Meditation.* New York: Weiser; 1962.
10. Goldstein J, Kornfield J. *Seeking the Heart of Wisdom.* Boston: Shambhala; 1987.
11. Goldstein J. *The Experience of Insight.* Boston: Shambhala; 1976.
12. Kornfield J. *A Path with Heart.* New York: Bantam; 1993.
13. Levine S. *A Gradual Awakening.* New York: Doubleday; 1979.
14. Suzuki S. *Zen Mind, Beginner's Mind.* New York: Weatherall; 1970.
15. Beck C. *Nothing Special.* San Francisco, CA: Harper Collins; 1993.
16. Beck C. *Everyday Zen.* San Francisco, CA: Harper Collins; 1989.
17. Osler W. *A Way of Life.* Baltimore: Remington-Putnam; 1932.
18. Osler W. *Aequanimitas: With Other Addresses to Medical Students, Nurses, and Practitioners of Medicine.* Philadelphia, PA: P. Blakiston; 1904: 363–388.
19. Thoreau H. *Walden.* New York: Random House; 1937:101.
20. Eliot T. From Little Gidding. *Four Quartets.* New York: Harcourt Brace; 1943: 59.
21. Rilke R. *Selected Poems of Ranier Maria Rilke,* translated by Robert Bly. New York: Harper & Row; 1981:31.
22. Kabat-Zinn J. *Wherever You Go, There You Are.* New York: Hyperion; 1994.
23. Epstein M. *Thoughts Without A Thinker.* New York: Basic Books; 1995: 146.
24. Goleman D. *Emotional Intelligence.* New York: Bantam; 1995.
25. Boorstein S. *It's Easier than You Think.* San Francisco, CA: Harper Collins; 1995.
26. Cassell E. The nature of suffering and the goals of medicine. *N Engl J Med.* 1982; 306:639–645.
27. Toombs K. *The Meaning of Illness.* Boston: Kluwer; 1993.

28. Kabat-Zinn J. Foreword. In: Lerner M, ed. *Choices in Healing*. Cambridge, MA: MIT Press, 1994: xi–xvii.
29. Levine S. *Who Dies?* Garden City, NY: Doubleday; 1982.
30. Levine S. *Healing into Life and Death*. Garden City, NY: Doubleday; 1987.
31. Stolbach L, Brandt V, et al. Benefits of a mind/body group program for cancer patients [abstract]. *Soc Behav Med*. 1988; 62(3).
32. Stolbach L, Lorman C. Further comments on counseling people with cancer: pursuing the perfect paradigm. *Advances*. 1994; 10:57–59.
33. Kabat-Zinn J. Psychosocial factors: their importance and management. In: Ockene J, Ockene I, eds. *The Prevention of Coronary Heart Disease: A Skills-Based Approach*. Boston: Little Brown; 1992:299–333.
34. Krishnamurti J. *Think on These Things*. New York: Harper & Row; 1964.
35. Kapleau P. *The Three Pillars of Zen*. Boston: Beacon; 1967:53.
36. Spiegel D, Bloom J, Kraemer H, Gotheil E. Effect of psychosocial treatment on survival of patients with metastatic breast cancer. *Lancet*. 1989; 2:888–891.
37. Beck A. *Cognitive Therapy and the Emotional Disorders*. New York: International Universities Press; 1976.
38. Clark D. A cognitive approach to panic. *Behav Res Ther*. 1986; 24:46–1–470.
39. Kabat-Zinn J, Lipworth L, Burney R. The clinical use of mindfulness meditation for the self-regulation of chronic pain. *J Behav Med*. 1985; 8:163–190.
40. Kabat-Zinn J, Lipworth L, Burney R, Sellers W. Four year follow-up of a meditation-based program for the self-regulation of chronic pain: treatment outcomes and compliance. *Clin J Pain*. 1986; 2:159–173.
41. Kabat-Zinn J, Chapman-Waldrop A. Compliance with an outpatient stress reduction program: rates and predictors of program completion. *J Behav Med*. 1988; 11(4):333–352.
42. Kabat-Zinn J, Massion A, Kristeller J, et al. Effectiveness of a meditation-based stress reduction program in the treatment of anxiety disorders. *Am J Psychiatry*. 1992; 149:936–943.
43. Miller J, Peterson L, Fletcher K, Kabat-Zinn J. Three-year follow-up of a meditation-based stress reduction intervention in the treatment of anxiety disorders. *Gen Hosp Psychiatry*. 1995; 17:192–200.
44. Kobasa S. Stressful life events, personality, and health: an inquiry into hardiness. *J Pers Soc Psychol*. 1979; 37:1–11.
45. Antonovsky A. Pathways leading to successful coping and health. In: Rosenbaum M, ed. *Learned Resourcefulness*. New York: Springer; 1990: 31–63.
46. Bernhard J, Kristeller J, Kabat-Zinn J. Effectiveness of relaxation and visualization techniques as an adjunct to phototherapy and photochemotherapy of psoriasis. *J Am Acad Dermatol*. 1988; 19(3):572–573.
47. Wrone-Smith T, Johnson T, Nelson B, et al. Discordant expression of *Bcl-x* and *Bcl-2* by keratinocytes in vitro and psoriatic keratinocytes in vivo. *Am J Pathol*. 1995; 146:1079–1088.
48. Epstein M, Lieff J. Psychiatric complications of meditation practice. In: Wilber K, Engler J, Brown DP. *Transformation of Consciousness*. Boston: New Science Library; 1986:53–63.
49. Shapiro D. Adverse effects of meditation: a preliminary investigation of long-term meditators. *Int J Psychosom*. 1992; 39(1–4):62–67.
50. Otis L. Adverse effects of transcendental meditation. In: Shapiro D, Walsh R, eds. *Meditation: Classic and Contemporary Perspectives*. New York: Aldine Publishing; 1984:201–208.
51. Miller J. The unveiling of traumatic memories and emotions through mindfulness and concentration meditation: clinical implications and three case reports. *J Transper Psychol*. 1993; 25:169–180.
52. Bandura A. Self-efficacy: toward a unifying theory of behavioral change. *Psychol Rev*. 1977; 84:191–215.
53. Beck A, Rush A, Shaw B, Emery G. *Cognitive Therapy of Depression*. New York: Guilford Press; 1979.
54. Wright J, Beckt A. Cognitive therapy of depression: theory and practice. *Hosp Commun Psychiatry*. 1983; 34(12):1119–1127.
55. Barlow D, Craske M, Cerny J, Kosko J. Behavioral treatment of panic disorder. *Behav Ther*. 1989; 20:260–282.
56. Moorey S, Greer S. *Psychological Therapy for Patients with Cancer: A New Approach*. Washington, DC: American Psychiatric Press; 1989.
57. Moorey S, Greer S, Watson M, et al. Adjuvant psychological therapy for patients with cancer: outcome at one year. *Psycho-Oncology*. 1994; 3:39–46.
58. Greer S, Moorey S, Baruch J, et al. Adjuvant psychological therapy for patients with cancer: a prospective randomized trial. *Br Med J*. 1992; 304:675–680.
59. Classen C, Hermanson K, Spiegel D. Psychotherapy, stress, and survival in breast cancer. In: Lewis C, O'Sullivan C, Barraclough J, eds. *The Psychoimmunology of Cancer*. Oxford: Oxford University Press; 1994: 123–162.
60. Spiegel D, Spira J. *Supportive-Expressive Group Therapy: A Treatment Manual of Psychosocial Intervention for Women with Recurrent Breast Cancer*. Stanford, CA: Psychosocial Treatment Laboratory, Stanford University School of Medicine; 1991.

APPENDIX 1: AWARENESS OF BREATHING MEDITATION

Sit quietly or lie down in a place where you will not be disturbed. If sitting, sit in a posture that embodies dignity, erect but not stiff. If lying down, lie on your back if possible, on a comfortable padded surface (bed or floor) with a pillow under your knees and your head supported. Allow the eyes to gently close, if that feels comfortable. Otherwise, leave them half-opened and focused on one point. When you are ready, bring your attention to the feeling of the breath flowing in and out of your body, moment by moment and breath by breath, without forcing the breath in any way. You can focus on it at the nostrils, or at your abdomen, where you can feel the expanding of the belly on each inbreath and the receding of your belly on each outbreath. As best you can, simply stay in touch with the feeling of the breath and/or the belly moving, as if your mind were "surfing" on the waves of the breath. As best you can, stay with the feeling of the wave of the breath for the full duration of the inbreath and the outbreath, allowing yourself to just dwell here, moment by moment, following the breath as it comes in and as it goes out. Each time you notice your mind has wandered off the breath, which it will certainly do many times, simply note where it went, (i.e. observe what is on your mind in this moment without pursuing it or rejecting it), and then, without judging it in any way, letting go of whatever captured your attention, and gently but firmly bring it back to your nostrils or your belly and to this breath, whether it is now coming in or going out. If your mind wanders off the breath 20 times, then each time, as soon as you are aware of it, you can note where it is, let go, and come back to the breath.

APPENDIX 2: FORMAL MEDITATION PRACTICES

All practices are done with the same orientation to the present moment described in Appendix 1.

The Body Scan Meditation. This is done lying on one's back if possible on a comfortable surface. In conjunction with a continuous awareness of breathing, the subject is guided to attend to the sensations in the body in a systematic order, starting from the toes of the left foot, and going up the left leg, over to the right foot, up the right leg, and then through the torso, the arms from the finger tips up to the shoulders, and then the neck and head.

Mindful Hatha Yoga. Poses are done standing, sitting, and lying on the floor in a variety of postures. The emphasis is on cultivating moment-to-moment awareness of sensations and an overall sense of the body as a whole. Each posture also has metaphorical significance that can be felt through the body. For instance, the "mountain" and the "warrior" are both standing poses that embody a sense of rootedness, steadfastness, dignity, and strength in the face of ever-changing life challenges.

Sitting Meditation. Described in Appendix 1.

Walking Meditation. As a formal practice, walking meditation is usually done slowly. Emphasis is on moment-to-moment awareness of the lifting, moving, placing of each foot, the shifting of the weight over the forward foot, the breath moving in the body, and a sense of the body as a whole moving, walking. When the mind wanders, the practitioner notes where the attention has gone, and intentionally lets go and returns the focus to the breath and moment-to-moment awareness of the elements of walking slowly.

67

Religion and Spiritual Beliefs

MARC A. MUSICK, HAROLD G. KOENIG, DAVID B. LARSON, AND
DALE MATTHEWS

Addressing the role of religion in medicine in the first decade of this century, William Osler wrote:

Nothing in life is more wonderful than faith—the one great moving force which we can neither weigh in the balance nor test in the crucible. Intangible as the ether, ineluctable as gravitation, the radium of the moral and mental spheres, mysterious, indefinable, known only by its effects, faith pours out an unfailing stream of energy while abating nor jot nor tittle of its potency (1).

These words were written in the context of an article which reviewed the state of faith in medicine in 1910. Osler concluded that not only did faith have important effects for health outcomes, but that practitioners should seek to encourage and incorporate faith as part of clinical care.

Over eight decades later, researchers are finding that religion and spirituality do indeed have significant effects on health. Some studies have found that they act as a coping mechanism to ward off mental illness, while others have found that certain religious activities lead to better physical health (2–5). This chapter reviews this literature, particularly as it pertains to cancer. It examines the relationship between religion and spiritual beliefs and behaviors which lower risk of cancer, as well as explores how they help patients and their caregivers cope with illness.

DEFINING AND MEASURING RELIGION AND SPIRITUALITY

Since spirituality and religion can be thought of in a range of ways, it is important to discuss the manner in which these concepts are usually defined and measured. Religion, as the term is typically used, involves traditional religious beliefs, attitudes, and practices. Spirituality, on the other hand, is a broader term that includes religion, but goes beyond (see Fig. 67–1). In a study of spirituality among the terminally ill, Reed (6) asserted, "[S]pirituality is defined in terms of personal views and behaviors that express a sense of relatedness to a transcendent dimension or to something greater than the self." She went on to say that religiosity is often an indicator of spirituality, but this is not always true. In a review of articles dealing with spirituality, Craigie et al. (7) also concluded that spirituality encompasses a number of beliefs and behaviors that relate to religion. They noted that the most common dimensions that make up spirituality are beliefs related to meaning, ritual activities, social support, and "encounters with the deity."

In contrast, Emblen (8) argued that the term spirituality often refers to ideas that do not necessarily involve religion. Rather, spirituality in this sense refers to beliefs involving meaning and purpose in life, regardless of their orientation (9,10). If one divorces religion from spirituality, however, it becomes a concept that is difficult to define, operationalize and measure. In fact, while the term "spirituality" has been used frequently in the published literature, it is almost always measured in terms of traditional religious beliefs, attitudes, or behaviors, (i.e., religion (11)).

For this reason, this chapter focuses on dimensions that have been measured and studied, (i.e., religious affiliation, beliefs, attitudes, or behaviors), referring to the broader term spirituality when it is appropriate. A number of specific behaviors have been used to test the linkages between religion and health. The two most common behaviors used in these studies have been attendance at worship services (12) and devotional activities (13). Beliefs relating to comfort or strength from religion have also been used (2). Finally, measures of religious affiliation have been employed to tap the normative dimension of religiosity (14,15).

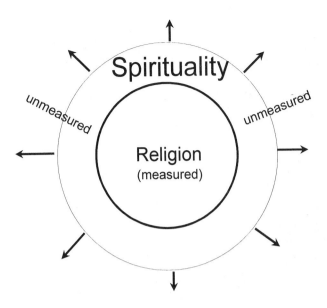

FIG. **67–1.** Defining and measuring religion and spirituality.

POTENTIAL MECHANISMS OF EFFECT

In an influential study of religion and health among the elderly, Idler (3) proposed four ways in which religion might influence health in general. First, religious groups may encourage their members to refrain from certain activities that might adversely affect health (alcoholism, smoking, unsafe sexual practices). Second, active participation in a religious group could provide certain types of instrumental and cognitive support that are beneficial to the individual. Third, a religious belief system may provide the individual with meaning in life and better enable them to cope with painful circumstances. Finally, certain religious worldviews may actually influence the ways in which individuals perceive and handle problems. Worldviews that encourage the individual to perceive problems in a more positive way may mitigate against the mental distress that would otherwise occur (16).

RELIGION AND GENERAL PHYSICAL HEALTH

Before embarking on a specific discussion of religion and cancer, it is important to note research which has linked religion to physical health, mental health, and well-being. Several investigators have found that certain types of religiosity influence physical health. McIntosh and Spilka (4) reported that intrinsic religious beliefs and prayer were associated with better physical health. Idler and Kasl (2) reported that public religious involvement was strongly related to improvement in functional ability over time among older adults

living in the community. Several other studies have shown that different aspects of religiosity, particularly church attendance, are positively related to persons' perceptions of their health status (subjective health) (17,18); however, when functional status has been controlled (e.g. the ability to get to church), these associations weaken. Finally, a more recent study has shown that elderly persons who draw strength or comfort from religion had lower mortality rates following cardiac surgery than those who did not report such feelings (19).

RELIGION AND MENTAL HEALTH

Williams et al. have found that while religious attendance does not directly enhance mental health, it is beneficial for buffering the deleterious effects of stressful life events (20). Likewise, in a study of hospitalized elderly men, Koenig et al. found that religious coping was related to lower levels of depression both cross-sectionally and longitudinally (21). Finally, Idler and Kasl (2) found that subjective religiosity and religious coping acted as a buffer against depression among newly disabled men.

Similarly, several authors have linked religion to higher levels of psychological well-being. Using a nationally representative sample, Ellison (22) found that greater religious faith was directly linked to higher levels of life satisfaction and happiness and also led to fewer psychological problems after traumatic stress. In a another study, Ellison et al. (23) reported that devotional activity and church attendance were positively associated with overall life satisfaction. Pollner (24) found that relationships with God or the Divine (i.e., regular prayer activity and feeling close to God) were better predictors of global happiness, life satisfaction, and life excitement than other sociodemographic variables commonly linked to these outcomes. He also showed that the effects of these relationships were stronger for persons with less education. Finally, Koenig et al. (25) found in a sample of over 800 midwestern older adults that those who were 75 years or older reported better morale if they were more actively involved in either public or private religious behaviors. Because many of these studies are cross-sectional, however, it is difficult to determine whether religious involvement leads to better morale or better morale leads to more religious involvement.

In short, previous research has demonstrated the importance of examining the linkages between health, well-being, and religion. In the remainder of this paper, we will examine these issues as they specifically relate to patients with cancer. Most of the religion–cancer studies in the United States are related to the over 90% of the population which is Christian. Thus, the reports overly represent members of this religious tradition. Furthermore, many studies utilize samples of elderly individuals, the group which is also at greatest risk for cancer.

With these caveats in mind, we discuss the prevalence of religious beliefs and behaviors in the general population and among persons with cancer. Next, we examine the evidence showing that behaviors among certain religious groups reduce the risk of cancer. Third, we discuss the role that religion may play in the lives of cancer patients, particularly as a coping strategy. Fourth, we discuss the importance of religion for the family of those with cancer, and how it may help them deal with grief after their loved one dies. Finally, we conclude with a discussion of clinical implications and research directions.

PREVALENCE OF RELIGIOUS BEHAVIORS

While religious participation rates vary by religious affiliation, gender, socioeconomic status, and race (26,27), discussion is limited to overall prevalence rates. Nationally representative data from the General Social Survey (28) collected during the late 1980s revealed that over 85% of Americans attended religious services at least once per year. Almost one-half reported attending more than once a month, and 29% attended once a week or more often. Similar results were found for prayer. Only 25% reported that they never pray, whereas 45% prayed at least once per week, and 22% prayed once a day or more. In sum, it would seem that religious behavior in the general population is quite common.

Using a sample of elderly individuals attending an outpatient geriatric clinic, Koenig et al. (29) examined the extent to which the respondents participated in religious activities and adhered to religious beliefs. They found that 54% attended church services at least once a week or more often, and 72% prayed at least once a day or more often. These results were consistent with those of Blazer and Palmore (30) who reported that 61% of an elderly community-dwelling sampled attended church at least once per week, and 74% reported praying at least once per day. Koenig et al. also examined religious behaviors of elderly outpatients with cancer. They reported that persons with cancer showed lower levels of both public and private religious activity (29) which may have been due in part to limitations of illness. In a sample of patients with advanced cancer who were terminally ill at home (ages 28–85 years), Yates et al. (31) found that only 37% of patients had attended church during the past month; frequent church attendance, however, was associated with significantly higher satisfaction with life, happiness, positive affect, and was related to better control of pain. In that study, intensity of religious belief and importance of church in life were also related to greater life satisfaction and better control of pain.

For church attendance, these findings may in part be related to the physical and mental limitations imposed by cancer and cannot be entirely attributed to being less religious. Many patients with cancer maintain strong religious beliefs (31) and religious involvement as much as they are able until death; in fact, as death approaches, at least two studies have demonstrated that patients become more religious (32,33).

CANCER PREVALENCE AMONG RELIGIOUS GROUPS

Early studies of serveral Jewish groups showed lower cancer risk related to tumors primarily associated with use of alcohol and tobacco (references in Table 67.1). Higher levels of some cancers among Jews are likely related to genetic risks for colon, breast, and ovary in particular. Other studies have shown that affiliation with certain religious groups, such as the Seventh Day Adventists and Mormons, reduces risk of cancer by encouraging behaviors which reduce exposure to carcinogens, particularly tobacco (Table 67.1). Troyer (34) conducted an indepth review of cancer rates among four religious sects: Mormons, Seventh-Day Adventists, Amish, and Hutterites. He showed that, while all groups had strong restrictions against alcohol and tobacco use, only Mormons and Seventh-Day Adventists were discouraged from consuming tea or coffee. The Seventh-Day Adventists were also expected to abstain from eating meat, and 40%–50% reported conforming to a lacto-ovo-vegetarian diet. Overall cancer rates were indeed lower in these religious groups than those of comparison groups. He concluded that a lower cancer rate could largely be attributed to those sites associated with smoking. He noted, however, that multiple factors were probably interacting to account for the lower rates of cancer in these religious groups.

Studying a large sample of California Seventh-Day Adventists, Phillips and Snowden (35) examined differences in cancer mortality rate from three sites of cancer unrelated to smoking: large bowel, breast, and prostate. They found that Seventh-Day Adventist mortality rates from these cancers, particularly large bowel cancer, was lower than that in the general national population and in a comparable population in California. They went on to examine whether Seventh-Day

TABLE 67.1. *Studies Demonstrating Reduced Cancer Risk Among Religious Groups*

Authors	Year	Subjects	Findings*
MacMahon (75)	1960	Jews in New York City	Lower mortality from tongue, buccal, pharynx, larynx, lung, prostate cancers in men, but higher mortality from stomach, intestine, pancreas, melanoma, glioma, lymphomas and leukemia. Lower mortality from cervical cancer in women, but higher mortality from cancer of ovary
Seidman (76)	1970	Jews in New York ($n = 36,342$)	Lower cancer mortality in men Higher mortality in women
Herman and Enterline (77)	1970	Jews in Pittsburgh	Lower mortality from lung cancer in men Higher mortality from lung cancer in women
Greenwald et al. (78)	1975	Jews in United States ($n = 789$)	Lower cancer mortality (men) from lung, higher from colon Lower cancer mortality (women) from cervix/breast, higher from stomach and lung
Enstrom (79)	1975	Mormons in California and Utah ($n = 3871$)	Lower mortality from lung, esophageal, stomach, colon, rectal, pancreas, prostate, bladder, kidney in men, and lung, breast, and uterus in women
Lyon et al. (36)	1976	Mormons in Utah ($n = 10,490$)	Lower cancer incidence (overall
Jarvis (37)	1977	Mormons in Canada ($n = 1116$)	Lower cancer mortality overall, especially cancer of lung
Lyon et al. (80)	1977	Mormons in Utah ($n = 10,490$)	Lower cancer mortality (overall)
Enstrom (81)	1978	Mormons in Utah and California ($n = 70, 500$)	Lower cancer mortality (overall)
Phillips et al. (82)	1980	Seventh-Day Adventists in California ($n = 135,666$)	Lower cancer mortality (overall), especially cancer of rectum, lung, and leukemia
Hamman et al. (83)	1981	Old order Amish in Indiana, Ohio, and Pennsylvania ($n = 59,227$)	Lower cancer mortality (overall) in men
Martin et al (84)	1980	Huterrites in South Dakota and Alberta, Canada ($n = 12,652$)	Lower cancer mortality (overall) in men, especially lung cancer (higher leukemia, though)
Phillips and Snowden (35)	1983	Seventh-Day Adventists in California	Lower mortality from cancer of bowel, breast, and prostate
Berkel and deWaard (85)	1983	Seventh-Day Adventists in Netherlands ($n = 482$)	Lower cancer mortality (overall)*
Zollinger et al (86)	1984	Seventh-Day Adventists in California ($n = 2304$)	Lower mortality from breast cancer
Dwyer et al. (38)	1990	Mormons, Catholics, liberal, moderate and conservative Protestants, Jews	Lower cancer mortality (overall) in Mormons and conservative Protestants

*When compared with general population or those not affiliated with particular religious group under study.

Adventist stipulations against meat and coffee consumption could account for this difference. They found that meat consumption accounted for little of the substantial difference in large bowel cancer rates, whereas coffee consumption was more contributory. Phillips and Snowden speculated that, since many Seventh-Day Adventists are vegetarians, they consume less cholesterol and more vitamins A and C, which had previously been found to reduce cancer risk.

Two studies focused on a group of Mormons living in Utah and in Alberta, Canada (36,37). Both found that Mormons had a lower risk of cancer mortality. The study based in Utah found lower rates for sites of cancer related to smoking and also for breast and cervical cancer. Lower cervical cancer could likely be explained by the likelihood of later onset of sexual behavior and fewer partners. The study based in Alberta reported similar findings in that overall cancer mortality for Mormons were lower than those for Alberta and all of Canada.

In a more recent study, Dwyer et al. (38) speculated that the dietary and behavioral restrictions placed on religious adherents not only benefit them, but also benefit others in the community who are not of the same faith. To test this hypothesis, they examined county level data to determine if religious concentration and affiliation had an effect on county-level cancer mortality rates. Counties with the highest concentrations of Mormons had the lowest cancer mortality rates, controlled for other risk factors. Higher concentrations of conservative or moderate Protestants were also associated with lower rates. In short, it would seem that the behavioral restrictions of certain religious groups tend to "spillover" and have preventative effects for others in the community not of the same faith.

In sum, mortality rates for certain religious groups are lower than for the population as a whole. Moreover, it seems that this effect spills over onto the surrounding populace who are not of the same religious affiliation. Much of the difference in mortality rates can be traced to restrictions against smoking, although diet, alcohol, and sexual behaviors may impact as well. It is interesting to speculate whether membership in cohesive, supportive religious groups may endow individuals with other as yet unidentified protective factors, stemming from the strong sense of community or a fulfilling spiritual life.

RELIGION AND COPING WITH CANCER

In this section, we will focus on the role that religion plays for the individual with cancer, exploring ways in which cancer patients use religion to cope with their illness. The cancer patient is faced with suffering associated with pain, anxiety about the future, fear of disability, and the spectre of death. As Osler (1) noted, religious beliefs serve many individuals as a reservoir of personal strength for confronting such issues. In a sample of 103 women with breast cancer, Johnson and Spilka (39) found that only two of the sample reported that religion was of no help in coping with their illness. In contrast, Carver et al. (40) studied women with breast cancer before and after surgery. They found that religious beliefs had little effect on optimism or level of distress. Their results also indicated that reliance on religion was highest presurgery, and declined thereafter over a 12 month follow-up period. Noting this exception, most of the studies we have examined (see below) have shown religion to have beneficial influences for the patient in terms of coping (39,41–48).

There are four specific ways in which persons may draw strength from their religious views, recognizing that here is significant overlap between the strategies:

(1) secondary control, (2) provision of spiritual worldview, (3) participation in a spiritual community, and (4) dealing with death and dying.

Secondary Control

In the presence of cancer, the patient may cope by relinquishing control of the situation to God. "It is in God's hands now." In this way, the patient may be comforted in knowing that, whatever happens, God's will is done. In studying the general population, Pollner (24) found that viewing God as being one who solves problems results in positive well-being. Similarly, in patients with cancer, Jenkins and Pargament (41) showed that persons who believed that God was in control of their situation showed lower levels of psychological disturbances and higher levels of self-esteem. Furthermore, the authors showed that the belief that God is in control (secondary control) had stronger effects on adjustment than did feelings of personal control over circumstances (primary control). Those who coped most effectively perceived God as working collaboratively with them in their efforts to help control the disease.

A comment from a woman in Johnson and Spilka's study (39) illustrates the importance of believing that God is in control: "No matter what happens, God is with me. I am never alone. He will give me the strength I need." Likewise, Koenig (42) found that when patients with cancer and other serious diseases were asked what enabled them to cope successfully with their condition, "turning it over to God" and "putting it in God's hands" were among the most frequent of responses.

The existential crisis posed by a cancer diagnosis sometimes causes feelings of hostility towards God for causing the disease or allowing it to happen: "Why me?", "Am I being punished?", "Is there a God?" While systematic research is absent, these feelings are often part of the initial shock and crisis of diagnosis or of an incurable stage of disease. In general, they abate but a skilled clergy or mental health professional may be needed. Johnson and Spilka (39) noted that many patients strongly indicated that God was not responsible for their having cancer and did not blame God for their illness.

Some patients perceive that cancer is a punishment for some prior behavior, though they may intellectually know it is not true. Significant depression can develop, especially if there has been some significant prior life problems. Evaluation by a skilled clergy or mental health professional may be indicated.

Religious or Spiritual Worldviews

The interpretive framework or worldview of the individual will influence how disease and treatment are perceived and tolerated. A strong religious tradition may provide meaning to the crisis of illness, and the meaning of potential pain and suffering. Religion can play a crucial role by giving meaning and explanations of illness and suffering.

Acklin et al. (43) found that cancer patients who expressed higher levels of transcendent meaning showed greater mental well-being than did a control group, although the two groups did not differ significantly in absolute levels of either meaning or mental well-being. They also found that meaning among both groups was correlated with personal religiosity and church attendance, underscoring the importance of religious activity for building cognitive resources to facilitate adaptation. Similarly, other authors have demonstrated that seriously ill patients who rely more on their religious beliefs or have greater spiritual well-being tend to report higher quality of life (6,44,45).

Private Religious Practices

The cancer patient may rely on private, personal forms of religious activity. Sodestrom and Martinson (46) found that the most frequently cited coping strategies by hospitalized cancer patients were personal prayer and prayers of others. The second most common activity was reading religious literature, such as the Bible, other religious books, and listening to religious broadcasts. Overall, 88% indicated using several types of religious activities to cope with their illness. Furthermore, those informed of their prognosis engaged in a significantly greater number of religious activities than those without such knowledge.

Mickley et al. (47) studied women with breast cancer to examine whether certain types of religiosity had an effect on spiritual well-being and hope. They found that women who engaged in personal religious activities, and who saw religion as the central focus in their lives, had better outcomes in terms of both spiritual well-being and level of hope. Likewise, in their study of breast cancer patients, Johnson and Spilka (39) noted the importance of prayer for creating a sense of well-being. They argued that not only does personal prayer act as a coping mechanism by increasing feelings of closeness to God, but prayer by others also brought comfort. Finally, Halstead and Fernsler (48) noted that prayer was the most frequently cited coping strategy in their sample of individuals diagnosed with cancer.

As noted before, there is significant overlap among religious coping strategies. Using interview data from cancer patients, Jenkins and Pargament (41) found that subjects frequently reported obtaining help or personal strength from God through prayer. This finding confirmed an earlier report by Pargament et al. (49) that the interactive style which results in feelings of God being in control is most beneficial for positive mental health outcomes. An active personal spiritual life, then, may be conducive to certain beliefs about God that are in turn beneficial to the individual. Moreover, the knowledge that others pray on their behalf may further bolster their feelings that God is in control.

Participation in Community

Perceiving oneself as a member of a community with others having similar beliefs provides important aspects of social support. Such participation may help the cancer patient by: (1) allowing more contact with others of a similar faith which in turn will bolster their own faith; (2) meeting with people and obtaining their promises to pray; (3) being part of a social group which may provide instrumental help; and (4) reminding the patient that she or he is part of a caring community. Indeed, one recent study of 4000 randomly selected older adults reported that those who attended church weekly or more often were only about one-half as likely to be depressed (odds ratio, 0.56: 95% confidence interval, 0.48–0.65), after controlling for age, sex, race, subjective and objective health, functional status, and social support (50). Berger (51) in his book, *The Sacred Canopy*, argued that individuals immersed in social groups tend to adopt the values and meaning structures of the group as their own. This tendency, he thought, was especially potent for religious groups.

Coping with Dying and Death

As persons with cancer face the possibility of death, existential and spiritual issues come to the forefront. Many patients are helped by a life review which gives positive meaning to their lives. Spiritual beliefs related to connection to something bigger than self will help the person to put their life in order, tolerate the difficulties of their illness, and come to grips with the meaning of death. Religious rituals are helpful, such as confession and the receiving and giving of forgiveness. Families and loved ones should be encouraged to reconcile differences and past hurts. Spiritual beliefs allow for a more positive reframing of circumstances, forgiveness, and tolerance of pain and suffering, providing a context of meaning (42,52). Belief in life after death in some religious traditions makes possible the hope of reuniting with loved ones who are dead and hope of an existence beyond death. Indeed, several studies have demonstrated lower death anxiety in persons who are more religious (53–56).

HELPING THE FAMILY COPE

Loved ones suffer as much as patients with cancer, particularly when caregiving responsibilities are heavy, the patient's pain and suffering is severe or protracted, and the patient is depressed, anxious, and often delirious in terminal stages. Studies have shown high rates of depression in caregivers of cancer patients (57). Religious beliefs and practices, as well as emotional and instrumental support (e.g., respite care offered by the religious community), may help to relieve caregiver burden. Rabins et al. (58) found that caregivers of patients with either Alzheimer's disease or metastatic cancer who had strong religious beliefs were more likely than those without a strong faith to be emotionally adjusted 2 years after the death. Other researchers have shown that caregivers tend to engage in religious behavior and seek spiritual guidance more often than noncaregivers (59,60).

A number of authors have linked religious and spiritual beliefs to successful grieving. In a study of bereaved persons, Martocchio (61) found that religious and spiritual beliefs were important factors which facilitated the grief process. Likewise, Cook and Wimberley (62), studying bereaved parents, found that bereavement theodicies (e.g., a belief that one will be reunited with loved ones in the afterlife) were instrumental for helping the parents to cope with the loss of a child. They went on to show that those parents who used their religious beliefs in coping with the death actually strengthened those beliefs.

In another study of parents with recently deceased children, McIntosh et al. (63) reported that both importance of religion or religious group participation led to greater social support and a greater ability to find meaning in the death of the child, which predicted better long-term adjustment. Thus, not only do spiritual beliefs help persons to adjust to the death of a loved one, but religious participation may play an additional role by facilitating access to others who provide comfort or instrumental support.

RELIGION AND LIVING WITH CANCER

As indicated above, religion plays an important role in the adaptation of individuals with cancer and that of their families. For older individuals, religion gives them a sense of strength, hope or meaning that may ward off despair and depression associated with poorer quality of life and reduced survival (64). By encouraging the individual to maintain a positive outlook and bolstering their support network, religion can help to promote the overall well-being of the patient living with cancer. In a provocative study by Spiegel et al. (65) (see Chapter 63), weekly group sessions over 1 year with women with advanced breast cancer led to better quality of life, pain control, and longer survival. Should these findings be replicated, it may be possible to identify the mechanism by which this life extension is gained. Spiegel hypothesizes that it was the positive impact of social support.

One could extrapolate that the social support given in a religious community might be similar and hence might offer benefits with regard to outcome and quality of life for cancer patients.

In addition to support from other church members (66,67), support by the patient's family and their clergy may also increase quality of life for those surviving with cancer. In a study of childhood adjustment to cancer, Spilka et al. (68) demonstrated the importance of family religious activities for the cancer patient. The authors reported that religious families appeared to bind more closely together under the stress of having a child with cancer. In summing up this finding, the authors stated that "a strong faith implies a close-knit family, the bonds of which are reinforced when the stress of life-threatening illness enters the picture." In another study by Spiegel et al. (69), they found that the family environment of breast cancer patients was important for their psychological adjustment. They showed that families characterized by more openness and less conflict tended to produce less mood disturbance in patients. However, they also reported that a moral-religious family element seemed to predict increased mood disturbance. These investigators were at a loss to explain this finding, but a selection effect may have been involved. That is, persons who used religion beyond the support they received from family may have been those who viewed their illness as more threatening, which could have resulted in more negative mood states. In any case, it appears that religion plays an important role in the cohesion of the family unit, which in turn aids the patient in adjustment to the disease.

Cancer patients also receive support from their clergy. Johnson and Spilka (39) examined the role that clergy played in the adjustment of women with breast cancer. They found that approximately 27% of the women were visited by their minister at home, and 56% were visited in the hospital. Most of the clergy either offered to or did pray with the individual. Women were pleased with these visits from clergy and many noted that the visit demonstrated to them that someone cared about them.

CLINICAL IMPLICATIONS

Medical and mental health specialists who care for persons with cancer should be aware of the important role that religion plays in the lives of many patients. For some, it provides a framework by which to understand and find meaning in their situation, helps them to cope with the uncertainty of their illness, instills hope, and brings comfort and support from others. Clinicians should always include questions about a religious history from patients and assess to what extent they use religion as a coping behavior; if done in a respectful and appreciative manner, this dialogue by itself validates this aspect of the patient's coping (see Chapter 68). Health care providers should support and encourage use of religion in coping by referring patients to the clergy of their faith who can provide them with religious resources according to their wishes. Integrating chaplains as part of the health care team will help to ensure that patients' spiritual needs are met and that health providers are familiar with religious issues.

RESEARCH DIRECTIONS

Research that includes religious variables in assessing health and health outcomes (particularly cancer) has been lacking despite the frequency and importance of religious beliefs in cancer patients, the potential for improved quality of life, and other evidence for clinically beneficial effects (70–72). Measures of spiritual and religious beliefs, however, are now being included in multidimensional quality of life instruments, such as the FACT by Cella et al. (73). Three areas of research are particularly in need of further development.

Cancer Prevention Research

Can religious communities be used to enhance cancer preventive and early detection behaviors? Experience in use of churches in black communities has been helpful in encouraging dietary changes and smoking cessation. Are there ways that faith communities confer attitudes through their practices, that impact on altered risk behaviors such as alcohol use? Intervention studies are needed.

Assessment Method Development

The accurate and reliable measurement of religiousness is of critical importance when conducting research on religion's effects on health outcomes in cancer patients. Religion is a multidimensional construct that includes attitudes, beliefs, public and private behaviors, experience, and knowledge. Typically, only one dimension is assessed. This is a mistake, because research has shown that different dimensions of religiousness may be differentially related to both physical and mental health outcomes (51).

Broader Studies of Religions and Spirituality

With few exceptions (74), most of the research involving religion and cancer patients has focused on the role of traditional religious behaviors, beliefs, and attitudes among Christians and Jews. The findings reported here, then, cannot be generalized to other religion's with different belief systems. Similar research is needed among members of other world religions — Buddhists, Muslims, Hindus, and other groups — to see whether these relationships generalize across faith traditions.

Furthermore, we have not yet been able to measure the broader concept of spirituality or been able to operationalize it sufficiently to assess its impact on health outcomes in cancer patients. As noted before, almost all the published research which has proported to measure "spirituality" in cancer patients has, in fact, assessed traditional religious beliefs and behaviors. The impact of spirituality by itself on health outcomes, independent and apart of traditional religious beliefs and behaviors, needs to be defined, assessed, and studied.

ACKNOWLEDGMENTS

Funding in part provided by the John Templeton Foundation, Radnor, PA, Monarch Pharmaceuticals, a division of King Pharmaceuticals, Bristol, TN, and the Program on Religion, Aging, and Health at Duke University Medical Center, Durham, NC.

REFERENCES

1. Osler W. The Faith that heals. *Br Med J*. 1910; 1:1470–1472.
2. Idler E, Kasl SV. Religion, disability, depression, and the timing of death. *Am J Sociol*. 1992; 97:1052–1079.
3. Idler E. Religious involvement and the health of the elderly: some hypotheses and an initial test. *Soc Forces*. 1987; 66:226–238.
4. McIntosh D, Spilka B. Religion and physical health: the role of personal faith and control beliefs. *Res Soc Sci Study Relig*. 1990; 2:167–194.

5. Mickley JR, Carson V, Soeken KL. Religion and adult mental health: state of the science in nursing. *Issues Ment Health Nurs.* 1996; 16:345–360.

6. Reed PG. Spirituality and well-being in terminally ill hospitalized adults. *Res Nurs Health.* 1987; 10:335–344.

7. Craigie FC Jr., Larson DB, Liu IY. References to religion in *The Journal of Family Practice. J Fam Pract.* 1990; 30:477–480.

8. Emblen JD. Religion and spirituality defined according to current usage in nursing literature. *J Prof Nurs.* 1992; 8:41–47.

9. Burkhardt MA. Becoming and connecting: elements of spirituality for women. *Holist Nurs Prac.* 1994; 8:12–21.

10. Miller MA. Culture, spirituality and women's health. *J Obstet Gynecol Neonatal Nurs.* 1995; 24:257–263.

11. Levin JS. Religion and health: Is there an association, is it valid, and is it causal. *Soc Sci Med.* 1994; 38:1475–1482.

12. Levin JS, Vanderpool HY. Is frequent religious attendance really conducive to better health? Toward an epidemiology of religion. *Soc Sci Med.* 1987; 24:589–600.

13. Ferraro KF, Koch JR. Religion and health among black and white adults: examining social support and consolidation. *J Sci Study Relig.* 1994; 33:362–375.

14. Koenig HG, George LK, Meador KG, et al. Religious affiliation and psychiatric disorder in Protestant baby boomers. *Hosp Commun Psychiatry.* 1994; 45:586–596.

15. Ferraro KF, Albrecht-Jensen CM. Does religion influence adult health? *J Sci Study Relig.* 1992; 30:193–202.

16. Wortman CB, Sheedy C, Gluhoski V, Kessler R. Stress, coping, and health: conceptual issues and directions for future research. In: Friedman HS, ed. *Hostility, Coping, and Health.* Washington, DC: American Psychological Association; 1991: 227–256.

17. Broyles PA, Drenovsky CK. Religious attendance and the subjective health of the elderly. *Rev Relig Res.* 1992; 34:152–160.

18. St. George A, McNamara PH. Religion, race and psychological well-being. *J Sci Study Relig.* 1984; 23:351–363.

19. Oxman TE, Freeman DH, Manheimer ED. Lack of social participation or religious strength and comfort as risk factors for death after cardiac surgery in the elderly. *Psychosom Med.* 1995; 57:5–15.

20. Williams DR, Larson DB, Buckler RE, et al. Religion and psychological distress in a community sample. *Soc Sci Med.* 1991; 32:1257–1262.

21. Koenig HG, Cohen HJ, Blazer DG, et al. Religious coping and depression among elderly, hospitalized medically ill men. *Am J Psychiatry.* 1992; 149:1693–1700.

22. Ellison CG. Religious involvement and subjective well-being. *J Health Soc Behav.* 1991; 32:80–99.

23. Ellison CG, Gay DG, Glass TA. Does religious commitment contribute to individual life satisfaction? *Soc Forces.* 1989; 68:100–123.

24. Pollner M. Divine relations, social relations, and well-being. *J Health Soc Behav.* 1989; 30:92–104.

25. Koenig HG, Kvale JN, Ferrel C. Religion and well-being in later life. *Gerontologist.* 1988; 28:18–28.

26. Davidson JD. Socio-economic status and ten dimensions of religious commitment. *Soc Sci Res.* 1977; 61:462–485.

27. Roof WC, McKinney W. *American Mainline Religion: Its Changing Shape and Future.* New Brunswick, NJ: Rutgers University Press; 1987.

28. Davis JA, Smith TW. *General Social Surveys, 1972–1993.* Chicago: National Opinion Research Center; 1993.

29. Koenig HG, Moberg DO, Kvale JN. Religious activities and attitudes of older adults in a geriatric assessment clinic. *J Am Geriatr Soc.* 1988; 36:362–374.

30. Blazer D, Palmore E. Religion and aging in longitudinal panel. *Gerontologist.* 1976; 16:82–85.

31. Yates J, Chalmer BJ, St. James P, et al. Religion in patients with advanced cancer. *Med Pediatr Oncol.* 1981; 9:121–128.

32. Reed PG. Religiousness among terminally ill and health adults. *Res Nurs Health.* 1986:9:35–41.

33. Reed PG. Spirituality and well-being in terminally ill hospitalized adults. *Res Nurs Health.* 1987: 10:335–344.

34. Troyer H. Review of cancer among 4 religious sects: evidence that life-styles are distinctive sets of risk factors. *Soc Sci Med.* 1988; 26:1007–1017.

35. Phillips RL, Snowden DA. Association of meat and coffee use with cancers of the large bowel, breast, and prostate among Seventh-Day Adventists: preliminary results. *Cancer Res.* 1983; 43:2403s–2408s.

36. Lyon JL, Klauber MR, Gardner JW, et al. Cancer incidence in Mormons and non-Mormons in Utah, 1966–1970. *N Engl J Med.* 1976; 294:129–133.

37. Jarvis GK. Mormon mortality rates in Canada. *Soc Biol.* 1977; 24:294–302.

38. Dwyer JW, Clarke LL, Miller MK. The effect of religious concentration and affiliation on county cancer mortality rates. *J Health Soc Behav.* 1990; 31:185–202.

39. Johnson SC, Spilka B. Coping with breast cancer: the roles of clergy and faith. *J Relig Health* 1991; 30:21–33.

40. Carver CS, Pozo C, Harris SD, et al. How coping mediates the effect of optimism on distress: a study of women with early stage breast cancer. *J Pers Soc Psychol.* 1993; 65:375–390.

41. Jenkins RA, Pargament KI. Cognitive appraisals in cancer patients. *Soc Sci Med.* 1988; 26:625–633.

42. Koenig HG. *Aging and God.* New York: Haworth Press, 1994.

43. Acklin MW, Brown EC, Mauger PA. The role of religious values in coping with cancer. *J Relig Health.* 1983, 22:322–333.

44. Kaczorowski JM. Spiritual well-being and anxiety in adults diagnosed with cancer. *Hospice J.* 1989; 5:105–116.

45. Reed PG. Religiousness among terminally ill and healthy adults. *Res Nurs Health.* 1986; 9:35–41.

46. Sodestrom KE, Martinson IM. Patients' spiritual coping strategies: a study of nurse and patient perspectives. *Oncol Nurs Forum.* 1987; 14:41–46.

47. Mickley JR, Soeken K, Belcher A. Spiritual well-being, religiousness and hope among women with breast cancer. *IMAGE.* 1992; 24:267–272.

48. Halstead MT, Fernsler JI. Coping strategies of long-term cancer survivors. *Cancer Nurs.* 1994; 17:94–100.

49. Pargament KI, Kennell J, Hathaway, et al. Religion and the problem solving process: three styles of coping. *J Sci Study Relig.* 1988; 27:90–104.

50. Koenig HG, Hays J, George LK et al. Modeling the cross-sectional relationships between religion, poor health, social support, and depression. Abstracts,

American Association for the Advancement of Science, 162nd Annual Meeting, Baltimore, MD.

51. Berger PL. *The Sacred Canopy: Elements of Sociological Theory of Religion.* New York: Doubleday; 1967.

52. Conrad, NL. Spiritual support for the dying. *Nurs Clin North Am.* 1985; 20:415–426.

53. Jeffers JC, Nichols CR, Eisdorfer C. Attitudes of older persons toward death: a preliminary study. *J Gerontol.* 1961; 16:53–56.

54. Swenson WM. Attitudes toward death in an aged population. *J Gerontol.* 1961; 16:49–52.

55. Koenig HG. Religion and death anxiety in later life. *Hospice J.* 1988; 4(1):3–24.

56. Thorson JA, Powell FC. Meanings of death and intrinsic religiosity. *J Clin Psychol.* 1990; 46:379–391.

57. Rabins PV, Fitting MD, Eastham J, et al. The emotional impact of caring for the chronically ill. *Psychosomatics.* 1990; 31:331–336.

58. Rabins PV, Fitting MD, Eastham J, et al. Emotional adaptation over time in caregivers for chronically ill elderly people. *Age Ageing.* 1990; 19:185–190.

59. Kaye J, Robinson KM. Spirituality among caregivers. *IMAGE.* 1994; 26:218–221.

60. Baines E. Caregiver stress in the older adult. *J Commun Health Nurs.* 1984; 4:257–263.

61. Martocchio BC. Grief and bereavement: healing through hurt. *Nurs Clin North Am.* 1985; 20:327–341.

62. Cook JA, Wimberley DW. If I should die before I wake: religious commitment and adjustment to the death of a child. *J Sci Study Relig.* 1983; 22:222–238.

63. McIntosh DN, Silver RC, Wortman CB. Religion's role in adjustment to a negative life event: coping with the loss of a child. *J Pers Soc Psychol.* 1993; 65:812–821.

64. Koenig HG, Shelp F, Goli V, et al. Survival and health-care utilization in elderly medical inpatients with major depression. *J Am Geriatr Soc.* 1989; 37:599–606.

65. Spiegel D, Bloom JR, Kraemer HC, et al. Effect of psychosocial treatment on survival of patients with metastatic breast cancer. *Lancet.* 1989; 8668:888–891.

66. Cohen S, Wills TA. Stress, social support, and the buffering hypothesis. *Psychol Bull.* 1985; 98:310–357.

67. George LK, Blazer DG, Hughes DC, et al. Social support and the outcome of major depression. *Br J Psychiatry.* 1989; 154:478–485.

68. Spilka B, Zwartjes WJ, Zwartjes GM. The role of religion in coping with childhood cancer. *Pastoral Psychol.* 1991; 39:295–304.

69. Spiegel D, Bloom JR, Gottheil E. Family environment as a predictor of adjustment to metastatic breast carcinoma. *J Psychosoc Oncol.* 1983; 1:33–44.

70. Larson DB, Pattison EM, Blazer DG, et al. Systematic analysis of research on religious variables in four major psychiatric journals, 1978–1982. *Am J Psychiatry.* 1986; 143:329–334.

71. Levin JS, Schiller PL. Is there a religious factor in health? *J Relig Health. 1987; 27:9–36.*

72. Koenig HG. *Research on Religion and Aging.* Westport, CT: Greenwood Press; 1995.

73. Cella DF, Tulsky DS, Gray G, et al. The functional Assessment of Cancer Therapy scale: development and validation of the general measure. *J Clin Oncol.* 1993; 11:570–579.

74. Jussawalla DJ, Jain DK. Breast cancer and religion in greater Bombay women: an epidemiological study of 2,130 women over a nine-year period. *Br J Cancer.* 1977; 36:634-638.

75. MacMahon B. The ethnic distribution of cancer mortality in New York City, 1955. *Acta Unio Int Contra Cancrum.* 1960; 16:1716–1724.

76. Seidman H. Cancer death rates by site and sex for religious and socioeconomic groups in New York City. *Environ Res.* 1970; 3:234–250.

77. Herman B, Enterline PE. Lung cancer among the Jews and Non-Jews of Pittsburgh, Pennsylvania, 1953–1967: Mortality rates and cigarette smoking behavior. *Am J Epidemiol.* 1970; 91:355–367.

78. Greenwald P, Korns RF, Nasca PC, Wolfgang PE. Cancer in United States Jews. *Cancer Res.* 1975; 35:3507–3512.

79. Enstrom JE. Cancer mortality among Mormons. *Cancer.* 1975; 36:825–841.

80. Lyon JL, Gardner JW, Klauber MR, et al. Low cancer incidence and morality in Utah. *Cancer.* 1977; 39:2608–2618.

81. Enstrom JE. Cancer and total mortality among active Mormons. *Cancer.* 1978; 42:1943–1951.

82. Phillips RL, Garfinkel L, Kuzma JW, et al. Mortality among California Seventh-Day Adventists for selected cancer sites. *J Natl Can Inst.* 1980; 65:1097–1107.

83. Hamman RF, Barancik JI, Lilienfeld AM. Patterns of mortality in the old order Amish. I. Background and major causes of death. *Am J Epidemiol.* 1981; 114:845–861.

84. Martin AO, Dunn JK, Simpson JL, et al. Cancer mortality in a human isolate. *J Natl Cancer Inst.* 1980; 65:1109–1113.

85. Berkel J, deWaard F. Morality pattern and life expectancy of Seventh-Day Adventists in the Netherlands. *Int J Epidemiol.* 1983; 12:455–459.

86. Zollinger TW, Phillips RL, Kuzma JW. Breast cancer survival rates among Seventh-Day Adventists and non-Seventh-Day Adventists. *Am J Epidemiol.* 1984; 119:503–509.

68

Spiritual Assessment, Screening, and Intervention

GEORGE FITCHETT AND GEORGE HANDZO

Research indicates that for many people religion plays an important role in health, well-being, and coping with stress. A number of helpful reviews have been published (1–3). The role of religion in reducing cancer risk through altered behaviors related to known risk factors, and supporting positive coping with cancer has also been documented (4–10). However, religion has also been associated with poor adjustment (4,11). This evidence points to the importance of including an assessment of religious needs and resources in a holistic assessment of cancer patients and their families.

Distinctions can be made between the religious and the spiritual aspects of life (4). Spirituality refers to the more personal search for meaning and purpose in life, while religion refers to beliefs and practices associated with organized groups such as churches or synagogues. These aspects of life overlap and we will use the terms interchangeably unless otherwise indicated.

We begin this chapter with a discussion of some background issues about spiritual assessment: what it is, why it is important, how to do it, and who may do it. This is followed by brief descriptions of several models for spiritual assessment and guidelines which can be used to evaluate these different models. Then we describe issues in research on religion and health and several instruments which can be used to measure religion in such research. Following this we discuss the application of this research to the development of tools for spiritual screening. Finally, our discussion will turn to characteristic spiritual interventions with cancer patients and their families.

BACKGROUND ISSUES IN SPIRITUAL ASSESSMENT

At this point in the evolution of spiritual assessment, most of the important models were not developed for specific patient populations, and no models specifically for use with cancer patients and their families have been published. The models for spiritual assessment we describe were developed for use in different contexts where spiritual care is provided; however, they are applicable for work with cancer patients and their families.

Spiritual assessment is the process of discerning the spiritual needs and resources of persons in various contexts where spiritual care is offered. Like diagnostic models in psychology and social work, spiritual assessment does not simply focus on a person's problems, but includes the resources the person brings to help them cope with those problems. As in other fields, it is possible to conduct brief spiritual screening, to identify patients at risk for spiritual crisis. However, this is not the same as spiritual assessment which is a more indepth and extensive process.

Spiritual assessment is important because it improves a caregiver's ability to be accountable for the spiritual care they provide. What are the goals of spiritual care with a particular person? How do we know if the care being provided is the care the person needs? How do caregivers guard against projecting their needs and assumptions onto the person being cared for? In order to answer these important questions we require a way to describe the spiritual care we think a person needs. Spiritual assessments provides caregivers with a way to talk with a patient, or other person with whom they are working, to see if they share their understanding of their spiritual needs and agree with the kind of spiritual care being suggested. Spiritual assessments also provide a way to talk with and consult with staff colleagues about our understanding of a patient's spiritual needs and our goals for spiritual care with them.

Many caregivers welcome the idea of being more explicit about the spiritual dimension of their work. They also welcome being more accountable for the goals of their spiritual care, but they do not like the idea of spiritual assessment. Four objections to spiritual assessment have been raised. First, some caregivers argue that the spiritual dimension of life is ineffable. To try to subject it to objective assessment is seen as either foolish or risking serious distortion of true spirituality. Second, some caregivers are concerned that spiritual assessment requires spiritual care to be impersonal, forcing chaplains and other spiritual caregivers to enter patient's rooms with a clipboard and a list of questions. Third, some caregivers believe spiritual assessment is incompatible with their use of intuition in caregiving. Finally, some caregivers are concerned that spiritual assessment will violate patient confidentiality.

The aim of spiritual assessment is not to exhaust the complexity or mystery of the spiritual dimension of life. The aim is to organize observations about people's spiritual beliefs, behaviors, and relationships in ways that enhance caregiving. Doing spiritual assessment need not alter a caregiver's use of open-ended conversations, or sensitive and empathic responses to the needs and feelings of the person with whom they are working. Nor does an interest in spiritual assessment require any compromise in building trusting relationships with those to whom spiritual care is offered. A caregiver's spiritual assessment is their summary of key issues in the patient's spiritual needs and resources, formulated according to a specific model, often after an open-ended or semistructured conversation.

Intuition, understood as the rapid and sometimes preconscious gathering of information, can be a resource for spiritual assessment. To be more effective in spiritual assessment, caregivers who rely strongly on intuition may need to practice taking time to recall and record the observations which contributed to their impressions. Finally, spiritual assessment does not require spiritual caregivers to report or chart everything a patient shares with them. The same judgment caregivers currently use in communicating important information and in protecting patient privacy and confidentiality can be employed in spiritual assessment.

As with assessment in other fields, spiritual assessment is an open-ended process. The pressure to provide spiritual care in a crisis or other critical situation often makes it impossible to learn all that we would like to know about a person or family before we must begin to offer spiritual care. In such cases we gather the information that is essential and we begin to offer the care that is needed. At the same time we look for an opportunity to gather additional helpful information. As we work with a patient over time we should continue to revise and develop our assessment and care plan based on the additional knowledge and understanding which emerges.

One need not be an ordained clergy person or chaplain, or a person of deep religious or spiritual conviction, in order to conduct spiritual assessments or offer spiritual care. In fact, as will be seen below, colleagues in psychology, nursing, and medicine have made important contributions to this subject. What is required is an understanding of the spiritual dimension of life and training in the process of spiritual assessment and care. This knowledge and skill can be obtained in a variety of academic and clinical training programs. One of the oldest organizations providing such training, for clergy, seminarians, and others, is the Association for Clinical Pastoral Education (1549 Clairmont Road, Suite 103, Decatur, GA 30033-4611, U.S.A. Tel: 404-320-1472). There are Association accredited training centers across the United States and programs accredited by cognate organizations worldwide.

EARLY MODELS FOR SPIRITUAL ASSESSMENT

Although discernment of signs of religious or spiritual maturity is probably as old as religion, the modern roots of spiritual assessment can be traced to the beginning of this century. In his *Varieties of Religious Experience* (12), the psychologist Williams James distinguished two fundamental approaches to religion, the healthy-minded or once-born and the sick soul or twice-born. James described the healthy-minded as congenitally happy persons who see everything in life as good. In contrast, he described the sick soul as "peculiarly sensitive to life's discordances. Struck by the precariousness of existence, the ubiquity of suffering, and the inevitability of death, an individual of this inclination finds evil to be an essential clue to the world's dimly perceived meaning" (13, p 485). While obviously oversimplified, James' description reminds us that religious people are not all identical. Further, his two types are often confirmed by our observations of ourselves and our colleagues. They have obvious significance for understanding some of the differences in how our patients and their families cope with the experience of having cancer.

A pioneer in the development of modern pastoral care, Anton Boisen (1876–1965), was one of the first to develop a formal method of religious assessment and apply it in his ministry and research with seriously ill psychiatric patients and in his pioneering clinical training program for seminarians (14,15). Boisen's assessment outline included: a medical and psychiatric history, a detailed background psychosocial history, and many questions regarding the patient's specific religious beliefs and practices (15,16). Later, the psychiatrist Edgar Draper demonstrated that a psychiatrist could make an accurate psychiatric diagnosis using only information about the patient's religious beliefs (17). The religious interview schedule Draper used in this study became somewhat popular and formed the basis of several models for religious assessment developed for both pastors and nurses (18–22).

SELECTED MODELS FOR SPIRITUAL ASSESSMENT

There was little further development in spiritual assessment until the psychologist Paul Pruyser published his important book, *The Minister as Diagnostician* (23). While Pruyser's intent was to convince clergy of the importance of spiritual assessment, rather than propose a definitive model for such assessments, the absence of other models for spiritual assessment led many interested chaplains to adopt Pruyser's seven guidelines for spiritual assessment (24–27). In his guidelines, Pruyser suggested that pastors attend to seven aspects of a person's religious life: awareness of the holy, providence, faith, grace or gratefulness, repentance, communion, and sense of vocation. Table 68.1 summarizes each of these seven areas.

Among the models for spiritual assessment based on Pruyser, the model developed by Stoddard et al. is one of the most useful (26,28). As can be seen from Table 68.2, the model focuses on four areas: concept of God, subjective meaning of illness; approach to hoping; and relation to support system. Stoddard et al. provide a helpful discussion of how assessment should be conducted and relate assessment to the other steps in the clinical care process. They also provide samples of the tools they developed for internal department use, for teaching, and for the patient's record. Allison (29) has developed an interesting graphic version of this model.

Several physicians have developed models for spiritual assessment (30–32). Kuhn's descriptive, multidimensional model employs a functional approach to defining the spiritual dimension of life. That is, Kuhn examines how a person makes meaning in their life rather than assessing their specific religious beliefs. Kuhn's inventory describes seven aspects of spirituality. For each aspect he offers a definition or description, provides some discussion of the salience of that aspect for the physician–patient relationship, and suggests five brief questions which may be asked to elicit information about this aspect of the patient's spiritual

TABLE 68.1. *Pruyser's Guidelines for Pastoral Diagnosis*

1. Awareness of the Holy
   What if anything is sacred, revered
   Any experiences of awe or bliss, when, in what situations
   Any sense of mystery, of anything transcendent
   Any sense of creatureliness, humility, awareness of own limitations
   Any idolatry, reverence displaced to improper symbols

2. Providence
   What is God's intention toward me
   What has God promised me
   Related to capacity for trust
   Extent of hoping versus wishing

3. Faith
   Affirming versus negating stance in life
   Able to commit self, to engage
   Open to world or constricted

4. Grace or Gratefulness
   Kindness, generosity, the beauty of giving and receiving
   No felt need for grace or gratefulness
   Forced gratitude under any circumstances
   Desire for versus resistance to blessing

5. Repentance
   The process of change from crookedness to rectitude
   A sense of agency in one's own problems or one's response to them being a victim versus being too sorry for debatable sins
   Feelings of contrition, remorse, regret
   Willingness to do penance

6. Communion
   Feelings of kinship with the whole chain of being
   Feeling embedded or estranged, united or separated in the world, in relations with one's faith group, one's church

7. Sense of Vocation
   Willingness to be a cheerful participant in creation
   Signs of zest, vigor, liveliness, dedication
   Aligned with divine benevolence or malevolence
   Humorous and inventive involvement in life versus grim and dogmatic

Source: Pruyser (23).

life. Kuhn suggests that sufficient information regarding the patient's spiritual life can be elicited by using a few of the questions for each item in the inventory. As can be seen from Table 68.3, the seven aspects of spirituality in Kuhn's model are: the attachment of meaning or purpose, belief and faith, love, forgiveness, prayer, capacity for quiet and meditation, and worship.

In contrast to the work of Kuhn is the model developed by another physician, McSherry (32–37). McSherry has emphasized the importance of a

TABLE 68.2. *Stoddard's Spiritual Assessment Instrument*

1. Concept of God (awareness of the holy)

    What has been most important for you in your life?

    What are the things that you have found most meaningful during the past year?

2. Subjective Meaning of Illness (sense of providence, grace, repentance)

    What does it mean to you that you've become ill?

    How have you been making sense of what has happened to you?

3. Approach to Hoping (faith, vocation)

    How have you kept a sense of hope in the past?

    What does having hope mean for you at the present time?

4. Relation to Support System (communion)

    How have you felt your family has been doing with this illness?

    Who have you felt has been able to be most supportive of you in this time?

Source: Stoddard and Burns-Haney (26).

quantitative approach to spiritual assessment to allow the impact of spiritual care to be measured. Her model was designed to take advantage of computerized record keeping. While her model employs some substantive categories of evangelical Protestantism (e.g., a personal relationship with God), and therefore may not be suitable for all patients, it demonstrates one approach to meeting the challenge of documenting changes resulting from spiritual care.

Chaplain Gary Berg, building on McSherry's work, developed a comprehensive computer program for spiritual assessment suitable for use with persons from a variety of religious backgrounds (38) (Chaplain Gary Berg, Living Water Software, 1203 7th Avenue North, St. Cloud, MN 56303, U.S.A. Tel: 320-253-5437). The program has seven sections. Four dimensions of religion are measured, including organizational religious activity, nonorganizational religious activity, intrinsic religiousness, and spiritual injury. The three other sections address ultimate values (based on Rokeach's Ultimate Values Test), loss and life changes (based on the Holmes–Rehe life stress scale as modified by Westberg), and whether the patient has or wishes to have advance directives.

The Spiritual Injury Scale in Berg's program is an original contribution and a fine example of a spiritual assessment scale which may be relevant for patients from a variety of religious traditions. It appears to have strong potential for separate use as a resource for spiritual screening or triage. As can be seen from Table 68.4, Berg's Spiritual Injury Scale focuses on seven areas: guilt, resentment, grief, despair, God being unfair, doubt, and fear of death.

Colleagues in nursing have a longstanding interest in spiritual assessment and have published a number of models (22,39,40). One of the most highly developed models for nursing spiritual assessment stems from the work of the North American Nursing Diagnosis Association (NANDA). Over a period of almost 20 years NANDA has developed a list of conditions which nurses are qualified to diagnose and treat. Spiritual distress is an approved nursing diagnosis. It is defined as "disruption in the life principle that pervades a person's entire being and that integrates and transcends one's biological and psychosocial nature." This model identifies two possible causal factors for spiritual distress, separation from religious and cultural ties and a challenged belief and value system. As can be seen from Table 68.5, over 20 specific defining characteristics are part of the diagnosis.

Other important approaches to spiritual assessment have also been published. For example, Steven Ivy has described a model based on the important concept of faith development (41), while Shulevitz and Springer (42) have proposed a model based on distinctive aspects of Jewish religious beliefs and practices. A helpful resource for exploration of different models for spiritual assessment is Fitchett (43), an annotated bibliography of 27 published models.

The 7 × 7 Model for Spiritual Assessment

The 7 × 7 model for spiritual assessment, developed by Fitchett, is widely used in spiritual care as well as in training chaplains and pastors (44). The 7 × 7 model employs a functional approach to spiritual assessment. A functional approach to spiritual assessment is concerned with how a person finds meaning and purpose in life and with the behavior, emotions, relationships and practices associated with that meaning and purpose. The functional approach to spiritual assessment can be contrasted to a substantive approach. The former inquires in an open-ended way about a person's ultimate concern. An example of the latter would be to ask whether or not a person believes in God. In a spiritually pluralistic context, such as a hospital, the functional approach to spiritual assessment is preferable. This approach permits spiritual assessment across a wide spectrum of religious beliefs and practices, including people who wrestle with spiritual issues while having no specific religious affiliation. The functional approach to spiritual assessment offers a greater possibility that a person can share their spiritual story using their own terms versus having to organize their story around the ideas of one particular substantive religious-spiritual world view or another.

TABLE 68.3. *Kuhn's Spiritual Inventory*

1. The Attachment of Meaning or Purpose

   Why do you think you have become ill now?
   Has this illness changed any attitudes you might have about the future?
   Is there anything more important to you than regaining your health?
   How does this illness interfere with your goals in life?
   What is the purpose of regaining your health?

2. Belief and Faith

   What things do you believe in or have faith in?
   Has this illness influenced your faith?
   How do you exercise faith in your life?
   How has your faith influenced your behavior during this illness?
   What role does your faith play in regaining your health?

3. Love

   Is there any person or group of people that you would say you truly love?
   What is the most loving things that you have ever done?
   What is the most loving thing ever done to you or for you?
   What is the significance of the Golden Rule to you?
   Is there any person or group for whom you would gladly give your life?

4. Forgiveness

   Are you able to forget about times when people offend you or do you hold a grudge?
   Do you feel guilty about anything in your life?
   Do you wish others to feel guilty about things they have done to you?
   What is meant by "let bygones be bygones"?
   How can a person make it up to another person when he has hurt or offended him?

5. Prayer

   Do you pray?
   When do you pray?
   What is your prayer?
   How are your prayers answered?
   What do you think is meant by "the power of prayer"?

6. Capacity for Quiet and Meditation

   Do you ever spend time just being quiet?
   Do you meditate?
   Do you enjoy being alone in a quiet place?
   Do you know how to relax your body completely?
   Have you ever tried to empty your mind of all thoughts for a brief time?

7. Worship

   What is the most powerful or important thing in your life?
   Upon what do you depend the most when things go wrong?
   What do you worship?
   Do you participate in any religious activities?
   What do you consider the most significant act of worship in your life?

Source: Kuhn (30).

TABLE 68.4. *Berg's Spiritual Injury Scale**

	Very often 4	Often 3	Sometimes 2	Never 1
1. How often do you feel guilty over past behaviors?				
2. Does anger or resentment block your peace of mind?				
3. How often do you feel sad or experience grief?				
4. Do you feel that life has no meaning or purpose?				
5. How often do you feel despair or hopeless?				
6. Do you feel that God/life has treated you unfairly?				
7. Do you worry about your doubts/disbelief in God?				
8. Do you worry about or fear death?				

* Chaplain Gary Berg, Living Water Software, 1203 7th Avenue North, St. Cloud, MN 56303, U.S.A. Tel: 320-253-5437.

The 7 × 7 model employs a multidimensional view of spirituality. This view reflects an understanding of the complexity of the spiritual dimension of life, encompassing beliefs, behavior, emotions, relationships, and practices. This view can be contrasted with a one-dimensional model of spirituality, for example, a model which describes what church a person is a member of, or a model which describes a person's beliefs about God.

The 7 × 7 model places spiritual assessment in the context of a holistic assessment. The spiritual dimension of life affects and is affected by other dimensions of life. A person's medical or psychological status can have a profound impact on their spirituality as can factors associated with their psychosocial or racial/ethnic background.

The 7 × 7 model for spiritual assessment has two broad divisions, a holistic assessment and a multidimensional spiritual assessment. The specific elements considered in the model are illustrated in Table 68.6.

In the holistic assessment, the 7 × 7 model examines the following six dimensions of a person's life:

TABLE 68.5. *Defining Characteristics for North American Nursing Diagnostic Association Diagnosis Spiritual Distress*

Expresses concern with meaning of life and death and/or belief system

Anger toward God (as defined by the person)

Questions meaning of suffering

Verbalizes inner conflict about beliefs

Verbalizes concern about relationship with deity

Questions meaning of own existence

Unable to choose or chooses not to participate in usual religious practices

Seeks spiritual assistance

Questions moral and ethical implications of therapeutic regimen

Displacement of anger toward religious representatives

Description of nightmares or sleep disturbances

Alteration in behavior or mood evidenced by: anger, crying, withdrawal, preoccupation, anxiety, hostility, apathy, etc.

Regards illness as punishment

Does not experience that God is forgiving

Unable to accept self

Engages in self-blame

Denies responsibility for problems

Description of somatic complaints

Source: Kim et al. (40).

TABLE 68.6. *The 7 x 7 Model for Spiritual Assessment*

Holistic Assessment	Spiritual Assessment
Biological (Medical) Dimension	Belief and Meaning
Psychological Dimension	Vocation and Obligations
Family Systems Dimension	Experience and Emotions
Psychosocial Dimension	Courage and Growth
Ethnic, Racial, Cultural Dimension	Ritual and Practice
Social Issues Dimensions	Community
Spiritual Dimension	Authority and Guidance

Source: Fitchett (44).

1. *Medical Dimension*. What significant medical problems has the person had in the past? What problems do they have now? What treatment is the person receiving?
2. *Psychological Dimension*. Are there any significant psychological problems? Are they being treated? If so, how?
3. *Family Systems Dimension*. Are there at present, or have there been in the past, patterns within the person's relationships with other family members which have contributed to or perpetuated present problems?
4. *Psychosocial Dimension*. What is the history of the person's life, including, place of birth and childhood home, family of origin, education, work history and other important activities and relationships? What is the person's present living situation and what are their financial resources?
5. *Ethnic, Racial or Cultural Dimension*. What is the person's racial, ethnic or cultural background? How does it contribute to the person's way of addressing any current concerns?
6. *Social Issues Dimension*. Are the present problems of the person created by or compounded by larger social policies, social institutions, or the absence of them?

The spiritual dimension is the seventh holistic dimension considered in the 7 × 7 model. The model examines the following seven dimensions of a person's spiritual life:

1. *Belief and Meaning*. What beliefs does the person have which give meaning and purpose to their life? What major symbols reflect or express meaning for this person? What is the person's story? Do any current problems have a specific meaning or alter established meaning? Is the person presently or have they in the past been affiliated with a formal system of belief (e.g., church, synagogue, mosque)?

2. *Duties and Obligations*. Do the persons' beliefs and sense of meaning in life create a sense of duty, vocation, calling or moral obligation? Will any current problems cause conflict or compromise in their perception of their ability to fulfill these duties? Are any current problems viewed as a sacrifice or atonement or are they otherwise essential to this person's sense of duty?
3. *Experience and Emotion*. What direct contacts with the sacred, divine, or demonic has the person had? What emotions or moods are predominantly associated with these contacts and with the person's beliefs, meaning in life and associated sense of vocation?
4. *Courage and Growth*. Must the meaning of new experiences, including any current problems, be fit into existing beliefs and symbols? Can the person let go of existing beliefs and symbols in order to allow new ones to emerge?
5. *Ritual and Practice*. What are the rituals and practices associated with the person's beliefs and meaning in life? Will current problems, if any, cause a change in the rituals or practices they feel they require or in their ability to perform or participate in those which are important to them?
6. *Community*. Is the person part of one or more, formal or informal, communities of shared belief, meaning in life, ritual or practice? What is the style of the person's participation in these communities?
7. *Authority and Guidance*. Where does the person find the authority for their beliefs, meaning in life, for their vocation, their rituals and practices? When faced with doubt, confusion, tragedy or conflict, where do they look for guidance? To what extent does the person look within or without for guidance?

As caregivers seek to be more explicit about the spiritual dimension of their assessment and care, the 7 × 7 model can be a helpful resource. It places spiritual assessment in a holistic context and focuses on a number of important dimensions in the spiritual aspect of life. It assists in elaborating a distinctly spiritual perspective regarding a person without ignoring insights from the behavioral sciences. Its functional approach to spirituality makes it suitable for work with people from diverse spiritual and religious backgrounds.

Guidelines for Evaluating Models for Spiritual Assessment

Pruyser's challenge to pastors and chaplains to bring pastoral diagnosis back into their ministry highlighted the need to find a language with which to name and address the spiritual dimension of life. That language must have four attributes. It must be useful in the spiritually pluralistic contexts in which spiritual care is offered. It must be dynamic, allowing caregivers to incorporate insights from other perspectives, especially psychology, into their assessments and treatment. It must be multidimensional, attending to behavioral and interpersonal aspects of spirituality, and not just the dimension of belief. Finally, it must be, as Pruyser urged, a distinct perspective, not just a restatement of the psychosocial perspective.

In evaluating different models for spiritual assessment which may be considered for clinical use, or in developing their own models, caregivers should consider six issues: applicable contexts, concept of spirituality, relation to other disciplines, concept of norms and authority, connection to caregiving, and user friendliness. We will elaborate briefly on each of these issues. (For the application of these guidelines in evaluating various published models for spiritual assessment, see Fitchett (43,44).)

1. *Applicable Contexts*—One of the first and most practical things we need to know about an assessment model is the context for which it was developed and any additional contexts in which it can be employed. Some models may have wide applicability across age, gender, faith group, and health status lines. Other models may have more restricted applicability. For example, Berg's model, mentioned above, was developed for spiritual care in a psychiatric hospital, but it can be used in many different contexts.

2. *Concept of Spirituality*—One of the most important features of a model for spiritual assessment will be its underlying concept of spirituality or theological framework. For some models, the author's theological beliefs gave explicit shape to his or her assessment model. For others the theological background is more implicit (e.g., Pruyser). One approach in this area is to use the beliefs of one confessional tradition to shape the assessment questions. This is sometimes referred to as a substantive approach. A contrasting approach takes a more functional look at *how* religious beliefs or practices serve a person, rather than specifically examining *what* the beliefs and practices are. In this area it is also important to see if the model treats spirituality as unidimensional: does it explore only beliefs or only practices for example, or does it have a multidimensional approach, looking at a number of the ways religion is manifest in human life. In a similar manner, we want to know if the model sees spirituality as static or as a process. If it has a process view of spirituality, does it have specific norms for how the spiritual life progresses? Finally, does the model take religious beliefs and behavior at face value, or does it support a hermeneutic of suspicion which allows for a dynamic exploration of their meaning?

3. *Relation to Other Disciplines*—What relation between religion and other aspects of human life is assumed or expressed in the model? Is religion treated in isolation from other aspects of life, or are the linkages between religion, culture, personality, family, and health, for example, considered in the model? If the model recognizes the linkage between the spiritual and the psychosocial dimensions of life, does it describe how they are distinct?

4. *Norms and Authority*—Every model of assessment expresses a set of norms against which a patient, counselee, or parishioner is being assessed. Are the norms explicit and how is the authority of the respective parties in the assessment process conceptualized? Does the patient or parishioner have a passive or more active role in focusing the process and defining its results?

5. *Connection to the Caregiving Process*—The purpose of assessment is to inform spiritual care. In looking at models of assessment we also want to look at how the model fits the caregiving process. Does it direct our attention to information we feel is important to inform and shape our caregiving? Does it provide direction for interpreting the information that is gathered or leave the interpretation to the judgment of the caregiver? Similarly, does it provide direction for developing a care plan based on the assessment or is that work left to the caregiver?

6. *User Friendliness*—Finally, we want to look at some very practical aspects of the assessment model. How much training is required to understand and use it? How long does it take to complete? Does it

summarize its conclusions in a manner that patients or counselees will be able to understand for themselves or in a way that professionals from other disciplines will be able to understand?

Using these guidelines caregivers can evaluate the suitability of different models for spiritual assessment for their setting or develop their own model.

MEASURING RELIGION IN RESEARCH

While many studies have documented the influence of religion on physical and mental health, much work remains in explicating and testing various theoretical models which may explain these complex relationships. In their review of the literature, Levin and Vanderpool (45) identified six theoretical possibilities to be considered: religiously prescribed behavior, psychosocial effects, psychodynamics of religious belief systems, psychodynamics of religious rites, psychodynamics of religious faith, and superempirical or supernatural influences. Additionally, several authors have tested the multiple influences of religion in a stress-coping model, a theoretical framework which may have important applications in work with cancer patients and their families (4,46–48). This work has been extended to test the specific model for the stress-buffering role of religion (suppressor, moderator, or distress-deterrent) (49).

There has been considerable methodological progress in the scientific study of religion in the past 20 years. It is no longer adequate to test whether a one-dimensional measure of religion, such as affiliation or frequency of attendance at public worship, is associated with adjustment to cancer. Investigators who wish to explore the relationship between religion and cancer risk or adjustment to cancer, using one or more of these models, must employ a multidimensional conceptualization of religion and select measures of the specific dimensions of religion which are appropriate for each study. A variety of instruments are available for investigators who wish to include one or more measures of religion in their research. (For a helpful discussion see ref. 4.) Six research instruments which can be useful in such research will be briefly described here.

1. *A Three-dimensional Measure of Religiosity.*
   Chatters et al. (50) have reported confirmation of a twelve-item, three dimensional model of religiosity. The model was tested with a sample of 446 Black Americans, age 65 and older. The three dimensions in the model are organizational religious activity ("How often do you usually attend religious services?"), non-organizational religious

activity ("How often do you read religious books or other religious materials?"), and subjective religiosity ("How religious would you say you are?"). The factor structure which emerged from this study is consistent with the findings from a number of other studies. The three dimensions of religiosity in this model are the three most important and the minimum number of dimensions which investigators should consider in any broad study of the effects of religion on cancer risk and adjustment to cancer.

2. *Systems of Belief Inventory.* Kash et al. (51) have reported the development of the fifteen item Systems of Belief Inventory (SBI). Two hundred and forty healthy individuals and 117 patients with malignant melanoma were given a fifty-four item version of this instrument. Factor analysis yielded two factors, beliefs and practices ("Religion is important in my day-to-day life." "I pray for help during bad times.") and social support from a religious community ("I seek out people in my religious or spiritual community when I need help."). Based on this analysis the scale was shortened to fifteen items. Social support from one's religious community has been suggested as an important factor in the association between religion and health. The inclusion of this factor in the SBI makes this an important tool with which to study the role of religion in coping with cancer and quality of life.

3. *Religious Problem-solving and Coping Activities.* Pargament et al. have conducted extensive research on religion and coping with stressful life events (46, 47,52,53). They have described three styles of religious problem solving: deferring, self-directing, and collaborative (54). Individuals with a deferring style defer responsibility for problem solving to God. Those with a self-directing style take an active problem solving stance in which God is not directly involved. In the collaborative problem solving style, responsibility for problem solving is held jointly by the individual and God.

   Pargament and colleagues have also described six types of religious coping activities. They are: spiritually based coping ("I trusted that God would not let anything terrible happen to me."), religious good deeds ("I provided help to other church members."), religious discontent ("I felt angry with or distant from God."), religious support ("I received support from other members of the church."), pleading ("I bargained with God to make things better."), and religious avoidance ("I prayed or read the Bible to keep my mind off of my problems.") (4,52). In more recent work Pargament reports a two factor model of positive and negative religious coping has emerged from a study of church members in Oklahoma City coping with the April, 1995 bombing of the federal building in that city (Pargament, 1996, personal communication).

The application of these instruments to religion and health research is just beginning. Bickel (55) examined the role of religious coping and depression in a sample of 245 adult church members. He found that in persons with high levels of perceived stress, higher levels of depression were associated with greater use of a self-directing religious coping style, and lower levels of depression were associated with greater use of a collaborative religious coping style. This is consistent with preliminary results from a study by Fitchett and colleagues which found that self-directed coping was positively associated with depression ($r = .31$, $P = .01$) and negatively associated with quality of life ($r = -.30$, $r = .03$) in a sample of 50 head and neck cancer patients. Jenkins also reports that greater use of plead and discontent coping activities was associated with higher levels of depression and loneliness in 422 persons with HIV infection (56).

Pargament et al. report that religious coping activity is predictive of psychological and religious adjustment to stressful life events, even when controlling for the effect of other dimensions of religiosity such as organizational religious activity or intrinsic religious orientation (52). Inclusion of measures of religious problem-solving style and coping activities in future research should expand our understanding of the role of religion in coping with cancer. Such research may also point to ways to include these constructs in spiritual assessment and screening instruments which may help identify persons whose religious problem-solving style or coping activities contribute to poor coping which might then become the focus of education or spiritual care interventions.

4. *Index of Core Spiritual Experience.* Kass (57) has developed a brief measure of core spiritual experiences (INSPIRIT). Kass theorizes that people who report a greater sense of closeness to God, or other similar spiritual experiences, will have decreased ontological anxiety and this will be associated with better health and adjustment to stress. Among patients in a 10 week behavioral medicine program, Kass reports that those who had core spiritual experiences had greater decreases in the frequency of stress-related medical symptoms than those who did not have such experiences. They also

reported higher increases in life purpose and satisfaction (58). Kass' work points to an often neglected dimension of spirituality which may play a role in adjustment to cancer. Kass' scale will appeal to investigators who are looking for a measure which focuses on the spiritual rather than the religious dimension of life.

5. *Religious Orientation.* One of the oldest and most widely used measures of religion focuses on religious orientation. As originally proposed by Allport and Ross (59), there were two religious orientations, intrinsic and extrinsic. They wrote that "the extrinsically motivated person uses his religion, whereas the intrinsically motivated person lives his religion" (59, p 434). Later, Batson proposed a third orientation, quest, "the degree to which an individual's religion involves an open-ended, responsive dialogue with existential questions raised by the contradictions and tragedies of life" (60).

These scales and their underlying theoretical formulations have been the subject of extensive debate (61,62). The most widely used versions of these measures are: intrinsic (63), extrinsic (64), and quest (60). Measures of intrinsic and extrinsic religious orientation have been employed in a number of studies with cancer patients. In general it appears that higher intrinsic orientation is associated with better psychological adjustment among cancer patients (4).

6. *Spiritual Well-being.* Ellison and Paloutzian's Spiritual Well-Being Scale (SWBS) has become a popular tool for research on the relationship of religion and health (65–67). The scale has two 10 item sub-scales, religious well-being and existential well-being. Religious well-being is conceptualized as one's relationship to God. A typical item is, "I have a personally meaningful relationship with God." Existential well-being is conceptualized as life purpose and satisfaction. A typical item is, "I believe there is some real purpose for my life."

Several studies have examined the role of spiritual well-being in quality of life for persons with cancer. In a study of 175 women with breast cancer, spiritual well-being was significantly associated with hope independent of prognosis ($r = .66$, $P < .001$) (8). Another study looked at the relation of spiritual well-being and anxiety in a sample of 114 persons with cancer. Subjects varied in the type of cancer they had and the length of time since diagnosis. There was a significant negative correlation between state-trait anxiety and spiritual well-being ($r = -.44$, $P < .001$) (7). In an unpublished study of 25 cancer inpatients, Fitchett and Cella found that spiritual well-being was positively associated with quality of life ($r = .53$, $P < .01$).

An examination of the psychometric properties of the SWBS reveals that the instrument has a ceiling effect and while able to discriminate those with low spiritual well-being, it is less effective in discriminating between subjects with average and high spiritual well-being (68). Further, the scale employs a conceptualization of religious well-being that is most consistent with evangelical Protestantism, a meaningful personal relationship with God. Thus it is not surprising that studies have shown that evangelical Christians—who identify themselves as "born again" score higher than ethical Christians, those who accept the moral teachings of Jesus (65). The SWBS may be best suited for research with populations who share its underlying view of spiritual maturity.

SPIRITUAL SCREENING

As noted above, spiritual assessment is not the same as spiritual screening or triage. Spiritual screening refers to the methods used to identify persons at risk for a spiritual crisis, those who request spiritual care, or those for whom more careful spiritual assessment should be completed. At present the simple models for spiritual screening which have been published are designed for general use in the inpatient context. Montonye (69) has described the development and use of a process in which, during the admitting process, nurses ask patients about their need for a chaplain's visit, for assistance in contacting their own clergy, receiving sacraments, or helping with other spiritual needs. Derrickson (70) has described a procedure in which trained volunteers visit and welcome newly admitted patients. After the visit the volunteers record their observations about the patient's stresses (potential effect of illness on changes in life; other concurrent life changes; gravity of prognosis), and resources (understanding of illness and hospital routines; support from family and friends; spirituality as a source of strength). These observations then permit the staff chaplains to prioritize their work schedules.

Carpenito (71) proposed a set of "Focus Assessment Criteria" for use by nurses as part of an overall psychosocial assessment (Table 68.7). These questions

TABLE 68.7. *Focus Assessment Criteria*

SUBJECTIVE DATA
Assess for defining characteristics
What is your source of spiritual strength or meaning?
How do you practice your spiritual beliefs?
Are there any practices that are important for your spiritual well-being?
Do you have a spiritual leader?
Has being ill or hurt affected your spiritual beliefs?
Assess for related factors
How can I help you maintain your spiritual strength (e.g. contact spiritual leader, provide privacy at special times, request reading materials)?
OBJECTIVE DATA
Assess for defining characteristics
Current practices
The presence of religious or spiritual articles (clothing, medals, texts)
Visits from spiritual leader
Visits to place of worship or meditation
Requests for spiritual counseling or assistance
Response to interview on spiritual needs
Grief
Anxiety
Doubt
Anger
Participation in spiritual practices
Rejection or neglect of previous practices
Increased interest in spiritual matters

Source: Carpenito (71).

both gather the data necessary for medical caregivers and signal to the patient that religion and faith can be discussed openly.

Building on early work by NANDA, Stoddard (72) has described four levels of increasing spiritual need: no spiritual concern, spiritual concern, spiritual distress, and spiritual despair (Table 68.8). Need-defining characteristics have been identified for each level. For example, the defining characteristics for spiritual concern are verbalizing inner conflict about beliefs with mild anxiety. For spiritual despair two defining characteristics are loss of hope and loss of spiritual belief. Stoddard has trained the staff in his hospital to screen patients and make referrals to the chaplain based on this framework.

Many hospital chaplaincy departments are in the process of developing and refining procedures for spiritual screening. At Memorial Sloan-Kettering Cancer Center, patients are asked on admission whether religion is part of their coping, whether they wish to see a chaplain, and whether there are any religious or cultural practices they wish to continue while in the hospital. Most patients are also visited by a volunteer who assesses their religious needs. A brief collection of these procedures has been published in the newsletter of the National Association of Catholic Chaplains (*Vision, The Newsletter of the NACC*, 1996; 6(3):10–24. National Association of Catholic Chaplains, 3501

South Lake Drive, Milwaukee, WI 53207-0473, U.S.A. Tel: 414-483-4898). Most of these procedures involve checklists of types of contact, spiritual needs, interventions, and patient responses listed either on data cards or computer screens. The checklists facilitate the documentation of an assessment and a care plan as well as data gathering. Berg's spiritual injury scale, noted above, could also easily be used for spiritual screening. Chaplains who have instituted procedures for spiritual screening report better referrals, more effective use of the chaplain's time, and, in some cases, increased referrals for spiritual care.

FUTURE DIRECTIONS IN SPIRITUAL ASSESSMENT AND SCREENING

Much work is needed in the area of spiritual assessment and screening, and research on religion and cancer. Spiritual assessment tools which reflect the specific spiritual challenges associated with cancer diagnosis for adults and children need to be developed and tested. Screening tools for cancer patients who are at risk for spiritual crisis or despair also need to be developed. Spiritual caregivers will need to document whether such tools assist in more accurate descriptions of the spiritual needs and resources of these patients and in more effective spiritual care.

TABLE 68.8. *Levels of Spiritual Need*

0	No spiritual concerns	No spiritual content expressed by patient or family concerning hospital stay.
1	Spiritual concerns — mild	Anxiety Concerns with God Anticipatory Grieving Questions of Meaning
2	Spiritual distress — marked	Conflicting beliefs Searching for alternative beliefs Struggling to find meaning in life or death Seeking spiritual aid Disturbed God concept Ethical dilemma Moderate/severe anxiety Disturbed sleep Grieving
3	Spiritual despair — marked	Social withdrawal Loss of meaning Severe depression Death wish
4	Crisis ministry	ONE CONTACT medical emergencies: "house staff" or "Code Blue"
5	Crisis ministry	Medical emergencies requiring follow-up beyond the crisis event

Source: Stoddard (72).

The development both of tools for spiritual assessment and tools for spiritual screening should take note of recent findings in open heart surgery patients. Research studies have found that open heart surgery patients with a low level of acceptance or who receive no strength or comfort from religion are at a greater risk for postoperative morbidity and mortality (73,74). These findings could be incorporated into a simple spiritual screening tool for heart surgery patients. Patients with low scores would be referred for further spiritual assessment and possible spiritual care. Since research in religious problem solving and coping suggests that certain religious problem solving styles and religious coping styles may be associated with poor adjustment to stressful events, further research should examine the role of these and other aspects of religion in the lives of cancer patients and their families.

SPIRITUAL AND RELIGIOUS INTERVENTIONS

Spiritual and religious interventions can and should be performed by all medical and mental health professionals. Any caregiver, no matter what their personal faith stance, can assist patients with spiritual issues. Some still believe that a caregiver can only discuss religion helpfully with a patient of the same belief. This logic is identical to saying that one can only help a patient who uses the same kinds of coping mechanisms that you do.

Working with religious and spiritual issues follows the same pattern. The question is not, "Do I think this person's beliefs are right or wrong?", but "Are this person's religious beliefs and practices helpful to him or her in coping with illness?" Our job is not to accept or reject these beliefs but to try to understand them and help the patient to use them to full advantage in coping with their illness. A number of resources are available for the caregiver who wishes to gain a greater understanding of the role of religious beliefs and practices in coping with cancer (6,75–83).

SELF-ASSESSMENT

As a first step, the caregiver must seek to understand his or her own religious beliefs, biases and feelings in order to avoid the transferences and countertransferences inherent in this process. In other words, we need to assess ourselves. The point of this introspection is not necessarily to decide definitely what we believe and do not believe. Religious faith is dynamic for most people. Our beliefs and doubts tend to change over time. It is as important to discover where our doubts and uncertainties are as to know what we definitely believe. It is critically important to discover what feelings we have about our beliefs or lack of them.

If we are anxious about a certain area of our belief, we will be much less able to affirm a patient who is confident in that same area. Conversely, if we are absolutely certain about something we believe, we may not want to hear that someone else has doubts. Our doubts or certainties may make it more difficult to accept a patient whose beliefs are different from those we are trying to hold.

We must take seriously how we regard the relationship of religious belief and truth. Most religious groups in our culture teach that their set of beliefs constitutes the truth about a supreme being and how that being interacts with the world. Some groups imply, and others state outright, that those who believe differently than they do are at least wrong, and at most subject to punishment by their God. Most of us are inculturated to believe that there is one correct set of religious beliefs and all others, including nonbelief, are wrong to some degree. This inculturation makes disagreements over religious belief different from disputes in other areas of our society. To affirm someone else's religious belief is to admit that one's own belief is wrong.

In talking to patients and families about religion, we must adopt the attitude that both we and the patient can be right. Since no-one can prove one belief or another, it is possible to affirm the patient's belief while not doubting one's own. Caregivers must move away from the idea that belief can be right or wrong and embrace the idea that persons have a right to their own beliefs without infringing on someone else (84).

There are several areas of belief that should be explored in personal assessment. What is holy? What has ultimate meaning? This question has to do with discovering the source of meaning and purpose in our lives and corresponds to Fitchett's assessment of belief and meaning described above (44). Is it a god? Is it our personal relationships, either in general or specific ones? Is our professional status that which we would do the most to protect? It is important to recognize that while we may not believe in the God of an organized religion, each usually has something to which we owe god-like devotion. If we know who or what our God is, it is easier to see the similarities and differences between what drives us and what motivates our patients.

Each of us needs to honestly assess what we think and feel about the supreme being variously known as God, Yahweh, or Allah by western religions. Caregivers frequently encounter patients for whom God is centrally important and to whom they attach strong positive or negative feelings. If the caregiver's feelings about their particular view of God prevent the patient from discussing God, an avenue of their coping is being limited by not affirming it. The caregiver's feelings about God are of no consequence.

Lastly, each caregiver should know what he or she thinks and feels about living by faith and trust rather than by scientific standards of proof. This distinction involves the basic question of what authority a person uses to establish that which is true in their lives. The person who lives by faith accepts as true whatever their God says is true without any further proof. A person trained to rely on scientific data to establish truth may find living by faith irrational and difficult to deal with. He or she may be frustrated trying to convince the believer of something because the believer does not respond to scientific argument. On the other hand, some caregivers may be in awe of the person who lives by faith or share this approach to some degree.

INTERVENTIONS TO SUPPORT EMOTIONAL ASPECTS OF FAITH

Removing personal barriers allows discussion of religion and faith in a supportive and nonjudgmental way. The simplest and most common strategy is to provide emotional support for these beliefs and practices creating an atmosphere in which the patient feels encouraged to talk about the role of religious faith in his or her life and feels affirmed and supported in using religion as a way of coping with illness. Asking a few simple questions about the patient's religious practice and belief, such as those suggested by Carpenito, will often free the patient to talk while supporting and affirming positive contributions from religion to coping. The patient who says, "I put my trust in the Lord" should be encouraged and told how positive this belief is for him or her. Likewise, the patients who say they rely on prayer for comfort or relaxation should be helped to continue their practice during their illness. The caregiver's basic goal is to affirm any kind of coping behavior that is positive.

Hope

One of those behaviors is the ability to hope in the face of overwhelming odds. Hope is a feeling which has been often misunderstood in relationship to terminal illness. It has been perceived as synonymous with inappropriate denial. However, according to Callan (85), "Denial is a defense mechanism that consists of avoiding the facts, whereas hope accepts painful facts but places them in a wider perspective that includes other,

more acceptable aspects of those facts. Hope, to be authentic, must be based on reality, taking into account the obvious meaning of a tragic event as well as additional meanings that a person finds more acceptable." Callan goes on to outline three developmental stages for hope. He calls the third stage, "transcendent hope based on meaning." This stage involves meaning which is not dependent on the present situation and which is unaltered by the course of the illness. Drawing from Frankl (86), Callan asserts that this meaning enhances the patient's sense of mastery and therefore improves coping.

A basic goal of spiritual interventions is to increase hope. A key is for caregivers to continually appreciate that patients can be simultaneously hopeful and realistic about their grim prognosis especially if their authority comes from faith rather than from facts as discussed earlier. The hope is not necessarily focused on a physical cure. It may be focused on finding a God who is more of a comforter than a judge. It may be focused on finding forgiveness or redemption from one's God. It may be focused on the promise of an afterlife. It is not the caregiver's job to try to plant or force hopefulness when the patient needs to grieve or be angry. However, the caregiver should verbally encourage this hope where it appears rather than being implicitly or explicitly disapproving because the hope does not seem to be consonant with the prognosis.

Guilt and Shame

Shame and guilt are also common feelings among cancer patients. Guilt is the feeling that one has committed some wrong act, either by commission or omission, whereas shame is a sense that one does not measure up or that one is not good enough as a person (87,88). In either case, most people suspect or believe that their cancer means that some misdeeds from their past have come back to haunt them.

Humanist psychology or psychotherapy deals with these feelings by helping people vent them and then by helping them see that there is nothing about who they are or what they have done that justifies these concerns. This strategy works for many people. However, many religious people will not be convinced that what they have done is not sin or that they are basically good people. Their illness may simply be further proof to them that they have fallen short of what their God expects of them. Traditional therapeutic technique will be frustrating for both the patient and therapist.

However, the caretaker can help the patient seek redemption or forgiveness as it is practiced in their faith tradition. Although Christian patients may be helped by a Christian caretaker sharing their own belief in forgiveness, these patients will likely require a referral to a clergyperson of their faith who has the authority in the patient's eyes to hear their confession and pronounce God's forgiveness. Other patients may believe that forgiveness and redemption comes from making direct restitution for their misdeeds or seeking forgiveness directly from the person they have wronged. Any caretaker can help the patient make plans for satisfying these requirements.

Patients who believe that suffering itself is redemptive may pose a major problem for the caregiver. These patients believe that the illness and pain are themselves gifts from their God which allow them to atone for past sins. They may underreport pain, not take advantage of pain relief available to them and even not rehabilitate themselves as quickly as they might. A referral to a chaplain is appropriate here to help the patient look for alternate ways to forgiveness. However, all caretakers need to be aware that some of these patients may experience less existential suffering if they remain in some pain than if they are pain free. Respect for the patient's beliefs dictates that we allow the patient to refuse comfort measures without being judgmental or coercive.

INTERVENTIONS IN SUPPORT OF INTELLECTUAL ASPECTS OF FAITH

Beyond emotional faith support, there is a need to support the patient's intellectual beliefs. The feeling a person has about illness and their ability to cope are largely dependent on what they believe about it and what they attribute it to. In this regard, the central question for people of faith is, How does God act in the world? How patients answer this question can dictate much of the feeling they have about their illness and, therefore, how well they cope with it. Although there are clearly a wide spectrum of answers to this question, they tend to break down into several categories.

God Will Heal Me
It is not uncommon for a patient to say to a caretaker, "God will take care of me" or "I've put the illness in God's hand" or "God will heal me". Caretakers often assume that these statements signify passivity on the part of the patient and that the patient may not be willing to comply with treatment. It is important not to make assumptions but to ask the patient or family member to explain this belief, what it means to him or her and how conventional medical treatment fits into

God's role. Often patients believe modern medicine is part of God's healing process. The patient may also understand "healing" to include death and going on to another life.

While most patients for whom faith is important will acknowledge that their God does not provide physical healing for everyone in every illness, some are convinced that their God is going to heal them. These patients should be encouraged to talk about their belief and what it would mean to them if they were not healed. Some patients will refuse to enter this dialogue believing that to even acknowledge the question is to express a doubt that will be an obstacle to healing. These patients should be referred to a chaplain for ongoing support, especially if they have a poor prognosis. Often when it becomes evident that they will die, many acknowledge that they may have misread God's intention for them. They become peacefully willing to accept that God's will is for them to die. Other patients may be willing to explore how "healing" might take various forms including inner peace or passage into an afterlife. This discussion may help the patient solidify their beliefs and make better use of them

God Caused My Illness as a Test
Some patients who believe that their God causes everything that happens in the world may focus on God as the cause of the illness rather that as an agent of cure. These patients view their God mainly as a judge rather than a potential healer. If these people also believe that their God is basically loving, they may accept illness and death as a part of God's beneficent plan or as a test of their faith. They may interpret the test as a sign of God's high regard for them. They must therefore prove themselves worthy of this honor by enduring the suffering without complaint. This patient's behavior may look much like the guilty patient described above. Again, caregivers need to allow patients to maintain their faith even if it means unnecessary physical suffering. However, the patient may also believe that passing the test means working as hard as possible to be well. In this case caregivers can support the belief as a positive motivation. In either case, a chaplaincy referral is appropriate.

God Caused My Illness as a Punishment
Patients who believe that God is basically judgmental may see their illness as a punishment. If they believe that this judgment is justified they may feel tremendously guilty or ashamed as discussed above. The patient who feels that the judgment is not justified may feel angry and abandoned by their God. It is

important to allow these feelings to be expressed and validated. Patients can be told that these feelings are completely normal under the circumstances. They should be encouraged to express their anger directly to God and helped to see that doing so will be a sign of the strength of that relationship. A referral to the chaplain is appropriate here although these patients may refuse chaplaincy intervention. They may transfer their anger at their God to the chaplain who they see as the agent of that God. A chaplain of a faith group different from the patient's may be able to avoid this transference and yet have the skills necessary to counsel the patient.

This circumstance in which patients feel punished and rejected by their God may lend itself to the caretaker sharing his or her own faith with the patient. They may be comforted to know that others believe differently. If the caretaker is a person of faith, it is helpful to simply say to the patient," I don't believe that God intentionally causes anyone pain or suffering." Sharing of this sort should be short and limited to a simply statement of belief. The patient who wants a further explanation will invite one. This kind of sharing is difficult for some caretakers since it is contrary to training. However, it may be extremely helpful to the patient in distress who is trying to find their way back to a supportive God.

Another strategy with patients in this position is to steer them away from a God who does or does not do things to a God whose main activity is to comfort and console. The popular "Footprints" tells the story of a person who, looking back over his life, sees two sets of footprints stretching out behind him except during the difficult times of his life when there is only one set of prints. He asks why, during these times of trial, he was abandoned by God. God responds that it was during these times of trial that God carried him. It is noteworthy that the god figure does not protect the person from trouble, but carries him when trouble occurs. Likewise, Psalm 23 is meaningful to many Christians and Jews, not because God promises to keep believers out of "the valley of the shadow of death," but because God promises to be with the believer and provide comfort. A God whose main task is to provide comfort and support will help a patient maintain the courage to grow no matter what happens. The caretaker can ask the patient if their God functions for them in this way and encourage them to explore this belief. A chaplain may also be helpful in suggesting practices which will help the patient draw more strength from the comforting and supporting side of their God.

RELIGIOUS RITUALS

Although many religious rituals and practices require the assistance of a chaplain, other caregivers have a definite role to play. Every person entering a health care facility should be asked about religious practices they want to continue. This process is probably most efficient if done as part of the overall initial assessment usually done by an admitting nurse. Again, Carpenito's questions are a good guide. Including these practices in any care plan gives the patient permission to continue them uninterrupted and without fear of disapproval from the staff. The most commonly practiced religious ritual is prayer. Many patients pray at set times of the day and are helped by having this practice included in their care plans so that this ritual is facilitated. As in faith sharing, there is a place for non-chaplaincy staff to pray with patients. Patients who are known to pray can be asked by caregivers who are comfortable doing it if they might pray with them. Prayers need not be formal, long or terribly articulate. They may include only a single thought or wish that the patient and caregiver have been talking about. The content may be agreed upon by the participants beforehand. The patient may be the one verbalizing the prayer while the staff member listens. The prayer may become a simple blessing in which the caregiver expresses his or her hope that God will be with the patient or grant them healing. A staff member who can pray with a religious patient offers an extremely important support to the patient and encourages a practice which is central to the patient's coping.

Reading sacred texts of the patient's faith tradition should be encouraged by caregivers. Patients who want to read at set times can have these times included in their care plans. In many traditions, it is considered important to hear the sacred texts read. The patient may be too ill to read to themselves. In virtually every tradition, the reader does not have to be from the same faith group as the patient. Patients who value hearing scriptures read will likely not care who the reader is. Staff can ask patients if they have special passages they would like read and how to find them.

Both prayer and scripture reading can function as important methods of relaxation for religious patients. Beyond these specific practices, religious patients who might benefit generally from relaxation and meditation can be encouraged to include religious images or words which carry special meaning for them. Incorporating religious practice into meditation can enhance the relaxation response and help patients learn it faster (89).

Religiously prescribed dietary practices can be problematic in a hospital because the proper foods are not available on the hospital menu especially for those on special diets. This circumstance can result in inadequate nutrition for the patient. Any initial assessment of a religious patient should inquire about religiously prescribed dietary restrictions. Fasting is prescribed in most major religions in observance of certain holidays or as a way of making a special appeal to God. Normally the prescription to fast on a holy day is waived for the ill and frail. However, patients may not know about this waiver or choose not to invoke it. These patients should be referred immediately to a chaplain of their faith group.

Rituals around the end of life often have tremendous importance to families but strain the limits of hospital policy and thus the relationships of family and staff. Many of these rituals are on the border between cultural practice and religious observance since they are typical of certain religious groups but not specifically prescribed by that religion. Thus, it is hard to anticipate what a specific family will want to do by simply knowing their religious affiliation. As with the rest of end-of-life planning, timely assessment and negotiation with the family is central to patient satisfaction. Ideally, this assessment would be done when the goals of the patient's care change to comfort only from active treatment. It also might be part of a discussion about resuscitation. Family members should be encouraged to talk about and share with the staff what they want to happen before and after their loved one's death. Who do they want to be there? Does a clergyperson of their faith group need to be present? What rituals need to be performed before or during the death? What do they want done or not done to the body and by whom? What difference would it make if the patient died on a religious holy day or sabbath? What do they believe about autopsy and organ donation? While these questions are often not easy to ask, knowing the answers may very well preclude significant conflict between family members and staff during the dying process. Knowing the answers also allows staff to examine practices which may be new to them or possibly in conflict with current hospital policy. Where a practice absolutely cannot be accommodated, family must be informed as soon as possible so that alternate arrangements can be made.

Finally, staff should be in touch with the patient's religious leaders. As inpatient stays become shorter and less frequent, helping the patient remain connected to his or her community becomes increasingly important. Religious communities are helpful to the patient in physical as well as spiritual ways. With the patient's consent, information can be shared by the medical staff with the local clergyperson which can enhance the care of the patient in the community through monitoring of physical care and provision of transportation as well as spiritual support.

SUMMARY

Spiritual assessment and intervention are important elements in the complete care of any patient. All health care professionals must be prepared to assess a patient's religious beliefs and practices as part of any total assessment. A number of schemas are available to assist the caregiver in this assessment process. Several reliable and valid research instruments have also been developed in this area. Religious belief and practice can be an important support to the patient or sometimes an impediment to cure. It is incumbent upon all caregivers to remove these impediments where they exist and maximize the patient's ability to use their religious resources in coping with their disease. Emotional faith support, intellectual faith support, and participation in religious ritual are important in this process.

REFERENCES

1. Levin JS, Schiller PL. Is there a religious factor in health? *J Relig Health.* 1988; 26(1):9–36.
2. Levin JS. Investigating the epidemiologic effects of religious experience: findings, explanations, and barriers. In: Levin JS, ed. *Religion in Aging and Health.* Thousand Oaks, CA: Sage Publications; 1994.
3. Pargament KI, Maton KI, Hess RE, eds. *Religion and Prevention in Mental Health: Research, Vision and Action.* Binghamton, NY: Haworth Press; 1992.
4. Jenkins RA, Pargament KI. Religion and spirituality as resources for coping with cancer. *J Psychosoc Oncol.* 1995; 13(1/2):51–74.
5. Jenkins RA, Pargament KI. Cognitive appraisals in cancer patients. *Soc Sci Med.* 1988; 26(6):625–633.
6. Johnson SC, Spilka B. Coping with breast cancer: the roles of clergy and faith. *J Relig Health.* 1991; 30(1): 21–33.
7. Kaczorowski JM. Spiritual well-being and anxiety in adults diagnosed with cancer. *Hospice J.* 1989; 5(3/4):105–116.
8. Mickley JR, Soeken K, Belcher A. Spiritual well-being, religiousness and hope among women with breast cancer. *Image.* 1992; 24(4):267–272.
9. Rabins PV, Fitting MD, Eastham J, Fetting J. The emotional impact of caring for the chronically ill. *Psychosomatics.* 1990; 31(3):331–336.
10. Reed PG. Spirituality and well-being in terminally ill hospitalized adults. *Res Nurs Health.* 1987; 10:335–344.
11. Peteet JR. Religious issues presented by cancer patients seen in psychiatric consultation. *J Psychosoc Oncol.* 1985; 3(1):53–66.

12. James W. *The Varieties of Religious Experience: A Study in Human Nature.* Cambridge, MA: Harvard University Press; 1985 (Original edition, 1902).

13. Wulff DM. *Psychology of Religion: Classic and Contemporary Views.* New York: John Wiley, 1991.

14. Boisen AT. *The Exploration of the Inner World: A Study of Mental Disorder and Religious Experience.* Philadelphia: University of Pennsylvania Press; 1976 (Originally published 1936).

15. Asquith GH Jr., ed. *Vision From a Little Known Country: A Boisen Reader.* Decatur, GA: Journal of Pastoral Care Publications, Inc.; 1992.

16. Asquith GH Jr. The case study method of Anton Boisen. *J Pastoral Care.* 1980; 34(2):84–94.

17. Draper E, Meyer GG, Parzen, Z, Samuelson G. On the diagnostic value of religious ideation. *Arch Gen Psychiatry* 1965; 13:202–207.

18. McKeever DA. Personal religious history as a pastoral tool. *Pastoral Psychol.* 1975; 24(228): 65–75.

19. Oates WE. Religious diagnosis and assessment of psychiatric patients. *The Religious Care of the Psychiatric Patient.* Philadelphia: Westminster Press, 1978; 87–100.

20. Oates WE. The pastor's understanding and assessment. *The Christian Pastor.* Philadelphia: Westminster Press; 1982. 167–189.

21. Richardson EA. The religious interview as a method for teaching psychodynamics. In: Holst LE, Kurtz HP, eds. *Toward Creative Chaplaincy.* Springfield, IL: Charles C. Thomas, 1973; 128–138.

22. Stoll, RI. Guidelines for spiritual assessment. *Am J Nurs.* 1979; 9:1574–1577.

23. Pruyser PW. *The Minister as Diagnostician.* Philadelphia: Westminster Press; 1976.

24. Malony HN. The clinical assessment of optimal religious functioning. *Rev Relig Res.* 1988; 30(1): 3–17.

25. Sackett G. Seven dimensions of spirituality. *CareGiver.* 1985; 1(2):27–30.

26. Stoddard G, Burns-Haney J. Developing an integrated approach to spiritual assessment: one department's experience. *Caregiver J.* 1990; 7(1):63–86.

27. Weiss FS. Pastoral care planning: a process-oriented approach for mental health ministry. *J Pastoral Care.* 1991; 45(3):268–278.

28. Stoddard GA, Sheffieck AH, Leonard G. The science of caring. *Health Prog.* 1990; March:66–70,79.

29. Allison D. Communicating clinical pastoral assessments with the healthcare team. *J Pastoral Care.* 1992; 46(3):273–280.

30. Kuhn CC. A spiritual inventory of the medically ill patient. *Psychiatr Med.* 1988: 6(2):87–100.

31. Maugans TA. The SPIRITual history. *Arch Fam Med.* 1996; 5:11–16.

32. McSherry E, Kratz D, Nelson W. Pastoral care departments: more necessary in the DRG Era. *Health Care Manage Rev.* 1986; 11(1):47–59.

33. McSherry E. Modernization of the clinical science of chaplaincy. *Caregiver.* 1987; 4(1):1–13.

34. McSherry E. The need and appropriateness of measurement and research in chaplaincy: its criticalness for patient care and chaplain department survival post 1987. *J Health Care Chaplaincy.* 1987; 1(1):3–41.

35. McSherry E, and Nelson W. The DRG era: a major opportunity for increased pastoral care impact or a crisis for survival? *J Pastoral Care.* 1987; 41(3):201–211.

36. Ciulla MR, Salisbury S, McSherry E. Quality assurance in DNR (do not resuscitate) decisions — the role of chaplaincy: a case report and a 92 patient group study. *J Health Care Chaplaincy.* 1988; 2(1):57–80.

37. Salisbury S, Ciulla M, McSherry E. Clinical management reporting and objective diagnostic instruments for spiritual assessment in spinal cord injury patients. *J Health Care Chaplaincy.* 1989; 2(2):35–64.

38. Berg GE. The use of the computer as a tool for assessment and research in pastoral care. *J Health Care Chaplaincy.* 1994; 6(1):11–25.

39. Highfield MF, Cason C. Spiritual needs of patients: are they recognized? *Cancer Nurs.* 1983; June: 187–192.

40. Kim MJ, McFarland GK, McLane AM. *Pocket Guide to Nursing Diagnosis,* 3rd ed. St. Louis; MO: CV Mosby; 1989.

41. Ivy SS. A faith development/self-development model for pastoral assessment. *J Pastoral Care.* 1987; 41(4):329–340.

42. Shulevitz M, Springer M. Assessment of religious experience — a Jewish approach. *J Pastoral Care.* 1994; 48(4): 399–406.

43. Fitchett G. *Spiritual Assessment in Pastoral Care: A Guide to Selected Resources.* Decatur, GA: Journal of Pastoral Care Publications, Inc.; 1993.

44. Fitchett G. *Assessing Spiritual Needs: A Guide for Caregivers.* Minneapolis: Augsburg; 1993.

45. Levin JS, Vanderpool HY. Religious factors in physical health and the prevention of illness. In: Pargament KI, Maton KI, Hess RE, eds. *Religion and Prevention in Mental Health: Research, Vision and Action.* Binghamton, NY: Haworth Press; 1992; 83–103.

46. Hathaway WL, Pargament KI The religious dimensions of coping: implications for prevention and promotion. In: Pargament KI, Maton KI, Hess RE, eds. *Religion and Prevention in Mental Health: Research, Vision and Action.* Binghamton, NY: Haworth Press; 1991; 65–92.

47. Pargament KI. God help me: toward a theoretical framework for the psychology of religion. *Res Soc Sci Study Relig.* 1990; 2:195–224.

48. McIntosh D, Spilka B. Religion and physical health: the role of personal faith and control beliefs. *Res Soc Sci Study Relig.* 1990; 2:167–194.

49. Krause N, Tran TV. Stress and religious involvement among older blacks. *J Gerontol Soc Sci.* 1989; 44:S4–S13.

50. Chatters LM, Levin JS, Taylor RJ. Antecedents and dimensions of religious involvement among older blacks. *J Gerontol Soc Sci.* 1992; 47(6):S269–S278.

51. Kash KM, Holland JC, Passik SD, et al. The System of Belief Inventory (SBI): a scale to measure spiritual and religious beliefs in quality of life and coping research. *Psychosom Med.* 1995; 57:62.

52. Pargament KI, Ensing DS, Falgout K, et al. God help me: I: Religious coping efforts as predictors of the outcomes to significant negative life events. *Am J Commun Psychol.* 1990; 18(6):793–824.

53. Pargament KI, Olsen H, Reilly B, et al. God help me II: The relationship of religious orientation to religious coping with negative life events. *J Sci Study Relig.* 1992; 31(4):504–513.

54. Pargament KI, Kennell J, Hathaway W, et al. Religion and the problem-solving process: three styles of coping. *J Sci Study Relig.* 1988; 27(1):90–104.

55. Bickel CO. *Perceived Stress, Religious Coping Styles, and Depressive Affect.* Ph.D. Dissertation, Loyola College in Maryland, Baltimore, 1993.

56. Jenkins RA. Religion and HIV: implications for research and intervention. *J Soc Issues.* 1995; 51(2):131–144.

57. Kass JD, Friedman R, Leserman J, et al. Health outcomes and a new index of spiritual experience. *J Sci Study Relig.* 1991; 30(2):203–211.

58. Kass JD. Contributions of religious experience to psychological and physical well-being: research evidence and an explanatory model. *Caregiver J.* 1992; 8(4):4–11.

59. Allport GW, Ross JM. Personal religious orientation and prejudice. *J Pers Soc Psychol.* 1967; 5:432–443.

60. Batson C, Ventis W. *The Religious Experience: A Social-Psychological Perspective.* New York: Oxford University Press; 1982.

61. Donahue MJ. Intrinsic and extrinsic religiousness: review and meta-analysis. *J Pers Soc Psychol.* 1985; 48:400–419.

62. Kirkpatrick LA, Hood RH Jr. Intrinsic-extrinsic religious orientation: boon or bane. *J Sci Study Relig.* 1990; 29(4):442–462.

63. Hoge D. A validated intrinsic religious motivation scale. *J Sci Study Relig.* 1972; 11(4):369–376.

64. Feagin J. Prejudice and religious types: a focused study of southern fundamentalists. *J Sci Study Relig.* 1964; 4(1):3–13.

65. Paloutzian R, Ellison CW. Loneliness, spiritual well-being and the quality of life. In: Peplau LA, Perlman D, eds. *Loneliness: A Sourcebook of Current Theory, Research and Therapy.* New York: Wiley; 1982; 224–237.

66. Ellison CW. Spiritual well-being: conceptualization and measurement. *J Psychol Theol.* 1983; 11:330–340.

67. Ellison CW, Smith J. Toward an integrative measure of health and well-being. *J Psychol Theol.* 1991; 19:35–48.

68. Bufford RK, Paloutzian RF, Ellison CW. Norms for the spiritual well-being scale. *J Psychol Theol.* 1991; 19:56–70.

69. Montonye M. Patient-centered caring: identifying religious needs. *Caregiver J.* 1994–1995; 11(1):33–37.

70. Derrickson PE. Screening patients for pastoral care: a preliminary report. *Caregiver J.* 1994–1995; 11(2):14–18.

71. Carpenito LJ. *Nursing Diagnosis: Application to Clinical Practice,* 6th ed. Philadelphia: Lippincott; 1995.

72. Stoddard GA. Chaplaincy by referral: an effective model for evaluating staffing needs. *Caregiver J.* 1993; 10(1):37–52.

73. Mills M, et al. Prediction of results in open heart surgery *J Relig Health.* 1975; 14(3):159–164.

74. Oxman TE, et al. Lack of social participation or religious strength and comfort as risk factors for death after cardiac surgery in the elderly. *Psychosom Med.* 1995; 57:5–15.

75. American Cancer Society. *Pastoral Care and Cancer.* Chicago: American Cancer Society, Illinois Division; 1988.

76. Burton LA, Handzo G, eds. *Health Care Chaplaincy in Oncology.* New York: Haworth Pastoral Press; 1993.

77. Campbell D, Baile W, Galloway A. Advanced training for clergy in psychosocial oncology. *Caregiver J.* 1992; 9(2):71–79.

78. Dawson J. *The Cancer Patient.* Minneapolis: Augsburg; 1978.

79. Sproull A. The voices on cancer care: a lens unfocused and narrowed. In: Holst L, ed. *Hospital Ministry: The Role of the Chaplain Today.* New York: Crossroads; 1985; 118–126.

80. Kerney L. Ministering to cancer patients. In: Dayringer R, ed. *Pastor and Patient.* New York: Jason Aronson; 1982: 159–165.

81. Stelling J. Outpatient ministry: three approaches. *Caregiver J.* 1988; 5:109–114.

82. Taylor E. Factors associated with meaning in life among people with recurrent cancer. *Oncol Nurs Forum.* 1993; 20(9):1399–1405.

83. Weisman A. *Coping With Cancer.* New York: McGraw-Hill; 1979.

84. Baldridge W Gleason J. A theological framework for pastoral care. *J Pastoral Care.* 1978; 32(4):232–238.

85. Callan D. Hope as a clinical issue in oncology social work. *J Psychosoc Oncol.* 1989; 7(3):31–46.

86. Frankl V. *The Unheard Cry for Meaning.* New York: Simon and Schuster; 1978.

87. Burton LA. Respect: response to shame in health care. *J Relig Health.* 1991; 30(2):139–148.

88. Burton LA. Original sin or original shame. *Q Rev.* 1988; 5(4):31–41.

89. Benson H, Proctor W. *Beyond the Relaxation Response.* New York: Berkley Publishing Group; 1985.

69

Bedside Interventions

JEANNIE V. PASACRETA AND RUTH McCORKLE

Dramatic changes in medical technology and health care delivery continue to impact on patient care at every level. New treatments have rendered previously fata diseases treatable with risk, however, of acute and long-term consequences to patients including lifelong symptomatic episodes and varying degrees of continuous functional impairment. These issues, although characteristic of chronic illness in general, are most apparent in cancer. Concurrent with medical advances are dramatic shifts in the delivery of health care. Patients are discharged from hospitals sooner than ever before, while experiencing a range of problems and requiring a range of services. The burden of care is increasingly shifted to families who are often ill-equipped to manage them. In the midst of these changes, consultants and support personnel such as psychiatrists, psychiatric liaison nurses, social workers and chaplains are being cut from many health care budgets. Consequently, nurses, on the "frontlines" of patient care, are increasingly in the position of managing the multiple problems presented by cancer patients and their families. This chapter highlights the role of nurses in managing patients' psychosocial problems, albeit often indirectly via interventions directed at providing information, managing physical symptoms, and functional impairments in the hospital and at home. Education and research is imperative to assist nurses in the management of psychosocial problems and to assess the utility and cost-effectiveness of nursing interventions in these changing times.

RELATIONSHIPS AMONG PHYSICAL SYMPTOM DISTRESS, PSYCHOLOGICAL DISTRESS, AND FUNCTIONING

The awareness that many cancer treatments have the potential to cause unpleasant and deleterious side effects has emphasized that quality of life issues should be as important a consideration of treatment as survi-

val and cure. Obviously since some cancers are not curable, nursing interventions become paramount, particularly when palliation and symptom control are the issues at hand. Padill and Grant (1) highlighted the crucial role of the nurse in assisting patients to cope with cancer treatment side effects and suggested that nursing interventions can impact positively on quality of survival, during both active treatment and palliative care.

At any stage of disease, psychological distress can exacerbate the effects of cancer treatment agents as demonstrated by the development of anticipatory chemotherapy-related nausea and vomiting (2). Conversely, treatment side effects can have a dramatic impact on the psychological profiles of its recipients (3). The impact of "bedside" nursing interventions are effective in diminishing such symptoms as pain and psychological symptoms related to cancer and its treatment (4,5).

Due to the expected and overlapping nataure of somatic and psychological changes secondary to cancer illness and treatment, understanding when psychological symptoms reach clinical significance is inherently difficult. Physical symptoms imposed by illness and treatment often coexist with psychological symptoms. In part, due to the fact that psychological issues may take a back seat to physical problems in the medical setting, a lack of understanding regarding the significance of psychological symptoms among cancer patients has lead to such common misconceptions as the assumption that excessive emotional distress is an appropriate response to a physically and emotionally disruptive chronic illness. In light of these issues, basic nursing education as well as staff development programs must do more to address psychological aspects of an increasing array of chronic illnessesd including cancer (see Chapter 93). Similarly, understanding the types of interventions that may reduce psychological distress in oncology settings is vital. For example, some studies have shown that educational interventions indirectly improve patients' and families' sense of control and thereby enhance functioning and well-being (4,6,7).

Particularly during the treatment phases, patients face a range of physical symptoms related to treatment side effects and toxicities. Intensive therapies produce severe and life-threatening side effects. The frequent somatic symptoms include chills, fever, stomatitis, pain, nausea, vomiting, alterations in mobility, inability to tend to self-care needs, and dependence on caregivers (8). Patients often rank their most distressing problems as hair loss, nausea, vomiting, fatigue, weakness, and diminished stamina interfering with personal and work obligations. Symptoms become most problematic when they interfere with the activities in which people want to engage (7).

Psychological distress, particularly depression, interferes with optimal functioning. Graydon found high rates of depression were predictive of poor functioning in lung and breast cancer patients following radiation therapy (9). Others have reported the converse, that diminished functioning enhances the potential for depression (10). Others reported that despite the relationship between affect and functioning the direction is unclear and causation cannot be concluded (11). Despite a lack of clear evidence regarding causality, these studies demonstrate the complex interrelationships among physical symptoms, psychological symptoms, and functioning. These issues highlight the notion that nursing interventions aimed at reducing physical symptoms and enhancing functioning can have a direct effect on improving psychological state.

Nagi found that level of functioning attained following a period of disability is determined not only by physical capacity but by the individual's assessment of their situation as well as the assessment of the situation by significant others (12). An interesting hypothesis is that cancer patients who perceive somatic symptoms and associated functional alterations as being permanent are more prone to psychological distress than those who view symptoms as transient. These issues have important implications in terms of tailoring nursing interventions aimed at mobilizing patients who are striving to maintain a quality lifestyle within the context of chronic health problems associated with their cancer and its treatment.

According to information derived from studies of psychological symptoms in patients with cancer, the potential for disturbance appears to increase in patients with advanced illness (13–18). Additionally, in a study that elicited information from nurses regarding psychiatric symptoms present in their patients,

almost twice as many patients with metastatic disease were reported to have prominent symptoms in contrast to those with localized disease (19). Investigators studying quality of life in cancer patients have demonstrated a clear relationship between an individual's perception of their quality of life and the presence of discomfort (7). As uncomfortable symptoms increase, perceived quality of life diminishes and psychological distress often increases. In patients with advanced cancer, the presence of increased physical discomfort combined with a lack of control and predictability regarding the occurrence of symptoms often enhances anxiety, depression and organic mental symptoms. Weissman and Worden, in their classic study of existential plight, found that patients with advanced cancer exhibited more vulnerability, were more distressed, had more mood disturbance, and were more concerned about existential, health, and work issues than those with less advanced cancer (20).

Diminishing ability to engage in physical activities and interact with others is associated with advanced stages of cancer (21). Focused interventions to support day-to-day activities of the ill person are particularly important. Consultation with family members may be critical during treatment and during clinical decline. Nail (22) found that 81% of subjects undergoing treatment experienced fatigue. Sarna (23) found that 56.5% of women with lung cancer had serious complaints of fatigue and a third had difficulty with household chores and ability to care for themselves. Difficulties in sleeping in this and other studies may contribute to feelings of lassitude (7). The utility of nursing interventions targeted to these problems is just beginning to be understood.

Although further study is needed to clarify the complex relationships among physical symtpoms, psychological distress and functioning, nurses are mindful that concurrent stresses may adversely affect patients' experience and overall quality of life. Nurses are in an ideal position to assess, treat and monitor distressing symptoms over time. As stated, trends in cancer treatment have increasingly produced patients who are acutely ill, and receive aggressive treatments in complex technological settings. Additionally, patients are often sent home with continuing acute care needs (24). The preceding factors leave patients increasingly vulnerable to emotional distress. A growing body of research is beginning to address the impact that trends in cancer treatment are having on the emotional adjustment of patients, and the utility and cost-effectiveness of nurses' interventions to deal with them.

NURSING INTERVENTIONS

Psychosocial Nursing Interventions

In diverse oncology settings, nursing care is an essential element of treatment since symptom control, information, and support are the cornerstone of effective therapy across the illness trajectory. Patients with cancer constitute a large group of nursing care recipients. The nature of nursing interventions include direct physical care, information/education, ongoing psychosocial support, and management of treatment side effects (see Table 69.1).

Caring. Caring is an essential and universal concept underlying nursing practice (25). Studies on nurses' caring behaviors have found different perceptions of caring by nurses, patients, and families. Nurses often identify their most caring activities as listening, talking, touching, and comforting (26,27). Patients, on the other hand, identified clinical competence and attention to physical care as most indicative of caring. Knowledge and skills, such as how to give an injection well, how to handle equipment, and when to call the physician, were consistently identified by patients as examples of caring behaviors (28–31). In one study, 57 cancer patients reported that caring was demonstrated by being accessible, monitoring, and following thought (26). In a study by Hull (32), families of patients with advanced cancer identified four areas of caring: 24 hour accessibility, effective communication, a nonjudgemental attitude, and clinical competence.

Enhancing, Coping, Counseling, and Referral. A primary role for oncology nurses is to facilitate a positive adjustment in patients under their care. The likelihood of intermittent emotional distress and coping problems should be kept in mind and monitored routinely due to the chronic nature of cancer and the many transitiions that can occur along the illness trajectory. The uniqueness of individual patients should always be kept in mind with awareness of the person's past coping style as well as the fact that an intense emotional reaction is not the same as maladaptive coping. Understanding an individual's unique circumstances can assist nurses in supporting coping abilities that work best. It is often helpful for nurses to focus on a specific stressor and the individual's response to it during therapeutic interactions and also try to reinforce positive self-care behaviors.

In addition to verbal communication with cancer patients about coping strategies, written materials can be used to teach patients new coping skills. Carey and Jevne (33) have developed an effective teaching program for postmastectomy patients to help them cope with breast cancer. The program includes specific guidelines on dealing with emotions, handling changes in family roles and relationships, encouraging family involvement in care, dealing with problems in sexuality, discussing cancer with other patients, communicating with physicians and family, and developing specific coping skills. The educational materials also advise patients to help friends and family to be comfortable with the cancer diagnosis by giving accurate information and by sharing their feelings and needs. The teaching program normalizes common emotional reactions to cancer. Suggestions are offered to patients for dealing with these emotions by distracting themselves through activity, by talking with someone with whom they feel comfortable, by solving everyday problems as they arise and not letting them buildup, and by learning specific relaxation techniques.

To enable health care providers to facilitate patients' coping, Weismann and Worden (20) suggest the following activities for nurses: clarify problems for the patient; help patients maintain control by encouraging them to exercise whatever options they have available to them; offer a willing and noncritical ear so that patients can relieve pent-up emotions; direct patient to constructive channels to reduce anxiety; help reduce a problem to a manageable size; discourage hasty actions; and be comfortable sharing periods of silence with a patient. Appropriate interventions include giving clear information about treatments and procedures, providing reassurance that symptoms will be managed, and using the patient's support system along with hospital chaplains and volunteers to offer comfort and reassurance.

Nurses should also encourage patients to seek out the many resources available for cancer patients: psychological and social work services, chaplains, patient to patient volunteers, services offered by the American Cancer Society and by local hospitals and community groups. Nurses should be able to provide information on such resources. Hospitalized patients should be given addresses and phone numbers of important local agencies available to serve their needs and be advised of the support groups available (both general and site or procedure specific groups). It should be kept in mind that patients may not be ready for outside support immediately and should be reminded periodically of what is available. Additionally, not all services are right for everybody; for instance, many individuals shy away from divulging personal feelings in a group

TABLE 69.1. *Selected Studies of Nursing Behaviors/Interventions Linked with Positive Psychosocial Outcomes*

Author	Research Design	Sample	Behaviors/Interventions	Measures	Outcomes
Dodd (1988)	Longitudinal, experimental	60 patients prior to initiating chemotherapy 30 received information about treatment 30 controls	Proactive information and education concerning self-care and side effect management related to chemotherapy provided to experimental subjects	Self-care behaviors, state trait anxiety, multidimensional health locus of control	More self-care activities performed by treatment group with significant improvement in function 6 weeks after intervention
Johnson et al. (1989)	Experimental	84 patients prior to RT 42 received intervention 42 controls	Informational intervention provided concrete descriptions of the RT experience prior to treatment planning, prior to the first treatment, at the fifth treatment and during the last week of treatment	Sickness Impact Profile Profile of Mood States	Experimental group had significantly less disruption in function during and for 3 months following RT than the controls
Hull (1989)	Qualitative/descriptive	10 families involved in a home care hospice program	24 hour accessibility, effective communication, nonjudgemental attitude, clinical competence	Semistructured interview during home visits	Families felt reassured that relatives were receiving competent care
Weintraub and Hagopian (1990)	Experimental	56 subjects receiving RT, randomly assigned to one of three groups: control, health education and nursing consultation	Nursing consultation intervention provided assistance for patients to manage side effects of treatment on their own	Side Effects Profie Spielberger's State-Trait Anxiety Inventory	Experimental group had significantly less anxiety than the control and health education group
Ferrell et al. (1993)	Longitudinal, descriptive	66 elderly patients	Structured pain education intervention during 3 home visits with audiotaped reinforcement message	Quality of Life self-care log Pain intensity and severity Knowledge and attitudes	Decreased pain intensity and severity, decreased anxiety, improved quality of life Improved attitudes to pain and use of drugs
McCorkel et al. (1994)	Longitudinal, descriptive	49 home care patients 11 no home care	Monitoring patient status/patient, family teaching, provision of direct care, communication with MD, emotional support, referrals	Symptom distress, enforced social dependency, health perceptions, mental health status	Significant improvements for patients receiving homecare on mental health and function when compared to no home care group

RT, radiotherapy.

setting whereas others thrive on the support (34). The individual needs and preferences of each individual must always be paramount.

Family-Focused Care. Cancer is a disease that affects not only the person diagnosed but the family as well (7,11,35). This is particularly true as the location of most care has moved to the home. Families are increasingly replacing skilled health care workers to give complex care to their loved ones, despite the other obligations and responsibilities. They must learn to deal with unfamiliar procedures and equipment within the context of limited support services in many geographic locations. Nurses are instrumental in the liaison role that they serve between the health care institutions and the family, as well as providing direct technical and psychological support. Research has shown that, whether relatives were hospitalized or being cared for at home, clear, honest information about all aspects of care was important to families (35). Pain control and assurance that relatives were receiving competent care were major concerns (36). Families usually do not want attention focused on them and often identify behaviors that encourage them to express their feelings as least supportive. The preference of most families is to be reassured that their relative is in competent hands (36–38).

Physically Oriented Nursing Interventions

Increased length of survival for patients from time of diagnosis has highlighted the need for nursing interventions to reduce physical distress and improve functioning both in the hospital and at home. While ongoing research is needed to document the impact of physically oriented interventions on psychoosicial outcomes, some important studies have documented the positive psychosocial outcomes associated with interventions aimed at providing information about physical problems, managing symptoms distress directly, and for nursing interventions carried out in home care settings.

Providing Information about Physical Symptoms. Johnson et al. examined the effects of providing an information intervention on the outcome of coping with radiation treatment (RT) for prostate cancer (5), giving a description of the RT experience in objective terms. Forty-two men received the intervention prior to treatment planning, prior to the first treatment, at the fifth treatment, and during the last week of treatment; forty-two received standard care only. The experimental group had significantly less disruption in function during and for 3 months following RT than the comparison group. Consistent with a self-regulation theory of coping based on an information processing perspective (39), expectations, experience, and understanding of the experience mediated the effect of the intervention on function (35).

Smith et al. (40) conducted a meta-analysis of 28 studies that tested the effects of a range of nursing interventions aimed at control of physical symptoms. The studies reviewed represented 10 years of nursing research published between 1981 and 1990. Nine studies addressed nausea and vomiting, five addressed pain, and four addressed anxiety. Alopecia, infection, and chemotherapy side effects were each addressed in two studies; mucositis, shivering, radiodermatitis, and anorexia were each addressed in one study. Categories of nursing interventions that emerged in the analysis included medication administration, teaching imagery, progressive muscle relaxation and self-hypnosis techniques, exercise, massage, and teaching of self-care management, to name a few. Significant effectiveness and improvement rates were noted for the interventions in each of the symptom groups. Significant effect variability, however, was related to differences in subject characteristics across studies, variability in the way interventions were administered, and variation on sociocultural orientation. Fewer studies addressed such common symptoms as sleep, mobility, elimination, ventilation, circulation, sexual function, and appearance. The authors also cited a need for research to test the effectiveness of specific nursing interventions on specific symptom profiles and to achieve specific psychosocial outcomes, such as enhanced quality of life.

A longitudinal, experimental study by Dodd (6) tested the efficacy of providing side effect management information proactively for chemotherapy patients. An experimental group received a nursing intervention that provided patients with information on all side effects that they were likely to develop, while a control group received standard information only. The experimental group performed significantly more self-care behaviors than the control group. Performance status increased significantly for the experimental group between interviews (at beginning of study and 6 weeks later).

Ferrell et al. (4) studied the effect of a pain management program on elderly cancer patients and documented the positive impact of a structured information intervention. Elderly subjects were randomly assigned to an experimental group that received a three part structured pain education program or a control group that received usual care. The pain education program was found to be effective in decreasing pain intensity and severity, decreasing fears of addiction, decreasing anxiety, and increasing the use of pain medication. The experimental group also repsorted improved sleep and enhanced knowledge of pain principles such as using pain medication on a schedule rather than an as needed basis.

Weintraub and Hagopian (41) examined the effect of nursing consultation sessions on anxiety, side effects experienced and self-care strategies used by patients receiving radiation therapy. Using an experiental design, 56 subjects were randomly assigned to one of three groups: control, health education, and nursing consultation. The nursing consultation intervention provided ongoing information and education for patients that fostered self-care behaviors in managing treatment side effects. An important finding in this study was that state anxiety scores were consistently lower for patients who received nursing consultation. Findings suggest that nursing interventions can have a positive impact on patient anxiety which is often high during the period of active treatment.

Home Nursing Care. Two home care nursing studies have demonstrated the vital role professional nurses play in providing quality home care to patients with cancer and their family caregivers, and specifically examined psychosocial outcomes associated with nursing interventions. The first study was a randomized clinical trail conducted to assess the efficacy of home care provided by oncology clinical nurse specialists in the community in Seattle (7). One hundred sixty-six patients with lung cancer were asigned to either an oncology home care group (OHC) that received care from community oncology clinical nurse specialists, a standard home care group (SHC) that received care from the traditionally prepared home care nurses, or an office care group (OC) that received the care they required except home care. Patients who received care from the OHC and SHC nurses remained physically and socially independent for a longer period of time than patients who did not receive such services. In addition, patients who received the specialized home care had relatively fewer hospital admissions for symptoms and complications of their cancer compared to the other two groups.

Family caregivers in the preceding study in all three groups had similar patterns of psychological symptoms before and after the death. They reported high symptoms during the 3 months preceding the death and for 1 year after the death, with symptoms peaking within the first 3 months. Findings indicated that, with time,

the unmet needs of caregivers overshadowed those of patients with complex problems. Caregivers are often burdened with daily care required to monitor patients' complex problems. A repeated measures comparison was used to examine psychological distress over time among 46 spouse caregivers using the Brief Symptom Inventory (BSI). Significant differences in the hostility and paranoid ideation subscales were found between the home care and no home care groups, with those receiving no home care receiving higher scores (42). Findings support the need for nursing interventions that assist families in transition from before a death through theperiod of bereavement in order to improve outcomes for survivors.

In a second study (34), home care and no homecare groups were compared on several measures. Ninety-nine percent of the home care group ($n = 49$) received their care from a registered nurse. Primary nursing activities included assessment and monitoring, patient/family teaching, hands-on care, communication with physicians, emotional support, counseling, and referral. Interviews were obtained on all patients at hospital discharge and approximately 3 months later. Scores were obtained for physical symptom distress, a mental health index, functional dependency, and health perceptions. Home care patients had more symptom distress and greater functional dependency at discharge. Three months later, home care patients showed significant improvements in mental health and dependency. The no home care group did not show significant changes in any area.

The results of the two home care studies cited above indicate that nursing behaviors are used by home care nurses to effect positive patient and family member psychosocial outcomes. Patients receiving home care had less symptom distress, improved functional status and more realistic health perceptions and mental health. Family caregives in the experimental groups had improved health perceptions and less caregiver burden over time, when compared with the control group.

The aforementioned studies illustrate the importance of nursing interventions aimed at patients' physical needs in improving psychosocial aspects of the cancer experience for patients and their families. Structured information and education, monitoring and managing distressing symptoms, and promoting control and independence are but a few of the nursing activities that have been shown to exert a positive effect on patient and family outcomes. (See Table 69.2 for guidelines on nursing interventions that can improve patients' psychosocial outcomes.) More research that documents and clarifies these issues is

TABLE 69.2. *Guidelines Regarding Nursing Interventions to Enhance Psychological Outcomes in Oncology Settings*

Assess each individual's unique circumstances

Assess and treat somatic symptoms in a timely fashion

Recognise patients who are at risk for excessive physical and/or psychosocial problems and refer promptly

Reinforce positive self-care and problem-solving behaviors

Provide information to normalize common emotional reactions to cancer and its treatment

Provide information about relaxation techniques and other avenues to reduce emotional distress

Offer a noncritical ear

Give clear information about treatments and procedures

Utilize available resources to assist with providing patient and family assessment and support

Inform patients and families of available community resources and assist them in using them

imperative as changes in the delivery of health care continue to dictate the realities of the workplace, particularly in terms of availability of psychosocial resources.

NEEDS AND FUTURE DIRECTIONS

Nurses need education and consultation to care for the complex, interrelated physical and psychosocial needs of the patients they care for. Information about control of symptoms such as pain, nausea, and vomiting, organic mental impairment, functionals tatus changes, and how those symptoms can impact on quality of life is needed. Education about signs, symptoms and interventions for quality of life problems, most common in patients with advanced illness, as well as appropriate use of resources (e.g., pain service, hospital chaplains, etc.) is essential.

Often nurses on the "frontlines" of patient care correctly perceive quality of life problems and ask physicians to make appropriate referrals. Despite these requests, these concerns often seem less important in the acute medical setting where death is ever-present, severe catastrophes happen often and the demand to attend to acute medical problems take the time and energy of house officers and attending staff. Since budget restrictions and program cutbacks are common in hospitals throughout the country, the existence of clinicians that specialize in symptom and quality of life management is usually limited. Since hiring of additional clinicians is usually not feasible, efforts should be directed toward increasing the level of nursing knowledge regarding assessment and management of quality of life issues in patients. When consultants are

available, providing education about "markers" that warrant outside consultations is indicated. Psychiatric and pain management consultations are but two examples of resources that can have an invaluable impact on improving quality of life of patients and their families. Examples of markers that warrant outside psychiatric intervention are a sudden change in the personality of a patient and/or depressive symptoms that are unresponsive to usual psychosocial support by family and staff. Short hospital stays demand more rapid assessment of day-to-day problems by nurses so that management does not fall exclusively to family members who are often ill equipped to manage them alone following discharge of the patient.

Despite the need for ongoing research that describes and clarifies specific nursing behaviors and interventions and their impact on selected outcomes, it seems clear within our current state of knowledge that providing information about what to expect to both patients and families is often instrumental in reducing distress and enhancing control. Keeping patients comfortable, promoting independence and offering avenues for questions when problems arise are key nursing behaviors that can significantly improve the psychosocial aspects of the cancer experience.

REFERENCES

1. Padilla GV, Grant MM. Quality of life as a cancer nursing outcome variable. *Adv Nurs Sci.* 1985; 8:45–58.
2. Andrykowski MA, Redd WH, Hatfield AK. The development of anticipatory nausea: a prospective analysis. *J Consult Clin Psychol.* 1985; 4:447–454.
3. Burish TG, Lyles JN. Effectiveness of relaxation training in reducing adverse reactions to cancer chemotherapy. *J Behav Med.* 1981; 4:65–78.
4. Ferrell BR, Rhiner M, Ferrell BA. Development and implementation of a pain education program. *Cancer.* 1993; 72S:3426–3432.
5. Johnson JE, Lauver DR, Nail LM. Process of coping with radiation therapy. *J Clin Consult Psychol.* 1989; 57:358–364.
6. Dodd MJ. Efficacy of proactive information on self-care in chemotherapy patients. *Patient Education Couns.* 1988; 11:215–225.
7. McCorkle R, Benoliel JQ, Donaldson G, et al. A randomized clinical trial of home health nursing care for lung cancer patients. *Cancer.* 1989; 64:199–206.
8. Sarna L, McCorkle R. Living with lung cancer: a prototype to describe the burden of care for patient, family and caregivers. *Cancer Pract.* 1996; 12:42–49.
9. Graydon FE. Factors that predict patients' functioning following treatment for cancer. *Int J Nurs Stud.* 1988; 25:117–124.
10. Cella DF, Orofiamma B, Holland JC, et al. The relationship of psychological distress, extent of disease and performance status in patients with lung cancer. *Cancer.* 1987; 60:1661–1667.

11. Northouse LL, Swain MA. Adjustment of patients and husbands to the initial impact of breast cancer. *Nurs Res.* 1987; 36:221–225.

12. Nagi SZ. A conceptual framework. In: Nagi SZ, ed. *Disability and Rehabilitation: Legal, Clinical and Self Concepts and Measurement.* Columbus: Ohio State University Press; 1969.

13. Craig TJ, Abeloff MD. Psychiatric symptomatology among hospitalized cancer patients. *Am J Psychiatry.* 1974; 26:133–136.

14. Plumb MM, Holland JC. Comparative studies of psychological function in patients with advanced cancer. I. Self-reported depressive symptoms. *Psychosom Med.* 1977; 39:264–272.

15. Plumb MM, Holland JC. Comparative studies of psychological function in patients with advanced cancer. II. Interviewer-rated current and past psychological symptoms. *Psychosom Med.* 1981; 43:243–254.

16. Peck A, Boland L. Emotional reaction to having cancer. *Am J Roentgenol Radiat Ther Nucl Med.* 1972; 114: 346–353.

17. Bukerb J, Penman D, Holland JC. Depression in hospitalized cancer patients. *Psychosom Med.* 1984; 46: 199–212.

18. Derogatis LR, Morrow GR, Fetting J, et al. The prevalence of psychiatric disorders among cancer patients. *J Am Med Assoc.* 1983; 249:751–757.

19. Pasacreta JV, Massie MJ. Psychiatric complications in patients with cancer. *Oncol Nurs Forum.* 1990; 17:19–24.

20. Weissman A, Worden JW. The existential plight in cancer: significance of the first 100 days. *Int J Psychiatry Med.* 1976–1977; 7(1):1–15.

21. McCorkle R. Terminal illness: human attachments and intended goals. In: Batey M, ed. *Communicating Nursing Research: Nursing Research in the Bicentennial Year.* Boulder, CO: WICHE; 1977: 9:207–221.

22. Nail L. Used and perceived efficacy of self-care activities in patients receiving chemotherapy. *Oncol Nurs Forum.* 1991; 18:883–887.

23. Sarna L. Women with lung cancer: impact on quality of life. *Qual Life Res.* 1992; 2:13–22.

24. Petitti DB. Sounding board, competing technologies, implications for the costs and complexities of medical care. *N Engl J Med.* 1986; 315:1480–1483.

25. American Nurses Association. *Nursing: A Social Policy Statement.* Kansas City, MO: American Nurses Association; 1966.

26. Larson PJ. Comparison of cancer patients' and professional nurses' perceptions of important nurse caring behaviors. *Top Clin Nurs.* 1987; 8:30–36.

27. Wolf ZR. The caring concept and nurse identified caring behaviors. *Top Clin Nurs.* 1986; 8:84–93.

28. Larson PJ. Important nurse caring behaviors perceived by patients with cancer. *Oncol Nurs Forum.* 1984; 11:46–50.

29. Brown L. The experience of care: patient perspectives. *Top Clin Nurs.* 1986; 8:56–62.

30. Cronin SN, Harrison B. Importance of nurse caring behaviors as perceived by patients after myocardial infarction. *Heart Lung.* 1988: 17:374–389.

31. Mayer DK. Cancer patients and families' perceptions of nurse caring behaviors. *Top Clin Nurs.* 1986; 8:63–69.

32. Hull MM. Hospice nurses, caring support for caregiving families. *Cancer Nurs.* 1991; 14:63–70.

33. Carey RL, Jevne R. Development of an information package for post-mastectomy patients on adjuvant therapy. *Oncol Nurs Forum.* 1986; 13:78–79.

34. Johnson JE. Psychological interventions and coping with surgery. In: Baum A, Taylor SE, Singer JE, eds. *Handbook of Psychology and Health,* vol 4. Hillsdale, NJ: Earlbaum; 1984.

35. McCorkle R, Jepson C, Malone D, et al. The impact of posthospital home care on patients with cancer. *Res Nurs Health.* 1994; 17:243–251.

36. Garland TN, Bass DM, Otto ME. The needs of hospice patients and primary caregivers: comparison of primary caregivers' and hospice nurses' perceptions. *Am J Hospice Care.* 1984; 3:40–45.

37. Hull MM. Family needs and supportive nursing behaviors during terminal cancer: a review. *Oncol Nurs Forum.* 1989; 16:787–792.

38. Skorupka P, Bohnet N. Primary caregivers' perceptions of nursing behaviors that best meet their need in a home care hospice setting. *Cancer Nurs.* 1982; 10:371–374.

39. Leventhal H, Johnson JE. Laboratory and field experimentation: development of a theory of self regulation. In: Wooldridge PJ, Schmitt MH, Skipper JK, eds. *Behavioral Science and Nursing Theory.* St Louis, MO: Mosby; 1983.

40. Smith MC, Holcombe JK, Stullenbarger E. A meta-analysis of intervention effectiveness for symptom management in oncology nursing research. *Oncol Nurs Forum.* 1994; 21:1201–1210.

41. Weintraub FN, Hagopian GA. The effects of nursing consultation on anxiety, side effects, and self care of patients receiving radiation therapy. *Oncol Nurs Forum.* 1990; 17:31–36.

42. McCorkle R, Robinson L, Lev E, Nuamah L. The effects of home nursing interventions provided to patients during terminal illness on the bereaved's psychological distress. Presented at the Second Annual Scientific Symposium, The Center for Advancing Care in Serious Illness, University of Pennsylvania, School of Nursing, March 1996.

70

Alternative and Complementary Therapies

BRIAN D. DOAN

How far the mind-cure movement is destined to extend its influence, . . . no one can foretell. It is essentially a religious movement, and to academically nurtured minds its utterances are tasteless and often grotesque enough. It also incurs the natural enmity of medical politicians, and of the whole trades-union wing of that profession. But no unprejudiced observer can fail to recognise its importance as a social phenomenon today, and the higher medical minds are already trying to interpret it fairly, and make its power available for their own therapeutic ends.

—Wm. James (1906, 1911)

The latter half of this century has featured tremendous technological advances in orthodox cancer medicine. Public surveys have shown corresponding shifts in beliefs about the causes, preventability, and treatability of cancer that seem to reflect changes in our scientific understanding of cancer (1–3). For example, there has been a gradually increasing acknowledgement of the role of smoking in cancer, and a waning of the belief that cancer is contagious (4). Up to the 1980's both health professionals and the public tended consistently to emphasize the seriousness and uncontrollability of the disease (4,5). Although cancer is still a leading cause of death in North America, roughly half of contemporary cancer patients will survive beyond 5 years after their diagnosis. Some will be completely cured (6). As a result, the last decade or so finds the popular press paying increasing attention to the possibilities for "beating" cancer. Among these possibilities, there has been a sustained and growing public interest in unconventional and unproven treatments. Lifestyle-oriented alternatives rank among the most popular unconventional approaches, along with beliefs that psychological and social variables can directly influence the development and course of cancer.

We tend to view current trends as unique to our age. But as the opening quotation from James' *The Energies of Men* (7) suggests, the idea that psychological and social factors can contribute to the onset and course of malignant disease is not new. Written nearly

a century ago, James' comments have a disturbingly contemporary ring. He was addressing the popularity of the healing movement of *his* day, yet his assessment could just as readily describe the prevailing stance in cancer medicine towards belief in psychological effects on cancer and the use of alternative healing methods. As Hurny (8) noted, " . . . harsh battles between 'believers' and 'nonbelievers' have been fought . . . discussion within and outside the medical community still goes on," and " . . . the emotional storms usually stirred up show that it is not strictly a scientific dialogue" (8, p 6).

The persisting popularity of unconventional cancer treatments continues to raise complex ethical and practical questions for caregivers. The purpose of this chapter is to consider some of the underlying reasons for the appeal of alternative healing practices. Our inquiry begins with some definitions and a historical context, followed by a brief review of the data on the prevalence of unconventional treatments today and how these data have been interpreted. We then consider contemporary beliefs regarding psychological influences on cancer, and the heroic response that such beliefs can evoke when a person has to face cancer in his or her own body. The entire phenomenon of alternative healing practices reflects spiritual and moral themes of great importance to patients—themes that have implications both for conventional cancer care and for our conceptions of mental health.

DEFINITIONS

The domain we are interested in encompasses healing practices of various kinds. It includes *adjuvant* and *complementary* approaches, as well as *alternative* and *unproven* treatments for cancer. These two broad classes of treatment can be distinguished in several ways. Complementary approaches are designed to enhance coping and adaptation. They are typically used by patients to supplement conventional cancer treatment, both curative and palliative. Examples include the use of relaxation and meditative techniques, prayer and church affiliation, stress management training, healthy nutrition and psychotherapy, as well as individual and group peer support programs. All are aimed at enhancing mental and general physical well-being (9).

Alternative treatments are aimed at affecting tumor growth. They are typically used by patients with hopes of directly slowing, halting, or reversing the spread of cancer, either with, or instead of, conventional treatment. There is overlap between complementary and alternative approaches because some complementary psychosocial interventions are advocated by some as capable of affecting cancer outcomes such as mortality, survival time and quality of life. Relaxation and guided imagery, for example, are complementary treatments when promoted as enhancing emotional control and psychological well-being. They are alternative treatments when promoted as an anticancer intervention. The rationale for using psychologically based techniques in cancer care has been made more ambiguous by

popular usage of the term "healing" in reference to both psychological and physical processes. Also included among the alternative approaches are a number of physical and biochemical interventions that are based on competing accounts of tumor growth. These are the controversial, unconventional treatments, each with their own toxicities and hazards, that routinely garner the most public attention: severe nutritional regimes in conjunction with purgative and other "cleansing" agents, metabolic and immunological treatments, and a variety of single agents or preparations such as laetrile, Essiac, shark cartilage, wheatgrass, mistletoe, and many others.

Complementary approaches are more likely to be accessed within the conventional cancer care delivery system, whereas alternative treatments are more likely to be accessed outside of conventional care, through naturopaths, homeopaths, chiropractors, and other providers of alternative medicine, and the health foods and supplements industry. Table 70.1 attempts to depict some of the relationships between conventional, adjuvant/complementary, and alternative/unproven treatments. The table is by no means exhaus-

TABLE 70.1. *A Conceptual Framework for Classifying Approaches to Cancer Treatment*

Conventional Therapies	Complementary or Adjunctive Therapies	Alternative Therapies
EXAMPLES		
Radiation treatment	Meditation/imagery	Homeopathy
Systemic treatment	Spiritual approaches	Naturopathy
Surgery	Psychotherapy	Osteopathy/chiropracty
	Nutrition	Essiac
	Stress management	Megavitamin therapies
		Shark's cartilage
		Koch's antitoxins
		Metabolic therapy
		Macrobiotics
		Wheatgrass
		Laetrile
CONCEPTUAL UNDERPINNINGS		
Biological and molecular approach to cancer	Holistic approach to health and illness	Cure and healing require purifying the body and strengthening its resources
	Unity of mind and body	
	Personal responsibility for health	
Medical Model*	Moral and Compensatory Models*	
POTENTIAL HAZARDS OR PROBLEMS		
Significant short- and long-term toxicities associated with conventional care	Adjunctive methods used for the effective management of psychological and emotional aspects of cancer are seen by some as able to control or cure tumor growth	Many demonstrated to be "inactive" or fraudulent
		Some may be toxic or harmful
	No firm confirmatory evidence	

*After Brickman et al. (57) and Northouse and Wortman (56).

tive, but it does provide a general framework for classifying any given cancer intervention.

HISTORICAL CONTEXT

Folk remedies for cancer have been used for centuries. During the past 150 years or more, cancer remedies typically have consisted of a combination of various quasi-medical treatments, dietary and lifestyle interventions and faith healing (10–13). Back at the turn of this century, in William James' day, American society was taken with homeopathy, naturopathy, osteopathy and chiropracty. The notion that health is best maintained through vegetarianism and natural foods was popular then. It persists today in approaches that seek to purify and cleanse the body through vegetarian diets and colonic irrigation—practices that harken back to the naturopathic movement of the late 1800s.

Tonics, pills, and ointments for a variety of ailments were among the most popular folk remedies of the early 1900s. From the 1940s on, a single, widely popular cancer cure has dominated each decade. In the 1940s, it was Koch's glyoxilide, a fraudulent product that was found to be distilled water. Hoxsey's herbal tonic gained national attention in the 1950s. It was made from ten herbs allegedly responsible for the cure of a horse's leg cancer. A 10-year court battle ultimately led to the sale of Hoxsey's tonic being declared illegal. It is still available in Mexico. In the 1960s Krebiozen was marketed as a product that would stimulate the body's inherent anticancer responses. It was found by the FDA to be a hoax (9). Laetrile followed in the 1970s as the main alternative treatment. Although the extract of apricot pits was found in NCI clinical trials to be of no benefit with respect to " . . . cure, improvement or stabilization of cancer, improvement of symptoms related to cancer or extension of the life span" (14), public pressure led to legislated assurance that laetrile could be obtained by patients with cancer who wanted it.

The American Cancer Society (ACS) has kept an accurate and continuous record of the 50–60 alternative cancer treatments that have emerged since the 1940s. A formal ACS committee has reviewed and provided thorough reports on the most popular alternatives over the decades, and constitutes an important resource on unproven methods for health care providers (9).

The 1980s and 1990s have been characterized by a departure from alternative therapies that rely on a single substance, and a reversion to the earlier, naturopathic concepts of health maintenance. Our society has increasingly come to value personal responsibility for health maintenance and to subscribe to a holistic approach to health and illness that includes the concept of the unity of body and mind. Consequently, the more prevalent alternative cancer care approaches today tend to reflect these social views.

PREVALENCE

Relatively consistent findings on the use of unconventional methods have been reported in a number of studies of cancer patients over the past 10 years (15–23). It appears that from 10% to 60% of cancer patients use some alternative treatment. McGinnis (22) reported that better educated patients with higher than average income are more likely to choose alternative therapies and are often supported by a physician in their choice. Downer et al. (18). reported that patients using complementary therapies tend to be younger, of higher social class, and female. Cassileth et al. (15) also noted that the majority of patients receiving unorthodox treatment were well-educated, usually asymptomatic, and in the early stages of disease.

Unconventional treatments are rarely adopted in the absence of conventional care. Cassileth et al. (15), for example, reported the use of unorthodox treatments alone at less than 8%. Others since then have reported even lower estimates (22). Typically, patients undergo conventional treatment first and adopt alternative approaches an average of 2 years after initiating conventional treatment. A proportion of patients discontinue conventional treatment in favour of alternatives, but what evidence there is suggests that the decision is usually reasonable given the patient's circumstances—i.e., advancing disease despite an average of 8 months of conventional treatment, adverse reactions to conventional treatments, etc.; see Lerner and Kennedy (20).

Downer et al. (18) observed that the most popular complementary therapies are healing, relaxation and visualization, diets, homeopathy, vitamins, and herbalism. Cassileth et al. (15) reported the most prevalent unorthodox therapies as being: metabolic and diet therapies, megavitamins, mental imagery, spiritual or faith healing, and immune therapy. In his recent comprehensive review, Lerner (21) also identified the more popular alternatives as being nutritional approaches, unconventional drugs and traditional Chinese medicine, physical therapies, and psychological/spiritual perspectives. To echo William James, "the ideas here are healthy-minded and optimistic" (7). Although contemporary alternative treatments differ in focus, they share a common, holistic, perspective (24). The aim of such treatments is to improve the patient's own biological and psychological ability to overcome the cancer illness. The mind–body emphasis of this perspective is intuitively appealing. Patients seem to welcome the opportunity to pursue lifestyle-oriented options and to assume a measure of control and active participation in regaining and maintaining their health.

In view of such findings, it is unclear why McGinnis (22) would attribute "a renaissance" of alternative therapies to "an anti-establishment, anti-intellectual climate," and an "increasingly mobile, rootless" society. Many patients pursue alternatives with the support of a physician during or after conventional treatment. Others avoid mentioning their decision because they expect a negative response from their oncologist. In either case, they believe that their cancer could have been prevented, that it is reversible, and that alternative treatments will help them achieve this by restoring rather than weakening the body's reserves and its capacity for healing. Cassileth et al. (15) did note that more than half of the patients in their study were of the opinion that the government and the medical establishment tend to restrict freedom of choice in cancer treatment. However, that opinion does not distinguish patients who pursue unconventional cancer care from those who do not. Patients who pursue alternative treatments do tend to be less satisfied with their experience of conventional care, usually because of side effects and the lack of hope of cure (15,18). But that is a long way from suggesting that such patients are rebellious, anti-intellectual, or rootless.

The difficulty, of course, is that for most health professionals, the terms "alternative," "unconventional," and "unorthodox" usually connote interventions of unproven effectiveness, often based upon questionable scientific rationales, and frequently with claims of benefits that outweigh the evidence. Sometimes, alternative treatments are presented in ways that explicitly challenge conventional approaches to treatment.

The bulk of the recent scientific literature on alternative cancer treatments has focused on the evaluation of the more "biological" varieties of unorthodox treatments: the nutritional therapies, including macrobiotic and other similar dietary regimens, metabolic therapies, vitamin and herbal therapies, and "immunoaugmentative" therapies (17,19,22,25–29). By most conventional assessments, many of these questionable therapies have been found to be harmless or inexpensive, although some are also potentially harmful or toxic, and some can be costly. More important, none have scientifically demonstrable efficacy, and the ACS routinely advises that such treatments be avoided.

In contrast, complementary approaches—especially the psychological ones—have tended to fare better. A growing portion of the current scientific literature on adjuvant and complementary cancer treatments extols the various benefits of some form of relaxation therapy, taught individually or in groups, with or without visualization or guided imagery (30–39). Relaxation and meditative techniques have been shown to be useful in alleviating patient distress and in decreasing the experienced severity of physical symptoms such as nausea, vomiting, and pain arising both from the disease itself and from its treatment with chemotherapy or radiation. It bears noting here again that, although scientific demonstrations of the efficacy of relaxation in cancer care are a relatively new development, belief in the beneficial effects of relaxation is long-standing. The companion lecture to the one quoted above, in James' *On Vital Reserves*, is *The Gospel of Relaxation* (7). In it, James reviewed the Lange–James theory of emotions and the evidence of the day on the hazards of habitual tension. His conclusion: "We must change ourselves from a race that admires jerk and snap for their own sakes, . . . to one that, on the contrary, has *calm* for its ideal." (7, p 65)

In addition to the evaluation of nutritional, metabolic, and relaxation therapies, increasing attention in conventional cancer medicine is currently focused on the dilemmas posed for health care professionals by patient interest in alternative approaches (21,23,24,40–51). The main thrust of this literature has been to stress the practical, ethical and legal reasons for physicians and nurses to be better informed about alternative cancer treatments and more sensitive to patients' reasons for pursuing alternatives. However, the responses advocated for health professionals vary, from being supportive when it is not obviously against a patient's interests to pursue an unproven treatment (24,44), to adopting a strict and principled stance in promoting the scientific treatment of cancer and discouraging questionable treatment methods (46).

Montbriand (49) makes an interesting counterargument for those who maintain that the medical establishment seeks to limit patients' freedom of choice. She noted that patients who choose alternative therapies often do so on the basis of limited information from the lay literature. She therefore questioned their freedom of choice, arguing that since patients typically are not exposed to the biomedical assessment of alternative therapies, their poorly informed choice is less free. Montbriand (23,49) joins Fletcher (40) in suggesting that nurses can play a vital role in assisting patient access to the relevant scientific literature on alternative treatments and helping patients and families in choosing among treatment options.

Others are less certain about the most appropriate role for health professionals with respect to unconventional therapies (52). Kennedy (45) and Nwoga (53) each point to substantial discrepancies between the perspectives of patients and physicians, and Hufford (54) notes that these differences in perspective arise from differing assumptions and from patients crediting subjective experience over medical statistics. Jackson (44) cautions health professionals that there may not be "the right" response to patients seeking alternative therapies, only alternative appropriate responses. We shall return to this issue of how the health professional can best be helpful later.

BELIEF IN PSYCHOLOGICAL EFFECTS ON CANCER

The finding that generally well-educated patients will adopt alternative methods on the basis of limited information is itself quite telling. In the absence of evidence to the contrary, people are attracted to the notion that the state of the whole person can determine whether or not cancer can be overcome. Thus, any nutritional, herbal, physical or psychological intervention with a putative anticancer effect, and which also is purported to enhance a person's health and well-being, is a candidate alternative or complementary treatment of choice. When patients approach an alternative treatment in this way, as just one component of an altered lifestyle, information about the efficacy of that alternative by itself may well be seen as relatively unimportant, given the "total effect" they hope to achieve with the appropriate attitude, motivation, and various other health-promoting behaviors.

Central to the appeal of unconventional, holistic approaches to cancer treatment is the emphasis on personal responsibility for one's health and the belief that psychological states can affect the course of the illness. Recently, we surveyed 135 oncology caregivers and 442 university students to explore their views about psychological influences on cancer (55). The sampling was more purposive than representative: the students were a uniform group of young adults seeking higher education, and the health professionals were drawn from our own regional cancer center and from the membership of our national psychosocial oncology association. Thus, while the generalizability of our findings remains uncertain, the results were nonetheless illuminating.

The physicians in our sample were in general more reserved than other caregivers (nurses, social workers, psychologists, and others), and the health professionals

in general were more sensitive than the students to the potential danger of belief in psychological influences on cancer. Nevertheless, the majority of both groups agreed strongly that psychological factors can influence physical health and that stress and coping style can influence the course of cancer, including its curability. Both groups also rated various psychological strategies (e.g., a fighting spirit, positive thinking, relaxation) as very helpful physically to persons with cancer. Most indicated that they would adopt such approaches if they themselves had cancer.

The survey afforded an opportunity to test current models of belief regarding psychological effects on cancer. Northouse and Wortman (56) identified four such models, which differ with respect to whether or not patients are seen as responsible for causing and/or for resolving a cancer illness. Following Brickman et al. (57), Northouse and Wortman cite a "medical model," which views patients as neither responsible for causing, nor for resolving, health problems. In effect, the medical model characterises nonbelievers. Only 7% of our sample of students and health professionals fit the medical model. They disagreed that psychological variables can influence health and they disagreed that either personal stress or coping style could be causal factors in the development or course of cancer.

Among the majority who responded as believers, 44% of both the students' and health professionals' responses corresponded to what Northouse and Wortman called the "moral model." Not only did they agree strongly that psychological factors can influence health, they also agreed strongly that stress and coping style can both cause and affect the course of cancer. This "moral model" is the one exemplified by the holistic health movement. The work of theorists such as LeShan and Gassman (58), Pelletier (59), Simonton (60,61), and Siegel (62,63), are examples of this model.

Equally popular among the believers in our sample was a set of responses that corresponded to Northouse and Wortman's "compensatory model." The compensatory model characterizes the position typically adopted by cancer education programs such as "Reach to Recovery," "CANSURMOUNT," and "I Can Cope." It attributes low responsibility to the patient for causing health problems, but high responsibility for resolving them. Of the caregivers and students in our sample, 40% agreed that psychological factors can influence health. However, they disagreed that stress or coping can be contributing causes of cancer, and many expressed concern about the harmful effect of believing that how one coped with stress might have brought cancer on. At the same time, they clearly placed a high value on the use of psychological strategies to enhance the health of persons with cancer, and agreed strongly that stress and coping style could alter the course of the disease.

If our findings are any indication, the idea that psychological factors can influence the course of a cancer illness is believed by a majority of people, including many health professionals who work in oncology. Their beliefs are largely consistent with a moral and a compensatory model of helping and coping described by Northouse and Wortman (56) and Brickman et al. (57). The popularity of such beliefs should come as no surprise. Contemporary notions about psychological effects on cancer are consistent with the more general—and quite respectable—health promotion focus in Western society on taking personal responsibility for health maintenance through physical fitness, proper nutrition and an improved mental attitude.

THE HEROIC STANCE

There is something deeper than current trends in health promotion motivating many cancer patients' interest in alternative treatments. A diagnosis of cancer is arguably a tragedy; at a minimum, it constitutes one of life's most dreaded personal crises. It is one of those fundamental life crises that—if it does not overwhelm—can galvanize a person into action. To the person with cancer, the prospects for survival may seem highly uncertain. The ambiguity of being given even odds of surviving beyond 5 years typically raises questions for patients about what they can do to improve those odds. Naturally, most people with cancer feel a strong need to regain control of their lives (56,57,64–72). But the response of many people to the crisis of cancer goes far beyond merely striving for personal control. For them, cancer calls for a heroic response, an all-out effort to alter the course of their illness by changing who they are. Journalist David Steen, writing about time spent with his brother and his dying wife, put it most eloquently: "Being up close and personal with death makes you ask who you are, where you are going, and what really counts." (73)

Gray and Doan have described the heroic stance as an attempt to control the course of cancer illness through psychological self-transformation (41,74). According to popular belief, the path to self-healing lies in becoming a more effective, more expressive, more loving, more positive, and more courageous person. The media and popular press routinely feature stories about heroic individuals who have battled cancer in this way and survived. The slogan "Cancer can

be beaten!" has become a rallying cry for the individual to engage in a heroic fight against his or her illness in the tradition of the archetypal hero.

Historically, hero myths have taken various forms. A familiar and recurrent one is of the warrior hero who has to face a devouring monster and is subjected to a series of trials and intense suffering (75–77). This is a powerful metaphor for the predicament of the patient with a spreading tumor and dealing with invasive treatment. Through great courage and virtue, and much learning, the mythical hero usually vanquishes the monster and returns home victorious and transformed.

The person with cancer who focuses on self-transformation and survives—even for the time being—dramatically fulfils the criteria for archetypal heroism. According to analytic psychologists and anthropologists, hero myths symbolize our urge for self-transcendence—our wish to be more than what we are, to be larger than life. The heroic urge is, according to Becker (76) our most common defense against death. For the person with cancer, adopting a heroic stance can provide security, a sense of identity, and a way to endure hardship and an uncertain future.

We have noted a number of benefits to a heroic stance towards cancer (41,74). It can be a healthy counterresponse to the sense of loss of control and helplessness that typically characterizes the experience of being a cancer patient. Those who believe that their health will improve by keeping fit, by practicing visualization and relaxation, by changing their relationships and by redefining life priorities, frequently feel an enhanced sense of mastery over their lives and their illness, even when long-term survival is out of the question.

Adoption of a heroic stance can also provide some patients with a way of understanding their illness so that it has some positive personal meaning. We have encountered several patients, for example, who interpreted their illness as a serious *warning* that important elements of their life and relationships with others had to change. Believing that cancer has this kind of personal relevance has motivated many such patients to undertake important life changes which, they claim, they would not have otherwise, and even to feel grateful in some measure for having developed cancer.

Faced with the possibility of an imminent death, it is natural to reflect harder on the meaning of one's life, and to question "Who am I?" and "How shall I face this?" Patients often answer: "I believe I am basically a good person, and it's important to me to deal with my illness and potential demise in an exemplary way," that is, with a good measure of poise and fortitude, courage, and dignity. Adopting a heroic stance can help focus the person with cancer in setting priorities and in taking action to remedy life problems.

We have also noted attempts to adopt a heroic stance that have brought a burden of guilt or a sense of failure to the person with cancer, or impaired relationships with family and friends. Sometimes, this occurs because the patient interpreted being heroic in a way that led them either to assume blame for being ill or to protect others from the illness; sometimes, because loved ones put undue pressure on the patient to be heroic and positive and will not tolerate expressions of anxiety or despair. Often in such cases, there is an underlying fear that anxiety or sadness might promote disease progression. Such hazards—often brought about by misinterpretations of the heroic stance or by generalizations and misleading claims in the popular literature on the influence of the psyche on disease—more often than not can be resolved with effective psychological support.

The point is, attempts to adopt a heroic stance are not always helpful to a patient's emotional well-being, let alone his or her chances for survival. Everyone has their own interpretation of what it might take to respond heroically in the face of a cancer illness. Each person brings to the task preexisting anxieties about his or her self-worth, integrity, courage, and maturity. Sometimes those anxieties lead to unfortunate and problematic attempts at heroism, difficulties that call for the most sensitive and thoughtful response possible from health professionals.

IMPLICATIONS FOR CLINICAL CARE

For many cancer patients, the use of alternative and complementary treatments is just a small part of a larger journey they have undertaken—namely to regain their health by embracing life and facing their cancer heroically, with courage, hope and optimism, intelligence, and exemplary conduct. Seen in this way, a patient's expressed interest in pursuing alternatives should be greeted by any health professional with respect and the utmost sensitivity. Health professionals are well advised to inform themselves about popular alternative approaches and to be prepared to assist patients seeking information about alternatives. Reservations about a given alternative can be expressed without undermining a patient's hope or determination to fight the disease. When there are no obvious grounds for concern about the use of an alternative or complementary treatment, health professionals are well advised to support the patient's interest.

It is now well documented that a cancer patient's emotional well-being is likely to be enhanced when the patient actively participates in getting well and is able to maintain a positive, survival-oriented attitude towards the illness and its treatment (66–70,78). What is lacking is convincing evidence that psychological change of the sort that is involved in adopting a heroic stance can alter or halt the course of cancer. We have noted some inherent risks for health professionals who either advocate a heroic stance unreservedly or dismiss it out of hand (41). The unreserved advocate who takes on the role of "hero's guide" can compromise his ability to assist the cancer patient emotionally when the disease recurs or progresses. In contrast, the complete sceptic risks undermining the patient's hope and increasing the patient's sense of helplessness through his or her failure to support the patient's attempts to go beyond conventional care.

The conflict for a conscientious health professional between maintaining scientific and professional integrity and maintaining a patient's emotional well-being arises in part because the patient's and the caregiver's perspectives are so divergent. The health professional, not having cancer, can afford to be sceptical about alternative treatments until all the relevant data are in. The cancer patient, however, has little choice about what to believe. His or her options are, to use William James' term (79), "forced". The patient's plight accordingly calls for a tolerant and compassionate response from the health professional, one that focuses less on whether patients hold "correct" beliefs about what can affect cancer, and more on the effects of those beliefs on the patient's mental and physical health.

The psychologically oriented alternative approaches in particular provide hope, control and mastery through self-help, and a focus and sense of concern for the whole person. All are features of health maintenance that are frequently seen as deficient within the conventional health care delivery system. A commitment by those who work in oncology to provide maximal emotional support in the context of conventional treatment, encompasses how the health professional deals with the issues raised by patients' interest in pursuing alternative care. Here are several guidelines that should be used in responding to patients and families regarding alternative treatments (see Table 70.2).

When health professionals adopt a flexible approach to patients' commitment to getting well, they are better able to address the unique circumstances of individual patients. When a patient's adoption of a heroic stance and complementary treatments seems to be enhancing their sense of personal control, hopefulness, and

TABLE 70.2. *Guidelines for Oncology Staff Regarding Alternative Treatments*

Be well informed about current alternative therapies

Evaluate the reasons for the patient's interest in an alternative therapy. Does it reflect emotional needs that are not being addressed within conventional care?

Provide accurate information about alternatives to patients and families

Encourage questions, take all questions seriously

Advise pro and con based on the alternative approach being discussed, its potential to interfere or not with conventional therapy and its possible adjunctive versus alternative use

Avoid moral judgments

Discuss risks and benefits thoroughly

Follow-up with questions over the ensuing weeks to monitor for any negative emotional or physical sequelae

Source: Adapted from Holland et al. (9)

emotional well-being, our recommendation to health professionals is to support and facilitate their efforts. When a patient's attempts at a heroic response or his/her pursuit of alternative therapies cause unnecessary distress, impairs the patient's coping ability, or results in increased isolation or alienation from loved ones, we are inclined to draw his or her attention to the difficulty and suggest an alternative course of action, taking care all the while to preserve the patient's sense of mastery, hope, and commitment to living.

Psycho-oncology staff are in an ideal position to serve as informed resources on alternative and complementary treatments for both patients and other health professionals. The guidelines recommended above for dealing with a patient's are also applicable in many instances in responding to oncology staff who are having difficulty with patients' interest in pursuing alternatives. Because the patient's decision to pursue alternatives will often arise in the context of advancing disease and perceived deficiencies in conventional care, the reaction of oncology staff to alternative treatments may reflect a number of emotional issues—including self-protective responses against feelings of powerlessness, failure and impending loss that can adversely affect the patient–provider relationship. The psycho-oncologist would do well to be informed about current alternatives, to carefully evaluate the reasons for the staff member's difficulty with the patient's decision to pursue alternatives, and to review with him or her the risks and benefits of the alternative therapy in question. Encourage open discussion, and avoid making moral judgments about the provider. Encourage staff to recognize the patient's motivation to be an active participant in his or her care, and explore ways in which he or she might take the opportunity to strengthen a collaborative patient–provider relationship.

It can be very difficult for oncology staff on those rare occasions when a patient decides to use a dubious alternative treatment to the exclusion of conventional treatment. Oncology staff should always consult a psycho-oncologist in such cases, and refer the patient and family, for these are invariably complex situations in which the patient has become very dissatisfied with conventional care and may even have contributed substantially to conflict with the health care delivery system, and/or is emotionally overwhelmed by his or her disease. It is important to remember in such cases that, provided the patient's capacity to consent to treatment is intact, his or her right to decide autonomously what treatments to have must be respected. This holds whether or not the patient's choice is seen by staff as in his or her "best interests." The psycho-oncologist can help oncology staff to maintain a constructive and caring approach with the patient—including the provision of effective palliative care—even if the patient rejects conventional treatment and opts for an alternative.

IMPLICATIONS FOR MENTAL HEALTH THEORY

All too often, the clinical and scientific literature on the subject of alternative treatment has focused rather narrowly on the unproved efficacy of given alternatives and the responsibilities (professional, moral, and legal) of the health care provider with respect to a patient's use of alternatives. In the few articles where the question of *why* patients pursue alternatives is addressed, the focus is invariably on beliefs and attitudes about unorthodox treatments and the implications for conventional health care systems and practitioners (15,22). This is a regrettable myopia, for the popularity of alternative and complementary treatments in cancer and concomitant beliefs about the importance of a heroic stance in combating the disease go right to the heart of how we conceive of mental and physical health.

Frank recently discussed the concept of "illness as a moral occasion." (82) A recurring theme in Frank's writing is the patient as person. His focus in this particular paper was the propensity among the ill to want to "rise to the occasion" and "do the best or the right thing" (see also Hoffmaster (83) and Zaner (84,85) cited in Frank (82)). This is precisely what is involved when persons with cancer adopt a heroic stance towards their illness and venture off to explore alternatives. Questions about who we are, and how we should conduct ourselves in the face of a life-threat, involve *ideals*, and, as such, are moral questions. Our collective sense of the heroic, and our myths and tales of heroes and heroines embody and personify the values and ideals that are implicated in major personal crises. Adoption of a heroic stance by a person with cancer involves contact with idealizations of what it means to be human and idealizations of the proper attitude towards a life crisis. It follows from this that to the extent that illness can be viewed as a moral occasion, then so too is health, in part, a moral concern.

A similar set of points about mental health was made recently by John Macnamara in an entirely different context (86). Reflecting on the failure of psychoanalytic theory to inform us about mental health, Macnamara argued that there is "a surprisingly close link between mental health and ethics." His thesis warrants some attention. Macnamara contends that mental health theory has suffered without a focus on normalcy in mental health.

When people study the normal knee or lung, they seek to delimit what its states and operations are when it fulfils its normal functions. The corresponding study of human persons and their behavior would seek to delimit what persons ought to be and how they ought to behave if they are to fulfil their functions. But what might these functions be? . . . those . . . that most closely touch one's status as a person. (86, p 16)

According to Macnamara, mental health "includes the ability to deal with life's successes and disappointments in a balanced manner, to rejoice over good fortune and have compassion with bad," and it includes the inclination to try our best "to be wise and good;" hence the surprisingly close link between mental health and ethics.

The importance of Frank's (82) and Macnamara's (86) positions is driven home when we consider the popular view that self-improvement and personal growth can promote healing, even of cancer. Suppose you have cancer and your heroic attitude and actions enhance your emotional well-being, leaving your chances for survival uncertain. Are you "healthier"

believing that you have control over your life even if you don't? Are you better adjusted believing that you will survive, even if it turns out that you won't? Note that these are not empirical questions. The answers depend crucially on fundamental values and beliefs about what it means to be a healthy, well-adjusted person.

The evidence suggests that the initial reason for adopting a heroic stance, or for pursuing an alternative treatment, is the person's conviction that he or she can do something to beat the cancer. For some, that fight for their own life evolves into a principled fight on their own and others' behalf for such things as the dignity and autonomy of patients, and fairness in the health care delivery system and on the part of health care providers. These are matters that go far beyond a single-minded concern for one's own survival. Many such patients actively engage in volunteerism, to provide emotional support and serve as advocates for fellow cancer patients, or to participate in cancer research. Most of them would maintain that these more altruistic activities are critical to their adjustment to cancer, and, hopefully, to the maintenance of their physical health as well. They become heroes in a way that cannot be measured merely in terms of their longevity or survival. Any measure of their heroism has to take into account what they have accomplished as individuals in moral, human terms. And for that, we need a theory of mental health that encompasses ethics.

CONCLUDING REMARKS

In this chapter, I have cast the pursuit of alternative or complementary cancer treatments as a minor part of a larger journey undertaken by the person with cancer. The use of alternative approaches is often just one outcome of a heroic stance adopted by the patient that involves a concerted attempt at self-transformation and personal growth. Health professionals have a delicate balance to maintain between expressing legitimate reservations about particular alternatives they consider to be hazardous, and respecting and supporting the patient's underlying reasons for pursuing them. Their reasons not infrequently include ethical and spiritual considerations about what it means to be healthy and well-adjusted, and how best to confront a life-threatening illness. All health professionals who care for people with cancer face a great deal of pain and loss. Health professionals in oncology also routinely encounter persons whose response to cancer is to aspire to make the best of their circumstances and be the best that they can be, in spite of their suffering. We desperately need a theory of mental health that can do justice to those aspirations, a theory that will encourage in the health care provider compassion, respect, caring and intelligence—qualities that enhance courage, independence, and a sense of worth in those to whom they are directed.

ACKNOWLEDGMENTS

This chapter is dedicated to the memory of Professor John Macnamara (1931–1996).

REFERENCES

1. Lieberman Associates. *Report for the American Cancer Society*, vols I and II. New York: American Cancer Society; 1966.
2. Knopf A. Cancer: *Changes in Opinion after 7 Years of Public Education in Lancaster*. Manchester: Manchester Regional Committee on Cancer; 1974.
3. Wakefield J. ed. Public education about cancer. *UICC Technical Report Series*, vol. 24. Geneva: UICC; 1968.
4. Brooks A. Public and professional attitudes towards cancer: A view from Great Britain. *Cancer Nurs.* 1979; 2:453–460.
5. Box V. Cancer: myths and misconceptions. *J Res Sociol Health.* 1984; 104:161–166.
6. American Cancer Society. *Cancer Facts and Figures.* New York: American Cancer Society; 1994.
7. James W. *On Vital Reserves: The Energies of Men; The Gospel of Relaxation.* New York: Henry Holt & Co.; 1911.
8. Hurny C. Psyche and cancer: odyssey of an old idea in the troubled waters of modern science. *Ann Oncol.* 1990; 1:6–8.
9. Holland JC., Geary N., Furman A. Alternative cancer therapies. In: Holland JC. Rowland JR., eds. *Handbook of Psychooncology*. London: Oxford University Press; 1989: 508–515.
10. Cassileth B. Unorthodox cancer medicine. *Cancer Invest.* 1986; 4:1482–1484.
11. Gavitz N. Sectarian medicine. *J Am Med Assoc.* 1987; 255:505–507.
12. Geary N. Indian explanatory models of illness and cancer. Honors Thesis, Harvard University, Boston, 1985.
13. Whorton JC. Traditions of folk medicine in America. *J Am Med Assoc.* 1987; 257:1632–1635.
14. Moertel CA, Fleming TR, Rubin J, et al. A clinical trial of amygdalin in the treatment of human cancer. *N Engl J Med.* 1982; 306:201–206.
15. Cassileth BA, Lusk EJ, Strouse TB, Bodenheimer BJ. Contemporary unorthodox treatments in cancer medicine: a study of patients, treatments and practitioners. *Ann Intern Med.* 1984; 101:105–112.
16. Cassileth BA, Brown H. Unorthodox cancer medicine. *CA Cancer J Clin.* 1988; 38:176–186.
17. Curt GA. Unsound methods of cancer treatment In: DeVita V, Hellman S, Rosenberg SA, eds. *Cancer: Principles and Practices of Oncology*, 4th ed. Philadelpha: JB Lippincott; 1993: 2734–2747.

18. Downer SM, Cody MM, McCluskey P, et al. Pursuit and practice of complementary therapies by cancer patients receiving conventional treatment. *Br Med J.* 1994; 309:86–89.
19. Dwyer JT. Unproven nutritional remedies and cancer. *Nutr Rev.* 1992; 50:106–109.
20. Lerner IJ, Kennedy BJ. The prevalence of questionable methods of cancer treatment in the United States. *CA Cancer J Clin.* 1992; 42:181–191.
21. Lerner M. *Choices in Healing: Integrating the Best of Conventional and complementary Approaches.* Cambridge: MIT Press; 1994.
22. McGinnis LS. Alternative therapies, 1990: an overview. *Cancer.* 1991; 67(suppl. 6):1788–1792.
23. Montbriand MJ. An overview of alternate therapies chosen by patients with cancer. *Oncol Nurs Forum.* 1994; 21:1547–1554.
24. Hauser SP. Unproven methods in cancer treatment. *Curr Opin Oncol.* 1993; 5:646–654.
25. Anonymous. Questionable methods of cancer management: 'nutritional' therapies. *CA Cancer J Clin.* 1993; 43:309–319.
26. Herbal Roulette. Consumer Rep. 1995; 60(11):698–705.
27. Houston RG. Immunoaugmentative therapy. *J Am Med Assoc.* 1994; 271:1319–1320.
28. Hunter M. Alternative dietary therapies in cancer patients. *Rec Results Cancer Res.* 1991; 121:293–295.
29. Moss RW. Immunoaugmentative therapy. *J Am Med Assoc.* 1994; 271:1319–1320.
30. Arathuzik D. Effects of cognitive-behavioral strategies on pain in cancer patients. *Cancer Nurs.* 1994; 17: 207–214.
31. Baider L, Uziely B, De-Nour AK. Progressive muscle relaxation and guided imagery in cancer patients. *Gen Hosp Psychiatry.* 1994; 16:340–347.
32. Burish TG, Jenkins RA. Effectiveness of biofeedback and relaxation training in reducing the side effects of cancer chemotherapy. *Health Psychol.* 1992 11:17–23.
33. Burish TG, Snyder LS, Jenkins RA. Preparing patients for cancer chemotherapy: Effect of coping preparation and relaxation interventions. *J Consult Clin Psychol.* 1991; 59:518–525.
34. Decker TW, Cline-Elsen J, Gallagher M. Relaxation therapy as an adjunct in radiation oncology. *J Clin Psychol.* 1992; 48:388–393.
35. Greene PG, Seime RJ, Smith ME. Distraction and relaxation training in the treatment of anticipatory vomiting: a single subject intervention. *J Behav Ther Exp Psychiatry.* 1991; 22:285–290.
36. Larsson G, Starrin B. Relaxation training as an integral part of caring activities for cancer patients: effects on wellbeing. *Scand J Caring Sci.* 1992; 6:179–185.
37. McIllmurray MB, Holdcroft PE. Supportive care and the use of relaxation therapy in a district cancer service. *Br J Cancer.* 1992; 67:861–864.
38. Sloman R, Brown P, Aldana E, Chee E. The use of relaxation for the promotion of comfort and pain relief in persons with advanced cancer. *Contemp Nurse.* 1994; 3:6–12.
39. Vasterling J, Jenkins RA, Tope DM, Burish TG. Cognitive distraction and relaxation training for the control of side effects due to cancer chemotherapy. *J Behav Med.* 1993; 16:65–80.

40. Fletcher DM. Unconventional cancer treatments: professional, legal and ethical issues. *Oncol Nurs Forum.* 1992; 19:1351–1354.

41. Gray RE, Doan B.D. Heroic self-healing and cancer: clinical issues for the health professions. *J Palliat Care.* 1990; 6:32–41.

42. Guzley GJ. Alternative cancer treatments: Impact of unorthodox therapy on the patient with cancer. *South Med J.* 1992; 85:519–523.

43. Isaacs R. Questionable methods of cancer treatment: time to face the facts. *NZ Med J.* 1993; 106:379–380.

44. Jackson J. Unproven treatment in childhood oncology–how far should paediatricians co-operate? *J Med Ethics.* 1994; 20:77–79.

45. Kennedy BJ. Use of questionable methods and physician education. *J Cancer Educ.* 1993; 8:129–131.

46. Lerner IJ. The physician and cancer quackery: the physician's role in promoting the scientific treatment of cancer and discouraging questionable treatment methods. *NY State J Med.* 1993; 93:96–100.

47. Lynoe N. Ethical and professional aspects of the practice of alternative medicine. *Scand J Soc Med.* 1992; 24: 217–225.

48. Monaco GP, Green S. Recognising deception in the promotion of untested and unproven medical treatments. *NY State J Med.* 1993; 93:88–91.

49. Montbriand MJ. Freedom of choice: an issue concerning alternate therapies chosen by patients with cancer. *Oncol Nurs Forum.* 1993; 20:1195–1201.

50. Stoll BA. Can unorthodox cancer therapy improve quality of life? *Ann Oncol.* 1993; 4:121–123.

51. Zaloznik AJ. Unproven (unorthodox) cancer treatments: a guide for healthcare professionals. *Cancer Pract.* 1994; 2:19–24.

52. Yeoh C, Kiely E, Davies H. Unproven treatment in childhood oncology–how far should paediatricians co-operate? *J Med Ethics.* 1994; 20:75–76.

53. Nwoga IA. Traditional healers and perceptions of the causes and treatment of cancer. *Cancer Nurs.* 1994; 17:470–478.

54. Hufford DJ. Epistemologies in religious healing. *J Med Philos.* 1993; 18:175–194.

55. Doan BD, Gray RE, Davis CS. Belief in psychological effects on cancer. *Psycho-Oncology.* 1993; 2:139–150.

56. Northouse LL, Wortman CB. Models of helping and coping in cancer care. *Patient Educ Couns.* 1990; 15: 49–64.

57. Brickman P, Rabinowitz VC, Laiiza K, et al. Models of helping and coping. *Am Psychol.* 1982; 37:368–384.

58. LeShan LL Gassman M. Some observations on psychotherapy with patients suffering from neoplastic disease. *Am J Psychother.* 1958; 12:723–734.

59. Pelletier K. *Mind as Healer, Mind as Slayer.* New York: Dell; 1977.

60. Simonton OC. *The Healing Journey.* New York: Harper & Row; 1993.

61. Simonton OC, Mathews-Simonton S, Creighton J. *Getting Well Again.* Los Angeles: JP Tarcher; 1978.

62. Siegel BS. *Love, Medicine and Miracles.* New York: Harper & Row; 1986.

63. Siegel BS. *Peace, Love and Healing.* New York: Harper & Row; 1989.

64. Dennis KE. Dimensions of client control. *Nurs Res.* 1987; 36:151–156.

65. Hilton BA. The phenomenon of uncertainty in women with breast cancer. *Issues Mental Health Nurs.* 1988; 9: 217–238.

66. Seeman M, Seeman TE. Health behavior and personal autonomy: a longitudinal study of the sense of control in illness. *J Health Soc Behav.* 1983; 24:144–160.

67. Smith RA, Wallston BS, Wallston KA, et al. Measuring desire for control of health care processes. *J Pers Soc Psychol.* 1984; 47:415–426.

68. Taylor SE. Adjustment to threatening events: a theory of cognitive adaptation. *Am Psychol.* 1983; 38:1161–1172.

69. Taylor SE, Brown JD. Illusion and well-being: a social psychological perspective on mental health. *Psychol Bull.* 1988; 103:193–210.

70. Taylor SE, Lichtman RR, Wood JV. Attributions, beliefs about control and adjustment to breast cancer. *J Pers Soc Psychol.* 1984; 46:489–502.

71. Thompson SC. Will it hurt less if I can control it? A complex answer to a simple question. *Psychol Bull.* 1981; 90:89–101.

72. Turk DC, Salovey P. Chronic pain as a variant of depressive disease: a critical reappraisal. *J Nerv Mental Dis.* 1988; 172:398–407.

73. Steen D. Time is short: get started living by your own agenda. *The Toronto Star.* 1995; 19 November; Sec. E7.

74. Doan BD, Gray RE. The heroic cancer patient: a critical analysis of the relationship between illusion and mental health. *Can J Behav Sci.* 1992; 24:253–266.

75. Becker E. *The Denial of Death.* New York: The Free Press; 1973.

76. Jung CG. *Modern Man in Search of his Soul.* Princeton, NJ: Princeton University Press; 1968.

77. Pearson C. *Awakening the Heroes Within: 12 Archetypes that Help us Transform our Lives.* San Francisco: Harper Collins; 1991.

78. Derogatis LR. Psychology in cancer medicine: a perspective and overview. *J Consult Clin Psychol.* 1986; 54:632–638.

79. James W. *The Will to Believe and Other Essays in Popular Philosophy.* New York: Dover; 1956: 1–31.

80. American Society of Clinical Oncology (ASCO), Subcommittee on Unorthodox Therapies Ineffective cancer therapy: a guide for the layperson. *J Clin Oncol.* 1983; 1:154–163.

81. Ontario Breast Cancer Information Exchange Project (OBCIEP). *A Guide to Unconventional Therapies*; 1995.

82. Frank AW. Illness as moral occasion: The other side of clinical ethics. Paper presented at the University of Michigan Conference on the Sociology of Medical Ethics, September 1995.

83. Hoffmaster B. Can ethnography save the life of medical ethics? *Soc Sci Med.* 1992; 35:1421–1431.

84. Zaner R. *Troubled Voices: Stories of Ethics and Illness.* Cleveland: The Pilgrim Press; 1993.

85. Zaner R. Experience and moral life: a phenomenological approach to bioethics. In Dubose E, Hamel R, O'Connell LJ, eds. *A Matter of Principles? Ferment in US Bioethics.* Valley Forge, PA: Trinity Press International; 1994.

86. Macnamara J. The freudian conspiracy. *The Literary Review of Canada.* 1994; December: 15–16.

71

Rehabilitation

RICHARD TUNKEL AND STEVEN D. PASSIK

Physical medicine and rehabilitation is a medical specialty whose primary aim is to maximize the patient's neuromusculoskeletal function. The ultimate goal of rehabilitation is to approach functional independence as close as is allowed by underlying impairments. Many nonneuromusculoskeletal impairments interfering with function, such as cardiac and pulmonary problems, are also within the scope of rehabilitative intervention.

Impairment is generally defined as the loss of use of, or derangement of physiologic or anatomic structure or function. The World Health Organization includes psychological loss or abnormality as well (1). It defines disability as the loss or restriction of the ability to perform a particular activity resulting from an impairment. Handicap is defined as a limitation or loss of the ability to perform a role normal for the individual, resulting from an impairment or disability.

REHABILITATION AND CANCER

Rehabilitation specialists must address specific concerns when evaluating the patient with cancer. The effect of the cancer can directly impact upon the patient's level of function. The mass effect of a tumor is location and size dependent. For example, a mass in the upper lobe of a lung may initially be clinically silent. As the mass increases in size, it may first be manifest as dyspnea upon significant exertion. As it enlarges, the amount of physical activity required to cause shortness of breath may decrease. If the tumor grows upward, it can put pressure on the neurovascular bundle entering the ipsilateral arm. Resulting symptomatology may lead to impaired function of the arm because of motor and sensory deficits as well as pain and possibly edema. Should this occur in the dominant upper limb, even greater difficulty with activities of daily living (ADLs) will be seen. Lack of use of the limb may lead to joint stiffness and eventually contracture.

Metastatic cancer can produce various problems that are distant from the primary tumor. Of special concern are those that may involve bone, the central nervous system, and the cardiopulmonary system. Bone metastases threaten to disturb the integrity of the bony matrix responsible for weight-bearing. The presence of fracture requires appropriate intervention, and the presence of impending fracture often necessitates a change in the weight-bearing status upon the particular bone or bones involved. Tumors within the bony confines of the spine or cranium may require fairly urgent intervention, especially if they are producing neurologic sequelae. Pulmonary metastases may significantly impair pulmonary capacity. This can be a primary concern or it may complicate other underlying impairments.

Paraneoplastic disease is much less common than metastasis but may also affect physiologic functions distant from the primary tumor. Most commonly, these are of endocrinologic or neurologic importance (2). These, too, may have a deleterious effect on the patient's function.

Cancer treatment itself is a major contributor to functional impairment. Surgical intervention may necessitate the sacrifice of neurologic, muscular, bony, pulmonary, or other tissues. Resulting impairments must be addressed by the rehabilitation team. Chemotherapeutic agents are generally more toxic towards less well-differentiated tissues, including neoplasms. Various agents have specific neurologic, cardiac, pulmonary, and other toxicities. Radiation therapy also tends to have more effect upon less mature cell lines. Postradiation fibrosis which occurs some time later is related to tissue ischemia. The specific detrimental effect depends upon the site irradiated, the fractional dose, and the total dose.

Both the effects of cancer and treatment themselves may result in prolonged bed rest. Significant weakness and muscle wasting can occur after only a short period of immobility. Endurance is compromised by decreased aerobic capacity of muscle tissue (3). Decubitus ulcers may develop in those who lack the strength for bed mobility. Prolonged venous stasis predisposes especially the deep veins of the lower limbs to thrombosis, thus potentially predisposing the patient to pulmonary embolism. The patient's heart rate at rest slowly increases, compensating for decreased left ventricular stroke volume (4). Especially with prolonged bed rest there is more restriction to full inspiration. This can further contribute to decreased endurance. The patient's ability to tolerate an upright position can become compromised because of resulting orthostatic hypotension (5).

All of the above problems may be further complicated by other comorbid processes. For example, a patient with a history of emphysema would have further pulmonary impairment with primary or metastatic neoplasia in the lung, pulmonary fibrosis from bleomycin or prior lung irradiation, or from the deconditioning effects of prolonged bed rest (6,7). Another example might be in the patient with diabetes mellitus with a history of paresthesias in the toes secondary to diabetic neuropathy. Further insult to the peripheral nervous system from vincristine neurotoxicity, paraneoplastic neuropathy, or compressive neuropathy of the peroneal nerve resulting from loss of cushioning because of cachexia and muscle atrophy, may all exacerbate the preexisting neuropathy (8–10).

The goal of cancer rehabilitation is dependent upon the underlying impairment or disability of the patient. Each type of rehabilitative effort implies a slightly different role for the psycho-oncologist. Dietz has described four levels of the rehabilitation of cancer patients (11). The psychoncologist can interface with the rehabilitation team and provide a different function or role in each instance, as outlined below.

1. *Preventive rehabilitation* tries to limit anticipated functional impairment, as in implementation of an exercise and mobility program to prevent deconditioning from prolonged bed rest. In this type of rehabilitation, the psycho-oncologist can be instrumental in assisting the patient to anticipate the psychological and physical effects of being immobilized for a prolonged period of time, planning coping strategies and helping with the setting of appropriate goals.

2. *Restorative rehabilitation* attempts to restore premorbid function when permanent impairment is

not anticipated, as in implementation of a progressive strengthening program to recover from weakness during a prolonged hospital stay. Patients may become frustrated, discouraged, and depressed by their deconditioned state. Psycho-oncologists can facilitate the continuation of strength conditioning by providing support, helping the patient set intermediate goals that are reachable as they seek the restoration of physical functioning and diagnosis, and treat conditions (fatigue, pain, depression) that may hinder the attainment of these goals.

3. *Supportive rehabilitation* maximizes function when permanent impairment exists, as in training a lower limb amputee with a prosthesis. Recent amputees face a number of difficult psychological issues regarding quality of life, especially grief associated with the loss of their limb. The psycho-oncologist should assist the patient in facilitating communication with medical staff, in particular to help in exploring options regarding prosthetics, dealing with psychosocial issues of disfigurement and stigma, and the diagnosis and treatment of psychiatric or physical problems (i.e., "phantom limb" pain) that hinder efforts to maximise function.

4. *Palliative rehabilitation* gives comfort and support, and decreases dependence in ADLs in the patient with advance malignancy. This population of patients faces multiple psychiatric and physical problems that may lead to hopelessness, anticipatory grief, and despair. Helping the patient with cognitive deficits or depression can help them better attend to rehabilitative efforts, diminish dependency, and engender hope that maximizes quality of life. The psycho-oncologist can help in addressing these issues with patients and families to facilitate their efforts on enhancing quality of life.

Patients with cancer often have special needs different from other rehabilitation candidates. For example, the patient requiring above-knee amputation for osteogenic sarcoma is usually much younger than the more commonly seen dysvascular amputee. Rehabilitation efforts may be modified or compromised because of required chemotherapy or radiation treatments (12,13). Additionally, existence of metastatic diseases further complicate rehabilitation efforts. In the older osteosarcoma survivor, chronic postradiation changes, including radiation-induced sarcoma, as well as later metastatic disease, may create a new need for rehabilitation.

Malignancy involving the central nervous system often presents as a dynamic process. For example, epidural metastatic disease causing spinal cord compression is by no means a static lesion. It requires appropriate aggressive initial management which can help minimize permanent neurologic sequelae (14). Frequently, epidural disease will be present in other areas of the spine. Therefore, subsequent episodes of paraparesis or tetraparesis may occur during the remainder of the patient's life. Obviously, the rehabilitation needs of such a patient may radically change over a short period of time, unlike the more commonly seen spinal cord injured patient who generally has a static lesion. Neoplasia within the cranial vault may present with stroke-like symptomatology reminiscent of that developing after occlusion of the middle cerebral artery. On the other hand, often the single or multiple lesions cause manifestations quite dissimilar from involvement of a particular arterial territory.

The psychological needs of the patient with cancer need to be seen in the context of the individual patient and the level of rehabilitation intervention. Psychological factors may limit rehabilitation and the ultimate functional attainment of the patient. Various emotional states as well as organic mood disorders resulting from brain metastases, high dose corticosteroids, or electrolyte abnormalities may be responsible. Obviously dementia, delirium or other organic mental syndromes can severely restrict participation in rehabilitation. Lack of attainment of functional independence may contribute to a patient's depressed mood. Conversely, there is a good amount of literature suggesting that activities such as exercise may have quite positive benefits on the patient, including enhanced sense of self and diminished depression and anxiety. The diagnosis and treatment of psychiatric disorders such as depression, cognitive disorders, and adjustment problems are vital to compliance and ultimately the success of rehabilitative efforts. In our clinical experience at Memorial Sloan-Kettering Cancer Center, we have found that inpatient oncology requests for rehabilitation tend to focus on patients with advanced disease as physical impairments accrue with disease progression. This is also the time in the course of disease when psychiatric comorbidity is highest and thus intensifies the need for collaboration between physiatrists and psycho-oncologists.

The rehabilitation team caring for the patient with cancer must be multidisciplinary to deal with what can be multidimensional problems (15). The physiatrist is the medical specialist who directs and coordinates the rehabilitation intervention. In the oncologic setting, the physical therapist concentrates on the patient's gross motor function and mobility. The occupational therapist focuses more on fine motor function and skills of daily activities as well as cognitive and perceptual abilities. Additionally, the occupational therapist is often called upon to supply adaptive equipment and certain limb splinting, and may be requested to help with functional impairments of swallowing. The speech therapist specializes in anatomic and physiologic impairment of both speech and swallowing. The prosthetist/orthotist appropriately fits and constructs braces and limb prostheses, whereas the prosthodontist is responsible for oral prostheses. The nurses working with the patient, even if not specialized in rehabilitation care, are also an important part of the rehabilitation of the patient. They are often the first to mobilize the patient and assist in ADLs. Important psychosocial support and a range of psychological and psychopharmacological interventions can be provided by the psychologist, psychiatrist and social worker, the latter helping coordinate discharge planning for the patient. Psycho-oncologists may be called upon to help with the management of various psychiatric problems, when pharmacologic intervention is required, or when psychological and behavioral interventions are needed to maximize compliance and remove barriers to rehabilitative efforts. For example, the treatment of depression might involve pharmacologic intervention tailored to the oncologic rehabilitation patient, such as use of both psychostimulants and antidepressants as fatigue is such a ubiquitous and formidable barrier to improved function. The depressed or discouraged patient may also need to help in setting reachable goals that are challenging enough so that when reached they build self-esteem, but no so difficult to attain that they engender a sense of failure. The recreational therapist provides the patient with recreational and functional activities which may be helpful in providing psychological support. A chaplain may provide both emotional and spiritual support to the patient. A vocational counselor, when appropriate, can help the patient with the transition to a previous or new occupation. Below we discuss in detail the special roles of the psycho-oncologist in rehabilitative efforts, and give some specific examples from the Memorial Sloan-Kettering Cancer Center liaison experience.

REHABILITATION INTERVENTIONS

Various categories of intervention are described below. They should not be viewed in isolation from one another. Not only is rehabilitation a multidisciplinary approach but it is also multifaceted or multilayered by design. The effects of various interventions employed are often complementary and interdependent.

Therapeutic exercise is most commonly used to strengthen weakened musculature. Of equal importance are aerobic exercises and activities that are necessary to increase endurance (16). Devices that may be used to assist in exercise include elastic bands that may provide low to moderate resistance, bicycle pedals with variable resistance, weights for progressive resistive exercises, and isokinetic devices in the later stages of rehabilitation of specific joints. Various forms of active range of motion exercises can help prevent loss of muscle strength and endurance. These will also help maintain range of motion of the involved joints. Neuromuscular reeducation techniques may be helpful in cases where increased muscle tone, as in upper motor neuron lesions, interferes with motor movement. Antispasticity agents as well as physical modalities such as ice, electrical stimulation, and electromyographic biofeedback may be beneficial in such patients (17,18). In selected cases, when function is impaired because of focal spasticity, motor point block, neurolysis or tenotomy may be required (19).

Sustained stretching of muscles may be useful in certain cases of spasticity. Such sustained terminal stretch is also employed when joint contracture has occurred (20). When feasible this is done in conjunction with deep heating of the local soft tissues of the joint to increase the distensibility of collagen fibers (21). If joint contracture is severe, serial casting or dynamic splinting may be required, especially if the patient is incapable of activities that would discourage the contracted posture (22).

Muscle incoordination such as found in disorders involving the cerebullum or its tracts is difficult to address with physical rehabilitation. Coordination exercises are a form of neuromuscular reeducation which may be helpful. The use of a weighted walker or the use of weights on the lower limbs may be helpful in gait training (23).

In the severely debilitated, bedridden patient, mobility training typically is initiated at the level of bed mobility. Activities as simple as changing one's position in bed are initiated and may be helpful in preventing deleterious effects of bed rest such as pressure sores. Transfer training is necessary to help the patient achieve independence in moving from one surface to another. An over-bed trapeze may be helpful to the patient in positioning for transfers. Other devices such as a sliding board or walker may be necessary. For the patient who has difficulty tolerating an upright posture or is prohibited from sitting, a tilt table may be employed. This would allow gradual movement from a supine posture to an inclined and eventually standing posture (24).

Out of bed mobility for some patients will require a wheelchair, and transfer training will be necessary (25).

Initial ambulation training may utilize a wheelchair for the patient to walk behind, a walker with or without wheels, or an IV pole. The patient can then be progressed as tolerated to less restrictive assistive devices. All assistive devices help widen the patient's base of support and involve the arms in weight-bearing (26). In the case of sensory ataxia, an assistive device allows the upper limb to receive sensory information from the surface upon which the patient is walking.

Various orthoses may be used to maintain proper limb positioning and thus enhance function. An ankle foot orthosis (AFO) can reposition a foot and ankle that have an equinovarus position, such as in spastic hemiparesis. A double metal upright AFO or a custom molded plastic AFO may be utilized (27). Each will assist in foot clearance during the swing phase of gait. An AFO can also be quite helpful in cases of "foot drop," again to enhance foot clearance.

Orthoses are also commonly used for the distal upper limb as well. A wrist cock-up splint holds the wrist in mild extension, enhancing hand function. A resting hand splint prevents finger flexion contracture in cases of spasticity and aids in hygiene.

Thoracic and lumbar spine orthoses are helpful in preventing pain provoked by movement (28). Mechanical pain is often provoked by forward flexion. This is because the weight-bearing portion of the vertebrae, the vertebral bodies, are most commonly affected by bone metastases. Thus, discouraging forward flexion may discourage vertebral compression deformity and fracture. Lumbosacral corsets and lumbosacral and thoracolumbosacral orthoses can be employed. The cervical spine is only minimally restricted in its movements by a soft cervical collar. The Philadelphia collar offers some additional restriction, in particular, in flexion and extension. The sterno-occipital mandibular immobilizer offers greater limitation of motion and may be donned in a supine position (29). A halo vest is necessary when more complete immobilization is required (30).

Lower limb prostheses following amputation are fabricated in hopes of returning the patient to more independent ambulation. In general the more proximal the level of amputation, the greater the energy expenditure required for reciprocal gait. Today's lighter weight components, "energy-storing feet," and improved socket designs have improved available prostheses (31,32). Adequate training with the prostheses is absolutely necessary to maximize the patient's new compensated gait. Upper limb amputations are much less common than lower limb. The terminal devices of an upper limb prosthesis may be cosmetic or volitionally controlled by the patient. Control can be either mechanical or "myoelectric" (33). Extensive therapy is necessary, especially in the case of the myoelectric prosthesis, in order to integrate the prosthesis into the patient's ADLs.

ADL training by an occupational therapist relies on a combination of therapeutic exercise, compensatory techniques, and adaptive equipment. Bimanual activities may be helpful, and fine motor retraining may be required. If there is severe weakness or amputation of the dominant arm, the patient will require dominance retraining. This is necessary for the relearning of performance of certain ADLs, such as writing.

Various physical modalities can be used in the treatment of pain. When pain is of muscular or myofascial origin, ice or heat, electrical stimulation, massage and treatment of trigger points may all be utilized. Heat can increase local blood flow and metabolic rates. Heat may be contraindicated depending upon the location of the malignancy (34). This may also be true of massage and vigorous electrical stimulation. Trigger points may be treated by "spray and stretch" technique, when involved muscle is stretched after vapocoolant spraying, or by local constant pressure maintained over a trigger point. Trigger point injection or dry needling may also be quite effective (35). With or without treatment of trigger points, reconditioning of local muscle to increase both strength and range of motion are strongly recommended.

Superficial heat and cold may also serve as local counterstimulants, inhibiting transmission of pain signals up the spinal cord (36). Various forms of mechanical stimulation can also be utilized. Transcutaneous electrical nerve stimulation (TENS) is perhaps the most widely recognized application of counterstimulation. It has also been postulated that TENS may increase release of endogenous opioids (37).

Neurogenic bladder or bowel disorders are also addressed by the rehabilitation team. Initial indwelling catheters for urinary incontinence are often gradually replaced by either clean intermittent catherization techniques or bladder retraining (38). The latter is often dependent on a scheduled voiding regimen and assisted by Valsalva maneuver or suprapubic tapping or pressure (Credé). Pharmacologic intervention may also be helpful (39). Constipation is by far the most common form of bowel dysmotility seen. Increased mobility often enhances bowel motility. Initial management of constipation begins with increased fluid or fiber intake, stool softeners, and oral laxatives as needed (40). Suppositories, digital stimulation, or enemas may be required, and digital extraction in the case of fecal impaction may be necessary (41,42).

Swallowing disorders can result from anatomic disruption or neurologic dysfunction. Various interventions for dysphagia are available depending upon the level of disorder. Limiting the texture or bolus size of food or liquids, or altering head or body position may improve swallowing. Different therapeutic swallowing techniques are also utilized. Prosthodontic appliances may be needed following resection of a portion of the oral swallowing mechanism (43).

Disorders of language occur following lesions of the central language processing areas of the brain. Resulting aphasias, or less common verbal apraxia, are addressed by the speech therapist using techniques such as melodic intonation therapy and different communication devices (44,45). Speech disorders may result from neurologic dysfunction or anatomic lesion. Dysarthria may benefit from pausing or rate control of speech. A palatal lift may decrease hypernasal speech. Dysphonia following unilateral vocal cord lesion may be improved by vocal cord adduction exercises. Following laryngectomy, an artificial larynx, tracheoesophageal puncture, or esophageal speech may all be approaches to the patient's resulting aphonia (46,47).

Chest physical therapy enhances gas exchange in the lungs by assisting in mobilization of secretions. Postural drainage, often in combination with chest vibration or percussion, assist in clearing specific areas of the lungs (48). Secretions may be loosened prior to therapy with the use of a nebulizer. Reconditioning exercises for the muscles of ventilation may also be helpful (49).

Lymphedema is a frequent cause of limb swelling in the cancer patient. Limb elevation may be helpful in its early stages. Static compression garments help contain limb volume and enhance the "muscle pump" action of muscle contraction of the limb. Gradient pressure elastic sleeves or stockings are most commonly employed. Bandaging techniques and specific legging orthoses are also available (50,51). Specific therapeutic exercises can be helpful when utilizing the "muscle pump." Pneumatic compression pumps have been available to deliver dynamic limb compression; more contemporary pumps inflate in a distal to proximal direction, thus "milking" the limb (52–54). Manual lymph drainage (MDL) facilitates the flow of lymph fluid through residual lymphatic channels (50). Bandaging the limb between MLD sessions helps to maximize treatment results (55,56). Active disease may contraindicate either pneumatic pumping or MLD.

THE INTERFACE OF REHABILITATION AND PSYCHO-ONCOLOGY

Assessment and Treatment of Psychiatric Disorders

As was mentioned at various points above, the psycho-oncologist plays an integral role in the multidisciplinary approach to the successful rehabilitation of the cancer patient. At Memorial Sloan-Kettering Cancer Center, a significant number of requests for physical rehabilitation are for complications related to advanced disease. Upon consultation, these patients are typically found to be badly deconditioned and very symptomatic (e.g., pain). These conditions may be attributable to either prolonged bed rest, aggressive treatment modalities and/or advanced stage of disease. Unfortunately, the presence of advanced cancer significantly increases the patient's risk for the development of a variety of different disorders on the psychiatric spectrum. Our experience in the Psychiatry Service at Memorial Sloan-Kettering Cancer Center suggests that depression and organic mental disorders (e.g., delirium, dementia) are the most prevalent psychiatric disorders among patients with advanced stage neoplasms. Patients presenting with organic mental syndrome are often very fatigued, mildly confused and/or have memory deficiencies that can severely impede the implementation of successful rehabilitation efforts. The psycho-oncologist should assess the patient and develop an appropriate intervention to improve outcome. Stimulants and neuroleptics, either alone or in combination, are useful in decreasing levels of fatigue and improving mental status. Patients who are able to actively comprehend and remember the nature and goals of the rehabilitation process will ultimately enjoy much improved chances of maximizing their function and quality of life.

In addition to pharmacological approaches, there are a variety of psychotherapeutic interventions that are very beneficial in facilitating treatment compliance with rehabilitative efforts. Having evaluated and treated for any existing mental disorders, the psycho-oncologist should evaluate the patient's motivation for rehabilitation. Motivation is a significant component of a successful physical rehabilitation plan. Some patients may not wish to "go it alone," which can be a recipe for failure and lowered self-esteem and motivation, while individuals with advanced malignancies may feel that rehabilitation is futile given their poor prognosis. Behavioral interventions that foster an increased level of motivation in the patients are very beneficial in maximizing compliance with the rehabilitation process and minimizing frustration. In addition, the involvement of family in the planning of the reha-

bilitation program is also very helpful. Interventions such as appropriate goal setting, journal keeping, self-monitoring and reinforcement principles are very instrumental facilitating a level of motivation conducive to successful physical rehabilitation. An example of the interface of psychiatry and rehabilitation is the "Road to Fitness Program," developed at Memorial Sloan-Kettering Cancer Center, which represents a comprehensive, multidisciplinary approach to rehabilitation in cancer patients involving psychiatry, rehabilitation, nutrition, patient education, and posttreatment services. Survivors of cancer received group support, counseling about proper nutrition and supervised exercise instruction. Frequently, patients will become discouraged by the apparent lack of progress they are making in posttreatment rehabilitation simply because they are not able to achieve the unrealistic goals they have set for themselves. To help minimize this phenomenon, patients were also provided counseling on how to establish appropriate treatment goals for themselves. Food logs were kept by all patients and reviewed each week by both the nutritionist and psychologist. Through the use of these logs, both clinicians were able to show patients their progress from week to week, reinforce positive dietary intake, and identify areas in need of improvement. Thus, the "Road to Fitness" program allowed patients to: (1) see concrete improvements in their physical state; (2) develop a sense of enthusiasm and motivation towards their rehabilitation program; and (3) correct problems through the use of self-reinforcement.

Psycho-oncologists provide a unique dimension to the rehabilitation process not afforded by other members of the rehabilitation team. The implementation of psychotherapeutic, such as cognitive-behavioral techniques, and psychopharmacological interventions that directly address deficits commonly present in the patient requiring rehabilitation (e.g., pain, insomnia, anxiety) are of significant benefit. The use of relaxation techniques, possibly in combination with some form of pharmacological treatment, are beneficial in minimizing the symptoms of panic commonly expressed in patients with pulmonary complications. Anxiety and psychological distress related to difficulties breathing (e.g., shortness of breath) are frequently encountered and may discourage the patient from complying with rehabilitation efforts. Other direct cognitive behavioral interventions that focus on the reduction of pain, insomnia, and difficulties with food consumption are equally important and beneficial.

Psycho-oncologists have a variety of pharmacological tools available that address the symptomology commonly found within this patient population. Clinicians should consider the implementation of a psychotropic drug intervention that is directly aimed at decreasing the patient's level of fatigue and pain and facilitates improvement in sleeping. Because all of these symptoms negatively impact the patient's rehabilitation program and overall quality of life, psychotropic drugs (e.g., tricyclic antidepressants) that directly address deficits and improve levels energy and motivation will permit the patient to benefit from the proven efficacy of physical rehabilitation.

Staff Education

Because of the relatively recent development of the field of psycho-oncology, there are relatively few large psycho-oncology services outside of academic cancer centers. Therefore, a key role of psycho-oncologists is in educating junior rehabilitation medicine staff about the psychological aspects of cancer patients in need of their services and the interventions that they might adopt from psycho-oncologists that will maximize rehabilitative efforts. The staff will be able to utilize these techniques early in their training and subsequently carry this knowledge to future positions at other institutions. The use of case focused conferences and multidisciplinary rounds for staff are very beneficial in facilitating discussion of the psychological aspects of cancer rehabilitation. Similarly, work-related support groups allow for staff to share their perspectives on patient management and should help to increase morale and decrease levels of frustration and burnout.

COMBINED REHABILITATIVE AND PSYCHO-ONCOLOGY EFFORTS TO DOCUMENT AND OVERCOME COMMON PROBLEMS IN QUALITY OF LIFE

Disease-related complications and treatment side effects frequently impact upon the patient's quality of life and require the implementation of restorative rehabilitation. Upper extremity lymphedema is a disfiguring and sometimes painful complication of the treatment for breast cancer. Thus, the psycho-oncology and rehabilitation medicine services at Memorial Sloan-Kettering Cancer Center began clinical and academic work to clarify quality of life issues and intervene effectively to reduce the distress and disability associated with this condition. Our combined studies have documented the impact of upper extremity lymphedema in women treated for breast cancer and highlighted predictors of those patients most vulnerable to functional, sexual, and social problems. The group also

highlighted the neglected problem of pain in this group (57,58). Clinically, individual psychiatric consultations and supportive group therapy for women with upper extremity lymphedema have helped to facilitate adjustment, and help women comply with their often arduous rehabilitative efforts. The most common reasons for referral have been depression, anxiety, and social and sexual problems. The presence of pain, lack of social support, avoidant coping, and dominant affected extremity have been shown to be significant predictors of difficulties in areas of sexual, physical, and psychosocial functioning.

Psychiatric consultation that provides support, assessment, and treatment contributes to compliance with rehabilitative treatment. Indeed, it is clear rehabilitation in cancer patients is inclusive of a variety of physical and psychosocial components that necessitates the collaborative efforts of psycho-oncology and rehabilitation medicine.

REFERENCES

1. World Health Organization. *International Classification of Impairments, Disabilities, and Handicaps.* Geneva: World Health Organization; 1980: 1–205.
2. Posner JB. Paraneoplastic syndromes. *Neurol Clin.* 1991; 9(4):919–936.
3. Halar EM, Bell KR. Rehabilitation's relationship to inactivity. In: Kottke FJ, Lehmann JF, eds. *Krusen's Handbook of Physical Medicine and Rehabilitation.* Philadelphia: WB Saunders; 1990: 1113–1133.
4. Taylor HL, Henschel A, Brozek J, Keys A. Effects of bed rest on cardiovascular function and work performance. *J Appl Phys.* 1949; 2(5):223–239.
5. Halar EM, Bell KR. Contracture and other deleterious effects of immobility. In: DeLisa JA, ed. *Rehabilitation Medicine — Principles and Practice*, 2nd ed. Philadelphia: JB Lippincott; 1993: 681–699.
6. Collis CH. Chemotherapy-related morbidity to the lungs. In: Plowman PN, McElwain TJ, Meadows AT, eds. *Complications of Cancer Management.* Oxford: Butterworth Heinemann; 1991: 250–271.
7. Travis EL. Lung morbidity of radiotherapy. In: Plowman PN, McElwain TJ, Meadows AT, eds. *Complications of Cancer Management.* Oxford: Butterworth Heinemann; 1991: 232–249.
8. Sandler SG, Tobin W, Henderson ES. Vincristine-induced neuropathy. *Neurology.* 1969; 19:367–374.
9. Patchell RA, Posner JB. Neurologic complications of systemic cancer. *Neurol Clin.* 1985; 3(4):729–750.
10. Lachmann EA, Rook JL, Tunkel R, Nagler W. Complications associated with intermittent pneumatic compression. *Arch Phys Med Rehabil.* 1992; 73:482–485.
11. Deitz JH Jr. *Rehabilitation Oncology.* New York: Wiley; 1981: 1–180.
12. Lewis RJ, Marcove RC, Rosen G. Functional effects of radiation therapy. *J Bone Joint Surg.* 1977; 59A:325–331.
13. McElwain TJ. Cardiac morbidity of chemotherapy. In: Plowman PN, McElwain TJ, Meadows AT, eds.

Complications of Cancer Management. Oxford: Butterworth Heinemann; 1991: 184–192.

14. Rodichok LD, Harper GR, Ruckdeschel JC, et al. Early diagnosis of spinal epidural metastases. *Am J Med.* 1981; 70:1181–1188.

15. DeLisa JA, Martin GM, Currie DM. Rehabilitation medicine past, present and future. In: DeLisa JA, ed. *Rehabilitation Medicine—Principles and Practice*, 2nd ed. Philadelphia: JB Lippincott; 1993: 3–27.

16. DeLorme TL. Restoration of muscle power by heavy-resistance exercises. *J Bone Joint Surg.* 1945; 27(A): 645–667.

17. Bajd T, Gregoric M, Vodovinik L, Benko H. Electrical stimulation in treating spasticity resulting from spinal cord injury. *Arch Phys Med Rehabil.* 1985; 66:515–517.

18. Basmajian JV. Biofeedback in rehabilitation medicine. In: DeLisa JA, ed. *Rehabilitation Medicine—Principles and Practice*, 2nd ed. Philadelphia: JB Lippincott; 1993: 425–439.

19. Little JW, Massagli TL. Spasticity and associated abnormalities of muscle tone. In: DeLisa JA, ed. *Rehabilitation Medicine—Principles and Practice*, 2nd ed. Philadelphia: JB Lippincott; 1993: 666–680.

20. Steinberg FU. *The Immobilized Patient: Functional Pathology and Management.* New York: Plenum Medical Books; 1980: 1–156.

21. Lehmann JF, Masock AJ, Warren CG, Koblanski JN. Effect of therapeutic temperatures on tendon extensibility. *Arch Phys Med Rehabil.* 1970; 51:481–487.

22. Zander CL. Healy NL. Elbow flexion contracture treated with serial casts and conservative therapy. *J Hand Surg (Am).* 1992; 17(4):694–697.

23. Hewer RL, Cooper R, Morgan MH. An investigation into the value of treating intention tremor by weighting the affected extremity. *Brain.* 1972; 95:579–590.

24. Nagler W. *Manual for Physical Therapy Technicians.* Chicago: Yearbook Medical Publishers; 1974: 1–181.

25. Trombly CA. Activities of daily living. *Occupational Therapy for Physical Dysfunction*, 2nd ed. Baltimore: Williams & Wilkins; 1983: 458–479.

26. Joyce BM, Kirby RL. Canes, crutches and walkers. *Am Fam Pract.* 1991; 43(2):535–542.

27. Corcoran PJ, Jebsen RH, Brengelmann GL, Simons BC. Effects of plastic and metal leg braces on speed and energy cost of hemiparetic ambulation. *Arch Phys Med Rehabil.* 1970; 51:69–77.

28. Fidler MW, Plasmans CMT. The effect of four types of support on the segmental mobility of the lumbosacral spine. *J Bone Joint Surg.* 1983; 65A:943–947.

29. Fisher SV. Cervical orthotics. *Phys Med Rehab Clin North Am.* 1992; 3:29–43.

30. Koch RA, Nickel VL. The Halo-Vest: an evaluation of motion and forces across the neck. *Spine.* 1978; 3: 103–107.

31. Micheal J. Energy storing feet: a clinical comparison. *Clin Prosthet Orthop.* 1987; 11:154–168.

32. Leonard JA Jr, Meier RH III. Upper and lower extremity prosthetics. In: DeLisa JA, ed. *Rehabilitation Medicine—Principles and Practice*, 2nd ed. Philadelphia: JB Lippincott; 1993: 507–525.

33. Sears HH. Approaches to prescription of body-powered and myoelectric postheses. *Phys Med Rehabil Clin North Am.* 1991; 2(2):361–371.

34. Lehmann JF, deLateur BJ. Diathermy and superficial heat, laser, and cold therapy. In: Kottke FJ, Lehmann JF, eds. *Krusen's Handbook of Physical Medicine and Rehabilitation*, 4th ed. Philadelphia: WB Saunders; 1990: 283–367.

35. Travell JG, Simmons DG. *Myofascial Pain and Dysfunction: The Trigger Point Manual*, vol. I. Baltimore: Williams & Wilkins; 1983: 1–713.

36. Melzack R, Wall PD. Pain mechanisms—a new theory. *Science.* 1965; 150:971–979.

37. Rodriguez E, Meizoso MJ, Garabal M, et al. Effects of transcutaneous nerve stimulation on the plasma and CSF concentrations of beta-endorphin and the plasma concentrations of ACTH, cortisol and prolactin in hysterectomized women with post operative pain. *Rev Esp Anestesiol Reanim.* 1992; 39:6–9.

38. Cardenas DD. Neurogenic bladder evaluation and management. *Phys Med Rehabil Clin North Am.* 1992; 3(4):751–763.

39. Wein AJ. Practical uropharmacology. *Urol Clin North Am.* 1991; 18(2):269–281.

40. Portenoy RK. Constipation in the cancer patient. *Med Clin North Am.* 1987; 71:303–311.

41. Lennard-Jones JE. Clinical aspects of laxatives, enemas, and suppositories. In: Kamm MA, Lennard-Jones JE, eds. *Constipation.* Petersfield: Wrightson Biomedical; 1994: 327–341.

42. Wrenn K. Fecal impaction. *N Engl J Med.* 1989; 321:658–662.

43. Davis JW. Prosthodontic management of swallowing disorders. *Dysphagia.* 1989; 3:199–205.

44. Sparks RW. Melodic intonation therapy. In: Chapey R, ed. *Language Intervention Strategies in Adult Aphasia.* Baltimore: Williams & Williams; 1981: 265–282.

45. Bennett J. Talking about low technology. In: Enderby P, ed. *Assistive Communication Aids for the Speech Impaired.* Edinburgh: Churchill Livingstone; 1987: 112–132.

46. Prater RJ, Swift RW. *Manual of Voice Therapy.* Boston: Little, Brown and Co.; 1984.

47. Wenig BL, Mullooly V, Levy J, Abramson AL. Voice restoration following laryngectomy: the role of primary versus secondary tracheoesophageal puncture. *Ann Otol Rhinol Laryngol.* 1989; 98 (1 Pt 1): 70–73.

48. Helmholz HF Jr, Stonnington HH. Rehabilitation for respiratory dysfunction. In: Kottke FJ, Lehmann JF, eds. *Krusen's Handbook of Physical Medicine and Rehabilitation*, 4th ed. Philadelphia: WB Saunders; 1990: 858–873.

49. Coffin Zadai C. Therapeutic exercises in pulmonary disease and disability. In: Basmajian JV, Wolf SL, eds. *Therapeutic Exercise*, 5th ed. Baltimore: Williams and Wilkins; 1990: 405–427.

50. Casley-Smith JR. Modern treatment of lymphedema. *Mod Med Aust.* 1992; 32:70–83.

51. Vernick SH, Shapiro D, Shaw FD. Leg orthosis for venous and lymphatic insufficiency. *Arch Phys Med Rehabil.* 1987; 68:459–461.

52. Zanolla R, Monzeglio C, Balzarini A, Martino G. Evaluation of the results of three different methods of postmastectomy lymphedema treatment. *J Surg Oncol.* 1984; 26:210–213.

53. Zelikovski A, Haddad M, Reiss R. The "Lympha-Press" intermittent sequential pneumatic device for the treat-

ment of lymphoedema: five years of clinical experience. *J Cardiovasc Surg*. 1986; 27:288–290.

54. Klein MJ, Alexander MA, Wright JM, et al. Treatment of adult lower extremity lymphedema with Wright linear pump: statistical analysis of a clinical trail. *Arch Phys Med Rehabil*. 1988; 69:202–206.

55. Weiselfish S. Manual lymph drainage: a total body approach. *Phys Ther Forum*. 1987; 6:2–4.

56. Foldi E, Foldi M, Weissleder H. Conservative treatment of lymphedema of the limbs. *Angiology*. 1985; 36:171–180.

57. Passik S, Newman M, Brennan M, Holland J. Psychiatric consultation for women undergoing rehabilitation for upper-extremity lymphedema following breast cancer treatment. *J Pain Symptom Manage*. 1993; 8:226–233.

58. Newman ML, Brennan M, Passik S. Lymphedema complicated by pain and psychological distress: a case with complex treatment needs. *J Pain Symptom Manage*. 1996; 12:376–379.

XI

PERSONS WITH SPECIAL NEEDS

EDITOR: RUTH McCORKLE

72

The Older Patient

BETTY R. FERRELL AND BRUCE FERRELL

THE EPIDEMIOLOGY OF CANCER AND AGING

The United States has the third largest population of elderly (age 60 and older) in the world, behind China and India. The U.S. is second only to China in the size of the population aged 80 and older (1). The elderly comprise a significant portion of the U.S. population and a challenge to a burdened health care system.

Growth in the U.S. population in the future will be less than for underdeveloped nations but greater than average for developed countries. The projected percentage increase in the population aged 60 and above by the year 2020 is 159% in less developed countries, 59% in developed countries, and 69% in the United States (1).

Cancer is one of the major chronic illnesses in all adults and of special significance to the elderly. Cancer is predominantly a disease of the elderly that is associated with substantial physical and psychological sequelae. Barraclough (2), in his classic study of suicide in the elderly, found a significant excess of terminal malignancies (often undiagnosed before death) compared with matched controls dying through accidental death.

The incidence of cancer increases with age, with only a slight moderation among those over age 85. Some exceptions to this pattern exist, such as with lung and uterine cancer, for which peak incidence occurs earlier, in the ages of 75 to 79. Cancer incidence rates in general have risen over time and, with the growing population of the elderly, are a major geriatric concern.

PSYCHOSOCIAL PROBLEMS AND THE NEEDS OF THE ELDERLY

The proportion of the population with functional impairments caused by physical and dementing diseases increases with age. The rate of impairments in managing the basic activities of daily living and keeping mobile more than doubles in each decade after age 65 (3). Almost half (43%) of the population over age 85 have a functional impairment impacting daily living. It is not uncommon to find a close association between physical impairments and psychological sequelae such as chronic depression or anxiety.

The older adult population is increasing and will continue to increase significantly in the United States, where about 2.1 million people are added to the older population (over age 65) each year. This age group numbered 32.3 million in 1992 and represented 12.7% of the United States population. It is estimated that in the years 2010 to 2030, the older population will grow 73%. It is also predicted that by the year 2040 there may be more people aged 65 or older than persons under 20 years of age. These projections have significant implications for the health care system since the fastest growing age groups are those 85 years old, the poor, and minority elders.

Minority populations are projected to constitute 25% of the older population in 2030, which is almost double the 13% figure cited in 1990. Between 1990 and 2040 the Caucasian population aged 65 and older is projected to increase by 93%, compared with 328% for minorities. There is also special interest in the population labeled as the "oldest-old," or those over the age of 85. The centenarian groups more than doubled during the 1980s. In 1990, there were 35,808 individuals over the age of 100 years (2,3).

The number of older adults is made more significant by considering their use of health care resources. While older adults represent 13% of the U.S. population, they account for over 30% of the health care expenditures and use over half of the acute and chronic hospital beds in the nation (4).

Geriatric patients are often known for their physical limitations but they also have significant psychiatric disorders. Older adults have a higher rate of psychiatric illness, behavioral stress, and adjustment problems than younger adults. The incidence of suicide, depression and paranoid states, and organic brain disease increases with age. The suicide rate is four times higher for the older Caucasian man than it is for younger adults (5–7). Table 72.1 summarizes major mental health problems of older persons.

Depression is the most common psychiatric disorder in the elderly and is estimated to occur in 10% to 15% of individuals over the age of 65 (8). The prevalence of depression increases in medically ill older people to a rate of 20% to 35% (8). Table 72.2 summarizes problems related to the mental health of older adults. It is evident that physical as well as psychological demands of aging greatly influence the management of pain or other symptoms in the elderly.

The nursing home setting is a common environment for the elderly and is often neglected in the literature as a setting of care. There are 16,000 Medicare–Medicaid eligible nursing homes in the United States with 1.6 million older people residing in these facilities. It has been estimated that 843,000 of these residents have a mental, social, behavioral, or emotional disorder, but that only 2% have contact with a mental health

TABLE 72.2. *Unique Problems Relating to the Mental Health of Older Adults*

Multiple pathologies (comorbidity)
Atypical or nonspecific presentation of illness
Delay in reporting problems
Underreporting of symptoms
Polypharmacy
Substance abuse and mental illness
Diabetes and depression
Selected cancers and depression
Sleep disturbances and substance abuse
Hypertension and diabetes
Myocardial infarct and diabetes
Dementia and depression

Source: Adapted from Harper (48).

professional (9). In 1990, the Department of Veterans Affairs reported that 72% of all residents of their nursing homes had a primary or associated psychiatric diagnosis (10). Similar findings have been reported in community-dwelling elderly indicating that psychiatric disorders are common while support services are few (11).

Elderly patients transferred from the community or nursing homes to inpatient hospital settings often exhibit extreme anxiety. Depression, agitation, and disorientation are common upon hospital admission. Admission to a hospital may imply impending death to an older patient.

TABLE 72.1. *Major Mental Health Problems of Older Persons*

Delirium
Dementia
Depression
Agitation
Emotional problems associated with poor physical health
Crying spells
Irritability
Pacing
Wandering
Assaultiveness
Expressions of feelings of unworthiness, hopelessness
Diminished memory, orientation, and judgment
Apathy
Withdrawal
Suicidal impulses and/or attempts
Loneliness/lonesomeness
Paranoid delusions
Demanding behavior
Anxiety disorders
Alcohol abuse
Impaired concentration
Short attention span
Tendencies to hoard personal items, including feces
Stress incontinence
Disorientation

Source: Adapted from Harper (48).

PAIN AND PSYCHOSOCIAL ISSUES IN THE ELDERLY PERSON WITH CANCER

Psychosocial consequences of cancer are widespread in the elderly population. More than any other population, elderly patients with cancer require aggressive symptom management and psychosocial support. Depression (12–14), decreased socialization (15,16), sleep disturbance (14), impaired ambulation (15,16), and increased use of health care services (16) have all been associated with the presence of uncontrolled symptoms among elderly people with cancer. Gait disturbances, falls, slow rehabilitation, polypharmacy, cognitive dysfunction, and malnutrition are among many other geriatric conditions potentially worsened by the presence of cancer and treatment. Psychosocial care and symptom management have major implications for quality of life and quality of care, especially for terminal patients (17). Residents of long-term-care facilities (15), the frail elderly, those over the age of 75 or those with chronic illness, are particularly vulnerable.

The psychosocial demands of cancer on the elderly are accompanied by the burdens of physical symptoms such as pain. Pain is extremely common among older people. Population-based studies have estimated that 25% to 50% of community-dwelling elderly people have chronic pain problems (18,19). Thus, the elderly person with cancer may have concurrent sources of moderate to severe discomfort. In a survey by Crook et al. (18) of 500 randomly selected households in Ontario, the incidence of pain was twice as great (250 per thousand vs 125 per thousand) in those over age 60 than in those 60 and under. Estimates range from 45% to 80% among nursing home residents (15,20) with a predominance of musculo-skeletal causes of pain, especially osteoarthritis. Thus, a diagnosis of cancer in the elderly is often an added burden to existing physical or psychosocial demands of aging.

The multiple chronic illness demands of the elderly create psychosocial challenges beyond any other population. It is estimated that arthritis may affect 80% of people over age 65, and most suffer significant pain (21). A number of other specific pain syndromes are known to affect the geriatric population disproportionately, including herpes zoster, temporal arteritis, polymyalgia rheumatic, and atherosclerotic peripheral vascular disease (22).

There continues to be diverse opinion regarding the influence of gender on pain. General consensus is that pain tolerance and sensitivity do not differ between men and women, although many gender characteristics influence the pain experience. Cultural influences on gender, such as the need for stoicism, are an example of the effect of gender when combined with other variables. In the elderly population, pain data is also influenced by longevity as women have longer lifespans.

PSYCHOSOCIAL ASSESSMENT IN THE ELDERLY

The literature has documented an association between psychological conditions and physical symptoms in chronic illnesses such as cancer (15). Most patients with chronic pain will have significant depressive symptoms at one time or another and may benefit dramatically from psychological or psychiatric intervention. Likewise, anxiety may be a significant psychological factor affecting the management of physical symptoms. However, care providers should avoid assigning a psychological cause to an elderly patient's pain. Needless suffering may result from attributing pain complaints only to depression rather than acting aggressively to recognize the source of pain.

There are important issues in assessment of the elderly with regard to the relationship between cognitive impairment and symptom assessment. Cognitive impairment in elderly patients may present special problems in the assessment and management of pain and other symptoms. Clinical evidence suggests that cognitive impairment may be exacerbated by uncontrolled symptoms and also by their treatment. Symptom assessment in the cognitively impaired patient is challenging because of limitations with the use of existing assessment tools, which depend on the patient's active participation and self-report (23).

Psychological assessment should include a thorough mental status examination and evaluation for depression. Tools such as the Folstein Mini Mental State examination for cognitive impairment and the Hamilton, Beck, or Yesavage inventories for depression are easily utilized. Formal psychological tests such as the Minnesota Multiphasic Personality Inventory, which has been validated for use in older populations, may be useful in identifying personality traits that may benefit by specific psychological or psychiatric therapy.

Assessment of pain includes an evaluation of the effect of pain on the patient's quality of life. Cancer pain is a multidimensional experience affecting the entire person and therefore cannot be viewed as a single symptom of illness. Pain influences many aspects of a patient's world, including physical well-being, psychological well-being, social concerns, and spiritual well-being. Even mild or moderate pain in an elderly nursing home patient may be significant enough to interfere with important daily activities such as participating in social outings or religious activities (24, 25).

A multidimensional approach to symptom assessment is usually required for all patients, but may be particularly important for the elderly. Physical, functional, and psychological evaluation should be combined to ensure accurate assessment. There are standardized comprehensive psychosocial assessments used at Cancer Comprehensive Centers, e.g. the City of Hope National Medical Center. Evaluation begins with a thorough history and physical examination. Special attention should be directed toward the musculo-skeletal and nervous systems. The history is important to establish a baseline description of symptoms. For the frail elderly, any history of trauma should be thoroughly evaluated. Sudden changes in the character of pain may indicate deterioration or new injury and should be carefully evaluated.

It is important to remember that elderly patients may present special problems in obtaining an accurate history. Failures in memory, depression, and sensory impairments may hinder history-taking. The elderly may also under-report symptoms because they expect pain associated with aging and their diseases. Cancer patients may not report pain because they fear the meaning of pain or because they think pain cannot be relieved. Many elderly patients may not report pain because they "just don't want to bother anyone." The importance of family and caregivers as a source of information about elderly patients cannot be overemphasized.

Because elderly patients suffer concurrent illness, care must be taken to avoid attributing new symptoms to pre-existing chronic illness. Making this problem worse is the fact that symptoms are usually not constant. Both the character and intensity of chronic pain may fluctuate with time. Injuries due to trauma, as well as other acute problems are easily overlooked in this population. Only astute questioning and comprehensive evaluation will avoid these pitfalls.

Additionally, a thorough neurologic examination should be conducted, including attention to signs of autonomic, sensory, and motor deficits suggestive of neuropathic conditions and nerve injuries (26). Evaluation of function is important so that mobility and independence can be maximized for elderly patients (27). Functional assessment may include information from the history and physical examination as well as several available functional assessment scales. Scales frequently used in routine geriatric evaluation, such as the Tinetti gait evaluation scale (28) and the Lawton (29) and the Katz (30) activities of daily living scales may be useful. However, at least two studies in elderly people have suggested that advanced activities of daily living and "elective" activities such as ambulation and psychosocial functions, may correlate better with the presence and severity of pain.

ELDERLY CARE IN NURSING HOMES

Supportive care has been neglected in geriatric medicine and especially among nursing home residents. However, symptom management is greatly needed in this setting. In one study of 97 subjects from a 311-bed multilevel teaching nursing home, patient interviews and charts were reviewed for pain problems and management strategies. Functional status, depression, and cognitive impairment were also evaluated. Results indicate that 71% of residents had at least one pain complaint (range, 1–4). Of subjects with pain, 34% described constant (continuous) pain and 66% described intermittent pain. Of 43 subjects with intermittent pain, 51% described pain on a daily basis. Major sources of pain included low back pain (40%),

arthritis of appendicular joints (24%), previous fracture sites (14%), and neuropathies (11%).

Pain-management strategies in this study consisted of analgesic drugs, physical therapy, and heating pads. Only 15% of patients with pain had received medication within the previous 24 hours. The findings suggest that pain is a major problem in long-term care. Important barriers were identified that influence the reporting and management of pain in this setting (15). Related problems such as anxiety, depression, diminished mobility, and increased dependence were also apparent in this setting.

Functional correlates of pain have been described for only a few specific conditions in the elderly. The Iowa Rural Health Survey (16) found that older people were more likely to have functional impairment and increased health-care utilization associated with low-back pain. A pain survey by Roy and Michael (31) reported that 83% of selected residents from a Canadian multilevel long-term care facility had a pain "problem." In this study of residents with little functional impairment, no significant correlations were found between pain and activity level, living arrangements, or depression.

The National Nursing Home Survey of 1977 reported that 36.6% of residents were receiving analgesic medications (32). This study also reported analgesic use in several chronic conditions. Forty-eight percent of residents with arthritis or rheumatism were receiving analgesics. The National Hospice Study suggested that elderly patients required fewer analgesic medications for terminal cancer pain than did younger patients (33). Most studies have failed to demonstrate distinct relationships between age and variables such as pain, anxiety, or depression. Rather, investigators have concluded that it is a combination of variables, of which age is one factor, that influence physical or psychological symptoms in illness.

THE ROLE OF FAMILY CAREGIVERS IN CARE OF THE ELDERLY

While the family is often cited as a significant source of support for the patient with cancer, few studies have examined family caregiver roles for cancer care of the elderly patient. Family members become active caregivers, often with minimal training or support, and assume the caregiver role whether or not they feel competent to do so (34–36). Family caregiving requires adjustments in daily schedules, imposes financial burdens, and causes individual members to re-evaluate their relationships with the patient (37–41).

Researchers have consistently found symptom management to be a major source of concern for family caregivers. The impact of pain on patients and their families has been cited in the literature (42,43). Patients and their caregivers experience helplessness, coping by denying feelings, and wish for death as an end to the suffering. Family members caring for a physically ill person in the home need skills in making decisions, planning care, and assessing the need for care.

Several recent studies have focused on pain management at home (44). Family members often fear addiction and respiratory depression or drug tolerance and lack knowledge regarding chronic pain and pain management. These problems are especially intensified in the elderly; therefore, family caregivers may undermedicate the elderly patient, even though the patient continues to experience unrelieved pain.

Pain management has become very complex with the use of multiple medications, including adjuvant drugs, and the use of complex delivery systems such as patient controlled analgesia (PCA) devices, epidural catheters, or continuous parenteral infusions. Patients are cared for in increasing numbers at home by family members who, despite their negative attitudes to drugs and lack of knowledge about pain management, assume responsibility for pain relief. Several authors (34) have stressed the need to educate family caregivers to manage this complex and often "high tech" care provided in the home.

Research data confirm that in the majority of situations the family has the responsibility for managing pain for the individual with cancer. Families assess pain, make decisions regarding the amount and type of medication, and determine when the dose of medication is to be taken. Family members may deny that the patient is in pain to avoid acknowledging that the cancer is progressing. Research has demonstrated that the family is greatly affected by the diagnosis of cancer in one of its members and, furthermore, the family can and does influence the patient's adjustment to the illness. Although these studies cite pain as a major concern of family caregivers, research specifically focusing on the caregivers' role in pain management is limited.

CONCLUSION

The elderly represent a growing population in society and a particular challenge to the health care system. Chronic illnesses such as cancer impose strain on the patient and family. Physical symptoms, as well as psychosocial demands, are common in cancer and greatly diminish quality of life (45–48).

There is a need for psychological evaluation which respects the specific concerns of the elderly. Caution is advised against accepting psychiatric problems as "normal" components of aging. The elderly patient with cancer deserves aggressive palliative care.

REFERENCES

1. United States Bureau of the Census Current Population Reports, Special Studies. *Sixty-five Plus in America.* Washington, DC: US Government Printing Office; 1992: 23–178.
2. Barraclough BM. Suicide in the elderly. In Kay SWK, Walk AA, eds. *Recent Developments in Psychogeriatrics.* Ashford, Kent, UK: Headley Bros; 1971.
3. US Department of Health and Human Service, National Center for Health Statistics, Public Health Services. *Americans needing help to function at home. Advance Data from Vital and Health Statistics of the National Center for Health Statistics*, No. 92. Washington, US Government Printing Office; 1983.
4. Miller LS, Kelman DS. Estimates of the loss of individual productivity from alcohol and drug abuse, and mental illness. In Frang RG and Manning WG, eds. *Economics and Mental Health.* Baltimore: The Johns Hopkins University Press; 1992: 91–129.
5. Osgood NJ, Brant BA. Suicide among the elderly in institutional and community settings. In Harper MS, ed. *Management and Care of the Elderly.* Newbury Park, CA: Sage; 37–71.
6. Riley BB. Mental disorders. In Hogstel MO, ed. *Nursing Care of the Older Adult.* 3rd ed. New York: Delmar, 1994: 204–233.
7. Wasylenki D. The psychogeriatric problem. *Can Mental Health.* 1982; 30(3):16–19.
8. Ruegg RG, Zisook S, Swerdlow NR. Depression in the aged: An overview. *Psychiatr Clin N Am.* 1988; 11(1): 83–97.
9. Burns BJ, Wagner HR, Taube JE, et al. Mental health service use by the elderly in nursing homes. *Am J Pub Health.* 1993; 83(3):331–337.
10. Kelly J, Urquhart A. *A Report on Caring for the Mentally Ill Nursing Home Patient: Introduction and Care Planning.* Washington DC: US Department of Veterans Affairs; 1993.
11. Regier DA, Myers JK, Kramer M, et al. The NIMH epidemiologic catchment area programs, historical context, major objectives and study population characteristics. *Arch Gen Psychiatry.* 1984; 41:934–944.
12. Dworkin SF, Von Korff M, LeResche L. Multiple pain and psychiatric disturbance: An epidemiologic investigation. *Arch Gen Psychiatry.* 1990; 47:239–244.
13. Magni G, Fabrizio S, De Leo D. Pain as a symptom in elderly depressed patients. *Eur Arch Psychiatry Neurol Sci.* 1985; 235:143–145.
14. Roy R. A psychosocial perspective on chronic pain and depression in the elderly. *Soc Work Health Care.* 1986; 12(2):27–36.
15. Ferrell BA, Ferrell BR, Osterweil D. Pain in the nursing home. *J Am Geriatr Soc.* 1990; 38(4):409–414.
16. Lavsky-Shulan M, Wallace RB, Kohout FJ, et al. Prevalence and functional correlates of low back pain

in the elderly: The Iowa +65 rural health survey. *J Am Geriatr Soc*. 1985; 33(1):23–28.

17. Ferrell BR, Wisdom C, Wenzel C. Quality of life as an outcome variable in management of cancer pain. *Cancer*. 1989; 63(11):2321–2327.

18. Crook J, Rideout E, Browne G. The prevalence of pain complaints among a general population. *Pain*. 1984; 18:299–314

19. Brattberg G, Mats T, Anders W. The prevalence of persistent pain in a Danish population. In: *Proc. 5th World Congress on Pain. Pain Suppl*. 1987; 4:S332.

20. Lau-Ting C, Phoon WO. Aches and pains among Singapore elderly. *Singapore Med J*. 1988; 29:164–167

21. Davis MA. Epidemiology of osteoarthritis. *Clin Geriat Med*. 1988; 4(2):241–255.

22. Ferrell BR, Ferrell BA. Pain in the elderly. In McGuire, Yarbro & Ferrell, eds. *Cancer Pain Management*. St Louis: Jones & Bartlett; 1995.

23. Ferrell BA, Ferrell BR, Rivera L. Pain in Cognitively Impaired Nursing Home Patients. *J Pain Symptom Manage*. 1995; 10(8):591–598.

24. Ferrell BR, Cohen MZ, Rhiner M, Rozak A. *Pain as a metaphor for illness, part II: Family caregivers' management of pain*. Oncol Nurs Forum. 1991; 18:1315–1321.

25. Ferrell BR, Ferrell BA. Comfort, in Corr DM, Corr CA, eds. *Nursing Care in an Aging Society*. New York: Spring; 1990: 67–91.

26. Ferrell BA, Ferrell BR. Assessment of chronic pain in the elderly. *Geriatr Med Today*. 1989; 8(5):123-134.

27. Rubenstein LZ, Campbell LJ, Kane RL, eds. *Clinics in Geriatric Medicine*; vol 3. Philadelphia: WB Saunders; 1987.

28. Tinetti ME. Performance oriented assessment of mobility problems in elderly patients. *J Am Geriatr Soc*. 1986; 34:119–126.

29. Lawton MP, Brody EM. Assessment of older people: Self-maintaining and instrumental activities of daily living. *Gerontologist*. 1969; 9:179–186.

30. Katz S, Ford AB, Moskowitz RW, et al. Studies in the aged. The index of ADL: A standardized measure of biological and psychosocial function. *J Am Med Assoc*. 1963; 185:914–919.

31. Roy R, Michael T. A survey of chronic pain in an elderly population. *Can Fam Physician*. 1986; 32:513–516

32. *Characteristics of Nursing Home Residents, Health Status, and Care Received: National Nursing Home Survey, 1977.* (National Health Survey Series 13, No. 51. DHHS Publication #(PHS) 81-1712, April 1981).

33. Goldberg RJ, Mor V, Wiemann M, et al. Analgesic use in terminal cancer patients: report from the national hospice study. *Chronic Dis*. 1986; 39:37–45.

34. Hinds C. The needs of families who care for patients with cancer at home: Are we meeting them? *J Ad Nurs*. 1985; 10, 575–581.

35. Germino B. The impact of cancer on the patient, the family, and the nurse. *Living with Cancer: The Fifth National Conference on Cancer Nursing*. Arlington, VA: American Cancer Society; 1987.

36. Hull MM. Family needs and supportive nursing behaviors during terminal cancer: A review. *Oncol Nurs Forum*. 1989; 16:787–792.

37. Ferrell BR, Ferrell BA, Rhiner M, Grant M. Family factors influencing cancer pain management. *Postgrad Med J*. 1991; 67(suppl. 2), S64–69.

38. Ferrell BR, Johnston Taylor E, Sattler GR, et al. Searching for the meaning of pain: Cancer patients', caregivers', and nurses' perspectives. *Cancer Pract*. 1993; 1:185–194.

39. Ferrell BR, Rhiner M, Cohen MZ, Grant M. Pain as a metaphor for illness. Part I: Impact of cancer pain on family caregivers. *Oncol Nurs Forum*. 1991; 18: 1303–1309.

40. Ferrell BR, Schneider C. Experience and management of cancer pain at home. *Cancer Nurs*. 1988; 11:84–90.

41. Ferrell BR, Ferrell BA. *Pain in the Elderly*. London: International Association for the Study of Pain (IASP); 1996.

42. Johnston Taylor E, Ferrell Br, Grant M, Cheyney L. Managing cancer pain at home: The decisions and conflicts of patients, caregivers, and their nurses. *Oncol Nurs Forum*. 1993; 20:919–927.

42. Lewandowski W, Jones SL. The family with cancer: Nursing interventions throughout the course of living with cancer. *Cancer Nurs*. 1988; 11:313–321.

43. Northouse L. The impact of cancer on the family: An overview. *Int J Psychiatr Med*. 1984; 14:215–242.

44. Ferrell BR, Grant M, Chan J, et al. The impact of cancer pain education on family caregivers of elderly patients. *Oncol Nurs Forum*. 1995; 22(8):1211–1218.

45. Finch EJL, Ramsay R, Katona CLE. Depression and physical illness in the elderly. *Clin Geriatr Med*. 1992; 8(2):275–284.

46. Gurland B. The impact of depression on quality of life of the elderly. *Clin Geriatr Med*. 1992; 8(2):377–385.

47. Guttmann D, Lowenstein A. Psychosocial problems and the needs of the elderly in mental health. In Turner FJ, ed. *Mental Health and the Elderly: A Social Work Perspective*. New York: The Free Press.

48. Harper MS. An overview of mental health and older adults. In Hogstel MO, ed. *Geropsychiatric Nursing*. St Louis: Mosby.

73

Underserved Patients

R. ERIC WESTON, BRUCE D. RAPKIN, RANDOLPH G. POTTS, AND
MEREDITH Y. SMITH

Advances in cancer treatment have led to prolonged survival for many individuals who are diagnosed with cancer (1). Nearly half of all newly diagnosed cancer patients will survive longer than five years. Survival rates are most encouraging for individuals diagnosed and treated for certain primary tumor sites, particularly when identified at an early stage in the disease process (1). Thus, for many patients, cancer is no longer considered to be an acute illness resulting in imminent death but rather a chronic disease which requires long-term treatment and follow-up care.

It is in this context that health promotion has taken on an increasingly important role. The World Health Organization Working Group (1984), as quoted by Glanz, Lewis, and Rimer, p. 8 (2), define health promotion as, "a process of enabling people to improve their health by synthesizing personal choice and social responsibility." The results of this emphasis on positive lifestyle choices have been noticeable: decreases in morbidity and mortality have been noted for "mainstream" Americans in a number of diseases, including cancer (3).

CANCER AMONG THE UNDERSERVED

Over the past decade, research efforts have identified significant discrepancies in cancer incidence and mortality among certain sectors of the population in the United States despite targeted intervention efforts (4–6). Such discrepancies suggest that there are those within our society who have not benefited in equal measure from ongoing advances in cancer care.

In this chapter, we argue that psycho-oncologists have a critical role to play in alleviating existing inequities in the delivery of oncology services. Moreover, we contend that this role extends to not only redressing inequities in the distribution of cancer prevention and treatment services, but to securing more equal access to

participation in cancer clinical trials, and to ensuring that health professionals in the field of oncology, including practicing clinicians, administrators, and other policy makers, are more representative of underserved populations as well.

We begin our discussion by exploring the definition of the term "underserved." Notably, there is no consensus in the literature concerning a definition of this term, especially within the context of cancer. Second, we provide a brief historical overview of the delivery of health care, particularly oncology services, within the United States. Third, we summarize the current distribution patterns of cancer care in this country today. Fourth, we enumerate and discuss the barriers to obtaining adequate cancer services, Fifth, we critique the efficacy of oncology interventions designed to target the underserved, with a special emphasis on cancer health promotion and prevention efforts. Sixth and finally, we conclude by highlighting new directions for the field of psycho-oncology in addressing issues concerning the underserved and cancer.

DEFINING UNDERSERVED CANCER POPULATIONS

While the term "medically underserved" is frequently used in the health care literature, the phrase has rarely been explicitly defined. In a 1991 publication, the National Institutes of Health defined the underserved as consisting of society's most "vulnerable" members, including visible racial and ethnic groups as well as "school drop-outs, gang members, the homeless, migrant workers, prostitutes, children of drug users, recent immigrant groups, the unemployed or the working poor, the elderly, veterans, incarcerated adults and juveniles, the mentally ill, or other vulnerable groups" (7). A specific example of the relationship between these characteristics and cancer is provided by a review of oral cancer. The characteristics associated with the incidence of oral cancer include: unemployment in adults, blue collar workers, self perception of health as fair or poor, no private insurance, low socioeconomic status (SES); older age, non-white, less than 12 years education, no perceived symptoms, lower rates of health service utilization; male gender; low educational attainment; and frequent use of alcohol and other drugs, including tobacco (8–10). Moreover, these characteristics define those segments of the population least likely to participate in community health promotions efforts. Thus, those individuals who are most vulnerable to oral cancer are also least likely to participate in health promotion/disease prevention activities.

The role of gender has been equivocal in its relation to the status of underserved. While the majority of health promotion efforts have been targeted towards males, the message has been received to a greater extent by women, as evidenced by the high number of women who participate in health fairs, and other health promotion initiatives (11). This has been so evident in the literature that male gender is often included as a risk factor for disease (11).

Other more specific definitions have focused on additional sociodemographic characteristics such as:

• young adulthood (aged 18–44);
• low socioeconomic status;
• low educational level;
• non-English-speaking;
• other than Western European heritage (11–14).

A third approach has been to describe the underserved exclusively in terms of service utilization and access to care. According to this definition, the underserved include those who have not had equal access to state-of-the-art primary, secondary and tertiary oncology services (8). As we will see the question of equal access is confounded by many of the sociodemographic characteristics discussed above.

Our final definition of the underserved evokes a sociopolitical perspective. Historically, the term underserved refers to a relationship between certain groups in the U.S. that are underrepresented as recipients of services from facilities providing state-of-the-art cancer detection and treatment, and who have not shared the benefits of health promotion and cancer control campaigns. These groups have been underrepresented in health research, underrepresented as health professionals in oncology, and underrepresented in determining health policy (15–17). For example, the number of African American cancer research and clinical profes-

sionals directly involved in National Cancer Institute (NCI) programs is marginal and has decreased (18). The proportion of physicians that are African American is minuscule and has declined since 1960–from 4.4% to 3.7% (19).

Among the underserved are a disproportionately high number of people who have faced similar inequities in employment, housing and education, e.g., people of African descent, Latinos and Native Americans. The asymmetries in U.S. oncology are consistent with the asymmetrical power relationships within U.S. society generally. A social dichotomy between "privileged" and "underprivileged," "advantaged" and "disadvantaged" (well-served and underserved) reflects the resource asymmetry that accompanies oppression (20–23).

In summary, our review suggests the existence of a group, or groups, that have been consistently excluded from the health benefits enjoyed by their European American counterparts. This group is largely defined by specific sociodemographic characteristics including:

• visible racial or ethnic group status;
• low SES, unemployed or underemployed;
• poor self perception of health;
• absence of private insurance;
• less than 12 years education;
• lower rates of health service utilization;
• male gender;
• frequent use of alcohol and other drugs, including tobacco.

In general, there has been a paucity of research on this group and there is a growing consensus that there is an urgent need to address the issues of this special population (24,25). This interest has been contiguous with improvements in medical knowledge and technology that has extended life beyond the limits of the nineteenth and twentieth centuries and accompanying expectations for an improved quality of life. This group(s), has been called by many names in the literature depending on the specific risk factor(s) under investigation, e.g., hard to reach populations, culturally disadvantaged, socially alienated, the underclass (12–14). The current designation used to describe this group is the medically underserved.

HISTORICAL PERSPECTIVE OF THE UNDERSERVED

There is evidence of a clear relationship between under service in medical and other areas in society (14,18, 26–28). In order to review this relationship, we have chosen to focus on a specific visible racial and ethnic group, people of African descent. This choice was largely a function of the relative greater amount of available research and literature on this group. We believe, however, that many of the elements that arise from this review are pertinent to other visible racial and ethnic groups.

Slavery Period

Underservice in communities of African descent must be viewed in the wake of 400 years of legally sanctioned separate and inferior health care in the U.S. Historical accounts show that African slaves in the U.S. experienced the worst health status and outcome of any racial or ethnic group in North America (29–31).

Post Civil War Period

After the Civil War the inferior slave health system gave way to total neglect—approximately one-third of the newly emancipated died in the first five years after the Civil War (18). It was not until the mid 1960s that there were legal incentives for hospitals to alter racist practices. Title VI of the Civil Rights Act made racial discrimination by institutions receiving federal funds illegal.

Post-1964 Period

During the first decade after segregated health care was declared illegal, African Americans were still being used in medical research so deadly and abusive to subjects that in 1974 a national commission was formed to develop standards for biomedical research ethics (32, 33). This commission published the Belmont Report on Ethical Principles for the Protection of Human Subjects of Research (32).

Current Period

The long-term incidence and prevalence of cancer among non-traditional populations is not well documented as a result of inadequate record-keeping practices. In a review of U.S. cancer mortality using data obtained from the National Center for Health Statistics for the period 1950–1967, Burbank and Fraumeni (34) reported a dichotomous categorization system: White, i.e., White, Mexican, Puerto Rican, and Cuban; and Nonwhite, i.e., all other races. Even using a classification system that would be considered inadequate by current standards, Burbank and Fraumenti reported a trend towards increased cancer related mortality for the non-white population beginning in 1950 for men and 1956 for women. The investigators cited the difficulties with identifying the causes of this trend owing to the aforementioned classification system,

inadequate record keeping among the nonwhite group, and socioeconomic and environmental differences.

In an early study of the differences in the prevalence of squamous carcinoma of the cervix and related atypias between women of African descent, and women of European descent, Christopherson and Parker (35) reported no significant difference in occurrence between these groups (35). These investigators suggest that these findings highlight the importance of controlling for socioeconomic level when conducting intergroup research.

There was little effort directed toward assessing or improving black cancer status and outcomes until the research of Lefall (36,37) brought national attention to the African American cancer crisis. Lefall's research showed that, despite the giant strides in U.S. oncology, African Americans were falling farther and farther behind whites in cancer survival.

In 1984, the Secretary of Health commissioned a task force to evaluate the health status of visible racial and ethnic groups. The minorities in question consisted of people of African descent Latinos, Native Americans and Asian/Pacific Islanders (38). The results of the Task Force's investigation identified six causes of death responsible for more than 80% of the excess mortality of the visible racial and ethnic groups in comparison to people of European descent. Cancer related deaths ranked high on this list. The specific sites of excess death identified for each visible racial and ethnic group are found in Table 73.1.

Freeman (14) and others have pointed out that many of the current cancer education programs have not been designed to target underserved racial and ethnic groups (14). In developing interventions that are more culturally grounded, oppression is an important construct to consider in that it addresses historical inequalities in access to valued resources, such as quality health care and the psychological and behavioral consequences of such long-term denial of resources. Certain health related behaviors among oppressed groups (such as suspicions and distrust of the health care system and use of alternative remedies) may not be simply manifestations of cultural traditions and preferences, but adaptations to a history of oppression (39–40). Indeed, from craniometry to eugenics to theories on intellectual and linguistic deficits among oppressed groups, mental health practitioners have provided an aura of science in justifying race and class stratification (41–42). Nobles (43) has described psychological research relationships with the black community as "scientific colonialism": the community is exploited as a source of data (raw material), which is

TABLE 73.1. *Leading Sites of Excess Cancers-Related Death by Racial Group*

Type	African descent	Latino	Asian/Pacific Islander	Native American
Lung	X†		X	X
Prostate (male)	X†	X†		
Corpus uteri	X‡			
Breast	X‡		X‡	
Esophagus	X	X		
Esophageal	X			
Stomach	X		X	
Multiple myeloma	X		X	
Stomach	X	X†	X	
Cervix	X‡	X‡	X‡	X‡
Pancreas		X	X‡	
Ovarian			X‡	
Gall bladder				X
Liver				X
Nasopharyngeal			X	
Colon			X	

Source: Secretary's Task Force on Black and Minority Health (38). † Male. ‡ Female.

then processed and marketed as books and articles (finished goods) by white professionals in predominantly white institutions.

In summary, the technological and theoretical advancements that have effectively lowered the incidence and prevalence of cancer in the United States for people of traditional populations have not been universally effective. We have identified multiple populations that have not shared the benefits of improved cancer care and, to the contrary, have experienced a deterioration in health status. Moreover, for cancer survivors who are members of the underserved, the range of potential physical and social sequelae of cancer diagnosis and treatment may be compounded by other chronic factors. In the following section, we will review these factors that contribute to the maintenance of the status quo for the medically underserved, despite efforts from health professionals to narrow this ever increasing gap.

BARRIERS TO ADEQUATE CANCER DETECTION AMONG THE UNDERSERVED

Several factors have been implicated in the failure of cancer control efforts in underserved communities, including cultural differences, poverty, accessibility of health care, inappropriate programs, lack of knowledge, low frequency preventive behavior, and inadequate monitoring of high risk individuals. Each of these factors is reviewed below.

Cultural Differences

In some communities, the understanding of cancer is influenced by non-western cultures and traditions. These deeply-held folk beliefs may impact health care choices. For example, Snow (44) noted that some segments of the African American community hold health views that are in sharp contrast to the public health messages and methods of modern western medicine, e.g., illness as a punishment from God (44). In order to be effective in reaching underserved populations, public education must bring these traditions together (45). Failure to achieve a working alliance between these beliefs may serve to create what Orlandi (46) calls the Barrier of the Inappropriate Target: that is, members of underserved groups are further alienated from public health services and information by the perception that they were never intended to participate or benefit from mass-oriented education or prevention programs.

Poverty

Health care statistics indicate that health care is least accessible to persons who are uninsured, unemployed or underemployed, and who utilize hospital emergency rooms as the primary source for health care (14). These indicators are characteristic of low SES, a category in which the underserved are overrepresented (3,7–9). Laveist (47) highlights the complexity of the relationship between socioracial status and SES by alluding to the practice of using the racial designation of a visible racial or ethnic group member as an indicator of poverty. Freeman (14) summarizes the complex relationship among race, poverty, and cancer through the following statistics:

- Americans over the poverty level report a lower incident rate of cancer and five-year survival rates 10–15% greater than Americans at or under the poverty level;
- visible racial and ethnic group members are at greater risk for poverty in the U.S.A.

Accessibility of Health Care

Access to health services has been defined as a function of three elements, availability, affordability, and convenience (48). Medical care has been severely cut in urban communities, the environment of a significant proportion of the underserved, within the past decade (48). Moreover, Mettlin et al. (49), in a review of prostate cancer reports from hospital cancer registries across the U.S., concluded that men of African descent receive different types of interventions than do men of European descent. In addition to accessibility, the rising cost of health care has created a wave of concern from even the most affluent of the population of this country. Currently, the lion's share of health care cost is paid by either employers or through federal initiatives such as Medicaid/Medicare. Underserved populations are overrepresented among the ranks of the unemployed, underemployed, and uninsured, and the cutbacks in federal eligibility programs have forced many families to choose between health care and other basic needs.

Inappropriate Intervention Programs

The deteriorating health status of the underserved is evidence of the inability of traditional intervention approaches to meet the special needs of this population. Factors leading to this failure include theoretical concerns, inappropriate material, lack of knowledge on the part of the target audience, low frequency of preventive behavior, and inadequate monitoring of high risk individuals. Each of these factors is reviewed below.

Theoretical Deficits. Most intervention efforts are guided by theoretical constructs, and efforts in underserved communities are no exception. However, several limitations of the current theoretical models have been raised, such as the use of Eurocentric models with non-European populations and the failure to identify both intergroup and intragroup differences existing among underserved populations (46,50–53).

Inappropriate Educational Material. Another barrier to successful intervention is the lack of educational instruments targeted towards the underserved. The 1989 American Cancer Society Report (45) declared that the majority of cancer education programs lack cultural sensitivity and are viewed as largely irrelevant to visible racial and ethnic groups. Additionally, the reading level of the educational material is an important consideration. Poverty has been identified as a characteristic of the underserved population, and low literacy and illiteracy are highly correlated with low SES (14). While the average reading level of many of the educational materials regarding cancer is above the eighth grade level, between 20% and 40% of Americans (45 to 70 million individuals) do not possess the reading skills required to function adequately in our society (usually defined as the ability to read at an eighth grade level) (14).

Lack of Knowledge. Cancer is the second leading cause of death in the U.S. for most groups, yet data suggests that people in underserved communities are less knowledgeable regarding cancer risks than their mainstream American counterparts (54). For example, the report of the Secretary's Task Force on Black and Minority Health (38), stated that persons of African descent underestimate cancer prevalence, have a lower knowledge of the warning signs of cancer, are more pessimistic regarding survival of people with cancer and accept myths regarding cancer.

Low-Frequency Preventive Behavior. The current statistics suggests that people of African descent have the highest age-adjusted rates of cancer related incidence and mortality of any racial group in the United States (1,54). However, early detection strategies such as breast self-examination, mammographies, and prostate specific antigens are low (54–65). Factors that may contribute to the low frequency of preventive health behavior include perception of risk, beliefs regarding efficacy of early detection methods, beliefs regarding the effects of radiation and misunderstanding about the necessity of screening in the absence of symptoms (54).

Delayed Presentation of Symptoms. A critical element in the disproportionate morbidity and mortality among the underserved is the delay in seeking health care. Issues of access and poverty are key factors in this underutilization of medical services (14,66–69). Another important factor is the multilevel stressors that exist in underserved communities.

Individuals in these communities are routinely subjected to stressful events and circumstances that demand their attention and energy, e.g., family problems, poor housing conditions, inadequate transportation, unsafe neighborhoods, more imminent or pressing health problems, and stressors associated with aging (68). These stressors may lead individuals in underserved communities to ignore their own risk of cancer, even when signs and symptoms are evident. Other delay related factors include emphasis on self care, fear and stigmatization, mistrust of the health care system, and concern regarding racism among health care professionals (13,47,70–73).

Inadequate Monitoring of Families at Increased Risk.
Improved understanding of the genetics of cancer has prompted intensive efforts to reach and monitor individuals at genetic high risk (74). Close surveillance can help to ensure that cancer is detected as early as possible, greatly reducing morbidity and mortality. Unfortunately, lack of information about risk factors, lack of resources, and poor access to health services often result in an absence of aggressive follow-up of genetic risk.

INTERVENTIONS TARGETING THE UNDERSERVED IN CANCER

The failure of traditional intervention programs to respond effectively to these alarming statistics has led to a call for new and innovative strategies for public and mental health promotion in underserved communities (3,75). These innovative strategies must be both culturally and community syntonic, i.e., they must be anchored by an understanding of the cultural mores, community values, and ethnic values of the population that they seek to serve (76–78). Jackson (13) has stressed the need for a sophisticated view of these differences, that is, a recognition of the differences that exist among visible racial and ethnic groups, as well as the difference between such groups and European Americans (13).

Bowman (32) has operationalized this concept into two guiding principles which he terms significant involvement, and functional relevance:

Significant involvement—Bowman states that the principle of significant involvement , ". . . calls for members of the group under study to have a central role in the entire research process". (p. 755). Bowman asserts that this involvement must go beyond using community workers and conducting

key community informants. Truly significant involvement will incorporate participation in the planning, implementation, and evaluation of the intervention.
Functional relevance—According to Bowman, the second guiding principle, functional relevance, requires that interventions, ". . . should operate to promote the expressed needs and perspectives of the study population" (p. 755). While many projects give lip service to these principles, the operationalization from theory to practice is often difficult. Potential areas of conflict between the intervention team and the community sometimes threaten to doom the project prior to its implementation. These issues must be addressed, however, if successful strategies are to be initiated.

Several programs have addressed issues of outreach, education, and intervention among the medically underserved. Three such programs will be reviewed below, with a special focus on the strategies used to insure significant involvement and functional relevance.

The Harlem Health Connection
An example of a project that successfully utilized the principles of significant involvement and functional relevance is provided in a cancer prevention project conducted in the community of Harlem (79). The specific aims of this program were

- to develop strategies to promote smoke free lifestyles in the Harlem community;
- to develop an effective strategy to educate African Americans to the need for smoke free lifestyles;
- to identify effective channels to disseminate smoking cessation information;
- to evaluate the results of the smoking cessation initiative.

The community analysis phase of the project identified that housing, employment, and access to concrete services were high on the community priority list. The specific needs of the community were met through the development of a component of the overall project called the Harlem Health Connection. The Harlem Health Connection was composed of five core components:

1. A health newsletter designed specifically to address the health concerns of the community of Harlem.
2. A panel of speakers made up of the consortium of organizations comprising the project was made

available to make health related presentations to participating organizations.

3. Access to the Harlem Health Connection Information line, a Health and Human Services referral system that provides a participant with the information to access health related and concrete services.

4. A cash award to each of the participating sites of up to $500.00 for each person recruited into the research project.

5. A Closing Event for representatives of each participating organizations in which information gained from the project was disseminated to the community.

These components assured that the needs of the community were addressed while allowing the research component to conduct much needed research on the efficacy of cancer prevention strategies in African American communities.

La Programa Latino para Dejar de Fumar (Latino Program to Quit Smoking)

An example of a project that followed these basic premises in a Latino community is provided by *La Programa Latino para Dejar de Fumar* (80). This project was designed specifically for Latinos living in San Francisco. The community analysis phase of the project focused on attitudes, norms, expectancies, and values of the Latino community. Once collected and

analyzed, this information was used to develop messages regarding tobacco-related cancer and to identify the most effective channels for delivery of these messages to the target population. The messages were developed in a fashion that was consistent with cultural mores such as *familialism*, the importance of the family and the need to protect it from the dangers of tobacco-related diseases.

The specific needs of the community were addressed through the inclusion of personal consultants, *consultas,* among the dissemination strategies, and the use of monetary awards, in the form of raffles, as rewards for quitters.

Pathways to Freedom Community Demonstration Project

Another example within communities of African descent is provided by the *Pathways to Freedom Project* (81). The aims of this project was to lower the prevalence of cigarette smoking. The project was conducted in eight local units of the American Cancer Society. The community analysis suggested the importance of the family, the strong sense of communalism, and the desire to protect the community from hostile outside forces. Based upon this information, the project developed a manual and a video, which featured persons of African descent, and stressed the concept of community responsibility as a reason for quitting.

Other model cancer programs targeting underserved populations can be found in Table 73.2.

TABLE 73.2. *Model Cancer Intervention Programs Targeting Underserved Populations*

Type of Cancer	Type of Intervention	Target Population	Goals and Objectives
Breast and cervical	Early detection	Women of African descent	To increase the use of mammography, clinical and self-examination of the breast and cervical pap smear through culturally based screening project (6)
Breast and cervical cancer	Early detection	Women of African descent	To increase the use of mammography, clinical and self-examination of the breast and cervical pap smear through community based information and screening programs (84)
Breast cancer	Early detection	Women of African descent	To increase breast cancer screening awareness and provide a referral of free breast screening for women 50 and over through educational materials disseminated in community hair salons (85)
General	Prevention	Lower SES population	To establish a multidisciplinary, continuity-of-care-based comprehensive cancer prevention, education and early detection clinic within existing inner city health centers (86)
Prostate cancer	Men of African descent	Men with following risk factors: • family histroy of breast cancer • family history of prostate cancer • Age >40	To identify high risk individuals and administer prostate-specific antigen test, and digital rectal examinations (87)

THE ROLE OF PSYCHO-ONCOLOGISTS IN ALLEVIATING THE PROBLEMS OF THE UNDERSERVED

The above description of the status of the medically underserved sets an agenda of action for psycho-oncology. The role of psychology/oncology in the creation and maintenance of the underserved cannot be ignored. It is important that psycho-oncologists, both delivering oncology services and conducting research in underserved communities, remain mindful of historical ties between psychology/psychiatry and the status quo. An appreciation of these ties can direct psycho-oncologists to a path leading to the provision of services to all populations. In order to achieve this goal, psycho-oncologists must possess an understanding of the racial, cultural, economic, and political forces that impact these populations. Towards this end basic suggestions for the development of health related programs in underserved communities are provided below:

1. *Reject the myth of homogeneity regarding underserved populations.* There are differences among the groups that comprise the traditionally underserved. As we have indicated, these differences are often reflected in the types of cancer that present the greatest risk to specific groups. Equally important, however, are the differences within each of these groups in regard to their beliefs, values and behavior (82, 83). Psycho-oncologists must be knowledgeable about the differences between and within underserved populations in order to develop effective cancer intervention programs.

2. *Be responsive to the non-cancer needs of the population.* Psycho-oncologists must demonstrate a respect for the needs of the communities that they wish to serve. This respect is operationalized through the development of programs that address the concrete as well as the cancer related needs of the community. For example, in a lower socioeconomic community where child care is a pressing need, cancer screening programs could provide free child care services to all participants.

3. *Develop partnerships with the underserved.* Although most institutions give lip service to the concept of forming partnership with the community, the issue of sharing power is often difficult to negotiate. How much power is appropriate to cede to the community when developing cancer intervention programs? When is it professionally inappropriate to cede control? These are questions that psycho-oncologists must face before instituting programs in under-

served communities. However, it is clear that the mutual fear and mistrust that often exist between institutions and underserved communities must be addressed before programs can be successfully implemented.

4. *Develop strategies to overcome identified barriers to participation.* Although the literature is replete with identified barriers faced by interventionists in underserved communities, many such programs are developed as if they were targeting traditional populations. For example, in communities where the target population reads at less than a sixth grade level, advertising the program in the local paper may be less than effective. The use of dissemination channels that are popular in the target community, such as radio or hair salons is often more effective.

5. *Be honest with the community regarding future programs.* Many underserved populations view psycho-oncologists conducting research in their communities as outsiders who are interested in collecting data, rather than in meeting the needs of the community. This image is reinforced each time a research project enters the community with promises of continuing services and leaves at the end of the funding period. Programs must be planned in a way that maximizes the potential for continuity of services, and the community must be informed of the potential failure of efforts to generate funds for long term community service. While this declaration may dampen the enthusiasm of potential participants, it will avert charges of deception and betrayal at the end of the funding cycle.

Guided by these principles, psycho-oncologists can play a powerful role in promoting health and reducing morbidity and mortality among the medically underserved. It is useful to envision some of the roles psycho-oncologists can play all along the continuum of care; as in the following sections.

Health Promotion

Beyond identifying culturally appropriate ways to assist individuals and families in achieving healthy lifestyles, psycho-oncology must continue to play a critical role in public policy as it affects public health. It is easy to blame the victim when we focus on individual behavior change, but psycho-oncologists must also study how context effects behavior. For example, what are the implications of new federal welfare policies for health promotion? How well can families follow health promotion guidelines, no matter how culturally sensitive, without access to adequate nutrition, stable housing, and clean, safe neighborhoods? What are the psychological and biological effects of lifelong stress due to chronic poverty and discrimination, and what role does this chronic stress have in producing the excess cancers seen in the underserved? How likely are underserved patients to heed a health provider's recommendations when those recommendations are made in a most hurried fashion, in a setting that is uncomfortable and unwelcoming? Balancing the budget on the backs of the poor may have serious implications for future cancer morbidity and mortality among the underserved. Psycho-oncology has the tools to raise these concerns to public awareness. Public policy makers are an important audience for our research findings, but it is up to us to be sure that research highlights the implications of policy for the medically underserved.

Early Identification

Reaching at risk populations for screening requires partnerships between health providers and communities. Providers and community representatives must work together to provide clear pathways to screening and care. Psycho-oncology can help to ensure that the ingredients of a successful partnership are available. These ingredients include:

1. providing information to raise awareness about risk and screening provided in a culturally appropriate fashion;
2. creating opportunities for individuals to seek information they want and need at a time it becomes relevant to them;
3. providing pre-test counseling, to help individuals understand their risk and the implications of testing at a personal level;
4. identifying and reducing barriers to screening;
5. post-test counseling for individuals with negative as well as positive findings, to help them understand the meaning of their test results, and what they need to do next;
6. help accessing care, when needed.

At each step of the process, psycho-oncologists can help to identify and address other health and nonhealth related concerns that impede underserved individuals' ability to take advantage of methods for early detection.

Entry into Treatment

As we have addressed, psycho-oncology must be concerned with overcoming barriers to care experienced by the medically underserved. Beyond the more general points enumerated above, the issues of access take on special significance in regard to the underrepresentation of patients of color in cancer clinical trials research. Psycho-oncologists can play a valuable role in helping medical colleagues keep special issues of underserved patients in mind as they design and implement trials. How can the benefits and risks of a particular trial best be communicated to underserved patients? Are certain inclusion or exclusion criteria more likely to impede participation of underserved patients? Is the recruitment strategy one that is likely to reach underserved populations? Are appropriate provisions made available to support underserved patients' participation? In addition, psycho-oncologists must address the legacy of exploitation and mistrust that affects many underserved patients' willingness to take part in medical experiments. The informed consent process is more than a mere formality. Psycho-oncologists must help to ensure that patients truly understand their treatment options and their rights as a patient.

Treatment Adherence

As more and more care shifts to the ambulatory setting, patients are required to take a greater role in effecting treatment. This may pose special difficulties to underserved patients. Underserved patients may not receive adequate attention to management of pain, nausea, fatigue, and other side effects. Without proper management, patients may decide to skip a chemotherapy infusion rather than deal with these side effects. In some instances, patients or family members may need assistance working treatment requirements around other demands of work and family life. In addition, patients may need assistance with practical barriers that make treatment adherence more difficult, including lack of transportation and child care. As is the case with many aspects of care, psycho-oncology's greatest contribution may lie in conducting research to document factors that interfere with adherence, and designing model interventions to help underserved patients overcome these problems.

Survivors

Medically underserved patients may experience unique difficulties after completion of treatment. Psycho-oncologists have an important part to play in documenting and addressing these difficulties. For example, re-entry to the workplace may present different challenges for individuals employed as unskilled laborers or with more transient work histories. Given new "workfare" requirements, many underserved patients may be under considerable pressure to return to work after illness.

Psycho-oncologists must also address the needs of patients' families, who may have difficulty providing care for patients who experience prolonged disability after treatment. The emotional impact of cancer on survivors and their families is also a key concern for psycho-oncologists. Underserved patients in particular may enter into care with more fatalistic attitudes, and may need assistance coping with fears of recurrence. Factors which can predispose patients to symptoms of trauma may be more prevalent among underserved survivors, including poorer management of symptoms and treatment side effects, poorer prognosis, psychiatric comorbidity, inadequate social support, and experience of other major stressors. In many cultures, cancer remains a stigma and patients and families may feel embarrassed, ashamed or guilty about expressing their feelings and needs. Interventions to address these issues during and after treatment are critical to the well-being of underserved cancer survivors and their families.

Palliative Care

Effective palliative care requires open communication and collaborative decision-making involving patients, families, and providers. This takes on particular importance in working with underserved patients. We have a role in helping providers recognize unique cultural and family issues, and to develop the necessary skills to communicate effectively and sensitively about death and dying. The medical options we give to patients have emotional, economic, and spiritual implications for patients and families, and underserved patients may need special assistance in making these decisions. Once again, psycho-oncologists must be mindful of the social and economic factors that affect the underserved. These patients and their families often believe that care might be withheld because they cannot afford it. At times, their belief may be well founded. Thus, a recommendation that active treatment be discontinued may be met with considerable suspicion. Conversely, end-of-life decisions may be compounded if pain, depression, and other symptoms are not well controlled. Psycho-oncologists can help to ensure that patients and families have access to the information and care they need to make decisions throughout the course of treatment, so that decisions around the end of life emerge out of a clear and well-understood plan, rather than a pronouncement from the provider.

In summary, this chapter has outlined the historical, cultural, economic, and political factors that have contributed to the development and maintenance of the medically underserved; the current statistics that demonstrate higher rates of cancer related morbidity and mortality among underserved populations; and programs that have successfully addressed the barriers to serving this population. It is our hope that those psycho-oncologists currently working with underserved populations, as well as those who may work with this population in the future, will use this chapter as a starting point for the development of programs that will make the term underserved population an anachronism in the twenty-first century.

REFERENCES

1. Clayton LA, Byrd, WM. The African American cancer crisis, Part I: The problem. *J Health Care Poor Underserved.* 1993; 4(2):83–101.
2. Glanz K, Marcus-Lewis, F, Rimer BK. The scope of health education: Parameters of a maturing field. In: Glanz K, Marcus-Lewis F, Rimer BK, eds. *Health Behavior and Health Education: Theory, Research and Practice.* San Francisco: Jossey-Bass; 1990.
3. Hardy RE, Hargreaves MK. Cancer prognosis in Black Americans: A mini-review. *J Nat Med Assoc.* 1991; 83(7):574–579.
4. Lacey L. Cancer prevention and early detection strategies for reaching underserved urban, low-income Black women: Barriers and objectives. *Cancer.* 1993; 72: 1078–1083.
5. McCoy CB, Nielsen BB, Chitwood DD, et al. Increasing the cancer screening of the medically underserved in South Florida. *Cancer.* 1991; 67:1808–1813.
6. Gregg J, Curry RH. Explanatory models for cancer among African-American women at two Atlanta neighborhood health centers: The implications for a cancer screening programme. *Soc Sci Med.* 1994; 39(4):519–526.
7. Wohlford P. *Trends in NIMH Support for Clinical Training for Ethnic Minorities.* American Psychological Association: Washington, DC; 1991.
8. Adany LA, Forthofer RN. A profile of Black and Hispanic subgroups' access to dental care: Findings from the National Health Interview Survey. *J Public Health Dent.* 1992; 52(4):210–215.
9. Newman JJ, Gift HC. Regular pattern of preventive dental services—A measure of access. *Soc Sci Med.* 1992; 35(8):997–1001.
10. Day GL, Blot WJ, Austin DF, et al. Racial differences in risk of oral and pharyngeal cancer: Alcohol, tobacco, and other determinants. *J Nat Cancer Inst.* 1993; 85(6): 465–473.
11. U.S. Department of Health and Human Services. *Recommendations Regarding Public Screening for Measuring Blood Cholesterol.* NIH Publication 1989; No. 89-3045.
12. Jackson JS. Conducting health behavior research in ethnic and racial minority communities. *Health Behavior Research in Minority Populations: Access, Design, and Implementation.* U.S. Department of Health and Human Services NIH Publication; 1992; No. 92-2965.
13. Baquet CR, Horm JW, Gibbs T, Greenwald P. Socioeconomic factors and cancer incidence among

Blacks and Whites. *J Nat Cancer Inst.* 1991; 83(8): 551–557.

14. Freeman HP. Editorial: Race, poverty, and cancer. *J Nat Cancer Inst.* 1991; 83(8):526–527.

15. Larson E. Exclusion of certain groups from clinical research. *Image—J Nurs Scholarship.* 1994; 26(3): 185–190.

16. Robertson NL. Clinical trial participation: Viewpoints from racial/ethnic groups. *Cancer.* 1994; 74(9 Suppl.): 2687–2691.

17. Millon-Underwood S, Sanders E, Davis M. Determinants of participation in state-of-the-art cancer prevention, early detection/screening, and treatment trials among African Americans. *Cancer Nurs.* 1993; 16(1):23–25.

18. Byrd WA, Clayton LA. The African American cancer crisis. Part II: A prescription. *J Health Care Poor Underserved.* 1993; 4(2):102–116.

19. Hacker A. *Two Nations: Black and White, Separate, Hostile, Unequal.* New York: Ballantine Books; 1995.

20. Prilleltensky I, Gonick LS. The discourse of oppression in the social sciences: past, present, and future. In: Trickett EJ, Watts RJ, Birman D, eds. *Human Diversity: Perspectives on People in Context.* San Francisco: Jossey-Bass, 1994:145–177.

21. Watts RJ. Paradigms of diversity. In: Trickett EJ, Watts RJ, Birman D, eds. *Human Diversity: Perspectives on People in Context.* San Francisco: Jossey-Bass; 1994:145–177.

22. Serrano-Garcia I, Lopez-Sanchez G. Asymmetry and oppression: Pre-requisites of power relationships. Unpublished manuscript; 1992.

23. Bulhan HA. *Franz Fanon and the Psychology of Oppression.* New York: Plenum; 1985.

24. Burish TG. Behavioral and psychosocial research building on the past, preparing for the future. *Cancer.* 1991; 67:865–867.

25. Freeman HP. Cancer in the socioeconomically disadvantaged. *CA—J Clin.* 1989; 39:263–295.

26. Williams DR, Lavizzo-Mourey R, Warren RC. The concept of race and health status in America. *Public Health Rep.* 1994; 109(1):26–41.

27. Airhihenbuwa CO. Health promotion and disease prevention strategies for African Americans: A conceptual model. In: Braithwaite RL, Taylor SE, eds. *Health Issues in the Black Community.* San Francisco: Jossey-Bass; 1992:267–320.

28. Braithwaite RL. Coalition partnerships for health promotion and empowerment. In: Braithwaite RL, Taylor SE. eds. *Health Issues in the Black Community.* San Francisco: Jossey-Bass; 1992:321–337.

29. Savitt TL. *Medicine and Slavery: The Diseases and Health Care of Blacks in Antebellum Vriginia.* Urbana, IL: University of Illinois Press; 1987.

30. Sheridan RB. *Doctors and Slaves: A Medical and Demographic History of Slavery in the British West Indies, 1680–1834.* Cambridge: Cambridge University Press; 1985.

31. Kiple KF, King VH. *Another Dimension to the Black Diaspora: Diet, Disease, and Racism.* Cambridge: Cambridge University Press; 1981.

32. Bowman PJ. Race, class and ethics in research: Belmont principles to functional relevance. In: Jones RE, ed.

Advances in Black Psychology. Berkeley: Cobb and Henry; 1991.

33. Jones JH. *Bad Blood: The Tuskeege Syphilis Experiment.* New York: The Free Press; 1981.

34. Burbank F, Fraumeni JF. U.S. cancer mortality: Nonwhite predominance. In: Shiloh A, Cohen Selavan I, eds. *Ethnic Groups of America: Their Morbidity, Mortality and Behavior Disorders:* vol. II The Blacks. Springfield: Charles C. Thomas; 1974.

35. Christopher WM, Parker JE. A study of the relative frequency of carcinoma of the cervix in the Negro. In: Shiloh A, Cohen Selavan I, eds. *Ethnic Groups of America: Their Morbidity, Mortality and Behavior Disorders:* vol. II The Blacks. Springfield: Charles C. Thomas; 1974.

36. Lefall LD Jr. Cancer mortality in blacks. *Cancer.* 1974;24:42–46.

37. Lefall LD Jr. The challenge of cancer among Black Americans. In: *Proceedings of the American Cancer Society National Conference on Meeting the Challenge of Cancer among Black Americans.* New York: American Cancer Society, 1979.

38. *Report of the Secretary's Task Force on Black & Minority Health: Cancer VII.* U.S. Department of Health and Human Services; 1986.

39. Watts RJ. Elements of a psychology of human diversity. *J Community Psychol.* 1992; 20:116–131.

40. Watson WH, ed. *Black Folk Medicine: The Therapeutic Significance of Faith and Trust.* New Brunswick, NJ: Transaction Books; 1987.

41. Sarason SB. *Psychology Misdirected.* New York: Free Press; 1981.

42. Gould SJ. *The Mismeasure of Man.* New York: W.W. Norton; 1983.

43. Nobles WW. Extended self: Rethinking the so-called Negro self-concept. In: Jones R, ed. *Black Psychology.* New York: Harper; 1980.

44. Snow L. Folk medical beliefs and their implication for care of patients. *Ann Intern Med.* 1974; 81:82–96.

45. American Cancer Society. *Annual Report 1989: Catalyst for change—Targeting cancer in the poor.* Atlanta, GA; 1989.

46. Orlandi MA. Community-based substance abuse prevention: A multicultural perspective. *J School Health.* 1989; 56:394–401.

47. Laveist TA. Segregation, poverty, and empowerment: Health consequences for African Americans. *Milbank Q.* 1993; 71(1):41–50.

48. Cornelius LJ. Access to medical care for Black Americans with an episode of illness. *J Nat Med Assoc.* 1991; 83(7):617–626.

49. Mettlin CJ, Murphy GP, McEnck HR. The National Cancer Data Base report on prostate cancer. *Cancer.* 1995; 76(6):1104–1112.

50. Cochran SD, Mays VM. Applying social-psychological models to predicting HIV-related sexual risk behaviors among African Americans. *J Black Psychol.* 1993; 19(2):142–154.

51. Orlandi MA, Weston RE, Epstein LG. *Cultural Competence for Evaluators: A Guide for Alcohol and Other Drug Abuse Prevention Practitioners with Ethnic/Racial Communities.* U.S. Department of Health and Human Services, Public Health Services, Office for

Substance Abuse Prevention; DHHS Publication No. 1992; (ADM)92-1884.

52. Weston RE, Rapkin BD, Ortiz-Torres B, Mantell JE, Tross SE, Potts R. Reference group orientations, racial identity and tobacco and alcohol use in African American women: Data from the Cultural Network Project. New York: unpublished manuscript; 1995.

53. Ortiz-Torres B, Rapkin B, Mantell JE, Tross SE. The relationship between transculturation and HIV risk behaviors among immigrant latinos in the United States. New York: unpublished manuscript; 1993.

54. Office of Minority Health Resource Center. *Closing the Gap: Cancer and Minorities.* Washington DC; 1989.

55. Jacob TC ,Penn NC, Brown M. Breast self-examination: Knowledge, attitudes, and performance among black women. *J Nat Med Assoc.* 1984; 81:769–776.

56. Long E. Breast cancer in African-American women. *Cancer Nurs.* 1993; 16:1–24.

57. Bastani R, Marcus A, Hollatz-Brown A. Screening mammography rates and barriers to use: A Los Angeles county survey. *Prev Med.* 1991; 20(3):350–363.

58. Fink R, Stein S, Roestner R. Impact of efforts to increase participation in repetitive screenings for each breast cancer detection. *Am J Public Health.* 1972; March:328–336.

59. Rimer BK. Understanding the acceptance of mammography by women. *Ann Behav Med.* 1992; 14(3):197–203.

60. Kaplan KM, Weinberg GB, Small A, Herndon JL. Breast cancer screening among relatives of women with breast cancer. *Am J Public Health.* 1991; 81(9): 1174–1179.

61. Caplan LS, Wells BL, Haynes S. Breast cancer screening among older racial/ethnic minorities and whites: Barriers to early detection. *J Gerontol.* 1992; 47:101–110.

62. Freeman HP, Wasfie T. Cancer of the breast in poor black women. *Cancer.* 1989; 63(12):2562–2569.

63. Stein JA, Fox SA. Language preference as an indicator of mammography use among Hispanic women. *J Nat Cancer Inst.* 1990; 82(21):1715–1716.

64. Massie MJ, Holland JC. The older patient with cancer. In: Holland JC, Rowland JH, eds. *Handbook of Psychooncology: Psychological Care of the Patient with Cancer.* Oxford: Oxford University Press; 1989.

65. Rowland JH, Holland JC, Chaglassian T, Kinne D. Psychological response to breast reconstruction: Expectations for and impact on post-mastectomy functioning. *Psychosomatics.* 1993; 34:241–250.

66. Antonovsky A, Hartman H. Delay in the detection of cancer: A review of the literature. *Health Educ Monog.* 1974; 2(2):98–127.

67. Weissman J, Epstein AM. Case mix and resource utilization by uninsured hospital patients in the Boston metropolitan area. *J Am Med Assoc.* 1989; 261(24):3572–3576.

68. Blake JH. Doctor can't do me no good: Social concomitants of health care attitudes among elderly blacks in isolated rural populations. In: Watson WH ed. *Black Folk Medicine: The Therapeutic Significance of Faith and Trust.* New Brunswick, NJ: Transaction Books; 1984.

69. Stein JA, Fox SA, Murata PJ. The influence of ethnicity, socioeconomic status, and psychological barriers on use of mammography. *J Health Soc Behav.* 1991; 32:101–113.

70. Ellmer R, Olbrisch ME. The contribution of a cultural perspective in understanding and evaluating client satisfaction. *Eval Program Plann.* 1983; 6:275–281.

71. Bloom JR, Hayes WA, Saunders, F, Flatt S. Cancer awareness and secondary prevention practices in Black Americans: Implications for intervention. *Fam Commun Health.* 1987; 10:19–30.

72. Perez-Stable E, Sabogal F, Otero-Sabogal R, et al. Misconceptions about cancer among Latinos and Anglos. *J Am Med Assoc.* 1992; 268(22):3219–3223.

73. Wiley C, Sillman RA. The impact of disease on the social support experiences of cancer patients. *Psychosoc Oncol.* 1990; 8(1):79–96.

74. Powell IJ. Early detection issues of prostate cancer in African American men. *In Vivo.* 1994; 8(3):451–452.

75. Braithwaite R, Lythcott N. Community empowerment as a strategy for health promotion for Black and other minority populations. *J Am Med Assoc.* 1989; 261:282–283.

76. Orlandi MA. The challenge of evaluating community-based prevention programs: A cross cultural perspective. In: Orlandi, MA, Weston RE, Epstein LG, eds. *Cultural Competence for Evaluators: A Guide for Alcohol and Other Drug Abuse Prevention Practitioners Working With Ethnic/Racial Communities.* U.S. Department of Health and Human Services, Public Health Service, Office for Substance Abuse Prevention; DHHS Publication No. (ADM)92-1884; 1992.

77. Weston RE, Ray K, Landers C, et al. Mobilization and Educational Strategies in a Model Community Cholesterol Education Program. *Health Values,* 1992; 16(4):8–21.

78. Damond ME, Breuer NL, Pharr AE. The evaluation of setting and a culturally specific HIV/AIDS curriculum: HIV/AIDS knowledge and behavioral intent of African American adolescents. *J Black Psychol.* 1993; 19(2): 168–189.

79. Resnicow K, Futterman R, Weston RE, et al. Smoking prevalence in Harlem, New York. *Am J Health Promotion,* 1996; 10(5):343–346.

80. Marin Van Oss B, Perez-Stable EJ, Marin G, Hauck WW. Effects of a community intervention to change smoking behavior among Hispanics. *Am J Prev Med.* 1994; 10(6):340–347.

81. Robinson RG. Evaluation of a Tobacco Education Video Developed for African Americans. Personal communication, 1992.

82. Cross WE. *Shades of Black: Diversity in African-American Identity.* Philadelphia: Temple University Press; 1991.

83. Landrine H, Klonoff EA. *African American Acculturation: Deconstructing Race and Reviving Culture.* Los Angeles: Sage; 1996.

84. Aansell D, Lacey L, Whitman S, et al. A nurse-delivered intervention to reduce barriers to breast cancer and cervical cancer screening in Chicago inner city clinics. *Public Health Rep.* 1994; 109(1):104–111.

85. Forte DA. Community-based breast cancer intervention program for older African American women in beauty salons. *Public Health Rep.* 1995; 110(2):179–183.

86. Renne Ker M, Lim N, Wheatley B, et al. An inner city cancer prevention clinic in West Oakland, California. *Cancer Pract.* 2(6):427–437.

87. Sartor O. Early detection of prostate cancer in African American men with an increased familial risk of disease. *J La State Med Soc.* 1996; 148(4):179–185.

74

The Patient from a Different Culture

MARIA DIE-TRILL

Culture refers to learned patterns of behaviors, beliefs and values shared by individuals in a particular social group. It provides human beings with both their identity and a framework for understanding experience (1,2).

Cultural factors and their influence on behavior acquire special importance in the medical setting. Cultural groups define their own ideas about health, illness and health care practices in such ways that patients bring with them preconceived ideas and expectations about their physical condition and the ways to treat. Complex cross-cultural issues are usually not manifested overtly by patients or their families. However, there is evidence that culture shapes responses to pain (3); identification and selection of medical care (4); value attached to specific body parts (1); compliance with prescribed treatments (5); support networks utilized during medical illness (6), and meaning attached to physical symptoms (7,8).

Cancer is one of the most feared diseases in every culture. As in other diseases, the experience of cancer is not immune to the influence of cultural factors. Psychosocial differences determined by cultural background can make a major difference in the responses of individuals to the disease, even though medical advances can be applied with little change to culturally diverse people (9). Because cancer is a disease not well understood by many, it is likely to have different meanings attached to it, all of which are shaped by the values and beliefs of particular cultural groups. In addition, because optimal cancer treatment is often highly specialized and not always available, cancer patients frequently need to cross geographical barriers in order to receive it, facing the double challenge of undergoing cancer therapy and understanding a culturally foreign environment.

The care of cancer patients becomes increasingly complex and may result in culturally based conflicts as both patients and staff need to find ways to communicate with individuals whose worlds of symbols and beliefs are different from their own. Although value differences exist among subgroups within the same culture (e.g., across class, caste or gender), cross-cultural conflicts may be more deeply rooted between cultures, since such differences embody not just different opinions or beliefs, but different ways of daily living and different systems of meaning (10). The combination of medicine and social sciences, as well as the accurate identification and understanding of cultural factors influencing illness behavior, should facilitate the development of ways to resolve such conflicts.

This chapter is a recognition of the fact that medical care increasingly takes place in pluralistic settings where interaction with individuals from different cultures requires sensitizing oneself to cultural issues related to medicine. It describes cross-cultural issues that are relevant in the medical and psychological care of the patient with cancer including beliefs about cancer causation, communication patterns, disclosure of medical information and family roles in cancer care. Specific issues that arise with immigrant patients, patient–physician relationships, and death, dying and bereavement are discussed in a cultural context as well. Recommendations to optimize patient care are provided.

BELIEFS ABOUT CANCER CAUSATION

Explanatory models of disease describe what disease is, how it is caused, why it exists, what can be done to prevent it, control it or cure it, and why it attacks some people and not others. These models alleviate anxiety and fears that accompany otherwise inexplicable events. Culturally defined beliefs about illness causation affect responses to illness. Treatment of the "immediate cause" of a disease (e.g., pathogens) may be sought at the same time that a healer who will deal with the "ultimate cause" (e.g., bad luck) is consulted, because different medical systems are directed to different levels of cause (11).

Many cultures have supernatural explanations for disease causation (12–18) and in some instances these factors may be viewed as more significant than the natural ones in the understanding of illness. Causes of disease have also been categorized into internal or external. Emphasis on external causes of disease (e.g., germs) has been described among British and North Americans, while Germans and French are said to regard disease more frequently as a failure of internal defenses (19).

Research has specifically addressed culturally determined beliefs about cancer causation. Late stage cancer patients in the United States believed past behavior (e.g., smoking) was clearly associated with the development of the disease (20). Dodd et al. (21) surveyed 45 cancer patients in Taiwan, 60% of whom reported not knowing what had caused their disease. The remaining 40% identified long-term stress, physical discomfort, drinking and smoking, having too many children, poor hygiene, and a "bad" personality as etiologic factors. A similar study performed in Egypt revealed that over 90% of the cancer patients surveyed reported not knowing what had caused their disease (22). Psychological and genetic factors were identified as causing cancer by almost 50% of a sample of Swiss oncology patients. However, doubts were often added when discussing behaviors such as smoking as a probable etiologic factor, even in the case of lung cancer patients (23). Healthy Hispanics have been found to develop more misconceptions about causes of cancer than their Anglo-Saxon counterparts, and more frequently identified sugar substitutes, bruises from cuts, microwave ovens, eating pork or spicy foods, breast-feeding, and antibiotics as causing cancer (24).

Beliefs about cancer causation have significant clinical implications since they influence preventive behaviors and decisions about treatment. Four out of five healthy adults interviewed in Australia believed that individuals can take steps to reduce their risk of cancer including not smoking, dietary measures and solar protection (25). Similar beliefs have been found among British (26) and other European communities (27), suggesting an increased sense of control over health among members of these cultural groups. On the other hand, cultures which ascribe supernatural or internal causes to cancer will most likely believe that there is little they can do to prevent or treat it, and will be likely to adopt more passive attitudes during the course of the disease.

Beliefs about cancer causation affect the psychological adjustment to the disease as well.

CASE 1

ND, an 18-year-old Caribbean female with an osteogenic sarcoma in the left tibia, was referred for psychological services because of severe depressive symptoms which she attributed to separation from significant family members. ND, whose parents were estranged, lived with her mother, Mrs D. Her father lived with his second wife and their two young children to whom ND was very attached but had been unable to see in several months. Mrs D. did not allow ND to visit her father because she believed that ND's cancer was a result of her stepmother's voodoo practices.

Beliefs about the cause of specific cancer symptoms are equally important.

CASE 2

RS was a 48-year-old male Hispanic patient with a brain tumor. RS experienced severe nausea and vomiting throughout treatment of the tumor. However, he consistently refused anti-emetic therapy. When questioned by a Spanish speaking staff member, RS reported believing that "little pieces of the brain tumor" were eliminated through the vomiting and therefore thought it best to continue experiencing this symptom.

COMMUNICATION PATTERNS

Cultural differences in the oncology setting are usually most evident when communication barriers between patient and members of the healthcare team exist. Health care providers have been found to communicate differently with culturally different patients (28) and to develop poorer relationships with them (29).

Cultural factors influence how disease is discussed and how physical symptoms and psychological distress are reported. A tendency to express vague symptoms and generalized descriptions of one's health status, to avoid disclosure of detailed personal information during the initial encounter, and to dislike health care staff who do not take time to establish a relationship with the patient, have been described in certain Middle Eastern cultures (30). Patients' tendency to exaggerate symptoms in order to obtain optimal care has been reported among Russian immigrants (31) and may complicate history taking and symptom follow-up. Other cultural groups hold the belief that discussing negative and unpleasant events will make them happen and therefore they avoid such conversations.

Language barriers contribute to ineffective communication between patient and physician or psychotherapist in a variety of ways. They may interfere with accurate assessments of the patient's physical and mental status.

CASE 3

TW was a four year old Hispanic girl with a supratentorial glioma whose unresponsive behavior was considered to be due to a language barrier by the medical staff. Upon psychological evaluation in the patient's language, she was found to exhibit autistic symptoms including limited communication skills, impaired play, lack of speech and eye contact, and abnormal social interactions.

Language barriers also interfere with the patient's ability to organize the distressing experience that cancer imposes and with the establishment of alliances between the patient and physician or psychotherapist (32).

Using a family member or friend of the patient to translate medical information, although expedient, is not the ideal solution to overcome communication barriers. Patients may be reluctant to transmit personal or embarrassing information through these individuals, who may also find it difficult, if not impossible at times, to transmit painful information to the patient. The use of interpreters is particularly useful if they have experience in medical settings. Failure of the interpreter to translate information accurately or to communicate empathic expressions by either patient or staff must be considered (33,34).

Non-verbal patterns of communication also vary culturally. Etiquette, modesty, touching, and spatial distance when talking convey significant non-verbal messages about relationships and traditions. Hand-shaking and smiling have been described as essential ingredients of productive medical interactions with Hispanic and Black patients but signs of frivolity and immaturity in certain Russian émigrés (11).

DISCLOSURE OF MEDICAL INFORMATION

Truth-telling practices in the cancer setting vary enormously among cultures. In many cultural groups open discussions of cancer diagnoses and prognoses are thought to be inhumane and cruel and are avoided at all costs. In other cultural groups concealing medical information is considered illegal and unethical. Patients' rights movements and the need to provide informed consent to undergo medical procedures or treatment have both contributed to disclosure of relevant medical information to patients. In yet other situations, both patient and family will receive diagnostic information, but only family members will learn about the patient's prognosis, especially if poor.

Disclosure of medical information in oncology varies widely not only across cultural groups but historically as well (35). The development in recent years of specialized cancer centers and the rapid propagation of cancer-related information through the media make it harder to conceal information from patients. In addition, the burden of revealing medically relevant information to cancer patients is currently reduced, given that new therapeutic developments make it easier to transmit hope to patients. Studies performed in the United States 40 years ago reveal that despite cancer patients' stated preferences for being informed of their disease (36,37), only 10% to 35% of physicians disclosed the diagnosis of cancer to their patients (38,39). Personalities, feelings and physician attitudes played a major role on the manner in which they communicated with and treated patients, and feared reactions to telling (e.g., patient suicide) could rarely be substantiated. Even though such practices and their rationale are no longer in vogue in Northern European countries or the United States (40,41), they are still described in Southern Europe (42,43), Japan (44), India (45), Africa and Latin America (40), although significant trends in all countries towards increasingly providing patients with diagnostic information are consistently reported (40,41). Patient's information preferences also seem to vary cross-culturally. Significantly more healthy Hispanics have been found to prefer not knowing if they have incurable cancer when compared to a matched sample of Anglo-Saxons (24).

One of the largest cross-cultural studies on truth-telling practices is currently being performed by the International Psycho-Oncology Society through its National Representation Committee. Over 500 physicians practicing oncology in 28 different countries have been surveyed on the type of information they disclose to cancer patients and their families. Preliminary results corroborate an increased variability in disclosure of medical information and a significant trend towards truth-telling worldwide.

Truth-telling practices have important clinical implications. In the first place, physicians must be responsive to the expectations of patients and their families as to what may be revealed in a particular culture. However, both patient and physician are determined by their own cultural norms and what may be considered necessary for one, may not be so for the other. Second, conflicts may arise when diagnostic and prognostic information is not shared between family members.

CASE 4

GL was a 14-year-old Middle Eastern female with an abdominal tumor who traveled to the United States with her father in order to receive chemotherapy, which was initially expected to be of short duration. The diagnosis of her malignancy had been confirmed in their home country, after she had undergone initial surgery. However, it had been kept from GL's mother. It was Mrs L's understanding that GL would receive brief post-surgical rehabilitation. The patient developed numerous unexpected treatment-related complications which required prolonged hospitalizations and caused significant delays in therapy administration. In addition to the emotional pain caused by the treatment and separation from loved ones, father and daughter had to deal with the burden of lying to Mrs L during their frequent telephone conversations in order to account for the delay in returning home.

Third, the important bond between patient and physician is determined by the way the information is transmitted and the meaning that is conveyed, rather than by what is being transmitted (41).

In addition, it may be necessary to reveal diagnostic information for the purpose of secondary prevention, as in the case of children of cancer patients. Disclosure of certain types of medical information to patients is becoming increasingly complicated as advances in biotechnology have made it possible to identify carriers of genetic abnormalities that predispose individuals to developing tumors. Anxiety and depression may result when individuals learn that they are carriers of such genetic abnormalities. On the other hand, not revealing this type of information may keep them from engaging in the preventive measures necessary for early detection and treatment. In countries such as the United States, identifying carriers of genetic abnormalities in the cancer setting has complex implications. An individual may encounter difficulties obtaining medical coverage if insurance companies learn about the individual's condition, and may have to confront emotional difficulties that are likely to arise in the work, family and social settings if the information is shared. The need for genetic counseling to take place within a cultural context has been discussed (46) and reported in a Navajo population (47).

FAMILY ROLES IN CANCER CARE

Understanding how a patient defines a family acquires significant relevance when working with culturally diverse populations, because the nature and extent of family relationships influence the interpretation of physical malaise, its treatment, and the use of coping strategies throughout an illness episode (1). Culture provides unwritten definitions of what constitutes a family and how families respond to illness. In Anglo-Saxon cultures, a family consists primarily of parents and their children (48). Members of these families value autonomy and individual responsibility and set distinct boundaries between themselves and others. They tend to assume full responsibility over their

needs, and lack of control over their bodies, actions, and emotions may be guilt-provoking (49). When diagnosed with cancer, they do not necessarily share the burden of medical decision-making with other family members. These individuals' perceived control over their disease results in part from their active participation in their medical care. Autonomy and independence may be anxiety-provoking when important treatment decisions must be made with limited family involvement.

On the other hand, Hispanics and Middle Easterners define families as extended networks of uncles, aunts, cousins, and grandparents. For Blacks, families usually consist of wide networks of kin and community (48, 50). Certain Asian groups include ancestors and all their descendants as family members. These families are usually characterized by intense emotional connections and constant affective exchanges between their members (51,52). Dependency rather than autonomy, is a valued trait. Loyalty to family members has been described as more important than individual rights and needs. Losing one's sense of self by immersion in social and family obligations is a potential problem that these individuals encounter (53). When an individual is diagnosed with cancer, all family members are expected to participate in different levels of patient care and medical decision-making. Such familial involvement provides the oncology patient with a useful support system but may at times interfere with the patient's wishes regarding cancer therapy as well as with a sense of control over the disease and its treatment. Extended family involvement during illness has been described in Hispanics (54,55); Koreans (56); Vietnamese (9); Japanese (57,58); Chinese (59); and Middle Eastern cultures (30,60).

Culture addresses how different family members' advice is valued during illness (61). In most cultural groups, leadership roles are assumed by elder family members. The oldest male is thought to be more capable of coping with bad news in some Middle Eastern and Asian cultures (30). Communication and treatment planning may be more effective when key members of the family are included in the process (62).

Sources of support within the family vary culturally as well. Mexican mothers have been found to rely on one another rather than on their husbands for support in dealing with childhood cancer (9). Middle Easterners and Hispanics rely on members of their extended family, all of whom are expected constantly to exhibit attention and care towards the patient (30,50).

Cultural norms also describe children's role during illness by addressing when a child is considered mature enough to learn about a cancer diagnosis and participate in medical care. Cultures that focus on achieving autonomy and independence encourage children to actively participate in their medical care (62). The pediatric bill of rights developed by the Association for the Care of Children's Health in the United States (63) refers to the possibility of children describing how they want to take part in their treatment and to make treatment-related choices whenever possible. Other pediatric cancer patients come from cultural backgrounds that predispose them to comply with the recommendations agreed upon by their physicians and parents without questioning them. Direct communication about illness with these children is usually seen as inappropriate.

IMMIGRATION

Migration is a disruptive event and readjustment to a new culture is by no means a single event but a prolonged developmental process of adjustment that will affect family members differently. Depending on the conditions in which migration takes place, it may be experienced as a more or less isolating and disorganizing process. Best adjustment is achieved when individuals keep in touch with their own culture as they integrate in the new culture. However, this is not always the case. While some immigrants bury their past entirely, others tend to block off the new culture (64).

The diagnosis of cancer in an immigrant may trigger a variety of responses related to specific cultural issues. While in some cases it will inspire them to reconnect with their culture and traditions, in others disability may prevent them from doing so.

CASE 5
AD was a 49-year-old male who had immigrated from Eastern Europe nearly 20 years before the diagnosis of his Hodgkin's disease had been confirmed. He had always remained in contact with his family of origin and had always expressed a wish to die at home. AD's shame over his deteriorated physical appearance and inability to function, as well as his fears of not being recognized by family members, interfered with his wishes to return to his native country before dying.

For others, losses caused by the disease may trigger intense feelings about those related to the migration, given that immigrants experience losses ranging from mild to most profound. Other individuals may seek support from patients with similar cultural backgrounds. Psychotherapeutic groups in Spanish with female Hispanic cancer patients at the Memorial Sloan-Kettering Cancer Center in New York were highly successful in providing support and coping strategies in ways that were culturally acceptable.

"Temporary immigrants," those who travel to another country in search of optimal medical care, are confronted with different issues. Their sometimes unrealistic expectations of cure may interfere with medical decision-making and may delay termination of treatment to which the disease is not responding. Feelings of guilt and shame that arise if the expected therapeutic response has not been obtained may be exacerbated by the elevated financial and emotional investment that traveling in search of treatment has required.

Attempts to understand a new medical system may become a burden for some immigrant patients. Adjusting to the team approach characteristic of some Western health care systems may be confusing to families that are mostly familiar with medical systems that operate through patient–physician dyads.

Differences in the degree of acculturation between young cancer patients and their more traditional parents during the course of an illness may intensify intergenerational conflicts. This may be exacerbated by the fact that the meaning of cultural traditions increases as we age.

PAIN

Even though there appear to be no ethnic differences in the ability to discriminate painful stimuli (65), culture is widely acknowledged as contributing to variations in pain responses (66,67). Culture teaches us how to express pain behaviorally and how to interpret it at an unconscious, symbolic level (68). Italians have been found to exhibit a greater dramatization about their pain than Irish, who tend to handle it by denial (7). Hindu's quiet acceptance of pain (45) may prevent accurate pain assessments and efficient management.

Strategies to cope with pain also vary interculturally. Anglo-Americans are said to prefer internally applied therapies such as oral medication and injections, while Orientals tend to use external agents for pain control (e.g., salves, massages and oils). Some prefer sedation and others tend to avoid it (69,70). There is also evidence attesting to differences in drug response and disposition among certain ethnic groups (71). Hawaiians and Caucasians were found to require significantly more post-operative analgesics than Filipinos, Japanese or Chinese who underwent similar surgical procedures (72).

The need for awareness of culturally shaped reactions to pain stems from the fact that individuals tend to regard their own responses to pain as normal and those differing from their own as wrong, improper or abnormal.

PATIENT–PHYSICIAN RELATIONSHIPS

Culturally patterned medical roles influence physician–patient relationships by establishing guidelines for what is considered appropriate clinical responsibility and communication (11). Adequate patient–physician interactions are important in the cancer setting because they may enhance treatment compliance, a most important ingredient of successful cancer therapy. Because health professionals generally have greater authority and power than patients, and patients are frequently confused and distressed by their illness, the risk of patients unjustly being coerced is heightened when staff members represent the dominant culture and the patient is from a minority group (73).

Different models of patient–physician relationships are appropriate not only under particular clinical circumstances (74), but also within specific cultural groups. The basic form of patient–physician relationship in the United States is egalitarian and consensual rather than obligatory, based on a contractual agreement between patient and physician; one in which patient participation is crucial and heavily influenced by the ideological emphasis on individualism and autonomy as well as by consumerism (75). The central role of the physician in this model is to offer expertise, maintain updated knowledge and skills, and use consultation referrals appropriately. Patients are expected to be responsible for their own welfare as well as to protect their own rights and be compliant. In contrast, physician–patient relationships in other cultural groups are hierarchical, characterized by interconnectedness and interdependence, with full expectation of reciprocity and highly empathic sensitivity to one another's feelings and needs without explicitly expressing them. Patients from these cultures may tend to seek informal relationships with their physicians rather than strictly professional ones (76). Successfully treating Hispanics requires a personal and open approach. Hispanic patients are generally inclined to relate to and trust persons rather than institutions and dislike formal impersonal structures and organizations (54). The authority of a physician is never questioned in certain cultural groups (e.g., Russians, Vietnamese and Middle Easterners) and patients are not likely to ask or provide information that would contradict or be considered disrespectful (9,30). In other cultures, physician expectations of patient involvement in medical care indicate to the patient that the physician does not know what he is doing. In other instances, a physi-

cian's youth is suspect: age, wisdom and experience go together and are valued more or as much as knowledge and skills (31).

A cultural "blind spot" syndrome addresses the perception that similarities in background between patient and physician will maximize communication leading to an improved compliance (59). On the other hand, cultural differences may be used by healthcare staff as mechanisms to distance themselves from patients and to avoid, in this way, identifying and engaging emotionally with them.

The most powerful force that has been described in the doctor-patient relationship is the patient's perception of the doctor's degree of concern (77), a concept that may be applied cross-culturally.

DEATH, DYING, AND BEREAVEMENT

Culture shapes the experience of loss and the rituals around it. Among the culturally determined attitudes towards death and dying that have been identified are those that are death accepting and those that are death-denying (32,78). Death-accepting cultures view death as part of the life cycle. Death here gives a meaningful coherence to an individual's life. Death-denying cultures tend to view death as an intrusion into a scientific quest for eternal existence, given that medical technology is generally devoted to the preservation of life. This attitude is reflected in the United Stated in the hiding of morgues in hospitals and in the existence of funeral homes that are ultimately in charge of making the dead person's body look alive.

Fears of death occur in every culture (79). However, how these fears are dealt with varies from one culture to another. In some Asian cultures children are taught at very early ages to avoid the use of words that are remotely associated with the "misfortune" of death in order to avoid attracting it (80). Western expressions such as "Passing away" or "Going to meet one's Maker" reflect similar death-avoidant attitudes. Beliefs in a life after death also aid in avoiding confrontation with the fears and anxieties that a permanent loss may elicit.

Profound cultural variations exist in mourning rituals. Chinese burn firecrackers in order to scare the evil spirits of death away, as well as make paper money, paper clothes, paper cars and paper houses so that the dead can use them once the smoke has reached the heavens. Failure to produce a proper funeral for one's deceased parent may be considered a great source of shame, with funeral ceremonies becoming at times so extravagant that they impose a severe financial burden on the survivors (51). In the Jewish culture, burial within 24 hours of the death, a week of "sitting Shiva" during which family members mourn and friends and family visit, certain prayers which are said for a year, and the celebration of a memorial service all aid in the mourning process (48). Among Hispanics death is a family event and, more than in other cultures, individuals openly express their desire to spend their last days with their loved ones. Women are usually designated the primary mourners and, as in Mediterranean cultures, wear black clothing for extended periods of time after the death has taken place. White middle-class people tend to hold a modernist approach to life, emphasizing goal directedness, efficiency and rationality, all of which suggest that people need to recover from loss, emotionally detach from the deceased, and return to normal functioning as quickly and efficiently as possible (81).

Emotional expressions of grief vary culturally as well. While in some groups displays of intense emotions may be expected around death, stoic reactions to it or the development of somatic symptoms may be more appropriate among members of other groups (82).

Awareness of death beliefs and rituals is important in the cancer setting because of cancer patients' frequent confrontation with the possibility of dying. Lack of acknowledgment and respect for such traditions will interfere with our ability to aid the dying and the bereaved, and prevent a mourning process with resolution.

IMPROVING PATIENT CARE

The care of culturally diverse cancer populations does not require members of the health care team to become familiar with every cultural issue related to medicine, but rather to be increasingly sensitive to the role that different cultural beliefs and traditions play in the health care setting. Patient and health care staff share the responsibility for achieving a mutually satisfying interaction by recognizing and resolving obstacles that may result from cultural diversity. Denial of cultural and ethnic differences does not foster positive interactions with the patient. Acknowledgment of such differences may facilitate open and honest discussions about them, in addition to enhancing an understanding of the patient's needs.

Cultural stereotyping must be avoided at all times. Patients should be treated as members of a particular culture only after they are approached as individuals. Patient behaviors that do not conform to the health professional's cultural norms or recommendations are usually attributed to differences in cultural background. This is rarely the case when culturally different patients are well adjusted and compliant with prescribed therapies.

Health care professionals must be aware of how their own cultural background influences their behaviors and decisions in the medical setting. Effort should be made to recognize the manifestations of transference and countertransference that may be affected by race, ethnicity, and culture (83).

Detailed cultural assessments should ideally take place in the patient's language and include ethnic affiliation, an understanding of why the patient seeks medical care, what the patient believes has caused the illness, and what the most concerning symptoms are to him or her. Family involvement in patient care and religious beliefs and practices should be well understood. Patient expectations regarding treatment outcome are equally important. The use of non-conventional treatments should be investigated, given that they tend to be underreported out of shame and fear of physician disapproval (56,61). Judgmental approaches to non-conventional forms of treatment will inhibit the patient from openly discussing them with the staff.

Effective medical and psychological intervention with cancer patients may be aided by consultation with and inclusion of native healers relevant to the patient's cultural group and will facilitate compliance with treatments. Including key family members in patient care will enhance patient adjustment as well.

Attempts should be made to facilitate communication and exchange of important medical information between patient and health professionals in cases where linguistic barriers exist. Concerns about having reported their symptoms accurately or having understood medical prescriptions are usually expressed by patients. Cards containing commonly used hospital words in the patient's language may be kept at the bedside. Interpreters from the appropriate Embassy or Consulate should be contacted if not available at the health care facility.

SUMMARY

Culture influences health care practices in ways that operate outside our awareness. It shapes responses to disease, treatment planning and compliance with medical care. As in other diseases, the experience of cancer does not escape the influence of cultural factors. Beliefs about the causes of cancer and its symptoms may affect the types of treatment sought. Differences in communication patterns may interfere with the establishment of an alliance between patient and health care staff. Language barriers only add to the already chaotic experience of cancer, interfering with adequate patient evaluations. In the disclosure of medical information, health care staff needs to be sensitive to the type of information that may be revealed in a particular society and attempt to adjust to it as much as their own cultural norms permit. Attention should be paid to how information is transmitted to the patient, rather than how much is provided. Families play an important role in the disease process. The degree of involvement of family members in patient care and medical decision-making is, in great part, a function of cultural artifacts.

As a result of a cancer diagnosis, immigrant patients may experience identity conflicts which may interfere with adaptive responses to the disease. The identification of culturally shaped pain behaviors is required in order to assess pain accurately and to manage it effectively. Attitudes towards death and bereavement vary profoundly and definitions of normalcy in assessing a family's response to death should be made carefully.

Recognition and sensitivity to cultural diversity is increasing in the medical setting and will lead to new, improved conceptual models of clinical intervention.

REFERENCES

1. Marshall P. Cultural influences on perceived quality of life. *Semin Oncol Nurs.* 1990; 6(4):278–284.
2. Olweny C. The ethics and conduct of cross-cultural research in developing countries. *Psycho-Oncology.* 1994; 3:11–20.
3. Zborowski M. *People in Pain.* San Francisco: Jossey-Bass; 1969.
4. Chrisman NJ. The health-seeking process: An approach to the natural history of illness. *Cult Med Psychiatry.* 1977; 1:351–377.
5. Wood PR, Zeltzer LK, Cox AD. Communicating with adolescents from culturally varied backgrounds: A model based on Mexican-American adolescents in South Texas. *Semin Adolesc Med.* 1987; 3:99–108.
6. Sarell M, Baider L. The effects of cultural background on communication patterns of Israeli cancer patients. *Psychopathology.* 1984; 17:17–23.
7. Zola IK. Culture and symptoms: An analysis of patients presenting complaints. *Am Soc Rev.* 1966; 31:615–630.
8. Kleinman A, Eisenberg L, Good B. Culture, illness and care. Clinical lessons from anthropologic and cross-cultural research. *Ann Intern Med.* 1978; 88:251–258.
9. Spinetta J. Measurement of family function, communication and cultural effects. *Cancer.* 1984; 53:2330–2337.
10. Ware NC, Kleinman AR. Culture and somatic experience: The social course of illness in neurasthenia and chronic fatigue syndrome. *Psychosom Med.* 1992; 54:546–560.
11. Clark MM. Cultural context of medical practice. *West J Med.* 1983; 139:806–810.
12. Gould-Martin K, Ngin C. Chinese-Americans. In: Harwood R, ed. *Ethnicity and Medical Care.* Cambridge, MA: Harvard University Press; 1981: 130–171.
13. Namboze JM. Health and culture in an African society. *Soc Sci Med.* 1983; 17(24):2041–2043.
14. Mitchell MF. Popular medical concepts in Jamaica and their impact on drug use. *West J Med.* 1983; 139:841–847.
15. Castro FG, Furth P, Karlow H. The health beliefs of Mexican, Mexican-American and Anglo-American women. *Hispan J Behav Sci.* 1985; 6(4):365–383.
16. Kunitz SJ. *Disease Change and the Role of Medicine: The Navajo Experience.* Berkeley, CA: University of California Press; 1983.
17. Bailey E, Urban S. *African-American Health Care.* Lanham, MD: University Press, 1991.
18. Klonoff EA, Landrine H. Culture and gender diversity in commonsense beliefs about the causes of six illnesses. *J Behav Med.* 1994; 17(4):407–418.
19. Payer L. How medical practice reflects national culture. *The Sciences* 1990; Jul–Aug:38–42.
20. Linn MW, Linn BS, Stein SR. Beliefs about causes of cancer in cancer patients. *Soc Sci Med.* 1982; 16:835–839.
21. Dodd MJ, Chen SG, Pipe B, Lindsey AM. Attitudes about cancer and its treatment of cancer patients living in Taiwan. *Cancer Nurs.* 1985; 8(4):214–220.
22. Dodd MJ, Ahmed N, Piper B, Lindsey AM. Attitudes of patients living in Egypt about cancer and its treatment. *Cancer Nurs.* 1985; 8(5):278–284.
23. Kesserling A, Dodd MJ, Lindsey AM, Strauss AL. Attitudes of patients living in Switzerland about cancer and its treatment. *Cancer Nurs.* 1986; 9(2):77–85.
24. Perez-Stable EJ, Sabogal F, Otero-Sabogl R, et al. Misconceptions about cancer among Latinos and Anglos. *J Am Med Assoc.* 1992; 268(22):3219–3223.
25. Hill D, White V, Borland R, Cockburn J. Cancer-related beliefs and behaviors in Australia. *Aust J Public Health.* 1991; 15(1):14–23.
26. Cancer Relief MacMillan Fund. *Public Attitudes to and Knowledge of Cancer in the UK.* London: Cancer Relief MacMillan Fund, 1988.
27. Commission of European Communities. *Survey: Europeans and the Prevention of Cancer.* Brussels: Commission of the European Communities; 1987.
28. Jones DC, van Amelsvoort-Jones GM. Communication patterns between nursing staff and the ethnic elderly in a long-term care facility. *J Adv Nurs.* 1986; 11:265-272.
29. Levy DR. White doctors and black patients: Influence of race on the doctor–patient relationship. *Pediatrics.* 1985; 75:639–643.
30. Lipson JG, Meleis AI. Issues in health care of Middle Eastern patients. *West J Med.* 1983; 139:854–861.
31. Wheat ME, Brownstein H, Kvitash V. Aspects of medical care of Soviet Jewish émigrés. *West J Med.* 1983; 139:900–904.
32. Die Trill M, Holland J. Cross-cultural differences in the care of patients with cancer. A review. *Gen Hosp Psychiatry.* 1993; 15:21–30.
33. Thompson WL, Thompson TL, House RM. Taking care of culturally different and non-English speaking patients. *Int J Psychiatry Med.* 1990; 20(3):235–245.

34. Vazquez C, Javier RA. The problem with interpreters: Communicating with Spanish-speaking patients. *Hosp Commun Psychiatry*. 1991; 42(2):163–165.

35. Weil M, Smith M, Khayat D. Truth-telling to cancer patients in the Western European context. *Psycho-Oncology*. 1994; 3:21–26.

36. Branch CH. Psychiatric aspects of malignant disease. *Ca Bull Ca Prog*. 1956; 6:102–104.

37. Samp RJ, Curreri AR. Questionnaire survey on public cancer education obtained from cancer patients and their families. *Cancer*. 1957; 10:382–384.

38. Fitts WT, Ravdin IS. What Philadelphia physicians tell patients with cancer. *J Am Med Assoc*. 1953; 153:901–904.

39. Oken D. What to tell cancer patients. *J Am Med Assoc*. 1961; 175:1120–1128.

40. Holland JC, Geary N, Marchini A, Tross S. An international survey of physician attitudes and practice in regard to revealing the diagnosis of cancer. *Cancer Invest*. 1987; 5(2):151–154.

41. Thomsen OO, Wulf HR, Martin A, Singe PA. What do gastroenterologists in Europe tell cancer patients? The *Lancet*. 1993; 341:473–476.

42. Mosconi P, Meyerowitz B, Liberati MC, Liberati A. Disclosure of breast cancer diagnosis: Patient and physician reports. *Ann Oncol*. 1991; 2:273–280.

43. Surbone A. Truth-telling to the patient. *J Am Med Assoc*. 1992; 268(13):1661–1662.

44. Long SO, Long BD. Curable cancers and fatal ulcers. Attitudes towards cancer in Japan. *Soc Sci Med*. 1982; 16:2101–2108.

45. Francis MR. Concerns of terminally ill adult Hindu cancer patients. *Cancer Nurs*. 1986; 9(4):164–171.

46. Weil J, Mittman I. A teaching framework for cross-cultural genetic counseling. *J Genet Couns*. 1993; 2(3):159–169.

47. Lynch HT, Drouhard T, Vasen HFA, et al. Genetic counseling in a Navajo hereditary nonpolyposis colorectal cancer kindred. *Cancer*. 1996; 77:30–35.

48. McGoldrick M, Hines P, Lee E, Preto NG. Mourning rituals. How culture shapes the experience of loss. *Network*. 1986; Nov–Dec.:29–36.

49. Varma VK. Cultural psychodynamics in health and illness. *Indian J Psychiatry*. 1986; 28(1):13–34.

50. Meleis AI. The Arab American in the health care system. *Am J Nurs*. 1981; 81:1180–1183.

51. Chen CL. Bereavement in Chinese-Americans. In: Chen CL, Lowe WC, Ryan D, Kutscher AH, Halporn R, Wang HH, eds. *Chinese-Americans in Loss and Separation. Social, Medical and Psychiatric Perspectives*. New York: Foundation of Thanatology, 1992:57–76.

52. Roland A. *In Search of Self in India and Japan*. New Jersey: Princeton University Press, 1988.

53. Doi T. *The Anatomy of Dependence*. Tokyo: Kodashna International; 1973.

54. Maduro R. Curanderismo and Latino views of disease and curing. *West J Med*. 1983; 139:868–874.

55. Arruda EN, Larson PJ, Meleis AI. Comfort: Immigrant Hispanic cancer patients' views. *Cancer Nurs*. 1992; 15(6):387–394.

56. Sawyers JE, Eaton L. Gastric cancer in the Korean-American: Cultural implications. *Oncol Nursi Forum*. 1992; 19(4):619–623.

57. Kobayashi JS. Depathologizing dependency: Two perspectives. *Psychiatr Ann*. 1989; 19:653–658.

58. Lock M. *East Asian Medicine in Urban Japan: Varieties of Medical Experience*. Berkeley: University of California Press; 1980.

59. Lin EH. Intraethnic characteristics and the patient-physician interaction: "Cultural blind spot syndrome". *J Fam Prac*. 1983; 16:91–98.

60. Racy J. Death in an Arab culture. *Ann NY Acad Sci*. 1969; 164:8717–8880.

61. Olness K. Cultural issues in primary pediatric care. In: Hoekelman RA, Friedman SB, Nelson NM, Siedel HM, eds. *Primary Pediatric Care*. St. Louis, Mosby Year Book, 1992:138–145.

62. De Trill M, Kovalcik R. The child with cancer: Influence of culture on truth-telling and patient care. *Ann NY Acad Sci*. 1997; 809:197–210.

63. Association for the Care of Children's Health. *A Pediatric Bill of Rights*. Bethesda, MD: Association for the Care of Children's Health; 1991.

64. McGoldrick M. Ethnicity and the family life cycle. In: McGoldrick M, Pierce JK, Giordano J, eds. *Ethnicity and Family Therapy*. New York: Guilford Press, 1982: 69–90.

65. Wolff B. Behavioral measurement of human pain. In: Sternbach R, ed. *The Psychology of Pain*. New York: Raven Press, 1986:121–152.

66. Wolfe B, Langley S. Cultural factors and the response to pain: A review. *Am Anthropol*. 1968; 70:494–501.

67. Weisenberg M. Pain and pain control. *Psychol Bull*. 1977; 84:1008–1144.

68. Zatzick DF, Dimsdale JE. Cultural variations in response to painful stimuli. *Pychosom Med*. 1990; 52:544–557.

69. Moore R. Ethnographic assessment of pain coping perceptions. *Psychosom Med*. 1990; 52:171–181.

70. Swerdlow M, Stjernsward J. Cancer pain relief—An urgent problem. *World Health Forum*. 1982; 3:325–330.

71. Mendoza R, Smith MW, Poland RE, et al. Ethnic psychopharmacology: the Hispanic and native American perspective. *Psychopharm Bull*. 1991; 27:449–461.

72. Streltzer J, Wade JC. The influence of cultural group on the undertreatment of postoperative pain. *Psychosom Med*. 1981; 43:393–403.

73. Jecker NS, Carrese JA, Pearlman RA. Caring for patients in cross-cultural settings. *Hastings Cent Rep*. 1995; Jan–Feb:6–14.

74. Emanuel EJ, Emanuel L. Four models of the physician-patient relationship. *J Am Med Assoc*. 1992; 267(16):2221–2226.

75. Brody DS. The patient's role in clinical decision-making. *Ann Inter Med*. 1980; 93:718–722.

76. Nilchaikovit T, Hill J, Holland JC. The effects of culture on illness behavior and medical care. *Gen Hosp Psychiatry*. 1993; 15:1–50.

77. Platt F. "I just don't want to know". *Patient Care*. 1992; 26:164.

78. Pattison EM. The experience of dying. *Am J Psychother*. 1967; 21:32–43.

79. Kubler-Ross E. *Death: The Final Stage of Growth*. Englewood Cliffs, NJ: Prentice Hall; 1975

80. Huang WWC. Attitudes towards death: Chinese perspectives from the past. In: Chen CL, Lowe WC, Ryan D, et al., eds. *Chinese-Americans in Loss and Separation*.

Social, Medical and Psychiatric Perspectives. New York: Foundation of Thanatology; 1992:1–5.

81. Stroebe M, Gergen MM, Gergen KJ, Stroebe W. Broken hearts or broken bonds. Love and death in historical perspective. *Am Psychol.* 1992; 47(10): 1205–1212.

82. Kleinman A, Good B. *Culture and Depression. Studies in the Anthropology and Cross-cultural Psychiatry of Affect and Disorder.* Berkeley: University of California Press; 1984.

83. Varghese FT. The racially different psychiatrist— Implications for psychotherapy. *Aust NZ J Psychiatry.* 1983; 17:329–333.

75

Psychosocial Sequelae of Perceived Environmental Exposures

KAROLYNN SIEGEL

In recent years, the public has grown increasingly concerned about potential environmental hazards such as toxic chemicals, ionizing radiation, and electromagnetic fields (1). Typically these concerns center on fears about the health risks posed by exposure to these substances, especially the fear of developing cancer (2). The myriad laws and regulations that the federal and state governments have enacted in an effort to reduce the public's exposure to potential environmental carcinogens reflect the unique threat attached to cancer by the public.

Individuals who believe they have suffered a dangerous environmental exposure confront the difficult adaptational challenges of living with the open-ended threat that they may experience future significant health consequences due to their exposure, and of managing (i.e., reducing, tolerating) their own sense of helplessness to affect the consequences (3). Moreover, these individuals experience significant ambiguity about issues that usually cannot be resolved, i.e., the dose of radiation they experience, what constitutes a dangerous level of exposure, the latency of radiation-related illness, the probability of future health problems (3). According to Lazarus (4), when an individual has situational grounds for feeling threatened, "ambiguity concerning the significance of a stimulus situation will usually intensify the threat because it limits the individual's sense of control or increases his sense of helplessness over the danger" (p. 117). When a threat is poorly defined it is difficult to appraise and choose an appropriate coping response (3–9). Thus, to the extent that ambiguity remains unresolved, the potential for successful coping will be limited (8).

This chapter identifies the sources of psychosocial distress associated with a perceived exposure to a health threatening environmental hazard and common strategies for coping with the stress of such exposures. Three case examples of such exposures are reviewed—Three Mile Island (TMI), Chernobyl, and Love Canal. Finally, suggestions for future research on the psychosocial sequelae of perceived environmental exposures are offered.

SOURCES OF PSYCHOSOCIAL DISTRESS

The concern of individuals that they may have suffered an exposure to an environmental hazard often follows notification of a technological disaster or industrial accident, or an awareness that a cluster of cancers has occurred in a discrete geographic area. In many such instances, it is unclear whether a real exposure has occurred or not. Even when exposure is certain, it frequently remains ambiguous whether the level of exposure experienced was a potentially harmful one. Yet from a psychosocial perspective, these distinctions are often unimportant in terms of the psychological distress that results. A growing body of literature suggests that, as a class, technological disasters are inherently more stressful than natural disasters and tend to have more enduring psychosocial sequelae (10–13) and, further, that within the category of human-made technological disasters, those involving environmental/biospheric contamination by an invisible potentially hazardous substance share features that pose particularly difficult adaptational challenges for their victims and complicate the psychological mastery of the event (3).

Chronic Stress

Vyner (3) has argued that "adaptation to a palpable threat presents a person or persons with a considerably different set of problems than does adaptation to an uncertain and impalpable threat" (p. 75). Individuals exposed to potentially hazardous levels of radiation or toxins often live for many years with the perpetual fear of future illness since the health problems associated with exposure may require a long period (i.e., 10–20 years) to develop. Thus their exposure poses a persistent threat that may become a chronic stressor (14–17). The inability to perceive the noxious agent only heightens the ambiguity of the situation and complicates resolution of the "invisible trauma" because the stressor is not an event that can be processed by the senses (3,18).

As a result of the open-ended threat characteristic of this class of disasters, there is no identifiable "low point" after which victims may assume the "worst is over" and recovery, restoration and normalization can proceed (10,19). Rather, Baum (11) argues, that this characteristic extends the period of victimization. Similarly, Erikson (12) has asserted that, in a sense, the consequences of toxic disasters are interminable in that contaminants are absorbed into the landscape, body tissues and even the genetic material of victims, threatening generations to come.

Loss of Control

Technological disasters also tend to undermine people's sense of control (10) since usually little can be done to alter the consequences that one will suffer (e.g., of radiation exposure). Thus victims feel powerless to adequately protect themselves or their families or influence their fates (20,21). In a study of TMI area residents Houts, Cleary and Hu (22) found that people's perceived inability to protect themselves, or evaluate what harm they may have experienced, created fear and uncertainty, as well as feelings of frustration and helplessness. Other researchers (20,23) have reported similar findings regarding feelings of helplessness in residents living near a toxic waste dump.

While people generally accept that natural forces, and thus natural disasters, are not controllable, technology is generally assumed to be under human control (10). Consequently, people experience technological disasters as a loss of control or violation of the expectation of control. They have shown that natural disasters tend to be associated with reactance and stress-like arousal; while technological disasters tend to be associated with more helpless-like and passive responses.

Stigmatization

Finally, much of the stress inherent in disasters involving environmental contaminants may be due to the perception that such disasters pollute, befoul, or taint rather than merely damage (12). Social rejection and stigma have been suggested to be among the most sig-

nificant post-disaster sources of stress for Chernobyl survivors (24). Furthermore, environments can become stigmatized because of their perceived contamination and individuals associated with these environments become secondarily devalued and acquire spoiled identities (25). These individuals may become socially and emotionally removed from their communities and avoided, causing them to experience a social rejection that may evoke high levels of victim alienation, a well established cause of psychological distress (21). Victims may also engage in more negative self-appraisals regarding their bodies as damaged, poisoned, or altered for the worse (13).

Event Implications

There is considerable evidence that the psychological impact of negative life events is accounted for, at least in part, by the life changes they bring about that can become persistent sources of stress or strain (26–28). These life changes may relate, for example, to negatively viewed alterations in social roles, financial security or changes in the quality of social relationships. They may also relate to perceived losses (literal or symbolic), e.g., lost opportunities, wishes and aspirations for the future that the event is perceived as precluding, or the loss of a valued aspect of the victim's pre-event world (27).

Network Member's Responses

The responses of people in the victims' social network and environment can be another source of psychological after effects. Network-induced distress has a number of common sources (28–32). First, people around the victims tend to, at least implicitly, blame them for their plight. Derogating or blaming the victims allows network members to feel relieved of a sense of responsibility to aid them and confers a sense of protection against the same fate; that is, if one can believe that the victims brought their fate upon themselves, then one can feel that by avoiding similar action one can avoid a similar fate. It also permits one to maintain a belief in a just world (33,34); that is, if individuals get what they deserve, then the world is just and purposeful.

Network members may also impede recovery by discouraging the victims from talking about the traumatic or stressful event and from expressing their distress. Such actions may be motivated by a network member's desire to avoid the demands for emotional support that would ensue if victims openly expressed their distress. Or more benignly, such actions may be related to the widespread belief that it is best to deflect the victim's attention away from the traumatic event and its negative consequences

(32,35). By depriving the victims of the opportunity to discuss the event and their reactions to it; others may be impeding a necessary process for psychological resolution of the trauma (27).

COPING WITH AMBIGUITY AND FEELINGS OF LOSS OF CONTROL

Above we have suggested that victims of disasters involving invisible trauma face particular adaptational dilemmas. The extant research literature suggests that victims tend to use four principal coping strategies:

- hypervigilance;
- the construction of symbolic belief systems;
- a reliance on primarily emotion-focused coping;
- self-blame.

Hypervigilance

People may tend to become hypervigilant in response to a high level of threat or fear (36). Hypervigilance is also a common adaptive response to exposure to invisible contaminants that pose the threat of uncertain future health consequences (3). One strategy for managing uncertainty is to assume that the threat will materialize and to optimize vigilance as a way of maximizing the possibility of discovering any information that might aid adaptation, as well as detecting any signs of impending danger, at the earliest possible moment (36). While this strategy may possess some utility, it carries the danger that individuals will become so focused on the threat that their life becomes severely constricted by this preoccupation (3,36,37). Additionally, constant preoccupation with a potential danger about which little can be done creates rumination that may lead to psychological fixation and chronic stress (21).

Construction of Symbolic Belief Systems

The psychological need of individuals exposed to an invisible contaminant to reduce what is typically a very distressing, if not intolerable, uncertainty leads them to construct a nonempirical belief system about the threat (3,21). Vyner (3) identifies common themes across belief systems concerning environmental contamination:

- the certainty that the environment or a portion of it is now dangerous and to be avoided;
- the certainty that the bodies of the believers (in the threat) and of their children are being poisoned;

- victims can expect little empathy or assistance from neighbors and government;
- escape or relocation is the only reasonable way to avoid further damage.

These belief systems, which actually become the content of the cognitive appraisals, serve the function of conferring a certainty on reality and thus make adaptation possible (3).

Reliance on Emotion-Focused Coping

Lazarus and Folkman (5,38,39) have described problem-focused coping and emotion-focused coping as two general strategies for coping with stressful circumstances. Problem-focused coping involves action directed at removing or circumventing the threatening stimulus, thus allowing the individual to move toward the attainment of goals. Emotion-focused coping involves the attempt to reduce or eliminate the emotional distress associated with or cued by the stressful situation. Although not mutually exclusive, problem-focused coping tends to be used when the person believes that something constructive can be done about the stressor while emotion-focused coping is more common when an individual believes that the situation is one which must be endured (38). There is evidence that emotion-focused coping is more likely to be invoked in illness-related contexts of ambiguity or uncertainty (40,41).

Self-Blame

Evidence suggests that attributions of self-blame for misfortune suffered may be associated with more effective coping because such attributes promote the perception of control (42–45). However, other research indicates that self-blame may result in guilt and self-recriminations and higher levels of somatization (46,47). Janoff-Bulman and Frieze (43) offer a resolution for this seeming inconsistency by distinguishing between behavioral self-blame and characterological self-blame. The former can be adaptive because it allows victims to believe that they can avoid future victimization by altering their behavior, thus promoting a sense of control. Characterological self-blame, on the other hand, is often associated with depression and helplessness and a sustained sense of vulnerability because it explains one's victimization in terms of enduring personality characteristics that are assumed to be generally unalterable.

PSYCHOSOCIAL SEQUELAE OF PERCEIVED ENVIRONMENTAL EXPOSURES: CASE EXAMPLES

Three Mile Island

Background. The nuclear power plant accident at Three Mile Island (TMI) in central Pennsylvania began at 4 a.m. on March 28, 1979 when several cooling water pumps malfunctioned, resulting in damage to the radioactive core of one of the two reactors (TMI Unit 2), generation of tremendous heat, leading to the release of radioactive gas and water, and possible exposure of nearby residents to low levels of radiation. The amount of radiation released into the environment was not reliably measured or reported, thus leaving residents with unanswered questions about their radiation exposure and continuing plant emissions.

Over the next few days, the crisis was compounded by equipment failures, conflicting reports, and human errors. On the third day, the Governor in consultation with the Nuclear Regulatory Commission (NRC), issued an advisory of health risk to all pregnant women and preschool children to leave the five-mile area, closed all area schools for two weeks, and advised residents within 20 miles to remain indoors. During the two-week emergency, approximately 60% of the residents living within five miles of the plant and 45% within 20 miles evacuated the area. These were primarily families with preschool children (48,49).

In the years that followed, the accident at TMI was transformed from an acute event into a situation of long-term chronic stress. Intermittent radiation leaks, persistent difficulties with cleanup, media reports about presumed health effects and plant-related problems, varying and contradictory estimates of escaped radiation, and erosion of the credibility of involved officials were all important factors in residents' prolonged stress reactions to the accident (50). The TMI crisis did not end with any announcements but remained an episodic stressor with residents subject to the distress of uncertainty and vulnerability. Ventings over the next several years and 150 tons of debris served as continual reminder of what had occurred and what still remained, extending the sense of threat and stress for many residents. In one report on cancer rates in the TMI area, chronic stress, not radiation exposure, was identified as the probable cause of observed increases in rates of illness and cancer following the nuclear accidents at TMI and Chernobyl (51).

Public health officials concluded that despite serious damage to the TMI plant, the actual release of radio-activity would have a negligible health effect on area residents and that mental stress would be the main effect (52). Nevertheless, radiation's emotional associations with the atomic bomb, nuclear war threats, and frightening reproductive health risks created significant anxiety and controversy (53). Because of the unusual nature of the stresses endured by the community, federal [NRC, National Institute of Mental Health (NIMH)] and state agencies supported investigations into possible mental health consequences, beginning with the President's Commission on the Accident at Three Mile Island (54).

Psychosocial Sequelae. Numerous longitudinal studies provide convergent evidence of acute and long-term psychological or psychophysiologic consequences, particularly chronic stress among TMI residents. The TMI incident provided an opportunity to study the ways people perceived, evaluated, and responded to a unique, if somewhat ambiguous, disaster situation that persisted over an extended period. However, because many of the studies of the psychosocial consequences of the accident are based on residents' self-reports, it is important to acknowledge that some residents may have exaggerated distress in order to influence the permanent closing of the plant, while plant proponents may de-emphasize any problems they experienced (55).

The Task Force on Behavioral Effects of the President's Commission examined immediate and short-term effects on "the mental health of the public" (48). Interview data on mental health symptoms were collected from probability samples of high-risk groups in the general population and control groups (i.e., male and female heads of households living within 20 miles of the plant and controls; mothers of preschool children and comparison group mothers; TMI workers and a comparison group of nearby nuclear power plant workers; TMI adolescents; and clients from community mental health centers in the TMI area, who provided a criterion group to assess demoralization). The Task Force found that, while early high levels of distress decreased within 6 months, levels of distrust in authorities remained elevated (48,49).

Baum and colleagues (52,53,55–60) have carried out the most extensive research on the psychological sequelae of the TMI incident for area residents, starting 15 months after the accident and extending ten years after the accident. They compared small samples of TMI residents living within five miles and three comparable control groups near another nuclear reactor, near a fossil-fuel plant, and not near a power plant. In all of their studies, TMI residents performed more poorly on all measures than controls short-term and up to five years after the accident. At 16 months after the accident (when decisions were made to vent radioactive gas into the atmosphere), TMI-area residents showed greater stress as indicated by their reports of more symptoms, their performance on proofreading tasks, and their exhibited higher concentrations of catecholamine in urine reflecting levels of sympathetic nervous system activity relative to controls (55). Stress was highest before venting and decreased six weeks after venting (60).

Two years after the accident, researchers found persistent stress responses psychologically, behaviorally, and biochemically (59). Residents living within five miles of TMI had higher levels of norepinephrine than controls (52). Higher levels of support were associated with less stress; coping by denial was associated with more stress, and emotion-focused coping led to more effective handling of the situation.

Five years after the accident, TMI residents exhibited greater symptoms of stress overall than did a control group matched for age, education, and socioeconomic status (SES). Specifically, TMI residents experienced greater depression, anxiety, and psychosomatic symptoms. They also evidenced a decreased sense of well being, increased blood pressure and neuroendocrine stress markers, and decreased persistence and problem solving abilities. Researchers (58) also found that TMI residents showed more symptoms of post traumatic stress disorder (e.g., hyperarousal and exaggerated startle responses, withdrawal, and intrusive thoughts or dreams about stressors). On most stress measures, the TMI-area populations began to recover seven or eight years after the accident. They gradually accommodated to the threats that persisted. Ten years after accident, differences between TMI and controls were no longer significant.

In a series of longitudinal studies from shortly after the accident to the tenth anniversary in 1989, Bromet and colleagues (54,61–63) focused on three at-risk groups—mothers of young children living near the plant, workers employed at TMI, and community mental health center clients living near the plant. The studies generally indicated that, although initially high distress levels apparently diminished over time for the majority of the population, some subgroups, particularly mothers of young children living within five miles, experienced mental difficulties as long as five years after the accident (54). At a follow-up after the undamaged unit was restarted in 1985, mothers who felt that TMI was dangerous were more likely to have experienced an episode of clinical depression compared to mothers perceiving the plant as less dangerous, and

mothers living within five miles of the plant were more likely to experience a clinical episode during the previous year compared to mothers living farther away.

At the tenth anniversary of the accident in 1989, Bromet and colleagues (61) found that only a minority of mothers had no concerns about the safety of living within ten miles of a nuclear power plant or were not worried about their children's health. Overall, the women became more symptomatic over time with the major increase occurring at the time of the restart. In 1989, women perceiving TMI as dangerous had significantly more symptoms of depression, anxiety and hostility compared to women who believed the plant was safe or were unsure (61).

Chernobyl

Background. The nuclear power plant accident at Chernobyl took place seven years after TMI. In the early morning of April 26, 1986 a reactor sustained an initial explosion and fire followed by a graphite fire that combined to produce gases and aerosols containing large quantities of radioactive material (64). According to Ginzburg and Reis (65), Soviet estimates of the numbers of people with significant exposure to radiation from the Chernobyl accident vary from 9 to 17.5 million people (including 2.5 million children under 7 years). Two plant operators died immediately, 29 others (including fire fighters) died shortly later of radiation sickness (66); eventually about 250–320 deaths (67) were directly attributed to radiation exposure, primarily plant operators and emergency workers (65).

Soviet authorities claim that about 400,000 to 600,000 people were involved in the enormous cleanup in the three republics from 1986 to 1989 (64,66,67). When mechanical robots became stuck in the debris, human volunteers worked with radioactive debris "by hand" (67). The clean-up people or "liquidators" were apparently not provided with dosimetry devices or protective clothing and radioactive waste water from the cleanup was not contained (67). During the ten days required to contain the fires, clouds of radioactive material were dispersed by wind and rain throughout the world. Approximately 825,000 people lived in the areas of Russia (primarily Byelorussia) where contamination levels from radioactive cesium were considered harmful (64). Over 100,000 people were evacuated (66). Pripyat, home of plant workers and the largest city in the zone with a population of 45,000, became a ghost town (65). Potassium iodine prophylaxis was administered to 5.4 million people including 1.7 million children. The degree of risk was a function of where family members worked and their food sources (fresh fruit, vegetables, milk, milk products, and meat products) (64). Soviet officials withheld much information about the reactor damage and contamination areas for several years.

Psychosocial Sequelae. While psychosocial consequences of the TMI incident are well documented, similar information about the population affected by the Chernobyl accident is limited. Two themes emerged from early examination of the psychological effects of the accident by Soviet officials:

- change to the community (e.g., significant changes in many lives including relocation, activity modifications because of continued high radioactivity levels, parental concerns about children becoming ill, attribution of all unexplained illness to exposure, distrust of central government to monitor radioactivity);
- change to individuals with numbers of people being labelled "radiophobic," defined as inappropriately afraid of radioactive material, even if they had appropriate concerns about potential long-term effects of low dose radiation on their small children or themselves (65).

Interviews conducted in 1990 indicated that people worried about the effects of radiation on their health and impressions that diseases have increased since the accident; about threats to the future health of children; and about effects on their everyday lives including food purchases, cultivation of their land, and activities such as collecting wild mushrooms (66). Because pre-accident morbidity data are unavailable, exposure effects are difficult to assess. A Russian psychiatrist examined 1572 persons living in the immediate vicinity of the plant who had complaints about their mental state (68). Most of these people were found to be in a state of alarmed tension associated with a fear of getting radiation injury through contaminated foodstuffs or to be anxious about radiation-induced genetic defects in their newborns.

Ginzburg and Reis (65) have reported that Soviet researchers who investigated the psychological impact of Chernobyl on survivors identified problems of "psycho-emotional tension and radiophobia". The researchers, they note, attributed these problems primarily to the lack of adequate and understandable information about the low-dose radiation provided by scientists and the media, lack of scientific agreement about the probability of developing cancer, inadequate measurement equipment, and a lack of a sense of personal control. While still other Soviet researchers, Ginsburg and Reis (65) note, contended that the

immediate evacuation of 150,000 people living near Chernobyl was accompanied by high tension, stress, and radiophobia and that these conditions cause a greater threat to health than actual radiation exposure.

Three years after the Chernobyl accident, the Soviet government requested that the International Atomic Energy Agency evaluate the medical and psychological health of residents of areas contaminated with radioactive fallout (64). The researchers conducted structured interviews and gathered clinical data from 1350 residents of 13 villages in three republics and researchers concluded that no health disorders in either contaminated or nearby uncontaminated control villages "could be attributed directly to radiation exposure" (64). No differences were found, for example, in immune system functioning, thyroid tumors, leukemia, or blood lead levels (64). Levels of anxiety and stress of the villagers were found to be disproportionate to the biological significance of the measured radioactive contamination. About 45% of adults living in the contaminated villages believed that they had a radiation-related illness, compared to 30% of those in the control villages. A full 70% of persons in contaminated villages wanted to move away; and approximately 83% believed the government should relocate them (64). In both the contaminated and control villages general morale and confidence in the future were low as a result of a "multitude of life-changes" including significant changes in their government, as well as concerns about the future health of their children and themselves because of the accident. The IAEA study concluded that "radiophobia" (a Soviet psychiatric term that had been used to describe an inappropriate or pathological fear of radioactive material) seems inappropriate; rather it concluded that concerns and anxiety among exposed individuals were understandable given the inconsistent and incomplete data they were receiving.

Collins (67) suggests that the worst aspect of Chernobyl may be the pervasive invisible threat and "continuing fear that the future is marred by irreversible cancer or genetic defects." The UN International Atomic Energy Agency assessment (200 scientists from 25 countries) found that anticipatory stress was readily apparent and that stress-related illnesses were caused by lack of public information about the disaster and the subsequent mass evacuations.

A report by Torubarov (69) concludes that "data have shown that for the vast majority of people, the psychological consequences play the most important role" (p. 81). Sensational publication in the mass media induced and sustained anxiety in the victims, so that the majority of the population was convinced that living in contaminated regions would result in terrible harmful effects. Some problems were self-serving with people trying to resolve their complex social and economic problems by qualifying for privileges given to emergency workers and people in contaminated areas (69).

Love Canal

Background. The Love Canal disaster differs from the accidents at TMI and Chernobyl because the Love Canal disaster unfolded more slowly and residents were not aware of their exposure until informed by officials. Technical information about Love Canal remains limited, making it difficult to establish causal relationships between the environmental toxins and damage to people or property (70).

Love Canal events began in 1953 when Hooker Chemical Company sold the abandoned Love Canal property to the Niagara Falls, New York school board for a token $1. In 1955, an elementary school opened that had been built atop the covered-over canal, into which Hooker had dumped tons of residue from the manufacture of chemical compounds (70). Eventually 1000 families, including 250 tenants of federally subsidized housing, settled in the ten-block area surrounding the canal. "By the mid-1970s it was apparent that chemicals were leaking from the disposal site" (70). Following two years of preliminary governmental studies, residents were suddenly alerted to environmental dangers in the spring of 1978. Within weeks, air samples from area basements and materials from basement pumps and storm sewers revealed the presence of highly toxic chemicals (benzene, lindane, trichloroethylene). In August, the State Commissioner of Health stated that "Love Canal was a great and imminent peril to the health of the general public residing at or near the site" (70) and ordered temporary closing of the elementary school, implementation of a remedial plan for toxic substances, and further environmental and health studies. It was also recommended that pregnant women and children under 2 years immediately move from the canal area and that all residents avoid their basements and refrain from eating their garden vegetables (70). A citizens' action group formed immediately. President Carter declared an emergency and the Governor of New York personally told residents that the state would buy 239 homes in the inner ring and would assist families in their move. The Governor's ten-agency task force set up headquarters and "the Department of Health distributed hundreds of health questionnaires and took thousands of blood samples" (70). In October huge machines began to recap and partially drain the canal.

The citizen's group helped inner-ring residents to move out of their homes and then during a two-year period began to address the needs of outer-ring residents, including the closed school, health threats, worthless homes, and problems with agencies that minimized health risks and offered conflicting advice. State officials announced abnormal liver function tests among some young boys and men in November 1978 and in December announced at a public meeting that dioxin had been found in storm sewers, nearby creeks, and some properties. Residents received the conflicting message that the area was a health hazard, but that specific individuals were not harmed (70). In February 1979, the State Health Commissioner issued a supplemental health order after finding excessive miscarriages and low-birth-weight babies in some outer-ring families and recommended that pregnant women, children under 2 yr, and their families should be moved out at state expense until the youngest child was 2 yr old. In June 1980, chromosome damage was found in 11 of 36 persons tested and the government decided to help relocate 710 families living near Love Canal, but the decision did "little to dissipate the miasma of fear and anger that envelopes the area" (71).

Psychosocial Sequelae. Some studies indicate that perceived exposure is a better predictor of response than actual exposure (23). A geneticist providing counseling services stated that "when the smoke has cleared, it may turn out that the greatest damage to health will be psychological and social" (71). Levine interviewed residents in the midst of the collective stress situation, in Fall, 1978 (after the formation of citizens' group and after inner-ring residents began to leave) and again in the Spring, six months later when outer-ring residents were offered relocation help (70). Using an informal snowball recruitment design and an open-ended, semi-structured format, Levine interviewed people with a wide range of views and social characteristics, including both people who moved and stayed. The most frequent problems mentioned in the first interview were physical health and worry/anxiety. Many felt loss of control of major aspects of their lives, expressed uncertainty about whether or not to move, whether illnesses were related to exposures, and whether their families would have future chemical-related illnesses; felt distrust of the advice of authorities, and concerns about finances and to a lesser extent property values (70). In Fall 1978, shortly after the crisis began, most respondents (63%) reported that they felt their health had worsened during last few years; these were primarily younger heads of households, families with younger children, and inner-ring homeowners. Complaints (e.g., fatigue, headaches, allergies, dizziness, nausea, weakness, insomnia) were vague (70,71). By Spring, however, when many had moved, 39% said their health had improved since the Fall (compared with 26% reporting worse health). The emotional impact of loss of their homes and decisions about leaving their neighborhoods were particularly anguishing (70). In response to questions about perceived stigma, 56% of residents felt negative attitudes from people in government and about one-fourth felt that other Niagara Falls residents resented the adverse publicity for an area based on the chemical industry and tourism (70). The situation and subsequent relocation caused tension and many divorces and separations with the wife leaving with the children and the husband staying because of his work and his investment in the home (71). People "feel betrayed by all levels of government" (p. 1243) and worn down by the uncertainty of living in hotels and apartments with insurance running out, and household belongings in jeopardy of vandalism while waiting for government decisions (71).

Levine (72) also describes observations over a three-year period about the trust and confidence held by Love Canal residents towards government and scientific professionals. Residents expected useful, comprehensible information, yet realized that researchers were politically and financially involved and influenced decisions rather than remaining impartial. The initial interaction set the stage for ambiguity, lack of confidence, rush, and disorganization: the Commission's health warning in August was issued in Albany and residents of Love Canal heard the news from the media (72).

FUTURE DIRECTIONS FOR RESEARCH

Research needs to be undertaken that would further extend our understanding of coping with perceived exposures to environmental hazards. In research on technological disasters, surprisingly little inquiry into coping has been undertaken to date. What little has been done has primarily focused on examining the adaptational consequences of a tendency to make greater use of either emotion-focused or problem-focused coping. While the weight of the limited data would suggest that emotion-focused coping is of greater benefit in the case of disasters involving technological accidents and accompanying biospheric con-

tamination, where little can be done to modify the nature of the stressor, the findings have not been consistent. This may be attributable to the failure of this research to link coping strategies with specific adaptational tasks. That is, typically, the respondent is simply asked to report (using a standardized coping inventory) on how he/she has coped with the "event." Since disasters or major stressful or traumatic life events are inevitably complex and pose many adaptational challenges, this information would seem to be of limited value. Summary coping measures averaged across tasks may obscure coping efforts rather than illuminate them (73). Since certain adaptive tasks may be central to one's goals and commitments, the coping effectiveness of the strategies employed to master those tasks will probably assume greater weight in determining adaptational outcomes.

Research on the psychosocial consequences of a perceived exposure to environmental contaminant has also been characterized by conspicuously little phenomenological research. Yet the personal meanings that victims assign to these events are clearly a critical determinant of their psychological impact and the coping responses enacted. Lazarus (74) has recently written, "I am confident that personal meanings are the most important aspects of psychological stress with which the person must cope, and they direct the choice of coping strategy" (p. 244). Similarly, Horowitz (75) has emphasized "that life events are always combined with internal meanings to create a situation that may or may not traumatize the individual" (p. 147). By understanding these events from the perspective of the individuals involved we can develop new insights that have not been accessible through more traditional survey research methods.

Finally, Silver and Wortman (76) have noted that most stage models of reactions to undesirable life events have postulated a final stage of resolution or adaptation. They and others (27,77) however, have questioned the validity of this conceptualization and argued that prevailing notions of recovery need to be re-evaluated as there is sufficient empirical data to suggest that a substantial minority of individuals experience distress or involuntary event-related ruminations for very extended periods of time or re-experience the crisis in some sense for the rest of their lives. What is needed, they have argued, is a more extensive investigation into what is normative with respect to long-term adaptation to major stressful life events. Such information could then become an appropriate basis for judging what constitutes (in relative terms) good and poor adaptation to a particular kind of stressor.

REFERENCES

1. Wandersman AH, Hallman WK. Are people acting irrationally?: Understanding public concerns about environmental threats. *Am Psychol*. 1993;43:681–686.

2. Freudenberg, N. Action for environmental health: report of a survey of community organizations. *Am J Public Health*. 1984;174:444–448.

3. Vyner H. *Invisible Trauma: The Psychosocial Effects of the Invisible Environmental Contaminants*. Lexington, MA: D.C. Heath; 1988.

4. Lazarus RS. Coping and the process of secondary appraisal: degree of threat and factors in the stimulus configuration. In: *Psychological Stress and the Coping Process*. New York: McGraw Hill; 1966: 150–209.

5. Lazarus RS. Cognitive and personality factors underlying threat and coping. In: Appley MH, Turnbull R, eds. *Psychological Stress, Issues in Research*. New York: Appleton-Century-Crofts; 1967: 151–181.

6. Lazarus RS, Averill JR, Optom EM. The psychology of coping: issues of research and assessment. In: Coelho GV, Hamburg DA, Adams JE, eds. *Coping and Adaptation*. New York: Basic Books, 1974: 249–315.

7. Mishel MH. The measurement of uncertainly in illness. *Nurs Res*. 1981; 30:258–263.

8. Shalit B. Structural ambiguity and limits to coping. *J Hum Stress*. 1977; 3:32–45.

9. Weiner H. The concept of stress in the light of studies on disasters, unemployment, and loss: a critical analysis. In: Zales MR, ed. *Stress in Health and Disease*. New York: Brunner/Mazel; 1985: 24–96.

10. Baum A, Fleming R, Davidson LM. Natural disaster and technological catastrophe. *Environ Behav*. 1983; 15:333–354.

11. Baum A. Toxins, technology, and natural disasters. In: VandenBos GR, Bryant BK, eds. *Cataclysms, Crises, and Catastrophes: Psychology in Action*. Washington, DC: American Psychological Association; 1987:5–54.

12. Erikson K. A new species of trouble. In: Couch SR, Kroll-Smith JS, eds. Communities at Risk: *Collective Responses to Technological Hazards*. New York: Peter Lang; 1991:12–29.

13. Kroll-Smith S, Couch SR. Technological hazards, adaptation and social change. In: Couch SR, Kroll-Smith JS, eds. *Communities at Risk: Collective Responses to Technological Hazards*. New York: Peter Lang; 1991:293–320.

14. Baum A, Schaeffer MA, Lake CR, et al. Psychological and endocrinological correlates of chronic stress at Three Mile Island. In: Williams RB, ed. *Perspectives on Behavioral Medicine*. Vol. 2. San Diego, CA: Academic Press; 1985.

15. Baum A, Fleming I, Israel A, O'Keeffe MK. Symptoms of chronic stress following a natural disaster and discovery of a human-made hazard. *Environ Behav*. 1992; 24:347–365.

16. Fowlkes MR, Miller P. *Love Canal: The Social Construction of Disaster* (Project No. 6441E). Washington, DC: Federal Emergency Management Agency; 1982.

17. Pijawka KD, Cuthbertson BA, Olson RS. Coping with extreme hazard events: emerging themes in natural and technological disaster research. *Omega*. 1987–1988;18:281–297.

18. Green BL, Lindy JD, Grace MC. Psychological effects of toxic contamination. In: Ursano R, McCaughey B, Fullerton C, eds. *Individual and Community Responses to Trauma and Disaster*. Boston: Cambridge University Press; 1994:154–178.

19. Bolin R. Response to natural disasters. In: Lystad M, ed. *Mental Health Response to Mass Emergencies: Theory and Practice*. New York: Brunner/Mazel; 1988:22–51. (Brunner/Mazel Psychosocial Stress Series; No. 12).

20. Gibbs MS. Psychopathological consequences of exposure to toxins in the water supply. In: Lebovits AH, Baum A, Singer JE, eds. *Advances in Environmental Psychology*. Vol. 6: *Exposure to Hazardous Substances: Psychological Parameters*. Hillsdale, NJ: Lawrence Erlbaum Associates; 1986.

21. Kroll-Smith S, Couch SR. Technological hazards: social responses as traumatic stressors. In: Wilson JP, RaphaelB, eds. *International Handbook of Traumatic Stress Syndromes*. New York: Plenum Press; 1993:79–92.

22. Houts PS, Cleary PD, Hu T. *The Three Mile Island Crisis: Psychological, Social, and Economic Impacts on the Surrounding Population*. State College, PA: Pennsylvania State University Press; 1988.

23. Fleming I, O'Keefe MK, Baum A. Chronic stress and toxic waste: the role of uncertainty and helplessness. *J Appl Soc Psychol*. 1991; 21:1889–1907.

24. Bertazzi PA. Industrial disasters and epidemiology: a review of recent experiences. *Scand J Work Environ Health*. 1989; 15:85–100.

25. Edelstein M. Ecological threats and spoiled identities: Radon gas and environmental stigma. In: Couch SR, Kroll-Smith JS, eds. *Communities at Risk: Collective Responses to Technological Hazards*. New York: Peter Lang; 1991:206–225.

26. Siegel K, Christ GH. Hodgkin's disease survivorship: Psychosocial consequences. In: Lacher MJ, Redman JR, eds. *The Consequences of Survivial*. Philadelphia: Lea & Febiger; 1989:383–399.

27. Tait R, Silver RC. Coming to terms with major negative life events. In: Uleman JS, Bargh JA, eds. *Unintended Thought*. New York: Guilford Press; 1989:351–382.

28. Thoits PA. Dimensions of life events that influence psychological distress: an evaluation and synthesis of the literature. In: Kaplan HB, ed. *Psychosocial Stress: Trends in Theory and Research*. New York: Academic Press; 1983:33–104.

29. Pagel MD, Erdly WW, Becker J. Social networks: we get by with (and in spite of) a little help from our friends. *J Pers Soc Psychol*. 1987; 53:793–804.

30. Rook KS, Pietromonaco P. Close relationships: ties that heal or ties that bind? *Adv Pers Relationships*. 1987; 1:1–35.

31. Siegel K, Raveis VH, Karus D. Psychological well-being of gay men with AIDS: Contributions of positive and negative network interactions. *Soc Sci Med*. 1994; 23:217–230.

32. Wortman CB, Dunkel-Schetter C. Interpersonal relationships and cancer: a theoretical analysis. *J Soc Issues*. 1979; 35:120–155.

33. Lerner MJ. The desire for justice and reaction to victims. In: Macaulay J, Berkowitz L, eds. *Altruism and Helping Behavior*. New York: Academic Press; 1970.

34. Lerner MJ, Simmons CH. Observer's reactions to the "innocent victim": Compassion or rejection? *J Pers Soc Psychol.* 1966; 4:203–210.

35. Peters-Golden H. Varried perceptions of social support in the illness experience. *Soc Sci Med.* 1982; 16:483–491.

36. Janis IL. Decisionmaking under stress. In: Goldberger L, Breznitz S, eds. *Handbook of Stress: Theoretical and Clinical Aspects.* 2nd ed. New York: The Free Press; 1993:56–76.

37. Breznitz S. A study of worrying. *Br J Soc Clin Psychol.* 1971; 10:271–279.

38. Folkman S, Lazarus RS. An analysis of coping in a middle-aged community sample. *J Health Soc Behav.* 1980; 21:219–239.

39. Lazarus RS, Folkman S. *Stress, Appraisal and Coping.* New York: Springer; 1984.

40. Redeker NS. The relationship between uncertainty and coping after coronary bypass surgery. *West J Nurs Res.* 1992; 14:48–68.

41. Webster KK, Christman NJ. Perceived uncertainty and coping post myocardial infarction. *West J Nurs Res.* 1988; 10:384–400.

42. Bulman RJ, Wortman CB. Attributions of blame and coping in the "real world": Severe accident victims react to their lot. *J Pers Soc Psychol.* 1977; 35:351–363.

43. Janoff-Bulman R, Frieze IH. A theoretical perspective for understanding reactions to victimization. *J Soc Issues.* 1983; 39:1–17.

44. Miller DT, Porter CA. Self-blame in victims of violence. *J Soc Issues.* 1983; 39:141–154.

45. Thompson SC. Will it hurt less if I can control it: A complex answer to a simple question. *Psychol Bull.* 1981; 90:89–101.

46. Abrams RD, Finesinger JE. Guilt reactions in patients with cancer. *Cancer.* 1953; 6:474–482.

47. Solomon SD, Regier DA, Burke JD. Role of perceived control in coping with disaster. *J Soc Clin Psychol.* 1989; 8:376–392.

48. Dohrenwend BP, Dohrenwend BS, Warheit GJ, et al. Stress in the community: a report to the President's Commission on the Accident at Three Mile Island. *Ann NY Acad Sci.* 1981; 365:159–174.

49. Dohrenwend BP. Psychological implications of nuclear accidents: the case of Three Mile Island. *Bull NY Acad Med.* 1983; 59:1060–1076.

50. Goldsteen R, Schorr JK, Goldsteen KS. Longitudinal study of appraisal at Three Mile Island: implications for life event research. *Soc Sci Med.* 1989; 28:389–398.

51. Hatch MC, Wallenstein S, Beyea J, et al. Cancer rates after the Three Mile Island nuclear accident and proximity of residence to the plant. *Am J Public Health.* 1991; 81:719–724.

52. Collins DL, Baum A, Singer JE. Coping with chronic stress at Three Mile Island: psychological biochemical evidence. *Health Psychol.* 1983; 2:149–166.

53. Baum A. Stress, intrusive imagery, and chronic distress: presidential address. *Health Psychol.* 1990; 9:653–675.

54. Bromet EJ, Parkinson DK, Dunn LO. Long-term mental health consequences of the accident at Three Mile Island. *Int J Ment Health.* 1990; 19:48–60.

55. Baum A, Fleming I, Singer JE. Stress at Three Mile Island: Applying psychological impact analysis. In: Bickman L, ed. *Applied Social Psychology Annual 3.* Beverly Hills, CA: Sage; 1982:217–248.

56. Baum A, Fleming I. Implications of psychological research on stress and technological accidents. *Am Psychol.* 1993; 48:665–672.

57. Collins DL. Stress at Three Mile Island: altered perceptions, behaviors, and neuroendocrine measures. In: Ricks RC, Berger ME, O'Hara FM Jr, eds. *The Medical Basis for Radiation-Accident Preparedness. III: The Psychological Perspective.* New York: Elsevier; 1991:71–79.

58. Davidson LM, Baum A. Chronic stress and posttraumatic stress disorders. *J Consult Clin Psychol.* 1986; 54:303–308.

59. Davidson LM, Baum A, Fleming I, Gisriel MM. Toxic exposure and chronic stress at Three Mile Island. In: Lebovits AH, Baum A, Singer JE, eds. *Advances in Environmental Psychology. Exposure to Hazardous Substances: Psychological Parameters.* Vol. 6. Hillsdale, NJ: Erlbaum; 1986:35–47.

60. Gatchel RJ, Schaeffer MS, Baum A. A psychophysiological field study of stress at Three Mile Island. *Psychophysiology.* 1985; 22:175–181.

61. Bromet EJ. Psychologic effects of the radiation accident at TMI. In: Ricks RC, Berger ME, O'Hara FM Jr, eds. *The Medical Basis for Radiation-accident Preparedness. III: The Psychological Perspective.* New York: Elsevier; 1991:61–70.

62. Dew MA, Bromet EJ. Predictors of temporal patterns of psychiatric distress during 10 years following the nuclear accident at Three Mile Island. *Soc Psychiatry Psychiatr Epidemiol.* 1993; 28:49–55.

63. Dew MA, Bromet EJ, Schulberg HC. A comparative analysis of two community stressors' long-term mental health effects. *Am J Commun Psychol.* 1987; 15:167–184.

64. Ginzburg HM. The psychological consequences of the Chernobyl accident—findings from the International Atomic Energy Agency study. *Public Health Rep.* 1993; 108:184–192.

65. Ginzburg HM, Reis E. Consequences of the nuclear power plant accident at Chernobyl. *Public Health Rep.* 1991; 106:32–40.

66. Giel R. The psychosocial aftermath of two major disasters in the Soviet Union. *J Traumatic Stress.* 1991; 4:381–392.

67. Collins DL. Behavioral differences of irradiated persons associated with the Kyshtym, Chelyabinsk, and Chernobyl nuclear accidents. *Mil Med.* 1992; 157:548–552.

68. Spivak LI. Psychiatric aspects of the accident at Chernobyl nuclear power station. *Eur J Psychiatry.* 1992; 6:207–212.

69. Torubarov FS. Psychological consequences of the Chernobyl accident from the radiation neurology point of view. In: Ricks RC, Berger ME, O'Hara FM Jr, eds. *The Medical Basis for Radiation-Accident Preparedness. III: The Psychological Perspective.* New York: Elsevier; 1991:81–91.

70. Levine AG, Stone RA. Threats to people and what they value: residents' perceptions of the hazards of Love Canal. In: Lebovits AH, Baum A, Singer JE, eds. *Advances in Environmental Psychology. Exposure to*

Hazardous Substances: Psychological Parameters. Vol. 6. Hillsdale, NJ: Erlbaum; 1986:109–130.

71. Holden C. Love Canal residents under stress. *Science.* 1980; 208:1242–1244.

72. Levine A. Psychosocial impact of toxic chemical waste dumps. *Env Health Perspect.* 1983; 48:15–17.

73. Oberst MT. Response to "coping amid uncertainty: An illness trajectory perspective." *Schol Inq Nurs Pract.* 1993; 7:33–35.

74. Lazaruz R. Coping theory and research: Past, present, and future. *Psychosom Med.* 1993; 55:234–247.

75. Horowitz MJ. Disaster stress studies: conclusions. In: Shore JH, ed. *Disaster Stress Studies: New Methods and Findings.* Washington, DC: American Psychiatric Press; 1986:142–149.

76. Silver RL, Wortman CB. Coping with undersirable life events. In: Garber J, Seligman MEP, eds. *Human Helplessness: Theory and Applications.* New York: Academic Press; 1980:279–340.

77. Wortman CB, Silver RL. The myths of coping with loss. *J Consult Clin Psychol.* 1989; 57:349–357.

XII

THE CHILD WITH CANCER

EDITOR: JIMMIE C. HOLLAND

76

Biology of Childhood Cancers

PETER G. STEINHERZ AND JOSEPH SIMONE

Malignancy in children is relatively rare, yet it is in this population that many of the advances in cancer therapy over the last four decades were first conceived and implemented. Advances in the treatment of children have contributed to the understanding and management of cancer in adults. Today, with intensive therapies utilizing the concerted efforts of the pediatric oncologists, surgeons, radiotherapists immunotherapists and the vast resources of a medical center for supportive care and rehabilitation, it is possible to cure cancer in a majority of children (1–3).

EPIDEMIOLOGY

The control of infectious disease with immunizations and antibiotics, and better prenatal care to reduce congenital abnormalities, has left cancer as the leading cause of death from disease in children in the economically advantaged nations of the world. In the United States in 1987 (4), 10.4% of all deaths in children under 15 years of age were due to malignancies (Table 76.1). However, malignant tumors are still rare. The annual incidence for all histologic types was 133/million children from 1979–1989 (5), with considerable variation in the age-specific incidence rates (Fig. 76–1). Boys had a higher annual incidence than girls: 141 cases per million boys compared to 125 in girls. It has been estimated that an average practicing pediatrician diagnoses a new case of leukemia, the most common childhood malignancy, less than once every ten years. Yet the economic and social impact and the number of person-years of potential life saved by the successful treatment of pediatric malignancies is surpassed only by that of breast cancer (Fig. 76–2) (3,6,7). There has been a slow, steady increase in the incidence of cancer in all age groups over the last two decades. Unfortunately, the decrease in cancer mortality with better therapies during the same period was confined to the younger age groups (Fig. 76–3).

Although almost any variety of cancer can occur in children, the common types that occur in childhood differ sharply from those found in adults. Epithelial tumors, carcinomas—which comprise the majority of adult malignancies—are rare in childhood. Leukemias, lymphomas, neural tumors and sarcomas are the tumors most frequently seen in children (Table 76.2 and Fig. 76–4). Each childhood neoplasm has its own age, sex and racial pattern. Leukemia, neuroblastoma and Wilms' tumor have a pre-school age peak incidence. Hodgkin's disease and the bone tumors peak in the teenage years, while rhabdomyosarcoma has a biphasic incidence. Non-Hodgkin's lymphoma and many of the brain tumors occur at similar rates throughout the pediatric age groups. Most pediatric malignancies occur at similar rates in boys and in girls. The predominant male incidence of non-Hodgkin's lymphoma is a notable exception. There are a few racial differences in childhood cancer incidence in the United States. The peak incidence of acute lymphoblastic leukemia (ALL) is not seen in black children at 2–4 years of age and the incidence of ALL is less frequent in African Americans. Leukemias comprise 24% of cancers in blacks while leukemias are 32% of the tumors seen in whites. Ewing's sarcoma and testicular cancer are extremely rare in the black population, while retinoblastoma is more frequent in non-whites. The predominant pediatric cancers by age and site are depicted on Table 76.3.

ETIOLOGY

The causative agent for neoplastic growth in the majority of children and adults is still unknown. It now seems apparent that a complex interaction of host, environmental and genetic factors causes cancer. Current belief is that no single agent causes cancer, but a variety of environmental and host factors in combination (8–12). Multiple factors might cause a single

TABLE 76.1. *Ten Leading Causes of Death in the United States, 1987*

	All Ages			Ages 1–14	
	Males	Females		Males	Females
1. Heart disease	385,217	375,136	Accidents	4,712	2,407
2. Cancer	254,653	222,274	Cancer	970	716
3. Accidents	64,818		Congenital anomalies	757	615
CVA*		90,774			
4. CVA*	59,061		Homicide	410	331
Pneumonia, influenza		35,663			
5. COPD†	47,039	31,341	Heart disease	346	300
6. Pneumonia, influenza	33,562		Suicide	199	
Accidents		30,204	Pneumonia, influenza		139
7. Suicide	24,272		Pneumonia, influenza	154	
Diabetes		22,295	Cerebral palsy		119
8. Cirrhosis	17,051		Cerebral palsy	126	
Atherosclerosis		14,046	Meningitis		74
9. Diabetes	16,237		COPD†	103	
Nephritis		11,180	HIV		65
10. Homicide	15,855		Meningitis	102	
Septicemia		10,947	COPD†		65
All causes	1,107,958	1,015,365		9,840	6,376

*CVA, cerebrovascular accident. †COPD, chronic obstructive pulmonary disease.
Source: Ref. 4.

malignancy and a single agent might cooperate to cause different malignancies in different individuals under similar circumstances. It is known that certain environmental factors lead to an increased incidence of cancer.

1. *Radiation*: Atom bomb survivors, radium miners, radium-watch-dial painters, those exposed to high levels of radon and radiologists, all have a higher risk of developing cancer than control populations. Children given radiotherapy for leukemia, lymphoma, tinea capitis, acne, thymic enlargement and lymphadenopathy have an increased risk of subsequent cancer. About 80% of teenagers who develop thyroid cancer have had radiation to the neck, usually in early childhood.

2. *Drugs and chemicals*: Phenytoin therapy for epilepsy may cause lymphoproliferative disorders that progress to malignancy. Tumors may develop many years after a drug has been used. Teenage girls whose mothers have had stillbesterol during pregnancy have an increased incidence of adenocarcinoma of the vagina. Patients who had androgen hormones for aplastic anemia have an increased incidence of liver tumors. Smoking, asbestos and arsenic exposure can lead to lung cancer, mesothelioma and skin cancers, respectively. Naturally occurring zeolite fibers in certain parts of Turkey lead to a high incidence of mesothelioma. A high rate of lung cancer has been linked to cooking oil vapors in some areas in China. Drugs and chemicals that damage the marrow are often potential carcinogens. Benzene can cause bone marrow failure which after an interval of years may transform into leukemia.

3. *Viruses*: Since viruses cause cancer in animals, there is no reason to doubt that viruses also cause cancer in humans. Burkitt's lymphoma, hepatoma and nasopharyngeal carcinoma have been associated with the presence of the Epstein–Barr virus.

The incidence of specific types of cancer varies widely in different geographic locations. Diverse social and dietary habits suggest a number of factors that may contribute to carcinogenesis. The rate of esophageal cancer is high in China and varies more than a

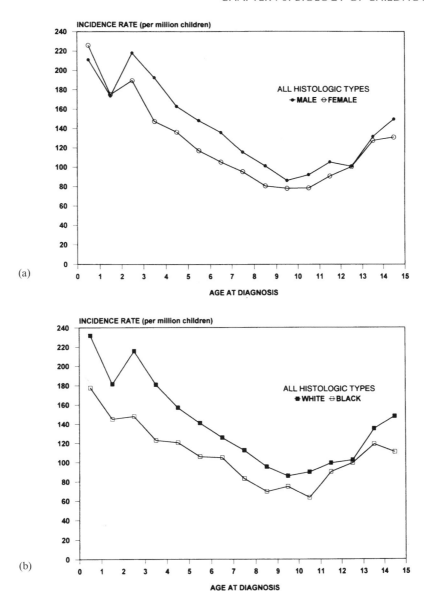

FIG. 76–1. (a) Age- and sex-specific incidence rates of all histologic types combined among U.S. children younger than 15 years of age. (b) Age-specific incidence rates of all histologic types combined among U.S. white and black children younger than 15 years of age. (Reprinted with permission from Gurney JG, Severson RK, Davis S, Robison LL. Incidence of cancer in children in the United States, Sex-, race-, and 1-year age specific rates by histologic types. *Cancer.* 1995; 75:2186–2195.)

hundredfold between different provinces, possibly related to a chronic deficiency of nutritional factors or the extensive use of pickled food. Americans of Chinese ancestry do not have this propensity for esophageal cancer. Nitrosamines in salted fish have been linked to nasopharyngeal carcinoma and aflotoxins from fungus-contaminated food are related to increased liver cancer. While high dietary fat intake may increase the risk of breast or colon cancer, high dietary fibers or indole found in some vegetables can

decrease the incidence of colon carcinoma. Salty food increases the risk of gastric carcinoma while allyl sulfide in garlic or onions decreases its incidence. Children with tyrosinemia, an inborn error in the metabolism of tyrosine and phenylalanine, accumulate succinyl acetoacetic acid, a toxic metabolite that causes liver cirrhosis, leading to hepatocellular carcinoma at an unusually early age. Post cirrhotic hepatoma can also complicate the course of children with hemochromatosis.

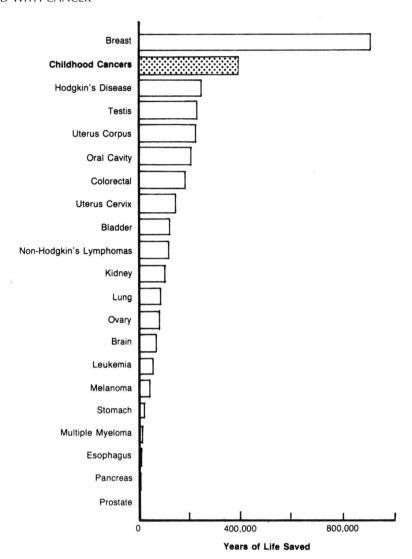

FIG. 76–2. Number of person-years of potential life saved annually in the United States among persons diagnosed with cancer, all races, both sexes, 1990. Derived from an expected life span of 72 years, the median age at diagnosis and the maximum number of patients surviving cancer each year. Person-years = (number of survivors) × (72 − [median age at diagnosis in years]). The maximum number of survivors per year was estimated from the "differential survival". For childhood cancer, this estimate assumes that children who are diagnosed with cancer at 0 to 14 years of age and who survive past their 15th birthday will live a normal life span. The SEER data for 1982 to 1986 were used for the adult data. (Reprinted with permission from Bleyer WA. The impact of childhood cancer on the United States and the world. *CA Cancer J Clin.* 1990; 40:355–368.)

Some studies in children suggest an increased risk due to maternal or paternal occupation or drug intake (13–17). A good example is maternal marijuana use during pregnancy, which can lead to an increased risk of monoblastic leukemia in the infant (18). However, while a majority of the malignancies seen in adults may be due to environmental factors, the long latency period and different features suggest that this mechanism is not likely to play a major role in childhood cancers.

Genetic, congenital and familial determinants of childhood cancer have been observed. Occasionally, leukemia clusters occur in families by chance, but sibling leukemia is much higher in families with parental consanguinity. There is also a high concordance of acute lymphoblastic leukemia in identical twins during infancy, especially in the first few months of life. A familial cancer syndrome has been described by Li and Fraumeni (22). Various members of the family develop sarcomas, breast, bone, brain, lung, larynx

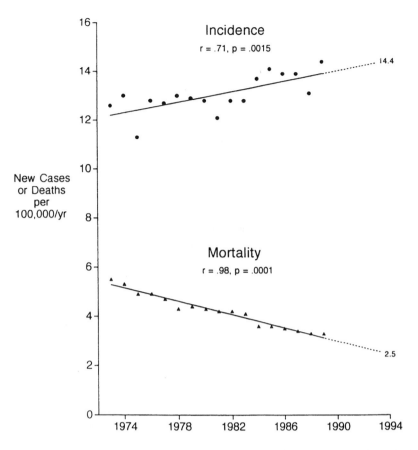

FIG. 76–3. Increasing incidence and declining mortality of cancer during childhood (0–14 years), United States, all races, both sexes, 1973–1989, with linear extrapolation to 1994. The rates are standardized on age distribution younger than 15 years of 1970 US census population. Data from United States SEER program, as reported in *Cancer Statistics Review*, 1973–1989. Values of statistical significance are based on the F-test applied to linear regression of the data with 13 degrees of freedom. (Reprinted with permission from Bleyer WA. The past and future of cancer in the young. *Pediatr Dent.* 1995; 12:285–290.)

TABLE 76.2. *Mortality from the Five Leading Cancers in the United States, 1987*

	All Ages			Under 15	
	Males	Females		Males	Females
1. Lung	87,261	42,748	Leukemia	402	293
2. Colon, rectum	27,889		Brain and CNS*	214	176
Breast		40,899			
3. Prostate	27,864		NHL†	73	
Colon, rectum		28,445	Connective tissue		44
4. Pancreas	14,550	12,187	Connective tissue	65	
			Bone		32
5. Leukemia	9,387		Bone	40	
Ovary		12,020	Kidney		27
All cancer	254,653	222,274		1,021	766

*CNS, central nervous system. †NHL, non-Hodgkin's lumphoma.
Source: Ref. 4.

TABLE 76.3. *Predominant Pediatric Cancers by Age and Site*

Tumors	Newborn (< 1 yr)	Infancy (1–3 yr)	Children (3–11 yr)	Adolescents and Young Adults (12–21 yr)
Leukemias	Congenital leukemia	ALL	ALL	AML
	AML	AML	AML	ALL
	AMMoL	CML, juvenile		
	CML, juvenile			
Lymphomas	Very rare	Lymphoblastic	Lymphoblastic Undifferentiated	Lymphoblastic Undifferentiated, Burkitt's, Hodgkin's
SOLID TUMORS				
Central nervous system	Medulloblastoma Ependymoma Astrocytoma Choroid plexus papilloma	Medulloblastoma Ependymoma Astrocytoma Choroid plexus papilloma	Cerebellar astrocytoma Medulloblastoma Astrocytoma Ependymoma Craniopharyngioma	Cerebellar astrocytoma Astrocytoma Craniopharyngioma Medulloblastoma
Head and neck	Retinoblastoma Rhabdomyosarcoma Neuroblastoma Multiple endorcine neoplasia	Retinoblastoma Rhabdomyosarcoma Neuroblastoma	Rhabdomyosarcoma Lymphoma	Lymphoma Rhabdomyosarcoma
Thoracic	Neuroblastoma Teratoma	Neuroblastoma Teratoma	Lymphoma Neuroblastoma Rhabdomyosarcoma	Lymphoma Ewing's Rhabdomyosarcoma
Abdominal	Neuroblastoma Mesoblastic nephroma Heptabolastoma Wilms' (> 6 mos)	Neuroblastoma Wilms' Hepatoblastoma Leukemia	Neuroblastoma Wilms' Lymphoma Hepatoma	Lymphoma Hepatocellular carcinoma Rhabdomyosarcoma
Gonadal	Yolk sac tumor of testis (endodermal sinus tumor) Teratoma Sarcoma Botryoides Neuroblastoma	Rhabdomyosarcoma Yolk sac tumor of testis Clear cell sarcoma kidney	Rhabdomyosarcoma	Rhabdomyosarcoma Dysgerminoma Teratocarcinoma, teratoma Embryonal carcinoma of testis Embryonal cell and endothermal sinus tumors of ovary
Extremity	Fibrosarcoma	Fibrosarcoma Rhabdomyosarcoma	Rhabdomyosarcoma Ewing's	Osteosarcoma Rhabdomyosarcoma Ewing's sarcoma

Reprinted with permission from Pizzo PA, Miser JS, Cassidy JR, Filler RM. Solid tumors of childhood. In: DeVita VT Jr, Hellman S, Rosenberg SA, eds. *Cancer: Principles and Practice of Oncology*, 4th ed. Philadelphia: JB Lippincott; 1993: 1740.

and adrenocortical neoplasms. Li–Fraumeni syndrome is often suspected after diagnosis of childhood sarcomas. The mothers are at high risk of early breast cancer. Some of the affected families have a mutation in the p53 gene on chromosome 17 (20). Other diseases that predispose children to cancer include neurofibromatosis, immune-deficiency states, ataxia telangiectasia, Down's syndrome and Fanconi's anemia (Table 76.4) (19). Perturbations of normal host physiology can result in an increased incidence of certain tumors. For instance, the time of rapid bone growth in puberty coincides with increased risk of developing osteogenic sarcoma. The interaction of environmental with genetic factors may also increase the risk of cancer, as shown in Table 76.5.

Inborn cytogenetic abnormalities predispose patients to an increased risk of cancer (Table 76.6) (23). Many solid tumors have abnormal chromosomes (Table 76.7) (23). A large number of nonrandom cytogenetic abnormalities have been described in leukemia, the best known being the Philadelphia chromosome in the adult type of chronic myelogenous leukemia. These observations suggest that all cancers have genetic aberrations, whether due to a preexisting or acquired mutation, a combination of mutations or a series of mutations involving multiple agents.

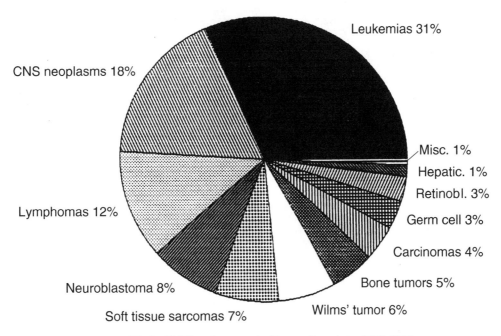

FIG. 76–4. Childhood cancer incidence: Seer data, 1973–1987.

Based on clinical and epidemiological observations, Knudson (21) suggested a two step process in the development of retinoblastoma. The subsequent discovery of oncogenes and tumor suppressor genes proved him correct and demonstrated a similar genetic mechanism in the development of other childhood cancers, including Wilms' tumor, hepatoblastoma, rhabdomyosarcoma and other tumors as well (Table 76.8).

BIOLOGIC DIFFERENCES BETWEEN CANCER IN CHILDREN AND ADULTS

The common cancers in children differ from those seen in adults in their tissue type, embryonic origin and in the presumed causative factors (Table 76.9). Pediatric cancers respond better to therapy and have much higher cure rates. Although the reason is not always evident, a tumor of identical histology in an adult or a child has a better prognosis in the latter; one explanation is that children can tolerate more intensive therapy (24).

CLINICAL MANIFESTATIONS

Signs and symptoms of cancer may mimic those of many other diseases. Cancer in children is rare, thus always unexpected and rarely high on a physician's list of differential diagnoses. Other possibilities, including psychosomatic disorders, are often pursued for a prolonged period of time. Because early diagnosis may prolong survival, the physician must always have a high index of suspicion. Patients may present with evident tumor, usually a lump, with symptoms caused by the tumor, such as severe anemia, or with non-specific symptoms, such as fever or vomiting. Some conditions that resemble cancer are so likely to be benign that they may safely be observed, such as inflammatory large lymph nodes, hemangiomas, or tumors whose characteristic location reveal a benign nature, such as benign pubertal gynecomastia in boys, thyroglossal duct cyst or ganglions. All other masses should be considered malignant until proven otherwise by excision biopsy.

Even more important for rapid diagnosis is to have the possibility of cancer in mind in patients with non-specific symptoms, such as hematuria from a urinary tumor, weight loss, or fever of unknown origin. Prolonged pain after trauma should alert the physician, and appropriate radiographs should be obtained promptly. Children cannot always localize pain or express what bothers them. For example, the only manifestation of bone pain may be limping, the inability to bear weight or irritability. Children with leukemia or neuroblastoma with bone metastasis are often misdiagnosed as having rheumatoid arthritis or "growing pains" because of apparently migratory bone or joint pain.

TABLE 76.4. *Selected Single Gene Traits Associated with Childhood and Adolescent Neoplasia*

Gene Trait, Neoplasm, or Disorder	Inheritance Chromosome* (if known)	Associated Neoplasms
PHAKOMATOSES		
von Recklinghausen's neurofibromatosis 1	AD[†] 17q11.2	Sarcoma, neuroma, schwannoma, meningioma, optic glioma, pheochromocytoma, nonlymphocytic leukemia
Tuberous sclerosis	AD[†] 9q11q	Adenoma sebaceum, periungual fibroma, glial tumors, rhabdomyoma of heart, renal tumor, lung cysts
von Hippel–Lindau syndrome	AD[†] 3p	Retinal angioma, cerebellar hemangioblastoma, other hemangiomas, pheochromocytoma, hypernephroma, cysts, gliomas
Sturge–Weber syndrome	AD	Angioma of numerous organs
NERVOUS SYSTEM		
Retinoblastoma	AD[†]; 13q14	Sarcoma, pinealoblastoma, early radiogenic tumors
Neurofibromatosis 2	AD[†]; 22q	Bilateral acoustic neuromas, meningioma, spinal neurofibroma
Neuroblastoma	AR; AD	
Macroencephaly	AD[†]	Ganglioneuroblastoma
ENDOCRINE		
Multiple endocrine neoplasia 1 (Wermer's syndrome; MEN-1)	AD[†] 11q13	Adenomas of islet cells, parathyroid, pituitary, and adrenal glands; malignant schwannoma; nonappendiceal carcinoid
Multiple endocrine neoplasia 2 (Sipple's syndrome; MEN-2)	AD[†] 10p	Medullary carcinoma of thyroid, parathyroid adenoma, pheochromocytoma
Multiple mucosal neuroma syndrome	AD[†] 10p	Pheochromocytoma, medullary carcinoma of the thyroid, neurofibroma, submucosal neuromas of tongue, lips, eyelids
Paraganglioma (Chemodectomal)	AD[†]	Pheochromocytoma
Pheochromocytoma	AD[†]	Parathyroid adenoma, chief cell hyperplasia
Thyroid goiter and dyshormonogenesis, including Pendred's syndrome	AD	Benign goiter
Arrhenoblastoma-thyroid adenoma	AD	
MESODERM (SOFT TISSUE)		
Nevoid basal cell carcinoma syndrome (Gorlin's syndrome)	AD[†] q31	Basal cell carcinoma, ovarian fibroma, medulloblastoma
Leopard syndrome	AD[†]	Multiple lentigines
Gingival fibromatosis ± hypertrichosis or other anomalies	AD[†]	
Juvenile fibromatosis	AR[†]	Multiple subcutaneous
Familial cutaneous collagenoma	AR	Multiple skin nodules
Multiple lipomatosis, sometimes site specific, neck or conjunctiva	AD[†]	Skin cancer
Goldenhar's syndrome	AR	Lipodermoid of conjunctiva, hemangioma
Macrosomia adiposa congenita	AR	Obese soon after birth, eosinophilia, adrenocortical adenoma
Multiple hamartoma (Cowden's) syndrome	AD[†]	Papillomatosis of lip; benign and malignant tumors of breast, colon and thyroid, meningioma
ALIMENTARY TRACT		
Familial polyposis coli and Gardner's syndrome	AD[†] 5q21	Carcinoma of colon; hepatoblastoma, intestinal polyps, osteomas, fibromas, sebaceous cysts, carcinomas of ampulla of Vater, pancreas, thyroid, and adrenal
Peutz–Jeghers syndrome	AD[†]	Intestinal polyps, ovarian (granulosa cell) tumor
Turcot syndrome	AR[†]	Brain tumor, intestinal polyposis
Hereditary pancreatitis	AD[†]	Carcinoma of pancreas
Tylosis with esophageal cancer	AD[†]	Carcinoma of esophagus
Familial, juvenile, and neonatal cirrhosis	AD[†] AR[†]	Hepatocellular carcinoma
Hemochromatosis	AD[†] AR[†]; 6p	Hepatocellular carcinoma

(continued)

TABLE 76.4. — *Continued*

Gene Trait, Neoplasm, or Disorder	Inheritance Chromosome* (if known)	Associated Neoplasms
UROGENITAL		
Gonadal dysgenesis, hermaphroditism, Reifenstein's syndrome, testicular feminization	AR† AR XR†	Gonadoblastoma, dysgerminoma
Wilms' tumor	AD†; 11p13, 11p15	
Neprhoblastomatosis (Perlman syndrome)		
VASCULAR		
Multiple glomus tumors	AD†	
Hereditary hemorrhagic telangiectasia of Rendu-Osler-Weber	AD†	Angioma
Lymphedema with distichiasis	AD†	Lymphangiosarcoma of edematous limb
SKELETAL		
Multiple exostosis	AD†	Osteosarcoma, chondrosarcoma
Cherubism	AD†	Fibrous dysplasia of jaws, giant cell tumor
Fibro-osseous dysplasia	AD	Osteosarcoma, medullary fibrosarcoma
Paget's disease of bone	AD	Osteosarcoma
Enchondromatosis (Ollier's syndrome)	AD	Bone tumors, hemangioma (Maffucci's syndrome)
OSLAM syndrome	AD	Osteosarcoma
LYMPHATIC AND HEMATOPOIETIC		
Histiocytic reticulosis generalized or neural only (Letterer–Siwe disease)	AR† AR XR†	
Familial lipochrome histiocytosis	AR†	
X-linked hyperproliferative syndrome of Purtilo	XR†	Burkitt and other lymphomas
Kostmann infantile genetic agranulocytosis	AR†	Acute monocytic leukemia (chromosomal breaks)
Polycythemia rubra vera	AR	Acute myelogenous leukemia
Glutathione reductase deficiency	AR†	Leukemia (chromosomal breaks)
Leukemia	AD	
Other lymphoproliferative disorders	AD	
Familial eosinophilia	AD†	
IMMUNODEFICIENCY		
Bruton agammaglobulinemia	XR†	Leukemia, lymphoreticular
Wiskott–Aldrich syndrome	XR†	Lymphoreticular
Ataxia-telangiectasia	AR† 11q22	Lymphoreticular, leukemia, carcinoma of stomach, brain tumors (chromosomal breaks)
Chediak-Higashi syndrome	AR†	Pseudolymphoma
MULTIPLE SYSTEM		
Bloom's syndrome	AR†	Leukemia, intestinal cancer (chromosomal breaks)
Fanconi's pancytopenia	AR† 20q	Acute monomyelogenous leukemia, squamous cell carcinoma of mucocutaneous junctions, hepatic carcinoma and adenoma (chromosomal breaks)
Dyskeratosis congenita	XR†	Leukoplakia with squamous cell carcinoma, including of cervix
Zinsser–Cole–Engman's syndrome	AD	
Nijmegen (Seemanova) syndrome	AR	Lymphoreticular malignancy (chromosomal breaks)
Beckwith-Wiedemann's syndrome	AR† 11p15	Visceromegaly, cytomegaly, macroglossia, adrenocortical neoplasia, Willms' tumor, hepatoma
Rothmund–Thomson's syndrome	AR†	Squamous cell carcinoma
Werner's syndrome	AR†	Sarcoma
Osteopoikilosis	AD†	Nevi
Noonan's syndrome	AD†	Schwannoma
Focal dermal hypoplasia (Goltz's syndrome)	AD†; 17p	Sarcomas of bone and soft tissue; young age breast carcinoma, brain tumors; leukemia; lung, and laryngeal cancer; adrenal corticla neoplasia

(continued)

TABLE 76.4. *Selected Single Gene Traits Associated with Childhood and Adolescent Neoplasia — Continued*

Gene Trait, Neoplasm, or Disorder	Inheritance Chromosome* (if known)	Associated Neoplasms
INBORN ERRORS OF METABOLISM		
Angiokeratoma diffusa (Fabry's syndrome)	XR[†]	
Tyrosinemia, hypermethioninemia, galactosemia, Wilson's disease, glycogen storage disease IV	AR[†] AR	Postcirrhotic hepatoma
Alpha-1-antitrypsin deficiency	Codominant; 14q31	Hepatoma, hepatocellular carcinoma
Vitamin D-resistant rickets	XR[†]	Parathyroid adenoma

*AD = autosomal dominant; AR = autosomal recessive; XD = X-linked dominant; XR = X-linked recessive.
[†]Mode of inheritance considered proved.
Reprinted with permission from Pizzo PA, Poplack DG, eds. *Principles and Practice of Pediatric Oncology*, 2nd ed. Philadelphia: JB Lippincott, 1993: 21–22.

TABLE 76.5. *Genetic–Environmental Interactions (Ecogenetics) in Tumors of the Young*

Environmental Agent	Genetic Trait	Tumor or Outcome
Ionizing radiation	Ataxis-telangiectasia with lymphoma	Radiation toxicity
	Retinoblastoma	Sarcoma
	Nevoid basal cell carcinoma syndrome	Basal cell carcinoma
		Medulloblastoma
Ultraviolet radiation	Xeroderma pigmentosum	Skin cancer, melanoma
	Cutaneous albinism	Skin cancer
	Hereditary dysplastic nevus syndrome	Melanoma
Stilbestrol	Turner syndrome	Adenosquamous endometrial carcinoma
Androgen	Fanconi pancytopenia	Hepatoma, benign and malignant
Iron	Hemochromatosis	Hepatocellular carcinoma
Tyrosine	Tyrosinemia	Hepatocellular carcinoma
Monosaccharides	Glycogen storage disease type 1	Hepatic adenoma
Epstein–Barr virus	Purtilo X-linked lymphoproliferative syndrome	Burkitt and other lymphomas
Papillomavirus type 5	Epidermodysplasia verruciformis	Skin cancer
Hepatitis B virus	Virus integration site	Hepatocellular carcinoma

Reprinted with permission from Pizzo PA, Poplack DG, eds. *Principles and Practice of Pediatric Oncology*, 2nd ed. Philadelphia: JB Lippincott, 1993: 12.

TABLE 76.6. *Childhood and Adolescent Neoplasms in Constitutional Cytogenetic Disorders*

Chromosome	Abnormality	Neoplasms
8	Trisomy	Preleukemia
11	Deletion q13	Miller's syndrome or sporadic aniridia with and without Wilms' tumor
13	Deletion q14	Sporadic retinoblastoma with and without birth defects; osteosarcoma; early radiogenic sarcomas; pinealoblastoma
21	Trisomy	Acute leukemia in Down's syndrome
X	Monosomy	Endometrial adenosquamous carcinoma in estrogen treated Turner's syndrome; possibly neural tumors
X	Extra	Breast carcinoma; extragonadal germ cell tumors in Klinefelter's syndrome
Y	Present	Gonadolbastoma in gonadal dysgenesis syndromes

Reprinted with permission from Pizzo PA, Poplack DG, eds. *Principles and Practice of Pediatric Oncology*, 2nd ed. Philadelphia: JB Lippincott, 1993: 19.

TABLE 76.7. *Selected Chromosomal Aberrations Associated with Pediatric Solid Tumors*

Ewing's sarcoma	t(11; 22) (q24; q12)
Germ cell tumors ovarian	i(12p)
	6q breaks
Glioma	del(9p)
	DMs
Medulloblastoma	i(17q)
	DMs
Neuroblastoma	del(1) (p32–36)
	DMs, HSRs
Osteosarcoma	del(13) (q14) or 13q14 alteration
Peripheral PNET	t(11; 22) (q24; q12)
Retinoblastoma	del(13) (q14) or 13q14 alteration
	1p or 1q aberrations
	i(6p)
Rhabdomyosarcoma	
Alveolar	t(2; 13) (q35; q14)
Embryonal	11p15.5 alterations
Synovial sarcoma	t(X; 18) Op11.2; q11.2)
Wilms' tumor	del(11) (p13) or 11p13/11p15 alterations
	1p or 1q alterations
	+12

Reprinted with permission from Pizzo PA, Poplack DG, eds. *Principles and Practice of Pediatric Oncology*, 2nd ed. Philadelphia: JB Lippincott, 1993: 40.

TABLE 76.8. *Cancer-Associated Genes Implicated in Selected Pediatric Malignancies*

Leukemia
  P53, *abl, fms, K-ras, myb, myc,* N-*ras, src*

Lymphoma
  bcl, myb, myc, ras

Glioma
  P53, *erb* B, *fes, myb, myc, neu,* N-*ras, raf, ros, sis*

Wilms' Tumor
  WT-1, *myb,* N-*myc*

Neuroblastoma
  myb, myc, N-*myc,* N-*ras, src*

Retinoblastoma
  RB, N-*myc, src*

Germ cell tumors
  hst, *myc,* N-*myc*

Rhabdomyosarcoma
  P53, *fos, K-ras, myb, myc,* N-*ras, rel, src*

Osteogenic sarcoma
  RB, *met, sis, sc*

Ewings' sarcoma
  dbl, ets, myc, raf, src

PNET
  ets, myc, raf, src

Reprinted with permission from Pizzo PA, Poplack DG, eds. *Principles and Practice of Pediatric Oncology*, 2nd ed. Philadelphia: JB Lippincott, 1993: 74.

TABLE 76.9. *Biologic Differences, Childhood and Adult Cancers*

	Pediatric	Adult
Incidence	133/million/yr (5)	4,041/million/yr (22)
New Cases/Year	9,308/million/yr (25)	1,100,000/million/yr
Mortality/Year	1,686/million/yr	520,000/million/yr
Median Age	7 years	65 years
Common Tumors	Leukemia/Sarcoma/CNS*	Carcinoma
Cell Type	Mesenchymal	Epithelial
Tissue of Origin	Mesoderm	Ectoderm
Embryonal Origin	Frequent	Rare
Congenital Anomalies	Frequent	Rare
Environmental Etiology Likely	Rare	Frequent
Genetic Etiology Likely	Frequent	Rare
Familial Incidence	Variable	Rare
Latency Period	Short	Long
Response to Therapy	> 90%	Variable†
Cure Rate	> 60%	Variable†

*CNS, central nervous system. † The control and cure of most adult cancers depend largely on complete surgical resection—thus, success varies within each tumor type.

Once the diagnosis of cancer has been considered seriously, a vigorous and rapid work-up should be initiated. If the local facilities are inadequate for a complete evaluation, the patient should be referred to a center with extensive experience in childhood cancer. Inadequate medical evaluation may result in unsatisfactory, incomplete or inappropriate surgery, further delays, possibly a second surgical procedure and, most important, loss of the chance of cure.

PROGNOSTIC FACTORS

With rare exceptions, no child with cancer should be considered incurable no matter the type of tumor or how advanced the disease is at diagnosis. Generally, cancer in children is far more sensitive to chemotherapy than cancer in adults. Children also tolerate therapy much better and rarely have co-morbid diseases that complicate treatment, such as diabetes or heart disease. Therefore, more intensive therapy is possible.

The identification of prognostic factors provides essential data for the design of proper therapy. Therapy that may be adequate for localized disease, could be insufficient for widespread involvement. Therapy that is necessary for the eradication of widespread metastases may be excessive for localized disease exposing the patient to unnecessary risks. Overaggressive therapy could unnecessarily suppress the patient's immune defenses, which may help eradicate the last vestiges of cancer and protect against opportunistic infections. Therefore, the treatment and its duration must be tailored to the specific type of cancer, its extent and prognosis. Important prognostic factors vary with the specific cancer and include: stage, which describes the anatomic extent of the tumor, its site, histology, and immunologic, cytogenetic and molecular features (24). For some cancers, age at diagnosis is a prognostic factor. Infants with neuroblastoma or Wilms' tumor have a better outcome than older patients while infants with acute lymphoblastic leukemia have a worse prognosis. Prognostic factors are treatment specific. Improved therapy can minimize or abolish the influence of even the most powerful prior predictors of outcome (23).

Once treatment is initiated, the rate of the tumor's response to therapy can further divide patients into good and poor prognostic categories. The faster the response, the better the prognosis. After one week of therapy for acute lymphoblastic leukemia, one can separate patients on the basis of the residual leukemia in the bone marrow or blood into those that have a 25% and those that have a 75% chance of cure, even though both groups will be in complete remission after one month of therapy (26).

SPECIAL CONSIDERATIONS IN THE MANAGEMENT OF THE PEDIATRIC PATIENT

Caring for the child with cancer is heart-rending, time-consuming and often frustrating. The physician is put in the awkward position of being the family doctor, marriage counselor, patient advocate, and protector of a family in turmoil. At the same time, he must provide excellent medical care and maintain the entire family's confidence and trust. Profound patience in the face of provocation and reproach from frightened and frustrated parents and patients is an absolute requirement. Beyond these, the physician must deal with his own anxieties.

Facilities Required for Optimal Results

For optimal results in the care of children with cancer the pediatric oncologist must carefully orchestrate a team that must include a pediatric surgeon, nurse, social worker, radiologist, radiotherapist, pathologist, pharmacist, and a variety of other subspeciality consultants. Data from nuclear medicine and various clinical and research laboratories has to be incorporated into the treatment plan. Psychosocial issues often emerge because parents, siblings, grandparents, and the numerous friends of the family all try to help but unintentionally may do as much harm as good by raising doubts about the diagnosis or suggesting inappropriate alternatives. Psychologic supportive care, rehabilitation, services of nutritionists, respiratory therapists, play, occupational therapists, and physiotherapists need to be integrated into the overall plan. Teachers and tutors are required to help the patient keep up with the work missed in school. The major pediatric cancer centers possess the multidisciplinary facilities that are required for good long-term results.

It has been shown that patients cared for in centers who participate in formal nationally approved clinical trials have a better chance of survival (27–29). Even though many of today's chemotherapy protocols seem like cookbook recipes, the end result depends a great deal on the experience and expertise of the chef. Also, one of the greatest sources of emotional support for the patient and the family is other patients and families with similar experiences. The fact that they are not the only ones burdened with this ordeal makes it more bearable. Sharing similar experiences reduces the feeling of isolation.

Discussion of the Disease with the Patient

Cancer occurs at every age. The wide spectrum of age, body size, understanding and maturity requires a different approach tailored to each child's personality and ability to comprehend. Children and adolescents with cancer continue to have the same problems of childhood and adolescence as do their peers without cancer. The particular problems caused by the disease and its treatment compound and magnify the universal ones. How the child deals with the disease will depend greatly on the age, specific cancer, symptoms, personality, intelligence, previous experience, and background, as well as interactions with his parents and physician. The parents and the physician together must decide what the child will and will not be told and what will be divulged to other family members and friends. Experience shows that children, especially adolescents, should be told in understandable terms the name and nature of the cancer and what it is likely to mean. If this is not done, they will sense the conspiracy of silence around them and they become hostile, resentful, isolated, distrustful, uncooperative, and antagonistic. When they are told the truth, they can talk about the disease and thus create avenues for more meaningful relationships with the doctor and parents. If the parents insist on silence, then the explanation will have to be good enough to justify repeated blood tests, radiation therapy, bone marrow aspirations, lumbar punctures and intravenous medications, and their attendant side effects, such as alopecia, severe nausea and vomiting, and peripheral neuropathy. The terms "anemia," "infection in the blood" or "tumor" are frequently used by parents, but children often learn of their diagnosis from siblings or peers.

Today's children tend to be more knowledgeable about human biology than their parents and, if motivated, can learn the truth in their school or community library in a few minutes. However, the information in most general libraries is almost always outdated and inaccurate. It is much preferred that the patient learn the truth from their physician. Prearmed with this knowledge, they will most likely be more informed about their disease than anyone they will encounter. They will then be able to refute with facts any comments that could otherwise be very destructive. It is not uncommon for a patient to be told by classmates that "you have leukemia and you are going to die." When the parents decide that they are going to "protect" the patient, the patient plays along and in the end it is the child who protects the parents, themselves unable to accept the diagnosis. This leads to unnecessary loneliness and the isolation of the patient. When children are told that they have leukemia, they accept it without untoward reactions, many with surprising relief. The truth is frequently better than the possibilities conjured up by an unbridled imagination.

Family Considerations

Parents may want to restrict discussion of the diagnosis to close family members and friends. In some instances, wide dissemination of the information leads to community isolation of the family. Even when it is known that the cancer is not contagious, the family is avoided because friends and neighbors are uncomfortable with the disease. They feel sorry for the patient, but the patient does not want to be pitied or to feel different. He wants to be normal and should be treated as normally as possible. Relations with grandparents can also be difficult. Often, instead of giving support to the family, they are the ones who need the help. With good intentions and trying to help, they may raise doubts about the diagnosis, suggest "shopping" for alternatives or the "magic cure" and may even create a disruptive aura of tension, guilt and anger. The diagnosis should be shared with siblings old enough to understand; otherwise they will resent the seemingly special treatment accorded the patient. Clergy can be of help to the family, but only if meaningful relations existed before the onset of the illness.

The parents should be told, even if they do not ask, that their action or inaction had nothing to do with causing the cancer or its prevention. Parents want to be reassured that the malignancy is not infectious and that their other children are not susceptible. It is a good policy to reassure them—even in cases of leukemia when it is virtually though not technically, true—that their other child has the same small chance of developing leukemia as any other unrelated child. The parent should be reassured that the latest and best medical care will be provided and that new developments in the field will be constantly monitored. After the parents have heard that their child has cancer, everything that is related thereafter may be heard with only half an ear. They frequently hear, but do not comprehend, what is said so that most of the points must be restated at a later date, usually several times. Parents should be urged to write down any questions that they might have in the future.

Child–Physician Interaction

The child must form a positive relationship with the physician. The success of the therapy will depend, especially with teenagers, on how well the adolescent relates to the physician. They must feel that the doctor is trustworthy and interested, and will be available to provide continuous and personalized care. Patients should be told at least that they have a "tumor" or "leukemia," and that the condition is serious, that it requires prompt treatment and that effective therapy is available. They should be reassured that patients much sicker have been cured. A basic understanding of the disease process, its treatment and its possible complications should be presented. The child should be prepared for the upcoming hardships, inconvenience and disruption of normal life style. It should be stressed that utmost cooperation will be needed. They should be reassured that the physician will always explain what will be done beforehand so that the patient can be prepared. The child needs to be reassured that they will be warned in advance if a painful procedure is to be done so that they can trust and believe when told that a test will be pain-free. Whenever possible, painful or frightening procedures should be done under brief general anesthesia, with sedation or effective local anesthesia.

The child wants to know and must be told before surgery exactly what will be done and what to expect once they awaken, the anesthetic to be used, the length of the incision, the severity and duration of postoperative pain, the anticipated degree of disability and the need for rehabilitation. Cooperation will be difficult to elicit unless the patient is informed and prepared. In many hospitals, specialized nurses aid in the pre-operation preparation. When amputation is contemplated, the fact has to be told. It is best if the adolescent can meet a patient who has successfully undergone a similar procedure so that they will not feel isolated and alone. Seeing a patient with a functioning prosthesis can be a very reassuring experience. Adolescents cannot tolerate dishonesty. The doctor–patient relationship could be destroyed at the outset if proper care in preoperative preparation is not taken.

Extraordinary Chemotherapy Issues

Special needs of children have to be considered in the design and administration of chemotherapy. The doses of chemotherapy are generally calculated for the patients size based on body surface area. For some agents, this method can overestimate the drug tolerance of infants for whom doses based body weight can be more appropriate. In young children, the head to body size ratio is much greater than in adults. The head and cerebrospinal fluid volume reaches adult size by three years of age, while adult height is not reached until the teens. Thus, intrathecal medications calculated according to body surface will underdose younger children. Adults' body surface area changes little during chemotherapy or may actually decrease if there is significant weight loss. Children on the

other hand can grow significantly during the two to three year period of treatment and unless the chemotherapy is adjusted periodically, therapy may be inadequate. It is important to keep in mind that small children cannot swallow tablets and that some medications do not come in liquid form; the closest one can reliably divide a tablet is in half and capsules cannot be subdivided. Teenagers often fail to comply with self administered prescriptions; when possible, one should rely more on observed parenteral drug administration than on oral medications taken at home.

Late Effects of Therapy

Children successfully treated for cancer have many decades of life expectancy (3). This success has created a new set of potential problems, the late effects of therapy (30–40). The inability of irradiated normal tissues to develop properly can lead to some growth failure, occasional learning disabilities, or hormone deficiencies. Even when the total dose of daunomycin and adriamycin has been kept under what was considered to be a safe level to prevent short-term cardiotoxicity, with long-term follow-up, aging, and atherosclerosis, the myocardial function of these patients may continue to deteriorate (33). Cyclophosphamide, ifosfamide and carboplatin uncommonly have long-term deleterious effects on the urinary bladder. Pulmonary fibrosis has been described on rare occasions with methotrexate, BCNU, busulfan, bleomycin, and cyclophosphamide. Methotrexate and ifosfamide at times may cause lasting neurotoxicity. Platinum compounds and repeated courses of some antibiotics can lead infrequently to permanent hearing loss and nephrotoxicity. Alkylating agents, epipidophyllotoxins, procarbazine and topoisomerase inhibitors are carcinogenic and may cause second malignancies in less than 5% of very intensively treated patients. Fertility is always a concern. While it is reasonable to expect that some cancer therapies impair the ability to conceive, the majority of the babies born to survivors of cancer have been normal. One must remember that these potential problems have come to light only because of the success in curing patients and the pediatrician's special concerns about the delayed consequences of therapy in a growing patient with a long life expectancy. While the study of these problems will aid the design of better therapies in the future, it should be remembered that the vast majority of survivors of childhood cancer are doing well, leading normal productive lives.

Specific Tumors

A detailed description of the common pediatric cancers is beyond the scope of this chapter. Recent reviews of the most common pediatric malignancies are listed in the references: acute lymphoblastic leukemia (41–44); acute myelogenous leukemia (45–47), brain tumors (48), lymphoma (49–53), neuroblastoma (54), Wilms' tumor (55–57), rhabdomyosarcoma (58), osteogenic sarcoma (59–61), Ewing's sarcoma (62–64).

REFERENCES

1. Hammond GD. Keynote Address, The cure of childhood cancer. *Cancer.* 1986; 58:2:407–413.
2. Pediatric Oncology Group. Progress against childhood cancer: The Pediatric Oncology Group Experience. *Pediatrics.* 1992; 89:597–600.
3. Bleyer WA. What can be learned about childhood cancer from "Cancer Statistics Review 1973–1988." *Cancer.* 1993; 71:3229–3236.
4. Boring CC, Squires TST, Tong T. Cancer Statistics. *CA Cancer J Clin.* 1991; 41:19–36.
5. Gurney JG, Severson RK, Davis S, Robison LL. Incidence of cancer in children in the United States, Sex-, race-, and 1-year age specific rates by histologic type. *Cancer.* 1995; 75:2186–2195.
6. Bleyer WA. The impact of childhood cancer on the United States and the world. *CA Cancer J Clin.* 1990; 40:355–368.
7. Bethesda MD. Division of Cancer Prevention and Control Surveillance Program. Cancer Statistics Review, 1973–1986. NIH Publication No. 89-2789. Bethesda MD: National Cancer Institute; May 1989.
8. Mulvihill JJ. Exogenetic origins of cancer in the young; Environmental and genetic determinants. In: Levine AS, ed. *Cancer in the Young.* New York: Masson; 1982: 13–17.
9. Doll R. The epidemiology of cancer. *Cancer.* 1980; 45:2475–2485.
10. Schwartzbaum JA, George SL, Pratt CB, Davis B. An exploratory study of environmental and medical factors potentially related to childhood cancer. *Med Pediatr Oncol.* 1991; 19:115–121.
11. Higginson J. Environmental carcinogenesis. *Cancer.* 1993; 72:971–973.
12. Pitot HC: The molecular biology of carcinogenesis. *Cancer.* 1993; 72:962–970.
13. Buckley JD, Hobbie WL, Ruccione K, et al. Maternal smoking during pregnancy and the risk of childhood cancer. *Lancet.* 1986; 2:519–520.
14. Bunin GR, Meadows AT, Emanuel BS, et al. Pre- and post-conception factors associated with sporadic heritable and nonheritable retinoblastoma. *Cancer Res.* 1989; 49:5730–5735.
15. Olshan AF, Breslow NE, Falletta JM, et al. Risk factors for Wilms tumor: Report from the National Wilms Tumor Study. *Cancer.* 1993; 72:938–944.
16. Goldhaber MK, Selby JV, Hiatt RA, Quesenberry BR. Exposure to barbiturates in utero and during childhood and risk of intracranial and spinal cord tumors. *Cancer Res.* 1990; 50:4600–4663.

17. Bunin GR, Buckley JD, Boesel CP, et al. Risk factors for astrocytic glioma and primitive neuroectodermal tumor of the brain in young children: A report from the Children's Cancer Group. *Cancer Epidemiol Biomarkers Prev.* 1994; 3:197–204.
18. Robinson LL, Buckley JD, Diagle AE, et al. Maternal drug use and risk of childhood acute non-lymphoblastic leukemia: An epidemiologic investigation implication marijuana. *Cancer.* 1989; 63:1904–1911.
19. Mulvihill JJ. Childhood cancer, the environment, and heredity. In Pizzo PA, Poplack DG, eds. 2nd ed. Philadelphia: JB Lippincott; 1993: 11–27.
20. Malkin D, Li FP, Strong LC, et al. Germ line p53 mutations in a familial syndrome of breast cancer, sarcomas, and other neoplasms. *Science.* 1990; 250:1233–1238.
21. Knudson AG Jr. Mutation and cancer: Statistical study of retinoblastoma. *Proc Nat Acad Sci USA.* 1971; 68:820–823.
22. Fraumeni JR Jr, Hoover RN, Devesa SS, Kinlen LJ. Epidemiology of cancer. In: DeVita VT Jr Hellman S, Rosenburg SA. eds. *Cancer Principles & Practice of Oncology.* 4th ed. Philadelphia: JB Lippincott, 1993: 150–181.
23. Pizzo PA, Poplack DG, eds. *Principles and Practice of Pediatric Oncology.* 2nd ed. Philadelphia: JB Lippincott; 1993.
24. Miller DR. Childhood acute lymphoblastic leukemia. 1. Biological features and their use in predicting outcome of treatment. *Am J Pediatr Hematol Oncol.* 1988; 10:163–173.
25. Miller RW, Young JL Jr, Novakovic B. Childhood cancer. *Cancer.* 1994; 75:385–405.
26. Steinherz PG, Gaynon PS, Breneman JC, et al. Cytoreduction and prognosis in acute lymphoblastic leukemia: The importance of rapid early response. Report from the Childrens Cancer Group. *J Clin Oncol.* 1996; 14:2703–2706.
27. Tefft M, Brown A, Burke BA, et al. American academy of pediatrics: Guidelines for the pediatric cancer center and role of such centers in diagnosis and treatment. *Pediatrics.* 1986; 77:916–917.
28. Kramer S, Meadows AT, Pastore G, et al. Influence of place of treatment on diagnosis, treatment and survival in three pediatric solid tumors. *J Clin Oncol.* 1984; 2: 917–923.
29. Meadows AT, Kramer S, Hopson R, et al. Survival in childhood acute lymphocytic leukemia: Effect of protocol and place of treatment. *Cancer Invest.* 1983; 1:49–55.
30. Hoffman B. Current issues of cancer survivorship. *Oncology.* 1989; 3:85–88.
31. Mulhern RK, Abby L, Wasserman AL, et al. Social competence and behavioral adjustment of children who are long-term survivors of cancer. *Pediatrics.* 1989; 83:18–25.
32. Green DM, Zevon MA, Hall B. Achievement of life goals by adult survivors of modern treatment for childhood cancer. *Cancer.* 1991; 67:206–213.
33. Steinherz LJ, Steinherz PG, Tan CTC, et al. Cardiac toxicity 4–20 years after completing anthracycline therapy. *J Am Med Assoc.* 1991; 266:1672–1677.
34. Neglia JP, Meadows AT, Robison LL, et al. Second neoplasms after acute lymphocytic leukemia in childhood. *N Engl J Med.* 1991; 325:1330–1336.

35. Feeny D, Furlong W, Barr RD, et al. A comprehensive multiattribute system for classifying the health status of survivors of childhood cancer. *J Clin Oncol.* 1992; 10:923–928.

36. Feeny D, Leiper A, Barr RD, et al. The comprehensive assessment of health status in survivors of childhood cancer: application to high-risk acute lymphocytic leukemia. *Br J Cancer.* 1993; 67:1047–1052.

37. Hays DM. Adult survivors of childhood cancer—Employment and insurance issues in different age groups. *Cancer.* 1993; 71:3306–3309.

38. Neglia JP: Childhood cancer survivors—Past, present, and future. *Cancer.* 1994; 73:2883–2885.

39. Nicholson HS, Fears TR, Byrne J. Death during adulthood in survivors of childhood and adolescent cancer. *Cancer.* 1994; 73:3094–3102.

40. Robertson CM, Hawkins MM, Kingston JE. Late deaths and survival after childhood cancer: implications for cure. *Br Med J.* 1994; 309:162–166.

41. Greaves M. A natural history for pediatric acute leukemia. *Blood.* 1993; 82:1043–1051.

42. Pui C-H, Crist WM. Biology and treatment of acute lymphoblastic leukemia. *J Pediatr.* 1994; 124:491–503.

43. Miller DR: Hematologic malignancies: leukemia and lymphoma. In: Miller DR, Baehner RL, Miller LP, eds. 7th ed. *Blood Diseases of Infancy and Childhood in the Tradition of C.H. Smith.* New York: Mosby; 1995: 660–804.

44. Rivera GK, Pinkel D, Simone JV, et al. Treatment of acute lymphoblastic leukemia. Thirty year's experience of St. Jude Children's Research Hospital. *N Engl J Med.* 1993; 329:1289–1295.

45. Creutzig U, Ritter J, Zimmermann M, Schellong G. Does cranial irradiation reduce the risk for bone marrow relapse in acute myelogenous leukemia? Unexpected results of the childhood acute myelogenous leukemia study BFM-87. *J Clin Oncol.* 1993; 11:279–286.

46. Nesbit ME Jr, Buckley JD, Feig SA, et al. Chemotherapy for induction of remission of childhood acute myeloid leukemia followed by marrow transplantation or multiagent chemotherapy: A report from the Childrens Cancer Group. *J Clin Oncol.* 1994; 12:127–135.

47. Wells RJ, Woods WG, Buckley, JD, et al. Treatment of newly diagnosed children and adolescents with acute myeloid leukemia: A Childrens Cancer Group Study. *J Clin Oncol.* 1994; 12:2367–2377.

48. Cohen ME, Duffner PK, Eds. Brain Tumors in Children—Principles of diagnosis and treatment. 2nd ed. New York: Raven Press; 1994.

49. Link MP, Donaldson SS, Berard CW, et al. Results of treatment of childhood localized non-Hodgkin's lymphoma with combination chemotherapy with or without radiotherapy. *N Engl J Med.* 1990; 322:1169–1174.

50. Anderson JR, Jenkin RDT, Wilson JF, et al. Long-term follow-up of patients treated with COMP or LSA$_2$L$_2$ therapy for childhood non-Hodgkin's lymphoma: A report of CCG-552 from the Childrens Cancer Group. *J Clin Oncol.* 1993; 11:1024–1032.

51. Maity A, Goldwein JW, Lange B, D'Angio GJ. Comparison of high-dose and low-dose radiation with and without chemotherapy for children with Hodgkin's disease: An analysis of the experience at the Children's Hospital of Philadelphia and the Hospital of the University of Pennsylvania. *J Clin Oncol.* 1992; 10: 929–935.

52. Mendenhall NP, Cantor AB, Williams JL, et al. With modern imaging techniques, is staging laparotomy necessary in pediatric Hodgkin's disease? A Pediatric Oncology Group Study. *J Clin Oncol.* 1993; 11: 2218–2225.

53. Hudson MM, Greenwald C, Thompson E, et al. Efficacy and toxicity of multiagent chemotherapy and low-dose involved-field radiotherapy in children and adolescents with Hodgkin's disease. *J Clin Oncol.* 1993; 11:100–108.

54. Bonilla MA, Cheung N-K V. Neuroblastoma. *Cancer Invest.* 1994; 12(6):644–653.

55. Bonaiti-Pellie C, Chompret A, Tournade MF, et al. Genetics and epidemiology of Wilms' tumor: The French Wilms' tumor study. *Med Pediatr Oncol.* 1992; 20:284–291.

56. Breslow N, Sharples K, Beckwith JB, et al. Prognostic factors in nonmetastatic, favorable histology Wilms' tumor. *Cancer.* 1991; 68:2343–2353.

57. Green DM, Breslow NE, Beckwith JB, et al. Treatment outcomes in patients less than 2 years of age with small, Stage I, favorable-histology Wilms' tumors: A report from the National Wilms' Tumor Study. *J Clin Oncol.* 1993; 11:91–95.

58. Pappo AS, Shapiro DN, Crist WM, Maurer HM. Biology and therapy of pediatric rhabdomyosarcoma. *J Clin Oncol.* 1995; 13:2123–2139.

59. Meyers PA. Malignant bone tumors in children: Ewing's sarcoma. *Hematol Oncol Clin N Am.* 1987; 1:667–673.

60. Damron TA, Pritchard DJ. Current combined treatment of high-grade osteosarcomas. *Oncol.* 1995; 9:327–340.

61. Meyers PA, Heller G, Healey J, et al. Chemotherapy for nonmetastatic osteogenic sarcoma: The Memorial Sloan–Kettering experience. *J Clin Oncol.* 1992; 10:5–15.

62. Oberlin O, Habrand J-L, Zucker JM, et al. No benefit of ifosfamide in Ewing's sarcoma: A nonrandomized study of the French Society of Pediatric Oncology. *J Clin Oncol.* 1992; 10:1407–1412.

63. Burgert EO, Nesbit ME, Garnsey LA, et al. Multimodal therapy for the management of nonpelvic, localized Ewing's sarcoma of bone: Intergroup Study IESS-II. *J Clin Oncol.* 1990; 8:1514–1524.

64. Picci P, Rougraff BT, Bacci G, et al. Prognostic significance of histopathologic response to chemotherapy in nonmetastatic Ewing's sarcoma of the extremities. *J Clin Oncol.* 1993; 11:1763–1769.

77

Psychological Problems of Curative Cancer Treatment

MARIA DIE-TRILL AND MARGARET L. STUBER

Treatment for pediatric malignancies has changed dramatically over the past 30 years. More aggressive treatment has significantly improved the prognosis while increasing the complications. For example, acute lymphoblastic leukemia (ALL), the most common form of childhood malignancy, had a six month survival rate of 4% in 1966; now 65% of children with ALL live at least 5 years after diagnosis (1,2). However, repeated hospitalizations, radiation, and steroids are extremely stressful and can interfere with normal development, resulting in physical, social, academic, and emotional difficulties.

Children are also more actively involved in treatment than they were in the past. Increasing knowledge of children's affective cognitive and behavioral development and greater participation of mental health professionals in the pediatric oncology setting have changed the approach from one of protective secrecy to open communication at developmentally appropriate levels. Children are now seen as capable of understanding the severity and chronicity of their condition and being active participants in their treatment.

In this chapter, we will first briefly consider developmental and psychiatric responses to pediatric cancer treatment. We will then examine behavioral difficulties that arise during active cancer therapy, such as non-adherence, treatment refusal, responses to treatment side-effects, and difficulties with school and social adjustment. Pre-existing psychological difficulties which interfere with treatment administration are examined. Because cancer in a child affects the entire family system, parent and sibling adjustment issues during cancer therapy will be discussed throughout.

PSYCHIATRIC PROBLEMS DURING CURATIVE CANCER TREATMENT

Issues of control and competence are challenged by almost every aspect of cancer treatment. From infancy onward, the child's development progresses toward greater control of self, of relationships and of the surrounding environment. Cancer therapy poses a threat to achieving greater mastery of the world in the toddler and pre-school child, of one's own body during the school years, and the formation of a sense of identity in adolescents (3). Eating problems are not unusual in children with cancer and may be used by them as a means of gaining control over the situation. Restriction and impairment in mobility and activity due to medical procedures and administration of blood, fluids, medications, or nutrients are added to physical restrictions secondary to surgeries, pain, or vomiting. These limitations can interfere with the infant's normal development. For older children, being bed-ridden or remaining in a bed with side-rails has clear regressive implications (3). Restrictions of activity and contact may suggest to children that their illness is very serious, as well as creating social isolation.

Several investigators have reported behavioral and emotional disturbances manifested in increased anxiety, depression, regression and withdrawal among children in treatment for cancer (4–6). One study found diagnosable DSM-III axis I disorders in 98% of pediatric cancer patients 2 to 16 years after diagnosis, most of these being adjustment disorders (52%). Patients with primary depressive features were found to be significantly older than those with anxious features (7). Some investigators examined the types and frequencies of psychological problems experienced by children with various types of cancer diagnosed 3 to 57 months earlier (8). Parent ratings revealed a significant number of patients who had difficulties in adjustment, with somatic concerns and problems in academic functioning. Greater frequencies of adjustment problems were reported among boys compared with girls. Extreme separation anxiety and pathological attachment have also been observed (9).

Other investigators, however, have reported few emotional or behavioral problems in children with cancer and demonstrate normal psychosocial functioning during treatment administration (10). Questioning, cheerfulness, denial, talkativeness, depression, humor, withdrawal, optimism, and low energy level may be the initial responses to therapy, but tend to change over time. Individuals alternating between sadness and cheerfulness, anger and acceptance, reality and denial may be seen as demonstrating coping, rather than psychopathology (11). Older children appear to use more adaptive cognitive behavioral and affective strategies than their younger counterparts (12).

Methodological discrepancies between the studies may explain the differences in findings. While some studies on the psychosocial adjustment in pediatric cancer patients evaluate only patients who are in active phases of cancer treatment, others include patients who are in remission or receiving only maintenance therapy. In addition, there are some problems with instruments that have been employed to evaluate psychosocial adjustment. For example, commonly used pediatric psychological tests and scales, such as the somatic scale of the Children's Behavior Checklist, are not appropriate in an oncology population, given that such instruments were standardized for use with healthy children (13).

Problems commonly seen in adults undergoing cancer treatment are relatively rare in children. Delirium is infrequently noted. It is not clear that this represents a true decreased incidence, as delirium is more difficult to detect in children, who are inclined to fantasy and have little concern with dates or time. When clinical withdrawal is more carefully assessed, however, confusion and hallucinations may be evident. Treatment has not been extensively researched in this population, but can generally be approached similarly to that of adults, while controlling dosages for size. Interactions between pain, delirium and depression should be evaluated, as is done with adults.

IMPEDIMENTS TO TREATMENT ADMINISTRATION

Non-adherence to prescribed treatments constitutes one of the most frequently encountered impediments to therapy administration in children with cancer. Non-adherence can take many forms (9): refusal of a procedure or treatment, failure to keep an appointment, or choice of alternative "unorthodox" treatment modalities. In general, studies in pediatrics have found an overall rate of non-adherence with home medication to be about 50% (14). In the cancer setting, non-adherence with outpatient oral medication has been reported to be 33% in children under 13 years of age, and 59% in adolescents (15). These findings have been replicated by other investigators (16–19). The increased rates of non-adherence among adolescent cancer patients may be due to greater parental involvement in young children's medical care, as well as to conflict over control between parents and adolescents, and adolescent denial of the life-threatening nature of the illness (20).

Research has been unable to reliably predict which patients are at risk for non-adherence with oral medication. Although it might be expected that patients with more severe or life-threatening illness would be at lower risk for treatment non-adherence, there is no consistent evidence to support this conclusion. Lansky and her colleagues (21) observed that, while rates of adherence were equal in boys and girls, psychological correlates of adherence differed between sexes. In girls, the child's own level of anxiety was the best predictor of adherence. In boys, parental levels of anxiety, anger and obsessive–compulsive behavior correlated positively with adherence. Patients' knowledge about oral medications has not been found to increase medication adherence in the pediatric cancer setting (22,23). However, non-adherent adolescents have less insight into the causality of their illness and prognosis and exhibit a greater tendency to use denial as a defense in the context of health-related issues than adherent adolescents (23).

Health locus of control, the degree to which individuals perceive that they have the ability to control factors affecting their health, has been studied in the context of pediatric treatment compliance. While some studies show medication compliance to be inversely correlated with a sense of external health locus of control in pediatric oncology patients (24), other studies have found no such relationship (18). Inverse correlations have also been described between medication intake and number of siblings (18), and poor self-image (24) in adolescents with cancer.

Cultural differences between patient, family and medical staff may interfere with treatment administration. Culture defines a family's response to an ill child and may explain behaviors such as non-adherence to prescribed therapies, degree and quality of parental involvement in patient care, and the family's relationship with health care staff (25). More aggressive treatments, parental depressive symptoms and general child behavior problems have been associated with greater non-adherence (26). Common problems reported by parents were administration of oral medications, mouth care, and getting the child to eat and drink sufficiently. Child age was correlated with missed mouth care administration, with older children missing more mouth care doses.

Some evidence exists of a direct causal relationship between treatment adherence and prognosis. Five of eleven adolescents with ALL who were non-adherent to prescribed prednisone relapsed, compared to one of ten who were adherent. Adherence has been found to decline over the course of therapy (27). Therefore, it is necessary to avoid underestimating non-adherence in the pediatric oncology setting and to monitor accurately adherence to treatment.

Treatment refusal is another form of treatment non-adherence. Refusing treatment may be seen as a means of regaining a sense of control over one's life. Pediatric patients who refuse treatment for cancer are most often adolescents. They may profoundly dislike treatment side effects, be overwhelmed with feelings of hopelessness, find alternative methods as the solution to their disease, or deny the seriousness of their condition. Adolescent cancer patients who refused treatment for leukemia have been shown to score lower than consenting adolescents on measures of state anxiety and subjective distress, but higher on characterologic or trait anxiety, religiosity, and external locus of control (27).

Increased participation of children and adolescents in medical decision-making and treatment planning in some Western countries raises ethical questions regarding an adolescent's right to request medical care without parental consent or to refuse potentially life-saving treatment. In general, under the age of 18 years, parental consent must be obtained in the United States except in the cases of medical emergency or emancipated minors (minors who are married, in military services, or who have left the family home and are self-supporting). Courts rarely intervene when parents support a youth's refusal of medical care (28).

Currently, a parent's failure to provide "adequate" medical care for a child is a criminal offense under all states' child neglect laws. Pediatric oncologists caring for children whose parents reject prescribed treatments and contemplating a court order petition must decide whether the benefit to the child is worth the emotional trauma to patient and parents of asking the court to place the patient in foster care during the treatment phase. Only when there is a belief that the treatment will be curative, or at least there is a fairly certain expectation of a long-term remission, can this course of action be justified (29).

DISTRESS ASSOCIATED WITH MEDICAL PROCEDURES

Pediatric cancer treatment often involves multiple administrations of highly aversive medical procedures such as lumbar punctures, bone marrow aspirations and venipunctures over a prolonged period of time. Because of the pain and distress caused by such invasive procedures and many children's limited understanding of treatment, patients often actively resist them or become apprehensive in anticipation of the procedures (30). Distress is usually manifested by crying, screaming, requesting emotional support or physical contact, verbal resistance, verbal expression of fear, information seeking, and requesting delays in the administration of the procedure. Common fears include disfigurement, losing all their blood or being overloaded with it during transfusions, and death. Shame for not being able to control oneself is frequently experienced by older children.

Overt manifestations of distress by the child have a significant impact on other pediatric patients in the clinic, who often have frightening fantasies about the situation and fear regarding what they may at some point have to undergo themselves. Parents often feel helpless and guilty as they watch their child suffer. Witnessing and performing invasive medical procedures in pediatrics is also stressful on the medical staff. Turnover rates of 50% have been described among nurses whose primary job is to perform venipunctures (31). At times procedural distress can be so severe that additional sedation or postponement of the procedure is required. However, physicians tend to avoid pharmacological interventions because of possible long-term neurological side-effects, as well as the brevity and frequency of most medical procedures administered during pediatric cancer treatment.

Younger children have been found to exhibit more distress than older ones (32). The occurrence of child distress and coping behaviors varies by phase of procedure and is closely related to specific adult prompts, which also appear to be phase specific (33). However, child behavior seems to be more stable across time than that of adults. Children engaged in more coping during the anticipatory period of the procedure continued to cope, and children distressed and crying at the onset were likely to continue doing so during the procedure (34).

Parent's presence may result in reductions of distress or may actually worsen the situation. Explanations by the parents at the beginning of the medical procedure have been associated with reductions in distress later in the procedure in children who were distressed at the outset. For those not distressed at the beginning, explanations were associated with increased distress (34). In another study, children separated from their parents displayed less distress during painful medical procedures than those with their parents (35). However, most children reported preferring having their parents present during painful medical events even though they could not specify what the parent could do to help them. Agitation by mothers has also been associated with increase in child distress (36).

ANTICIPATORY SYMPTOMS

Nausea and vomiting have been described as the most troublesome and debilitating side-effect of cancer treatment (37). In addition to the distress directly produced by frequent episodes of nausea and vomiting, patients generally feel ashamed of experiencing them and often avoid contact with peers. Some children develop nausea and vomiting prior to treatment administration. This phenomenon is known as anticipatory nausea and vomiting and has been conceptualized as the result of a classical conditioning process (38). Through repeated associations with chemotherapy and its aftereffects, certain environmental stimuli (e.g., smells and sights of the clinic) that are initially neutral, come to elicit symptoms (e.g., nausea and vomiting) similar to those induced by chemotherapy. As many as 29% of pediatric cancer patients receiving chemotherapy develop anticipatory nausea and 20% develop anticipatory vomiting during treatment (39). The most consistent medical predictor of anticipatory nausea and vomiting is the emetic potential of the chemotherapy regimen (40,41). Parents of patients with anticipatory nausea and vomiting have been found to rely more heavily on threat of punishment and less on modeling and reassurance when managing their children in fearful situations than parents of patients without anticipatory nausea and vomiting (42).

ALTERATIONS IN PHYSICAL APPEARANCE

An altered physical appearance is a constant visual reminder not only of the disease but also of how different the child is from peers. Children, and especially adolescents, with cancer who are physically disfigured or exhibit external signs of disease have difficulty finding a place in a society where healthy, attractive looks are highly valued. Weight changes, hair loss, amputations, placement of catheters to facilitate treatment administration, surgical scars, and alterations in skin coloration and texture not only make the child feel different from peers, but may represent frightening changes in the body to the child and may impact self-esteem adversely (42). Fear that the body will never return to its original appearance, fears of not being recognized by others, or of being mistaken for an individual of the opposite sex (frequently experienced by adolescent girls who lose their hair) often lead to shame, social isolation, and regressive behaviors. Alopecia has been described as a traumatic side effect of chemotherapy (43). Some children adjust well to hair loss. Others fear teasing and find it extremely painful and anxiety-provoking. Significant changes in body image have been reported in cancer patients with alopecia (44). Sudden alterations in body image such as that caused by hair loss are perceived by patients as a threat to their well-being, causing anxiety (45). Children's responses to baldness vary along cognitive developmental lines. Preschoolers rarely experience hair loss as a disability because of a lack of any preoccupation with appearance. School-age children are more disturbed by baldness because they have an increasing self-awareness and social outlook and this affects how others perceive the child and how the child perceives him- or herself. Adolescents, for whom personal appearance and peer group acceptance are of primary importance, often experience baldness with the highest level of anxiety (46). Much focus is placed on the visible loss of hair on the head, but adolescents rarely mention the impact of loss of pubic hair. Yet, as a perceived threat to a newly emerging sexual identity, this may constitute a more devastating loss and handicap in the development of sexuality (47).

Coping with alterations in physical appearance may be equally distressing for the child's parents, even in cases where such alterations are temporary. Parental reactions to disfigurement strongly affect how the child views him or herself. Parental acceptance of deformity and their consistent support play fundamental roles in the patient's global psychological adjustment and acceptance of continued treatment (48).

SCHOOL ADJUSTMENT

One criterion of adequate adjustment to illness in the pediatric oncology population is how long it takes a child to return to school following initiation of treatment. School represents the continuation of children's normal life as well as the primary source of social activity. Regular school attendance is vital to foster normal development and to prevent isolation from peers and social regression (49). Early school return is an important part of a child's successful rehabilitation. Positive school experiences can reduce children's maladaptive emotional response to the disease and its treatments by helping them feel academically accomplished and socially accepted.

Even though most patients are able to resume school activity in early outpatient phases of the treatment, some develop increased anxiety and phobic reactions. Fear of falling behind, or of being unable to catch up, fatigue, fear of the negative social reactions from peers and school staff to treatment side-effects, and shame stemming from the need to depend on school staff (e.g., the school nurse) are frequently encountered in the pediatric oncology setting. Complexity of treatment regimens, frequency of routine follow-up, disease status, neutropenia, infection, and chicken pox in the classroom can contribute to school difficulties (50). It is for these reasons that high rates of school absenteeism have been reported in pediatric cancer patients (51). More than half of 83 young cancer patients aged 13 to 23 were found to experience cancer-related problems in returning to school after diagnosis (52). Patients on treatment have been reported to experience greater difficulties than those off therapy (53).

School problems fall into four categories in pediatric cancer patients (54):

1. Patients exhibit school anxiety secondary to the illness or its treatment-induced side-effects (hair loss, weight changes, nausea and vomiting, surgical disfigurement).
2. Patients, parents and schools have difficulty reintegrating the patients into school after prolonged absences.
3. Patients have illness-related learning disabilities requiring psychological evaluation and possible school arrangements.
4. Newly diagnosed patients require preventive intervention and guidance to be reintegrated.

Neuropsychological deficits may result from either primary treatment modalities involving the central nervous system (CNS), as in the case of brain tumors (55), or of prophylactic therapies used in the prevention of CNS involvement, as in the case of childhood leukemias (56).

Peer reactions to the ill child and teachers' limited understanding of cancer may also interfere with proper school reintegration. Peers may tease children with cancer because of their appearance or may avoid them for fear of contagion. Teachers may either give the child "special" treatment, reinforcing the differences with peers, or may place excessive academic demands on a cognitively impaired child. Chronic illness or physical disabilities may be so severe that academic success and adaptation to the school environment are unrealistic and highly stressful goals. It is important for children that their school experiences do not become still another source of frustration and failure.

SOCIAL ADJUSTMENT

The examination of peer relationships of children with chronic illnesses is an essential component in understanding their current emotional and social functioning (57). Children with cancer may develop significant social adjustment difficulties and social skills deficits. Changes in physical appearance, separation from peers as a result of repeated hospitalizations or functional restrictions, restrictions on physical activity and athletic competition, and reactions of peers, parents and other adults may result in a heightened sense of social isolation and inadequacy (58). Physical weakness and restrictions on activity may also interfere with the discharge of aggressive drives through physical activity.

Studies of the social adaptation of children with cancer report conflicting results. Some researchers describe increased isolation and a reduced number of friends in children with cancer, as perceived by their classmates and teachers (59–61). Pediatric cancer patients whose teachers rated them as less socially competent and whose parents reported fewer effective coping responses were found to exhibit greater adjustment difficulties (8). Compared to healthy controls, pediatric cancer patients played less with children their age, spent more time alone, and had greater feelings of isolation. However, few differences were found between cancer patients and controls in teacher and parent reports (58). Other studies indicate that the social reputation of children with chronic illness such as cancer is not necessarily denigrated by the disease or its treatments (57). Conflicting results are due to the lack of appropriate controls when evaluating psychosocial morbidity and chronic illness, to the assessment of patients receiving cancer treatment at different ages, to the inclusion of children on and off treatment, and to the use of an inconsistent number of informants (58).

FAMILY ADAPTATION TO PEDIATRIC CANCER

Hearing about the diagnosis of cancer in a child is often devastating news for parents. Family activities are disrupted by the disease and treatment and are now planned around the ill child. Walker (62) has described the coalition that develops between care-taker–parent and ill child and how such a coalition will organize the entire family into roles relative to this central relationship. Parents experience an increased sense of isolation. They must resolve the dilemma of how much time to devote to the illness and how much to their healthy children. They may lose confidence in their parenting skills and blame themselves for the illness.

Raising a child with cancer may alter a parent's ability to parent effectively (63–65). Patterns that emerge suggest problems related to overprotectiveness, difficulty with consistent discipline, and expression of appropriate anger towards the child, as well as concerns about "spoiling" the child. In a study assessing differences in child-rearing practices of parents of children with cancer and controls, self-report data suggested that parents of pediatric cancer patients did not differ from other parents in their communities in their basic orientation to child rearing. These findings were not consistent with professionals' predictions, who believed there were differences in areas of over-involvement, discipline, and nutritional concerns (66).

Having their child undergo painful medical procedure, repeated hospitalizations, and dealing with the possibility of death challenges the parents' emotional stability. Lack of familiarity with the disease and the medical system is another source of parental stress. Parents are expected to cope with a life-threatening illness in their child as they learn to understand medical jargon and to manage a health care system in many ways unknown to them. Taking a child home from the hospital following diagnosis also involves many stressors. Parents may question their capacity to provide adequate home care. Outpatient care requires transportation to and from the hospital and sometimes moving to a different geographical location in order to receive optimal medical care, as well as additional financial burdens and re-arrangement of family roles.

Two models have been used to describe parental reactions to having a chronically ill child (67). Time bound models suggest that parents progress through sequential stages when coping with their child's condition. Fortier and Wanlass (68) have labeled the stages in this model as

1. *Impact*: this first stage marks the beginning of a crisis for parents and usually occurs at the time of diagnosis. It is characterized by anxiety and disorganization.
2. *Denial*.
3. *Grief*: manifested through anger, guilt and sadness.

4. *Focusing attention*: parents demonstrate coping measures appropriate for their situation.
5. *Closure*: parents accept that the illness disrupts normal family life and mechanisms to accommodate the disease into the family life are incorporated.

The second model used to explain parental reactions to a child's illness is one of chronic sorrow, in which mourning for the loss of the complete child and grief for their long-term aspirations for the child can occur (69).

Pre-existing family problems are newly stressed by the child's illness and treatment. Histories of psychiatric illness in either parent, of child abuse or neglect, of child–parent conflicts, of parental divorce or marital discord, cultural and language barriers, multiple family losses, or other stressors place families at risk for adaptation problems (12).

Some families appear to be strengthened by the illness and adapt successfully. In others, high rates of psychiatric and psychological disturbance have been reported. Observations of families where there was a leukemic child found that most families cope well during the first six months post diagnosis (70). While some families coped through the expression of emotions, others were self-contained; some optimistic, others fatalistic; some stoically self-reliant, others seeking support from family and friends. Parental reactions tended to change over time with people alternating between sadness and cheerfulness, anger and acceptance, optimism and pessimism, reality and denial. Coping style at the time of diagnosis and initial weeks of treatment was predictive of coping over a six-year period. Family and friends' support systems and similarities in coping among family members, as well the lack of additional stressors, facilitated coping with the illness and treatments. Although studies generally show that global family adjustment appears to be satisfactory, more subtle psychosocial sequelae may exist and warrant further examination (12).

Other studies have described a number of problems and pathologies in families as a result of pediatric cancer (71). For example, Magni and his colleagues (72) provided a longitudinal evaluation of psychological distress in parents of children affected by ALL and Hodgkin's disease. Initial parental reactions to the disease included shock and general alarm. Diagnosis generated profound anxiety of separation from the loved one. Over 50% of parents had increases in anxiety, depression, sleeping disturbances, and obsessive–compulsive symptoms at diagnosis. Eight months later, during periods of remission, relatively high incidences of psychological distress persisted: even though reductions in obsessive–compulsive symptoms were found, anxiety and depression remained high. Twenty months post-diagnosis more subjects had psychological distress, manifested mainly in sleeping disturbance and depression. Others have found almost one fourth of mothers of leukemic children to be clinically depressed and anxious one to eighteen months post diagnosis (64).

Yet other investigators describe problematic behaviors and reactions, but do not view them as pathological (73). One possible explanation of these discrepancies in results may be that families are frequently studied at one point in the illness and treatment process, rather than throughout the course of the disease. Data are collected retrospectively in some studies, and there may be differences between professionals regarding their definitions of coping (70). Parents' coping responses can be expected to vary with the child's diagnosis and medical status. For example, more adaptive family coping evidenced by greater levels of family organization, cohesion, emotional expressiveness, and marital satisfaction has been observed in families off treatment than on therapy (12). However, there is accumulating research evidence that adjustment to chronic illness in general, and to cancer in particular, is independent of its type or severity (74). Family support, marital satisfaction, fewer concurrent stressors, and open communication have been associated with good adjustment to illness (75,76). Family expressiveness with less conflict and more moral–religious emphasis have also been found to correlate positively with the patients' adjustment (77,78).

Despite the intense distress caused by childhood cancer in a family, divorce rates are no higher in these families than in the general population (79). Marriages appear to remain stable regardless of the child's chronic illness (80,81). Consistency in these results may lead to the belief that even in cases where there might be pre-existing marital difficulties, parents may decide to remain together throughout treatment in what they believe to be the ill child's best interest. Differences between the couple may be dissipated by their focus on the illness and treatment rather than on their relationship, but may be exacerbated once therapy ends.

Because childhood cancer affects the entire family system, how families adjust to it will depend not only on how they use their resources, but also on how they handle the differing reactions of each family member. Siblings of a pediatric cancer patient require special attention. Loss of parental attention, changes in family roles, structure and activities, and fear of death consti-

tute major stressors (82). Guilt may arise regarding having escaped the disease themselves and for feeling angry and resentful towards the ill child. Dramatic physical changes in the patient's appearance may facilitate young siblings' understanding of the disease but may induce feelings of shame for having a "different" brother or sister. Siblings may become quite anxious and concerned about their own health. They may develop frequent somatic concerns, at times to gain parental attention, due to an identification with the ill child, or because they may not find an explanation for their not being the ill member of the family. Behavioral changes may occur, as well as reductions in academic performance and isolation from peers. They often feel left out of the ill child's medical care and may develop worries that a parent—or themselves—will die. In addition, siblings of pediatric cancer patients must learn to deal with the practical limitations placed on their lives by the child's cancer.

SUMMARY

The diagnosis of cancer in a child is devastating for patients and families. Because of the development of more complex and aggressive therapeutic modalities, treatment may constitute as significant a stressor as the disease itself. Non-compliance with medical recommendations, aversive reactions to invasive medical procedures, school phobias, learning disabilities and social skills are not uncommon and may result in significant reductions in the child's self-esteem and psychological well-being. Cultural barriers and pre-existing psychopathology may complicate treatment administration. The experience is equally distressing for the patient's parents and siblings, who struggle to organize the chaotic events taking place in their lives.

REFERENCES

1. American Cancer Society. *Cancer Facts and Figures*. New York: American Cancer Society; 1994.
2. Chauvenet AR, Wofford MM. Cures in childhood cancer. *Pediatr Rev.* 1990; 11(10):311–317.
3. Brunquell D, Hall M. Issues in the psychological care of pediatric oncological patients. *Am J Orthopsychiatry.* 1982; 52(1):32–44.
4. Kashani J, Hakami N. Depression in children and adolescents with malignancy. *Can J Psychiatry.* 1982; 27:474–477.
5. Eiser C. Choices in measuring quality of life in children with cancer: a comment. *PsychoOncology.* 1995; 4:121–131.
6. Van Dongen-Melman JEW, Sanders-Wondstra JAR. Psychological aspects of childhood cancer: A review of the literature. *J Child Psychol Psychiatry.* 1986:145–180.

7. Rait D, Jacobsen PB, Lederberg M, Holland JC. Characteristics of psychiatric consultations in a pediatric cancer center. *Am J Psychiatry*. 1988; 145(3):363–364.

8. Sanger MS, Copeland DR, Davidson ER. Psychosocial adjustment among pediatric cancer patients: A multidimensional assessment. *J Pediatr Psychol*. 1991; 16(4):463–474.

9. Pfefferbaum B. Common psychiatric disorders in childhood cancer and their management. In: Holland JC, Rowland JH, eds. *Handbook of Psychooncology. Psychological Care of the Patient with Cancer*. New York: Oxford University Press; 1989.

10. Allen L, Zigler E. Psychological adjustment of seriously ill children. *J Am Acad Child Psychiatry*. 1986; 25:708–712.

11. Kupst MJ, Schulman JL, Maurer H, et al. Psychosocial aspects of pediatric leukemia: From diagnosis through the first six months of treatment. *Med Pediatr Oncol*. 1983; 11:269-278.

12. Brown RT, Kaslow NJ, Hazzard AP, et al. Psychiatric and family functioning in children with leukemia and their parents. *J Am Acad Child Adolesc Psychiatry*. 1992; 31(3):495–502.

13. Perrin EC, Stein REK, Drotar D. Cautions in using the Child Behavior Checklist: Observations based on research about children with a chronic illness. *J Pediatr Psychol*. 1991; 16(4):411–421.

14. Dunbar J, Dunning EJ, Dwyer K. The development of compliance research in pediatric and adolescent populations: Two decades of research. In: Krasnegor N, Johnson S, Epstein 1, Jaffe S, eds. *Developmental Aspects of Health Compliance Behavior*. Hillsdale, NJ: Lawrence Erlbaum Associates; 1992.

15. Smith SD, Rosen D, Trueworthy RC, Lowman JT. A reliable method for evaluating drug compliance in children with cancer. *Cancer*. 1979; 43:169–173.

16. Lansky S, Smith ST, Cairns NU, Cairns GF. Psychological correlates of compliance. *Am J Pediatr Hematol Oncol*.1983; 5(1):8792.

17. Dolgin MJ, Katz ER, Doctors SR, Siegel SE. Caregivers' perceptions of medical compliance in adolescents with cancer. *J Adolesc Health Care*. 1986; 7:22–27.

18. Tebbi CK, Cummings KM, Zeron MA, Smith L, Richards M, Mallon J. Compliance of pediatric and adolescent cancer patients. *Cancer*. 1986; 58:1179–1184.

19. Festa R, Tamaroff MH, Chasalow F, Lanzkowsky P. Therapeutic adherence to oral medication regimens by adolescents with cancer: 1. Laboratory assessment. *J Pediatr*. 1992; 120:807–811.

20. Zeltzer L. The adolescent with cancer. In: Kellerman J, ed. *Psychological Aspects of Childhood Cancer*. Springfield, IL: Charles C. Thomas; 1980.

21. Lansky SB, Smith SD, Cairns NV. Refusal of treatment. *Am J Pediatr Hematol Oncol*. 1983; 10:1007–1013.

22. Richardson JL, Marks G, Johnson C, et al. Path model of multidimensional compliance with cancer therapy. *Health Psychol*. 1987; 6:183–207.

23. Tamaroff MH, Festa RS, Adesman AR, Walco GA. Therapeutic adherence to oral medication regimens by adolescents with cancer: 11 Clinical and psychologic correlates. *J Pediatr*. 1992; 120:812–817.

24. Jamisson RN, Lewis S, Burish TG. Psychological impact of cancer on adolescents: Self image, locus of control, perception of illness and knowledge of cancer. *J Chronic Dis*. 1986; 39:609–617.

25. Die Trill M, Kovalcik R. The child with cancer: Influence of culture on truthtelling and patient care. In A Surbone, M Zwitter, eds. Communication with the cancer patient: Information and truth-telling. *Ann NY Acad Sci*. Aug. 1996; 809:197–210.

26. Manne SL, Lesanics D, Meyers P, Redd W. Psychological predictors of pediatric cancer compliance. *Proceedings of Annual Meeting of the Society of Behavioural Medicine*, Boston, MA; 1994.

27. Blotcky AD, Cohen DG, Conatser C, Klopovich P. Psychosocial characteristics of adolescents who refuse cancer treatment. *J Consult Clin Psychol*. 1985; 53:729–731.

28. Holder AR. Disclosure and consent problems in pediatrics. *Law, Med Health Care*. 1988; 16(3–4):219–228.

29. Holder AR. Childhood malignancies and decision-making. *Yale Biol Med*. 1992; 65:99–104

30. Jacobsen P, Manne S, Gorfinkle K, et al.. Analysis of child and parent activity during painful medical procedures. *Health Psychol*. 1990; 9:559–576.

31. Manne S. Behavioral treatment of children's distress during invasive medical procedures. *Proceedings of the Annual Meeting of the Association for Advanced Behavioral Therapy*. New York; 1988.

32. Blount RL, Landolf-Fritsche B, Powers SW, Sturges JW. Differences between high and low coping children and between parent and staff behaviors during painful medical procedures. *J Pediatr Psychol*. 1991; 16(6):795–809.

33. Blount RL, Sturges JW, Powers SW. Analysis of child and adult behavioral variations by phase of medical procedure. *Behav Ther*. 1990; 21:33–48.

34. Manne SL, Bakeman R, Jacobsen P, et al. Adult–child interaction during invasive medical procedures. *Health Psychol*. 1992; 11(4):241–249.

35. Gonzalez JC, Routh DK, Saab PG, et al. Effect of parent presence on children's reactions to injections: Behavioral, psychological and subjective aspects. *J Pediatr Oncol*. 1989; 14:449–462.

36. Bush JP, Melamed BG, Sheras Pi, Greenbaum PE. Mother–child patterns of coping with anticipatory medical stress. *Health Psychol*. 1986; 5:137–157.

37. Aapro MS. Controlling emesis related to cancer chemotherapy. *Eur J Cancer*. 1991; 27:356–362.

38. Redd WH, Andrykowski A. Behavioral interventions in cancer treatment: Controlling aversion reactions in cancer therapy. *J Consult Clin Psychol*. 1982; 50:1018–1029.

39. Dolgin MJ, Katz ER, McGinty K, et al. Anticipatory nausea and vomiting in pediatric cancer patients. *Pediatrics*. 1985; 75:547–552.

40. Morrow GR. Prevalence and correlates of anticipatory nausea and vomiting in chemotherapy patients. *J Nat Cancer Inst*. 1982; 68:585–588.

41. Dolgin M, Katz ER. Conditioned aversions in pediatric cancer patients receiving chemotherapy. *J Dev Behav Pediatr*. 1988; 9:82–85.

42. Varni JW, Ruberfield LA, Talbot D, Setoguchi Y. Stress, social support and depressive symptomatology in chil-

dren with congenital/acquired limb deficiencies. *J Pediatr Psychol.* 1989; 14:515–530.

43. Holmes W. Alopecia from chemotherapy: Can nursing measures help? *Am Nurs Assoc. Clin Sessions.* 1979; 1:223–232.

44. Baxley KO, Erdman LK, Henry EB, Roof BJ. Alopecia: Effects on cancer patients' body image. *Cancer Nurs.* 1984; 7:499–503.

45. Wagner L, Bye MG. Body image and patients experiences. Alopecia as a result of cancer chemotherapy. *Cancer Nurs.* 1979; 2:365–369.

46. Moore DC, Hotton CP, Marten GW. Psychologic problems in the management of adolescents with malignancy. *Clin Pediatr.* 1969; 8:464–473.

47. Sourkes B. *Armfuls of Time: The Psychological Experience of the Child with a Life-Threatening Illness.* Pittsburgh: University of Pittsburgh Press; 1995.

48. Die Trill M, Straker N. Psychological adaptation to facial disfigurement in a female head and neck cancer patient. *Psycho-Oncology.* 1992; 1:247–251.

49. Spinetta JJ. Behavioral and psychological research in childhood cancer. An overview. *Cancer.* 1982; 50:1939–1943.

50. Klopovich P, Vats TS, Butterfield G, et al. School phobia. *J Kansas Med Soc.* 1981; 82:125–127.

51. Lansky SB, Cairns NV, Zwarties W. School attendance among children with cancer: A report from two centers. *J Psychosoc Oncol.* 1983; 1:75–82.

52. Feldman FL. *Work and Cancer Health Histories: Work Expectations and Experiences of Youth with Cancer Histories (Ages 13–23).* New York: American Cancer Society, California Division; 1980.

53. Mancini AF, Rosito P, Canino R, et al. School related behavior in children with cancer. *Pediatr Hematol Oncol.* 1989; 6(2):145–154.

54. Katz ER, Kellerman J, Rigler D, et al. School intervention with pediatric cancer patients. *J Pediatr Psychol.* 1977; 2:72–76.

55. Danoff BF, Cowchock FS, Marquette C, et al. Assessment of the long-term effects of primary radiation. Therapy for brain tumors in children. *Cancer.* 1982; 49:1580–1586.

56. Moss HA, Nannis ED, Poplack DG. The effects of prophylactic treatment of the CNS on the intellectual functioning of children with acute lymphocytic leukemia. *J Am Med Assoc.* 1981; 71:47–52.

57. Noll RB, Ris MD, Davies WH, et al. Social interactions between children with cancer or sickle cell diseases and their peers: Teachers' ratings. *J Deviant Behav Pediatr.* 1992; 13:187–193.

58. Spirito A, Stark LJ, Cobiella C, et al. Social adjustment of children successfully treated for cancer. *J Pediatr Psychol.* 1990; 15(3):359–371.

59. Noll RB, LeRoy SS, Bukowski W, et al. Childhood cancer: The impact on cnildren's friendships. *Proceedings of the Annual Meeting of the American Psychological Association.* Atlanta, GA: American Psychological Association; 1988.

60. Noll RB, Bukowski WM, Rogosch FA, et al. Social interactions between children with cancer and their peers: Teachers' ratings. *J Pediatr Psychol.* 1990; 15:43–56.

61. Noll RB, LeRoy SS, Bukowski WM, et al. Peer relationships and adjustment of children with cancer. *J Pediatr Psychol.* 1991; 16:307-312.

62. Walker G. The pact: The caretaker–parent/ill child coalition in families with chronic illness. *Fam Syst Med.* 1983; 1(4):6–29.

63. Chesler MA, Barbarin GA. *Childhood Cancer and the Family: Meeting the Challenge of Stress and Support.* New York: Brunner/Mazel; 1987.

64. Maguire GP. The psychological sequelae of childhood leukemia. In: Duncan W, ed. *Pediatric Oncology.* Berlin: Springer-Verlag; 1983.

65. Powacek M, Payne JS, Goff JR, et al. Psychosocial ramifications of childhood leukemia: One year post diagnosis. In: Schulman JL, Kupst MJ, eds. *The Child with Cancer: Clinical Approaches to Psychosocial Care Research in Psychosocial Aspects.* Springfield IL: Charles C. Thomas; 1980.

66. Davies WH, Noll RB, Destefano L, et al. Differences in the child-rearing practices of parents of children with cancer and controls: The perspectives of parents and professionals. *J Pediatr Psychol.* 1991; 16(3):295–306.

67. Clubb RL. Chronic sorrow: Adaptation patterns of parents with chronically ill children. *Pediatr Nurs.* 1991; 17(5):461–466.

68. Fortier LM, Wanlass RL. Family crisis following the diagnosis of a handicapped child. *Fam Relations.* 1984; 33:13–24.

69. Buschmann PR. Pediatric orthopedics: Dealing with loss and chronic sorrow. *Loss Grief Care* 1988; 2:39–44.

70. Kupst MJ, Schulman JL, Mauser H, et al. Psychosocial aspects of pediatric leukemia: From diagnosis through the first six months of treatment. *Med Pediatr Oncol.* 1983: 269–278.

71. Kaplan DM, Grobstein R, Smith A. Predicting the impact of severe illness in families. *Health Soc Work.* 1976; 1:71.

72. Magni G, Carli M, Deleo D, et al. Longitudinal evaluations of psychological distress in parents of children with malignancies. *Acta Pediatr Scand.* 1986; 75:283–288.

73. Susman EJ, Hollenbeck AR, Nannis ED, Strope BE. A developmental perspective on psychosocial aspects of childhood cancer. In: Schulman JL, Kupst MJ, eds. *The Child with Cancer: Clinical Approaches to Psychosocial Care. Research in Psychosocial Aspects.* Springfield, IL: Charles C. Thomas; 1980: 129–142.

74. Arpin K, Fitch M, Bohn Brown G, Corey P. Prevalence and correlates of family dysfunction and poor adjustment to chronic illness in specialty clinics. *J Clin Epidemiol.* 1990; 43(4):373–383.

75. Kupst MJ, Schulman JL, Mauner H, et al. Coping with pediatric leukemia. *J Pediatr Psychol.* 1984; 9:149–163.

76. Cassileth B, Lusk EJ, Strouse TB, et al. A psychological analysis of cancer patients and their next of kin. *Cancer.* 1985; 55:72–76.

77. Spiegel D, Bloom JR, Gollheil E. Family environment as a predictor of adjustment to metastatic cancer. *J Psychosoc Oncol.* 1983; 1(1):33–44.

78. Barbarin OA, Chesler M. The medical context of parental coping with childhood cancer. *Am J Commun Psychol.* 1986; 14(2):221–235.

79. Lansky SB, Cairns NV, Hassanein R, et al. Childhood cancer: Parental discord and divorce. *J Pediatr.* 1978; 62:184–188.

80. Barbarin O, Hughes D, Chesler M. Stress, coping and marital functioning among parents of children with cancer. *J Marriage Fam.* 1985; 47:473–480.

81. Stehbens A, Lascani AD. Psychological follow-up of families with childhood leukemia. *J Clin Psychol.* 1974; 30:394.

82. Walker C. Stress and coping in siblings of childhood cancer patients. *Nurs Res.* 1988; 37(4):208–212.

78

Pediatric Palliative Care and Pain Management

GERRI FRAGER AND BARBARA SHAPIRO

Palliative care of children requires an understanding of how this specialized care is best integrated with the comprehensive care of the critically ill child. With recognition of the special needs of dying patients, initiatives have developed and shaped the basic principles of "palliative care." "Palliate" as defined by the *Concise Oxford Dictionary* (1) means "to alleviate without curing." Traditional palliative care services developed from this concept, which is represented diagrammatically in Figure 78–1 (2).

Care has been delivered using several different models, including designated palliative care teams, within free-standing hospices, geographically defined community-based units, and allocated beds within hospitals. Access to these services generally requires that the recipients be identified as "terminally ill." The palliative care framework, which has traditionally provided options to critically ill individuals at the end of their lives, needs re-working to eliminate the concepts of "cure" and "care" as being mutually exclusive.

Children confronted with significant life-threatening disease, such as cancer, their families, and caregivers may feel forced to make a difficult, if not impossible, transition to care that is exclusively "palliative." Such a construct restricts access to essential "palliative care" services from which these children could clearly benefit (3). Creative modification can offer universal access to comprehensive care that is initiated at diagnosis and integrated throughout the child's disease course, regardless of whether the outcome is cure or death. The following definition by the World Health Organization (4) broadens the boundaries and permits a more expanded and inclusive view of palliative care:

Control of pain, of other symptoms, and of psychological, social and spiritual problems, is paramount. The goal of palliative care is achievement of the best quality of life for patients and their families. Many aspects of palliative care are also applicable earlier in the course of illness in conjunction with anticancer treatment.

This model is represented schematically in Figure 78–2.

Initiating such a service at diagnosis provides the needed on-going support and ensures continuity of care. Components should include expert pain and symptom management, and psychological support for the child's family, teachers, classmates, and others affected. Such comprehensive care should be portable and accessible, whether the child happens to be in the tertiary care hospital, in the rural community hospital, or at home. However, the age, developmental level and diverse malignancies of childhood make it extremely unlikely that any individual health professional will have the experience or expertise to provide all elements of such specialized care. Therefore, a multidisciplinary team can be the model for a pediatric palliative care service, with designated individuals providing anticipatory grief counselling and formal bereavement follow-up in the case of a dying child. In children diagnosed with a significant life-threatening disease, loss-related issues present at diagnosis need to be addressed early and throughout the course of the illness.

ETHICAL DILEMMAS IN THE CARE OF CRITICALLY ILL CHILDREN

It is essential to have clear and open dialogue early between health professionals and families caring for critically ill children. Reassessment and clarification of goals of care throughout the course of the child's illness help shape the treatment plan. For example, a review of the goals of care for a child with end-stage leukemia admitted with distressing breathlessness might prevent the initiation of monitoring of blood gases and oxygen saturation. By contrast, interventions taken could be directed to symptom control

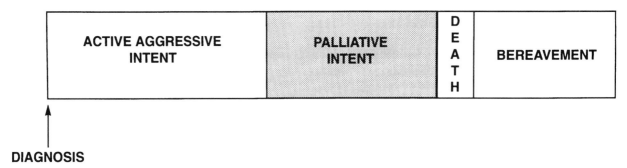

DIAGNOSIS

FIG. **78–1.** Traditional palliative care services, modified from *Palliative Care Services Guidelines*, Health and Welfare Canada (2) (with permission of publisher).

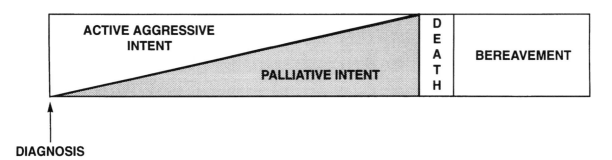

DIAGNOSIS

FIG. **78–2.** Proposed palliative care services, modified from *Palliative Care Services Guidelines*, Health and Welfare Canada (2) (with permission of publisher).

and comfort. No measures would be undertaken which could cause discomfort unless relief was an obvious outcome. Such clarification serves to unite the staff, child, and family in the effort to relieve the child's distress.

Frequently, in such circumstances, questions are raised about initiation or withdrawal of life-saving or life-preserving treatments, euthanasia, and physician-assisted suicide. Difficulty in dealing with the care of a dying child frequently presents itself as disagreement over goals of care between parents and health care professionals and these beliefs should be explored carefully. It is helpful to point out that the process of ethical deliberation is followed and the guiding principles are the same whether initiation or withdrawal of life-sustaining interventions is being considered. Similarly, there is no ethical or medico-legal distinction between the use of interventions considered "extraordinary" or "heroic," such as cardiopulmonary resuscitation, or "ordinary" measures, such as providing for antibiotics or hydration. The essential ethical imperative is to consider all actual and potential benefits and burdens from the perspective of the child as patient (5).

The principle of medical futility must also be considered when evaluating potential outcome. Futility refers to those situations where a given intervention has a limited effect without the capacity to restore the "whole." A clinical example would be the effect of mechanical ventilation on reversing carbon dioxide retention in a child with refractory neuroblastoma without being able to stop the progression of the cancer. In such a case, it would be "medically futile" to attempt resuscitation for the secondary problem as the primary pathology will, unfortunately, remain unchanged. Schneiderman, Jecker and Jonsen (6) emphasized that futility should not be equated with hopelessness, as futility and hope can co-exist for the same situation and in the same individual. It is more that the goals have shifted significantly and assumed a new perspective.

The concepts of withdrawal of treatment and medical futility are different from euthanasia and physician-assisted suicide. Euthanasia is the act of terminating a life, with death as the intended outcome. It is based on the premise of ending a life to end suffering. In physician-assisted suicide a physician provides the tools, either medication or other means, to terminate an individual's life. In this circumstance, the physician knows exactly how these resources will be used and condones their use for a given patient.

In the course of treating terminally ill children, one may encounter those with refractory pain or other symptoms, including profound psychological distress. In some instances medical intervention includes symptom control through administration of large doses of opioids and other centrally acting agents, such as barbiturates, neuroleptics, and benzodiazepines. These medications may need to be given in very large doses to provide comfort, even at the risk of potential compromise of the sensorium, or of respiratory or cardiac function. This "principle of double effect" differs from euthanasia. Aggressive symptom management including providing for terminal sedation is appropriate and is recognized legally and justified ethically in the care of the terminally ill (7,8). The primary goal is to provide comfort with the understanding that a potential secondary, although unintended, consequence may be the hastening of death. However, it is important to appreciate and provide a debriefing opportunity for health professionals to help defuse the feelings, at times the sense of guilt, when a medication given for symptom relief is temporally associated with a patient's death.

Symptom Management

Symptom management must be addressed throughout the course of treatment of children with cancer. It is essential that how the child feels is valued and that symptom management is initiated at the onset of symptoms. An unacceptable and inappropriate practice is the conscious attempt to "save" or "reserve" comfort-based interventions for the terminal phase of the disease. Such actions are generally based on misperceptions about the use of medications used for symptomatic relief, such as opioids. Although certain symptoms tend to occur exclusively or primarily in the terminal phase, many occur throughout the child's illness and the same management principles can apply at any stage.

PAIN MANAGEMENT

The Meaning of Pain

The significance and the perception of pain are modified by the clinical context. The pain sustained by a healthy adolescent fracturing his femur while skiing is different from the pain experienced by a teenager with a fracture from osteogenic sarcoma. Not only is the etiology obviously different, but the meaning of the pain experience is interpreted through the distorting filter of illness, experience, and meaning. Severe or continuing pain is a powerful experience and its meaning goes beyond its physiology. In children's ways of thinking, the existence of pain may be justified because of their guilt and "bad thoughts" (9). Thus cognitive explanations of the pain are important, even for the very young child.

Older children, like adults, appreciate that pain can herald cancer recurrence or progression. They also associate pain with tests, all of them unwanted and some producing distress and pain (10). Even very young children, who may not fully understand their condition, witness their parent's anxious response to their report or expression of pain. As a consequence, the child may elect to deny, minimize, or hide the pain. Similarly, children often strive gallantly to protect their parents and other adults from the grief of progressive disease.

The manner in which meaning and context interface with sensation is well demonstrated in procedure-related pain. Children with cancer often cite procedure-related pain as the worst part of their illness (11). However, pain related to disease can certainly be as severe, and is apt to be continuing rather than intermittent. Procedure-related pain is particularly onerous. Anticipatory anxiety and distress are high as most children fear and hate needles, and most have had experience with needles before they developed cancer. Procedures are discrete, highly visible events and as such may serve as repositories for the pervasive but more elusive reactions to the entire experience of having cancer. Despite being in a position to support the child, health care professionals and parents are often inadequately prepared to deal with procedural pain and sometimes minimize procedural distress. As a result, children are inadequately prepared and treated. As children usually do not consent to procedures, the procedure can be experienced as a total loss of control over their bodies, a loss of autonomy.

Pain also can have various meanings for the parents. Their child's suffering induces feelings of helplessness, grief, and anger, and fear that the pain is a sign of progressive illness. Some parents may deny the severity of the pain in a futile attempt to deny the seriousness of their child's illness. Pain can exacerbate pre-existing dissent between parents, with each blaming the other for not being able to help the child adequately. Even mild pain may become the total focus of attention for both parents and children, serving as a diversion and displacing more difficult concerns. Their unresolved anxiety, untold grief, and depression can further escalate the pain. Siblings, who may previously have wished for illness or death of their brother or sister, can be overcome with grief and remorse while witnessing their pain and suffering.

A component of the comprehensive assessment of the child with pain requires that the health care professional elicit and understand the personal meaning of pain for the child and parents. Then, the child's fears can be addressed and alleviated through appropriate interventions directed to help the child be more comfortable and less distressed.

The meaning of unrelieved pain for the child and family also requires examination. Pain can be unbearable, by virtue of its intensity, chronicity, or both. Pain that might be experienced as mild if it lasted only a few hours becomes unbearable when present day after day, or when occurring unpredictably. Intolerable pain threatens the integrity of the child and family. All energies go toward managing the pain, diverting them from other tasks facing the child and family. Thus, it is crucial for the well being of the child and the family that pain be recognized and that the intervention be appropriate, empathetic, and timely (10,12).

THE ETIOLOGY OF PAIN IN CHILDREN WITH CANCER

Pain in children with cancer can be classified as related to:

1. disease;
2. procedures;
3. treatment.

All three kinds of pain may be experienced during the course of illness.

Pain related to disease occurs in response to the underlying tumor biology. Generally, childhood cancers are responsive to primary disease-related interventions, such as radiation or chemotherapy. However, when they are refractory to treatment, they will often have rapid dissemination of disease and a short terminal phase. Pain may be somatic, visceral, or neuropathic in nature, or occur in combination resulting from infiltration, obstruction, or pressure on surrounding structures.

Diagnostic and therapeutic procedures cause procedure-related pain which is particularly difficult for children (13). Common pain syndromes related to treatment are mucositis, peripheral neuropathy, and obstipation. These are rarely chronic, except occasionally for the neuropathies.

Pain also varies by phase of disease:

1. pain with diagnosis and initial treatment;
2. pain during relapses;
3. pain associated with terminal disease and dying;
4. chronic pain as a late effect of successful treatment.

Pain during diagnosis and initial treatment can be very severe, but usually responds to non-opioid and opioid analgesics, and resolves with response to treatment. Anxiety and uncertainty are mixed with the hope that the child is going to live. Relapse undermines hope, and depression and demoralization can erode the child's ability to cope with pain. Chronic pain as a late effect of treatment can be particularly troublesome reminding the child and the parents of the previous suffering, and the possibility of recurrence.

PRINCIPLES OF PAIN MANAGEMENT

There are several basic principles for management of pain in children:

1. Consider and involve the child and the family, separately and together.
2. Regard pain as an emergency. Initiate treatment rapidly, and titrate analgesics to optimal effect in a timely manner.
3. Treat all components of pain—physiologic, emotional, and social.
4. Assess and reassess the pain frequently. Adjust the treatment based on the assessment in a timely manner.
5. Help the parents help the child.
6. Starting with the first procedure, anticipate and treat procedure-related pain and anxiety.
7. Utilize pharmacologic and non-pharmacologic methods of pain management as complementary strategies.
8. Anticipate, assess and treat side effects.

PAIN ASSESSMENT

The initial pain assessment consists of a comprehensive history and physical examination. A history includes a detailed discussion of all temporally related factors, location, quality, intensity of pain, and inventory of coping strategies. This section is an overview of the measurement and management of pediatric pain. There are excellent sources for more detailed information (14–17).

Pain assessment starts with determining the child's status along his or her dynamic developmental spectrum. Allowance should be made for possible illness-related regression (18). The measurement methods should match the child's developmental level, not the chronologic age. There are few tools available for use in a child with chronic pain since most were developed for measuring acute procedural or post-operative pain. Changes of blood pressure, pulse, and other physiologic parameters are inaccurate for chronic pain measurement since they dissipate with time (19). Similarly, the behavioral correlates typical of acute pain, such as facial grimacing and crying, may also not be apparent in a stoic or exhausted child with chronic pain. However, their absence does not mean the absence of pain.

Self-report is the gold standard for pain measurement; with chronic pain, it assumes even greater importance. Verbal children at the developmental age of 3–4 years and older can use a visual-analogue scale such as Beyer's "Oucher" Scale available with multiethnic representation (Fig. 78–3) (20) or a diagrammatic representation of a scale such as the Bieri Faces Pain Scale (21). For all facial scales the child is asked in their own age-appropriate language to point to the face that helps us know how much "owie" or "hurt" they are having. They can also be asked if their pain is "a little or a lot," or similar words illustrative of a categorical scale.

Most older children can use a visual-analogue scale such as a ruler with numbers from 0 to 5 or 10. Behavioural measures such as the Gauvain-Piquard (DEGR) (22) are helpful for those who cannot answer, who are regressed, or who have cognitive impairment. A rating is assigned to such items as to how the child sleeps, plays or interacts, the time they take to console, and body position with movement. The input of someone who knows the child and their baseline behavior, such as the parent or primary nurse, is very helpful in this regard. In fact, unless there is severe family dysfunction, their input in the assessment process is of primary importance.

If the child's report is ambiguous, it is appropriate to give a therapeutic analgesic. A follow-up assessment may help to confirm the clinical impression and scheduled analgesia can then be continued regularly as part of the treatment plan.

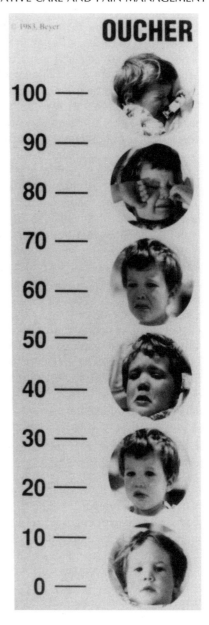

FIG. **78–3.** The Oucher: self-report pain assessment scale. Caucasian version, developed and copywrited by Judith E. Beyer, RN, PhD (20) (reprinted with permission of author).

NON-PHARMACOLOGIC INTERVENTIONS

Pain is a multifaceted, complex subjective experience and must be addressed with a combination of pharmacologic and non-pharmacologic approaches. There are many non-pharmacologic interventions. The most powerful interventions, which enhance the effectiveness of all the other approaches, are:

1. Listening to, respecting, and validating the child's perceptions and concerns, ideas, and strengths.
2. Doing the same for the parents.
3. Establishing a trusting and honest therapeutic alliance.
4. Helping the parents to be helpful to their children.
5. Understanding that children have their own inner life.

With these as a base, other interventions can be added. Explanations tailored to the cognitive ability and emotional style of the child are crucial, as children's fantasies are often worse than reality. Relaxation, self hypnosis, and imagery can be used by many children, and their parents (23–25). Art therapy and play therapy can help the child to express and work through concerns. Supportive psychotherapy is sometimes indicated.

Pain can exacerbate thoughts and fears of death (10–12). These vary with the developmental age of the child. Preschool children understand that animals and people die, and that when someone dies, they are not seen again, though they may not understand death as a permanent state. They may have thoughts about what happens in the grave and fear that they or a parent or sibling might die, triggering anxieties of abandonment and bodily mutilation. School age children have more sophisticated concepts; they begin to understand that death is final. Adults need to provide the opportunity for a child to ask questions and discuss concerns even though it may be uncomfortable, otherwise the child may be left to struggle with these difficult issues alone.

The child should have adequate privacy during diagnostic and therapeutic procedures. They should also have "safe times" when no procedures are performed (with the exception of emergencies). There is well documented benefit to having a parent present throughout procedures. Even the most severe pain is more bearable when a trusted adult is present, adding to the child's sense of security and decreasing the fear of abandonment. A parent should be encouraged to be present for almost all such interventions (10,26,27) and provide transitional objects and telephone calls when absent. However, this can be very difficult for many parents and there needs to be a formal way of guiding the parent through this experience by providing information and modeling of concrete tools to support the child. These include preparation and story telling, pop-up books, bubbles, and other options tailored to the child's preferences used before and during procedures (25). Children should not be left in their rooms alone for long periods when they may dwell on their worries and their pain. Parents also fear abandonment, especially when it is clear that the cancer is not responding to treatment. Health care professionals should provide continuity of care throughout all stages of the child's illness and continue to be available regardless of prognosis.

The physical environment is important. The child should be comfortable and secure, with familiar stuffed animals and pictures. Music, video games, and television can be powerful distracters. Judicious use of touch can be of much benefit. Another physical method is transcutaneous electrical nerve stimulation (TENS), which can be of benefit although of variable success. Physical therapy can decrease secondary myofascial pain and prevent the cycle of progressively less activity leading to increased pain with any subsequent mobilization.

PHARMACOLOGIC TREATMENT OF PAIN

Most of the principles underlying the pharmacologic treatment of pain are similar in children and adults (26, 28,29). Pharmacologic agents available for patients of all ages are the non-steroidal anti-inflammatory drugs (NSAIDs) and acetaminophen, opioids, tricyclic antidepressants, stimulants, corticosteroids, and topical agents. The WHO ladder for cancer-pain management in children parallels that used for adults, with the exception of NSAIDs which are often contraindicated owing to the frequent thrombocytopenia accompanying the chemotherapy for childhood cancers and in children with refractory disease (Fig. 78–4) (30). Although initial doses for children are given on a mg per kg basis according to the child's size, titration to effect can result in very large doses. Intramuscular administration should be avoided. Many children would choose to have pain rather than receive an intramuscular injection (31). Young children are also unable to associate the pain of injection with eventual pain relief.

Appropriate intervention for pain associated with terminal disease is likely to involve the use of opioids and adjuvant analgesics. Adjuvants refer to that class of drugs with a primary indication other than pain, but can have analgesic properties in some conditions.

NSAIDs and Acetaminophen
NSAIDs are useful for many kinds of pain, particularly when inflammation is involved. Acetaminophen can be used when NSAIDs are contraindicated. The four hourly dosing interval for acetaminophen can be problematic, especially when a child is taking many other medications. On their own, these agents are indicated for mild pain but are also helpful as adjuvants and can be continued with opioids and the other compounds used for moderate to severe pain.

Opioids
Opioids are the mainstay of treatment for moderate to severe pain (32). Table 78.1 can be referred to alongside the text. The oral route should be used whenever possible. Codeine, oxycodone, morphine, and hydromorphone are some of the short half-life opioids available

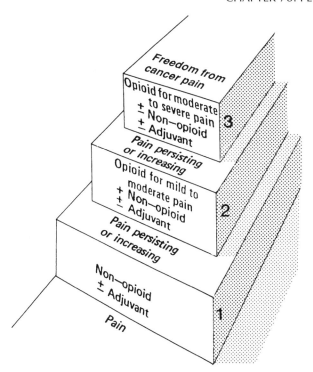

FIG. **78–4.** WHO three-step analgesic ladder. Reproduced from *Cancer Pain Relief*, 2nd ed. Geneva: World Health Organization (30) (with permission of publisher).

for enteral administration. Methadone is readily available, but its long half-life requires a skilled clinician to titrate the dose to prevent respiratory depression.

Many pills can be pulverized and suspended in palatable concoctions, some in elixir form. Children who can take pills can be given dose-appropriate sustained release preparations. Some areas have morphine available as capsules of timed-release beads. These capsules can be opened and sprinkled onto food or put through feeding tubes without destroying their slow-release property.

In certain situations, oral administration is impossible or ineffective. The child who is nauseated, vomiting, or who has a partial or complete bowel obstruction cannot be given oral medication. Severe pain requires rapid titration, and this is more easily accomplished by the parenteral route. For children requiring very large doses of opioids, the sheer number of tablets can be prohibitive. The depressed or dying child may be unwilling to take oral medication. In these situations intravenous access may already be established and can be used for the administration of analgesics such as morphine, hydromorphone or fentanyl. If IV access is not available or is problematic, an alternative is subcutaneous administration via small,

indwelling "butterfly" needles [#25 or 27 Gauge] changed every five days (33). Alternatively, the transdermal route is indicated if the child has trouble taking pills and has persistent pain that has stabilized. Rectal administration can be used occasionally, but is generally disliked by children and is relatively contraindicated by severe thrombocytopenia or neutropenia.

Meperidine is not recommended for chronic pain management since its metabolite, nor-meperidine can cause neurotoxicity. Mixed agonist–antagonists generally have limited analgesic effects, but may be useful in the treatment of pain associated with obstipation because they interfere less with intestinal motility than the agonists (34,35). Their use is restricted to initial therapy as they can precipitate withdrawal and are contraindicated in opioid tolerant patients.

Pain medication should be given around the clock, unless the pain is truly intermittent and unpredictable. Providing rescue doses for breakthrough pain using a continuous delivery system is more effective than intermittent dosing. Continuous delivery may be via sustained release preparations, regular dosing with immediate release medications, or infusions. Patient controlled analgesia (PCA) can be used for children old enough to trigger the device themselves and those who are not overwhelmed by depression and fatigue (26,36). For some children, judicious use of such a device by the parent can be helpful, especially to facilitate care at home. Hospitalized adolescents able to use oral medication may benefit from oral bedside PCA, to which the adolescent patient has access and therefore control of when and how often they take their analgesics (37).

Starting opioid dose is by weight, with 0.1 mg/kg IV/SC of morphine or its equivalent as the usual starting dose for moderate-to-severe pain. Initial doses in babies less than 6 months of age should be reduced to about one fourth to one third of the usual starting dose. The dose is then titrated to effect. Infants and children can require very large doses of opioids such as greater than 50 mg/kg/h of parenteral morphine. As with adults, there is no limit to the dose that can be used, as long as the increases are performed in a timely manner, balancing pain relief against side effects that are bothersome to the child. With escalating pain associated with terminal disease, doses may need to be doubled or tripled rapidly.

Children may refuse medication if they experience bothersome side effects, such as nausea, pruritus, and dysphoria. A bowel regimen to prevent constipation is part of appropriate opioid management.

Tolerance and physiologic dependency is differentiated from psychological dependency or addiction.

TABLE 78.1. *Opioids*

Drug	Equianalgesic Dose Parental	Usual Starting Dose IV/SC[a]		IV/SC:PO Ratio	Usual Starting Dose PO[a]		Biologic T1/2 Half-life (h)
		< 50 kg	> 50 kg		< 50 kg	> 50 kg	
SHORT-HALF-LIFE OPTIOIDS							
Codeine	130 mg	0.5 mg/kg q3–4 h	130 mg q3–4 h	1:1.5	1 mg/kg q3–4 h	15–30 mg q3–4 h	2.5–3
Morphine	10 mg	0.05–1 mg/kg q3–4 h	5–10 mg q3–4 h	1:3	0.3 mg/kg q3–4 h	10 mg q3–4 h	2.5–3
Hydromorphone	1.5 mg	0.015 mg/kg q3–4 h	1–1.5 mg q3–4 h	1:5	0.06 mg/kg q3–4 h	2 mg q3–4 h	2–3
Oxymorphone	1 mg	0.02 mg/kg q3–4 h	1 mg q3–4 h	N/A[b]	N/A[b]	N/A PO 5mg PR equianalgesic with 1 mg IV	1.5
Fentanyl	Single dose: 100 μg Continuous infusion: 100 μg/h = 2.5 mg/h morphine	0.5–1.5 μg/kg q30 min	25–75 μg q30 min	N/A[c]	N/A[c]	N/A[c]	IV 3–12 TD:IV/SC = 1:1[d]
LONG-HALF-LIFE OPIOIDS—Caution: Biologic T1/2 may not match analgesic T1/2[e]							
Methadone	10 mg	0.1 mg/kg q4–8 h	5–10 mg q4–8 h	1:2	0.2 mg/kg q4–8 h	10 mg q4–8 h	12–50
Levorphanol	2 mg	0.02 mg/kg q4–8 h	2 mg q4–8 h	1:2	0.04 mg/kg q4–8 h	2 mg q4–8 h	15

Source: ©Modified from Neuro Pain Service, Memorial Sloan–Kettering Cancer Center.

[a] "Usual" starting doses are often empiric and *not* necessarily calculated according to equi-analgesic principles (i.e., the usual starting dose for hydromorphone may be 2 mg PO even though the Parenteral : PO Ratio = 1:5). [b] N/A = not available. [c] NR = not recommended. [d] Transdermal:Parenteral ratio is based on clinical experience. [e] When converting to long-half-life opioids, particularly methadone, the dose should be reduced by at least 75% of the calculated equi-analgesic dose (based on clinical experience). [f] Meperidine is *not recommended* for cancer pain. It has a toxic long-acting metabolite, nor-meperidine.

914

Physiologic dependence can develop if treatment with opioids has been maintained for more than 5–7 days. Therefore, once the pain has improved, the dose is weaned slowly to prevent symptoms of withdrawal. The rate of the taper may vary from 10% to 25% every other day, depending on the length of time on opioids, the total dose, and the status of the pain. Tolerance is a physiologic response when a larger dose of opioid is needed to provide the same intensity and duration of pain relief. Some patients fear taking opioids because they will be ineffective at a later time. In fact, this is not a problem since the opioid dose can be increased as needed. Also, change to an alternate opioid can be made. Increasing opioid requirements are most often related to disease progression rather than opioid tolerance.

The use of opioids for the treatment of pain does not result in any increased incidence of psychologic dependence or addiction in children or adults over and above that known for the general population (38–42). Therefore, opioids can be used whenever necessary, with doses as high as needed, and for as long as needed, without fears of long-term sequelae. Undertreated pain may cause unnecessary suffering in the short term and adverse emotional sequelae in the long term. Parents and children are often fearful of opioids' addictive qualities and require education and repeated explanations to resolve this misconception. Parents can understand the concept that energy spent fighting the pain is not available for the child to use in coping with the illness and getting well.

OPIOID THERAPY SUMMARY

A "Baker's Dozen" Principles of Opioid Dosing and Titration

1. Ask the child about the presence of pain. Children may have many reasons for not volunteering information about their pain, even when it may be severe.
2. Use the oral route when possible. Avoid noxious options, such as the intramuscular route, even if it ultimately provides analgesia.
3. There is no "maximum" dose limit for opioids. The opioid dose should be adjusted to provide the best possible pain relief with the least amount of side effects.
4. Provide an opioid on a "scheduled" basis unless the pain is truly intermittent and so infrequent that the patient would be unlikely to benefit from regular "around the clock" dosing.

5. When calculating the dose of a continuous IV/SQ infusion of a short-half-life opioid, whatever dose was required to "load" the patient to achieve at least 50% pain relief can then be divided by twice the biologic half-life of the opioid. For example: if a patient required 30 mg of morphine over 1 hour to achieve pain relief, her hourly morphine infusion rate would be 5 mg/h (30 ÷ (2 × 3), the denominator made up of twice the half life of the opioid (for morphine = 3)].
6. Provide "rescue" or as needed doses in a form that provides rapid onset of action. These should be available in between and in addition to the scheduled doses. This allows the patient to achieve comfort without having to wait until the next scheduled dose.
7. The breakthrough or rescue doses should be provided as needed on a half- to one-hourly basis for most short-half-life opioids.
8. The quantity of each rescue dose can be estimated as representing 10–15% of the 24 hour opioid requirements. An alternative method is to provide a rescue dose that represents 50–200% of their calculated hourly opioid dose. For example: the patient who is receiving a 5 mg per hour morphine infusion should have rescue doses of 2.5–10 mg of IV morphine offered q30–60 minutes.
9. When four to six rescue doses are required in a 24 hour period, pain relief is inadequate and the continuous preparation should be increased. Either the amount of additional opioid taken in the prior 24 hours could be added to the continuous dose or a 30–50% increment could be made in the continuous preparation.
10. Any adverse effects noted with one opioid may occur with an alternate opioid. However, there is great variability between opioid groups and within an individual patient.
11. When a patient has reached dose limiting toxicity with one opioid, the adverse effects can be reduced by the following manoeuvres:
    - add an adjuvant as a co-analgesic, which may allow a reduction in opioid dose;
    - change to an alternate opioid to make use of the principle of incomplete cross tolerance and variability with individual opioids.
12. When changing from one short-half-life opioid to another, it is prudent to reduce the new opioid by 50% of the calculated equianalgesic dose (to account for incomplete cross-tolerance). If the patient has poorly controlled pain and adverse effects, a 25% or 0% reduction may be appropriate; see Table 78.1.

13. Ensure that the frequent misperceptions about opioid use have been discussed openly with the patient and his or her family.

Adjuvants

Tricyclic antidepressants are useful adjuvants to opioids for pain, and for treating insomnia and nightmares. They are particularly indicated as co-analgesics for the dysesthetic quality of neuropathic pain, often described as "pins and needles" and exacerbated by light touch. The starting dose for children is 0.2 to 0.3 mg/kg of amitriptyline or its equivalent, titrating up to the recommended antidepressant range using clinical response and serum levels to guide treatment. When used as a co-analgesic, the dose achieving pain relief is generally 2–3 mg/kg, compared with the higher dose range often required if used as an anti-depressant. An electrocardiogram (EKG) should be obtained before starting these agents (43). The EKG should be repeated and a blood level drawn once a dose of 100–150 mg/day is reached, or lower, if antracyclines have been used in chemotherapy. The EKG may be impractical and intrusive for the child who is dying, and in such situations clinical judgement and concern for the child's comfort and well being should guide the clinician's actions. Side effects such as dry mouth and daytime sedation can be troublesome, especially if the initial dose is large. Use of alternative agents, such as desipramine, may have a more acceptable side-effect profile, with less anticholinergic activity.

The psychostimulants dextroamphetamine, methylphenidate, and pemoline are mentioned in the order of most to least cardiotonic. They are used to increase alertness and reduce sedation. The initial dose of 0.1–0.2 mg/kg of either dextroamphetamine or methylphenidate, or approximately 0.2 mg/kg of pemoline, can be given in the morning and early afternoon and the dose titrated to effect. Pemoline, a chewable tablet, has the advantage of transmucosal absorption. Some children may experience an increase in anxiety or agitation requiring discontinuation of the agent.

Other adjuvants can be selected based to some extent on the etiology of the pain. When neuropathic pain is described as intermittent lancinating or shooting, it may be most responsive to anticonvulsants, such as phenytoin, carbamezepine, or clonazepam. The dose range matches that used for anti-seizure activity.

Methotrimeprazine, a phenothiazine, can help with pain and agitation. As it is very sedating, it can be helpful in patients with intractable terminal pain or agitation. Corticosteroids increase the sense of well being and appetite and can have a direct effect on pain. Because of side effects, unless required for treat-ment of the cancer, they should be used after careful consideration and most often only in the terminal phase. Anxiolytics, such as benzodiazepines, are useful to relieve anxiety and muscle spasm. Barbiturates provide no analgesia, but can be used in conjunction with analgesics when sedation is required in a dying child.

Topical Agents

Topical agents, such as a eutectic mixture of local anesthetics (EMLA) are useful for procedures. They are applied for a minimum of 1 hour and a maximum of 4 hours before a procedure involving needles, such as a lumbar puncture, bone marrow biopsy, venipuncture, access of an indwelling central line, or before a subcutaneous injection (44,45). Its use must be explained to the child, especially when the child is already anxious about procedures. It may require sequential applications over time for the child to become confident of the effect.

Anesthesiologic Approaches

Epidural anesthesia is recommended for focal pain (rare in childhood cancer), when the pain cannot be controlled with titrated doses of parenteral opioids or when the side effects are not able to be controlled with adjuvants.

TREATMENT OF PROCEDURE-RELATED PAIN

For children, procedures are the worst part of having cancer. They are anticipated with fear and remembered with emotions ranging from distaste to horror. There is no reduction of anxiety over time. In fact, the child who starts out anxious may end up phobic. However, with intervention, procedures need not be such distressing experiences.

Both pharmacologic and non-pharmacologic interventions are available and should be used together, as they are of greatest benefit in combination than when used in isolation. In most cases, non-pharmacologic methods are insufficient to manage severe pain and distress and pharmacologic agents do not address a child's fears. For example, the child undergoing a lumbar puncture could receive several interventions: preparation, explanation, a eutectic local anesthetic cream (EMLA), self hypnosis or distraction with coaching by the parents, an anxiolytic, an opioid analgesic, and local anesthetic. Discussion afterwards of how things went and what was helpful promotes trust.

Intervention must be tailored to the procedure, the degree of anticipatory anxiety, the expected anxiety and pain during the procedure, and the coping skills of the child. For some procedures, such as fingersticks in an adolescent, self-hypnosis may be sufficient (46).

For procedures like bone marrow aspiration in a phobic or unprepared child, general anesthesia may be necessary and should be the standard for all first procedures involving bone marrow aspiration. Coping skills should not be equated with behavior. The distress of children who act out or cry and struggle is clear. However, some children do not complain or cry, and are compliant with the demands of their parents and the health care professionals. Such children may be quietly experiencing considerable distress. As an example, a child who is very depressed and who has given up hope may evidence little reaction to procedures.

Analgesics are used to decrease the pain. Anxiolytics are used for anxiety and are appropriate on their own for non-painful procedures that require the child to be sedated. They have no effect on pain and, if used for a painful procedure, an opioid analgesic should be used in addition. Analgesics and anxiolytics can be given either by mouth or intravenously, although titration to effect is easier with the intravenous route. When analgesics and anxiolytics are used, short acting agents are preferable. Proper monitoring is necessary with a designated individual providing close monitoring of the child's airway, vital signs, and oxygen saturation. Equipment for resuscitation must be readily available with a person skilled in airway management in attendance (47). Such arrangements can be made safely on the patient's unit without necessitating a trip to the operating room.

OTHER SYMPTOMS

Nausea and Vomiting

There are many classes of antiemetics (Table 78.2). Some act centrally, others are more locally selective.

In the absence of adverse effects, it is best to increase each anti-emetic to the maximum dose tolerated and then add one or more anti-emetics from another class with a different mode of action, rather than changing anti-emetics. It may be that for problematic nausea and vomiting, a child may be on two to four anti-emetics in combination. Specific agents may be preferred when the child's nausea or vomiting has a fairly clear source or trigger.

When the gastro-intestinal distress is related to movement, then scopolamine or a similar anticholinergic agent is indicated. Clinicians should be aware of the possibility of bilateral or particularly unilateral pupillary dilatation with the transdermal scopolamine preparation. If gastric stasis is a factor, a prokinetic agent such as metoclopramide is the best choice. Cisapride, an alternative to metoclopramide, carries an improved side-effect profile notable for absence of central nervous system (CNS) effects. A steroid, such as dexamthasone, is generally helpful and is indicated when the vomiting is caused by increased intracranial pressure. Some children develop anticipatory nausea and vomiting when they have received repeated chemotherapy drugs. For such children, the addition of a benzodiazepine, such as lorazepam, should be tried in combination with a psychological based intervention. Ondansetron, a 5-HT3 receptor agonist, is an extremely useful agent for chemotherapy-related emesis. Other medications are antihistamines, such as diphenhydramine and hydroxyzine, or a neuroleptic such as haloperidol, chlorpromazine or prochlorperazine. Nabilone, an agent similar to cannabis, is more socially acceptable than acquiring illicit preparations, but it carries the same propensity for dysphoric reactions.

TABLE 78.2. *Antiemetics*

Medication	Usual Starting Dose	Comments
Scopolamine	0.5 mg q72 Transdermal patch	May have CNS effects
Metoclopramide	0.1–0.2 mg/kg IV/PO q6 h	Watch for possible dystonia
Cisapride	0.2 mg/kg PO qID	
Dexamethasone	0.2 mg/kg IV/PO 2–4x/daily	Side effects of steroids
Lorazepam	0.05 mg/kg IV/PO q4 h	Side effect profile of benzodiazepines
Ondansetron	0.15 mg/kg q4 h IV/PO	Used in chemotherapy
Diphenhydramine or Hydroxyzine	0.5–1 mg/kg IV/PO q4 h	Anti-histamine (dry mouth)
Haloperidol	0.01–0.1 mg/kg IV/PO q8 h	Max of 30 mg/day
Chlorpromazine	0.5–1 mg/kg q6 h IV/PO	Watch for possible dystonia with all neuroleptics
Prochlorpromazine	0.1–0.2 mg/kg IV/PO q6 h	
Nabilone	0.5-1 mg TID	Potential dysphoria

Dyspnea

Dyspnea, like pain, is a subjective experience. Terminal breathlessness may be one of the most difficult sensations to experience, manage, and witness. The cause of the breathlessness can sometimes be treated with management directed to the etiology. For example, in certain circumstances, it may be helpful to consider antibiotic therapy for pneumonia or the draining of a large pleural effusion for symptomatic relief.

However, it is imperative that treatment also be directed to relief of the sensation. It is important that attempts at treating the cause not be responsible for potential or actual distress to the dying child. Environmental modifications, such as air blown towards the face, cool circulating air, oxygen, and use of the child's favourite scent, such as strawberry fragrance, in the room may be helpful. Where oxygen by face mask or nasal prongs increases the sensation of feeling constricted, blow-by oxygen or room air is preferable.

In addition, morphine and other opioids can be very helpful for symptomatic relief of breathlessness. The appropriate dose is that needed to achieve relief. This intervention requires on-going assessment and aggressive titration to therapeutic effect. The addition of an anxiolytic can potentiate the beneficial effect of the opioid and help reduce the fear associated with dyspnea. Aerosolized or inhaled opioids have been used empirically as an alternative method of opioid delivery for dyspneic patients and are currently being formally studied (48). The effect is thought to be locally mediated via opioid receptors in lung tissue. A mixture of 79% helium and 21% oxygen has been helpful in the case of tracheal obstruction, an uncommon event in childhood cancers (49).

Patients and their families need discussion about what the process of dying may be like and need reassurance that comfort will be ensured. In children who are able to describe their symptoms and level of distress, their self-report determines management. Because dyspnea is a subjective experience, interventions should be used only if they are found useful by the child. When children cannot give information, the child should be treated empirically if there is presumed breathlessness. It is important to manage the family's distress as they may be disturbed by how the child is breathing. The family should be reassured that, although the child may be looking as if "they are working hard to breathe," the effect of the medication is helping them not to mind it. Bruera studied morphine's effect on the relief of dyspnea in terminally ill adults, and noted that the subjective relief reported by the patient was not necessarily evident to the observer (50).

It can also be distressing to those who wish to be in the room with an unconscious dying child, to listen to the child's noisy breathing, termed "death rattle." The meaning of this pattern of breathing should be explained, noting that it is not bothersome to the child. However, reducing this noise through scopolamine or glycopyrolate administered via the transdermal, IV/SC, or gastrostomy route can be of relief to those who are staying with the child (51).

Seizures

Seizures are very difficult for the families of a terminally ill child to witness. While potentially reversible and treatable causes are pursued as appropriate, the family can be instructed to administer rectal diazepam or lorazepam. It is useful, as in other aspects of palliative care management, to anticipate symptoms and discuss and plan for them with the family (52). Such pro-active rather than crisis-oriented interventions give the family a measure of control in a situation in which they feel anxious and powerless. This can also help the family continue to care for the child at home. The parenteral preparation of diazepam can be given rectally via a feeding tube or a needleless, plastic IV cannula at a dose of 0.5 mg/kg to a maximum of 10 mg. This can be repeated at 10 minute intervals to a total of three doses per episode.

Depression and Anxiety

Getting through the experience of cancer is very difficult. It is amazing that children cope as well as they do. Depression and anxiety may exist alone or, more frequently for the child with cancer, together. They are treatable and, like pain, without treatment, result in unnecessary suffering. Sometimes children make it clear that they are depressed or anxious, by words or by overt and unmistakable behaviors (see Chapter 83). However, often children mention nothing about their feelings and may indeed not be aware of their depression and anxiety, in addition to possible anger, irritation, or fatigue. It is incumbent on the health care professional to maintain vigilance for these symptoms and to instruct parents in recognizing the symptoms and to intervene early.

The depressed child may have low energy, withdraw from others, and play or interact less than their physical state allows. They may be slow to answer questions, or may turn away, letting their parent answer all the questions. At the other extreme are depressed children who are irritable, pick fights, and go joylessly from activity to activity. Such a child may be depressed, anxious, or both. Anxiety may manifest with clear symptoms, but at times is more difficult to discern. For example, an anxious child may be labeled as "difficult." Panic disorders are not uncommon and may present as somatic symptoms only. Anxiety and depression are both accompanied by a variety of somatic symptoms and can also worsen coexisting pain and other symptoms. A child may be sad because of inadequately treated pain or the pain may be difficult to treat with analgesics alone because the child is sad and has pain, and the two interact.

For many children with cancer who are depressed and/or anxious, non-pharmacologic treatment is adequate. However, the intervention must be carefully tailored to the situation and to the needs of the child and the family. Although pharmacologic agents should not be used in isolation, their addition can be helpful in some cases. Tricyclic antidepressants may help with both pain and depression. Other antidepressants can be used when indicated, although there is less evidence for other antidepressants as adjuvants in pain management. Anxiolytics must be used judiciously. If the child is depressed, they have the potential for increasing the depression (see Chapter 83).

Disturbed Sensorium: Restlessness, Agitation, and Confusion

With the approach of death, the child may experience restlessness, agitation, and confusion as a consequence of the metabolic derangements accompanying progressive organ failure. Some of the medications for symptom control, such as opioids for pain and dyspnea, benzodiazepines for anxiety, or neuroleptics for nausea and vomiting, can be responsible for a disturbed sensorium. When precipitated by renal or hepatic compromise, decreasing the dose or lengthening the interval of these centrally acting medications can reduce these adverse effects as long as pain relief is still well controlled. At times, when a medication is clearly implicated in the absence of organ failure, a change to an alternate opioid or benzodiazepine in the same class, can have fewer or more tolerable side effects, while remaining effective for the target symptom.

Simple environmental measures can help reduce nightmares and mild restlessness. Old night-time rituals should be re-instituted. For example, if the child was accustomed to being rocked and read a favourite story, this could be done. A warm bath, massage, or soothing music comforts and helps the child relax before sleep. Relaxation tapes for children, with descriptions of their favourite places and music, may be of much benefit. It may be helpful to add a neuroleptic for control of agitation and to enhance sleep. Although there is frequently concern voiced about causing dystonic reactions with neuroleptics in children, this has not been common in wide clinical experi-

ence. The selection of which neuroleptic is geared to the degree of sedation needed. Haloperidol produces little and methotrimeprazine produces more sedation. In the case of severe unresponsive agitation, the child may require aggressive pharmacologic management, as described in the next section.

TREATMENT OF REFRACTORY SYMPTOMS

There are occasions, albeit rare, when the combined goals of comfort, an intact sensorium and relative absence of side effects, cannot be achieved. In such a situation, it is appropriate to consider terminal sedation to allow the child "to sleep through the experience." Terminal sedation should not be offered until all viable alternatives have been explored. In reaching the decision to discuss terminal sedation as an option, it is prudent to ensure that several conditions have been met. The first is a comprehensive evaluation of the potential for relief through invasive and non-invasive techniques, assuring relief within a reasonable time. Such a perspective is best approached through consultation with an individual with expertise in pain and symptom management. This can be done by telephone in areas with limited access to such resources. The interventions themselves must be tolerable to the child and balanced against the risk of distress to the child (53). In discussing goals with the patient, family, and staff, what is being offered and what the process involves must be made absolutely clear. This avoids the confusion that sometimes accompanies these desperate situations. When the patient finally rests comfortably after a period of significant distress, the preceding period of intolerable distress can recede in the family's memories. In their need to interact with the patient, family members may request that sedation be withdrawn. On some occasions, it is best to allow the child's sedation to diminish so that the family can assure themselves that continuous sedation is the only tolerable option.

When carefully considered and gently discussed with the terminally ill child and family, the option of terminal sedation can be extremely helpful. The patient and family are assured freedom from the anguish of refractory symptoms. In addition, the impact of the child's comfort on the family, friends, and staff is profound.

The pharmacologic options for providing terminal sedation are varied (54). Regardless of physicians' individual preferences, the principles remain the same: any symptom which the patient finds intolerable is refractory. The primary goal of care is to provide for comfort, recognizing that a secondary unintentional, but possibly unavoidable, consequence may be the hastening of death.

Once the decision has been reached to provide terminal sedation, the first line of approach is generally to increase the opioid dose when the patient is already being treated with opioids. At times, opioid tolerance compounded by the stimulating drive of the symptom, such as severe pain, may make sedation with this pharmacologic intervention impossible. At other times, the adverse effects with escalation of the opioid dose may prove problematic. An example is the precipitation of agitation or severe myoclonus. In such instances, a second agent, such as a neuroleptic, benzodiazepine, or barbiturate, should be added.

A sedating neuroleptic, such as methotrimeprazine or chlorpromazine, should be started at a dose of approximately 0.1 mg/kg or 0.5 mg/kg, respectively. These agents can be given at this dose parenterally or, when possible, orally. Options include diazepam or lorazepam, the latter being more useful since it can be given sublingually or as a continuous infusion. Midazolam is also an option, but can be prohibitively expensive. Again, the usual starting doses parallel those used for anxiolysis, in the range of 0.1 mg/kg for diazepam and 0.02–0.05 mg/kg for lorazepam. Agitation can sometimes occur as a paradoxical reaction with benzodiazepines. Alternatives to these agents are the barbiturates with an initial loading dose of 4 mg/kg of pentobarbital, then maintained via infusion or repeated boluses. For some children, the use of several of these agents in combination may be required.

Initial starting doses suggested here serve as a rough guideline. Escalation can be aggressive and patients in great distress can require monumental doses to produce sedation. Titration should be carried out while monitoring the patient for breakthrough symptoms. Dose augmentation should be made by at least 50% increments.

BEREAVEMENT

Bereavement is characterized by feelings of loss, deprivation, sadness, and loneliness and may be particularly profound when the impending death is that of a child. The sense of loss begins in anticipation of the death. Several basic principles of bereavement support are outlined.

Principles of Anticipatory Grief and Bereavement Support

1. Support must be a formal part of the care provided to the child and the family, given by a designated person who carries the responsibility.

2. The service needs to begin at the time of diagnosis and continue through the course of the child's illness.

3. Support must be continued for the family following the death of the child.

4. All individuals affected by the child's illness should be considered, including brothers and sisters and extended family. Friends, schoolmates, teachers, and religious and community members need a forum in which to share and express their grief and best support the family.

5. Staff providing care for terminally ill children and their friends and family require their own psychological and spiritual support.

The personnel providing anticipatory grief and bereavement counselling should have experience and skill in dealing with issues of loss and death. Although potentially from diverse backgrounds, these individuals provide a service sharing the following basic principles. These are that counseling is done in a private place; that information is shared in an age-appropriate, gentle and honest manner; that there are no rules for the best way to grieve and counsellors help the individual to find their best way through this tragic event (see Chapter 88).

SUMMARY

Children with a life-threatening disease follow a very difficult path. In fact, this path is traveled by all those in contact with the critically ill child: the family, friends, health professionals, and the school, religious and social communities. A strong framework is provided by the principles of palliative care applied throughout the child's illness. The provision of aggressive pain and symptom management, emotional support, and bereavement follow-up cushions the distress of the child, the family, and others. In cases in which the child dies, there is a legacy and memory left. It is a huge opportunity to shape the way the child's life is remembered. The tools of palliative care provide health professionals with the capacity to make a difference.

REFERENCES

1. *Oxford Concise Dictionary of Current English.* Ninth ed. Oxford: Clarendon Press; 1995.
2. *Palliative-Care Services.* Report of the Subcommittee on Institutional Program Guidelines. Health Services and Promotion Branch, Health and Welfare, Ottawa, Canada; 1989.

3. Frager G. Pediatric palliative care: Building the model, bridging the gaps. *J Palliative Care*. 1996; 12(3):9–12.

4. *Cancer Pain Relief and Palliative Care*. Technical Report Series 804. Geneva: World Health Organization; 1990.

5. Solomon M, O'Donnell J, Jennings B, et al. Decisions near the end of life: professional views on life-sustaining treatments. *Am J Public Health*. 1993; 83(1):14–21.

6. Schneiderman LJ, Jecker NS, Jonsen AR. Medical futility: its meaning and ethical implications. *Ann Intern Med*. 1990; 112(12):949–953.

7. American Nurses Association. *Position Statement on Promotion of Comfort and Relief of Pain in Dying Patients*. Kansas City, MO: American Nurses Association; 1985.

8. Wanzer SH, Federman DD, Adelstein SJ, et al. The physician's responsibility toward hopelessly ill patients: a second look. *N Engl J Med*. 1989; 320:844–849.

9. Gaffney A, Dunne EA. Children's Understanding of the Causality of Pain. Pain 1987; 29:91-104.

10. Shapiro B. The Suffering of Children and Families. In: Ferrell B, ed. *Suffering*. Sudbury, MA: Jones & Bartlett; 1996: 67–93.

11. Weekes DP, Savedra MC. Adolescent cancer: coping with treatment related pain. *J Ped Nurs*. 1988; 3:318–328.

12. Foley GV, Whiten EH. Care of the child dying with cancer. Part 1. *CA Cancer J*. 1990; 40:327–354.

13. Miser AW. Management of pain associated with childhood cancer. In: Schechter NL, Berde CB, Yaster M, eds. *Pain in Infants, Children, and Adolescents*. Baltimore: Williams and Wilkins; 1993:411–424.

14. Schechter NL, Berde CB, Yaster M. *Pain in Infants, Children and Adolescents*. Baltimore, MD: Williams and Wilkins; 1993.

15. McGrath JA. *Pain in Children: Nature, Assessment and Treatment*. New York: Guilford Press; 1990.

16. McGrath PJ, Unruh AM. *Pain in Children and Adolescents*. Amsterdam: Elsevier, 1987: 73–104.

17. Ross DM, Ross SA. *A Study of the Pain Experience in Children: Final Report*. Ref No. 1 ROI HD 13672-01. Bethesda: National Institute of Child Health and Human Development; 1982a.

18. McGrath PJ, Craig K. Developmental and psychological factors in children's pain. *Pediatr Clin N Am*. 1989; 36:823–836.

19. Chapman CR, Casey KL, Dubner R, et al. Pain measurement; an overview. *Pain*. 1985; 22:1–31.

20. Beyer JE. The Oucher: self-report pain assessment scale. In: *The Oucher: A User's Manual and Technical Report*. Evanston, IL: Judson Press; 1984: 1–12.

21. Bieri D, Reeve RA, Champion GD, et al. The Faces of Pain Scale for the self-assessment of the severity of pain experienced by children: development, initial validation, and preliminary investigation for ratio scale properties. *Pain*. 1990; 41:139–150.

22. Gauvain-Piquard A, Rodary C, Rezvani A, Lemerle J. Establishment of a new rating scale for the evaluation of pain in young children (2 to 6 years) with cancer. *Pain*. 1983; Suppl 2:S25.

23. Hilgard L, LeBaron S. *Hypnotherapy of Pain in Children with Cancer*. Los Angeles: William Kaufman; 1984.

24. Zeltzer L, LeBaron S. Hypnosis and nonhypnotic techniques for reduction of pain and anxiety during painful procedures in children and adolescents with cancer. *J Pediatr*. 1982; 101:1032–1035.

25. Kuttner L, Bowman M, Teasdale M. Psychological treatment of distress, pain, and anxiety for young children with cancer. *J Dev Behav Pediatr*. 1988; 9:374–381.

26. Jacox AK, Payne R, eds. *Clinical Practice Guideline: Management of Cancer Pain*. Washington DC: US Department of Health and Human Services, Agency for Health Care Policy and Research; March 1994.

27. Bauchner, H. Commentaries: procedures, pain and parents. *Pediatr*. 1991; 87:563–565.

28. Max M, Payne R, eds. *Principles of Analgesic Use in the Treatment of Acute Pain and Cancer Pain*. 3rd ed. Skokie, IL: American Pain Society; 1992.

29. Schechter NL, Altman A, Weisman S. Report of the consensus conference on the management of pain in childhood cancer. *Pediatr*. 1990; Supplement 86.

30. *Cancer Pain Relief*. 2nd ed. Geneva: World Health Organization; 1996.

31. Eland JM. Minimizing injection pain associated with pre-kindergarten immunizations. *Issues Compr Pediatr Nurs*.1982; 5:361–372.

32. Yaster M, Deshpande JK. Management of pediatric pain with aped analgesics. *J Pediatr*. 1988; 113:421–429.

33. Miser AW, Davis DM, Hughes CS, et al. Continuous subcutaneous infusion of morphine in children with cancer. *Am J Dis Child*. 1983; 137:383–385.

34. Yukioka H, Rosen M, Evans KT, et al. Gastric emptying and small bowel transit times in volunteers after intravenous morphine and nalbuphine. *Anaesthesia*. 1987; 42:704–710.

35. Gawrisch E, Cheng E. Buprenorphine sedation of intensive care unit patients and ileus reversal. *Crit Care Med*. 1990; 18:1034–1036.

36. Berde CB, Lehn BM, Yee JD, et al. Patient-controlled analgesia in children and adolescents: A randomized prospective comparison with intramuscular administration of morphine for postoperative analgesia. *J Pediatr*. 1991; 118:460–466.

37. Litman R, Shapiro B. Oral PCA in Adolescents. *J Pain Sympt Manage*. 1992; 7:78–81.

38. Perry S, Heidrich G. Management of pain during debridement:A survey of U.S. burn units. *Pain*. 1982; 13:267–280.

39. Kanner RM, Foley KM. Patterns of narcotic drug use in a cancer pain clinic. *Ann NY Acad Sci*. 1981; 362: 161–172.

40. Morrison RA. Update on sickle cell disease: incidence of addiction and choice of opioid in pain management. *Pediatr Nurs*. 1991; 10:7–8.

41. Porter J, Hick H. Addiction rare in patients treated with narcotics. *New Engl J Med*. 1980; 302:123.

42. Weissman DE, Haddox JD. Opioid pseudoaddiction - an iatrogenic syndrome. *Pain*. 1989; 36:363.

43. Pfefferbaum B, Hagberg CA. Pharmacologic management of pain in children. *J Am Acad Child Adol Psychiatry*. 1993; 32:235–242.

44. Steward DJ. Eutectic mixture of local anesthetics (EMLA): What is it? What does it do? *J Pediatr*. 1993; 122(5), Part 2:S21–S23.

45. Koren G. Use of the eutectic mixture of local anesthetics in young children for procedure-related pain. *J Pediatr*. 1993; 122(5), Part 2:S30–S35.

46. Kuttner L. Management of young children's acute pain and anxiety during invasive medical procedures. *Pediatrician.* 1989; 16:39–44.

47. American Academy of Pediatrics. Guidelines for the elective use of conscious sedation, deep sedation, and general anesthesia in pediatric patients. *Pediatrics.* 1985; 76:317–321.

48. Davis CL. The therapeutics of dyspnea. *Cancer Surv.* 1994; 21:85–98.

49. Regnard C, Ahmedzai S. Dyspnea in advanced cancer: a flow diagram. *Palliat Med.* 1990; 4:311–315.

50. Bruera E, Macmillan K, Pither J, MacDonald N. Effects of morphine on the dyspnea of terminal cancer patients. *J Pain Sympt Manage.* 1990; 5(6):341–344.

51. Twycross RG, Lack SA. *Therapeutics in Terminal Cancer.* London: Pitman; 1984: 120–121.

52. Frager G. Relieving suffering in children with malignant disease. In: Arbit E, ed. *Management of Cancer-related Pain.* New York: Futura Publishing; 1993: 193–205.

53. Cherny NI, Portenoy RK. Sedation in the management of refractory symptoms: guidelines for evaluation and treatment. *J Palliat Care.* 1994; 10(2):31–38.

54. Kenny NP, Frager G. Refractory symptoms and terminal sedation of children: ethical issues and practical management. *J Palliat Care.* 1996; 12(3):40–45.

79

Long-Term Adaptation, Psychiatric Sequelae, and PTSD

JAMES M. HILL AND MARGARET L. STUBER

It has been estimated that as many as one of every thousand twenty-year old Americans is a childhood cancer survivor (1). This number is due in large part to the excellent survival rates of many forms of childhood cancer. However, long-term survival after childhood malignancies is a relatively recent phenomenon. As recently as the 1960s, acute lymphocytic leukemia (ALL), the most common childhood cancer, had a six month survival rate of 4% (2). Technical advances in treatment rapidly changed the prognostic picture, such that by the early 1990s ALL in children had an overall five year survival of approximately 65%.

The intensive chemotherapy and radiation treatments which led to these greatly improved results were known to have physical sequelae in children. In the early 1900s researchers had become aware that the negative sequelae of radiation might have a more severe impact on developing children than on adults (3). Subsequent work identified an increased incidence of second malignancies (20 times expected) (4), organ defects (5), growth retardation (6–8), and infertility (9).

Mental health professionals have carefully examined the cognitive and neuropsychological impact of two specific kinds of treatment, cranial irradiation and intrathecal chemotherapy (see Chapter 81). Based on clinical impressions of stress and distress, behavioral scientists have also conducted investigations of psychopathological sequelae of childhood cancer treatment, as well as the impact on survivors' parents and siblings. Much of the psychosocial research has not been systematic and has been complicated by design issues which make it difficult to compare studies to one another. Varying sample sizes, diagnoses, inclusion criteria, treatment differences, time from treatment to study, and choice of instruments for assessing psychosocial functioning have contributed to an ambiguity

regarding the long-term adaptation of childhood cancer and their families.

This chapter will review what is known about the long-term adaptation of childhood cancer survivors and their families. We will first examine the differences that have been found in the psychiatric or psychosocial functioning of childhood cancer survivors and their families compared to those who have not experienced cancer. We will then discuss possible causes of these differences, as well as factors which might predict who would be most susceptible. We will conclude with some discussion of interventions that have been found to be of use for survivors and their families.

PSYCHOSOCIAL SEQUELAE

Despite the sometimes serious medical sequelae, few significant differences have been found when childhood cancer survivors were compared to the general population regarding their overall emotional development, their employment, or their marital status (5, 10–20). However, specific problems have been identified that would be expected to impact social functioning of a subset of survivors. Preoccupation with their physical condition and problems with body image have been found in approximately a fourth of adolescent survivors (10), and were noted to be more common, the older the adolescent was at the time of diagnosis (19). The growth retardation seen in survivors of ALL who received craniospinal radiation (6–8) may result in heights as much as two standard deviations below the mean (21), contributing to problems of body image.

Survivors of pediatric malignancies who are now young adults are denied health insurance more often than their siblings (20) and have more difficulties with educational achievement, employment, and workplace relationships (16). Young adult survivors perceive themselves to be more vulnerable to negative health behaviors than their siblings (22), although they generally saw themselves as coping well and achieving the same lifestyle goals (23). Although survivors of acute lymphocytic leukemia were more likely than their siblings to require special or learning-disabled education, they appeared generally able to finish school and get equivalent employment (24). Eighty-four percent of blue-collar workers and 54% of white-collar workers reported work-related problems that they attributed to their childhood cancer (19). One study found that 32% of male survivors were rejected from job opportunities, compared to only 19% of their male siblings. No such differences were found between female survivors and their siblings (13).

An early study found that 88% of the unmarried adult survivors of childhood cancer attributed their single status to having had cancer (11). More recent research found that the effect of the cancer experience on later marriage was viewed as generally positive by spouses and negative by the young adult survivors (25). A recent study of 580 young adult survivors of childhood leukemia found that survivors report more tension, depressive symptoms, anger, and confusion than their siblings, using the Profile of Mood States as a self-report instrument. These symptoms were predicted by the perceived negative impact of the treatment on their school and work performance, but not by treatment variables, such as dose of radiation or intrathecal methotrexate (Zeltzer, 1996, unpublished presentation).

PSYCHOLOGICAL AND PSYCHIATRIC SEQUELAE

Repeatedly, studies have found there to be a normal overall level of psychological adjustment among childhood cancer survivors (26). However, there appears to be a subset of survivors who are at risk for psychological and psychiatric symptoms. In their early groundbreaking effort, Koocher and O'Malley (27) found moderate-to-severe psychological problems in 21% of their sample of 117 survivors. Other studies have noted evidence of depression and hypochondriasis (28), behavioral adjustment problems (29), and a preoccupation with somatic concerns (10,29,30). Some survivors appear to do better than controls, reporting significantly fewer depressive symptoms and lower levels of overall anxiety (31). Sixty percent of adolescents in one study reported a greater sense of well-being than their peers; and perceptions of greater empathy, maturity, and goal direction as a result of their experience (10). However, some researchers are concerned that these

studies may represent coping through denial rather than actual improvements in coping (31, 32).

Curative treatments for childhood cancer involve intensive regimens that are frequently experienced as physically and emotionally traumatic. Although the observation that some ill children demonstrate symptoms similar to those of victims of other traumas (e.g., war veterans) is not a new one (33); only recently has there been work to document the presence of post-traumatic stress symptoms in survivors. Changes in the criteria for Post-traumatic Stress Disorder in the *Diagnostic and Statistical Manual* of the American Psychiatric Association (34) have opened the possibility of such a diagnosis for both childhood cancer survivors and their families. Interviews with children before and after bone marrow transplantation have found evidence of continuing post-traumatic stress symptoms (35–38). In a questionnaire study of 64 pediatric leukemia survivors, 12.5% reported symptoms consistent with a severe level of post-traumatic stress. (39). However, a study of 130 childhood leukemia survivors compared to 155 healthy controls found no significant differences in post-traumatic stress symptoms (40).

FAMILY ADAPTATION TO CHILDHOOD CANCER

Acknowledging that the impact of cancer goes well beyond the sick child, researchers have focused on familial adaptation to the cancer experience. Some of these efforts have studied the functioning of the family as a unit, while other authors have specifically addressed effects on siblings or parents. Family problems that have been identified include: financial concerns (41-44); an increase in family stress (45), changes in family cohesion (46), and an increase in fear about the survivor's future health (47). Although these studies indicate that there are many potential problems facing the family of the cancer survivor, other studies have demonstrated apparent positive effects of the cancer experience. Some have found that these families experience an increase in cohesion (46) and that there is a greater sense of compassion and shared experience perceived by family members (48).

Studies of siblings of pediatric cancer patients have found them to be vulnerable to distress and feelings of not having their needs met (48), with negative behavioral change (49) during the acute illness. Parents report positive changes in siblings, as well as behavioral and emotional problems. In one of the largest studies of siblings of pediatric cancer patients, parents of 254 siblings reported improvements in the siblings' maturity, supportiveness, and independence (50). The degree to which either positive or negative effects are lasting is unclear as sibling survivor issues have not been formally studied.

Most of the literature on problems with parental coping focuses on the period of cancer diagnosis and treatment or after a child dies. A new area of research into long-term adaptation of parents has examined the possibility of post-traumatic stress responses. Parents, having been exposed to both the threat to their child's life of a cancer diagnosis and the stress of cancer treatment, appear to be at risk for symptoms of post-traumatic stress (51). A questionnaire study of 64 survivors of pediatric leukemia and their parents found that 39.7% of the mothers and 33.3% of the fathers reported symptoms of severe post-traumatic stress up to five years after the completion of successful cancer treatment (39). When 130 mothers and 96 fathers of childhood leukemia survivors were compared to 148 mothers and 80 fathers of healthy controls, mothers and fathers of survivors were significantly more likely to report symptoms of post-traumatic stress than control parents (40).

Limitations of Research on Long-Term Sequelae

The conflicting data and interpretations in the studies of long-term psychological and psychiatric sequelae of childhood cancer for survivors and their families reflects the relative newness of this field of study. There has been insufficient use of common standardized measures to allow comparison across studies. Definitions of psychological health and morbidity differ between studies. Many studies have been limited by small samples and inadequate control groups. The measures and methodology may also have been insufficiently specific to identify the concerns of the diverse group of survivors and parents. When these studies are viewed as a group, there is evidence of "enduring psychological consequences" (10, p. 713) of being treated for childhood cancer, which are problematic for a subset of the survivors and their families. We await the results of studies such as the large epidemiologic study currently ongoing through the National Cancer Institute to give us a clearer sense of the prevalence of these adaptive difficulties.

CAUSES OF ADAPTATION PROBLEMS

Although researchers are unable to predict with any reliability which survivors and families will experience adaptation difficulties, there is a growing literature on potential contributors to these problems which suggests that long-term adaptation is a multi-determined phenomenon. Specific factors of interest include the role of medical sequelae, treatment intensity, age, family environment, and coping style.

Medical Sequelae

The presence of medical and physical sequelae of cancer treatment in survivors has been suggested as a possible contributor to long-term stress and adaptation difficulties. Survivors with obvious physical changes or deformities have been studied by researchers who hypothesized that they would have greater adjustment problems. As a whole, this work has failed to demonstrate significant relationships between the presence of physical changes or abnormalities and adjustment problems or psychiatric symptoms (52).

Prophylactic cranial radiation, either alone or in combination with intrathecal chemotherapy has been associated with long-term school related functional difficulties (53-58). Unlike visible physical changes and abnormalities, these functional difficulties have been related to psychosocial adjustment problems. Long-term negative consequences of cranial radiation upon psychosocial adjustment and academic achievement have been demonstrated in survivors of childhood ALL who had been treated approximately 15 years ago by Hill and colleagues. Given the significant neuropsychological problems, academic achievement effects, and functional impairments associated with cranial irradiation, intrathecal chemotherapy, and brain tumor resections, children whose illness or treatment directly involves CNS functioning may be at higher risk for psychological distress and adaptation difficulties (59). The underlying mechanism for this is unclear, but it is apparent that survivors with functional difficulties are more susceptible to psychosocial adaptation problems.

Treatment Intensity

At present it is not clear whether the life-threat of the cancer itself or the intrusive treatment is the more significant contributor to post-traumatic symptoms, although these appear to vary with age at diagnosis or time of treatment. The utility of a post-traumatic stress model is evident in the ability of the model both to describe some of the survivor phenomena and to suggest possible interventions to manage or treat the post-traumatic psychological sequelae. No other models in the childhood cancer survivor field provide both of these features. Future work in this arena will likely be fruitful in further elucidating the problems, and in establishing and evaluating specific psychological treatment approaches.

Age

Some of the studies discussed above (6–8,19) suggest that age, particularly age at the time of diagnosis and treatment, is a potential mediator of distress. It appears that adolescents at the time of diagnosis and treatment might have more difficulty with later psychosocial adaptation than younger children. Children under the age of 6 years at the time of diagnosis also appear to have fewer symptoms of post-traumatic stress. Although there is no clear explanation for these findings in the existing research, these age differences may be due to differences in ability to understand and process the experience at the time of diagnosis and treatment. If the older child or adolescent is more acutely aware of what is at risk during their treatment, the distress that is engendered by this understanding may have a longer and more severe impact than for the younger child with less understanding. The developmental tasks of older children and adolescents also differ from those of younger children and the impact of cancer on these tasks may be more disruptive for the older child (see chapter 77).

The observation that older age at the time of treatment is more predictive of greater adaptation difficulty may not be true for neuropsychological sequelae. There is some evidence (52) that children treated with cranial radiation prior to the ages of 4-6 may suffer greater neuropsychological sequelae in the future than older children.

FAMILY ENVIRONMENT

Having supportive families has correlated with better adjustment in several studies of childhood cancer survivors (27,53). In these studies measures of family functioning and psychological state were based on patients' reports of their current status, making interpretations of causality difficult. The cancer patient and his/her family are in an interactive relationship, influencing each other. However, in keeping with much of the social support literature (54,55), the effect of the family environment likely has greater impact upon the survivor's psychological state, rather than the reverse. The appraisal of the life threat posed by the illness and self-reported symptoms of post-traumatic stress of childhood cancer survivors appear to be related to the anxiety and symptoms of their parents, especially mothers (56,57).

COPING STYLE

The manner in which the survivor handles the cancer experience psychologically may also mediate the occur-

rence of future sequelae. A recurrent theme discussed by many cancer survivors is a feeling of loss of control over their lives as a consequence of the illness (30,59, 60). Serious illness changes a child's daily life and imposes restrictions on his or her ability to choose from available options. This experience usually occurs over a lengthy period and can result in a sense of learned helplessness (30). From this perspective, the task of survivorship in part becomes a struggle to regain a sense of control over their life. Findings from studies at Memorial Sloan-Kettering by Hill and colleagues demonstrated the opposite of this assumption and found that survivors' psychological state was not significantly influenced by their perceptions of control over their own physical well-being and health, and that those who did psychologically better were those who felt less personal responsibility for their illness. Having cancer controlled by their doctors and/or chance or fate was preferable to feeling that they were personally in control. These findings are contrary to another study demonstrating a positive relationship between a better sense of control and adjustment (60). There appear to be significant individual differences in the optimal way of approaching the illness and treatment. For some a greater sense of personal control may be more adaptive, whereas less personal control over illness factors may work better for others. Some work has even suggested that the use of denial and repression by childhood cancer patients may result in less distress and psychiatric symptoms (32,61).

INTERVENTIONS TO IMPROVE PSYCHOSOCIAL ADAPTATION

Despite the extensive study of the psychosocial sequelae of childhood cancer, only a few recent efforts at intervening and addressing these adaptation problems have been initiated. These have primarily focused on efforts to treat psychosocial, neuropsychological, or psychological sequelae.

Treatment of Psychosocial Sequelae

As discussed earlier, childhood cancer survivors must not only cope with psychological late effects but with job-related and insurance difficulties. With the passage of the Americans With Disabilities Act of 1990, cancer survivors have a foundation on which to build cancer-based employment discrimination legal actions. These problems can cause significant distress for both survivors and their families. Legislation to combat discrimination based on cancer history, education of survivors regarding their rights, and survivor advocacy programs are all essential components to addressing these potential barriers and stressors (62,63).

Approaches to Cognitive and Neuropsychological Sequelae

Efforts to address the neuropsychological, cognitive, and school-related sequelae have included neuropsychological rehabilitation aimed at improving the underlying functions that have been impaired by the illness or treatment (64). This treatment occurs in the clinical setting and involves attempts to strengthen deficits and teach survivors approaches to circumventing their specific cognitive problems. Other treatments have been proposed for the school setting. Greater use of individualized instruction and tutoring (65), social skills training in conjunction with school reintegration efforts (66), and behavioral management efforts to assist parents in working with their children (67) have been recommended to address cognitive and school related sequelae. The social skills training components of these programs are also designed to help survivors with cancer-related interpersonal difficulties by providing supportive counseling for the child and parent, and educational presentations for school personnel and classmates concerning cancer.

Efforts Designed to Treat Psychological Sequelae

Psychological interventions targeted for childhood cancer survivors and their families are rare. Some authors have suggested that such efforts should be an integral part of general oncology services and should focus on facilitating communication between survivors in group settings (55). These authors further suggest the need to decrease the emphasis on possible psychopathology in these treatment groups and to increase the emphasis on adaptive coping. Others have argued that family focused groups and groups of multiple survivor families are the best intervention modality (58). However, few data are yet available to assess the relative value of various interventions.

SUMMARY

Survivors of childhood cancer are becoming a larger part of the adult population of the United States. Although it appears that the majority of the survivors will do well, it is clear that the cancer experience has a significant impact on the lives of not only the survivors but also their parents and siblings. Both negative and positive effects can be seen in the psychological, interpersonal, social, academic, and physical functioning of survivors and their families. Although we are beginning to understand the quality and nature of the seque-

lae associated with childhood cancer, we are not yet able to predict those at risk with any accuracy. Even less is known about how to intervene to assist troubled survivors and families establish the best adaptation possible. Future energies need to be directed towards such endeavors on both research and clinical fronts.

REFERENCES

1. Meadows AT, Hobbie W. The medical consequences of cure. *Cancer*. 1986; 58:524–528.
2. American Cancer Society. *Cancer Facts and Figures*. New York: American Cancer Society, 1994.
3. D'Angio GJ. An overview and historical perspective of late effects of treatment for childhood cancer. In: Green DM, D'Angio GJ, eds. *Late Effects of Treatment for Childhood Cancer*. New York: Wiley–Liss, 1992: 1–6.
4. Byrd BL. Late effects of treatment of cancer in children. *Pediatr Ann*. 1983; 12:450–460.
5. Li FP, Stone R. Survivors of cancer in childhood. *Ann Intern Med*. 1976; 84:551–553.
6. Thompson E, Fairclough D, Crom D. Normal physical and psychosocial function in the majority of childhood cancer patients surviving 10 years or more from diagnosis. *Proc Ann Meet Am Soc Clin Oncol*. 1987; 6:A1013. [Abstract].
7. Schriock EA, Schell MJ, Carter J. Abnormal growth patterns and adult short stature in 115 long-term survivors of childhood leukemia. *J Clin Oncol*. 1991; 9:400–405.
8. Sklar C, Mertens A, Walter A. Final height after treatment for childhood acute lymphoblastic leukemia: comparison of no cranial irradiation with 1800 and 2400 centigrays of cranial irradiation. *J Pediatr*. 1993; 123:59–64.
9. Byrne J, Mulvihill JJ, Myers MH. Effects of treatment on fertility in long-term survivors of childhood or adolescent cancer. *N Engl J Med*. 1987; 317:1315–1321.
10. Fritz GK, Williams JR. Issues of adolescent development for survivors of childhood cancer. *J Am Acad Child Adolesc Psychiatry*. 1988; 27:712–715.
11. Holmes HA, Holmes FF. After ten years, what are the handicaps and lifestyles of children treated for cancer? *Clin Pediatr*. 1975; 14:819–823.
12. Tebbi CK, Bromberg C, Piedmonte M. Long-term vocational adjustment of cancer patients diagnosed during adolescence. *Cancer*. 1989; 63:213–218.
13. Teta MJ, Del Po, Kasl SV, et al. Psychosocial consequences of childhood and adolescent cancer survival. *J Chronic Dis*. 1986; 39:751–759.
14. Wasserman AL, Thompson EI, Wilimas JA, Fairclough DL. The psychological status of survivors of childhood/adolescent Hodgkin's Disease. *Am J Dis Childhood*. 1987; 141:626–631.
15. Hays, DM, Landsverk J, Sallon SE, et al. Educational, occupational, and insurance status of childhood cancer survivors in their fourth and fifth decades of life. *J Clin Oncol*. 1992; 10:1397–1406.
16. Hays DM. Adult survivors of childhood cancer. Employment and insurance issues in different age groups. *Cancer*. 1993; 71(10 Suppl.):3306–3309

17. Meadows AT, McKee L, Kazak AE. Psychosocial status of young adult survivors of childhood cancer: A survey. *Med Pediatr Oncol.* 1989; 17:466–470.

18. Madan-Swain A, Brown RT, Sexson SB, et al. Adolescent cancer survivors: Psychosocial and familial adaptation. *Psychosomatics.* 1994; 35:453–459.

19. Feldman F. *Work and Cancer Health Histories: Work Expectations of Youth with Cancer Histories (Ages 13–23).* Oakland, CA: American Cancer Society, California Division; 1982.

20. Vann JC, Biddle AK, Daeschner CW, et al. Health insurance access to young adult survivors of childhood cancer in North Carolina. *Med Pediatr Oncol.* 1995; 25(1):389–395.

21. Schriock EA, Schell MJ, Carter J, et al. Abnormal growth patterns and adult short stature in 115 long-term survivors of childhood leukemia. *J Clin Oncol.* 1991; 9:400–405.

22. Mulhern R, Fairclough D, Ochs J. A prospective comparison of neuropsychologic performance of children surviving leukemia who receive 18 Gy, 24 Gy, or no cranial irradiation. *J Clin Oncol.* 1991; 9:1348–56.

23. Evans SE, Radford M Current lifestyle of young adults treated for cancer in childhood. *Arch Dis Child.* 1995; 72(5):423–426.

24. Haupt R, Fears TR, Robison LL, et al. Educational attainment in long-term survivors of childhood acute lymphoblastic leukemia. *J Am Med Assoc.* 1994; 272(18):1427–1432.

25. Ruccione K, Landsverk J, Schoonover D, et al. Marriage and family decisions among long-term survivors of childhood cancer. Presentation at the 3rd International Conference on the Long-Term Complications of Treatment of Children and Adolescents for Cancer, 1994.

26. Kazak A. Implications of survival; Pediatric oncology patients and their families. In: Bearison DJ, Mulhern RK, eds. *Pediatric Psychooncology: Psychological Perspectives on Children with Cancer.* New York: Oxford University Press; 1994: 171–192.

27. Koocher GP, O'Malley JE. The Damocles syndrome: Psychosocial consequences of surviving childhood cancer. New York: McGraw-Hill, 1981.

28. Fritz GK, Williams JR, Amylon M. After treatment ends: Psychosocial sequelae in pediatric cancer survivors. *Am J Orthopsychiatry.* 1988; 58:552–561.

29. Mulhern RK, Wasserman AL, Friedman AG, Fairclough D. Social competence and behavioral adjustment of children who are long-term survivors of cancer. *Pediatrics.* 1989; 83:18–25.

30. Madan-Swain A, Brown RT. Cognitive and psychosocial sequelae for children with acute lymphoblastic leukemia. *Clin Psychol Rev.* 1991; 11:267–294.

31. Canning EH, Canning RD, Boyce WT. Depressive symptoms and adaptive style in children with cancer. *J Am Acad Child Adolesc Psychiatry.* 1992; 31:1120–1124.

32. Phipps S, Fairclough D, Mulhern R. Avoidant coping in children with cancer. *J Pediatr Psychol.* 1995; 20:217–232.

33. Levy DM. Psychic trauma of operations in children. *Am J Dis Children.* 1945; 69:7–25.

34. American Psychiatric Association. *Diagnostic and Statistical Manual of the Mental Disorders.* 4th ed. Washington, DC: American Psychiatric Association; 1994.

35. Pot-Mees CC. *The Psychosocial Effects of Bone Marrow Transplantation in Children.* Delft: Eburon; 1989.

36. Stuber ML, Nader K, Yasuda P, et al. Stress responses after pediatric bone marrow transplantation: Preliminary results of a prospective, longitudinal study. *J Am Acad Child Adoles Psychiatry.* 1991; 50:407–414.

37. Stuber ML, Nader K. Psychiatric sequelae in adolescent bone marrow transplant survivors: Implications for psychotherapy. *J Psychother Pract Res.* 1995; 4(1):30–42.

38. Stuber ML, Nader K, Houskamp BM, Pynoos RS. Acute trauma responses of children undergoing bone marrow transplantation. *J Traumatic Stress.* [In press.]

39. Stuber ML, Christakis D, Houskamp BM, et al. Post trauma symptoms in childhood leukemia survivors and their parents. *Psychosomatics.* 1996.

40. Kazak AE, Barakat LP, Meeske K, et al. Posttraumatic stress symptoms, family functioning, and social support in survivors of childhood leukemia and their mothers and fathers. *J Clin Consult Psychol.* [In press.]

41. Murinen JM. The economics of informal care: Labor market effects in the national hospice study. *Med Care.* 1986; 24:1007–1017.

42. Bodkin CM, Pisott TJ, Mann JR. Financial burden of childhood cancer. *Br Med J.* 1982; 284:1542–1544.

43. Bloom BS, Knorr RS, Evans AE. The epidemiology of disease expenses: The costs of caring for children with cancer. *J Am Med Assoc.* 1985; 253:2393–2397.

44. McCubbin HI, Figley C, eds. Stress and the Family. Vol. 2. Coping with Catastrophe. New York: Brunner/Mazel; 1983.

45. Turk DC, Kerns RD. The family in health and illness. In: Turk DC, Kerns RD, eds. Health, Illness and Families: A Life-span Perspective. New York: John Wiley; 1985: 1–22.

46. Gonzalez S, Steinglass P, Reiss D. Putting the illness in its place: Discussion groups for families with chronic medical illnesses. *Fam Proc.* 1989; 28:69–87.

47. Leventhal-Belfer L, Bakker AM, Russo C. Parents of childhood cancer survivors: A descriptive look at their concerns and needs. *J Psychosoc Oncol.* 1993; 11:19–42.

48. Sargent JR, Sahler OZ, Roughmann KJ, et al. Sibling adaptation to childhood cancer collaborative study: Siblings perceptions of the cancer experience. *J Pediatr Psychol.* 1995; 20:151–164.

49. Breyer J, Kunin H, Kalish LA, Patenaude AF. The adjustment of siblings of pediatric cancer patients: A siblings and parent perspective. *PsychoOncology.* 1993; 2:201–208.

50. Barbarian OA, Sargent JR, Sahler OZ, et al. Sibling adaptation to childhood cancer collaborative study: Parental views of pre- and postdiagnosis adjustment of siblings of children with cancer. *J Psychosoc Oncol.* 1995; 13(3):1–20.

51. Pelcovitz D, Goldenberg B, Kaplan S, et al. Posttraumatic Stress Disorder in mothers of pediatric cancer survivors. *Psychosomatics.* 1996; 37:116–126.

52. O'Malley JE, Foster D, Koocher G, Slavin L. Visible physical impairment and psychological adjustment among pediatric cancer survivors. *Am J Psychiatry.* 1980; 137:94–96.

53. Rait DS, Ostroff JS, Smith, K. Lives in a balance: Perceived family functioning and the psychosocial adjustment of adolescent cancer survivors. *Fam Proc.* 1992; 31:393–397.

54. Bloom JR, Kang SH, Romano P. Cancer and stress: The effect of social support as a resource. In: Cooper CL, Wason M, eds. *Cancer and Stress: Psychological, Biological and Coping Studies.* Chichester, UK: John Wiley; 1991: 95–124.

55. Chesler MA, Weigers M, Lawther T. How am I different? Perspectives of childhood cancer survivors on change and growth. In: Green DM, D'Angio GJ, eds. *Late Effects of Treatment for Childhood Cancer.* New York: Wiley–Liss; 1992:1–6.

56. Stuber ML, Meeske K, Gonzalez S, et al. Posttraumatic stress after childhood cancer II: A family model. *PsychoOncology.* 1994; 3:313–319

57. Stuber ML, Stress responses to pediatric cancer: a family phenomenon. *Fam Syst Med.* 1995; 13(2):163–172

58. Ostroff J, Steinglass P. Psychosocial adaptation following treatment: A family systems perspective on childhood cancer survivorship. In: Baider L, Cooper CL, Kaplan De-Nour A, eds. *Cancer and the Family.* New York: John Wiley; 1995.

59. Van Dongen-Melman JE, Sanders-Woustra JA. Psychosocial aspects of childhood cancer: A review of the literature. *J Child Psychiatry.* 1986; 27:145–180.

60. Nannis ED, Susman EJ, Strope BE. Correlates of control in pediatric cancer patients and their families. *J Pediatr Psychol.* 1982; 7:75-84.

61. Worchel FF, Rae WA, Olson T, Crowley S. Selective responsiveness of chronically ill children to assessment of depression. *J Pers Assess.* 1992; 59:605–615.

62. Hoffman B. Legal remedies to job and insurance discrimination against former childhood cancer patients. In: Green DM, D'Angio GJ, eds. *Late Effects of Treatment for Childhood Cancer.* New York: Wiley-Liss; 1992: 165–170.

63. Hays DM, Landsverk J, Ruccione K, et al. Employment problems and workplace experience of childhood cancer survivors. In: Green DM, D'Angio GJ, eds. *Late Effects of Treatment for Childhood Cancer.* New York: Wiley–Liss; 1992: 171–178.

64. Butler RW, Rizzi, L The remediation of attentional deficits secondary to treatment for childhood cancers. *Newslett Soc Pediatr Psychol.* 1995; 19:5–13.

65. Peckham VC, Meadows AT, Bartel N. Educational late effects in long-term survivors of childhood acute lymphocytic leukemia. *Pediatrics.* 1988; 81:127–133.

66. Katz ER, Rubenstein CL, Hubert N. School and social reintegration of children with cancer. *J Psychosoc Oncol.* 1988; 6:123–140.

67. Varni JW, Katz ER, Colegrove R. The impact of social skills training on the adjustment of children with newly diagnosed cancer. *J Pediatr Psychol.* 1993; 18:751–767.

80

Psychosexual Sequelae

KAROLYN WOOLVERTON AND JAMIE OSTROFF

From the first caresses given to a newborn, to discovery of one's sexual organs and a child's first "crush" on the playground at school, the groundwork needed for adult psychosexual functioning is being established. Psychosexual well-being in adulthood is epitomized by a capacity for satisfying sexual functioning within the context of an intimate relationship. Healthy psychosexual development encompasses physical, psychological, and interpersonal processes that begin in infancy and extend into adulthood. If any of these processes are seriously compromised, psychosexual well-being is at risk. When a child or adolescent experiences the traumatic procedures and the overwhelming threat that accompany a diagnosis of cancer, hugs may be replaced by restraining arms during painful venipunctures, sexual self-exploration by repeated physical examinations, and a promising future by anxious uncertainty. Though a cancer diagnosis and its treatment may potentially compromise psychosexual adjustment in all patients, cancer's impact during childhood may be more subtly problematic. Young patients must concurrently manage normative developmental tasks that serve as precursors to adult psychosexual health and the demands of their illness and its treatment. The illness experience may be deeply and intractably assimilated into their psychosexual development (1).

Formal research efforts examining the psychosexual adjustment of cancer survivors are hampered by the private nature of the subject (2), although studies of survivors of adult cancers have documented sexual difficulties (3,4). For young survivors of childhood cancer, psychosexual issues have been virtually ignored (5), with research focusing instead on more easily measurable long-term outcomes such as educational achievement or mood (6). The remarkable resiliency of children is illustrated by this empirical literature, given general findings that survivors of childhood cancer, as a group, achieve adequate global psychosocial

adjustment (7). Furthermore, anecdotal evidence exists suggesting benefits a cancer experience can bring to a young person's life (8), such as an appreciation for life or a reordering of priorities. However, investigators often caution that anecdotal evidence also exists for subtle disruption in specific areas: psychosexual functioning is such an area of concern (9–11).

After a brief overview of normative psychosexual development, this chapter will review the impact of childhood cancer on the three main components (physical, psychological, interpersonal) of healthy adult psychosexual functioning, integrating empirical findings with clinical impressions. Following this review, psychosexual interventions for survivors of childhood cancer will be discussed.

NORMATIVE PSYCHOSEXUAL DEVELOPMENT

"Healthy adult sexuality" is a complex notion including the physical capacity to engage in and enjoy sexual activity and the psychosocial resources to develop and maintain an intimate relationship. While sex is something we do, sexuality is something we are (12). Sexuality is expressed in a broad range of activities, from conversation to sexual intercourse. Establishment of one's sexuality is a developmental process that begins at birth and continues through the life span. We are not born with the necessary prerequisites for healthy adult sexuality; rather they *develop* in the context of one's physical and psychological self, family, peers, and society. Though adolescence has become synonymous with "sexual unfolding" (13), research and clinical observations support the belief that psychosexual development actually begins with infancy. Signs of sexual behavior and interest are readily noted in children through age 5 or until a child learns to conceal such behaviors as a result of cultural taboos and values. For example, erections are observed in male infants, masturbation in preschoolers is not atypical, and children aged 3-6 years old can be "outrageously flirtatious and seductive" (14). Psychological features of infancy and early childhood critical to psychosexual development include establishment of confidence and trust in one's bodily self and one's environment followed by healthy attachment to and subsequent anxiety-free separation from, a primary caregiver.

Overt sexual behaviors diminish during the elementary school years and are replaced by modesty and inhibition (15). During these years, a need for privacy in the bathroom or while dressing is expressed. Psychological energies are highly focused on achievement and control and the development of friendships becomes paramount as a precursor to intimate relationships in later life. Overt sexuality re-emerges during adolescence, as epitomized by preoccupation with one's attractiveness and physical appeal to peers, flirtatiousness, and varying degrees of sexual activities ranging from hand holding and masturbation to sexual intercourse. Psychological energies are focused on questions of self and gender identity, crucial processes to later adult sexuality.

When the developmental context includes a chronic and/or potentially life-threatening physical illness, such as cancer, the likelihood of alterations in this developmental trajectory increases greatly (16). Because development occurs in a succession of stages, one building upon another, disruption at an earlier stage may have a profound impact on subsequent development (17). For example, serious illness during infancy and early childhood may compromise the basic sense of trust necessary for healthy intimate adult relationships as a result of separations from primary caregivers, the infliction of bodily pain as part of treatment, and/or lack of consistency in the environment. Serious illness during middle childhood, a period of mastery and competence for most children, disrupts friendship patterns and sense of self-control, crucial building blocks to later adult psychosexual functioning. More obvious disruptions caused by serious illness are apparent during adolescence as the child begins to make the transition to adult sexual functioning. Cancer and its treatment (typically, multimodal therapies including chemotherapy, radiation therapy, surgery, and/or bone marrow transplant) have the potential to disrupt physical, psychological, and social processes throughout childhood, all of which are crucial processes in the unfolding of the sexual adult. Currently, developmental theory and clinical practice, coupled with a limited empirical research literature in this area, best guide our understanding of the impact cancer in childhood has on psychosexual adjustment in survivors.

PHYSICAL FUNCTIONING AND PSYCHOSEXUAL ADJUSTMENT

Puberty heralds an individual's physical transition into adult sexual responsivity and performance. Visible changes such as the development of secondary sex characteristics and enormous growth spurts are coupled with invisible, yet equally profound, changes such as attainment of reproductive capacity and a qualitative alteration in libido and sexual arousal. Puberty in healthy children can both positively and negatively impact adult psychosexual functioning (18). Specifically, pubertal status (changes experienced by every individual as he or she matures physically) and pubertal timing (timing of these changes relative to same-aged peers) have been associated with psychosexual functioning. Problems related to puberty can lead to diminished psychosexual functioning in adulthood.

Since the 1970s, cures for children with cancer have been achieved through the use of multimodal treatments that have documented toxic effects on the hypothalamic–pituitary–gonadal axis. Depending on a complex interaction of factors including the patient's age and sex, Tanner stage of development, cancer diagnosis and type, dosage, and duration of treatment, effects range from negligible to profound (19). The impact of these potential late effects on the healthy psychosexual functioning of survivors of childhood cancer can be divided into two general categories: cancer and its treatment may alter *pubertal timing*, and, in post-pubertal children, may cruelly "reverse" *pubertal status*.

Alterations in Pubertal Timing

Cancer and its treatment may alter the timing of puberty, thus resulting in a puberty that occurs out of synchrony with one's peers. The pre-pubertal gonad, once hypothesized to be relatively resistant to cytotoxic agents, is now known to be quite sensitive to their effects (20). For example, early onset of puberty is noted in girls treated with chemotherapy for ALL (21), who must then deal with both the ill effects of chemotherapy and the documented negative effects of early puberty (22). In boys, reproductive capacity can be compromised (23). Toxic effects of cancer treatment to the hypothalamic–pituitary–gonadal axis can also result in delayed growth in young patients (24). Although once treatment is completed, average adult height is commonly attained (25), a memory of being small, and so less "grown-up," as compared to peers commonly persists in the survivor. Whether due to early or delayed physical maturation, the experience of "being different" can have profound effects on psychosexual development in any child, healthy or ill.

"DON'T MAKE ME GROW UP"

Frank is a 19-year-old survivor of Hodgkin's disease diagnosed when he was five years old. Successful treatment for cancer proved toxic to Frank's hypothalamic–pituitary–gonadal axis. By the age of 15, Frank had not yet entered puberty and still resembled a pre-pubertal boy. Though hormone replacement began to induce the development of secondary sexual characteristics, Frank was very non-compliant with the treatment. While exploring with Frank his non-compliance, he revealed "It doesn't feel right. I'm not ready." Frank's delayed physical transition to "adulthood" seriously impacted his psychological development such that he felt more comfortable being his mother's "little boy," having younger friends, and avoiding the adult world of dating and sexuality.

"Reversal" of Pubertal Status

Post-pubertal children have endured the "physiological revolution" often equated with puberty (25). Their physically adult bodies, their appearance and functioning, are still new to them. Tragically, treatments for many childhood cancers can rob teenagers of their newly earned sexuality. Depending on their treatment protocol, adolescents may experience numerous psychosexual *losses* including fertility, menses, sexual libido, erections, and pubic hair (26).

"I'M A GIRL, NOT A WOMAN"

Anne is a 26 year old survivor of Hodgkin's disease for which she received chemotherapy during her late adolescent years. Struggling with her status as a virgin, she reported the following incident she experienced during treatment: "I had a chance to have sex with a boy I cared about a lot who was real understanding about my illness and its treatment. He was great and he wanted to be with me. But how could I have sex with him? He may have been okay with me being bald, but he had no idea that I had lost *all* the hair on my body, I mean, all of it. I looked, and felt, like a little girl. Now, even though I've "matured" again, it's like I can't shake that little girl feeling."

The losses experienced by the post-pubertal child not only include changes in physical appearance but losses in physical functioning. For example, the potential for loss of reproductive capacity may have an enormous impact on psychosexual functioning. In male childhood cancer patients, sperm banking, while viewed as a crucially important option by parents, frequently poses difficulty for developing boys.

"MY FIRST TIME"

Bob, a young adult survivor of acute leukemia diagnosed in adolescence, recalls being given the option of sperm banking. "Sperm banking? One minute I was a regular kid and the next minute I was trying to masturbate into a cup, with my mother in the next room well aware of what I was doing. And guess what? It was my 'first time.' I had never even masturbated before. Kind of a weird introduction to sex if you ask me."

PSYCHOLOGICAL FUNCTIONING AND PSYCHOSEXUAL ADJUSTMENT

How one's body works is only one aspect of adult psychosexual functioning. The desire and capacity for intimacy is another hallmark of healthy psychosexual adjustment. As complex as the notion of sexuality, the capacity for intimacy begins to develop in middle to late adolescence as a result of the process of separation/individuation and involves far more than physical intimacy. Likened to "commitment," sexual intimacy includes a mixture of "eroticism, emotional closeness, mutual caring, vulnerability, and trust" (27) with minimal anxiety or defensiveness.

Individuals can have sexual feelings and engage in sexual activities, but true intimacy is possible only once an individual's identity is fully established (28), autonomy from family has been achieved, and a vision of the future is beginning to form. Thus, three domains of psychological functioning are particularly relevant to the capacity for intimacy and will be reviewed in this chapter:

1. self-concept, specifically sexual self-concept and body image;
2. sense of autonomy;
3. future orientation.

Self-Concept and Psychosexual Adjustment

The term self-concept is "a phenomenological organization of individuals' experiences and ideas about themselves in all aspects of their lives" (29). Self-concept is a multidimensional construct encompassing functioning in various physical, social, and psychological domains. How individuals see themselves is not always evident, as self-concept not only manifests in overt behaviors but is experienced in unspoken thoughts and hidden feelings as well. Perhaps most unavailable to outsiders is a person's sexual self-concept. Overt sexual behaviors are not always most revealing about the sense an individual has of him/herself as a sexual being, because this incorporates not only sexual experience but issues related to body image, generativity, and the experience of one's masculinity/femininity. As children, we learn whether we are a boy or girl and how our bodies work, but it is only as adolescents that the physical changes of puberty force us to search for a new self-image that incorporates the new physical self as well (30). A child's physical self-concept, imbued with the qualitatively different libidinal urges of puberty, develops into a sexual self-concept. Healthy psychosexual functioning hinges on our knowing ourselves and our bodies intimately in order then to share our self-experiences with others. The perception of having a body that has "failed," as childhood cancer patients often describe their illness experience, can be incorporated into the young child's physical self-concept or the developing adolescent's sexual self-concept.

Empirical Findings

The overall self-concept of survivors of childhood cancers has been documented in numerous studies as being quite robust and well-developed (9,31). The physical changes and chronic hardships of cancer seem to force an "identity crisis" (32), requiring intense self-scrutiny. Such scrutiny often results in a sense of mastery and achievement in having successfully completed treatment and battled cancer. However, empirical research also suggests that encapsulated difficulties in self-concept do exist. A number of studies highlight the devastating effects in a generally well adjusted survivor that treatment for cancer during childhood can have on sexual self-concept and body image; these include concerns about physical attractiveness and somatic hypervigilance (9), and heightened worries about their body, its functional status, and its appearance (33). Disruptions in sexual self-concept in young survivors with otherwise adequate self-concepts is the typical finding (31,34,35).

Clinical Impressions

Experiencing a chronic, life threatening illness during childhood introduces obstacles to exploring one's sexuality. The disease and its treatment result in the nearly universal side effects of nausea, fatigue, hair loss, weight gain or loss, and acute and/or chronic pain. Illness may provoke an "identity crisis" (32). Children and adolescents report looking in a mirror and seeing someone else, although feeling that they look the same as all the other kids. They feel bald and genderless, dissociated from their bodies during painful procedures, and choose to disavow their bodies entirely. Alterations in sexual self-concept continue beyond the treatment phase as survivors are forced to remain vigilant over body changes. As they mature, survivors confront issues such as premature menopause and infertility. Not surprisingly, many survivors report being unable to shake deeply embedded feelings about themselves related to treatment.

"MY BODY REMEMBERED FOR ME"

Sam is a 32-year-old long-term survivor of acute leukemia. Treated as a young child, Sam remembers very little about his treatment, which was completed prior to the age of five. Sam reports that he is one of the "lucky" ones: he has minimal residual side effects from his disease and/or treatment, he has a good job, a loving wife, and two children. In fact, he had stopped seeing his oncologist for check-ups many years ago and returned recently only to say farewell to a retiring staff member. As the staff member discussed her memories with him of how he would "howl and scream" during BMAs and LPs, Sam began to cry. "All these years, I thought I was a 'cold' person—I couldn't stand having people, even my wife, touch me, particularly my back. I know she feels rejected when I tense up. Don't you see? It's not that I'm physically cold. Even though my mind doesn't remember what happened to me, my *back* does!"

Not surprisingly, a common concern of people who have not been sexually active prior to their diagnosis is that cancer means they will never begin a sexual life (2). Sexuality gets put on hold and young survivors may defer a sex life until they have successfully resolved other issues facing them, such as returning to school or work full time, regaining a healthier appearance, and figuring out when and how to discuss the cancer treatment with a potential partner. This reluctance to address sexual issues stems not only from survivors. The denial of sexuality may be unintentionally reinforced by parents and staff treating young patients (30) through failure to respect privacy in an environment that readily denies it, by necessarily being involved in the intimate physical activities of young people, and by reinforcing more adult priorities such as health and compliance over more youthful priorities such as worry about physical appearance or quest for self-control and determination.

"WHO ME?"

Lisa had spent much of her early adolescent years hospitalized, battling a rhabdomyosarcoma. Currently ten years post-treatment she reported being unable to even consider herself as a candidate for a romantic relationship. "You have to understand, I spent a huge portion of my life being poked and prodded by strangers, mostly men, some of them really handsome, whose interest in me didn't extend past my tumor. My mom and I stopped doing 'girl things' with each other because we had to do medical stuff. I guess one of the crowning blows was when my friends stopped telling me about dances at school. The message seemed to be that I wasn't supposed to be interested in that sort of stuff while *battling cancer*. I guess I listened more closely than I realized because now, years later, I can't believe someone would find me appealing. When a guy says, 'hey, you look great,' my knee-jerk response is 'who me?'"

Autonomy and Psychosexual Adjustment

Historically, autonomy in adulthood was conceptualized as being achieved through a turbulent, often painful, disconnection from parents resulting in an individual independent of his or her family of origin. More recently, developmental researchers have re-articulated adult autonomy as a process achieved through greater differentiation of self throughout the childhood years without rupturing enduring family bonds (36,37). Autonomous functioning develops (or is thwarted) from birth to adulthood. As originally described by Bowlby (38), "self-reliant", autonomous young adults know who they are, how to care for themselves, and whom they can count on. Psychosexual functioning is optimized when an individual is truly autonomous. A capacity for individuated relationships, characterized by both separateness and mutuality, is a prerequisite for intimacy (36). Independence is normally marked by ambivalence, a conflict which may be all the more heightened in the child with a chronic illness (16,30).

Empirical Findings. In western society, signposts of impending adulthood and autonomous functioning include graduation from high school/college, getting a driver's license, serving in the military, starting a job, marrying or becoming a parent (39). Empirical findings, though scant, offer preliminary support for the hypothesis that childhood cancer alters the development of autonomy in the survivor. The literature suggests that the mechanism for this alteration may be due to changes in the former patient, changes in family affective bonds, and/or limitations imposed by society as a result of the survivor's medical history. Illness, and the hospital environment, can have an enormously regressive pull on children and adolescents. For example, adolescents with cancer have been shown to depend on others for direction rather than having their sense of direction emanate from within (40), remain at home longer than age matched peers (41), and siblings (42), and report ill-defined long-term goals (41). Lower rates of marriage in childhood cancer survivors (43) particularly in survivors of central nervous system (CNS) tumors (44,45), have been found. In an overview of autonomy in childhood cancer survivors, Zeltzer (46) stated that researchers attributed the general tendency of survivors to marry less frequently and at a later age to "parental overprotectiveness during treatment, resulting in a delay in achieving adult maturity, combined with a delay in leaving the parental home to achieve independent residence." Socioeconomic inequities serving as barriers to autonomy have also been identified in childhood cancer survivors. Most notably, Teta (47) examined the occupational and educational status of approximately 2500 survivors of childhood cancer and found, particularly in male survivors, alarming inequities in the areas of employment, education, and military service. Despite academic parity (48), survivors experience poorer occupational performance and report a higher frequency of employment rejections. Finally, preliminary findings from our study of relationships in young adult survivors of childhood cancer suggest that autonomy is an enormously complex issue for these young people. They report experiencing being both more independent and mature than their peers, while also feeling an enormous tug from and more dependence upon family (49).

Clinical Impressions. During clinical interviews (49), young adult survivors of childhood cancer frequently describe both enjoying and suffering from intensely close relationships with their family of origin, particularly their mothers, and the conflict this poses to outside relationships. Having counted on parents, rather than peers during their treatment, young adults find it hard to relinquish both the intensity and safety of the parent–child relationship, sometimes to the exclusion of allowing peers and romantic partners into their lives.

"IT'S LIKE MY MOTHER WAS RIGHT THERE WITH ME"

Ted completed treatment for osteogenic sarcoma when he was 17 years old. During his treatment, which involved extensive chemotherapy coupled with multiple surgeries, he formed a very close attachment with his mother. "She was really wonderful throughout my treatment, was there when I needed her and would get lost when she was bugging me. She was the one person I could truly count on. I got so use to telling my mom everything—and believe me, during treatment they know and see everything—that I didn't, or couldn't, stop doing so after treatment. After my first sexual experience, my mom was the first to know. I told her all about that relationship. When my friends would say to me 'You told your *mother* about that?', I felt lucky to be so close to my mom. Now, though, I'm beginning to see that the relationship failed because it had a very "crowded" bed— my girlfriend, my mother, and me. To this day, it's still hard for me to hold things back from mom."

Future Orientation and Psychosexual Adjustment

A third psychological process crucial to the development of intimacy and healthy psychosexual adjustment is the development of a future orientation. Planning for the future, dreaming about its possibilities, and having a clarity about its existence are all building blocks to developing and maintaining an intimate relationship. When the future is in doubt, closeness in relationships may be threatened.

Empirical Findings. Perhaps the most profound piece of evidence for alteration in future orientation is fear of recurrence. Nearly half of all young survivors of childhood cancer express worry about recurrence (10,33,50) and acknowledge an ominous sense of uncertainty. This fear may directly translate into being reluctant to marry and worry about health of progeny (45).

Clinical Impressions. Survivorship is an ambiguous period characterized by the Damocles Syndrome: the desire to embrace life, coupled with a fear of what life holds (51). This ambiguity and uncertainty may mark the survivor's life for years or for a lifetime (52). Survivors may wonder when, or if, it's safe to begin living beyond the one day at a time philosophy typically developed during treatment. "Young survivors express concern over a wide range of issues related to the future such as relapse, death, marriage, and career" (5). Young cancer survivors and those who love them realize the uncertainty of their future.

"COULDN'T YOU DUMP ME AFTER I'M GONE?"
Fran, a 26-year-old survivor of acute leukemia, had finally found the "man of her dreams." She was unprepared for his reaction when she told him about her past cancer history. "Initially he was silent, then he became very overprotective. I felt like I was going to drop dead any minute. Finally, he told me he couldn't stand to lose me if my cancer returned, and, despite my reassurances that my cancer had been gone for over 15 years, he dumped me. How ironic."

INTERPERSONAL FUNCTIONING AND PSYCHOSEXUAL ADJUSTMENT

Psychosexual functioning is poignantly personal and private. However, the social/interpersonal context has a crucial role in both psychosexual development and psychosexual expression. Though historically sexual behavior has been characterized as the manifestation of instinctual drives (i.e., Freud and other drive theorists), recent research supports a view of sexual behavior as socially shaped, learned behavior (53). For example, social or peer pressure determines the onset of dating in adolescents to a far greater influence than degree of sexual maturation. Individual rates of maturation that deviate from the norm for that age have little impact on dating patterns (54). *Perceptions* of what is normative in one's peer group are powerful influences on sexual behavior (55). Thus, peers exert their influence on each other's sexual behavior not only through direct socialization but also through comparisons with perceived norms. Increasingly, social psychologists concur that individuals are not neutral observers of themselves and their worlds but active constructors of the social realities with which they compare themselves. The hoped-for yield from this comparison for children and, even more so, adolescents is to fit in with peers.

Children and adolescents need to be with their peers. Having friends and feeling their support is highly associated with feeling good about oneself (56). Feeling a sense of belonging with similar others is crucial to child development, particularly for adolescents seeking to expand their worlds (57) and to find models of behavior. Furthermore, having friends may help to promote romantic and sexual socialization (58). So important is the need to be a part of a peer group that being different, as in having cancer, constitutes developmental deprivation in that it blocks access to peers (57). Minimal contact with few peers limits choices from the rich "supermarket" of attributes, qualities, and skills that a larger group of age mates offers. Limited exposure implies that choices in friendships, experiences, and role models may be made prematurely. Furthermore, lack of exposure to peers increases the likelihood that perceptions of peers will be inaccurate as the isolated child spends increased amounts of time imagining how peers act, think, and feel rather than directly experiencing these phenomena. Thus, opportunities for socializing and social development are restricted, leading some researchers to suggest that social disability related to chronic illness can be far more serious than the effect of the physical condition (16).

Empirical Findings. For cancer survivors, the diagnosis of a life-threatening illness has rendered them different from their peers. The stated goal of many newly diagnosed patients is to return to "normal" as soon as possible, and, once off treatment, to "be like everyone else." Having missed up to two or more years of school while on treatment, and being unable to participate in "normal" activities with peers, a distortion of what is "normal" may occur. As they return to school, usually the first step in the process of "normalization," differences between self and others may become crystallized. Though others may see no visible signs of the adolescent survivor's illness, as is particularly the case with hematologic malignancies, the adolescent may feel those differences acutely as comparison with peers begins.

Empirical literature on the maintenance and quality of social relationships during and after treatment for childhood cancer supports the hypothesis that chronic illness alters peer relationships; the question is just to what degree and through what mechanism. Some studies suggest that peers do the "rejecting" (8), while others have identified a lowered interest in interpersonal relationships and social withdrawal on the part of the cancer survivor (41,59,60), and still others have examined the interaction between these two mechanisms (49). Despite the undetermined mechanism, peer disruption, social isolation, interpersonal sensitivity, and/or disappointment and dissatisfaction with peer support as negative consequences of childhood cancer, both during and after treatment, are typically reported (5,8,11,41,61–64).

Few studies have examined the impact of childhood cancer on dating and romantic relationships. Notable studies (11,9,49) have identified romantic relationships in young survivors of childhood cancer as particularly problematic. For example, Fritz and Williams (9) found that 50% of their sample of adolescent cancer survivors acknowledged extreme discomfort with and avoidance of dating relationships. These same adolescents reported having "intimate confidantes" (i.e., close, though platonic, relationships with opposite sex peers). Similarly, we have found that young adult survivors of adolescent cancer struggle with romantic relationships in that dating becomes a process of testing others to see if they can handle the survivor's "secret." However, having experienced intensely emotional relationships with parents, staff, and occasionally peers during the life-and-death context of their illness and treatment, often the young adult survivors report disappointment in their inability to capture this intensity with romantic partners. Many survivors wonder how they can truly feel close with someone who did not experience this life-changing event with them (49). Similar expectations and disappointments were noted by Gray et al. (11) as well.

Clinical Impressions. Although little information is currently available on actual sexual activity in childhood cancer survivors, it is highly plausible that young survivors may become uncomfortable with sexual activity (65). Having developed misperceptions and unrealistic expectations of sexual relationships and sexual partners as a result of limited socialization and experience, sexual activity becomes less a function of intimacy and sexuality and more a function of dependence and need for physical comfort and reassurance. Sexual activity may become a means of affirming life (66) or of "fitting in."

Particularly for the survivor who reports feeling "out-of-step," sexual activity may be an avenue for re-entry.

"OKAY, SO MAYBE I WAS WRONG"

Sue finished treatment just before her nineteenth birthday. She missed her last two years of high school—'the party years' as she called them. Her one solid friend was male; they had been best friends since grade school. Repeatedly and insistently, Sue pressured her friend to have sex with her. She wanted to make sure that everything was working right. Besides, she hated thinking she was the only high school graduate in town who was a virgin and she just wanted to "get it over with." When he finally relented, Sue was overwhelmed by how emotional she felt about their having had sex. He was right not to want to do it just to do it."

All children need exposure to both "vertical" and "horizontal" relationships (56) in order to develop skills necessary to deal with the world. "Vertical" relationships are attachments with individuals, typically adults, who have greater knowledge and power. "Horizontal" relationships are attachments with individuals who are more or less *similar* to, and equal with, oneself. Childhood cancer survivors have experienced an abundance of "vertical" relationships, as they maneuver the sophisticated environment of the medical setting. These relationships may become idealized, often at the expense of "horizontal" connections with similar others, thereby influencing psychosexual well-being.

"NO ONE WILL EVER UNDERSTAND THE WAY MY DOCTOR DOES"

Leslie considered her survivor status to be a miracle. Treated at a very young age for non-Hodgkin's lymphoma with a lengthy, experimental protocol that led to the first cures for this disease, Leslie spent much of her childhood in hospitals and with medical personnel. She was the staff darling, representing the heralding of the medical professions' ability to cure childhood cancer. She had begun to date, but no one seemed to "measure up." 'They are all so immature, they haven't experienced life the way I have. So many people don't understand this. Thank goodness my doctors do.'

For new relationships, survivors must struggle with a multitude of disclosure issues. They must decide who they will tell, when they will tell, what they will tell, and so on. Until a survivor divulges his/her history, the survivor has an enormous responsibility as s/he balances his/her feelings and needs must be balanced with the feelings and needs of the other person. Not surprisingly, young survivors frequently report dating people who knew them, or knew of them, prior to and during their treatment.

"I WISH THERE WERE A COOKBOOK I COULD FOLLOW"

Ted survived ALL as a child. Though otherwise healthy, treatment left him infertile. "If it weren't for the infertility, I wonder if I'd even tell potential partners about my past. It's like this, if I say something too soon, the woman acts like I am being presumptuous. Yet I've also been accused of 'holding back' by women who think I should have said something sooner. I feel they have a right to know about my past, but don't I have rights too? Isn't there some tried and true recipe to follow for talking about all this?"

PHYSICAL, PSYCHOLOGICAL, AND INTERPERSONAL FUNCTIONING AND PSYCHOSEXUAL ADJUSTMENT

In summary, though overall adjustment of childhood cancer survivors is quite good, adult psychosexual adjustment in childhood cancer survivors is affected through alterations in physical, psychological, and interpersonal functioning. A crucial developmental task of the first two decades of life is to progress to young adulthood, having reduced the developmentally normal self-absorption of childhood and adolescence. By decreasing self-focus, the capacity for respect of and empathy for others can grow. This necessarily requires a movement from the arena of family to that of peers and romantic partners, both of whom serve as catalysts for the diminishment of self-involvement. However, owing to the physical, psychological, and interpersonal hardships of cancer and its treatment, this developmental trajectory may be derailed. As such, the cancer experience induces an "iatrogenic self-absorption." For example, both during and post treatment, young cancer patients are urged to be hypervigilant about their bodies and physical responses. They receive abnormal yet necessary attention, often to the detriment of others. Their courage and bravery are praised even as they report being demanding and mean. In essence, successful treatment and post-treatment care nurtures a self-absorption in young patients, a stance which, if maintained, interferes with relationships and cruelly sets the former patient up for disappointment.

CLINICAL IMPLICATIONS AND INTERVENTION APPROACHES

There is no universal response to childhood cancer and so there is no one psychosocial intervention for all survivors (9). However, research and clinical impressions support the presence of significant post-treatment disruptions in childhood cancer survivors ability to have fully developed, satisfying intimate relationships.

Owing to the complex interaction of residual physical, psychological, or social sequelae, many young survivors appear to struggle with a conflict of unbalanced development: they present as mature and competent in many domains of their lives while feeling a lag in their intimate lives. As one childhood cancer survivor stated, "It's like I'm older than my friends, but younger than my friends. Does that make sense? How can that make sense?" As a result of their treatment, survivors are necessarily self-absorbed with their bodies and their health; however, interest in their sexual well-being has not been nurtured.

Post-treatment interventions include individual and group supportive psychotherapies. Young-adult survivor support groups prove to be a comfortable format for young survivors who need support in addressing relationship issues and are reluctant to burden their existing support network, which they feel may already be strained from the pressures of active treatment. By creating groups that address particular development groups, such as young adults, relevant milestones and issues are more easily discussed. Thus, these groups typically focus on young adults' feelings of being socially isolated and out of step with the life events of their peers (67) and questions about disclosure of medical history. Sessions focusing specifically on mourning the loss of one's fertility are often requested. By using a group format, the particularly powerful curative factor of interpersonal learning (68) can be capitalized upon.

Preventive intervention programs must acknowledge the myriad ways cancer and its treatment may ultimately impact psychosexual functioning in order to minimize the consequences. When planning preventive intervention programs, developmental issues remain the most influential guiding factor. When intervening with young children to minimize future psychosexual consequences of cancer, modalities include play therapy designed to address preverbal subconscious issues, coupled with staff and parent awareness. Aggressive treatment of acute and chronic pain, use of anesthesia during painful medical procedures, and age-appropriate explanation of physical examinations serve to minimize a child's protective need to dissociate from his/her body. School interventions to inform classmates about a child's treatment and its sometimes disfiguring side effects have been found to decrease teasing by peers (69) and so reduce the beginnings of potentially long-lasting social disruption. Preparing pre-pubertal children for the onset of puberty, whether early or on schedule, helps children deal with the "physiological revolution" that is affecting their bodies even as treatment is making its mark.

For adolescents undergoing active treatment, modalities for enhancing relationship adjustment and body image include peer groups (supportive, psychoeducational and/or social skills training), individual therapy, and staff and parent awareness. These groups provide practical solutions for managing appearance, opportunities to practice handling difficult situations with peers, and a feeling of support. Additionally, support groups allow opportunities for frank discussions about sexual activity and sexuality. Such a format allows for anticipatory guidance and education, and a setting in which "normalcy" can be both validated and promoted (65). The use of role-playing techniques allows for the practicing of strategies prior to their implementation in the "real world." A crucial feature of adolescent groups is that adolescent issues are central; only secondarily are the participants ill.

The impact of cancer in childhood is ongoing, and therefore the need for information and support in dealing with its impact extends beyond treatment into the post-treatment years. As childhood cancer patients grow, the issues important to them mature and develop as well. Though they will address many challenges post treatment, young survivors would benefit from guidance in developing satisfying, intimate relationships. Only then will the field of pediatric cancer have achieved "total cures" (70).

REFERENCES

1. Greydanus D, Gunther M, Demarest D, Sears J. Sexuality of the chronically ill adolescent. In: Sugar M, ed. *Atypical Adolescence and Sexuality*. New York: W.W. Norton, 1990: 147–156 .
2. Auchincloss, S. Sexual dysfunction in cancer patients: Issues in evaluation and treatment. In: Holland J, Rowland J, ed. *Handbook of Psychooncology: Psychological Care of the Patient with Cancer*. New York: Oxford University Press; 1989: 383–413.
3. Anderson BJ. Sexual functioning morbidity among cancer survivors. *Cancer*. 1985; 55:1835–1842.
4. Moadel A, Ostroff J, Lesko L. Fertility and sexuality issues. In: Whedon M, Wujcik D, eds. *Blood and Marrow Stem Cell Transplantation: Principles, Practice, and Nursing Insights*, 2nd ed. Boston: Jones & Bartlett; 1997: 377–399.
5. Ettinger RS, Heiney SP. Cancer in adolescents and young adults: Psychosocial concerns, coping strategies, and interventions. *Cancer Suppl*. 1993; 71:(10)3276–3280.
6. List M, Ritter-Sterr C, Lansky S. Cancer during adolescence. *Pediatrician*. 1991; 18:32–36.
7. Kazak A. Implications of survival: Pediatric oncology patients and their families. In: Bearison DJ, Mulhern RK, eds. *Pediatric Psycho-Oncology: Psychological Perspectives on Children with Cancer*. New York: Oxford University Press; 1994: 171–192.
8. Wasserman AL, Thompson EI, Wilimas JA, Fairclough DL. The psychological status of survivors of childhood/adolescent Hodgkin's disease. *Am J Dis Child*. 1987; 141:626–631.
9. Fritz GK, Williams JR. Issues of adolescent development for survivors of childhood cancer. *J Am Acad Child Adolesc Psychiatry*. 1988; 27(6):712–715.
10. Meadows AT, McKee L, Kazak AE. Psychosocial status of young adult survivors of childhood cancer: A survey. *Med Pediatr Oncol*. 1989; 17:466–470.
11. Gray RE, Doan BD, Shermer P, et al. Psychological adaptation of survivors of childhood cancer. *Cancer*. 1992; 70:2713–2721.
12. Selekman J, McIlvain-Simpson G. Sex and sexuality for the adolescent with a chronic condition. *Pediatr Nurs*. 1991; 17:(6)535–538.
13. Sarrel LJ, Sarrel PM. Sexual unfolding in adolescents. In: Sugar M, ed. *Atypical Adolescence and Sexuality*. New York: W.W. Norton; 1990:18–43.
14. Money J, Ehrhardt A. *Man and Woman, Boy and Girl*. Baltimore: Johns Hopkins University Press; 1972.
15. Friedrich WN, Grambsch P, Broughton D, et al. Normative sexual behavior in children. *Pediatrics*. 1991; 88:(3)456–464.
16. Strax TE. Psychological issues faced by adolescents and young adults with disabilities. *Pediatr Ann*. 1991; 20(9):507–511.
17. Perrin EC, Gerrity PS. Development of children with a chronic illness. *Pediatr Clin N Am*. 1984; 31(1):19–31.
18. Petersen AC. Adolescent development. *Ann Rev Psychol*. 1988; 39:583–607.
19. Byrne J, Mulvihill J, Myers M, et al. *N Engl J Med*. 1987; 317:1315–1321.
20. Meyers S, Shilsky R. Prospects for fertility after cancer chemotherapy. *Semin Oncol*. 1992; 19:597–604.
21. Robison LR. Issues in the consideration of intervention strategies in long-term survivors of childhood cancer. *Cancer Suppl*. 1993; 71(10):3406–3410.
22. Brooks-Gunn J, Reiter E. The role of pubertal processes. In: Feldman S, Elliott G, eds. *At the Threshold: The Developing Adolescent*. Cambridge, MA: Harvard University Press; 1990:16–53.
23. Jaffe N, Sullivan M, Ried H, et al. Male reproductive function in long-term survivors of childhood cancer. *Med Pediatr Oncol*. 1988; 16:241–247.
24. Sklar CA. Growth and pubertal development in survivors of childhood cancer. *Pediatrician*. 1991; 18:53–60.
25. Petersen AC, Spiga R. Adolescence and stress. In: Goldberger L, Breznitz S, eds. *Handbook of Stress*. 1993:515–528.
26. Chambas K. Sexual concerns of adolescents with cancer. *J Pediatr Oncol Nurs*. 1991; 8(4):165–172.
27. Grant LM, Demetriou E. Adolescent sexuality. *Pediatr Oncol Nurs*. 1988; 35(6):1271–1289.
28. Greydanus DE, Gunther MS, Demarest DS, Sears JM. Sexuality of the chronically ill adolescent. In: Sugar M, ed. *Atypical Adolescence and Sexuality*. New York: W.W. Norton Company; 1990: 147–156.
29. Coombs A. Some observations of self-concept theory and research. In: Lynch M, ed. *Self-Concept: Advances in Theory and Research*. Cambridge, MA: Ballinger; 1981.

30. McAnarney ER. Social maturation: A challenge for handicapped and chronically ill adolescents. *J Adolesc Health Care*. 1985; 6:90–101.

31. Anholt UV, Fritz GK, Keener M. Self-concept in survivors of childhood and adolescent cancer. *J Psychosoc Oncol*.1993; 11(1):1–16.

32. Moos R, Tsu V. The crisis of physical illness. In: Moos R, ed. *Coping with Physical Illness*. New York: Plenum Press; 1977.

33. Smith (Woolverton) K, Ostroff J, Tan C, Lesko L. Alterations in self-perceptions among adolescent cancer survivors. *Cancer Invest*. 1991; 9(5):581–587.

34. Smith (Woolverton) K. *Measurement of Self-concept in Adolescent Cancer Survivors*. Dallas, TX: University of Texas Southwestern Medical School; 1992.

35. Stern M, Norma S, Zevon M. Adolescents with cancer: Self-image and perceived social support as indexes of adaptation. *J Adolesc Res*. 1993; 8:124–142.

36. Powers SI, Hauser ST, Kilner LA. Adolescent mental health. *Am Psychol*. 1989; 44(2):200–208.

37. Gilligan C. Adolescent development reconsidered. In: Irwin C, ed. *Adolescent Social Behavior and Health*. San Francisco: Jossey-Bass, 1987: 63–92.

38. Bowlby J. *A Secure Base*. New York: Basic Books, 1988.

39. Diamond M, Diamond GH. Adolescent sexuality: Biosocial aspects and intervention strategies. *J Soc Work Hum Sex*. 1986; 5(1):3–13.

40. Kellerman J, Zeltzer L, Ellenberg L, et al. Psychological effects of illness in adolescence: Anxiety, self-esteem, and perception of control. *J Pediatr*. 1980; 97:126–131.

41. Chang P, Nesbit ME, Youngren N, Robison LL. Personality characteristics and psychosocial adjustment of long-term survivors of childhood cancer. *J Psychosoc Oncol*. 1988; 5(4):43–51.

42. Lansky S, List M, Ritter-Sterr C. Psychosocial consequences of cure. *Cancer*. 1986; 58:529–533.

43. Zevon MA, Neubauer NA, Green DM. Adjustment and vocational satisfaction of patients treated during childhood or adolescence for acute lymphoblastic leukemia. *Am J Pediatr Hematol Oncol*. 1990; 12(4):454–461.

44. Byrne J, Fears TR, Steinhorn SC, et al. Marriage and divorce after childhood and adolescent cancer. *J Am Med Assoc*. 1989; 262(19):2693–2699.

45. Teeter MA, Holmes GE, Holmes FF, Baker AB. Decisions about marriage and family among survivors of childhood cancer. *J Psychosoc Oncol*. 1987; 5(4):59–67.

46. Zeltzer LK. Cancer in adolescents and young adults: Psychosocial aspects. *Cancer Suppl*. 1993; 71(10):3463–3468.

47. Teta J. Socioeconomic sequelae of childhood and adolescent cancer survival. In: Barofsky I, ed. *Work and Illness: The Cancer Patient*. New York: Praeger, 1989: 49–69.

48. Haupt R, Fears TR, Robison LL, et al. Educational attainment in long-term survivors of childhood acute lymphoblastic leukemia. *J Am Med Assoc*.1994; 272(18):1427–1432.

49. Sklar C, Lesko L, Ostroff J, et al. A preliminary examination of the psychological and psychosexual adjustment of young adult patients successfully treated for pediatric cancer. Unpublished manuscript, Memorial Sloan-Kettering Cancer Center, New York; 1997.

50. Lozowski S. Views of childhood cancer survivors. *Cancer*. 1993; 71:3354–3357.

51. Koocher G, O'Malley J. *The Damocles Syndrome: Psychological Consequences of Surviving Childhood Cancer*. New York: McGraw-Hill; 1981.

52. Cincotta, N. Psychosocial issues in the world of children with cancer. *Cancer*. 1993; 71(10):3251–3259.

53. Miller BC, Fox GL. Theories of adolescent heterosexual behavior. *J Adolesc Res*. 1987; 2(3):269–282.

54. Dornbusch SM, Carlsmith JM, Gross RT, et al. Sexual development, age, and dating: A comparison of biological and social influences upon one set of behaviors. *Child Dev*. 1981; 52:179–185.

55. Brooks-Gunn J, Furstenberg FF. Adolescent sexual behavior. *Am Psychol*. 1989; 44(2):249–257.

56. Hartup W. Adolescents and their friends. In: Laursen B, ed. *Close Friendships in Adolescence*. San Francisco: Jossey-Bass; 1993: 3–22.

57. Seltzer VC. *The Psychosocial Worlds of the Adolescent: Public and Private*. New York: John Wiley; 1989.

58. Laursen B. *Close Friendships in Adolescence*. San Francisco: Jossey-Bass, Inc. 1993.

59. Cella D, Tross S. Psychological adjustment to survival from Hodgkin's disease. *J Consult Clin Psychol*. 1986; 54:616–622.

60. Hodges MH, Graham-Pole J, Fong ML. Attitudes, knowledge, and behaviors of school peers of adolescent cancer patients. *J Psychosoc Oncol*. 1984; 2(2):37–46.

61. Carr-Gregg M, White L. The adolescent with cancer: A psychological overview. *Med J Aust*. 1987; 147:496–502.

62. Noll RB, Bukowski WM, Rogosch FA, et al. Social interactions between children with cancer and their peers: Teacher ratings. *J Pediatr Psychol*. 1990; 15(1):43–56.

63. Mulhern RK, Wasserman AL, Friedman AG, Fairclough D. Social competence and behavioral adjustment of children who are long-term survivors of cancer. *Pediatrics*. 1989; 83(1):18–25.

64. Tebbi CK, Stern M, et al. The role of social support systems in adolescent cancer amputees. *Cancer*. 1985; 56:965–971.

65. Heiney SP. Adolescents with cancer: Sexual and reproductive issues. *Cancer Nurs*. 1989; 12(2):95–101.

66. White SD, DeBlassie RR. Adolescent sexual behavior. *Adolescence*. 1992; 27(105):183–191.

67. Zampini K, Ostroff J. The Post-Treatment Resource Program: Portrait of a program for cancer survivors. *Psycho-Oncology*. 1993; 2:1–9.

68. Yalom I. *The Theory and Practice of Group Psychotherapy*. New York: Basic Books, 1978.

69. List M, Ritter-Sterr C, Lansky S. Enhancing the adjustment of long-term survivors: Early findings of a school intervention study. In: Green D, Dangio G, eds. *Late Effects of Treatment for Childhood Cancer*. Wiley-Liss; 1992: 159–164.

70. Friedman HL. Changing patterns of adolescent sexual behavior: Consequences for health and development. *J Adolesc Health*. 1992; 13:345–350.

81

Cognitive Sequelae of Treatment in Children

SUSAN E. WALCH, TIM A. AHLES, AND ANDREW J. SAYKIN

Improvements in pediatric oncology survival rates have allowed a greater focus on the quality of survival following successful treatment for cancer in children. The neurocognitive functioning of pediatric cancer patients has received increasing attention of the past 15 years. Cognitive functioning plays a critical role in quality of life for cancer patients and survivors (1). Cognitive impairment in pediatric cancer patients may be of particular concern because of the potential negative impact of cancer and treatment on the developing brain. The causes of adverse neuropsychological outcomes may be multifactorial, including such factors as central nervous system (CNS) tumors, metastases, and treatments, as well as infections, fever, medications, and other complications of treatment (2).

Brain tumors and leukemia represent the most common forms of pediatric malignancies. The survival rates for pediatric brain tumors and childhood leukemia have improved dramatically, primarily as a function of cranial irradiation and systemic chemotherapy. However, the potential for neurological complications from these cancers and the neurotoxicity of the common forms of treatment have generated considerable concern. This chapter reviews the literature examining the neuropsychological and cognitive functioning of pediatric patients with brain tumors and leukemia.

PEDIATRIC BRAIN TUMORS

Pediatric brain tumors are a relatively common form of pediatric malignancy, second only to childhood leukemias. The overall five-year survival rate is approximately 50% but varies widely according to the type of tumor (e.g., brainstem glioma five-year survival = 18%; cerebellar astrocytoma five-year survival = 95%). Surgery plus cranial irradiation has been the most common form of treatment for pediatric brain tumors, regardless of age and type of tumor (3). Risk for cognitive or neuropsychological impairment may

be posed by therapies directed at the CNS as well as a direct result of tumor characteristics such as location and size. Neuropsychological status, intellectual development, academic achievement, and psychosocial adjustment may be negatively impacted by brain tumors and their treatment. A variety of factors may influence these outcomes, including: tumor location, extent of surgical resection, presence of hydrocephalus/ventricular shunting, extent of radiation therapy, extent of chemotherapy, age at treatment, and time elapsed since completion of therapy (4).

A variety of impairments have been described among children treated for pediatric brain tumors, including: impaired or declining IQ scores (5–12), sensorimotor or motor dysfunction (6-8,11,13,14), psychological/emotional or adaptive sequelae (6,7,13, 15), memory impairment (8), and impaired attentional processes (7,10). Language abilities were found to be intact in the few studies that have specifically examined this function (8,13). Additionally, several studies have noted the presence of epilepsy/seizure disorder (6,11, 15).

Most empirical examinations of cognitive or neuropsychological functioning of children with brain tumors rely on intelligence scores or academic performance as an index. Early studies (prior to 1985) put forth estimates of the incidence of intellectual deficits in children treated for brain tumors that ranged between 30% (16) and 89% (17). The wide variation in these estimates may result from several factors. Differing cutoff values for a "normal" IQ score have been used; some have defined normal as ≥ 90 (16–19), while others have defined normal as ≥ 80 (20). Different means of assessing intellectual functioning have been used, most often via standardized IQ tests (16–19) or educational performance (20–22). The time of assessment has varied greatly within and across studies (e.g., assessed months to years post treatment). Furthermore, there has been heterogeneity of tumor type/location and treatment type within and across studies, as well as an absence of baseline measures of functioning and control or comparison groups in these early studies. In spite of the difficulties in interpreting such global estimates of intellectual deficit, it appears clear that a substantial proportion of children with pediatric brain tumors will experience some form of cognitive impairment. Subsequent studies have attempted to address some of the methodological issues noted above and provide some explanation for the variability in incidence and severity of deficits.

Numerous studies have suggested that the age at which a child is diagnosed and treated for a primary brain tumor is critical to subsequent neuropsychological performance (5–9). Each of these studies reported that children treated at younger ages fared worse than their older counterparts. Lannering and colleagues (6) found a strong linear relationship ($r = 0.70$) between age at which CNS radiation therapy (RT) was received and IQ. Studies utilizing serial assessments of children have found that performance scores may decline over time, particularly in younger children. Mulhern and Kun (7) noted that 63% of younger children (< 6 yr) versus 11% of older children displayed deterioration from before irradiation to six months post irradiation. Packer et al. (8) found an overall decline in IQ from before irradiation to one and two years post irradiation, with a median decline of 25 points in full scale IQ at two years for children under the age of seven. A significant decline in scores was not found for children treated with RT over the age of ten and a comparison group of children who were treated for cerebellar astrocytomas with surgery alone showed no significant decline in IQ. Ellenberg and colleagues (5) reported similar findings: young children receiving whole brain RT had the lowest mean IQ scores over the one to four-year follow-up, older children receiving whole brain RT showed a trend toward decline as well, but those receiving less than whole brain RT, regardless of age, remained stable over the four year follow-up period. This study also examined the impact of tumor location, hydrocephalus, and chemotherapy (not methotrexate). The authors concluded that hemispheric tumors posed greater risk for deficits than third- or fourth-ventricle tumors; acute hydrocephalus did not appear to be related to long-term IQ changes; and chemotherapy was not related to cognitive outcome. Duffner and colleagues (12), however, concluded that chemotherapy (particularly methotrexate) appeared to be a significant factor in treatment associated dementia. These findings highlight the importance of age at treatment and implicate cranial irradiation in younger children as a critical risk factor for impairment. Cognitive impairment appears to progress over time and may stabilize at two years (9); however, stabilization may take as long as three to four years (12).

Many studies have been performed in an effort to elucidate the impact of primary brain tumors and their treatments upon cognitive/neuropsychological outcomes. This body of literature has several methodological limitations, including: small samples; infrequent use of comparison/control groups; heterogeneity of patients studied (e.g., type/location of tumor, extent of tumor resection, extent of RT/ chemotherapy, age at diagnosis/treatment, time since treatment completion, age at evaluation); frequent non-random or continuous selection of patients; frequent absence of baseline assessment; variation in assessment measures across studies, and frequent use of retrospective or cross-sectional designs. In addition, there are inherent limitations in the use of such clinical samples, such as high attrition rates as a consequence of death and disease progression and difficulty defining an appropriate control group (e.g., well siblings, age-matched peers, children with other types of cancer who do not receive CNS treatments). Furthermore, other factors, which have received little attention, may be operating to influence outcome, such as the interruption of educational opportunities that may result from intense and long-term medical treatment, the psychosocial stress of being diagnosed and treated for a life-threatening illness, and socioeconomic status (23). In spite of the methodological limitations, this body of literature strongly suggests risk for adverse neuropsychological consequences for children with pediatric brain tumors. Mulhern and colleagues (4) put forth several overall conclusions based upon a thorough review of the literature (based on 22 studies, $N = 403$ patients):

1. On average, there was mild intellectual decline (overall mean IQ score = 91).
2. Treatment at a younger age was associated with lower IQ.
3. The effect of radiation treatment was dose-related.
4. Three of four studies that examined chemotherapy effects found that chemotherapy was associated with neurocognitive impairment.
5. Tumor location and extent of surgery did not appear to be reliably associated with outcome; however, these variables are not easily separated from the effects of other variables.
6. Most studies that have examined psychosocial functioning have found social-emotional or adaptive impairment.

CHILDHOOD LEUKEMIA

Childhood leukemia represents the most common form of pediatric malignancy. While systemic therapies have been very useful in promoting disease remission, the introduction of CNS prophylaxis, usually consisting of cranial irradiation and/or intrathecal methotrexate, has been responsible for increasing the five-year survival rate from virtually 0% to 50%. Neurological complications have been associated with both of these forms of treatment, including: microangiopathy; demyelination; cerebral necrosis; somnolence syndrome; seizure disorder; and cerebrovascular accident (23). Deficits on measures of neuropsychological functioning, IQ, school achievement, and job performance have been found in samples of children given CNS prophylactic treatment for leukemia (24–29). Because most of the studies of the neuropsychological impact of childhood leukemia have used samples of children in complete continuous remission, without evidence of CNS disease, impairments that are detected are *presumed* to be a result of treatment, rather than disease. Unlike the literature on pediatric brain tumor, the effects of disease and treatment may be more easily disentangled in the childhood leukemia population.

In contrast to the literature on pediatric brain tumor, neuropsychological examinations of patients treated for childhood leukemia have often included comparison/control groups of children without leukemia (22,30–38) or made comparisons between leukemic children treated with and without cranial irradiation for CNS prophylaxis (24,29,39–42). Control groups typically consist of children who were not treated with CNS prophylaxis, such as unrelated matched controls, siblings, or children treated for solid tumors. The ability to make comparisons between groups allows for more confidence in the interpretation of findings; however, results have been inconsistent across studies. Some studies have found that children treated with CNS prophylaxis for leukemia have lower IQ scores (particularly performance IQ) than controls (27,31,35,37,38,42), even though the mean IQ scores for treated children often fall within the normal range. Other studies have not found a significant difference between experimental and control groups (30,33).

Overall, the research implies that a younger age at treatment, particularly with greater doses of cranial irradiation, is associated with greater impairment (27, 31,35,37,38,42,43). Some studies have not found age- or dose-related effects for cranial radiation therapy (24,29). IQ scores are, however, overall measures of cognitive functioning: studies examining more specific neuropsychological functions have often found deficits in focal functions such as attention, short-term memory, reaction time, visuomotor coordination, speed of processing (26,27,30,34) and EEG correlates of cognitive processing speed (32).

Although the exact nature, incidence, and severity are unclear, the studies reviewed above suggest that CNS prophylaxis for childhood leukemia may result in neuropsychological impairment. Several pathophysiological mechanisms have been postulated to explain the neurotoxic effects of irradiation and chemotherapy, including:

1. vascular injury resulting in obstruction, thrombosis, ischemia/infarction, and parenchymal necrosis;
2. direct injury to the cerebral parenchyma, including the microglia, ogliodendrocytes, and axons;
3. immunologic response resulting in autoimmune vasculitis (44).

Several studies have assessed the structural integrity of the brain following CNS prophylaxis for childhood leukemia, although the underlying pathophysiological mechanism(s) responsible for such structural changes is yet unclear. Several cross-sectional imaging studies have suggested a frequency of structural abnormalities (cerebral atrophy, intracranial calcification, ventricular dilation, subarachnoid space dilation, decreased attenuation coefficient) as high as 41–53% in survivors of childhood leukemia treated with CNS prophylaxis (30,45–47). One study reported that abnormalities were found in 10% of children at the time of diagnosis/prior to therapy (48), while another detected transient white matter changes in 68% of children during consolidation chemotherapy (49). Serial, prospective imaging studies have yielded lower rates of structural abnormality. Ochs and colleagues (50) found CT abnormalities in 9% of irradiated patients and 19% of patients treated with intrathecal methotrexate and many of these abnormalities reverted to normal across the 24 month evaluation period. Riccardi et al. (51) noted that ventricular dilations and subarachnoid space dilations tended to remain over a seven-year follow-up period, while decreased attenuation coefficients resolved over the follow-up period and intracerebral calcifications tended to develop between five and seven years following cessation of therapy.

Neuropsychological, intellectual, and academic deficits have been documented in children treated with prohylactic cranial irradiation for childhood leukemia. As a result of this line of research, modifications have been made in treatment protocols in an effort to reduce the cognitive impact of treatment while maintaining clinical outcomes (52,53). Studies in the literature on childhood leukemia often have one or more methodological strengths, including; control/comparison groups; prospective or longitudinal designs; homogeneity of disease and treatment variables; and use of well standardized measures. The preponderance of individual studies have found various intellectual and/or neurocognitive impairments in children treated for leukemia; however, some sound investigations have not detected such impairments. Two comprehensive reviews of the literature have reached different conclusions regarding the inconsistencies in findings. While Fletcher and Copeland (54) concluded that the vast majority of studies have suggested that CNS prophylaxis (particularly cranial irradiation) impairs cognitive development, Williams and Davis (23) concluded that the discrepancies in findings may be due, in part, to methodological artifact. Chi-square analysis performed by the latter reviewers revealed that selection method was significantly related to positive or negative findings: 84% of studies that did not use consecutive patients found positive results in contrast to 38% of studies that did use consecutive sampling methods. These authors also note that the mean IQ scores of children treated for leukemia usually fall within the normal range, even for younger children, and that factors such as school attendance are rarely accounted for in such studies.

SUMMARY

Interest in the neuropsychological sequelae of cancer and cancer treatments has grown tremendously over the past 15 years. Empirical reports of children with pediatric brain tumors and childhood leukemia have suggested that there are significant intellectual and adaptive consequences for these children. Pediatric brain tumor patients may be at risk for intellectual deficits as a function of both the disease and its treatment. The impairments associated with childhood leukemia appear to be mild overall and linked to younger age at treatment, particularly with cranial irradiation. As a result of these findings, modifications have been made to treatment protocols in an effort to reduce the adverse neurocognitive consequences of treatment while maintaining clinical outcomes (52). While much of the research in pediatric populations has methodological merit, IQ has been the typical focus of attention. The IQ tests that have been used are well standardized and may be more sensitive than a gross neurological examination; however, these may not capture more subtle or focal cognitive deficits that may also be present. Finally, research that has examined

cognitive rehabilitation in other pediatric populations needs to be extended to children with cancer (55).

REFERENCES

1. Oxman TE, Schnurr PP, Silberfarb PS. Assessment of cognitive function in cancer patients. *Psychosoc Assess Terminal Care*. 1986; 2:99–128.
2. Silberfarb PS, Oxman TE. The effects of cancer therapies on the central nervous system. *Adv Psychosom Med*. 1988; 18:13–25.
3. Duffner PK, Cohen ME, Myers MH, Heise HW. Survival of children with brain tumors: SEER program, 1973-1980. *Neurology*. 1986; 36:597–601.
4. Mulhern RK, Hancock J, Fairclough D, Kun L. Neuropsychological status of children treated for brain tumors: A critical review and integrative analysis. *Med Pediatr Oncol*. 1992; 20:181–191.
5. Ellenberg L, McComb JG, Siegel SE, Stowe S. Factors affecting intellectual outcome in pediatric brain tumor patients. *Neurosurgery*. 1987; 21:638–644.
6. Lannering R, Marky I, Lundberg A, Olsson E. Long-term sequelae after pediatric brain tumors: Their effect on disability and quality of life. *Med Pediatr Oncol*. 1990; 18:304–310.
7. Mulhern RK, Kun LE. Neuropsychologic function in children with brain tumors: III. Interval changes in the first six months following treatment. *Med Pediatr Oncol*. 1985; 13: 318–324.
8. Packer RJ, Sutton LN, Atkins TE, et al. A prospective study of cognitive function in children receiving whole-brain radiotherapy and chemotherapy: 2 year results. *J Neurosurg*. 1989; 70:707–713.
9. Radclifffe J, Packer RJ, Atkins TE, et al. Three- and four-year cognitive outcome in children with non-cortical brain tumors treated with whole-brain radiotherapy. *Ann of Neurol*. 1992; 32:551–554.
10. Riva D, Pantaleoni C, Milani N, Belani FF. Impairment of neuropsychological functions in children with medulloblastomas and astrocytomas in the posterior fossa. *Child Nerv Syst*. 1989; 5:107–110.
11. Mulhern RK, Kovnar EH, Kun LE, et al. Psychologic and neurologic function following treatment for childhood temporal lobe astrocytoma. *J Child Neurol*. 1988; 3:47–52.
12. Duffner PK, Cohen ME, Parker MS. Prospective intellectual testing in children with brain tumors. *Ann Neurol*. 1988; 23:575–579.
13. Horowitz ME, Mulhern RK, Kun LE, et al. Brain tumors in the very young child: Postoperative chmotherapy in combined-modality treatment. *Cancer*. 1988; 61:428–434.
14. Bordeaux JD, Dowell RE, Copeland DR, et al. A prospective study of neuropsychological sequelae in children with brain tumors. *J Child Neurol*. 1988; 3:63–68.
15. Mulhern RK, Horowitz ME, Kovnar EH, et al. Neurodevelopmental status of infants and young children treated for brain tumors with preirradiation chemotherapy. *J Clin Oncol*. 1989; 7:1660–1666.
16. Eiser C. Psychological sequelae of brain tumors in childhood: A retrospective study. *Br J Clin Psychol*. 1981; 20:35–38.

17. Hirsch JF, Renier D, Czernichow P, ET AL. Medulloblastoma in childhood. Survival and functional results. *Acta Neurochirurg.* 1979; 48:1–15.

18. Kun LE, Mulhern RK, Crisco JJ. Quality of life in children treated for brain tumors: Intellectual, emotional, and academic function. *J Neurosurg.* 1983; 58:1–6.

19. Kun LE, Mulhern RK. Neuropsychologic function in children with brain tumors : II. Serial studies of intellect and time after treatment. American Journal of Clinical Oncology: Cancer Clinical Trials 1983; 6:651–656.

20. Duffner PK, Cohen ME, Thomas P. Late effects of treatment on the intelligence of children with posterior fossa tumors. *Cancer.* 1983; 51:23–237.

21. Bamford FN, Jones PM, Pearson D, et al. Residual disabilities in children treated for intracranial space occupying lesions. *Cancer.* 1976; 37:1149–1151.

22. Chin, HW Mruyama Y. Age at treatment and long-term performance results in medulloblastoma. *Cancer.* 1984; 53:1952–1958.

23. Williams JM, Davis KS. Central nervous system prophylactic treatment for childhood leukemia: Neuropsychological outcome studies. *Cancer Treat Rev.* 1986; 13:113–127.

24. Mulhern RK, Wasserman AL, Fairclough D, Ochs J. Memory function in disease-free survivors of childhood acute lymphocytic leukemia given CNS prophylaxis with or without 1,800 cGy cranial irradiation. *J Clin Oncol.* 1988; 6:315–320.

25. Peckham VC, Meadows AT, Bartel N, Marrero O. Educational late effects in long-term survivors of childhood acute lymphocytic leukemia. *Pediatrics.* 1988; 81:127–133.

26. Brouwers P, Riccardi R, Poplack D, Fedio P. Attentional deficits in long-term survivors of childhood acute lymphoblastic leukemia (ALL). *J Clin Neuropsychol.* 1984; 6:325–336.

27. Giralt J, Ortgea JJ, Olive T, et al. Long-term neuropsychologic sequelae of childhood leukemia: Comparison of two CNS prophylactic regimens. *Int J Radiat Oncol Biol Phy.* 1992; 24:49–53.

28. Mulhern RK, Ochs J, Fairclough D, et al. Intellectual and academic achievement status after CNS relapse: A retrospective analysis of 40 children treated for acute lymphoblastic leukemia. *J Clin Oncol.* 1987; 5:933–940.

29. Mulhern RK, Fairclough D, Ochs J. A prospective comparison of neuropsychologic performance of children surviving leukemia who received 18-Gy, 24-Gy, or no cranial irradiation. *J Clin Oncol.* 1991; 9:1348–1356.

30. Schuler D, Bakos M, Borsi J, et al. Neuropsychologic and CT examinations in leukemic patients surviving 10 or more years. *Med Pediatr Oncol.* 1990; 18:123–125.

31. Said JA, Waters BG, Cousens P, Stevens MM. Neuropsychological sequelae of central nervous system prophylaxis in survivors of childhood acute lymphoblastic leukemia. *J Consult Clin Psychol.* 1989; 57:251–256.

32. Heukrodt C, Powazek M, Brown WS, et al. Electrophysiological signs of neurocognitive deficits in long-term leukemia survivors. *J Pediatr Psychol.* 1988; 13:223–236.

33. Soni SS, Marten GW, Pitner SE, et al. Effects of central nervous system irradiation on neuropsychologic functioning of children with acute lymphocytic leukemia. *N Engl J Med.* 1975; 293:113–118.

34. Cousens P, Ungerer JA, Crawford JA, Stevens MM. Cognitive effects of childhood leukemia therapy: A case for four specific deficits. *J Pediatr Psychol.* 1991; 16:475–488.

35. Jannoun L. Are cognitive and educational development affected by age at which prophylactic therapy is given in acute lymphoblastic leukemia? *Arch Dis Child.* 1983; 58:953–958.

36. Rowland JH, Glidewell OJ, Sibley RF, et al. Effects of different forms of central nervous system prophylaxis on neuropsychologic function in childhood leukemia. *J Clin Oncol.* 1984; 2:1327–1335.

37. Moss HA, Nannis ED, Poplack DG. The effects of prophylactic treatment of the central nervous system on the intellectual functioning of children with acute lymphocytic leukemia. *Am J Med.* 1981; 71:47–52.

38. Meadows AT, Massari DJ, Fergusson J, et al. Declines in IQ scores and cognitive dysfunctions in children with acute lymphocytic leukemia treated with cranial irradiation. *Lancet.* 1981; 2:1015–1018.

39. Eiser C. Intellectual abilities among survivors of childhood leukemia as a function of CNS irradiation. *Arch Dis Child.* 1978; 53:391–395.

40. Pfefferbaum-Levine B, Copeland DR, Fletcher JM, et al. Neuropsychologic assessment of long-term survivors of childhood leukemia. *Am J Pediatr Hematol Oncol.* 1984; 6:123–128.

41. Kramer JH, Crittendon MR, Halberg FE, et al. A prospective study of cognitive functioning following low-dose cranial radiation for bone marrow transplantation. *Pediatrics.* 1992; 90:447–450.

42. Dowell RE, Copeland DR, Francis DJ, et al. Absence of synergistic effects of CNS treatments on neuropsychologic test performance among children. *J Clin Oncol.* 1991; 9:1029–1036.

43. Robison LL, Nesbit ME, Sather HN, et al. Factors associated with IQ scores in long-term survivors of childhood acute lymphoblastic leukemia. *Am J Pediatr Hematol Oncol.* 1984; 6:115–121.

44. Ball WS, Prenger EC, Ballard ET. Neurotoxicity of radio/chemotherapy in children: Pathologic and MR correlation. *Am J Neuroradiol.* 1992; 13:761–776.

45. Peylan-Remu N, Poplack DG, Pizzo PA, et al. Abnormal CT scans of the brain in asymptomatic children with acute lymphocytic leukemia after prophylactic treatment of the central nervous system with radiation and intrathecal chemotherapy. *N Engl J Med.* 1978; 298:815–818.

46. Kingma A, Mooyaart EL, Kamps WA, et al. Magnetic resonance imaging of the brain and neuropsychological evaluation in children treated for acute lymphoblastic leukemia at a young age. *Am J Pediatr Hematol Oncol.* 1993; 15:231–238.

47. Paako E, Talvensaari K, Pyhtinen J, Lannin M. Late cranial MRI after cranial irradiation in survivors of childhood cancer. *Neuroradiaology.* 1994; 36:652–655.

48. Vainionpaa L, Laitinen J, Lanning M. Cranial computed tomographic findings in children with newly diagnosed acute lymphoblastic leukemia: A prospective follow-up study during treatment. *Med Pediatr Oncol.* 1992; 20:273–278.

49. Wilson DA, Nitschke R, Bowman ME, et al. Transient white matter changes on MR images in children undergoing chemotherapy for acute lymphocytic leukemia:

Correlation with neuropsychologic deficiencies. *Radiology*. 1991; 180:205–209.

50. Ochs JJ, Parvey LS, Whitaker JN, et al. Serial cranial computed-tomography scans in children with leukemia given two different forms of central nervous system therapy. *J Clin Oncol*. 1983; 1:793–798.

51. Riccardi R, Brouwers P, DiChiro G, Poplack D. Abnormal computed tomography brain scans in children with acute lymphoblastic leukemia: Serial long-term follow-up. *J Clin Oncol*. 1985; 3:12–18.

52. Wingard JR. Historical perspectives and future directions. In: Whedon, MB, Wujcik D, eds. *Bone Cell and Marrow Transplantation: Principles, Practice, and Nursing Insights*. Boston: Jones and Bartlett; 1991: 3–19.

53. Hasle H, Helgestad J, Christenson JK, et al. Prolonged intrathecal chemotherapy replacing cranial irradiation in high-risk acute lymphatic leukemia: Long-term follow up with cerebral computed tomography scans and endocrinological studies. *Eur J Pediatr*. 1995; 154:24–29.

54. Fletcher JM, Copeland DR. Neurobehavioral effects of central nervous system prophylactic treatment of cancer in children. *J Clin Exp Neuropsychol*. 1988; 10:495–538.

55. Sohlberg MM, Mateer CA. *Introduction to Cognitive Rehabilitation: Theory and Practice*. New York: Guilford Press; 1989.

82

Psychotherapy

BARBARA M. SOURKES

I felt much better because I knew that I had somebody to talk to all the time. Every boy needs a psychologist! To see his feelings! (1, p. 3)
—*six-year-old child*

You don't look at me like other people do and judge my behavior. Instead you analyze my behavior and try to get to the root of it. Mostly you helped *me* to get to the root of it, and helped *me* handle it on my own. You can ask for your family's support, wisdom, experience; but it's not fair to burden them . . . I know that when I first met you, I didn't want to talk about it. I wanted to handle it on my own. But that faded so quickly because you're so helpless. You really do need somebody that can come in and help you. I think it takes awhile for people . . . (2, p. 113)
—*adolescent*

Psychotherapy with the child who has cancer attests powerfully to the struggle toward survival. Within its framework, the child seeks to express the experience of living with the threat of loss and to reintegrate the shattered facets of his or her life. Most children enter psychotherapy because of the stress engendered by the illness, rather than more general concerns. A comment by Lindemann referring to the polio epidemic of the 1950s bears striking parallels to the child or adolescent with cancer:

These are young people who suddenly have become quite a bit older; they are facing possible death, or serious limitation of their lives; and they will naturally stop and think about life, rather than just live it from day to day. A lot of what they say will be reflective—and you might respond in kind. It would be a mistake . . . to emphasize unduly a psychiatric point of view. If there is serious psychopathology, you will respond to it, of course; but if those children want to cry with you, and be disappointed with you, and wonder with you where their God is, then you can be there for them . . . (3, p. 101)

Lindemann thus reminds the therapist to "bear witness" to the child's extraordinary situation, and to respond within the context of that reality.

Much of this chapter is adapted from Barbara M. Sourkes. *Armfuls of Time: The Psychological Experience of the Child with a Life-threatening Illness*, ©1995 by permission of the University of Pittsburgh Press.

With a psychodynamic conceptualization as the overarching framework, this chapter addresses issues specific to psychotherapy with the child with cancer. In certain instances, special considerations for the adolescent will be mentioned. (A discussion of psychotherapeutic framework issues such as time and space (2) may be found in Chapter 60.) As Terr states: "Even though the therapy of childhood trauma is often modeled upon psychoanalytic principles, the treatment will work out quite differently" (4, p. 308). The psychic and physical demands on the child or adolescent translate into enormous challenges for the therapist.

REVIEW OF THE LITERATURE

Discussion of psychotherapy with the child with cancer is still somewhat uncharted territory in the literature. Many authors identify the clinical issues faced by the child and family, thus providing an essential foundation for understanding the universalities of the illness experience. Coping strategies for particular milestones and stressors are delineated. However, in general, psychotherapy is not considered as a context for the child's adaptation (5–14). Other authors focus more on psychological/psychiatric issues in the child with implications for psychotherapeutic or consultative intervention. To varying degrees, the vicissitudes of the therapeutic process throughout the spectrum of the illness are addressed (15-23). Two books focus exclusively on the psychotherapy of the child facing death (24,25).

THE CONCEPTUAL FRAMEWORK

Trauma

Therapist: If you could choose one word to describe the time since your diagnosis, what would it be?
Child: PAIN.

The concept of psychic trauma lends itself to understanding the experience of life-threatening illness in childhood. Terr (4, p. 8) offers the following definition:

"Psychic trauma" occurs when a sudden, unexpected, overwhelmingly intense emotional blow or a series of blows assaults the person from outside . . . but they quickly become incorporated into the mind. A person probably will not become fully traumatized unless he or she feels utterly helpless during the event or events.

Winnicott (26, p. 44) defined trauma as

an impingement from the environment and from the individual's reaction to the environment that occurs prior to the individual's development of mechanisms that make the unpredictable predictable.

These descriptions certainly relate to the overwhelming sense of loss of control experienced by the child with cancer: the shock of diagnosis, the indelible imprint of the sustained assault on the body and psyche, and the uncertainty of the outcome.

While illness does not literally originate in the environment, its devastating impact on the child more than qualifies it as trauma. In fact, the illness goes beyond what Winnicott (27, p. 44) referred to as "unthinkable anxieties" in its *actual* threat of death. The child with cancer stands unshielded from pain, terror and the ultimate threat of loss of life. In this sense, it is no exaggeration to state that he or she loses a critical aspect of childhood in the moment of diagnosis. The adolescent loses a sense of the open horizons of the future.

It takes a lot of days to be grown up, doesn't it . . . (2, p. 28)
—*five-year-old child*

I guess what summarizes my feelings is that as a teenager you're supposed to feel immortal, and I don't feel immortal.
—*adolescent*

Normal Development/Psychopathology

The therapist's knowledge of normal development is essential in evaluating the impact of cancer on the child. Cognitive, affective and social perspectives intersect at every juncture. The child's cognitive comprehension enables emotional mastery, while, reciprocally, the lived experience allows for conceptualization that would ordinarily lie beyond his or her grasp. Social factors (interpersonal and cultural) provide the framework, either facilitative or hindering, for the child's adaptation. In complementary ways, the developmental theories of Piaget (27) and Erikson (28) provide a context for understanding the child's experience; however, passage through the stages is

challenged to the utmost by the presence of life-threatening illness.

Although most psychological problems of the child with a life-threatening illness may be categorized as adjustment reactions, more severe psychopathology can emerge. This is especially true in the child with pre-existent vulnerabilities, or when there is a prior psychiatric history in the child or a family member. While it is important not to overemphasize pathology in the child, there is also a risk in minimizing or not recognizing it. Furthermore, any psychological response, however benign initially, can freeze into a traumatic reaction under sustained stress. Thus, the therapist must be able to assess the severity of symptoms, particularly in terms of intensity and duration, relative to the child's current reality. For example, if reactive depression or anxiety (which resolve relatively easily) develop into major clinical disorders, more intensive psychotherapy and psychotropic medication may be required. Disordered eating that originates as a secondary effect of the illness and treatment can develop into an eating disorder unto itself, or indicate significant depression. Difficult behaviors in a child may result in his or her becoming a "behavior problem" in settings beyond the medical center. Such clinical situations require careful differentiation by the therapist.

In addition to the knowledge of normal development and psychopathology, the therapist must be well informed of medical facts and their implications. The latter requirement grounds the therapist in the reality of the child's life situation, and thus is crucial for the psychotherapy to be effective.

Play

In child psychotherapy, play is the crucial vehicle of communication. The overwhelming nature of the illness cannot be approached by reality alone. Through play, the child can advance and retreat, draw near and pull away from the intense core. These tentative forays allow the child to contain and master the experience. Disturbances in play occur primarily in children with developmental disorders, severe psychopathology, or deprivation. However, the trauma of life-threatening illness can extinguish—at least temporarily—some children's capacity for play, or erode its range of expression into rigid patterns. Within the context of psychotherapy, a certain restoration is marked when the child's play reveals its former vitality. The therapist's willingness and ability to enter into the play are of utmost importance. Shared imaginative play enables the child to confront the realities of life and death. The psychotherapy session described here is a cameo of such "collaboration."

In the weeks following the death of his friend on the ward, a six-year-old child grappled with the concepts of life and death. He had recently acquired a rubber axe as a gift. He pretended that there was a whale swimming alongside the bed. (The whale was invisible).The child was vehemently trying to kill the whale with the axe, because one of his stuffed animals, Wally Skubeedoo Walrus, wanted to eat it for supper. The child kept asking: "Is the whale dead yet?" The therapist would look over the side of the bed and report that it was still swimming or blowing bubbles. Finally, the therapist suggested that the child check whether the whale was alive or dead. The child said: "I'll listen to his heart." He pretended to use a stethoscope and said: "Th-thump, th-thump . . . . He's still alive because his heart is beating." The therapist commented: "If the whale's heart is beating, then he isn't dead yet." The child looked startled and said: "But I don't want him to be dead." It appeared that he had not associated the fact of killing the whale with the whale being dead. The child leaned over the side of the bed to ask the whale how he was feeling. The whale answered (in the therapist's voice) that his back was sore from all the hitting, but that he would like to be friends. The child agreed, and named him "Mr. Whaley Whale Friend." He then threw down his axe in disgust. The therapist wondered aloud how the child might use his axe in a more constructive way. He decided that when he raised his axe, it would mean that all his stuffed animals must pay attention. The child then asked his animals the following riddle: "What did the big axe say to the little axe?" Triumphant answer: "Don't kill whales!"

Inextricably linked with play is the child's use of symbolic language. The words themselves (not simply the thematic content) often reveal images that are idiosyncratic to a particular child and consistent over time. They provide windows into his or her experience.

Images of cold (winter, ice water, ice age) were associated with fear and death in one child's stories and play. The dichotomous "up–down" was his indicator of whether or not things were going well. For example, "my heart was down" was his description of a medical crisis from which he had just emerged. Another child relied on this polarity as well. One day in the clinic, she informed the therapist: "Playing is up, but school is down." For both children, "up–down" may have been associated originally with blood counts or mood; it then generalized in their usage.

Psychotherapy with the adolescent, at least in its use of words as the vehicle of the process, more resembles work with adults. However, in the trauma of cancer, the potential role of expressive techniques, particularly art, and even in some instances play (the latter with younger adolescents), should not be overlooked.

THE THERAPIST'S ROLE

It is important that simple, non-threatening explanations be offered to the child. Terms such as "the talking doctor" provide a functional description that clearly distinguish the therapist from other professionals on the medical team. The anxiety about seeing a therapist can be allayed by explaining that all children who are ill have worries and that the therapist can help with these problems. Over time, even if not articulated, the child comes to understand the therapist's role in his or her care.

On one of her clinic visits, a child's physician asked her how she was feeling. She answered: "Medically I'm fine, but psychologically I'm not so fine, but I'll discuss that with my psychologist."

Although the explanation of the therapist's role to the adolescent can be quite straightforward, his or her acceptance of that role is often fraught with ambivalence and testing. In this age group, not only is there increased concern of "stigmatization" about seeing a therapist, but there is also often initial (if not ongoing) resistance to admitting the need for the support offered. Given that the rigors of the medical treatment and the ensuing impact on daily life strip the adolescent, at least temporarily, of much autonomy, he or she often perceives psychological treatment as additional confirmation of vulnerability and dependence. Thus, the process of psychotherapy must be explained as empowering in the thrust toward autonomy and control, even if bound by the confines imposed by the illness.

Maintaining confidentiality can be particularly complex in dealing with children and adolescents (2). It is critical that the therapist not become a divisive wedge between parents and child or be viewed with a sense of threat as the bearer of secrets which cannot be shared. The child must be secure in the "safety" of the therapeutic relationship, while at the same time understanding the rationale and need for contact between the therapist and parents. Most children express relief at knowing of this communication and even feel an increased security, provided that their own relationship with the therapist remains intact.

As long as a child's psychotherapy sessions were kept separate, he did not protest the therapist's meetings or telephone contact with his parents. He knew that these discussions focused on his coping with the illness. Interestingly, when his mother was upset one day, the child suggested that she talk to the *other* psychologist in the clinic (2, p.12).

Adolescence is a time when privacy and confidentiality are paramount concerns. This is especially true for the adolescent who feels physically and emotionally exposed by serious illness. For this reason, a team of cotherapists to work with the patient and the parents can be ideally effective. Although there is ongoing communication between the two therapists, the adolescent appreciates the less direct link between his or her own therapist and the parents. The therapist can thus provide a sense of emotional sanctuary for the adolescent. When no possibility exists for a cotherapist, the therapist must delineate with exquisite clarity for the adolescent what—if anything—will be communicated to the parents. The adolescent may agree to such contact if there is assurance that the therapist will serve as a resource for the parents in *their* dealing with the situation, and that disclosure of his or her therapeutic content will be minimal. A compromise that can be offered in some instances is that the adolescent be present for the therapist's meetings with the parents. In other cases, another professional on the team who is not specifically designated a therapist may provide the liaison to the parents.

The definition of the therapist's role relates directly to the therapeutic alliance and transference. For the child who lives under threat, the establishment of a secure therapeutic alliance is an intervention in and of itself. While transference is always a crucial vehicle for the exploration of feelings, the therapist must be vigilant to contain its intensity. The psychotherapeutic relationship itself should not take up an inordinate amount of "space" in the child's limited psychic reserves. Rather, the transference can fuel the child's available energy for relationships and activities outside the boundaries of the illness.

PSYCHOTHERAPEUTIC ISSUES

The content of the psychotherapy with the child with cancer can be conceptualized in three distinct, yet overlapping domains:

1. the illness and treatment;
2. the impact of the illness on "normal" life of family, school and peers;
3. life–death awareness/anticipatory grief.

By definition, the core issues are those around the illness and treatment: the child's comprehension and integration of the diagnosis; adaptation to bodily changes (both temporary and permanent) in the emergence of an altered body image; coping with painful medical procedures and hospitalization; facing subsequent milestones in the illness of either a positive (e.g., elective cessation of treatment) or negative (e.g., relapse) nature.

The impact of the illness on the child's daily life—family, school, peers—is pervasive, and provides much grist for the psychotherapeutic process. The longing to return to a "normal" life is counterbalanced by the realization that the profoundly "abnormal" presence of cancer cannot be erased, nor its psychological effects reversed. "Normal" as a taken-for-granted presumption of the child's daily life has been shattered by the diagnosis and its life-threatening implications. Thus, within the intertwined spheres of family, school and peers, the child must pursue pathways that include, but are not limited by, the illness. To achieve this re-entry and re-integration is an extraordinary challenge.

Most complex, and undergirding the entire illness experience, are the child's conscious and unconscious levels of awareness of the life-threatening nature of the illness, and the attendant vulnerability. Awareness is a fluid, not a static, state; thus, dependent on current medical status or related to a significant life event, the child's expressions will reflect different facets at different times. Comments may be expressed in both cognitive and emotional terms, and may be phrased matter-of-factly or cloaked in allusion. Whatever their form, they indicate the thought that the child has given to his or her life status. References to time, separations, remembered dreams, and spiritual concerns often emerge. Expressions of anticipatory grief—loss that is felt to be threatening or lurking around the edges of awareness—are the most powerful testimony to the child's recognition of his or her life-threatened situation.

All the above issues pertain to both the child and the adolescent with cancer. However, for the adolescent, there are added dimensions. For example, the effects of illness and treatment can have major impact on the young person's emerging sexual development (both physical and psychological), including concerns about fertility. Identity formation—a core task of adolescence—is immeasurably complicated by the illness. Premorbid plans regarding educational goals, career and relationships are now subject to question. Most basic, the adolescent who is striving for autonomy and control in his or her life must contend with the enforced dependence wrought by the illness.

PSYCHOTHERAPEUTIC TECHNIQUES

Psychotherapy with the seriously-ill young child demands that unstructured associative communication be combined with highly focused interventions. Given the specific focus on the emotional reverberations of the illness, the materials necessary for the psychotherapy can be highly selective. Absolute essentials include one or more stuffed animals or dolls, art materials, and an array of medical supplies related to the child's treatment. Most children are not intrigued by a plastic doctor's kit; it is too simplistic and innocent in light of their experience. In contrast, the opportunity to handle the real medical objects in a non-threatening context facilitates desensitization and mastery. The portability of these essential supplies extends the range of the therapist's office. Thus, for example, if the child is hospitalized, the therapist can "bring" his or her office to the child. The familiarity of the objects facilitates the transfer of the psychotherapy to a different setting.

A second tier of toys includes a dollhouse and family figurines, play hospital settings, and selected picture books related to illness and hospitalization in childhood. The classic *Curious George Goes to the Hospital* (29) is enduringly popular, especially in combination with a Curious George stuffed animal. Beyond these core supplies, each therapist develops his or her own selection to enable the child's creative expression in the psychotherapeutic setting.

Several psychotherapeutic techniques that the author has found to be particularly evocative include: the therapeutic stuffed animal, lists, letter-writing, the incomplete sentence story, creation of a book and the therapist's monologue; these techniques are elaborated in detail, with many examples, in Sourkes (1).

The *therapeutic stuffed animal* may be introduced into the psychotherapeutic process either simply as one of the therapist's toys or with a more focused agenda. In the latter instance, the therapist draws attention to the animal and discloses that it is being treated for the same illness as the child. Through this commonality, an alliance between the child and animal is formed. For a child who is receptive to this form of play, the identification with the animal and the projective process do not take long to establish.

Therapist: Look at Poly Polar Bear. He looks very sad and he is not playing.
Child: Is he sad because Johnny died?
Therapist: I guess so. What shall we do?
Child: He should play, because playing makes time go faster . . . . When Poly is sad, I am sad.

In certain ways, the animal comes to resemble Winnicott's "transitional object," a special possession adopted by the infant or young child that becomes vitally real and important. Within the psychotherapy, the stuffed animal "lives" in the relationship between the child and the therapist. The animal belongs to the therapist; yet by naming it and sharing identical experiences, the child comes to "own" it. The therapist's animal becomes vital to the child, and (in the child's mind), he or she to the animal, thus indirectly strengthening the therapeutic alliance. Through the authority of actual ownership, the therapist can impute feelings, or comment assertively about the "animal's" experience.

A technique that enables the child to focus on illness-related problems without undue stress is the compilation of a *list* entitled: "All the things I don't like about being sick" or "about treatment," or "about the hospital." With the title at the top of a page, the child either writes or dictates the list. The therapist elicits specific details. Issues identified and prioritized by the child become targets for intervention, whether through discussion and play or through relaxation and hypnosis techniques. The child feels a sense of mastery in the amelioration of problems or change in attitude over time. Topics most often addressed include: medical procedures; nausea; hair loss; hospitalization; school and peer problems, and general worry about medical status. The child can use lists effectively to formulate questions ahead of time for the caregivers, particularly at a critical juncture in treatment. The questions are often unpredictable, affording clues into the child's concerns and priorities. In the child's ability to pose the questions, he or she asserts a degree of control.

Letter-writing within the session can be an interesting and playful alternate route of communication. The letters may be between the child and the therapist, or involve a stuffed animal. The therapist can often phrase questions or observations through the letter that the child receives with less threat than if directly confronted. Even if the child does not reply to the questions, he or she is made aware that the therapist "knows."

The *incomplete sentence story* is particularly useful with the child who does not yet write and who enjoys dictating his or her thoughts. The therapist proposes telling a story together and provides the beginning of each sentence, as well as occasional questions. The topics relate to issues currently relevant to the child. A main character for whom the child chooses a name enhances the story's projective quality.

The child is often intrigued by the idea of *writing* (or *dictating*) *and illustrating a book* about his or her experience of the illness. As with many interventions, the book becomes an intermediary between the child and the therapist, allowing more threatening material to be discussed than might be possible directly. Such books range from the simple to the sophisticated, and may deal either implicitly or explicitly with the illness. Details such as choosing a title, decorating the cover and stapling the pages together are all important in the child's experience of a book that is complete unto itself.

In the *therapist's monologue*, the therapist articulates what he or she believes the child is thinking or feeling, without any demand on expression. The monologue should be used extremely selectively, reserved for those situations where the therapist judges that the child simply cannot form the words on his or her own, yet is longing to be understood. These are times when the child is withdrawn; either too exhausted physically to talk, or paralyzed by intense vulnerability. Unspeakable terrors are often holding him or her hostage. However, through the therapist's musings, he or she hears the actual "unsayable" words framed into a context, feels understood, and thus experiences re-connection and relief. These therapeutic effects are often manifested dramatically through words, body language, or behavior. The therapist may talk about the child directly, allude in more general terms to how "some children feel . . . ," or use a therapeutic stuffed animal as the subject. The therapist should speak slowly, calmly and repetitively, not emphasizing any one point over another. He or she should proceed from peripheral to core issues in successive approximations, allowing the child time to absorb each level. The child need only listen, or answer "yes" or "no" to questions.

ART TECHNIQUES

Art techniques can be a powerful tool to facilitate the child—and adolescent's—expression and integration of complex experiences (30). Drawings enable the emergence of profound disclosures. Structured art techniques—in addition to spontaneous drawing—allow the therapist to pose questions earlier in the process, and with more specificity than might be done through verbal means alone. Although these art techniques are simple to administer, they evoke complex and powerful responses. The therapist must be prepared for the conscious and unconscious material that the pictures reveal. Techniques include the mandala, the change-in-family drawing, and the "scariest" image; these techniques are elaborated in detail, with many illustrations, in Sourkes (1).

The *mandala*—a graphic symbolic pattern or design in the form of a circle—is used in art therapy today, when a person is asked to fill in a blank circle to reflect "how you are feeling now." In a more structured version of this projective technique. the therapist defines a topic around which the mandala will be focused. An example would be: "How I felt when I heard that I had cancer." The therapist begins by providing the child with a brief guided visualization:

Close your eyes and think about the day you were diagnosed with cancer. Remember where you were (hospital, doctor's office, clinic), who was with you, who told you the diagnosis, what words were used. Remember how you felt. You may open your eyes.

The visualization sets the stage for the concrete task that follows:

Now I am going to give you the names of feelings which other children have told me they felt when they heard the diagnosis. I want you to think about each feeling and see if it fits for you.

The therapist then presents a set of feelings that are commonly attributed to the experience. Each feeling should be written on a separate file card and arranged randomly on the table to avoid the order bias of a vertical list. The feelings for this topic might include: shock, scared, sad, angry, lonely, hopeful. A category called "other feelings" should also be included. It is best to limit the number of feelings to a maximum of eight. The therapist then gives the child a set of felt-tip markers and a sheet of paper with the outline of a circle on it:

Now, choose a color to match each feeling . I want you to color in a part of the circle for each feeling. If the feeling was big, then make it a big part of the circle; if it was small, color in a small area (proportion). You may use the same color for more than one feeling as long as you label it clearly. If you had other feelings that I have not mentioned, put them in. When you are all finished, we can talk about the feelings and the colors you have chosen.

Because the mandala requires little time and minimal exertion or coordination, it can be used even with a child who is very ill. Most children find the technique non-threatening and enjoyable, and often express relief at having an array of feelings already articulated for them. Interpretation of the mandala is based on the child's choice of feelings, colors, proportions, order, overall design, and verbal associations. At its simplest, the mandala is a tool for facilitating expression; at its most complex, it is powerful in its symbolism and depth.

The *Change-in-Family Drawing* is based on the Kinetic Family Drawing (31) technique. The child is asked to draw a picture of the entire family and to show each member engaged in an activity. In an added step after the child has completed the basic family portrait, the therapist asks: "What changed in your family after you got cancer? Show the change in your drawing, either in picture or in words." The responses to this simple question are often dramatic, and can be used for any "before and after" situation.

In *the scariest image,* the therapist asks: "Think of the scariest experience, thought, feeling or dream that you have had since you became ill . . . Draw it." Through this technique, the therapist invites the child to bring out the extreme fear, often the very image that he or she is most afraid to express. The drawings tend to focus on medical procedures, being alone, and death. They often represent a blend of actual and imagined experiences.

WORK WITH PARENTS

From the outset, an ongoing alliance between the child's therapist and the parents optimizes the outcome of the work. Because the parents must sustain the therapeutic work in the child's day-to-day encounters with both physical and emotional stresses, their role cannot be underestimated. In working with both sides of the parent–child dyad, the therapist is aware of emerging developments and concerns, and of issues that should be addressed with the child. Terr, in her work with traumatized children (4, p. 307), comes to similar conclusions.

It is almost impossible for a . . . [therapist] to treat a child without providing some access to parents . . . who participate in the child's life. Parents need the reassurance of visiting the . . . [therapist]. They need to know what the . . . [therapist] is doing, to know how the child is faring in treatment, and to know what specific plans for the child they must put into operation themselves. Once the . . . [therapist] is out of the picture, the family has to take over. Much of the therapeutic process consists of preparing for that time.

If two therapists are involved with the family, the child's therapist must carve out a route of access to the parents that is acceptable to everyone. This includes: having the parents' therapist alert him or her to significant developments; keeping the parents' therapist well informed of the child's progress; and scheduling occasional joint meetings to enable direct contact among all the adults.

The range and depth of work with parents can vary greatly, from a concentrated focus on child-management issues, to more traditional psychotherapy of the individual or the couple. Whatever the framework, the parents' reactions to the child's illness, and the impact on their marriage and family are the organizing themes. A crucial aspect of the work with parents is discussion of the well siblings.Too often, the siblings stand outside the spotlight of attention, even though they live through the illness experience with the same intensity as the patient and parents. At times, the therapist may work directly with the siblings, or refer them to another therapist at the medical center or in the community (32,33). In their own extreme state, the

parents must find the strength to care for their even more vulnerable child and the siblings: a formidable challenge to psychic resilience. Over time, the therapist's support becomes a resource from which the parents can draw.

The therapist facilitates and empowers the parents' interaction with medical professionals. In addition, and with the parents' consent, the therapist may share selective aspects of the therapeutic material that bear directly on the care of the child. The therapist can also enhance the parents' understanding of, and competence with, their child. By sharpening their observation and listening skills, they become associates in the therapeutic process. In keeping the parents informed about the direction of the child's therapy, their grasp of his or her experience is further deepened. Pain control techniques are valuable for the parents to learn with the child, so that eventually they can help him or her through medical procedures or at home. Any means of intervention that the therapist can provide for the parents to use with the child is an antidote for their helplessness.

COUNTERTRANSFERENCE

The affectively laden work of psychotherapy with the child with cancer demands of the therapist a heightened awareness and monitoring of his or her countertransference (34). The therapist comes face to face with the relentlessness of illness, if not with the specter of death itself, and his or her reactions pivot around the life-threatening situation of the child or adolescent. The therapist must be able to witness the child's experience, while containing and channeling the onrush of his or her own emotion in order to allow the child full access to expression. The therapist's own loss history—particularly loss during childhood—has enormous impact on work with the child with cancer. Guilt at his or her own health (and that of loved ones) and anxiety about illness can peak unexpectedly, and intrude upon the therapeutic process. Exposure to suffering is a given in work with the child with cancer and the therapist must develop a tolerance for witnessing physical, as well as psychic, pain. Psychotherapy with the child with cancer demands the therapist's use of self to an extraordinary degree, and the therapist must be prepared for more disclosure—intimately linked to the child's experience—than is typical in other therapeutic encounters. Most importantly, the therapist must recognize his or her responsibility in becoming a crucial anchor, a consistent and abiding presence, for the child in a precarious life situation.

REFERENCES

1. Sourkes B. Armfuls of Time: *The Child's Psychological Experience of Life-threatening Illness.* Pittsburgh: University of Pittsburgh Press; 1995.

2. Sourkes B. *The Deepening Shade: Psychological Aspects of Life-threatening Illness.* Pittsburgh: University of Pittsburgh Press; 1982.

3. Lindemann E. Quoted in: Coles R. *The Spiritual Life of Children.* Boston: Houghton-Mifflin; 1990.

4. Terr L. *Too Scared to Cry.* New York: Basic Books; 1990.

5. Kellerman J, ed. *Psychological Aspects of Childhood Cancer.* Springfield, IL: Charles C. Thomas; 1980.

6. Spinetta J, Deasy-Spinetta P, eds. *Living with Childhood Cancer.* St Louis: CV Mosby; 1981.

7. Van Dongen-Melman J, Sanders-Woudstra J. Psychosocial aspects of childhood cancer: a review of the literature. *J Child Psychol Psychiatry.* 1986; 27: 145–180.

8. Chesler M, Barbarin O. *Childhood Cancer and the Family.* New York, NY: Brunner/Mazel; 1987.

9. Adams D, Deveau E. *Coping with Childhood Cancer.* Hamilton ON: Kinbridge Publications; 1988.

10. Rowland J. Developmental stage and adaptation: child and adolescent model. In: Holland J, Rowland J, eds. *Handbook of Psychooncology.* New York: Oxford University Press; 1989: 519–543.

11. Katz E, Dolgin M, Varni J. Cancer in children and adolescents. In: Gross A, Drabman R, eds. *Handbook of Clinical Behavioral Pediatrics.* New York and London: Plenum Press; 1990: 129–146.

12. Bearson D. *"They Never Want to Tell You": Children Talk about Cancer.* Cambridge, MA: Harvard University Press; 1991.

13. Ettinger R, Heiney S. Cancer in adolescents and young adults. *Cancer Suppl.* 1993; 71:3276–3280.

14. Gibbons M. Psychosocial aspects of serious illness in childhood and adolescence. In: Armstrong-Dailey A, Goltzer S, eds. *Hospice Care for Children.* New York: Oxford University Press; 1993: 60–74.

15. Geist R. Onset of chronic illness in children and adolescents: psychotherapeutic and consultative intervention. *Am J Orthopsychiatry.* 1979; 49:4–23.

16. Brunquell D, Hall M. Issues in the psychological care of pediatric oncology patients. *Am J Orthopsychiatry.* 1982; 52:32–44.

17. Adams-Greenly M. Psychosocial interventions in childhood cancer. In: Holland J, Rowland J, eds. *Handbook of Psychooncology.* New York: Oxford University Press; 1989: 562–572.

18. Pfefferbaum B. Common psychiatric disorders in childhood cancer and their management. In Holland J, Rowland J, eds. *Handbook of Psychooncology.* New York: Oxford University Press; 1989: 544–561.

19. Emanuel R, Colloms A, Mendelsohn A, et al. Psychotherapy with hospitalized children with leukemia: is it possible? *J Child Psychother.* 1990; 16:21–37.

20. Glazer J. Psychiatric aspects of cancer in childhood and adolescence. In: Lewis M, ed. *Child and Adolescent Psychiatry: A Comprehensive Textbook.* Baltimore: Williams and Wilkins; 1991: 964–977.

21. Koocher G, Gudas L. Grief and loss in childhood. In Walker C, Roberts M, eds. *Handbook of Clinical Child Psychology.* New York: John Wiley; 1992: 1025–1034.

22. Lansky S, List M, Ritter-Sterr C, Hart M. Psychiatric and psychological support of the child and adolescent with cancer. In: Pizzo P and Poplack D, eds. *Principles and Practice of Pediatric Oncology.* 2nd ed. Philadelphia: JB Lippincott; 1993: 1127–1139.

23. Stuber M, Meeske K, Gonzalez S, et al. Post-traumatic stress after childhood cancer I: the role of appraisal. *Psycho-oncology.* 1994; 3:305–312.

24. Kubler-Ross E. *On Children and Death.* New York: MacMillan; 1983.

25. Bertoia J. *Drawings from a Dying Child: Insights into Death from a Jungian Perspective.* London and New York: Routledge; 1993.

26. Davis M, Wallbridge D. *Boundary and Space: An Introduction to the Work of D.W. Winnicott.* New York: Brunner/Mazel; 1981.

27. Piaget J, Inhelder B. *The Psychology of the Child.* New York: Basic Books; 1969.

28. Erikson E. *Childhood and Society.* New York: Norton; 1963.

29. Rey M, Rey HA. *Curious George Goes to the Hospital.* Boston: Houghton Mifflin; 1966.

30. Sourkes B. Truth to life: art therapy with pediatric oncology patients and their siblings. *J Psychosoc Oncol.* 1991; 9:81–96.

31. Burns R, Kaufman S. *Kinetic Family Drawings.* New York: Brunner/Mazel; 1970.

32. Sourkes B. Siblings of the pediatric cancer patient. In: Kellerman J, ed. *Psychological Aspects of Childhood Cancer.* Springfield, IL: Charles C. Thomas; 1980: 47–69.

33. Sourkes B. Siblings of the child with a life-threatening illness. *J Child Contemp Soc.* 1987; 19(3/4):159–184.

34. Sourkes B. The child with a life-threatening illness. In: Brandell J, ed. *Countertransference in Psychotherapy with Children and Adolescents.* Northvale, NJ: Jason Aronson; 1992: 267–284.

83

Pediatric Psychopharmacology

LADD SPIEGEL

Psychotropic medications contribute importantly to the quality of life of the child with cancer. Given the widespread use of psychiatric medications in pediatric oncology, however, there are remarkably few published studies of these treatments. This reflects, in large part, the general state of pharmacologic research in child and adolescent psychiatry, where controlled drug studies are rare. There are additional difficulties specific to research in pediatric oncology, where the clinical heterogeneity of cancer patients makes systematic drug study problematic.

In pharmacologic treatment studies, Pfefferbaum-Levine (1) described the successful use of tricyclic antidepressants for depressed and anxious children with cancer. In a later study (2), she reported the use of alprazolam for anticipatory and procedural anxiety. Maisami et al. (3) described three cases in which a combination of a tricyclic and a neuroleptic relieved symptoms of anxiety and depression in terminally ill children with cancer.

Psychiatric and psychological aspects of cancer in childhood were reviewed by Pfefferbaum (4) and by Kellerman (5). Mrazek discussed the care of terminally ill children and their families, and issues relating to liaison with the pediatric staff (6). Pfefferbaum-Levine et al. (7) addressed the use of pharmacologic agents in childhood cancer. Recent reviews of general psychopharmacology in children and adolescents are by Werry and Aman (8) and Green (9).

BASIC STRATEGIES OF PHARMACOLOGIC MANAGEMENT IN PEDIATRICS

Psychopharmacologic treatments are an integral part of the overall medical and psychological care of the child. They complement—but do not replace—psychotherapy, behavioral interventions, and emotional support. Pharmacologic interventions will rarely succeed without discussions with both the family and the pediatric staff about the benefits and side-effects of a particular medication. Since the pediatric staff may be unfamiliar with the dosing of psychotropic medications, "PRN" (as the child requests it) dosing schedules for psychiatric medications frequently lead to significant under use of psychiatric medications.

Psychiatric symptoms in pediatric oncology are often multiply determined and rapidly changing. Physical pain, neurologic dysfunction, and psychological distress are closely linked, and sometimes inseparable, making definitive psychiatric diagnoses often elusive. Pediatric psychopharmacology, as a result of these diagnostic ambiguities, proceeds on the basis of the management of specific symptoms, rather than the treatment of (presumed) underlying psychiatric disorders.

The standard mental-status examination for children is by necessity abbreviated for the acutely ill hospitalized child. Medical procedures, physical pain, and lack of privacy, among other factors, place limitations on the psychiatrist's ability to interview and examine the child appropriately. Multiple brief examinations, coupled with the observations of the pediatric staff and the family, are often more instructive than a single prolonged session with a physically ill child. Since the pediatric staff may underestimate "organic" aspects of a child's psychiatric presentation, the psychiatric consultant independently assesses the degree of both physical pain and of cognitive impairment. In many cases, psychiatric assessment can not be performed until pain management and/or treatment of delirium is addressed (see Pfefferbaum for a detailed discussion of the assessment process in children with cancer) (10).

The pharmacologic consultant in pediatric oncology often utilizes medications that have not been studied for use in children and adolescents. Many psychiatric medications, particularly the newer ones, are not approved for use in children. They lack, therefore, standardized doses and modes of administration.

Doses for the pediatric patient are often extrapolated from the adult schedules, with allowances made for body weight and overall physical condition. Pediatric psychopharmacology in oncology is further hampered by the lack of specific studies in debilitated or immunologically compromised children. Very little is known, for example, about the interactions of psychotropics with the chemotherapeutic agents routinely used in cancer treatment. In fact, even the psychiatric side effects of common medications remain largely unstudied in pediatrics. (The author has limited discussion of specific medication to approved and/or commonly used agents, except where noted.)

ANXIETY

Anxiety has long been associated with cancer and other potentially fatal childhood disorders, Spinetta [11], for example, in a ground-breaking study of children with leukemia found significant death-related anxiety in children, regardless of whether or not they were informed of their diagnoses. Katz [11] described anxiety symptoms in children undergoing stressful and/or painful procedures. Children and adolescents undergoing cancer treatment displayed generalized phobic symptoms that appeared to generalize from anxiety related to specific procedural phobias, according to studies by Redd [13]. Nir [14] reported evidence of post-traumatic stress disorder in 50% of pediatric cancer patients *not referred for psychiatric evaluation.*

"Anxiety" in physically ill children represents a widely diverse group of developmentally appropriate and pathological coping responses. Separation-anxiety, for example, may represent a normal developmental regression associated with trauma, or it may be a sign of an emerging phobia. Children who are provided with inadequate or contradictory information about their diagnosis or prognosis may also exhibit anxiety in a wide range of forms. Undertreated or intermittently treated pain may appear symptomatically as procedural phobias, and a sleep deprived child may become anxious, irritable, and agitated. Pre-existing or latent anxiety disorders, such as an obsessive–compulsive disorder, become exacerbated with the stress of illness. Post-traumatic stress disorder, and procedural phobias may develop during the course of treatment. Delirium in a child may initially present with anxiety or agitation.

Anxiety in children with cancer frequently results from physical and physiological factors. For example, infections, metabolic abnormalities, and central nervous system tumors may present with agitation. Medications which have side-effects of anxiety include sympathomimetic drugs (eg theophylline, isoprenaline, adrenaline), and steroids [15]. Importantly, and paradoxically, benzodiazepines may cause a disinhibition syndrome even at therapeutic doses, in many children, and this resembles anxiety (see below). Similarly, "rebound" anxiety may occur associated with the discontinuation of benzodiazepines.

Pharmacologic treatments for anxiety in children utilize a wide range of agents, including antihistamines, benzodiazepines, antidepressants, neuroleptics, and narcotic analgesics [16]. The choice of agents depends on the severity and chronicity of the anxiety and on associated diagnoses, specifically including depression and delirium. Since children often experience sedation as anxiolysis, sedating agents, regardless of their class, can be utilized in the treatment of anxiety symptoms in children.

Post-traumatic stress disorder (PTSD) requires particular attention, because of its association with pediatric cancer. Treatment strategies in childhood PTSD associated with cancer, as with other presentations of the disorder, are focused on specific co-existing anxiety and affective symptoms, rather than the underlying disorder. These associated symptoms include generalized anxiety and phobias, and the depressive symptoms of anhedonia and social withdrawal. Treatments vary as the symptoms of PTSD evolve; frequently, benzodiazepines are used in the acute setting and antidepressants for chronic treatment. Even with treatment, the disorder is chronic, with long-term sequelae [17].

Antihistamines

Antihistamines are helpful in sleep induction, sedation for procedures, and for generalized anxiety. The ease of administration, relative safety, and the comfort of the medical staff make antihistamines a common first step in the treatment of mild anxiety in hospital settings. They are routinely administered to children without psychiatric consultation. The mechanism of their anxiolytic action is not known, although it is presumed that their sedating anticholinergic properties are responsible. Antihistamines are safely administered to infants and young children.

Antihistamines are not, however, entirely without risks in children. As with other anticholinergic medications, antihistamines cause slowed mentation and confusion (which can contribute to the progression to delirium). Antihistamines react synergistically with other sedating agents, including alcohol, benzodiazepines, barbiturates, narcotics, and tricyclic antidepressants. For this reason, antihistaminic agents are not generally recommended for the treatment of anxiety in cognitively impaired or delirious children.

The commonly prescribed antihistamines, diphenhydramine, hydroxyzine, and promethazine, are available in tablet, capsule, oral elixir and injectable forms. Low doses of diphenhydramine (1 mg/kg/dose) are recommended in the treatment of insomnia and anxiety in pre-school children. Typical doses in older children and adolescents are 25–50 mg/dose, administered every 6 hours. Higher doses of antihistamines are not successful in the treatment of anxiety in children and adolescents. If the symptoms are unresponsive to the recommended doses, other pharmacologic and psychotherapeutic measures are indicated.

Benzodiazepines

Benzodiazepines are potent anxiolytic agents which, used judiciously, are beneficial for the short-term, symptomatic treatment of anxiety in children and adolescents with cancer. The benefits of benzodiazepines are the ease of administration, rapid onset, and relative safety. Specific indications for benzodiazepines in pediatric cancer are procedural anxiety, insomnia, and, under certain conditions, generalized anxiety. Short-acting benzodiazepines (lorazepam, alprazolam) are particularly successful in the prevention of procedural-related distress when used aggressively early in a child's course, in conjunction with relaxation and other behavioral treatments. Clonazepam, the long acting antiepileptic benzodiazepine, is highly effective both as a simple anxiolytic agent and as an adjunctive treatment for obsessive ruminations and compulsive symptoms in children (18).

Benzodiazepines can cause excessive sedation, confusion, and frank delirium in physically ill children and must be used with particular caution in the presence of pre-existing central nervous system (CNS) dysfunction. Withdrawal is a serious risk of chronic benzodiazepine treatment, particularly with hospitalized patients, whose medications may be abruptly terminated, when they are moved, for example, into an intensive care unit. Agents with longer half-lives (e.g., diazepam, clonazepam) should be substituted for rapid acting medications (e.g., alprazolam, lorazepam) if benzodiazepines are required on a continuous basis.

Behavioral disinhibition, clinically resembling intoxication, is particularly relevant in pediatric oncology. It is characterized by regressive behavioral outbursts and can occur with initial benzodiazepine doses. This loss of control may be misinterpreted and mistreated as increased "anxiety," leading to overmedication with benzodiazepines to the point of frank delirium. Patients who become disinhibited with benzodiazepines are treated instead with other classes of medication, or with nonpharmacologic treatments.

Benzodiazepines are administered both orally and parenterally. Oral preparations of the short-acting benzodiazepines are rapidly absorbed, taking effect within 15 min. Of major importance in young children, who may have difficulty swallowing pills is the sublingual application of alprazolam, with an almost immediate onset. Lorazepam, with a slightly longer half-life, is available as an oral elixir. Intramuscular preparations of lorazepam, midazolam, and diazepam are available. Intravenous diazepam is used in hospitalized children when no other routes of administration are available. Clonazepam is the preferred benzodiazepine for longer-term administration. The long half-life and the apparent absence of euphoric effects limit the abuse risks in adolescents.

Dosages of benzodiazepines are highly variable, and must be closely monitored for excessive sedation and other side-effects. Typical alprazolam dosages in children are 0.125–0.5 mg per dose, which can be repeated every 3–4 hours. Lorazepam doses commonly range from 0.25–1.0 mg per dose, repeated at 4–6 hour intervals. Recommended doses of diazepam, which is approved for infants and very young children, are 0.07–0.5 mg/kg per day (or 2–20 mg per day) Dosages of clonazepam up to 5mg per day in healthy children have been described in published studies, but higher doses are safely used in adolescents with cancer with severe symptomatology.

Antidepressants and Anxiety

Antidepressants, while not generally considered to be anxiolytic agents, have a long history in child psychiatry in the treatment of chronic anxiety disorders. Generalized anxiety, separation anxiety, panic disorder, and a variety of phobic and somatization disorders have been treated with tricyclics and, more recently, selective serotonin reuptake inhibitors (SSRIs) (19). Such diverse childhood conditions as enuresis, chronic pain, eating disorders, and attention-deficit disorder are additionally treated with tricyclic antidepressants (TCAs), with varying results. Antidepressants, as a group, may be more effective in the treatment of anxiety than they are for depression in children. Tricyclics appear to relieve both subjective anxiety (perhaps due in part to simple sedation) and specific somatic symptoms, particularly insomnia and panic attacks. Tricyclics are utilized in combination with neuroleptics for severly ill children with a mixed clinical picture of anxiety, depression and delirium. While SSRIs have not been studied specifically in association with childhood cancer, early reports suggest that they are safe and effective in a variety of disorders in physically healthy children. In particular, fluoxetine has been demonstrated to be an effective treatment for obsessive compulsive disorder (OCD) in children (20).

DEPRESSION

Depression in childhood—even without the complications of physical illness—remains poorly understood. The diagnosis and treatment of depression in children with major medical illnesses is even more complex, in large part because both physical and psychological factors are prominent. The uncertainty in the diagnosis of depression in children with cancer was demonstrated by Heigelenstein and Jacobsen (21) and by Kashani and Hakami (22). The functional impairments directly caused by physical factors in pediatric oncology patients are difficult to distinguish from the somatic symptoms used to diagnose depression in physically healthy populations. For example, apathy, irritability, and social withdrawal may result from undertreated pain, weakness and sedation. Subclinical delirium is common in pediatric patients referred for evaluation of depression. PTSD may also present clinically with symptoms of depression, including anhedonia, blunted affect, and isolation. Psychological struggles with separation, loss, and personal mortality may cause or contribute to depressive symptomatology in children (see Chapter 82).

Tricyclic Antidepressants

While tricyclic antidepressants (TCAs) have not been demonstrated to improve mood disorders directly in children, they remain useful for selected "depressive" symptoms which accompany pediatric cancer. For example, sleep disorders, including difficulty initiating sleep, disrupted sleep, and early morning awakening, respond well to low doses of TCAs. Similarly, TCAs increase appetite in children, usually within several days of initiating treatment. Often social withdrawal and irritability lessen as the child becomes generally more physically comfortable as a result of improved sleep and appetite.

The adverse effects of TCAs relate to their anticholinergic properties, and, particularly at high doses, these effects (sedation, dry mouth, and constipation) can be problematic. As in adults, both benign EKG changes and clinically significant cardiac arrhythmias have been reported. Delirium, as with all anticholinergic agents, is the most worrisome psychiatric side effect but is unlikely to occur at low dosage levels.

Selection of TCA agents in pediatric oncology is made on the basis of desired side effects. Of the generally used TCAs in children, amitriptyline is more sedating than imipramine although there is marked individual variation. Nortriptyline is available as an oral elixir, and amitriptyline is available in parenteral solution. Desipramine, which is the least sedating tricyclic, has been implicated in published reports of cardiac "sudden death" in children and is therefore not currently recommended by many pediatric pharmacologists (23).

Typical initial TCA doses for children with cancer are 10 mg, with maintenance doses of 25–50 mg per day, depending on the weight of the child. Adolescents may require a full adult dose of 100–200 mg. When difficulties with sleeping are primarly the focus of treatment, the lower dosage, administered as a single night-time dose, is used. EKGs and blood level monitoring are recommended with chronic or high-dose TCA administration, but are not necessary with the low doses used in the routine treatment of insomnia or appetite suppression. Physiologic parameters (sleep, level of sedation) are closely followed and used to determine appropriate doses for the individual patient.

Selective Serotonin Reuptake Inhibitors

Although conclusive studies are incomplete at present, selective serotonin reuptake inhibitors (SSRIs) are increasingly being utilized in the treatment of children and adolescents with depression. Clinical experience suggests that children and adolescents tolerate SSRIs well, but the use of SSRIs for treatment of depression in children and adolescents remains unapproved. Overall, children and adolescents appear to respond to SSRIs in a similar way to adults. In contrast to TCAs, SSRIs appear to elevate mood, at least in adolescents, and therefore may prove to be superior to TCAs, which primarily relieve the asssociated somatic symptoms, in the treatment of depression in children with cancer. SSRIs may prove to be useful for the treatment of long-term sequelae of PTSD in pediatric cancer survivors, as in adults.

Fluoxetine, the most widely studied SSRI in children and adolescents, is available in an oral elixir, which allows a flexible low dose strategy. Side effects of fluoxetine of particular relevance in oncology are insomnia and appetite disturbances. Dosages in published studies of fluoxetine in physically healthy patients are 5–20 mg per day in children, and 20–40 mg per day in adolescents (the higher doses are reserved for the treatment of OCD). SSRIs have been used successfully at higher doses in adolescents with refractory organic affective syndromes, but these patients have required benzodiazepines and other sedatives to counteract the associated sleep disturbances.

Stimulants

Stimulants, which are widely used in the treatment of attention deficit disorder, have applications within pediatric oncology as adjunct agents in the treatment of depressive symptoms. They are increasingly used for depressed adults with cancer and other debilitating medical illnesses, particularly with patients who cannot tolerate antidepressants. In pediatric oncology, stimulants are used to decrease lethargy in debilitated patients, both alone and in combination with standard antidepressants. They are additionally utilized to counteract the sedation associated with narcotic analgesics. Stimulants appear clinically to be more effective in adolescents and young adults than in younger children, reflecting, perhaps, a developmental aspect of mood regulation. There are no controlled studies of stimulants as antidepressants in pediatric cancer.

The benefits of stimulants include rapid onset and relative safety. The adverse effects, which may be significant in oncology, are insomnia and decreased appetite. One stimulant, pemoline, has been associated with fatal liver disease in children and is therefore not currently considered to be a first-line treatment. In outpatients, the potential for abuse of stimulants must be considered. Dosages for the treatment of children with cancer are lower than those recommended for attention deficit disorder in healthy children. Initial doses of methylphenidate of 5 mg in the morning, with gradual increases to 10 mg twice a day (second dose at noon) are typical. Stimulants may be combined with TCAs, SSRIs, and other psychotropic medications, with the exception of MAO inhibitors.

PSYCHOSIS AND ORGANIC BRAIN SYNDROMES

Delirium, dementia, and other neuropsychiatric syndromes which present with perceptual and cognitive disturbances constitute a clinical challenge in pediatric oncology. Delirium in particular is thought to be under-reported in pediatrics, because of both the striking lack of research and the clinical difficulties in diagnosis (24). A wide range of psychological and behavioral symptoms, from simple anxiety to frank psychosis,may be directly caused by neurologic dysfunction. Children are thought to be developmentally more inclined to experience psychotic symptoms than are adults, and are therefore at higher risk than adults for the development of delirium secondary to physical factors. In fact, stress can produce transient hallucinations in heathy preschool children (25). Cancer treatments, including chemotherapy and radiation, have direct and indirect effects on the central nervous system which predispose to neuropsychiatric dysfunction.

Metabolic changes, fever, sleep deprivation, and pain cause or contribute to delirium in children. Numerous medications can produce a toxic delirium in a child, including the commonly used agents and steroids. Among psychotropics, antihistamines, benzodiazepines and narcotic analgesics are notorious in their disorienting effects. Tricyclic antidepressants, which have anticholinergic actions, at high dosages can also produce delirium in pediatric patients.

There is no standardized reliable mental status screening examination that detects "organicity" in children. When time permits, neuropsychological testing is essential in the identification of chronic cognitive deficits (see Chapter 81). Delirium in a child may produce anxious, oppositional, and violent behavior. The symptoms may be strikingly intermittent. Amnesia is common. Delirium is suspected whenever aggressive behavior is encountered in pediatric cancer patients. as a result of the uncertainties in the diagnosis of delirium in pediatrics, CNS impairment may need to be inferred from the medical history and clinical presentation. The best clinical guide may be the family members, who may sense, but be unable to describe specifically, personality changes. Pharmacologic treatment is frequently initiated without determining a definitive causative factor. In fact, a trial of a neuroleptic agent may be helpful in confirming a suspected diagnosis of delirium.

Pharmacologic Management of Psychosis and Delirium

Neuroleptics are an essential part of the humane management of pediatric patients undergoing treatment for cancer. Psychotic reactions and other aspects of delirium in cancer patients generally respond rapidly to doses of neuroleptics well below those recommended in physically healthy psychiatric patients. Low-dose neuroleptics are additionally used in pediatric oncology for the treatment of anxiety and insomnia, particularly for children with neurologic dysfunction, and to counteract psychotic symptoms in patients with severe pain requiring high doses of narcotic analgesics. They are routinely and safely used in combination with other psychotropic medications.

The choice of specific neuroleptic in pediatric patients is made primarily according to the desirability of sedation for the particular patient. Additionally, the familiarity of the pediatric staff with a particular agent may help determine the specific agent. Among the neuroleptics approved for children, which include haloperidol, chlorpromazine, and thioridazine, haloperidol is preferred for simple delirium with a somnolent patient. When delirium is accompanied by insomnia or agitation, the sedating properties of chlorpromazine or thioridazine are beneficial. The benefits of neuroleptics are ease of administration and rapid onset. Tablets, capsules, elixirs, and rectal suppositories are available. Neuroleptics are rapidly and reliably absorbed parenterally. Intravenous haloperidol, while not an approved treatment, is safely used with cancer patients who cannot tolerate other forms of administration. Typical doses of chlorpromazine and thioridazine are of 10–25 mg every 4–6 hours. Initial haloperidol doses in debilitated pediatric patients are 0.25 mg per dose.

Neuroleptics are viewed with suspicion in pediatrics because of their well-known side effects and their association with serious mental disorders. When used at low doses for short periods in the treatment of delirium and other organic states, they are well tolerated by pediatric oncology patients. The potential adverse effects of neuroleptics are numerous and include sedation, hypotension and a variety of anticholiergic actions. The side effects of particular relevance in oncology are the "extrapyramidal effects," including acute dystonic reactions (which can be mistaken for seizure activity), parkinsonism, and akathisia (motor restlessness, often misdiagnosed as anxiety). These effects, more common with haloperidol and the other non-sedating neuroleptics, are significantly diminished with the use of antihistamines and antiparkinsonian agents. The lowering of seizure threshold is of limited clinical significance in relation to the low doses utilized in pediatric oncology. Reliable data is lacking concerning the effect of neuroleptics on the bone marrow, although there are isolated cases reports of leukopenia in patients treated with high doses of neuroleptics (26). Agranulocytosis has been repeatedly described in association with clozapine, an atypical antipsychotic agent used in only refractory psychosis. It is therefore not recommended for use in pediatric oncology.

SPECIFIC CLINICAL PROBLEMS

Insomnia
Insomnia in pediatric oncology is usually multidetermined. Environmental factors and developmentally appropriate anxiety coexist with chronic anxiety disorders, depression, and "organic" states of excitation. Uncomplicated insomnia in the newly hospitalized child is initially treated with antihistamines. Sedating antidepressants (e.g., amitriptyline in 10–50 mg in a single night-time dose), along with behavioral interventions, are recommended for chronic sleep difficulties. Short-acting benzodiazepines, such as lorazepam or alprazolam, may be judiciously used for short-term treatment in children and adolescents who have diffi-

culties initiating sleep, but may cause disruption of sleep "architecture" after only 2–3 weeks of daily use. Insomnia with delirium responds well to sedating neuroleptic (chlorpromazine or thioridazine, 10–100 mg). Benzodiazepines should be minimized or avoided in cognitively impaired patients, as these agents exacerbate confusion and can lead to delirium. Insomnia secondary to undertreated pain is best treated with higher dosages of narcotic analgesic.

Pain
Psychiatric consultation is frequently requested to assist in the treatment of physical pain. The consultant first makes an independent assessment of the adequacy of the pain treatment, and may, in certain cases, need to advocate more aggressive treatment. Anxiety frequently accompanies pain, and the relationship is complex and subtle (27). The fear of pain may persist, for example, after early traumatic experiences with painful procedures, and the younger child may confuse simple touch with physical pain. Benzodiazepines, especially the short-acting agent alprazolam, are useful for procedural pain, in conjunction with topical anesthesia. Used early in the course of illness, by limiting the psychological trauma, benzodiazepines and topical anesthetics may inhibit the development of a later phobic pattern. Tricyclic antidepressants (e.g., amitriptyline in dosages of 0.5–1.5 mg/kg) have been described as reducing anxiety, improving sleep and potentiating narcotics in patients with chronic pain; the effects may relate to simple sedation. Methylphenidate (dose 2.5–10 mg bid), which counteracts the sedating effects of narcotic analgesics, may permit a child to remain socially related while receiving adequate pain control.

Neuroleptics are important in the treatment of delirium secondary to narcotics. The non-sedating neuroleptic haloperidol in low doses (0.25–0.5 mg/dose) is an excellent adjunct to pain treatment. Neuroleptics (e.g., chlorpromazine 50–100 mg/dose) are additionally used for simple sedation in a delirious patient with pain, replacing antihistamines and benzodiazepines, both of which worsen delirium. Neuroleptics additionally provide amnesia for traumatic procedures when administered with anesthesia.

Violence and Aggression
Self-destructive or violent behavior in children represents a diagnostic and therapeutic challenge for the child and adolescent psychiatrist (28). Common causes of aggressive behavior in pediatric cancer patients are delirium (often undiagnosed), withdrawal from prescribed or self-administered medications, and drug-induced mania. Intermittent or inadequate

pain treatment may be a contributory factor. Acute pharmacologic interventions for violent behavior after review of organic causes are neuroleptics and, if pain is a factor, narcotic analgesics. Because neuroleptics are rapidly absorbed orally, parenteral administration is not always required. Haloperidol is administered to hospitalized patients via intravenous infusion when no other routes of administration are feasible, although this is not an approved use (see Neuroleptics, above). Benzodiazepines are generally avoided with violent patients as they promote further disinhibition. In oncology, where patients may have low platelet counts resulting from cancer treatment, physical restraining must be performed with great care, particularly with adolescent and young adults.

For patients who exhibit recurrent or chronic aggressive behavior, neuroleptics at lower maintenance doses are prescribed. Lithium carbonate, which has not been specifically studied in pediatric cancer, has been demonstrated to be effective in selected populations of neurologically impaired chronically aggressive adolescents (29). When aggressive behavior appears to be associated with pre-existing impulse dyscontrol in a patient with a developmental history suggestive of attention deficit disorder, psychostimulants (e.g., methylphenidate 5–20 mg bid) may be effective. The centrally acting antihypertensive clonidine is at this time a speculative treatment for chronic aggression, but has not been studied in 'physically ill children.

Survivorship

Long-term survivors appear to be at high risk for dysthymia and depression. Cognitive deficits, disfigurement, physical disabilities, and delayed social development are common in both chronically ill patients and in cancer survivors (see Chapters 79 and 81). These late effects often occur when the psychological support that accompanies cancer treatment is lacking. These difficulties impact significantly on self-esteem, increasing the risk of depression. In addition, the late sequelae of post-traumatic stress disorders (rumination, chronic sleep disorder, phobias) inhibit social and occupational functioning. Aggressive pharmacologic treatment of depressive symptomatology is indicated in survivors. SSRI agents appear clinically to be the most successful agents, although here again research is currently lacking.

Survivors are at increased risk for learning and attentional problems relating to the neurotoxic side effects of cancer treatments. Even without a formal diagnosis of Attention Deficit Disorder (ADD), school-age and adolescents cancer survivors may benefit from a trial of psychostimulants or antidepressants, both tricyclic and SSRI classes, which are utilized as adjunctive treatments for ADD (30).

Terminal Care

There are two specific goals in the pharmacologic treatment of a child in the terminal phases of care. First, short-acting benzodiazepines (e.g., alprazolam, lorazepam), which cause rebound panic when administered intermittently, are replaced with longer-acting agents (e.g., diazepam). Whenever possible, anxiety in the terminally ill patient, who is likely to have CNS dysfunction from infections and/or metabolic irregularities, is treated with low doses of neuroleptics rather than benzodiazepines, which increase confusion..

Second, neuroleptic management is required of the delirium that accompanies narcotic treatment and/or CNS disease. It is essential that narcotic analgesics *not* be discontinued in the terminal patient, even if delirium is present . Less sedating neuroleptics (e.g., haloperidol) are preferred to maintain alertness and assist in communications with family and staff. Later in the terminal phase, a sedating neuroleptic (e.g., chlorpromazine) provides comfort by providing an overall lower state of arousal and awareness. The pediatric psychiatrist needs to be aware of the emotional responses of the family and staff in order to assist them in the terminal phase, and to ensure adequate and appropriate medications for a dying child.

SUMMARY

Psychopharmacology in pediatric oncology is hampered by the paucity of research and the diagnostic uncertainties inherent in this population. Therefore treatments are oriented toward specific symptoms rather than underlying disorders. Anxiety in children with cancer is treated with antihistamines, benzodiazepines, and, when chronic, antidepressants. Depressive symptoms respond to both tricyclic and SSRI antidepressants, although the latter have not been extensively studied in children. Stimulants have some utility as an adjunctive treatment of depression. Neuroleptics are important agents in the treatment of delirium, which may be significantly underdiagnosed in children undergoing cancer treatment. Psychotropics may be additionally useful in the treatment of insomnia, pain and aggression. Specific pharmacologic treatments are recommended for survivors and in terminal care settings.

REFERENCES

1. Pfefferbaum-Levine B, Kumor K, Cangir A, et al. Tricyclic antidepressants for children with cancer. *Am J Psychiatry*. 1983; 140:1074–1076.
2. Pfefferbaum B, Overall JE, Boren HA, et al. Alprazolam in the treatment of anticipatory and acute situational anxiety in children with cancer. *J Am Acad Child Adolesc Psychiatry*. 1987; 26:532–535.
3. Maisami H, Sohmer BH, Coye JT. Combined use of tricyclic antidepressants and neuroleptics in the management of terminally ill children: a report of three cases. *J Am Acad Child Adolesc Psychiatry*. 1985; 24:487–489.
4. Pfefferbaum B. Common psychiatric disorders in childhood cancer and their management. In: Holland J, Rowland JH, eds. *Handbook of Psychooncology*. New York: Oxford University Press; 1989; 544–561.
5. Kellermen J, ed. Psychological Aspects of Childhood Cancer. Springfield: Charles C. Thomas; 1980.
6. Mrazek D. Child psychiatric consultation and liaison to pediatrics. In: Rutter M. Hersov L, eds. *Child and Adolescent Psychiatry*, 2nd ed. Oxford: Blackwell Scientific; 1985: 888–899.
7. Pfefferbaum-Levine B, De Trinis MA, Young MA, van Eys J. The use of psychoactive medication in children with cancer. *J Psychosoc Oncol*. 1984; 2:65–71.
8. Werry JS, Aman M, eds. *Practitioner's Guide to Psychoactive Drugs for Children and Adolescents*. New York: Plenum Press; 1993.
9. Green WH. *Child and Adolescent Clinical Psychopharmacology*. 2nd ed. Baltimore: Williams & Wilkins; 1995.
10. Pfefferbaum B. Common psychiatric disorders in childhood cancer and their management. In: Holland J, Rowland JH, eds. *Handbook of Psychooncology*. New York: Oxford University Press; 1989: 544–561.
11. Spinetta JJ. The dying child's awareness of death: A review. *Psychol Bull*. 1974; 81:256–260.
12. Katz ER, Kellerman J, Siegel SE. Behavioral disorders in children with cancer undergoing medical procedures: Developmental considerations. *J Consult Clin Psychol*. 1980; 48:356–365.
13. Redd WH. In: Holland J, Rowland JH, eds. *Handbook of Psychooncology*. New York: Oxford University Press; 1989: 573–584.
14. Nir Y. Post-traumatic stress disorder in children with cancer. In: Eth S, Pynoos RS, eds. *Post-Traumatic Stress Disorder*. Washington, DC: American Psychiatric Press; 1985: 121–132.
15. Waters B, Milch A. Psychoactive effects of medical drugs. In: Werry JS, Aman MG, eds. *Practitioner's Guide to Psychoactive Drugs for Children and Adolescents*. New York: Plenum Press; 1993: 35–80.
16. Allen AJ, Leonard H, Swedo SE. Current knowledge of medications for the treatment of childhood anxiety disorders. *J Am Acad Child Adolesc Psychiatry*. 1995; 34:8–12.
17. Amaya-Jackson L, March JS. Post-traumatic stress disorder in children and adolescents. In: Leonard HL, ed. *Anxiety Disorders*. (Lewis M, ser. ed. *Child and Adolescent Psychiatric Clinics of North America*.) Baltimore: WB Saunders; 1993: 2: 639–654.
18. Graafe F, Milner J, Rizzotto L, Klein RG. Clonazepam in childhood anxiety disorders. *J Am Acad Child Adolesc Psychiatry*. 1994; 35(3):372–376.
19. Ambrosini PJ, Bianchi MD, Rabinovich H. Elia J. Antidepressant treatments in children and adolescents. II. Anxiety, physical, and behavioral disorders. *J Am Acad Child Adolesc Psychiatry*. 1993; 32(3):483–493.
20. Riddle MA, Hardin MT, King R, et al. Fluoxetine treatment of children and adolescents with Tourette's and obsessive compulsive disorders: Preliminary clinical experience. *J Am Acad Child Adolesc Psychiatry*. 1990; 29:45–48.
21. Heiligenstein E, Jacobsen PB. Differentiating depression in medically ill children and adolescents. *J Am Acad Child Adolesc Psychiatry*. 1988; 27(6):716–719.
22. Kashani J, Hakami N. Depression in children and adolescents with malignancy. *Can J Psychiatry*. 1982; 27:474–477.
23. Sudden death in children treated with a tricyclic antidepressant. *Med Lett*. 1990; (June 1):32–53.
24. Platt MM, Perlmutter I, Williams D, et al. Pediatric delirium: underdiagnosed and undertreated? Meeting abstract. American Academy of Child and Adolescent Psychiatry; 1995.
25. Rothstein A. Hallucinatory phenomena in childhood: a critique of the literature. *J Am Acad Child Adolesc Psychiatry*. 1981; 20:623–625.
26. Volkmar FR. Childhood and adolescent psychosis: A review of the past 10 years. *J Am Acad Child Adolesc Psychiatry*. 1996; 35(7):843–851.
27. Green WH, Kowalik SC. Psychopharmacologic treatment of pain and anxiety in the pediatric patient. In: Lewis M, King RA, eds. *Consultation-Liaison in Pediatrics*. (Lewis M, ser. ed. *Child and Adolescent Psychiatric Clinics of North America*.) Baltimore: WB Saunders; 1994: 3:465–483.
28. Werry JS. Pharmacotherapy of disruptive behavior disorders. In: Greenhill LL, ed. *Disruptive Disorders*. (Lewis M, ser. ed. *Child and adolescent psychiatric clinics of North America*.) Baltimore: WB Saunders; 1994: 3: 321–341.
29. Alessi N, Nayor MW, Ghaziuddin M, Zubieta JK. Update on lithium carbonate therapy in children and adolescents. *J Am Acad Child and Adolesc Psychiatry*. 1994; 33(3):291–304.
30. Cantwell DP. Attention Deficit Disorder: A review of the past 10 years. *J Am Acad Child Adolesc Psychiatry*. 1996; 35(8):978–987.

84

Behavioral Interventions in Pediatric Oncology

KATHERINE N. DuHAMEL, SUZANNE M. JOHNSON VICKBERG, AND
WILLIAM H. REDD

The development of more effective treatment methods for childhood cancer has been associated with an increase in the aversiveness of almost every aspect of diagnosis, treatment and rehabilitation. Fortunately, these advances in medicine have been paralleled by a rapid expansion in the application of behavioral principles to reduce distress and to control pain during medical procedures, along with better analgesia and anti-emesis by medications. The purpose of this chapter is to review the application of behavioral interventions with children and adolescents undergoing comprehensive cancer treatment and rehabilitation. The chapter begins with an overview of behavioral procedures used with children. The focus then shifts to a review of the major treatment difficulties (i.e., invasive medical treatments and post-treatment psychosocial and cognitive readjustment) and an assessment of the efficacy of behavioral interventions for specific aspects of treatment and rehabilitation. The chapter ends with a discussion of future directions.

OVERVIEW OF BEHAVIORAL INTERVENTIONS

In 1988, a World Health Organization Consensus Conference was convened to establish guidelines for the management of pain in childhood cancer. Participants at that conference endorsed the use of behavioral procedures in pediatric cancer treatment. Their recommendation was that for children over the age of five undergoing repeated diagnostic and treatment procedures, psychological preparation and behavioral intervention, in addition to or without pharmacological intervention, is the treatment of choice (1).

Behavioral interventions that are used to reduce distress and increase cooperation are based on behavior theory. The principal components of such interventions include:

1. contingency management;
2. cognitive/attentional distraction;
3. hypnosis;
4. systematic desensitization;
5. modeling;
6. behavioral rehearsal;
7. multimodal intervention packages

(see Chapter 62).

Contingency management is derived from Thordike's Law of Effect (2) and essentially involves structuring facets of the patient's social environment (i.e., the patient's interaction with family and staff) so as to provide concrete reinforcers (i.e., social and material rewards) contingent on the child's positive behavior (e.g., holding still during medical procedures, cooperating with routine mouth care). In many cases contingency management programs are developed such that the child earns points, stars or special privileges for cooperation (3,4).

Cognitive/attentional distraction procedures seek to involve the child's attention in a pleasurable or challenging task in order to block his/her attention to the stressful procedure. It is often used to reduce distress and promote cooperation. We have hypothesized (5) that cognitive or attentional distraction involves blocking the patient's perception of pain or nausea by refocusing the child's attention. A commonly used distraction task is playing video games. For example, in our clinical research we used video games to reduce nausea associated with chemotherapy (5). Children's ratings of nausea were at least 50% lower when they were playing video games than when they were passively sitting and focusing on the intravenous transfusion. Another method of cognitive or attentional distraction is storytelling or fantasy in which the child is "cognitively engaged." When the strategy involves storytelling, it is quite similar to hypnosis and relies on the child's ability to engage in fantasy. The goal is to engage the child in an activity that distracts his/her attention and/or physically blocks the actual distress behavior. Manne and colleagues (6,7) found that giving a child a simple party blower (a paper whistle-like toy that expands like the truck of an elephant and makes noise when you blow it) reduced both child and parent distress. The premise was that the party blower serves to distract the child and the parent from the invasive procedure. Using the blower makes crying and resistance less likely and, at the same time, promotes relaxation through paced breathing.

A related technique is hypnosis. There are theoretical controversies about what constitutes hypnosis, and interventions employing "hypnosis" vary in their treatment strategies (8–11). For the purposes of this review, hypnosis is defined as a relatively simple process in which patients learn to focus their attention on thoughts or images that are unrelated to the source of distress. With children, imaginative involvement is often gained though storytelling and relaxation, and is similar to distraction. Hypnosis and distraction rely on many of the same skills. For example, hypnosis involves the ability to become highly absorbed. Hypnosis may be particularly useful for children, as research has shown that children have a greater capacity for hypnosis, i.e., are more hypnotizable, when compared to adults (12). Hypnosis (a combination of imagery and relaxation) or imagery alone is often used to distract children while they are undergoing diagnostic procedures (13,14), or receiving chemotherapy treatment (15–19).

In the case of extreme phobic-like anxiety, a structured systematic desensitization intervention is often required. The goal of systematic desensitization is the gradual introduction of the individual to a feared stimulus (in the case of cancer treatment, a procedure or diagnostic instrument) in the context of low levels of anxiety. According to behavioral theory, fear is gradually diminished with repeated exposures to the feared stimulus. One method of desensitization used with children is emotive imagery (4). Similar to distraction and hypnosis, emotive imagery takes advantage of the child's openness to fantasy. After establishing rapport with the child, the therapist determines the child's favorite storybook hero and tells the child a series of stories involving the child and his/her hero. Each subsequent story brings the child closer to the feared setting, while the hero helps the child to master the situation. This procedure is similar to systematic desensitization procedures used to treat phobias in adults. The rationale is that the elicitation of strong anxiety-inhibiting emotive images in the context of the feared stimuli will reduce the anxiety reactions to those stimuli. By hearing a story that involves favorite story book heros interacting with the phobic or distressing stimulus, the child comes to associate these stimuli with positive feelings of self-assertion and pride. Emotive imagery has been effectively used to reduce cancer related distress in children (4,20,21).

Behavioral rehearsal is another procedure often employed. It involves taking the child through all phases of the diagnostic procedure or treatment during training sessions. For the child, this reduces the fear of the unknown. During these sessions the child assumes each role: the doctor, nurse, and patient. The child carries out with a doll each aspect of the treatment and may also practice giving a procedure, for example a bone marrow aspiration, to a doll and then the therapist. While carrying out the diagnostic procedure or treatment, the child practices giving proper instructions, such as breathing exercises or emotive imagery. Often a component of interventions is deep breathing and/or progressive muscle relaxation. These techniques are used to help reduce the anxiety of the child, reduce physiological arousal, and increase relaxation.

Filmed modeling is also employed in the management of distress during pediatric cancer treatment. Unlike behavioral rehearsal, in filmed modeling the patient does not practice the procedure, but rather watches a film of another child going through the procedure. For example, the child is shown a film of another child their age undergoing bone marrow aspiration and describing his/her thoughts and feelings while using different behavioral techniques (such as breathing exercises) to cope (4). In the studies reviewed, filmed modeling was also used to help the parents of patients cope. For example, an intervention for parents had parents watch a video which portrayed a mother successfully coping as she witnessed her child receiving bone marrow aspiration and lumbar puncture (22).

The behavioral techniques outlined above are often employed in combination to create what is called a multimodal behavioral intervention. Multimodal interventions integrate specific behavioral procedures such as hypnosis, distraction, and positive reinforcement with the aim to reduce distress in children who may benefit differently from different procedures. For example, younger children undergoing bone marrow aspiration may benefit greater benefit from hypnosis than they do from distraction and older children may benefit from both (13). Multimodal intervention packages may also incorporate cognitive methods (i.e., helping the child see the situation as less frustrating). Cognitive therapy techniques, such as making positive self-statements, are based on the theory that changing the internal dialogue that people have with themselves can change their emotional responses (23). Multimodal intervention packages have been found to reduce distress in pediatric cancer patients (4,20,21).

FACTORS INFLUENCING CHILDREN'S REACTIONS

Children react in various ways to cancer diagnosis, treatment, and post-treatment challenges. Unfortunately, the factors that affect the nature and intensity of children's reactions are not well understood. Recent research has found that the child's age (24), anxiety level (25), prior experience with the procedure (26), procedure invasiveness (27), and parental distress (28), are relevant.

Younger children report greater distress with medical procedures (27–29). The younger child often thinks the doctor and nurse are punishing him/her for some wrong deed (26). Moreover, many children believe that they may die from such procedures (27,30). Misattributions regarding the purpose of treatment and cause of illness appear to be related to the child's level of cognitive development. For example, research has shown that children's casual attributions regarding health and illness are consistent with predications based on Piaget's theory of cognitive development (31). Interestingly, in regard to treatment side effects, adolescents have been found to report more severe nausea than younger children (25), but this result has not been consistently documented (16) making conclusions difficult.

The child's level of anxiety can be the result of both painful medical procedures and treatment side effects, as well as a cause of these difficulties. Research has indicated that anxiety is associated with pain, such that pain tends to increase as the individual's anxiety increases (23). In addition, the level of anxiety has been associated with treatment side effects. For example, children who demonstrate greater anxiety than other children when receiving chemotherapy, are at greater risk for nausea and emesis (25).

The child's previous experience with a procedure also influences the child's procedural distress. Children's distress levels have been found to increase as their exposure to a medical procedure increases (32,33), but the results have been inconsistent (3). In addition, when an intervention is not provided, the number of children developing treatment side effects

(anticipatory nausea and vomiting) increases as the number of treatments increases (16). Invasiveness of procedure is also a contributing factor to children's distress levels, as bone marrow aspirations have been reported to be more distressing than venipuncture (27).

Parental distress can influence children's distress (27,28). In the face of threat and uncertainty, the young child often looks to his or her parents for emotional support and for guidance in understanding what is happening. The child is keenly aware of the parents' reactions and quickly responds to any sign of anxiety on the parents' part. Parental tone of voice, posture, and eye gaze are subtle but powerful cues for the child during stressful events (34). For example, during an invasive procedure, if the parent is calm and relaxed, the child is more likely to believe that the situation is safe. If on the other hand, the parent is clearly anxious, the child's anxiety is fueled. Research suggests that a complex feedback loop exists between the parent and child, with each being exquisitely sensitive to the other's emotional reaction (35). Parents' own level of distress may also influence how they understand or view their child's anxiety. For example, in a study of pediatric cancer patients distress during bone marrow aspiration Manne et al. (29) found that parents who were more anxious reported their child as having experienced greater pain and distress.

The child's coping style may also affect the child's pain and distress as well the effectiveness of the behavioral intervention (36–39). To date, however, the results regarding the influence of a child's coping style on his/her psychological reactions have been mixed leading to lack of clear conclusions (see Refs. 9 and 10 for review).

All of these factors, described above, have the potential to influence a child's reaction to cancer-related events. Furthermore, different types of cancer-related events elicit different reactions from children. There are three major areas related to cancer and its treatment which challenge the resources of pediatric patients: the experience of invasive diagnostic and treatment procedures, treatment side effects, and social and academic re-integration.

STRESSFUL DIAGNOSTIC AND TREATMENT PROCEDURES AND BEHAVIORAL INTERVENTIONS

The diagnosis and treatment of cancer in children involves a series of medical procedures that may be painful and, in the case of chemotherapy, may be debilitating. Depending upon the disease the children may have to undergo repeated bone marrow aspiration, lumbar puncture, and chemotherapy. Bone marrow aspirations are reported by patients and parents to be the most traumatic and painful events in the therapeutic regimen, followed by lumbar puncture and then venipuncture (9,27).

Bone Marrow Aspiration and Lumbar Puncture

Bone marrow aspiration is a diagnostic procedure in which a needle is inserted into a bone, usually in the lower back, in order to extract marrow. Bone marrow aspiration is used to diagnose leukemia and other cancers, to determine if the cancer has metastasized, and to evaluate chemotherapy effectiveness (40). Bone marrow aspiration is extremely painful and often requires physical restraint of the child to complete the procedure if inadequate local anesthesia or sedation are used. Lumbar puncture involves the insertion of a needle into the spinal canal and the removal of spinal fluid. It is used to diagnose infections, brain hemorrhage, tumors, or other obstructions (40). Like bone marrow aspiration, many children become anxious and uncooperative during lumbar puncture.

Unfortunately, in many cases both of these procedures must be administered repeatedly, creating, for some children, near phobic reactions. Depending on the child's age and cognitive understanding of the procedure, bone marrow aspiration sometimes resembles torture to the child (26). Because of the anxiety and pain caused by such invasive treatments and many children's limited understanding of why treatment is necessary, young patients often become noncompliant and actively resist these procedures. Indeed, between 38% and 84% do not cope well during bone marrow aspiration and lumbar puncture (9).

Pharmacological interventions can reduce pain and anxiety during bone marrow aspiration and lumbar puncture, but many clinicians try to limit their use because of feared long-term neurological side effects. In addition, some children report that sedation makes them feel out of control (9), further supporting the use of behavioral interventions in lieu of, or in addition to, pharmacological intervention.

Hypnosis/Imagery and/or Distraction Strategies with Bone Marrow Aspiration and Lumbar Puncture

Although hypnosis has been used for over a century, most of the research regarding its effectiveness is anecdotal or based on case reports (9–11,41,42). Despite imprecision in definitions, a general lack of standardized interventions, and few controlled studies, hypnosis has been found to be effective in alleviating distress associated with a number of cancer treatment procedures. (Systematic studies of behavioral interventions

with pediatric oncology patients undergoing bone marrow aspiration and lumbar puncture are reviewed in Table 84.1—abbreviations given in Table 84.2).

In a pioneer study, Hilgard and LeBaron (43) found that hypnosis reduced distress during bone marrow aspiration in a group of 6–19-year-old patients. After one hypnosis treatment session, patients experienced a 30% reduction in self-reported pain. Treatment effects were found to vary by patients' level of hypnotizability, with more hypnotizable patients experiencing greater reductions in pain and anxiety.

In a more methodologically rigorous, randomized controlled study, Kuttner, Bowman and Teasdale (13) investigated the relative efficacy of imaginative involvement/hypnosis as compared to both distraction and standard care. Participants were 3–10-year-old children identified by medical staff as having difficulty tolerating bone marrow aspirations. After one intervention session, imaginative involvement/hypnosis was determined to be better (in terms of reduction in distress) than standard care.

In summary, hypnosis can be an effective, practical, transportable intervention for reducing procedural distress in children with cancer. Although results clearly indicate that hypnosis is more effective than standard care, research to date does not permit us to draw firm conclusions regarding the relative effectiveness of hypnosis as compared to other behavioral interventions. Future research needs to include both two intervention groups (hypnosis and an alternative behavioral intervention) and a standard-care treatment group.

Multimodal Strategies with Bone Marrow Aspiration and Lumbar Puncture

Jay and her colleagues (4,20,21) have developed a comprehensive intervention package which employs a range of techniques to reduce the pain and suffering of pediatric oncology patients during medical procedures. Their intervention package incudes various strategies such as breathing exercises, reinforcement in the form of a trophy (a prize) for lying still and doing the breathing exercises, emotive imagery, behavioral rehearsal, and modeling. Although there have been other multimodal intervention packages for reducing distress associated with lumbar puncture (32), the intervention developed by Jay and colleagues has been the most thoroughly evaluated. In a series of studies Jay and colleagues found their intervention to be effective in reducing procedural stress for children with cancer and their parents (4,20,22).

With 3–13-year-old children with cancer, Jay and her colleagues (4) compared their multimodal intervention to a low risk pharmacological intervention (oral

TABLE 84.1. *Behavioral Interventions for Pediatric Oncology Patients (see Table 84.2 for Abbreviations Used)*

Medical Procedure with Reference	Sample	Research Design	Intervention	Variables	Major Results/Significant Findings
BMA(63)	$N = 24$, 6–19 years old "chiefly forms of leukemia"; 24 had 1 intervention session, 19 had 2 or more	Baseline post-test	Hypnosis (e.g., imaginative involvement through story telling)	Self-reported Pain (scale of 0–10 or FACES) Observer-rated Pain and anxiety (scale of 0–10). Hypnotizability (SHCSC)	1. After 1 session reduction in: self-report pain, observer rated pain, and observer rated anxiety. 2. High hypnotizablility associated with greater decreases in pain and anxiety. 3. Additive effects of session 2 not significant. 4. Overall, the higher initial distress (pain and anxiety), the greater the likelihood of patients to participate in the intervention.
BMA & LP (14)	$N = 33$, 6–17 years old; 28 L, 3 NHL, 2 Neural tumors	Repeated measures factorial	Hypnosis (e.g., imagery, fantasy & deep breathing) vs. Nonhypnotic behavioral techniques (e.g., distraction & deep breathing)	Self-reported pain and anxiety (scale of 1–5). Observer-rated pain and anxiety (scale of 1–5).	1. BMA pain decreased in both groups, greater reductions in hypnosis group. 2. BMA anxiety reduced in hypnosis group. 3. LP pain decreased in hypnosis group. 4. LP anxiety reduced in both groups.
BMA & LP & Chemotherapy Injection (64)	$N = 16$, mean age 14.0 years, Sd $\pm$ 1.6, 8 ALL, 3 AML, 2HD & Ewing's sarcoma, 1 NHL, 1 Neurobl, 1 Osteogenic sarcoma	Baseline post-test	Hypnosis (e.g., fantasy and relaxation)	Self-reported anxiety and discomfort (scale of 1–5). Trait anxiety STAI. Self-esteem RSES. HLOC II.	1. Reductions in anxiety and discomfort 2. Reduction in trait anxiety
BMA (65)	$N = 36$, 6–12 years old; 36 ALL	Repeated measures factorial	Hypnosis (e.g., imagery, muscle relaxation, suggestion for mastery, and reentering hypnosis) vs. nondirected play	Observer-rated procedural distress (PBRS-r). Nurses rating of child's anxiety (scale 1–5). Self-reported fear (FACES 1–7) and pain (scale 0–100). Therapist rating of rapport and responsiveness to hypnosis (scale 1–5).	1. Self-rated pain and fear decreased after intervention in both groups 2. Children who were rated as responding to the hypnosis training tended to report less fear and pain during procedure.
BMA (13)	$N = 48$, 3–10 years old; 48 had ALL or AML. 48 had one intervention session, 30 had second session	Repeated measures factorial	Hypnosis/imaginative involvement (e.g., imagery & direct suggestions for analgesia) vs. distraction (e.g., younger children instructed in bubble blowing and older children in deep breathing) vs. standard medical practice (control group)	Observer-rated procedural distress (PBRS-r). Observed-rated anxiety (1–5). Observed-rated pain (1–5). Self-reported pain and anxiety (FACES 1–5).	1. At 1st intervention sessions, younger children (3–6 years old) who received hypnosis treatment had lower observer-rated distress as compared to the other two groups. 2. For older children (7–10 years old) both interventions resulted in less observer rated pain and anxiety vs. the control group.. 3. At second intervention session, all three groups showed reductions in distress, pain, and anxiety, and medical staff were observed using distraction with the control group.

(continued)

Medical Procedure with Reference	Sample	Research Design	Intervention	Variables	Major Results/Significant Findings
BMA & LP (66)	$N = 20$, 5–18 years old; no information on cancer diagnosis	Repeated measures factorial	Hypnosis (e.g. imagery & relaxation) and procedural information vs. active cognitive strategy (e.g. distraction techniques) and procedural information	Self-reported anticipatory anxiety, procedure anxiety, and procedural pain (scale 1–20). State anxiety (STAI). MPQ; for 12+ year old patients. Hypnotizability (SHCSC). Level of imaginative involvement (scale 1–4). Observer-rated procedural pain and anxiety (scale 1–20). Heart rate. Peripheral temp. (in finger).	1. Reductions in self-reported and observer-rated pain in both groups. 2. Observer-rated anxiety decreased in both groups.
LP (32)	$N = 14$, 3–11 years old; AML or ALL	Baseline post-test	Information, distraction, "hypnotic-like" suggestions for analgesia, imagery, relaxation, and modification of children's expectations of fear, anxiety, or pain	Parent and nurses rated anxiety (not at all anxious to extremely anxious), pain (no pain to intense pain), behavioral distress (e.g., crying), and relaxed behaviors (e.g., playing, remaining calm). Self-reported pain, and strength and unpleasantness of pain (FACES). Children were interviewed extensively about the procedure (e.g., about their perceived ability to control their pain and about their pain coping strategies).	1. Reductions in anxiety, pain, and distress behaviors. 2. Reductions in anxiety and pain at three-month and six-month follow ups.
BMA (4)	$N = 56$, 3–13 years old; 56 L	Repeated measures counterbalanced	Multimodal, see Jay et al. (24) vs. diazepam vs. minimal treatment-attention control	OSBD. Self-reported Pain (scale 0–100). Pulse rate. Blood pressure.	1. Reductions in observer-rated distress, self-report of pain, and pulse rates in the behavior therapy condition as compared to the attention control condition. 2. Reductions represent 18% less behavioral distress, and 25% less self-reported pain in the behavioral treatment as compared to the attention control condition. 3. Reductions in diastolic blood pressure in the diazepam condition as compared to the attention control condition.

(continued)

TABLE 84.1. *Behavioral Interventions for Pediatric Oncology Patients—continued*

Medical Procedure with Reference	Sample	Research Design	Intervention	Variables	Major Results/Significant Findings
BMA & LP (22)	$N = 72$ parents of L or lymph patients 3–12 years old	Repeated measures factorial	Stress inoculation (e.g., filmed modeling and education, self-statement training, muscle relaxation and imagery) vs. child-focused intervention (accompanying child in a multimodal condition or multimodal and valium condition)	Observer-rated parent behavior (PBS). STAI. Pulse rate. Blood pressure. Self-reported anxiety and coping difficulty. Self-statements (SSIMP).	1. Lower state and trait anxiety, and higher positive self-statement scores were found for parents in the stress inoculation condition as compared to parents in the child-focused condition.
BMA & LP (20)	$N = 83$, 3.5–12 years old; 83 L or lymph	Repeated measures factorial	Multimodal, see Jay et al. (21) vs. multimodal and diazepam	OSBD. Self-rated pain and fear (FACES 1–5). Pulse rate.	1. Reductions in behavioral distress, pain ratings, and heart rate found for both groups. 2. Although not significant, reduction in behavioral distress was greater in the multimodal intervention vs. multimodal and valium.
VP (44)	$N = 3$, 11–13 years old; 3 Lymph or Osteosarcoma	Baseline post-test	Multimodal (e.g., muscle relaxation, positive coping statements and positive reinforcement)	OSBD. Parent-rated child's distress. Medical-personnel-rated child's distress. Self-reported distress (scale 1–7).	1. 46–68% reduction in observer-rated distress. 2. 9–22% reduction in medical-personnel-rated distress. 3. 0–67% reduction in self-rated distress.
VP (7)	$N = 23$, 3–9 years old; 1 Neurobl, 13 L, 6 Embryonic rhabdo-myosarcoma, 1 Wilms' tumor, 1 Congenital immune disorder, 1 Eosinogranuloma	Repeated measures factorial	Multimodal involves both the child and the parent (e.g., distraction, paced breathing, and reinforcement for the child, and instruction in behavioral coaching for the parents) vs. attention control	Observer-rated procedural distress (modified PBRS). Self-reported pain and fear (FACES). Parents' self-report of their anxiety and their child's pain. Nurses report of needle insertion difficulty, his/her own distress, and the child's distress (five point scales).	1. Decreased observed child's distress, parents' rating of child's pain, and parents' own anxiety only in the intervention group. 2. Intervention was associated with reductions of physical restraint.

(*continued*)

Medical Procedure with Reference	Sample	Research Design	Intervention	Variables	Major Results/Significant Findings
VP (6)	$N = 35$, 3–8 years old; 19AL, 5 Neurobl, 2 Wilms' tumor, 2 Glioma, 2 Kostman's syndrome, 1 Embryonic rhabdo-myosarcoma, 1 HD, 2 Wiscott Aldrich syndrome, 1 Hepatoblastoma	Repeated measures factorial	Multimodal, see Mann et al. (7) and IV nurses' coaching of parents to coach the child vs. multimodal without nurses' coaching	Observer-rated child's distress (e.g., pain or fear, procedure noncompliance), child's coping (e.g., non-procedure-related activity), and parents' coping (scale developed by authors based in part on CAMPIS). Child's use of intervention procedure. Parents' coaching behaviors and parents' praise. Nurses' coaching of parent, coaching of child, and praise.	1. Most parents and children used the intervention, and intervention use was associated with less child crying. 2. Specific directions by parents predicted the child's use of the intervention more strongly than global encouragement. 3. Nurses in the no-coach condition were instructed to not coach parents, but parents in the no-nurse coaching condition were coached by the nurses. 4. Nurses in both conditions were instructed not to coach children directly, but most did. 5. Children who were older and less distressed during procedure preparation were more likely to accept the intervention.
Chemotherapy (17)	$N = 8$ (three additional participants rejected hypnosis and one participant did not display chemotherapy-related symptoms), 10–20 years old; 4 HD, 2 ANLL, 1 Neurobl, 1 Ependymoma, 1 Astrocytoma, 1 Ovarian carcinoma, 1 Brain stem astrocytoma, and 1 Osteogenic sarcoma	Baseline post-test	Hypnosis (e.g., symptom specific suggestions during imagery for "notice the cool, clean air and taste the snow," and posthypnotic suggestions for relaxation and re-entering an hypnotic state)	Self-reported frequency, duration, and intensity of emesis episode (scale 1–10). Trait anxiety (STAI). Self-esteem (RSES). HLOC. Observer-rated (parents and nurses) frequency, duration, and intensity of emesis episode (scale 1–10).	1. Reductions in self-reported frequency on emesis ranging from 19–100%. 2. Duration of emesis was reduced in six of the eight participants. 3. Reductions in trait anxiety six months post-intervention. 4. Four of the five participants who had taken an antiemetic (chlorpromazine) discontinued its use.
Chemotherapy (67)	$N = 19$, 6–17 years old; 11 L, 3 Lymph, 5 Bone tumors	Repeated measures factorial	Hypnosis (e.g., imagery, and posthypnotic suggestion to have a good appetite) vs. supportive counseling (e.g., distraction, deep breathing, and instruction to avoid thinking about his/her symptoms)	Self-reported nausea, vomiting, and extent of bother caused by these symptoms (scale of 0–10). Parent-rated child's nausea, vomiting, and bother (scale 0–10). Hypnotizability (SHCSC).	1. Reductions in nausea, vomiting, and bother in both groups. No differences between intervention groups. 2. Hypnotizability was not related to symptom reduction in the hypnosis group.

(continued)

Medical Procedure with Reference	Sample	Research Design	Intervention	Variables	Major Results/Significant Findings
Chemotherapy (68)	$N = 8$, 10–17 years old; 5 L, 1 Lymph, 2 Bone tumors	Baseline post-test	Hypnosis, distraction (e.g., playing games), relaxation, reassurance and information	Self-reported nausea, vomiting, and extent of bother and disruption of activities caused by these symptoms (scale of 0–10). Parent-rated child's nausea, vomiting, bother, and disruption of activities (scale 0–10).	1. Reductions in nausea, vomiting, bother, and disruption of activities.
Chemotherapy (18)	$N = 12$, 10–18 years old; 8 Sarcomas, 1 Testicular seminoma, 1 Neurobl, 2 ALL	Repeated measures factorial	Hypnosis (e.g., imagery, fantasy, suggestions for safety, feeling thirst) vs. standard procedure control group (e.g., comfort, deep breathing, and distraction)	Self-reported nausea and vomiting (e.g., severity 0–100). Nurse-rated nausea and vomiting (e.g., duration, amount of vomiting). Psychophysical scaling of child's severity and intensity of nausea (adapted PPP). Oral intake.	1. Reduction in frequency, amount, severity and duration of vomiting in the hypnosis group. 2. Children in the hypnosis group reported being "less bothered" by chemotherapy. 3. Children in the hypnosis group tended ($p = 0.071$) to have greater oral intake 24 hours post-infusion.
Chemotherapy (50)	$N = 3$, 11–17 years old; 3 ALL	Combined multiple-baseline and ABAB withdrawal	Distraction (i.e. played video games)	Self-reported anticipatory distress (24 h symptom checklist e.g., bit nails, insomnia). Self-reported and observer-rated distress due to side effects (e.g., distress, scale 0–4 due to dizziness, nausea). State Anxiety (STAI). Observer-rated distress (modified PBRS).	1. Reductions in anticipatory symptoms and state anxiety with video game use. The effect was replicated on the withdrawal and reintroduction of video game use. 2. Reductions in observer-rated distress with video game use. The effect was replicated on the withdrawal and reintroduction of video game use. 3. The introduction and withdrawal of video games produced changes (reductions and exacerbations) in post-chemotherapy side effects.
Chemotherapy (5)	Study 1: $N = 26$, 9–20 years old; 7L, 6 Lymph, 11 Sarcoma, 1 Teratoma, 1 Brain tumor	Study 1: Repeated measures factorial	Distraction (played video games), vs. control (no attempts to limit or change children's behavior)	Study 1: Self-reported nausea (no nausea to nausea as bad as it could be). Observed-rated nausea-related behaviors.	Study 1: 1. Reductions in nausea for the intervention group. 69% of the children who played video games reported a sizable decrease in nausea vs. 23% of the children in the control group reported a similar decrease.

(continued)

Medical Procedure with Reference	Sample	Research Design	Intervention	Variables	Major Results/Significant Findings
Chemotherapy (5) continued	Study 2: $N = 15$ initial 26, 9–18 years old; 6 L, 4 Lymph, 1 Brain tumor, 4 Sarcoma	Study 2: Combined ABAB withdrawal and repeated measures		Study 2: Self-reported nausea (same format as Study 1). Self-reported anxiety (no anxiety to anxiety as bad as it could be). Pulse rate. Blood pressure.	Study 2: 1. The introduction and withdrawal of the opportunity to play video games produced changes (reduction and exacerbation, respectively) in nausea. 2. In one instance (of nine comparisons) a physiological measure changed significantly, video game playing was associated with an increase in physiological arousal (i.e., increase in systolic blood pressure). 3. Contrast groups (based on the use of antiemetics) indicated that the group receiving antiemetics tended to rate their nausea as more severe and to report greater changes in nausea with the withdrawal and introduction of video games.
Chemotherapy (16)	$N = 54$, 5–17 years old; 20 L, 34 Solid tumor	Repeated measures factorial	Hypnosis (e.g., fantasy, suggestions for feeling good, security, feeling hungry and wanting to socialize) vs. Active cognitive distraction/ relaxation (e.g., counting dots on a father's tie, deep breathing), vs. equal amount of therapist attention (control group)	Self-reported anticipatory nausea and vomiting (yes or no). Parent-reported post-chemotherapy side effects (e.g., severity in terms of duration of nausea and vomiting on a scale 0–10). Distress (indicated by how much chemotherapy bothered the child. Functional dysfunction (e.g., days of disruption of school and social activities).	1. Shorter duration of nausea in both intervention groups vs. the control group. 2. Shorter duration of vomiting in the hypnosis vs. control group. 3. In general, side effects for the hypnosis group improved over time, for the active cognitive distraction/ relaxation group side effects improved slightly or stayed the same, and for the control group they got worse. 4. Functional dysfunction (e.g., in school, social, eating and sleeping) was determined by emetic potential of chemotherapy and total symptom score was predicted by emetic potential and prophylactic antiemetics.
Chemotherapy (15)	$N = 20$, 6–18 years old; 5 L, 8 HL, 7 Solid tumors	Repeated measures factorial	Hypnosis (e.g., imaginative involvement, suggestions for feeling safe and well, for turning off the vomiting-control center in the brain) and p.r.n. antiemetics vs. equal amount of therapist attention and standard antiemetic regimen (control group).	Self-reported nausea (five faces). Vomiting (frequency scale 0–9). Practice of hypnosis (for the intervention group). Antiemetic medication use (from medical records).	1. The hypnosis group used less p.r.n. medication. 2. At 1 to 2 months post-diagnosis, the hypnosis group experienced less anticipatory nausea, but no significant differences were found at 4–6 months post-diagnosis.

(continued)

TABLE 84.1. *Behavioral Interventions for Pediatric Oncology Patients—continued*

Medical Procedure with Reference	Sample	Research Design	Intervention	Variables	Major Results/Significant Findings
Social Reintegration (54)	$N = 64$, 5–13 years old; 36 ALL, 7 HD, 2 NHL, 2 Wilm's tumor, 3 Neurobl, 4 Rhabdomyo-sarcoma, 1 Osteogenic sarcoma, 1 Ewing's sarcoma, 2 Brain tumor, 5 Other	Repeated measures factorial	Multimodal behavioral (e.g., modeling and cue-controlled relaxation) and standard intervention vs. standard intervention	Self-reported depression (CDI), anxiety (STAIC), general self-esteem (SPPC), and perceived social support (SSSC). Parent-reported behavioral and emotional problems and social competence (CBCL).	1. Nine months post-intervention the behavioral intervention group displayed fewer behavioral problems, experienced increased school competence, and reported greater social and emotional support from classmates and teachers compared to pre-intervention. No such differences were found in the standard intervention group.

diazepam) and to a minimal treatment condition in which support and reassurance was provided. The results indicated that diazepam was helpful in lowering anticipatory distress, but the multimodal intervention was most helpful during the procedure and was most

TABLE 84.2. *Abbreviations used in Table 84.1**

DISEASE
L	Leukemia
AL	Acute leukemia
ALL	Acute lymphocytic leukemia
AML	Acute myelogenous leukemia
ANLL	Acute nonlymphocytic leukemia
HD	Hodgkin's disease
Lymph	Lymphoma
Neurobl	Neuroblastoma
NHL	Non-Hodgkin's lymphoma

PROCEDURES
BMA	Bone marrow aspiration
LP	Lumbar puncture
VP	Venipuncture

MEASURES
Anx	Anxiety
CAMPIS	Child–Adult Medical Procedure Interaction Scale
CDI	Children's Depression Inventory
CBCL	Child Behavior Checklist
FACES	Faces Scale, a set of face drawings
HLOC	Health Locus of Control Scale
II	Illness Impact
MPQ	McGill Pain Questionnaire
OSBD	Observation Scale of Behavioral Distress
PBRS	Procedural Behavior Rating Scale
PBRS-r	Procedural Behavior Rating Scale-Revised
PBS	Parent Behavior Scale
RSES	Rosenberg Self-Esteem Scale
SHCSC	Stanford Hypnotic Clinical Scale of Children
SSIMP	Self-Statement Inventory for Medical Procedures
SSSC	Social Support Scale for Children
SPPC	Self-Perception Profile for Children
STAI	State-Trait Anxiety Inventory
STAIC	State-Trait Anxiety Inventory for Children

*When appropriate, abbreviations from Chapter 20 were employed.

helpful overall. The authors noted the clinical significance of these results, such that, with their multimodal intervention, procedure pain scores were 25% less than those obtained during attention control.

Medical procedures are not only potentially distressing for the children who experience them, but may also cause distress for the parents who watch their children undergo these invasive procedures. Because some parents become distressed when their children undergo medical procedures and parents influence the distress experienced by their children (27), Jay and Elliot (22) designed and evaluated the efficacy of a multimodal intervention for parents. Parents were assigned either to accompany their child as he/she received one of two child-focused interventions or to receive stress inoculation training themselves. The stress inoculation program employed by Jay and Elliot (22) included three components: modeling and education; positive self-statements; and relaxation training combined with suggestions for coping. As compared to parents in the child focused conditions, parents in the stress inoculation group reported lower state and trait anxiety and higher positive self-statements.

The work of Jay and her colleagues (4,20,21) has indicated that a multimodal intervention is effective in reducing children's distress during bone marrow aspiration and lumbar puncture. In addition, their multimodal intervention was found to be more effective than a pharmacological intervention or an attention control condition in reduction of children's behavioral distress and pain during bone marrow aspiration (4). Adding a pharmacological treatment to the psychological intervention did not enhance the effect of the psychological intervention in reducing children's distress during bone marrow aspiration and lumbar puncture (20). Finally, an intervention for parents based on a stress inoculation training model was found to reduce parents' distress associated with their child's medical procedure (22). It is important to point out that these studies did not address which aspects of the multimodal intervention package were most effective nor which components were effective for which children. The question "Which intervention, and for whom?" needs to be addressed.

Venipuncture

Venipuncture is a frequent medical procedure required for diagnostic blood tests, transfusions, bone marrow aspiration, lumbar puncture, and chemotherapy. Up to 77% of children find venipuncture distressing (28). Children's apprehension concerning venipuncture can lead to muscle rigidity, making the procedure more difficult (and painful) to perform. The recent development of a local anesthetic (EMLA) may make the entire procedure less painful, thereby diminishing the need for behavioral intervention with venipuncture. However, until EMLA is more widely assessed in randomized clinical trials with children, behavioral interventions remain an important treatment option for distress associated with venipuncture. (Systematic studies of behavioral interventions with pediatric oncology patients undergoing venipuncture are reviewed in Table 84.1).

Multimodal Strategies with Venipuncture

Building on the work of Dahlquist and colleagues (44). Manne and colleagues (6,7) have obtained strong support for the efficacy of behavioral interventions in reducing distress associated with venipuncture. Their three-session intervention package involves both the child and the parent and includes a combination of distraction, paced breathing, and reinforcement for the children, and instructions in behavioral coaching for the parents. During venipuncture, the child is distracted by using a party blower while the parent coaches. The parent counts out loud to pace the child's breathing into the blower and encourages him/ her to use it. Positive reinforcement consists of the child "winning" stickers for holding their hand still while the venipuncture is performed and for using the party blower. In randomized controlled studies, Manne and her colleagues (6,7) have found that these behavioral interventions effectively reduce distress during venipuncture. Particularly important for clinicians is that they demonstrated that this cost-effective (e.g., use of a party blower and parent coaching) intervention reduced both children's and parents' distress. There are, however, several remaining questions, including which behavioral strategy is most effective

for reducing venipuncture distress, an intervention package such as that developed by Manne and colleagues or an intervention such as those used with bone marrow aspiration and lumbar puncture which also included hypnosis.

TREATMENT SIDE EFFECTS AND BEHAVIORAL INTERVENTIONS

Nausea and Vomiting

In addition to pain and anxiety associated with medical procedures, patients often have problems related to treatment side effects. Aggressive treatments using multimodal therapy such as surgery, radiation, and chemotherapy can lead to a variety of aversive side effects. With several chemotherapeutic agents and radiation, patients often experience fatigue, diarrhea, hair loss, and post-treatment nausea. The most common side effects associated with cancer chemotherapy are nausea, vomiting and dysphoria. After repeated chemotherapy treatments some patients develop anticipatory nausea, that is they become nauseated in anticipation of treatment. Like the conditioned reflex of Pavlov's dogs (45), the patient's nausea in response to conditioned stimuli such as the site of the clinic, can be as intense as unconditioned responses elicited by actual treatment (46). Although the prevalence of nausea and vomiting reported in the literature varies, up to 71.2% of children receiving chemotherapy have been found to report having nausea during chemotherapy, and up to 76% of children have been reported to have anticipatory nausea (15,16,47,48). In addition, up to 43% of children have been reported to have anticipatory vomiting (16). Although anti-emetic medications have had some success in treating nausea and vomiting during chemotherapy, they are not effective for anticipatory symptoms. Further, anti-emetic use can result in multiple side effects such as headache and extrapyramidal reactions (15). In young children, severe nausea and vomiting can also lead to dehydration, electrolyte imbalance, and weight loss (47). Compounding the issues surrounding side effects and quality of life, some patients' treatment can be so aversive that they become noncompliant with treatment regimes, leading to increased morbidity and mortality (49).

Hypnosis and/or Distraction Strategies for Nausea and Vomiting

There have been many studies published on the use of behavioral interventions such as hypnosis, progressive muscle relaxation training, systematic desensitization, and distraction for reducing nausea and vomiting during and in anticipation of chemotherapy treatment (see Chapter by 40). Most studies have focused on adult cancer patients, while studies with children are few. In addition, the behavioral methods studied with children have been generally limited to hypnosis and/or distraction and most involve a single participant, not comparisons of intervention groups (41). (Systematic studies of behavioral interventions for treatment side effects with pediatric oncology patients are reviewed in Table 84.1).

In a group of 10–17-year-old patients, LeBaron and Zeltzer (12) assessed the efficacy of a behavioral intervention for reducing nausea and vomiting during chemotherapy. The behavioral intervention package included directing the child's attention away from thoughts about the chemotherapy by playing games, focusing on a object in the room, telling stories, and using muscle relaxation. Reassurance and information were also provided. The results indicated that, after the intervention, there were reductions in children's disruption of activities, nausea, vomiting, and the bother these symptoms caused. However, the lack of a control group makes the benefits of the behavioral strategies over nonspecific factors, such as reassurance or simply the passage of time, difficult to evaluate. Despite this study limitation, this classic study provided preliminary results suggesting that a behavioral intervention package was effective in reducing treatment side effects.

Cognitive/attentional distraction through video game playing to control anticipatory nausea in a group of 9–20-year-old cancer patients was assessed in two studies conducted by Redd et al. (5). In both studies there was a marked (up to 69%) reduction in nausea for those children who received the intervention; see also (50). In a subsequent study Zeltzer et al. (16) investigated the relative efficacy of a hypnosis intervention as compared to a nonhypnotic distraction/relaxation intervention, and a standard control group in children 5–17 years of age. Their results suggested that hypnosis was superior to the nonhypnotic distraction/relaxation intervention in reducing chemotherapy side effects.

A recent study by Jacknow and colleagues (15) evaluated the efficacy of hypnosis to control nausea and antiemetics in a group of 6–18-year-old newly diagnosed cancer patients. Not only did the children in the hypnosis group experience less anticipatory nausea than those in the standard care comparison group, but they also used less antiemetic medication prescribed to be taken as they felt it was needed. The results also indicated the need to maintain active patient intervention throughout the child's treatment course. Beneficial

effects were observed at one and two month post hypnotic intervention, but not at six months.

It is difficult to draw clear conclusions regarding the relative efficacy of hypnosis versus distraction in the control of chemotherapy side effects in children. The problem is that the procedures (i.e., counting the dots on their father's tie and completing arithmetic problems) used by Zelter and colleagues (16) may be far less effective for distracting children than the video games procedures used by Redd and colleagues (5). Further research is needed to define the parameters of hypnosis, cognitive/ attention distraction, and relaxation training in the control of treatment side effects.

POST-TREATMENT READJUSTMENT AND BEHAVIORAL INTERVENTIONS

In addition to coping with the distress associated with medical procedures and treatment side effects, children with cancer must confront other challenges such as re-entering the school environment after diagnosis. Returning to school and resuming normal interactions with peers is an important process for the child who has been diagnosed with cancer. Based on the notion that an early return to school can "normalize" the child's life in the midst of coping with cancer, thus promoting optimal rehabilitation, several authors have recommended re-entry into the school environment as soon as possible for pediatric cancer patients (33,51,52). In addition to normalizing life and encouraging rehabilitation, a prompt return to school can provide opportunities for social support (from peers and teachers) and exposure to socialization processes typically experienced by school-aged children. Such access to social support and socialization experiences may be crucial for proper adjustment. Indeed, positive peer relationships and perceived social support are associated with several positive corollaries, such as increased stress resistance, improved academic achievement, decreased levels of behavioral problems, and pro-social behaviors in general (53,54).

Clinical researchers have only recently begun to explore the use of multimodal interventions to promote post-treatment adjustment. Varni and his colleagues (54) assessed the relative efficacy of a social skills training intervention as compared to a standard school reintegration program with 5–13-year-old children with cancer. Both groups received the Standard Intervention which included: education for patients, parents, school and medical staff emphasizing the importance of an early return to school; school conferences and classroom presentations intended to demystify the cancer experience for both teachers and classmates; and regular follow-ups with patients, parents, teachers, classmates, and medical staff. The Behavioral Intervention Group also received the multimodal social skills training (e.g., modeling and cue-controlled relaxation), while the Standard Care Intervention Group spent equal time in individual play interaction with the research assistant. Results indicate that nine months after completing the intervention, pediatric cancer patients in the Behavioral Intervention condition experienced fewer behavioral problems and increased school competence (as reported by their parents). In addition, these children reported experiencing greater emotional and social support from their classmates and teachers after completing the multimodal intervention. Children receiving standard care did not experience these positive changes. Results of this initial study are quite important as they indicate that behavioral techniques are useful tools for teaching social skills and that the acquisition of such skills has a positive effect on pediatric adjustment.

FUTURE DIRECTIONS

The clinical research reviewed in this chapter clearly indicates the utility of behavioral interventions to reduce the pain and suffering of children with cancer. Hypnosis, distraction, and multimodal interventions have been found to effectively reduce distress associated with medical procedures, and hypnosis and distraction were found to reduce treatment side effects. In addition, a multimodal behavioral intervention has been effectively used to improve adjustment of pediatric cancer patients returning to school.

It is difficult to predict future advances in behavioral intervention in pediatric oncology. However, there are a number of important new trends. The first is the shift towards greater sophistication in research methodology. For example, the earlier studies generally lacked appropriate comparison groups, making the effect of the specific intervention, as compared to nonspecific factors or time, difficult to assess. More recent studies have included standard care comparison groups, in addition to two treatment groups making examination of the mechanisms underlying treatment effectiveness possible (e.g., comparing distraction through hypnosis as compared to distraction thorough focusing on objects in the room). Second, there has been an increased interest in making training in behavioral interventions available to family members and other health care providers in the hopes of adding to the benefits of an intervention provided by trained professional. Third, behavioral interventions are also being applied to new areas outside symptom management, for example to facilitate school reintegration. In addition, there is recent work involving the application of both behavioral interventions and cognitive remediation for neuropsychological (attention difficulties) deficits (55).

There also are new problem areas currently being identified which may benefit from application of behavioral interventions. These include as other medical procedures (i.e., bone marrow transplant—BMT), cancer-related fatigue, and symptoms of Post-traumatic Stress Disorder (PTSD), such as night terrors.

There has been research documenting that BMT is a stressful experience for pediatric oncology patients and their families and that BMT may be associated with PTSD (56,57) (see also Chapter 51). In addition, PTSD and fatigue have been documented in adult cancer survivors (58,59) and behavioral interventions are being used to help adults cope with these difficulties (60,61). Pediatric oncology patients with PTSD symptoms and/ or fatigue may also benefit from behavioral intervention to reduce these difficulties; this is an area for future research.

One of the main thrusts of future work may well be the application of behavioral theory and research to prevent problems. For example, how can chemotherapy be given so as to reduce the development of aversive side effects, such as food aversions? We do not mean to suggest that behavioral interventions are a panacea for all the challenges faced by pediatric oncology patients. Nor are we suggesting that behavioral interventions be used exclusively, but rather as adjunctive treatments to other biological and psychosocial interventions. Indeed, there are limits to the application of behavioral principles, such as challenges to family adaptation. As noted by Ostroff and Steinglass (62), there are challenges experienced by most families of children with cancer, such as the family's need to change and adjust to the different stages of the child's illness (e.g., from illness focus during acute phase to post-treatment readjustment). These areas of potential difficulty faced by the families of children with cancer are outside the realm of behavioral interventions and may be more effectively treated by family therapy interventions designed specifically to address them (62). In addition, there are many factors (i.e., cultural influences) which may contribute to the patient's and their families adjustment, or lack thereof, which are also outside the realm of behavioral principles. Given the limits in theory and application, it is clear that behavioral researchers and clinicians have made a significant contribution to our understanding of patients' responses to cancer diagnosis, treatment, and rehabilitation and to the design of effective methods for reducing pediatric patients' distress. The strength of the work that has been conducted leads one to expect important advances in the future.

REFERENCES

1. Zeltzer LK, Altman A, Cohen D, et al. Report of the subcommittee on the management of pain associated with procedures in children with cancer. *Pediatrics.* 1990; 86:826–831.

2. Thorndike EL. Animal intelligence: An experimental study of the associative processes in animals. *Psychol Rev.* 1898; 2:28–31.

3. Manne S. Couples coping with cancer: Research issues and recent findings. *J Clin Psychol Med Settings.* 1994; 4:317–330.

4. Jay SM, Elliott CH, Katz E, Siegel SE. Cognitive-behavioral and pharmacological interventions for children's distress during painful medical procedures. *J Consult Clin Psychol.* 1987; 55:860–865.

5. Redd WH, Jacobsen PB, Die-Trill M, et al. Cognitive/attentional distraction in the control of conditioned nausea in pediatric cancer patients receiving chemotherapy. *J Consult Clin Psychol.* 1987; 55:391–395.

6. Manne S, Bakeman R, Jacobsen P, et al. An analysis of an intervention to reduce children's distress during venipuncture. *Health Psychol.* 1994; 13:556–566.

7. Manne SL, Redd WH, Jacobsen PB, et al. Behavioral intervention to reduce child and parent distress during venipuncture. *J Consult Clin Psychol.* 1990; 58:565–572.

8. Kirsch I, Lynn SJ. The altered state of hypnosis: Changes in the theoretical Landscape. *Am Psychol.* 1995; 50:846–858.

9. Ellis JA, Spanos NP. Cognitive-behavioral interventions for children's distress during bone marrow aspirations and lumbar punctures: A critical review. *J Pain Sympt Manage.* 1994; 9:96–108.

10. Rape RN, Bush JP. Psychological preparation for pediatric oncology patients undergoing painful procedures: A methodological critique of the research. *Child Health Care.* 1994; 23:51–67.

11. Manne S, Andersen B. Pain and pain-related distress in pediatric cancer patients. In: Bush J, Harkins S, eds. *Pain in Children: Clinical and Research Issues from a Developmental Perspective.* New York: Springer-Verlag; 1991.

12. Hilgard JR, LeBaron S. *Hypnotherapy of Pain in Children with Cancer.* Los Altos, CA: William Kaufmann; 1984.

13. Kuttner L, Bowman M, Teasdale M. Psychological treatment of distress, pain, and anxiety for young children with cancer. *J Dev Behav Pediatr.* 1988; 9:374–382.

14. Zeltzer L, LeBaron S. Hypnosis and nonhypnotic techniques for reduction of pain and anxiety during painful procedures in children and adolescents with cancer. *J Pediatr.* 1982; 101:1032–1035.

15. Jacknow DS, Tschann JM, Link MP, Boyce WT. Hypnosis in the prevention of chemotherapy-related nausea and vomiting in children: A prospective study. *J Dev Behav Pediatr.* 1994; 15:258–264.

16. Zeltzer LK, Dolgin MJ, LeBaron S, LeBaron C. A randomized, controlled study of behavioral intervention for chemotherapy distress in children with cancer. *Pediatrics.* 1991; 88:34–42.

17. Zeltzer L, Kellerman J, Ellenberg L, Dash J. Hypnosis for reduction of vomiting associated with chemotherapy and disease in adolescents with cancer. *J Adolesc Health Care.* 1983; 4:77–84.

18. Cotanch P, Hockenberry M, Herman S. Self-hypnosis antiemetic therapy in children receiving chemotherapy. *Oncol Nurs Forum.* 1985; 12:41–46.

19. Genuis ML. The use of hypnosis in helping cancer patients control anxiety, pain, and emesis: A review of recent empirical studies. *Am J Clin Hypn.* 1995; 37:316–25.

20. Jay SM, Elliott CH, Woody PD, Siegel S. An investigation of cognitive-behavior therapy combined with oral Valium for children undergoing painful medical procedures. *Health Psychol.* 1991; 10:317–322.

21. Jay SM, Elliott CH, Ozolins M, et al. Behavioral management of children's distress during painful medical procedures. *Behav Res Ther.* 1985; 23:513–520.

22. Jay SM, Elliott CH. A stress inoculation program for parents whose children are undergoing painful medical procedures. *J Consult Clin Psychol.* 1990; 58:799–804.

23. Gatchel RJ, Baum A, Krantz DS. *An Introduction to Health Psychology.* New York: Random House; 1989.

24. Manne SL, Jacobsen PB, Redd WH. Assessment of acute pediatric pain: Do child self-report parent ratings and nurse ratings measure the same phenomenon? *Pain.* 1992; 48:45–52.

25. Tyc VL, Mulhern RK, Fairclough D, et al. Chemotherapy induced nausea and emesis in pediatric cancer patients: External validity of child and parent emesis ratings. *J Dev Behav Pediatr.* 1993; 14:236–241.

26. Katz ER, Kellerman J, Siegel SE. Behavioral distress in children with cancer undergoing medical procedures: Developmental considerations. *J Consult Clin Psychol.* 1980; 3:356–365.

27. Jay SM, Ozolins M, Elliott C, Caldwell S. Assessment of children's distress during painful medical procedures. *J Health Psychol.* 1983; 2:133–147.

28. Jacobsen PB, Manne SL, Gorfinkle K, et al. Analysis of child and parent behavior during painful medical procedures. *Health Psychol.* 1990; 9(5):559–576.

29. Manne SL, Bakeman R, Jacobsen PB, et al. Adult and child interaction during invasive medical procedures. *Health Psychol.* 1992; 11:241–249.

30. Spinetta JJ, Maloney J. Death anxiety in the outpatient leukemic child. *Pediatrics* 1975; 56:1034–1037.

31. Perrin E, Gerrity S. There's a demon in your belly: Children's understanding of illness. *Pediatrics,* 1981; 67:841–849.

32. McGrath PA, de Veber LL. The management of acute pain evoked by medical procedures in children with cancer. *J Pain Sympt Manage.* 1986; 1:145–150.

33. Katz ER, Dolgin MJ, Varni JW. Cancer in children and adolescents. In: Gross AM, Drabman RS, eds. *Handbook of Clinical Behavioral Pediatrics.* New York: Plenum Press, 1990: 129–146.

34. Bloom K. Social elicitation of infant vocal behavior. *J Exp Child Psychol.* 1975; 20:51–58.

35. Bloom K. Patterning of infant vocal behavior. *J Exp Child Psychol.* 1977; 23:367–377.

36. Manne SL, Bakeman R, Jacobsen PB, Redd WH. Children's coping during invasive medical procedures. *Behav Ther*. 1993; 24:143–158.

37. Broome ME, Bates TA, Lillis PP, McGahee TW. Children's medical fears, coping behaviors, and pain perceptions during a lumbar puncture. *Oncol Nurs Forum*. 1990; 17:361–367.

38. Smith KE, Ackerson JD, Blotcky AD. Reducing distress during invasive medical procedures: relating behavioral interventions to preferred coping style in pediatric cancer patients. *J Pediatr Psychol*. 1989; 14:405–419.

39. Hubert NC, Jay SM, Saltoun M, Hayes M. Approach-avoidance and distress in children undergoing preparation for painful medical procedures. *J Clin Child Psychol*. 1988; 14:194–202.

40. Gambino SR. Diagnostic tests and procedures. In: Tapley DF, Morris TQ, Rowland LP, et al., eds. *The Columbia University College of Physicians and Surgeons Complete Home Medical Guide*. New York: Crown; 1989.

41. Carey MP, Burish TG. Etiology and treatment of the psychological side effects associated with cancer chemotherapy. A critical review and discussion. *Psychol Bull*. 1988; 104:307–325.

42. Zeltzer L, LeBaron S. The hypnotic treatment of children in pain. *Adv Dev Behav Pediatr*. 1986; 7:197–234.

43. Palmer AG, Tucker S, Warren R, Ader R. Understanding women's responses to treatment for cervical intra-epithelial neoplasia. *British Journal of Clinical Psychology*. 1993; 32:101–112.

44. Dahlquist LM, Gil KM, Armstrong D, et al. Behavioral management of children's distress during chemotherapy. *J Behav Ther Exp Psychiatry*. 1985; 16:325–329.

45. Pavlov IP. *Conditioned Reflexes: An Investigation of Physiological Activity of the Cerebral Cortex*. Lecture III. Oxford, Oxford University Press; 1927.

46. Redd WH, Andresen GV, Minagawa RY. Hypnotic control of anticipatory emesis in patients receiving cancer chemotherapy. *J Consult Clin Psychol*. 1982; 50:14–19.

47. Hockenberry-Eaton M, Benner A. Patterns of nausea and vomiting in children: Nursing assessment and intervention. *Oncol Nurs Forum*. 1990; 17:575–584.

48. Dolgin MJ, Katz ER, McGinty K, Siegel SE. Anticipatory nausea and vomiting in pediatric cancer patients. *Pediatrics*. 1985; 75:547–552.

49. Burish TG, Carey MP, Krozely MG, Greco A. Conditioned side effects induced by cancer chemotherapy: Prevention through behavioral treatment. *J Consult Clin Psychol*. 1987; 55:42–48.

50. Kolko DJ, Rickard-Figueroa JL. Effects of video games on the adverse corollaries of chemotherapy in pediatric oncology patients:A single-case analysis. *J Consult Clin Psychol*. 1985; 53:223–228.

51. Deasy-Spinetta P, Spinetta JJ. The child with cancer in school: Teacher's appraisal. *Am J Pediatr Hematol Oncol*. 1980; 2:89–94.

52. Lansky SB, Cairns NU, Zwartjes W. School attendance among children with cancer: A report from two centers. *J Psychosoc Oncol*. 1983; 1:72–82.

53. Green KD, Forehand R, Beck SJ, Vosk B. An assessment of the relationship among measures of children's social competence and children's academic achievement. *Child Dev*. 1980; 51:1149–1156.

54. Varni JW, Katz ER, Colegrove RJ, Dolgin M. The impact of social skills training on the adjustment of children with newly diagnosed cancer. *J Pediatr Psychol*. 1993; 18:751–767.

55. Butler R. Cognitive remediation of attentional deficits and non-verbal learning disabilities following childhood CNS disease. *J Int Neuropsychol Abstr*. 1996; 2:18.

56. Lee ML, Cohen SE, Stuber ML, Nader K. Parent–Child interactions with pediatric bone marrow transplant patients. *J Psychosoc Oncol*. 1994; 12:43–59.

57. Stuber ML, Nader K, Yasuda P, et al. Stress responses after pediatric bone marrow transplantation: Preliminary results of a prospective longitudinal study. *J Am Acad Child Adolesc Psychiatry*. 1991; 30(6):952–957.

58. Alter CL, Pelcovitz D, Axelrod A, et al. Identification of PTSD in cancer survivors. *Psychosomatics*. 1996; 37:137–143.

59. Piper BF. Measuring fatigue. In: Stromborg M, Olson S, eds. *Instruments for Clinical Research in Health Care*. 2nd ed. Philadelphia: W.B. Saunders, 1996.

60. Shalev AY, Bonne O, Eth S. Treatment of Posttraumatic Stress Disorder: A review. *Psychosom Med*. 1996; 58:165–182.

61. Piper BF. Hints on how to combat fatigue. In: Dollinger M, Rosenbaum EH, Cable G, eds. *Everyone's Guide to Cancer Therapy*. 2nd ed. Kansas City: Somerville House, 1994.

62. Ostroff J, Steinglass P. Psychosocial adaptation following treatment: A family systems perspective on childhood cancer survivorship. In: Baider L, Cooper CL, Kaplan De-Nour A, eds. *Cancer and the Family*. New York: John Wiley; 1996.

63. Hilgard JR, LeBaron S. Relief of anxiety and pain in children and adolescents with cancer: Quantitative measures and clinical observation. *Int J Clin Exp Hypn* 1982; 4:417–442.

64. Kellerman J, Zeltzer L, Ellenberg L, Dash J. Hypnosis for the reduction of acute pain and anxiety associated with medical procedures. *J Adoles Health Care*. 1983; 4:85-90.

65. Katz ER, Kellerman J, Ellenberg L. Hypnosis in the reduction of acute pain and distress in children with cancer. *J Pediatr Psychol*. 1987; 12(3):379–394.

66. Wall VJ, Womack W. Hypnotic versus active cognitive strategies for alleviation of procedural distress in pediatric oncology patients. *Am J Clin Hypn*. 1989; 31:181–190.

67. Zeltzer LK, LeBaron S, Zeltzer P. The effectiveness of behavioral intervention for reducing nausea and vomiting in children receiving chemotherapy. *J Clin Oncol.*. 1984; 2:683–689.

68. LeBaron S, Zeltzer LK. Behavioral intervention for reducing chemotherapy-related nausea and vomiting in adolescents with cancer. *J Adolesc Health Care*. 1984; 5:178–182.

XIII

PSYCHOLOGICAL ISSUES FOR THE FAMILY

Editor: MATTHEW LOSCALZO

85

The Family of the Cancer Patient

MARGUERITE S. LEDERBERG

The interdependence of family members in both health and disease was, until recent decades, an unexamined assumption. Of course, the family will care for its patient! And indeed the family has done so, often under heroically taxing circumstances.

In the 1950s, the Sutherland group described cancer patients in a family context drawing attention to the intimate reciprocity of suffering (1). It followed that psychologically, family members should be considered what Lederberg has called "second order patients." This observation gained importance in the medical setting as personnel could observe its association with impaired patient management. Family therapy was in its infancy during this time. Its interventions address the family system, rather than any individual and, as it matured, it addressed the effect on the family of a member's illness. In the 1980s and 1990s family-centered studies have flourished, in association with many conceptual analyses and several lines of research (2–7).

Thus, three possible approaches to the family have emerged. They are cumulative, not mutually exclusive, and all need to be considered for a thorough understanding of the family. All three will be addressed below, after a brief survey of the insights contributed to understanding the family by bereavement and survivor studies. Additional emphasis will be placed on exploring the family's interface with the medical establishment since that is the greatest intervention access point. Referral issues, evaluation models, and corresponding interventions will be discussed.

BEREAVEMENT AND SURVIVOR PERSPECTIVES

Studies of bereavement have given a strong impetus to the importance of family studies. Beckwith (8) has identified high risk factors to predict problems in bereaved spouses. Bass's group found that a difficult care-giving history does not result in relief after the patient's death, but rather in a more painful bereavement, and that perceived support while the patient was alive is more important to care-giver adjustment than post-mortem support (9,10). In their review of family grief, Kissane and Bloch (10,11) reaffirm the importance of pre-mortem variables, and the pivotal role of support, especially professional support during the illness. The Melbourne group (12,13) has described a typology of families (supportive, hostile and sullen) which predicts poor outcomes and can be used to identify high-risk families pre-mortem.

Studies of families of cancer survivors (14–16) also point to a lengthening shadow of illness disruptions extending far into the future, in particular, the importance of parental coping on long-term adjustment of both parents and children, and the high incidence of post-traumatic symptoms in parents, especially mothers. The importance of psychosocial factors is repeatedly observed, sometimes overshadowing illness factors (14,17–19). Spinetta has documented the consistency of suicides over time in both survivor and bereaved families (20).

Family Studies During the Illness

Studies on the family during the course of the cancer illness provide further support. A significant number of families are seen to function more poorly than other families in the same community. They do not improve over time, and worsen even in the face of patient improvement (14,15,17,21–23). Several outcome studies show that personal and psychological factors play a more important role in family well-being than do illness factors, even with procedures as rigorous as bone marrow transplants (17,20,24). All of them support the importance of early identification of psychological risk factors, especially as the need for triage is generally accepted (8,9,11–13,17,21,25,26). Empirical studies before 1982 are reviewed by Northouse (5) and later ones by Kissane, Bloch, Burns et al. (27). The latter's own study used "caseness" to define individuals scoring high enough on depression or anxiety scales to warrant clinical attention. They found 35% caseness in spouses and 28% in offspring, using the Beck Depression Inventory, confirming the family's need for attention. Family-centered approaches are powerful tools for diagnosing families in ways that more traditional approaches have failed to do, and they have led to on-going intervention studies in several centers.

THE FAMILY AS A PROVIDER OF PATIENT CARE

Throughout most of world history, patients have been cared for at home. In developed countries, political and financial considerations are conspiring to return patients home at a rapidly increasing rate, and more is being demanded of families than ever before. Their wide-ranging contributions can be subsumed under seven headings.

The Provision of Emotional Support and Containment

This is an abstract yet compelling family role. Although emotionally stunned, family members expect themselves, and are expected by others, to contain their feelings, and support the patient. As noted above, such support plays a crucial role, not only in patient well-being, but in outcome as well.

Informational Needs and Shared Responsibility for Decision-making

A cancer diagnosis makes immediate decisional demands on patients when they are least able to meet them. Family members routinely step in do the work needed to explore and evaluate a sea of new information. Often a patient abdicates decision-making altogether, but there may be overt conflict, creating a delicate situation for medical staff. Family members are not just willing, but have a deep need to receive information and share in decision-making which continues throughout the illness (28,29)

Family decision-making may stem from contradictory motives. While families have a more intimate knowledge of the patient's mood, level of pain, feelings about treatment and about the treating staff, they may blatantly deny the patient's reality, usually because they wish to maintain hope untarnished by that reality (30). Many studies on family surrogacy demonstrate significant disagreement between the patient's wishes and surrogate decisions (31,32). Family members are expected to use substituted judgment, that is, do what the patient would have wished, but they often follow their own desires. However, patients themselves often defer to the family, and sometimes put family welfare ahead of their own. An increased and accurate knowledge base has been shown to relieve family anxiety and improve problem-solving and overall emotional outcome, while also appearing to have a positive effect on many patient health variables (33). When effectively provided, it is experienced as a mark of staff involvement and respect, and contributes to family satisfaction (34).

Concrete Care-giving

Even in the days when housewives were automatic care-givers, the demands of nursing a sick patient could be disruptive. Today, several trends make the situation much worse. First, women have entered the workplace and their financial contribution is no longer discretionary. Second, many patients are in non-traditional families: split families in which responsibilities can be disowned by individuals, single parent families in which the demands easily overwhelm the supply, elderly households whose adult children are geographically distant. Third, sicker patients are going home sooner and sicker and for longer. They often need tube feeding, oral, intramuscular, subcutaneous and even intrathecal medication. In addition, a bedridden patient needs help just to stay clean and comfortable. Even in hospitals, staff are leaner and families often stay to give bedside care. Thus, political and social trends are throwing a growing part of the practical and financial burden back onto the family. Faced with necessity and driven by love and/or obligation, families strive to meet the need, but at what cost?

Meeting Financial Costs

The staggering financial burden on families has been amply documented, even in socialized medicine systems. As many as 25% of primary care-givers give up or lose their job, one third of families lose all their savings or their major source of income. Sixty percent of the remaining care-takers register a significant loss in income due to absenteeism or a shift to lesser paid work (35–37). Minorities and poorer families experience greater losses, and these are associated with poorer disease outcomes (38). It is clear that today's financial savings represent a cost-shifting from third party payors to individual families, a reality which is blatantly ignored. As commercial interests thrive, families suffer, beggaring themselves to provide better care, feeling forever guilty, anxious, and resentful that they might not have done enough.

Meeting Social Costs

No-one has quantified the permanent career disruption and overall loss of social mobility of care-givers and siblings, which may be as great as the survivor's. Care-givers abort their careers, children develop school problems, adolescents act out destructively, and the family cannot make long-term plans. Social abandonment by friends is well described, but families isolate themselves during this period. They are too involved and disrupted to socialize. They avoid friends out of depression, shame, or resentment. They ignore community resources out of fatigue and demoralization (39). All these behaviors cumulate and become irreversible, resulting in enormous long-term human cost.

Maintaining Stability

Throughout all this, the family must endure. It must maintain itself in many ways and at many different levels:

1. *Filling in for the lost role and contribution the sick member* can be overwhelming, when the patient is a breadwinner, a young mother or a patriarch.
2. *Coping with the demands and losses* goes far beyond the immediate care-giving tasks, difficult as those are, and includes mourning and surviving the many losses described above.
3. *Meeting the increased emotional needs of members* in the crisis is a spotty task. Some family members rise to the occasion, others regress and have more insistent needs. Overtly or not, children fall in the latter category; this does not imply psychopathology, but is inherent in the child's cognitive and developmental limitations.
4. *Continuing to perform standard family functions*, such as feeding, education, socialization, emotional containment, nurture of development, spiritual guidance, and financial maintenance, is taken for granted throughout.

These activities are not direct patient care, but their continuity is essential to patient well-being. Medical costs for every family member rise significantly for three years after the index hospitalization (40).

Adapting to Change

Paradoxically, the maintenance of stability requires a capacity for change since task performance requires major adaptation. Change may be the only constant, since the course of cancer presents continually changing demands. The needs of the diagnostic period are different from those of ongoing treatment. Remission, relapse, deterioration, and long-term survival all present the family with special requirements for patient

care and support. Hospital versus home is a particularly important distinction. Different types of cancer create very different emotional climates; witness the "roller-coaster" course of acute leukemia versus the slow progression of colon cancer. Northouse (5) divided the trajectory according to three major phases: initial, adaptive and terminal. Rait and Lederberg (41) adapted this to acute, chronic, and resolution phases (Table 85.1), where the resolution phase includes long-term survivorship as well as death and bereavement. (These are discussed in Chapters 20, 79 and 88.)

CHARACTERISTICS OF ACUTE PHASES (Table 85.2)

In the face of cancer, family members react in characteristic ways that are not always compatible with each other or with the needs of the moment. Some family members may be more acutely distressed than the patient. They may hide it, paying a high price, as they become more and more resentful of being "ignored." However, this is also a time of rallying and mobilization by extended family and friends, which is welcome and helpful. The availability of accurate information at this time is critical in helping the family move from an affective to an effective response (42). In trying to protect themselves and the patient, many families create a "conspiracy of silence" with far-reaching negative effects on family relationships and individual well-being. These require prompt intervention if they are not to crystallize. A contemporary dynamic stems from the relentless demand on the

TABLE 85.1. *Principal Phases of Adaptation*

ACUTE PHASES	CHRONIC PHASES
Diagnosis	Long period at home
First treatment	Long hospitalization
Relapse	Lengthy treatment
Unexpected complication	Remission

RESOLUTION PHASES
Long-term survivorship
Death and bereavement

TABLE 85.2. *Characteristics of the Acute Phases*

Asynchronous individual responses

Effective initial mobilization

Need for information

"Conspiracy of silence"

patient to have a "positive" attitude, when family helplessness is disowned and the responsibility for changing the unchangeable is shifted onto the patient! The subtle callousness associated with this easily blends into a "blame the victim" psychology and, indeed, the hapless patient begin to feel guilty and responsible for his or her disease. On the other hand, bitter patients have been known to leave behind a legacy of anguish by angrily accusing family members of having "caused the cancer."

The mechanisms of the "acute" period extend to initial treatment, relapse, and unexpected complications.

CHARACTERISTICS OF CHRONIC PHASES
(Table 85.3)

Different mechanisms characterize "chronic" periods, such as return to home, lengthy courses of treatment, long hospitalizations, and periods of remission. During these consolidation times, the family must juggle the needs of the patient with the needs of other family members and focus on resumption of normal developmental tasks for all. This can be very problematic. The problem of focusing efforts on family preservation versus the sometimes contradictory needs of individuals is the one of the most frequent ethical problems reported by family therapists (43). Family members may disagree on goals, as when a primary care-giver remains overly protective while others feel the necessity has passed. As more time passes, members acknowledge and manifest their anger, jealousy, and need, leading to a paradoxical increase in psychological symptoms. Extended family and friends decrease their support, paralleling the emotional withdrawal of the family, and the family finds itself more isolated while it still needs help. During this time the family still remains illness-oriented and puts off major decisions. What started as a stress response may become a "habit" as family homeostats remain at their new setting.

TABLE 85.3. *Characteristics of the Chronic Phases*

Resumption of normal development tasks
Conflict between needs of patient and family members
Paradoxical increase in psychological symptoms
Social and emotional isolation of the family
"Neutral time"

FAMILY MEMBERS AS SECOND ORDER PATIENTS

Spouses of Cancer Patients

Recent studies, reviewed by Northouse (44), Haddad (45), Baider (46), and Kaye (47) reaffirm that spouses show levels of emotional and functional disruption as great or greater than the patient's and that these often worsen with time, independent of patient mood or health. In stable couples, patients underestimated their spouses' distress at their pain, and spouses underestimated the value patients placed on their support (48). Male spouses are more distressed than female ones, but male patients are less distressed than female patients, which is in keeping with what has been called women's relatedness function (46). Spouses of mastectomy patients were found to be deeply emotionally engaged but hiding it, and minimizing it in a way they thought was most supportive (49). Their wives interpreted this as rejecting and insensitive, leading to increased distance in the relationship. Many other studies confirm the desirability of open communication, even at the deathbed (50,51). A positive relationship has been reported between social support and immune functions (52).

Parents of Cancer Patients

The anguish of parents losing a child to cancer and the impact of parental coping on the child patient have been well described. They are reviewed in Chapters 77 and 79. and continue to be confirmed by recent reports, in two of which post-traumatic symptoms, which were found in 39.7% of mothers and 33.3% of fathers in one study, and in 54.5% of mothers and 25% of fathers in another (15,16,53). Effects can continue for years after the end of treatment and are correlated with the inability to establish and maintain social ties (14,18). In the parents of adult cancer patients, poor outcomes were associated with longstanding ambivalence in the relationship (54).

Children of Cancer Patients

Young children of cancer patients were, in the past, a high-risk group, whose problems were minimized by overwhelmed parents and invisible to the medical staff who did not meet them. It is now recognized that they show vegetative disturbances, psychological symptoms, acting-out behaviors, and school problems, as well as long-term changes in cognitive performance and personality attributes, such as self-esteem, much of which is mediated through family relationships. All children experience guilt about their possible causative role, grief and yearning for lost parenting from both parents, fear for themselves, and anger and resentment about being abandoned or shunted aside. The latter can be reality-based as young children are often sent away and are almost always by-passed in the illness-communication network. Thus facts are replaced by fantasies that are more tormenting than the grim reality. It is crucial to include children in the family communication and support system. It often needs outside help since mothers seem to be poor informants about their children's mental states (55). Children who were told about a parent's terminal illness showed less anxiety than children who were not (56). Studies of adolescent daughters of mastectomy patients found no increased acting-out but increased psychosomatic problems (57). Some showed impaired sexual functioning as well as a sense of their mothers being sexually impaired as well (58). They may take on increased maternal duties with resentment in some cases and increased self-esteem in others. Inability to discuss the illness with the parent was one of the risk factors for high anxiety in the adolescent children of cancer patients (59), while the adult children of cancer patients have many concerns about the parent–child relationship and about altered role behavior (60). They must take on a care-giver role, in which some overshoot into overprotectiveness, depriving patients of a chance to use their strengths and threatening them with dreaded dependency, while others regress and make demands for continued parenting even from a very ill patient. Looking back on this period, adult children universally view it as profoundly stressful, sometimes leaving permanent scars.

Siblings of Cancer Patients

Siblings are a troubled group who show a similar range of problems to the youngsters described above, with the addition of disturbances in the sibling relationship which, given the potential for strong identification and severe rivalry, cut very deep, especially when the patient does not survive (61–63). Siblings have fared as badly or worse than patients, on selected measures such as self-esteem, social isolation and fear of confronting family members. One report found better outcomes in families with larger numbers of children (64,65).

THE FAMILY-CENTERED APPROACH

The field of family therapy has sheltered many different models of family functioning that are discussed further in the next chapter; this discussion flags a few of the concepts that seem most useful, regardless of theoretical orientation (see Table 85.4)

TABLE 85.4. *Aspects of the Family-Centered Approach*

Developmental family life cycle
Family history, myths and beliefs
Structural model of family organization
Circumplex model of family functioning
The family/staff interface: a new temporary family system

Family Developmental Stages

Families, like individuals go through a life cycle with different stages that present characteristic tasks:

1. *The youngest family.* The newly married couple must create a new system, while still dealing with issues of separation from their families of origin. Cancer in one of them may shatter the union, propelling the patient back into dependency on parents, with frequent frictions and a tendency to exclude the spouse. Acute problems may arise when the family wants to assume decision-making prerogatives that legally belong to the spouse.

2. *The young family.* The parents of young children juggle child-rearing duties with the needs of the marriage and the individual, while establishing a financial base and negotiating the interfaces with families of origin and with friends. Cancer in any member saps the available energy and disrupts the balance of relationships in the direction of least resistance, rather than greatest usefulness. For example, in a shaky marriage where the mother turns to a child for consolation, the stress of the cancer may well increase the marital distance and the mother's dependency on the child. It may also shatter appropriate boundaries between nuclear and extended families while paradoxically increasing overall family isolation.

3. *The family with adolescents and young adults.* The main task of this stage is parental promotion of gradual yet steady separation, a brittle task given the expected recrudescence of powerful emotional issues. The younger generation must move toward peer intimacy, while consolidating identity and goals. Cancer inevitably disrupts these processes. Cancer in a child may arrest normal development abruptly, as well as that of his or her siblings, forcing regression and creating severe dependence/autonomy conflicts. Cancer in a parent may place demands on adolescents which slow down, or arrest their separation process, whether they react with overt engagement and acquiescence or with withdrawal and acting out. Parental tasks are equally disrupted.

4. *The aging family*. Parents in the aging family must profoundly refocus their concerns and goals in the direction of old age, letting children consolidate their own adult role while anticipating a time of need and dependency. Often the generations live apart and there may be no care-giving adult available, creating a stressful care vacuum. Even in healthy families, adult children, accustomed to self-containment and support from their parent, are emotionally unprepared to find in their own parent the regression and self-involvement characteristic of the ailing elderly. Guilt is an inevitable consequence.

Family History and Family Beliefs

Each family has a cumulative history of important events, and a rich corpus of family myths and traditions that grow up around the emotional impact of that history. Much of it relates to illness and loss, and to management of pain and enforced dependency, providing the blueprint for present responses to the cancer diagnosis. Past behavior guides present crisis appraisals, resources management, role assignment and expectations of success—or failure. Family histories also define family assumptions about cancer and the prognosis. It has been said that, in seeking professional help, families are almost purely seeking "corroboration and continuation of existing family values" (66). This may explain patient and family behaviors that appear irrational. Family myth can cause intrafamilial conflict since individual members' beliefs are related to their own families of origin and not always compatible in the current family. If implicit assumptions are made explicit and the past and present disentangled, tensions decrease and behaviors become more appropriate.

Family Organization

All families, even seemingly chaotic ones, have a complex structure. Each is a system made up of functionally defined subsystems, such as spouses or siblings, who maintain dynamic boundaries and who relate to each other along hierarchical lines. A stable organization that promotes predictability, security, and cohesiveness is highly valued by family members, who go to great lengths to protect it. Cancer is a major destabilizer. Many families try to deny this as a way of denying the impact of the cancer and cling rigidly to their previous structure, forcing inefficient, even destructive, behaviors on the members. Others dissolve under the impact, leaving members needlessly disoriented and bereft of structure. Even flexible families show signs of stress and change their patterns by "overshooting

in the direction of their dominant style," putting too much reliance on familiar patterns because that is the easiest, although not always the best, thing to do. Experimenting with new patterns is valuable, but often associated with transient signs of strain as well. From a family-process point of view, the pathology lies not in the actual pattern of behavior of any given family, but in whether or not the family shows a capacity to change and adapt under stress. Thus a family may appear quite strange to staff members, but may be structurally "healthy" if it is changing to meet the needs of the situation and the members.

The Olson Circumplex Model and Related Measures

A growing body of work analyzes family functioning and outcomes using measures such as the Family Adaptability and Cohesion Scale (FACES III), the Family Environment Scale (FES) and the Family Relationship Index (FRI) (12,13,27,67). Communication surfaces universally as a strong positive determinant of family functioning. Other findings are less consistent, possibly as a result of methodological problems.

FAMILY/TREATMENT INTERFACE

The family-system viewpoint has also given theoretical support to what most health professionals know from direct observation, namely the important relationships that develop between family members and the health care team. This has important implications for patient compliance, case management, and staff morale.

Intensity of the Relationship

One cannot overestimate the intensity of the relationship families develop with the treatment staff and the institution where they are based. Illness related issues become the "prime referent" for the family's thinking and medical care-givers become endowed with enormous significance (68).

Statements are repeated and behaviors are scrutinized for covert messages about the patient's condition. In a more subtle process, the family adopts unspoken beliefs and rules from the treatment team and is effectively socialized to the medical system. The resulting "good fit" between team and family has obvious advantages, but the pressure to conform may be detrimental if the family's style is too foreign or if the team philosophy is discrepant. In the case of a "bad fit" between family and staff, the treatment is fraught with recurrent complications and the family may be scapegoated by frustrated care-givers. This underlies many problems incurred when there is no congruence between the dominant medical culture and socially, ethnically, or religiously discrepant families.

Staff Behaviors Affecting Families

Despite undergoing unintentional "socialization," families may be easily intimidated by the large number of specialized professionals who play a role in modern treatment. When they receive, as often happens, conflicting reports from different people, they feel intellectually stymied, anxious, and angry. It is difficult, in today's large treatment teams, to give a steady flow of information without occasionally being confusing or inconsistent. The staff may not accurately gauge the family's capacity. They may underestimate it and make them more passive than is necessary, or overestimate it, casually expecting the family to perform tasks for which they are not emotionally or practically prepared. Explicit problems can be dealt with; covert ones cause ongoing stress in the family and difficulties with case management.

Family Reaction to Staff Behaviors

What families lack in medical knowledge and decisional power, they make up for in intensity and commitment. Hence, they wield considerable influence on the treatment team and the course of treatment. The "good" families are acquiescent and identify deeply with the treatment team. Some acquiesce on the surface but remain very ambivalent, ready to explode with disappointment, anger, and blame, which may seem exaggerated and unrealistic and is not amenable to discussion. This shift is less likely to occur when there is a previously established base of open communication and trust, but has been known to take even seasoned doctors by surprise. The "exhausting" families never acquiesce to anything, arguing and negotiating at every step. Some families find the experience so painful that they avoid it altogether, either abandoning the patient or convincing the patient to abandon the treatment. Some compromise by "doctor shopping" or seeking alternative treatments. When family dissatisfaction or anxiety are too great, even a well-motivated patient may be convinced to stop treatment. Not understanding the terror and anguish that drive such families, staff label them as "irresponsible." It should be admitted that a few families truly deserve the label of "impossible" families, and others create a climate of subtle menace that invariably has a toxic effect on case management.

Family Dynamics in the Treatment Setting

Even with the best of care, the family brings its own dynamics into the medical situation, and staff members are subtly co-opted into pre-existing family conflicts. Witness the ward power struggles around managing a child whose parents have always disagreed on discipline. Families that are overenmeshed and have poor boundaries will induce staff members to become overinvolved with them. Families that are closed and suspicious will induce a distant, guarded stance in their care-givers, thus confirming the family members in their belief about the lack of support to be received from outsiders.

The "Hybrid System"

The family/treatment setting is an intense, complex one, a web of complementarities in which the medical system and the family system join to form a new ad hoc "hybrid system." During acute periods, the shape of the old family system may be almost submerged by the hybrid. During chronic periods it reassumes primacy. But once cancer has occurred in a family, the system is never the same again and, in some families, the need to remain hybridized may be very great, to the detriment of the original family system. It behooves caregivers to understand their awesome emotional power and to use it well. When family members look back on their medical experience, it is colored intensely and unremittingly by their feelings about the kind of human relatedness they experienced. Every individual wants to feel that his/her uniqueness is being acknowledged, but, in the staff/family setting, this should not be understood as a demand for extraordinary care and personal affection. It is an expression of a basic human need to feel that one's humanity is in play. In fact, most families can be satisfied, and many experienced care-givers can provide this satisfaction, in a reasonable amount of time and without an excessive blurring of boundaries. However, this requires teaching, modeling and valuing the skill, which are best provided by senior medical role models, but, de facto, mental health professionals also have a crucial role to play.

REFERRAL ISSUES

The occurrence of a major cancer in a family is catastrophic enough that every such family could ideally benefit from a family evaluation early in the course, since that is when patterns of coping and communication are set which solidify during the course and may result in permanent alterations of family structure. While this is not a practical option and would not do full justice to the resilience of many families, it is a strong argument for educating medical staff to look for problems involving family members and to refer the family or any member of the family promptly when necessary. It also argues that all mental health professionals in this field should learn to "think family," even if they do not call themselves family therapists.

There are two entries to family problems. One is through referrals from the medical staff, the other is through active screening for high risk families. Table 85.5 outlines reasons for which a referral is called. A family that fails significantly in its patient care functions, provokes serious non-compliance, or disrupts the unit through conflicts with staff or among its members, rapidly occasions a request for psychosocial intervention from medical staff who are directly involved. Obvious psychiatric dysfunction or breakdown in a visible family member also occasions a referral, as do the variety of behaviors listed in Table 85.5 and any obvious patient/family conflict. Unfortunately the same problems may be occurring in unseen family members, such as children sent to their grandparents or a spouse who works long hours. Unknown to the medical staff, these can wreak havoc just as effectively as the more visible problems.

FAMILY EVALUATION MODELS

With expanding interest, several approaches to family evaluation have been developed. They have included predicting high-risk families (8,13,27,69,70) invulnerable families (26), and families likely to develop conflicts with the treating staff (71). Many of them utilize quality-of-life measures and family-therapy methods and concepts (see Chapter 86). A group of studies addresses needs assessment, the more extensive ones covering not only the concrete aspects of care-giving, but also the psychology of family members and the

TABLE 85.5. *Family-Based Reasons for Medical Staff Referrals*

1. Breakdown of patient care and support
2. Treatment non-compliance
3. Disruptive family behaviors on the unit
4. Staff/family conflict
5. Obvious psychiatric problems and/or substance abuse problems in a visible family member
6. Bizarre or inappropriate behaviors in a member
7. Signs of extreme anxiety or depression in a member
8. Severe somatic complaints in a member
9. Sudden marked changes in a member's mental state
10. Visible conflict between patient and family

structure of the family as it relates to the provision of patient care (4,23,72,73).

Although these approaches overlap, it is useful to think of them as falling into three broad categories according to their central focus. The first prescribes a response to an acute consultation request (41), the second orients itself to the ability of the family to care for the patient at home and reviews the many determinants of instrumental behaviors, and the third seeks to evaluate the family's dynamic functioning. Together, they represent a thorough analysis of family issues over the whole illness cycle. Each center or clinical group can create its own amalgam, to screen for the highest-risk families and identify what are, for them, the most efficient avenues of intervention.

The Acute Family Evaluation

As described in Table 85.6, the on-site consultant must explore disease-based issues, assess psychopathology in individual family members, identify the most immediate factors in family functioning, and understand the staff/family interface. This should enable the individual to understand what is driving the majority of observable family behaviors and to delineate the way in which the family is most currently functioning as a system of support for the patient and all its members.

Instrumental Assessment of the Family Resources

Instrumental assessments can be very sophisticated and address coping strategies, defensive style and family structure, as well as concrete care-giving resources, but they all share the fact that the goals are organized around the patient and/or the primary caregiver. Table 85.7, adapted from Given's work (72), outlines the main headings of her detailed care-giver needs assessment. As one fleshes them out, it becomes easier to see why care-giver health declines over time. In what has been called earlier the "chronic" phases of the illness, the overt emphasis is on meeting the patient's ongoing medical care needs, tests, follow-up visits, emotional adjustment and adaptation to losses. During the terminal phase, the need for readily available medical consultation becomes prominent. The family's questions are very real, but they often have an intensity that points to their being a metaphor for questions about death.

Analysis of Dynamic Family Functioning

The family-centered evaluation is described in Chapter 86.

TABLE 85.6. *Components of an Acute Family Consultation*

DISEASE FACTORS

Understand the facts of the disease, diagnosis, treatment and prognosis

Assess the family's understanding of the disease

Explore the meaning of the disease to the family

SCAN FOR ACUTE OR SEVERE INDIVIDUAL PSYCHOPATHOLOGY IN A FAMILY MEMBER

BRIEF FAMILY ASSESSMENT

Establish structure of the functional family unit

Identify immediate emotional coalitions and rifts

Review main care-giving strengths and deficits

Inquire about the family's previous experiences with cancer, other major illness, loss and trauma

STAFF TREATMENT INTERFACE

Identify staff contribution if any, and staff misperceptions, if present

Delineate the ways in which the family may be handicapping care

---

INTERVENTIONS

Given the complexity of families and their tasks, the overall purpose of interventions is not to find the "right" solution, but to approximate the best fit between complex and conflicting requirements—while staying within the range of available resources. For purposes of clarity, the interventions too will be divided into three broad categories which roughly correspond to the three types of evaluations:

1. The optimization of the immediate situation and the provision of immediate emotional comfort.
2. The creation of an extended, flexible and long-lasting system of support in response to the instrumental assessment

3. The resetting of family homeostats and challenging of dysfunctional family patterns in response to the dynamic assessment (see Chapter 86).

The Immediate Response

Family members need to be supported and empowered from the very first encounter. It is important to legitimize their feelings, as they often feel they have no right to them because they are "healthy"; they may also feel that their family customs have no standing, and may think that the stress and negative feelings they are experiencing are unique and shameful; lastly, they keep many thoughts and feelings unstated, not only to staff, but among themselves. It provides immediate relief for the implicit to be made explicit

TABLE 85.7. *Components of a Family Needs Assessment*

ASSESSMENT OF FACTORS RELATED TO DIAGNOSIS AND TREATMENT

Facts surrounding disease treatment and prognosis

Family expectation and knowledge

Care plan

ASSESSMENT OF PATIENT AND FAMILY'S ROLE

Analysis of pre-existing roles and required changes for impacted members of the family

ASSESSMENT OF CARE REQUIREMENTS

Description of expected symptoms and the care required

Functional status and related patient needs, especially around activities of daily living

Detailed analysis of practical emotional and cognitive needs of family and patient

RESOURCES AVAILABLE FOR CARE

Detailed analysis of family capacity and available outside resources

---

and for family members to hear that disruption and ambivalence are commonplace, that they, as individuals, have a right to complex needs at this time, and that, as a family, they are acknowledged and respected. An important focus at this time should be to acknowledge and support the family's distinctiveness and strengths. This enhances self-esteem, which lowers anxiety. It also models open, non-traumatic communication and the acceptance of many ways of behaving and feeling.

If the staff/family interface is problematic, this too should be addressed immediately. Blurred boundaries should be clarified without creating embarrassment for the staff or a sense of abandonment for the family. Inappropriate negativity or scapegoating should be defused by giving the staff some understanding of the family's dynamics. Hostile and abusive families should be unequivocally contained or even removed. The consultant's methods will include direct work with the family, but may extend to direct intervention and modeling for the staff, detailed behavioral guidelines, didactic sessions about the family issues in play, and emotional validation of staff feelings, combined with reinforcements of professional behaviors.

Providing information during acute periods is particularly important since events move quickly and many decisions need to be made. Carmody (29) describes an informational program for families awaiting the outcome of surgery, which has been appreciated by both families and surgeons.

The Creation of an Extended System of Support

Families will have to support themselves emotionally and practically over the course of the illness. Interventions can be broken down into five major areas:

Education. The family's need for detailed information has been repeatedly documented, as well as the lower anxiety levels, improved problem-solving and better coping associated with meeting this need. Many modalities, such as audio-visual materials, reading matter, and didactic programs, are welcome, although nothing ever replaces the human encounter with an authoritative professional. A teaching component is often built in to other modalities such as support groups, home care training, and home visitation programs in which nursing plays a major role; Conatser (74) has reviewed the educational requirements for families of children with cancer.

Improving Family Communication. The value of improving communications in the family continues to

be demonstrated. Open channels of frank discussion should be encouraged among all members. Two axes of communication should be especially bolstered: the marital axis, the problems of which have been described above, and the parent–child axis because children's ways of reacting are often misinterpreted negatively by parents with destructive consequences that are easily avoidable. Support groups are also useful to promote better communication.

Smoothing the Family/Treatment-Team Interface. Just as it is helpful to explain children's behaviors to parents, it can be helpful to explain distraught families' behavior to staff members, after which the latter usually treat them less defensively and with more accurate empathy. Consultants can serve as role model for staff or act as an adjunct on the health care team, attending staff–family meetings and ensuring that the full range of issues is discussed adequately. The importance and effectiveness of the family conference is underestimated by non-mental health staff. Its mutative power sometimes surprises mental health professionals as well. Atkinson describes a service in which family conferences are a routine part of patient care and staff processing (75).

Sometimes families are being affected by, and are contributing to a destructive ward climate. The staff must be aware of this and must take action when informal coalitions of families are meeting in the hall and visitors' lounge, upsetting each other rather than performing their more usual function of support. Usually one or more troubled families can be identified and their effect defused through personal intervention. Family group meetings have become commonplace in many cancer units and outside organizations.

Provision of Services. While the patient's needs are being met in the hospital, families may be overburdened by many old and new needs and benefit greatly from instruction and guidance on available resources. Knowledge about what is locally available and the availability of personnel to transmit this knowledge is as important as what specific model is selected. Nevertheless, it is best to have a structured approach since surprising gaps are often revealed.

Mobilizing of Social Supports. Some of the interventions above relate to periods of acute illness, but the mobilization of social support is important throughout the course and becomes especially so during chronic and recovery phases. Families must be encouraged to re-open their connections to the broadest number of community institutions so as to counteract subtle trends towards ever-more entrenched isolation. If the connection is not friends, clubs, churches or other pre-existing social institutions, it should be cancer-related groups or societies, such as Cancer Care, the American Cancer Society or the Leukemia Society of America, all of which are running family groups in increasing numbers (76–78). Groups have emerged in the last decade as a very powerful modality for patients, but most of the group factors apply to families as well, and family groups have a long history (79,80). Baider (46) reports on a ten-session theme-based group intervention for couples and retreats have been reported (81), as have group programs that address the needs of children and siblings of cancer patients (82–84). Art therapy and day-long programs that include tours of the hospital, play-acting and single-session groups have also been used, with the children divided into developmentally homogeneous groups (85).

A number of unusual interventions have been reported, such as family therapy when a member is on the death bed (86) and incidental family benefit from behavioral interventions designed for child patients (87). The evaluation of the family for the use of behavioral techniques has been described by Finney and Bonner (88). Hypnosis has been used as part of a cognitive-behavioral intervention for families, where the intent was to help families change negative beliefs and perception, and music therapy has been offered to the children of cancer patients (89,90).

SUMMARY

This chapter has reviewed the important role of the family in providing care for the cancer patient, as well as the enormous impact on the family of cancer in one of its members. The short- and long-term human cost to all members has been described, and conceptual points of view have been outlined that highlight the active and adaptive role of the family. Different types of evaluations have been described, together with a range of interventions to respond to them.

To do justice to the family, one must be able to entertain complex, and at times contradictory, hypotheses; one must support both change and stability; one must label and encourage strengths, reframe symptoms in a constructive mode, and yet be unflinching in recognizing and addressing conflicts and dysfunctions.

One must make hard choices between conflicting needs without being co-opted by, or needlessly arousing guilt in, any part of the system. The effort is eminently worth while, given the level of distress of the human beings involved and given the remarkable benefit that can ensue from even brief interventions.

REFERENCES

1. Sutherland AM. Psychological impact of cancer and its therapy. *Med Clin N Am*. 1956; 40:705–720.
2. Siegel K. Psychosocial oncology research. *Soc Work Health Care*. 1990; 15(1):21–43.
3. Quinn WH, Herndon A. The family ecology of cancer. *J Psychosoc Oncol*. 1986; 4(1/2):45–59.
4. Pederson LM, Valanis BG. The effects of breast cancer on the family: a review of the literature. *J Psychosoc Oncol*. 1988; 6(1/2):95–118.
5. Northouse L. The impact of cancer on the family: an overview. *Int J Psych Med*. 1984; 14(3):215–242.
6. Kazak AE, Nachman GS. Family research on childhood chronic illness: pediatric oncology as an example. *J Fam Psychol*. 1991; 4(4):462–483.
7. Lewis FM. Strengthening family supports. *Cancer*. 1990; 65:752–759.
8. Beckwith BE, Beckwith SK, Gray TL, et al. Identification of spouses at high risk during bereavement. A preliminary assessment of Parkes and Weiss' risk index. *The Hospice J*. 1990; 6(3):35–45.
9. Bass DM, Bowman K. The transition from caregiving to bereavement: the relationship to care-related strain and adjustment to death. *Gerontologist*. 1990; 30(1):35–42.
10. Bass D, Bowman K, Noelker L. The influence of caregiving and bereavement support on adjusting to an older relative's death. *Gerontologist*. 1991; 31:32–38.
11. Kissane DW, Bloch S. Family grief. *Br J Psychiatry*. 1994; 164:728–740.
12. Kissane DW, Bloch S, Dowe DL, et al. The Melbourne Family Grief Study I: Perceptions of family functioning in bereavement. *Am J Psychiatry*. 1996; 153:650–658.
13. Kissane DW, Bloch S, Onghena P, et al. The Melbourne Family Grief Study II: Psychosocial morbidity and grief in bereaved families. *Am J Psychiatry*. 1996; 153:659–666.
14. Overholzer JC, Fritz GK. The impact of childhood cancer on the family. *J Psychosoc Oncol*. 1990; 8(4):71–85.
15. Stuber ML, Christakis DA, Houskamp B, et al. Posttrauma symptoms in childhood leukemia survivors and their parents. *Psychosomatics*. 1996; 37:254–261.
16. Pelcovitz D, Goldenberg B, Kaplan S, et al. Posttraumatic stress disorder in mothers of pediatric cancer survivors. *Psychosomatics*. 1996; 37:116–126.
17. Greenberg HS, Meadows AT. Psychosocial impact of cancer survival on school-age children and their parents. *J Psychosoc Oncol*. 1991; 9(4):43–56.
18. Speechley KN. Surviving childhood cancer, social support, and parents' psychological adjustment. *J Pediatr Psychol*. 1992; 17(1):15–31.
19. Fritz G, Williams J, Amylon M. After treatment ends: Psychosocial sequelae in pediatric cancer survivors. In: Chess S, Hertzig ME, eds. *Annual Progress in Child*

Psychiatry and Child Development: 1989. New York: Brunner/Mazel; 1990: 239–252.

20. Spinetta JJ, Murphy JL, Vik PJ. Long-term adjustment in families of children with cancer. *J Psychosoc Oncol.* 1988; 6(3–4):179–191.

21. Ell K, Nishimoto R, Mantell J, Hamovitch M. Longitudinal analysis of psychological adaptation among family members of patients with cancer. *J Psychosomat Res.* 1988; 429–438.

22. Sawyer MG, Antoniou G, Toogood I, Rice M, Baghurst PA. A prospective study of the psychological adjustment of parents and families of children with cancer. *Pediatr Child Health Watch.* 1993; 29(5):352–356.

23. McCorkle R, Yost LS, Jepson C, et al. A cancer experience: relationship of patient psychosocial responses to care-giver burden over time. *Psycho-Oncology.* 1993; 2:21–32.

24. Northouse LL, Swain MA. Adjustments of patients and husbands to the initial impact of breast cancer. *Psychiatr Ment Health Nurs.* 1987; 36(4):221–225.

25. Sales E, Schulz R, Biegel D. Predictors of strain in families of cancer patients: A review of the literature. *J Psychosoc Oncol.* 1992; 10(2):1–26.

26. Barbarin CA. Psychosocial risks and invulnerability: A review of the theoretical and empirical bases of preventive family-focused services for survivors of childhood cancer. *J Psychosoc Oncol.* 1987; 5(4):25–41.

27. Kissane DW, Bloch W, Burns I, et al. Psychological morbidity in the families of patients with cancer. *Psycho-Oncology.* 1994; 3:47–56.

28. Derdarian AK. Informational needs of recently diagnosed cancer patients. *Nurs Res.* 1986; 35:276–281.

29. Carmody S, Hickey P, Bookbinder M. Perioperative needs of families. *AORN J.* (Official publication of The Association of Operating Room Nurses, Inc.) 1991; 54(3):561–567.

30. Ferrell BR, Rhiner M, Cohen MZ, et al. Pain as a metaphor for illness. Part 1: Impact of cancer pain on family caregivers. *Oncol Nurs Forum.* 1991; 18(8):1303–1309.

31. Suhl J, Simons P, Reedy T, Garrick T. Myth of substituted judgment: surrogate decision-making regarding life support is unreliable. *Arch Intern Med.* 1994; 154:90–96.

32. Layde PM, Beam CA, Broste SK, Connors AF. Surrogates' predictions of seriously ill patients; resuscitation preferences. *Arch Fam Med.* 1995; 4:518–524.

33. Stewart MA. Effective physician–patient communication and health outcomes. *Cancer Med Assoc J.* 1996; 152:1423–1433.

34. Roter D, Hall J, Katz N. Relations between physicians' behaviors and patients' satisfaction, recall, and impressions: An analogue study. *Med Care.* 1987; 25:399–412.

35. Murinen JM. The economics of informal care: labor market effects in the national hospice study. *Med Care.* 1986; 14:1007–1017.

36. Glajchen M. Psychosocial consequences of inadequate health insurance for patients with cancer. *Cancer Pract.* 1994; 2(2):115–120.

37. Covinsky KE, Goldman L, Cook EF, et al. The impact of serious illness on patients' families. *J Am Med Assoc.* 1994; 272(23):1839–1844.

38. Cella DF, Orav E, Kornblith A. Socioeconomic status and cancer survival. *J Clin Oncol.* 1991; 9(8):1500–1509.

39. Hinds C. The needs of families who care for patients with cancer at home. Are we meeting them? *J Adv Nurs.* 1985; 10:575–581.

40. Patrick C, Padgett DK, Schlesinger HJ, et al. Serious physical illness as a stressor: Effects on family use of medical services. *Gen Hosp Psychiatry.* 1992; 14:219–227.

41. Rait D, Lederberg M. The family of the cancer patient. In: Holland JC, Rowland JH, eds. *Handbook of Psychooncology: Psychological Care of the Patient with Cancer.* New York: Oxford University Press; 1989: 585–597.

42. Sargent J. Physician–family therapist collaboration: Children with medical problems. *Fam Syst Med.* 1985; 3:454–465.

43. Green SL, Hanson JC. Ethical dilemmas in family therapy. *J Marital Fam Ther.* 1986; 12(3):225–230.

44. Northouse LL. The impact of cancer in women on the family. *Cancer Pract.* 1995; 3(3):134–142.

45. Haddad P, Pitceathly M, Maguire P. Psychological morbidity in the partners of cancer patients. In: Baider L, Cooper CL, De-Nour AK, eds. *Cancer and the Family.* New York: John Wiley; 1995: 257–269.

46. Baider L, Cooper CL, De-Nour AK. *Cancer and the Family.* New York: John Wiley; 1995.

47. Kaye JM, Gracely EJ. Psychological distress in cancer patients and their spouses. *J Cancer Educ.* 1993; 8(1):47–52.

48. Dar R, Beach CM, Barden PL, Cleeland CS. Cancer pain in the marital system: A study of patients and their spouses. *J Pain Sympt Manage.* 1992; 7(2):87–93.

49. Sabo D, Brown J, Smith C. The male role and mastectomy: Support groups and men's adjustment. *J Psychosoc Oncol.* 1986; 4(1.2):19–31.

50. Hinton J. Sharing or withholding awareness of dying between husband and wife. *J Psychosom Res.* 1981; 25:337–343.

51. Gritz ER, Wellisch DK, et al. Long-term effects of testicular cancer on marital relationships. *Psychosomatics.* 1990; 31(3):301–312.

52. Baron RS, Cutrona CE. Social support and immune functions among spouses of cancer patients. *J Person Soc Psychol.* 1990; 54(2):344–352.

53. Koch U, Harter M, Jakob U, et al. Parental reactions to cancer in their children. In: Baider L, Cooper CL, De-Nour AK, eds. *Cancer and the Family.* New York: John Wiley; 1995: 149–171.

54. Shanfield SB, Benjamin AH, Swain BJ. Parents' reactions to the death of an adult child from cancer. *Am J Psychiatry.* 1984; 141:1092–1094.

55. Lewis FM. The impact of breast cancer on the family: Lessons learned from the children and adolescents. In: Baider L, Cooper CL, De Nour AK, eds. *Cancer and the Family.* New York: John Wiley; 1996: 271–288.

56. Rosenheim E, Reicher R. Informing children about a parent's terminal illness. *J Child Psychol Psychiatry Allied Disc.* 1985; 26:995–998.

57. Rosenfeld A, Caplon G, Yaroslavsky A, et al. Adaptation of children of parents suffering from cancer: A preliminary study of a new field for primary prevention research. *J Prim Prev.* 1983; 3(4):244–250.

58. Wellisch DK, Schains W, Gritz ER, et al. Psychological functioning of daughters of breast cancer patients. Part III: Experiences and perceptions of daughters related to

mother's breast cancer. *Psycho-Oncology.* 1996; 5:271–281.

59. Nelson E, Sloper P, Charlton A, et al. Children who have a parent with cancer. *J Cancer Educ.* 1994; 9:30–36.
60. Germino BB. Cancer and the partner relationship: What is its meaning? *Semin Oncol Nurs.* 1995; 11(1):43–50.
61. Sourkes B. Siblings of the pediatric cancer patient. In: Kellerman J, ed. *Psychological Aspects of Childhood Cancer.* Springfield, IL: CC Thomas; 1980; 47–69.
62. McKeever P. Siblings of chronically ill children: A literature review with implications for treatment and practice. *Am J Orthopsychiatry.* 1983; 53:209–217.
63. Banks SP, Kahn MD. Siblings are survivors: Bond beyond the grave. In: Bank SP, Kahn MD, eds. *The Sibling Bond.* New York: Basic Books; 1982: 271–295.
64. Spinetta JJ. The sibling of the child with cancer. In: Spinetta JJ, Deasy-Spinetta P, eds. *Living with Childhood Cancer.* St. Louis, MO: CV Mosby; 1981; 133–142.
65. Madanswain A, Sexson RT, Ragab A. Family adaptation and coping among siblings of cancer-patients, their brothers and sisters, and non-clinical controls. *Am J Fam Ther.* 1993; 21(1):60–70.
66. Miller M, Bernstein H, Sharkey H. Denial of parental illness and maintenance of familial homeostasis. *J Am Geriatr Soc.* 1973; 21:278–285.
67. Zabora JR, Smith ED. Family dysfunction and the cancer patient: Early recognition and intervention. *Oncology.* 1991; 5(12):31–38.
68. Cassileth BR. *The Cancer Patient: Social and Medical Aspects of Care.* Philadelphia: Lea and Febiger; 1979.
69. Hill DR, Kelleher K. Shumanker SA. Psychosocial interventions in adult patients with coronary heart-disease and cancer. *Soc Sci Med.* 1993; 36(5):693–701.
70. Kupst MJ. Family coping—supportive and obstructive factors. *Cancer.* 1993; 71(10):3337–3341.
71. Zabora JR, Fettig JH, Shanley VB, et al. Predicting conflict with staff among families of cancer patients during prolonged hospitalizations. *J Psychosoc Oncol.* 1989; 7(3):103–111.
72. Given BA, Given CW. Family home care for individuals with cancer. *Oncology.* 1994; 8:77–88.
73. Adams-Greenly M. Psychosocial assessment and intervention at initial diagnosis. *Pediatrician.* 1991; 18(1):3–10.
74. Conatser C. Preparing the family for responsibilities during treatment. *Cancer.* 1986; 58:508–511.

75. Atkinson JH, Stewart N, Gardner D. The family meeting in critical care settings. *J Trauma.* 1980; 20(1):43–46.
76. Baider L. Psychological intervention with couples after mastectomy. *Support Care Cancer.* 1995; 38:239–243.
77. American Cancer Society, 1599 Clifton Road, N.E., Atlanta, GA 30329.
78. Leukemia Society of America, 600 Third Avenue, New York, NY 10016.
79. Wellisch DK, Mosher MB, Van Scoy C. Management of family emotion stress: Family group therapy in a private oncology practice. *Int J Group Psychother.* 1978; 28:225–231.
80. Ringler KE, Whitman HH, Gustafson JP. Technical advances in leading a cancer patient group. *Int J Group Psychother.* 1981; 31:329–344.
81. Walsh-Burke K. Family communication and coping with cancer: Impact of the We-Can weekend. *J Psychosoc Oncol.* 1992; 10(1):63–81.
82. Adams-Greenley M, Shiminski-Maher T, McGowan N, et al. A group program for helping siblings of children with cancer. *J Psychosoc Oncol.* 1986; 4(4):55–67.
83. Smith KE, Gotlieb S, Gurwich RH. Impact of a summer camp experience on daily activity and family interactions among children with cancer. *J Pediatr Psychol.* 1987; 12(4):533–542.
84. Greening K. The "Bear Essentials" program: Helping young children and their families cope when a parent has cancer. *J Psychosoc Oncol.* 1992; 10(1):47–61.
85. Sourkes BM. Truth of life: Art therapy with pediatric oncology patients and their siblings. *J Psychosoc Oncol.* 1991; 9(2):81–96.
86. Acworth A, Bruggen P. Family therapy when one member is on the death bed. *J Fam Ther.* 1985; 7:379–385.
87. Burish TG, Snyder SL, Jenkins RA. Preparing patients for cancer chemotherapy: Effect of coping preparation and relaxation interventions. *J Consult Clin Psychol.* 1991; 59(4):518–525.
88. Finney JW, Bonner MJ. The influence of behavioural family intervention on the health of chronically ill children. *Behav Change.* 1992; 9(3):157–170.
89. Negley-Parker E. Hypnotherapy with families of chronically ill children. *Int J Psychosom.* 1986; 33(2):9–11.
90. Slivka H, Magill L. The conjoint use of social work and music therapy in working with children of cancer patients. *Music Ther.* 1986; 6A(1):30–40.

86

Family Therapy: A Systems Approach to Cancer Care

JANE JACOBS, JAMIE OSTROFF, AND PETER STEINGLASS

Families exert critical influence on the treatment and recovery process of cancer patients at a time when they must also shoulder the emotional demands of the disease. The central premise of family-based interventions is that helping family members to identify shared interests, prioritize problems, and work collaboratively toward solutions is a remarkably powerful and efficient form of psychotherapy. Family interventions focus on the relationship between family dynamics and individual behavior, mobilizing family members' inherent strengths and functional resources in the service of collaborative problem solving and restructuring of maladaptive behavioral styles. Methods of helping families who face a serious medical crisis fall into two general areas:

1. *Supportive or preventive interventions*, designed for families without major symptoms, which help family members expand and adapt their own successful problem solving methods to the demands of the cancer episode.
2. *Family therapy*, recommended when dysfunctional behavioral patterns are preventing family members from managing essential cancer-related tasks (1,2).

There are also opportunities at critical junctures in the treatment process for clinicians to provide help through informal, focused contacts with family members.

Current family interventions encompass a wide variety of theoretical concepts and therapeutic techniques that focus on the interplay between family beliefs and behavioral patterns and individual development (3,4). Although they have primarily been applied to situations of acute and chronic psychiatric illness, childhood behavior disorders, and marital conflict, their usefulness in the medical setting is by now well established (5–7). Nevertheless, most psycho-oncology clinicians continue to view families as ancillary to their more central focus on the psychological reactions of the cancer patient. In doing so, they miss the opportunity to understand the impact of the cancer episode on family members, and to mobilize the family as an ally and resource in cancer care.

In this chapter, we will provide a conceptual overview of family systems therapy concepts germane to medical settings; describe family-focused intervention strategies that address the family systems issues most likely to present in a clinical oncology setting; and highlight new opportunities for family therapists in a cancer setting.

CONCEPTUAL OVERVIEW OF FAMILY SYSTEMS THERAPY IN MEDICAL SETTINGS

In contrast to individually oriented therapists who focus attention almost exclusively on the role of intra-individual cognitions and emotions on behavior, family therapists are interested as well in the relationship between individual psychological processes and the *interactional field* within which the behavior or emotion is expressed. This relationship has been called the "context" for behavior. The family therapist is particularly interested in combinations of behaviors and contexts for behaviors that occur repeatedly in a particular family, because focusing on patterns of interactional behavior is critical to an understanding of how families function. The underlying rationale for this approach is encompassed in a set of constructs collectively referred to as "family systems theory" (8).

Family Systems Theory

Family systems theory, the application to family functioning of general systems theory, has long been the dominant theoretical model in the family therapy field (8). Family systems theory is not, in the usual sense, a theory at all, but rather a descriptive model of how families are organized and function. It is a dynamic model, viewing families as organized around two major forces—a morphogenetic (developmental) force that is reflected in the universal tendencies of families to become organizationally more complex over time, and a morphostatic (regulatory) force reflected in the capacity of families to maintain stability, order, and internal constancy over time. These two forces are not only in constant interaction with each other, but must balance each other if the family is to function in a healthy fashion. Further, it is the dynamic interplay of regulatory and growth forces that gives shape to the organizational characteristics manifested by a particular family. Although families are thought to be responsive to both these forces, morphostatic mechanisms, insofar as they serve a regulatory function, tend to balance and shape the weight and direction of morphogenetic (growth) characteristics.

Thus, within this model, the dynamism of families derives from a constant interactive jockeying between regulatory and growth forces within the family. Family functionality/dysfunctionality is seen as deriving from the type of balance existing between these forces. In some families, the need for stability seems to win out and change occurs only in response to tremendous pressures. These families are often described as "rigid," "enmeshed," or "fragile." In other families, alterations and changes seem always to be occurring. Such families are described as "chaotic," "disorganized," or "out of control." The "healthy" or "resilient" family is one that has developed an appropriate balance between morphogenesis and morphostasis, the key being a coherent fit of regulatory mechanisms and developmental themes (9,10).

However, when challenged by a serious medical illness, most families react by trying to gain mastery over the situation (11,12). Typically, adaptive mechanisms include a heightening of what family therapists call family regulatory behaviors (13). However, once these coping styles are put into place, they can easily take on a life of their own. For example, organizing daily routines around illness-related needs (diet; maintaining stable routines; modification of physical activities; hypervigilance) can easily become a semipermanent way of life, even though the acute crisis has long since passed and these behaviors may no longer be medically necessary. Thus, in examining issues associated with transitions from one illness phase to another, one factor to track is whether family regulatory behaviors are also shifting in synchrony with changing illness needs and demands (14).

In other words, one can assume that one of the consequences of *all* medical illnesses for families is increased order and regularity in daily life. However, for most illnesses this overregulation of family life in the service of illness management is a temporary need. Once the illness has stabilized, a more balanced pattern of illness/non-illness activities can be restored. If that re-balancing process does not occur, we can conclude that the family has become "stuck" around illness issues. In relation to cancer, a metaphor that helps bring this phenomenon alive is to think about cancer as having *invaded* family life and, as a consequence, created a *distortion* or imbalance in family priorities (15).

What are these family regulatory mechanisms? Although a wide-ranging series of constructs have been introduced to describe parameters of family functioning that serve to regulate family life, one can conveniently organize them into two main sets. The first set of constructs describe ways in which families develop shared and implicit views of their social world. Variously called family world views (7), or family paradigms (1,16), families develop shared ideas or hypotheses about how their world operates and how the family should cope with these external environmental characteristics. One family might develop a shared view of the world as masterable, best approached with an open and continuously changing perspective, an exciting place in which to live. Another family might see the world as largely unfathomable, as potentially hostile and alien, as a place that calls for extreme caution and a steady and unchanging course based on long tradition.

These shared views of the external environment in turn would then play an important role in shaping behavior whenever the family is interacting with its social world. For example, the nature of family paradigms might in turn provide the guidelines for the assumptions families bring to their interactions with health care systems. From the vantage point of the physician or nurse, these differences would then translate into whether the family was perceived of as cooperative, compliant, receptive to medical information (i.e., a "good family"), or suspicious, combative, unduly demanding, unappreciative (i.e., a "bad family").

A second set of constructs focus not so much on how the family construes its environment, but rather on how the family sees *itself* in relation to its larger world. Variably called the family's *identity* (17,18), *sense of coherence* (19,20), or its *organizing principle* (9), this set of constructs refers to a family's shared values and priorities, that is, the way the family might think about itself and describe itself to outsiders. A particularly important point here is that most families tend to pick a delimited number of themes around which to organize their identities, and these themes in turn play major roles in shaping family behavior (21).

FAMILY-FOCUSED INTERVENTIONS IN AN ONCOLOGY SETTING

Specific situations around which family-focused approaches may be useful in working with the cancer patient can be roughly divided into those in which interventions are aimed at (a) *correcting regulatory imbalances* created by cancer challenges and management issues versus; and (b) those in which the primary goal of the intervention is to help the family *deal more effectively with clinical course issues* (that is, family/illness developmental conflicts). Dependent on the severity and frequency of illness-related stressors and the multiple crucial supportive roles played by family members, a range of family interventions may be indicated to assist families dealing with cancer. At one end of the spectrum, preventive interventions are used to support and expand family members' natural coping abilities. Preventive interventions can occur informally or as part of an organized psychosocial intervention program. Formal programs serving groups of families allow clinicians to normalize the crises of the cancer episode and to encourage families to advise and support one another (15,22). At the other end of the continuum, when a family clearly loses its ability to conduct necessary functions, or when one of its members develops psychiatric symptoms, it may be appropriate to suggest a referral to a family therapist, ideally one who has expertise in working with families dealing with serious or terminal illness.

Although families clearly influence and are influenced by cancer (23), clinical referrals for family therapy in traditional cancer care settings are surprisingly rare. Most often the clinician will be called by the oncology care team to consult on an individual patient and will determine that inclusion of and collaboration with the patient's family is indicated. In our clinical experience, we have observed five common scenarios that may serve as catalysts for family consultations:

1. onset of medical crises;
2. poor performance by the family of patient care functions;
3. conflict and/or communication difficulties among patient, family, and staff;

4. current psychiatric symptomatology of a family member having difficulty coping with the illness;
5. the transition from active treatment to the chronic phase of cancer survivorship.

In the following section, we will describe these reasons for family consultation in an oncology setting. Case examples will illustrate how family-focused interventions can help families to explore their system of beliefs, to understand how those beliefs have constrained them, and to generate new perspectives and behavioral strategies for coping with cancer.

Medical Crises

From a family's perspective, cancer can be viewed as a series of medical crises that profoundly challenge its emotional, physical, and financial resources. While the exact nature, frequency and severity of these crises is highly dependent upon the type of tumor, the specific treatment regimen, the overall prognosis for long-term survival, and the family life cycle phase, families typically experience a predictable series of crises at key transition times in the disease course. Facing the initial diagnosis, handling treatment complications, completing treatment, and, for some, facing disease progression and death are nodal points when families are most vulnerable and may benefit from family-focused interventions.

For example, in the aftermath of cancer diagnosis, one of the earliest challenges for families is the disclosure of the diagnosis, that is, the "who," "when," and "what" to tell of the initial medical crisis. The following questions serve as a guide for the clinician in assessing a family's ability to achieve tasks associated with managing the initial diagnosis:

- Do family members understand the diagnosis?
- Are they informing key members of the patient's social network?
- Are family members taking the steps necessary for making sound treatment decisions?
- After the initial shock is over, are any family members visibly struggling with guilt, denial, anger, depression or anxiety?
- Are family members making realistic plans for the treatment phase?

CASE EXAMPLE

A 48-year-old married man diagnosed with laryngeal cancer was referred to an oncology surgeon at a distant city and underwent a total laryngectomy. He and his wife had decided that they did not want to worry either their two teenage children or the patient's 77-year-old mother, so they left their hometown and went cross country without describing either the extensiveness of the disease or the functional losses anticipated with the surgical treatment.

The surgery went well and the patient had a steady four-week recuperation, although, as expected, the surgery resulted in significant facial disfigurement and functional disability, including loss of speech, difficulty swallowing, partial facial paralysis and pain. Although the patient and his wife had been able to maintain their "minimalist front" during his hospital stay by stating that Mr L was busy with the doctor or sleeping whenever other family members telephoned, as the date of hospital discharge neared, the patient and his wife became increasingly anxious about how to break the news of the losses associated with head and neck surgery to the rest of the family. Consequently they requested a consultation for assistance in preparing their adolescent children for their homecoming. After exploring the pros and cons of disclosure approaches, the family therapist encouraged the couple to identify and implement ways of both supporting their teen-age children and including their help as members of the patient's "recovery team."

Another crisis point for families occurs if the patient's clinical course deteriorates (24). The following questions serve as a guide for the clinician in assessing a family's ability to achieve tasks associated with coping with disease progression:

- Do family members understand the changes in prognosis and the course of cancer progression?
- Are they taking the necessary steps for making sound decisions about further treatment or palliation?
- Are family members having end-of-life discussions about preferences for life sustaining procedures?
- Are family members anticipating major changes in the family's arrangements or plans that may occur after the patient's death?

CASE EXAMPLE

Nearly five years after her cancer diagnosis, Mrs G was diagnosed with recurrence of her breast disease and referred for psychological consultation. During the evaluation, the clinician focused on obtaining the family's "telling of the story" of the initial cancer episode, Mrs G's recovery, and the recurrence of the disease. Following the initial diagnosis, the family had rallied their resources to "battle the disease." It was a source of much family pride that they had seemingly "won their private war on cancer." In contrast, following this recurrence and with her prognosis for long-term survival poor, Mrs G and her family members seemed depressed, anxious, and isolated.

After noting the centrality of the "battle" theme, the clinician explored this theme as a potential organizing principle in the family's history. In fact, four years prior to Mrs G's initial diagnosis, Mr G had been dismissed from naval service because of his longstanding heavy drinking. This episode was a disgrace to him and the family. He eventually sought intensive alcohol treatment, and had been able to maintain sobriety and find a new civilian job. However, when his wife was diagnosed, Mr G embarked on a "special mission" to provide emotional support to his wife and children and to take charge of everyday family routines. At the completion of

treatment, Mr and Mrs G felt united in their triumph over cancer. Over the next few years, they repeatedly invoked their "victory" as the hallmark of their renewed marital bond and commitment. When the recurrence was confirmed, their apparent strength seemed "to crumble before their eyes."

In drawing this story from the family, the clinician began to see how the initial cancer diagnosis had provided a welcome opportunity for Mr G to transform himself from "loser" to "winner." In addition, the family's adherence to a rigid belief system focused on the theme of "doing battle with adversity" precluded not only an appreciation for the uncertainty of cancer, but also the ability to develop an effective coping strategy for this new phase of the disease. As the 14-year-old daughter commented, "We weren't able to even think about a recurrence. That would have been treason."

The clinician helped the family to understand the origin of the family belief system and appreciate the core values that characterize the G family. As they gained a broader perspective of the illness beliefs that had constrained them, the G family began to develop different ways of thinking about their experience with cancer. When they no longer viewed the recurrence as a defeat, they reported feeling less isolated as they experienced the sadness of entering the terminal phase of the illness.

Poor Performance by Family of Supportive Care during Active Treatment

Families serve as the primary referent and emotional support group for family members who become medically ill (25). The role of family support in the adjustment of pediatric and adult cancer patients has also been extensively studied (26), with a wide variety of studies suggesting that family social support is a significant factor in patients' psychosocial adjustment and medical course. For example, families who are described as highly cohesive have been shown to promote patient's overall psychosocial adjustment (27–30). Families provide essential, instrumental supportive functions that enable patients to adhere to the arduous treatment protocols and manage the debilitating side effects associated with modern cancer treatment.

Health care providers expect a great deal from families. Families are routinely expected to provide emotional support, share responsibility for treatment-related decision making, handle financial concerns, participate in many at-home medical procedures, and maintain some semblance of stability and attention to non-illness-related needs. During the active phase of cancer treatment, the illness and its treatment demand an inordinate amount of the family's physical, emotional, social, and financial resources. As cancer care is delivered increasingly in an ambulatory care setting, even greater care-taking responsibilities are expected of family members. For instance, families are expected to provide many treatment-related tasks, such as transportation to and from medical visits, monitoring oral medications, preparing special diets, giving injections, and wound cleaning. Typically, family members must make several rapid adjustments, such as shifting authority and responsibility to other family members, suspension of or reduction in employment and/or financial resources, reduced contact with work and social networks, postponement of non-illness-related plans, less attention to the needs of other family members, and integration into the hospital culture in order to facilitate the treatment of the illness.

When the scope of these caregiving responsibilities and concomitant changes in daily family life is considered, it is somewhat surprising that families are typically able to manage as well as they typically do. Nonetheless, when staff observe that family members are not providing expected practical or emotional support, requests for psycho-oncology consultations often ensue. Cancer diagnosis and the accompanying appreciation of "life being short" may encourage making long-contemplated positive changes, such as seeking marital therapy to address long-standing marital problems. As such, cancer creates opportunities for evaluation and change of long-standing dysfunctional family patterns.

Family therapists may also need to help families detoxify patterns of scapegoating and blame in those situations in which the patient's lifestyle is thought to be a contributing factor to the etiology of the disease. For example, the spouse of a patient with lung cancer who has been a heavy, long-standing smoker or the mother of a patient with melanoma who has ignored warnings of excessive sun exposure often must struggle with strong feelings of anger and resentment. Similarly, in those cases in which a family members perceives that non-adherence to the treatment regimen may have contributed to disease progression, social support may be limited and problematic.

The following questions serve as a guide for the clinician in assessing a family's ability to perform patient care tasks associated with the active phase of treatment:

- Is the patient adhering with the treatment regimen?
- Are family members actively supporting implementation of the treatment?
- Are communications between the family and the medical staff clear and useful?
- Is the family generally prepared to deal with the acute side effects of the medical treatment?
- Do family members seem to be coping successfully with the disruptions associated with the treatments?

Often in-patient staff are the best source of information about these questions. For example, in-patient staff are privy to information about who and how often given patients are being visited by family members (and by which family members), and how these visits are going. These observations in turn provide a window into how well family–patient relationships are working, data that are obviously invaluable to a family-oriented psycho-oncologist. The next example illustrates this process.

CASE EXAMPLE
A recently married, 27-year-old man was admitted to the hospital for colorectal surgery. In preparation for his in-patient stay, his parents relocated to be nearby during his hospitalization and at-home recuperation. In addition to being a former nurse, his mother was a very dynamic woman with an upbeat attitude. In contrast, the patient's wife was rather overwhelmed by the diagnosis and treatment. While she made several attempts to support her husband, she lacked his mother's fluency in "post-op talk" and her confidence about dealing with medical illness.

During the weeks of his hospitalization, the patient's wife visited the hospital infrequently and, when she did visit, both the patient, his mother, and some of the staff complained about the quality of the care provided. Much of the work with this family focused on helping the patient and his wife deal better with their strong emotional reactions to his illness by normalizing their experiences of fear, anger, and sadness, and by encouraging them to take a "crash course" from both the staff and the patient's mother in coping with medical crises. Gradually, the patient benefited from the support and greater cooperation of his wife, parents and extended family members.

When clinicians are attuned to family process and are aware of the normative tasks required of families during the cancer crisis, they can respond in ways that support adaptive changes taking place in the family. These interventions are simple and at times almost imperceptible but they give momentum to efforts initiated by the family. The following case example illustrates an informal family intervention performed by a nurse to assist a family adapting to the treatment phase.

CASE EXAMPLE
Mrs C, an outgoing, confident woman, was diagnosed with skin cancer. Her husband, a quieter man, clearly needed to take charge of family affairs during Mrs C's treatment and recovery. Mrs C encouraged Mr C to take over the decision-making role, but he was used to following her lead and their two boys looked for their mother's approval as Mr C tentatively began to assert more leadership. Mrs C's primary nurse noticed Mr C's efforts and, knowing she had Mrs C's support, took a variety of subtle actions to reinforce this family's adaptive changes. During Mrs C's hospitalization the nurse made a point of complimenting Mr C on his management of family routines in front of his children and, when she informed them of upcoming medical events, she made as much eye contact with Mrs C as with her husband. Gradually both Mr C and his children became more comfortable with his assertiveness.

Conflict and/or Communication Difficulties among Patient, Family, and Staff

Families clearly play an important role in determining compliance with treatment and in shaping the perception of health professionals toward particular patients (31). The complexities of cancer treatment protocols and the need to build effective partnerships between patients, families, and medical treatment teams all point to the importance of a family-systems perspective in cancer treatment. For example, there is a greater likelihood of staff–family conflict on issues such as pain control or treatment refusal when there is a wide divergence in either ethnic/cultural background or religious beliefs between family and hospital staff members (32).

Given the complementary roles of patient, family, and health care providers, it is clear that the patient's health is best served under conditions of good communication and mutually shared goals. One common role for the psycho-oncology clinician is to support the collaborative relationship among patient, family and health care provider. This collaborative framework may be jeopardized in response to deteriorations in the patient's medical status. The following questions serve as a guide for the clinician in assessing systemic issues interfering with health care provider and family collaboration:

- What is the family's understanding of the current treatment plan?
- Do the health care providers have a realistic expectation of the family's strengths, limitations, and goals regarding patient care?
- What role do differences in cultural and spiritual beliefs play in the current conflict?
- What are the potential barriers for conflict resolution?

CASE EXAMPLE

When the diagnosis of recurrent bladder cancer was confirmed in a 62-year-old man, the patient began questioning whether he could handle another round of aggressive chemotherapy. He gathered as much information as he could regarding conventional therapies for metastatic disease. Unfortunately, clinical trials had been encouraging but inconclusive as to whether the proposed combination chemotherapy regimen recommended by his doctors was likely to be efficacious. A friend had told him about a doctor who claimed miraculous results with a currently unapproved therapy. He told his family that he wanted to try this non-conventional approach. His family was quite ambivalent about his preferred plan. On the one hand, they were pleased that he was hopeful and displaying a strong will to live; however, they were also concerned about the safety of this alternative treatment and wondered whether his primary physician would later refuse to treat him if he elected this alternative

therapy. In this case, an office appointment was scheduled for the patient, his family members, and his primary physician to review and discuss treatment options. The family therapist participated in this meeting and facilitated consensus on the treatment approach and acceptance of the patient's preferences for complementary treatment.

Current Psychiatric Symptomatology of a Family Member Having Difficulty Coping with Illness

Studies examining the impact of cancer on family members have demonstrated that stress levels may justify referring to close family members as "second-order patients" (33). In our work with adolescent cancer patients, for example, we observe heightened levels of sibling and parental emotional distress both during treatment and many years after treatment has ended. Being the intimate partner of a cancer patient is considered to be as stressful as being the cancer patient (34,35). Adolescents and young adults whose parents are diagnosed with cancer may also experience heightened emotional distress (1,36–38). Elevated levels of depression and anxiety and physical signs of stress, including fatigue and headaches, have consistently been reported by family members of cancer patients (39). In addition, family members have been shown to underutilize support programs and may not be likely to request support and assistance from health care providers (16). These findings underscore the need to consider family members not only as the primary providers of support for patients, but also as potential recipients of supportive interventions. However, there is no universal family response to the diagnosis and treatment of cancer. In addition to the numerous stresses experienced by non-patient family members, many families also report cancer having a positive impact on family relationships, as they become aware of strengths that had been under-appreciated and grow closer as a result of their cancer experience.

Given that the family members's most likely to be most psychologically vulnerable are those with a history of psychiatric illness, a thorough psychiatric evaluation and mental status examination should be performed for family members presenting with psychiatric symptoms. Other questions to include in an assessment are:

- What role does this family member play in the management of the disease?
- What sorts of coping strategies have helped with this problem?
- How have other family members responded to psychological symptoms?
- Is the family member currently receiving psychological services in their local community?

CASE EXAMPLE

Shortly after being diagnosed with breast cancer, Mrs R noticed that her five-year-old son, Ryan, became oppositional and withdrawn. At first, she and her husband attributed his behavior to "one of those stages of growing up," but his disruptive behavior during school, preoccupation with blood and gory scenes, frequent tantrums, and refusal to sleep anywhere but in his parents' room continued, and they began to explore the impact of cancer on Ryan and daily family life. As a family, they had made great efforts to normalize cancer and its treatment. In fact, Ryan's teacher recalled overhearing the boy ask a schoolmate "when his presumably healthy mother goes to the hospital for treatment." Mr and Mrs R had tried to keep the household running smoothly by maintaining the children's after-school activities, arranging sleepovers after each chemotherapy cycle and only discussing disease-related concerns after the children were asleep. But clearly, for Ryan these efforts were not working as intended. Ryan and his family were therefore referred to a family support group program for young children whose parents have been diagnosed with cancer. Through child-friendly lectures by medical professionals, tours of the hospital, storytelling and interactive art projects designed to help children express their thoughts and feelings, Ryan began to share his questions and concerns. These activities were designed to foster family cohesion and reduce children's sense of isolation, confusion, and fear. In addition to the group sessions, the car ride home and the frequent stop for ice cream proved to be an important time for family unity amidst the crisis of cancer.

Transition from Acute Treatment to Chronic Post-treatment Phase

Families are given minimal guidance about how to make the transition from the active phase to the off-treatment, survivorship phase of cancer. For many families, this transition is challenging in that, for months or even years, the acute illness and the demands of cancer treatment have virtually governed daily family life. Families often report that typical responsibilities (e.g., job duties, community involvement) and routines (e.g., extracurricular activities, leisure time, holidays) have been either suspended or greatly altered during the active phase of treatment. Re-integrating non-illness activities, routines, priorities, and goals is a vital reorganization task that involves flexibility and accommodation to the changing demands of cancer. Families engage in this re-entry process while simultaneously remaining "on guard" for disease recurrence or late complications of the treatment. Understandably, it may be quite challenging to balance the ongoing demands of an illness with an unpredictable course while maintaining efforts to meet the broader needs of

family members (15). While many families do not display obvious signs of distress during the acute treatment period, serious problems, such as depression, anxiety, substance abuse, or marital conflict, may emerge months after the patient has completed cancer treatment.

Family members often claim that they do not stop to think about the ordeal they have been through until the initial crisis of diagnosis and the active phase of treatment are completed. Certainly, cancer remains an indelible memory for families, as evidenced by several reports of post-traumatic stress responses among the parents of childhood cancer survivors (40–42). Families repeatedly report a high degree of psychological distress, intrusive thoughts about the illness and persistent fears of an uncertain future. While many families state that the experience of cancer has resulted in increased closeness, these persistent feelings of emotional distress may also strain relationships within the family (e.g., marital, sibling, parent–child). In recognition of the primacy of family factors in post-treatment adaptation, we have developed a Multiple Family Discussion Group (MFDG) program (15). The MFDG brings together four to six families who, with two group facilitators, explore the impact of cancer on daily family life and examine strategies for dealing with post-treatment issues. A central metaphoric theme in these short-term structured groups is the balancing of the need to "honor the illness" and "put the illness in its place."

The following questions serve as a guide for the clinician in assessing a family's ability to achieve tasks associated with completing active treatment and making the transition to the chronic phase of cancer survivorship:

- Do family members understand the proper post-treatment management of the patient's health?
- Does the family seem ready to loosen the support of the hospital?
- Do family members seem excessively preoccupied with the illness?
- Have they been able to reshape family roles to meet the requirements of family life after discharge?
- Are there emotional, financial, or physical repercussions from the illness that are interfering with family members' adjustment?
- Can family members raise lingering illness-related concerns or are discussions about the disease and treatment now off-limits?
- Are there "sleeper" issues that were ignored during active treatment?

CASE EXAMPLE

Mrs N, was known by the hospital staff to have earned "the purple medal of honor" for her devotion to her 17-year-old daughter while she was undergoing bone marrow transplantation (BMT) for treatment of recurrent leukemia. She had an optimistic attitude about the success of the BMT and had managed well to support her daughter during the arduous conditioning regimen and BMT hospitalization. She witnessed her daughter's suffering from painful medical procedures and the acute toxicities associated with BMT. It was said that "she threw herself into her daughter's treatment and recovery." Fortunately, the BMT was successful and her daughter had a slow but steady period of recuperation. While her daughter, other family members and even the health care team were celebrating the completion of treatment, Mrs N was reporting frequent flashbacks regarding the BMT ordeal, intrusive thoughts about death, and hypervigilance to physical sensations. Daily thoughts of disease recurrence impaired her attention to even short-range planning. For instance, when her daughter raised the issue of planning a high school graduation party, her mother would "freeze" as she was "stung" by her fears of disease recurrence. Mrs N also became quite adamant about restricting her daughter's activities, stating that she felt extremely anxious when her daughter was "out of range" for more than a few hours. Despite efforts by other family members "to shake the gloom and doom," Mrs N continued to feel out of control and unable to resume non-illness roles and activities. Family members complained that she was "stuck in a cancer mode." Following a routine follow-up medical appointment, the family was referred to a multiple family discussion group designed to facilitate family members' post-treatment adjustment by helping family members to balance the chronic demands of the illness with the activities of daily family life.

NEW OPPORTUNITIES FOR FAMILY THERAPISTS IN AN ONCOLOGY SETTING

Cancer diagnosis often functions as a "wake-up call" that prompts family members to be more cognizant of their physical vulnerability, their risks of developing certain diseases, and the critical role of preventive health behaviors. As such, there are numerous opportunities to broaden the scope of cancer prevention efforts to include a family-focused approach.

In our work, we have found that families often seek information about cancer risk of other family members. Many families make efforts to adopt salient health-promoting behaviors in order to restore a sense of perceived control and physical well-being (e.g., reducing dietary fat intake, using sunscreen, stopping smoking). Following the diagnosis of cancer, the risks of certain lifestyle behaviors are personalized and family members, particularly adolescents who are most likely to have an optimistic health bias (43,44), may be most likely to adhere to health recommendations. Follow-up medical appointments provide numerous opportunities for staff both to teach families new health behaviors and to support the maintenance of these life-style changes over time.

Likewise, burgeoning advances in cancer genetics have heralded new opportunities for cancer prevention, as well as profound challenges for families as they consider the impact of having knowledge of cancer risk (45). For instance, women with a strong family history of breast cancer typically report heightened anxiety and an exaggerated sense of their own cancer risk (46). These psychological reactions may interfere with adherence to cancer detection and screening guidelines, such as performing breast self-examinations and mammography (47–49). Cancer risk counseling focusing on making informed decisions about undergoing genetic susceptibility testing should include attention to the disclosure of genetic risk information to other family members (e.g., daughters, sisters) as well as making recommendations for family-wide cancer screening and preventive health behavior change (50). Further study is needed to prepare families to cope with the knowledge of heightened vulnerability to certain genetically determined cancers and to adopt precautionary health behaviors that facilitate early detection and cancer prevention efforts.

The central argument is that placing both patient and family within a systemic frame of reference allows one to see more clearly the needs not only of the patient, but also of the rest of the family and of the medical care team as well. Further, it helps identify situations in which competing needs (demands) exist between patient, family, illness, *and* medical care team and leads the clinician to suggest ways to alter these situations in the service of effective treatment planning and implementation. Finally, a family-systems approach to cancer care provides a useful framework for promoting the psychosocial adaptation of patients and their families throughout the course of cancer.

REFERENCES

1. Compas BE, Worsham NL, Epping-Jordan JE, et al. When Mom or Dad has cancer: Markers of psychological distress in cancer patients, spouses, and children. *Health Psychol.* 1994; 13(6):507–515.
2. Cohn LD, MacFarlane S, Yanez C, et al. Risk-perception: Differences between adolescents and adults. *Health Psychol.* 1995; 14(3):217–222.
3. Steinglass P. Family therapy. In: Kaplan HJ, Sadock BJ, eds. *Comprehensive Textbook of Psychiatry.* VI. Baltimore, MD: Williams and Wilkens; 1994.
4. Compas BE, Worsham NL, Ey S, Howell DC. When Mom or Dad has cancer: II. Coping, cognitive appraisals,

and psychological distress in children of cancer patients. *Health Psychol.* 1996; 15(3):167–175.

5. Campbell TL, Patterson JM. The effectiveness of family interventions in the treatment of physical illness. Special Issue: The effectiveness of marital and family therapy. *J Marital Fam Ther.* 1995; 21:(4):545–583.

6. Akamatsu J, Stevens MA, Hobfoll S, Crowther J. *Family Health Psychology.* Washington, DC: Hemisphere Publishing; 1992.

7. Ransom DC. The family in family medicine: Reflections on the first 25 years. *Fam Syst Med.* 1993; 11(1):25–29.

8. Steinglass P. A systems view of family interaction and psychopathology. In: Jacob T, ed. *Family Interaction and Psychopathology: Theories, Methods, and Findings.* New York: Plenum Press; 1987: 25–65.

9. Steinglass P, Bennett LA, Wolin SJ, Reiss D. *The Alcoholic Family.* New York: Basic Books; 1987.

10. Walsh F. The concept of family resilience: Crisis and challenge. *Fam Proc.* 1996; 35:261–282.

11. Rolland JS. Families, *Illness, and Disability: An Integrative Treatment Model.* New York: Basic Books; 1994.

12. Steinglass P, Horan ME. Families and chronic medical illness. *J Psychother Fam.* 1987; 3:127–142.

13. Wood B. Beyond the "psychosomatic family:" A biobehavioral family model of pediatric illness. *Fam Proc.* 1993; 32:261–278.

14. Reiss D, Steinglass P, Howe G. The family's organization around the illness. In: Cole RE, Reiss D, eds. *How Do Families Cope with Chronic Illness?* Hillsdale, NJ: Erbaum; 1993: 173–213.

15. Ostroff JS, Steinglass P. Psychosocial adaptation following treatment: A family systems perspective on childhood cancer survivorship. In: Baider L, Cooper CL, Kaplan De-Nour A, eds. *Cancer and the Family.* New York: John Wiley; 1996: 129–147.

16. Davis-Ali SH, Chesler MA, Chesney BK. Recognizing cancer as a family disease: Worries and support reported by patients and spouses. *Soc Work Health Care.* 1993; 19(2):45–65.

17. Wolin SJ, Bennett LA. Family rituals. *Fam Proc.* 1984; 23:401–420.

18. Pentecost RL, Zwerenz B, Manuel JW. Intra-family identity and home dialysis success. *Nephron.* 1976; 17:88–103.

19. Antonovsky A. *Health, Stress and Coping.* San Francisco: Jossey-Bass; 1979.

20. Antonovsky A, Sourani T. Family sense of coherence and family adaptation. *J Marriage Fam.* 1988; 50:79–92.

21. Papp P, Imber-Black E. Family themes: Transmission and transformation. *Fam Proc.* 1996; 35:261–282.

22. Gonzalez S. Putting the illness in its place: Discussion groups for families with chronic medical illnesses. *Fam Proc.* 1989; 28:68–87.

23. Campbell TL. *Families Impact on Health: A Critical Review and Annotated Bibliography.* Washington, DC: U.S. Government Printing Office; 1986. [(adm):86-1461: National Institute of Mental Health Series DN6, DHHHS PUB.]

24. Wellisch DK, Welcott DL, Pasnau RO, Fawzy FI, et al. An evaluation of the psychosocial problems of the homebound cancer patient: Relationship of patient adjustment to family problems. *J Psychosoc Oncol.* 1989; 7(1–2): 55–76.

25. Litman TJ. The family as a basic unit in health and medical care: a sociobehavioral overview. *Soc Sci Med.* 1974; 8:495–519.

26. Neuling SJ, Winefield HR. Social support and recovery after surgery for breast cancer. Frequency and correlates of supportive behaviors by family, friends, and surgeon. *Soc Sci Med.* 1988; 27:385–392.

27. Bloom JR. Social support, accommodation to stress and adjustment to breast cancer. *Soc Sci Med.* 1982; 16(14):1329–1338.

28. Friedman LC, Baer PE, Nelson DV, et al. Women with breast cancer: perception of family functioning and adjustment to illness. *Psychosomatics.* 1988; 50:529–540.

29. Rait DS, Ostroff JS, Smith K, Cella DF. Lives in a balance: Perceived family functioning and the psychosocial adjustment of adolescent cancer survivors. *Fam Proc.* 1992; 31(4):383–397.

30. Bolger N, Foster M, Vinokur AD, Ng R. Close relationships and adjustment to a life crisis: The case of breast cancer. *J Pers Soc Psychol.* 1996; 70(2):283–294.

31. Reiss D, Kaplan De-Nour A. The family and medical team in chronic illness: A transactional and developmental perspective. In: Ramsey C Jr, ed. *Family Systems in Medicine.* New York: Guilford; 1989:

32. Griffith JL, Griffith ME. The Body Speaks: Therapeutic Dialogues for Mind-Body Problems. New York: Basic Books, 1994:

33. Rait D, Lederberg M. The family of the cancer patient. In: Holland JC, Rowland JH, eds. *Handbook of Psychooncology: Psychological Care of the Patient with Cancer.* New York: Oxford University Press; 1989: 585–597.

34. Baider L, Perez T, Kaplan De-Nour A. Gender and adjustment to chronic disease: A study of couples with colon cancer. *Gen Hosp Psychiatry.* 1989; 11:1–8.

35. Northouse LL, Swain MH. Adjustment of patients and husbands to the initial impact of breast cancer. *Nurs Res.* 1987; 36(4):221–225.

36. Wellisch DK, Gritz ER, Schain W, Wang H. Psychological functioning of daughters of breast cancer patients: I. Daughters and comparison subjects. *Psychosomatics.* 1991; 32(3):324–336.

37. Wellisch DK, Gritz ER, Schain W, et al Psychological functioning of daughters of breast cancer patients. *Psychosomatics.* 1992; 33(2):171.

38. Ell KO, Nishimoto RH, Mantell JE, Hamovitch MB. Longitudinal analysis of psychological adaptation among family members of patients with cancer. *J Psychosom Res.* 1988; 32(4–5):429–438.

39. Stuber ML, Nader K, Yasuda P, et al. Stress responses following pediatric bone marrow transplantation: preliminary results of a prospective, longitudinal study. *J Am Acad Child Adolesc Psychiatry.* 1991; 30:952–957.

40. Stuber ML, Christakis DA, Houskamp B, Kazak AE. Posttrauma symptoms in childhood leukemia survivors and their parents. *Psychosomatics.* 1996; 37:254–261.

41. Pelcovitz D, Goldenberg B, Kaplan S, et al. Posttraumatic stress disorder in mothers of pediatric cancer survivors. *Psychosomatics.* 1996; 37:116–126.

42. Hoorens V, Buunk BP. Social comparisons of health risks: Locus of control, the person-positivity bias, and unrealistic optimism. *J Appl Soc Psychol.* 1993; 23(4):291–302.

43. Lerman C, Rimer BK, Engstrom PF. Cancer risk notification: Psychosocial and ethical implications. *J Clin Oncol.* 1991; 9:1275–1282.

44. Lerman C, Kash KM, Stefanek M. Younger women at increased risk for breast cancer: Perceived risk, psychological well-being, and surveillance behavior. *J Nat Cancer Instit Monogr.* 1994; 16:171–176.

45. Vogel VG, Schreiber Graves D, Vernon SW, et al. Mammographic screening of women with increased risk of breast cancer. *Cancer.* 1990; 66:1613–1620.

46. Kash KM, Holland JC, Halper MS. Psychological distress and surveillance behaviors of women with a family history of breast cancer. *J Nat Cancer Instit.* 1992; 84: 24–30.

47. Lerman C, Daly M, Sands C, et al. Mammography adherence and psychological distress among women at risk for breast cancer. *J Nat Cancer Instit.* 1993; 85:1074–1080.

48. Lerman C, Lustbader E, Rimer BK, et al. Effects of individualized breast cancer risk counseling: A randomized trial. *J Nat Cancer Instit.* 1995; 87(4):286–292.

87

Palliative Home Care—Impact on Families

SHERRY R. SCHACHTER and NESSA COYLE

Although most patients with cancer die in an institution, the day-to-day living with advanced cancer is largely at home (1). This chapter addresses the impact of palliative home care on the family and factors that influence and contribute to its being either a life-fulfilling or life-draining experience. "Family" is used to refer to those individuals who are either relatives or persons who are important to the patient and provide key support (2). Palliative care is defined as "the active total care of patients whose disease is not responsive to curative treatment" (2). The goal of palliative care is achievement of the best possible quality of life for patients and families. Table 87.1 outlines some of the key elements of palliative care.

WHERE PEOPLE DIE

Where people die has varied considerably in the last century. Data indicate an increase in the proportion of deaths in the hospital in the United States beginning in the late 1940s and continuing into the late 1970s (3). However, by the 1980s, a trend away from hospital care has led to an increase in deaths at home or hospices, particularly of patients with cancer and AIDS. Although most deaths continue to occur in a hospital setting, home is where most care is given to the terminally ill for the longest periods of time (4). The increase in home deaths is the result of several medical and social factors. The recent rapid advances in medical technology have prolonged life, regardless of the quality. For some, the knowledge of this possibility is viewed with ambivalence, because it evokes fears of dependency and lack of autonomy. The person dying at home with their family feels more in control of decision making. Of equal importance in the United States was the passage of the Medicare Hospice benefit in 1983. This led to an increase in the number of hospice programs and

home health agencies and provided a system of care and support for those individuals who wanted to die at home. As a result of these factors, the option of end-of-life care at home is once again gradually becoming part of the "norm" of our social fabric.

OPTION AND CHOICES FOR THE PROVISION OF PALLIATIVE CARE IN THE HOME

Mapping out a path for the patient and family with the knowledge that there is no "one right way," and no "one right place" to die, begins the discussion around end-of-life palliative care in the home (5–7). Clear, concise, and open communications are potent tools in initiating and maintaining effective interventions. The readiness to seek an understanding of the concerns of the patient and family, and to deal honestly with them, is pivotal. A high level of clinical flexibility, careful listening, and offering a sense of cooperating with them helps the patient and family in making decisions (8). Families are expected to "be there" for the patient and to supply concrete care and support. They are on the "front lines," bearing witness to their family member's suffering or comfort; the effectiveness of symptom control and palliative care is greatly enhanced by them.

Meetings involving the patient, family and health care professionals are useful both in identifying unresolved issues or problems and in reviewing the plan of care (9). These periodic meetings will vary depending on the situation (or crisis) and the needs of the individual.

Hospice programs are the centerpiece for helping families care for dying members at home. The hospice concept pre-dates the Middle Ages. In the 1960s, evolving in response to the unmet needs of the terminally ill, the modern-day hospice movement re-emerged in England through the St Christopher's

TABLE 87.1. *Key Elements of End-of-Life Palliative Care*

Provided by an interdisciplinary team

Affirms life and regards dying as a normal process

Neither hastens nor postpones death

Provides relief from pain and other distressing symptoms

Integrates psychological and spiritual aspects of patients care

Offers a support system to help the family cope during the family member's illness and in their own bereavement

Source: Adapted from the Report of a WHO Expert Committee on Cancer Pain Relief and Palliative Care. Geneva: World Health Organization; 1990: 11.

Hospice. The first American hospice opened in New Haven, Connecticut in 1974 and the National Hospice Organization was founded in 1977. In 1983, after evaluation of government-sponsored demonstration projects on the efficacy and cost of hospice care, hospice services became a Medicare benefit (3). Hospice programs are run by both profit and not-for-profit organizations and are becoming part of the standard of care offered to patients with a life expectancy of six months or less.

A hospice program, as defined by the National Hospice Organization, is a centrally administered program of palliative and supportive service which provides physical, psychological, and spiritual care for dying persons and their families. Services are provided by a medically supervised interdisciplinary team of health professionals and volunteers (10). Core team members include physicians, nurses, social workers, the clergy, and volunteers. Although hospice care is available on both an in-patient and out-patient basis, in the United States the focus is on home care. Brief periods of hospitalization are utilized for symptom control or respite for the family.

Because of the range of models of hospice programs, levels of sophistication, and depth of services offered, a particular program must be evaluated carefully before a patient is referred (11). If the dying person is hospitalized, knowledgeable nurses and social workers are helpful in initiating the application process, as well as clarifying information for the patient and family. However, even if the dying person is at home when hospice is first considered, individuals can contact their local hospice to arrange a meeting to explore hospice options and insurance benefits. Most hospice programs offer on-site meetings to help acquaint people with their program. Individuals can call the National Hospice Organization to identify the hospice closest to them.

Although individuals may have specific concerns, some helpful questions to ask the hospice personnel include:

- What services does the agency offer?
- Will I be able to continue under my doctor's care or will I have to change physicians?
- What is the availability of home health aids?
- Will I have the same home health aide every day?
- What if I don't like the home health aide? Can I interview them first?
- What is the average length of nursing visits?
- Who will organize and supervise the home health aides?
- Are all medications covered under hospice?'
- How does the hospice deliver prescriptions and needed supplies—an agent who will deliver at any time or are deliveries dependent on volunteers?
- If an emergency occurs in the middle of the night, will an answering machine take my message, or will a person answer my call and provide help at home?
- What if we change our minds, and decide we want to return to the hospital to die?
- Can I sign off the hospice benefit and sign back on—what are the implications?''

Families may, however, care for a dying member at home without the support of a hospice program. Reasons for this are varied and can include:

1. Hospice programs are not available in their community;
2. The patients themselves chose not to follow such a program;
3. The insurance hospice benefit provides insufficient services to meet the patient's required or desired needs, and it is possible to access more care via a different venue, including a more general community nursing service such as the Visiting Nurses Association, provisions for privately paid home health aides or private duty nursing care at home.

Provisions for insurance coverage are so varied that each policy must be reviewed beforehand to help the family in their decision making process and to evaluate which option(s) would be the most appropriate. Similar to the process of exploring hospice programs, a knowledgeable social worker can be a valuable asset to the patient and family seeking guidance. Sometimes the needs of the dying patient and their family are best served by a joint effort between the cancer center, community, and hospice agency. Emphasis must focus on continuity of care, home management, and community education and support. This need to foster the concept of continuity of care, bridging the gap between hospital and community, and using the expertise of comprehensive cancer centers as a resource in care of the dying at home is becoming more widely recognized (12).

PLANNING APPROPRIATE END-OF-LIFE HOME CARE: ASSESSMENT OF NEEDS

In order to plan for both appropriate end-of-life home care for the advanced cancer patient, and adequate support for the family, it is essential to address and complete a medical, psychological, spiritual, social, financial, and community assessment. For home care to be successfully managed, the complexity of the patient's needs must be matched with the ability of the family and supportive networks to meet those needs (11,13). The areas that need to be evaluated as part of this initial assessment process include:

1. medical variables in the patient, family, and available community medical system;
2. psychological variables in the patient, family, and psycho-social community supports;
3. spiritual dimension;
4. social and financial variables in the patient and family (11,14–16).

Each variable will be reviewed separately.

Medical Variables
Medical variables are evaluated in relation to the patient, the family, and the community. These are outlined in Table 87.2. Variables that must be assessed in the patient include the disease status, expected disease progression (i.e., the dying trajectory), the patient's present functional level, distressing symptoms, and the effectiveness of the current management approach (5,11).

Of particular importance is the patient's functional level, reflecting his or her mobility (e.g., fully bed bound to fully mobile without aids), ability to communicate (from severely impaired to minimal impairment), ability to perform activities of daily living, bowel and bladder functions (from incontinence to self-care), and level of alertness (from coma to full alertness) (11,17). Since changes may occur frequently and rapidly, this must be an on-going assessment. As the patient becomes more debilitated and his or her needs change, the family needs to be given concrete information about what is occurring, what to expect, and what to do. In this way the family's knowledge gaps are filled in, achievements are reinforced, and the care-taking role is optimized. Additional help in the form of home health aides to assist in the physical care of the patient or volunteers to provided additional assistance may be indicated.

It needs to be remembered that the emotional and physical cost to family members in supplying support and care to a dying family member at home is great as they attempt to maintain stability in the midst of change. Adequate control of symptoms is essential for successful care of the dying at home. Uncontrolled symptoms, such as pain, dyspnea, nausea and vomiting, and delirium, can make the burden of home care an intolerable nightmare for the family. One's prior experiences with death (either at home or in a hospital) will also influence the dying experience.

It's very difficult for me to see her this way, it's very difficult for me to go into her room. It brings my mother's death back to me, I was 10 and my brother was 6. It was terrible. (18, p. 50)

However, when symptoms are well controlled and the family willingly engage in the care of the dying person at home, the personal rewards can be enormous. In the words of a sister caring for her 40-year-old sibling dying of breast cancer:

Nothing that I have done has been more worthwhile than this. All else pales in comparison. (18, p. 56).

The family participating in end-of-life care should be considered as the "second order patient." Sensitivity to their needs is essential (8). Concurrent medical problems in a family member, particularly the primary care-giver, need to be known because the family member's ability to participate is pivotal to the ability to carry out the home care plan (11). Recurrence of an old problem, for example, back pain or a return to excessive drinking of alcohol, may be the first sign that the care provider is becoming overwhelmed and needs respite.

Mrs G wanted to keep her husband home, knowing his desire was to die at home. Her ability to care for him would wax and wane, depending on his physical and mental condition. Mrs G's fatigue increased as her husband's physical demands increased. Her own health deteriorated as her arthritis and diabetes became exacerbated. She was physically exhausted; unable to sleep at night, often waking to change Mr G, who was incontinent of both urine and stool. Identifying, addressing, and maintaining her own health needs were paramount in supporting her ability to care for Mr G at home.

TABLE 87.2. *Evaluation of Medical Variables*

PATIENT
Present functional level
Level of need in activities of daily living
Disease status and expected progression
Symptoms and management approaches

FAMILY
Concurrent medical problems

COMMUNITY
Community physician's willingness to make home visits and to assume responsibility for end-of-life home care
Community nurses—types of nursing available: visiting-nurse services; private duty nursing agencies; ability to handle complexity of patient needs
Community supports: e.g. American Cancer Society, Cancer Care, support groups, social service agencies, etc.; religious groups; hospital-based out-patient support and/or educational programs; volunteers
Community pharmacy: whether it carries or will obtain necessary medications in a timely manner (especially opioids)

Source: Adapted (with permission) from Table 48-2 of Coyle N, Loscalzo M, Bailey L. Medical variables in the assessment process of patient, family, and community. In: Holland JC, Rowland JH, eds. *Handbook of Psychooncology*. New York: Oxford University Press; 1989: 602.

In assessing the community medical support network, attention must be focused on the availability of a local physician to assume medical responsibility for end-of-life home care, as well as the availability of that physician to make home visits. Additional community assessments include the presence of a hospice in that community (and, if so, what level of care it offers), familiarity of the community nurses with pain management and symptom control, and their willingness to use expert resources if needed. It is also important to determine whether the community pharmacy will be able to obtain the necessary medications for the patient (especially opioids). This assessment establishes both the specific care needs for the patient and the level of support available in the community. These data will help match patient needs to the resources available (11).

Psychosocial Variables

The key psychosocial variables relevant to family function are outlined in Table 87.3. This assessment is an ongoing process that allows for a continuous evaluation of the family's response to the rapid changes caused by advancing disease and their level of fatigue. The process of assessment is designed to lead the health care practitioner to an understanding of the medical and psychosocial situation of the family system so that effective interventions can be developed (11). It is essential that the perceptions of the family be explored and understood prior to any interventions being implemented. Not only does this quickly establish in the mind of the care provider that their input is

valued, but it also increases the probability that interventions will be acceptable to the patient and family. The family needs to be secure that they will have the necessary knowledge and support to care for the person at home. Hospitalization is offered as an option if home care becomes too difficult or respite is need. This possible need for re-hospitalization should not be viewed as a failure, and therefore is built into the plan of care. The families "shared responsibility" in decision-making can be highly frustrating if they lack accurate information and a sense of ongoing involvement and respect from the medical and nursing staff for what they have to say.

They didn't hear me, this isn't going to work if I can't bring him into the hospital if I have to. I shouldn't have to beg. (18, p. 44).

Early on, it is necessary to gain from the family an adequate understanding of their major concerns: both individually and as a system. This enables the practitioner to engage the family as active participants in the team and to create an environment of effective problem solving. Conflicts among the patient, family and friends may surface, and their goals and expectations may differ dramatically from those of the medical staff. Recognition of these differing expectations is the first step in a problem-solving approach. The issue of control is of major importance in working with the family. For many families, having a sense of control may lessen the impact of not being able to slow down the disease process in any meaningful way. Prior coping strategies used, and their effectiveness, are

TABLE 87.3. *Evaluation of Psychosocial Variables*

PATIENT

Major concerns at this moment: ability to integrate this experience; control issues (e.g., perception of loss of control, life–death issues, environment); expectations of disease process (experience with illness and cancer); work; self image, independence–dependence issues; significant losses (e.g., activities, role change, social supports); goals and desires

Ability to communicate effectively: feelings, concerns, fears, needs, fantasies (e.g., life–death issues, causality, pain)

Developmental process: age-appropriate behavior (relationships, work hobbies, aspirations, etc.), life experience (as it influences how one sees things and acts)

Mood (e.g., calm, anxious, depressed): trait (consistent behavioral pattern); state (reaction to recent events)

Pre-existing psychopathology: psychiatric illness; psychiatric hospitalizations; substance abuse (use of drugs and/or alcohol causing significant impairment in social functioning); history of suicide attempts; mental illness in family; inadequate coping skills

Coping strategy: tackling, rationalizing, avoiding

FAMILY

Same variables as for patient

Pre-existing family structure and functioning

Present family structure and functioning

Presence of children at home (age-related ability to comprehend changes caused by the illness process)

Ability to reconcile differences (e.g., belief systems, coping styles, treatment decisions)

COMMUNITY SUPPORTS

Religious affiliation, volunteer group, friend network, counselors, hospice team, clubs

Source: Adapted (with permission) from Table 48-3 of Coyle N, Loscalzo M, Bailey L.. Psychosocial variables in the assessment of patient, family and community. In: Holland JC, Rowland JH, eds. *Handbook on Psychooncology*. New York: Oxford University Press; 1989: 603.

important for the practitioner to know. This can be assessed by interviewing the patient and family and exploring how the family as a unit coped in the past. When stressful things happened in the past, how did the family pull together to resolve the problem? Will that approach work in this situation? What things did the family do that were not effective? What can we do now to avoid the ineffective behavior? Exploring issues of spirituality, religion, and cultural beliefs need to be addressed in order for the health professional to identify and recognize how the individual views illness and death, potential resources, and the impact on the patient's/family's quality of life.

In general, successful coping strategies ordinarily used by the family should be supported. However, such strategies may be inappropriate or ineffective in the current situation. A family with a rigid, inflexible coping style is apt to be troubled by episodes of emotional crisis, as compared to one with more flexible coping. In addition, increased stress frequently leads to increased rigidity among family members and may lead to conflicts between health professionals and the family members. The family's opinion needs to be heard, listened to, and respected.

End-of-life home care, especially if prolonged over a period of months, places enormous stress on any family and most community health care providers.

I have a feeling of suspended animation, waiting for something to happen. It's difficult to continue to live actively and engage with each day. I'm overwhelmed with sadness. It's all so sad. (18, p. 46–47)

If this time period extends into a year or longer, there is a danger that the significance of the mounting strain on the part of the family may be missed. Although assessment is an ongoing process, patients and families require a more formal re-evaluation of their medical, psychological, social, and financial status by the home care team at a minimum of every few weeks. The family may be torn between whose needs to meet first, the patient or other members of the family, such as children or spouses.

I am so torn. My husband is sick, my baby is little, who do I take care of first? Both are calling me, who do I go to first? (18, p. 44)

Spiritual Dimension

Spirituality refers to those aspects of human life relating to experiences that transcend sensory phenomena. For the family caring for someone who is dying at home, spiritual struggle or spiritual ease may center on the meaning of this experience. The search for meaning is a universal phenomenon. There is a need to recognize that care-givers can have parallel or divergent needs to those of their sick family member, and may be dealing with the same or widely opposed spiritual issues and values. Not all spiritual issues are problematic: many families find that caring for a sick loved one at home adds a dimension to their lives that was missing. The intensity of the spiritual experience in caring for a family member who dies at home can leave a void after the event. For some, this is a difficult void to fill. Chaplains or other spiritual counselors can be helpful to the family in re-gaining their equilibrium and in integrating the experience into their life.

Social and Financial Variables

Outlined in Table 87.4 are a number of social and financial variables that must be considered in end-of-life home care. Essential features should include who lives with the patient, who will be contributing to their care, the number of actual hours the primary care provider is unable to spend with the patient (for which coverage must then be planned), and whether there is active, consistent, and reliable help from other family members and/or friends to assist in the patient's care. This accurate initial assessment of the patient's care will help to avoid later problems with the family, whose members genuinely want to care for their relative but who overestimated their ability to meet the required investment of time and energy (11).

The financial impact of advanced disease is widely accepted to have the potential for catastrophic proportions to patient and family members alike (2,8). It is important that health professionals understand the financial situation of the family so that planning and appropriate interventions be developed. The social work member of the hospice team plays a major role

in this area. The psychological, medical, and financial concerns are so interrelated that they can become indistinguishable as families perceive these three distressing aspects as one overwhelming dimension. The team looks at this "overwhelming dimension," identifies key areas of distress, and initiates interventions.

One purpose of this initial assessment is to identify strengths and weaknesses in the ability of the family to provide end-of-life care to a family member in the home, and to help them achieve their goal. The most critical ingredient, however, is a genuine desire and ability on the part of the family to manage the situation at home (11).

WHAT MAKES DYING AT HOME DIFFICULT FOR THE CARE PROVIDERS

There are several factors that contribute to care-provider stress when someone chooses to die at home. These stresses can be viewed from the perspective of the family as well as from that of the health care team. Without question, uncontrolled symptoms can make a home death impossible and indeed cruel for all concerned. In addition, stressors can include, but are not limited to the patient's cognitive impairment, fear of being a burden to loved ones, and the physical and emotional demands placed on the family members. To provide needed support for families wishing to facilitate end-of-life care at home, it is essential that the health practitioner be cognizant of these stressors and intervene appropriately and in a timely manner.

TABLE 87.4. *Evaluation: Social and/or Financial Variables*

PATIENT

Living arrangements (how altered to accommodate the dying family member)

Work status (e.g., retired, disability)

Finances (e.g., income, savings, debts)

Insurance coverage for hospital care

Insurance coverage for home care (partial or total), hospice; home health aides; private duty nurses; community nursing; equipment; medications

Medicare or Medicaid eligibility

FAMILY

Availability as primary care-provider (family, friends)

Consistency, reliability of family or friend: commitment of time

Actively involved friend network

Income other than patient (none, spouse, other)

Structural setup of the home (steps, elevator, number of rooms, bathroom, space for equipment, wheelchair accessibility, telephone)

Source: Adapted (with permission) from Table 48-4 of Coyle N, Loscalzo M, Bailey L. Psychosocial variables in the assessment of patient, family and community. In: Holland JC, Rowland JH, eds. *Handbook on Psychooncology*. New York: Oxford University Press; 1989: 604.

Family Stressors

Although many patients with their families make the decision and prefer to die at home, it is not an easy task. For most, caring for a dying family member or being present at the moment of death is a new experience and can be a frightening or "spiritual" one. Although caring for family members at home can usually be managed for short periods of time, when this care requires weeks and months, physical and emotional exhaustion take over. There are several factors that can contribute to this family exhaustion, making it difficult to care for dying persons at home.

Families often underestimate the physical aspects of home care, thinking, perhaps, only of the emotional upheavals and the anticipation of death. They may not, for example, consider the mountain of laundry that must be washed daily. Nor may the family caregivers be aware of the amount of physical care required of them, including night time care and the emotional fragility of the dying person. Lack of sleep, unless addressed, can lead to tension, anger, and a sense that no-one cares or understands and that a caregiver is "on their own." A family's perception that they are not being supported can correlate closely with a high level of physical exhaustion in the family caregiver (4).

The drain of the physical aspects of care is often made worse by the psychological stresses that the family unit incurs (4). Jensen and Given (19) have noted that physical exhaustion is compounded by the anxiety and uncertainty about the timing of death and the way it may occur. Patients may be humiliated by new feelings of dependency, fear of being a burden, and their sense of losing control. Family care-givers can become overwhelmed by unfamiliar new roles and the demands they face. Roles that were once the foundation of the family's structure (such as homemaker or breadwinner) may now crumble, often causing conflict and discord at the very time when closeness is most important. These roles are often taken over by other family members, who may or may not be prepared for them. In addition, the patient may be unable to accept the loss of prior positions and roles. The burden of families trying to cope with impending death is increased. The following case illustrates difficulties with role reversals:

Mr and Mrs H were professional writers. When he was diagnosed with cancer of the tongue, they had no idea how profoundly his disease would affect their professional and private lives. Numerous surgeries left him disfigured and speechless. Mr H became more passive, not willing or able to resume his former assertive role and responsibilities. Mrs H tried not to "damage his autonomy" when she was forced to assume more of the decision-making responsibilities, and she felt guilty about doing so. She described the remaining months as very stressful and she was resentful at being forced to assume roles that she had given up earlier in their marriage. (20, p. 62)

Contemplating and facing one's own mortality can be frightening and stressful. However, for individuals with prior psychiatric disorders these stresses have the potential to exacerbate the previous psychological problem (such as alcohol, substance abuse or personality problems). Life-threatening illness can produce anxiety, depression and acute confusional states that are extremely stressful and frightening to families. It is particularly difficult for families to understand that paranoid delusions and hallucinations are organic in origin and are not based on reality or external events; nor should they be seen as a result of the family's care of the patient (4). Therefore, it is imperative that health professionals anticipate and explain to family members potential problems and how they will be managed. Delirium occurred in 75% of dying patients studied by Massie et al. (21). Hull (22) also noted considerable distress at the high frequency of cognitive and memory problems that families did not expect or understand. This was particularly true with changes in mental status, especially confusion (22,23).

Physical symptoms that are not adequately managed can be the most difficult aspect of home care (24). Studies by Brown et al. (25) reported physical problems as being the major focus of stress. Often family stress is increased by the demands of having to give nursing care without medical knowledge and expertise. Intractable pain has been identified as one of the most stressful physical symptoms in dying cancer patients (12). The distress of seeing a loved one in pain is difficult and may make the family wish for an early death so that the patient does not have to continue suffering. This increases the stress for both patient and family care-giver (26). On one hand the family fears that giving too much medication will cause a reduction in the level of alertness, often over-sedating the patient and even hastening their death. On the other hand, the family is often reluctant and afraid to give too little medication in fear of not controlling their loved one's pain. These feelings of self doubt, guilt, and ambivalence are common in family members (4). Brown et al. (25) noted that the primary reason for the re-hospitalization of home care patients was inadequate pain management and control. Shortness of breath, anorexia, nausea, and constipation are other common troublesome symptoms that contribute to making home care stressful and difficult (27). Pain and other symptoms can be controlled at home, but patients and families need to know this. If pain and other symptoms are being inadequately controlled expert resources must be utilized by the community care providers—telephone consultation is not uncommon. For some families, however, the feeling of ongoing responsibility for a dying member is too much.

AB, an elderly retired teacher had metastatic adenocarcinoma of the stomach. Her only support was her younger brother, aged 68. Both individuals had been previously successfully treated with antidepressants for depression; the brother also had a history of generalized anxiety attacks. The patient's chief complaints were abdominal pain with severe bouts of nausea and vomiting. The patient was started on morphine, via a continuous infusion pump (patient controlled analgesia—PCA) The home-care nurse was able to instruct AB and her brother in the use of the PCA. With continued instruction he became more comfortable and knowledgeable. However, he was fearful of giving his sister "too much medication." Despite repeated instruction and reassurance, his own anxieties and feelings of inadequacy resulted in frequent trips to the hospital for re-evaluation and assessment.

Despite daily telephone calls and 24-hour availability of the health care team, this family member was giving us the non-verbal message that caring for his dying sister at home was too hard for him. He needed our acknowledgment and our permission to re-admit his sister into the hospital and have her die there.

Although most end-of-life care does not involve high technology, for a few this is required. In these circumstances, an additional stressor associated with home care is the fear of turning a home or bedroom into a mini ICU or hospital room. Brown et al. (25) have stressed the importance of not allowing the home environment to become "eroded" and cite the problems of maintaining "normalcy" in the home—trying to protect the patient's independence while filling the home with supplies and equipment.

Learning that his bladder cancer had spread to his larynx, Mr R stated that he wished to commit suicide because of the pain. During a psychiatric evaluation he stated that if symptoms were controlled, he would like to live for as long as he was comfortable and then die at home. He wanted pain control, his infection treated, and nutrition. An infusion pump was initiated for analgesia control, a gastrostomy tube was inserted for feeding, and intravenous antibiotics were administered for treatment of an abdominal wound. His wife welcomed his care at home, but quickly found that they often viewed the 24-hour private duty nurses, when they could afford, as an intrusion. Mrs R expressed feeling excluded from her bedroom, which became a "mini ICU." The sounds of repeated tracheostomy suctioning reached her in the other room, causing her much discomfort and distress. Mr R received aggressive palliative care with a good outcome for comfort, however, the loss of privacy and intimacy with her husband were negatives in an otherwise positive experience of end-of-life care. (20, p. 63)

After Mr R's death his wife repeatedly told the health care team that caring for her husband and having him die at home had been, for the most part, a positive and rewarding experience. Mrs R took great comfort that she had been an active participant in his care and felt her efforts were rewarded in that she was able to support her husband in the way he desired.

Sometimes when immediate symptoms are controlled and effectively managed, the focus of the family changes. This is the time when the family may look ahead and become distressed and fearful about the actual dying process. It is not unusual for families to ask: "What can I expect? What will happen? What will I see? Will my loved one die suddenly? Will I know what to do? Whom do I call?" It is imperative that health care professionals address these questions and assure the family that the available 24-hour on-call person will be there for them. This is crucial in guiding family members and reducing their anxiety (12). Health care professionals must repeatedly review and instruct the family members when to call, whom to call, and how to access the health care team; also sometimes how to use a long-range beeper. Printed directions are very helpful, especially if they are posted near the telephone. Along with this information, families should be encouraged to post important phone numbers (nurse, hospice team, physician). Families may use this area (by the telephone) to post the patient's Home Do Not Resuscitate Form (Fig. 87–1).

End-of-life home care is not the best choice for everyone. For some families it is so stressful that their distress level can exceed that of the patients (28,29). Some studies suggest that a strong interaction exists between the family's psychological state and successful coping and that of the patient's. Personal characteristics of the family that shows optimism and emotional maturity are associated with better outcomes for both patients and care-givers (28). It has also become apparent that "helping the helper" programs may be beneficial and are worth further study and investigation. This again reinforces the concept of the family as second-order patients.

Patient/Family/Team Stressors

It is not unusual for conflicts between family members and the dying person to arise at home. Additionally, members of the health care team may experience frustration and conflicts with the patient and/or family. Although conflicts can arise at numerous times in the dying trajectory, there are specific events that seem to trigger added stresses and conflicts, thereby making dying at home difficult. One such time has been identified as occurring during the period of changing, re-

Memorial Hospital for Cancer and Allied Diseases

 DNR ORDER

Patient Identification

State of New York Department of Health

Nonhospital Order Not to Resuscitate
(DNR Order)

Person's Name _____

Date of Birth _____/_____/_____

Do not resuscitate the person named above.

Physician's Signature _____

Print Name _____

License Number _____

Date _____/_____/_____

It is the responsibility of the physician to determine, at least every 90 days, whether this order continues to be appropriate, and to indicate this by a note in the person's medical chart. The issuance of a new form is **NOT** required, and under the law this order should be considered valid unless it is known that it has been revoked. The order remains valid and must be followed, even if it has not been reviewed within the 90 day period.

56-08393   A27   CIMC Approval Date: 6/9   ORIGINAL - Patient   COPY - Medical Record   00/01.010.07

FIG. 87–1. Example of Home Do Not Resuscitate form.

defining, and explaining appropriate goals of care. Another is when symptoms are poorly controlled. A third is when health care teams change.

Once the goals of care have been defined and agreed upon, patients and families need the reassurance that the confidence and trust that had been established during treatment will not be terminated if the patient is dying at home. It is imperative that the health professional understands, believes, and "buys into" the concept that palliative care does not mean "do nothing" or "no care." It is aggressive care, albeit not aggressive for cure but rather focusing on controlling symptoms and maximizing quality of life. The family members need to have their questions and concerns answered and to continue to have access to their physicians and nurses during the transition to home hospice care. In order to facilitate this process, it is helpful if the nurse, with his or her colleagues, can establish and organize a system that will work best for the patient, the family, and the health care team.

GL, was a 62-year-old professional gambler with lung cancer. His wife had a long, undocumented history of panic attacks and compulsive behaviors. She was hesitant to take him home from the hospital, fearing she would be "a prisoner at home." A multidisciplinary family meeting was held, at which discharge options and a plan of care were discussed. The wife believed "we were giving up" on her husband and closing the door on them. Palliative care was clarified and a plan of care was agreed upon allowing the patient to return home with the services of a home hospice and the psychiatry home care program making daily telephone calls and weekly home visits. Logistical problems of home care were discussed and the family was also given written directions on whom to contact in emergency situations.

A frequent concern voiced by both the dying patient and their family members is the problem of having "strangers in the house;" so much so, that the house no longer feels like their own and all sense of privacy is abandoned. This has been observed with prolonged care at home, necessitating visits from either physical therapists, home health aides, or private duty nurses. Even the around-the-clock presence of family members can be troublesome.

GM, was a 47-year-old Hispanic woman with breast cancer. She and her husband had three daughters and a large network of supportive family members. As GM's physical and mental condition deteriorated the family took turns cooking, cleaning and caring for the family. In addition to the numerous family members present throughout the day and night, there was a steady stream of "traffic:" a home health aide (eight hours a day), a nurse who monitored the patient (three times a week), the physical therapist who came twice a week, and weekly visits by the social worker. The youngest daughter became resentful and angry: "I can't bring my friends home anymore. There are always too many people here. I have no privacy." Even the presence of her aunts, with whom she previously had close relationships, was no longer a source of comfort.

Required home visits, when possible, were scheduled for the mornings. Efforts were made to provide "quiet time" in the afternoons when the patient's daughter was home from school. The daughter felt "listened to" and was able to become involved in her mother's care.

DEATH IN THE HOME

During the final stage of a person's illness at home, the family care-provider may become overwhelmed with the feeling of responsibility: "what ifs" are frequent: "What if I miss something? What if an emergency occurs? What is an emergency? What do I do if he stops breathing? Hemorrhages? Stops eating? Goes into a coma?" Each of these "what ifs" must be dealt with, usually repeatedly, in a concrete way. Although the manner of death and potential symptom constellation can be predicted for many patients, for some it cannot. Family members and home care staff may feel, in the abstract, that they can manage any situation, but, when reality strikes, they may become overwhelmed, the demands made being in excess of the family and staff's physical and emotional strength and general capabilities. Sometimes a home death is not possible, or best for the patient or family. The barriers are too great, and the patient is best cared for in an in-patient hospice setting or in a hospital that cares for the dying. However, with the provision of good palliative care, when symptoms are well controlled, the family well supported, and the home care team well trained and adequately staffed, a home death can be extremely rewarding (11).

Intense emotional involvement on the part of the primary care provider in end-of-life care is frequent, with the constant anticipation of something monumental and dramatic about to happen. Just before the patient dies, his or her final words are given special meaning. If these words are not heard, or the primary care-provider is not there at the moment of death, a sense of being cheated may be felt. This is especially true if there is unfinished business. The actual moment of death, so long anticipated and feared, is sometimes anticlimactic, with the family feeling "is that all there is?" (11).

After the death, the family may feel an intense void and loneliness. This may be expressed as a sense of loss of purpose, the most important work they have ever done has been taken from them. Work and everyday life pale in comparison. The "what ifs" become "if onlys" as normal guilt begins to surface. "What if I lacked sensitivity?" "Maybe I thought too much about myself." "Did I do everything I could have done?" Guilt may also be expressed in relation to the feeling of relief and freedom after death has occurred. "I didn't think I could live without him and yet I am doing so." Another fear sometimes expressed may be that of forgetting the deceased, or fear that the family will only remember the last days of the illness and not the earlier, happier times. Because these feelings are so common among families caring for a dying member at home, discussion prior to the death of the likelihood that such feelings will emerge can be very helpful (11).

CONCLUSION

The impact of home death on the family is powerful. For some, it can be a very positive and growing experience; with others, the experience is negative. Part of the skill of the home care team is to help the family sort out the best place for end-of-life care. This is very individualized and decisions may change. The team and family identify their strengths and vulnerabilities with a recognition of how these interactions play out at home. A home death is not the end goal, which is to facilitate what would work best, in the fullest sense of the word, for both patient and family. There needs to be fluidity in the decision making process which enables and supports the dying patient and those caring for them at home.

The experience of a family member dying at home becomes part of the narrative of the whole family (18). It becomes integrated into the family, part of their myth, of how it was. Although frequently the process of caring for a dying family member at home interrupts life, the myth of "how it was" re-integrates the experience back into the life of the family. The death is no longer separate from the family, but part of the family (18).

REFERENCES

1. Cherny NI, Coyle N, Foley KM. Suffering in the advanced cancer patient: a definition and taxonomy. *J Palliative Care*. 1994; 10:(2)57–70.
2. World Health Organization. *Cancer Pain Relief and Palliative Care*. Geneva: World Health Organization; 1990: 804.
3. Mor V, Greer DS, Kaastenbaum R. *The Hospice Experiment*. Baltimore: Johns Hopkins University Press; 1988.
4. Schachter S, Holland JC. Psychological, social and ethical issues in the home care of terminally ill patients. In: Arras JD, ed. *Bringing the Hospital Home: Ethical and Social Implications of High-Tech Home Care*. Baltimore: John Hopkins University Press; 1995.
5. Cherny N, Coyle N, Foley KM. Guidelines in the care of the dying cancer patient. In: Cherny N, Foley KM, eds. *Hematology Clinics of North America (Palliative Care)*. Philadelphia: WB Saunders; 1996: 269.
6. Hinton J. Can home care maintain an acceptable quality of life for patients with terminal cancer and their relatives? *Palliative Med*. 1994; 8:183–196.
7. Hinton J. Which patients with terminal cancer are admitted from home care? *Palliative Med*. 1994; 8: 197–210.
8. Rait D, Lederberg MS. The family of the cancer patient. In: Holland JC, Rowland JH, eds. *Handbook of Psychooncology*, 1st ed. New York: Oxford University Press; 1990: 585–597.
9. Walsh TD. Continuing care in a medical center: The Cleveland Clinic Foundation Palliative Care Service. *J Pain Symptom Manage*. 1990; 5:273–278.
10. Mor V, Masterson-Allen S. *Hospice Care Systems Structure, Process, Costs and Outcome*. New York: Springer Publishing Company; 1987.
11. Coyle N, Loscalzo M, Bailey L. Supportive home care for the advanced cancer patient and family. In: Holland JC, Rowland JH, eds. *Handbook of Psychooncology*, 1st ed. New York: Oxford University Press; 1990: 589–606.
12. Coyle N. Continuity of care for the cancer patient with chronic pain. *Cancer*. 1989; 63:2289–2293.
13. Baird SB. Nursing roles in continuing care: home care and hospice. *Sem Oncol*. 1980; 7:28–38.
14. Sykes NP, Pearson SE, Chell S. Quality of care of the terminally ill: the caregiver's perspective. *Palliative Med*. 1992; 6:227–236.
15. Ferrell BR, Rhiner M, Cohen MZ. Pain as a metaphor for illness. Part I: Impact of pain on family caregivers. *Oncol Nurs Forum*. 1991; 18:1303–1309.
16. Ferrell BR, Cohen MZ, Rhiner M. Pain as a metaphor for illness. Part II: Family caregivers' management of pain. *Oncol Nurs Forum*. 1991; 18:1315–1321.
17. Coyle N, Layman M, Passik S. Development and validation of a patient needs assessment tool (PNAT) for oncology clinicians. *Cancer Nurs*. 1996; 18.
18. Coyle N. Suffering in the first person. In: Ferrel B, ed. *Suffering*. Boston: Jones and Barlett; 1996.
19. Jensen S, Given B. Fatigue affecting family caregivers of cancer patients. *Cancer Nurs*. 1991; 14:181–187.
20. Schachter S. Quality of life for families in the management of home care patients with advanced cancer. *J Palliative Care*. 1992; 8:61–66.
21. Massie MJ, Holland JC, Glass E. Delirium in terminally ill cancer patients. *Am J Psychiatry*. 1983; 140:8–9.
22. Hull MM. Coping strategies of family caregivers in hospice homecare. *Oncol Nurs Forum*. 1992; 19:1179–1187.
23. Hull MM. Sources of stress for hospice caregiving families. *Hospice J*. 1990; 6:29–54.
24. Grobe ME, Iistrup DM, Ahmann DL. Skills needed by family members to maintain the care of an advanced cancer patient. *Cancer Nurs*. 1996; 371–375.
25. Brown P, Davies B, Martens N. Families in supportive care. Part 2: Palliative care at home: a viable care setting. *J Palliative Care*. 1990; 96:2127.

26. Ferrell BR, Ferrell BA, Rhiner M. Family factors influencing cancer pain management. *J Postgrad Med.* 1991; 67:9.

27. Portenoy, RK, Thaler HT, Kornblith AB, et al. Symptom prevalence, characteristics and distress in cancer population. *Qual Life Res.* 1994; (3):183–189.

28. Given CW, Stommel M, Given B, et al. The influence of cancer patients, symptoms and functional state on patient's depression and family caregivers' reaction and depression. *Health Psychol.* 1993; 12:277–285.

29. Overst MT, Thomas SE, Glass KA, Ward SE. Caregiving demands and appraisal of stress among family caregivers. *Cancer Nurs.* 1989; 12:209–215.

88

Bereavement: A Special Issue in Oncology

HARVEY M. CHOCHINOV, JIMMIE C. HOLLAND, AND
LAURENCE Y. KATZ

There is a pain – so utter –
It swallows substance up –
Then covers the abyss with Trance –
So memory can step
Around – across – upon it –
As one within a Swoon –
Goes safely – where an open eye –
Would drop Him – Bone by Bone

—Emily Dickinson

The experience of losing a loved one by death is an inevitable part of adult life; the frequency of such losses increases as an individual grows older. In fact, the annual incidence of bereavement in the population is estimated between 5% and 9% (1,2). This large bereaved group is composed annually of those who have lost a parent (most often an older parent), a spouse, a child, or a sibling. While grief has certain universal characteristics, regardless of the cause of death, it is still true that the circumstances of an illness or accident colour the experience of the bereavement.

The likelihood of cancer being the cause of death is quite high, because 20% of all deaths are the result of some form of cancer (3). This means that one to two percent of the population are experiencing bereavement as a result of cancer. A substantial portion of these newly bereaved individuals will have been intimately involved as a next of kin or family member of the deceased during treatment for cancer. It is a salient aspect of grief resulting from cancer that there is usually a period of anticipatory grieving preceding the death. This fact presents both an opportunity and an obligation for oncologic specialists and their teams, because they are in a unique position to combine care and comfort of the patient with assessment and guidance of the family through the phases of terminal illness and death (4). Done with concern and sensitivity, this can substantially affect the subsequent grieving in a positive way. In particular, the survivor remembers the details of the last days and how the

painful issues were handled, how the grave prognosis was conveyed, how sensitive the staff were to family wishes to be present at the bedside, and how the news of death was conveyed. The survivor also has intense but mixed feelings about the oncologist and support staff because of the special role they have had, and the memories that seeing them evokes. Because they knew the deceased and appreciated him or her as an individual during the fatal illness, they are the recipient of grateful feelings; yet they are also the sole source for answers to the nagging questions that accompany normal grief: "Was everything done?" "What happened?" "Could it have been prevented?" "Were mistakes made?" (5)

It is important that oncologists be able to identify the patterns of normal grief, to expedite its expression, and to guide the individual toward the return of normal activities. They should also be able to identify abnormal patterns of grieving for which professional help is indicated. The differentiation is not always easy. This chapter outlines some explanatory models of grief, including the nature and phases of grieving, types of complicated grief reactions, the complexity of bereavement-related depression, and the physical morbidity and mortality associated with grief. The unique aspects of bereavement following death by cancer are discussed, as well as interventions that have been found effective.

While this chapter deals with bereavement from a medical paradigm, one must put into perspective that religion is the spiritual and social institution that has been and remains the paramount source of solace and understanding of the meaning of loss by death for the majority of people. Each culture has its own religious practices and rituals that bring comfort. It is important that they also give meaning to a state after death that mitigates its finality. For many individuals, therefore, it is the solace given by the clergy that provides the most important support through painful grieving. The chaplain's role and consultation are critically important in assessing this aspect of a relative's needs in relation to impending or actual bereavement (6).

For clarity of communication in an area where the terms grief, mourning, and bereavement have been used interchangeably, definitions of the relevant terminology may be helpful.

Bereavement refers to the loss of a person as a result of death (7).

Grief describes the feelings and behaviors resulting from loss. The grieving process refers to the changing feelings and behaviors that occur over time (8).

Mourning refers to the social expressions in response to loss and grief, including rituals and behaviors that are specific to each culture and religion (8).

Anticipatory grief refers to the psychological and emotional reactions to the anticipation of loss (7).

Complicated grief is the failure to return to pre-loss levels of performance or states of emotional well-being (9).

MODELS FOR UNDERSTANDING BEREAVEMENT

Attempts to explain the phenomenology of normal bereavement and complicated grief have resulted in the development of several different models that provide a conceptual framework for understanding the spectrum of grief reactions and interventions. The theoretical models are largely empirically derived; they occasionally overlap with one another in describing the same phenomena from different perspectives, and clinicians often find it easiest to use an eclectic approach in applying them (8). The models also suggest an increasing convergence of concepts between the psychodynamic, cognitive-behavioral, and psychobiological, again supporting a conceptual approach to bereavement that does not adhere to a single rigid viewpoint.

The most thoroughly developed model is the psychodynamic one (see Table 88.1), based on psychoanalytical theory, which focuses on the intrapsychic process of grief. According to this theory, the grieving process is accomplished by gradual withdrawal of emotional energy (libido) from the lost love object (10). Because relinquishing the tie is emotionally painful, symptoms of grief can be understood as an initial denial of the loss followed by a period of preoccupation with thoughts of the deceased person. The memories are recalled and reviewed, permitting ties to the deceased to be gradually withdrawn. The grief work is completed when the individual has released emotional energy from the lost object, thus allowing engagement in new relationships.

The interpersonal model of bereavement is based on Bowlby's attachment theory (11). He viewed the formation of attachment bonds as instinctual and the psychosocial consequences of breaking them as resulting in grieving symptoms. After observing children who were separated from their parents in institutional settings, he viewed grieving symptoms as a reflection initially of protest, followed by searching behaviors in an attempt to recover the lost object. The children then experienced despair and disorganization from the unsuccessful attempts, and, finally, resolution and reorganization through forming new ties (12,13). Parkes (7,14) used attachment theory to describe similar phases. These begin with numbness, followed by yearning for the person and efforts to achieve reunion through fruitless searching, resulting in motor restlessness, irritability, and tension. The repeated failures lead to disorganization, depression, disinterest, and despair, which signals the acceptance of the loss as permanent. Reorganization occurs as attachment to the deceased diminishes and new ties to others are established.

Bereavement has also been examined in light of crisis theory in which it is recognized as one of the major stresses of life with both psychological and physiologi-

TABLE 88.1. *A Comparison of Theological Models Staging Bereavement*

Psychoanalytic	Interpersonal		Post-traumatic
(Freud, Abraham)	(Bowlby)	(Parkes)	(Horowitz)
Denial	Protest phase	Numbness and blunting	Outcry
Preoccupation with thoughts of the deceased	Searching	Pining and yearning	Denial intrusion
Libido gradually withdrawn	Despair, disorganization, withdrawal	Disorganization and despair	Working through
Libido available for new relationships	Resolution, reorganization	Reorganization and recovery	Completion

cal consequences (8,15). In this context, Horowitz et al. (16) have also presented a model delineating the nature and phases of grief. Their model is based on one previously prepared by Horowitz et al. (17) as a model for understanding stress responses and, in particular, post-traumatic stress disorder. They suggest that an individual progresses through a sequence of phases which results in adaptation to the loss. They describe the sequence as consisting of loss, followed by an outcry of emotions, denial, intrusion, working through, and finally completion.

Studies of separation in animals have produced a psychobiological model of grief, which builds on attachment theory and has relevance for understanding the psychological symptoms of bereavement (18). Hofer (19) viewed attachment bonds as important regulators of internal biological systems throughout life. The behavioral and psychological symptoms of grief, especially the chronic ones, as opposed to the acute waves of distress, represent the withdrawal of the internal regulators that were the result of the emotionally meaningful and constant interactions with an individual to whom there was significant attachment.

These models provide explanations for the clinical features of normal grief. Complicated grief and bereavement-related depression are associated with an arrest in the progress through, or a magnification of, the phases of grief.

CLINICAL FEATURES OF BEREAVEMENT

Let us first look at the nature of "normal" bereavement. Most considerations of the clinical picture of grief begin with the actual loss. However, it is important in discussing the bereavement of those in whom the loss is the result of cancer, to give particular attention to the anticipatory period of grieving and the actual immediate responses to the death. This is important because terminal care in a hospice, hospital, nursing home, or at home allows an opportunity for interventions with family members, which can have a long-lasting impact on the survivor's grief when they are given by staff members who understand bereavement and its management. Thus, clinical features of normal responses are described in the following paragraphs with relevance to the phases in which they appear in survivors of a relative's death by cancer—that is, anticipatory grief, responses to news of death, acute grief, and grieving reactions over time.

Anticipatory Grief
Anticipatory grief was first described by Lindemann (20) in reference to instances where spouses (or par-

ents) becomes so concerned with their adjustment in the face of a potential death, that they go through all the phases of grief prior to the actual death. While this reaction was felt to be a safeguard against the impact of a sudden death, it can be problematic when patients follow a more protracted terminal course than originally anticipated. Since Lindemann's first description, there has been significant debate over the nature of anticipatory grief.

The period of time when death is expected or appears highly likely is clearly a time of intellectual preparation for loss by the next of kin and for attempts at resolution of conflicts. While some observers feel the emotional responses of actual bereavement begin at that time (13,21), others report observations that the true grieving for the loss does not begin until the death has occurred (22,23). The attachment is actually transiently enhanced by threat of approaching death. Many who work in oncology frequently see the strong efforts made by a relative to avoid facing the impending loss. Some simply refuse to believe it may happen and become angry when efforts to inform are made; many more hear the message but cannot truly encompass it. They are emotionally unable to anticipate the loss. This period can be marked by defiant optimism, interspersed with periods of fear and despair that the death will actually occur.

Circumstances also alter the extent of anticipatory response. Relatives who keep their ill family member at home during terminal illness may experience the reality of impending death most intimately because they participate in physical care of the person and see the progressive changes in the body. Care at home and in a hospice also permits early bereavement counselling by the home care nurse or hospice staff. Irrespective of circumstances, advanced stage of cancer is the time when relatives are told about the grave prognosis (24). Increasingly today, they and the patient participate in discussions of their wishes about the use of heroic measures. Such discussions make impending death more real. In some cases of prolonged illness or pain, the death is seen rationally as a relief for the deceased from intolerable distress; death is a "blessing," and a religious perspective may help in accepting the outcome as "God's will."

Whether or not individuals experience anticipatory grief, the outcome of grief in which the loss is or is not anticipated is of interest here. There is agreement that sudden death, with little or no warning, has greater impact and produces a longer-lasting disorganization in the survivor than does death that follows warning and a prolonged terminal illness. Parkes (25) compared a group of survivors who had had less than two weeks warning of the seriousness of their spouse's condition and a terminal illness of less than three days, with another group who had had two weeks or more advance warning of impending death and longer than three days of terminal illness. He found much more intense psychological disturbance in those who had had little time to prepare; they remained more socially withdrawn and self-reproachful throughout the first year of bereavement. At two to four years later, the majority were still "trapped in a vicious cycle of emotional disturbance and withdrawal." Nearly three-fourths or 72% had a moderate to severe level of anxiety and difficulties coping. Only 28% had a positive view of the future. By contrast, those who had anticipated the loss were more likely to have seen the death as a relief from a painful or prolonged illness, and they found less cause for self-reproach during bereavement. By four years, 90% were ready to date, and several had remarried. It is of interest that in a study of thirty young widows, of the five women who had considered suicide, none had had a chance for anticipatory grieving (26).

Finally, Hays et al. (27) recently looked at the course of psychological distress following threatened and actual conjugal bereavement. They found that the pre-mortem psychological symptoms in the weeks and months prior to the death were not reliably distinguishable from the earliest and most intense experiences of post-mortem grief. There were non-significant differences in mean depression scores and hopelessness/helplessness measures. Thus, given the contrasting opinions and studies described above, there remains considerable disagreement in the literature regarding the nature of anticipatory grief.

Responses to News of Death

Ideally, a family should be present at the time of death if they wish to be. However, when they are not present, they should be notified as soon as possible. Informing them by telephone is not desirable and usually leaves strong negative feelings. There is no easy way to give news of death, and physicians and nurses receive little instruction in how to handle such sensitive communications. It is usually learned by on-the-job training. There are some caveats in handling the situation that make the bad news easier to hear. It is important because the details of the encounter will be remembered and recounted in great detail for years to come by the bereaved relative, expressing gratitude for a caring manner or anger at perceived insensitivity.

Ideally, the news should be conveyed by the physician who cared for the patient during the illness and who knows the surviving relatives well enough to be able to frame the news in a manner that anticipates the likely responses. Because it is not always possible for the responsible physician to be present, another physician, preferably one who is also known to the family, should convey the information. Taking the family member to a quiet place where expression of emotion will not be embarrassing is helpful. Having a relative present is also desirable, so that the person has someone to turn to for comfort. The immediate reaction is usually one of shock and disbelief, even when the death was expected, reflecting the initial phase of bereavement. The range of emotions elicited varies from the stoic and unemotional to hysteria. After the initial response has subsided, it is important that the relative or family be offered time alone with the body of the deceased. This may be comforting and also reinforces the reality of the loss. Further discussion should answer medical questions. A full and clear explanation of medical circumstances surrounding death should be given by the responsible doctor present. Open responsiveness to questions and discussion allow the bereaved to understand intellectually the circumstances that led to death and may alleviate misconceptions of personal responsibility (e.g., "If I had only not agreed to the surgery"). These facts may need to be stated again later when the family is calmer, can absorb the facts, and wish another discussion of the circumstances around the death.

One of the most controversial and sensitive issues when death occurs in the hospital is the request for autopsy. This task has traditionally been assigned to the house officer, although it should ideally be done by the responsible physician, with great sensitivity for the feelings of the grieving family. While autopsy rates have declined alarmingly because far fewer efforts are made to obtain permission, it is still important with respect to when cancer is the cause of death, and extent of disease or response to treatment may be unclear. The information obtained will be of value to the doctor and may clarify for the family the facts leading to death. Neoplasms that have hereditary patterns may be of interest for autopsy study to inform a family better about familial risk. These positive aspects should be emphasized, but the families' decision should be emphatically accepted, regardless of their choice (29).

It is important that the physician follow through by meeting with the family to discuss the results of the autopsy and to provide an opportunity for further questions when the full pathology report is available. Relatives sometimes are tormented by questions that can only be answered with these data. This discussion also allows a follow-up visit with the bereaved during which normal grieving feelings can be explored (30).

Pathological responses occur infrequently at the time of learning of the death of a relative. They are usually transient but, for some extreme reactions that occur, require immediate intervention to assure comfort and safety. The poignancy of the moment complicates the ability to manage the situation expeditiously at times. However, prior psychiatric problems may be exacerbated at this time and result in threat of harm to self or others. Several case reports demonstrate pathological responses that occur.

CASE REPORTS

Inability to separate. Following the death of her 10-year-old boy in the intensive care unit after lengthy treatment for osteogenic sarcoma, the mother clutched her son's body, appearing in a reverie state that responded little to attempts by the staff to encourage her to leave. After half an hour, the staff found it difficult to continue with other routine care. It was clear that attempts to insist that she leave were not heard. She was told she could remain and family members sat with her for another hour. She slowly emerged from her dazed state as family gradually persuaded her to return home with them.

Homicidal intent. A 45-year-old father with a history of emotional instability and erratic behavior appeared more and more disturbed during the vigil in his child's room as the child's condition worsened. He began to make menacing overtures toward the doctor, whom he blamed for the downward turn of the illness. When he was told that the child was dead, he became angry, found the doctor, verbally threatened his life, and attempted to hit him. Relatives forcibly held him and took him home. Over the following days, the father recovered and recognized that his anger was at the death itself, not the doctor who had done his best for the child. He later returned to the hospital and apologized for his behavior. Until then, however, the young doctor traveled to and from the hospital with an escort, because the history of prior violent episodes in the father was cause for concern for impulsive violent behavior.

Suicidal intent. The wife of a 35-year-old painter had indicated her strong wish to die with her husband. As his illness from cancer progressed and death was near, she took an overdose of diazepam (Valium) in his room. She was found lethargic, the bottle of pills empty. She received emergency treatment for drug intoxication and was hospitalized. Several days later, she recovered and said that she was glad the attempt had failed because she had failed her husband. With relatives accompanying her, she maintained her place at her husband's bedside. She accepted the news of his death with distress, but expressed that she felt the need to carry out several projects that her husband had been unable to complete.

Acute Grief

The first systematic study of acute grief was reported in 1944 by Lindemann (20), based on his observations of the grief of those who had lost relatives in the Boston Coconut Grove nightclub disaster. He described the clinical course of acute grief and major symptoms of somatic distress, preoccupation with the image of the deceased, guilt, hostility, loss of usual patterns of conduct, and assumption of symptoms or traits of the deceased. The behavior and physiological symptoms described by Lindemann were used by Hofer (19) to present a psychological hypothesis of bereavement (Table 88.2). Initially, numbness may be continuously present, following which waves of distress triggered by reminders of the deceased occur, characterized by agitation, crying, aimless activity, preoccupation with images of the deceased, tears, sighing respirations, choking, and a sense of muscular weakness. In fact, the bereaved person begins to try desperately to avoid stimuli that will precipitate a wave of acute distress.

There is a constant background disturbance which develops under the superimposed acute-distress episodes, characterized by behavioral changes of social withdrawal, decreased concentration, restlessness, anxiety, altered appetite, sad appearance, depressed mood, illusions of the presence of the deceased, dreams, and even hallucinations of hearing or seeing

TABLE 88.2. *Bereavement in the Human Adult*

Behavior	Physiology
ACUTE: WAVES OF DISTRESS, LASTING MINUTES	
Agitation	Tears
Crying	Sighing respiration
Aimless activity–inactivity	Muscular weakness
Preoccupation with image of deceased	
CHRONIC: BACKGROUND DISTURBANCE, LASTING WEEKS TO MONTHS	
Social withdrawal	Decreased body weight
Decreased concentration, attention	Sleep disturbance
Restlessness, anxiety	Muscular weakness
Decreased or variable food intake	Cardiovascular changes
Postures and facial expressions of sadness	Endocrine changes
Illusions, hallucinations	Immunological changes
Depressed mood	

Source: Reprinted with permission from Hofer MA. Relationships as regulators: a psychobiologic perspective on bereavement. *Psychosom Med.* 1984; 46:184.

the deceased. Cardiovascular, endocrine, and immunological changes develop concurrently with the behavioral changes. Preoccupation with events surrounding the death, searching for mistakes, or feeling guilt for not doing enough are typical. The bereaved feels distant from others, lacking in emotional response to them, and may express anger and envy at seeing others together. This period of acute distress is often structured for the individual by the mourning rituals of receiving friends, preparing for the funeral, and burial. The individual is seldom left alone, and the sense of numbness may persist as the person goes mechanically through the funeral and expected activities. Families who choose to forego any rituals sometimes suffer more because normal activity is emotionally impossible, and absence of social rituals, such as the funeral, can add to the sense of unreality and disbelief that a death has occurred.

Acute grief, with its characteristic waves, difficulty concentrating and functioning, was noted by Lindemann (20) to last for about six weeks. However, the manifestations of grief vary greatly from person to person and moment to moment. Thus, any attempt at staging the grieving process must not be taken too literally. Grief is a fluid process which ebbs and flows over time. Acute grief may be extended in spouses who were extremely dependent on their partners and in whom steps to function independently require an entirely new and unfamiliar set of activities. It may be prolonged, continuing with acute symptoms unabated, in a parent who loses a child. A birthday or holiday will result in marked exacerbation of the first days of grief; in fact "special days" come to be dreaded for the pain they cause (31).

Concerned relatives will usually seek help for the bereaved person in the first six weeks of acute grief if an abnormal response appears. Reasons for consultation may be due to a troubled psychological response, psychiatric symptoms or adverse physical sequelae. When the deceased died of cancer, it is not uncommon for the bereaved to fear that they have also developed it. A transient cancerophobia may ensue, confirming the observations of Zisook and colleagues (32) on the bereaved person's identification with the deceased's disease and symptoms. Psychological symptoms may become cause for alarm if weight loss is extreme, agitation precludes rest, or sleeplessness produces chronic fatigue. Reynolds et al. (33), in a controlled study of sleep disturbance during "normal" bereavement, found REM sleep abnormalities in the bereaved compared with non-bereaved controls. It appears these REM sleep abnormalities were distinct from those found in major depression. Medication to re-establish patterns of sleep each night may be important. If the daytime is experienced with high anxiety, irritability, and agitation, a low dose of a benzodiazepine may allow rest. While medication should be given judiciously, a low dose to control distressing symptoms may expedite the bereavement process rather than inhibiting its expression. (See the following intervention).

CASE REPORT

Julia, a 35-year-old married Italian woman, appeared for psychiatric consultation following her younger sister's death from disseminated lung cancer. She had appeared to cope very well initially. She arranged the funeral, settled outstanding financial and legal matters, and became guardian of her sister's two preschool children. Within two weeks, however, she could not cope with daily routines. Everything was a reminder of her sister, eliciting waves of overwhelming grief. Irritability, anxiety, restlessness, and insomnia also made carrying on daily tasks more difficult. She reluctantly spoke of an occasional feeling that she could hear her sister's voice calling her name; fear that she might be losing her mind resulted in her seeking psychiatric consultation. At this time, a brief course of sedative-hypnotics was begun. Over the next three months she expressed her great sense of loss, came to understand that her responses were normal, and slowly regained full activity.

Grieving Reactions Over Time

The initial phase of denial of the loss, followed by acute stress episodes, superimposed on the chronic background disturbance is finally followed by the phase of coming to terms with the loss over the succeeding months. It is during this period of time that symptoms of grief most resemble depression, and, indeed, it may be impossible immediately to differentiate them. Clayton and colleagues (34) found crying, depressed mood, and sleep disturbance as the cardinal symptoms during the first year of bereavement. Depression was a problem for 45% of the survivors at some time during the first year, and 13% were still depressed at a year. Clayton (34) found that when the symptoms in 34 bereaved individuals were matched with those of an equal numbers of depressed patients, they could not be differentiated on objective criteria for depression. Byrne and Raphael (35) found that 76.5% of bereaved elderly men had intrusive memories of their spouses at thirteen months; 49% reported feelings of distress, 43% were preoccupied with mental images of their spouse, 41% were still yearning for their spouses, and 25% had looked for their spouse in familiar places. Hays, Kasl, and Jacobs (27) found that bereavement produced a significantly elevated level of distress (i.e., depression, hopelessness/

helplessness, anxiety) over a control group at six months. They also found that the best prediction of duration and severity of grief was the intensity of initial distress, which correlated closely with distress over the next two years. Other studies (36,37) have documented significant distress as much as two years into the bereavement course.

A four-year follow-up of widows and widowers by Zisook and Schuchter (38) provided useful information by pointing out that individual variability is great and chronicity of bereavement is not uncommon. In fact, the time course for grief in their observations was much more prolonged than is generally expected. Affective distress reduced over time, but several widows were still tearful and depressed at four years. Guilt diminished, but anger toward those held responsible for the loss persisted in almost 10% of survivors. A continued relationship to the deceased, consisting of thoughts and visual images, was not infrequently found. Despite this, 23% were remarried by four years and 40% were living with someone of the opposite sex. At four years, 44% rated an excellent adjustment, but 20% saw their adjustment as fair to poor. Their physical health was unimpaired, except for aging. Most saw themselves and the world in positive terms. These findings suggest that normal grief may often be an ongoing lifelong process, bringing into question the concept that normal grief is a process in which resolution by loss of attachment to the deceased occurs in a circumscribed time period. These observations of the spouse's slow recovery are evidence that our concepts of normal grief need to be re-examined and extended.

COMPLICATED GRIEF

Distinguishing between normal and morbid forms of grief is difficult because the abnormal responses largely reflect a greater intensity, a prolongation, or an aberration of normal grief (30,40).

Parkes and Weiss (22) developed a typology to allow for classification of those grief reactions which are unduly influenced by the nature of the relationship or the type of bereavement. Once again, this typology is a fluid structure with frequent overlap amongst the different types of complicated grief (41). The *unexpected loss syndrome* may occur with deaths which are sudden and unexpected, associated with multiple losses, mutilation, or situations where the survivor's life was also threatened. It is a pattern of grieving in which attempts to avoid, repress, and delay grief continue for months or years, but do not prevent high levels of anxiety and tension (7,42). These reactions can be viewed as a type

of post-traumatic stress disorder (9,41). This is a syndrome which is divisible into three symptoms clusters (43). The first cluster involves intensive recollections of the dying, e.g., flashbacks, nightmares, intrusive memories. The second cluster includes feelings of detachment, restricted affect, sense of a foreshortened future, decreased interest in activities, and avoidance of feelings, thoughts or activities which arouse recollections of the event. The final cluster is related to persistent hyperarousal exemplified by difficult sleeping, irritability, and difficulty concentrating. This syndrome persists for extended periods of time and interferes with the normal grieving process, as the bereaved often attempts to maintain a fantasy relationship with the deceased who is now seen as ever present and watching over the living (7). This syndrome represents a distortion of the "normal" grieving process. Many aspects of "normal" early grief become fixed and magnified, making progress slow or impossible.

Chronic Grief/Dependent Grief Syndrome

This common grief reaction, also called unresolved grief, is marked by continuous symptoms of grief typical of early stages of loss that continue unchanged as grief fails to resolve (22,44). The *dependent grief syndrome* results from the end of a relationship in which one member was dependent on the other. Although initially believed to be a syndrome which occurred when the survivor was dependent on the deceased, it is now thought that it can also occur when the deceased was dependent on the survivor (7). The self-esteem, confidence, and identity of one or both partners was dependent on the relationship; when this system is disrupted, the survivor is left with a gaping wound. Horowitz et al. (45) believe that this results in the re-activation of an image of the self as weak, abandoned, and needy, with intense fear that rescue will never occur. Once the breakdown of the relationship has occurred, severe grief may be perpetuated by the everyday gains associated with this process. Overt mourning allows withdrawal from social and other responsibilities and often dignifies the mourner in the eyes of others (7). This may provide a needed boost to the self-esteem and also provides an identity within which to function. This admixture results in a chronic grief syndrome, marked by continuous symptoms of grief typical of early phases of loss that continue unchanged as grief fails to resolve (9,22,44,46).

As mentioned previously, these categories of complicated grief are not necessarily mutually exclusive. In fact, Prigerson et al. (9) describe a "complicated grief factor" which is a blend of the unexpected loss syndrome and the dependent grief syndrome. The symptoms which composed the complicated grief factor included feelings of disbelief, being stunned by the loss, decreased acceptance of the death, crying, preoccupation with thoughts of the deceased, yearning, and searching. This complicated grief factor was predictive of future functional impairment and was different from uncomplicated grief and bereavement-related depression.

The final element of the Parkes and Weiss typology is the *conflicted grief syndrome*. The nature of this syndrome is not as clear and its validation and placement on the spectrum of grief reactions has been debated in the literature. This syndrome was first proposed by Freud (10) and Abraham (47), and was thought to be a product of relationships in which the survivor had ambivalent feelings toward the deceased. The angry component of the ambivalence is turned inward resulting in guilt, self-blame, and self-derogation. Freud and Abraham saw this dynamic as leading to depression. Parkes (7) believes that this dynamic may sometimes result in delayed grief. While an initial reaction may be one of relief, in time the relationship is reviewed and there is a feeling of unfinished business. The bereaved find themselves having intrusive memories and associated feelings of anger and guilt. Some authors (41) do not believe that this construct has held up or been empirically validated; it thus remains a controversial explanation for understanding certain grief reactions.

Bereavement-Related Major Depression

Studies of predictors of poor bereavement outcome vary with regard to both the prevalence of mental disorders complicating bereavement outcome and the specific predictors. An association between bereavement and psychiatric hospitalization and care has been shown (48–50). However, it appears overall that about 20% of bereaved individuals (estimates vary from 10% to 36% in individual studies) will develop a psychiatric disorder, primarily depression. Most of those can be expected when one or more of the known predictors of poor outcome are present. These include poor social support, prior psychiatric history, unanticipated death, other significant stresses or losses, high level of initial distress with depressive symptoms, and death of a child (Table 88.3). The perception that there is no one to talk to or lean on, with the environment failing to meet emotional needs, appears to be a reliable predictor of poor outcome in several studies (51,52).

Not unexpectedly, prior mental health problems predict poor outcome. A history of alcoholism increases the suicide risk and likelihood of psychiatric hospitalization shortly after bereavement (53,54). Prior

TABLE 88.3. *Predictors of Poor Bereavement Outcome*

Perception of poor social supports
Prior psychiatric history
High initial distress with depressive symptoms
Unanticipated death
Other significant life stresses and losses
Prior high dependency on the deceased who provided key support
Death of a child

dependence on alcohol, drugs (especially tranquillizer or hypnotic medication), and tobacco predicts increased consumption during bereavement. Mortality data confirm the adverse effects of abuse of these substances on physical health by the increased risk of death by suicide, cirrhosis, and cardiovascular disease. High initial distress with many depressive symptoms is a predictor of depression at a year (51,55). Depressive symptoms can appear at any point during a bereavement course (37,56) and raise the clinical question of when these symptoms constitute a disorder requiring treatment. Opinion regarding this distinction has changed over the years as the high prevalence and serious consequences of depression have been delineated. Most investigators have found a significantly higher prevalence of major depression in widows and widowers than in control groups. The rates for major depression peak at approximately one month postmortem, reaching nearly 50% (57), then decline at two months to 27–30% (9,58,59) and continue to drop to 16% at one year (59), following which it stabilizes at this level for up to two years (36,37).

In the past, despite the frequent occurrence of syndromal magnitude depressive symptoms, the diagnosis of major depression was not made in the context of bereavement. It was felt that this reaction was understandable given the extenuating circumstances. Currently, DSM-IV (43) stipulates that a diagnosis of major depression should only be made when the symptoms are not better accounted for by bereavement, i.e., after the loss of a loved one, the symptoms persist for longer than two months or are characterized by marked functional impairment, morbid preoccupation with worthlessness, suicidal ideation, psychotic symptoms or psychomotor retardation. Recent investigators (37,58,60) have found that bereavement-related depressions tend often to be chronic and lead to protracted biopsychosocial dysfunction.

Karam (60) found that bereavement meeting criteria for major depression does not differ from major depression in the community with respect to age of onset, degree of dysfunction, visits to doctors or taking medication. Zisook (37) found that, despite its high prevalence and evidence that bereavement-related depression is as debilitating as major depression, 83% of bereaved spouses who met criteria for a major depression received no anti-depressant medications. This means that a highly disabling and potentially life-threatening illness is either not being diagnosed or not being treated. Zisook thus believes (37) that severe major depressive syndromes at any time, and all major depressive syndromes beyond the second month of bereavement, should be carefully evaluated and treated as aggressively as other non-bereavement-related depressions.

"Normal" grief is an intense psychological response to a catastrophic event. It is easy to attribute many symptoms and incapacities to such catastrophes and lose sight of the presence of significant illness and disability. The nature of the relationship, the circumstances of the death, the bereaved's personality, coping style, and predisposition to psychiatric illness may cumulatively be predictive of future complicated grief or prominent depressive symptoms.

HEALTH CONSEQUENCES OF BEREAVEMENT

It has been widely assumed that bereavement predisposes individuals to exacerbation of existing disease and places them at increased risk of death. The psychosomatic diseases were particularly considered to be exacerbated by threatened or actual loss. Anecdotal reports of onset of a range of diseases, including cancer, have readily identified a recent loss in the individual's history.

There are several physiological systems thought to be affected by bereavement, including abnormalities in the cardiovascular (8,61), endocrine (62), and immunological (63,64) systems. These were thought to lead to increased morbidity and mortality from cardiac disease (8,61), certain cancers (65), and a non-specific decline in general medical health (8). Questions still exist as to the clinical significance of changes in these systems in relation to altering vulnerability to disease (66,67). Whether change comes about by altered behaviors and loss of normal life-style patterns that occur with grieving, such as altered diet, drinking, and smoking, or whether some psychophysiological changes occur that enhance risk is unclear and remains of great research interest. The question whether grief might serve as an initiator or promoter of a malignant process has been asked repeatedly and as yet remains unanswered.

The psychobiological model of bereavement proposed by Hofer (19) is of interest in considering the effects on health. Table 88.2 outlines the physiological consequences, which include effects on the cardiovascular, endocrine, and immunological systems. The concept of interruption of an ongoing relationship causing disruption of biological homeostasis and, thereby, vulnerability to disease—particularly through the endocrine and immune systems—is intriguing in light of the morbidity associated with bereavement.

The seminal psychoendocrine studies by Hofer and colleagues (62) of parents during the fatal illness and death of their child from leukemia provided the first information on psychological and pituitary-adrenocortical system response to a stressful life event and bereavement. They found that the effectiveness of the psychological defenses modulated the level of cortisol. At six months and two years after death, cortisol levels generally related to the extent of active grieving, although not all parents fit this pattern.

Two studies have examined immunological function during bereavement. Bartrop and colleagues (63) in Australia studied the stimulation responses of phytohemagglutinin and concanavalin A on the lymphocytes of widows and widowers, as well as age-matched non-bereaved individuals. Lymphocyte response to the mitogens was significantly lower at two months after the loss. Schleifer and co-workers (68) examined mitogen responses in men before and after the death of their wives from breast cancer. The depressed lymphocyte response was seen only in the bereavement period and was apparent within one month. It is of interest, however, that in neither study did perturbations reach levels consistent with clinical immunosuppression.

Irwin, Daniels, and Weiner (64) extended these studies to examine bereavement, depressive symptoms, NK cell activity, and T cell subpopulations in three groups of women: those who anticipated their husbands' death from lung cancer, women who were bereaved, and a control group. NK cell activity was significantly lower in the group anticipating the loss and those studied after the death. Severity of depressive symptoms correlated with reduced NK cell activity and changes in the ratio of T helper to T suppressor cells, suggesting that the role of depressive symptoms may be more important than the loss per se. Cortisol, elevated only during bereavement, could not be solely responsible for the changes.

Questions still exist as to the clinical significance of the changes in immune function in relation to altering vulnerability to disease. For example, despite the stress of their child's illness and death, parents do not develop new illnesses nor do they develop frequent colds or minor illnesses (69). It would, however, appear that they smoke and use alcohol and drugs excessively to reduce tension.

Immune changes during grief must be interpreted with particular caution about their clinical relevance in light of these prospective data, which revealed no increased risk of cancer of any site among widowed individuals. In fact, immunosuppressed individuals, with AIDS or chemically induced immunosuppression (to reduce rejection or organ and bone marrow transplants), experience increased risk of only specific malignancies that include lymphomas and Kaposi's sarcoma. They do not develop other neoplasms with greater frequency.

The actual health consequences of bereavement that are known are interesting in light of the associated endocrine and immune changes. They can be summarized into the major areas of increased psychological distress, increased physical symptoms, increased use of health services, and increased reliance on self-medication for distress (by evidence of increased smoking, drinking and use of drugs—each contributing to the adverse health consequences). (See Table 88.4.)

The epidemiological studies of mortality following bereavement are based largely on ten major studies that are described in the review by Osterweis, Solomon, and Green (8). The most definitive studies on mortality after bereavement were reported by Helsing and colleagues in 1981 and 1982 (70,71). The 1963 health census of 91,909 persons was followed for twelve years, with the widowed population during that period matched to a married demographically similar population at the time; both were followed prospectively for mortality. Table 88.5 outlines the findings for both sexes, which showed no elevated mortality in the first year (suggesting failure to confirm increased mortality from existing disease), but greater mortality in both sexes among those living alone or having moved to a nursing home.

TABLE 88.4. *Summary of Major Morbidity and Mortality Associated with Bereavement*

Morbidity	Mortality
↑ Psychological distress	↑ Mortality, largely in older men
↑ Physical symptoms	
↑ Use of health services	Causes of death nonspecific except for infectious diseases, cirrhosis, suicide, and accidents
↑ Self-medication for distress (alcohol, smoking, drugs)	
Poor outcome in 20% of bereaved; most predictable by high-risk factors	

TABLE 88.5. *Mortality after Widowhood, 1963–1975**

Sex	Mortality influences
Men	Higher for widowed (age 55–74)
	Lower after remarriage
Women	Same for widowed and married
	Same after remarriage
Both	Higher living alone
	Higher moving to nursing home
	Not elevated in first year

*$n = 4032$.
Source: From Helsing and Szklo (70).

Women had no greater mortality, irrespective of being widowed or remarrying. Men, however, had an increased mortality that was confined to older ages 55–74, unless remarriage occurred, which return them to the same risk as their married counterparts (70) (see Fig. 88–1).

Table 88.6 outlines their findings on causes of death among 777 widowed and 604 married individuals. There was greater mortality among the widowed, but this was remarkably nonspecific as to its cause. Several diseases were individually significant in cause of death, but they represented only a small portion of the overall

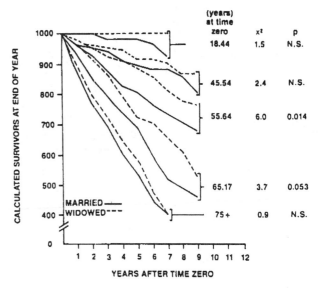

FIG. **88–1.** Calculated survivorship of widowed (broken lines) and married (solid lines) by years after time zero, for white males of ages indicated: Washington County, Maryland, 1963–1975. Note that χ^2(1 *df*) calculations are for entire 12 years of study by procedure suggested by Peto et al.). N.S., not significant. *Source*: Reprinted with permission from Helsing KJ, Szklo M. Mortality after bereavement. *Am J Epidemiol.* 1981; 114:49–50.

TABLE 88.6. *Causes of Death (777 Widowed, 604 Married)*

More deaths occurred among widowed than among married subjects.

Significant causes of disease-related death, though representing only a small portion of overall excess: men—infectious diseases, accidents, suicide; women—cirrhosis.

"Greater mortality is remarkably nonspecific as to its causes."

Widowed with chronic disease did not show earlier mortality after bereavement.

Source: From Helsing et al. (71).

excess: infectious diseases, accidents, and suicide in men; and cirrhosis in women. The absence of any over-representation of cancer is important to note in this large prospective study.

Li (72) has also found increased rates of suicide in bereaved men over controls. In a recent, large, prospective, longitudinal study Schaeffer et al. (73) found that mortality after bereavement was significantly increased in both men and women. The highest risks were in the first year, but rates remained elevated for more than two years after bereavement.

Levav and colleagues (66) have reported a nine-year follow-up study of Israeli parents who lost a son either in the Yom Kippur War or by an accident, to determine their mortality. Neither group of parents had a greater mortality when compared to that of the Israeli general population. There was a subset of parents, those who were widowed or divorced, who had an increased mortality; however, significance was reached only in mothers. Another large and well-designed study by Jones and co-workers (67) did not find greater mortality among the surviving spouses of those whose partners' death was due to cancer. More studies are needed to clarify the concurrent physiological changes with bereavement and their clinical implications.

BEREAVEMENT FOLLOWING SPECIFIC LOSSES

Other specific losses that warrant particular attention are loss of a parent, sibling, or child during adulthood and loss of a parent or sibling during childhood.

Loss of Parent in Adulthood

The loss of a parent, particularly an older parent, is a loss that is expected in adult life. In one study, 5% of the population had lost one parent in the prior year (74). Although it has been studied less than other losses of adulthood, it appears that adults have usually made other attachments and have busy lives that may make

the bereavement brief. However, bereavement can be more pronounced and the death more traumatic than what is usually assumed, especially for the daughter or son who has been physically and emotionally close to the deceased. Loss of the mother may be particularly difficult. A lengthy illness of the parent from cancer, requiring extensive care by a son or a daughter, may result in a more severe bereavement. The death may mean the loss of security, loss of the child role, and assumption of the role of oldest and most responsible family member. It may therefore sometimes result in a new level of maturation for the adult child.

Loss of Sibling in Adulthood

Attachment to siblings usually continues into adulthood, which means that death may result in severe bereavement. It often forces an examination of the relationship to other members of the family, resulting in increased sensitivity and concern for surviving members. In neoplasms with high familial incidence, such as in familial polyposis, colon cancer, and breast cancer, the meaning of death of a sibling may carry guilt that another sibling carried the trait and died, but also anxiety about the vulnerability of the survivor to the same disease.

Loss of a Child

While few systematic comparisons have been made between the bereavement following the loss of a spouse and a child, Sanders (75) noted that those who had lost a child had more intense grief reactions with more somatic symptoms, greater depression, anger, guilt, and a loss of meaning and purpose in life. Such a loss is tragic at any age, but the sense of unfairness of a life unfulfilled enhances the sense of anger. A longer and slower recovery period should be expected as well; in fact, grief sometimes intensifies over time. Even so, in a study of 263 bereaved parents, mothers grieved more than fathers, healthy children were grieved far more than ill children, and boys more than girls (76).

Because death by leukemia and childhood tumors, especially brain tumors, accounts for 18% of childhood deaths, understanding the bereavement of a parent, irrespective of the age of the child, is important.

CASE REPORT

Protracted but normal grief. A mother of a 17-year-old daughter who died of Hodgkin's disease experienced an inability over the first year to share the loss or any pleasures with her husband. He also grieved quietly, but attempted to hide it from his wife. He felt abandoned and unable to reach her. Psychotherapy with this couple diminished the wife's withdrawal, as she realized her husband's pain. She improved but did not return to her prior outgoing manner. Resigning herself to a loss that she would always feel, she put her grief aside to allow her to give emotionally to her husband. At three years she was functioning, with the exception of anniversaries, birthdays, and holidays, which were dreaded and spent away from home when possible.

Participation in the care of a terminally ill child appears to help parents cope, as well as a sense that they communicated closely with the child about the reality of the situation. Rando (77) found that, as shown with the loss of a spouse, parents who lost a child fared better when the loss was not sudden and death from cancer followed 6–18 months of illness. Deciding about home versus hospital care is an important task for parents (69). The place chosen is less important than their commitment to the choice, because good and poor outcomes occur with both. The impact on siblings at home, though largely positive, has not been fully assessed. The prevalence of overprotection of surviving siblings by the anxious parents, with later hypochondriacal fears of illness and death, is high.

Spinetta and colleagues (78) found that parents who coped better with their child's death had a philosophy of life (religious or not) and could find some meaning for their loss. Divorce does not appear to be more prevalent, but the differential rate of recovery of the parents (with the grief of fathers being briefer than mothers) can reduce the expected supportive communication and sharing of the loss. Replacement children are never a true replacement of the lost child, and advice about postponing a pregnancy until grieving for the child is diminished, if not resolved, should be part of counseling.

The age at which a child dies has an impact on the bereavement, whether as a young child, adolescent, or young adult. The loss appears equally severe at all ages, and bereavement is different but not less painful. Much less studied is the response to the loss of an adult child by middle-aged or older parents. Not protected by their child's presence, and severed from their hope of a future through their child, grief may be similarly intense and protracted.

Bereavement During Childhood

The most painful losses for a child are those of a parent or sibling during childhood. The immediate and long-term consequences have been studied more for parental loss. The age of the child at the time of the loss is of primary importance, because age determines the understanding of death. Briefly, it is believed that prior to age three, death is seen as reversible. From ages five to nine, the child comprehends a finality but views it more in terms of a separation. After ages nine to ten, a more mature understanding of death and its biological finality develops (79). It may be, however, that just as is observed with children with severe illness who seem to mature more rapidly in the understanding of death, presence of an ill parent or sibling during a lengthy illness with obvious physical deterioration may hasten awareness of death as a cessation of life.

As described with adult bereavement, the anticipation of death from cancer sometimes allows an opportunity for the preparation of a child for a parent's death. Many parents request advice at this time about how much to tell and when they should tell their children about their impending death. Intervention with a family at this time is helpful to monitor reactions and assure that the family is dealing with all members in a constructive way.

A program at Memorial Sloan-Kettering Cancer Center (MSKCC) has provided support for children of terminally ill parents to help them and the family face the impending loss. Especially helpful for the parents is guidance in handling information with the child by a social worker experienced in grief counseling, and counseling about decisions that bear long-term consequences on the child's adjustment after the death (80).

Bereavement symptoms in children are variable, but usually include sadness, a sense of vulnerability and insecurity, anxiety, and may include behavioral and disciplinary problems. Anger, guilt, and disorganization occur as well. Longitudinal observations indicate that a significant number of children have maladaptive symptoms, which continue for several years and interfere with academic and social performance (81).

The long-term effects of childhood bereavement are not clearly known because many studies have focused retrospectively on patient samples rather than community samples. However, the risk of adult major depressive disorder increases in those who had an early parental loss. There is no link established to manic-depressive illness. Tennant, Bebbington, and Hurry (82), on reviewing childhood parental death studies, felt that other considerations, such as quality of relationship to subsequent caretakers, may be more significant in determining the outcome than the loss itself. Because the surviving parent is bereaved, the care may be less consistent, interspersed with irritation and annoyance with the children, which contributes to a sense of insecurity. Extended family may play a critical stabilizing role.

For adults with cancer, having lost a parent to the same disease is a powerful early experience that complicates their adjustment to illness and often predisposes them to greater depression. Sometimes identification is seen in their assumption that someday they too would develop cancer.

Loss of Sibling During Childhood

Cancer is the second leading cause of death in childhood, after accidents. Because children are kept at home more during illness today, even during terminal stages, the impact on siblings is greater; however, the outcome of grieving appears better when families share in terminal care, including siblings (77,78). The long-term effect of this more intimate association is not clear as yet. The parents are focused on the ill child, and after the death they may grieve to the point that surviving children continue to receive little attention (83). The efforts of the surviving child to try to replace the dead child and diminish the parent's pain are often seen. The surviving child may also feel intense secret guilt because he or she harbored wishes for the sibling's death or imagines that he or she contributed to the death. Parents often become hypervigilant about the health of surviving children. Hypochondriasis and anxiety disorders in adulthood may result from the emphasis on physical symptoms and fears of cancer.

Interventions for bereaved children need to address the child, the parents, and the family generally. The child has three common questions, even if not articulated: Did I cause it? Will it happen to me? Who will take care of me? Interventions must deal with these questions (8). In anticipation of death, visits with the ill parent or sibling are helpful as long as meaningful interaction can occur. They help to reduce the potential for irrational guilt. However, a child should not be forced to visit.

Preventive intervention by counseling with the surviving child, alone or with other family members, may result in a better outcome (84). Counseling with parents about the child's impressions and questions expedites communication and guides management (5).

Decisions about informing the child of the death should be consistent with the family's culture, religion, and beliefs. The most important caveat is to avoid keeping the death a secret while the child senses the altered mood and behavior in the home. An explanation of the death with regard to the illness and reassurance about his or her own security are adequate, with the offer of answers to questions as they arise. Sharing grief and memories with family members confirms the child's worth and role in the family.

The decision about the child's attending the funeral should be made after explaining what will happen there, again giving permission but not forcing the child to attend. If he or she attends, it may serve positively to make the death more real. Children as well as adults experience the loss again on special days. Sharing the occasion with family support marks it as an expected normal sadness.

In a review of present understanding of childhood bereavement, it is clear that children should be kept informed of illness and death. They should be told in a way that is consistent with their age and understanding. They should be encouraged to participate in events as they are able to tolerate them. Grieving has expected symptoms of sadness, restlessness, and behavioral changes that benefit from counseling for unusual distress; counseling for all children may be helpful to encourage a healthy response (8).

INTERVENTIONS FOR ADULT BEREAVEMENT

It is important to recognize first that most bereaved individuals recover from their loss without any professional assistance. When efforts are made to offer counseling and support to a large group of recently bereaved individuals, many do not want it and, indeed, likely do not need it. Adequate support is gleaned from family, friends, and spiritual resources. When intervention is attempted, it should be directed toward those who are at known high risk of poor bereavement outcome (Table 88.3). When added support is needed, the two models that are beneficial are the professional interventions (consisting of psychotherapeutic and psychopharmacological approaches) and mutual support through nonprofessional sources.

Psychotherapy

While most bereaved do well, individuals with persistent anxiety or depression, which is the most common form of pathological grief, should be referred for evaluation and treatment (85). The individual often responds to six or eight psychotherapeutic visits to assist expression of grief and confrontation with the loss. Sometimes family therapy is the best approach, which includes all the survivors in the family who may be receptive to this approach that enhances their communication with one another. Individuals at high risk, however, may require much more protracted psychotherapeutic intervention, which is not always successful (41). Hospitalization is sometimes needed for treatment of severe depression or suicidal intent.

Marmar and colleagues (86) reviewed the few controlled intervention studies of spousal bereavement and noted that studies which targeted patients with high distress showed benefit to both physical and psychological health. Those that studied unselected subjects, however, showed less benefit. They conducted a trial that compared twelve brief dynamic psychotherapy sessions to a mutual-help group treatment in widows with unresolved grief. While there was a greater attrition rate in the group treatment, the two treatments both caused significant reduction in symptoms to an equal degree. Both had less effect on work and interpersonal relations. These interesting findings suggest that the more cost-effective treatment by mutual-support should be considered further, with efforts to train the leaders to deal with the more distressed individuals who might be most prone to drop out.

Bereavement counseling requires that the therapist know the clinical features of normal and abnormal bereavement, and that the therapist has skills in dealing with the problems of loss, which are so much a part of work with cancer patients and their loved ones. As in dealing with terminal illness, the therapist must be empathic to an individual experiencing great pain; exploring it in repeated sessions can be draining. It requires that the therapist have a good understanding of personal limitations and awareness of personal responses to prior losses that might affect care (see Chapter 60 on psychotherapy). Zisook and Schuchter (38) offered several key tasks in bereavement counseling: giving permission for expression of feelings and recounting of details of the experience, assessing defenses for dealing with the painful affect, integrating the continuing relationship with the deceased spouse with the present, encouraging healthy functioning, handling altered relationships, and achieving a new view of the personal world and the self in it, with a willingness to try new experiences.

Psychopharmacology

Medication is best used in combination with psychotherapy and for a limited time (87). Anxiolytics, mostly commonly the benzodiazepines, are used frequently during the early weeks of grief for insomnia. Daytime use reduces the feeling of tension, anxiety, and irritability. Although the use of medications in the bereaved has been controversial in the past—based on excessive use of barbiturates to sedate the bereaved during the early period of grief (88)—cautious use of mild sedation to reduce intolerable anxiety symptoms makes it easier to deal with working through the grief. Similarly, depressive symptoms associated with bereavement-related depression, especially the vegetative signs of insomnia and agitation, may be relieved by an antidepressant. A pilot study of a four-week open trial of desipramine by Jacobs, Nelson, and Zisook (89) showed moderate to marked improvement

of depressive symptoms in seven of ten bereaved, depressed spouses. Despite the absence of controlled trials with grieving persons, clinical experience is positive (38).

Mutual Help

There is no greater immediate alliance than that which is felt between two individuals who have shared the same stressful experience (see Chapter 61). This is particularly true for the sharing of grief with another who has experienced it. In fact, the Widow-to-Widow program was developed on the premise that the person best qualified to understand and help with the problems of a bereaved person is another bereaved person (22,90). To help widows through the critical transitions precipitated by bereavement, the multifaceted program offers one-to-one emotional support by an individual who herself presents a positive model of coping. Fundamental information about practical concerns and about bereavement are discussed. Groups promote the personal examination of coping and offer alternative ways that may be more effective. As an advocacy group, they become a source of identification with a group of individuals facing similar problems. The widow who resolves her own grief reinforces the gain by in turn helping others.

Such programs are located throughout the United States, Canada, and the United Kingdom. In a study examining the efficacy of the widow-to-widow model, Vaccine and colleagues (91) randomly assigned widows to the program. Follow-up assessment at 1, 6, 12, and 24 months showed better psychological adaptation by the women using the Widow-to-Widow program. By 24 months, they were better on all measures assessed. Women in the treatment group who were at high risk for poor outcome were significantly better than those at high risk who got no help. Mutual support interventions have also been shown to reduce physician visits during bereavement (92).

The Candlelighters and Compassionate Friends are two outstanding organizations that have developed mutual help programs for parents who have a child with cancer and for those who have lost a child from any cause. Chapters in many cities and in other countries have been formed. They have become sources of information, referrals, and advocacy for parents with these experiences. The Candlelighters particularly have had an impact on both the medical and humane aspects of pediatric cancer care. Compassionate Friends offer support to many bereaved parents through their chapters.

Hospice

Hospice care is unique in that it offers both professional and mutual support for the bereaved. Geared to maximal attention to the emotional, social, and spiritual needs of patients, the hospice offers support to many families of cancer patients who constitute the majority of those served (93). Most programs assign a bereavement counsellor to the families when the patient enters the program. They offer assistance through the terminal phase of the illness and into the bereavement period with home visits, phone calls, letters, support groups, counseling, and referrals to other needed support services.

SUMMARY

Management of the bereaved family is a common clinical problem faced by the oncology staff. Knowing the symptoms of normal grief and its stages allows support for normal grief and identification of abnormal reactions. Most individuals will recover from acute grief within one to two months, and it will be largely resolved within a year, usually without professional help. The anticipatory grieving period that is common with cancer may make the bereavement easier. However, about 20% of individuals will have trouble and will need help. Individuals likely to have trouble include those who have a history of emotional problems, are dependent, have experienced sudden death of the deceased, have poor support, are beset by other stresses and losses besides the death, have high initial distress, or have lost a child. Professional and mutual support are helpful in those who are at high risk or who have unusually intense initial symptoms. Medication may be efficacious if used cautiously for a limited time as an adjunct to psychotherapy. Assumptions about the risk of exacerbation of physical illness and mortality have likely been exaggerated in the distant past. However, in the most extensive studies, mortality was increased among older widowers from suicide, accidents, and infectious diseases. However, there was no over-representation of other diseases. It is of interest that, in epidemiological studies, there was not an increased risk of death by cancer. The clinical significance of the perturbations of the endocrine and immune system functions, demonstrated in psychoimmune studies of bereavement, remain unclear. Given the substantial medical and psychiatric morbidity and mortality, it is imperative that palliative care teams make every effort to include assessment and management of bereavement as part of their treatment mandate.

REFERENCES

1. Imboden JB, Canter A, Cliff L. Separation experiences and health records in a group of normal adults. *Psychosom Med.* 1963; 25: 433–440.
2. Frost NR, Clayton PS. Bereavement and psychiatric hospitalization. *Arch Gen Psychiatry.* 1977; 34: 1172–1175.
3. American Cancer Society. *Cancer Facts and Figures.* New York: American Cancer Society, 1986.
4. Koocher GP. Coping with a death from cancer. *J Consult Clin Psychol.* 1986; 54:623–631.
5. Pasnau RO, Fawzy RI, Fawzy N. Role of the physician in bereavement. *Psychiat Clin North Am.* 1987; 10: 109–120.
6. Rome HP. Personal reflections: Those who remain. *Psychiatr Ann.* 1986; 16:268–71.
7. Parkes CM. Bereavement. In: Doyle D, Hanks GWC, Macdonald N. (eds.) *Oxford Textbook of Palliative Medicine.* Oxford University Press, 1993: 663–678.
8. Osterweis M, Solomon F, Green M. (eds.). *Bereavement: Reactions, Consequences and Care.* Washington, D.C.: National Academy Press, 1984.
9. Prigerson HG, Frand E, Kasl SV, et al. Complicated grief and bereavement-related depression as distinct disorders: Preliminary empirical validation in elderly bereaved spouses. *Am J Psychiatry.* 1995; 1: 22–30.
10. Freud S. Mourning and melancholia. In: Strachey J. (ed. and trans.) *The Complete Psychological Works*, std. ed. Vol. 14. New York: Norton, 1976: 243–258 (original work published 1923).
11. Bowlby J. The making and breaking of affectional bonds, I: Aetiology and psychopathology in the light of attachment theory. *Br J Psychiatry.* 1977; 130: 201–210.
12. Bowlby J. Process of mourning. *Int J Psychoanal.* 1961; 42:317–340.
13. Bowlby J. *Attachment and Loss.* Vol 3, *Loss: Sadness and Depression.* New York: Basic Books, 1980.
14. Parkes CM. *Bereavement: Studies of Grief in Adult Life.* Madison, Conn: International Universities Press, 1972.
15. Elliott GR, Eisdorfer G. *Stress and Human Health: Analysis and Implications of Research*: A study by the Institute of Medicine/National Academy of Sciences. New York: Springer, 1982.
16. Horowitz MJ, Bonanno GA, Holen A. Pathological grief: Diagnosis and explanation. *Psychosom Med.* 1993; 55: 260–273.
17. Horowitz MJ. *Stress Response Syndromes*, 2nd ed. Northvale, NJ: Aronson, 1986.
18. Lewis JK, McKinney WT, Young LLD, Karemer GW. Mother-infant separation in rhesus monkeys as a model of human depression—a reconsideration. *Arch Gen Psychiatry.* 1976; 33: 699–705.
19. Hofer MA. Relationships as regulators: A psychobiologic perspective on bereavement. *Psychosom Med.* 1984; 183–197.
20. Lindemann E. Symptomatology and management of acute grief. *Am J Psychiatry.* 1944; 101:141–148.
21. Brown JT, Stoudemire A. Normal and pathological grief. *JAMA.* 1983; 250(3): 378–382.
22. Parkes CM, Weiss RS. *Recovery from Bereavement.* New York: Basic Books, 1983.
23. Vaccine MLS. Predictors and correlates of adaptation in conjugal bereavement. *Am J Psychiatry* 1982; 139: 998–1002.

24. Cassen NH. The dying patient. In: Hackett TP and Cassem NH (eds.) *Massachusettes General Hospital: Handbook of General Hospital Psychiatry.* St. Louis: C.V. Mosby, 1978: 300–318.

25. Parkes CM. Determinants of outcome following bereavement. *Omega J Death Dying.* 1975; 6: 303–323.

26. Blanchard DG, Blanchard EB, Keeker JL. The young: Depressive symptomatology throughout the grief process. *Psychiatry.* 1976; 39: 394–399

27. Hays JC, Kasl SV, Jacobs SC. The course of psychological distress following threatened and actual conjugal bereavement. *Psychol Med.* 1994; 24: 917–927.

28. Engel GL. Grief and grieving. *Am J Nursing.* 1964; 64: 93–98.

29. Reynolds R. Autopsies: Benefits to the family. *Am J Clin Pathol.* 1978; 69(Suppl. 25): 220–222.

30. Green M. Roles of health professionals and institutions. In: Osterweis M, Solomon F, Green M (eds.). *Bereavement: Reactions, Consequences, and Care.* Washington, D.C.: National Academy Press, 1984: 215–236.

31. Barton D. *Dying and Death: A Clinical Guide for Caregivers.* Baltimore: Williams and Wilkins, 1977.

32. Zisook S, Devaul RA, Click MA. Measuring symptoms of grief and bereavement. *Am J Psychiatry.* 1982; 139: 1590–1593.

33. Reynolds CF, Hoch CC, Buysse DJ, et al. Sleep after spousal bereavement: A study of recovery from stress. *Biol Psychiatry.* 1993; 34: 791–797.

34. Clayton P. Mourning and depression: Their similarities and differences. *Can J Psychiatry.* 1974; 1: 309–312.

35. Byrne GSA, Raphael B. A longitudinal study of bereavement phenomena in recently widowed elderly men. *Psychol Med.* 1994; 24: 411–421.

36. Harlow SD, Goldberg EL, Comstock GW. A longitudinal study of the prevalence of depressive symptomatology in elderly widowed and married women. *Arch Gen Psychiatry.* 1991; 48: 1065–1068.

37. Zisook S, Schuchter SR. Uncomplicated bereavement. *J Clin Psychiatry.* 1993; 54: 365–372.

38. Zisook S, Schuchter SR. The first four years of widowhood. *Psychiatr Ann.* 1985; 16: 288–294.

39. Volkan V. Normal and pathological grief reactions. A guide for the family physician. *Va Med Monthly.* 1966; 93: 651–656.

40. Worden W. *Grief Counselling and Grief Therapy: A Handbook for the Mental Health Practitioner.* New York: Springer, 1982.

41. Rynearson EK. Psychotherapy of pathologic grief. *Psychiatr Clin N Am.* 1987; 10(3): 487–499.

42. Lundin T. Morbidity following sudden and unexpected bereavement. *Br J Psychiatry.* 1984; 144: 84–88.

43. American Psychiatric Association. *Diagnostic and Statistical Manual of Mental Disorders,* 4th ed. Washington, D.C.: American Psychiatric Association, 1994.

44. De Vahl R, Zisook S. Unresolved grief: Clinical considerations. *Postgrad Med.* 1976; 59: 267–271.

45. Horowitz M, Wilner N, Marmar C. Pathological grief and the activation of latent self-images. *Am J Psychiatry.* 1980; 137: 1157–1162.

46. Raphael B, Middleton W. What is pathologic grief? *Psychiatr Ann.* 1990; 20: 304–307.

47. Abraham K. Notes on the psychoanalytical investigation and treatment of manic-depressive insanity and allied conditions. In: Gaylin W. (ed.) *The Meaning of Despair.* New York: Jason Aronson, 1968: 26–49.

48. Parkes CM. Effects of bereavement on physical and mental health: A study of the case records of widows. *Br Med J.* 1964; 2:274–79

49. Parkes CM. Bereavement and mental illness: A clinical study of the grief of bereaved psychiatric patients. *Br J Med Psychol.* 1965; 38:1–12.

50. Stein ZJ, Susser MW. Widowhood and mental illness. *Br J Prevent Soc Med.* 1969; 23:106–110.

51. Vaccine MJ, Sheldon AR, Lance WJ, Lyall WA, Rogers J, Freeman SJ. Correlates of enduring distress patterns following bereavement. Social network, life situations and personality. *Psychol Med.* 1982; 12:783–788.

52. Maddison DC, Walker W. Factors affecting the outcome of conjugal bereavement. *Br J Med Psychol.* 1967; 113: 1057–1067.

53. Murphy GE, Robins E. Social factors in suicide. *JAMA.* 1967; 199: 303–308.

54. Robins LN, West PA, Murphy GE. The high rate of suicide in older white men: A study testing ten hypotheses. *Soc Psychiatry.* 1977; 12: 1–20.

55. Bornstein PE, Clayton PJ, Halikas JA, Maurice WL, Robins E. The depression of widowhood after thirteen months. *Br J Psychiatry.* 1973; 122: 561–566.

56. Lieberman PB, Jacobs SC. Bereavement and its complications in medical patients: A guide for consultation-liaison psychiatrists. *Int J Psychiatry Med.* 1987; 17(1): 23–39.

57. Clayton PJ. Bereavement and depression. *J Clin Psychiatry.* 1990; 51: 34–38.

58. Zisook S, Shuchter SR. Depression through the first year after the death of a spouse. *Am J Psychiatry.* 1991; 148: 1346–1352.

59. Zisook S, Shuchter SR, Sledge PA. The spectrum of depressive phenomena after spousal bereavement. *J Clin Psychiatry.* 1994; 55 (4, Supp): 29–36.

60. Karam EG. The nosological status of bereavement-related depressions. *Br J Psychiatry.* 1994; 165: 48–52.

61. Engel GL. Is grief a disease? A challenge for medical research. *Psychosom Med.* 1961; 23: 18–22.

62. Hofer M, Wolff C, Freedman S, Mason J. A psychoendocrine study of bereavement: Parts 1 and 2. *Psychosom Med.* 1972; 34: 481–507.

63. Bartrop R, Lazarus L, Luckhurst E, Kiloh LG, Penny R. Depressed lymphocyte function after bereavement. *Lancet.* 1977; 1: 834–836.

64. Irwin M, Daniels M, Weiner H. Immune and neuroendocrine changes during bereavement. *Psychiatr Clin N Am.* 1987; 10: 449–465.

65. Schmale AHS, Iher HP. The affect of hopelessness and the development of cancer. I, Identification of uterine cervical cancer in women with atypical cytology. *Psychosom Med.* 1966; 28: 714.

66. Levav I, Friedlander Y, Kark S, Peritz E. An epidemiologic study of mortality among bereaved parents. *N Engl J Med.* 1988; 319: 457–461.

67. Jones DR, Goldblatt PO, Leon DA. Bereavement and cancer: some data on death of spouses from the longitudinal study of Office of Population Censuses and Surveys. *Br Med J.* 1984; 289:461–464.

68. Schleifer SJ, Keller M, Camerino J, Thornton C, Stein M. Suppression of lymphocyte stimulation following bereavement *JAMA*. 1983; 250:374–377.

69. Martinson IM, Moldow DG, Henry WF. *Home Care for the Child with Cancer*. Final report, Grant CA19490, HHS, National Cancer Institute. Minneapolis: University of Minnesota School of Nursing, 1980.

70. Helsing KJ, Szklo M. Mortality after bereavement. *Am J Epidemiol*. 1981; 114: 41–52.

71. Helsing KJ, Comstock G, Szklo M. Causes of death in a widowed population. *Am J Epidemiol*. 1982; 116: 524–532.

72. Li G. The interaction effect of bereavement and sex on the risk of suicide in the elderly: An historical cohort study. *Soc Sci Med*. 1995; 40(6): 825–828.

73. Schaefer C, Quesenberry CP, Sorra W. Mortality following conjugal bereavement and the effects of a shared environment. *Am J Epidemiol*. 1995; 141: 1142–1152.

74. Pearlin L, Lieberman M. Social sources of distress. In: Simmons RG (ed.) *Research in Community and Mental Health: an Annual Compilation of Research*, Vol 1. Greenwich, Conn: JAI Press, 1979: 217–249.

75. Sanders C. A comparison of adult bereavement in the death of spouse, child, and parent. *Omega J Death Dying*. 1979; 10:303–322.

76. Littlefield CH, Rushton JP. When a child dies: The sociobiology of bereavement. *J Pers Soc Psychol*. 1986; 51: 792–802.

77. Rando TA. An investigation of grief and adaptation in parents whose children have died of cancer. *J Pediatr Psychol*. 1983; 8:3–20.

78. Spinetta JJ, Swarner J, Shepost J. Effective parental coping following death of a child from cancer. *J Pediatr Psychol*. 1981; 6:251–263.

79. Nagy M. The child's theories concerning death. *J Genet Psychol*. 1948; 73:3–12.

80. Adams-Greenly M, Moynihan RT. Helping the children of fatally ill parents. *Am J Orthopsychiatry*. 1983; 53: 219–229.

81. Kaffman M, Elizar E. Children's bereavement reactions following death of father. The early months of bereavement. *Int J Her*. 1979; 1:203–229.

82. Tennant C, Bebbington P, Hurry J. Parental death in childhood and risk of adult depressive disorders: A review. *Psychol Med*. 1980; 10:289–299.

83. Pollack GH. Childhood sibling loss: A family tragedy. *Psychiatr Ann*. 1985; 16:309–314.

84. Rosenheim D, Ichilou Y. Short-term preventive therapy with children of fatally ill parents. *Israel Ann Psychiatr Rel Dis*. 1979; 17:67–73.

85. Raphael B. *The Anatomy of Bereavement*. New York: Basic Books, 1983.

86. Marmar CR, Horowitz MJ, Weiss DS, Wilner NR, Koltreider NB. A controlled trial of brief psychotherapy and mutual-help group treatment of conjugal bereavement. *Am J Psychiatry*. 1988; 145: 203–209.

87. Hollister L. Psychotherapeutic drugs in the dying and bereaved. *J Thanatol*. 1972; 2:623–629.

88. Morgan D. Not all sadness can be treated with antidepressants. *W Va Med J*. 1980; 76(6): 136–137.

89. Jacobs SC, Nelson JC, Zisook S. Treating depressions of bereavement with antidepressants: A pilot study. *Psychiatr Clin N Am*. 1987; 10: 501–511.

90. Silverman PR. The widow as caregiver in a program of preventative intervention with other widows. In: Killelie CG (ed.) *Support Systems and Mutual Help*. New York: Grune and Stratton Inc, 1976: 233–243.

91. Vaccine MLS, Sheldon AR, Lancee WJ, et al.: A controlled study of self-help: Intervention for widows. *Am J Psychiatry*. 1980; 137: 1380–1384.

92. Tudiner F, Permaul-Woods JA, Hilditch J, Harmina J, Saini S. Do widowers use the health care system differently? Does intervention make a difference? *Can Fam Physician*. 1995; 41: 392–400.

93. Gaetz D. The case for hospice from a hospital perspective. *Am Protestant Hosp Assoc Bull*. 1981; 45:33–40.

XIV

STAFF SUPPORT AND TRAINING IN PSYCHO-ONCOLOGY

EDITORS: MARGUERITE S. LEDERBERG AND
MARY JANE MASSIE

89

Oncology Staff Stress and Related Interventions

MARGUERITE S. LEDERBERG

SOCIETAL PERSPECTIVES

Public perception of medical caregivers has undergone major shifts in the last three decades. Particularly after WWII, the religiously inspired physician of the previous century gave way to the idealized secular caregiver, knowledgeable enough to harness the promises of modern scientific progress for the patient's benefit. Within three decades, a post-modern backlash became prominent, and doctor-bashing became a popular sport, as the public struggled with the dashing of unreal hopes for prolonged life, and coped instead with prolonged aging, and often prolonged suffering as well (1). One consequence has been the growth of the medical consumer movement resulting in more demanding, more knowledgeable patients who expect to play an active role in decision making. Another has been the growth of a grassroots movement that supports not only the right to die, but also the right to assisted suicide and voluntary euthanasia. At the same time as their authority and expertise is under attack, caregivers are also being asked to participate in bringing about death, which is, for many, the ultimate betrayal of their calling (2).

A new facet of staff stress relates to the massive changes sweeping health care delivery as many countries experience a slowly dropping level of general affluence, and are severely restricting their health care expenditures. Thus, caregivers in all settings are experiencing the helplessness already so familiar to professionals in developing countries where the long-standing gap between two-tier levels of care yawns ever wider. During transitions, uncertainty reigns and salaries drop, in the face of larger workloads, less flexibility and greater cross-coverage. Redefined jobs lead caregivers to feel vulnerable and ethically torn when they feel unable to deliver their previous care, while patients and families become suspicious, angry or desperate at being denied interventions that might be of benefit.

However, starting with the description of burnout in the early seventies, there has been a parallel movement which examines the plight of caregivers with curiosity and compassion (3–8). Reinforced by an increased awareness of post-traumatic disorders, researchers exploring the psychological consequences of disasters now study health care workers alongside the identified victims, sometimes finding comparable levels of stress in both groups (9–10).

OCCUPATIONAL RISKS FOR HEALTH CARE WORKERS

Exposure to radiation and the handling of chemotherapeutic drugs before strict safety procedures were put into place, have been implicated in an increased risk of thyroid cancer (11), leukemia, lymphoma, birth defects (12), and fetal loss (13–16). Growing public awareness of "the era of emerging infections" reminds caregivers that they face higher risks from infections found in immuno-compromised hosts such as HIV, hepatitis, tuberculosis, and cytomegalovirus (17–21). Some of these have emerged under the umbrella of AIDS (tuberculosis and sexually transmitted diseases), others have become resistant to previously effective treatments, (drug resistant tuberculosis, *Clostridium diffi-cile*). In some cases infected workers lose their jobs and their insurance coverage even when they are still physically well.

Some infections like HIV are particularly frightening, others, like Hepatitis B, are more common, yet seldom discussed. The level of concern on a well-run unit may be more a function of staff–administration relations than of concrete risk or staff beliefs about contemporary environmental dangers. For example, when radiation badges for monitoring risk are developed and found to show no exposure, a contented staff will be relieved. An angry staff may wonder if they have been tampered with. Effective responses to the latter must deal with the root problem and with the irrational, as well as the rational aspects of staff behavior.

CURRENT RESEARCH ON STAFF STRESS

Issues of Conceptualization and Methodology

Delvaux and Razavi (1988) (22) and Zevon (1990) (23) have pointed out that the literature on staff stress is bedeviled by confusion between stress as a stimulus and stress as a response. It is, rather, an individualized response to a stimulus, suggesting a more complicated model than is used in most psychosocial studies. Furthermore, van Servellen (1993) (24) has pointed out that rigorous studies may be too difficult to do, because of the dependence on self-reports, the small opportunistic samples and the cross-sectional designs. Zevon, Donnelly and Starkey (1990)'s longitudinal study (23) illustrates the possibilities. Following the unexpected closing of a bone marrow transplant unit, they found a wide divergence between individual responses. Caregivers who were in an initially high-stress state became more involved in their work as their control diminished, while the low-initial-stress workers became less involved, and felt less additional stress. This suggests that cross-sectional studies with indefinite or contradictory findings may reflect a wash-out of significant subgroups. However, psychosocial research proceeds by successive approximations, and the findings of numerous studies are consistent enough across countries, diseases, and caregiver populations that they should be taken seriously despite their many methodological problems

Summary of Recent Studies

Many studies have documented the high incidence of burnout and/or clinically significant anxiety or depression in oncology staff (25–29). Catalan et al., (1996) (30) found 44% cases in oncology and 40% in HIV staff. In the largest available sample, Whippen and Canellos (1991) (29) reported a 56% incidence of burn-out in a questionnaire of 1000 American oncologists, with the lowest score among academicians and the highest scores having a positive relationship to the amount of direct patient care. They received a 60% response to their questionnaire, most of it within 2 weeks, and often enriched by lengthy handwritten comments. Clearly the subject is one that has great

meaning and importance to professionals. Bram and Katz (1989) (31) compared nurses in hospital and hospice settings, finding that hospice nurses showed less burnout than hospital ones ($P < 0.05$). Beck-Friis, Strang and Sjoden (1993) (32) compared working conditions in hospital-based home care and in hospital care; while both were stressful, the home-based group fared better than the hospital group. Hospice staff, and staff on units where they feel more free to express their views and have a sense of solid relationships, score lower on stress measures (33–34). The quality of an individual's social support system at work was found to be one of the strongest predictors of job satisfaction (31,35). In Cronin-Stubs' study (36), the impact of affection was stronger than that of recognition. All of these findings are reminiscent of the original study that defined "the Hawthorne effect," namely the fact that workers who felt cared about had greater productivity (37). They are further reinforced by repeated findings documenting the positive effects of social support in living creatures, animal and human, patients and non-patients.

A major area of research has grown from the observation that patient and family dissatisfaction often revolve around communication issues. Patients can tolerate bad outcomes with less anger at caregivers when the latter are experienced as humane and available for explanation and comfort (38). Lack of staff know-how is an important factor, and caregivers respond to their inadequacy not only with tension, anxiety, and avoidance, but with low self-esteem and decreased job satisfaction as well (27–28,39).

A disconcerting group of studies reveals that staff do not evaluate their performance well, thus perpetuating a cycle of inadequacy unless active interventions are undertaken (27–28,40). They have been found to underestimate patient pain and anxiety, to overestimate the success of their DNR discussions as well as patient family satisfaction with ethics consultations (40–42). They do not predict patient advance directive preferences well (43), but it should be said that family members do not predict those any better (44). Fortunately, it has been shown that communication and listening skills can be taught (45).

ANATOMY OF STRESS

The following sections will outline the different kinds of stresses that impinge on caregivers. Work-based stressors that are independent of the medical setting will be discussed in the intervention section. Medical stressors will be divided into those which are unique to oncology, those which are a function of patient reactions, and those which are inherent in high technology.

Stresses Specific to Cancer

Stresses specific to cancer (see Table 89.1) can be thought of as those that are inherent in the nature of the disease, to the nature of the treatment, and lastly to the nature of patient psychological responses.

Disease-related. Since Susan Sontag's groundbreaking personal book about her experience with breast cancer, many public figures have described their struggles in the media, promoting greater public awareness of cancer as a potentially curable, or chronic illness. Nevertheless, cancer remains a ubiquitous disease that strikes the young and old, rich and poor, strong and weak, cheerful and gloomy. . . It remains unpredictable in its course and its response to treatment; the most seasoned personnel talk sadly among themselves about an unexpectedly fulminant course, or derive pleasure and encouragement from the unexpected remission. Difficult cancer deaths are frequent enough to have a greater impact than the less dramatic trajectories, and the many cancers that continue to have a poor prognosis insure that a profound emotional fear of cancer is very much alive. It has been reinforced by the explosion of knowledge about the genetic basis of cancer, which has not yet resulted in therapeutic advantages, but has created a large population of the "worried well," individuals at high risk for cancers whose special problems are outlined in Chapters 17 and 18.

Self-selected as they are, caregivers focus on constructive actions and observable results. They do not adopt quack theories or dubious treatments, but they do need defenses against especially upsetting cases. Hence they develop a private system of special meanings, associations, and omens that helps them to predict the course of subsequent difficult cases, and as such, is helpful to them. However, because of its idiosyncratic, irrational nature, this private code can also

TABLE 89.1. *Stresses Specific to Cancer*

---

1. INHERENT IN THE NATURE OF THE DISEASE

2. TREATMENT-RELATED
    a. The nature of the treatments
    b. Treatment side-effects
    c. Decisional stressors
    d. Interstaff disagreements

3. PATIENT RESPONSES

---

be a burden. For example, a young physician had become very involved with a leukemia patient who had died after an unusual presentation and a stormy course. Subsequently, characteristics of this patient's illness remained vividly present, and often colored the physician's expectations when similarities occurred in subsequent cases.

Treatment-related.

NATURE OF THE TREATMENTS. The mainstays of cancer treatment, radiation and chemotherapy, were hailed with enthusiasm during the post-WWII era, but in the current, post-modern era, they are associated with mankind's deepest fears of nuclear contamination and environmental degradation. The growing use of bone marrow transplants has breathed new life into treatment, but has not escaped this fearful aura. Ablative surgery remains a crucial and often successful form of treatment, but when it is disfiguring or extremely radical, it is also experienced as fundamentally damaging. The large array of new biological treatments gives rise to great hope but the results have not yet been dramatic or consistent enough to significantly alter public or staff perception.

The ethical issues associated with high-technology care, and the even more poignant ones associated with terminal care, such as discontinuation of life supports, hydration, nutrition, or assisted suicide and euthanasia, are played out in cancer patients far more often than in other diseases. These are more fully discussed elsewhere (see Chapters 37 and 96) but are flagged here because of their anxiety-provoking effects on staff. This is due to their intrinsically complex nature, compounded by public attention and external interventions at the bedside, so-called "limelight medicine."

TREATMENT SIDE-EFFECTS. The management of ever-present side-effects is a constant reminder to patient and staff of the cytotoxic nature of cancer treatment. They range from transient cosmetic ones such as hair loss to life-threatening nadir sepsis or graft-versus-host-disease. Caregivers feel anguish over iatrogenic complications, which is exacerbated because these feelings are generally repressed and unavailable for discussion. Even transient side-effects such as hair loss and nausea can be distressing to staff, because they are so difficult for some patients to tolerate. Disfigurement affects caregivers, even seasoned ones, as it affects all human beings. Severe complications grieve them, sexually related problems always have a special impact. Less obvious long-term effects such as infertility are very significant for caregivers in child-bearing years.

Treatment procedures that carry a significant mortality, like bone marrow transplantation, have an ever-present emotional tension and potential for anguish. As McCue (1982) (6) put it, modern technology can put physicians (and other staff) in "absurdly stressful" situations. Unacknowledged guilt about life-threatening complications often underlies aggressive overtreatment, although it is not readily admitted by the caregiver who remains unaware of it even while stating the contrary.

DECISIONAL STRESSORS. Decision making has become more complicated as modalities have multiplied and patients have become more active participants. Patient difficulties with decision-making have been described, but there are dissensions in the staff as well. Choices may be less ambiguous, very early or very late in the disease, but much of the course is spent in the middle, trying to chart a course without reliable coordinates. As treatment moves through successive phases, the shift from curative to palliative intent may be very difficult to negotiate. It engenders anxiety, confusion, depression, and many negative reactions in patients and families which are often diverted onto staff, in ways which are widely acknowledged to generate further strain and dissension.

INTERSTAFF ISSUES. Staff members vary widely in their degree of comfort with this delicate transition, and in their philosophy of when and how it should occur. This is especially so in institutional settings with large medical teams and multiple missions that sometimes coexist uneasily. Depending on their background, discipline, and role on the team, staff members have different ways of reducing stress. Each team, each discipline, or each individual may focus on its own facet of care with little sympathy for the other's viewpoint. This can be exacerbated in research settings where ethical and philosophical conflicts between research and clinical care commitments can readily occur, even in objectively well-managed cases. Whether acknowledged or not, these conflicts intensify other sources of division. Some differences are discipline-based. Doctors have the most detailed information about the natural history of the disease, its likely course and prognosis in a given patient, on the basis of which they generate the treatment plan. It is most natural for them to assume an intellectual approach for which they are already pre-selected. Having the ultimate responsibility for decisions enhances the commitment to the treatment, and the ability of the physician to accept partial results. In fact, working in oncology requires the ability to maintain dedication and energy

in the face of all outcomes. Many oncology nurses now also assume a high level of responsibility, and self-select for the use of "the doctor stance", i.e., the same intellectual approach in dealing with the stresses. However, a number of nurses do not identify with this approach and view themselves more as "nurturers." There is definitely no incompatibility or absolute distinction between the two stances, but a primary identification with one or the other dictates a set of emotional responses and sources of professional satisfaction. Failure to acknowledge the existence of these two stances, or valuing one at the expense of the other can create tensions on units or within a team.

Besides doctors and nurses, cancer care today involves many other disciplines such as medical secretaries, aides, ward clerks, and technicians. Many of their patient interactions have a strong emotional impact and resonate with their personal feelings about cancer, and about the institution. Some feel closely identified with it and derive a sense of pride and security from their association. Others feel alienated and captive due to lack of job mobility. These conflicts can erode the quality of life for the staff member and quality of care they deliver. This is worsened by the fact that training rarely equips them for the troubled patient and family interface they negotiate repeatedly. They may feel inappropriately devalued, as they are often the recipients of displaced anxieties and resentments. Self-esteem suffers and attempts to protect it often translate into anger toward patients and bitterness toward superiors, with further harm to worker and patient.

Stresses Related to Patient Morbidity and Patient Psychological Responses

There are many stresses at the staff-patient interface (Table 89.2).

Patient Reactions to Severe Illness. Patient responses to cancer outlined in Table 89.3 include regressive behavior which may require great patience

TABLE 89.2. *Stresses at the Patient Interface*

1. Patient reaction to severe illness
2. The "difficult" patient
3. The "special" patient
4. Responses to severe debilitation and disfigurement
5. Responses to death and dying: fear, grief, survivor guilt
6. Responses to suicidal ideation
7. Adjustment to poor outcomes
8. Injustice of human suffering

TABLE 89.3. *Possible Patient Responses to a Cancer Diagnosis*

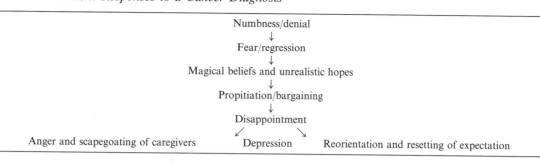

from staff; numbness and inappropriate denial, which staff must judiciously confront when it is interfering with needed treatment; panic and grief, which staff must tolerate while continuing to treat the patient; a powerful need to propitiate and bargain, which staff must recognize and gently discourage while understanding the unrealistic expectations that underlie it; disappointment and anger, which staff must endure without altering their efforts; and depression, which can be the most draining of all. Overall, this is a difficult set of projections to handle with professional demeanor. The required steadfastness of personal behavior demands much strength and maturity.

The "Difficult" Patient. Patients with characterological disorders are notorious for creating chaos around them. A cancer diagnosis does not impair that ability, and the staff can become angry and unempathic. Yet the illness still endows the patient with pathos, and caregivers may feel guilty about their hostile feelings. It is helpful to normalize staff emotions while tempering their behaviors.

The "Special" Patient. This patient arouses deep involvement in the caregiver, usually because of personal experiences. Such a patient can become "special" for a whole team or unit, as the team's "child," or the team's "special survivor" or "bravest patient," resulting in overinvolvement, impaired judgment, interstaff disagreements, and undigested grief.

Exposure to Severe Debilitation and Disfigurement. Intense and repeated exposures to mutilation and suffering lead to pain and sadness, but also fear and revulsion. These, in turn, engender shame and guilt with avoidance or compensatory overinvolvement.

Responses to Death and Dying. Frequent exposure to death leads to a premature loss of the sense of invulnerability and a painful awareness of personal mortality. For young staff members, the first confrontation with death may be a shattering experience. This is not helped by the practice that requires staff members to go on, without any opportunity to digest their emotional responses or express grief. Even seasoned staff will react with tension and the need to escape, when deaths are too frequent, unexpected, or difficult. The fear of death is a permanent subtext that is never fully confronted by the caregiver whose grief is for ever aborted. Their survivor guilt is equally universal and unexpressed. It underlies overtreatment, overinvolvement, and the inability of some staff to allow themselves to fully escape from their work.

Responses to Suicidal Ideation. Patients' suicidal statements frighten staff, who often mistake extreme frustration for active suicidality. Faced with the latter, caregivers totally committed to "fighting" cancer react with incomprehension and negative judgments. Others are gripped by inner agreement, which they cannot express or act upon, leaving them feeling torn and inauthentic.

Adjustment to Poor Outcomes. Much has been said about the need of doctors to "win the fight" but less about other aspects of their subjective experience with repeated losses. Foreseeable declines, patients' struggles to come to grips, family desperation, all create a climate of dull pain, suppressed sadness and regret, if not outright guilt. Learning to come to terms with this, and to replace these sapping emotions with acceptance of the inevitable coupled with trust in one's best efforts and maintenance of self-esteem is far more demanding than is realized by the many facile critics who have never faced the task. The adjustment must engage both the caregiver's personality and previous experience, as well as his work environment and colleagues.

Injustice of Human Suffering. No caregiver can maintain a simplistic belief in terrestrial justice. Religious staff members find comfort in their beliefs about another life. Others become cynical, but many more remain engaged and upbeat by molding their hopes and desires to be more flexible. For young people, the confrontation shapes a lifelong attitude. Support of colleagues is crucial in weathering this existential crisis, and a few do well to leave.

Stresses Related to Modern Treatment

High tech oncology settings demand a high level of intellectual acuity for rapid decision-making based on a thorough understanding of complex techniques and algorithms (Table 89.4). These requirements are enmeshed in the emotional freight of human tragedies, the responsibility of life–death decisions, the ambiguity of terminal care discontinuation issues, and the increasing immediacy of assisted suicide legislation.

As long as caregivers felt trusted and given autonomy to do their best, these demands were often experienced as stimulating challenges. But current changes have undermined morale significantly and challenges have become burdens. The future is unclear, but eventual stability may allow more positive adaptations.

The Psychodynamics of Caregivers

The range of staff reactions is demonstrated in Table 89.5.

There are different levels of caregiver responses. Their conscious adaptation reflects a professional ego-ideal with its intellectual mastery, rejection of irrationality, reliable emotional controls, and the ability to remain effective and action-oriented under all conditions. Underlying this are contradictory attitudes, idiosyncratic, fear-laden, and anchored in their emotional past. If unconscious, they lead to involuntary behaviors which are puzzling to others, and are rationalized by the individual. If conscious, they feel shameful and are kept hidden. Widespread dissimulation confirms caregivers in the belief they are alone or unusual in having such feelings, and results in emotional isolation in the workplace.

This self-imposed isolation is often compounded by isolation in personal life, since friends and family often cannot, or will not, share in the sad events of the workday. They respond with humor, silence, avoidance, sometimes frank annoyance or rejection. Unrealistic admiration is more pleasant but just as distancing.

TABLE 89.4. *Stresses Related to the Modern Medical Environment*

1. High cognitive demands of technology and science
2. Increasing difficulty of choice of treatment
   a. Greater number of choices
   b. Greater ambiguity of outcomes
3. Increasing problem of iatrogenic disease
4. Increasing patient expectations and assertiveness
5. Increasing regulation and outside regulation of care
6. Intensity and repetitiveness of difficult emotional situations.
7. Need to make life/death decisions
8. Terminal care medical, ethical and emotional controversies (discontinuation of life supports, fluids or nutrition, requests for assisted suicide)
9. Ethical conflicts
10. "Limelight" medicine
11. Stresses associated with altered delivery of medical care

TABLE 89.5. *Psychodynamics of Caregivers*

1. CONSCIOUS ADAPTATION
   a. Intellectual grasp of the situation
   b. Rejection of superstition
   c. Problem-solving stance
   d. Reliable emotional controls
   e. Good functioning under pressure

2. UNCONSCIOUS BELIEFS
   a. Idiosyncratic, fear-laden, irrational
   b. If unconscious: lead to involuntary behaviors, mystifying or rationalized
   c. If conscious: self-labeled as weakness and kept hidden

3. UNCONSCIOUS MOTIVATIONS
   a. Establishing mastery over feared events
   b. Propitiating unconscious guilt
   c. Satisfying voyeuristic, sadistic, or masochistic impulses
   d. Acting out powerful family scenarios

4. ISOLATION FACTORS
   a. Characteristics of personal life / work interface
   b. Self-imposed workplace isolation
   c. Externally imposed social isolation
      – Distancing from painful topics
      – Humor, silence, avoidance
      – Unrealistic admiration

5. REWARDS OF MEDICAL WORK: THE "FLIP" SIDE OF THE COIN
   a. Emotional excitement
   b. Intellectual challenge
   c. Being part of a valued social enterprise
   d. Playing a positive role in profound human experiences
   e. Existential "initiation"
   f. Sense of being special

Caregivers, in turn, may find their loved ones callous, naive, or self-indulgent in their reactions to the work, and in their unquestioning focus on their daily concerns. The latter may seem trivial to the caregiver who may not respond empathically to family, any more than they responded to him/her. Alternatively, caregivers may focus with more intensity on their family members, especially parents on young children, for they have lost much of the automatic obliviousness to risk that eases daily life for many individuals. Lastly, caregivers can be cancerophobic in varying degrees. New employees almost all go through such a period, rather like medical students.

The factors underlying caregivers' unconscious motivations include establishing mastery over feared events, propitiating unconscious guilt, satisfying voyeuristic, sadistic, or masochistic impulses, and acting out family scenarios. The mental health consultant needs insight into these issues, but should never interpret them unless it is clearly the only way to alter poor practices.

Anxiety and fatigue can create a vicious cycle that further exacerbates fear of failure and saps self-esteem. Increasing numbers of ethical dilemmas force staff to confront ambiguity and irreducible conflicts. A growing sense of personal risk can lead to fear and anxiety, translated into anger and bitterness or, in abreaction, shame and overinvolvement.

The emphasis to date has been on difficulties, but one must never forget all the positive experiences which keep caregivers working with relish for many years (34,46–47). Many thrive on emotional excitement and intensity, many love the intellectual challenge especially in the context of interacting with people in a helpful way. They gain satisfaction from being part of a valued social enterprise, from playing a positive role in profound human experiences, from having survived a form of existential initiation. In brief, they feel like valuable, constructive human beings. Even when there is not much outside socializing with co-workers, caregivers derive sustenance from being surrounded by people who share these commitments and experiences with them, even if it is unexpressed much of the time.

Course of Initial Adaptation. The naive caregiver's first reaction to the acuteness and severity is severe dysphoria, held at bay by repressive mechanisms that numb the individual so that s/he can focus on developing competence. After three to four months, there is a sense of relief that competence is within grasp, which is often mistaken for full adaptation. But it takes several months for the personal meaning and impact of the work to make itself felt, as the

worker's past experiences with disease and loss are brought into play. Only then can the pain and uncertainty be more fully acknowledged. Only then can caregivers confront serious doubts about their sense of purpose, about the purpose of the endeavor itself, or even about the meaning of life itself, in a world so rife with suffering and injustice. Support can be crucial at this time, but a caregiver who emerges from this period with continued motivation will have a satisfying career, given minimally adequate working conditions.

Dysfunctional Responses

1. *Reactive anxiety and depression*: Dysfunctional responses can occur at any point in a staff member's career. They are usually associated with a precipitant such as the loss of a loved one, acute marital strife, or cancer in a family member. The caregiver experiences acute dysphoria reminiscent of the early adaptation stages, and may react with unexpected tearfulness, or uncharacteristic anger and resentment. These symptoms are usually transient, but available support can be needed, or a vacation, a leave, or a brief change of venue. Rarely is a permanent change necessary. The loss of "special" patients to whom the caregiver was emotionally attached may give rise to a milder form of the same reaction, or to an unexpected outburst of overt grief, when the attachment was unacknowledged.

2. *Psychiatric problems in staff*: Occasionally, an individual develops a clinical disorder, usually in the presence of a previous history or pre-existing vulnerability. Prompt referral is desirable, but well-meaning or intimidated co-workers will often protect their colleague. This response may be a facet of the qualities that make for empathic, supportive caregivers, but it is inappropriate and unhelpful in the long run.

INTERVENTIONS

Table 89.6 outlines a possible schema for organizing interventions.

Principles of Staff Selection

Beyond the usual wish-list—intelligence, competence, integrity, good interpersonal skills, energy, and reliability—there are few guidelines to insure that caregivers are well-suited to a kind of work whose demands cannot be understood a priori. Vachon's emphasis on the importance of assessing the individual's social network has been borne out by later work, but it may not be legal to explore this in some

TABLE 89.6. *Issues Related to Managed Care*

1. ALTERED WORK CONDITIONS
    a. Fewer jobs
    b. Harder work for less pay
    c. Loss of autonomy
    d. Insecurity

2. DOWNSIZING AND MERGING
    a. Turf issues
    b. In the lifeboat? Or each man for himself?

3. JOB REDEFINITION
    a. Adaptability
    b. Previous marginality exposed
    c. Age, gender, race, and cultural factors

4. SURVIVORS AND INTERLOPERS
    a. Problems of each
    b. Task of re-integration

5. PSYCHOLOGICAL RESPONSES
    a. Shared equally by facilitator, leader, and participants
    b. Danger of defeatist reverberations
    c. Speakable and unspeakable fears
    d. Ethical, professionalism, and self-esteem issues

jurisdictions (48). She also noted that staff self-select for previous experiences with death and cancer, although there are no formal data on the subject. Its presence does not predict success or failure, but it gives some clue to the emotional issues the individual will be facing.

Organizational Interventions

The second category pragmatically divides the environmental interventions that lie outside the power of unit leaders (and outside the scope of this discussion), from those within their sphere of autonomy. The distinction is not always obvious to a demoralized staff that feels hopeless, or an angry staff that believes their unit leader could fix it all, if s/he only tried hard enough. Developing a clear awareness in this area helps the unit leader defend against inappropriate projections and demands, and helps both leader and staff to identify what is feasible.

Table 89.7 outlines some of the areas in which the unit leader can play a significant role. The first five are standard measures that promote competence, self-esteem, and self-care. The next set, educational and career-enrichment opportunities, plays a large role in sustaining interest, and supporting the prevalent intellectualizing coping style.

Leadership traits which help staff maintain clear boundaries about work expectations *and* work limitations, assume special importance in the oncology setting. Helping unit leaders develop their own clarity in this arena, generally through one-on-one contact, is an efficient intervention. Setting realistic expectations includes keeping tasks reasonable and helping with priority setting in ambiguous situations. But it also refers to controlling the unstated expectations, the ill-defined humanitarian goals that emanate from the leader's own semi-conscious rescue fantasies which develop a life of their own in the unit's culture.

Modeling open communications is also important. Several studies have noted the positive effect of being able to express one's feelings, as might be expected from the isolation dynamics described above (49–51). It improves patient care and contains covert scapegoating or destructive norms. Being an interpreter and a buffer between the unit and the larger parent systems is very difficult, but a unit leader who is an honest interpreter will minimize the splitting and negative projections associated with an angry, passive, suspicious staff.

The team approach has several advantages. First and foremost, it results in better care, but it also promotes the use of social support, sustains group cohesion, encourages older staff to mentor younger ones, and, lastly, prevents any individual from becoming too indispensable.

TABLE 89.7. *Desirable Leadership Traits*

1. Good orientation procedures
2. Unambiguous work assignments
3. Clear lines of authority
4. Respect for time-off and vacations
5. Provision for positive feedback
6. Educational or career enrichment opportunities
7. Realistic expectations
    amount
    goals
8. Open communications about:
    work issues
    burnout issues
    interface with the larger system
9. Team approach
10. Encouragement of group cohesion
11. Leader self-awareness and self-control

Staff-based Interventions

There are several ways of conceptualizing staff-based interventions. Delvaux and Razavi (1988) (22) divide them into cognitive, behavioral, and emotional approaches. Lederberg has divided them into organizational, individual and group approaches (52–54). These schemata are complementary, one focused on the content, the other on the target of the intervention, but these distinctions are not always reflected in the literature.

Content. Cognitive approaches involve in-service teaching about human responses under stress, patient psychological responses and symptoms, through lectures or case presentations, allowing staff to improve their skills and learn something about their own reactions without personal exposure. Behavioral ones involve teaching anxiety management techniques, and occasionally some role play and rehearsal. Emotionally based interventions refer to experiential learning, and various forms of individual or group counseling and support, as in support groups, retreats, and workshops. When too removed from the work setting, they tend not to carry over to work, hence it is best to stay near the workplace. Some of the most fruitful techniques involve several categories at once, most particularly the workshops aimed at improving staff communication skills that are being widely pursued at this time. Razavi and Delvaux have reported on psychological training workshops that improve staff attitudes and feelings but may not be maintained beyond one year (55–57) in the absence of booster mechanisms. Roter and colleagues in the United States, and Faulkner, Maguire, and Fallowfield in the United Kingdom, and the psychosocial group in Hamburg, Germany, have used a range of approaches with caregivers in oncology (58–60). They have included interventions for individuals, small groups, and extensive retreats for interested staff. These efforts have often integrated teaching communication skills with self-awareness and stress management in a mix which shows great promise.

Target Population

1. *Individuals:* Individually based support can come from the unit leader or co-workers, but a more distant person is often required. This can be a psychiatric nurse clinician, social worker, consultation/liaison psychologist, or psychiatrist. The consultations should be rapid, flexible, and confidential, and, if necessary, lead to more formal evaluation and referral, discreetly and without stigmatization.

2. *Groups:* Group-based interventions, either free-standing or embedded in larger organizational programs are widely reported in the literature.

FREE-STANDING SUPPORT GROUPS. These are the earliest interventions, and have been reviewed by Lederberg (61) and by Moynihan and Outlaw (54). The first groups were often run by psychoanalytically oriented psychiatrists (62–63). When sensitive to the need for controlling group anxiety and preventing regression, they promoted group cohesion and increased psychological awareness. But failures were common, and can be better understood if one reviews the differences between therapy and support groups outlined in Table 89.8 and realizes how easy it is to overlook them. Weiner, Caldwell and Tyson (64) analyzed their experience with three nursing groups, two successes and one failure, pointing out the crucial effect of many environmental and cultural factors. Two developmental models of group development have been described. The Lederberg model will be described below. In 1983, Collins and Grobman (65), described a four-stage model of group development: during the first, the leader takes a didactic approach; during the second, group members take more responsibility for running the group, and began to share some personal responses to patients. During the third stage, the leader begins to teach about transference, but only in relation to patients, not within the group. Countertransference is the last concept to be introduced, and requires the most sensitivity given the leader's goal of avoiding personal disclosure. In the fourth stage, the staff moves from patient–staff material to staff–staff interactions. Only then do the authors call it a "nursing support group," and alter the contract to make it a closed group with much more explicit contracts about confidentiality and attendance. They give no indication of how often and under what conditions different groups proceed to the later stages.

There are many anecdotal reports of successfully run groups, including some which include enough practical details to be quite useful to the beginning leader. A few evaluations have been done, questionnaires using self-reports, burnout scores, sick call frequency, or the creation of buddy systems and intershift projects (62–63,66–70). One study that attempted more rigorous methods worked hard to design a good methodology, but gave disappointing results, giving some insight into the difficulty of the task (35). Nevertheless reports still appear and there is continuing interest in the modality.

TABLE 89.8. *Differences Between Therapy Groups and Support Groups*

Issue	Therapy Group	Support Group
1. Contact	yes	no
2. Payment	yes	no
3. Regular attendance	yes	no
4. Confidentiality	yes	no
5. Outside subgroup socializing	no	yes
6. Presenting complaints	yes	no
7. Personal psychological goals	yes	no
8. Therapeutic use of anxiety	yes	no
9. Areas of members' reactions and associations brought into play	all	only as work-related
10. Encouragement of member-to-member confrontation	yes	only occasionally, if at all
11. Interpretation of transference to leader	yes	no
12. Focus on outsiders and outside events	not without returning it to the group	yes—working through case material
13. Tolerance for regression	some	none
14. Leader stance a. activity b. transparency	less directive less	more direction—frequently channels group affect minimize anxiety, fantasy and intensity in the transference
15. Authenticity and reality checks	yes	yes

GROUPS EMBEDDED IN LARGER PROGRAMS. Given the extreme state of flux that exists in many health care systems at this time, it is not surprising that several programs have addressed broader issues. Only a few have been evaluated, but they, too, may be useful for individuals faced with the need to develop programs of their own (71–72).

PRACTICAL ISSUES IN RUNNING STAFF SUPPORT GROUPS

Given the continuing interest, there follows a practical description of support groups based on the Lederberg developmental model. It is a generic description and needs to be adapted to each setting.

Leadership requirements include sensitivity to systems issues and a good understanding of individual and group dynamics, coupled with the ability to restrain one's tendency to demonstrate all these skills. One must never forget that the small group is completely permeable to all the issues active in the parent group. Hence the group leader must learn about them if s/he is to understand the group, even if they are not to be confronted directly in the group. Any small group generates anxiety, and can lead to emotion-driven behaviors, hence the group leader must establish a climate of safety from the very beginning. Goals must be made clear, confidentiality and the boundaries of disclosure must be discussed, as well as the emphasis on work issues. Cognitive structure must be provided as

needed, and open-ended sharing must develop spontaneously, not by probing. It is best to honor a group's refusal about unit leader attendance. Groups in which the unit leader attends are less spontaneous, especially about authority and discipline, but the attendance demonstrates approval, promotes attendance and can result in more efficient translation of group insights into policy. Whether or not they attend, it is crucial to establish a good relationship with unit leaders, since members will respond to their underlying disapproval with disinterest and absenteeism.

The group may be described as a workshop, psychosocial rounds, interdisciplinary meeting. Pizza lunches or breakfast meetings are welcome. While this partly reflects leadership style, it also highlights the fact that in many situations, the staff feel so overworked and deprived that they will not readily attend extra meetings without some concrete gratification. The setting should be private yet convenient.

Timing is critical since it will dictate attendance of particular members or shifts, which may, in turn, accentuate certain problems if it is not well thought through. Weekly meetings may be desirable, but much useful work can be done in bimonthly meetings, or time-limited groups ranging from four to twelve weekly meetings. The time limit tends to relieve the anxiety of members who fear too much exposure or intimacy, and may help to focus the group. If desired, subsequent groups can be renegotiated at the end of the first one.

Keeping in mind that the issue of belonging is universally important, the group leader must make an individualized decision about whether to include different disciplines or shifts. For example, one should make sure that certain patterns of exclusion are not perpetuated by the group. Membership negotiations may be the early group agenda.

CONTENTS AND DYNAMICS OF STAFF SUPPORT GROUPS

Staff support groups with stable membership, if they are not too rigidly structured, go through developmental stages which recur in a cyclical way (52–54). (See Table 89.9.)

Early Stages of Group Dynamics

The early group complains about overwork, under staffing and problems with authority, co-workers and other disciplines, with much projection and externalization, and a sense of passivity and helplessness. Ventilation is welcome, but must be followed by further analysis of the emotionally loaded issues. This defuses the negative effect and often uncovers component parts that are amenable to intervention. Focusing on selected and achievable goals mitigates the sense of passivity.

Internalized doubts about treatment lead to guilt and lowered self-esteem. Externalized and projected ones create corrosive schisms between co-workers and contaminate many other issues. Groups are an excellent setting in which to develop more understanding of the professional and ethical beliefs that drive others and to discuss relevant institutional developments. They are also a place to let down and complain about difficult patients, to normalize unconscious responses, reinforce conscious ones, discourage scapegoating, and support realistic goals and norms.

Staff confrontations with death are a quasi-universal topic, in all group stages and at all levels of staff. The group can be an effective holding environment in which caregivers support and validate each other, around the grief, fear, and sense of inadequacy which can overwhelm them unpredictably in their demanding work lives.

Middle Stage of Group Dynamics

As a group meets over time, more trust is developed, and members bring up the "special" cases connected to personal experiences. The group leader must help the group acknowledge the universality of human emotions and prevent the member from feeling isolated by his/her openness, modeling if necessary. S/he must

TABLE 89.9. *Developmental Stages of Staff Support Groups*

EARLY STAGE

Overwork, hectic pace, understaffing, sense of exploitation

Conflicts among staff: intra shift or team, intershift or team

Conflicts between disciplines and services

Problems with authority

Treatment scruples

"Difficult" cases

Confrontations with death

MIDDLE STAGE

Less projection and scapegoating

More trust and introspection

"Special" patients

Questions of professional self-definition

Interest in personal style of coping and confrontation

LATE STAGE

High morale and cohesion

Ambivalent thrust toward deeper personal issues (the pseudo-therapy group)

Increased intensity and vulnerability

Increased anxiety and acting-out

Threat of disruption in the work place

The group disbands—or—returns to safer levels

also shield the member from overexposure when the group responds more intensely than the member can handle. When the unit leader is present, the members may cautiously confront, and the group leader must modulate the interaction and encourage a constructive outcome. The group members reflect on their professional identity and acknowledge their strengths and vulnerabilities. Interpersonal conflicts are less smothered in anger and blame, as protagonists recognize coping patterns in themselves and others, a stance associated with more tolerance.

Late Stage of Group Dynamics

Many of the middle stage concerns are very meaningful to the members and are on the boundary between work and personal issues. Members feel less isolated, less anxious, with better self-esteem and better communication. Unit morale is higher and patient care always benefits. In the group, the sense of intimacy may lead some members to feel anxious, while others want to blur the boundaries even further. The latter course is bound to fail because a more therapeutic focus brings more vulnerability, hence more anxiety, and usually some acting-out, none of which can be contained in the group under its existing (and necessary) ground rules. The threat of workplace disruption is unacceptable to all, hence the group self-destructs or returns to safer levels of discourse, thus accounting for the episodic, cyclical quality often described by leaders who have long experience. This also explains why some leaders choose to maintain a purely educational focus. The few members who insist on the emotive focus may approach the leader privately and be referred for treatment, since this thirst for emotional confrontation often reflects a broader psychological need.

Effects of Contemporary Changes on the Group

The acute dislocation of medical delivery has a powerful effect on both the group and the leader. Sharing the negative feelings is useful to a point, but the group leader must not let his/her own feelings lead to a defeatist climate. Personal fears are harder to share because they bring up questions about who will be fired, who will be transferred, who will remain, issues which create a tension between co-workers that the usual support group is not equipped to handle. When the dissolution of a unit is expected, plans may be made to absorb as many people as possible on other units, by not filling vacancies in the preceding months. The transfers come to a unit that has been covering their positions for some time, causing resentment and making it integration more difficult. Units appear to be composed of survivors and interlopers. In the group, these questions may be brought up and the feelings identified and discussed but as a general issue, modulating as always the degree of individual focus.

It has been observed that under these conditions, caregivers express a greater and greater need for continued training and for concrete stress management techniques, such as relaxation and hypnosis, and turn to less traditional methods such as "healing touch." They use these both for themselves and for their patients, who are also more stressed by their shorter hospital stays and more limited follow-up. The caregiver's need to work with grief and loss is being recognized with the development of memorial services and related educational programs around bereavement (73–75). Chaplaincy participation gives some staff members the unusual experience of receiving spiritual support in the work setting. Given that the dedication of many medical professionals has the intensity of a vocation independent of any religious affiliation, these new programs are very welcome, and this broader response to the health professional's humanity is long overdue. In association with the more traditional training programs currently under development, they will go a long way toward improving patient care.

SUMMARY

The psychological stresses on medical caregivers, particularly in the field of oncology, are being increasingly recognized and documented. As they have been better understood, they have given rise to an increasingly sophisticated and broad-based group of interventions. They include cognitive measures to improve competence and communication skills, and emotional ones in the form of group-based experiences geared to improving self-awareness, cohesiveness, and understanding of their own and their patients' psychological experiences. It is not unreasonable to expect that helping caregivers stay in touch with their own humanity is a sine qua non of expecting them to remain sensitive to the human experience of their patients.

REFERENCES

1. Siegler M. Falling off the pedestal: what is happening to the traditional doctor–patient relationship? *Mayo Clin Proc.* 1993; 68:461–467.
2. Miles SH. Physician-assisted suicide and the profession's gyrocompass. *Hastings Center Rep.* 25. 1995; 2(3):17–19.
3. Freudenberger HJ. Staff burnout. *J Soc Issues.* 1974; 30, 159–165.
4. Maslach C. The Burn-Out Syndrome and Patient Care. In: Garfield CA, ed. *Stress and Survival: The Emotional Realities of Life-Threatening Illness.* St. Louis, MO: C V Mosby, 1979: 111–120.
5. Fox RC. *The Human Condition of Health Professionals.* Distinguished Lecture Series, School of Health Studies, University of New Hampshire. Durham, NH: University of New Hampshire, 1980: 11–39.
6. McCue JD. The effects of stress on physicians and their medical practice. *N Engl J Med.* 1982; 306:458–463.
7. Starrin B, Lareson G, Styrborn S. A review and critique of psychological approaches to the burn-out phenomenon (Review). *Scand J Caring Sci.* 1990; 4(2):83–91. (Review)
8. Creagan ET. Stress among medical oncologists: the phenomenon of burnout and a call to action. *Mayo Clinic Proc.* 1993; 68:614–615.
9. Wilkinson CB. Aftermath of a disaster: the collapse of the Hyatt Regency Hotel skywalks. *Am J Psychiatry.* 1983; 140:1134–1139.
10. Vachon MLS, Lyall WAL, Freeman SJJ. Measurement and management of stress in health professionals working with advanced cancer patients. *Death Education.* 1978; 1:365–375.
11. Antonelli A, Silvano G, Bianchi F, et al. Risk of thyroid nodules in subjects occupationally exposed to radiation: a cross sectional study. *Occup Environ Med.* 1995; 52(8):500–504.
12. Matte TD, Mulinare J, Erickson, JD. Case control study of congenital defects and parental employment in health care. *Am J Indust Med.* 1993; 24(1):11–23.
13. Skov T, Maarup B, Olsen J, et al. Leukemia and reproductive outcome among nurses handling antineoplastic drugs. *Br J Indust Med.* 1992; 49(12):855–861.

14. Selevan S, Lindbohm ML, Hornung R, Hemminki K. A study of occupational exposure to antineoplastic drugs and fetal loss in nurses. *N Engl J Med.* 1985; 313: 1173–1178.

15. Babich H. Reproductive and carcinogenic health risks to hospital personnel from chemical exposure—a literature review. *J Environ Health.* 1985; 48:52–56.

16. Bingham E. Hazards to health workers from antineoplastic drugs. *N Engl J Med.* 1985: 1220–1221.

17. Geberding JL. Prophylaxis for occupational exposure to HIV (Review). *Ann Intern Med.* 1996; 125(6):497–501.

18. Dunlap NE, Kimerling ME. Drug resistant tuberculosis in adults: implications for the health care worker. *Infect Agents Dis.* 1994; 3(5):245–255.

19. Meredith S, Watson JM, Citron KM, et al. Are health-care workers in England and Walas at increased risk of tuberculosis? *BMJ.* 1996; 313(7056):522–525.

20. Jereb JA, Klevens RM, Privett TD, et al. Tuberculosis in health care workers at a hospital with an outbreak of multidrug resistant mycobacterium tuberculosis. *Arch Intern Med.* 1995; 155(8):854–859.

21. Brennan T. Transmission of the human immunodeficiency virus in the health care setting—time for action. *N Engl J Med.* 1990; 324:1504–1509.

22. Delvaux N, Razavi D, Farvacques C. Cancer care—a stress for health professionals. *Soc Sci Med.* 1988; 27:159–166.

23. Zevon MA, Donnelly JP, Starkey EA. Stress and coping in the medical environment: a natural experiment. *J Psychosoc Oncol.* 1990; 8:63–77.

24. van Servellen G, Leake B. Burn-out in hospital nurses: A comparison of acquired immunodeficiency syndrome, oncology, general medical, and intensive care unit nurse samples. *J Prof Nurs.* 1993; 9(3):169–177.

25. Barni S, Mondin R, Nazzani R, Archili C. Oncostress: evaluation of burnout in Lombardy. *Tumori.* 1996; 82:85–92.

26. Hershbach P. Work-related stress specific to physicians and nurses working with cancer patients. *J Psychosoc Oncol.* 1992; 10(2):79–99.

27. Ramirez AJ, Graham J, Richard MA, et al. Burnout and psychiatric disorder among cancer clinicians. *Breast J Cancer.* 1995; 71:1263–1269.

28. Ullrich A, FitzGerald P. Stress experienced by physicians and nurses in the cancer ward. *Soc Sci Med.* 1990; 31(9):1013–1022.

29. Whippen DA, Canellos GP. Burnout syndrome in the practice of oncology: results of a random survey of 1,000 oncologists. *J Clin Oncol.* 1991; 9(10):1916–1920.

30. Catalan J, Burgess A, Pergami A, et al. The psychological impact on staff of caring for people with serious diseases: the case of HIV infection and oncology. *J Psychosom Res.* 1996; 40(4): 425–435.

31. Bram PJ, Katz LF. A study of burnout in nurses working in hospice and hospital oncology settings. *ONF.* 1989; 16(4):555–560.

32. Beck-Friis B, Strang P, Sjoden PO. Caring for severely ill cancer patients. A comparison of working conditions in hospital-based home care and in hospital. *Support Care Cancer.* 1993; 1(3):145–151.

33. Woolley H, Stein A, Forrest GC, Baum JD. Staff stress and job satisfaction at a children's hospice. *Arch Dis Childhood.* 1989; 64:114–118.

34. Peteet JR, Murray-Ross D, Medeiros C, et al. Job stress and satisfaction among the staff members at a cancer center. *Cancer.* 1989; 64:975–982.

35. Gray-Toft P, Anderson JG. Organizational stress in the hospital: development of a model for diagnosis and prediction. *Health Ser Res.* 1985; 19:753–774.

36. Cronin-Stubbs D, Rooks CA. The stress, social support, and burnout of critical care nurses: the results of research. *Heart Lung.* 1985; 14:31–39.

37. White KL. Hospitals and health services enterprises as social systems. *Bull NY Acad Med.* 1996; 73:430–432.

38. Suchman AL, Roter DL, Green M, Lipkin M. Physician satisfaction with primary care office visits. *Med Care.* 1993; 31:1083–1092.

39. Ford S, Fallowfield LJ, Lewis S. Can oncologists detect distress in their out-patients and how satisfied are they with their performance during bad news consultations? *Breast J Cancer.* 1994; 70:767–770.

40. Tulsky JA, Chesney MA, Lo B. See one, do one, teach one? House staff experiences discussing do-not-resuscitate orders. *Arch Intern Med.* 1996; 156:1285–1289.

41. Lampic C, Nordin K, Sjoden PO. Agreement between cancer patients and their physicians in the assessment of patient anxiety at follow-up visits. *Psycho-Oncology.* 1995; 4:301–310.

42. McClung JA, Kramer RS, DeLuca M, Barber HJ. Evaluation of a medical ethics consultation service: opinions of patients and health care providers. *Am J Med.* 1996; 100:456–460

43. Morris BA, Van Niman SE, Perlin T, et al. Health care professionals' accuracy in predicting patients' preferred code status. *J Fam Practice.* 1995; 40:41–4.

44. Emanuel EJ, Emanuel LL. Proxy decision-making for incompetent patients: an empirical and ethical analysis. *JAMA.* 1992; 267:2067–2071.

45. Kern DE, Grayson M, Barker LR, et al. Residency training in interviewing skills and the psychosocial domain of medical practice. *J Gen Intern Med.* 1989; 4:421–431.

46. Sigurdardottir V, Bolund C, Nilson B. Quality of life and ethics: opinion about chemotherapy among patients with advanced melanoma, next-of-kin and care providers. *Psycho-Oncology.* 1995; 4(4):287–300.

47. Haberman MR, Germino BB, Maliski S, et al. What makes oncology nursing special? Walking the road together. *ONF.* 1994; 21(8):41–47.

48. Vachon, MLS. Motivation and stress experienced by staff working with terminally ill. *Death Education.* 1978; 2:113–l22.

49. Gaynor SE, Verdin JA, Bucko JP. Peer social support: a key to care giver morale and satisfaction. *J Nurs Adm.* 1995; 25(11):23–28.

50. Astrom G, Jansson L, Norberg A, Hallberg IR. Experienced nurses' narratives of their being in ethically difficult care situations. The problem to act in accordance with one's ethical reasoning and feelings. *Cancer Nurs.* 1993; 16(3):179–187.

51. Browner CH. Job stress and health: The role of social support at work. *Res Nurs Health.* 1987; 10:93–100.

52. Lederberg MS. Stresses on cancer staff: the uses of group to mitigate them. In: Holland JC, ed. *Current Concepts in Psychosocial Oncology.* New York, Robert Gold & Associates, 1982.

53. Lederberg, MS. Psychological problems of staff and their management. In Holland JC, Rowland JH, eds. *Handbook of Psycho-Oncology*. Oxford University Press, New York, 1989.

54. Lederberg M. Group support for medical staff in high-stress setting. In: Alonzo A, Swillel HI, eds. *Group Psychotherapy in Clinical Practice*. APA Press, Inc., 1993:171–183.

55. Razavi D, Delvaux N, Farvacques C. Cancer care—a stress for health professionals. *Soc Sci Med*. 1988; 27:159–166.

56. Razavi D, Delvaux N, Farvacques C, Robaye E. Brief psychological training for health care professionals dealing with cancer patients: a one-year assessment. *Gen Hosp Psychiatry*. 1991; 13:253–260.

57. Razavi D, Delvaux N, Marchal S, et al. The effects of a 24hr psychological training program on attitude, communication skills and occupational stress in oncology: a randomized study. *Eur J Cancer*. 1993; 29A(13):1858–1863.

58. Roter DL, Hall JA, Kern DE, et al. Improving physicians' interviewing skills and reducing patients' emotional distress: a randomized clinical trial. *Arch Intern Med*. 1995; 155:1877–1884.

59. Faulkner A, Argent F, Jones A, Keeffe CO. Improving the skills of doctors in giving distressing information. *Med Ed*. 1995; 29:303–307.

60. Fallowfield LJ. Communication skills of oncologists. *Forum: Trends in Experimental Medicine*. 1995; 5(1): 99–103.

61. Moynihan RT, Outlaw E. Nursing support groups in a cancer center. *J Psychosoc Oncol*. 1984; 2:33–47.

62. Mohl PC. A systems approach to liaison psychiatry. *Psychosomatics*. Jun, 1980; 21(6):457–61.

63. Eisendrath SJ. Psychiatric liaison support groups for general hospital staffs. *Psychosomatics*. 1981; 22:685–694.

64. Weiner MF, Caldwell T, Tyson J. Stresses and coping in ICU nursing: why suppress groups fail. *Gen Hosp Psychiatry*. 1983; 5:179–183.

65. Collins AH, Grobman J. Group methods in the general hospital setting. In: Kaplan HI, Sadock BJ, eds. *Comprehensive Group Psychotherapy*, 2nd ed. Baltimore, MD: Williams & Wilkins; 1983: 289–293.

66. Scully R. Staff support groups: helping nurses help themselves. *J Nursing Adm*. March, 1981; 81:48–51.

67. Hover D. Development of a hospice staff support group. *Am J Hospice Care*. Sept–Oct 1986: 39–41.

68. Silberfarb, PM, Levine PM. Psychosocial aspects of neoplastic disease: group support for the oncology nurse. *Gen Hosp Psychiatry*. 1980; 3:192–197.

69. Kunkler J, Whittick J. Stress-management groups for nurses: practical problems and possible solutions. *J Adv Nurs*. 1991; 16(2):172–6.

70. Guillory BA, Riggin OZ. *Clin Nurs Spec*. 1991; 5(3): 170–173.

71. Cull A. Staff support in medical oncology: a problem-solving approach. *Psychol Health*. 1991; 5:129–136.

72. Kash KM, Holland JC. Reducing stress in medical oncology house officers: a preliminary report of a prospective intervention study. In: Hendrie HD, Lloyd C, eds. *Educating Competent and Humane Physicians*. Bloomington, IN: Indiana University Press; 1990: 183–195.

73. Granger CE, George C, Shelly MP. The management of bereavement on intensive care units. *Intens Care Med*. 1995; 21(5):429–36.

74. Heiney SP, Hasan L, Price K. Children's Center for Cancer and Blood Disorders of Richland Memorial, Children's Hospital of Richland Memorial, Columbia, SC 29203. Developing and implementing a bereavement program for a children's hospital. *J Ped Nurs*. 1993; 8(6):385–391.

75. Anderson B, McCall E, Leversha A, Webster L. A review of children's dying in a pediatric intensive care unit. *NZ Med J*. 1994; 107(985):345–347.

90

Establishing a Psycho-oncology Unit in a Cancer Center

JIMMIE C. HOLLAND

The past two decades have seen a remarkable increase in interest in the "human" side of cancer: the psychological, social, behavioral, psychiatric, ethical, and spiritual dimensions. These aspects were often condensed in cancer under the term "psychosocial," and more recently, quality of life. It is of interest that though these issues are involved in the care of *every* patient by *every* oncology staff member, and in *every* encounter, they have received few resources and minimal support for developing a clinical and scientific base. The field of psycho-oncology, or psychosocial or behavioral oncology (as it is also called), has evolved in spite of this environment (1). The program at Memorial Sloan-Kettering, begun twenty years ago, has not only survived, but has expanded to include a large training and research program. In fact, the training program has produced many of the leaders of many developed programs. As such, it has served as a model for some to guide the development of psycho-oncology in a cancer center. As founder of the Memorial program in 1977, I am often asked to serve as consultant in advising about setting up a division in a cancer center, and to identify the components of a fledgling program that predict success or failure.

Provided below are suggested steps in establishing a unit, based largely on our own trials and errors and observations of the experience of others at other centers. Some of the principles are appropriate for establishing any new program in a larger administrative structure. Others, however, are related to the pitfalls to which psycho-oncology is particularly vulnerable, and to the barriers that are more apt to affect development of services in this area.

This is an unusually challenging time in which to establish a psycho-oncology unit in a cancer center. The crisis of economics-driven medicine bodes ominously for psychological care of patients which many would identify as a "luxury." Yet, the crisis is also occurring at the time when the concept of patient-centered care is becoming an accepted fact. The evaluation of health care will increasingly depend upon patients' own perceptions and their satisfaction with the care they receive. The evaluation of new cancer agents has already incorporated patient self-report of the impact of treatment on health-related quality of life (HRQL). Assessment of HRQL is an integral part of treatment outcome research today (2). Thus, this may be the best and the worst of times for psycho-oncology, providing both challenge and opportunity (3).

BACKGROUND FOR DEVELOPING A PROPOSED PSYCHO-ONCOLOGY UNIT

Developing a proposal should not be undertaken until several facts are clarified: Is the Director of the cancer center or oncology division supportive of the idea? Who is fiscally and administratively responsible for the development of the psycho-oncology unit? These two questions must be addressed before any efforts are undertaken toward developing a concrete proposal. Oncologists and administrators vary widely in their interest and enthusiasm for the psychological dimension of care. It is essential that a supportive person be present in the administrative structure who will assure fiscal support and parity in the table of organization and in budget planning. Without this in place, the development of a more definite plan should not be undertaken. However, with the presence of support by oncology, the steps outlined in Table 90.1 should be undertaken. Table 90.2 gives the outline for a proposal to form a new unit and the areas which should be included in a negotiation to establish a psycho-oncology unit. Table 90.3 outlines the barriers to development of

TABLE 90.1. *Steps in Developing a Psycho-Oncology Unit*

1. Develop a proposal containing mission, rationale, functions, table of organization, and staffing pattern

2. Recruitment of staff:
   Director
   Multidisciplinary staff

3. Recruitment of community resources
   Psychosocial
   Cancer-related

4. Plan to sustain morale
   Individual
   Group

5. Educational and research ties

6. Advocacy, ethical issues, and interface with oncologic specialties

TABLE 90.2. *Proposal*

A. Mission statement

B. Rationale
   1. Identified focus
   2. Central triage for clinical needs
   3. Central resources for teaching
   4. Nucleus for response to changing needs
   5. Focus of multi-center programs

C. Range of functions
   1. Clinical
   2. Training of medical staff
      Training of psycho-oncologists
   3. Clinical research

D. Table of organization

a unit and interventions which should be undertaken to overcome them.

STEP 1. DEVELOP A PROPOSAL CONTAINING THE RATIONALE FOR THE UNIT, ITS MISSION, FUNCTION, TABLE OF ORGANIZATION, AND THE MULTIDISCIPLINARY STAFF REQUIRED

Mission Statement

The mission statement is important since it states succinctly the thrust of the effort. It must convey the passion and enthusiasm in a short statement as to why a single integrated unit is important and how it will impact upon patients' quality of life and contribute to the overall humanistic approach and effectiveness of the center in providing clinical care.

Rationale

The rationale describes the need for the program, based on literature citations and experience. Justification for the integrated unit of psycho-oncology services should address several issues: (*1*) it will provide an identified focus and advocacy within the cancer center for psychosocial activities; (*2*) it will provide a single entity for receiving requests for consultations and services which can then refer them to the appropriate staff member or discipline, avoiding costly and inefficient use of staff; (*3*) it will provide a *central resource* to accept requests for teaching and training in the range of issues (e.g. doctor–patient communication, in-service training in psychological aspects of care of patients); (*4*) it will provide a nucleus for developing new programs and identifying needs and gaps in clin-

TABLE 90.3. *Barriers to Developing a Unit and Interventions to Overcome Them*

Barriers	Interventions
No clearly defined role in clinical care; potential for conflict is increased	Define a clinical role and demonstrate value in clinical care
Administrative lines may be blurred due to multidisciplinary team	Negotiate clear lines of reporting; table of organization
Staff of unit must represent several disciplines; interstaff tensions occur	Recruit team members who have a concept of a multidisciplinary unit
Conflict of new psycho-oncology unit staff with preexisting psychosocial staff giving psychosocial care	Define role as complementary to, not competitive with, existing psychosocial staff
Psychosocial issues may be devalued in planning (budget, space, expansion)	Assume a strong advocacy role for unit and quality of life issues
Morale may be difficult because of small staff, stress of patient care	Maintain morale with group cohesion, group/ individual support
Support for training may be absent, with a lack of potential for sustaining the unit staff through trainees who join the staff	Build training into the negotiations for the psycho-oncology unit
Support for research and inclusion of QOL measurement in outcome evaluation may be absent	Build research potential into initial negotiations for the unit
Psycho-oncology unit staff feel isolated from their parent disciplines	Develop ties in community to universities, and training sites (e.g. psychology, social work, nursing)

ical services; and, (5) it will constitute an identified unit which can accept requests for collaboration in research within the center.

Functions

The functions should firstly describe the expected range of psychosocial *clinical services* to be offered. Ideally, the unit should provide services not only to hospitalized but also to ambulatory patients since cancer care is increasingly being given in outpatient settings. Ideally, there should be continuity of psychosocial care by the same professional to patients, whether they are in the hospital or at home. In a large academic center where continuity of *medical care* may be compromised, this is particularly important. The services to be provided will need to be defined and the request for staff should be based on a thoughtful estimate of need, as well as the staff required and the space needed by them, in order to provide the services. As more care is given in the ambulatory clinics and offices and less in the hospital, the mental health professional(s) should be housed within the outpatient oncology space to assure informal, ready interaction with the oncology staff, and to better fulfill a liaison function.

The second function described in the plan should be the nature of *training and teaching* to be provided and the staff needed to provide it. This should have two dimensions: first, the training of oncology staff in psychological aspects of care, with emphasis on physicians and nurses; and second, the training of individuals in psycho-oncology per se (4). The latter activity provides an academic focus to clinical care which assures attention to supervision, group discussion of observations, and attention to relevant literature and scholarly pursuits. It also provides the potential to identify outstanding trainees for appointment to staff whose skills are known, who bring a background of experience within the center, and who are known to the oncologic staff.

The third area of function to be described should be a plan for *clinical research*. This might, initially, be a simple follow-up of clinical observations, or a collaboration with other cancer center investigators, or seeking a consultation about developing a formal research program. The psycho-oncology unit should include this function, especially in an academic center where multidisciplinary research is the mode.

Table of Organization

The plan should include a proposed table of organization that clearly defines the person to whom the director of the unit reports administratively. In addition, the

reporting pattern of the psycho-oncology unit staff should indicate that their primary responsibility for daily tasks is to the unit's director. This is important because most cancer centers have had little or no experience with such a unit. They do not understand the range of functions outlined above; the potential for misunderstanding is great.

The director should report in exactly the same manner as other departments: to the director of the cancer center. The multidisciplinary staff will represent the range of disciplines, each of which may be represented already by separate departments in the institutions (e.g., nursing, social work). The staff must report to the director of psycho-oncology for their clinical work and research. They will need dual reporting to the department of their own discipline for purposes of academic and career development and identification with colleagues of like background.

Inter-Institutional Role

It is important that the director and the psych-oncology unit staff convey at the outset that their activities will be complementary to, and not competitive with, other existing psychosocial services. The new psycho-oncology unit is vulnerable to interstaff conflicts which arise because of the overlap of counseling and psychotherapeutic services offered by nursing, social work, psychology, psychiatry, and chaplaincy. While each brings a different perspective, collectively they have a "core" of support services that overlap. Attention to screening of patients by a central mechanism and triage of patients to the right discipline for help can be a useful activity in which the multidisciplinary psycho-oncology unit can be helpful, since the unit should represent all disciplines. A task force or council within an institution would be useful to guide in the delivery of psychosocial care. Attention to this issue early on can prevent serious and long-term conflicts about "turf" which can potentially hamper the development of the unit. Consultation and planning with existing staff providing similar services can prevent awkward and trying situations.

STEP 2. RECRUITING STAFF

First, the choice of the director for the psycho-oncology unit is critical. In terms of professional background, thus far, directors have largely come from the mental health disciplines of psychology and psychiatry. They have usually had experience or (more recently) actual training in psycho-oncology. A background in mental health is helpful, but persons from nursing or social work, the other disciplines usually represented, can be equally effective and should be equally considered. The second point related to qualifications is more personal: (*1*) the candidate must be able to forcefully represent and advocate for the unit within the administrative structure of the cancer center; (*2*) the candidate must have sufficient qualifications to command respect from those in oncology and in mental health for clinical and/or research areas; and, (*3*) the person must have an acute awareness of the multidisciplinary nature of psycho-oncology, being able to represent all disciplines in a fair and unbiased manner.

The recruitment of staff members is important after the director is chosen. The psycho-oncology group should have representation from the mental health disciplines (psychology and psychiatry), and from nursing, social work, and clergy. Volunteers should be included in the staff itself, or they should be available as an affiliated group. Any professional recruited should have had experience or training in psycho-oncology, beyond the basic training of their discipline or specialty. However, again, the personal qualities of full commitment to multidisciplinary approach is essential. The potential for conflict is great between members of the psycho-oncology unit staff, since there is an overlap in skills and expertise. Roles and job descriptions must be defined at the outset, since some functions, such as counseling and psychotherapy, are conducted by all the disciplines. The overlap in function, along with recognition of the unique skills and function of each discipline, must be acknowledged. Clinical case conferences can be used to clarify the staff member best suited to be assigned particular types of cases. Special expertise for specific areas will develop in the group and serve, over time, to develop a range of services (e.g. sexual or grief counseling). Since the division of clinical tasks is poorly defined in social and psychological areas, without careful attention, conflicts will arise, often to the detriment and limitation of the unit's effectiveness.

With limited resources, the staff will likely be composed of one or two full-time members and the rest will be part-time, due to economic constraints. The important issue is to have all disciplines represented, at least as consultants. A psychiatrist is needed particularly to advise about serious psychiatric disorders, suicidal risk, and psychopharmacological interventions. Similarly, clergy or chaplains should be either part of the unit or available on a consultative basis to the unit. Today, nurses and social workers with training in psychiatry or psycho-oncology often constitute a key part of full-time staff.

STEP 3. RECRUITMENT OF COMMUNITY RESOURCES AND ORGANIZATIONS

The psycho-oncology unit staff often serves as an important liaison to cancer support organizations and psychological support services in the community. It also often is the locus within the center for information about community services. The director and staff should seek ties to these organizations, requesting the participation of representatives to seminars and educational activities. Clinical case conferences, discussion of research studies, and shared review of pertinent literature are all activities that can be enriched by participation from the community. This activity can serve well in bringing together information about the range of resources in the community, providing an updating mechanism, and assuring that information is gathered from all disciplines in the community as identified by the multidisciplinary staff.

STEP 4. PLAN TO SUSTAIN MORALE

Often, psycho-oncologists feel professionally isolated since they represent a small group in a cancer center whose mission and background is quite different from the majority of the psycho-oncology staff. Often, oncology staff members do not understand the role of psycho-oncology in the center, nor are they familiar with the methods of clinical or research work, or the background information and literature on which they are based. This leads at times to the devaluing of psycho-oncology, based on unfamiliarity with the area, and the common persisting stigma that exists around psychological and emotional areas. These negative attitudes may cause the psycho-oncologist to feel defensive. The initial steps taken by the psycho-oncology unit staff are critically important (5). They must concentrate on showing a willingness to learn the problems faced by oncologists and participate in the activities of the medical staff by being a part of clinical ward rounds, outpatient clinics and discussions of patients in clinical and research conferences. Learning the nurses' problems and attending their conferences, as well as social work and multidisciplinary rounds, makes for a collegial relationship. The stance should be "I've come to learn about your work and your patients," not "I've come to teach you about psychosocial issues." The teaching role will evolve only after the person has proven him or herself by being helpful in the management of a few patients which proves credibility to a sometimes skeptical staff. After the "initiation," the psychosocial professional becomes one of the team.

Indeed, it is better not to expect "too much too soon." Prejudicial views of some medical staff require lengthy education and psycho-oncology staff must be cautioned to expect slow progress in being accepted as an equal discipline. It is important that the staff have ample opportunity to discuss the distress of feeling underaccepted. Persons who do consultation–liaison psychiatry often describe the need for a particularly resilient personality to be able to tolerate the stresses of poor appreciation at times by staff and also by patients who may not have wanted to be seen in consultation. In addition, the clinical work is at times stressful since it requires the person to empathize with patients and situations in which they must come to grips repeatedly with threatened and actual loss (see Chapter 60). Staff members being recruited should be queried about their experience and perceived ability to handle these stresses. Importantly, they should have ample opportunity for discussion of cases with a supervisor from the senior staff who has a thorough knowledge of clinical issues in care of cancer patients. The potential for distress is great, especially when interactions with a patient bring up prior personal issues. For these reasons, psychological support for the group must be planned from the beginning, provided by a skilled person in both individual and group support in a medical setting (see Chapter 89).

STEP 5. ARRANGING OF EDUCATIONAL AND RESEARCH TIES

It will advantageous to develop ties to the local training programs in medicine, nursing, psychology, social work, and chaplaincy so that interaction with them is an integral part of the unit's philosophy and activity. These ties are intellectually stimulating and they provide a source of young individuals for training and opportunities for research collaborations. For example, schools of nursing often have master's programs in psychiatric nursing, whose students may be interested in psycho-oncology. Social work doctoral students and those in psychology graduate programs may choose to pursue psychosocial issues in oncology. Theological seminaries welcome the opportunity for their students to learn pastoral care issues in an oncology setting.

STEP 6. ADVOCACY, ETHICAL ISSUES, AND INTERFACE WITH ONCOLOGIC SPECIALTIES

Within the cancer center, the psycho-oncology unit should be viewed as the advocate of patient-centered care. Its mission is to pursue maximal quality of life for all patients at all stages of illness. Advocacy and concern may lead some members of the unit to develop an interest in the management of ethical conflicts in the center through serving on an Ethics Committee. Conflicts between staff, families, and patients often present a range of issues which may represent cultural or social problems, but they may also have religious, psychological, or psychiatric origins. Lederberg has written about the difficulties in separating the ethical issues from these common problems seen in patients or families (6) (see Chapter 98)

Likewise, interface with the chaplaincy and community clergy should be active since, especially in end-of-life care, religious, spiritual, and psychological issues are often intertwined. Palliative care staff and those in pain management are apt to share patient problems with psycho-oncology staff, leading to a need for joint conferences and interactions.

Cancer prevention, early detection, and compliance are areas in which behaviors and psychological issues are important. Interface with cancer control and epidemiology units must be developed. Programs to alter lifestyles in relation to smoking, alcohol, sun exposures, and diet depend heavily on behavioral intervention for their success. Clinics offering help for smoking cessation are often part of the outpatient services of a psycho-oncology unit.

The clinical oncology disciplines of surgery, radiation, and medical oncology, all involved in active treatment aimed at cure, contain colleagues with whom an alliance must be developed. Trust and mutual respect usually develop through the interactions on shared clinical rounds and in combined conferences (7). These opportunities provide a way for the oncology staff to come to know the psycho-oncology consultant as colleague. It is helpful to encourage this direction by having one staff member serve as liaison to a particular staff or unit. This promotes the mental health professional learning the particular clinical problems which that staff faces and the social environment of the unit, including the personalities of key individuals and the administrative structure. It also allows the medical staff to become familiar with one individual's style and to feel comfortable discussing emotional problems with that person. There is less reluctance on the part of an oncologist in requesting a psychiatric consultation when the consultant is someone who is well known to the individual. Requests for help with particular patients occur more often when a personal as well as a professional relationship has been established.

SUMMARY

Thoughtful attention must be given to developing a proposal to establish a psycho-oncology unit which outlines its rationale, its mission, functions, staffing, and table of organization (8,9). Recruitment of staff must involve assessment of professional and personal qualifications to integrate well in a multidisciplinary unit. Sustaining of high morale, interface with other units of the cancer center, community organizations, and volunteer groups are equally important issues to the development and sustaining of an effective team.

REFERENCES

1. Holland JC. Psycho-oncology: overview, obstacle and opportunities. *Psycho-Oncology*. 1992; 1:1–13.
2. Kornblith A, Holland JC. Model for quality of life research from the cancer and leukemia Group B experience: the telephone interview, conceptual approach to measurement and theoretical framework. *J Nat Cancer Inst Monogr*. 1996; 20:55–62.
3. Holland JC. Psycho-oncology in the new millennium. *Int Med* . 1995; 2:255–257.
4. Die Trill M, Holland, JC. A model curriculum for training in psycho-oncology. *Psycho-Oncology*. 995; 4:169–182.
5. Lederberg M. Psychological problems of staff and their management. In: *Handbook of Psycho-Oncology*, JC Holland and JH Rowland (eds.), pp. 631–646. Oxford University Press, 1989.
6. Lederberg M. The interface of psychiatry, the law, and ethics. In: *Handbook of Psycho-Oncology*, JC Holland and JH Rowland (eds.), pp. 694–702. Oxford University Press, 1989.
7. Holland JC. Stress on mental health professionals. In: *Handbook of Psycho-Oncology*, JC Holland and JH Rowland (eds.), pp. 678–682. Oxford University Press, 1989.
8. Heiney SP, Dunaway NC, Slade M, et al. Planning and organizing a multidisciplinary psychosocial oncology service. *Cancer Practice*. 1995; 3(6):343–350.
9. Zabora JR, Loscalzo MJ. Comprehensive psychosocial programs: a prospective model of care. *Oncol Issues*. 1996; 1:14–18.

91

Training Psychiatrists and Psychologists in Psycho-oncology

STEVEN D. PASSIK, CHARLES V. FORD, AND MARY JANE MASSIE

The past twenty years has seen emerging interest in the psychological dimensions of cancer from both clinical and research perspectives (see Chapter 90). Contributions have come from many disciplines, though psychology and psychiatry have made seminal contributions to the field, and have been central to its development. As in any new area, training issues become apparent only after the new field is somewhat established. Psycho-oncology itself is less than twenty years old, and psychologists and psychiatrists who helped to establish the field brought diverse backgrounds to the area, which had no core of shared knowledge in the beginning. However, sufficient information has developed in the past ten years, and clinical experience in cancer centers has grown so that one can begin to outline what a person entering the field should learn and what their training experiences should be. It is likely that psychologists and psychiatrists will continue to carry a heavy burden of the research and clinical care in psycho-oncology and in helping in training other disciplines. For these reasons, this chapter is devoted to outlining the key issues in training of these two disciplines. Overriding all training, however, is the requirement in psycho-oncologic work, that a trainee learn from the beginning the critical need to respect all other disciplines and their work, and to be able to work collaboratively with other disciplines (see Chapter 90).

The largest psycho-oncology training program in the United States was established in 1977 at Memorial Sloan-Kettering Cancer Center (MSKCC). This two-year program, which prepares both psychiatrists and psychologists for academic careers, is approved by the Academy of Psychosomatic Medicine and has been viewed as a model training program in psycho-oncology. Over the past 19 years, this service has had a significant role in defining and developing the sub-specialty of psycho-oncology. Graduates of this training program have developed psycho-oncology training programs in the U.S. and internationally. Many of the observations described here are derived from this experience.

APPLICANT VARIABILITY

One of the challenges for psycho-oncology training programs is accommodating trainees with variable past experiences. As a rule, post-residency psychiatrists have less intragroup variability in past training than do psychologists. However, there are large differences in the consultation–liaison experience of residents from different programs (e.g., based on settings, exposure to oncology patients, length of rotation), which lead to the need to evaluate their level of expertise.

Psychologists often have had a widely varied training experience, holding either a Ph.D. in Clinical or Health Psychology or a Doctorate in Psychology. Psychology graduate schools vary tremendously in philosophy (psychodynamic *vs.* cognitive behavioral) and the amount of didactic course work that they offer in the area of behavioral medicine. To further complicate the situation, psychology internship training varies in length and in the amount of interaction with medically ill populations, including oncology patients (1). Special "remediation" is required in some settings to help applicants of varying backgrounds begin their training in psycho-oncology. A "core" course involving basic information at the beginning of a training year is an effective way to provide all with a singular knowledge base.

LACK OF STANDARDIZATION OF PSYCHO-ONCOLOGY PROGRAMS

Basic components of a curriculum in psycho-oncology have been reported (2–5). However, there is as yet no consensus or standardization of what constitutes a curriculum or clinical training as a psycho-oncologist. There are basic issues, such as minimum amount of time spent in psycho-oncology training, content of the training program, and credentialing that are just now under discussion. The following sections discuss the goals, curriculum, and evaluation components of psycho-oncology training for psychologists and psychiatrists.

GOALS

The broad goals of training in psycho-oncology are to teach clinical skills, fundamentals of research in psycho-oncology, and the necessary communication and administrative skills to foster professional growth and to help advance the field. Table 91.1 outlines the goals of psycho-oncology training for psychiatrists and psychologists. They fall into several categories: clinical (to be able to carry out a comprehensive psychiatric evaluation on cancer patients; appropriately apply a range of psychiatric interventions for cancer patients; work

effectively in a liaison role), research and communication (communicate psycho-oncology information to others; be able to critically evaluate and understand and/or conduct research in psycho-oncology) and administrative (learn organizational and administrative skills needed to administer a psycho-oncology program).

Clinically, graduates of psycho-oncology programs must be able to recognize common psychiatric syndromes and disorders in cancer patients and distress; must be aware of cancer-site and treatment-specific psychiatric problems. They must also know when and how to apply interventions to appropriate situations. These interventions include individual, family, group, dynamic, supportive, crisis intervention, sexual, bereavement counseling and cognitive behavioral forms of psychotherapy and psychopharmacology (both M.D.s and Ph.D.s need to know the indications for the use of medications and the ways medications affect cancer patients); Ph.D.s need to learn how to interact meaningfully with psychiatric medical backup, non-psychiatric physicians and nurses.

In addition, psycho-oncologists must have a basic knowledge of cancer sites, treatment, and the clinical course of cancer of different sites. Within the liaison role, they must be able to provide support to oncology

TABLE 91.1. *Goals of Psycho-oncology Training*

Graduates of training programs should be able to:

1. Carry out comprehensive psychiatric evaluations of cancer patients
   recognize common psychiatric syndromes, disorders, distress
   be aware of cancer-site and treatment-specific psychiatric problems

2. Appropriately apply a range of psychiatric interventions for cancer patients
   psychotherapy
   individual, family, group
   dynamic, supportive, crisis intervention, sexual, bereavement, cognitive-behavioral
   psychopharmacology
   M.D./Ph.D. – indications for medications and ways medications affect cancer patients
   Ph.D. – interact meaningfully with psychiatric medical backup, oncologists, nurses

3. Work effectively in a liaison role
   provide support to oncology staff
   facilitate the understanding of patient and families by oncology staff members
   know ins and outs of specific cancers

4. Communicate psycho-oncology information to others
   write clinically based or research-oriented scholarly papers
   teach medical students, psychiatric interns, residents
   oral presentation

5. Be able to critically evaluate and understand and/or conduct research in psycho-oncology

6. Learn organizational and administrative skills needed to administer a psycho-oncology program

---

staff; facilitate the understanding of patients and families by oncology staff; and know some of the facts about prognosis, treatment and side effects of specific cancers. Psycho-oncologists need to be skilled in communication with members of other disciplines and with one another. Graduates of training programs must develop their skills in writing clinically based or research-oriented scholarly papers, teaching medical students, psychology interns, and psychiatry residents, and in oral presentation. Finally, the further growth of psycho-oncology as a discipline necessitates that graduates of training programs be able to critically evaluate and understand and/or conduct research in psycho-oncology and must learn organizational and administrative skills which are needed to administer a psycho-oncology program.

DIDACTIC CURRICULUM AND TRAINING

Apart from direct clinical and research experience, psycho-oncology training for psychiatrists and psychologists necessitates extensive didactic course work. (See Table 91.2.) Such courses should necessarily include an introductory or "core" course that covers basic areas within psycho-oncology, such as depression, anxiety, organic mental disorders, adjustment disorders, normal reactions to the stress of cancer, substance abuse, management of emergencies, and suicidal patients. Offering an introductory course at the beginning of training provides basic knowledge to the trainees and contains the anxiety of trainees.

An academic conference, such as a grand rounds, helps trainees and faculty to keep abreast of recent developments in the field of psycho-oncology, consultation–liaison (C-L) psychiatry, and behavioral medicine and psychiatry in general. If the C-L service is part of a larger department of psychiatry, trainees should attend departmental grand rounds. By featuring visiting speakers when possible, trainees can be exposed to differing viewpoints on relevant topics. Faculty should assure that areas, such as cancer medicine, epidemiology, psycho-neuroimmunology and behavioral medicine are covered by speakers from these disciplines.

Another important aspect of the didactic curriculum is clinically oriented rounds. The format of such rounds may be case conferences, professors' rounds, and ongoing psychotherapy seminars. A favorite of trainees at MSKCC has been "a counter-transference rounds" in which emotional reactions to working with cancer patients are explored.

Another format is short specialty conferences that cover a wide range of issues, including pain, bereavement, palliative care, cross-cultural psychiatry, pediatric issues, family issues, psycho-neuro immunology, spirituality, research methods, writing, genetics, prevention and early detection of cancer. Finally, trainees should be encouraged to pursue areas of research or articles of special interest in trainee-run journal clubs.

Table 91.3 shows the suggested timing of emphasis in several areas of training. Clinically, the broadest exposure should be sought early on under circumstances that can be closely supervised. The inpatient oncology setting is ideal for this purpose and affords opportunities to learn about a broad range of psychiatric syndromes (especially organic mental syndromes and issues related to advanced illness). Subsequently, the balance can begin to shift to the addition of ambulatory patients and the conduct of outpatient psychotherapy groups. Once the trainee has mastered the basic aspects of consultation work, guidance by the trainee's mentor should be toward the development of an ongoing liaison to a specific clinical group.

TABLE 91.2. *Forums in Which to Deliver Good Training in Psycho-oncology*

Introductory ("core") course	Acclimate/contain anxiety (basic training)
Grand rounds	Visiting speakers
in psycho-oncology	Updates on topics relevant to cancer
in psychiatry/psychology	Epidemiology, psycho-oncology, C-L in general
in oncology/palliative care/rehabilitation/cancer prevention and control	
Clinically oriented rounds (case conferences, professors rounds, psychotherapy seminars)	
Specialty conferences	Pain, bereavement, palliative care, cross-cultural psychiatry, psychoneuroimmunology, spirituality, research methods, writing, genetics, cancer prevention, early detection, pediatric/family rounds
Journal club	

TABLE 91.3. *Suggested Timing of Emphasis in Training*

Clinical liaison and clinical specialty	Inpatients	Outpatients	Group therapy
Didactic core curriculum	Clinical conferences	Ongoing seminars	Specialty seminars
Supervision	Observed interviews	Traditional supervision work rounds	Discussion of how to supervise site rounds
Academic	Mentoring/teaching medical students	Scholarly writing and presenting	Research assistantships
→ Time			

Table 91.3 also suggests the timing of supervisory modes to help provide close monitoring and support of the trainee early in the process and greater autonomy later in training. The goal is to prepare the graduating trainee to assume the role of supervisor in the future.

The development of the trainees' academic identity and abilities might begin with mentoring medical students and other junior staff and gradually progresses through scholarly writing and presentation of research and apprenticeship and, perhaps ultimately, independent research.[1]

FACULTY

Psycho-oncology faculty members should have extensive experience with the multi-disciplinary approach to cancer care. They should have in-depth clinical experience with cancer patients and their families and have knowledge of the principles related to the medical, psychiatric, and psychological care of the cancer patient. Having faculty with extensive experience in direct patient care has been found critical in the acceptance of the training program by medical staff (6). Psycho-oncology faculty members should have extensive consultation–liaison and/or behavioral medicine experience, a commitment to teaching and training or the knowledge and skills required to carry out research projects in psychosocial oncology. Since psychiatrists and psychologists will be trained, faculty members should be of both of these disciplines. Role-model mentoring by each discipline and cross-fertilization by full-time faculty and part-time volunteer supervising faculty is important. They have expertise in analytically oriented psychotherapy, group therapy, psychopharmacology, behavioral interventions, child psychology/psychiatry, research design and methodology, psychiatric disorders of cancer patients (delirium, pain), ethics, or supportive and palliative care; many

have overlapping areas of expertise. Teaching and training efforts by faculty and trainee expertise, as well as interests and needs of both, should be considered when making supervisory assignments. Under the direction of the training director, a training committee which has as its goals selecting and monitoring the progress of the trainees helps foster their career interests.

EVALUATION

The periodic evaluation of the curriculum, trainees, and faculty should be an integral part of the training program. Every six months supervisors should complete written evaluations of fellows; and fellows meet with their supervisors, the Director of Training and the Service Chief to discuss their performance and curriculum for the next six months.

TRAINING

In some institutions, organizational structure, departmental philosophies, and prejudices preclude combined training of M.D.s (psychiatric physicians, medical oncologists) and Ph.D.s. Professional society and intra-institutional battles lead to the development of separate training tracks for students of psychiatry and psychology. Psychological testing, developmental psychology, behavioral techniques and cognitive psychology have been viewed as the purview of the Ph.D.; the psychiatrist had sole responsibility to monitor patients' medical progress and prescribe drugs. In oncology, it has been easier to avoid the conflicts and maintain training together to the benefit of both groups.

From its inception, the MSKCC program has trained medical students, psychiatry residents and fellows, psychology interns, post-doctoral psychologists, and a few internists and medical oncologists. A goal of the program was to provide opportunities for M.D.s to acquire clinical and basic research skills in psycho-oncology. For non-psychiatrists, they must acquire

---

1. At MSKCC we have a clinical and a research training track. In the research track, the vast majority of the time spent is in research activity.

knowledge of the complexities of the medical complications of individuals with cancer and the interdisciplinary cooperation necessary to serve their mental health needs. The "cross-pollination" that has resulted has led to the mutual enhancement of trainees from all backgrounds. A blurring of boundaries of professional roles was neither a goal nor a result of the training. Rather, individuals from different disciplines have been able to expand their knowledge base about medicine, behavioral medicine, oncology, psychiatry and psychology, and to learn how combining professional "strengths" and approaches in a service can lead to opportunities for novel research and clinical program development.

Many in the field of psycho-oncology recognize that the psychosocial needs of patients are so vast that the need for collaboration is great and there is less potential for interdisciplinary conflict than other areas of mental health care (see Chapter 90).

FUTURE ISSUES

The Interface of Psycho-oncology and Palliative Care

An accepted discipline in Canada, Europe, and elsewhere, palliative medicine has a large psychiatric and psychosocial component. A future challenge for psycho-oncology educators may be that of training highly medically knowledgeable individuals from palliative care backgrounds who nonetheless lack formal training in psychiatric consultation, psychotherapy, and therapeutic process. Considerable changes in core curriculum will be required to meet the training needs of this growing group of physicians that are likely to seek fellowships in psycho-oncology.

Many psycho-oncologists have already begun the process of academic collaboration with hospice physicians and others in the field of palliative medicine (7). The potential of training psychologists and psychiatrists alongside these physicians (many of whom are from Canada, Australia, and the United Kingdom and bring a cross-cultural dimension) is the enhancement of psycho-oncologists' abilities in the area of symptom management. The potential benefit is worth the effort in tailoring our programs to meet the needs of these trainees.

The Shift of Care of Cancer Patients to Ambulatory Care Settings

The care of oncology patients is shifting rapidly to ambulatory care settings due to multiple advances in the control of cancer treatment side effects. And the emphasis is on cost-saving. The training of psycho-

logists and psychiatrists in psycho-oncology will require the imparting of skills suited increasingly to the ambulatory setting. Considerable challenges exist in the areas of the development of group and other ambulatory programs and the ability to work along with those who provide home care. Many such programs will likely be geared toward health promotion (smoking cessation, exercise, nutritional counseling) and the patient populations that are not in need of more traditional types of psychiatric consultation.

Health Behaviors and Prevention

An equally strong element as palliative care is the importance of mental health professionals in changing health behaviors. Psycho-oncologists have led the way in smoking cessation research and behavioral issues in health. Psycho-oncologists will need in the future to be able to carry out behavioral interventions not only for symptom control, but for cancer preventative behaviors involving smoking, alcohol use, and sexual practices which are associated with cancer risk. The preventable cancer agenda has grown as part of the Healthy People 2000 initiative. It will likely continue to grow and the psycho-oncologist of the future should be at the forefront of behavioral science research and application.

The Changing Health Care Environment

The economic realities that confront psycho-oncologists in the 1990s have already begun to force changes in the ways in which psychologists and psychiatrists are trained. Graduates of psychology internships and psychiatry residencies have accumulated significant debt and are unable to entertain the possibility of continuing as trainees for prolonged periods of time (i.e., 1–2 years). This may force psycho-oncology education to be completed in a shorter period of time. Fewer medical school graduates are choosing psychiatry as a medical specialty, and this is likely to cause shortages of psychiatrists that can be recruited into psycho-oncology.

Another repercussion of changes in the health care environment is the mandate issued by third-party payers to reduce cost and demonstrate cost efficiency of services. Psychiatrists and psychologists entering the field of psycho-oncology will require training in research methodologies that will allow them to meet this challenge and assure the continuation of psycho-oncology as a discipline.

REFERENCES

1. Jellineck MS, Die-Trill M, Passik S, et al. The need for multi-disciplinary training in counseling the medically ill. *Gen Hosp Psychiary.* 1992; 14s:3s–10s.
2. Die-Trill M, Holland JC. A Model curriculum for training in psycho-oncology. *Psycho-Oncology.* 1995; 4:169–182.
3. Marin RS, Foster JR, Ford CV, et al. A curriculum for education in geriatric psychiatry. *Am J Psychiatry.* 1988; 145(7):836–843.
4. Pollin IS, and Attendees, Linda Pollin Foundation/NIHM Workshop. Model curriculum in medical crisis counseling. *Gen Hosp Psychiatry.* 1992; 14s:11s–27s.
5. Razavi D, Delvaux N, Farvacques C, et al. Brief psychological training for health care professionals dealing with cancer patients: A one-year assessment. *Gen Hosp Psychiatry.* 1991; 13:253–260.
6. Rainey LC, Wellisch DK, Fawzy Fl, et al. Training health professionals in psychosocial aspects of cancer: A continuing education model. *J Psychosoc Oncol.* 1983; 1(2):41–60.
7. Breitbart W, Passik S. Psychiatric aspects of palliative care. In: Doyle D, Hanks G, McDonald N (eds.), *Oxford Textbook of Palliative Medicine.* New York: Oxford University Press, 1993: 607–626.

92

Principles of Training Social Workers in Oncology

ELIZABETH D. SMITH, KATHERINE WALSH-BURKE, AND
CHRIS CRUSAN

The complexity and variability of psychosocial issues associated with cancer has created the demand for highly skilled practitioners who are trained to provide multilevel assessment and intervention throughtout the illness continuum. Oncology social workers are primary providers of psychosocial services in major oncology treatment centers and community health care settings throughout the world, both because of their knowledge about cancer and its psychosocial impact, and because of their practice versatility. Oncology social workers are trained in prevention, education, advocacy, research, and counseling. Their role has evolved to a central role in oncology care for several reasons.

1. Social work was established early in the 20th century as an essential component of the interdisciplinary health care team when Ida Canon became the first hospital social worker at Massachusetts General Hospital in Boston in 1919. The hospital social work role was initiated as it was recognized that "the sources of illness are not exclusively biological; disease onset and recovery and resumption of function are influenced by social forces . . . Integration of social work in medical care shifts the emphasis away from an exclusively biologic to a biopsychosocial model in which the patient is viewed as an individual with a personal, not only medical, history; with human strengths and frailties and with obligations, responsibilities, and preferences." (1)

In the seventy years succeeding the initiation of medical social work, oncology social workers have practiced in outpatient as well as inpatient health care settings, public and private social service agencies, and community organizations (such as the American Cancer Society and Leukemia Society) which provide service to a wide spectrum of people affected by cancer.

This experience, and the empirical study of this work, has enabled social workers to accumulate a vast body of knowledge about the interactions of people with cancer in their environments. As a member of the interdisciplinary team, the oncology social worker focuses on the psychosocial effects of cancer and cancer treatment as well as the effectiveness of various coping strategies of individuals, families and groups. Oncology social workers also intervene with other oncology professionals who experience significant levels of stress in providing care to this population (2–4).

2. The biopsychosocial model of social work practice necessitates broad exposure in social work training to the variety and breadth of biopsychosocial theories that social workers incorporate into their practice. This ecological perspective uniquely equips the social worker to both assess and intervene to assist patients and families with the multiple effects of cancer. The person-in-environment ecological framework of social work (5) clearly emphasizes both psychological and sociological theories which prepare the social worker to design and implement interventions aimed at simultaneously strengthening individual adaptation and strengthening environmental responsiveness to the needs of persons affected by cancer (6–7). The theoretical models introduced in Master of Social Work (MSW) training include developmental theories, psychodynamic theories, family systems theory, and cultural theory as well as theories of oppression, social policy, administration, and community organization.

3. The requirements of masters level training ensure that social workers are prepared, through both this broad theoretical foundation and field practicum experience, to practice in a wide variety of settings with culturally diverse and vulnerable populations.

Specialized continuing education and training is required for oncology social workers to acquire the necessary skills and expertise relevant to this field of practice. These are offered through agency or hospital-based programs such as the oncology social work clinical skills training courses offered in major cancer centers throughout the U.S., fellowships in oncology social work provided through the Rustaccia Foundation and the American Cancer Society, and conferences and programs offered by the Association of Oncology Social Workers and other social work organizations. Social workers are among the psychosocial care providers whose practice is regulated through professional licensure in almost every state in the U.S., which ensures a high level of professional training and practice.

The fundamental task of oncology social work is to facilitate patient and family adjustment to a cancer diagnosis, its treatment and rehabilitation. This chapter describes the roles and tasks in oncology practice which this multilevel training prepares the social worker to perform on behalf of patients and families. Included are the roles oncology social workers perform in training and supervising other social workers, and supporting other staff members. Collaboration with volunteer programs which serve as an adjunctive resource in the broad system of cancer care will also be discussed.

PSYCHOSOCIAL CARE PROVIDER

Basic Tenets

The primary role of the oncology social worker is that of psychosocial care provider. In this role, the oncology social worker is trained in a philosophy of care which is framed by the following basic tenets.

First, the patient and family are viewed as a unit of care (8). Social work theory supports a systems focus through its emphasis on working with a person-in-environment approach. This view maintains that all individuals are part of an intricate web whose central ties begin with the family. Understanding this allows for an enhanced assessment of the psychosocial dynamics of the patient's illness and its effects on the family. Training in the biological, psychological, and social theories of development and adaptation, therefore, best prepares social workers to assist individuals and families in the ways described elsewhere in this book (see Chapters 17, 60 and 85). Social work's focus on the larger system of community and society extend the role beyond that of individual counselor or family therapist to ensure that the health care system

and the larger community are responsive to the needs of individual units (9–10). Outreach prevention programs, community-based psycho-educational groups, and church-based health fairs for cancer screening are but a few examples of the ways oncology social workers work collaboratively to intervene at the community level.

Second, the biopsychosocial model ensures an understanding that the continuum of psychosocial care is necessarily affected by the medical condition of the patient. An intervention that might be appropriate at one particular stage of the illness may actually be detrimental at another. Comprehending this fundamental principle is at the core of the oncology social worker's ability to listen to and to follow the patient's needs. Starting where the patient is, is a core social work value.

Third, psychosocial needs change over time and are influenced by many factors. The medical condition of the patient is not the only factor influencing the type of care that would be most effective. Life events such as marriages, divorces, births, graduations, etc. have an impact on the cancer patient and the patient's family, which change the type or level of psychosocial care actually needed by the patient. Social work's systems perspective allows for the consideration of the effects of such life events.

Fourth, individual differences require multi-modal approaches for support, problem solving, and rehabilitation. Awareness of diversity is at the heart of social work practice. Social workers understand that patient receptivity to treatment is influenced by psychological and social factors. Cultural and developmental factors influence the patient/family's view of the patient role, their reactions to illness, and the meaning they make of asking for or accepting help. Focus in training on multiculturalism prepares social workers to address the broad spectrum of people affected by cancer, particularly ethnic, gender, or cultural groups that may not receive as much attention in the training of other professional groups (11–12).

Social Work Tasks

The oncology social worker is attentive to the psychological, social, spiritual/existential, and practical concerns of patients and families. Thus, the tasks of oncology social work are multi-faceted and must be comprehensively framed at each stage of illness. In the realm of direct service, these tasks include:

1. screening, evaluation, and assessment;
2. adjustment to illness counseling, and individual, family, or group psychotherapy;

3. discharge planning;
4. referral;
5. advocacy.

Table 92.1 details the tasks of oncology social work in the provision of psychosocial care of the cancer patient.

Screening, Evaluation, and Assessment. Social workers utilize a multi-modal approach to assessment. The use of screening instruments on a triage basis identifies the level of urgency of psychosocial need, and facilitates the design of appropriate intervention. Rapid assessment tools and self-report instruments add informative data to the evaluation process (13–14). When risk factors are identified, interviews allow for a more in-depth understanding of the patient's adaptive capacities through a comprehensive psychosocial assessment. Many social workers utilize both the DSM IV (*Diagnostic and Statistical Manual IV*, American Psychiatric Association) multiaxial assessment or the PIE (person-in-environment) system which provides a system of brief, uniform descriptions of a patient's interpersonal, environmental, mental, and physical health problems and includes an assessment of the patient's ability to deal with these problems. Use of the DSM IV provides the oncology social worker with a diagnostic language with which to communicate with other mental healthcare providers.

Individual, Family, and Group Psychotherapy and Counseling. Through field practicums and academic coursework in MSW graduate programs, the theories and skills of psychotherapy are acquired that allow the social worker to effectively function in the role of psychotherapist or counselor in the oncology setting. Oncology-specific internships and post-graduate training equips the oncology social worker with expertise in the psychosocial issues most relevant to

medically ill patients and their families (15). This enables the oncology social worker to distinguish, for example, depressive reactions to chemotherapy from endogenous depression and can help the patient and family anticipate and manage commonly experienced effects of treatment.

Oncology social workers have been instrumental in organizing and facilitating patient psychotherapy and support groups in hospital and community settings. As a result, many of these groups have helped launch the growing number of self-help groups and organizations which provide patients and families with an additional source of social support, recognized to be an essential component to longevity in cancer (16).

Discharge Planning. Dating back to the days of Ida Canon at Massachusetts General Hospital, medical social workers have been engaged in facilitating the discharge of the patient from the hospital. The social worker has acted as an interface between the hospital and home, intervening where necessary to aid in the transition from medical patient to healthy family/community member. Often these interventions have been practical in nature, i.e transportation, home medical supplies or equipment, home-making services, or meals (17). Like their general medical colleagues, oncology social workers are also actively engaged in discharge planning. However, with the development of high-tech equipment and advanced medical treatments as well as hospice and palliative care programs and complicated insurance modifications, homecare and nursing home care has changed dramatically. With these changes, discharge planning has become extremely intricate. In the case of cancer, the tasks of discharge planning often involve complicated coordination of services, detailed planning, and a comprehensive enviromental assessment. The role includes helping the patient and family to make crucial decisions regarding their care,

TABLE 92.1. *Oncology Social Work Tasks: Psychosocial Care of the Patient*

Screening, Evaluation, and Assessment	Adjustment to Illness Counseling, Individual, Family, and Group Psychotherapy	Discharge Planning	Referral	Advocacy
Use of rapid assessment tools (screening), self-report instruments, interviews, PIE and the DSM IV	Psychodynamic psychotherapy, cognitive–behavioral approaches, relaxation techniques, guided imagery, transpersonal and/or existential psychotherapy, supportive psychotherapy.	Assessment, information sharing, patient education, resource linkage, concrete services, practical help, family aid, environmental interventions.	Psychiatric, psychological, social, and spiritual resources. Information sharing, resource linkage.	Advocating for patient and family needs, inpatient, outpatient, at home, and in the community with staff, extended family, and friends. Patient advocacy at the policy level on healthcare legislation.

particularly regarding quality of life. Assessing patient and family values and philosophy as well as their capability and resistance to assistance requires a high level of skill, especially if language or cultural differences are a factor. An ability to empathically and assertively advocate for patients in a community care system that may have scarce resources is also essential. While some tasks may be relatively straightforward, because of its complexity, discharge planning has been and continues to be an important social work role (18).

Referral. Social workers are a conduit for the referral process as referrals are both received and made on behalf of the patient. Knowing when to refer is critical to the effective oncology social worker in providing psychosocial care to cancer patients and their families. The referral process is a key component of psychosocial care as social workers are called upon to provide clinical intervention in the form of individual, couples, family, or group psychotherapy, and/or to link patients with other appropriate resources to match their concrete service needs. Referrals are received by social work from all members of the multidisciplinary team. As a primary psychosocial care provider, the social worker then determines the treatment plan, manages the case, and/or refers to adjunctive services such as nutrition, financial services, AA, support groups, chaplaincy, psychiatry. Social workers are uniquely trained through the person-in-environment model to understand the specialized process of referring. They have a clear understanding of the types of referrals appropriate for social work intervention, as well as how to skillfully refer the patient to other specialty sources. (See Table 92.2.)

Advocacy and Social Change. Patient and family advocacy is another task in psychosocial caregiving for which the oncology social worker is uniquely prepared. Coursework and training at the master's level equips social workers with macro skills that allow them to integrate the specialized needs of patients and families with larger systems issues. Acting as an advocate with schools, churches, communities, neighborhoods, etc. on behalf of the cancer patient and family moves psychosocial caregiving out of the realm of psyche to the social environment. A person-in-environment perspective provides many points of intervention and different forms of advocacy efforts (19).

Irrespective of the form of intervention – community organization, casework, administration, or political activity – the resource most needed for advocacy is information. Through research, publication of clinical literature, education and training, oncology social workers are actively engaged in acquiring and sharing information which leads to making communities, and society in general, more responsive to the needs of persons with cancer. The Council on Social Work Education's 1982 policy statement pertaining to advocacy states: "The knowledge and skills students accumulate in social welfare policy and services should prepare them to exert leadership and influence as legislative and social advocates, lobbyists, and expert advisors to policy makers and administrators." The 1992 policy statement adds, "The pursuit of policies, services and programs through legislative advocacy, lobbying and other forms of social and political action, including providing expert testimony, participation in local and national coalitions and gaining political office." (20–21)

TABLE 92.2. *Types of Referrals*

Usual Referral	Urgent Referral	Emergent Referral
Durable medical equipment	Patient distress related to:	Suicidal ideation
Hospice	Poor prognosis	Substance abuse
Homecare	Deteriorating condition	Homicidal ideation
Transportation	Test results	Signing out AMA
Housing	Procedures	Treatment refusal
Adjustment to illness counselling	Diagnostic tests	Fear of death
Support group	Unconrollable anxiety	
Psychoeducational group	Depression	
Medical insurance	Noncompliance with Tx	
Entitlements	Family Distress	
Grief/bereavement		

Social workers, unlike many other psychosocial care providers, are trained in community organization and human rights advocacy which enables them to facilitate collaborative or other efforts on the part of groups, organizations, and communities to effect social action and social change. The National Breast Cancer Coalition and the National Coalition of Cancer Survivors include many oncology social workers among their members, many of whom have been instrumental in improving funding and legislation related to cancer. Oncology social workers serve as expert advisors to policy makers and bear influence on federal and state health care reform initiatives to insure comprehensive psychosocial care of persons affected by cancer. Effecting change at the policy level strengthens the social worker's ability to impact the individual healthcare of patients and is viewed as a necessary role of oncology social work.

ADMINISTRATION AND CLINICAL SUPERVISION

In addition to serving in the primary role of psychosocial care provider for patients and families with its multiplicity of tasks, oncology social workers are, at times, also called upon to serve as administrators and clinical supervisors. As such, they address the clinical training needs of students and beginning workers, as well as experienced workers through a variety of methods including: the tutorial model of a one-to-one relationship, peer supervision, group supervision, and case consultation. Through these specific educational, administrative, and supportive techniques oncology social workers at the administrative/supervisory level strive to enhance worker performance and job satisfaction (22). While there are certain stressors inherent in the nature of social work unique to hospital settings, there are needs universal to all oncology social workers which are held in common.

Perhaps the most difficult of these is the inevitable close identification the worker has with the cancer patient and his family. The possibility that the worker or a relative can develop cancer is real. Concomitantly, there is a confrontation with and recognition of one's own mortality which must be dealt with by the worker, often at an earlier age than is 'normal' for the general population. There is the traumatic exposure to mutilation and a constant sense of loss. (22)

These pressures, and many others, accompany social work practice in an oncology setting, and require a high level of skill and training on behalf of the social worker in the administrative or supervisory role. Fortunately, oncology social workers at all levels are

continuously developing their clinical expertise through ongoing inservice training, attendance at and participation in professional conferences, and clinical practicums at the master's, postmaster's and doctoral level.

STAFF INTERVENTION AND SUPPORT

The pressures oncology social workers experience as inherent in the oncology setting are shared by all the members of the multidisciplinary team. While mutual support among the team members is readily available, oncology social workers, as designated psychosocial care providers, are often called upon to take the lead in supportive interventions with staff. Oncology social workers often lead staff support groups, do critical incident stress debriefings (CISD), and meet one-on-one with individual oncology staff members, both formally and informally to defuse work-related stressors and offer psychosocial support.

TRAINING, SUPERVISION, AND COLLABORATION WITH VOLUNTEERS

Recognizing that the effective use of volunteers can significantly enhance patient care, social workers have regularly been involved in their training and supervision in addition to making referrals to them. Volunteers provide a range of services from practical assistance to social support. In fact, they can serve in a variety of functions to aid cancer patients across the disease continuum to include: assistance in screening, orientation, diversionary activities, education, fundraising, peer counseling, transportation, and research activities. (See Table 92.3.)

Volunteers are actively involved with cancer prevention and screening programs through health fairs and other educational efforts sponsored by a variety of health care and community organizations. At the time of diagnosis, volunteers with specialized training in the reactions and needs of newly diagnosed patients can orient patients and families to the health care setting, can help provide information, and offer companionship. During the treatment phase volunteers often offer help with practical concerns including transportation, work in residential facilities specifically designed to house patients and families, and provide diversionary activities for inpatients and companionship to visiting family members. Sometimes during the remission phase, cancer patients and their family members become volunteers, utilizing their accumulated experience to help others who are facing the same life-threatening illness. They

TABLE 92.3. *Volunteer Services Across the Disease Continuum*

Prevention	Diagnosis	Treatment	Remission	Recurrence	Palliative
Breast cancer screening	New patient orientation	Diversionary activities	Patient educators	Peer counselling	Bereavement program
Community health fairs	Peer counseling	"Lood Good, Feel Better"	Fundraising	Peer support	Research activities
Research activities	Inpatient/outpatient companion	Residential care	Advocacy	Research activities	
	Tour guides	Transportation	Research activities		
	Research activities	Research activities			

become patient educators, fundraisers and advocates for positive change. Volunteer peer counselors often provide crucial support to patients and their families following the recurrence of a patient's disease. Similarly, volunteers play an important role in assisting patients and families experiencing palliative care, particularly in residential and home-based hospice programs.

As economic considerations deplete the availability of some services, such as transportation, the effective use of volunteer services becomes more significant. Some volunteer tasks, such as providing patients with information about hospital and community programs, may require limited training, but many tasks require in-depth orientation to the psychosocial impact of cancer and the health care system in order for the volunteer to provide service sensitively and efficiently. Social workers are often instrumental in the training and supervision of volunteers in all of these roles. They serve as facilitators and instructors in comprehensive volunteer training programs which prepare volunteers to help patients both in the hospital and in the community and provide ongoing supervision and consultation to those volunteers involved in peer support. Programs such as Reach to Recovery, Man to Man, and Patient to Patient provide enhanced patient care through peer support. Because social workers have recognized that "much of the impetus for self-help participation is the attraction of comparing notes with like-minded people who have faced similar situations . . . and that self-help groups can provide a range of examples of how others have faced difficult lifestyle issues" (23), they have been instrumental in facilitating the development of such volunteer groups. Ongoing consultation, training, and supervision is then provided to assist these volunteers in coping with the challenges of providing this kind of peer support (24).

MULTIDISCIPLINARY TEAM MEMBER

The oncology social worker is a vital member of the multidisciplinary team. They recognize the interconnectedness of the patient's internal and external environmental systems and are uniquely qualified to help the team address the patient's pyschological and social well-being in relation to his or her illness. Oncology social workers assist the team in moving beyond the disease process, to attend to very practical matters that may effect the patient's quality of life. They serve as a conduit between patient and staff to facilitate optimum responsiveness to treatment goals. Issues related to adjustment to illness and discharge planning are designated clinical tasks of the oncology social worker. In this important role, the social worker becomes a valued team member.

As a multidisciplinary team member, oncology social workers are not only skilled in providing clinical services, but are also cognizant of the explicit and implicit obligations they may have to other team members, the social work profession, and to the patient and family. They are taught the parameters of teamwork, which include the team composition, purpose, member roles and responsibilities, value bases, and processes. As ethical dilemmas may result from conflicts of competing values in fulfilling obligations to equally entitled sources, responsibility and accountability for decisions made by the team are shared by the oncology social worker (25–26).

"Informed consent for treatment and patient participation in decision-making implicate social workers because of their role in facilitating communication and mutual understanding between patient and family and professional caregivers." (27) Since the advent of the Patient Self-Determination Act of 1990, which requires hospitals and health agencies to develop policies on advance directives, social workers have been involved not only in helping patients and families to understand the mandates of the law but also to prepare advance directives and deal with decisions when advance directives have not been completed. Schools of social work routinely include ethics in their curriculum, making social workers a valuable resource for patients, families, and the oncology health care team in ethical decision-making.

PATIENT/STAFF/COMMUNITY EDUCATOR

Oncology social workers not only support their own education through the annual national conference of the Association of Oncology Social Work (AOSW), and participation in a vast array of international conferences and workshops, but also play a key role in the education of medical, nursing, and other allied health professionals regarding the psychosocial impact of cancer (27–28). Social workers are frequently facilitators of the widely disseminated I Can Cope education and support series sponsored by the American Cancer Society and have authored numerous patient-education materials including those published by the National Cancer Institute, the American Cancer Society, the Leukemia Society, the Wellness Community, and many other organizations which provide patient and professional education regarding psychosocial issues and cancer.

RESEARCHER

Research is a required component of MSW training as it facilitates the development and teaching of professional knowledge and skills required to practice social work. The Institute for the Advancement of Social Work Research, created in 1992, reflects the profession's recognition of the importance of research in both evaluating practice and furthering knowledge of people and their problems (29–31). The leading interdisciplinary journal of psychosocial oncology care, the *Journal of Psychosocial Oncology*, which is published by AOSW, serves as a forum for sharing research and clinical data. Many of the articles published in this quarterly journal reflect the prevailing practitioner–scholar model, adopted by the oncology social work field, which underscores the need for empirically informed practice (32).

In addition, in 1994, AOSW created the Social Work Oncology Research Group (SWORG), which promotes research relevant to oncology social work through multi-institutional collaboration and function. Ongoing projects include an exploration of the prevalence of distress across the disease continuum from diagnosis to terminal illness, and an examination of the psychosocial needs of high-distress patients, which constitute one-third of all cancer patients.

CONCLUSION

Oncology social workers perform many roles and functions in inpatient and outpatient health care settings to assist persons with cancer on the micro and macro levels. These roles and functions serve to enhance both patient care and the smooth and efficient functioning of the health care systems in which they are cared for. They also require intensive training beyond the masters degree which addresses the specific psychosocial issues associated with cancer. In the past three decades, the social work profession has produced some of the most expert psychosocial clinicians working in the field of oncology today.

These clinicians, in conjunction with their professional organization, AOSW, have developed a wide variety of interventions and programs to facilitate coping with cancer. Their empirical studies have documented the efficacy and cost-effectiveness of these interventions, and their future research and clinical literature will continue to contribute to our understanding of how to prevent as well as manage the devastating effects of this life-threatening illness (33,34).

REFERENCES

1. Ross J. Hospital Social Work. In: *Encyclopedia of Social Work*, 19th edn, Washington, D.C. NASW Press, 1995.
2. Supple-Diaz, L, Mattison D. Factors affecting survival and satisfaction: navigating a career in oncology social work. *J Psychosoc Oncol.* 1992; 10:111–131.
3. Weisman, AD. Understanding the cancer patient: the syndrome of caregiver's plight. *Psychiatry.* 1981; 44:157–167.
4. McGrath FJ, Dodds-Waugh A. Support group for nurses in an oncology ward. *Aust Soc Work.* 1989; 42:29–34.
5. Germain C. An ecological perspective on social work practice in health care. *Soc Work Health Care.* 1977; 3:67–76.
6. Black RB. Challenges for social work as a core profession in cancer services. *Soc Work Health Care.* 1989; 14:1–13.
7. Berkman B. Knowledge base needs for effective social work practice in health. *J Ed Soc Work.* 1981; 17:85–90.
8. Tolley NS. Oncology social work, family systems theory, and workplace consultations. *Health Soc Work.* 1994; 19: 227–230.
9. Barg F, McCorkle R, Jepson C, et al. A statewide plan to address the unmet psychosocial needs of people with cancer. *J Psychosoc Oncol.* 1993; 10:55–77.
10. Norman AD, Brandeis L. Addressing the needs of survivors: an action research approach. *J Psychosoc Oncol.* 1992; 10:3–18.

11. LaRosa M. Health care needs of Hispanic Americans and the responsiveness of the health care system. *Soc Work*. 1989; 34:104–107.

12. Glajchen M, Blum D, Calder K. Cancer pain management and the role of social work: barriers and interventions. *Health Soc Work*. 1995; 20(3):200–206.

13. Sam H, Koopmans J, Mathieson C. The psychosocial impact of a laryngectomy: a comprehensive assessment. *J Psychosoc Oncol*. 1991; 9:37–58.

14. Zabora J, Smith E, Baker F, et al. The family: the other side of bone marrow transplantation. *J Psychosoc Oncol*. 1992; 10:35–46.

15. Loscalzo M, Amendola J. Psychosocial and behavioral management of cancer pain. *Adv Pain Res Therapy*. 1990; 16:429–442.

16. Spiegel, D. Psychosocial interventions with cancer patients. *J Psychosoc Oncol*. 3(4):83–93.

17. Bryan J, Greger H, Miller M, et al. An evaluation of the transportation needs of disadvantaged cancer patients. *J Psychosoc Oncol*. 1991; 9:23–36.

18. Lurie A, Pinsky S, Tuzman L. Training social workers for discharge planning. *Health Soc Work*. 1981; 6:12–18.

19. Mickelson J. Advocacy. In: *Encyclopedia of Social Work*. Washington, D.C., 1995 p. 96.

20. Council on Social Work Education. Curriculum Policy Statement. Washington, D.C., 1982.

21. Council on Social Work Education. Curriculum Policy Statement. Washington, D.C., 1992.

22. Blum D. Clinical supervisory practice in oncology settings. *Clin Supervisor*. 1983; 1:17–27.

23. Self-help groups. In: *Encyclopedia of Social Work*. Washington, D.C., 1995.

24. Hill H. Patient to patient, heart to heart: a peer support program that works. *Picker/Commonwealth Report*. 1(3): Winter 1992.

25. Roberts CS. Conflicting professional values in social work and medicine. *Health Soc Work*. 1989; 14:211–218.

26. Downs S. Ethical issues in bone marrow transplantation. *Sem Oncol Nurs*. Feb 1, 1994; 10(1):58.

27. Zayas LH, Dyche LH. Social workers training primary care physicians: essential psychosocial principles. *Soc Work*. 1992; 37:247–252.

28. Hunsdon S. The impact of illness on patients and families: Social workers teach medical students. *Soc Work Health Care*. 1984; 10:41–52.

29. Glajchen M, Magen R. Evaluating process, outcome and satisfaction in community based cancer support groups. *Soc Work Groups*. 1995; 18:27–40.

30. Rathbone-McCuan E, Herbert EL, Fulton JR. Evaluation as an imperative for social services preservation: a challenge for the Dept. of Veteran Affairs. *J Soc Work Ed*. 1991; 22:114–124.

31. Siegel K. Psychosocial oncology research. *Soc Work Health Care*. 1990; 15:21–43.

32. Meyer C. Integrating research and practice. *Soc Work*. 1985; 29:323.

33. Massachusetts Chapter, National Association of Social Workers. Managed Care Information and Resource Packet. 1992. Boston, Mass.

34. U.S. House of Representatives Committee on Post Office and Civil Service Report No. 99-710, 99th Congress, 2nd Session, p. 5 (July 24, 1986).

93

Education of Nurses in Psycho-oncology

RUTH McCORKLE, MARILYN FRANK-STROMBORG, AND
JEANNIE V. PASACRETA

In oncology practice, regardless of the setting, nurses are usually on the "front line" of patient care. On inpatient units, in outpatient clinics, and in homecare situations, nurses are responsible for the assessment and referral of the psychosocial problems demonstrated by patients and their families. Nurses often receive the most concentrated exposure to intense emotions in terms of number of hours and number of cases when compared with other professional groups. Despite these realities of the workplace nurses receive little in the way of formal education regarding the psychological aspects of cancer. It is the intent of this chapter to describe the education of nurses, particularly as it pertains to psycho-oncology and to offer some innovative ways to address some of the deficiencies that currently exist.

NURSING EDUCATION

The formalization of cancer nursing education in the United States has evolved during the second half of the twentieth century. The first college course in cancer nursing was offered at Columbia University Teachers College by Katherine Nelson in 1947. The practice of cancer requires knowledge from a wide range of disciplines, including nursing, epidemiology, pathophysiology, sociology, pharmacology, medicine, nutrition, and psychology. In 1980, the members of the Oncology Nursing Society passed a resolution declaring that a baccalaureate degree be recognized as the entry level to practice oncology nursing to facilitate the continuous commitment to learning required to stay current. Three levels of nursing education – undergraduate, graduate, and doctoral education – prepare nurses for practice, advanced practice, and research roles respectively. An associate degree and diploma certificate also prepare an individual for RN licensure but are not university-based degrees and are

thought by some to minimize the need for developing critical thinking and problem-solving skills. Around the time when the Oncology Nursing Society (ONS), was assuming leadership and establishing education standards for oncology nursing, educational institutions were making drastic changes in their curricula. In the 1980s, curricula were changed at the undergraduate level from a medical model approach to an integrative approach. During that time, nurse educators re-evaluated the meaning of nursing, delineated recurring themes in nursing, and developed new strategies to transmit nursing knowledge (1).

Traditionally, cancer nursing has been taught in a limited number of hours of didactic instruction within a medical–surgical rotation, and clinical experiences with cancer patients may or may not have been planned concurrently. As part of the new integrated curriculum, oncology nursing content and clinical experiences in the undergraduate curriculum ranged extensively across programs (2) and continues to vary today. Because cancer is such a common diagnosis, it the rare undergraduate student who does not care for a cancer patient before graduating. However, the integrated curriculum allows little time to study the specific psychosocial responses of individuals and their families to a life-threatening diagnosis such as cancer (3). Undergraduate nursing students are often exposed to psychological responses as broad psychiatric concepts and diagnoses such as depression and anxiety. Exposure to these phenomena often occur during a first psychiatric clinical experience on a "locked" unit or in a community-based mental health facility. Unfortunately, the basic nursing curricula allows little to no time to expose the student to in-depth didactic content related to psychological distress in medically ill patients, especially during times of transition and crisis. Pope (4) found that in schools where the oncology hours were too integrated into the program and were allocated no distinct place of their own, many students experienced frustration, and some were not even aware that they had any instruction in this area.

In the mid 90s, the American Cancer Society (ACS) Professors of Oncology Nursing recommended oncology curriculum content that they believed was essential for students to learn during their basic nursing education. The psychosocial content recommendations of the ACS Professors included:

- Patient and family psychosocial responses
- Sexuality
- Referral to psychosocial resources

Clinical competencies recommended by the ACS professors in cancer care upon graduation from a baccalaureate program in nursing related to psychooncology include:

- Ability to describe the major psychosocial responses of the individual and family to cancer
- Ability to communicate effectively with people with cancer and their families

While it is recognized to be unlikely that all important psychosocial content specific to cancer will be addressed, the ACS Professors' argue that some of it can be presented with other illness-related situations. For example, all students need content related to dying patients and to the anxiety and depression associated with a life-threatening diagnosis. This content is certainly applicable to a variety of patient populations. However, as it stands, the content is not presented adequately in any format. In general, basic nursing education inadequately prepares nurses in cancer nursing and gives them a limited understanding of the theoretical content related to psycho-oncology (5).

At the graduate level, students in oncology nursing are exposed to didactic and clinical experiences underlying psycho-oncology. Nurses receive education regarding assessment and screening of cancer patients to determine if they need referrals to psychosocial resources. In addition to providing an advanced knowledge base in oncology nursing, graduate-level education also provides preparation in the theoretical basis of nursing practice, the trends and issues that have an actual or potential impact on nursing, the process of nursing research, and the theories that influence advanced nursing practice such as conflict, role, change, stress, learning, organizational management, and system theories (6).

GAPS IN KNOWLEDGE REGARDING PSYCHO-ONCOLOGY

An important role of the nurse is to enhance the ability of patients and families to cope with alterations in a health status. The emotional distress that individuals experience with the diagnosis of cancer has been documented by multiple researchers (7–9). Corner and Wilson-Barnett (10) report that newly graduated nurses ranked their highest needs to be for more educational training to help them communicate with cancer patients as well as to receive information on the social and psychological problems of cancer patients. The nurses in Corner and Wilson-Barnett's study did not perceive that they were competent to address the psychosocial aspects of patient care.

This study has highlighted the extent to which newly registered nurses . . . hold very deep concerns about caring for patients with cancer, and felt ill-prepared for this aspect of their role. They also held mixed or negative attitudes towards the disease and associated cancer with inevitable death regardless of stage of the disease or cancer site. (p. 188)

It is acknowledged that nurses need to know how to assess these psychosocial problems and to then make the appropriate community-based referrals. All nurses should be prepared to address the basic psychosocial needs of patients, to accurately assess and screen patients, and to make timely referrals based on their assessments and screening activities. Lack of relief from the emotional suffering associated with cancer has been linked to such problems as unrelenting depression, anxiety, family dysfunction, lack of compliance with treatment, and suicide, to name just a few (11). Thus, the importance of helping nurses, who are on the "front line" of patient care, to recognize and address unmet psychosocial needs is clear.

To compound the deficiencies in nursing education regarding psychosocial aspects of cancer care are trends in healthcare that have led to numerous changes in the characteristics of hospitalized and home-based cancer patients. Patients are hospitalized for shorter periods, are more acutely ill, and receive increasingly aggressive treatments in advanced technological settings (12). It is well established that psychiatric problems are most prevalent in the seriously ill (13). Oncology nurses who place a high value on their ability to support patients and families through the stresses of cancer are often ill prepared to adequately manage patients' psychosocial problems.

A survey by Pasacreta and Massie (14) asked nurses to identify psychiatric symptoms exhibited by 475 cancer inpatients on one particular day. Few patients had major psychiatric problems which antedated cancer illness, and a similar number had developed psychiatric problems after their cancer diagnosis. The nature and prevalence of psychiatric problems that nurses reported are fairly consistent with reports by others. Situational depression and anxiety are the most common psychiatric problems encountered in patients (13, 15), and were the most frequently reported symptoms in this study. The authors' work concluded that psychiatric problems were most prevalent in the seriously ill (16). Almost twice as many acutely ill patients received reports by nurses of having psychiatric symptoms than did less acutely ill patients. Nurses reported an inability to intervene themselves for one or more of the following reasons: insufficient time to provide emotional support, and insufficient information about supportive interventions which could be helpful, or lack of objectivity.

Nurses state that they often put management of emotional problems aside because of short staffing, lack of information about what to do, lack of objectivity, or a need to manage more pressing and acute medical issues. Education regarding psychosocial management may have important implications for new staff nurses who may lack competence in this area because they are in the process of learning many other skills. One result of insufficient education in the psychosocial domain is that patient problems may become extreme before they receive attention or they may receive no attention at all. This leads to greater patient distress as well as greater distress on the part of the nursing staff who feel ill-equipped to manage emotional problems in a growing number of individuals.

It has been the experience of some psychiatric consultants working in the oncology setting that referrals are often of patients who have a poor prognosis and acute medical problems. Appropriate psychosocial interventions include giving clear information about treatments and procedures, providing reassurance that symptoms will be managed, normalizing the patients' and families' distress and using the patients' existing support systems in addition to available hospital and community resources to offer comfort and reassurance. Teaching the nurse to differentiate normal from pathologic reactions is also paramount. We can certainly teach nurses to identify patients who will respond to these interventions while assisting them to set realistic goals and clarify personal boundaries so that patient involvement does not become overwhelming.

Another situation encountered by psychiatric consultants is that some patients with severe psychiatric syndromes are not referred for psychiatric consultation or they are referred when problems become severe and cause major disruption on a unit. The patient with a full-blown delirium who showed subtle but intensifying signs and symptoms for a week and is now climbing over siderails and pulling out life-sustaining equipment is a familiar scene for the psychiatric consultant responding to an emergency call. It is possible that at times nurses refer patients who cause them the most distress as opposed to referring those who exhibit objective psychopathology. Undoubtedly, underreferring for psychiatric consultation occurs in many settings and may result from: nurse, physician, and patient concern that psychiatric referrals stigmatize patients; the belief that all psychiatric symptoms are normal responses to cancer and that there are no effective treatments; the belief that psychiatric problems will resolve on their own or, concern that psychiatric intervention will make the patient worse by "unleashing" feelings. Often nurses on the "front line" of patient care correctly perceive psychiatric problems and approach physicians to make psychiatric referrals. Despite these requests, psychiatric concerns may seem less important within the context of a life-threatening illness. Since budget restrictions and program cutbacks are common in hospitals and outpatient settings throughout the country, and the presence of psychiatric clinicians is often not a reality, efforts should be directed toward increasing the level of nursing knowledge regarding assessment and management of psychiatric complications in patients.

An important component of new educational programs for nurses will be an effort to teach them to realistically appraise goals for psychiatric intervention. For example, severe and long-standing character pathology is not a fixable problem; however, learning to set limits with disturbed patients and families is a realistic goal. Providing education about "markers" which warrant psychiatric consultation is also indicated. In addition, information about indications, contraindications, desired effects, side effects, and paradoxical reactions to psychotropic medications should be given to all nursing staff. Information about control of symptoms such as pain, nausea, and vomiting, and how those symptoms can intensify psychiatric symptoms is needed. Education about signs, symptoms, and interventions for delirium, most common in patients with advanced illness, as well as appropriate use of resources (e.g., pain service, hospital chaplains, etc.) is essential.

Weisman (8,17–18) developed a model of stress and coping for cancer patients. He identified four psychosocial stages in coping with cancer, each with differing characteristics, concerns, and implications for interventions for nurses. Weisman suggested that health professionals can facilitate patients' coping by accomplishing the countercoping tasks of clarification, collaboration, relief, and cooling off. Specifically, he suggested activities for nurses to help cancer patients cope, such as: clarify problems for patients, help patients maintain control by encouraging them to exercise whatever options they have available to them, and try to discourage emotional extremes by offering a willing and noncritical ear so that patients can relieve pent-up tensions without fear of retribution (19). Thus, Weisman saw a very definite role for nurses in assisting cancer patients to cope more effectively with their illness and its treatment. Nurses are one of the most significant professional support systems available to the patient with cancer because the nurse has the most frequent contact with the patient and family.

Unfortunately, as this review has shown, undergraduate nursing programs in the United States do not contain the educational content that will give the average nurse the skills to conduct psychosocially oriented assessment/screening activities. Presently, this type of content is limited to specialized graduate programs. Further compounding the problem is the rapidly changing health care system. Patients are routinely discharged from the hospital as soon as possible, leaving nurses little time to evaluate the patient's problems. Because hospital stays have been dramatically curtailed, to be effective, the nurse must have the skills and knowledge to rapidly ascertain the psychosocial needs of the patient and family and design cost-effective community-based referrals. To make cost-effective community-based referrals, nurses need to be aware of the psycho-oncology resources that are available for cancer patients and how best to access these resources.

SUCCESSFUL CONTINUING EDUCATION PROGRAM FOR NURSES

Recognizing that the average nurse does not possess the needed skills and knowledge to address the cancer patient's psychosocial needs, several successful continuing education programs have been instituted in the United States to remedy this situation (20–23).

Barg and her colleagues (20) developed a model statewide, standardized, continuing education program for health professionals who care for cancer patients. This program was presented in 19 different locations in southeastern Pennsylvania. The justification for this program was based on the research conducted by Houts et al. (21). Houts and his research team interviewed 629 people with cancer to assess unmet psychological, social, and economic needs. The most

frequently mentioned unmet need was for help in dealing with emotional problems. They concluded that more effectively screening for psychosocial problems and referral to supportive services was needed.

The content of the curriculum was designed to last three $6\frac{1}{2}$-hour days. On Day 1, the concept of unmet psychosocial needs and the process of psychosocial assessment were introduced. The themes of loss and interdisciplinary team approach to cancer care were emphasized. On Day 2, physical and psychosocial interventions were addressed, and on Day 3 the skills that caregivers can use to help patients and families make decisions about the patients' care was introduced.

One unique aspect of the continuing education offering was to have a *gaps and contracts strategy*. Sixty-seven per cent of the participants developed contracts during the three-day program to implement changes in their practice. Four months later, the participants were asked whether they had made any progress in implementing these changes. Of the 67 per cent who had written contracts, 118/274 said they had made progress (23). The types of primary goals the participants established for themselves included: *system-oriented assessment* – institute pain and psychosocial assessment tools and procedures, establish standards of care, monitor systems for plans of care; and *system-oriented interventions* – coordinate psychosocial resources, enhance patient/professional communication, facilitate communication with the team, educate team, distribute resource manuals to team, and enhance referral procedures (23, p. 410).

This standardized continuing education program for health providers working with cancer patients had a profound effect on the development of services for patients and their families. The state-coordinated effort not only educated over 400 health providers in southeastern Pennsylvania concerning the care of people with cancer, it also established lasting structure by creating a network for health providers who are interested and educated in the psychosocial aspects of cancer care. The researchers write that the "opportunity for reaching patients who have unmet needs is exponential". (p. 76)

REFERENCES

1. Pennington EA. The integrated curriculum: a 15 year perspective. In: Pennington EA (ed.), Curriculum revisited: an update of curriculum design (NLN Pub. No. 15-2165). New York: National League for Nursing; 1986: 37–38.
2. Kruse LC. Undergraduate cancer nursing education. In: McCorkle R, Hongladaron G (eds.), *Issues and topics in*

cancer nursing. Norwalk, CT: Appleton-Century-Crofts; 1986.

3. McCorkle R, Preston F, Volker D. Cancer nursing education today. In: McCorkle R, Grant M, Frank-Stromborg M, Baird S (eds.), *Cancer Nursing* (2nd edn). Philadelphia, PA: W.B. Saunders; 1996.

4. Pope S. Fundamentals for a new concept of oncology nursing in the professional nursing education program. *Cancer Nurs*. 1992; 15(2):137–147.

5. Brown JK. Survey of cancer nursing education in U.S. schools of nursing. *Oncol Nurs Forum*. 1983; 10:82–83.

6. Cooley ME, Spatz DL, Yasko J. Role implementation in cancer nursing. In: McCorkle R, Grant M, Frank-Stromborg M, Baird S (eds.), *Cancer Nursing* (2nd edn). Philadephia, PA: W.B. Saunders; 1996.

7. Frank-Stromborg M. Reaction to the diagnosis of cancer questionnaire (RDCQ): development and psychometric evaluation. *Nurs Res*. 1986; 38:364–369.

8. Weisman AD. *Coping with Cancer*. New York: McGraw-Hill Book Co; 1979.

9. Woods NF, Lewis FM, Ellison ES. Living with cancer: family experiences. *Cancer Nurs*. 1989; 12:28–33.

10. Corner, J, Wilson-Barnett, J. The newly registered nurse and the cancer patient: educational evaluation. *Int J Nurs Stud*. 1992; 29:177–190.

11. Holland J. Clinical course of cancer. In: Holland JC, Rowland JH (eds.), *Handbook of psychooncology: psychological care of the patient with cancer*. New York: Oxford University Press; 1989: 75–100.

12. Pettitti DB. Sounding board, competing technologies, implications for the costs and complexities of medical care. *N Engl J Med*. 1986; 315:1480–1483.

13. Plumb M, Holland JC. Comparative study of psychological function in patients with advanced cancer, I: Self-reported depressive symptoms. *Psychosom Med*. 1977; 39:264–275.

14. Pasacreta JV, Massie MJ. Nurses' reports of psychiatric complications in patients with cancer. *Oncol Nurs Forum*. 1990; 17:347–353.

15. Cassileth BR, Lusk E, Hutter R. Concordance of depression and anxiety in patients with cancer. *Psychol Rep*. 1984; 54:588–590.

16. Bukberg J, Penman D, Holland JC. Depression in hospitalized cancer patients. *Psychosom Med*. 1984; 46: 199–212.

17. Weisman AD. Early diagnosis of vulnerability in cancer patients. *Am J Med Sci*. 1976; 271:187–196.

18. Weisman AD. A model for psychosocial phasing in cancer. In: Moos RH (ed.), *Coping with physical illness*. New York: Plenum; 1984; 2:107–122.

19. Jalowiec A, Dudas S. Alterations in patient coping. In: Baird S, McCorkle R, Grant M (eds.), *Cancer Nursing*. Philadelphia, PA: W.B. Saunders; 1991: 806–820.

20. Barg FK, McCorkle R, Jepson C, et al. A statewide plan to address the unmet psychosocial needs of people with cancer. *J Psychosoc Oncol*. 1993; 10(4):55–77.

21. Houts PS, Yasko JM, Kahn SB et al. Unmet psychological, social, and economic needs of persons with cancer in Pennsylvania. *Cancer*. 1986; 58:2355–2361.

22. Barg FK, McCorkle R, Robinson K, et al. Gaps and contract: evaluating the diffusion of new information. *Cancer Nurs*. 1992; 15(6):401–406.

23. Robinson K, Barg FK, McCorkle R, et al. Gaps and contract: evaluating the diffusion of new information. Part II. The measurement of the strategy. *Cancer Nurs*. 1992; 15(6):406–414.

94

Principles of Training Medical Staff in Psychosocial and Communication Skills

DEBRA ROTER AND LESLEY FALLOWFIELD

The post World War II period has been identified as the pivotal moment in the modern transformation of medicine (1). The discovery of new drugs and the rapid burgeoning of medical technology revolutionized medical care. However, the importance of these discoveries was not so much in the prescription of particular drugs or use of tests, but in their impact on defining the molecular and biochemical paradigms so central to medicine. The drug revolution led medicine into a new and complex world of chemistry-oriented sciences which demanded ever finer medical training and specialization.

Thus, the "biomedical" model of disease and medicine's focus on the internal workings of the patient's biochemistry, supplanted the broader vision of the patient and his/her experience of illness. Almost immediately, the shortcomings of the biomedical model on doctor–patient relationship was apparent (2). The loss of the patient's perspective, and indeed loss of the person of the patient, has come to characterize the worst of high-technology medicine (2–5). Nowhere is the extreme of the biomedical model more evident than in the treatment of cancer patients with the rapid evolution of technological intervention and simultaneous decline of patient-centered care.

Incorporation of the patient's perspective into the medical system is not simply a return to the relationships of a previous era. As pointed out by Wilson and Cleary (6), the patient-centered alternative to the biomedical model incorporates a "quality-of-life" paradigm, focusing on complex behaviors and feelings which reflect dimensions of functioning and overall well-being. With its foundations in sociology and psychology, the patient-centered approach is sometimes as foreign to physicians as biomedicine is to patients. As such, medical training for patient-centered medicine requires a departure from traditional approaches,

broadening the biomedical view to one which "sees through the patient's eyes" and appreciates the web of relationships and contexts within which a patient suffers (7–9). Patients need their physicians' help in defining their own medical goals, actively participating in management and treatment considerations, and building confidence in judgments regarding their own functioning and well-being (7).

Communication skills at the heart of a more patient-centered medicine are not unlike the many other technical skills which comprise the basis of medical practice and for which proficiency is demanded. Nonetheless, the clinically technical skills belong to a domain which has traditionally been afforded "scientific" status, while communication skills belong to a domain which has not (9). The two realms, however, in practice represent a single and integrated approach in which the clinical reasoning process proceeds through both observation and dialogue concurrently, allowing the physician to understand both the disease and the patient (8).

Arguments for a more patient-centered medicine are not limited to societal demand and ethical deliberations, although these are indeed present and convincing (10). Patient-centered medicine and its associated communication skills are important because they are linked to both patient and physician well-being, and this is particularly relevant for both oncologists and cancer patients.

PATIENT-CENTERED COMMUNICATION SKILLS AND PHYSICIAN OUTCOMES

As many as one-third of oncologists suffer emotional exhaustion and a sense of low personal accomplishment, with as many as one-quarter having a psychiatric disorder (11). Extraordinary expectations may contribute to the stress burden these oncologists carry; they are expected to be scientifically expert providers, who are both technologically competent and empathic communicators, able to deal with patients' physical and psychological distress. Significant minorities of oncologists recognize that they are insufficiently trained in both communication and management skills and that the lack of training contributes to their stress (12). Nevertheless, few physicians have received systematic training in communication skills, with many adopting idiosyncratic strategies, largely through a process of trial and error (13, 14).

Dealing with patients' emotional reactions to cancer has emerged as one of the primary areas of communication difficulty for senior cancer clinicians attending training courses in England (15). Between 25% and 30% of patients with cancer experience anxiety and/or depression significantly severe to warrant psychological intervention (16). Unfortunately, several studies have shown that oncologists frequently fail to recognize these problems in their patients (17–19). Poor recognition of patients' emotional distress has been linked to inadequate training and poor counseling and assessment skills (20). Lacking formal training, many of these doctors develop cold, detached styles of communication. While detachment may provide some emotional protection, it appears more illusory than real. It is the emotional connection with patients which allows doctors to establish the sorts of therapeutic relationship that is a source of satisfaction for oncologists (12,21). Not surprising, the nature of the interpersonal relationship developed between patient and physician is the primary contributor to overall physician satisfaction with medical visits for primary care physicians (22).

PATIENT-CENTERED COMMUNICATION SKILLS AND PATIENT OUTCOMES

The consequences of patient-centered communication skills for patient outcomes is convincing. Stewart's recent comprehensive review of physician-patient communication interventions (23) found strong supporting evidence linking patient-centered communication elements with a variety of patient health outcomes, including emotional health, symptom resolution, function, physiologic measures (i.e., blood pressure and blood sugar level), and pain control. The review of interventions was organized around the communication functions within the visit, distinguishing studies examining history-taking, discussion of the management plan, and presentation of diagnostic information. Positive associations between communication elements

and health outcomes were evident in many of these visit segments. Table 94.1 reviews key communication elements as predictive of health outcomes identified in the Stewart review.

Several of the studies reviewed by Stewart specifically targeted oncology patients and linked aspects of enhanced communication or information delivery to improved health outcomes. (The communication elements associated with oncology visits are marked with an asterisk on Table 94.1.) Most notable among these, is the intervention study designed to affect actual communication between patient and physician in the medical visit conducted by Kaplan et al. (24). In separate trials, diabetic, hypertensive, peptic ulcer, and breast cancer patients were coached in methods designed to improve patient participation in clinical decision making through enhanced information-seeking and communication skills. The patient's medical record was reviewed with them prior to seeing their doctor following an algorithm to identify the relevant medical decision likely to arise during the current visit. The patient was encouraged to focus on treatment issues that could be affected by his or her lifestyle and preferences (i.e., dosage or timing of medication, diet restrictions, or exercise recommendations) and which could be reasonably negotiated with the physician. Negotiation skills were rehearsed with the patient according to a standardized script, and patients were encouraged to ask focused questions of their physicians. Patients rehearsed simple techniques for overcoming obstacles to negotiation such as embarrassment, forgetfulness, and intimidation, and after the coaching session, proceeded directly to the physician's office for their medical visit.

The medical visits were audiotaped and analyzed by a system which categorized medical conversation based on whether it was aimed at controlling the behavior of the other party, communicating information, or conveying emotion (positive or negative). The intervention had a significant impact on physician–patient communication and, subsequently, on treatment-related symptom experience reported by patients. The breast cancer study sample findings paralleled those of the chronically ill study populations of diabetic, hypertensive, and peptic ulcer patients. A symptom experience checklist over a 6-month course of adjuvant chemotherapy demonstrated fewer symptoms for cancer patients when they participated in the communication intervention, and their medical visit audiotape indicated greater patient communication control (and less physician communication control), greater expression of negative affect by both patients and physicians,

TABLE 94.1. *Communication Elements of Effective Medical Visits*

Physician Communication	Patient Outcome Affected
Asks many questions about the patient's understanding of the problem, concerns, and expectations, and about his or her perception of the impact of the problem on function.	Patient anxiety Symptom resolution
Asks patient about feelings.	Psychologic distress
Shows support and empathy.	Psychologic distress Symptom resolution
Physician gives clear information along with emotional support.	Psychologic distress Symptom resolution Blood pressure
Physician is willing to share decision making.	Patient anxiety*
Physician and patient agree about the nature of the problem and the need for follow-up.	Problem resolution Symptom resolution

Patient Communication	
Full patient expression, in regard to feelings, opinions and information	Role and physical limitations (21) Health status, functional status and blood pressure*
Patient perceives that a full discussion of the problem has taken place.	Symptom resolution
Patient is encouraged to ask more questions	Role and physical limitations Anxiety
Patient is successful at obtaining information	Functional status Physiological status
Patient is provided with information packages/programs	Pain Function Mood and anxiety*

*Oncology studies.
Source: Adapted from M. Stewart (1995). Effective Physician–Patient Communication and Health Outcomes: A Review. *Canadian Medical Association Journal*, 152: 1423–1433.

and more information provided by physicians during the office visit.

The authors suggest that these aspects of communication reflect "healthy friction" or role tension between physicians and patients. On the one hand, patients' assertions of control through more effective information-seeking, and perhaps disagreements, transform an otherwise physician-dominated monologue into a two-way exchange in which the patient has an active role and an obvious stake. The patient thus engaged is invested, perhaps more than otherwise, in the process as well as the outcome of the visit. On the other hand, expressions of frustration by the physician with a patient who is not progressing as expected may be interpreted by the patient as an expression of caring on the part of the physician. Other investigations have found that when physicians sound angry and anxious, their patients are more satisfied and compliant (25). The effective mechanism here may be an attribution

of greater concern and sincerity to a physician who is emotionally engaged than to one who appears emotionally neutral.

Investigating another aspect of participation in clinical decision making, both Morris et al. (26) and Fallowfield et al. (27) found a significant effect on patients' psychologic adjustment when women with breast cancer were offered choice in regard to surgical treatment. This appears evident in a reduction in median scores for psychologic and physical complaints (26) and in the reduction of patients' anxiety and depression (27). Choice in itself, however, was not the only factor influencing psychiatric morbidity. Fallowfield et al. conclude that satisfaction with the information given at the time that the diagnosis was confirmed and treatment options discussed was more important than choice alone to womens' psychologic adjustment (27–28). Doctors who offered choice whenever possible were perceived as better communicators with more satisfied patients. Some patients with cancer want greater autonomy, others prefer the doctor to be more directive, but both groups need to have options and reasons for recommendations about treatment explained in a way that either assists and supports them with the choice they make, or helps them to understand the doctor's advice.

For some patients a greater feeling of control may come with confidence that they are fully informed of their condition. Two clinical trials in which audiovisual information was provided to patients undergoing radiation therapy resulted in improved emotional status, as measured by anxiety level and mood disturbance (29), and improvement in patient functioning, as measured by the Sickness Impact Profile (30). Consistent findings were also reported by Butow et al. (31) in a descriptive study of the visits of an oncologist and 142 of her cancer patients attending their first consultation. The investigators found that patients whose questions were answered showed better psychological adjustment at the 3-week follow-up than those who asked questions but did not receive a response.

Answering questions, or fully disclosing the biomedical details of the patient's condition, however, may not be enough to assure positive patient outcomes. Even very experienced and well-informed patients perceive themselves to be poorly informed. In referring to radiation patients who had previously experienced radiation therapy (and were presumably knowledgeable about the process) Cassileth (32) reports that many felt they were "not being told enough." The feelings of information inadequacy, the author notes, may be attributed to insecurity due not to insufficient frankness about their exact diagnosis or the long-term prognosis, but to a need to confirm their physicians' sustained interest in their symptoms, support for their hopes, and confirmation of the validity of what they thought they knew.

Indeed, information exchange conveys more than just substantive meaning. Research suggests that patients attribute positive affective motivation to a physician who is informative. The physician who takes time to inform patients fully is regarded as sincere, concerned, interested, and dedicated (33). There is also evidence that physicians attribute positive characteristics to patients who are more verbally active in their visit, viewing them as more interested, concerned about their health, and intelligent. A patient who has truly heard distressing and often very complicated information about his or her medical condition, is likely to feel more knowledgeable, to ask more intelligent questions, be treated more as a partner, and adopt

a more directive role in his or her own medical care in subsequent medical visits.

While direct communication with cancer patients often reflects positive elements of biomedical informativeness, it does not often include the more comprehensive aspects of psychological and social adjustment. Using content analysis techniques to describe the cancer consultation, Ford and colleagues (34) examined the structure and content of 117 consultations with newly referred cancer patients who were receiving bad news, such as confirmation of their diagnosis or recurrence. Applying the Roter Interaction Analysis System (RIAS), the investigators showed that discussion within these visits was overwhelmingly biomedical, emphasizing information giving from both patients and physicians. Patients received a large amount of information from their doctors about diagnosis, prognosis, and treatment options, with much reassurance and counseling on biomedical topics. Nonetheless, the authors concluded that the level of patient-centeredness was very low. Patients asked few questions, and while physicians often asked whether or not they understood what was being conveyed to them, patients were rarely given the opportunity to respond fully to these queries. Most disappointing, was the very low levels of psychological probing and counseling; there was little attention paid to patients' psychosocial concerns and issues related to psychological and social adjustment to cancer.

The lack of discussion devoted to feelings and emotions is all the more troubling considering evidence that breast cancer patients' perceptions of the physician as caring were especially important to subsequent psychologic adjustment to cancer, even more so than their perception of physician informativeness (35). The authors conclude that provision of information needed for decision making appears to be valued by patients largely within the context of a caring physician–patient relationship. Specific surgeons' behaviors identified as facilitating patient adjustment (in order) included the expression of empathy, allowing the patient time to absorb the cancer diagnosis, provision of information, and engagement of the patient in treatment decision making.

While not specific to cancer visits, a meta-analysis of patient–physician communication found consistent relationships between physicians' communication and patient outcomes (36). The meta-analysis concluded that three dimensions of communication—informativeness, interpersonal sensitivity, and partnership building—were consistently associated with patient satisfaction, compliance, and recall of medical information. These aspects of communication appear equally as relevant to cancer patients as general medical patients.

PHYSICIAN TRAINING IN COMMUNICATION SKILLS

While it is clear from the earlier discussion that patient-centered communication skills are associated with positive patient outcomes, fewer than 10% ($n = 18$) of the continuing medical education (CME) interventions meeting rigorous methodological criteria reviewed by Davis and colleagues (37), address communication. Among the select group of studies meeting these criteria, only slightly more than half of counseling-type interventions reported a positive result in terms of physician performance or health outcomes, with the remainder reporting mixed or negative results. In contrast to other areas of CME, these results are weak. For instance, interventions to improve prevention and screening activities demonstrated a positive outcome in 83% of trials, and improvements in prescribing and resource utilization reported success rates exceeding 70% of trials. The authors suggest that effective behavior-change strategies used in these programs differ; the challenges of changing discrete behaviors related to screening or immunizations demand less complicated interventions than those associated with so broad a set of behaviors as communication and counseling. Among the effective lifestyle and counseling intervention strategies were the use of peer discussion (38) and rehearsal (39), which allow physicians to practice the targeted communication skills. Formal CME conferences that do not allow practice- reinforcing strategies had relatively little impact.

At least part of the variation in intervention efficacy may be attributable to physicians' readiness to change (37,40). Readiness is a reflection of the learner's motivation, knowledge of a problem, and the perception of a gap between current knowledge and skills and those needed for adequate performance. Indeed, success in the reviewed studies was directly related to investigators' attention to these aspects of their CME intervention. Readiness to change is perhaps more problematic in regard to communication skills than many other areas of CME. Despite general agreement that interviewing skills are critical and that prior training has been inadequate, there is little consensus on any gold-standard criteria for adequate performance. Relatively little attention has been directed to the development of standardized assessment methodologies of the medical dialogue, and the medical interview has remained largely outside of the quality of care revolution (41). Few physicians have systematically analyzed their own performance nor are they generally aware of what standard practice is, let alone ideal practice. It is unusual for a medical student or resident to directly observe medical visits, especially ambulatory care, with a focus on communication dynamics (42).

This is not to say that the field of communications research has not progressed. An encouraging observation noted in regard to the CME literature is that it is substantially increasing in number and quality each year (37). As evidenced by the list of elements of communication related to health outcomes in Table 94.1, there is considerable evidence of efficacy.

In contrast to the far fewer studies which have linked specific skills directly to performance or health outcomes in rigorously evaluated clinical trials, many studies have established that specific communication skills can be taught (42). Trials of such educational interventions, however, have been generally characterized by relatively small numbers of participants, limited measures of effectiveness, and unstated or unclear theoretical assumptions. Moreover, many of these studies have been conducted within the context of medical school or physician training curriculums which are too time-consuming for most busy practitioners.

PROTOTYPES OF SUCCESSFUL COMMUNITY-BASED TRAINING PROGRAMS IN COMMUNICATION SKILLS

Addressing the need for communication skills training among oncologists in the United Kingdom, a model program was developed by Fallowfield et al. (15). The program was directed toward enlisting the support and enthusiasm of senior oncologists for their own training in communication skills, and designed to encourage these senior doctors to help with the introduction of these skills to their juniors. Inasmuch as senior doctors provide the most credible role-models for physicians in training and medical students, it was seen as crucial to harness their co-operation and enthusiasm if the program was to succeed (43).

Based on the conceptual teaching model developed by Lipkin and colleagues (44), the key principle of the program was the integration of learner-centered, self-directed learning, with core human values such as unconditional positive regard for others and attention to affect. Consistent with adult learning precepts, the Lipkin model builds upon the work of educational philosophers Paulo Friere (45) and Malcolm Knowles (46). The guiding principles of the model recognize that the learning experience must be defined by the learners themselves, be relevant to daily experience, and provide opportunities to practice skills and knowledge, while reflecting upon the effects of that experience.

In this light, the communication course was designed by Fallowfield and her colleagues (15) focusing on the critical role of oncologists' prior experience as the major source of motivation for learning and use of problem-centered, rather than subject-centered, approaches. The course attempted to provide change in three major spheres of learning: knowledge acquisition, skill development, and personal awareness. Knowledge and skills were developed through task-oriented work groups, demonstrations, and exercises. Work on attitudes and personal awareness was integrated with other parts of the course and explored through further group discussion wherever appropriate. Although courses had a clear pre-determined structure with respect to exercises and demonstration workshops, participants set their own agendas regarding the topics included in skills group sessions. In practice most participants focused on problem areas identified in their pre-course self-assessment forms.

Over a two and a half year period 178 senior residents and attendings working within cancer medicine attended 1½-day or 3-day courses. Subjective improvements in many communication problems were reported post-course and appeared to be maintained at 3 and 12 months follow-up. Based on these results, the investigators conclude that most doctors recognize that their practice of medicine is hampered by the inadequacies of their previous training in communication skills. However, if the format is right, they will devote time and effort to correct this and attend communication skills courses.

Taking a somewhat different approach to the training of established physicians in communication skills, an 8-hour, short course was developed and tested in a randomized trial (47). While geared toward primary care physicians and their patients, the training curriculum would be equally relevant to oncologists. The curriculum emphasized aspects of doctor–patient communication relevant to the identification, discussion, and management of patients' emotional distress. The kinds of interviewing skills thought to be effective in recognizing patients' emotional distress, whether these are diagnosable conditions or lower order psychological problems, were broadly characterized as falling within two skill domains. The first of these was affective in focus, based on the physicians' feeling-oriented or emotion-handling skills, broadly reflecting the theories of Rogers (48), while the second was cognitive, emphasizing the physicians' question-asking, probing, and problem-solving skills, as described by Lesser (49).

Training programs of both types have reported success in the teaching of these skills (50–59). Moreover, several of these studies have found that use of particular communication skills led to greater patient disclosure of sensitive psychosocial information to physicians. (50,58). Others have found that training family medicine residents in interviewing skills improved their ability to detect emotional distress among their patients (59). The consequences of detection appear far reaching. Detection of emotional distress has been associated with shorter duration of psychiatric symptoms following detection and shorter duration of total medical symptoms throughout the year (60), as well as decreases in psychopathology and social disability as long as 14 months after initial interviews (61).

The study by Roter and colleagues was a randomized clinical trial of 69 practicing physicians in non-university settings with some 700 of their patients. Each physician was assigned to one of two study groups which received 8 hours of training in either problem-solving or emotion-handling skills, or to a control group which did not receive training until completion of the study. The educational intervention was identical for the two experimental groups, except in the specific skills taught, which were distinguished as loosely fitting two conceptually discrete models of interpersonal communication. As presented in Table 94.2, the first set of 8 skills reflected the Rogerian model of emotion-handling (48) while the second set of 8 skills reflected a more cognitive approach to problem definition based generally on the work of Lesser and associates (49). Faculty helped focus discussion on role play and audiotaped material that illustrated use of, or opportunities for use of, each of the designated skills; however, no attempt was made to suppress discussion of other skills that were identified by participants as relevant to the situation. The faculty were interdisciplinary, consisting of practicing and academic general internists, an academic family practitioner-psychiatrist, and a social scientist. All were experienced instructors in communication skills who strove to create safe, supportive environments for the participants that encouraged risk taking, self-assessment, and the elicitation of feedback from colleagues.

Evaluation of the skills training intervention was based on audiotape analysis of all study physicians' visits with 10 actual patients, as well as a simulated patient. Patient outcomes, based on repeated administration over a 6-month period of the General Health Questionnaire (GHQ), a standardized measure of general emotional distress, were assessed through telephone follow-up.

TABLE 94.2. *Targeted Communication Skills*

EMOTION-HANDLING SKILLS

Signaling Receptivity by:

1. Asking patients about their feelings

2. Listening more, talking less

3. Following-up on signs of patients' emotional distress

Showing positive regard by:

4. Complimenting patient efforts

5. Making statements of legitimation (explicitly stating that patients' feelings/views are normal or understandable)

Expressing mutuality by:

6. Expressing empathy (accurately acknowledging an emotion expressed by the patient)

7. Making explicit statements of partnership or support

8. Providing appropriate reassurance

PROBLEM-DEFINING SKILLS

Eliciting the full-spectrum of patient concerns by:

1. Resisting immediate follow-up of the patient's first expressed concern

2. Asking the patient explicitly about other problems or concerns ("anything else"), including problems of daily living and stressors

3. Prioritizing with patients (negotiating use of time)

Delineating the patient's problem by:

4. Starting with open-ended questions

5. Using facilitative statements to help patients tell their story in their own words

6. Assessing the impact of the patient's problem on psychosocial functioning

Understanding the patient's perspective by:

7. Probing explicitly for patients' understanding/concerns related to their problem(s)

8. Clarifying patient expectations for the visit

There were four findings of importance in the study. First, physicians' use of communication skills in their practices changed as a result of a modest 8-hour CME program. This was evident in visits with physicians' actual patients audiotaped at least a month after the training, as well as in the simulated patient visits. Second, physicians trained in specific communication skills recognized more psychosocial problems in their patients and employed more strategies to manage emotional problems in their patients than did untrained physicians. Furthermore, trained physicians demonstrated greater clinical proficiency in the management of a standardized patient compared with control group physicians. Third, the patients of trained compared with untrained physicians demonstrated greater reduction in emotional distress for as long as 6 months following their medical visit. Fourth, these results were not associated with significantly longer medical visits or increased utilization.

The communication skills training helped the physicians engage more effectively in the process of psychosocial exploration. This was not only important for problem recognition, but may in itself be therapeutic.

In noting a direct effect of recognition on patient outcome, Ormel and associates (61) concluded that the benefits cannot be wholly attributed to specific mental health treatments. Rather, other effects of the recognition process, such as acknowledgment, reinterpretation of signs and symptoms, and social support may be contributing the "active element" to the recovery process. The mechanism by which even limited attention to psychosocial problems may alleviate distress is also proposed by Stoeckle and others (62). The authors suggest that "active listening" can assist a patient in more appropriate attribution of distress, alleviate feelings associated with helplessness and isolation, and create a sense of support and partnership.

CONCLUSION

The supportive function of communication may be seen at the intersection of the patient's experience and the physician's expertise. The physician's appreciation for how a patient integrates and interprets biomedical information into their everyday experience, as well as the physician confirmation of what that experience is, is critical. Without this intersection, Mishler maintains (3), the medical dialogue proceeds as two parallel and largely separate monologues. It is likely that both the substantive content of communication—the degree of specificity and detail associated with medical explanations—as well as an affective appreciation for the life context within which the information is placed, are necessary for effective communication between patients and their physicians.

As articulated by McWhinney (8), medicine is in the midst of a transformation from the traditional clinical method and social relations it fosters between doctor and patient to a new patient-centered clinical method. This transformation is not a trivial refinement in the practice of medicine; it defines new goals and methods for medicine. While the traditional method diagnoses disease, it does not aim to understand the meaning of the illness for the patient. However, it is exactly the meaning of illness which should stand at the heart of a more humane medicine. This will continue to be the most meaningful of the training challenges the medical profession will face in future years, regardless of how dramatic the changes become in the structure, form, or financing of medicine.

REFERENCES

1. Shorter E. *Bedside Manners.* New York, NY: Simon and Schuster; 1985.
2. Engel GL. The need for a new medical model: a challenge for biomedicine. *Science.* 1977; 196:129–136.
3. Mishler EG. *The Discourse of Medicine: Dialectics of Medical Interviews.* Norwood, NJ: Ablex; 1984.
4. Cassell EJ. *Talking with Patients: Volume 2. Clinical Technique.* Cambridge, MA: MIT Press; 1985.
5. Kleinman A, Eisenberg L, Good B. Culture, illness and care: Clinical lessons from anthropologic and cross-cultural research. *Ann of Inter Med.* 1978; 88:251–258.
6. Wilson IB, Cleary PD. Linking clinical variables with health-related quality of life: A conceptual model of patient outcomes. *JAMA,* 1995; 273:59–65.
7. Maloney T, Paul B. Rebuilding public trust and confidence. In: Gerteis M, Edman-Levitan S, Daley J, Delbanco T (eds.), *Through the Patient's Eyes: Understanding and Promoting Patient-centered Care.* San Francisco, CA: Jossey-Bass; 1993.
8. McWhinney I. The need for a transformed clinical method. In: Stewart M, Roter D (eds.), *Communicating With Medical Patients.* Newbury Park, CA: Sage; 1989.
9. Engel GL. How much longer must medicine's science be bound by a seventeenth century world view? In: White, K (ed.), *The Task of Medicine: Dialogue at Wickenburg.* Menlo Park, CA: The Henry J. Kaiser Family Foundation; 1988.
10. President's Commission for the Study of Ethical Problems in Medicine and Biomedical and Behavioral Research, Volume I: *Making Health Care Decisions.* Washington, DC: U.S. Government Printing Office; 1982.
11. Ramirez AJ, Graham J, Richards MA, et al. Mental health of hospital consultants: the effects of stress and satisfaction at work. *Lancet.* 1996; 347:724–728.
12. Ramirez AJ, Graham J, Richards MA, et al. Burnout and psychiatric disorder among 'cancer clinicians'. *Br J Cancer.* 1995; 71:1263–1269.
13. Byrne JM, Long BEL. *Doctors Talking to Patients.* London: HMSO; 1976.
14. Fallowfield LJ. Giving sad and bad news. *Lancet.* 1993; 341:476–478.
15. Fallowfield LJ. Communication skills of oncologists. *Forum: Trends Experi Med.* 1995; 5(1):99–103.
16. Derogatis LR, Morrow GR, Fetting J, et al. The prevalence of psychiatric disorder among cancer patients. *JAMA.* 1983; 249:751–757.
17. Derogatis LR, Abeloff MD, McBeth CD. Cancer patients and their physicians in the perception of psychological symptoms. *Psychosomatics.* 1976; 17:197–201.
18. Hardman A, Maguire P, Crowther D. The recognition of psychiatric morbidity on a medical oncology ward. *J Psychol Res.* 1989; 33:235–239.
19. Ford S, Fallowfield LJ, Lewis S. Can oncologists detect distress in their out-patients and how satisfied are they with their performance during bad news consultations? *Br J Cancer.* 1994; 70:767–770.
20. Hopwood P, Maguire P. Priorities in the psychological care of patients. *Int Rev Psychol.* 1992; r:35–44.
21. Fallowfield LJ. Can we improve the professional & personal fulfilment of doctors in cancer medicine? *Br J Cancer.* 1995; 71:1132–1133.
22. Suchman AL, Roter DL, Green M, Lipkin M, Jr. Physician satisfaction with primary care office visits. *Med Care.* 1993; 31:1083–1092.
23. Stewart MA. Effective physician–patient communication and health outcomes: a review. *Can Med Assoc J.* 1996; 152:1423–1433.
24. Kaplan SH, Greenfield S, Ware JE Jr. Assessing the effects of physician-patient interactions on the outcomes of chronic disease. *Med Care.* 1989; 27:S110–S127.
25. Hall J, Roter D, Rand C. Communication of affect between patients and physicians. *J Health Soc Behav.* 1981; 11:18–30.
26. Morris J, Royle GT. Offering patients a choice of surgery for early breast cancer: a reduction in anxiety and depression in patients and their husbands. *Soc Sci Med.* 1988; 26:583–585.
27. Fallowfield LJ, Hall A, Maguire GP, Baum M. Psychological outcomes of different treatment policies in women with early breast cancer outside a clinical trial. *BMJ.* 1990; 301:575–580.
28. Fallowfield LJ, Hall A, Maguire P, et al. A question of choice: Results of a prospective 3 year follow-up study of women with breast cancer. *Breast J Cancer.* 1994; 3: 202–208.
29. Rainey LC. Effects of preparatory patient education for radiation oncology patients. *Cancer.* 1985; 56:1056–1061.
30. Johnson JE, Nail LM, Lauver D, et al. Reducing the negative impact of radiation therapy on functional status. *Cancer.* 1988; 61:46–51.

31. Butow PN, Dunn SM, Tattersall MHN, Jonew QJ. Computer based interaction analysis of the cancer consultation. *Br J Med.* 1995; 71:1115–1121.

32. Cassileth BR, Volckmar D, Goodman RL. The effect of experience on radiation therapy patients' desire for information. Inter. *Int J Radiation Oncol Biol Phys.* 1980; 6:493–496.

33. Roter D, Hall J, Katz N. Relations between physicians' behaviors and patients' satisfaction, recall, and impressions: an analogue study. *Med Care.* 1987; 25:399–412.

34. Ford S, Fallowfield LJ, Lewis S. Doctor–patient interactions in oncology. *Soc Sci Med.* 1996; 42:11:1511–1519.

35. Roberts CS, Cox CE, Reintgen DS, et al. Influence of physician communication on newly diagnosed breast patients' psychologic adjustment and decision-making. *Cancer.* 1994; 74:336–341.

36. Hall JA, Roter DL, Katz NR. Meta-analysis of correlates of provider behavior in medical encounters. *Med Care.* 1988; 26:657–675.

37. Davis DA, Thomson MA, Oxman AD, Haynes B. Changing physician performance: A systematic review of the effect of continuing medical education strategies. *JAMA.* 1995; 274:700–705.

38. Davidoff F, Goodspeed R, Clive J. Changing test ordering behavior: A randomized controlled trial comparing probalistic reasoning with cost-containment education. *Med Care.* 1989; 27:45–58.

39. Kottke TE, Brekke ML, Solberg LI, Hughes JR. A randomized trial to increase smoking intervention by physicians: Doctors helping smokers, round I. *JAMA.* 1989; 261:2101–2106.

40. Fox RD, Mazmanian PE, Putnam RW. *Changing and Learning in Lives of Physicians.* New York, NY: Praeger; 1989.

41. Starfield B. *Primary Care: Concept Evaluation and Policy.* New York, NY: Oxford University Press; 1992.

42. Kern DE, Grayson M, Barker LR, et al. Residency training in interviewing skills and the psychosocial domain of medical practice. *J Gen Intern Med.* 1989; 4:421–431.

43. Fallowfield LJ, David H. Organization and training issues. In: David H, Fallowfield LJ (eds.), *Counseling and Communication in Health Care.* Chichester England. John Wiley & Sons Ltd; 1991: 319–340.

44. Lipkin M, Kaplan C, Clark W, Novack DH. Teaching medical Interviewing: the Lipkin model. In: Lipkin M, Putnam S, Lazare A. (eds.), *The Medical Interview: Clinical Care, Education, and Research.* New York: Springer-Verlag, 1995: 422–435.

45. Friere P. *Pedagogy of the Oppressed.* New York, NY: Continuum; 1986.

46. Knowles MS. *The Modern Practice of Adult Education: From Pedagogy to Androgogy.* New York, NY: Adult Education Company; 1980.

47. Roter DL, Hall JA, Kern DE, et al. Improving physicians' interviewing skills and reducing patients' emotional distress: A randomized clinical trial. *Arch Intern Med.* 1995; 155:1877–1884.

48. Rogers CR. *Client-Centered Therapy.* Boston: Houghton Mifflin, 1951.

49. Lesser AL. Problem-based interviewing in general practice: A model. *Med Ed.* 1985; 19:299–304.

50. Putnam SM, Stiles WB, Casey Jacob M, James SA. Teaching the medical interview: An intervention study *J Gen Intern Med.* 1988; 3:38–47.

51. Bensing JM, Sluijs EM. Evaluation of an interview training course for general practitioners. *Soc Sci Med.* 1985; 20:737–744.

52. Maguire P, Fairbairn S, Fletcher C. Consultation skills of young doctors: I. Benefits of feedback training in interviewing as students persist. *BMJ.* 1986; 292:1573–1576.

53. Stillman P, Sabers D, Redfield D. Use of trained mothers to teach interviewing skills to first year medical students: A follow-up study. *Pediatrics.* 1977; 60:165–169.

54. Gask L, Goldberg A, Lesser L, Miller T. Improving the psychiatric skills of the general practice trainee: An evaluation of a group training course. *Med Ed.* 1988; 22: 132–138.

55. Gask L, McGrath G, Goldberg A, Miller T. Improving the psychiatric skills of established general practitioners: Evaluation of group teaching. *Med Ed.* 1987; 21:362–368.

56. Maguire P, Roe P, Goldberg D, et al. The value of feedback in teaching interviewing skills to medical students. *Psychol Med.* 1978; 8:695–704.

57. Levinson W, Roter D. The effects of two continuing medical education programs on communication skills of practicing primary care physicians. *J Gen Intern Med.* 1993; 8:318–324.

58. Cox A, Holbrook D, Rutter M. Psychiatric interviewing techniques. VI. Experimental study: eliciting feelings. *Br J Psychiatry.* 1981; 139:144–152.

59. Marks J, Goldberg D, Hiller V. Determinants of the ability of general practitioners to detect psychological illness. *Psychol Med.* 1979; 9:337–353.

60. Johnstone A, Goldberg D. Psychiatric screening in general practice: A controlled trial. *Lancet.* 1976; March: 605–608.

61. Ormel J, VanDen Brink W, Koeter MWJ, et al. Recognition, management and outcome of psychological disorders in primary care: A naturalistic follow-up study. *Psychol Med.* 1990; 20:909–923.

62. Stoeckle J, Barsky A. Attributions: Uses of social science knowledge in the doctoring of primary care. In: Eisenberg and Kleinman (eds.), *The Relevance of Social Science for Medicine.* New York, NY: Reidel Publishing Co.; 1980.

XV

ETHICAL ISSUES IN ONCOLOGY: A PSYCHOLOGICAL FRAMEWORK

Editor: Marguerite S. Lederberg

95

Truth Telling and Informed Consent

NANCY NEVELOFF DUBLER AND LINDA FARBER POST

Informed consent is the concept that has animated discussion between doctors and their patients over the last several decades. It is an amalgam of philosophical notions of autonomy and respect for persons, legal principles of self-determination and liberty, and administrative concepts of prudent and careful procedure. Historically, discussions of informed consent have provided the fulcrum for shifting the balance of power from physician paternalism to shared physician–patient responsibility (1–7). At least that is the mythical explanation. In reality, informed consent is more often equated with a piece of paper that permits the next hospital intervention to proceed smoothly or a risk-management technique for attempting to limit possible future liability.

Nonetheless, the rigor of the paradigm and its distance from actual practice should not discourage physicians from attempting communication with patients, even if the conversation falls short of meeting some idealized notion of informed consent. Some patients have the intellectual and emotional capacity to weigh alternative care plans and measure them against personal needs and preferences. Almost all patients have some ability to make choices if the options and their consequences are sketched out clearly. Likewise, some physicians have the temperament for and commitment to careful explanation of the available choices. But all physicians understand the broad differences among multiple care plans and can place an outline of the various options before the patient. In this area, as in other bioethical quagmires, the best should not become the enemy of the good. Although they will not always achieve the ideal result, physicians must struggle constantly to work as effectively as they can with each individual patient.

The ethical and legal roots of the informed consent doctrine provide the basis for its power. The legal history begins with the medieval concept of assault and battery at the time when physicians were barbers. On

the theory that any unconsented-to touching constituted an unlawful act, the patient's contemporaneous consent to the barber's touching precluded a later charge of assault and battery (8–12). The subsequent legal trend toward negligence rather than battery as a measure of a physician's duty reflected judicial dissatisfaction with the artificial notion that consent either did or did not happen (13–15).

The doctrine of negligence permits nuanced examination of whether the discussion reflects the risks and benefits that are material to this patient. It provides a range of possibilities in determining when and what physicians should disclose to patients (3,9). More recently, support for the right of the patient to make knowledgeable health care decisions has been found in doctrines of privacy, autonomy, and liberty (5,8,16). Finally, in the current litigious climate of malpractice, cost containment, and managed care, informed consent has become a defensive risk-management weapon. Indeed, risk managers advise physicians that risks that have been adequately disclosed to patients cannot be the basis for later claims. The problem with this logic lies in the fact that malpractice suits have more to do with the strength of the provider–patient relationship than with the content of the communication.

During the past approximately 30 years since the explosion of the various "rights" movements, the ethical principle of autonomy has gained increasing currency as the major support for individual empowerment and self-determination. In virtually every social sphere, notably the civil rights and feminist movements, the activist agenda has been to level the playing field by eliminating imbalances of power caused by differences in race, class, gender, and education. In the health care setting, the twin notions of patient as partner in therapeutic decision making and patient as informed health care consumer were reflected in the increasing importance of the concept of patient autonomy. Simultaneously, changes in the standards for judging malpractice litigation put patient wishes, rather than conventions of physician practice, at the core of the duty to disclose. Over time, patients came to see informed consent as their security against physician overreaching, while doctors perceived it as a defensive protection against charges of malpractice—the medical equivalent of a prenuptial agreement. The unfortunate result is an adversarial rather than therapeutic climate, with informed consent as the weapon of choice.

The tension between the theory and the reality of informed consent has been explored by scholars in medicine, philosophy, law, and psychiatry (9,14). Problems in implementing the concept arise from the social, informational, and intellectual power imbalance that generally exists between physicians and patients, the resulting discomfort in patient-physician communication, the want of structural supports in the medical culture for sharing authority, and the lack of reimbursement for the time that discussion would require (17–22)—the last, a very real factor in the lives of physicians driven harder by managed care organizations to increase productivity and decrease consultant referrals. Psychological factors also have impact on communication. The physician's compassion and sense of powerlessness in the face of the pain and suffering of fatal illness may result in overidentification with the patient and loss of objectivity, which can significantly impede communication. Finally, education in medical school and residency curricula, or the lack thereof, ill prepares physicians for the task of ensuring that the consent the patient gives is both voluntary and informed. Arrayed against this formidable set of barriers and disincentives are exhortations of ethicists, clear dictates of courts, guidelines for professional behavior, and the advice of risk managers (8,12,23–24).

Having identified this gulf between theory and practice, many commentators insist that the choice is between capitulating to the reality of paternalistic practice or insisting on the utility of a doctrine that is clearly honored more in the breach than in the observance. This chapter proposes a middle ground: first, another attempt to understand the ongoing physician reluctance to discuss choices and options with patients; and second, an effort to fashion a mid-level position that embodies the centrality of patient autonomy, while recognizing the difficulties and disincentives in the care system for implementing a full and robust notion of informed consent.

REASONS SUPPORTING THE PROCESS OF INFORMED CONSENT

Information about and involvement in the informed consent process create the basic understanding that helps patients to withstand the pain and suffering of treatment (25–28). The resulting stake in the decision provides both the illusion and the reality of control, creating a sense of active participation in and cooperation with treatment, rather than passive compliance with directed behavior. It is the most ostensible symbol of the partnership between physicians and patients, and forms the ethical bedrock of care plans (10,23). It is the personal convenant through which patients pledge their efforts to stay fast to the treatment despite pain and suffering, and physicians dedicate themselves to pursue the best interest of their patients.

As the history of informed consent followed changes in legal rules and ethical perceptions, so too it reflected developments in science and medicine. Thus, informed consent became important only as choice became possible. For centuries, medicine could offer comfort consistently, diagnosis occasionally, and cure rarely. The ability of medical science to intervene and affect the quality of life and longevity changed for cancer patients with improved surgical techniques early in the century, radiation therapy in the 1940s, chemotherapy in the 1950s, and the use of biologicals in the 1980s. These developments took place against the backdrop of discoveries that can sustain organ systems and support renal, pulmonary, and cardiac function that may be compromised by treatment. These miraculous discoveries provided oncology with a set of interventions that could reverse disease processes and repair bodies, but only for a certain percentage of patients and always at the cost of pain and suffering. Thus, in addition to their other skills, oncologists are required to develop the ability to communicte hope in the context of uncertainty and determination in the face of despair. If, as new data indicate, 50% of each year's cohort of new cancer patients will be alive in five years (29), the process of productive hope and protective denial must proceed simultaneously.

Prognosis has become more complicated. Even promising interventions are not assured of success. In cancer, almost no treatment—especially radiotherapy and chemotherapy—comes unaccompanied by negative, and potentially life-threatening, side effects. The complex series of choices presented by modern science and technology demands a new paradigm; uncertainty becomes the unacknowledged companion of medical advice. It is difficult for a physician to choose, let alone advise, about the possible options for care in early breast cancer. The available data do not provide an unequivocal choice between mastectomy or lumpectomy, and it is nearly impossible to gauge the significance of greater deformity from mastectomy against the greater intellectual and emotional comfort that aggressive surgery might provide. In many other cancers, there is no certain choice among the various combinations of radiation and chemotherapy currently available. Cytotoxicity is the hallmark of cancer treatment and, despite efforts to render its effects tumor-specific, present techniques leave the patient open to occasionally disastrous outcomes. Notwithstanding efforts at intellectual candor and empathy, the physician's guidance must rest primarily on the attitudes and needs of patient and family. As the range of therapeutic options grows, so does the honest and responsible doctor's recognition that no single choice is indicated in every instance, and that patients must assume a more active role in the selection (30). These choices become particularly poignant when advancing disease permits only noncurative options.

The existence of choices demands the identification of a person to choose. The nominees include the physician, the capable patient, or some coalition of family members or close friends to whom the patient has turned for advice and decision. For the patient who is not able to exercise choice because of physical or mental incapacity or because of deep-seated psychological aversion, the possible surrogate deciders include the patient's legally appointed proxy; a close family member or friend, in those states with surrogate choice legislation or case law; or an ethics committee, judge or court-appointed surrogate (31).

The physician is, in many but not all cases, the least attractive of the optional decision makers, particularly in tertiary academic medical centers. She is often a stranger to the patient and likely to be unaware of the important themes and values in the patient's life. Medical choices are basd on scientific data interpreted in the light of personal experience. The physician possesses the knowledge base and the professional skills to evaluate these data and communicate the results to the patient. The patient, in turn, brings to the discussion a set of personal values and philosophies, emotional needs and strengths, and an individual history that has created sensitivity to some behaviors and antipathy to others (32). The patient also brings a style of deciding that is somewhere on the continuum between solitary and communal. Empirical studies reveal that a notion of patient autonomy that "premises that all people desire the same things and attempt to get them in similar ways" is not reflected in clinical practice (33,12,34). Indeed, the issue has been framed in

terms of the ownership of the decision. Jay Katz notes the multifaceted nature of treatment decisions, which he describes as "a combination of medical, emotional, aesthetic, religious, philosophical, social, interpersonal, and personal judgments[.]" Katz then asks, "Which of these judgments belong to the physician and which to the patient?" (9) Yet, in the end it is the patient who will suffer the consequences of the decision, including the benefits of effective treatment and the disabilities of treatment failure. The decisional balance between the patient and the physician is clear—ultimately, the patient must decide. This analysis might not apply to a well-known and fondly regarded primary care physician who has treated the patient and family for decades. However, tertiary care specialists, a term applied to the vast number of oncologists, almost never have this close long-standing relationship with a patient. In any event, the familiar general practice of Marcus Welby, if he exists at all, will likely be ended by managed care.

DECISIONS BY PERSONS OTHER THAN THE PATIENT—CAPACITY AND SURROGATE CHOICE

But what if the patient cannot or will not decide? The first must be determined and the second accommodated.

Despite its complexity, the allocation of decision-making authority does not relegate the physician to a passive role at the sidelines of the process. It requires knowledge, skill, and compassion to decide what specific information the patient needs to know, how much he wants to know, and when he needs to know it. There are times when the patient elects to shield himself from some kinds of information (35–37) and only an understanding relationship with the patient can ground the physician's decision to support or challenge denial that may be protective or destructive. Trust and empathy are needed to guide the patient in relating the relevant material to his particular needs and goals. Rather than informed consent, the process might better be called advised consent, because it requires all the professional and personal skills of the physician to present and evaluate the data and offer guidance that the patient may elect to follow.

Decisional capacity is determined by evaluating the patient's decision-making ability in light of the risks and complexity of the particular choice and the possible or likely consequences of the intervention or of nonintervention. Although the terms "capacity" and "competence" are often used interchangeably, for bioethics purposes there are important distinctions that go beyond semantics. "Competence" is technically a legal designation made only by a court, whereas health care decisions are a matter of medical determination. Because the legal system is rarely involved in decision making in the clinical setting, it has become customary to refer to the patient's "capacity" to make health care decisions and to refer to the decisionally "capacitated" or "capable" individual (38,28). The classic definition of decisional capacity is from the President's Commission:

Decision-making capacity requires, to greater or lesser degree: (*1*) possession of a set of values and goals; (*2*) the ability to communicate and to understand information; and (*3*) the ability to reason and to deliberate about one's choices. (10)

This definition of informed consent presupposes, and most scholars agree, that decisional capacity is decision specific. It is not an on/off switch, but rather reflects a continuum of abilities, also known as a sliding scale, needed to evaluate choices of escalating complexity, risk, and consequences. This means that the greater the complexity of the decision and the more serious the consequences, the greater must be the patient's ability to marshal his intellectual and emotional resources (39). The benefit of this formulation is that it requires that the patient or a surrogate actually be up to the task of deciding about whether treatment should be consented to or refused. It demands that the pleasant, socially appropriate but demented patient, who may be fully capable of deciding whether to have fish or chicken for lunch, not be empowered to decide whether to agree to or refuse chemotherapy for leukemia. Honoring a capable patient's decision demonstrates respect for the individual and deference to his autonomy. Following the direction of a patient who is without the ability to address the complex issues and appreciate their implications constitutes abandonment.

Somewhat separate problems arise when seeking surrogate consent and acting in opposition to a patient's refusal of care. Any initial patient refsual should signal the beginning, rather than the end, of conversation exploring the patient's understanding, confusion, fears, trust, and sense of isolation. Consistent refusal, however, even on the part of a decisionally compromised patient, should never be overridden by caregivers alone. This is one of the few instances in which petition to a court is both morally and legally mandatory.

The problem with decision-specific capacity assessment is that it revives notions of paternalism and imports them back into the decision-making process through the obligation to evaluate the capacity of the patient. Disagreement with the physician, seen through the lens of differing values, can be taken to reflect diminshed capacity rather than dissimilar priorities, and can be used as the basis for challenging decisional ability. As such, capacity determinations are potent tools to disempower patients and should be used carefully and respectfully to address concerns about the process of deciding, not disagreements with the decision itself. For this reason, in addition to capacity, a morally and legally valid informed consent process must provide for consent that is voluntary, not coerced directly by persons or indirectly by circumstances, and is based on disclosure of all facts that are material to the patient's decision. The danger of physicians wittingly or unwittingly exerting undue influence on patient's decision making, especially acute in the context of clinical research, is discussed below.

However, some patients have the capacity to decide, but refuse to exercise it. Pathological denial that precludes consideration of the prognosis and its likely consequences renders a patient decsionally incapacitated. More commonly, patients ask physicians to decide—"I'll do whatever you say is best"—or to involve other family members in the decision. It is not unusual to hear an elderly patient request that the physician talk to her daughter or son and be guided by that person's judgment. Whereas the physician may continue to approach the patient and attempt to involve her in choosing, decision-making patterns developed over time are unlikely to be revised in times of stress. If the patient's tendency has been to rely on the advice of a physician or the judgment of an adult child, that pattern is likely to survive exhortations to independent choosing.

Patients exercise autonomy in very different ways. Some plunge headlong into the minutiae of the decision and require masses of specific data, references to articles, and responses to myriad questions. Others request summaries of complex analyses that identify the probability of various outcomes. Some prefer discussion with the physician alone, while others are far more comfortable if family and loved ones are present. All these variations are permissible—and, indeed, recommended—for the patients who need them. The conept is guided by the particular needs and goals of the individual with all the peculiarities that attach. Patients cannot be dragged into the sorts of autonomous behaviors that some physcans may prefer or be forced to face issues directly if their habit is to defer to others.

Recent objections to standard analyses of autonomy and informed consent criticize the doctrines as reflecting Western, male, gender-biased, individualistic values. Studies have demonstrated repeatedly that patient autonomy, firmly enshrined as one of the central concepts of biomedical ethics, is almost exclusively a product of the Western preoccupation with individuality and self-control. Increasingly, commentators have charged that, whereas American bioethics attempts to cloak its principles in universal terms, in fact their Western slant results in articulations of informed consent that rarely meet the varieties of patient needs. Pellegrino and others argue that this biased view of autonomy prevents caregivers from recognizing that some patients may not want to make health care decisions, and that beneficence and respect include adapting to multicultural considerations and not imposing an unwanted burden of decision making (12,32,40).

To some degree, all patients process information and deal with life and death issues based on oblique rather than direct manipulation of information. In addition to personality factors, characteristic modes of decision making are heavily influenced by culture, gender, and economic status (32,41–43). The literature demonstrates that Asian cultures, for example, place great value on family consensus and communal decision making, in contrast to the Western emphasis on individual decisions (44–45). In some native American cultures, talk of death is avoided as a self-fulfilling prophecy, so a forthright discussion about a prognosis may only force the patient into emotional retreat (37). Cultural insensitivity, demonstrated by an insistence on the patient's exercise of personal autonomy, may in fact constitute pressure to relinquish valued traditions. Gostin even suggests that legal reform may be needed to promote cultural diversity in health care decision making, and proposes a standard of disclosure based on patient values, including the right to decide whether to receive medical information at all (34).

What the critics of the generic informed consent do not provide is guidance for physicians whose patients are not accommodated by a one-size-fits-all mode of ethical analysis. Just as treatment care plans are based on the specific medical or surgical needs of the patient, so too must the information disclosure and consent process conform to the individual's intellectual and emotional make-up. Only in this way will the physician–patient partnership achieve the best possible therapeutic outcome.

Some patients, because of age, disease process, dementia, disability, or personality disorder, cannot decide about appropriate care. For these individuals there is a range of solutions providing morally and legally adequate informed consent. Regarding chil-

dren, the general rule is that parents are empowered to provide consent to care, but may not have co-equal rights to refuse treatment. A series of cases has established that parental refusal of potentially life-sustaining or health-restoring care, where there is a high likelihood of successful treatment, can be considered medical neglect, justifying judicial intervention to order treatment over parental objection. The courts reason that, while capable adult patients may refuse care for themselves even when the result is likely to be death, they ordinarily should not be permitted to deprive their children of life-sustaining treatment. Balancing the interests of the child, the parents, the physicians, and the state, courts regularly order blood transfusions for children whose parents refused consent based on the tenets of the Jehovah's Witness religion (46). Judges have also ordered chemotherapy treatments for children with cancer when the chance of remission or cure was statistically promising, regardless of whether the parents' objections were based on religious or personal reasons (47).

For adult patients who are not capable of making decisions about their care, physicians and hospitals look for ethical guidance to what the patient would want. The range of surrogate deciders for an incapable patient may include: (*1*) a proxy or health care agent appointed by the patient while still capacitated; (*2*) a surrogate identified by statue or under the case law pattern of the state; (*3*) an institutional ethics committee; (*4*) a judge; or (*5*) a court-appointed guardian. There may also be a living will, executed when the patient was capacitated, that provides specific guidance for the choice under consideration.

All these possible deciders for an incapacitated patient must engage in a decision-making process that most closely reflects and implements the patient's express wishes. First, the surrogate seeks to implement the prior explicit written instructions or statements made by the patient when capacitated. Second, absent prior spoken or written directives, the surrogate invokes the doctrine of "substituted judgment" that extrapolates insights from the patient's past behavior, statements, or choices to determine what her likely position would be on the treatment plan under consideration. Finally, when there is no way to know what the patient would have decided if capable, the surrogate looks to the "best interest" standard and decides what course most appropriately meets the patient's present interests and needs. Legal opinions, scholarly bioethics commentaries, and most religious analyses agree that, under certain conditions, death may be in the best interest of the patient (48).

LIVING WILLS AND PROXY APPOINTMENTS

The best indication of prior patient wishes is a living will, a written document detailing the possible treatments that the patient, when capable, either consented to or refused. Living wills were developed, largely in the 1980s, as a way for individuals to indicate prospectively which interventions they would refuse. These instruments evolved in reaction to the popular perception that, at the end of life, patients were being kept alive long after they would have wished by an unstoppable medical juggernaut. In an effort to avoid unwanted future care, living wills identified trigger events, such as, "If I am terminally ill" or—in our preferred formulation-"If I am unable to recognize and relate to family and friends, and my physicians say that I will not recover," then certain interventions are not authorized. In most living wills, those refused treatments include cardio-respiratory resuscitation, dialysis, surgery, antibiotics, and other life-prolonging interventions. Living wills also make clear, however, that their directives do not preclude any care that is solely for the comfort of the patient. Unfortunately, pieces of paper are not good advocates, especially in complicated situations where the outcome is unclear. Pieces of paper cannot challenge assumptions or argue for a particular option. Therefore, despite their legal support, living wills are often ineffective in guiding care decisions.

While living wills are traditionally used to prospectively refuse care, they are actually value-neutral instruments. Increasingly, they are used by Orthodox Jews and Catholics to request future care because many in these groups believe it is their religious obligation to support life as long as possible. Using a living will to request care is also increasingly common for many patients motivated not by religious docstrine or resistance to the imposition of unwanted care, but rather by concern about managed care decisions to allocate or ration care. As the financial incentives for withholding care rise in the market revolution of consumer choice and managed care, patients are increasingly apprehensive about inappropriate restrictions of care and are using living wills to protect themselves from this perceived danger.

Living wills were the first mechanisms designed to be executed by decisionally capable patients to address care issues in the future when incapacity might have extinguished the opportunity for meaningful choice. Experience with these documents, however, has been discouraging. Although the language may be clear, the directions are too inflexible and unresponsive to the nuance and uncertainty of care. So, for example,

what most living wills *say* is that the individual refuses mechanical ventilation. However, what most people *mean* is that they do not want to be on a ventilator indefinitely; they *do not* mean that they would not want to be on a ventilator for a few hours if it meant recovery. The subtle but enormously important difference that gets lost between intention and articulation can have tragic consequences.

As the defects of living wills became apparent, most commentators agreed that a preferable mechanism was the appointment by a capacitated person of a health care agent or proxy who knew the individual's values and wishes and could act on her behalf. This legally appointed and empowered person could talk with physicians at the moment of deciding, consent to a plan of care, and agree to alterations in that plan if the patient's condition changed or the prognosis became more certain. The key to the success of the proxy, however, is choosing an agent who can and will decide as the *patient* would have decided, *not* as the *agent* would decide for him- or herself. What is invoked in the proxy situation is the combination of trust, explicit direction, and substituted judgment before descending to reliance on the standard of best interest.

While these advance patient directives are far preferable to the alternatives (decisions by unappointed surrogates, hospital committees, or courts, all of whom are strangers to the patient), studies show that, despite efforts by staff, no more than 25% of patients are likely to execute these generic instructions or specific appointments. The Patient Self-Determination Act (49) passed by Congress and effective since December 1991, requires that hospitals, long-term care facilities, and health maintenance organizations receiving federal funds inform patients of their right to complete advance directives and offer them the opportunity to do so. Unfortunately, even this federal mandate has had little impact on the low rate of advance directive execution.

Scholars hypothesize and data confirm that reluctance to execute advance directives comes from the inability of American society to initiate or conduct discussions about dying, the specific reluctance of certain ethnic groups to address death, the fear of those medically underserved that this is one more plot to deprive them of care, and the advice of some clergy that religious dictates prohibit prospective refusals of care. Studies also identify the disinclination of physicians to devote the necessary time to the discussion of advance directives and a general lack of enthusiasm for the enterprise (50). Most important, the existential dilemma for human beings is that the consideration of our own death always complicates and often destroys rationality. Despite our best efforts, death can be contemplated by mortals only in fear and trembling.

INFORMED CONSENT FOR RESEARCH

Today, a well-established consensus exists about the ethics of the use of human subjects in research. This consensus includes wide agreement that medical and other health professions engaged in research are obligated to have norms and practices of consent for all human subjects, whether sick or well. (51)

Many of the treatments provided in oncology departments and special cancer centers are classified as clinical research, implying open questions about the efficacy of the proposed treatment in addressing the patient's condition. Whether it is called research, experimental treatment or innovative therapy, the net result is the same in terms of informed consent—the physician presenting this option to the patient is uncertain about the effectiveness of the intervention. Given this uncertainty, research is always ethically problematic because no unproven intervention can confidently be presented as serving the best interest of the patient.

Research is also problematic in that it risks making the patient a means to an end rather than an end in himself. In contrast to clinical practice, where the sole goal is to benefit the individual patient, research is designed to benefit the patient and expand the body of knowledge that will benefit the general population. In clinical research, the twin goals of the physician are to provide treatment that improves the condition of the individual patient and also to prove or disprove the scientific hypothesis that undergirds the research. This benevolent use of the patient as a vehicle to the end of greater knowledge to benefit the greater number is ultimately defensible in a society that respects science, but always places the physician in the uncomfortable position of divided loyalty. It is always ethically problematic.

The ethical complexity of research is intensified further by the fact that the investigator may have an independent interest in pursuing clinical research as part of her career. In this case, if there are two competing protocols that might be appropriate for the patient, the choice of one over the other may be determined more by the interests of the physician–researcher than by the needs of the patient (52).

Finally, clinical research is ethically sensitive because, despite the researcher's efforts to be clear and candid about possible conflicting loyalties, patients always assume that the doctor is acting in their best interest. This phenomenon, known as the "therapeutic fallacy," means that, even in research protocols, each patient thinks that the suggested plan of care is based exclusively on what the physician thinks will promote the patient's therapeutic good (53–55).

The ethical dilemmas posed by the dual obligations of the doctor–researcher are perhaps more significant in oncology than in other medical specialties. In most clinical situations, therapeutic intervention is based on established regimens, tested and proven to be safe and effective. While there is never complete certainty about the efficacy of any treatment, doctors are generally able to offer a patient one or more well-accepted options with fairly high success rates and fairly low risks. Informed consent in these situations is relatively straightforward: although the physician may weight the presentation to favor a preferred course of treatment, there are few unknowns or potential conflicts of interest.

In contrast, oncology depends to a large extent on pushing back the frontiers of the unknown and advancing experimental techniques. Like AIDS, cancer does not easily expose its vulnerable side and effective treatment demands aggressive and innovative efforts. Every advance is the product of data from previous protocols and each documented success is immediately incorporated into the design of the next attack. Thus, finding the cure for cancer proceeds apace with caring for the cancer patient and the two endeavours are inextricably linked. Experimental protocols and randomized clinical trials have become the standard of care. The cancer specialist does not choose between being a clinician and a researcher; she is, by virtue of the disease, both.

This duality has profound implications for the informed consent process. Especially in large, academic tertiary care centers, the intellectual atmosphere places the accumulation of knowledge on the same high plane as the achievement of technical proficiency. Scientific data are vital weapons, not only in the treatment of the individual patient, but in the treatment of the countless others who will benefit from the therapeutic innovations. The underlying message is that, by coming to a research and teaching hospital, the patient has already signaled his willingness to participate in the latest scientific projects; the problem is that most patients fail to grasp the implications of their choice. Even without the inevitable desire to increase their patient–subject cohorts, oncologists committed to scientific progress believe that aggressive and creative therapies offer the best hope for their patients. Precisely because of this institutional and intellectual bias, oncologists should temper enthusiasm with the recognition that informed consent in this context can easily become coerced, persuaded, or manipulated consent. Disclosure of the benefits, risks, and burdens of various therapies must be balanced, with scrupulous attention paid to the filter through which cancer patients are likely to hear and process the information. Studies have shown that the kind and amount of information patients focus on and retain is influenced by various factors, including the severity of the illness, the personal values and preferences of the patient, and the enthusiasm of the physician in providing the patient with relevant information (56–59). The very diagnosis of cancer carries its special burden of fear and despair, making patients excruciatingly vulnerable to the suggestion of new discoveries or possible cures. Oncologists must be mindful of their responsibility to guide as well as cure, care as well as innovate, and of their ethical obligation to empower their patients at a time when they are feeling most powerless.

A BRIEF HISTORY OF THE REGULATIONS GOVERNING RESEARCH

It is ironic that the system of regulations governing research dedicated to beneficence is the legacy of history's most notorious episode of maleficence. Following the second world war and especially during the Nuremberg trials, world attention was focused on the terrible experiments of Nazi doctors and the grotesque violations of human rights they represented. Testimony at Nuremberg led to the Declaration of Helsinki, a multi-national agreement stipulating that only subjects who had provided capable and uncoerced consent could be included in research protocols (60).

This international soul searching provided the background for investigations and exposés in the United States during the 1970s. In the Tuskegee experiments beginning in 1932, the United States Public Health Service followed a cohort of poor black men in Alabama to gather data on the natural history of syphilis. When effective treatments were developed, they were deliberately not offered to the subjects. In the Brooklyn Hospital for Chronic Diseases, very disabled patients were injected with live cancer cells. Finally, and perhaps most egregiously, retarded children in the Willowbrook State School were given hepatitis as a way of developing a vaccine for the disease. While none of these rose even close to the level of the terrible tortures that Nazi doctors inflicted on their victims, they all indicated that patients had been coerced or deceived into participating in research without adequate attention to issues of autonomy and informed consent, much less decency (61–62).

As a result of these revelations, the federal government convened the National Commission for the Study of Problems in Biomedical and Behavioral Research. During the late 1970s and early 1980s, this commission produced the documents and reports that were codified as the Federal Regulations Governing Research with Human Subjects (63). Since their adoption, these regulations and the Belmont Report (64), which spelled out the underlying philosophical principles of research, have been the foundation for designing, conducting, and evaluating research. The regulations provide that research can proceed only with the voluntary informed consent of the capable adult subject. They also set forth special sets of concerns that must be addressed before research can be done with prisoners or children, and before experiments can be conducted in the area of in vitro fertilization. Running parallel to the development of regulations governing research, a small line of cases has shaped judicial law regarding informed consent in research (65–69).

The process outlined in the regulations requires that the research protocol be presented to and approved by an Institutional Review Board (IRB) with responsibility for and authority over research in a particular institution. This review body must determine that the possible therapeutic benefit of the experiment to the particular subject and the possible scientific benefit to society together outweigh the risk to the patient. If this risk–benefit ratio favors research, then the IRB must approve both the process and the documents that secure the informed consent of the patient. These rules, as first developed, were assumed to apply to major academic medical centers where peer review obtains and scientific discoveries are openly reported. As medicine becomes increasingly corporate and as discoveries are hidden umder protective patents, the ability of single institutional watchdog committees must be reexamined (70).

The regulations that govern the informed consent process require that a capable adult selected as a possible research subject be offered the opportunity to consent or refuse to participate in the research. In order to make this decision, the potential subject must be presented with the diagnosis, prognosis, alternative treatments, the risks and benefits of the proposed treatments, plus the likely consequences of nontreatment. She must be told about the compensation policy of the institution that will apply if she is injured as a result of the research. Finally, she must be assured that her treatment by the facility and its doctors will not be affected by her decision whether to participate in the research.

Because considerable research is conducted on patients with Alzheimer's disease and those disabled by strokes or other catastrophic events, there exists a scholarly literature to help IRBs protect decisionally incapable patients in an ethically appropriate research setting (71–72). Despite publication in the early 1980s of draft regulations in the Federal Register that would have provided a clear process for research with patients of diminished or fluctuating capacity, these regulations were never adopted and there seems little likelihood of their passage anytime soon. Until clear regulations are in place to provide the needed guidance, protocols should offer a significant promise of benefit, research should be monitored closely, and only patients with actively involved family or close friend should be considered as subjects (73).

Eligibility to participate in research is further affected in pharmaceutical clinical trials by the stage of testing. Phase I protocols, testing toxicity, can never be open to children or adults without the capacity to make decisions. Phase II protocols, testing safety and efficacy, may be appropriate for children or decisionally incapable persons if they provide the only or best hope for cure and thus promise a direct therapeutic benefit. Phase III protocols, seeking to develop dose/response data for interventions of proven effectiveness, are the least ethically problematic. These pharmaceuticals are really part of proven treatment and need only comply with Food and Drug Administration (FDA) requirements.

In recent years, the arguments of AIDS activists have caused the FDA to open "parallel track" access to many drugs in Phase III testing. After some years with this system, most researchers and activists think that it has compromised accumulation of data without providing a huge benefit to patients.

SPECIAL DILEMMAS OF ONCOLOGICAL RESEARCH

Given the growth of research cooperatives and the enormous numbers of subjects necessary to support statistically meaningful data, most cancer patients are treated within some sort of protocol. It is often the case that, for otherwise fatal conditions, these protocols offer innovative and promising therapies that are not accessible outside the research setting. The fact that access to certain kinds of care is only available within the experimental setting is not consistent with the claim that care will not be compromised by the patient's decision whether to participate in research.

More important, these protocols establish the norm for treatment as an integral part of research and the result of this linkage may work to support or undermine patient autonomy. Some patients see hope in the possibility of joining a protocol, even if it is a Phase I trial with many dangers and very little promise of benefit. For many patients, participation in research is a reflection of the possibility physicians see of symptom amelioration, remission, or cure. Participation in research enables these patients to bolster their spirits and marshal their energy. Even if denial or delusion is the basis for hope, the patient's psyche reworks these psychological phenomena as the support for some feelings of well-being. For patients who choose this route, the process yields important psychological and emotional dividends.

Other patients, less committed to slim hopes, choose to forego participation in Phase I protocols that offer little promise of benefit. For those who have entered the terminal phase of illness for which no real treatment exists and who continue to receive experimental therapy, the demands of the protocol may conflict with desired end-of-life care. For example, in some protocols cardiac or pulmonary arrest may be among the predictable side effects of the treatment. For patients who do arrest, researcher–physicians may feel obliged to resuscitate, despite the fact that the patient may have expressed a contrary desire. Critics of this practice have suggested that it derives from the desire to compile all possible results of patient treatment. This may be true, but aggressive care at the end of life may also result from the physician's feelings of complicity in providing the treatment carrying the possible secondary result of arrest.

Whatever motivates aggressive behavior in the face of terminal illness, the specific wishes of the patient may not be the sole determinant of care. The notion of informed consent works only if the patient is kept informed, permitted to express her wishes, and provided the respect that honoring her wishes affords. Whereas oncologists are often criticized for overly aggressive end-of-life treatment, they justify their fierce fight for their patients as the counterbalance to other medical specialties that respond to the diagnosis of cancer as a death warrant. The behavior of oncologists compensates—and perhaps overcompensates—for the perception that other branches of medicine fail to treat cancer patients with hope and determination.

CONCLUSION

Informed consent in oncology must accommodate both the realistic desires and the vain delusions of patients desperate for some hope of remission in the face of uniformly discouraging data, as well as the determination of oncologists trained in medical settings where patients with cancer are not seen as curable. Informed consent is an expression of trust forged in the doctor–patient partnership that has as its primary goal the cure or comfort of the patient. Despite challenges to this venerated relationship, informed consent arises to secure the patient's freedom to question and the security to believe the answers provided by the physician. It is this trust that facilitates discussion and permits decision in the face of uncertainties and barely comparable risks, and it is this trust that gives the informed consent process special application in the oncology setting where patients are particularly vulnerable.

ACKNOWLEDGMENTS

This chapter incorporates material that appears in other published work, including Post LF, Blustein J, Gordon E, and Dubler NN. Pain: Ethics, Culture, and Informed Consent to Relief. *The Journal of Law, Medicine & Ethics*. 1996; 24(4): 348–359.

REFERENCES

1. *Mohr* v. *Williams*, 95 Minn. 261 (1905).
2. *Pratt* v. *Davis*, 224 Ill. 300 (1906).
3. *Natanson* v. *Kline*, 86 Kan. 393 (1960).
4. *Salgo* v. *Leland Stanford University Board of Trustees*, 154 Cal. App.2d 560 (1970).
5. *Canterbury* v. *Spence*, 464 F.2d 772 (D.C. Cir.), *cert denied* 409 U.S. 1064 (1972).
6. *Moore* v. *Regents of the University of California*, 51 Cal.3d 120 (1990).
7. *Arato* v. *Avedon*, 5 Cal.4th 1172 (1993).
8. Kiev A. A history of informed consent doctrine. *Applied Clin Trials*. 1993; 2:51–69.
9. Katz J. Informed consent: ethical and legal issues. In: Arras JD, Steinbock B, eds. *Ethical Issues in Modern Medicine*. Mountain View, CA: Mayfield Publishing Co., 1995: 87–97.
10. President's Commission for the Study of Ethical Problems in Medicine and Biomedical and Behavioral Research. *Making Health Care Decisions: A Report on the Ethical and Legal Implications of Informed Consent in the Patient–Practitioner Relationship*. Washington, DC: U.S. Government Printing Office; 1982.
11. Faden R, Beauchamp T. *A History and Theory of Informed Consent*. New York: Oxford University Press; 1986.
12. Pellegrino ES. Patient and physician autonomy: conflicting rights and obligations in the patient–physician relationship. *J Contemp Health Law Policy*. 1993: 47–68.
13. Rozovsky FA. *Consent to Treatment: A Practical Guide*, 2nd ed. Boston: Little Brown & Co., 1990; §1.3.
14. Katz J. Informed consent: must it remain a fairy tale? *J Contemp Health Law Policy*. 1994: 10:69–91.
15. Dworkin R. Medical law and ethics in the post-autonomy age. *Indiana L J*. 1993; 68:727–742.
16. *Cruzan* v. *Director, Missouri Dep't Health*, 497 U.S. 261 (1990).
17. Baum M. Do we need informed consent? *Lancet*. 1986; 2 (Oct. 18): 911–912.
18. Schain WS. Barriers to clinical trials part II: knowledge and attitudes of potential participants. *Cancer Suppl*. 1994; 74:2666–2671.
19. LaCombe MA. The quality of consent. *Am J Med*. 1996; 100:258–260.
20. Schoene-Seifert B, Childress JF. How much should the cancer patient know and decide? *CA-A Cancer J Clinicians*. 1986; 36:85–93.
21. Patterson E. The therapeutic justification for withholding medical information: what you don't know can't hurt you, or can it? *Neb L Rev*. 1985; 64:721–771.
22. Jones CJ. Autonomy and informed consent in medical decision making: toward a new self-fulfilling prophecy. *Wash & Lee L Rev*. 1990; 47:379–430.
23. Katz J. *The Silent World of Doctor and Patient*. New York: Free Press; 1984.
24. Schultz MM. From informed conset to patient choice: a new protected interest. *Yale L J*. 1985; 95:219–299.
25. Cassell EJ. The nature of suffering and the goals of medicine. *N Eng J Med*. 1982; 306:639–645.
26. Angell M. The quality of mercy. *N Eng J Med*. 1982; 306:98–99.
27. Quill T. "You promised me I wouldn't die like this!" a bad death as medical emergency. *Arch Intern Med*. 1995; 155:1250–1254.
28. Wanzer SH, et al. The physician's responsibility toward hopelessly ill patients, a second look. *N Eng J Med*. 1989; 320:844–849.
29. NCI surveillance epidemiology and end results program, 1995. *CA-A Cancer J Clinicans*. 1996; 46:21.
30. Ganz PA. Treatment options for breast cancer – beyond survival. *N Eng J Med*. 1992; 326:1147–1149.
31. The New York Task Force on Life and the Law. *When Others Must Choose: Deciding for Patients Without Capacity*. 1992.
32. Blackhall LJ, et al. Ethnicity and attitudes toward patient autonomy. *JAMA*. 1995; 274:820–825.
33. Schneider CE. Bioethics with a human face. *Indiana L J*. 1994; 69:1075–1104, 1076.
34. Gostin LO. Informed consent, cultural sensitivity and respect for persons. *JAMA*. 1995; 274:844–845.
35. Meisel A. The "exceptions" to the informed consent doctrine: striking a balance between competing values in medical decision making. *Wisconsin L Rev*. 1979; 1979:413–488.
36. Meisel A. Entrapment, informed consent, and the plea bargain. *Yale L J*. 1975; 84:683–703.
37. Carrese JA, Rhodes LA. Western bioethics on the Navaho reservation: benefit or harm? *JAMA*. 1995; 274:826–829.
38. Lo B. Assessing decision-making capacity. *J Law, Med & Ethics*. 1990; 18:193–203.
39. Buchanan AE, Brock DW. *Deciding for Others: The Ethics of Surrogate Decision Making*. Cambridge: Cambridge University Press; 1989.
40. Jecker NS, Carrese JA, Pearlman RA. Caring for patients in cross-cultural settings. *Hastings Center Rep*. 1995; 25:6–13.

41. Helman G. *Culture, Health and Illness*. Oxford: Butterworth-Heinemann Ltd; 1994.
42. Spector RE. *Cultural Diversity in Health and Illness*, 3rd ed. East Norwalk, CN: Appleton-Century-Crofts; 1991.
43. Wolf SM. Shifting paradigms in bioethics and health law: the rise of a new pragmatism. *Am J Law Med.* 1994; 20:395–415.
44. Kimura R. Conflict and harmony in Japanese medicine: a challenge to traditional culture in neonatal care. In: Pellegrino ES, et al., eds. *Transcultural Dimensions in Medical Ethics*. Frederick, MD: University Publishing Group, Inc., 1992: 145–153.
45. Henderson G, Primeaux M. *Transcultural Health Care*. Menlo Park, CA: Addison-Wesley Publishing Co., 1981.
46. *Jehovah's Witnesses of Washington* v. *Kings County Hospital*, 278 F.Supp. 488 (W.D. Wash. 1967), *aff'd*, 390 U.S. 598, *reh'g denied*, 391 U.S. 961 (1968).
47. *Custody of a Minor*, 378 Mass. 732 (1979).
48. The New York Task Force on Life and the Law. *Life-Sustaining Treatment: Making Decisions and Appointing a Health Care Agent*, 1987.
49. 42 U.S.C.A. § 1395cc(f) (1992).
50. Simes RJ, et al. Randomised comparison of procedures for obaining informed consent in clinical trials of treatment for cancer. *BMJ.* 1986; 293:1065–1068.
51. Research ethics and the medical profession: report on the advisory committee on human radiation experiments. Advisory Committee on Human Radiation Experiments. *JAMA.* 1996; 276:403–415, 406.
52. Penman DT, et al. Informed consent for investigational chemotherapy: patients' and physicians' perceptions. *J Clin Oncol.* 1984; 2:849–855.
53. Prestifilippo J, et al. The ethical treatment of cancer: what is right for the patient? *Cancer Suppl.* 1993; 72: 2816–2819.
54. Levine RJ. Ethics of clinical trials: do they help the patient? *Cancer Suppl.* 1993; 72:2805–2810.
55. Levine RJ. Referral of patients with cancer for participation in randomized clinical trials: ethical consierations. *CA-A Cancer J Clinicians.* 1986; 36:95–99.
56. Schaeffer MH, et al. The impact of disease severity on the informed consent process in clinical research. *Am J Med.* 1996; 100:261–268.
57. Schain WS. Barriers to clinical trials: part II: knowledge and attitudes of potential participants. *Cancer Suppl.* 1994; 74:2666–2671.
58. Markman M. Ethical difficulties with randomized clinical trials involving cancer patients: examples from the field of gynecologic oncology. *J Clin Ethics.* 1992; 3:193–195.
59. Lynn J. Choices of curative and palliative care for cancer patients. *CA-A Cancer J Clinicians.* 1986; 36:100–104.
60. Iserson KV, et al., eds. *Ethics in Emergency Medicine*. Baltimore: Williams & Wilkins; 1986.
61. Rothman D. Ethics and human experimentation: Henry Beecher revisited. In: Arras JD, Steinbock B, eds. *Ethical Issues in Modern Medicine*. Mountain View, CA: Mayfield Publishing Co., 1995: 525–531.
62. Donagan A. Informed consent to experimentation. In: Arras JD, Steinbock B, eds. *Ethical Issues in Modern Medicine*. Mountain View, CA: Mayfield Publishing Co., 1995: 531–537.
63. Code of Federal Regulations, Title 45, Part 46, Protection of human subjects, *revised* June 18, 1991, Washington, DC: U.S. Government Printing Office.
64. The National Commission for the Protection of Human Subjects of Biomedical and Behavioral Research. *Belmont Report: Ethical Principles and Guidelines for the Protection of Human Subjects of Research*. 44 Fed Reg 76 (April 19, 1979) Washington, DC: U.S. Government Printing Office, 1988.
65. *Fortner* v. *Koch*, 272 Mich. 273 (1935).
66. *Halushka* v. *University of Saskatchewan*, 52 W.W.R. 6088 (Sask. 1966).
67. *Whitlock* v. *Duke University*, 637 F.Supp. 1463 (M.D.N.C. 1986).
68. *Karp* v. *Colley*, 493 F.2d 408 (5th Cir. 1974).
69. *Moore* v. *Regents of the University of California*, 51 Cal.3d 120 (1990).
70. Rothman D, Edgar H. The institutional review board and beyond: future challenges to the ethics of human experimentation. *Millbank Q.* 1995; 73:489–506.
71. Rothman D. Human research: historical aspects. In: *Encyclopedia of Bioethics*. New York: Macmillan, 1995; 1:2248–2258.
72. Levine RJ. Research ethics committees. In: *Encyclopedia of Bioethics*. New York: Macmillan, 1995; 1:2266–2270.
73. Melnick VL, Dubler NN, Butler R. Clinical research in senile dementia of the Alzheimer type: suggested guidelines addressing the ethical and legal issues. *J Am Geriatr Soc.* 1984; 32:531–536.

96

Ethics of Treatment: Palliative and Terminal Care

EZEKIEL J. EMANUEL

ADVANCE DIRECTIVES

History

The living will was initially proposed by Louis Kutner in 1967 at a meeting of the Euthanasia Society of America (by complex genealogy, the forerunner of Choice in Dying). It expressed the growing view that heroic medical technologies should not be used to keep hopelessly ill patients alive. The following year a physician who was a state legislator introduced a bill to recognize the living will in Florida. The bill was defeated. Over the next 8 years similar living will bills were defeated in a number of states (1–3). In 1976, following the *Quinlan* case, California enacted the first natural death act that recognized living wills. In 1990, Congress for the first time recognized the importance of living wills by enacting the Patient Self-Determination Act which mandated that all health care facilities, including hospitals, nursing homes, and managed care organizations, ask patients whether they have a living will or other advance directive, and to inform them of their right to establish such directives at the time of admission or enrollment (4). Today, living wills are legally recognized in all states.

Definitions

There are three terms that are usefully distinguished. All refer to ways a person, when competent, can make preparation to make informed decisions about their medical care in the eventuality that they become incompetent or mentally incapacitated. The generic term is advance directive. An advance directive, or advance care directive, is any document in which a person specifies his or her wishes in anticipation of future incapacity. Broadly speaking, there are two types of advance directives: living wills and durable powers of attorney for health care. Living wills are directives in which a patient specifies his or her wishes regarding medical treatments in the event of incapacity. Living wills can be general statements of preferences; there are also living wills that elicit patients' preferences regarding specific treatments, such as artificial feedings or chemotherapy, in specific scenarios; and there are detailed "values histories." There are several standard living will forms available: the generic form most commonly available is the standard "Choice in Dying" living will form (5); the most commonly available treatment-specific document is the Medical Directive; and there are two commonly available values histories, the University of New Mexico's Values History and a Values History by Doukas and McCullough (6). (See Table 96.1).

Durable powers of attorney for health care or proxy decision-making forms are documents in which a patient appoints a proxy, another individual, to make decisions about medical treatments if the patient were to become incompetent.

It is important to recognize that living wills and durable power of attorney are not mutually exclusive, indeed they are complimentary since a written living will cannot provide for all eventualities and proxy decision-makers cannot speak for the patient without information about the patient's wishes. Consequently, it is becoming more common to have comprehensive advance directives that incorporate both living wills and durable power of attorney forms into one document. Finally, it is worth noting that sometimes people use the term living will as the generic term for advance directive. This is a result of historical accident because living wills were the first type of advance directive.

TABLE 96.1. *Types of Advance Directives*

Choice in Dying	General statements of preference	Choice in Dying 200 Varick Street New York, NY 10014
The Medical Directive	Treatment-specific preferences	The Medical Directive P.O. Box 6100 Holliston, MA 01746-6100
Values Histories	Health-related values	Department of Family Practice Program University of Michigan 1018 Fuller Street Ann Arbor, MI 48104

Ethical Aspects

The ethical basis for advance directives is an appeal to the principle of autonomy (3,7). Patients should have the power to determine what medical treatments they receive and which appropriate treatments they do not receive. This is the basis of informed consent. Advance directives are a mechanism to extend this control over medical interventions to times when a patient can no longer make contemporaneous, informed decisions regarding medical treatments. While competent patients make real-time decisions and express their current interests, advance directives express patients' surviving interests. Surviving interests refer to overriding interests people have in how they or their property are treated beyond the time when they can make real-time decisions. Estate wills are a common example of a mechanism by which individuals express their surviving interests for disposal of their property after their deaths. Organ donation cards are another example of how people express their surviving interests. Advance directives apply this same idea to medical treatments and the patient's body. What advance directives do then is not express real-time wishes; real-time wishes are an unhelpful illusion and fiction for mentally incapacitated patients. What advance directives do is express people's prior wishes for what treatments they should receive in a potential future circumstance. Thus, advance directives do not provide information on what the patient would want were he or she miraculously made competent; like estate wills, living wills provide the information on what the competent person wanted before he or she became incompetent, the competent person's surviving or prior interests.

Legal Aspects

As stated, the first living will law was enacted in California in 1976. Since then, 47 states and the District of Columbia have enacted living will laws. In the three states that have not enacted living will laws—Massachusetts, Michigan, and New York—courts have recognized the legality of living wills as a mechanism for patients to express their wishes. Indeed, in the 1990 *Cruzan* decision, the U.S. Supreme Court invoked the liberty interest of the 14th Amendment to recognize that people have a constitutional right to refuse medical treatments (8). The Court also recognized the importance of being able to effect this right through advance directives, including living wills. Therefore, advance directives are a mechanism for people to exercise their constitutional right to control their own medical care and refuse medical treatments they do not want; all forms of advance directives—living wills and durable power of attorney for health care—are therefore legally protected in all states.

Most state statutes have included specific living will documents in their laws. These are statutory living wills. Physicians who follow them are ensured the living will is legal and that they cannot be held liable for implementing them. Other advance directives, not specified in the statute, are advisory. Although it has never been tested in court, these advisory advance directives also carry legal authority assuming they clearly state the patient's preferences. To emphasize, clear advisory advance directives are legal, whether they are specifically mentioned in state laws or not, because they provide a mechanism to exercise a constitutional right and are protected by the Supreme Court's *Cruzan* ruling. Thus physicians can be assured that patient statements accurately recorded in any type of advance directive are legally binding; the distinction between legal and non- or illegal advance directives is erroneous. Indeed, many courts have given protection to patient's wishes that were verbally expressed, but never written down, as long as they were clear and reflected considered judgments. As recent cases suggest, physicians who do not follow patients' advance directives might be held liable.

It is also important to recognize that patients have the right to refuse all manner of medical treatments (9). Their right is not restricted to life-sustaining, or heroic treatments or just to cardio-pulmonary resuscitation. In advance directives, patients can refuse everything from high-technology interventions, such as mechanical ventilators and dialysis, to simple interventions such as antibiotics or even blood draws for routine laboratory tests. Cancer patients can refuse chemotherapy and radiation therapy (10). In the *Cruzan* decision, the Supreme Court recognized that artificial nutrition and hydration provided by intravenous or G-tube are like any other medical intervention and can be refused (8).

Empirical Data

There are three areas in which there has been important empirical research that should guide our understanding of advance directives. First, there has been some controversy over which living will forms are best. The initial documents were developed to enable patients to refuse high-technology interventions and used undefined, ambiguous phrases: "extreme physical or mental disability," "heroic measures," "artificial means," "irreversible condition that will cause my death within a relatively short time." (5) The problem is that while we often use these phrases in talking, they are not self-defining and mean different things to different people. Indeed, court cases are filled with illuminating debates illustrating the divergence in interpretations of these various phrases. Consequently, beginning as early as 1976 there have been efforts to make advance directives more specific (11–12). The developments have progressed along two lines: to better describe patient's health-related values (values histories) and to specify the treatments in distinctive, commonly encountered scenarios (treatment-specific directives such as The Medical Directive) (5–6).

Research has indicated that general statements of preference—e.g., not wanting heroic measures—cannot predict patients' wishes regarding specific interventions (13). That is, just knowing a patient wants quality rather than quantity of life does not significantly assist in determining whether the patient would want mechanical ventilation or chemotherapy or antibiotics. Since decisions at the end of life frequently entail determinations about what orders to write, what interventions to stop or not start, treatment-specific instructions seem most helpful to the clinician. In addition, research has suggested that physicians are more willing to follow specific advance directives rather than general statements of preference (14). This research suggests that these two modalities are not mutually exclusive; having values and specific-treatment directives combined is probably the best available option. Consequently over the years, even the generic forms, such as Choice in Dying's living will form, have

become more specific, including lists of treatments that should specifically be accepted or rejected and specific scenarios for treatment cessation.

More importantly, the advance directive used needs to be rigorously evaluated. Just because these documents are not high-technology interventions does not mean they should not be subject to the same rigorous standards of reliability that we apply to other medical interventions. We rightly expect quality of life assessments to meet standards of validity and reliability if they are to guide medical decision-making; similarly we should expect advance directives to be held to the same standards of validity and reliability. The reason to use validated forms is clear; non-validated forms may misrepresent the true wishes of patients and may not cover the relevant domains, confusing decision making at critical junctures. Unfortunately, only a few living wills have been subject to evaluations of validity and reliability (3,6).

Second, studies and public opinion polls have consistently shown that the vast majority of Americans endorse living wills and would want one for themselves. Despite this endorsement and all the attention concentrated on living wills, few people have actually completed them. Prior to 1990 studies had consistently shown that only 10% or so of Americans had completed living wills. With all the media attention after the *Cruzan* decision, the proportion of Americans completing advance directives increased to between 20% and 25% of the population in 1991 (9,15). Polls of the public and studies of hospitalized patients have shown that the proportion has not budged; in 1996 still only 20%-25% of Americans have advance directives.

Studies have attempted to identify patients that might be inclined to greater use of advance directives. One reliable finding is that patients with cancer complete advance directives at a much higher rate than other patients. Over 40% of cancer patients have completed advance directives, double the general population rate (16). Another fairly consistent finding is that white patients tend to complete living wills at a higher rate than non-white, minority patients. Some, but not all studies have shown that patients with higher formal education tend to complete advance directives at a higher rate. But most other demographic factors, age, sex, religion, income, etc., have not consistently correlated with use of advance directives (9,17–18).

What are the barriers to greater use of living wills? There are two main actors in completing and implementing advance directives: physicians and patients. Most interventions have targeted patients by providing them with more information about advance directives, providing them with actual living will forms, or encouraging them to complete the living will forms. The most extensive intervention tried has been passage of the Patient Self-Determination Act (PSDA). The premise of the PSDA is that patients lack information about living wills and that if hospitals and other health care facilities provide information and even living will forms, more people would complete documents. Unfortunately, despite significant—and costly—efforts by hospitals and other health care facilities to inform patients about advance directives, the PSDA has not had a measurable impact in increasing the proportion of Americans who completed living wills (9,15,19–20). One reason for the failure of the PSDA, supported by much evidence, is that patients do *not* lack information about living wills (21–22). Another explanation is that patients entering a hospital are more focused on their illness and getting out than on completing another form. In addition, data suggest that many patients, especially patients admitted through emergency rooms, do not even recall being told about advance directives (9). The failure of the PSDA has led many people to conclude that hospital admission is not the optimal time to introduce and discuss advance directives.

Another large intervention was the SUPPORT study which employed a "specially trained nurse . . . [to talk with patients and their families] to elicit preferences, improve understanding of outcomes, encourage attention to pain control, and facilitate advance care planning." The SUPPORT intervention also failed; specially trained nurses in hospitals failed to improve elicitation of preferences or increase the use of living wills or advance care planning (23).

Other studies directed at patients have reported mixed results. Some have reported that mailing living wills to patients in advance of hospitalization has increased use of advance directives (24). Others have reported that giving people living wills and stamped envelopes to mail them in has not increased use of living wills (25). Some have distributed educational brochures or placed messages about living wills on the hospital TV (26–28). Again, the results are inconsistent and do not strongly suggest these interventions will dramatically increase completion of advance directives.

Many fewer interventions have been directed at physicians encouraging them to discuss advance directives with their patients. One reason to think targeting physicians is important is that patients are frequently waiting for their physicians to introduce the topic (29–30). In this regard it should be noted that most data suggest that physicians and other health care professionals are not more likely to complete living wills than their

patients. However, just as oncology patients are more likely to complete living wills than other patients, oncologists also complete living wills at about twice the national average (16). The low level of completion of living wills among physicians may suggest a certain hesitancy on the part of physicians to confront end-of-life care issues themselves, which translates into aversion to having these discussions with their patients (31). One intervention that encouraged physicians to offer advance directives to their patients resulted in significant increase in use of the advance directive (13). Similarly some studies suggest that training physicians to discuss end-of-life care issues have also resulted in increased completion of living wills (32). Training physicians or providing them a direct incentive to discussing living wills remains an area that still needs to be more fully studied to see if it can increase use of advance directives.

There has been some important research in documenting the stability of wishes expressed in advance directive forms (33). In general the studies document a very high degree of stability. Danis and colleagues demonstrated that patients' wishes were stable 85% of the time (34). Similar results were found by Emanuel et al., who also documented that wishes regarding invasive treatments, such as ventilation and dialysis, were significantly more stable than wishes regarding less invasive treatments, such as antibiotics (35). Importantly, wishes regarding cardiopulmonary resuscitation (CPR)—and therefore "do-not-resuscitate" (DNR)— were not particularly stable. Indeed, there is some evidence that as patients get more sick and closer to death they are more inclined to want CPR. Finally some, albeit conflicting evidence suggests that patients who change their views—i.e. are unstable—are more likely to be depressed (36,37).

Finally, there are several studies documenting that physicians and hospitals are not implementing advance directives and living wills well (38). Frequently they are not in patients' charts, when they are in the charts some staff, especially covering staff, do not know about their existence, and they are not always honored. It certainly takes time for hospitals and other health care institutions to develop and implement new policies. It took over a decade for hospitals to develop and implement well DNR policies. These studies show there is plenty of room for improving how advance directives are implemented once completed.

Practical Recommendations

One of the most important recommendations in relation to advance directives may be for practicing physicians to complete one themselves. Confronting one's own preferences while healthy and recording them in a formal advance directive form may grant physicians insights about advance care planning and may make it much easier for them to discuss end-of-life care issues with patients.

Another very important recommendation to practicing physicians is to view living wills more as a part of a process of discussion about care at the end of life rather than an event (39–41). Living wills can facilitate the process. In this sense having a patient complete a living will is part of a longitudinal process that should be integrated into clinical practice and discussions about care. One useful way to think about this process and the appropriate use of living wills is to follow the five steps proposed by Emanuel and colleagues (34,39). (See Table 96.2.) It is useful to delineate these steps for heuristic purposes although they may not be so discrete in actual practice.

The first step is to introduce the topic of advance care planning and end of life care. This is frequently the most difficult, because physicians worry that patients might interpret discussing living wills as an ominous sign of adverse medical news or a poor prognosis. One way to counteract this fear in the patient is for the physician to inform the patient that he or she has personally completed an advance directive and that he or she holds discussions about advance care planning with all patients, those who will be cured and those who are terminal. Directly and openly confronting the latent fear that having a discussion about living wills is a "bad omen" can be an effective way to help introduce the topic.

After the topic of advance directives is introduced, the second step is actually having a structured or detailed discussion to cover the main points about a living will and elicit the patient's specific wishes. To accomplish this it may be easiest for the physician and patient to go through an actual advance directive form provisionally completing it. The intent of this discussion is to obtain clear instructions for interventions the patient definitely wants and does not want and to identify areas in need of further reflection,

such as the use of pain medications even if they cause premature death. If the patient will have a proxy decision-maker as well as completing a living will (and this should be encouraged), the proxy should be present for this discussion to ensure he or she understands the patient's wishes and is not relying on intuition when required to make decisions. It is often helpful to urge the patient to take the provisionally completed living will home and think about the choices.

The third step then is for the physician to finalize the living will document with the patient. Having the patient, the proxy, and the physician all sign the final document is an important way to communicate the message that decisions about end of life care are made jointly and that all three parties will work together as partners to ensure the patient gets the care he or she wants.

The fourth step is to up-date the document either at routine intervals—e.g., every year or so—with any significant change in health status, or with other seminal life events, such as marriage. The fifth step involves implementing the advance directive when it becomes appropriate. Having a treatment-specific living will accompanied by a discussion should help in making choices that reflect the patient's wishes. Implementing these documents also entail ensuring that there are good systems and procedures in the hospital to implement them. For instance, ensuring there is a mechanism to inform all staff about the living will's existence and its provisions.

PROXY DECISION-MAKING

History

Beginning in 1983, states recognized decision-making by a proxy through the durable power of attorney for health care (42). This gave patients the authority to designate a person to make decisions for them regarding health care issues if they became incompetent. By 1996, 48 states and the District of Columbia had durable power of attorney for health care (proxy or health

TABLE 96.2. *Practical Recommendations for Use of Advance Directives*

1. Physician should initiate discussion of advance care planning and end-of-life with patient.
2. Formally document the patient's end-of-life care wishes.
3. Finalize the legalize the final document with signatures by the patient, the proxy, and the physician.
4. Up-date the document at regular intervals in order to ensure the patient's wishes are accurately and currently reported.
5. Implementation of the document at the appropriate time.

Source: Adapted from References 39 & 41.

care agent) laws. In the 1990 *Cruzan* case the Supreme Court recognized the appointment of a proxy an essential mechanism to give expression to a person's constitutional right (8).

Definitions

A durable power of attorney for health care is a mechanism by which a patient can appoint someone else to make health care related decisions if the patient becomes mentally or physically unable to make informed and competent decisions. The designated person is sometimes called a proxy, surrogate, or health care agent. These all mean the same thing. Proxy forms are the forms to designate such a person. Frequently they are combined with a living will form into a single, comprehensive advance care directive as in the Medical Directive (5). However, it is possible for people only to designate a proxy without completing a living will.

Ethical Aspects

The general ethical arguments for proxy decision-making have traditionally been that the proxy knows the patient well and will make "the decision that the incompetent patient would make if he or she were competent." (42–43) Thus the proxy decision-maker is justified in exercising the patient's right to refuse care to the extent that he or she can "don the mental mantle" or "stand in the shoes" of the incompetent patient (10,44). This justification is called substituted judgment. It is often bolstered by noting that the incompetent patient's family will usually be the proxy and that families have unique and personal understanding of the patient's values and preferences (7,8, 43–45). This intimate understanding allows families to make decisions as the patient would.

A secondary justification is practicality. The proxy can make real-time decisions with all the nuanced medical information about prognosis. In this way a proxy is more "flexible and responsive to actual circumstances [and it] covers a wider range of health care decisions than living wills" that use vague terms and cannot anticipate all eventualities (44).

It should be noted that not all commentators are so sanguine about proxy decision-makers. Many have raised two basic ethical objections to proxies. First, just because someone is a family member does not ensure that he or she really knows what the patient wants (42). Having a general sense of a person's values does not translate into real knowledge about their preferences for specific life-sustaining treatments unless there is a discussion about these treatments (13). In addition, it may not be accurate to portray families

as simply loving and devoted to the patient. Family members may have many of the usual conflicts with patients, including emotional friction and unresolved issues (7). And there may be additional conflicts especially since caring for incompetent patients can be both emotionally and financially stressful (46). These conflicts and stresses can cloud and distort a proxy's judgments, making it less than an unbiased attempt to do what the patient wanted.

Legal Aspects

In 1983 California became the first state in the U.S. to formally enact a durable power of attorney for health care decisions. Currently 48 states and the District of Columbia have legislation that recognizes the appointment of a health care proxy. The exceptions are Alabama and Alaska. However, as with living wills, the U.S. Supreme Court in the *Cruzan* case appeared to recognize proxies as an essential mechanism for people to exercise their constitutional right to refuse medical care. As Justice O'Connor wrote:

> I also write separately to emphasize that the Court does not today decide the issue of whether a State must also give effect to the decisions of a surrogate decisionmaker. In my view, such a duty may well be constitutionally required to protect the patient's liberty interest in refusing medical treatment (8).

In addition many state courts have added their endorsement and recognition of proxy decision-makers. As the New Jersey Supreme Court wrote:

> Where an irreversibly vegetative patient like Mrs. Jobes has not clearly expressed her intentions with respect to medical treatment, the Quinlan "substituted judgment" approach best accomplishes the goal of having the patient make her own decision. In most cases in which the "substituted judgment" doctrine is applied, the surrogate decisionmaker will be a family member or close friend of the patient. Generally it is the patient's family or other loved ones who support and care for the patient, and who best understand the patient's personal values and beliefs. Hence they will be best able to make a substituted judgment for the patient (43,47).

As with living wills, there is important and widespread legal approval for proxy decision-makers. Physicians who ignore duly appointed decision-makers do so at some personal risk.

Empirical Data

There is a growing body of empirical data about the decisions of proxies that casts doubt on the practices of proxies and their ability to effect patients' wishes. Studies have shown that proxies and patients have discussed issues and values surrounding end-of-life decisions only infrequently (42,48–49). While they do have general discussions of end-of-life care, only a minority of patients, indeed frequently less than 25% of patients, report having discussed their wishes regarding specific life-sustaining treatments with their families (9). It appears that just as there is an aversion to having such discussions with physicians, patients have an aversion to such discussions with their family.

Not discussing preferences for end-of-life care means that family members and proxies cannot accurately predict patients' preferences for life-sustaining treatments. Indeed, all studies demonstrate that while proxies can predict patients' preferences regarding medical interventions for current states of health, they are no better than chance in predicting what treatments patients would want if they became incompetent either through dementia or stroke. These data undermine the idea that family members' intimacy lends them special insight into patients' views and preferences regarding life-sustaining treatments. (See Table 96.3.)

New evidence from the SUPPORT study raises additional concerns about proxy decision-makers. The study suggests that proxies who are experiencing financial burdens from care of the patients may be more willing to forgo life-sustaining treatments (50). While this study cannot prove a causal connection between financial burdens and the wish to have patients die, it does raise concerns about the factors which might influence and bias proxy decision-making. Evidence which goes in the opposite direction suggests that the emotional burden of making end-of-life choices for a patient, makes proxies hesitant to terminate care.

Surveys indicate that proxies are more reluctant to terminate care for a family member than they are to terminate care for themselves (51). This probably reflects, conscious or unconscious, reluctance to assume the moral and psychological responsibility for terminating life-sustaining treatments and letting a loved one die, even when the family knows this is the right thing to do. This growing body of evidence about the motivation of proxies casts significant doubt on the claim that family members and proxies have special knowledge that empowers them to give voice to the patient's wishes; the proxy's own views and preferences may be more important than the patient's.

Practical Recommendations

There are two important practical recommendations regarding proxies. The first is to include them in advance care planning with patients, to be sure they do understand the patient's general values for care and specific treatment preferences (39). Having the proxy present at the time of initial structured discussion of advance directives (the second step delineated in the practical recommendations regarding living wills) to listen to the discussion between the patient and physician and to witness the final advance care document are excellent ways to ensure the proxy understands the patient's wishes. In addition, having the proxy present whenever the advance directive is updated (the fourth step delineated in the practical recommendations regarding living wills) is also helpful. Finally, having the proxy present to hear the discussion when the patient makes some other critical medical care decision, such as forgoing chemotherapy or opting for a

TABLE 96.3. *Concordance Between Patients and Proxies on Life-Sustaining Interventions**

Authors/Reference	Scenario	Intervention	% Agreement	K Statistic	# Pairs
Seckler et al. (105)	Current health	CPR	88	0.30	57
	Dementia	CPR	68	0.27	57
Uhlmann et al. (48)	Current Health	CPR	90	0.35	90
	Stroke with aphasia and functional dependence	CPR	53.4	0.08	90
Zweibel and Cassel (106)	Coma	Ventilation	67	NA	42
	Dementia	Amputation	33	NA	36
Gerety et al. (104)	Current health	CPR	56	0.05	52
		Ventilator	64	0.19	52
		Tube feedings	77	0.39	52
	Vegetative State	Feedings	77	0.39	52
		IV antibiotics	67	0.28	52
Covinsky et al. (50)	Current health	Goals of care	72.5	0.45	1684

*CPR indicates cardiopulmonary resuscitation; and NA, not available.

Phase I protocol, can also be helpful in providing them insight into the patient's decision-making process regarding health care. Obviously, finding a way to have the proxy present at such discussion can be logistically difficult and meet with resistance. In addition, just having him or her present to hear the discussion is no guarantee the proxy will understand the patient's wishes and have the fortitude to make decisions as the patient would. Nevertheless, including the proxy in the advance care planning process is the best we have to ensure accurate proxy decisions.

The second recommendation is for physicians and others to be sensitive to influences and factors that might potentially distort the proxies decisions. Physicians should be aware of conflict between the proxy and patient, tensions between different family members, financial burdens, or other stresses that might intrude on the proxy. If the physician suspects such conflicts then they need to be sensitively and carefully addressed. One way is for the physician to emphasize to the proxy decision-maker the overriding moral and practical claim of doing what the patient wanted and, therefore, strongly recommending that the proxy put aside other motives and influences.

EUTHANASIA AND PHYSICIAN-ASSISTED SUICIDE

History

Discussions and debates about euthanasia and physician-assisted suicide (PAS) are as old as medicine. In ancient Greece, the Hippocratic injunction against euthanasia was an effort to counteract the common practices of physicians who routinely provided people with euthanasia or assisted suicide for ailments ranging from uncontrollable pain to loss of honor (52–54). It was not just in ancient Greece that euthanasia and PAS were topics of intense debate. In 1870, S.D. Williams spoke before the Birmingham (England) Speculative Club advocating euthanasia with ether or chloroform for patients with intense unremitting pain (52,55–56). Williams' speech sparked an intense debate in both the U.S. and Britain about euthanasia (56–58). His controversial views were discussed in the pages of London's leading literary and political journals and became the subject of meetings of the Pennsylvania, Maine, South Carolina medical societies as well as editorials in the *Boston Medical and Surgical Journal* and other leading medical journals (59–60). This intense debate culminated in 1905 when a bill was introduced into the Ohio state legislature proposing the legalization of euthanasia. Debate over the Ohio proposal was reported in *The New York Times* and sparked significant public attention (55,61–62). Ultimately the bill was defeated.

Subsequently, the debate about euthanasia and PAS was quiescent in the U.S. and Britain, but was begun in Germany after World War I when Hoche and Binding, renowned psychiatrist and lawyer, respectively, published *The Permission to Destroy Life Unworthy of Life* (63). They advocated euthanasia for people leading "unworthy lives," that is, people with incurable diseases, the mentally defective, and deformed children. In Lifton's words, Hoche and Binding were the "prophets of direct medical killing" in Germany (64). In the 1930s, prominent physicians launched an effort to legalize euthanasia in Britain through the Voluntary Euthanasia Legislations Society (65–66). A bill was introduced into the Parliament in 1935, but was defeated in the House of Lords, 35 to 14.

This brief historical review suggests that interest in euthanasia and PAS is not new and pre-dates the development of modern life-sustaining technologies, such as respirators, artificial nutrition, and even the widespread use of antibiotics (52). Thus it is fair to say that the current debate is less a result of advances—or failures—in medical technology and more a reflection of (1) the general acceptance of terminating life-sustaining care and interest in testing the limits; (2) the struggle over decision-making authority and whether the physician or patient should control decision-making at the end of life; and (3) the change in social values which celebrates efficiency and productivity and views the old, infirm, and dying as burdens and costs (52).

Definitions

The debate about euthanasia and PAS has been fraught with difficulty because of the use of ambiguous terms that mean different things to different people. Table 96.4 provides standard definitions that should be used (55). In this chapter the term euthanasia will only refer to active voluntary euthanasia because this is the practice that is under discussion. In addition, both active involuntary and active non-voluntary euthanasia are neither widely advocated nor being proposed in referenda or statutes. It should be noted that both "indirect euthanasia" and terminating life-sustaining treatments are widely endorsed as ethical and legal. (See Table 96.4.)

Ethical Aspects

The debate about euthanasia and PAS has focused on four ethical arguments: (1) autonomy; (2) beneficence; (3) the distinction between withdrawing life-sustaining

TABLE 96.4. *Definitions of Euthanasia and Physician-Assisted Suicide*

Term	Definition
Voluntary active euthanasia	Intentionally administering medications or other interventions to cause the patient's death at the patient's explicit request and with full informed consent.
Involuntary active euthanasia	Intentionally administering medications or other interventions to cause patient's death when patient was competent but without the patient's explicit request and/or full informed consent; e.g., patient may not have been asked
Non-voluntary active euthanasia	Intentionally administering medications or other interventions to cause patient's death when patient was incompetent and mentally incapable of explicitly requesting it; e.g., patient might have been in a coma
Terminating life-sustaining treatments (passive euthanasia)	Withholding or withdrawing life-sustaining medical treatments from the patient to let him or her die
Indirect euthanasia	Administering narcotics or other medications to relieve pain with incidental consequence of causing sufficient respiratory depression to result in patient's death
Physician-assisted suicide (PAS)	A physician providing medication or other interventions to a patient with understanding that the patient intends to use them to commit suicide

treatments and actively, intentionally ending a patient's life; and (*4*) slippery slope considerations (55).

Advocates of euthanasia and PAS argue that autonomy justifies euthanasia (55,67–70). Individuals can choose their goals in life and, similarly, should be able to choose when their life is no longer worth living. To respect individual choices we must permit individuals to choose whether they want to use euthanasia or PAS or not. Second, advocates argue that in many situations life is a burden and even worse than death. For lives filled with unremitting pain or total debility, euthanasia and PAS can actually be a relief and a good thing (67–68). Third, advocates argue that euthanasia and PAS are really no different from withdrawing or withholding life-sustaining treatments. After all for both euthanasia and PAS and terminating life sustaining care, the end result is the same—a dead patient; the physician's intention is the same—to end the patient's life; and the patient's goal is the same—to end his or her own life (67–68). So if terminating care is ethical then so should euthanasia and PAS be. Finally, advocates of euthanasia and PAS argue that there is no slippery slope and that any adverse consequences to these interventions are speculative and have not materialized. After all in the Netherlands, where these have been practiced for over 15 years, medicine is still the same as it always has been.

Opponents of euthanasia and PAS counter these arguments contending first that individual autonomy does not permit everything and anything a person wants to do (71–74). After all people cannot sell themselves into slavery or engage in dueling even if they want to. Anything which irreversibly forsakes autonomy itself is not permitted by the principle of autonomy. Indeed, even Kant, the greatest philosopher of autonomy, held that suicide was ethically wrong. Second, opponents argue that the medical system does not now provide adequate care to the dying and if it did there would be very few cases in which patients with unremitting pain or debility would choose to be relieved by death (75). And it is not at all clear that permitting euthanasia or PAS in these handful of cases would be beneficial to dying patients in general. Improving the well-being of a few might not improve the well-being of the majority. Third, it is claimed that there is an important difference between terminating life-sustaining treatments and euthanasia and PAS. In the former case physicians are removing (or not starting) invasive treatments, and death comes as a consequence of the patient's underlying illness. In the case of euthanasia and PAS the physician's invasion is for the purpose of ending life. Moreover, the intentions of the physicians and patients in terminating life-sustaining treatments are to remove the invasive intervention, with death occurring as incidental, not intentional. And differences in intentions are key to ethical evaluation of actions (76). Finally, opponents claim legalization of euthanasia and PAS is "perilous public policy" (73). It would undermine the trust necessary for the physician–patient relationship; it would lead to coercion of terminally ill patients to utilize euthanasia or PAS; it would lead to intrusion of courts and lawyers into end-of-life decisions; and ultimately it would lead to the slippery slope permitting euthanasia and PAS not just for competent adults but also for the incompetent, the comatose, children, and mentally ill.

These ethical arguments appear inconclusive. Reasonable people can find euthanasia and PAS both ethical and unethical. Much of the debate revolves around the practical consequences where there is currently significant uncertainty about the implications of legalizing euthanasia and PAS. It is important, however, to distinguish between finding these interventions ethical and thinking they should become legalized and a socially sanctioned practice. That one finds them ethical in particularly poignant cases does not necessarily entail that they should be legalized and widely available.

Legal Aspects

As of 1 July, 1996 euthanasia and PAS are legal in the Northern Territory of Australia (77). They remain illegal in Britain and Canada. In the United States, the legal situation is much more confusing. In November 1994 voters in Oregon passed the "Death with Dignity Act," which permits PAS but not euthanasia, by a margin of 51.3% to 48.7% (78). This Act has just been implemented. In March 1996, the 9th Circuit Court ruled that there is a constitutional right to euthanasia and PAS: "Court cases provide persuasive evidence that the Constitution encompasses a due process liberty interest in controlling the time and manner of one's death—that there is a constitutionally recognized 'right to die.'" (79) Just after this ruling the 2nd Circuit Court issued a more narrow ruling which rejected the 9th Circuit Court's analysis but argued that PAS should be permitted because there is no substantive difference between patients who want PAS and patients refusing life-sustaining medical treatment; therefore permitting one but not the other violates the equal protection clause of the 14th Amendment (80). Juries have failed to convict Jack Kevorkian for murder in his euthanasia and PAS cases. In June 1997, the U.S. Supreme Court ruled that a right to euthanasia and PAS was not constitutionally guaranteed. For the moment one can only say that the legality of euthanasia and PAS are unclear, and different states will be free to develop different laws.

Two things regarding the legal aspects of euthanasia and PAS, however, are worth noting. First, no physician, even Jack Kevorkian in some of his most questionable cases, has been successfully prosecuted for assisting in euthanasia or PAS. Juries are unlikely to convict a physician who acts in good conscience for the care of his or her patient, especially if the patient's family concurs in the intervention. Second, all proposals to permit euthanasia or PAS contain a "conscience

clause" which permits a physician to refuse to participate if he or she finds euthanasia or PAS morally wrong (78). Thus, even if euthanasia or PAS are permitted, physicians will not be required to fulfill patients' wishes. Interestingly, the Oregon statute does not have a conscience clause for pharmacists who would provide the medications and has been criticized for this lacuna.

Euthanasia and PAS in the Netherlands

The Dutch experience with euthanasia and PAS is worth studying in more detail because while these interventions remain illegal they have been permitted for almost two decades and subject to rigorous study (55,81–83). In the 1970s there were several legal cases involving physicians who administered lethal doses of medications to patients. These cases, along with statements by the Royal Dutch Medical Society, recognized that in some cases physicians could have a conflict of interest between their duty to preserve life and their duty to relieve suffering; in such circumstances euthanasia and PAS were permissible to relieve suffering.

Through court cases and agreements with public prosecutors, it evolved that if four conditions were complied with euthanasia and PAS would be permitted—that is, not prosecuted as a violation of Article 293 of the Dutch Penal Code that prohibits taking another person's life even at his or her explicit and serious request. These four conditions include the following (55,82). First, the patient must take the initiative in requesting euthanasia and the request must be made repeatedly, consciously and voluntarily. Second, the patient must be experiencing excruciating suffering that can only be relieved by euthanasia—the suffering need not be only physical, mental suffering is permitted. In addition, the patient need not be terminally ill; patients without terminal illnesses but with excruciating suffering can have euthanasia or PAS. Third, another physician must be consulted to confirm that euthanasia is acceptable. Fourth, the euthanasia case must be reported to the coroner.

In September 1991 the Remmelink Report, the first detailed empirical study of the practice of euthanasia and PAS in the Netherlands, was published. Recently this report was updated (84,85). The report demonstrates four important findings. First, there are approximately 9,000 explicit requests for euthanasia and PAS in the Netherlands each year, but only 3,000 cases of euthanasia and PAS. Overall 2.4% of all deaths in the Netherlands are by euthanasia and 0.3% are by PAS. The vast majority of euthanasia and PAS deaths, 80%, are for patients with cancer.

Indeed, almost 6% of all cancer deaths are by euthanasia or PAS (85).

Second, according to the physicians who performed euthanasia or PAS, the most common reason for requesting these interventions was loss of dignity (57%). Pain was any part of the rationale in fewer than half of cases (32%) and was the sole reason for requesting euthanasia or PAS in only 9% of cases (85). Third, among Dutch physicians, 54% had participated in euthanasia and almost 25% had done so in the previous two years. Just 12% of Dutch physicians claimed they would never perform euthanasia under any circumstances (85). Importantly, nursing home physicians perform euthanasia and PAS rarely; mostly it is primary care physicians and oncologists.

Finally, the Remmelink Report found that 0.7% of deaths, almost 1,000 deaths per year, were cases of euthanasia in which there was no explicit and repeated request by the patients mainly because the patients were no longer competent when the life-ending drugs were administered (85). This means that for nearly 25% of all euthanasia and PAS cases the conditions established for permitting euthanasia are being violated. In addition, a recent study of nursing homes revealed that in only 41% of euthanasia cases are all rules actually followed. The majority of euthanasia cases seem to violate at least one rule. There have also been recent cases which have raised questions about adherence to the conditions for permissible euthanasia. A depressed woman without a terminal condition who refused medications or psychotherapy for her depression was given medications for PAS (16). Several neonates with complex genetic defects, including trisomy 18, were also given euthanasia (16).

Empirical Data on Euthanasia and PAS

The amount of empirical data on attitudes and practices toward euthanasia and PAS is growing. Among physicians there have been many surveys including more than 20 surveys of American physicians alone (55,86–95). And there is a survey of nurses regarding practices related to euthanasia or PAS (96). For almost 50 years public opinion surveys have asked a few general questions about euthanasia; there have only been a small number of in-depth surveys of the general public on euthanasia and PAS. Over the last few years researchers have begun to interview terminally ill patients on the subject.

We need to be cautious when analyzing and interpreting these survey data because they tend to have many methodological problems. First, many surveys use ambiguous terms and questions that make interpretation problematic. For instance, some surveys do not clearly distinguish euthanasia or PAS from withdrawing life-sustaining treatment; therefore positive answers may not reflect endorsement of euthanasia or PAS. Other surveys conflate euthanasia and PAS with interest in a quick end to life, as if the process by which one died made no difference. Second, respondents to many surveys are unrepresentative either because the response rates are low or respondents were accrued in ways which are known to bias the sample, such as advertising for participants. Third, respondents tend to be localized in one city or state.

Acknowledging these limitations, there are several conclusions regarding the attitudes and practices related to euthanasia and PAS that seem to be emerging. First regarding attitudes it appears clear that about one third of the American public strongly supports euthanasia and PAS in almost any conceivable circumstance and about one-third of the public opposes euthanasia and PAS in almost any conceivable circumstance. The remaining one third will support euthanasia and PAS when it is described most abstractly or for patients with unremitting pain or debility, but are unwilling to endorse these interventions for other reasons such as being a burden (16). This means that for select circumstances about 60%–70% of Americans endorse euthanasia and PAS. Interestingly, this high level of support has been present for almost two decades, almost 15 years before the vigorous campaigns to legalize euthanasia and PAS began in the U.S., Canada, and other countries (97). Support is much less among physicians. Most surveys suggest that fewer than half of physicians endorse euthanasia even for patients with unremitting pain. And support is almost non-existent—less than 10%—for euthanasia for patients who feel themselves to be a burden on their families (16). Interestingly it appears that physicians who routinely care for terminally ill patients, such as oncologists, are significantly less willing to endorse euthanasia than physicians who are not primary providers for such patients, such as psychiatrists (94).

Second, patients and the public do not distinguish euthanasia from PAS; an equal proportion endorse euthanasia as endorse PAS (16). Indeed, if anything they seem to favor euthanasia slightly more frequently than PAS. Conversely, physicians consistently favor PAS more than euthanasia. In some surveys a majority of physicians endorse PAS in some circumstances (94); most surveys, however, find only a minority of physicians endorses PAS even for patients in pain (16). These differences may reflect the clarity and precision of the questions. In any case, it is clear that physicians prefer to avoid the ultimate responsibility, giving the choice and action to patients, while patients and the public do not seem to emphasize the difference between euthanasia and PAS.

Third, physicians, patients, and the public all clearly distinguish euthanasia and PAS from the acts of terminating life-sustaining treatments or increasing morphine to ease pain even with the consequent risk of premature death (16). Surveys consistently show that a significantly higher proportion of respondents—usually over 90%—endorse terminating treatments or increasing morphine while far fewer—around 60%-70%—endorse euthanasia or PAS.

Fourth, these attitudes toward euthanasia and PAS are consistently associated with religious beliefs. Respondents who identify themselves as very religious or Catholics are consistently opposed to euthanasia and PAS. Conversely, respondents who claim to be non-religious tend to favor euthanasia and PAS.

When it comes to the practice of euthanasia or PAS there is also growing data. Surveys of physicians indicate a wide varition in the proportion who have received requests for euthanasia or PAS. Surveys of internists indicate that as few as 13.2% have received requests for euthanasia whereas surveys of oncologists suggest as many as 57% have received requests for euthanasia or PAS (55,90–91). This range may reflect who is being asked; physicians who do not routinely care for a large number of terminally ill patients may receive fewer requests compared with oncologists. Surveys of oncology patients indicate that as many as 12% of American patients have discussed euthanasia or PAS for themselves (16). Interestingly, however, most of these discussions are not with their physicians but are with their family and friends. A survey of AIDS patients in the U.S. found that 55% had considered PAS for themselves (98). A survey of Australian oncology patients found even less interest in euthanasia and PAS (95). (See Table 96.5.)

Surveys of physicians regarding the actual performance of euthanasia and PAS reveal interesting results. This data indicates that in countries that have not legalized euthanasia and PAS, less than 5% of

TABLE 96.5. *Euthanasia/Assisted Suicide Surveys*

Study Authors and Dates	Country	Patient Numbers and Types	Interest in Suicide or PAS	Interest in Euthanasia	Predictors of Interest in Euthanasia or PAS	Factors Not Associated with Interest in Euthanasia or PAS
Brown et al. (101) 1986	Canada	44 oncology patients in hospice	23% (desire for hastened death)	Not reported	Depression	Not reported
Owen et al. (107) 1992	Australia	100 oncology patients	20%	33%	Good prognosis Past psychiatric history	Worse prognosis
Owen et al. (95) 1994	Australia	100 oncology patients	4% in current health 14% in worsening health	1% in current health 18% in worsening health	Past psychiatric history Younger age	Not reported
Breitbart et al. (98) 1996	USA	378 AIDS patients	55%	Not reported	Depression and psychological distress Experience with terminal illness in family member Non-religious White Few social supports	Pain Pain-related functional impairment Overall distress from physical symptoms
Emanuel et al. (16) 1996	USA	155 oncology patients	20% – interest 11.7% – discussed PAS, hoarded drugs or read *Final Exit*	16.7% – interest in euthanasia	Depression or psychological distress Poor physical functioning Non-religious Higher incomes	Pain

physicians have performed euthanasia (16,66). A higher proportion of physicians, possibly as high as 12%–15% have performed PAS. Importantly, surveys of physicians and patients re-affirm the Dutch data indicating that pain is *not* the major factor motivating interest in euthanasia (16). Surveys suggest that the primary reasons motivating interest in euthanasia or PAS are to avoid being a burden on family or to avoid loss of dignity. Indeed, surveys of patients indicate that patients who are depressed are significantly more likely to take active steps toward euthanasia or PAS (16,98). Conversely, almost all surveys indicate that oncology and AIDS patients experiencing pain are not very interested in euthanasia (16,98). And pain is much less frequently given as the reason for wanting euthanasia and PAS. For instance, a survey of Washington state physicians who had performed euthanasia or PAS found that among reasons given for interest in these interventions were, "future loss of control" 77%; "being a burden" 75%; "being dependent on others for some or all personal care" 74%; and "loss of dignity" 72% (3). And, a survey of oncology patients found that those who were depressed were significantly more likely to discuss euthanasia and PAS for themselves, hoard drugs, or read *Final Exit*, the Hemlock Society's suicide manual (16).

This data on attitudes and practices points out three important conclusions. First, there seems to be a tension—if not direct conflict—between when people find euthanasia and PAS acceptable and the circumstances in which these interventions are actually performed. Physicians, patients, and the public all find euthanasia and PAS most acceptable for patients with unremitting pain; only about a third find these interventions acceptable for patients who feel they are a burden to their family. However, consistent with the results of the Remmelink Report, surveys of physicians and patients indicate pain is not the main motivating factor behind requests for euthanasia or PAS. If anything, patients in pain are opposed to euthanasia and PAS. Conversely, it is depressed patients—not those in pain—who are interested in euthanasia and PAS.

Second, even in countries where euthanasia and PAS are illegal, physicians frequently receive requests for and do perform them. Indeed by some estimates as many as one in seven oncologists have performed euthanasia or PAS. Physicians seem more comfortable with PAS than with euthanasia and participate in PAS significantly more frequently than euthanasia.

Finally, like many other highly controversial issues, such as abortion, proponents and opponents are divided by religion. Those who are religious and Catholic tend to oppose euthanasia and PAS, while those who are not religious endorse these interventions. This religious divide might be reinforced by conflicts on other social issues, making it hard for people to compromise and to find consensus on euthanasia and PAS.

Practical Advice

What should oncologists do when patients express interest in euthanasia or PAS? It is important for physicians to understand that few requests culminate in actual performance of euthanasia or PAS. According to the data from the Netherlands, only about one-third of requests culminate in actual interventions (85). The rate is probably lower in countries where euthanasia is not permitted since, according to some surveys, in the U.S. 57% of physicians have received requests but fewer than 15% have engaged in such actions (16, 66). Furthermore, expressing interest in euthanasia or PAS may be a signal or request from the patient unrelated to actual interest in receiving euthanasia or PAS.

Thus, no matter what one's personal views about the ethics of euthanasia or PAS, two responses seem in order. The first response should be reassurance. Patients should be reassured that they will be provided optimal palliative care and maximal pain control; latent or explicit fears about being left with significant pain or debilitated should be addressed with information about the ability to alleviate pain and willingness to provide all needed pain medications. Similarly, patients should be reassured that they will not lose control and that their wishes regarding care at the end of life will be respected. In this context, it may be appropriate to discuss these issues with the patient completing a living will and selecting a proxy decision-maker, if such discussions have not already occurred. Such discussion would serve as concrete manifestations of this assurance.

In addition to reassuring the patient about providing palliative care and maintaining control over decision making, physicians should probe the reasons for the patient's interest in euthanasia and PAS. Since depression appears to be associated with interest in euthanasia and PAS, physicians should probably rigorously evaluate patients for depression or refer patients to a psychiatrist or other therapist for evaluation of depression and, if necessary, treatment. It is too common for physicians treating terminally ill patients to believe that their depression or psychological distress is "appropriate" and not treat it (99–103). Depression is not a necessary concomitant to terminal illness; it must be treated by appropriate psychotherapy or medications in these patients just as in patients who are not dying. Similarly, physicians should explore whether the patient's interest in euthanasia or PAS is a result of the patient's fears about being a burden on others. Frank discussions with family members may indicate that such fears are projections or misplaced. It is also possible that the fear of being a burden could be mitigated with provision of additional support services, such as visiting nurse or homemaker services.

Despite reassurance, psychiatric care, and provision of additional support services, some patients may still express a desire for euthanasia or PAS. This is likely to be a small minority of patients—even in the Netherlands only 3% of people who die each year utilize euthanasia or PAS (85). Nevertheless, physicians will confront this situation and must be prepared for their response. While it might not be appropriate for the physician to inform the patient about his or her willingness or reluctance to participate in euthanasia or PAS at the first request—since few requests are likely to culminate in actual interventions and since reassurance, better pain management, and evaluation for depression need to be implemented—it is important for the physicians to be honest with patients. If the patient repeatedly requests euthanasia or PAS after reassurance is provided, living wills and proxies are discussed, the pain regimen is adjusted, a referral to psychiatrists has occurred, then physicians must tell patients what they are willing to do and what they cannot, in good conscience, do. To come to this decision, it is worth remembering that all proposals for permitting euthanasia and PAS have a "conscience clause" that permits physicians who personally object to performing euthanasia or PAS to refuse to participate. Similarly, no physician has been successfully prosecuted in the U.S. for providing euthanasia or PAS.

REFERENCES

1. Society for the Right to Die, *Handbook of Living Will Laws.* New York, Society for the Right to Die; 1987.
2. Society for the Right to Die, *The First Fifty Years;1938–1988.* New York, Society for the Right to Die; 1988.
3. Emanuel EJ, Emanuel LL. Living wills: past, present and future. *J Clin Ethics.* 1989; 1:9–19.
4. The Patient Self-Determination Act. Congressional Record. October 26, 1990: 12638.
5. Emanuel LL, Emanuel EJ. The Medical Directive. a new comprehensive advance care document. *JAMA.* 1989; 261:3288–3293.
6. Doukas DJ, Lipson S, McCullough LB. Value History. In: Reichel W, ed. *Clinical Aspects of Aging,* 3rd ed. Baltimore, Williams and Wilkins; 1989.
7. Buchanan AE, Brock DW. *Deciding for Others: the Ethics of Surrogate Decision Making.* Cambridge University Press; 1989.

8. *Cruzan v Director, Missouri Department of Health,* 110 S.Ct. 2841 (1990).
9. Emanuel EJ, Weinberg DS, Gonin R, et al. How well is the patient self-determination act working?: an early assessment. *Am J Med.* 1993; 95:619–628.
10. *Superintendent of Belchertown State School v Saikewicz,* 373 Mass 728 (1977).
11. Bok S. Personal directions for care at the end of life. *N Engl J Med.* 1976; 295:367–369.
12. Relman AS. Michigan's sensible "living will." *N Engl J Med.* 1979; 300:1270–1272.
13. Schneiderman LJ, Pearlman RA, Kaplan RM, et al. Relationship of general advance directive instructions to specific life-sustaining treatment preferences in patients with serious illness. *Arch Intern Med.* 1992; 152:2114–2122.
14. Mower WR, Baraff LJ. Advance directives. Effect of type of directive on physician's therapeutic decisions. *Arch Intern Med.* 1993; 153:375–381.
15. General Accounting Office. Report to the Ranking Minority Member, Subcommittee on Health, Committee on Ways and Means, House of Representatives. Patient Self-Determination Act: providers offer information on advance directives but effectiveness uncertain. August 1995.
16. Emanuel EJ, Fairclough DL, Daniels ER, Clarridge BR. Euthanasia and physician-assisted suicide: attitudes and experiences of oncology patients, oncologists, and the public. *The Lancet.* 1996; 347:1805–1810.
17. McClung JA. Time and language in bioethics: when patient and proxy appear to disagree. *J Clin Ethics.* 1995; 6:39–43.
18. Haas JS, Weissman JS, Cleary PD, et al. Discussion of preferences for life-sustaining care by persons with AIDS. *Arch Intern Med.* 1993; 153:1241–1248.
19. Robinson MK, DeHaven MJ, Koch KA. Effects of the Patient Self-Determination Act on patient knowledge and behavior. *J Fam Practice.* 1993; 37:363–368.
20. Silverman HJ, Tuma P, Schaeffer MH, et al. Implementation of the Patient Self-Determination Act in a hospital setting. An initial evaluation. *Arch Intern Med.* 1995; 155:502–510.
21. Schneiderman LJ, Teetzel H. Who decides who decides? When disagreement occurs between the physician and the patient's appointed proxy about the patient's decision-making capacity. *Arch Intern Med.* 1995; 155:793–796.
22. Roe JM, Goldstein MK, Massey K, Pascoe D. Durable power of attorney for health care. A survey of senior center participants. *Arch Intern Med.* 1992; 152:292–296.
23. The SUPPORT Principal Investigators. A controlled trial to improve care for seriously ill hospitalized patients. The study to understand prognoses and preferences for outcomes and risks of treatments (SUPPORT). *JAMA.* 1995; 274:1591–1598.
24. Rubin SM, Strull WM, Rialkow MF, et al. Increasing the completion of the durable power of attorney for health care. *JAMA.* 1994; 271:209–212.
25. Stelter KL, Elliott BA, Bruno CA. Living will completion in older adults. *Arch Intern Med.* 1992; 152:954–959.

26. Meier DE, Gold G, Mertz K, et al. Enhancement of proxy appointment for older persons: physician counselling in the ambulatory setting. *JAGS*. 1996; 44:37–43.

27. Reilly BM, Wagner M, Ross J, et al. Promoting completion of health care proxies following hospitalization. A randomized controlled trial in a community hospital. *Arch Intern Med*. 1995; 155:2202–2206.

28. Cugliari AM, Miller T, Sobal J. Factors promoting completion of advance directives in the hospital. *Arch Intern Med*. 1995; 155:1893–1898.

29. Emanuel LL, Barry, MJ, Stoeckle JD, et al. Advance directives for medical care – a case for greater use. *N Eng J Med*. 1991; 324:889–895.

30. Emanuel LL. Structured advance planning. Is it finally time for physician action and reimbursement? *JAMA*. 1995; 274:269–273.

31. Morrison SR, Morrison EW, Glickman DF. Physician reluctance to discuss advance directives. An empiric investigation of potential barriers. *Arch Intern Med*. 1994; 154:2311–2318.

32. Markson LJ, Fanale J, Steel K, et al. Implementing advance directives in the primary care setting. *Arch Intern Med*. 1994; 154:2321–2327.

33. Everhart MA, Pearlman RA. Stability of patient preferences regarding life-sustaining treatments. *Chest*. 1990; 97:159–164.

34. Danis M, Patrick DL, Garrett J, Harris R. Stability of choices about life-sustaining treatments. *Ann Intern Med*. 1994; 120:567–573.

35. Emanuel LL, Emanuel EJ, Stoeckle JD, et al. Advance directives: stability of patients' treatment choices. *Arch Intern Med*. 1994; 154:209–217.

36. Rosenfeld KE, Wenger NS, Phillips RS, et al. Factors associated with change in resuscitation preference of seriously ill patients. *Arch Intern Med*. 1996; 156: 1558–1564.

37. Silverstein MD, Stocking CB, Antel JP, et al. Amyotrophic lateral sclerosis and life-sustaining therapy: patient's desires for information, participation in decision making, and life-sustaining therapy. *Mayo Clin Proc*. 1991; 66:906–913.

38. Danis M, Southerland LI, Garrett JM, et al. A prospective study of advance directives for life-sustaining care. *New Engl J Med*. 1991; 324:882–888.

39. Emanuel LL, Danis M, Pearlman RA, Singer PA. Advance care planning as a process. *JAGS*. 1995; 43:440–446.

40. Emanuel LL. Appropriate and inappropriate use of advance directives. *J Clin Ethics*. 1994; 5(4):357–359.

41. Emanuel LL. Structured deliberation for medical decision making. *Hasting's Center Rep*. 1995; 25(6):S14–18.

42. Emanuel EJ, Emanuel LL. Proxy decision making for incompetent patients. *JAMA*. 1992; 267:2067–2071.

43. *In re Jobes*, 108 NJ 394 (1987).

44. *Life-Sustaining Treatment: Making Decisions and Appointing a Health Care Agent*. New York, NY: New York State Task Force on Life and the Law; 1987.

45. President's Commission for the Study of Ethical Problems in Medicine and Biomedical and Behavioral Research. *Deciding to Forego Life-Sustaining Treatment*. Washington DC: US Government Printing Office;1983.

46. Covinsky KE, Goldman L, Cook EF, Oye R, et al. The impact of serious illness on patients' families. *JAMA*. 1994; 272:1839–1844.

47. *In re Peter*, 108 NJ 365 (1987).

48. Uhlmann RF, Pearlman RA, Cain KC. Physicians' and spouses' predictions of elderly patients' resuscitation preferences. *J Gerentol*. 1988; 43(suppl):M115–M121.

49. Gamble ER, McDonald PJ, Lichstein PR. Knowledge, attitudes, and behavior of elderly persons regarding living wills. *Arch Intern Med*. 1991; 151:277–280.

50. Covinsky KE, Landefeld S, Teno J, et al. Is economic hardship on the families of the seriously ill associated with patient and surrogate care preferences? *Arch Intern Med*. 1996; 156:1737–1741.

51. Steiber SR. Right to die: public balks at deciding for others. *Hospitals*. 1987; 61:72.

52. Emanuel EJ. The history of euthanasia debates in the United States and Britain. *Ann Intern Med*. 1994;121:793-802.

53. Edelstein L. The Hippocratic Oath: text, translation and interpretation. In: Temkin O, Temkin CL, eds. *Ancient Medicine: Selected Papers of Ludwig Edelstein*. Baltimore, Md: Johns Hopkins Press; 1967:4–63.

54. Amundsen DW. The physician's obligation to prolong life: a medical duty without classical roots. *Hastings Center Rep*. August 1978; 8:23–30.

55. Emanuel EJ. Euthanasia: historical, ethical and empiric perspectives. *Arch Intern Med*. 1994; 154:1890–1901.

56. Williams SD. *Euthanasia*. London, England: Williams and Norgate; 1872.

57. Essays of the Birmingham Speculative Club. *Saturday Rev*. 1870; 30:632–634.

58. Euthanasia. *Spectator*. 1871;44:314-315.

59. Permissive euthanasia. *Boston Med Surg J*. 1884; 220:19–20. Editorial.

60. The moral side of euthanasia. *JAMA*. 1885; 5:382–383. Editorial.

61. To kill suffering persons. *New York Times*. January 24, 1906:2. Editorial.

62. Euthanasia and Civilization. *New York Times*. February 3, 1906:8. Editorial.

63. Binding K, Hoche A. Permitting the destruction of unworthy life: its extent and form. *Issues Law Med*. 1992; 8:231–265.

64. Lifton RJ. *The Nazi Doctors: Medical Killing and the Psychology of Genocide*. New York, NY: Basic Books Inc; 1986.

65. Millard CK. The legalization of voluntary euthanasia. *Public Health*. 1931; 45:33–34. Editorial.

66. Voluntary euthanasia: propaganda for legislation. *BMJ*. 1935; 2:856. Editorial.

67. Brock DW. Voluntary active euthanasia. *Hastings Center Rep*. 1992; 22:10–22.

68. Rachels J. *The End of Life: Euthanasia and Morality*. New York, NY: Oxford University Press; 1986.

69. Foot P. Euthanasia. *Philos Public Affairs*. 1977; 6: 85–112.

70. Cassel CK, Meier DE. Morals and moralism in the debate over euthanasia and assisted suicide. *N Engl J Med*. 1990; 323:750–752.

71. Callahan D. When self-eetermination runs amok. *Hastings Center Rep*. 1992; 22:52–55.

72. Kass LR. Is there a right to die? *Hastings Center Rep.* 1993; 23:34–43.
73. Singer PA, Siegler M. Euthanasia – a critique. *N Engl J Med.* 1990; 322:1881–1883.
74. Mill JS. *On Liberty.* Indianapolis, Ind: Hackett Publishing Co Inc; 1978.
75. Teno J, Lynn J. Voluntary active euthanasia: the individual case and public policy. *J Am Geriatr Soc.* 1991; 39:827–830.
76. Wolf SM. Holding the line on euthanasia. *Hastings Center Rep.* 1989; 19:13–15.
77. Ryan CJ, Kaye M. Euthanasia in Australia – the Northern Territory Rights of The Terminally Ill Act. *N Engl J Med.* 1996; 334:326–328.
78. Emanuel EJ, Daniels E. Oregon's physician-assisted suicide law. *Arch Intern Med.* 1996; 156:825–829.
79. *Compassion in Dying v. Washington.* 79 F.3d 790 (9th Cir. 1996).
80. *Quill v. Vacco*, 80 F.3d 716 (2nd Cir. 1996).
81. Pence GE. Do not go slowly into that dark night: mercy killing in Holland. *Am J Med.* 1988; 84:139–141.
82. DeWachter MAM. Euthanasia in the Netherlands. *Hastings Center Rep.* 1992; 22:23–30.
83. Gevers JKM. Legislation on euthanasia: recent developments in the Netherlands. *J Med Ethics.* 1992; 18:138–141.
84. Van der Maas PJ, van der Wal G, Haveskate I, et al. Euthanasia, physician-assisted suicide, and other medical practices involving the end of life in the Netherlands 1990–1995. *N Engl J Med.* 1996; 335:1699–1705.
85. Van der Maas PJ, van Delden JJM, Pinjnenborg L, Looman CWM. Euthanasia and other medical decisions concerning the end of life. *The Lancet.* 1991; 338:669–674.
86. Washington State Medical Association. *Initiative 119 WSMA Membership Survey.* Seattle, Wash: Washington State Medical Association; March 1991.
87. Overmyer M. National survey: Physicians' views on the right to die. *Phys Manage.* 1991; 31:40–60.
88. Crosby C. Internists grapple with how they should respond to requests for aid in dying. *Internist.* 1992; 33:10.
89. Caralis PV, Hammond JS. Attitudes of medical students, housestaff, and faculty physicians toward euthanasia and termination of life-sustaining treatment. *Crit Care Med.* 1992; 20:683–690.
90. Fried TR, Stein MD, O'Sullivan PS, et al. The limits of patient autonomy: physician attitudes and practices regarding life-sustaining treatments and euthanasia. *Arch Intern Med.* 1993; 153:722–728.
91. Shapiro RS, Derse AR, Gottlieb M, Schiedermayer D, Olson M. Willingness to perform euthanasia: a survey of physician attitudes. *Arch Intern Med.* 1994; 154:575–584.
92. Hellig S. The SFMS euthanasia survey: results and analysis. *SF Med.* 1989; 61(5):24–26, 34.
93. Back A, Wallace J, Starks H, Pearlman R. Physician-assisted suicide and euthanasia. *JAMA.* 1996; 275:919–925.
94. Cohen J, Fihn S, Boyko E, et al. Attitudes toward assisted suicide and euthanasia among physicians in Washington State. *N Engl J Med.* 1994; 331:89–94.
95. Owen C, Tennant C, Levi J, Jones M. Cancer patients' attitudes to final events in life: wish for death, attitudes to cessation of treatment, suicide and euthanasia. *Psycho-Oncology.* 1994; 3:1–9.
96. Asch DA. The role of critical care nurses in euthanasia and assisted suicide. *N Engl J Med.* 1996; 334:1374–1379.
97. Blendon RJ, Szalay US, Knox R. Should physicians aid their patients in dying? *JAMA.* 1992; 267:2658–2662.
98. Breitbart W, Rosenfeld MD, Passik SD. Interest in physician-assisted suicide among ambulatory HIV-infected patients *Am J Psychiatry.* 1996; 153:238–242.
99. Chochinov HM, Wilson KG, Enns M, et al. Desire for death in the terminally ill. *Am J Psychiatry.* 1995; 152:1185–1191.
100. Eisenberg L. Treating depression and anxiety in primary care: closing the gap between knowledge and practice. *N Engl J Med.* 1992; 326:1080–1084.
101. Brown JH, Henteleff P, Barakat S. Is it normal for terminally ill patients to desire death? *Am J Psychiatry.* 1986; 143:208–211.
102. Winokur G, Tsuang M. The Iowa 500: suicide in mania, depression and schizophrenia. *Am J Psychiatry.* 1975; 132:650–651.
103. Schulberg HC, McCelland SM, Ganguli M, et al. Assessing depression in primary medical and psychiatric practices. *Arch Gen Psychiatry.* 1985; 42:1164–1170.
104. Gerety MB, Chiodo, LK, Kanten, DN, et al. Medical treatment preferences of nursing home residents: relationship to function and concordance with surrogate decision-makers. *J Am Geriatr Soc.* 1993; 41:953–960.
105. Seckler AB, Meier DE, Mulvihill M, Cammer Paris BE. Substituted judgment: how accurate are proxy predictions? *Ann Intern Med.* 1991; 115:92–98.
106. Zweibel NR, Cassel CK. Treatment choices at the end of life: a comparison of decisions by older patients and their physician-selected proxies. *Gerontologist.* 1989; 29:615–621.
107. Owen C, Tennant C, Levi J, Jones M. Suicide and euthanasia: patient attitudes in the context of cancer. *Psycho-Oncology.* 1992; 1:79–88.

97

Global Issues of Resource Allocation in Health Care

CHARLES L. M. OLWENY

The World Health Organization (WHO) defines health as the state of complete physical, mental. and social well-being, and not merely the absence of disease or infirmity (1). This definition embraces the main functional domains of the multidimensional construct we currently refer to as quality of life (QOL). Health can either be a means or an end. Being healthy is an appealing goal and yet, health is a means towards fulfilling other life goals, including QOL. Callahan (2) suggests that the proper goals for health care are a normal life span for all and relief of suffering for those who live beyond that life span. Knowingly or unknowingly, Callahan is arguing for a health care system whose goal is to prolong life (quantity) and to prevent pain and suffering (quality). When, for instance, we combine the measures of quantity with those of quality-adjusted life years (QALYs), it is possible to evaluate healthcare not only from the perspective of the patient, but the information is usable by the health care provider for discussion of options with patients. QALYs can be costed and are then useful to policy makers, health planners, and financiers (3). This concept, first proposed by an economist at York University, is more relevant than the crude use of premature death rates (4).

Sickness and disability are major impediments to happiness and flourishing in human society and are often caused by poverty, ignorance, and unemployment. Health cannot, therefore, be viewed in isolation because wealth (or lack of it) and education (or lack of it) have a significant impact on health. Health is not a finite concept. Budgets on the other hand are, and therefore, the problems posed by economic restraints are inescapable while considering health. The cost of maintaining good-quality health care in an era of diminishing fiscal resources is the most pressing issue facing all governments today.

RESOURCE ALLOCATION

Resources have always been scarce and the issues that surround their allocation are as old as mankind. In the past, health care resource allocation was left almost entirely in the hands of health care providers, without any recourse to the community. The debate on health care resource allocation is now more visible than previously and politicians as well as the general public are equally concerned with the issues at stake.

Medical need in the context of technological innovations is inherently elastic and tends to be open-ended (5). Relying entirely on medical needs as a guide to what is actually good for patients or what doctors are obligated to provide can be unreliable. Vigorous management of scarce health care resource is not only necessary, but also unavoidable (6). Resource allocation is fundamental to improving health and delivery and to improving QOL for individuals and the community.

The main issue of concern in health care delivery in the 1980s was that of access. There was universal agreement that all individuals should have access to at least an "adequate level" or "decent minimum" of health care. The WHO, together with 66 other United Nations bodies at the Alma Ata Conference in 1978, coined the utopian slogan of "health for all by the year 2000" (7).

The paradigm has clearly shifted in the 1990s from health care access to allocation and rationing (8). Because the total amount of resources available for programs and services is limited, resource allocated in one sector leaves less and less to be allocated to others. Money spend on the purchase of new computerized tomographic scanning or magnetic resonance imaging is money not available for defense, education, roads, and other social programs. The 1990s is clearly a decade of cost containment in medicine, with one of the most controversial issues to have emerged being rationing on the basis of age (2,9–11).

Budget deficit policies of the 1970s and 1980s that enabled health facilities to expand are no longer sustainable. Revenues have been curtailed forcing severe fiscal restraints. The on-going world-wide recession with only a faltering recovery has mandated massive commercial, industrial, and financial restructuring on an unprecedented global scale. Businesses are relocating to where labour is cheap and exploitable. The North American Free Trade Agreement would have others believe that bigger is better. The dismantling of the former Soviet Union has suddenly made the world aware that all was not rosy behind the iron curtain. Structural adjustment policies in Africa and many other Third World countries seem to have placed economic priorities ahead of social health (12).

Because resources are limited and rationing unavoidable, we must attempt to distribute the little that is available as fairly as possible. Thus, the purpose of allocating resource is to help and to act in the best interest of both the individual and the population (13). This task is both very difficult and ambiguous but must not be overlooked.

STEPS IN RESOURCE ALLOCATION

Important steps in resource allocation include the following.

Determination of Outcome of Clinical Procedures or Treatment

Knowledge of the outcome and effectiveness of treatment is essential if we are to determine how resources should be allocated. One tool is the clinical audit process, a systematic evaluation of clinical procedures based on defined standards of quality and developing guidelines of good clinical practice. Through its use, procedures which are not effective or actually prove

TABLE 97.1. *Key Elements in Resource Allocation*

Outcome evaluation	Professional perspectives
	Patient perspectives
Economic appraisal	Is it cost effective?
Investment in research and development	New technologies
Public involvement	Patient
	Family
	Community

harmful are not applied beyond the experimental stage (Table 97.1). Unfortunately, not all outcomes of health care can be measured. For example, ethical values like justice, respect for human autonomy, dignity, and the qualitative aspect of caring cannot be measured easily. Besides, emphasis on outcome tends to ignore the importance of structure and process.

Economic Evaluation

Once efficacy of treatment has been demonstrated, the next step is to undertake a review of the financial implications. Although the treatment may be effective, it may not be cost effective when compared with other methods of treating the same condition. A classic example is the drug recombinant human erythropoietin (rHuEPO), an analogue of a naturally occurring hormone produced by the kidney which stimulates the marrow to produce red cells under hypoxic condition. rHuEPO has been shown to increase the haematocrit, reduce transfusion requirements, and improve QOL in several conditions including anaemia of chronic renal failure (14), and chemotherapy-induced anaemia (15). Patients at risk for blood transfusion are those who are anaemic prior to the initiation of cytotoxic chemotherapy, those receiving cisplatin- and anthracycline-based combinations, and those with lung cancer, lymphoma, and gynaecologic malignancies, especially ovarian cancer (16). The use of rHuEPO enables chemotherapy to be given while avoiding blood transfusions and eliminating its attendant side effects. The drug rHuEPO remains very expensive and may therefore be withheld from those likely to benefit from it. Before rHuEPO is made universally available, careful cost utility analysis must be carried out and guidelines for the selection of patients likely to benefit from its use established. What is said for rHuEPO is also true for other drugs such as interleukin-2 (17) for metastatic renal cell carcinoma, other cytokines like granulocyte colony stimulating factor (G-CSF), or programs such as marrow transplantation for epithelial solid tumours. These agents and programs are already at the heart of many controversies in the developed countries between providers and consumers on the one hand and third party payers on the other.

Research and Development

The third step relates to research and development leading to the changing and improving of technology. In oncology the greatest hope for progress lies with studies that will result in a better understanding of basic mechanisms of various malignancies alongside the search for new treatment methods (new cytotoxic agents and improved delivery of old agent). The key issue is how to identify new resources for such development. Resource allocation is an exercise in the management of uncertainty (13). This therefore calls for continued research to determine the unknown parameters.

LEVELS OF RESOURCE ALLOCATION

Three main levels of resource allocation are recognized (Table 97.2), and there are competing priorities at each level. At the macro-level, resource is allocated to programs and/or services such as health, which has to compete with other equally demanding priorities such as agriculture, defense, education, or transport. This level of allocation calls for political decision, and governments, especially in developing countries, have to make agonizing decisions in trying to assign priorities to the long list of developmental needs (12). At the macro-level, there is, in addition, the process of allocating resource within the health care system, i.e., one institution in preference to another. This is often done at the Ministry of Health level and again political overtones and ideologies play a part although many health bureaucrats are involved. In developed countries cancer has received a great deal of attention. In the developiping countries it has been relegated to second place, and in medicine leading priorities include the control of infectious and parasitic diseases and the provision of an adequate level of nutrition. However, adequate cancer pain management can have enormous impact on QOL and inexpensive solutions and options now exist.

The second level is allocating within an institution (meso-allocation). A given hospital or cancer centre has to apportion its global budget to salaries, equipment, drugs, telephones, housekeeping, etc. This is often done by the hospital board and administration in collaboration with health care professionals as members of Medical Staff Committees. The decisions reached often depend on the vagaries of local hierarchal status rather than rationally explored priorities.

Heart transplants may easily win over cancer pain control programs.

The last level is the allocation of resource to individual patients (micro-allocation) and deciding who should receive what treatment. Historically this has often been left to the health care professioinals, who were expected to give each patient without question the fullest access to all useful care. New social trends are beginning to impinge on that autonomy in ways that individual doctors and their patients find very troubling.

Both the macro- and meso-allocations have to do with availability, quality, and what services are offered. Micro-allocation, on the other hand, is concerned with access to services offered.

SCARCITY, WASTE, AND INEFFICIENCY

Most observers agree that there is considerable waste and inefficiency in most public health systems. Since waste means lost opportunities and cost to health care, reducing waste is morally obligatory, especially as scarcity is said to be at the root of moral issues in resource allocation. If we cannot afford to do everything, we have to prioritize our options. Options that are assigned low priority must be traded off for higher priority ones (18). Scarcity is not usually a matter of absolute lack of resources, but rather a decison by "society" (or the elected government as society's representatives) not to forgo other benefits so as to make adequate health care services available.

Ideally, rationing is the fair, reasonable, and systematic allocation of scarce resource. Although rationing is a term which may not be politically expedient, health care professionals, the health care industry, the public, and political leaders must be prepared to acknowledge the need for it and not to shirk the necessity (19). The criteria for providing everyone with a decent minimum of health care services is rooted in the premise that with limited resources the fairest and most politically feasible option is rationing in order to provide a basic minimum for all.

TABLE 97.2. *Levels of Resource Allocation*

Level	Who Allocates	Competing Priorities
1. Macro-allocation	Government	Programs, e.g., health, education, defence
2. Meso-allocation	Institutional administrators in collaboration with professionals	Salaries, drugs, laboratory tests, housekeeping
3. Micro-allocation	Health care professional	Other patients (who should receive a given treatment?)

In the course of resource allocation, it is proper to review the structure and the process to ensure efficiency. Structural efficiency endeavors to use the available facilities with a minimum of waste. Technical efficiency seeks to optimize output from the various components of a service. For example, shutting down a machine after 8 hours when it could operate continuously for 16 hours is indeed a technical inefficiency. On the other hand, running it longer may mean certain patients may be stressed by enduring procedures at inconvenient times. Allocative efficiency should address the mix of services best suited to meet the needs of the community and the disease in question. For example, a good understanding of the level of morbidity associated with different cancer diagnoses and treatments would allow for the best balancing of patient needs with efficiency in the scheduling of procedures and treatment.

Clinicians are best suited to understand the needs of patients and the effects of hospital decisions on them. Planners tend to see patients as rational economic agents, while pure bioethicists see them as autonomous moral agents. Patients, for their part, vary enormously in the degree of rationality and concerns for and about others that may conflict with their emotion and self-interest in decision making. In allocating resources it is imperative, therefore, to have a consultative forum that will bring together the various interest groups and highlight the concerns of all. In reality, decisions are a mixture of intuitioin, good sense, politics, and, above all, people.

DOCTORS' ROLE AND DILEMMA

Considerable concern has been expressed about the role of the doctor in priority setting, a role which Pellegrino describes as "medical gatekeeping" (20). Pellegrino and others argue that it is ethically perilous to move from the view that scarce health care resources need rationing to the conclusion that the individual practising doctor should be the designated guardian of society's resources. In the traditional model, the clinician acts as the agent or advocate for the patient. Since the time of Hippocrates, physicians have accepted the responsibility for maximizing the welfare of their patients through relief of suffering and cure of illness whenever possible. The physician has also been willing to work as an ally, partner, or ombudsman in obtaining the best medical treatment for his/her patient. However, contemporary changes in health care financing have raised the question of the physician's ability to remain a strong advocate for the patient when health care resources are limited.

Physicians are increasingly being called upon to expand their advocacy role beyong individual patients and recognize their responsibility to the population (21). In effect the physician is being told he/she also has a morally binding responsibility to function as a gatekeeper. There is thus growing conflict between the physician's role as the advocate of the best interest of his/her patient regardless of cost and the more recent role as gatekeeper of society's scarce health care resource. These conflicting roles pose an acute ethical dilemma.

Most physicians accept and see themselves as their patients' advocate, but they have trouble acknowledging the gatekeeper role. To some there is no dilemma as they have no choice in the matter. The decision is often made for them at a higher level (administration or staff committee). Some feel the role of gatekeeper is being forced on them by budgetary cutbacks which lead to greater competition among patients for the limited resources.

Both roles can be justified ethically (22). Arguments in favour of the physician doing everything possible for the patient include:

1. The patient and society expect this of the physician. To act otherwise would be a breach of trust.
2. The principle of patient autonomy implies that physicians should respond to the needs of their patients rather than those of the institution or society.
3. Given that each patient is unique, outside attempts to regulate medical decision-making result in anappropriate care for some patients.

An equally strong case can be made for the physician as gatekeeper:

1. The Canadian Medical Association Code of Ethics, for instance, clearly states that ethical physicians "will accept their share of the profession's responsibility to society in matters relating to the health and safety of the public . . ."
2. The responsibility of physicians to individual patients is not absolute: both as medical practitioner and as citizen the physician has duties to other patients and to society.
3. Physicians must be sensitive to the requirements of justice and some patients should not benefit unduly at the expense of others.

SOCIETAL ROLE

Decisions about criteria for rationing and the principle of justice to be followed should rest with society at large. This calls for an open debate of the issues in an environment where government acknowledges its own limitations. It is up to society to set the moral agenda (23). It is society's inescapable responsibility to set the moral parameters and it is for the doctor to decide where a particular patient fits in relation to the broader spectrum of available facilities and services.

Ethically, decisions should be made only with the involvement of those whom the decision will affect. It is inappropriate for political representatives, health care providers, and hospital administrators to make important decisions in isolation without recourse to patients. By ignoring those most likely to be affected, they will make elitist decisions that express only the values, perceptions, and interest of business and professional groups (24). Health care professionals, however, have the duty to determine the facts and make the needs of their areas of interest known to the other decision makers. With respect to cancer, the importance of cancer control measures and especially primary prevention and palliative care are areas where public education and subsequent commitment might have major positive impact.

THE OREGON INITIATIVE

In the state of Oregon USA, a procedure was developed for ranking health care services by polling the local community to seek their opinions regarding the relative contributions of each treatment procedure to QOL. Using this approach and after much public discussion, a comprehensive priority list was produced by applying a complex formula which took into account both cost and QOL benefits to be expected for a person receiving treatment for a specific condition. Each of the 709 treatments or procedures fell into one of three major categories: essential, very important, and valuable. This list was used as the basis for resource allocation decisions. Of the original 709 individual items which ranged from the most to the least important, it was agreed to fund 568 (25).

The Oregon initiative has made two important contributions to health care resource allocation:

1. Substantial public involvement at the grass root level is possible.
2. It has brought to the surface explicit recognition of the need to make painful choices.

The Oregon State Legislature's attempt to involve society is having its effect in the real world (26). It was possible to arrive at an index figure derived from cost, benefit, and public opinion. It was not perfect but at least it was a beginning and provided sets of guide-

lines of how to attempt to proceed in a rational manner.

Critics of the Oregon approach object to the use of consumer surverys (achieved by a detailed telephone interview of a sample of the electorate) to quantify outcomes on the grounds that it may lead to an impossible comparison such as treatment of a premature infant with, say, a hip replacement for an old person, or it may produce socially unacceptable results such as suggesting that all prenatal care should be provided before any organ transplants (27). Unfortunately decisions in health care cannot be made by following algorithms. It is always necessary to negotiate and to compromise. Action taken must be socially acceptable and ethically justifiable. Reference must be made at every stage to ethical values such as autonomy, justice, respect for human life, and integrity of the body, as well as being sensitive to the needs of minority groups. Whatever the critics might say, the experience in Oregon has brought to light some of the challenges and opportunities we are likely to encounter in attempting to involve the public in resource allocation.

ETHICAL PRINCIPLES

Ethics plays an important role in health care. It clarifies our thinking about the issues at stake; it assists in the analytical process and provides individuals and organizations with a way to support a particular course of action. Although ethical principles aid in rational decision making, no single principle is adequate for making health care decisions. Each principle emphasizes a specific moral value and a number of them tend to overlap and actually complement or even conflict with each other.

The basic principles of medical ethics include autonomy, confidentiality, dignity, justice, and truth telling, in addition to avoiding harm and producing benefit (28). Theories of justice and especially distributive justice provide the frame of reference most appropriate to the evaluation of resource allocation decisions. Justice deals with the notion of fairness; what one is legitimately entitled to and what one can claim. Justice may serve as a balance that limits personal autonomy. Decisions and actions that may seem morally compelling and appropriate for an individual may not be allowable to the wider community because of increasing risks. In the case of cancer patients, justice demands that they have access to care equal to others. This is not always the case. Some cancer patients may not be regarded as candidates for certain therapies which might be offered to patients with diseases that are deemed "curable." It should be stressed that once it is determined that patients with cancer are not responding to a given treatment or are dying, justice demands that a comprehensive cancer care programme be laid out for them, including palliative/hospice care, home care, pain and other symptom control measures. There are two major components of justice:

(a) substantive; and
(b) procedural.

The substantive principle of justice deals with the criteria used for distribution, while the procedural principle involves setting up committees to develop a priority list.

Substantive Principle of Justice

This principle embraces the key issue of need, equality, utility, liberty, and restitution. The egalitarian principle is based on the belief that being in need imposes on society an obligation to help meet the need. A just society is one that is compassionate and humane. However, not all needs can be met, and when there is more that one need to be met, the greatest need or the most urgent need should be given priority.

It should be borne in mind that the world is functionally shrinking and becoming one not only in the traditional areas of global communications and information transfer, but also in that interdependence is now seen in economic, environmental, demographic, and migration issues. In other words, the global village concept is fast becoming a reality and no single country or nation can afford to go it alone. In the health area there is a need to tackle major problems jointly (29). Equality in health care, which often means equality in access and equality in health status, is rooted in solidarity, a sense of oneness and being together with everyone else in the same boat; sharing a common destiny and a common humanity.

There is also the utilitarian principle based on the notion of the "greatest good for the greatest number." In applying this principle, decisions are guided by maximizing benefit and providing the greatest net utility possible. When two or more allocations are in competition, preference is given to the one with lowest cost–utility ratio. A recent study concluded that people place greater importance on equity than is reflected by cost–effectiveness analysis (30), and basing health care priorities on cost-effectiveness may not be possible without incorporating other values such as equity into the cost-effectiveness analysis equation.

Unfortunately the world is not a just place. There are many disadvantaged groups, for example the Blacks in the United States and the Aboriginal people in Australia and Canada. In such instances, the principle of restitution should perhaps be invoked to allow for a greater proportion of health care resource to be allocated to them in response to their greater need.

Lastly, one cannot talk of injustice without addressing the right of the individual to make choices. One such right is the right to dispose of one's personal resources as one sees fit. This is the libertarian principle. Libertarians object to the exercise of state power to distribute wealth by taking money from some people to subsidize the health of others. They contend that health resource ought to be allocated on the basis of what people are willing and able to pay for. In other words, they would like the free market approach of supply and demand to be applied in resource allocation. Those who subscribe to the egalitarian philosophy contend that the best possible medical care is a right for all. Libertarians disagree, and see the best possible care as a privilege rather than a right. They see it as something to be earned rather than given on a silver platter. The debate cannot be resolved in principle. Instead, the existing political and social systems dictate the response, with participatory democracies opting for one way and oligarchies opting for the other. Each cancer caregiver must situate himself or herself in this spectrum and act according to his/her conscience and courage.

Procedural Principle of Justice

The procedural principle of justice addresses the process by which decisions are made. It is concerned with the moral authority in decision making. In publicly funded systems such as the Canadian health care system, or several European ones, the public is the ultimate source of authority. The key elements are transparency and accountability. Those charged with the task of deciding must be open to public scrutiny and must be held accountable for all the decisions made. In the United States, market forces have been playing an increasing role, while in many countries, health is only one of many glaring needs for which governments feel no accountability can be expected.

ALLOCATION OF ORGANS FOR TRANSPLANTATION

The allocation of a very scarce non-renewable resource such as the liver or the heart for transplantation poses a real ethical dilemma. How are patients put on the waiting list and what criteria are used to allocate available organs? A recent review and ethical analysis of how livers are allocated in Canada (31) revealed the following: The primary justification for placing patients on the waiting list is the likelihood of a positive clinical outcome. The substantive criteria for allocating a liver to a person on the waiting list was need (severity of disease, urgency, and blood type). Thus the resource allocation decision-making model is grounded in egalitarian theories (severity and urgency), although utilitarian consideratons also played a role (blood type). It is gratifying to note that criteria such as age, social status, and geography did not feature at all. As for the procedure, most, if not all decision makers were health care professionals and there was little evidence of involvement of persons outside the health care team. The reviewers argue that, since donated organs represent a public resource, it would make sense to include representatives from the public or from donor families.

In the USA, the United Network for Organ Sharing (UNOS) applies similar criteria, namely urgency, blood type, length of time on the waiting list, and donor size. Each criteria is weighted. The patient with the most points receives the next available organ (32). The UNOS approach has the advantage of producing policies that are consistent, explicit, and open to public scrutiny.

GLOBAL INEQUALITY IN CANCER CARE

Lack of resources in some countries is one of the main reasons for global inequality in health care generally, and cancer control in particular. Treating cancer is an expensive high-technology process that few developing countries can afford. Resources and scarcity are relative. What might seem like scarcity in the USA would be described as an abundance in most Third World countries. The per capita expenditure on health in the USA is US$ 2050/annum and in Canada it is US$ 1230/annum. This is in stark contrast to Africa, where the per capita expenditure on health is at best US$ 25 in Botswana and in some countries such as Equatorial Guinea and Democratic Republic of Congo (former Zaire) is less than one US dollar. The rest of this chapter will review the ethics of health care and resource allocation in selected countries and continents.

HEALTH CARE AND RESOURCE ALLOCATION IN NORTH AMERICA

There are similarities and differences between the American and the Canadian health care systems. In both countries the standards of care and the availability of new technologies rank among the best in the world, and there end the similarities. The publicly funded Canadian system permits access to the health care system by all; the rich and the poor alike (33). In addition, the single payer system provides for efficiency and reduces costs considerably. The administration costs in Canada account for less than 10% of hospital costs while it is over 20% in the USA (34). Canadian patients are free to select both their primary health care as well as their specialist physicians. In contrast, many United States patients enroled in health maintenance organizations and managed health care plans do not have that freedom of choice. Although managed care has led to centralized planning and reimbursement for expensive procedures such as organ transplantation, the trend towards insurance-mandated medical decision-making in the United States is on the increase. Physicians have lost the autonomy to make decisions about what is in the best interest of their patients (35). The physicians in Canada also have the choice of remuneration methods and most choose fee for service. The shame of the American model is that over 40 million persons have no health insurance coverage and, therefore, have no access to the apparently sophisticated and perhaps the most technologically advanced system in the world. The Americans for their part criticize the Canadian system for creating long waiting lists. A number of Canadian patients cross the border into the United States to beat the queue.

The challenge is whether Canada can maintain its present health care at a level which is available, accessible, portable, and publicly administered. A case in point can be seen in the Province of Alberta. With deep funding cuts in Alberta, access to beds has become a real problem. No health care system has met the conflicting objectives of providing ready access to high-quality care at a low cost for everyone who needs it while at the same time granting the patients and health care professionals the freedom of choice (33).

THE AUSTRALIAN APPROACH

The Australian system appears to embrace some of both the Canadian and the American systems. In Australia everybody has a health insurance plan under medicare, making basic health care accessible to all Australians. However, those who want and can afford private coverage, purchase added insurance which provides for the freedom in choosing one's physician, private hospital room, private home nursing, or urgent investigations such as computerized tomography or magnetic resonance imaging. Because the private and medicare insurances are administered from the same office, the cost is considerably reduced.

In addition to unemployment, foreign policy, and republicanism, medicare was one of the main issues in the recent Australian elections. Both contenders agreed there should be no change in the existing medicare system except for some fine tuning. Labour (then in government) indicated they would allocate more money to enable families to pay for some services currently not covered by medicare. The Liberal–National Coalition (then in opposition; now in government) promised more money to enable families to purchase private health care insurance. It seems Australia is poised to maintain the current status quo.

THE BRITISH NATIONAL HEALTH SERVICE

The British National Health Service (NHS) established in 1948 is a publicly funded system that provides universal access to health care within a moderate and fixed budget. The advantages of the NHS system include universality and cost control. However, it lacks incentives for efficiency. The NHS accounts for 7.1% of the gross domestic product (GDP). This compares favourably with 9.9% of GDP in the other countries within the Organization for Economic Cooperation and Development (OECD), and is certainly much less than the 13.8% in USA (36). Management costs in 1992 accounted for about 7% of non-capital health care costs. Since health outcome in the UK is similar to other developed countries and the relative cost is low, it can be argued that the NHS is relatively cost efficient.

However, a centralized NHS with free universal coverages was inconsistent with the philosophy of the Thatcher government, which introduced reform in 1991. Reform was intended to contain cost, maintain equity, and introduce an element of efficiency in resource alloation. Some form of free market competition and institutional autonomy were encouraged. Five years later, the basic tenet of the NHS remains the same. The UK population has access to high-quality health care with a moderate wait for non-emergency procedures. However, there are disturbing reports of terminally ill cancer patients being denied palliative radiotherapy because of over-run budgets. Trusts running certain hospitals have decided to close down one linear accelerator in order to save money (37). Clinicians in making choices are giving higher priority to patients being treated with a curative intent, and those needing palliation are sent to their family physicians.

The British NHS (government on behalf of the people) has chosen to use time instead of the ability to pay as the tool for rationing access to medical care, a technique referred to as queuing (38). In comparing the British health care system to that of USA one might ask whether it is more just to provide universal access to primary care while rationing x-ray films, medical management of metastatic cancers, and renal dialysis or whether it is justifiable to engage in the extensive use of diagnostic and therapeutic services in chronic disorders like cancer, while "rationing" or failing to provide millions with prenatal care and immunizations (39)?

HEALTH CARE RESOURCE ALLOCATION IN AFRICA

Africa can be viewed as the epitome of the Third World. Poverty has proven Africa's most intractable problem. There is an unending cycle of poverty and the main reason why poverty is getting worse is poverty itself. Endemic poverty hangs like a millstone round Africa's neck, dragging its people into the abyss of helplessness where the day-to-day struggle for survival outstrips any chances to achieve economic progress. Money for health is simply not there. It is being diverted and spent on defense, purchase of consumer goods, and repair of roads, and, in some countries where drought is common, on importation of food (40).

The task of medicine is to promote health, to prevent disease, to treat the sick when prevention has broken down, and to rehabilitate the people after they have been cured (41). The right to essential health care for all is now recognized explicitly or implicitly by all, alongside the rights to justice before the law, basic education, and public security. There should therefore be a public health system which provides the basic essentials of water, shelter, and food and which encourages the prevention of ill health by immunization and health promotion (42). Perhaps funding utilities like clean water as well as agriculture and education may have a greater impact on health than spending money on health care facilities. Development is increasingly being viewed as a process which involves not just economic but also social values. In the context of good health, development entails universal education, good working conditions, and suitable amenities in the home and the environment.

In the atmosphere of abject poverty, what constitutes basic medical need? Is it right to provide radiotherapy in an environment with no clean water? Should emphasis be on infectious and parasitic diseases rather than cancer? Is the provision of a renal dialysis and kidney transplantation facility justified and can it be classified as a basic medical need? Is the high cost of locating donors and immunosuppression justifiable? If the facilities are provided, who decides what should be done? In India local committees are set up to review proposed transplants in the best interest of both parties (donor and recipient). There the wealthy are encouraged to underwrite the cost of health and social projects such as provision of clean water to a village or funding for another kidney donor. The wealthy recipients thus plough tangible resources back into the community, a practice referred to as "mandated philanthropy." (29)

A number of African countries have stood by and short-sightedly allowed the health of their citizens to deteriorate appallingly. Sooner or later every society reaches a point where the cost of doing nothing or not providing facilities becomes politically, socially, and economically too high to ignore.

Who will decide on macro- and meso-allocations in Africa? Unfortunately in most African countries, it is not even the local populations any more. The World Bank has recruited outside experts to work in the central banks and manage the local economies. Thus the foreigners will decide on priorities. Time is ripe to allow grassroot decisions to be made by the people likely to be impacted by such decisions. Allow the local community to decide whether it is water, schools, roads, or dispensaries that would best serve their needs. It is only if they participate in the decision that they will value what is being done. It is not only a question of who decides. Equally important is what criteria are applied to decide on priorities. The health professionals can and should play the pivotal educational role. The community can come up with appropriate criteria for priority setting only in the presence of a modicum of good and relevant information. This approach will lay the criteria open to public scrutiny.

The most troublesome aspect of resource allocation in Africa is the continued use of public funds to ferry away the privileged few (usually government ministers and their families) for treatment abroad even for simple ailments when the majority have no access to clean water, hospital linen, or aspirin for pain relief (12). In the distribution of limited health care resources, primary care, including basic preventive services, ought to be provided to everyone before any allocations are made to provide subsets of the population with more sophisticated medical care.

How else might limited health care resource be rationally allocated in Africa? One approach is the development of an essential drugs list. The author is a firm believer that one can practice "good" medicine in Africa with the constant provision and availability of five key drugs (Table 97.3). The inclusion of chlor-

TABLE 97.3. *Essential Drugs: Barest Minimum for Africa*

Aspirin or acetaminophen
Antimalarial, e.g., quinine or mefloquine
Broad spectrum antibiotic, e.g., chloramphenicol*
Broad spectrum antihelmithic, e.g., albendazole
Ferrous sulfate

* Chloramphenicol is cheap and has a broad spectrum of activity. The rare aplastic anaemia is outweighed by the advantages.

amphenicol on this list underscores the need to evaluate th risk/benefit ratio for each country separately. In a country with limited resources, chloramphenicol is cheap, affordable, and has a broad spectrum of activity. The rare aplastic anaemia resulting from its use is outweighted by the benefits. No chemotherapeutic agent is on this list, nor, needless to say, is radiation therapy. WHO has developed an essential drugs list for a number of diseases including cancer (43), and it encourages each country to use these as templates for the development of similar lists that are locally relevant. In addition, emphasis should be placed on the use of generic drugs rather than brand names, which are 5–10 times more expensive.

ACQUIRED IMMUNODEFICIENCY SYNDROME (AIDS)

AIDS poses a formidable challenge to African policy makers, health planners, and health care professionals. It is creating economic chaos and tremendous social disruption. Both the direct cost of prevention, diagnosis, and treatment as well as the indirect cost of lost wages and lost productivity continue to escalate. AIDS has destabilized many already precarious health institutions and has jeopardized the establishment of pressing health objectives. AIDS patients who contract tuberculosis (TB) require 2–3 times more drugs than non-AIDS TB patients. Consequently hospitals run out of drugs. TB goes untreated and continues to spread. Hospital beds are filling with AIDS patients and other medical problems are slowly being crowded out. Blood transfusion services deserve special mention. The search for donors and screening will all add to the unbearable cost of providing this service.

Few diseases have brought to light as many ethical questions as AIDS (8). Some of these include issues like quarantine, isolation, mandatory screening, mandatory reporting, the duty to warn, and the duty to treat. In the area of resource allocation, AIDS competes for the limited resource. It competes for a large share of drugs, hospital resources, and public education. The most important resource, the family volunteers, are having to make painful choices whether to place the sick in the health care facility or look after them at home.

GREATER GOOD AND EXPENDITURE OF RESOURCES

While the concept of greater good would seem theoretically appealing, society, no matter where, cannot view greater good in purely utilitarian terms, but in terms of a complex mix of competing philosophies (44). While society demands the wise spending of its resources, it is aware of its humane responsibility to all its members, and those responsibilities can only be met by the expenditure of resources. In other words, health care delivery expenditure must be reduced without infringing thoughtlessly on the dictates of justice, compassion, and dignity.

CONCLUSION

In conclusion, it ought to be reiterated that resource is limited, rationing is unavoidable, and resource must be distributed fairly. In the allocation of any public resource the principal concern is with justice, which involves giving each person his or her due. In allocating health care resource the main concern is largely with distributive justice (to distribute amongst members of the community those benefits and burdens due to them). The basis of distributive justice is the notion of fairness. Respect for life underlies the concern for distributive justice and is clearly a fundamental principle of any moral society. While governments have been given the mandate to balance books, that does not mean they have the mandate to be iron-fisted, callous, and indifferent to patients and those who care for them. Thus political representatives and government bureaucrats must resist any temptations to balance books at the expense of the poor, the sick, and the disadvantaged. In the case of cancer, those countries with very limited resources should lay emphasis on cancer prevention and palliative care. If cytotoxic drugs must be purchased, an essential drugs list should be prepared and adhered to.

REFERENCES

1. The Constitution of the World Health Organization. *WHO Chronicle*. 1947; 29.
2. Callahan D. *Setting Limits: Medical Goals in an Aging Society*. New York: Simon and Shuster, 1987;
3. Olweny CLM. Quality of life in cancer care. *Med J Aust*. 1993; 158,429–432.
4. William A. Health economies: the end of clinical freedom? *BMJ*. 1988; 297,1183–1186.
5. Goodman NW. Resource allocation: idealism, realism, pragmatism, openness. *J Med Ethics*. 1991; 17,179–180.
6. Maynard A., Occasional book: healthy competition? *Lancet*. 1990; 336,1305.
7. *Alma Ata Declaration: Health for All by the Year 2000?* International Conference on Primary Health Care. WHO and UNICEF, Alma Ata, USSR; 1978, Sept. 6–11.
8. Faden RR, Kass NE. Bioethics and public health in the 1980's: resource allocation and AIDS. *Annu Rev Publ Health*. 1991; 12,335–360.
9. Smeeding TM, Battlin MP, francis LP, Landesman BM. *Should Medical Care be Rationed by Age?* Ottawa NJ: Rowman and Littlefield; 1987.
10. Daniels N. *Am I My Parents' Keeper? An Essay on Justice between the Young and the Old*. New York: Oxford University Press; 1988.
11. Lewis RA, Charney M. Which of two individuals do you treat when only the ages are different and you can't treat both? *J Med Ethics*. 1989; 15,28–32.
12. Olweny C. Bioethics in developing countries: ethics of scarcity and sacrifice. *J Med Ethics*. 1994; 20,169–174.
13. Calman KC. The ethics of allocation of scarce health resources: a view from the centre. *J Med Ethics*. 1994; 20,71–74.
14. Eschbach JW, Egrie JC, Downing MR et al. Correcting of anaemia of end stage renal disease with recombinant human erythopoietin. *N Engl J Med*. 1987; 316,73–80.
15. Leitgeb C, Pecherstorfer M, Fritz E. Ludwig H. Quality of life in chroic anaemia of cancer during treatment with recombinant human erythropoietin. *Cancer*. 1994; 73,2535–2542.
16. Skillings JR, Sridhar FG, Wong C, Paddock L. The frequency of red cell transfusion for anaemia in patients receiving chemotherapy. *Am J Clin Oncol*. 1993; 16(1):22–25.
17. Healy D. Psychopharmacology and the ethics of resource allocation. *Br J Psychiatry*. 1993; 162,23–29.
18. Yeo M. Ethics and economics in health care resource allocation. Ottawa; Queen's University of Ottawa Economics Projects, Working Papers Series 93-07; 1993.
19. Veatch RM. Allocating health resources ethically: new roles for administrators and clinicians. *Front Health Admin*. 1991; 8.3–29.
20. Pellegrino ED. Rationing health care: the ethics of medical gatekeeping. *J Contemp Health Law Policy*. 1986; 2,23–45.
21. The physician as the patient's advocate (Editorial) *J Clin Oncol*. 1993; 11, 1011–1013.
22. Williams JR, Beresford EB. Physicians, ethics and allocation of health care resources. *Ann R Coll Phys Surg Can*. 1991; 24:305–309.
23. Kennedy I. Fron principles to practice in allocating resources. Australian Hospital Association Conference, Hobart, 1984. The ethics of resource allocation. *Med J Aust*. 1990; 153,437–438.
24. Higgins GL. The operation was successful but the patient died: reflections on health care cost and social support cuts. *Can Family Physician*. 1994; 40,421–423.

25. Hadorn DC. The Oregon priority-setting exercise: quality of life and public policy. *Bioethics News*. 1992; 11,38–48.

26. Dixon J, Welch HG. Priority setting: lessons from Oregon. *Lancet*. 1991; 337,891–894.

27. Welch HG, Larron EB. Dealing with limited resources: the Oregon decision to curtail funding for organ transplantation. *N Engl J Med*. 1988; 319,171–173.

28. Ruark JE, Raffin TA. The Stanford University Medical Centre Committee on Ethics: initiating and withdrawing life support. *N Engl J Med*. 1989; 15,25–20.

29. Olweny, C. The ethics and conduct of cross cultural research in developing countries. *Psycho-Oncology*. 1994; 3,11–20.

30. Ubel PA, DeKay ML, Baron J, and Asch DA. Cost-effectiveness analysis in a setting of budget constraints: is it equitable? *N Engl J Med*. 1996; 334,1174–1177.

31. Muller MA, Kohut N, Sam M, et al. Access to adult liver transplantation in Canada: a survey and ethical analysis. *Can Med Assoc J*. 1996; 154,337–342.

32. Singer PA. A review of public policies to procure and distribute kidneys for transplantation. *Arch Intern Med*. 1990; 150,53–527.

33. Lowy FH. Restructuring health care: rationing and compromise. *Humane Med*. 1992; 8,263–267.

34. Woolhander S, Himmelstein DV. The deteriorating administrative efficiency of the United States health care system. *N Engl J Med*. 1991; 324,1253–1258.

35. Weston B, Lauria M. Occasional notes. Patient advocacy in the 1990's. *N Engl J Med*. 1996; 334,563–564.

36. Maynard A, Bloor K. Occasional notes. Introducing a market to the United Kingdom's National Health Service. *N Engl J Med*. 1996; 334,604–607.

37. *Medical Post*. 19 March 1996; p. 4.

38. Brahams D. Enforcing a duty to care for patients in the National Health Service. *Lancet*. 1984; 2,1224–1225.

39. Miller FH, Miller GAH. The painful prescription: a procrustean perspective. *N Engl J Med*. 1986; 314, 1383–1386.

40. Olweny CLM. Global inequalities in cancer care. *Trans R Soc Trop Med Hyg*. 1991; 85,709–710.

41. Sigerist HE. *Civilization and Disease*. Chicago: University of Chicago Press, Phoenix Edition; 1962. (First published by Cornell University Press, 1943.)

42. Callahan D. *What Kind of Life: The Limits of Medical Progress*. New York: Simon and Schuster; 1990.

43. *The Selection of Essential Drugs*. WHO Expert Committee Technical Report Series No. 641. WHO: Geneva; 1979.

44. Whitaker P. Resource allocation: a plea for a touch of realism. *J Med Ethics*. 1990; 16,129–131.

98

Understanding the Interface Between Psychiatry and Ethics

MARGUERITE S. LEDERBERG

The inclusion of a bioethics section in a medical text-book is a comparatively recent phenomenon. Yet it is taken for granted, now that the paternalistic assumptions of physicians have been challenged, and the pervasiveness of value judgments in medical management has been effectively demonstrated. Indeed, the pendulum has swung the other way. The Joint Commission on Accreditation of Health Care Organizations now requires institutions to have a formal mechanism to address ethical issues (1). This has resulted in the rapid proliferation of ethics committees, accompanied by an increasing awareness of the limitations of the earlier "principlism" method of ethical analysis, as opposed to "narrative" ethics, a more pragmatic method, embedded in the unique nuances of each case, a stance which is naturally more compatible with medical management (2).

Meanwhile, many mental health professionals have viewed themselves as the guardians of a certain kind of humanism in medical care (3). In particular, psychiatrists have always been over-represented on ethics committees and many have worked hard to educate themselves and work constructively with bioethicists. Thoughtful participants from all disciplines now recognize that ethical dilemmas develop in a context of psychological stress and/or open conflict. The psychological complexity of the informed consent process came as a surprise to philosophers, while its philosophical complexity surprised clinicians. It took time to acknowledge that this complexity did not only reside in medical ineptitude, but that it was a poignant human response to barely tolerable anxiety and confusion. Terminal care decisions, organ transplantation, genetic testing, all present ever more bewildering problems in which philosophical complexity is inextricably bound up with psychological determinants.

In recognition of this, there follows a description of the clinical interface between consultation–liaison psychiatry and bioethics, with an emphasis on helping mental health professionals recognize the difference between psychiatric and ethical issues and on maximizing the accuracy and effectiveness of their contribution in both.

THE CONFLUENCE OF PSYCHIATRY AND ETHICS IN CONSULTATION-LIAISON PSYCHIATRY

The stresses of enduring cancer described throughout this text are frequently translated into increased interpersonal conflicts and dysfunctional reactions, especially when difficult decisions must be made. And the more difficult the decision, the more likely it is to have an ethical dimension.

It is hard to exaggerate the interconnectedness that exists between participants. Figure 98–1 describes a constant state of flux, in which:

1. Stress, dysfunctional responses, and ethical conflicts all flow into each other bidirectionally.
2. Patients, families, and staff all play a role.
3. The dysfunctional responses vary from minimal to severe.

Each component can affect and be affected by the others, and all parties are often too involved to understand their own role (4). With or without a significant ethical dilemma, patients and their families can become dysfunctional to the point of developing a DSM-IV axis-I disorder, especially when there are pre-existing vulnerabilities. But inappropriate psychiatric labeling may also occur, if the staff focuses too exclusively on psychological manifestations and misses the underlying ethical precipitants. Responses range from brief emotional reactions and cognitive distortions to more

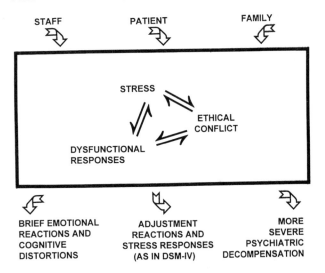

FIG. **98–1.** Schematic representation of interactions among participants in cancer treatment settings. (Adapted from Lederberg M. Making a situational diagnosis: educating psychiatrists to function at the interface of psychiatry and ethics. *Psychosomatics.* 1997; 38(4): 327–338.)

severe psychiatric decompensations. Generally the staff is only involved at the mildest level, but it takes little distortion or over-involvement to generate a complicated situation. In this fluid setting, calling a psychiatry or an ethics consult is often a matter of perception as much as a matter of substance. The consultant's task is to move beyond the initial request to a deeper analysis of the main problems.

REVIEW OF MAJOR STRESSORS

It is useful to review the major categories of stress among which the consultant must identify the operative ones. They are summarized in Table 98.1. The first three are reviewed elsewhere in this volume; this discussion will focus mainly on the last two.

Decisional Stressors

The new and difficult decisions that are now integral to the patient role have been semi-facetiously described as "the perils of being a modern patient," since they have a particularly contemporary cast (5).

Having to Choose Between Comparable Treatment Options. Patients such as those with early stage breast cancer are often given equivalent treatment options. For a vulnerable subgroup, this creates severe anxiety, leading to decisional paralysis, and a range of symptoms in the adjustment/anxiety disorder spectrum. With psychiatric intervention the

patient resumes a functional "patient role," but symptoms often last long after the end of treatment.

Deciding on Life-Threatening Treatment. Bone marrow transplantation is an example of an increasingly common procedure that is difficult for patients to accept or refuse. When parents must decide on treatment for their children, the anguish is even more acute. If the child dies, parents may be devoured by guilt at having "subjected the child to torture" and the already difficult mourning process may grind to a destructive halt. The negative effects can mark surviving siblings for life.

Making Decisions about Life-Sustaining Technology. Giving permission to withhold or withdraw life-sustaining treatments such as respirator support, nutrition, or fluids is a quintessential modern stressor. Patients who are not realistically informed, or have denied their prognosis, experience it as a betrayal or emotional assault. It is more difficult than generally realized to guide patients through this transition.

Patient Factors. Four years after the Federal Patient Self-Determination Act, only 15%–20% of patients prepared advance directives unless labor intensive programs were in place to increase their number (6–7). Patients themselves may have difficulty formulating advance directives that can be trusted to

TABLE **98.1.** *Major Categories of Stressors*

1. ILLNESS-RELATED FACTORS
2. PATIENT-RELATED PSYCHOLOGICAL FACTORS
3. FAMILY-RELATED FACTORS
4. DECISIONAL STRESSORS
   Choosing between comparable treatments
   Considering a life-threatening treatment
   Withholding or withdrawing life supports
   Withdrawing fluids and/or nutrition
   Patient factors
   Physicians as surrogates
   Family members as surrogates
5. ENVIRONMENTAL STRESSORS
   Lack of social, religious, or cultural congruence
   Social and financial inequities
   Legal intrusions into medical care
   Third-party intrusions into medical care
   Resource allocation

correspond to their choices in a time of crisis (8–9). Attempts are underway to improve methods of obtaining patient preferences (10–11), but for now, families and physicians play an important role in making decisions for patients who have not prepared advance directives.

Physicians as Surrogates. Physician claim to expert judgment in terminal care situations has been both strongly defended (12–13) and attacked (14). Several studies have found that physicians consider many factors in decision-making, some related to personal beliefs (15–16), others to unacknowledged evaluations of medical futility (17). Physician accuracy in guessing their patient's preferences has not been good (18). Most recently, the possibility that doctors "hasten" death surreptitiously has been extended to include ICU nurses (19), although the study methodology has been severely criticized (20). One recent study, the largest of its kind, has shown that doctors ignore even clearly stated patient preferences (21–22).

Family Members as Surrogates. Like the patient, family surrogates may feel that terminal care discussions are cruel and inappropriate. Their grief is usually accompanied by anxiety-provoking feelings, such as anger, ambiguous anticipations of the future, guilt-ridden reviews of the past, and a wish for the death to come. These may be balanced by a fierce determination to ensure that "everything is done" or accompanied by an equally strong determination to prevent "unnecessary" suffering. Even detachment and financial self-interest are rarely present without guilt and discomfort. Lastly one finds blind panic, a desperate refusal to consider life without the dying person. Even when a gentle physician outlines options realistically, the decision carries a symbolic meaning far beyond its practical implications. Unfortunately, the importance given to resuscitation decisions by lawyers, ethicists, and especially the media, has tended to perpetuate magical beliefs about a procedure which, in the setting of cancer, is so often a travesty of medical interventionism. Yet many family members carry away with them the feeling that they gave permission for death to occur. In addition, the accuracy of family surrogates in predicting patient choices has been no better than that of physicians (23–26). Hence, the whole concept of substituted judgment, the legal principle empowering surrogates, is being re-evaluated (27) (see Chapter 96).

Environmental Stressors

Environmental stressors arise spontaneously from existing circumstances and are often as troubling to the staff as to the patient and family.

Lack of Social, Cultural, or Religious Congruence Between the Patient and Family and the Medical Team. The problems in communication related to discrepancies between patients and providers are discussed in Chapter 94. Here, it suffices to say that these same families are repeatedly observed to be more frequently involved in ethical dilemmas as well.

Financial Limitations or Inequities of Social Class. The well-demonstrated negative impact of poverty on survival is discussed in Chapter 8. The inability to give oneself or one's loved ones available care is profoundly corrosive. It is worst when the discrepancy between expectation and availability is greatest, creating a climate of resentment and anger which health professionals must absorb without letting it undermine their self-esteem or drive them to alter their caregiving in negative ways.

In a very few nations, medical care is disbursed with some adequacy and equitability. But it has proved so costly that the best socialized medicine systems are in a process of retrenchment and partial privatization. In many more countries, there is so little of either equitability or adequacy that despair submerges active expectation. But caregivers must try not to internalize this hopelessness, since it affects their work and diminishes the effectiveness of their interactions with patients. Perhaps they can help each other remember the meaning inherent in each of their acts of care and nurture, a meaning whose value is ultimately beyond measure. They should also remember that fatalism can be a brittle seal over rage and grief, and not personalize the patient outbursts that occur when the seal is shattered.

Legal Intrusions into Care Decisions. Ethics and law are closely intertwined in practice, but not in fundamental substance, making for an uneasy marriage with many opportunities for conflict. Legalism may be used by staff and knowledgeable consumers to both obscure and resolve ethical dilemmas.

Conflicts between the law and ethical beliefs place professionals in difficult situations. The noble solution may place an enormous burden on the individual. Most ethical theories state that such personal sacrifices cannot be required. But the dilemma and the inner conflict remain, and the problem remains unsolved. The situation is exacerbated when patients or families make insistent demands, as for example, when a family demands discontinuation of life supports to diminish patient suffering, and the physician agrees with the humaneness of this privately but cannot act upon his conviction legally.

Third-Party Intrusions into Care Decisions. Patronage and institutionalized discrepancies between private and public sectors occur all over the world. Within a non-profit one-party-payor system, physicians know the care decisions forced on them are part of a plan to maximize overall benefits. Where a profit motive underlies the organization of care, ethical conflicts for doctors become massive (28), and consumers become angry and desperate. In the United States, this problem is in a bewildering stage of transformation, and little can be said about it, except to underline the psychological anguish endured by both consumers and providers (29).

Allocation of Scarce Resources. The previous issues viewed at a systemic level present different problems depending on available resources. Some hospitals have the luxury of deciding the number of bone marrow transplants. Others must decide whether to provide chemotherapy for curable patients or morphine for incurable ones, without enough of either. While it seems perverse to consider these extremes together, there is, in both cases, a corrosive emotional burden on staff who face insoluble ethical conflicts in their daily work. They bear it alone, but when patients are aware, the climate is one of intense conflict with both parties feeling abused and helpless.

SITUATIONAL DIAGNOSIS

Mislabeling of consult requests by the staff members requesting it can result in pseudo-psychiatric, pseudo-ethics, and mixed psychiatry/ethics consults which will be illustrated below (4).

Lederberg has described the process of probing beyond the initial consult request to understand the deeper questions and has called it "making a situational diagnosis." It is a four-step process that needs to be carried out before ethical issues can be addressed with some assurance that the right issues are under discussion. Table 98.2 outlines the components of each step. The first explores the contributions of patient and family dynamics. The second explores staff dynamics as they relate to case management. The third analyzes the interface between patient, family, and staff. The fourth reviews all the possible legal, regulatory, and institutional constraints that may bear upon the case. Only after these issues have been clarified can one isolate and analyze the underlying ethical conflicts, and understand whether they are driving the psychiatric symptoms, or whether the psychiatric symptoms are driving them. Accurate answers dictate the most effective hierarchy of interventions.

HIERARCHY OF INTERVENTIONS

It is useful to think of interventions as being hierarchically organized. They can be broadly classified into three categories, educational, psychiatric, and ethical analysis, with the first being almost universally required, the next often, but not always needed, and

TABLE 98.2. *Components of a Situational Diagnosis*

I. PATIENT/FAMILY ISSUES
1. Is there a psychological problem or treatable psychiatric disorder affecting the patient or any relevant family member?
2. Psychologically, what issues are driving the situation?
3. Whom do they involve?

II. STAFF ISSUES
1. Is there disagreement about medical management?
2. Is some other interstaff conflict being played out?
3. Is a legal or administrative requirement driving the situation?

III. JOINT ISSUES
1. What is the nature of the relationship between the staff and the patient and family?
2. What is the understanding and explicit labeling of the issues by different participants?

IV. LEGAL ISSUES
1. Are there laws or regulations, federal, state or local, that impinge upon the case?
2. Are there institutional constraints that impinge upon the case?
3. Could any of these create a potential conflict? What is the nature of that conflict?

V. ETHICAL ISSUES
1. Is there an ethical dilemma? a true conflict of values that cannot be reduced to any other problem or misunderstanding?
2. Is it driving the psychological symptoms? or are the symptoms generating it?
3. How can it be most usefully analyzed and shared?

with the last and most complex being addressed only after the others have been evaluated.

Educational Interventions

In the absence of significant psychopathology, simply sharing the situational diagnosis, in a non-judgmental way calculated to help participants understand their own role and that of others, can be a transforming intervention. Conflict resolution may begin to occur and moral dilemmas may become negotiable. If not, they are at least more clearly revealed, and stripped of many obscuring factors.

Psychiatric Interventions

In the presence of psychopathology, consultants must make an accurate diagnosis, recommend multimodal treatments, and implement them as promptly as possible. They should not be intimidated by the presence of ethical and legal controversies, as long as they stay clearly within their area of expertise. Careful self-awareness and discipline are required, because their training in interpersonal relations and conflict resolution makes it easier for them to inject value judgments into the process. Some of this is inevitable, but it should be minimal, and always in a self-aware fashion.

Ethics Interventions

Outside of their area of expertise, consultants must be humble and ready to call the appropriate experts. In the United States, hospitals are required to have a mechanism for the resolution of ethical disputes, hence help is always at hand, in the form of an ethics committee whose members represent several disciplines, or an ethicist acting alone with various methods of accountability (1,30–31). Ethicists need to have the same awareness of their limitations that is being recommended for mental health professionals. Few of them have psychiatric expertise, nor does training in conflict resolution address all the psychological concomitants of the situation. Lastly, they too are uniquely qualified to inject their own values into the process, although intellectual rigor can diminish the danger. They can best define and analyze the ethical issues, and identify the protagonists to whom responsibilities are owed. They help outline different options, and the moral implications and consequences of each one. They may make immediate recommendations or consult others, and do further research to bring back useful documentation. Occasionally some options become obvious; often they do not, but competing values will have been made clear, and participants will be empowered to act as effective moral agents in making difficult decisions.

Legal Input

In the United States, the law plays an on-going role in defining social ethics, both through case law, and regulations. But resorting to court proceedings guarantees adversarial polarization, the very climate one seeks to minimize. Good coordination of psychological and ethical input should make this outcome extremely rare.

In the next section three cases will be described. The first two were mislabeled, but were comparatively simple to disentangle. The third was quite complex and will be discussed in detail.

EXAMPLES OF MISLABELED CASES

The Pseudo-Psychiatry Consult

A psychiatry consultation was requested because of possible delirium in a 54-year-old businessman with advanced gastric cancer and pneumonitis, who required vasopressors and had become negativistic and irritable. On evaluation, he was cognitively intact, and revealed a deep desire to stop treatment which he felt his family was refusing to hear. As a result, he felt betrayed, abandoned, and angry. Meetings with his family and physician were arranged, during which his feelings were acknowledged and the family was educated about his options and helped to come to terms with him. During that time, the patient was quiet and cooperative with no change in medications. After three days, he elected to stop vasopressors, a decision which his family was now able to accept. He died quietly during the next day.

In this case there was no individual psychopathology driving the psychiatric symptoms in either patient or family. There were no staff disagreements and no problems at the patient/staff interface. There was a relevant legal issue, namely the absolute right of a competent patient to refuse treatment, even life-saving treatment. Hence the precipitant could be narrowed to an unacknowledged ethical conflict between the family, who would not entertain "suicide," and the patient, who felt, with some biological accuracy, that it was time to "let himself die."

Once this family was educated about the patient's rights and at the same time given psychological support, they were able to deal with the moral question. And once the patient's right to refuse treatment was addressed, the psychological symptoms resolved spontaneously. However, this case also highlights the confusion that develops when medical staff label an unhappy patient as "mildly delirious," or a mildly delirious patient as "hostile" or "a poor coper." Making these distinctions accurately can require a great deal of sophistication. The psychiatric consultant needed to be familiar with the ethical and legal status of stopping key treatments, as well as family dynamics and the symptoms of early delirium. While the deeper layers of the family's non-suicide stance were not explored, some insight into them enabled the discussions to proceed more smoothly and minimized the family's likelihood of stubbornly opposing him, or of feeling too guilty about giving in.

The Pseudo-Ethics Consult

An ethics consultation was called by a surgeon concerned about a patient's decision to refuse treatment. She was a 56-year-old female, scheduled for operation on a uterine cancer which had been canceled and delayed for 72 hours. The patient was now refusing the surgery to which she had previously agreed. The ethics committee members found a lucid, angry patient, who refused to discuss her decision. However, her nurse mentioned she had no visitors during the last three days. When this was noted, she burst out with feelings of hurt and fear that she would lack adequate family support to get through the experience. Family members were contacted and sounded out. Family conferences were arranged during which the patient was reassured and readily agreed to proceed.

At first glance, one might have wondered whether the patient's competence was under question only *because* she was refusing treatment, as had happened in decades past. But the surgeon was correct in questioning the patient's change of heart, and in good contemporary fashion, did not automatically put a psychiatric label on the problem, calling an ethics consult instead. Yet what was needed was an understanding of the patient's acute psychological state and again, of the family situation. The response was a standard psychiatric consultation–liaison intervention.

THE COMPLEX ETHICS/PSYCHIATRY CASE

In this case, it was necessary to use the full situational diagnosis scheme to disentangle many issues.

Ethics consultation was requested on a 21-year-old female with terminal cancer of the cervix because the staff felt the attending was going against the parents' wishes in not confronting the patient with the grimness of her prognosis. Three members of the ethics committee responded as a group, a Ph.D. ethicist, an oncologist, and a psychiatrist.

Situational Diagnosis

Patient/Family Issues. The patient was lucid and manifested no acute psychological symptoms. She was, however, immature and functioning psychologically at a younger level than her chronological age. She refused to talk about her illness, making small talk about unrealistic plans. The parents showed no unusual psychological symptoms, and seemed devoted to the patient. However, they revealed a profound state of emotional exhaustion related to their anticipatory grief, the length and arduousness of the illness, and the additional stress of dealing with a needy child–woman. As the end came near, their grief was resonating with their resentment of their daughter's denial. It made their dealings with her more uncomfortable as they realized she would leave them without ever having a real talk with them, without ever acknowledging their devotion, and without saying goodbye.

Staff Issues. There was no problem with medical management, but there was interstaff conflict, as the attending was seen by staff to avoid realistic prognostication, committing them to perform resuscitations that had no chance of success, an event they experienced as brutalizing to the patient. The staff's resentment made them readier to resonate with the parents' emotional state. They also had strong feelings about "truth-telling" for a patient over eighteen.

Joint Issues. The family had had a good relationship with the attending and the staff for years. The parents had begun to display uncharacteristic anger and bitterness. Staff resentment about the cardiopulmonary resuscitation (CPR) situation added to their emotional fatigue and sadness about this familar patient, and made them resonate with the parents' emotional state.

Legal Issues. In this jurisdiction, CPR was legally required for any patient, unless the patient agreed to a "do-not-resuscitate" (DNR) order after a formal discussion. This could be avoided by invoking a "therapeutic exception," in which a competent patient was not offered a choice about resuscitation when it was felt that the discussion would be destructive. Both the institution and the staff routinely scrutinized this exception closely, to insure it was not being used to circumvent the spirit of the law.

Ethical Issues. Many questions needed to be asked.

1. Was the patient's denial sufficiently entrenched and beneficial to her, to warrant the attending's avoidance of talking with her?
2. Would supporting him be a collusion and a denial of the patient's capacity for growth and meaningful contact?
3. Was it legitimate to consider her immaturity against her chronological age as having any bearing on the decision?

4. Would any confrontation deprive her of her right not to know?

5. Were the parents putting their emotional needs ahead of hers in pushing for a discussion?

6. Was the staff using the parents and the autonomy issue to play out their negative feelings about the physician, rather than attending to the patient's state? Or were they putting an appropriate emphasis on this competent and legally adult patient being given a full opportunity to exercise her options?

7. Would a therapeutic exception be appropriate or an evasion in this case?

These questions could be further narrowed to two fundamental issues:

(a) How could the patient's autonomy be best honored, and her best interests be optimally identified, in this particular situation?

(b) How could it be done with the least impact on the needs and rights of other participants?

Interventions

Educational. The members of the ethics committee reviewed and discussed the findings described above, and shared them with family and staff.

Psychiatric. Empathic attempts to explore the patient's attitude continued. The parents discussed their feelings and acknowledged the multiple factors impinging on them. These were normalized for them, validating the complexity and pain inherent in the issues they faced, in an effort to defuse the potential for guilt. The staff was given insight into the parents' feelings, and as a result, decreased their unconscious identification with them.

Ethics. All aspects of the right to know, and not to know, and their possible abuse, were discussed with parents and staff. The staff discussed the attending obligations about "truth-telling" as well as the supporting staff's responsibility to take action or stand by. Their right to honor their feelings was matched against the need for professional discipline. Legal, ethical, and psychological aspects of the therapeutic exception clause were explored.

Outcome

Throughout, the patient remained unchanged. Her parents resumed a more protective stance and no longer pushed for change in the management. Staff members were able to relinquish their negative attitude about the physician, accept the discomfort inherent in dealing with this patient, and support the parents'

change of heart. The consultants explored their own thinking and motivation in supporting this kind of exception. They reviewed their committee's past performance about the "therapeutic exception," and came to the conclusion that they had seldom used it and could probably trust themselves to support it in this case. The issue was put on the agenda for discussion at the next ethics committee meeting, so as to further review their decision, and discuss therapeutic exceptions in a broader context.

A purely psychiatric intervention reaching the same conclusion might have deprived the participants of a chance to explore so effectively the many ethical questions involved on the case. The parents were reassured by the thoroughness of the discussion. The staff learned much that would be of help to them in other cases. An intervention by an ethicist alone, though reaching the same conclusion, might have missed the dynamics of the parents' feelings and been less able to relieve them.

In any case, supporting the staff and parents in "truth-telling" and confronting the long-standing infantilization of the patient would have been difficult for the patient and would have contributed to the parents' subsequent guilt about their negative feelings. The staff would have been reinforced in covertly playing out their resentment of the primary physician.

Follow-up

There was no further controversy about the patient. The parents resumed their earlier stance, receiving more empathic support from the staff, who no longer felt so aggrieved. The use of the therapeutic exception clause to bypass a DNR discussion with the patient was accepted, and formal psychiatric intervention was never required.

GUIDELINES FOR THE EFFECTIVE USE OF PSYCHIATRIC INPUT

Patient care will benefit if professionals have a clear picture of the types of clinical/ethical situations in which mental health consultants can make a contribution, as well as a clear understanding of the range of interventions involved. This will encourage the appropriate use of their services, and will be an efficient contribution to the welfare of patients and their families. Relevant situations are outlined in Table 98.3.

The need to deal with diagnosable psychopathology in the patient is usually well understood. The role of problems in a family member is often less understood. The reverberations of dysfunctional family dynamics may be apparent to the staff and to the ethicist, but

TABLE 98.3. *Clinical Situations Calling for Psychiatric Input*

1. Diagnosable psychopathology in any participant
2. Unusually acute emotional distress or symptoms
3. Active conflict associated with emotional distress
4. Staff over-involvement or rejection
5. Intrastaff conflict or non-cooperation
6. Questions about a patient or a surrogate's decisional capacity

effective interventions at that level require more skill than these professionals usually possess. There is also a tendency to underestimate significant past events and their power to shape current patient and family attitudes. Their power cannot be diminished if it has not been recognized and dealt with. Psychological symptoms, if they are acute enough, may trigger a psychiatric consultation, especially if they are disrupting case management. But there is a tendency to wait much too long, because non-mental health participants often have an internal pre-conception of how much emotional distress is "reasonable" or, in the case of ethicist, "irrelevant" in a given situation. This also leads them to ignore the significance of mild reactions which may point the way to key factors in the resolution of an impasse.

Conflict per se is not an indication for psychiatric input, since an ethics consultation is, by definition, called because of an unresolved question. It is needed when a conflict generates enough heat to obscure issues, and significantly impairs the ability of key individuals to participate in the resolution process.

Decisional Capacity

Serious confusion has developed about the role of psychiatric input in establishing decision-making capacity. Medical staff, in a well-meaning attempt to honor patient autonomy, often couch management problems in ethical terms, overlooking the fact that the real issue is the patient's psychological state. Establishing capacity is a *psychiatric determination*, often a subtle and difficult one. Understanding the significance of a fluctuating mental state is a *psychiatric judgment*. Treating the patient to improve and stabilize capacity is a *psychiatric intervention*. A case which does not use all these inputs prevents the patient from being an effective moral agent on his own behalf. It is poor medicine and poor ethics.

On the other hand, the psychiatric consultant must remember there is a presumption of competence and that their determination must be specific to the matter at hand. A patient need not count backwards by sevens perfectly if he understands the reasons for, the consequences of, and the alternatives to, his decision (32).

Types of Psychiatric Interventions

The ways in which psychiatry can intervene are summarized in Table 98.4. The lists ranges from areas in which psychiatric input is uniquely required, to areas in which other disciplines play a major role. There can be, in all of them, a level of psychological complexity which benefits from a thorough understanding of psychodynamics.

CONCLUSION

The recent entry of bioethics into medical care is a welcome addition to the armamentarium of caregivers. It is hoped that the preceding discussion will give consultants a method for maximizing their contribution in this as well as their more traditional ways.

TABLE 98.4. *Types of Psychiatric Interventions*

1. Treating individual psychological problems.
2. Diagnosing decisional capacity, when in doubt.
3. Restoring, improving, or stabilizing mental capacity.
4. Improving dysfunctional family dynamics.
5. Diminishing the emotional aspects of the conflicts.
6. Using their insider status to efficiently involve other medical caregivers.
7. Diagnosing problems at the staff/patient/family interface, and working to resolve them.
8. Understanding the psychological/cultural/religious interface as it impacts on ethical decision making, and insuring that the decisional input is congruent with patient and family values, through their own efforts, or by enlisting appropriate guidance.
9. Evaluating the role of other external factors, and working with other hospital and community resources to make disposition plans that are as broad as possible.

ACKNOWLEDGMENTS

Parts of this chapter are adapted from an article that appeared in *Psychosomatics*.

REFERENCES

1. Joint Commission on Accreditation of Health Care Organizations, *Accreditation Manual*, 1992.
2. Hastings Center Report. *The Sources and Stories of Moral Knowledge*. 1996; 26(1).
3. Sider RC. Clements C. Psychiatry's contribution to medical ethics education *Am J Psychiatry*. 1982; 139(4): 498–501.
4. Lederberg M. Making a situational diagnosis: psychiatrists at the interface of psychiatry and ethics in consultation-liaison psychiatry. *Psychosomatics*. 1997; 38(4): 327–338.
5. Lederberg M, Massie MJ, Holland JC. Psychiatric consultation to oncology. In: Tasman SM, Goldfinger,. Kaufman CA, eds. *American Psychiatric Review of Psychiatry*, vol 9. Washington, DC: American Psychiatric Press; 1990: 491–514.
6. Federal Patient Self-Determination Act, Pub.L. 101–508, sections 420–6, 4751(OBRA), 42 U.S.C. 1395 cc(a) et seq (1990).
7. Emanuel LL, Danis M, Pearlman RA, Singer PA. Advance care planning as a process: structuring the decisions in practice. *JAGS*. 1995; 43:440–446.
8. Cohen LM, Germain M, Woods A, et al. Patient attitudes and psychological considerations in dialysis discontinuation. *Psychosomatics*. 1993; 34:395–401.
9. Sehgal A, Galbraith A, Chesney M, et al. How strictly do dialysis patients want their advance directives followed? *J Am Med Assoc*. 1992; 267:59–63.
10. Emanuel LL, Barry MJ, Emanuel EJ, Stoeckle JD: Advance directives: can patients' stated choices be used to infer unstated choices? *Med Care*. 1994; 32:95–105.
11. Lynn J. Procedures for making decisions for incompetent adults. *J Am Med Assoc*. 1995; 267:2082–2084.
12. Finster S, Theaker N, Raper R, Fisher M. Surrogates' decisions in resuscitation are of limited value. *Br Med J*. 1994; 309:953.
13 Curtis JR, Park DR, Krone MR et al: Use of the medical futility rationale in do-not-attempt-resuscitation orders. *J Am Med Assoc*. 1995; 273:124–128.
14. Nelson JL. Families and futility. *JAGS*. 1994; 42: 879–882.
15. Cook DJ, Guyatt GH, Jaeschke R, et al. Determinants in Canadian health care workers of the decision to withdraw life support from the critically ill. *J Am Med Assoc*. 1995; 273:703–708.
16. Asch DA, Lanken PN. Decisions to limit or continue life-sustaining treatment by critical care physicians in the United States: conflicts between physicians' practices and patients' wishes. *Am J Respir Crit Care Med*. 1995; 151:288–292.
17. Hanson LC, Danis M, Mutan E, Keenan NL. Impact of patient incompetence on decisions to use or withhold life-sustaining treatment. *Am J Med*. 1994; 97:235–241.
18. Morris BA, Van Niman SE, Perlin T, et al. Health care professionals' accuracy in predicting patients' preferred code status. *J Fam Practice*. 1995; 40:41–44.
19. Asch DA. The role of critical care nurses in euthanasia and assisted suicide. *N Engl J Med*. 1996; 334:1374–1379.
20. Scanlon, C. Euthanasia and nursing practice - right question, wrong answer. *N Engl J Med*. 1996; 334:1401–1402.
21. Anonymous. a controlled trial to improve care for seriously ill hospitalized patients. The study to understand prognoses and preferences for outcomes and risks of treatment (SUPPORT). The SUPPORT Principal Investigators. *J Am Med Assoc*. 1995; 274:1591–1598.
22. Phillips RS, Wenger NS, Teno J, et al. for the SUPPORT Investigators. Choices of seriously ill patients about cardiopulmonary rescucitation: correlates and outcomes. *Am J Med*. 1996; 100:128–137.
23. Emanuel EJ, Emanuel LL. Proxy decision-making for incompetent patients: an empirical and ethical analysis. *J Am Med Assoc*. 1992; 267:2067–2071.
24. Seckler AB, Meier DE, Mulvihill M, et al. Substituted judgment: how accurate are proxy predictions? *Ann Intern Med*. 1991; 115:92–98.
25. Hare J, Pratt C, Nelson C. Agreement between patients and their self-selected surrogates on difficult medical decisions. *Arch Int Med*. 1992; 152:1049–1054.
26. Layde PM, Beam CA, Broste SK, et al. Surrogates' predictions of seriously ill patients' resuscitation preferences. *Arch Fam Med*. 1995; 4:518-524.
27. Suhl J, Simons P, Reedy T, Garrick T. Myth of substituted judgment: surrogate decision-making regarding life support is unreliable. *Arch Intern Med*. 1994; 154:90–96.
28. Woolhandler S, Himmelstein DU. Extreme risk—the new corporate proposition for physicians. *N Engl J Med*. 1996; 333:1706-8.
29. Larson E. The soul of an HMO. *Time Magazine*, January 22, 1996; 44–52.
30. Ross JW, Glazer JW, et al. *Health Care Ethics Committees: The Next Generation*. American Publishing, Inc., 1993.
31. Fletcher JC. The consultant's credentials. *Hastings Center Rep*. 1995; 25:39–40.
32. Appelbaum PS, Grisso T. Assessing patients' capacities to consent to treatment. *N Engl J Med*. 319:1635–1638.

XVI

RESEARCH METHODS IN PSYCHO-ONCOLOGY

Editor: William Breitbart

99

Quality of Life

DAVID CELLA

The value of health care interventions, including those directed at people with cancer, is judged by their impact upon quantity of life and quality of life. That impact, measured against cost, determines value. It has always been easy to measure quantity of life. It has not always been easy to measure life's quality. In part due to this, quantity of life (survival time) emerged in oncology as the most frequent and comfortable indicator of treatment effectiveness. Recognizing that time without quality is of questionable value, cancer treatment investigators have historically been forced to assume that adding time would naturally add value. This assumption is frequently, but not always, correct.

Now, with the recent availability of valid and practical quality of life (QOL) questionnaires, we have the opportunity to measure quality alongside quantity of life when evaluating cancer treatment effectiveness. This allows us to confirm the assumption that the time added by therapy is of sufficient value to justify its cost, and to examine many other possibilities. For example, treatments that do not extend survival may be of significant value because they improve QOL. The critical trade-off is not always between toxicity and survival time; sometimes a treatment temporarily palliates tumor-induced symptoms without extending survival. Patients may find this desirable even in the face of competing toxicity. Only a careful evaluation of patient-derived QOL can allow one to evaluate these trade-offs between symptom relief and toxicity. It has been shown that some cancer treatments improve QOL even though they carry toxicity.

QOL evaluation entails a multidimensional quantification of patient functional status, usually as perceived by the patient. QOL evaluation differs from classical toxicity ratings in two important ways: *(1)* It incorporates more aspects of function (e.g., mood, affect, social well-being) than those which have typically been attributed to treatment; and *(2)* it focuses on the patient's perspective. Many practical and valid questionnaires are available. This chapter discusses core issues in defining and measuring QOL during and after cancer treatment, and follows with a summary of emerging research issues.

CORE ISSUES OF DEFINITION AND MEASUREMENT

Defining Quality of Life and Its Dimensions

Until one has a clear definition of the conception, one cannot fully determine whether a QOL questionnaire is valid. There is a long tradition of defining the term quality of life. The classic definition of Campbell and colleagues ("A vague and ethereal entity, something that many people talk about, but which nobody very clearly knows what to do about") (1) does not help the test developer, who must accept the tolerance inherent in pragmatism. The integrity of the term QOL has been challenged on the grounds that it cannot be validly measured because it means different things to different people. Some have suggested abandoning the term quality of life because it is too general to have meaning. Others have pointed out that because the current definition of the term is so vague, it has been exploited as a marketing tool (2). There is truth in both of these perspectives. It appears, however, that the term is here to stay, at least for the foreseeable future, and it is therefore most productive to derive a consensus on the definition, at least as it relates to medical outcome evaluation. Some degree of consensus is a prerequisite for moving research and understanding forward.

There is wide consensus that QOL is both subjective and multidimensional (2–6). We had earlier developed a working definition of quality of life which laid a groundwork for measurement: "Quality of life refers to patients appraisal of and satisfaction with their current level of functioning as compared to what they perceive to be possible or ideal" (4). This earlier definition was modified to explicitly incorporate the multidimensionality of QOL: "Health-related quality of life (QOL) refers to the extent to which one's usual or expected physical, emotional and social well-being are affected by a medical condition or its treatment" (7). This definition provides minimum requirements for QOL measurement: that it obtain the *patient's* perspective and that it capture physical, mental, and social well-being.

There are many QOL questionnaires available and appropriate for use with cancer patients. These questionnaires are described in detail and compiled for reference elsewhere (8–9). A review of the many available questionnaires revealed that over 30 different names for QOL dimensions were listed by various authors (9). Careful review of the descriptions of these dimensions and available factor analytic studies suggested *seven* QOL dimensions which are sufficiently distinct to warrant separate listing. They are: *(1)* Physical concerns (symptoms, pain); *(2)* Functional ability (activity); *(3)* Family well-being; *(4)* Emotional well-being; *(5)* Treatment satisfaction (including financial concerns); *(6)* Sexuality/intimacy (including body image); and *(7)* Social functioning. Two summary dimensions are also relevant but not always available with every QOL questionnaire: Global evaluation of QOL (i.e., a single question rating the patient's global or overall perception of QOL or health status); and Total score (i.e., the summation of dimension scores into an aggregate index of QOL (9).

Dimension Versus Aggregated Scores. There are at least three distinct QOL dimensions: physical, mental, and social. Factor analytic and aggregate index studies have suggested that the physical domain should be divided into symptom (i.e., physical experience) versus function (i.e., physical abilities and activities) (5), and perhaps even further, dividing gastrointestinal toxicity into a separate group (6,10). Mental well-being usually refers to mood, both positive and negative. The social aspects of QOL have been notoriously the most difficult to capture with brief measurement approaches. Unfortunately, because of issues of cost and burden, brief measurement approaches appear to be essential in contemporary health services research. As a result, the social well-being dimension has tended to be under-represented and is therefore poorly understood.

Quality of life is indeed multidimensional, but it does not necessarily follow that reported QOL scores should always remain disaggregated when being reported. There are benefits to reporting QOL data both ways. Disaggregated dimension scores give one a more detailed and precise estimation of the different areas of patient function and well-being. This is usually preferred by the clinician. Aggregated scores and summary indexes are critical, however, to enable decision makers to meaningfully adjust time for its quality. Summary scores, while they lost some precision, are preferred by treatment outcome evaluators and economists.

QOL dimension scores are not only more detailed than an aggregated score; they provide differential sensitivity in many cases. Compared with physically-based scales, psychosocial scales are less sensitive to change in a primarily physical rating (e.g., performance status) and less sensitive to differences in groups formed on the basis of physical characters (e.g., extent of disease). For example, the emotional functioning scale of the European Organization for Research and Treatment of Cancer (EORTC) Quality of Life Questionnaire was unable to detect change in Performance Status Rating (PSR) (3), or in extent of disease (11–12). It was also shown to be less sensitive than the physcial scales to differences in PSR groups (3,11,13). Similar findings have been reported for the Functional Assessment of Cancer Therapy (FACT) Measurement System (14–16). Also, the Profile of Mood States (POMS), a widely used measure of emotional distress, closely paralleled findings we have reported for the Emotional Well-Being (EWB) and Social Family Well-Being (SWB) scale in breast cancer (16). In fact, the POMS Depression, POMS Tension, and POMS Anger could not differentiate between any of the "extent of disease" subgroups (unpublished data (16)). Indeed, other studies have found no difference in emotional well-being between people diagnosed with cancer and those without cancer (17–18). Using the Functional Living Index-Cancer (FLIC), Ganz and Coscarellie reported that they found no difference in QOL by nodal status, adjuvant chemotherapy, and type of surgery (19). Ganz and colleagues (20) also found that the psychological distress scale of the Cancer Rehabilitation Evaluation System (CARES) was unable to distinguish among clinical disease status groups of HIV+ patients. Also, McHorney and colleagues (21), in their validity studies of the SF-36, present data demonstrating that measures of mental health are insensitive detectors of change in physical health. Ware and colleagues (22) also demonstrate that physical and mental health can diverge across time, as in an aging population. Indeed, once the physical components of mental well-being are extracted from measures of mental well-being, the relationship between the two is modest. A major problem encountered in using earlier measures of psychological distress in the medical population is that these measures are laden with physical symptoms (e.g., appetite, sleep, fatigue).

Notwithstanding the above point supporting separate reporting of QOL dimension scores, there remains strong and justifiable pressure to aggregate dimension scores into a summary index. Ultimate, "bottom line" decision making depends upon having a manageable summary of benefits and problems caused by treatments. We (16–18) and others (19–22) have aggregated dimension scores into summary indexes for practical application, and in an attempt to compare the usefulness of psychometric QOL evaluation with that of utility assessment (see later discussion of utilities) to determine patient preferences or valuations for their current health. We typically recommend using a physical Trial Outcome Index (TOI) as an efficient and precise summary measure of physical and functional well-being in clinical trials. We stress that we recommend this as an analytic strategy for purposes of enhancing measurement sensitivity, reducing data points and summarizing physical/functional outcomes. It is always recommended that the entire FACT be administered and evaluated, as the TOI will inadequately capture the psychosocial dimensions of QOL, dimensions which contribute significantly and uniquely to QOL.

Measuring Quality of Life

Selecting a Questionnaire. There are now many brief quality of life assessment instruments which are suitable for clinical trial and clinical database application. Many of them share some common features and content areas. Because of its ease of comprehension and flexibility (e.g., can be administered over the telephone), most questionnaires use an ordered category (Likert) item format. Most also cover at least two dimensions of quality of life: physical well-being and psychological well-being. Considerably more variability exists on the extent to which instruments cover two other important areas: social well-being and disease-specific problems/treatment concerns.

Disease-Specific and Generic Assessment. Generic and disease-specific instruments have competing advantages and disadvantages. Instruments which strike a balance between these two approaches have tended to become most popular in oncology. Disease-specific and treatment-specific questions are usually of benefit when added to a general measure of QOL. Together, they can provide comparability across diseases (types of cancer, in this context), and

sensitivity to specific issues or symptoms relevant to a given disease or treatment. For example, lymphedema is important to women who have had breast surgery, and should arguably be included in a breast cancer quality of life instrument. However, the question is irrelevant to other cancers. The availability of disease-specific questions which need not be asked of all patients is therefore an asset because it allows for the ideal combination of questionnaire length and content covered.

There is no single QOL questionnaire choice for every application. Often, a scale that is good in one setting is inappropriate in another. This leaves the investigator with the burden of scale selection. The frequent absence of a clearly superior questionnaire places the investigator in the uncomfortable position of worrying that important information may be untapped by an insensitive measure. This fear of missing what is most important can lead to a burdening of the patient with a wide array of measures given as a protection against the investigator's uncertainty. For many reasons (e.g., responder burden, statistical validity), investigators are advised to be judicious in their selection of measures. Typically, the best strategy is to pick the questionnaire which comes closest to asking the most clinically appropriate questions, confirm its reliability and validity, and supplement with a *few* additional questions targeted to the disease, condition, and/or treatment under study.

At times, investigators may wish to select specific items or sets of items from previously validated tests. Assuming one had the scale author's approval, it is important to confirm the reliability and validity of the extracted item set. That has been done by the Cancer and Leukemia Group B (CALGB), shortening the 65-item POMS to 11 items (23). It has also been used to shorten the Medical Outcomes Study (MOS) item set to 36 items (24), and subsequently to 20 items, and by the EORTC to shorten the Hospital Anxiety and Depression Scale from 14 to 8 items (25).

Multi-Method Approach. In QOL assessment, it is useful to assess function and change in more than one way. Multiple indicators of change in the same or similar endpoint can enhance reliability, which in turn can improve validity. If one is evaluating methods to improve self-care and general well-being in patients who have been discharged from the hospital, it is useful to obtain information from the patient, a family member, and a rating by an objective interviewer (not a core member of the investigative team). Each of these information sources provides different and potentially disparate data, so the omission of one or two of them could reduce the reliability of the data, thereby diminishing the validity of the claim that self-care and well-being were assessed.

A second reason for preference of multiple measures over single measures is breadth of coverage. It may be worthwhile to examine dependent variables that are peripheral to the central medical study, such as social support and well-being, because they may provide useful information when the more physical endpoints yield negative results. A good example of this is the assessment of quality of life in clinical trials that compare two or more different treatment regimens. Often, a large-scale clinical trial will contrast treatment regimens that possess different potentials for toxicity and medical risk. The advantage of adding quality of life measurement in such studies, besides the obvious advantages of random assignment to treatment arms, is that differences in QOL can be used as part of the evaluation of efficacy of treatment. This has been demonstrated in the treatment of lung carcinoma, for example, within the cooperative clinical trials setting (26), and in the treatment of breast cancer (27), as well as sarcoma (28).

The Use of an Interviewer. Failure to monitor data quality at the time it is collected is perhaps the most common reason for missing data and the resulting failure of the quality of life investigation. Use of an interview format would vritually eliminate this shortcoming. There are other adverse consequences of relying upon patient self-administration of QOL questionnaires (29–32). Missing items, misunderstood instructions, inconsistent responses, and language and reading barriers are some of the risks encountered when using patient self-administration. There is also evidence that patient self-administration is less sensitive than a probing interview in obtaining accurate QOL data (33). Therefore, it is advisable to supplement any questionnaire with a clarifying interview. At the very least, data received from patient self-report should be checked for completeness *before* acknowledging the end of the assessment.

Questionnaire Reliability and Validity

In general, a test cannot be considered valid until it has demonstrated satisfactory reliability. Reliability and validity are frequently expressed in the form of correlation coefficients, which can be squared to determine the proportion of shared variance between two measures (e.g., $r = .50$ indicates $(.5)^2 = .25$, or 25% shared variance).

Reliability. Synonyms for reliability are repeatability and consistency. Repeatability refers to the extent to which a questionnaire, applied two different times (test–retest), or in two different ways (alternate form and inter-rater), produces the same score. Consistency refers to the homogeneity of the items of a scale.

Test–retest reliability refers to the stability of a measure over time (i.e., the correlation between test scores at assessment 1 and those at assessment 2). The time interval between assessments should be relatively brief (e.g., 3–7 days), because it is hoped that true change in the patient's QOL will not have occurred during the interval. Any true change detected by the questionnaire will be interpreted as error and thereby incorrectly deflate the correlation coefficient. No QOL measure will ever achieve perfect reliability, expressed as a test–retest correlation coefficient of 1.0, but close approximations (e.g., correlations above .70) are important (34).

Internal consistency examines whether individual items within one test contribute consistently to the total score obtained. A measure's internal consistency is usually expressed in terms of Cronbach's coefficient alpha, because it is comprehensive and can be easily done with many computer statistical packages. If a test is made up of 20 items that purport to measure QOL, then responses to each of the 20 items should correlate with one another and the total score, if the scale is to have high internal consistency. However, since QOL is not a unidimensional construct, a high overall internal consistency coefficient might not be necessary to obtain valid measurement. In light of this, it may be acceptable to use scales with internal consistency (alpha) coefficients below the usual conventional value of .70. We have set .60 as an acceptable coefficient for group comparisons.

Inter-rater reliability refers to the association between ratings of two or more independent judges. Naturally, this is an issue only for observer-rated QOL scales. Pearson correlation coefficients above .70 are generally considered acceptable. When ratings are done on a noncontinuous (categorical) scale, the coefficient should be corrected for the likelihood of chance agreement between judges (Cohen's Kappa).

Most experts in assessment of patient function and symptoms agree that the patient's report is the gold standard (35–36). Providers typically underestimate patient symptoms and disability (36–38). In their excellent review, Sprangers and Aaronson (38) report that healthcare providers and significant others are equally inaccurate in terms of estimating patients' reports of QOL. Nevertheless, there are times when ratings from providers and family members are necessary due to patients' inability to respond for themselves (e.g., cognitively impaired patients and young children). Because of the difficulty in obtaining accurate proxy ratings of QOL, this important area of research remains extremely challenging, without a clear correct solution.

Reliability is not a fixed property of a measure, but rather a measure used with certain people under certain conditions. Because of this, reported reliability cannot be assumed to be generalizable and therefore should be reevaluated in later applications. This is not usually possible with test–retest reliability, because of the brief reassessment window. But internal consistency can (and should) easily be checked in any data set.

Validity. Validity refers to a scale's ability to measure what it purports to measure. A scale must be reliable in order to be valid, but it needn't be valid in order to be reliable. Validity has generally been subdivided into three types: content, criterion and construct.

Content validity is further divided into *face validity* (the degree to which the scale superficially appears to measure the concept in question) and true *content validity* (the degree to which the items accurately represent the range of attributes covered by the concept). With a multidimensional concept such as QOL, content coverage should cut across at least three broad domains (i.e., physical, psychological, and social) in order to be considered valid from the perspective of item content. The scale reviewer can evaluate this by examination of the development strategy for the scale as well as the actual content of the items themselves, which may or may not be separately reported as dimension scores.

Criterion-related validity is also subdivided into two types, *concurrent validity* and *predictive validity*. The distinction between the two is a function of when the criterion data are collected. Criterion data that are collected simultaneously with the scale data provide evidence of concurrent validity. Criterion data that are collected some time after the assessment (e.g., survival time; response to treatment; future answers to questionnaire) provide evidence for predictive validity.

Construct validity extends criterion-related validity into a broader arena in which the questionnaire is tested against a theoretical model, and adjusted according to results that can help refine the theory (39). There are many different approaches to construct validation. One is to examine a matrix of correlations between the scale in question and other measures of the same concept, measures of related concepts, measures of unrelated concepts, and different methods of data collection (e.g., self-report versus observer rating). This multitrait-multimethod matrix permits one to test for the presence of hypothesized high correlations (convergent validity) and hypothesized low correlations (discriminant validity).

Other contributions to construct validity can be derived from multidimensional scaling and factor analytic approaches which can confirm the presumed multidimensional nature of QOL. It might seem contradictory, but it may also help to conduct item analyses based upon a unidimensional scaling model for the overall measure as well as the component subtests, given the fact that QOL dimensions are intercorrelated.

The ability of an instrument to differentiate groups of patients expected to differ in QOL is also an important validation of its sensitivity. A "known groups technique" (40) can be employed in which patients with, for example, advanced disease are compared with those with limited disease to determine whether the QOL measure detects the differences known to exist between groups. The same could be done by comparing QOL scores of inpatients with outpatients, patients receiving adjuvant therapy with a clinically comparable group receiving no therapy, homebound patients with ambulatory patients, and so forth. Finally, the demonstration of an instrument's sensitivity or responsiveness to change over time, parallel to changes in clinical status, is an important feature of its validity (41).

Like reliability, validity should not be considered to be an absolutely achieved status of a measure. Validity data are cumulative and relative in that a given measure might be valid (i.e., sensitive) in one setting and not in another. Consider a measure which emphasiszes activities of daily living skills and physical sensations. Such a measure may be valid in the context of metastatic breast cancer, but insensitive in early stage disease, where virtually all patients will score at the top of the scale. The potential for sample-dependent ceiling effects such as this (and floor effects in the reverse case), suggest caution when selecting the best instrument for a given population.

EMERGING RESEARCH ISSUES IN QOL ASSESSMENT

Quality of life measurement in oncology has progressed to a point where challenges which have until now been elusive are being overcome by many groups of researchers. Some of these challenges include: (1) obtaining cross-culturally valid assessment; (2) standardizing scores across different instruments; (3) determining clinically significant differences; and (4) combining quantity with quality, especially in the analysis of clinical trials with missing (censored) data over time. These four challenges are somewhat hierarchical inasmuch as the later ones depend on successful accomplishment of the preceding ones.

Cross-Cultural Validity

Culture influences health behavior and perceptions by shaping explanations of sickness, social position and meaning of life. In any multicultural context, people with medical conditions possess attributes that create barriers to standard QOL evaluation, such as different language and low literacy. Most commonly-used QOL instruments were developed in the English language. EruoQol (42–44) and the Rotterdam Symptom Checklist (45–46) are two exceptions. There is increasing need for multilingual QOL instruments which are at least acceptable and preferably valid across cultures. Many groups have gone about translation and validation of questionnaires originally written in the English language. Translations are available and continuing for the CARES (19,47), EORTC-QLQ (3,11), FACT (13,48–49), FLIC (6,50) MOS 36-Item Short Form Health Survey (SF-36) (21–22,51), Sickness Impact Profile (SIP) (52–54), Nottingham Health Profile (NHP) (55–56), McMaster Health Index (57–58), and the Southwest Oncology Group (SWOG) questionnaire (59). Information about current status of translations for any questionnaire is best obtained from the scale developer, however, a good (1996) review can be found in Spilker (60).

Translation of an existing single-language document ideally involves an iterative forward–backward–forward sequencing and review of difficulties on an item-by-item basis. Decentering, or selective modification of the source document based upon problems encountered in this process, is ideal when possible. The final translated document should then be pretested for acceptability and content validity, and then implemented in multilingual clinical trials, where the derived data can then be tested statistically for cross-cultural equivalence or bias.

When an instrument developed in English with primarily Anglo-European patients is adapted to other languages or cultures, it is important to produce a culturally equivalent instrument. This is best understood not as an effort to make different groups of people look the same, but to ensure that different groups of people are evaluated without significant

bias. To expect any measure of QOL to be free of cultural influence is unrealistic. However, we must work toward constructing measures based on common cores of items which are not culture-biased, neither more attractive or repulsive to one group or another. Developing item equivalence across cultures does *not* imply that measures will show equivalent QOL levels across different groups of people. Indeed, it may be that levels of QOL differ across cultural or linguistic groups. This is an empirical question that should be addressed as such without making prior assumptions. "Equivalence" in this context refers to the absence of differential item functioning. In addition to language and culture is the issue of literacy. It is desirable to justify para-professional interview assessment of QOL as an equivalent (or at least equivalent with correction) form of QOL data collection. The demands of cost-efficiency in multicenter clinical trials precludes the administration of a QOL interview to all patients. Self-administered questionnaire is thus the method of choice. However, this carries the risk of excluding or at least confusing low-literacy patients who cannot complete the form. Because low-literacy patients *require* interviewer administration, and because most high-literacy patients in clinical trials will, for reasons of convenience and cost, be asked to self-administer, it is important to evaluate the comparability of self and interviewer administration. This requries a three (rather than two) facet psychometric analysis, in which not only patients and QOL items (the usual two facets) are specified and measured, but also a third facet in which interviewers themselves are also specified and measured for their influence on the response levels of the patients they assess.

Analyzing for statistical equivalence of measurement is a two-step process. The first step is at the measurement level, where the purpose is to determine whether a given rating scale works in the same manner with different groups of people. This step is crucial when one is interested in detecting systematic measurement bias and a particular rating scale is used with different groups of people (e.g., Hispanic vs Black non-Hispanic vs White non-Hispanic culture; Spanish vs English language; high vs low literacy) or administered in different ways (e.g., self vs interviewer). Then the extent to which each QOL item with which the rating scale is used performs similarly across different reference groups is of critical interest when determining which of the QOL items can be used to provide an unbiased basis for comparing groups. We need rating scale categories and QOL items that match across groups on both category step and item "difficulty." The measurement step of equivalence construction and testing provides that reassurance.

The second step after establishing and evaluating equivalence is the analysis level, in which we evaluate scale measure differences across reference groups and test conditions, to determine what real differences exist. We are seeking assurance that any detected group difference (as analyzed in the analysis step) is not based upon items which are systematically biased in favor of one of the groups.

Standardized Scores

Many current clinical trials have included QOL as a primary or secondary end point. Also, many clinicians would like to integrate knowledge about individual patients' QOL into their daily practice and clinical decision-making. While this increased interest has been encouraging, implementation of QOL measurement in clinical trials and in clinical practice has been hampered by the absence of a "gold standard" instrument. There are several QOL instruments which have been validated for use with cancer patients, each with its own set of questions and scoring rules. However, even the most ambitious of oncology clinicians can only be expected to master one of these many available instruments. As a result, we are creating a potiental "Tower of Babel" in which we lack a common language. An additional concern is that the use of raw scores is problematic because raw scores are not usually equal interval measures.

To correct these problems, one can test an algorithm which generates a common standard metric ("Q-score") for QOL (61–62). This score has the same meaning across instruments, as long as the instruments are shown to be equivalent. The procedure involves five steps: (1) simultaneously administer two quality of life questionnaires; (2) convert raw scores to logit measures; (3) assess the agreement (equivalence) of the logit measures; (4) obtain the functional relationship between the logit measures via orthogonal least squares regression; and (5) derive universal Q-scores from the logit measures. After this procedure, one can derive a Q-score conversion table ranging from 0 to 100 (mean = 50; SD = 10), so one can subsequently use either of the equated instruments and derive an equivalent Q-score which can be readily understood as having the same meaning to the clinician, regardless of which instrument was administered. This same five-step approach can be applied to any two instruments, including common subscales and higher order factors. Details of possible applications of equating methodology can be found elsewhere (62–63).

Determining Clinically Significant Differences

It is possible to achieve reliability and validity of measurement, and still be unable to interpret the data collected. Large clinical trials might easily obtain statistically significant differences between treatment arms; and these differences may reflect measurement of a true effect (i.e., the instrument was valid; it measured what it claimed to measure and detected a real difference). Still, because of the large sample size (and perhaps the small score difference), we might question the clinical meaning of the difference score (64). Is the difference clinically significant? What is the meaningful pattern of change that deserves clinical attention? There is little available guidance on how to address this problem. Some approaches that have been used include the statistical examination of effect size across different thresholds of quality of life (65), calibration of change/difference scores to an external criterion (3,14), direct longitudinal assessment of patients (41,66), determination of population weights or valuations (67–68), and utility/trade-off/willingness to pay interviewing (69). For seven-point Likert scaling of symptoms, Jaeschke et al. (66) have suggested a difference of approximately 0.5 units as a minimal clinically important difference. For other types of scaling (e.g., linear analogue), Jacobson and Truax (70) recommend a Reliable Change Index that estimates whether a change measured is real versus a consequence of imprecise measurement. Their suggestions are based upon data collected in such a way as to allow calibration of change scores to meaningful criteria.

All of these approaches offer some data about meaningful differences in quality of life scores within and across patients over time. It is this area of clinical significance which will ultimately determine whether people pay close attention to change in QOL over time and across treatment options. Considerably more research effort must be expended in this area before we have clear and convincing data about clinical significance and value attached to measured change.

Combining Quantity with Quality

In the evaluation of cancer clinical trials, this is the final common pathway of all of the above work. Life quantity (survival) analyses have emphasized the time-to-event approach, whereas in the past quality of life analyses have relied upon multivariate analysis of various models. The latter carry insurmountable hurdles with regard to informative censoring and other missing data problems; the former is problematic because it is unclear how to define an "event" in quality of life data. This is a problem in part because of the difficulty in knowing what is a significant difference. Furthermore, even if a significant difference score were known, a time-to-event analysis does not readily allow cases back into the analysis, which would be desirable because patients get better and worse over time.

Missing Data. Missing data poses the greatest challenge to the statistician attempting to make sense of a QOL data set from a clinical trial or clinical program database. The first issue to be addressed in an analysis is whether or not the data are missing at random. Data which are missing at random (both "missing completely at random" or "missing at random") can be reasonably well-imputed and replaced with estimation models that draw from available data. Data not missing at random cannot be so easily imputed; in fact, there are no good models for doing so. Patient disability and death, common reasons for missingness over time in a data set, are not random events with regard to the QOL data set. Therefore, unfortunately, non-randomly missing data will always be an analytic challenge. Random reasons for missing data (e.g., staff forgetting) are easier to handle. Of course, such reasons are best avoided in the first place. Since understanding missing data mechanisms is so important to later analyses, it is recommended that any data collection plan (e.g., in a clinical trial) include a reporting of why patients did not complete specific questions or entire questionnaires. The more detailed information is available, the more able will the investigator and statistician be to determine whether missing data encountered later are random or non-random. For this reason, planning of the reporting of reasons for missing data is best done in consultation with the statistician who will be doing the analysis.

Despite the problems associated with imputing missing values, imputation of missing data is superior to dropping cases with missing data and analyzing only those with all available data. This leads to greatly distorted conclusions, particularly in data sets which have patient drop off over time due to illness, death, or even reasons not clearly random or non-random (e.g., lost to follow up). Therefore, having imputed values for missing data, one must now conduct a QOL analysis where there is no clearly correct approach. Slope analysis is possible when there is a consistent (linear) direction of change and there are at least two assessments (71). Area under the curve analysis is another approach which has intuitive appeal in that it is conceptually similar to quality-adjusted time, summing areas under the sequence of trapezoids laid out over time (72). Mixed models (repeated measures analysis of

variance; growth curve models) (73) also have promise because they can use all available data, including incomplete cases. Joint mixed effects/survival models (74) have appeal because they offer the opportunity to jointly estimate survival and QOL.

Utilities, QALYs, and Q-TWIST. Related to the analysis problem is the recognition of the need to combine health status data with utility data in some way. Health status measurement approaches have the strength of descriptive accuracy and measurement sensitivity; utility approaches have the strength of a single index weight for a given period of time which is anchored to a 0 (death) to 1.0 (perfect health) scale tied to economic (utility) theory. Perhaps the best of these complementary approaches can be combined into a unified approach which will allow for simple, meaningful, and sensitive evaluation of quality of life in a clinical trial.

A technique first described by Bush and colleagues in 1973 (75), adjusts survival time downward to a degree proportional to the amount of disability or toxicity endured. Variations on this theme have been called "quality-adjusted life-years," or QALYs (76), "well-years" (77), and, most recently in the cancer-specific context, "quality-adjusted time without symptoms or toxicity," or Q-TWIST (78–79). These approaches are most useful in health policy decision-making, or where the effectivenss of two or more competing treatments or programs must be evaluated for relative efficacy. The utility approach to health status measurement evolved from a tradition of cost–benefit analysis, into cost-effectiveness approaches and, most recently, cost–utility approaches (80). The cost–utility approach extends the cost-effectiveness approach conceptually by evaluating the QOL benefit produced by the clinical effects of a treatment, thereby including the (presumed) patient's perspective. To be used this way, QOL must be measured as a utility since, by definition, utilities can be multiplied by time to produce an adjusted time which is less than or equal to actual survival time.

Two general cost–utility methods are the standard gamble approach and the time-trade-off approach (81). In the standard gamble approach, people are asked to choose between their current state of health and a "gamble" in which they have various probabilities for death or perfect health (cure). The time-trade-off method involves asking people how much time they would be willing to give up in order to live out their remaining life expectancy in perfect health. All utility approaches have in common the use of a 0–1 scale in which 0 = death and 1 = perfect health. In practice, most cost–utility analyses employ expert estimates of utility weights, or in some cases, weights provided by healthy members of the general public. It is often assumed that these weights are reasonable approximations of patient preferences. However, several studies have demonstrated that utilities obtained from patients are generally higher than those provided by physicians, which are, in turn, higher than utilities for the same health states obtained from healthy individuals (82). There are practical impediments to collection of utilities directly from patients, including the complexity of the concepts involved and the requirement for an interviewer-administered questionnaire (often unfeasible in the cooperative group setting). In addition, utility assessments provide little information on important disease- and treatment-specific problems and are probably less sensitive to changes in health status over time than psychometric data (83–84). Finally, the few studies that have been done involving simultaneous measurement of utilities and health status have found them at best to be moderately correlated, with measures of mood and depression correlating more highly than other measures with utilities (85).

A modified utility approach has been developed to evaluate the effectiveness of adjuvant therapy (78–79). This approach, the Quality-adjusted Time Without Symptoms and Toxicity (Q-TWIST), discounts survival time spent with toxicity or symptoms relative to disease-free survival off therapy. Thresholds for decision making were determined by modeling actual survival data, and judgments were made by the investigators regarding where patient preferences were likely to fall relative to these threshold values. There is no theoretical reasons that actual patient preference data could not be used in the Q-TWIST analyses or other studies of quality-adjusted survival. If the relationship between psychometric data and utilities can be established, it will become possible to collect psychometric data and base utility estimates on the reports of patients rather than the best guesses of others. This is a very significant area for further research, with many groups of assessment teams working on it.

SUMMARY AND CONCLUSION

Quality of life is a multidimensional, subjective, and fluid endpoint, so its measurement must be comprehensive, include the patient's perspective, and be sensitive to change over time. Given the challenges and burdens of most cancer treatment systems, QOL measurement must also be brief. There is no "gold standard" or "best" quality of life measure. It is important to be aware of the strengths and weaknesses of available questionnaires when setting out to study quality of life. While knowledge of the reliability of existing measures is necessary, it is not sufficient in planning study implementation. Other issues, like patient characteristics, cross-cultural validity, translation quality, standardized scores, and ultimate analytic plan must be considered early in the process.

Following are some concluding recommendations:

1. Avoid using the term quality of life when measuring only one dimension of function or well-being (e.g., pain, mood, vocational functioning, performance status, nausea). Measurement should usually include at least three of the generally accepted components of QOL.

2. Use caution when defining the study population and questions. The QOL questionnaire selected should derive from them, rather than vice versa.

3. Select the QOL questionnaire according to the characteristics of the population to be studied. The scale should be sensitive enough to detect subtle changes if people will be followed during treatment.

4. Supplement an existing, validated scale with relevant and specific items tapping areas not included in the selected scale. This will provide both standardized assessment for comparison across disease sites and treatments, and specific information about problems unique to the individual patient group under study. When analyzing these results, keep separate the selected scale and the additional items, thereby retaining the psychometric integrity of the standardized test.

5. When feasible, combine self-report with observer rating, since they often do not match, and provide complementary information.

6. Consider the burden on the patient and the study personnel. For most multicenter research it is advisable to use questionnaires that require less than 15 minutes on average to complete. Select the number of repeat assessments judiciously, and with attention to the treatment procedures within the institution.

7. Use QOL assessment as an adjunct to, rather than a replacement for, clinical decision-making. This will avoid the risk of QOL data being used against the interests of good medical treatment.

8. Attempt to integrate QOL data with other related data, such as survival time and cost. This effort will test the limits of our knowledge and in so doing challenge us to move this exciting field forward.

REFERENCES

1. Campbell A, Converse PE, Rodgers WL. *The Quality of American Life*. New York: Sage; 1976: 471.
2. Aaronson NK. Quality of life: What is it? How should it be measured. *Oncology*. 1988; 2(5):69–74.
3. Aaronson NK, Ahmedzai S, Bergman B, et al. The European Organization for the Research and Treatment of Cancer QLQ-C30: a quality of life instrument for use in international clinical trials in oncology. *J Nat Cancer Instit*. 1993; 85(5):365–376.
4. Cella DF, Cherin EA. Quality of life during and after cancer treatment. *Compr Ther*. 1988; 4(5):69–75.
5. Stewart AL, Ware JE, Brook RH. Advances in the measurement of functional status: construction of aggregate indexes. *Med Care*. 1981; 19:473–488.
6. Schipper H, Clinch J, McMurray A, et al. Measuring the quality of life of cancer patients. The Functional Living Index-Cancer: development and validation. *J Clin Oncol*. 1984; 2:472–483.
7. Cella DF. Measuring quality of life in palliative care. *Sem Oncol*. 1995; 22(2)Suppl 3:73–81.
8. Cella DF, Bonomi AE. Measuring quality of life: 1995 update. *Oncology 1995; 9*(Suppl 11):47–60.
9. Kornblith AB, Holland JC. *Handbook of Measures of Psychological, Social and Physical Function in Cancer*, Vol 1: *Quality of Life*. New York: Memorial Sloan-Kettering Cancer Center; 1994.
10. deHaes JCJM, Raatgever JW, van der Burg MEL, et al. Evaluation of the quality of life of patients with advanced ovarian cancer treated with combination chemotherapy. In: Aaronson NK, Beckman J, eds. *The Quality of Life of Cancer Patients*. New York: Raven Press; 1987.
11. Bergman B, Sullivan M, Sorenson S. Quality of life during chemotherapy for small cell lung cancer II. A longitudinal study of the EORTC core quality of life questionnaire and comparison with the Sickness Impact Profile. *Acta Oncol*. 1992; 31:19–28.
12. Osoba D, Zee B, Pater J, et al. Psychometric properties and responsiveness of the EORTC quality of life questionnaire (QLQ-30) in patients with breast, ovarian and lung cancer. *Qual Life*. 1994; 3:353–364.
13. Wisloff F, Eika S, Hippe E, et al. Measurement of health-related quality of life in multiple myeloma. *Br J Haematol*. 1996; 92:604–613.
14. Cella DF, Tulsky DS, Gray G, et al. The Functional Assessment of Cancer Therapy (FACT) Scale: development and validation of the general version. *J Clin Oncol*. 1993; 11(3):570–579.
15. Cella DF, Bonomi AE, Lloyd S, et al. Reliability and validity of the Functional Assessment of Cancer Therapy-Lung (FACT-L) quality of life instrument. *Lung Cancer*. 1995; 12:199–220.
16. Brady MJ, Cella DF, Mo F, et al. Reliability and validity of the Functional Assessment of Cancer Therapy-Breast (FACT-B) quality of life instrument. *J Clin Oncol*, in press.
17. Cella DF, Tross S. Psychological adjustment to survival from Hodgkin's disease. *J Consult Clin Psychol*. 1986; 54:616–622.
18. Andyrkowski MA, Brady MJ, Hunt JW. Positive psychosocial adjustment in potential bone marrow transplant recipients: cancer as a psychosocial transition. *Psycho-Oncology*. 1993; 2:261–276.
19. Ganz P, Coscarelli A. Quality of life after breast cancer: a decade of research. In Dimsdale JE, Baum A, eds. *Quality of Life in Behavioural Medicine Research*. New Jersey: Lawrence Erlbaum; 1995.
20. Ganz P, Coscarelli Schag CA, Kahn B, et al. Describing the health-related quality of life impact of HIV infection: Findings from a study using the HIV Overview of Problems-Evaluation Systems (HOPES). *Qual Life*. 1993; 2:109–119.
21. McHorney CA, Ware JE, Raczek AE. The MOS 36-item short-form health survey (SF-36): II. Psychometric and clinical test of validity in measuring physical and mental health constructs. *Med Care*. 1993; 31:247–263.
22. Ware JE, Kosinski MA, Bayliss MS, et al. Comparison of methods for scoring and statistical analysis of SF-36 health profile and summary measures: Summary of results from the medical outcomes study. *Med Care*. 1995; 33:AS264–AS279.
23. Cella DF, Jacobsen PB, Orva EJ, et al. A brief POMS measure of distress for cancer patients. *J Chronic Dis*. 1987; 40(10):939–942.
24. Stewart AL, Hays RD, Ware JE. The MOS short-form General Health Survey: reliability and validity in a patient population. *Med Care*. 1988; 26:724–735.
25. Aaronson NK, Bullinger M, Ahmedzai S. A modular approach to quality-of-life assessment in cancer clinical trials. *Recent Results in Cancer Research*. Berlin: Springer-Verlag; 1988: 111:231–249.
26. Silberfarb PM, Holland JCB, Anbar D, et al. Psychological response of patients receiving two drug regimens for lung carcinoma. *Am J Psychiatry*. 1983; 140:110–111.
27. Coates A, Gebski V, Bishop JF, et al. Improving the quality of life during chemotherapy for advanced breast cancer. *N Engl J Med*. 1987; 317:1490–1495.
28. Sugarbaker PH, Barofsky I, Rosenberg SA, et al. Quality of life assessment of patients in extremity sarcoma trials. *Surgery*. 1982; 91:17–23.
29. Yates JW, Edwards B. Practical concerns and pitfalls in measurement methodology. *Cancer*. 1984; 53(suppl 10):2376–2379.
30. Ganz PA, Haskell CA, Figlin RA, et al. Estimating the quality of life in a clinical trial of patients with metastatic lung cancer using the Karnofsky Performance Status and the Functional Living Index-Cancer. *Cancer*. 1988; 61:849–856.
31. Schipper H, Levitt M. Measuring quality of life: risks and benefits. *Cancer Treat Rep*. 1985; 69:1115–1123.
32. van Dam FSAM, Aaronson NK. Practical problems in conducting cancer-related psychosocial research. In: Aarsonson NK, Beckmann J, eds. *The Quality of Life of Cancer Patients*. New York: Raven Press; 1987.
33. Anderson JP, Bush JW, Berry CC. Classifying function for health outcome and quality of life evaluation: self-versus interviewer modes. *Med Care*. 1986; 24(5):454–469.
34. Nunnally JC. *Psychometric Theory*. New York: McGraw-Hill; 1967.
35. Moinpour CM, Savage M, Hayden KA, et al. Quality of life assessment in cancer clinical trials. In: Dimsdale JE, Baum A, eds. *Quality of Life in Behavioural Medicine Research*. New Jersey: Lawrence Erlbaum; 1995.

36. Slevin ML, Plant H, Lynch D, et al. Who should measure quality of life, the doctor or the patient? *Br J Cancer.* 1988; 57:109–112.

37. da Silva FC. Quality of life in prostatic carcinoma. *Eur Urol.* 1993; 24(suppl 2):113–117.

38. Sprangers MAG, Aaronson NK. The role of healthcare provders and significant others in evaluating the quality of life of patients with chronis disease: A review. *J Clin Epidemiol.* 1992; 45:743–760.

39. Campbell DT, Fiske DW. Convergent and discriminant validation by the multitrait-multimethod matrix. *Psychol Bull.* 1959; 56:85–105.

40. Bohrnstedt GW. Measurement. In: Rossi PH, Wright JD, Anderson AB, eds. *Handbook of Survey Research.* New York: Academic Press; 1983.

41. Guyatt G, Walter S, Norman G. Measuring change over time: assessing the usefulness of evaluative instruments. *J Chronic Dis.* 1987; 40:171.

42. The EuroQol Group: EuroQol—a new facility for the measurement of health-related quality of life. *Health Policy.* 1990; 16:199–208.

43. Brooks R, Jendteg S. Lindgren B, et al. EuroQol: Health-related quality of life measurement. Results from the Swedish questionnaire exercise. *Health Policy.* 1991; 18:37–48.

44. Nord E. EuroQol: health-related quality of life measurement. Valuations of health states by the general public in Norway. *Health Policy.* 1991; 18:25–36.

45. de Haes JCJM, van Knippenberg FCE, Neijt JP. Measuring psychological and physical distress in cancer patients: structure and application of the Rotterdam Symptom Checklist. *Br J Cancer.* 1990; 62:1034–1038.

46. Watson M, Law M, Maguire GP, et al. Further development of a quality of life measure for cancer patients: The Rotterdam Symptom Checklist (revised). *Psycho-Oncology.* 1992; 1:35–44.

47. Schag CA, Ganz PA, Heinrich RL. Cancer Rehabilitation Evaluation System-Short Form (CARES-SF): A cancer specific rehabilitation and quality of life instrument. *Cancer.* 1991; 68(6):1406–1413.

48. Cella DF, Bonomi AE. The Functional Assessment of Cancer Therapy (FACT) and Functional Assessment of HIV Infection (FAHI) quality of life measurement systems. In: Spilker B, ed. *Quality of Life and Pharmacoeconomics in Clinical Trials.* New York: Raven Press; 1996: 203–214.

49. Bonomi AE, Cella DF, Bjordal K, et al. Multilingual tranlsation of the Functional Assessment of Cancer Therapy (FACT) quality of life measurement system. *Qual Life Res.* 1996; 5:1–12.

50. Clinch J. The Functional Living Index-Cancer: ten years later. In: Spilker B, ed. *Quality of Life and Pharmacoeconomics in Clinical Trials.* New York: Raven Press; 1996: 215–226.

51. McHorney CA, Ware JE, Lu JFR, Sherbourne CD. The MOS 36-Item Short Form Health Survey (SF-36): III. Tests of data quality, scaling assumptions and reliability across diverse patient groups. *Med Care.* 1994; 32(1): 40–66.

52. Bergner M, Bobbit RA, Carter WB, et al. The Sickness Impact Profile: Development and final revision of a health status measure. *Med Care.* 1981; 19:787–806.

53. De Bruin AF, De Witte LP, Diederiks JP. Sickness impact profile: The state of the art of a generic functional status measure. *Soc Sci Med.* 1992; 8:1003–1014.

54. Chwalow AJ, Lurie A, Bean K, et al. A French version of the Sickness Impact Profile (SIP): Stages in the cross validation of a generic quality of life scale. *Fundamental Clin Pharmacol.* 1992; 6:319–326.

55. Hunt S, McKenna SP, McEwan J, et al. The Nottingham Health Profile: Subjective health status and medical consultations. *Soc Sci Med.* 1981; 15A:221–229.

56. Wiklund I. The Nottingham Health Profile—A measure of health-related quality of life. *Scand J Primary Health Care.* 1990; (suppl 1):15–18.

57. Chambers LW, Macdonald LA, Tugwell P, et al. The McMaster Health Index Questionnaire as a measure of quality of life for patients with rheumatoid disease. *J Rheumatol.* 1982; 9:780–784.

58. Chambers LW. The McMaster Health Index Questionnaire: An update. In: Walker SR, Rosser RM, eds. *Quality of Life Assessment: Key Issues in the 1990s.* London: Kluwer Academic Publishers' 1993: 131–149.

59. Moinpour CM. Quality of life assessment in Southwest Oncology Group clinical trials: Translating and validating a Spnaish questionnaire. In: Orley J, Kuyken W, eds. *Quality of Life Assessment: International Perspectives.* Berlin: Springer-Verlag; 1994: 83–97.

60. Spilker B, ed. *Quality of Life and Pharamcoeconomics in Clinical Trials,* 2nd ed. Philadelphia: Lippincott-Raven; 1996.

61. Cella DF, Gonin R, Lloyd S. The Q-Score: Scaling the Tower of Babel in quality of life (QL) measurement. *Proc ASCO.* 1995; 14:305 (Abstract 886).

62. Gonin R, Lloyd S, Cella DF. Establishing equivalence between scaled measures of quality of life. *Qual Life Res.* 1996; 5:20–26.

63. Cella DF, Lloyd SR, Wright BD. Cross-cultural instrument equating: Current research and future directions. In Spilker B, ed. *Quality of Life and Pharmacoeconomics in Clinical Trials.* New York: Raven Press; 1996: 707–715.

64. Braitman L. Statistical, clinical and experimental evidence in randomized controlled trials. *Ann Intern Med.* 1983; 98(3):407–408.

65. Kraemer H. Reporting the size of effects in research studies to facilitate assessments of practical or clinical significance. *Psychoneuroendocrinology.* 1992; 10:407–415.

66. Jaeschke R, Singer J, Guyatt GH. Measurement of health status: Ascertaining the minimal clinically important difference. *Controlled Clinical Trials.* 1989; 10:407–415.

67. Torrance G. Measurement of health state utilities for economic appraisal. *J Health Econ.* 1986; 5:1–30.

68. Torrance G, Feeny D. Utilities and quality-adjusted life years. *Int J Tech Assessment Health Care.* 1989; 5: 559–575.

69. Singer P, Tasch E, Stocking C, et al. Sex or survival: Trade-offs between quality and quantity of life. *J Clin Oncol.* 1991; 9(2):328–334.

70. Jacobson NS, Truax P. Clinical significance: A statistical approach to defining meaningful change in psychotherapy research. *J Consult Clin Psychol.* 1991; 59:12–19.

71. Korn EL, O'Fallon J (for the Statistics Working Group). Statistical considerations. In: Nayfield SG, Hailey BJ, McCabe M, eds. *Quality of Life Assessment in Cancer Clinical Trials: Report of the Workshop on Quality of*

Life Research in Cancer Clinical Trials. National Cancer Institute, US Department of Health and Human Services; 1990.

72. Cox DR, Fitzpatrick R, Fletcher AI, et al. Quality of life assessment: Can we keep it simple? (with discussion). *J Royal Stat Soc.* 1992; 155:353–393.

73. Diggle P. Liange K-Y, Zeger SL. *Analysis of Longitudinal Data.* Oxford: Clarendon Press; 1993.

74. Schluchter MD. Methods for the analysis of informatively censored longitudinal data. *Stat Med.* 1992; 11:1861–1870.

75. Bush JW, Chen M, Patrick DL. Cost-effectiveness using a health status index: Analysis of the New York State PKU screening program. In: Berg R, ed. *Health Status Index.* Chicago: Hospital Research and Educational Trust; 1973: 172–208.

76. Weinstein MC. Cost-effective priorities for cancer prevention. *Science.* 1983; 221(4605):17–23.

77. Kaplan RM, Bush JW. Health-related quality of life measurement for evaluation research and policy analysis. *Health Psychol.* 1982; 1:61–80.

78. Gelber RD, Goldhirsch A. A new end-point for the assessment of adjuvant therapy in postmenopausal women with operable breast cancer. *J Clin Oncol.* 1986; 4:1772–1779.

79. Gelber RD, Goldhirsch A, Cavalli F. Quality-of-life-adjusted evaluation of adjuvant therapies for operable breast cancer. *Ann Intern Med.* 1991; 114:621–628.

80. Drummond MF, Stoddart GL, Torrance GW. *Method for Economic Evaluation of Health Care Programmes.* Oxford: Oxford University Press; 1987.

81. Torrance GW. Measurement of health state utilities for economic appraisal: A review article. *J Health Econ.* 1986; 5:1–30.

82. Boyd NF, Sutherland HJ, Heasman KZ, et al. Whose utilities for decision analysis? *Medical Decision Making.* 1990; 10:58–67.

83. Tsevat J, Goldman L, Soukup JR, Lee TH. Stability of utilities in survivors of myocardial infarction. *Medical Decision Making.* 1990; 10:323.

84. Canadian Erythropoietin Study Group. Association between recombinant human erythropoietin and quality of life and exercise capacity of patients receiving hemodialysis. *Br Med J.* 1990; 300:573–578.

85. Tsevat J, Cook EF, Soukop JR, et al. Utilities of the seriously ill (abstract). *Clin Res.* 1991; 39:589A.

100

Pain and Physical Symptom Assessments

JANE INGHAM AND RUSSELL K. PORTENOY

The measurement of physical symptoms, including the quantification of specific symptom characteristics and global symptom distress, can guide therapy in the clinical setting and is essential in research. Surveys of symptom epidemiology, quality of life studies, and clinical trials of symptomatic therapies all require the ability to measure these inherently subjective phenomena in a valid and reliable manner. The process can be illuminated by reviewing the broader principles of symptom assessment, the measurement instruments for several common symptoms, and the application of symptom measures to the clinical setting.

PRINCIPLES OF SYMPTOM ASSESSMENT AND MEASUREMENT

Symptoms are, by definition, subjective perceptions (1) and must be distinguished from objective indicators of pathology, or signs, and from diagnoses. Diseases cause a spectrum of symptoms, each of which may or may not clarify a disease process or diagnosis. A comprehensive symptom assessment begins with the recognition that patient perception may or may not correspond with any overt physical pathology, and may or may not provide the specificity needed for diagnosis.

Both symptom assessment and measurement are complicated by the range of words used to describe related subjective phenomena. The words used to label a symptom may have many meanings for patients and a wide range of implications in the medical setting. This problem is well illustrated by the complexity of the language used to report "fatigue," "confusion," "breathlessness," and "pain." Fatigue may be used by some patients to describe a lack of vitality. Others apply the term to feelings of apathy or difficulty concentrating, or to sleepiness or muscle weakness. Confusion may refer to impaired concentration, disorganized thinking, forgetfulness, or even hallucinations.

"Breathlessness" may or may not be reported when other words used to denote dyspnea are endorsed (2). The nomenclature applied to pain is so voluminous that an international effort was undertaken to develop a formal taxonomy (3).

This inconsistent use of language may underlie the variability in the prevalence of identical symptoms when assessed by different instruments (Table 100.1) (4–7) and justifies the need for formal validation of symptom assessment instruments. It further underscores two fundamental characteristics of these instruments, subjectivity and multidimensionality.

Subjectivity

Self-report must be the primary source of information for subjective phenomena, including symptoms (8–14). Numerous studies have demonstrated that the accuracy of a clinician's assessment cannot be assumed. In a study of patient–physician concordance in the assessment of patients' pain, for example, correlations were especially poor in the subgroup with the most severe pain (8). This finding suggests that inferences about subjective states may be most uncertain at a level of patient distress that is most clinically relevant. Another study revealed that retrospective assessments by bereaved family members did not accurately depict patient symptoms at the end of life (10).

Although objective data can provide useful complementary information, symptom assessment and measurement should incorporate patient ratings, if possible. The measurement of oxygen saturation can illuminate the status of the dyspneic patient, for example, but cannot be used to determine the severity or distress of dyspnea. Nausea measurement may be supplemented by assessment of the frequency of emesis, and pain measurement may be clarified by functional assessment, but the objective data do not substitute for patients' ratings of their own experiences.

TABLE 100.1. *Varying Prevalence of Selected Symptoms in 200 Cancer Patients*

Symptom	ESAS (%)	FACT (%)	MSAS (%)
Pain	55.4	47.7	46.0
Nausea	26.6	22.4	21.5
Sadness	–	41.3	27.5
Nervous feeling	–	46.0	35.5

ESAS = Edmonton Symptom Assessment System
FACT = Functional Assessment of Cancer Therapy
MSAS = Memorial Symptom Assessment Scale
Source: Adapted from Table 1 in Ingham J, Portenoy RK. The measurement of pain and other symptoms. In: Doyle D, Hanks G, Macdonald N, eds. *Oxford Textbook of Palliative Medicine*, 2nd ed. Oxford: Oxford University Press, in press.

In some populations, such as demented or obtunded patients or pre-verbal children, it may not be possible to obtain self-reports. In this setting, the use of proxy data from family members or staff can be informative (15–20), but must be interpreted cautiously. In reporting such data, investigators should always acknowledge the source of information and describe the self-report and proxy data separately, if both are acquired (21).

Multidimensionality

Historically, symptom surveys have assessed prevalence rates or prevalence combined with a single descriptor, usually severity. Although this type of assessment can be sufficient in some cases, it is limited in scope. Symptoms are multidimensional phenomena and can be evaluated in terms of a broad range of descriptive information. Symptoms can be described in terms of varied characteristics, impact on different domains of function, or overall impact (22–25) (Table 100.2).

Symptom Characteristics. Although the utility of multidimensional assessment may be self-evident in the clinical setting, where history taking routinely inquires about symptom frequency, severity and distress, this approach has not been extensively applied in the research setting. Studies that have assessed different dimensions confirm the variability of these symptom descriptors (7,22,24,26). For example, a study of 215 patients with prostate, colon, breast, or ovarian cancer identified large variations in the frequency, severity, and distress associated with 32 physical and psychological symptoms (22). Although some of the symptoms were reported to be frequent or severe, not all of these were described as highly bothersome or distressing. These data confirm that the mere report of a symptom does not imply that it is burdensome or in need of treatment.

Multidimensional measurement of symptoms may provide the most information about the interactions between symptoms and overall quality of life (QOL). In one study of cancer patients, for example, measurement of symptoms using a distress scale combined with either a severity or frequency scale gave more information about quality of life than measurement of any single dimension; measurement of distress was the most informative dimension (7). These data suggest that distress, or, if possible, distress and another dimension, should be assessed if the goal of the evaluation is to clarify the interaction between symptoms and QOL.

Symptom Impact. In the setting of medical disease, the presence of multiple symptoms and other adverse influences on QOL can complicate efforts to define the impact of a particular symptom. For example, pain is often associated with depression, anxiety, social isolation, and impaired physical performance. Although these problems are often construed to be secondary, and can be assessed in such terms (e.g., as assessed by the pain interference items of the Brief Pain Inventory (27), correlations do not establish causation. The possibility that pain may have been worsened by a primary mood disturbance, or by social dysfunction caused primarily by another problem, cannot be dismissed. Symptom impact must be interpreted cautiously from correlational data.

Furthermore, the relationships between symptoms and the putative impact of these symptoms may not be intuitive, and are likely to be subject to large indi-

TABLE 100.2 *Multidimensional Characteristics of Symptoms*

Symptom characteristics	frequency
	severity
	distress
	desire for treatment
Symptom impact	other physical and psychological symptoms
	physical or psychosocial function
	family, social, financial, spiritual, and existential resources and concerns.
Related global constructs	global symptom distress
	health-related quality of life

Source: Adapted from Table 2 in Ingham J, Portenoy RK. The measurement of pain and other symptoms. In: Doyle D, Hanks G, Macdonald N, eds. *Oxford Textbook of Palliative Medicine*, 2nd ed. Oxford: Oxford University Press, in press.

vidual variation. Even if causation can be clarified, there is no means to anticipate the amount of symptom change that would be required to produce changes in any other functional sphere. Nonetheless, recent studies using the Brief Pain Inventory (BPI), which demonstrate a disproportionate impairment in function above a pain severity rating of 4 on a 10-point scale (28,29), suggest that simple guidelines for symptom interpretation may be possible if sufficient data can be collected. Such guidelines could be useful in identifying target ranges for the assessment of new pain therapies.

Global Constructs. Several studies have explored the utility of global symptom distress as a construct that denotes overall symptom burden in the cancer population (7,25,30). Unidimensional assessment of a small group of highly prevalent physical and psychological symptoms can validly indicate global symptom distress. The rating of global symptom distress correlates with both impairment in quality of life and declining performance status (7,22). Although multidimensional assessment probably has a greater potential for clarifying the impact of symptoms on QOL (7), the use of a brief measure, requiring limited evaluation time, can provide clinically relevant information with minimal effort.

Quality of life (QOL) is another multidimensional construct associated with symptom distress. QOL reflects the broad influence of many positive and nega-tive factors on perceived well-being (21,31–38). Physical and psychological symptoms may contribute to QOL, but the extent and character of this contribution are highly variable and often change over time. This complexity is particularly apparent in the setting of advanced medical disease, which is characterized by numerous physical and psychological symptoms (22,23,39–48) and extraordinary diversity in other factors—physical, emotional, social, spiritual, and others—that similarly contribute to overall QOL. Each of the latter concerns has the potential to independently influence QOL, and to augment or lessen the distress associated with specific symptoms. Assessment of these complex interactions may be facilitated by the use of valid multidimensional measures of QOL.

CLINICAL APPLICATIONS OF SYMPTOM MEASUREMENT

Although detailed symptom measurement could potentially be useful in the clinical setting (8,14,49–52), symptom measurement at the bedside historically has neglected formal measurement techniques. Rather, the emphasis has been on comprehensive symptom assessment that incorporates informal measurement of selected components. This approach to bedside evaluation is described in textbooks and reviews, and requires a detailed evaluation of symptom characteristics, pathogenesis, and impact (53–56) (Table 100.3).

TABLE 100.3. *Clinical Symptom Assessment*

MEDICAL HISTORY	PSYCHOSOCIAL ISSUES	CURRENT MEDICATIONS
Diagnosis	Family history	
Chronology	Social resources	
Therapies	Impact of disease and symptoms	
Patient expectations		
ASSESSMENT	GLOBAL SYMPTOM IMPACT	PATHOPHYSIOLOGY
Review of systems	Global symptom distress	For each symptom:
For each symptom:	• impact of overall symptom distress on quality of life	Inferred pathophysiology
• chronology and frequency		Relationship to other symptoms
• severity	Impact of symptoms on quality of life:	• differing pathophysiologies
• degree of distress	• physical condition	• same pathophysiology
• impact on function	• psychological status	• causal pathology induced by another symptom
• other clinical characteristics	• social interactions	• causal factor is treatment directed at another symptom
• prior treatment modalities	Factors that modulate global symptom distress, e.g., coping strategies and family supports	
• other factors that alleviate or modulate distress associated with specific symptoms, e.g., coping strategies and supports		
PHYSICAL EXAMINATION	ASSESS AVAILABLE LABORATORY AND IMAGING DATA	

Source: Adapted from Tables 1 and 2 in Ingham JM, Portenoy RK. Symptom assessment. In: Cherny N, Foley KM, eds. *Hematology/ Oncology Clinics of North America. Pain and Palliative Care.* Philadelphia: WB Saunders Company; 1996: 21–39.

Instruments for structured history taking are available, but are rarely used (57–59).

Although systematic symptom measurement is seldom used in the assessment of an individual patient, it may have promise as a technique to increase awareness of a clinical problem and implement quality improvement strategies. For example, systematic pain measurement may enhance caregiver understanding of pain status in hospitalized patients (60). In a cancer center, regular pain measurement using a modified bedside chart (Fig. 100–1) has been incorporated into a continuous quality improvement strategy; preliminary data suggest that nurse's knowledge and attitudes about pain, and patient satisfaction with pain management, have improved subsequently (51,61). Recent

guidelines from the Agency for Health Care Policy and Research (14) and the American Pain Society (50) endorse this regular use of pain rating scales to assess pain severity and relief in all patients who commence or change treatments.

The experience with pain measurement in the clinical setting could be expanded to the measurement of other symptoms. The simplest approach would be the use of symptom checklists, which indicate prevalence, or prevalence and a descriptor such as intensity. Unfortunately, these face-valid instruments have notable limitations, which include the lack of adequate validation and the inability to address more than one symptom dimension (5,62–65). Newer validated measures may supersede these simple checklists (see below)

PAIN MANAGEMENT PROGRAM
Charting Pain Intensity and Relief Measures

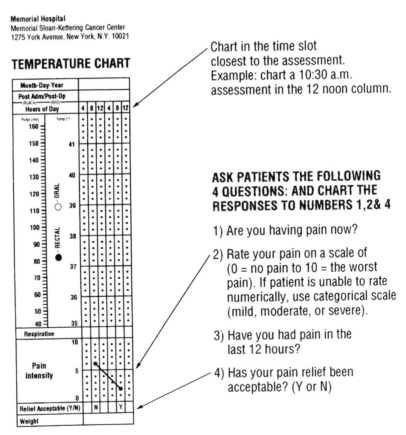

FIG. 100–1. Example of a modified bedside chart that includes pain measurements and has been incorporated into a continuous quality improvement strategy at a major cancer center. (From Ingham J, Portenoy RK. The measurement of pain and other symptoms. In: Doyle D, Hanks G, Macdonald N, eds. *Oxford Textbook of Palliative Medicine*, 2nd ed. Oxford: Oxford University Press, in press, with permission.)

(7,22,25,30,66–67). These instruments could also be used to monitor quality of care or evaluate barriers to symptom control (5,45,68–69).

In the clinical setting, symptom assessment could also assess the impact of specific symptoms on global symptom distress, overall QOL, or other quality of life concerns. Again, however, the development of valid instruments for the evaluation of global symptom distress (7,22,25,30) and QOL (6,38,70–73) has not been followed by their routine use in patient care or quality improvement.

RESEARCH APPLICATIONS OF SYMPTOM MEASUREMENT

Depending on the purpose of the study, symptom measurement can yield informative epidemiologic data or outcome data that can be either primary or secondary. As outcome data, symptoms can clarify treatment efficacy or toxicity. The scope of symptom measurement, and the rigor with which it is performed, should be planned to match the overriding goals of the investigation.

Historically, symptom measurement in cancer clinical trials has been used to assess treatment toxicity only. The approach has relied on the periodic administration of standardized toxicity scales, such as those recommended by the World Health Organization and the National Cancer Institute (62). This method provides some useful information, but has notable deficiencies that highlight the potential for improved symptom assessment. Standard toxicity scales include many items that are not patient-rated and some items that lack severity ratings. Distress ratings are not included and temporal characteristics are not explored. Data are commonly acquired at relatively long intervals. Although recent modifications to the standard approach recommend documentation of side-effect duration (74), conventional side-effect assessment in cancer clinical trials remains limited and may not accurately assess the severity of, and distress associated with, symptoms, particularly when the symptom is transitory.

Cancer clinical trials now frequently incorporate repeated assessment using a multidimensional QOL instrument, which provides some additional information about symptoms. The instruments that have been used for this purpose include the QLQ-C30 of the European Organization for Research and Treatment of Cancer (38), the Functional Living Index-Cancer (FLIC) (70,71), the Functional Assessment of Cancer Therapy Scale (6), the Cancer Rehabilitation Evaluation System (72), and the SF-36 of the Medical Outcome Study (73). Modified versions of some of these instruments have also been used in populations with HIV infection and other illnesses (75–79). All of these instruments assess a small number of prevalent symptoms, such as pain and fatigue (6,38,70,72). They do not clarify the prevalence rates or characteristics of a diverse array of physical and psychological symptoms. If a detailed symptom assessment is likely to be valuable, a specific instrument for this purpose must be co-administered with the QOL instrument. This method of "tailoring" the assessment by supplementing an instrument that screens many potential domains with instruments that assess more specific phenomena appears to be promising (6,32–33,38,80–81). Depending on the purpose of the assessment, such "tailoring" of the method can be focused on the specific measurement of one salient symptom, or on the evaluation of multiple symptoms or global symptom distress.

The utility of this "tailored" approach to symptom assessment was recently demonstrated in a survey of pain and QOL during a phase II trial of paclitaxel and recombinant human granulocyte-colony stimulating factor for breast cancer (81). Clinical observations had suggested that frequent short-lived episodes of pain were likely to occur during this treatment regimen and supplemental pain measurements were planned to capture this information. The assessment revealed a marked disparity between the pain data obtained during a routine QOL assessment performed at 3-week intervals and those acquired through the supplemental pain evaluation obtained twice weekly. In contrast to the decline in pain scores measured at the interval assessments, the supplemental assessment demonstrated transient acute and severe pains in almost half the patients. Careful selection of instruments and timing of measurement based on the anticipated outcomes is needed to optimize symptom measurement during clinical trials.

INSTRUMENTS FOR SYMPTOM ASSESSMENT

Instrument selection for symptom measurement must be guided by an understanding of the goals of assessment and the practicality, applicability, and acceptability of the instrument, or instruments, in the patient population. The burdens associated with assessment must be carefully considered. Measurement strategies that are simple and brief may limit patient burden and encourage compliance, but also preclude evaluation of complex and clinically meaningful phenomena. If the information is salient and would not be assessed otherwise, the increased burden may be warranted.

Measurement of Multiple Symptoms

Most studies that have incorporated systematic symptom assessment have relied on simple, face-valid measures, often in the form of symptom checklists (5,62,63). The development of new, validated measures may supersede these checklists.

Memorial Symptom Assessment Scale. The Memorial Symptom Assessment Scale (MSAS) is a validated, patient-rated measure that provides multidimensional information about 32 physical and psychological symptoms (7,22) (Fig. 100–2). Symptoms are characterized in terms of intensity, frequency, and distress. The MSAS provides a Global Distress Index (MSAS-GDI), a 10-item subscale that reflects global symptom distress, and separate subscales that measure physical (MSAS-PHYS) and psychological (MSAS-PSYCH) symptom distress, respectively. The MSAS may be a useful measure in a variety of research settings. Additional studies are needed to establish its reliability and validity with repeated administration, assess its utility as an outcome measure in cancer clinical trials, and confirm its value in patients with various types of cancer and other disease states.

Rotterdam Symptom Checklist. The Rotterdam Symptom Checklist (RSCL) is a validated, patient-rated measure that evaluates a spectrum of common symptoms in terms of patient-rated distress (66–67). Thirty physical and psychological symptoms are included and an additional 8 items specifically attempt to define the impact of symptoms on physical activity and function. The RSCL provides quantitative information about global symptom distress and subscales that distinguish physical and psychological symptom distress. Multidimensional assessment is not addressed by this instrument and information is not obtained about symptom intensity or frequency. Some symptoms that may be common in advanced disease, such as change in taste and appearance, are not evaluated and there are questions about pain in the head, back, abdomen and mouth, but no general pain item.

FIG. **100–2.** Memorial Symptom Assessment Scale.

DURING THE PAST WEEK, Did you have any of the following symptoms?	DID NOT HAVE	IF YES, How OFTEN did you have it?				IF YES, How SEVERE was it usually?				IF YES, How much did it DISTRESS or BOTHER you?				
		Rarely	Occas-ionally	Frequ-ently	Almost Cons-tantly	Slight	Moder-ate	Severe	Very Severe	Not At All	A Little Bit	Some-what	Quite A Bit	Very Much
Vomiting		1	2	3	4	1	2	3	4	0	1	2	3	4
Shortness of breath		1	2	3	4	1	2	3	4	0	1	2	3	4
Diarrhea		1	2	3	4	1	2	3	4	0	1	2	3	4
Feeling sad		1	2	3	4	1	2	3	4	0	1	2	3	4
Sweats		1	2	3	4	1	2	3	4	0	1	2	3	4
Worrying		1	2	3	4	1	2	3	4	0	1	2	3	4
Problems with sexual interest or activity		1	2	3	4	1	2	3	4	0	1	2	3	4
Itching		1	2	3	4	1	2	3	4	0	1	2	3	4
Lack of appetite		1	2	3	4	1	2	3	4	0	1	2	3	4
Dizziness		1	2	3	4	1	2	3	4	0	1	2	3	4
Difficulty swallowing		1	2	3	4	1	2	3	4	0	1	2	3	4
Feeling irritable		1	2	3	4	1	2	3	4	0	1	2	3	4

Continued on next page ....

SECTION 2:

INSTRUCTIONS: We have listed 8 symptoms below. Read each one carefully. If you have had the symptom during this past week, let us know how SEVERE it was usually and how much it DISTRESSED OR BOTHERED you by circling the appropriate number. If you DID NOT HAVE the symptom, make an "X" in the box marked "DID NOT HAVE."

DURING THE PAST WEEK, Did you have any of the following symptoms?	DID NOT HAVE	IF YES, How SEVERE was it usually?				IF YES, How much did it DISTRESS or BOTHER you?				
		Slight	Moderate	Severe	Very Severe	Not At All	A Little Bit	Somewhat	Quite A Bit	Very Much
Mouth sores		1	2	3	4	0	1	2	3	4
Change in the way food tastes		1	2	3	4	0	1	2	3	4
Weight loss		1	2	3	4	0	1	2	3	4
Hair loss		1	2	3	4	0	1	2	3	4
Constipation		1	2	3	4	0	1	2	3	4
Swelling of arms or legs		1	2	3	4	0	1	2	3	4
"I don't look like myself"		1	2	3	4	0	1	2	3	4
Changes in skin		1	2	3	4	0	1	2	3	4

** IF YOU HAD ANY OTHER SYMPTOMS DURING THE PAST WEEK, PLEASE LIST BELOW AND INDICATE HOW MUCH THE SYMPTOM HAS DISTRESSED OR BOTHERED YOU.

OTHER:	0	1	2	3	4
OTHER:	0	1	2	3	4
OTHER:	0	1	2	3	4

FIG. 100–2. Memorial Symptom Assessment Scale—*continued.* (From Portenoy RK, Thaler HT, Kornblith AB, et al. The Memorial Symptom Assessment Scale: an instrument for the evaluation of symptom prevalence, characteristics and distress. *Eur J Cancer.* 1994; 30A(9):1326-1336, with permission.)

Symptom Distress Scale. The Symptom Distress Scale (SDS) is a 13-item patient-rated scale that evaluates 11 symptoms, 9 physical and 2 psychological, in terms of either frequency, intensity, or distress (25,30). This scale has been widely used as a valid measure of global symptom distress. Recent studies suggest that the score can be an independent predictor of survival in patients with cancer (82).

Measurement of Specific Physical Symptoms

Although validated instruments exist for the assessment of some common symptoms, such as pain, there is a paucity of similar instruments for many other symptoms, including, for example, anorexia, dry mouth, and constipation. Moreover, many instruments have been validated in specific populations and may not be generalizable. For example, dyspnea measurement has been developed and validated for pulmonary and cardiac conditions (83–87), and there has been little exploration of the measurement of this symptom in patients with other systemic diseases such as cancer (88–90). The salient characteristics of the current symptom measures, including subjectivity, multidimensionality, and the importance of validation, may be illustrated by a discussion of pain, dyspnea and fatigue.

Pain Measurement. Pain intensity and relief are usually measured with unidimensional visual analogue, numerical, or categorical scales. Multidimensional instruments, which assess additional characteristics, include the McGill Pain Questionnaire (91–93) and an instrument that has been extensively validated in the cancer population, the Brief Pain Inventory (27).

The Memorial Pain Assessment Card (MPAC) is a brief, validated measure that uses visual analogue scales (VAS) to characterize pain intensity, pain relief, and mood, and an 8-point verbal rating scale (VRS) to further characterize pain intensity (94) (Fig. 100–3). The mood scale is a valid measure of global psychological distress. The brevity, simplicity, and reliability of the MPAC are strong advantages. Although it provides limited information, it has been useful in many analgesic clinical trials.

The Brief Pain Inventory (BPI) provides information about pain history, intensity, location and quality (27) (Fig. 100–4). Separate numeric scales rate pain intensity in general, at its worst, at its least, and right now. A percentage scale quantifies pain relief from current therapies. A body figure can be shaded to localize the pain and one item queries pain quality. Seven questions evaluate the degree to which pain interferes with function, mood, and enjoyment of life; the sum or average of these items is a useful indicator of overall pain interference with function. The BPI has been translated into numerous languages and is a widely used instrument for the multidimensional assessment of pain in cancer.

The McGill Pain Questionnaire (MPQ) evaluates the sensory, affective, and evaluative dimensions of pain using lists of verbal descriptors (91–93). It provides a global score and subscale scores for each of these dimensions. A 5-point VRS and a body figure are included to characterize pain intensity and location, respectively. The MPQ is multidimensional but does not assess the impact of pain on function. It has been used generally in studies of populations with chronic, non-malignant pain. The utility of the subscale scores has not been demonstrated for cancer pain (95).

Measurement of Fatigue. As discussed previously, the nomenclature applied to the common symptom of fatigue is inconsistent, and this may complicate assessment (2). To date, there has been no international consensus regarding the definition of fatigue. The report of fatigue may indicate a lack of vitality, cognitive disturbances (such as difficulty concentrating), sleepiness, mood disturbance (particularly depression), muscular weakness, or other problems. In some patients, fatigue is probably best understood as a multidimensional phenomenon that may be depicted according to a combination of these disturbances and other dimensions, including severity, frequency, and distress.

A small number of unidimensional fatigue scales have been used in research settings. These scales include single items in symptom checklists and the fatigue subscale of the Profile of Mood States (POMS) (25,67,96). These measures are simple to administer, but offer relatively little information.

The multidimensional perspective has generally been preferred in the measurement of fatigue (97–100). Instruments developed in the industrial setting have been applied to clinical assessment (99,101–105), and studies have usually relied on the evaluation of a range of symptoms associated with fatigue or the use of a validated multidimensional fatigue scale. The measurement of associated symptoms and signs, e.g., drowsiness and cognitive impairment, has been used effectively in clinical trials of psychostimulants for opioid-related fatigue (106–109); study patients completed a VAS to assess "drowsiness" and other scales to evaluate cognitive status.

Several multidimensional fatigue scales have been validated in the medically ill. The 41-item Piper Fatigue Self Report Scale (PFS) addresses the severity,

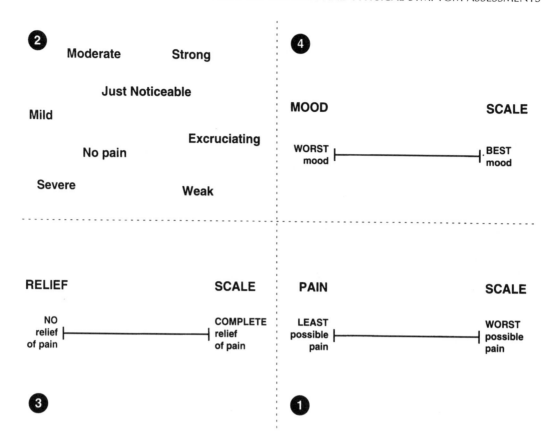

FIG. 100–3. Memorial Pain Assessment Card. (From Fishman B, Pasternak S, Wallenstein SL, et al. The Memorial Pain Assessment Card. A valid instrument for the evaluation of cancer pain. *Cancer.* 1987; 60(5):1151–1158, with permission.)

distress, and impact of fatigue, and can be administered as either a series of VASs or as numeric scales (110). This scale, which was developed to assess fatigue in patients receiving radiation therapy, has excellent reliability and moderate construct validity in this population. It is relatively lengthy, however, and the burden that some patients experience in completing it is a problem. In the initial validation study, for example, 24% of patients experienced difficulties in responding to the scales and almost half the patients approached for the study refused to participate.

A recently developed multidimensional fatigue scale, the Multidimensional Fatigue Inventory, has also been validated in the cancer population (radiotherapy patients), as well as other patient and non-patient populations (111). The validation study for this 20-item measure demonstrated the reliability of five subscales that assess varying dimensions of fatigue. Construct validity was indicated by confirming that group differences in measured fatigue corresponded with clinically expected variations. Experience with

this scale is yet limited, but it may prove useful in medically ill populations.

Other multidimensional fatigue measures have been validated, but have not been systematically assessed in populations with medical illness. The Visual Analogue Scale-Fatigue (VAS-F) is an 18-item instrument that was validated in a population with sleep disorders (112). It has high internal consistency and significant correlations with the POMS fatigue subscale and a sleepiness scale. The Chalder Fatigue Scale is an 11-item instrument that has subscales for physical and mental fatigue, as well as a total fatigue severity score (113). The brevity and multidimensionality of both these instruments suggest their potential utility in studies of patients with fatigue related to medical illness. Further experience will be needed, however, to clarify their advantages and disadvantages.

The problems encountered in the measurement of fatigue demonstrate some of the challenges inherent in symptom assessment. For example, the target population may have limited tolerance for assessment bur-

Brief Pain Inventory

Date: ___ / ___ / ___

Name: _____
　　　　　Last　　　　　　　First　　　　　　Middle Initial

Phone: (___) _____　　　Sex: ☐ Female　☐ Male

Date of Birth: ___ / ___ / ___

1) Marital Status (at present)
　　1. ☐ Single　　　3. ☐ Widowed
　　2. ☐ Married　　4. ☐ Separated/Divorced

2) Education (Circle only the highest grade or degree completed)
　　Grade　　0　　1　　2　　3　　4　　5　　6　　7　　8　　9
　　　　　　10　11　12　13　14　15　16　　M.A./M.S.
　　　　　　Professional degree (please specify) _____

3) Current occupation_____
　　(specify titles; if you are not working, tell us your previous occupation)

4) Spouse's Occupation_____

5) Which of the following best describes your current job status?
　　☐ 1. Employed outside the home, full-time
　　☐ 2. Employed outside the home, part-time
　　☐ 3. Homemaker
　　☐ 4. Retired
　　☐ 5. Unemployed
　　☐ 6. Other

6) How long has it been since you first learned your diagnosis? _____ months

7) Have you ever had pain due to your present disease?
　　1. ☐ Yes　　2. ☐ No　　3. ☐ Uncertain

8) When you first received your diagnosis, was pain one of your symptoms?
　　1. ☐ Yes　　2. ☐ No　　3. ☐ Uncertain

9) Have you had surgery in the past month?　1. ☐ Yes　　2. ☐ No

10) Throughout our lives, most of us have had pain from time to time (such as minor headaches, sprains, and toothaches). Have you had pain **other** than these everyday kinds of pain during the **last week?**　1. ☐ Yes　　2. ☐ No

IF YOU ANSWERED YES TO THE LAST QUESTION, PLEASE GO ON TO QUESTION 11 AND FINISH THIS QUESTIONNAIRE. IF NO, YOU ARE FINISHED WITH THE QUESTIONNAIRE. THANK YOU.

11) On the diagram, shade in the areas where you feel pain. Put an X on the area that hurts the most.

Front　　　　Back

Right ☺ Left　Left ☺ Right

12) Please rate your pain by circling the one number that best describes your pain at its **worst** in the last week.
　　0　1　2　3　4　5　6　7　8　9　10
　　No　　　　　　　　　　　　　Pain as bad as
　　Pain　　　　　　　　　　　　you can imagine

13) Please rate your pain by circling the one number that best describes your pain at its **least** in the last week
　　0　1　2　3　4　5　6　7　8　9　10
　　No　　　　　　　　　　　　　Pain as bad as
　　Pain　　　　　　　　　　　　you can imagine

14) Please rate your pain by circling the one number that best describes your pain on the **average.**
　　0　1　2　3　4　5　6　7　8　9　10
　　No　　　　　　　　　　　　　Pain as bad as
　　Pain　　　　　　　　　　　　you can imagine

15) Please rate your pain by circling the one number that tells how much pain you have **right now.**
　　0　1　2　3　4　5　6　7　8　9　10
　　No　　　　　　　　　　　　　Pain as bad as
　　Pain　　　　　　　　　　　　you can imagine

16) What kinds of things make your pain feel better (for example, head, medicine, rest)?
_____
_____

17) What kinds of things make your pain worse (for example, walking, standing, lifting)?
_____

18) What treatments or medications are you receiving for your pain?
_____
_____

19) In the last week, how much relief have pain treatments or medications provided? Please circle the one percentage that most shows how much relief you have received.

　　0%　10%　20%　30%　40%　50%　60%　70%　80%　90%　100%
　　No　　　　　　　　　　　　　　　　　　　　　　Complete
　　Relief　　　　　　　　　　　　　　　　　　　　Relief

20) If you take pain medication, how many hours does it take before the pain returns?
　　☐ 1. Pain medication doesn't help at all　☐ 5. Four hours
　　☐ 2. One hour　　　　　　　　　　　　　☐ 6. Five to twelve hours
　　☐ 3. Two hours　　　　　　　　　　　　☐ 7. More than twelve hours
　　☐ 4. Three hours　　　　　　　　　　　☐ 8. I do not take pain medication

21) Circle the appropriate answer for each item.
　　I believe my pain is due to:
　　☐ Yes　☐ No　　1. The effects of treatment (for example, medication, surgery, radiation, prosthetic device).
　　☐ Yes　☐ No　　2. My primary disease (meaning the disease currently being treated and evaluated).
　　☐ Yes　☐ No　　3. A medical condition unrelated to primary disease (for example, arthritis).

22) For each of the following words, check yes or no if that adjective applies to your pain.

Aching	☐ Yes	☐ No	Exhausting	☐ Yes	☐ No
Throbbing	☐ Yes	☐ No	Tiring	☐ Yes	☐ No
Shooting	☐ Yes	☐ No	Penetrating	☐ Yes	☐ No
Stabbing	☐ Yes	☐ No	Nagging	☐ Yes	☐ No
Gnawing	☐ Yes	☐ No	Numb	☐ Yes	☐ No
Sharp	☐ Yes	☐ No	Miserable	☐ Yes	☐ No
Tender	☐ Yes	☐ No	Unbearable	☐ Yes	☐ No
Burning	☐ Yes	☐ No			

23) Circle the one number that describes how, during the past week, **pain** has interfered with your:

A. General Activity
　　0　1　2　3　4　5　6　7　8　9　10
　　Does not　　　　　　　　　　　Completely
　　Interfere　　　　　　　　　　　interferes

B. Mood
　　0　1　2　3　4　5　6　7　8　9　10
　　Does not　　　　　　　　　　　Completely
　　Interfere　　　　　　　　　　　interferes

C. Walking ability
　　0　1　2　3　4　5　6　7　8　9　10
　　Does not　　　　　　　　　　　Completely
　　Interfere　　　　　　　　　　　interferes

D. Normal work (includes both work outside the home and housework)
　　0　1　2　3　4　5　6　7　8　9　10
　　Does not　　　　　　　　　　　Completely
　　Interfere　　　　　　　　　　　interferes

E. Relations with other people
　　0　1　2　3　4　5　6　7　8　9　10
　　Does not　　　　　　　　　　　Completely
　　Interfere　　　　　　　　　　　interferes

F. Sleep
　　0　1　2　3　4　5　6　7　8　9　10
　　Does not　　　　　　　　　　　Completely
　　Interfere　　　　　　　　　　　interferes

G. Enjoyment of life
　　0　1　2　3　4　5　6　7　8　9　10
　　Does not　　　　　　　　　　　Completely
　　Interfere　　　　　　　　　　　interferes

Pain Research Group, Department of Neurology, University of Wisconsin-Madison

FIG. **100–4.** Brief Pain Inventory. (Courtesy of the Pain Research Group, University of Wisconsin, Madison, Wisconsin, with permission.)

den. Specifically, patients with severe fatigue may be relatively less willing to participate in studies, or less able to complete multiple instruments or a lengthy multidimensional instrument. Further, the concern about respondent burden is compounded by problems of nomenclature, the complexity of the phenomena that may contribute to the symptom, and a lack of validated measures. Much research is needed to improve the measurement of fatigue.

Measurement of Dyspnea. The instruments for the measurement of dyspnea have, for the most part, been developed in populations with pulmonary or cardiac disease. In these populations, studies that have used adjectival checklists (2,114–115) reveal both commonalities and differences in the descriptors used by patients with different types of pathology. One study, for example, found that the descriptor "I feel short of breath" was used frequently by patients with diverse types of lung disease, whereas the descriptor "chest tightness" was more likely to be endorsed by asthmatics than others (114). Such studies demonstrate the complexity of nomenclature in symptom assessment and, further, the disease-specific characteristics emphasize the importance of selecting instruments for measurement that have been validated in the appropriate population.

Unlike other symptoms, dyspnea is usually measured in association with a dyspnea-producing task, usually standardized or graded exercise. Indeed, commonly used dyspnea measures, such as VASs and the Borg scale (116–117), have only been validated using this methodology. Although a lack of validation for dyspnea at rest may be an important limitation in some studies, an approach incorporating a task offers an opportunity to assess therapeutic interventions that may have little impact on baseline dyspnea but substantial effect on exercise-induced dyspnea. Measurement of dyspnea after a defined stress may enhance the clinical relevance of the result.

In addition to incorporating a standardized measure to assess the impact of a therapeutic intervention, some investigators have included standardized exercise protocols in study design to improve the reliability of dyspnea measurement using a VAS (118). Standard exercise has also been incorporated into methodologies with the aim of "calibrating" the VAS, such that the upper end of the scale is anchored to the breathlessness produced by the task (84–85); repeated testing with the calibrated scale may yield a more sensitive indicator of change. Although the measurement of dyspnea following a defined exercise task has not been adequately studied in populations with medical illnesses other than chronic lung and cardiac disease, it is likely that a design could be created that accommodates the specific characteristics of these populations. Further research is needed to define the most appropriate methodology.

Like other symptoms, dyspnea can be conceptualized as a multidimensional symptom, which could be assessed in terms of severity, frequency, associated distress, or other aspects (86). As noted, the most commonly used measures evaluate the severity of breathlessness in relation to a defined exercise task. Studies that have used VASs have generally demonstrated reliability that is very good during a brief time frame (83,118), but less when the same exercise task is repeated at longer intervals, such as two weeks (119). There is large between-subject variation and some patients appear to have difficulty in using the measure (120).

Verbal categorical scales and numerical scales have also been used to assess dyspnea (84–85,115,121). The modified Borg scale (116–117), for example, uses verbal ratings to describe dyspnea in comparison to that produced by a standard exercise.

Other instruments assess the degree of functional impairment caused by dyspnea. These instruments, which include the Modified Medical Research Council Dyspnea Scale (122), the American Thoracic Society Five Level Scale of Breathlessness (123), the Baseline Dyspnea Index (124), and the Transition Dyspnea Index (124), can be appropriate for patients who experience dyspnea as the sole or predominating symptom, but are clearly limited when impairment also relates to other symptoms such as pain or fatigue.

SYMPTOM MEASUREMENT IN SPECIAL POPULATIONS

Symptom measurement is particularly challenging in a number of subpopulations, including the pediatric population, the imminently dying, and those patients whose language or culture differs from that of the health care professionals involved in their care. With few exceptions, there is little systematic information that can be used to resolve the practical problems that arise in attempting to study these populations. In the absence of empirical data, decisions are usually based on clinical experience and extrapolation from other populations.

There has been little effort to evaluate methods to assess symptoms experienced by children with chronic illness. Although there have been many studies of pediatric pain, these have focused on acute pain related to surgery or procedures (125–128). These studies have demonstrated that children older than 6 years can usually indicate pain intensity using self-report measures, including the VAS and "faces" scales (129–133). Pain assessment in children 6 years and younger usually relies on behavioral observations. Instruments such as the Observational Scale of Behavioral Distress (134) and the Procedure Behavior Checklist (135) quantify the occurrence, intensity, and range of a child's pain. Although a behavioral observation scale for assessment of tumor-related pain in children aged 2–6 years has been developed (136), this has not, to date, been validated, and the items lack operational definitions. The assessment of chemotherapy-related nausea and vomiting has been undertaken using, for the most part, VASs and "face" scales (137–138).

Assessment of the imminently dying population has also usually relied on observer ratings, notwithstanding concerns about the validity of this approach. Self-report may be possible in these populations and should be explored further. In one large survey, for example, only 15% of 16,000 decedents were described by their relatives as disoriented in the hours or days prior to death (139). Although other surveys have suggested that the prevalence of impaired communication may be much higher in certain populations, for example, among cancer patients nearing death (45,98–99,140–141), a recent survey of inpatient and homecare cancer deaths found that approximately 33% of patients were able to interact 24 hours prior to death; 26% could interact 12 hours before, and 8% were communicative in the hour before death (142).

Additionally, symptom measurement may be difficult when the culture and language of the patients differ from the professionals involved in their care (143). Only a few instruments have been shown to be reliable and valid across cultures and languages (144–145) and translation and validation of other symptom measures is needed. In the clinical setting, simple, face-valid symptom measures may be devised to overcome language barriers. For example, the clinician may be able to use information provided by the patient through a translator to construct a simple, two-language verbal rating scale to keep by the bedside. Such a scale can focus on relevant symptoms and provide a means to monitor the level of distress and impact of interventions. Both intensity and relief should be recorded, if possible.

CONCLUSION

Comprehensive symptom assessment is a vital aspect of clinical practice. Valid symptom measurement is essential for research in the epidemiology of quality of life concerns and for clinical trials of interventions, including both primary and symptomatic treatments. Symptom measurement may also be applied in the clinical setting and further the goal of enhanced QOL. Substantial progress has been made in the development of a conceptual basis for the measurement of physical symptoms and the validation of specific instruments for highly prevalent symptoms. Further work is needed to validate current instruments in diverse medical illnesses, develop and validate new measures of common symptoms, and create valid multisymptom measures that may be useful for screening diverse patient populations.

REFERENCES

1. *The New Shorter Oxford English Dictionary*, Oxford: Clarendon Press; 1993.
2. Elliott MW, Adams L, Cockcroft A, et al. The language of breathlessness: Use of verbal descriptors by patients with cardiopulmonary disease. *Am Rev Respir Dis.* 1991; 144(4):826–832.
3. Merskey H, Bogduk N. *Classification of Chronic Pain*, 2nd ed, Seattle, WA: IASP Press; 1994.
4. Chang VT, Hwang SS. Symptom prevalence in a population of cancer patients in a Veteran's Administration hospital. *Proc.* Unpublished data.
5. Bruera E, Kuehn N, Miller MJ, et al. The Edmonton Symptom Assessment System (ESAS): A simple method for the assessment of palliative care patients. *J Palliat Care.* 1991; 7(2):6–9.
6. Cella DF, Tulsky DS, Gray G, et al. The Functional Assessment of Cancer Therapy scale: Development and validation of the general measure. *J Clin Oncol.* 1993; 11(3):570–579.
7. Portenoy RK, Thaler HT, Kornblith AB, et al. The Memorial Symptom Assessment Scale: An instrument for the evaluation of symptom prevalence, characteristics and distress. *Eur J Cancer.* 1994; 30A(9):1326–1336.
8. Grossman SA, Sheidler VR, Swedeen K, et al. Correlation of patient and caregiver ratings of cancer pain. *J Pain Symptom Manage.* 1991; 6(2):53–57.
9. Clipp EC, George LK. Patients with cancer and their spouse caregivers: Perceptions of the illness experience. *Cancer.* 1992; 69(4):1074–1079.
10. Higginson I, Priest P, McCarthy M. Are bereaved family members a valid proxy for a patient's assessment of dying? *Soc Sci Med.* 1994; 38(4):553–557.
11. Slevin ML, Plant H, Lynch D, et al. Who should measure quality of life, the doctor or the patient. *Br J Cancer.* 1988; 57:109–112.
12. Kahn SB, Houts PS, Harding SP. Quality of life and patients with cancer: A comparative study of patient versus physician perceptions and its implications for cancer education. *J Cancer Educ.* 1992; 7:241–249.
13. Osoba D. Lessons learned from measuring health-related quality of life in oncology. *J Clin Oncol.* 1994; 12:608–616.
14. Jacox A, Carr DB, Payne R, et al. *Management of Cancer Pain. Clinical Practice Guidelines.* No. 9., U.S.

Department of Health and Human Services, Public Health Service, Agency for Health Care Policy and Research; 1994.

15. Greer DS, Mor V, Morris JN, et al. An alternative in terminal care: Results of the National Hospice Study. *J Chron Dis.* 1986; 39(1):9–26.

16. Morris JN, Suissa S, et al. Last days: A study of the quality of life of terminally ill cancer patients. *J Chron Dis.* 1986; 39(1):47–62.

17. Reuben DB, Mor V. Dyspnea in terminally ill cancer patients. *Chest.* 1986; 89(2):234–236.

18. Mor V. Cancer patients' quality of life over the disease course: Lessons from the real world. *J Chron Dis.* 1987; 40:535–544.

19. Mor V, Masterson-Allen S. A comparison of hospice vs. conventional care of the terminally ill cancer patient. *Oncology.* 1990; 4(7):85–91.

20. Higginson IJ, McCarthy M. A comparison of two measures of quality of life: Their sensitivity and validity for patients with advanced cancer. *Palliat Med.* 1994; 8(4):282–290.

21. Aaronson NK. Quality of life research in cancer clinical trials: A need for common rules and language. *Oncology.* 1990; 4(5):59–66.

22. Portenoy RK, Thaler HT, Kornblith AB, et al. Symptom prevalence, characteristics and distress in a cancer population. *Qual Life Res.* 1994; 3(3):183–189.

23. Dunlop GM. A study of the relative frequency and importance of gastrointestinal symptoms and weakness in patients with far advanced cancer. *Palliat Med.* 1989; 4:37–43.

24. Welch JM, Barlow D, and Richardson PH. Symptoms of HIV disease. *Palliat Med.* 1991; 5:46–51.

25. McCorkle R, Young K. Development of a symptom distress scale. *Cancer Nurs.* 1978 1:373–378.

26. Portenoy RK, Hagen NA. Breakthrough pain: Definition, prevalence and characteristics. *Pain.* 1990; 41(3):273–281.

27. Daut RL, Cleveland CS, Flanery RC. Development of the Wisconsin Brief Pain Questionnaire to assess pain in cancer and other diseases. *Pain.* 1983; 17(2): 197–210.

28. Daut RL, Cleeland CS. The prevalence and severity of pain in cancer. *Cancer.* 1982; 50(9):1913-1918.

29. Serlin RC, Mendoza TR, Nakamura Y, et al. When is cancer pain mild, moderate or severe? Grading pain severity by its interference with function. *Pain.* 1995; 61(2):277–284.

30. McCorkle R, Quint-Benoliel J. Symptom distress, current concerns and mood disturbance after diagnosis of a life-threatening disease. *Soc Sci Med.* 1993; 17(7): 431–438.

31. Till JE, McNeil BJ, Bush RS. Measurements of multiple components of quality of life. *Cancer Treat Symp.* 1993; 1:177.

32. Aaronson NK, Bullinger M, Ahmedzai S. A modular approach to quality of life assessment in cancer clinical trials. In: Scheurlen H, Kay R, Baum M, eds. *Recent Results in Cancer Research*, Vol. 11. Berlin: Springer-Verlag; 1988: 231.

33. Moinpour CM, Feigl P, Metch B, et al. Quality of life end points in cancer clinical trials: review and recommendations. *J Nat Cancer Inst.* 1989; 81(7):485–495.

34. Moinpour CM, Hayden KA, Thompson IM, et al. Quality of life assessment in Southwest Oncology Group trials. *Oncology.* 1990; 4(5):79–84.

35. Cella DF, Tulsky DS. Measuring quality of life today: Methodological aspects. *Oncology.* 1990; 4(5):29–38.

36. Aaronson NK. Methodologic issues in assessing the quality of life of cancer patients. *Cancer.* 1990; 67(Suppl. 3):844–850.

37. Nayfield SG, Ganz PA, Moinpour CM, et al. Report from a National Cancer Institute (USA) workshop on quality of life assessment in cancer clinical trials. *Qual Life Res.* 1992; 1(3):203–210.

38. Aaronson NK, Ahmedzai S, Bergman B, et al. The European Organization for Research and Treatment of Cancer QLQ-C30: a quality-of-life instrument for use in international clinical trials in oncology. *J Nat Cancer Inst.* 1993; 85(5):365–376.

39. Curtis EB, Krech R, Walsh TD. Common symptoms in patients with advanced cancer. *J Palliat Care.*, 1991; 7(2):25–29.

40. Coyle N, Adelhardt J, Foley KM, Portenoy RK. Character of terminal illness in the advanced cancer patient: Pain and other symptoms during the last four weeks of life. *J Pain Symptom Manage.* 1990; 5(2): 83–93.

41. Dunphy KP, Amesbury BDW. A comparison of hospice and homecare patients: Patterns of referral, patient characteristics and predictors on place of death. *Palliat Med.* 1990; 4:105–111.

42. Brescia FJ, Adler D, Gray G, et al. Hospitalized advanced cancer patients: A profile. *J Pain Symptom Manage.* 1990; 5(4):221–227.

43. Grosvenor M, Bulcavage L, Chlebowski RT. Symptoms potentially influencing weight loss in a cancer population: Correlations with primary site, nutritional status, and chemotherapy administration. *Cancer.* 1989; 63(2):330–334.

44. Ventafridda V, DeConno F, Ripamonti C, et al. Quality-of-life assessment during a palliative care programme. *Ann Oncol.* 1990; 1(6):415–420.

45. Fainsinger R, Miller MJ, Bruera E, et al. Symptom control during the last week of life on a palliative care unit. *J Palliat Care.* 1991; 7(1):5–11.

46. Reuben DB, Mor V, Hiris J. Clinical symptoms and length of survival in patients with terminal cancer. *Arch Intern Med.* 1988; 148(7):1586–1591.

47. Levine PM, Silberfarb PM, Lipowski ZJ. Mental disorders in cancer patients: A study of 100 psychiatric referrals. *Cancer.* 1978; 42(3):1385–1391.

48. Derogatis LR, Morrow GR, Fetting J, et al. The prevalence of psychiatric disorders among cancer patients. *JAMA.* 1983; 249(6):751–757.

49. Jacox A, Carr DB, Payne R. New clinical practice guidelines for the management of pain in patients with cancer. *N Engl J Med.* 1994; 330(9):651–655.

50. Max M. American Pain Society quality assurance standards for relief of acute pain and cancer pain. In: Bond MR, Charlton JE, Woolf CJ, eds. *Proceedings VI World Congress on Pain.* Amsterdam: Elsevier; 1990: 185–189.

51. Bookbinder M, Kiss M, Coyle N, et al. Improving pain management practices. In: McGuire DB, Yarbo CH, and Ferrell BR, eds. *Cancer Pain Management*, 2nd

ed. Boston: Jones and Bartlett Publishers International; 1995: 321–363.

52. Foley KM. Pain relief into practice: Rhetoric without reform. *J Clin Oncol.* 1995; 13(9):2149–2151.

53. Ingham J, Portenoy RK. The measurement of pain and other symptoms. In: Doyle D, Hanks G, Macdonald N, eds. *Oxford Textbook of Palliative Medicine*, 2nd ed. Oxford: Oxford University Press; in press.

54. Cherny NI, Portenoy RK. Cancer pain: Principles of assessment and syndromes. In: Wall PD, Melzack R, eds. *Textbook of Pain*, 3rd ed. Edinburgh: Churchill Livingstone; 1994: 787–824.

55. Ingham JM, Portenoy RK. Symptom assessment. In: Cherny NI, Foley KM, eds. *Hematology/Oncology Clinics of North America. Pain and Palliative Care.* Philadelphia: WB Saunders; 1996: 21–39.

56. Sui AL, Reuben DB, Moore AA. Comprehensive geriatric assessment. In: Hazzard WR, Bierman EL, Blass JP, et al., eds. *Principles of Geriatric Medicine and Gerontology*, 3rd ed. New York: McGraw-Hill; 1994: 203–211.

57. Pecoraro RE, Inui TS, Chen MS, et al. Validity and reliability of a self-administered health history questionnaire. *Public Health Rep.* 1979: 94:231–238.

58. Brodman K, Erdmann AJ, Lorge I, Wolff HG. The Cornell Medical Index: An adjunct to medical interview. *J Am Med Assoc.* 1949; 140:530–534.

59. Coyle N, Layman-Goldstein M, Passik S, et al. Development and validation of a patient's needs assessment tool (PNAT) for oncology clinicians. *Cancer Nurs.* 1996; 19(2):81–92.

60. Au E, Loprinzi CL, Dhodapkar M, et al. Regular use of a verbal pain scale improves the understanding of oncology inpatient intensity. *J Clin Oncol.* 1994; 12(12): 2751–2755.

61. Bookbinder M, Coyle N, Thaler HT, et al. Implementing quality assurance standards for pain management: Program development and pilot study. *J Pain Symptom Manage.*, in press.

62. Miller AB, Hoogstraten B, Staquet M, Winkler A. Reporting results of cancer treatment. *Cancer.* 1981; 47:207–214.

63. Donnelly S, Walsh TD. The symptoms of advanced cancer. *Sem Oncol.* 1995; 22(2)(Suppl. 3):67–72.

64. Burgess AP, Irving G, Riccio M. The reliability and validity of a symptom checklist for use in HIV infection: A preliminary analysis. *Int J STD AIDS.* 1993;(4): 333–338.

65. Osoba D. Self-rating symptom checklists: A simple method for recording and evaluating symptom control in oncology. *Cancer Treat.* 1993; 19(Suppl. A):43–51.

66. de Haes JCJM, Raatgever JW, van der Burg MEL, et al. Evaluation of the quality of life of patients with advanced ovarian cancer treated with combination chemotherapy. In: Aaronson NK, Beckman J, eds. *The Quality of Life of Cancer Patients.* New York: Raven Press; 1987: 217–225.

67. de Haes JCJM, van Kippenberg FCE, Neijt JP. Measuring psychological and physical distress in cancer patients: Structure and application of the Rotterdam Symptom Checklist. *Br J Cancer.* 1990; 62:1034–1038.

68. Bruera E, MacMillan K, Hanson J, MacDonald RN. Palliative care in a cancer center: Results in 1984 versus 1987. *J Pain Symptom Manage.* 1990; 5(1):1–5.

69. Stiefel F, Fainsinger R, Bruera E. Acute confusional states in patients with advanced cancer. *J Pain Symptom Manage.* 1992; 7(2):94–98.

70. Schipper H, Clinch J, McMurray A, Levitt M. Measuring the quality of life of cancer patients: The Functional Living Index-Cancer: Development and validation. *J Clin Oncol.* 1984; 2(5):472–483.

71. Morrow GR, Lindke J, Black P. Measurement of quality of life in patients: Psychometric analyses of the Functional Living Index-Cancer (FLIC). *Qual Life Res.* 1992; 1:287–296.

72. Ganz PA, Schag CA, Lee JJ, Sim MS. The CARES: A generic measure of health related quality of life for patients with cancer. *Qual Life Res.* 1992; 1:19–29.

73. Stewart AL, Hays RD, Ware JE. The MOS short-form general health survey: Reliability and validity in a patient population. *Med Care.* 1988; 26:724–735.

74. Creekmore SP, Urba WJ, Longo DL. Principles of the clinical evaluation of biological agents. In: Devita VT, Hellman S, Rosenberg SA, eds. *Biologic Therapy of Cancer.* Philadelphia: JB Lippincott; 1991:67–86.

75. Kaplan RM, Anderson JP, Wu AW, et al. The Quality of Well-Being Scale: Applications in AIDS, cystic fibrosis, and arthritis. *Med Care.* 1989; 27:35–49.

76. Wu AW, Rubin HR, Mathews WC, et al. A health status questionnaire using 30 items from the Medical Outcomes Study. *Med Care.* 1991; 29(8):786–798.

77. Wachtel T, Piette J, Mor V, et al. Quality of life in persons with human immunodeficiency virus infection: Measurement by the Medical Outcomes Study instrument. *Ann Intern Med.* 1992; 116(2):129–137.

78. Cleary PD, Fowler FJ, Weissman J, et al. Health-related quality of life in persons with Acquired Immune Deficiency Syndrome. *Med Care.* 1993; 31(7):569–580.

79. Bozzette SA, Hays RD, Berry SH, Kanouse DE. A Perceived Health Index for use in persons with advanced HIV disease: Derivation, reliability and validity. *Med Care.* 1994; 32(7):716–731.

80. Bjordal K, Kassa S. Psychometric validation of the EORTC core quality of life questionnaire, 30-item version and a diagnosis-specific module for head and neck cancer patients. *Acta Oncol.* 1992; 31:311–321.

81. Ingham JM, Seidman A, Yao T-J, et al. The importance of frequent pain measurement in a cancer clinical trial: A lesson for quality of life assessment. *Qual Life Res.*, in press.

82. Kukull WA, McCorkle R, Driever M. Symptom distress, psychosocial variables and survival from lung cancer. *J Psychosoc Oncol.* 1986; 4:91–104.

83. Stark RD, Gambles SA, Lewis JA. Methods to assess breathlessness in healthy subjects: A critical evaluation and application to analyse the acute effects of diazepam and promethazine on breathlessness induced by exercise or by exposure to raised levels of carbon dioxide. *Clin Sci.* 1981; 61(4):429–439.

84. Stark RD. Dyspnoea: assessment and pharmacological manipulation. *Eur Respir J.* 1988; 1(3):280–287.

85. Cockcroft A, Adams L, Guz A. Assessment of breathlessness. *Quart J Med.* 1989; 72(268):669–676.

86. McCord M, Cronin SD. Operationalizing dyspnea: focus on measurement. *Heart Lung.* 1992; 21(2): 167–179.

87. Eakin EG, Kaplan RM, Ries AL. Measurement of dyspnoea in chronic obstructive pulmonary disease. *Qual Life Res.* 1993; 2(3):181–191.

88. Brown ML, Carrieri V, Janson-Bjerklie S, Dodd MJ. Lung cancer and dyspnea: the patient's perception. *Oncol Nurs Forum.* 1986; 13(5):19–23.

89. Bruera E, DeStoutz N, Velasco-Leiva A, et al. Effects of oxygen on dyspnoea in hypoxaemic terminal-cancer patients. *Lancet.* 1993; 342:13–14.

90. Roberts DK, Thorne SE, Pearson C. The experience of dyspnea in late-stage cancer: Patients' and nurses' perspectives. *Cancer Nurs.* 1993; 16(4):310–320.

91. Melzack R. The McGill Pain Questionnaire: Major properties and scoring methods. *Pain.* 1975; 1:277–299.

92. Graham C, Bond SS, Gerkovich MM, Cook MR. Use of the McGill Pain Questionnaire in the assessment of cancer pain: Replicability and consistency. *Pain.* 1980; 8:377–387.

93. Melzack R. The short-form McGill Pain Questionnaire. *Pain.* 1987; 30:191–197.

94. Fishman B, Pasternak S, Wallenstein SL, et al. The Memorial Pain Assessment Card. A valid instrument for the evaluation of cancer pain. *Cancer.* 1987; 60(5):1151–1158.

95. DeConno F, Caraceni A, Gamba A, et al. Pain measurement in cancer patients: A comparison of six methods. *Pain.* 1994; 57:161–166.

96. McNair D, Lorr M, Deoppleman LF. *Profile of Mood States Manual.* San Diego: Educational and Industrial Testing Service; 1971.

97. Irvine DM, Vincent L, Bubela N, *Thompson L, Graydon JA.* A critical appraisal of the literature investigating fatigue in the individual with cancer. *Cancer Nurs.* 1991; 14(4):188–199.

98. Smets EM, Garssen B, Schuster-Uitterhoeve AL, de Haes JCJM. Fatigue in cancer patients. *Br J Cancer.* 1993; 68(2):220–224.

99. Glaus A. Assessment of fatigue in cancer and non-cancer patients and in healthy individuals. *Support Care Cancer.* 1993; 1:305–315.

100. Winningham ML, Nail LM, Burke MB, Brophy L, Cimprich B Jones LS, et al. Fatigue and the cancer experience: The state of the knowledge. Oncol Nurs Forum 1994; 21(1):23-34.

101. Pearson PG, Byars GE. *The Development and Validation of a Checklist Measuring Subjective Fatigue.* Randolf AFB, Texas: School of Aviation, USAF; 1956.

102. Yoshitake H. Relations between the symptoms and feelings of fatigue. *Ergonomics.* 1971; 14:175–196.

103. Haylock PJ, Hart LK. Fatigue in patients receiving localized radiation. *Cancer Nurs.* 1979; 2(12):461–467.

104. Kogi K, Saito Y. Assessment criteria for mental fatigue. A factor-analytic study of phase discrimination in mental fatigue. *Ergonomics.* 1971; 14(1):119–127.

105. Kobashi-Schoot JAM, Hanewald GJFP, Van Dam FSAM, Bruning FP. Assessment of malaise in cancer patients treated with radiotherapy. *Cancer Nurs.* 1985; 8(6):306–313.

106. Bruera E, Chadwick S, Brenneis C, et al. Methylphenidate associated with narcotics for the treatment of cancer pain. *Cancer Treat.* 1987; Rep. 71(1): 67–70.

107. Bruera E, Brenneis C, Paterson AH, MacDonald RN. Use of methylphenidate as an adjuvant to narcotic analgesics in patients with advanced cancer. *J Pain Symptom Manage.* 1989; 4(1):3–6.

108. Bruera E, Fainsinger R, MacEachern T, Hanson J. The use of methylphenidate in patients with incident cancer pain receiving regular opiates: A preliminary report. *Pain.* 1992; 50(1):75–77.

109. Bruera E, Miller MJ, Macmillan K, Kuehn N. Neuropsychological effects of methylphenidate in patients receiving a continuous infusion of narcotics for cancer pain. *Pain.* 1992; 48(2):163–166.

110. Piper BF, Lindsey AM, Dodd MJ, et al. The development of an instrument to measure the subjective dimension of fatigue. In: Funk SG, Tornquist EM, Champange MT, Copp LA, Wiese RA, eds. *Key Aspects of Comfort. Management of Pain, Fatigue and Nausea.* New York: Springer Publishing Company; 1989: 199–208.

111. Smets EMA, Garssen B, Bonke B, de Haes JCJM. The Multidimensional Fatigue Inventory (MFI): Psychometric qualities of an instrument to assess fatigue. *J Psychosom Res.* 1995; 39:315–325.

112. Lee KA, Hicks G, Nino-Murcia G. Validity and reliability of a scale to assess fatigue. *Psychiatr Res.* 1991; 36:291–298.

113. Chalder T, Berelowitz G, Pawlikowska T, et al. Development of a fatigue scale. *J Psychosom Res.* 1993; 37:147–153.

114. Janson-Bjerklie S, Carrieri VK, Hudes M. The sensations of dyspnea. *Nurs Res.* 1985; 35(3):154–159.

115. Simon PM, Schwartzstein RM, Weiss JW, et al. Distinguishable sensations of breathlessness induced in normal volunteers. *Am Rev Respir Dis.* 1989; 140: 1021–1027.

116. Borg G. Perceived exertion as an indicator of somatic stress. *Scand J Rehab Med.* 1970; 2(2):92–98.

117. Borg G. Psychophysical bases of perceived exertion. *Med Sci Sports Exerc.* 1982; 14(5):377–387.

118. O'Neill PA, Stretton TB, Stark RD, Ellis SH. The effect of indomethacin on breathlessness in patients with diffuse parenchymal disease of the lung. *Br J Dis Chest.* 1986; 80(1):72–79.

119. Wilson RC, Jones PW. A comparison of the visual analogue scale and modified Borg scale for the measurement of dyspnea during exercise. *Clin Sci.* 1989; 76:277–282.

120. Stark RD, Morton PB, Sharman P, Percival PG, Lewis JA. Effects of codeine on the respiratory responses to exercise in healthy subjects. *Br J Clin Pharmacol.* 1983; 15(3):355–359.

121. Eakin EG, Kaplan RM, Ries A. Measurement of dyspnea in chronic obstructive pulmonary disease. *Qual Life Res.* 1993; 2:181–191.

122. Research Council Committee on the Aetiology of Chronic Bronchitis. Standardized questionnaires on respiratory symptoms. *Br Med J.* 1960; 2:1665.

123. American Thoracic Society. Recommended respiratory disease questionnaires for use with adults and children in epidemiological research. *Am Rev Respir Dis.* 1978; 118:7–53.

124. Mahler D, Weinberg D, Wells C, Feinstein A. The measurement of dyspnea: Contents, interobserver agreement, and physiologic correlates of two new clinical indexes. *Chest.* 85:751–758.

125. Karoly P. Assessment of pediatric pain. In: Bush JP, Harkins SW, eds. *Children in Pain: Clinical and Research Issues from a Developmental Perspective.* New York: Springer-Verlag; 1991:59–82.

126. Manne SL, Andersen BL. Pain and pain-related distress in children with cancer. In: Bush JP, Harkins SW, eds. *Children in Pain: Clinical and Research Issues from a Developmental Perspective.* New York: Springer-Verlag; 1991:337–372.

127. Matthews JR, McGrath PJ, Pigeon H. Assessment and measurement of pain in children. In: Schechter NL, Berde CB, Yaster M, eds. *Pain in Infants, Children and Adolescents.* Baltimore: Williams and Wilkins; 1993.

128. Porter F. Pain assessment in children: Infants. In: Schechter NL, Berde CB, Yaster M, eds. *Pain in Infants, Children and Adolescents.* Baltimore: Williams and Wilkins; 1993.

129. Jay S, Elliot C, Katz E, Seigal S. Cognitive-behavioral and pharmacologic interventions for childrens' distress during painful medical procedures. *J Consult Clin Psychol.* 1987; 55:860–865.

130. Katz E, Kellerman J, Ellenberg L. Hypnosis in the reduction of acute pain and distress in children with cancer. *J Ped Psychol.* 1987; 12:379–394.

131. LeBaron S, Zeltzer LK. Assessment of pain and anxiety in children and adolescents by self-reports, and a behavior checklist. *J Consult Clin Psychol.* 1984; 52(5):729–738.

132. Kuttner L, Bowman M, Teasdale M. Psychological treatment of distress, pain and anxiety for children with cancer. *Develop Behav Pediatr.* 1988; 9:374–381.

133. Manne S, Redd WH, Jacobson P, et al. Behavioral intervention to reduce child and parent distress during venipuncture. *J Consult Clin Psychol.* 1990; 58:565–572.

134. Jay S, Elliott C. Behavioral observation scales for measuring childrens' distress: The effects of increased methodological rigor. *J Consult Clin Psychol.* 1984; 52:1106–1107.

135. Elliott C, Jay S, Woody P. An observational scale for measuring childrens' distress during medical procedures. *J Ped Psychol.* 1987; 12:543–551.

136. Gauvain-Piquard A, Rodary C, Rezvani A, Lemerle J. Pain in children aged 2-6 years: A new observational rating scale elaborated in a pediatric oncology unit—a preliminary report. *Pain.* 1987; 31:177–188.

137. Zeltzer LK, LeBaron S, Richie DM, Reed D. Can children understand and use a rating scale to quantify somatic symptoms? Assessment of nausea and vomiting as a model. *J Consult Clin Psychol.* 1988; 56(5):567–572.

138. Tye VL, et al. Chemotherapy induced nausea and emesis in pediatric cancer patients: External validity of child and parent emesis ratings. *Develop Behav Pediatr.* 1993; 14(4):236–241.

139. Seeman I. National Mortality Followback Survey: 1986 Summary, United States National Center for Health Statistics. *Vital and Health Statistics.* 1992; 20:19.

140. Saunders C. Pain and impending death. In: Wall P, Melzack R, eds. *Textbook of Pain.* Edinburgh: Churchill Livingston; 1984: 472–478.

141. Hinton JM. The physical and mental distress of the dying. *Quart J Med.* 1963; 32(125):1–21.

142. Ingham JM, Layman-Goldstein M, Coyle N, et al. Unpublished data.

143. *Cross Cultural Caring: A Handbook for Health Professionals in Western Canada.* University of BC Press; 1990.

144. Cleeland CS, Ryan KM. Pain assessment: Global use of the Brief Pain Inventory. *Ann Acad Med Singapore.* 1994; 23(2):129–138.

145. Cleeland CS, Ladinsky JL, Serlin RC, Nguyen CT. Multidimensional measurement of cancer pain: Comparisons of US and Vietnamese patients. *J Pain Symptom Manage.* 1988; 3(1):23–27.

XVII

INTERNATIONAL ASPECTS

EDITORS: JIMMIE C. HOLLAND AND
ANTHONY MARCHINI

101

International Psycho-oncology

JIMMIE C. HOLLAND AND ANTHONY MARCHINI

The past two decades have seen the development of psycho-oncology on a worldwide basis. This development has made possible the opportunity to better identify and study the impact of different cultures and systems of health care on the treatment and quality of life of patients with cancer and their families' psychological adjustment. The International Psycho-Oncology Society (IPOS), formed in 1984, has been a helpful structure facilitating collaborative cross-cultural studies and educational activities by an international network of health care professionals devoted to global issues involving the psychological and social aspects of cancer (1). (See Chapter 1 on the History of Psycho-oncology.) This chapter reviews the current status of psycho-oncology at an international level. It particularly draws upon data collected by IPOS through several cross-cultural surveys of psychosocial management of patients (2–4). (For further information about IPOS on the Internet, see http://www.ipos.org.)

GLOBAL PATTERNS

Prior to the 1970s, psychological and social issues in cancer medicine were given little formal attention or study. Cancer equals death was so pervasive a concept that it was the routine management of patients not to discuss the diagnosis or prognosis, though it was recognized that patients "knew," but the social norms were that they didn't reveal that they knew to their family or doctor. It was not until there was greater openness of discussion and greater pressure from patients and consumer groups that this changed and opened the way for active study of psychological issues. Since the mid-seventies, however, there has been increasing emphasis placed on the psychological, social, and quality of life issues in patient care and on behavioral issues in cancer prevention and early detection. The changes in delivery of health care,

based on global economic restraints, and emphasis on quantitative outcome measures, has placed patient reported health-related quality of life as a legitimate and important domain in health outcomes research. These research areas which involve the psychological dimensions of care have evolved into a subspecialty called psycho-oncology, psychosocial oncology or sometimes, behavioral oncology (5). Its principles and practices are described in a textbook and there are two journals devoted to it, *Psycho-Oncology: A Journal of the Psychological, Social and Behavioral Dimensions of Cancer* and the *Journal of Psychosocial Oncology*. A curriculum for the basic knowledge needed to work in the field is available (6) as well as published literature with articles numbering more than a thousand.

In an attempt to find out developments in this subspecialty in different countries, IPOS National Representatives in each country were asked to provide data on the status of psycho-oncology in their countries. Information was provided from 25 countries and additional information has been provided by international colleagues from those countries that did not report.

Overall, the decade between 1975 and 1985 marks the beginning of psycho-oncology in most countries. During that short span of time, interest and work in psychosocial oncology emerge, at least to some degree, in most countries around the world. Sweden and the United States are historically the countries with the earliest efforts in this field, starting far back in the 1950s at the Karolinska Institute under Feigenberg and at Memorial Sloan-Kettering Cancer Center under Sutherland. The United Kingdom and Denmark also began work in the 1950s. The most recent beginnings, in the nineties, are found in such countries as Turkey, Portugal, and Spain. There are some, like the Philippines, who report still no concerted effort in psycho-oncology. It is encouraging that in Africa, the Pan African Psycho-Oncology Society has held congresses in 1994 and 1996. Many activities are beginning in India with the support of the Indian Psychooncology Society. The establishment of a national psycho-oncology group has usually heralded significant networking and educational activities. There are now almost twenty national psycho-oncology societies:

American Society of Psychiatric-Oncology/AIDS
Belgian Society of Psychosocial Oncology
Brazilian Psycho-Oncology Society
British Psychosocial Oncology Group
Canadian Association of Psychosocial Oncology
French Psycho-Oncology Society
German Psycho-Oncology Society
Hellenic Society of Psychosocial Oncology
Hungarian Psychooncology Group
Indian Psychooncology Society
Society of Psycho-Oncology in India
Israel Psycho-Oncology Association
Italian Society of Psycho-Oncology
Japanese Psycho-Oncology Society
Mexican Society of Psycho-Oncology
Polish Psycho-Oncology Society
Portuguese Society of Psycho-Oncology

An Australian group is forming within the national oncology organization.

The European Society of Psychosocial Oncology links activities in several countries in Europe, including the United Kingdom. The Nordic Society unites professionals in Scandinavia. The International Psycho-Oncology Society serves as an integrating force to link the societies internationally. The strength of the movement was demonstrated in 1996 when the Third World Congress of Psycho-Oncology was held in New York with nearly a thousand people attending from 49 countries. They represented the range of disciplines interested in the psychological aspects of cancer.

Progress in psycho-oncology, over the course of the past twenty years, varies geographically, but overall, there has been steady international growth of activity of both a practical and theoretical nature. There is a growing concern about quality of life issues which places greater emphasis on patients' reports of their symptoms and emotional distress. Nevertheless, surveys show that many more have severe distress that goes undiagnosed and an even smaller percent actually receive psychological help. Counseling was cited by all countries except Spain as the most common intervention used to alleviate distress. Behavioral interventions were rated first in Spain and were second in a third of the countries surveyed. The use of psychopharmacologic agents was rated third by all countries. Psychosocial support groups are increasingly used across cultural and geo-political boundaries. Reach to Recovery for breast cancer patients is the best known and was cited as the most widely used internationally.

While these services are available to more patients, in most countries, they are usually not provided through a designated psycho-oncology unit in general hospitals or cancer centers. At the present time, most cancer patients with psychological and social problems are managed by the nurse or social worker and only severe problems are referred by the oncologist to a mental health professional. In most countries, this would be a psychiatrist, psychologist, clinical nurse specialist or social worker, who work closely with clergy to assure attention to spiritual needs. However, we are beginning to see small psycho-oncology units comprised of an integrated multidisciplinary team which provides these services (see Chapter 90). Such units at present are limited to a few in the United States, United Kingdom, Canada, and Japan, where its first Psycho-Oncology Unit was established at the National Cancer Research Center under Uchitomi in 1995.

Opportunities for training in psycho-oncology and education for oncology staff in psychosocial issues are extremely limited on a global level. Indeed, a more basic need is for the development of training modules which provide the materials and curricular components that are tailored to the culture as well. Under the aegis of IPOS, a model international curriculum in psycho-oncology was developed and reported by Die-Trill and Holland in 1995 (6). The pioneering and internationally known programs in Europe, particularly those of Razavi in Belgium, Ratzak in Germany, Greer, Watson, and Maguire in the United Kingdom and in North America are based in hospitals or cancer centers, many of which relate to universities. New efforts are reported in Israel, Uruguay, Japan, and Greece, where they are based in clinical settings, or directed by cancer-related societies. In Turkey, the University of Istanbul has started a Master's program for psychologists and social workers and its goal is to develop understanding of the psychosocial issues in cancer care and to improve the communication skills of these caregivers. Efforts are now under way in Brazil to train mental health professionals in psycho-oncology. Worldwide, the trend is for cancer centers or hospitals with large cancer units to include psycho-oncology principles in the training of medical staff as well as the training of mental health professionals in this subspecialty. However, globally, efforts are modest compared with the need for these concepts and services to be incorporated into overall care.

The IPOS survey explored the degree to which oncologists believed that patients' pain and psychological distress in their country were recognized and treated. Sixty percent of the countries reported that pain was more likely to be recognized and treated than psychological distress, which was likely to remain unrecognized and untreated. This trend reflects the international effort put forth in the past decade by both national groups interested in pain and the World Health Organization, as well as the growing attention to palliative care and pain control. The United Kingdom, Canada, Australia and Italy have spearheaded much of these efforts to make narcotic analgesics more widely available and to educate oncology staff in simple treatment guidelines. The World Health Organization Pain Ladder has been a highly successful teaching tool. Similar efforts are needed to focus on the management of psychological distress.

In psycho-oncology research, small units in Sweden, the United Kingdom, and United States represented the total effort until the 1980s. Since then, other centers have been able to develop, but numbers remain small. Most psychosocial and behavioral research is done at academic medical centers or at cancer institutes. The three designated World Health Organization Collaborating Centers for Cancer Pain Relief and Study of Quality of Life are important identified efforts in Amsterdam, Winnepeg, and New York. Some cancer societies and public health institutes focus on psychosocial research. The WHO Center in Amsterdam represents an important pioneering effort directed since the late 1970s by van Dam. More recently, Aaronson, in the same center, has organized a major landmark effort involving other mental health professionals to provide valid quality of life measurement in the European Organization for Research in the Treatment of Cancer (EORTC) (see Chapter 1).

Oncologists taking part in the IPOS survey were asked to identify the principal barriers to the improvement of psychosocial care for cancer patients in their country. Negative attitudes toward psychological issues and economic constraints were noted as the major barriers. There was consensus that in institutions where the model is strictly biomedical, it has been hard to expand the psychological side of patient care and the study of interventions for treating patients' psychological distress. Limited economic resources have a vital impact in the developed countries and are an unrelenting drawback in poorer countries where neither adequate medical nor cancer care is available (see Chapter 97). The dynamism of these interacting forces also fuels the continuing lack of formal education programs in psycho-oncology and the absence of trained manpower to do the clinical and investigative work. Increased public awareness through education, more funding opportunities, more designated psycho-oncology units, undergraduate and postgraduate training programs, and support for increasing the body of research and scientific data are needed to change the status quo.

CROSS-CULTURAL RESEARCH

Despite the fact that incidence of cancers of specific sites varies across countries, the types of cancer, their biologic nature, and treatment options are similar around the world. However, the biologic similarity stands in contrast to the widely varying attitudes of people and physicians toward what patients should be told about their diagnoses, prognoses, treatment options and management of psychological issues. These attitudes reflect cultural and religious influences as well as attitudes toward the physicians's role, which is still strongly authoritarian in some cultures, while egalitarian in others. The International Society has, as part of its mission, cross-cultural research examining these cultural differences in cancer. The key cross-cultural issue which differentiates attitudes across countries has been the strong differences in the custom of revealing or withholding the diagnosis of cancer.

In 1984, IPOS conducted a cross-cultural study to see how attitudes and the use of alternative medicines varied internationally. The initial survey published by Holland and colleagues in 1987 revealed that, in much of the world, physicians did *not* tell the diagnosis to patients, though they usually told the families (2). Ninety oncologists from 20 countries participated and they reported that the use of the word "cancer" was usually avoided in discussions with patients. Other words were used implying a "swelling" or an "inflammation" or a pathophysiologic change. Countries in which revealing the diagnosis to the patient was under 40% were France, Hungary, Iran, Panama, Portugal, Spain, and the African states. By contrast, greater than 80% were estimated to be told in Austria, Denmark, Finland, Netherlands, New Zealand, Norway, Switzerland, and Sweden. However, in all countries, the majority of physicians told the family the diagnosis. Ninety percent of the oncologists believed a change was occurring toward more open disclosure of the diagnosis. Sixty-eight percent of the oncologists felt that the overall effect of telling the truth was positive (see Table 101.1).

TABLE 101.1. *Estimate of Disclosure of Diagnosis: 1984 versus 1995*

1984 n = 90 Oncologists		1995 n = 1407 Oncologists	
Low < 40%	High > 80%	Low < 50%	High > 90%
France	Austria	Nepal	Canada
Hungary	Denmark	Syria	Denmark
Iran	Finland	Greece	Switzerland
Kenya	Netherlands	Croatia	Finland
Panama	Norway	Turkey	United States
Spain	Switzerland		Australia
	Sweden		Germany
			Netherlands

A decade later, in 1995, a second survey was undertaken, under the direction of Koinuma, Die-Trill and the IPOS National Representation Committee, to see how attitudes and practices had changed (3–4). In this later survey, 1407 oncologists from 29 countries were surveyed. There was a significantly greater percentage of physicians who revealed the diagnosis to patients in western versus eastern countries ($p < 0.001$). The overall average across countries revealed that 50.8% of patients were given full disclosure of a cancer diagnosis; while 88% of family members were informed. When the diagnosis was coupled with a poor prognosis, there was a decrease to 34.0% in the likelihood of revealing it to patients and 76% for family members. The range of full disclosure varied from lowest in Greece to highest in Finland and Denmark. Sixty-one percent of the respondents indicated a trend was occurring in their country toward full disclosure.

Compared with a decade earlier, the findings in 1995 are similar. A majority continue to see a trend toward full disclosure of diagnostic and prognostic information. However, actual practice in these areas, as shown by the percentages revealed diagnoses in most countries, has not changed appreciably. In another independent survey in 1996, Loge and colleagues observed that physicians in northern and western Europe are more likely to fully disclose the diagnosis as compared with doctors in southern and eastern Europe, who withhold the diagnosis from the patient (7). Cultural and social factors clearly play a large role in these differences. Loge noted that when a society has accepted full disclosure, then the spotlight shifts to how best to reveal the diagnosis.

CONCLUSION

There is a growing concern for the quality of life of patients with cancer, and this includes their psychological state and well-being. Recognition of psychological issues in cancer prevention and detection is increasing worldwide. The development of hospice and palliative care medicine, coming from the United Kingdom in the 1960s to Australia and Canada, has provided an important shift in emphasis in education and clinical care. The psychological and spiritual dimensions have been given prominence there from the beginning, as well as pain control. Palliative care medicine continues to grow around the world and psycho-oncology has an important role to play in symptom control and management of psychological distress.

Progress is not even on all fronts and it takes time. On the one hand, we find in some areas, that things fail to advance, e.g., the widespread custom of not revealing the diagnosis and the paucity of training opportunities and funding sources. Yet, on the other hand, we find that the psychosocial needs of patients with cancer are similar across cultural and political boundaries rather than they are different. Also, the types of the interventions utilized are similar, but there are marked differences in their availability. The collection of quality of life data on patients, using the same instruments in different languages and cultures, is encouraging. Cella's work to develop standardized quality of life scores, so that comparisons of patients can occur across countries, disease site and stage, and specific quality of life instruments is important. Establishing the clinical meaning of the quality of life scores is important. These factors should also promote improvement in patient care and facilitate collaborative research on the international level.

In summary, the changes which have occurred in the short time frame of a little over a decade suggest that an optimistic outlook is appropriate and that the next decade will see more impressive gains as methods of assessment improve and oncology in general becomes more interested in outcomes research that includes survival, disease-free interval, and quality of life in its evaluation.

REFERENCES

1. Holland JC. Psycho-oncology: Overview, obstacles and opportunities. *Psycho-Oncology.* 1992; 1:1–13.
2. Holland JC, Geary N, Marchini A, Tross S. An international survey of physician attitudes and practice in regard to revealing the diagnosis of cancer. *Cancer Invest.* 1987; 5:151–154.
3. *IPOS Newsletter.* December 1995; 2, 5–6.
4. *IPOS Newsletter.* Summer 1996; 2, 9–10.
5. Holland JC. Historical overview. In: Holland JC, Rowland JH, eds. *Handbook of Psychooncology: Psychological Care of the Patient with Cancer.* New York: Oxford University Press; 1989: 3–12.
6. Die-Trill M, Holland JC. A model curriculum for training in psycho-oncology. *Psycho-Oncology.* 1995; 4: 169–182.
7. Loge JH, Kaasa S, Ekeberg O, et al. Attitudes toward informing the cancer patient—a survey of Norwegian physicians. *Eur J Cancer.* 1996; 32:1344–1348.

XVIII

POLICY ISSUES

EDITOR: JIMMIE C. HOLLAND

102

Bridging the Gap Between Research, Clinical Practice, and Policy

JESSIE C. GRUMAN AND RENA CONVISSOR

Psycho-oncology is entering an era in which there are tremendous opportunities to expand its influence but there are substantial challenges to overcome in order to do so. The contributions of psycho-oncology to improve the lives of cancer patients will only take place through the combined efforts of researchers, clinicians, and policy makers.

It is clear that merely treating the disease of cancer is not sufficient to ensure optimal health outcomes. For health care providers to ignore the context in which cancer occurs is neither humane nor effective, and certainly not medically responsible. A growing body of evidence confirms the impact of psychological, social, behavioral, economic, and environmental factors on the progression and management of cancer. Today, more and more health care providers recognize that the consideration of these factors as part of standard cancer care can lead to more efficacious disease management. There is also greater awareness that specific psychosocial interventions can limit cancer's negative impact on patient functioning in ways that are acceptable to patients and are often cost-effective for providers. For the first time in the history of psycho-oncology, changes in the structure of health care delivery may provide the opening for widespread integration of behavioral and psychosocial concerns in the prevention, detection, treatment, and rehabilitation of cancer.

The stunning successes in biomedical cancer research over the past two decades are part of a larger series of victories in preventing and treating diseases that have helped millions of people all over the world to live longer and healthier lives. These biomedical successes paradoxically present new challenges for the field of psycho-oncology:

- The more we know about cancer, the more complicated it becomes. For example, new information about the effects of social support, exercise, diet, smoking, and genetic factors on cancer has implications for how we intervene to prevent cancer and how cancer patients and their families are treated.
- As more and more people survive cancer, our understanding of the long-term physical and psychological effects of cancer and cancer treatment is enhanced. With this expanded knowledge, new areas and opportunities for treatment arise.

The challenge for psycho-oncology is to improve the quality and focus of research, to demonstrate the effectiveness and efficiency of interventions to improve the lives of cancer patients, and to train researchers and clinicians in the use of this knowledge to improve the lives of cancer patients.

WHERE ARE WE NOW?

Over 8 million people in the United States are cancer survivors. Each year, approximately 1.2 million more cases of cancer will be diagnosed. The growing ranks of cancer survivors are a tribute to gains in scientific knowledge and to improved diagnostic and therapeutic techniques.

Yet in fiscal year 1993, the National Cancer Institute and the American Cancer Society combined spent only $1.56 per cancer patient on psychosocial and behavioral research, compared with $270.22 per cancer patient for biomedical research (1). Further, a survey of the National Cancer Institute's 27 Comprehensive Cancer Centers, conducted in 1994 by the Center for the Advancement of Health, found that only 24% of the Centers offer some coordinated psychosocial oncology program to their patients.

The explanations for the lack of attention to behavioral and psychosocial concerns of cancer patients are many and include the traditional medical focus on pharmacologic, radiologic, and surgical interventions designed to curb tumor growth, the lack of training of health care providers to address these issues, and the absence of well-documented, transportable intervention protocols. Whatever the historical precedents, however, the psychosocial concerns of people with cancer are still considered by many physicians, hospital administrators, and health care payers to be irrelevant to treatment of the disease, and psychosocial services are often considered luxurious add-ons. Since most psychosocial services are typically not paid for by medical insurance, there have been few incentives for institutions to offer them as standard medical care. As a result, support for research addressing the psychosocial aspects of cancer has been of low priority.

The majority of research funding for cancer research generally and psycho-oncology research specifically currently derives from two sources: the National Cancer Institute and the American Cancer Society. Both sources devote the bulk of their resources to research on cancer etiology, diagnosis, treatment, and training. But both have recently made significant commitments to increasing their investment in research directed toward helping patients to cope with cancer and cancer treatment.

THE NATIONAL CANCER INSTITUTE

The National Cancer Institute (NCI), the largest institute within the National Institutes of Health, is the lead government agency responsible for cancer research. The NCI supports a comprehensive research program in basic cancer biology, etiology, prevention, diagnosis, treatment, and rehabilitation. In fiscal year 1996, the NCI's budget was approximately $2.25 billion. The Institute asked Congress to support a budget for fiscal year 1997 of $2.28 billion, and $2.4 billion for 1998 (2).

Beginning in 1990, both the Senate and House Appropriations Committees have expressed support for an interest in the NCI expanding efforts in the area of behavioral and psychosocial research (3). In 1992, the Senate Appropriations Committee Report for fiscal year 1993 (102-397) called on the NCI to, "further explore the impact on survival and quality of life of cancer patients from psychosocial counseling services and to give greater priority to counseling services as an integral aspect of medical care" (4). Since that time, a number of such short-term funding initiatives have been funded through earmarking legislation.

In 1996, the NCI raised the priority of research to "investigate how cancer affects quality of life and find ways to address survivors' needs so they can meet the

everyday demands of life and return to a productive lifestyle." To coordinate this effort, NCI established an Office of Cancer Survivorship within the Division of Cancer Treatment, Diagnosis and Centers in the Clinical Investigations Branch within the Cancer Therapy and Evaluation Program. The purpose of the Office is to explore the research issues and consequences of cancer survivorship. The placement of the Office within the Division of Cancer Treatment is meant to send a signal of NCI's commitment to and recognition of survivorship issues as an integral part of cancer care.

It should be noted that the NCI also serves as a resource for cancer patients and their families through its Cancer Information Service (1-800-4-CANCER) and its extensive library of free patient education materials.

THE AMERICAN CANCER SOCIETY

The American Cancer Society (ACS) is the country's largest non-governmental source of funding for cancer research. The ACS raises money for research through local affiliates (Units), which are responsible to State-level organizations (Divisions), which, in turn, participate in a national-level consortium. While some Divisions make resources available for research, most pass their public contributions along to the National ACS to disseminate through a peer review process.

The ACS research program "conducts basic research, epidemiological research, preclinical and clinical research." The first psychosocial grants from the ACS were awarded in 1983 and since then, more than $14 million in grant funds have supported behavioral and psychosocial research. Historically, approximately 2% of the Society's $75 million research budget was devoted to psychosocial, behavioral and policy research. Beginning in 1996, the Society increased this amount to at least 5% with an eye toward increasing that percentage over the coming years.

The American Cancer Society also provides information about cancer to the public through their Cancer Response Service (1-800-ACS-2345) and their extensive public education publications which are available through local ACS organizations. Additionally, many local Units of ACS provide patient services such as Reach to Recovery and Look Good, Feel Better.

OTHER FUNDING RESOURCES

Funding for psycho-oncology research is becoming available through other agencies and organizations.

The United States Army has a renewable Congressional mandate to support breast cancer research and has a growing interest in supporting behavioral and psychosocial research. CaP CURE was established by Michael Milken in 1995 to increase the focus on prostate cancer research, including a limited focus on its behavioral and psychosocial aspects. A number of foundations have provided limited grants for psychosocial research and cancer over the past decade, most of which are associated with a foundation focus, e.g., children and cancer, prayer and cancer. Such grants tend to be small and time-limited.

PSYCHOSOCIAL SERVICES

In 1994, the Center for the Advancement of Health conducted a survey of the National Cancer Institute's 27 Comprehensive Cancer Centers. The survey was conducted to assess the current status of psychosocial services and to try to determine to what extent current clinical activities reflect psychosocial research efforts and priorities. The survey found that roughly 24% of the Centers offer some coordinated psychosocial oncology program to their patients, most often through the Department of Social Work. The services most often provided include support groups, individual counseling, and cancer education. The survey also found that the Centers are disturbingly unaware of the level of utilization of services, the services provided at affiliated institutions, the staffing patterns, and any psychosocial research conducted within their own institutions, but in disparate departments and Center facilities.

The findings documented the sorry state of psychosocial services as part of the cancer care continuum: if in the most advanced cancer treatment institutions in this country, these concerns were being ignored, it was certain that the national norm was similar at best. But this survey took place in 1994, the year of the proposed, then defeated, national health care reform. Market-based reform has stimulated changes that have radically shifted the shape of health care delivery in ways that hold promise for psycho-oncology.

CHANGING HEALTH CARE ENVIRONMENT

. . . health system change and the building of the national information infrastructure—are transforming American health care and dramatically affecting the health of Americans. The specific shape and pace of this transformation are impossible to predict today, but our observations of early initiatives give us some modest confidence that present day concepts of what determines health and disease, and our methods of intervening, will be dramatically different in the not too distant future . . .

—(C. Everett Koop and Michael McDonald, 1995)

Three major forces are changing today's health care environment: the health care delivery system shift toward managed care, the increasing expectation on the part of purchasers and policy makers that health plans will deliver good health at a reasonable cost, and the expanding knowledge of patients and consumers who expect to be treated as partners in their health care.

The rapid changes in the health care delivery system and the growth of managed care have enormous implications for the way cancer care—in fact, all chronic disease care—is delivered in this country. Managed care is now the dominant form of health care delivery and financing in the United States. The shift from the traditional fee-for-service medicine to managed health care systems provides unprecedented opportunities for psychosocial and behavioral interventions in cancer care. Under capititated health care (as opposed to fee-for-service) there are incentives now for health care providers to work to prevent cancer, to detect and treat it early, and to help patients to manage their illness and maintain functioning.

The financial justification for managed care stems from its ability to control costs and offer comprehensive and coordinated care. While managed care organizations may not immediately adapt the labor-intensive assessment and counseling that should be integral to cancer care, the evidence in support of these interventions makes a strong case for their inclusion: many such interventions help patients manage their pain and recover from treatment more quickly. In addition, managed care companies need to market themselves to meet patient needs. If patients demand these services, and research shows that the services result in positive health outcomes, plans will have to deliver them.

Health plans now pay attention to both the health outcomes realized from the care they deliver and the health care costs that are deferred. In addition, there is greater accountability to purchasers, regulators, and consumers for delivering comprehensive care than ever before. Health plans are focused on "doing what works," which means delivering care that has more predictable and better outcomes. This is accomplished in part by better matching services and treatments to the needs of patients, helping people to use medical services appropriately, and improving functional status so that people can return to work as contributing members of society. Psycho-oncology has much to offer in reaching these objectives.

Purchasers of health care—be they individual consumers or employers or State Medicaid directors—compare plans on the basis of more than just their cost. As pricing of health care services stabilizes, the quality of the care delivered and consumer satisfaction with that care are becoming important criteria for plan choice. Report cards which allow for the comparison of plan performance increasingly include measures of consideration of patients' behavioral and psychosocial concerns, thus providing additional incentives for health plans to attend to the special needs of cancer patients.

Patients and consumers are also having a profound impact on the way health care is delivered. Many patients are no longer willing to sit back and follow the physician's orders. Over the past ten years, the HIV/AIDS advocacy community has been a model for expanding the role of patients as partners in their own health care. Breast and prostate cancer advocates have been successful in advocating for larger NCI budgets to address those specific cancers and demanding that patients and survivors be represented on advisory committees and other decision-making bodies. Patients' rights and self-care activists encourage others to recognize the link between emotional and psychological health and their physical health. And patients themselves are much more open to psychosocial interventions and programs, although they still face some difficulties because of the stigma associated with psychological difficulties.

WHERE DO WE GO FROM HERE?

The phenomenal successes of biomedical research have conquered many of the causes of early morbidity. As the population ages, the goals of medicine must expand beyond curing disease to helping those living with cancer live for as long and as well as they can. With ongoing changes in the health care delivery system and the rise in managed care, we gain increasing opportunities to deliver vital psychosocial services in innovative clinical settings. However, while there has been an increase in both dollars and attention for psychosocial research, federal budgets are shrinking and may continue to do so for many years. A growing number of researchers will be competing for a limited amount of funds. Only through creative, collaborative

efforts will we place psychosocial research at the top of the agenda.

Researchers and clinicians work actively to bridge the gap between what is known about psychosocial and behavioral factors related to cancer and the incorporation of this knowledge into health care practice and policy:

- involving more medical specialists and primary care professionals in behavioral and psychosocial research
- working with young investigators and clinicians to spark their interest in this field
- working to overcome the stigma that patients and clinicians often associate with needing and providing psychosocial care
- providing opportunities for patients to ask for psychosocial and support services.

As the health care system is changing, so too is cancer care. As more people are living longer with and after cancer, increasing psychosocial needs and services must be addressed and provided for. This will become especially true in settings outside of cancer centers and large academic and research institutions.

Behavioral and psychosocial factors influence the onset of some kinds of cancer, the progression of many, and the management of nearly all. There is sufficient evidence available for health care delivery systems to integrate these concerns into the provision of cost-effective care that seeks to improve health-related quality of life and functioning of cancer patients in the United States. The challenge for psycho-oncology is to produce high-quality research that is relevant to the daily delivery of cancer care and to actively work to ensure that findings from this research inform further research, clinician training, and health care delivery planning.

REFERENCES

1. *The Cancer Letter*, Vol. 19, No. 47, December 3, 1993 and No. 48, December 10, 1993.
2. National Cancer Institute, The Nation's Investment in Cancer Research: A Budget Proposal for Fiscal Years 1997/1998. May, 1996.
3. NIH Revitalization Act of 1993: Conference Report Language from House Report 103-100 and Senate Language, September 29, 1993.
4. Senate Appropriations Committee Report, 102-397, 1992.

Index

4-ABP-Hb adducts, 29
ABVD regimen, 232, 409
Acetaminophen, 454, 912
Acetylcholine (ACh), 135
Acquired immunodeficiency syndrome.
   See AIDS
ACTH, 135, 136, 137, 140, 274, 335, 639, 641,
   642
Activities of daily living (ADLs), 828, 830,
   832
Acute leukemia, 411
Acute lymphocytic leukemia (ALL), 68–69,
   409, 413, 881, 897, 923, 925, 931
Acute nonlymphocytic leukemia (ANLL),
   409
Acute stress disorder, 511
Acyclovir, 635
Adaptation
   cancer survivors, 223–254
   and coping issues, 212–213
   evidence concerning, 213
   literature review, 243
   personality differences in, 214
   problems in childhood cancer survivors,
     925
   psychological issues in, 211–222
   psychosocial, 926
   social factors in, 211–222
   social support in, 213–214
   theoretical framework, 237–238
Adenocarcinoma of the stomach, 325
Adenomatous polyposis coli (APC), 181
Adjustment disorders, 233–235, 509–517
   counseling/psychotherapy, 515
   criteria defining, 509–511
   diagnosis, 513
   diagnostic categories, 510
   epidemiology, 511
   evolution and course, 514
   International Classification of Disease-10
     (ICD-10), 511
   maladaptation, 513
   mechanisms precipitating, 511–512
   pharmacotherapy, 515–516
   treatment, 514
Adjuvant chemotherapy in fatigue, 486
Adjuvant hormonal therapy in breast cancer,
   391–392
Adjuvant psychotropic analgesics, 458–461
Adjuvant therapies, 817
Adrenal insufficiency, 641

β-Adrenergic agonists, 556
β-Adrenergic antagonists, 532
Adrenocorticostimulating hormone.
   See ACTH
Adrenocorticotropic hormone. *See* ACTH
Adriamycin, 70, 335, 356, 409, 414
African-Americans, 167, 168
Agency for Health Care Policy and Research
   (AHCPR), 32, 454
Aggression, 959–960
Aging, epidemiology, 839
Agitation, 919
Agoraphobia, 558
AIDS, 94, 1035
   cognitive disorders in, 420
   dementia in, 420
   neurologic complications, 420–422
   psychiatric disorders in, 419
   psychological sequelae, 417–426
   resource allocation, 1120
   surveillance case definition, 418
Akathisia, 309, 489, 556
ALARM model for risk prediction, 363
Alcohol consumption, 45–48
   biochemical pathways in cancer, 46–47
   and breast cancer, 46
   and colorectal carcinoma, 46
   and head and neck cancer, 45, 318
   and liver carcinoma, 46
   and pancreatic carcinoma, 46
   screening, 658
Alcohol withdrawal syndrome, 590–591
Alcoholism, 587–594
   aftercare, 593
   assessment, 589–590
   comorbid psychiatric disorders, 588–589
   defined, 587
   historical perspective, 587
   medical treatment of withdrawal, 591
   pharmacological approach, 592
   prevalence, 587, 589
   primary/secondary, 588–589
   psychotherapeutic approach, 591–592
   psychotherapeutic management of cancer
     patient, 589–593
   treatment modalities, 591–593
Alprazolam, 439, 444, 557, 558, 956, 959
Alternative therapies, 817–827
   belief in psychological effects, 821–822
   cancer of unknown primary (CUP),
     432–433

   definition, 818
   guidelines for oncology staff, 824
   heroic stance, 822–823
   historical context, 819
   implications for clinical care, 823–824
   implications for mental health theory,
     824–825
   prevalence, 819–821
American Cancer Society (ACS), 6, 8, 45, 46,
   52, 161, 162, 349, 1173, 1174
American Society for Control of Cancer, 6
American Society of Human Genetics, 186
American Society of Psychiatric-Oncology/
   AIDS, 11
Aminoglutethimide, 392
Amitriptyline, 460, 536, 617
Amoxapine, 535
Amphetamines, 632
Amphotericin B, 635
Analgesics, 454, 917
Anger suppression, 117–118
Animal cancer models, 126
Ankle foot orthosis (AFO), 831
Anorexia, 468
Anthracycline, 409
Antianxiety medications, 605
Antibiotics, 634–635
Antibody-dependent cellular cytotoxicity
   (ADCC), 128
Anticholinergic drugs, 566
Anticipatory nausea and vomiting (ANV),
   721–723
Antidepressant analgesics, 454
Antidepressant medications in advanced
   disease, 442
Antidepressants, 439, 440, 459, 534, 535, 556,
   593, 605, 617, 956
Antidiuretic hormone (ADH), 646
Antiemetics, 478, 479, 556, 630, 631
Antifungals, 634–635
Antigenicity, 127–128
Antihistamines, 439, 955
Anti-inflammatory agents, 635
Antineoplastic drugs, 632, 633
Antipsychotic drugs, 616, 617
Antisocial personality disorder, 628
Antivirals, 634–635
Anxiety
   acute symptoms, 552
   in childhood cancer, 919, 955
   chronic, preexisting, 552

Anxiety (*cont.*)
clinical presentation, 552
course and outcome, 556–557
demographic variables, 553
diagnosis, 548–549
in HIV, 420
disorders, 548–563
drug effects in, 556
etiologic factors, 553
management, 557
measurement, 549
medical conditions associated with, 555
organic factors, 554
pharmacological treatment, 557
premorbid adjustment, 553
prevalence, 550–552
psychological treatment, 558
in radiotherapy, 270, 554
role of treatment, 553–554
and stage of neoplastic disease, 553
substance-induced, 555
syndromes, fatigue, 488–489
in terminally ill patient, 438
treatment, 557
Anxiolytics, 412, 439, 592, 916, 956, 1029
Apoptosis, 16
Aromatherapy, 464
Art therapy, 464, 743–757
cancer patients with psychiatric symptoms, 748
childhood cancer, 951–952
cognitive-symbolic dimension, 744
communicative dimensions, 744
death and dying, 747
expressive-creative dimension, 743
future directions and lines of research, 755–756
groups, 745
historical roots, 743
hospitalized children, 745–746
individual, 745
interactive-analytic dimension, 744
interventions, 744–745
medical issues, 745–750
need for innovative interventions, 745
patients in isolation, 747
and psychological self-healing, 749–750
studio-based, 744–745
therapeutic factors, 750–754
tripolar field, 744
visual imagery in, 743–744
working with pain, fatigue, and stress, 746–747
working with staff, caregivers, and relatives, 749
Asparaginase, 409, 445, 642
Aspirin, 635
Association of Oncology Social Work (AOSW), 1067
Asterixis, 458
Asymptomatic illness, 163
Attitudes of society toward cancer, 4–7
Avoidant personality disorder, 627
Axillary mass, 429–430
Azidothymidine (AZT), 635

Basal cell carcinoma, 60–61
diagnosis, 372
etiology, 371–372
incidence, 371
mortality, 371

prevention, 372
prognosis, 373
treatment, 372
BCNU, 304, 414, 445
Beck Depression Inventory, 551
Bedside interventions, 809–816
needs and future directions, 815
Behavioral interventions, 203, 440, 559
in childhood cancer, 962–977
in stressful diagnostic and treatment procedures, 964
post-treatment readjustment in childhood cancer, 974
treatment side effects in childhood cancer, 973
Behavioral management in nausea and vomiting, 480–481
Behavioral manipulation, 412
Behavioral therapy, 514
Behavioral training, 558
Behavioral treatment in cachexia, 474
Benzodiazepines, 439, 444, 447, 479, 557, 558, 566, 591, 592, 593, 617, 916, 919, 956, 959, 1029
Bereavement, 115, 129, 981, 1016–1032
in childhood, 1027–1028
in childhood cancer, 920–921
clinical features, 1018
cultural factors, 862
definition, 1017
following specific losses, 1026
health consequences, 1024–1025
hospice care in, 1030
inability to separate, 1020
interventions, 1028–1030
loss of child, 1026–1027
loss of parent in adulthood, 1026
loss of sibling during childhood, 1028
loss of sibling in adulthood, 1026
models for understanding, 1017
morbidity and mortality associated with, 1025
mutual help, 1029
outcome prediction, 1023
psychopharmacology in, 1029
psychotherapy in, 1028–1029
Berg's Spiritual Injury Scale, 795
Biofeedback techniques, 464
Biologic modifiers, 635
Biologic pathways, 737–738
Biologic response modifiers, 504
Biology of cancer, 16–23
Biomarkers of carcinogenesis, 29
Biotherapy, 279
side effects, 279–280
Bladder cancer
diagnosis and management, 355–356
epidemiology, 355
sexual function in, 331, 355
Bladder disorders, 832
Bleomycin, 232, 409, 445, 478
α_1-Blockade, 441
Body dysmorphic disorder (BDD), 611
Body image, 225, 237, 469
Bone, sarcomas, 402–403
Bone marrow aspiration, 965
Bone marrow transplantation (BMT), 223, 231, 233, 234, 289–299, 392, 406, 409, 411, 414, 975
allogeneic, 289–291, 293
autologous, 289–291, 293

decision to undergo, 291–292
historical overview, 289
hospital discharge and early post-BMT recovery, 293
indications for, 290
involved in, 289–290
long-term recovery, 294
marrow donor, 296–297
medical overview, 289
medical staff, 297
neuropsychological impact, 503–504
patient, 291
patient's family, 294–296
post-BMT hospitalization, 292–294
pre-BMT preparation, 292
psychosocial and behavioral issues, 291–297
quality of life, 294, 415
syngeneic, 289, 293
Borderline personality disorder, 623–624
Bowel disorders, 832
Brain edema in radiotherapy, 273
Brain metastases, 304–305, 307
Brain tumors, 304, 500–501
pediatric, 940–941
BRCA1 testing criteria, 191
Breast cancer, 182, 190, 380–401, 429
adjuvant chemotherapy, 390
adjuvant hormonal therapy, 391–392
advanced disease, 392
and alcohol consumption, 46
chemotherapy, 390–391
computer risk counseling, 190–192
denial regarding, 197
diet in, 73–74
factors contributing to psychological responses, 381
genetic risk counseling, 191
incidence patterns, 81–82
inherited predisposition, 197
interventions, 392–393
limited resection and radiation (L-R), psychological response, 387
lumpectomy and irradiation, 386
mastectomy, 385
psychological response, 387
medical variables, 385–392
misconceptions and myths, 197
psychiatric evaluation, 385
psychological issues in risk, 196
psychological variables, 383–385
psychosocial factors, 380–392
public attitudes, 383
quality of life, 395–396
radiotherapy, 388
risk assessment, 190
risk counseling (BCRC), 201
role and care of family, 393–395
screening, 198
sexual functioning, 395–396, 495
sociocultural context, 380
special issues, 393–396
TNM classification, 19
treatment choices, 381–383
Breast Cancer Prevention Trial (BCPT), 200
Breast conservation, 388
Breast reconstruction, 388–390
immediate versus delayed, 390
Breast self-examination (BSE), 198
Breast surgery
psychosocial issues, 262–263

and sexual functioning, 233
See also Mastectomy
Brief Pain Inventory (BPI), 1149, 1154
Brief Symptom Inventory (BSI), 224, 655, 659
British Psychosocial Oncology Group, 12
Bronchodilators, 556
Bupropion, 444, 535
Butyrophenones, 479

Cachexia, 468–475
  behavioral treatment in, 474
  clinical features, 469–471
  definition, 468
  HIV-related, 472
  mechanisms of, 471–472
  nutritional supplementation in, 473–474
  pharmacologic treatment, 472–473
  psychological factors, 470–471
  social and cultural factors, 470
  systemic effects, 469
  treatment, 472–474
CAGE Questionnaire, 590
Calcium, 642–644
  formation, 62
  intake, 50
Caloric intake, 50, 51
Cancer
  attitudes of society toward, 4–7
  events altering perceptions of, 5–6
  family syndrome, 189
  prevention counseling, 189
  psychological adjustment to, 4
  risk counseling, 188–189
  societal views of, 1
Cancer and Leukemia Group B (CALGB),
    10, 1137
Cancer cells, 17
Cancer Information test, 683
Cancer Inventory of Problem Situations
    (CIPS), 686, 692
Cancer of unknown primary (CUP), 427–433
  alternative therapies, 432–433
  continuation of treatment, 431–432
  cytogenetic evaluation, 428
  dealing with anticipatory grief, 432
  definition, 427
  diagnostic evaluation, 427–428
  identification of treatable subgroups, 429
  oncologic therapy, 430
  pathologic evaluation, 428
  psychiatric aspects, 430–432
  psychological adjustment, 431
  psychosocial aspects, 430–432
  quality of life, 431–432
  solitary site of disease, 429
  treatable types, 429
  tumor markers, 428
Cancer-prone pedigree, 177
Cancer Rehabilitation Evaluation System
    (CARES), 1136
Cancer risk
  assessment
    in breast cancer, 190
    tumor markers, 151
  colon cancer, 82
  counseling, 190, 200
  lung cancer, 80–81
  prediction, ALARM model for, 363
  psychological issues in, 196–198
  reduction behaviors and childhood, 52–53
  and schizophrenia, 615

Cancer survivors. *See* Survival
Cancer susceptibility, 201
CANCERLIT, 341
Cannabinoids, 479
Carcinogenesis, biomarkers of, 29
Carcinoid tumors, 645–646
Carmustine, 479
Case-control studies, human stress, 112–114
Catharsis in art therapy, 750
Cefaclor, 634
Cell biology, 16
Cell cycle, 176
Cell genetics, somatic, 178–180
Center for Epidemiological Studies-
    Depression Scale (CES-D), 224
CentiMorgan (cM), 177
Central nervous system (CNS), 132
  drugs acting through, 631–632
  effects, 630, 632–635
  leukemia, 409
  lymphoma, 423, 424
  paraneoplastic disorders, 647
  prophylaxis, 413, 414
  radiotherapy, 501–502
  side effects, 413
  toxicity, 630
Central nervous system tumors, 303–313
  psychiatric and psychosocial aspects,
    305–307
  psychosocial impact on families, 310–311
  psychotherapeutic and
    psychopharmacologic interventions
    for patients' families and staff,
    307–308
  quality of life, 312
  See also Neuro-oncologic illnesses
Cephalexin, 634
Cephazolin, 634
Cervical cancer, 365–366, 423
Cervical Pap smears, 169
Chalder Fatigue Scale, 1155
Chemoprevention intervention trials, 72–73
Chemotherapy, 20–23, 277–278
  adjuvant, 20
  and anxiety disorders, 554
  aversive reactions, 721–723
  childhood cancer, 894
  cognitive-behavioral interventions, 721–723
  combination, 22, 277–278
  compliance with cancer treatment, 68–71
  fatigue, 486–488
  goals of, 278
  interpreting reports of side effects, 631
  introduction of, 8
  nausea and vomiting, 476–480
  neoadjuvant, 20
  neurologic and neuropsychological impact,
    502–503
  neuropsychiatric side effects, 630–638
  potential outcomes, 278
  psychological issues
    at end of and after treatment, 283–285
    before treatment, 280
    during treatment, 280
  psychological preparation, 391
  quality of life, 285
  side effects, 281–283, 486
  smoking cessation in, 30
  toxicity, 278
  See also under specific drugs

Chernobyl nuclear power plant accident,
    871–873
Child–physician interaction, 893–894
Childhood cancer, 881–896
  age factor, 926
  by age and site, 886
  alterations in physical appearance, 900
  anticipatory symptoms, 900
  anxiety, 919, 955
  art therapy, 951–952
  behavioral interventions, 962–977
  bereavement in, 920–921
  biologic differences between children and
    adults, 887
  chemotherapy, 894
  clinical manifestations, 887–892
  coping strategies, 946
  countertransference in, 952
  depression, 919, 957
  distress associated with medical procedures,
    899–900
  dyspnea in, 918
  epidemiology, 881
  ethical dilemmas, 907–909
  etiology, 881–887
  factors influencing child reactions, 964
  family adaptation to, 901–903
  family considerations, 893
  genetic–environmental interactions, 890
  impediments to treatment administration,
    898–899
  incidence, 887
  insomnia, 959
  late effects of therapy, 894
  long-term sequelae in, 925
  management, 892–895
  mortality, 885
  nausea and vomiting, 900, 917, 973
  pain management, 909–917, 959
  palliative care, 907–909
  play in, 947–948
  prognostic factors, 892
  psychological problems of curative
    treatment, 897–906
  psychopharmacology, 954–961
  psychosis, 958
  psychotherapeutic techniques, 949–951
  psychotherapist's role, 948
  psychotherapy in, 946–953
  PTSD, 955, 957
  refractory symptoms, 920
  risk reduction behaviors, 52–53
  school adjustment, 900–901
  seizures, 919
  single gene traits associated with, 888–890
  social adjustment, 901
  specific tumors, 895
  survivors. *See* Survival
  terminal care, 960
  work with parents, 952
Children
  of cancer patients, 984–985
  screening, 657–658
Children's Global Assessment Scale, 511
Chlordiazepoxide, 591
Chlorpromazine, 440, 446, 473, 532, 616, 920
Chondrosarcoma, 402
Chromosomal aberrations, 891
Chronic myelocytic leukemia (CML), 409,
    411
Chronic myelogenous leukemia (CML), 279

Chutzpah hypothesis, 131
Cigarette smoking. *See* Smoking cessation;
    Tobacco use
Cilastin, 635
Ciprofloxacin, 635
Cisplatin, 70, 356, 445, 478, 632–633
Claus model, 190
Claustrophobia, 559
Clinical breast examinations (CBE), 198
Clonazepam, 439, 440, 557, 956
Clotrimazole, 635
Clozapine, 473
Clozaril, 572
CMF treatment, 233
Co-analgesics, 460
Codeine, 632
Cognitive-behavioral interventions, 514, 605,
    717–729
    chemotherapy, 721–723
    emotional well-being, 723–726
    in pain, 462–463
Cognitive disorders, 565
    in AIDS, 420
    in HIV, 420
    in lung cancer, 341–342
Cognitive distraction in nausea and vomiting,
    481
Cognitive functioning, 500–505
    neuropsychological assessment, 283
Cognitive sequelae in childhood cancer
    survivors, 927, 940–945
Cohort studies, human stress, 114
Colon cancer, 181
    risk factors, 82
Colorectal cancer, 326–333
    and alcohol consumption, 46
    ostomies, 329–333
    prevention and early detection, 327
    quality of life, 333
    rehabilitation and psychosocial adaptation,
        333
    screening, 164
    sexual function in, 331
    sphincter saving versus sacrificing surgical
        procedures, 328
    treatment and rehabilitation, 327–328
    types of ostomies and possible sequelae and
        complications, 329–333
Colostomy, psychosocial issues, 263–264
Commitment versus disengagement, 212–213
Communicating risk concepts, 187
Communication barriers, 236
Communication in art therapy, 751–752
Community-based interventions, 168
Complementary therapies, 817–827
    belief in psychological effects, 821–822
    definition, 817–818
    historical context, 819
    implications for clinical care, 823–824
    prevalence, 819–821
Complex ethics/psychiatry case, 1128–1129
Compliance with cancer treatment, 67–77
    adolescent, 68–70
    adult, 70–72
    clinic appointments, 71
    control protocols, 72–74
    dietary interventions in breast cancer, 73
    follow-up recommendations after
        abnormal examination, 67–68
    pediatric, 68–70
    protocols, 68–72

radiation therapy, 68
research, 74–75
strategies to improve, 72
Compliance with medical treatment, 736–737
Compulsiveness, 624–625
Computer risk counseling, breast cancer, 190–
    192
Conditioned nausea and vomiting, 226
Conflicted grief syndrome, 1023
Confusion, 919
Connections in art therapy, 752–753
Consent issues, 261
Consolidated Omnibus Reconciliation Act
    (COBRA) of 1986, 229
Constitutional cytogenetic disorders, 890
Consultation-liaison psychiatry, 1123–1124
Containment, 982
    in art therapy, 752
Conversion disorder, 610–611
Coping, 91–94, 676
    with ambiguity and feelings of loss of
        control, 869
    and disease outcome, 92–93
    issues and adaptation, 212–213
    methodologic issues, 91–93
    styles, 93–94
    ultimate function of, 212
Coping responses, 215
    cross-sectional studies, 215
    and personality, 217
    and physical well-being, 217
Coping skills training, 203–204
Coping strategies, 735–736
    childhood cancer, 946
Coping style, childhood cancer survivors, 926
Corticosteroids, 469, 473, 479, 489, 916
Corticotropin-releasing factor (CRF),
    135–140
Corticotropin-releasing hormone (CRH), 335,
    642
Cortisol, 639–642
Counseling, cancer risk, 200
Countertransference, 699–700
    in childhood cancer, 952
Creativity in art therapy, 751
Crisis counseling, 662–675
    advancing disease, 670
    bereavement, 670
    diagnosis, 664–669
    guidelines, 672–673
    impact on patient and family, 664–670
    primary aims, 670–677
    recurrence, 669
    remission, 669
    terminal stage, 670
    treatment, 669
Cross-cultural research, 1167–1168
Cross-sectional studies, coping responses, 215
Cultural factors, 857–866
    beliefs about cancer causation, 858
    bereavement, 862
    communication patterns, 858–859
    cross-cultural research, 1167–1168
    death and dying, 862
    disclosure of medical information, 859–860
    family roles in cancer care, 860–861
    improving patient care, 863
    pain, 861
    patient–physician relationships, 862
Cushing's syndrome, 639–641
Cutaneous malignant melanoma (CMM), 61

Cyclin-dependent kinases (CDKs), 176
Cyclophosphamide, 70, 233, 354, 479
CYP2D6 genotype, 40
Cyproheptadine, 473
Cytarabine, 409
Cytogenetics, 187
    cancer of unknown primary (CUP), 428
Cytokines, 139, 140
    in fatigue, 489
Cytosine arabinoside (Ara-C), 414, 634
Cytoxan, 70

Dacarbazine, 232, 409
Dactinomycin, 414
Days after administration, 479
Death and dying, 1004
    art therapy, 747
    cultural factors, 862
    in the home, 1013–1014
    religion in, 785–786
    responses to news of death, 1019
    See also Bereavement
Decision-making, proxy, 1100–1103
Delirium, 305, 445–447, 564–575, 958
    arousal and cognition, 567–568
    assessment, 568
    chemotherapy-induced, 570
    clinical features, 564–565
    diagnostic criteria, 566–567
    etiologies/differential diagnosis, 569–570
    management, 570–572
    opioid-induced, 458
    and pain, 572
    pathophysiology, 565–566
    prevalence, 564
    in suicide, 543
    subtypes, 566, 572
Delirium tremens (DTs), 588, 590
Dementia, 305–306, 958
    in AIDS, 420
    in HIV, 420
Dependency, 623–624
Dependent grief syndrome, 1022–1023
Dependent personality disorder, 623–626
Depressed mood, 115–116
Depression, 310, 333, 441, 518–540
    anticancer drugs associated with, 532
    art therapy, 751–752
    bereavement-related, 1023
    biologic markers, 135–136, 520
    in cancer patients, 531
    in childhood cancer, 919, 957
    diagnosis in patients with cancer, 531
    drugs causing, 532
    in elderly patients, 533
    electroconvulsive therapy (ECT) in, 537
    evaluating, 519
    following surgery, 262
    in human immunodeficiency virus (HIV),
        417–420
    hypothalamic-pituitary-adrenal (HPA) axis
        in, 136–137
    in medical illnesses, 521
    measuring, 519–520
    in neurological diseases, 521
    nonpharmacologic treatment, 445
    prevalence in medically ill patients, 520–522
    prevalence in patients with cancer, 522–531
    prevalence in patients with cancer referred
        for psychiatric consultation, 522
    psychological treatment, 534

with psychotic features, 532
somatic therapies, 534
in suicide, 543
treatment, 534–537
Depression, Anxiety, and Global Severity Index, 683
Depressive personality disorder, 625–626
Desensitization intervention, 963
Desipramine, 536, 1029
Detachment, 627
Dexamethasone, 473, 479, 489
Dexamethasone suppression test (DST), 136, 138, 520
Dextroamphetamine, 458, 461, 489, 537, 556, 632, 916
Diagnosis, 18
Diagnostic and Statistical Manual of Mental Disorders (DSM-IV), 518
Diagnostic Instrument Scale, 511
Diazepam, 439, 956
Diet, 49–57
in breast cancer, 73–74
calorie intake, 50
childhood risk reduction, 52–53
excess calories, 51
excess intakes of carcinogens, 51
excesses, 50–51
fat intake, 50
fatty acids, 51
fiber intake, 49–50
inadequacies, 49–50
micronutrient deficiencies, 50
nonnutrient food components, 50
and nutritional strategies, 51–53
oils, 51
optimal cancer risk reduction, 53–54
public health measures, 51–52
specific guidelines, 53–54
Dietary Guidelines for Americans, 51
Digital rectal examination (DRE), 349
Diphenhydramine, 956
Disclosure of medical information, 859–860
Disclosure statements, 192
Disease continuum, 664, 665–667
Disease-free survival (DFS), 147
Disease outcome
and coping, 92–93
and psychiatric symptoms, 93
Disengagement versus commitment, 212–213
DNA, 16, 19, 47, 175–178
DNA damage, 60, 180
DNA mismatch repair proteins, 182
DNA-reactive agents, 51
Doxepin, 536
Doxorubicin, 70, 232
Dramatization, 625
Dronabinol, 473
Drosophila, 177
Drug abuse. *See* Substance abuse disorders
Drug effects
in anxiety disorders, 556
delirium, 570
Drug withdrawal symptoms, 582
Drug withdrawal syndromes, 556
Drugs
clinical screening for neurotoxicity, 635
depression caused by, 532
and their indications, 21–22
DSM-III, 511, 512, 519, 520, 522, 551
DSM-III-R, 512, 519, 549, 565, 595, 604, 611

DSM-IV, 510–513, 520, 531, 549, 565, 577, 578, 595, 598, 599, 603, 608, 609, 611, 615, 619, 620
Ductal adenocarcinomas, 333
Dying. *See* Death and dying
Dyspnea
in childhood cancer, 918
measurement, 1157

Ecogenetics, 188
Education, 11, 558, 676, 735
See also Training
Elderly patients, 839–844
care in nursing homes, 842
mental health problems, 840
pain, 840–841
psychosocial assessment, 841–842
psychosocial problems, 839–840
role of family caregivers, 842–843
Electrocardiogram (ECG), 916
Electroconvulsive therapy (ECT), 444–445, 537
Electroencephalographic (EEG) biofeedback-assisted relaxation, 464
Electromyographic biofeedback-assisted relaxation (EIVIG), 464
Emesis, anticipatory, 478
Emotion-focused coping, 869
Emotional distress, 518
and lung cancer, 341
Emotional support, 676, 982
Emotional suppression, 117–118
Emotional well-being, 1136
cognitive-behavioral interventions, 723–726
Employee Retirement and Income Security Act of 1974 (ERISA), 229
Employment discrimination, 228
Employment problems, 228
Endocrine effects in radiotherapy, 274
Endocrine therapy, 279
Endocrine tumors, 639
Endometrial cancer, 366
Energy management, psychological aspects, 488
Engagement versus giving up, 212
Environmental effects, 189
Environmental exposures, 870–874
Environmental manipulation, 412
Environmental stressors, 1125–1126
Epidural anesthesia, 917
Epidural spinal cord compression (ESCC), 306
Epstein-Barr Virus (EBV), 127
Esophageal adenocarcinomas, 325
Esophageal cancer, 325
initial symptoms, diagnosis and surgery, 325
recovery after surgery and rehabilitation, 325
Ethical issues, 1096–1111
childhood cancer, 907–909
genetic testing, 204–205
and psychiatry, 1123–1131
research, 1091
See also Euthanasia; Living wills; Palliative treatment; Physician-assisted suicide; Resource allocation; Terminal care; Truth-telling
Ethical, Legal and Social Issues (ELSI) unit, 192

European Organization for Research and Treatment of Cancer (EORTC), 10
Quality of Life Questionnaire, 1136
European School of Oncology, 11
European Society of Psychosocial Oncology (ESPO), 11
Eutectic mixture of local anesthetics (EMLA), 917
Euthanasia, 1103–1109
Event implications, 868
Ewing's sarcoma, 402

Factitious disorders, 612
Fallopian tube cancer, 367
False negatives, tumor markers, 153
False positives, tumor markers, 154
Familial aggregation, 188
Familial cancer syndromes, 180
Family
adaptation to childhood cancer, 901–903
adaptation to childhood cancer survivors, 924–925
beliefs, 986
considerations in childhood cancer, 893
consultation, 989
development stages, 985–986
environment in childhood cancer survivors, 926
evaluation models, 988
history, 189, 986
impact of cancer, 664–670
interventions, 989–991, 996
involvement, 981–993
acute phases, 983–984
chronic phases, 984
patient care, 982
as second order patients, 984
monitoring, 850
needs assessment, 989
organization, 986
reaction to staff behaviors, 987
referral issues, 987–988
role in cancer care, 860–861
role in care of elderly patients, 842–843
role in supportive care, 997
role of religion in, 786
as second-order patient, 999–1001
stressors in palliative home care, 1010–1013
therapy, 994–1003
new opportunities for, 1001
Family Adaptability and Cohesion Scale (FACES III), 986
Family Environment Scale (FES), 986
Family Relationship Index (FRI), 986
Family/treatment interface, 986–987
Fat intake, 50
Fatigue, 485–493
adjuvant chemotherapy in, 486
in advanced cancer, 489–490
anxiety syndromes, 488–489
in cancer survivors, 490
character and meaning of symptom, 485
and chemotherapy, 486–488
and cytokines, 489
emotional components, 488
measurement, 486, 1154
mechanisms related to chemotherapy, 487
and mood disorder, 488
and pain, 489
presentations, 486
in radiotherapy, 273, 487–488

Fatigue (*cont.*)
  in suicide, 543
  and surgery, 488
  treatment-related, 486–488
Fatigue Self Report Scale (PFS), 1155
Fatty acids in diet, 51
Fear of disfigurement or death, 197
Fear of loss of control of developmentally
    achieved functions, 622
Fear of loss of love and approval, 622
Fear of loss of or injury to body parts, 622
Fear of recurrence, 225
Fear of strangers, 621
Female first-degree relatives (FDRs), 198
  quality of life of, 395
Fertility/infertility effects, 231–233, 354,
    363–364
Fetal occult blood test (FOBT), 169
α-Fetal protein (AFP), 429
α-Fetoprotein (AFP), 354
Fiber intake, 49
Fighting spirit, 116–117, 214
First-degree relative (FDR), 196
Fluconazole, 635
Fluorouracil (5-Fu), 70, 233, 335, 445, 487,
    632
Fluoxetine, 460, 535, 556, 592, 605, 617
Fluphenazine, 461, 473, 532
Fluvoxamine, 443
Focus Assessment Criteria, 800–801
Food and Drug Administration (FDA), 372
Food aversions, 470
Food Guide Pyramid, 51
Foscarnet, 635
Functional Assessment of Cancer Therapy
    (FACT) Measurement System, 1136
Functional Living Index-Cancer (FLIC), 1136

Gail model, 191
Gamma-aminobutyric acid (GABA) systems,
    566
Gastrointestinal cancer, 324–339
  future investigations, 336
  prevalence, 324
  See also Colorectal cancer; Esophageal
      cancer; Pancreatic cancer; Stomach
      cancer
General health education (GHE), 201
General Health Questionnaire (GHQ), 224
General Hospital Questionnaire (GHQ), 657
Genes, 175, 187
  in rare familial cancers, 180
Genetic analysis, 175, 176–178
Genetic counseling
  application, 186
  definition, 186
  identifying patients and families for, 188
  role in psycho-oncology, 187
  standard protocol, 202
  training and standards, 186
Genetic screening, 183
Genetic testing, 190–192, 196–207
  attitudes to, 201
  decision counseling, 204
  ethical principles of, 204–205
  uptake of, 201
Genetics, 175–185
Genitourinary (GU) cancer, 349–358
  See also Bladder cancer; Prostate cancer;
      Renal carcinoma; Testicular cancer

Genitourinary surgery, psychosocial issues,
    264–265
Genotypic analysis, 183
Gentamicin, 635
Gestational trophoblastic disease (GTD), 367
Giving up versus engagement, 212
Glioblastoma multiforme (GBM), 304
Global dysfunction model, 566
Global Severity Index (GSI) Score, 659
Glucocorticoids, 304, 635
Glucocorticosteroids, 445
Glucose, 644–645
Glutamate-sensitive *N*-methyl-D-aspartate
    receptors, 566
Graft-versus-host disease (GVHD), 291, 293,
    409
Grief, 1017
  acute, 1020–1021
  anticipatory, 1017, 1018–1020
  chronic, 1022–1023
  complicated, 1017, 1022–1024
  reactions over time, 1021–1022
Griseofulvin, 635
Group education, 761
Group therapy, 701–716, 735
  applications to specific populations,
      711–714
  benefits, 701–702
  facilitating, 703–709
  format, 709–714
  medically ill, 703
  for psychosocial disturbance, 703
  versus individual treatment, 703
Growth hormone (GH), 413
Guilt, 197, 622, 803–804
Gynecologic cancer, 359–370
  issues affecting all sites, 360–364
  physical changes, 361
  psychosocial aspects of increased risk, 368
  quality of life, 367–368
  sexual function in, 331
  sexual function/dysfunction, 362, 495
  site-specific issues, 365–367
  special populations, 364
  stigma and loneliness, 360
  treatment, 359
  treatment effects, 361
  See also under site-specific cancers

Hallucinatory drugs, 566
Haloperidol, 440, 446, 461, 532, 919, 960
Hamilton Depression Rating Scale (HDRS),
    224, 686
Handbook of Psychooncology, 12
Harlem health connection, 850–851
Head and neck cancer, 68, 314–323
  and alcohol consumption, 45
  communication difficulties, 316
  factors affecting psychosocial adjustment,
      315–319
  health risk behaviors, 320
  medical and psychological staff issues,
      320–321
  physical disfigurement and dysfunction,
      316–318
  promoting psychosocial adjustment,
      319–320
  psychosocial adjustment, 314–315
  rehabilitation, 319–320
  social factors, 319
  surgery, psychosocial issues, 264

tobacco/alcohol use, 318
Health Belief Model (HBM), 162, 168
Health beliefs
  among high-risk populations, 165–167
  among individuals at average risk, 163
  among minority populations, 167–168
  and screening, 162–168
Health care, accessibility, 849
Health care workers, occupational risks for,
    1035–1036
Health maintenance organizations (HMOs),
    166
Health-related behavior, 736
Health-related quality of life (HRQL), 1049
Health status, and socioeconomic status
    (SES), 78, 85
Helplessness, 116–117
Hematologic malignancies
  clinical course, 407–408
  growth and organ failure, 413
  medical concerns, 412
  psychological concerns, 412
    associated with diagnosis and treatment,
        409
Hematopoietic dyscrasias, 406–416
  disease classifications, 407
  See also Leukemia; Lymphomas
Hepatitis B, 1035
Hepatitis C, 279
Hereditary nonpolyposis colon cancer
    (HNPCC), 181–182
Histrionic personality disorder, 625
HIV
  anxiety in, 420
  cognitive disorders in, 420
  dementia in, 420
  depression in, 417–420
  mental disorders in, 422–423
  neurologic complications, 420–422
  occupational risks, 1035
  psychiatric disorders in, 419
  psychological issues related to
      opportunistic cancers in, 423–424
  psychological sequelae, 417–426
HIV-Associated Dementia Complex
    (HIV-ADC), 421–422, 424
HIV cachexia, 472
Hodgkin's disease, 8, 70, 223–232, 283, 407,
    413, 558, 682, 881
  psychological concerns, 414
Hodgkin's lymphoma, 407
Home care, 814–815, 1004
  screening, 658
Homicidal intent, 1020
Hope in terminal illness, 803
Hopelessness, 116–117
Hormonal therapy, 279
  breast cancer, 391
Hormone precursors, 640
Hormone-secreting tumors and anxiety
    disorders, 555
Hospice care in breavement, 1030
Hospice programs, 1004–1005
Hospital Anxiety and Depression Scale
    (HADS), 224, 335, 549, 551, 657, 691,
    692
Human β-choriogonadotropin (β-HCG), 354,
    429
Human Genome Project, 192
Human immunodeficiency virus. *See* HIV
Human leukocyte antigen (HLA), 289

Human stress
  case-control studies, 112–114
  cohort studies, 114
Huntington's disease (HD), 201, 203
  model, 193
Hybrid system, 987
Hydrazine sulfate, 473
Hydrocodeine, 632
Hydromorphone, 458, 632
5-Hydroxytryptamine (5-HT, serotonin), 460,
    473, 477
Hydroxyzine, 440, 956
Hypercalcemia, 642–644
  clinical features, 643
  neoplasms associated with, 643
Hypercortisolism, 639–641
Hyperglycemia, 645
Hypermetabolic state, 468
Hyperprolactinemia, 274
Hyperthyroidism, 642
Hypervigilance, 869
Hypnosis, 963, 973
  in nausea and vomiting, 481
  in pain, 464
Hypocalcemia, 644
Hypochondriasis, 609
Hypocortisolism, 641
Hypoglycemia, 644–645
  neoplasms associated with, 644
Hypomagnesemia, 646
Hyponatremia, 646–647
Hypophosphatemia, 646
Hypothalamic-growth hormone (HGH) axis,
    135
Hypothalamic-pituitary-adrenal (HPA) axis,
    135
  in depression, 136–138
  and immune dysfunction in cancer patients,
    138
  stress-related hyperactivity and tumor
    growth, 138–139
Hypothalamic-pituitary-thyroid (HPT) axis,
    135
Hypothyroidism, 642

Ibuprofen, 635
Ifosfamide, 633
Illicit substances. See Substance abuse
    disorders
Image changing in art therapy, 753–754
Imagery/distraction techniques in pain,
    463–464
Imipenem, 635
Imipramine, 460, 536, 558
Immigration, 861
Immune system
  as defence against cancer, 126–129
  detection of cancer by, 127–128
  and HPA axis, 138
  and infectious disease, 131–132
  and protection against development and/or
    progression of cancer, 128–129
  and psychosocial factors, 129
  responses to cancer, 128
  and stress factors, 129–130
  See also Psychoneuroimmunology
Immunogenicity, 128
Immunotherapy in metastatic disease, 504
Incidence
  in breast cancer, 81–82
  and marital status, 102–103

and social integration, 104
and socioeconomic status (SES), 79–82
and support functions, 105–106
Index of Vulnerability, 677, 682
Infectious disease and immune system,
    131–132
Infertility. See Fertility/infertility effects
Informed consent, 192–193, 1085–1095
Inherited vs. sporadic cancer, 182–183
Insomnia, childhood cancer, 959
Insurance problems, 229
Interferon, 486, 504
Interferon-α (IFN-α), 279, 281, 282, 283
Interleukin-1 (IL-1), 139, 140
Interleukin-2 (IL-2), 279, 282, 486, 504
Interleukin-6 (IL-6), 139, 140
International Classification of Disease-10
    (ICD-10), 511
International Ostomy Association (IOA), 331
International Psycho-Oncology Society
    (IPOS), 11, 1165–1169
International Union Against Cancer, 8
International Working Group on Dying,
    Death and Bereavement, 10
Interpersonal therapy (ITP), 514
Interventions, 168–169
  community-based, 168
  educational, 1127
  ethics, 1127
  hierarchy, 1126
  physician-based, 169
  psychiatric, 1127
  studies, 218
  See also Nursing interventions; Psycho-
    social interventions
Intrathecal methotrexate, 414
Inventory of Current Concerns (ICC), 655,
    677, 682
Iodine intake, 50

Job discrimination, 227–228
Johns Hopkins Psychosocial Screening
    Program, 658–660
Journal of Psychosocial-Oncology, 12, 1165

Kaposi's sarcoma (KS), 423
Karnofsky Performance Status, 234, 683
Karnofsky Rating Scale, 522
Karyotypic studies, 179
Ketoconazole, 635
Know Your Body (KYB) program, 53
Knudsen's hypothesis, 179
Korsakoff's syndrome, 591
Kuhn's Spiritual Inventory, 794

Lactate dehydrogenase (LDH), 354
Language disorders, 832
Legal input, 1127
Leukemia, 8, 224, 406
  approximate annual incidence, 407
  central nervous system (CNS), 409
  chemical courses, 408
  childhood, 942–943
  classification, 407
  medical concerns, 412
  psychological adjustment to disease,
    410–415
  psychological concerns, 414
  relapse and second malignancies, 413
  survivorship, 412
  treatment, 408–409

Levorphanol, 632
Li-Fraumeni cancer family syndrome, 180,
    189, 886
Limited resection and radiation (L-R),
    psychological response, 387
Linkage analysis, 178
Lithium (carbonate), 260, 261, 534, 537, 960
Liver carcinoma and alcohol consumption, 46
Living wills, 1096–1100
LOD score, 178
Longitudinal studies, 236
Long-term sequelae in childhood cancer, 925
Lorazepam, 439, 446, 557, 558, 571, 591, 956
Loss of control, 868, 869
Loss of heterozygosity (LOH), 17, 179–180
Love Canal disaster, 873–874
Lumbar puncture, 965
Lumpectomy and irradiation, 386
Lung cancer, 70, 340–348
  cognitive disorders in, 341–342
  economic consequences, 345–346
  and emotional distress, 341
  family impact, 344
  functional decline, 344
  guilt and tobacco use, 345
  long-term survivors and emotional well-
    being, 345
  overview, 340
  psychosocial distress, 345–346
  quality of life, 344–345
  risk factors, 80–81
  and SES, 79–80
  symptom distress, 342–344
Luteinizing hormone releasing hormone
    (LHRH) analogues, 392
Lymphedema, 832
Lymphokine-activated killer cells, 504
Lymphomas, 407
  chemical courses, 408
  CNS, 424
  HIV-related, 424
  medical concerns, 412
  psychological adjustment to disease,
    410–415
  survivorship, 412
  treatment, 408–409
Lysergic acid diethylamide (LSD), 566

McGill Pain Questionnaire (MPQ), 1154
Magnesium, 646
Maladaptive reaction, 513
Malingering, 612
Mammography, 169
Manipulativeness, 628
Manual lymph drainage (MDL), 832
Maprotiline, 460, 535
Marital status
  and incidence, 102–103
  and mortality, 102
  and recurrence, 103
  and survival, 103
Mastectomy, 385–386, 495
  anxiety states in, 553
  psychological response, 387
  See also Breast surgery
Mechlorethamine, 223
Mediational studies, 130–131
Medical crises, 996–997
Medical decision-making, 200
Medical illnesses, depressive disorders in, 521
Medical Outcomes Study (MOS), 1137

Medical Outcomes Study Short Form Health Survey (MOS SF-36), 657
Medical sequelae in childhood cancer survivors, 925
Medical staff, training, 1074–1082
Meditation, 767–779
  applications in cancer, 771–772
  applications to pain and suffering, 769–770
  breathing, 778–779
  comparison with other interventions, 774
  in coping with cancer, 770–771
  definition, 768
  formal practices, 779
  implications for change in lifestyle and health behaviors, 776
  and insight, 769
  potential adverse effects, 776
  professional instructor qualifications, 773
  teaching approaches, 773–774
MEDLINE, 341
Megace, 392
Megestrol acetate, 392, 472, 489
Melanoma, 58, 59, 61, 62, 63, 182, 183, 279, 377
  diagnosis, 373
  etiology, 373
  incidence, 373
  major risk factors, 61
  mortality, 373
  prevention, 373
  prognosis, 375
  recurrence and survival, 375
  staging, 373, 375
  TNM classification system, 374
  treatment, 373–375
Memorial Delirium Assessment Scale (MDAS), 568–569
Memorial Pain Assessment Card (MPAC), 453, 1154
Memorial Symptom Assessment Scale (MSAS), 1152
Mental Adjustment to Cancer Scale, 691, 692
Mental disorders
  in HIV, 422–423
  in pancreatic cancer, 334–335
Meperidine, 632, 915
6-Mercaptopurine (6MP), 68–69
Metabolic disorders, 639–649
Metabolic state and anxiety disorders, 555
Metastasis, 17–18
Metastatic disease, immunotherapy in, 504
Methotrexate (MTX), 68, 233, 356, 445, 632
Methotrimeprazine, 440, 446, 461, 571, 916, 919, 920
Methylphenidate, 458, 461, 489, 537, 556, 632, 916, 959
Methylprednisolone, 473, 479, 489
Metoclopramide, 469, 479, 556
Metronidazole, 635
MHC class I molecules, 128
Mianserin, 460
Micrococcus luteus, 69
Micronutrient deficiencies, 50
Midazolam, 439, 446, 571, 591, 956
Mindfulness-based stress reduction (MBSR), 772–773
  research, 774–775
  training opportunities, 777
Mini-Mental-Status Exam (MMSE), 568
Minority populations, health beliefs among, 167–168

Mislabeled cases, 1127–1128
Mitomycin, 335
Molecular biology, 16–17
Molindone, 532
Monoamine oxidase inhibitors (MAOIs), 260, 261, 535, 537, 558, 605, 634
Mood disorder
  with depressive features, 531
  and fatigue, 488
MOPP regimen, 223, 231, 409
Morphine, 572, 632
Mortality
  among current and former smokers, 28
  and marital status, 102
  and social integration, 104
  and social support, 119
  and socioeconomic status (SES), 82–85
  and support functions, 105
  in smokers relative to nonsmokers, 28
Mourning, 1017
Multidimensional Fatigue Inventory, 1155
Multiple endocrine neoplasia (MEN) syndromes, 181, 644, 645
Music therapy, 464
Myoclonus, 458

Naltrexone, 593
Narcissistic integrity, 621
Narcissistic personality disorder, 626–627
National Cancer Institute (NCI), 8, 161, 164, 1173, 1174
National Cancer Plan, 10
National Coalition for Cancer Survivors (NCCS), 235
National Comorbidity Survey, 551
National Health Service (NHS), 1119
National Institutes of Health (NIH), 54
Natural killer (NK) cells, 47, 107, 128–130
Nausea and vomiting, 476, 557
  anticipatory, 478
  behavioral management, 480–481
  in chemotherapy, 476–480
  in childhood cancer, 900, 917, 973
  in cognitive distraction (CD), 481
  patient characteristics affecting, 478
  physiology, 477–478
  posttreatment, 478
  in radiotherapy, 272–273
Needle/blood phobia, 559
Nefazodone, 443
Negative psychological consequences, 227
Network-induced distress, 868
Network size and social integration, 104
Neuroendocrine differentiation, 430
Neuroendocrine window strategy, 135
Neurofibromatosis, 181
Neuroleptic drugs, 571
Neuroleptic malignant syndrome (NMS), 309
Neuroleptic medications, 616
Neuroleptics, 309, 439, 440, 447, 461, 532, 591, 617, 959, 960
Neurological diseases, depressive disorders in, 521
Neurological paraneoplastic syndromes, 639
Neuro-oncologic illnesses
  prevalence and presentation, 303–304
  psychopharmacology, 308–310
  psychosocial impact on staff, 311
  treatment approaches, 304
Neuropsychiatric disorders, 639–649

Neuropsychiatric side effects of radiotherapy, 273
Neuropsychological issues, 500–505
Neuropsychological sequelae in childhood cancer survivors, 927
Neuroticism, 214
Nicotine gum, 36
Nicotine nasal spray (NNS), 37–38
Nicotine replacement in general population, 35
Nicotine replacement therapy (NRT), 34–38
Nitrogen mustard, 409
Noncompliance. *See* Compliance with cancer treatment
Non-Hodgkin's lymphoma, 70, 407, 413, 423, 881
  and sun exposure, 62
Nonmelanoma skin cancers, 60, 62, 371, 377
Nonnutrient food components, 50
Nonopioid analgesics, 454–456
Nonsteroidal anti-inflammatory drugs (NSAIDS), 454–456, 912
Nordic Society, 11
Norepinephrine (NE), 135
Norfloxacin, 635
Normeperidine, 458
Nortriptyline, 441, 536
NSAIDS, 454–456, 912
Nurses, training, 1069–1073
Nursing interventions, 811–815
  needs and future directions, 815
  physically oriented, 813–815
  psychosocial, 811–813
Nutritional considerations, 468
Nutritional effects in radiotherapy, 274
Nutritional strategies, 51–53
  See also Diet
Nutritional supplementation in cachexia, 473–474

Obsessive compulsive disorder (OCD), 957
Obsessive-compulsive personality disorder, 624–625
Occupational risks for health care workers, 1035–1036
Office of Alternative Medicines (OAM), 54
Office of Cancer Survivorship, 235
Ofloxacin, 635
Oils in diet, 51
Olanzapine, 572
Older patient. *See* Elderly patients
Olson Circumplex Model, 986
Oncogenes, 17, 179, 184
Oncology, early studies, 9
Opiates, 630, 632
Opioids, 439, 440, 454, 456–458, 572, 586, 912–917
  side effects, 458
Optimism and pessimism, 214
Orderliness, 624–625
Organ transplantation, 1117–1118
Organic brain syndromes, 958
Osteosarcoma, 402
Ototoxicity, 633
Ovarian cancer, 366
  screening, 166
  treatment, 359
Overall survival (OS), 147
Overdemandingness, 623–624
Oxazepam, 439
Oxycodone, 572, 632

*P*53 tumor-suppressor gene, 17, 29
PAH-DNA, 29
Pain, 459–467, 611
  and anxiety disorders, 554
  assessment issues, 452–453
  barriers to treatment, 453–454
  childhood cancer, 909–917, 959
  cognitive-behavioral techniques, 462–463,
    718–721
  cultural factors, 861
  and delirium, 572
  elderly patients, 840–841
  and fatigue, 489
  guidelines for symptom management, 582
  hypnosis in, 464
  imagery/distraction techniques in, 463–464
  inadequate management, 453–454
  inpatient treatment, 584
  management, 454, 1150
  measurement, 1150, 1154
  meditation in, 769–770
  multidimensional concept, 450–451
  non-pharmacologic interventions, 911–912
  pharmacologic treatment, 912
  pharmacotherapies for, 454
  physical modalities used in treatment, 832
  prevalence, 450
  procedure-related pain, 917
  and psychiatric disorders, 451–452, 519
  psychiatric management, 461–464
  psychological factors, 451
  psychological management, 461–464
  and psychotherapy, 461–462
  relaxation techniques, 463
  as risk factor for suicide, 544
  and suicide, 452
Pain syndromes, 450, 611
Palliative care, 437–439
  basic principles, 437
Palliative home care
  family stressors in, 1010–1013
  impact on families, 1004–1015
  option and choices for provision of, 1004
  spiritual dimension in, 1008–1009
Pan African Psycho-Oncology Society, 11
Pancreatectomy, 336
Pancreatic cancer, 333–336
  and alcohol consumption, 46
  diagnosis and management, 335–336
  mental disturbance in, 334–335
  pain and symptoms of depression, 333–334
Pancreatitis, 336
Panic attacks, 558
Para-aminobenzoic acid (PABA), 372
Paraneoplastic neurological syndromes, 641
Paranoid personality disorder, 627–628
Parathyroid hormone-related protein
    (PTHrP), 643
Parents of cancer patients, 984
Parosteal sarcoma, 402
Paroxetine, 443, 460, 535
Passive-aggressive personality disorder,
    625–626
Pathological anxiety, 548–549
Patient care, family involvement, 982
Patient concerns, quality health care delivery,
    286
Patient controlled analgesia (PCA), 457, 843,
    915
Patient Evaluation of Psychosocial
    Intervention, 677

Patient participation, 161–172
Patient–physician relationships, 862
Patient-to-patient relationships, 236
Pearson-Byars Fatigue Feeling Checklist, 486
Pemoline, 461, 537, 556, 632, 916
Penicillin, 70
Pentamidine, 635
Pentobarbital, 920
Pentoxifylline, 473, 489
Perceived barriers, 163
Perceived benefits, 163
Perceived severity, 163
Performance Status Rating (PSR), 1136
Pernoline, 458
Perphenazine, 489
Personality, 94–96
  cancer-prone, 94–95
  and coping responses, 217
  in head and neck cancer, 318
  types, 623–628
Personality differences in adaptation, 214
Personality disorders (PD), 619–629
  diagnostic criteria, 620
  DSM-IV, 620
  prevalence, 620
Pessimism and optimism, 214
Pharmacologic treatment in terminal illness,
    439
Pharmacotherapies for pain, 454
Phencyclidine, 566
Phenelzine, 558
Phenothiazines, 479
Phenotype, 177
Pheochromocytoma, 645
Phosphate, 646
Physical Activity Scale (PAS), 486
Physical sequelae in childhood cancer
    survivors, 925
Physical well-being and coping responses, 217
Physician-assisted suicide (PAS), 1103–1109
Physician-based interventions, 169
Physiological symptoms, screening, 658
Pimozide, 461
Placebo response, 461
Play in childhood cancer, 947–948
Policy issues, 1173–1176
Polycyclic aromatic hydrocarbons (PAHs), 29
Positive psychological consequences, 227
Positive reinforcement, 559
Postoperative delirium, 262
Posttraumatic stress disorder (PTSD), 225,
    511, 595–607, 975
  application to cancer patients, 596–597
  assessment, 603–605
  characteristics, 598
  childhood cancer, 955, 957
  in childhood cancer survivors, 923–929
  diagnosis, 597–598
  etiology, 602–603
  future directions, 605
  mechanisms, 602–603
  prevalence, 598–602
  research studies, 601
  risk factors, 602–603
  stressor in, 596–597
  treatment, 605
Post-Treatment Resource Program (PTRP),
    235
Potential curability, 18
Prebiopsy, 121–122

Prednisone, 68, 69, 70, 223, 409, 414, 473
Premature menopause, 391
Preoperative panic, 261
Procarbazine, 223, 409, 445, 634
Prochlorperazine, 469, 556
Profile of Mood States (POMS), 334, 656,
    677, 679, 682, 683, 686–688, 691, 1136
Progesterone, 489
Progestins, 392
Prognosis
  determination of, 155
  tumor markers in, 150
Programa Latino para Dejar de Fumar, 851
Progressive muscle relaxation training
    (PMRT), 480–481
Prolonged depressive reaction, 511
Promethazine, 956
Prophylactic surgery, 204
Propofol, 446, 571
Prospective studies, coping responses,
    215–217
Prostate cancer, 182, 429
  diagnosis and medical work-up, 350
  epidemiology, 349
  management/treatment, 350–353
  radiotherapy, 274
  screening guidelines, 349–350
Prostate-specific antigen (PSA), 349, 429
Protein precursors, 640
Protriptyline, 441
Proxy decision-making, 1100–1103
Pseudo-ethics consultation, 1128
Pseudo-psychiatry consultation, 1127
Psychiatric diagnosis, 224
Psychiatric disorders, 437–438, 519
  in AIDS, 419
  assessment and treatment, 833–834
  comorbid, 582, 583, 610, 611
    and alcoholism, 588–589
  in HIV, 419
  and pain, 451–452, 519
Psychiatric management of pain, 461–464
Psychiatric symptoms, 438–439
  and disease outcome, 93
Psychiatric syndromes in surgical patients,
    260–262
Psychiatric taxonomic hierarchical spectrum,
    510
Psychiatrists, training, 1055–1060
Psychiatry
  consultation-liaison, 1123–1124
  early studies, 9
  and ethics, 1123–1131
  guidelines for effective use, 1129–1130
  liaison-consultation division, 10
Psychoeducational studies, 676–693
  1978–1980, 677–679
  1981–1985, 679–683
  1986–1990, 683–688
  1991–1994, 688–692
Psychological adaptation. *See* Adaptation
Psychological adjustment to cancer, 4
Psychological distress, 224–225
  cancer-specific, 225
  implications of, 198–200
Psychological issues
  in adaptation, 211–222
  in cancer risk, 196–198
Psychological management of pain, 461–464
Psychologists, training, 1055–1060
Psychology, early studies, 9

Psychoneuroendocrinology, 135–143
Psychoneuroimmunology, 125–134
  conventional view, 125
  perspective on, 132
  See also Immune system
Psycho-oncology
  challenges to, 11
  clinical programs, 11
  current status, 11
*Psycho-Oncology: Journal of the
  Psychological, Social and Behavioral
  Dimensions of Cancer*, 12, 1165
Psycho-oncology unit, 1049–1054
  background for developing, 1049–1050
  steps in developing, 1050–1053
Psychopharmacologic agents, 617
Psychopharmacology
  in bereavement, 1029
  childhood cancer, 954–961
Psychosexual development, 930–931
Psychosexual sequelae in childhood cancer
  survivors, 930–939
Psychosis, 116
  childhood cancer, 958
  in depression, 532
Psychosocial adaptation. *See* Adaptation
Psychosocial adjustment, 223–235
Psychosocial Adjustment to Illness Scale
  (PAIS), 683, 686, 691
Psychosocial Aspects of Oncology, 12
Psychosocial care provider, 1062–1065
Psychosocial Collaborative Oncology Group
  (PSYCOG), 10, 438
Psychosocial distress, 867–868
  screening, 653–661
Psychosocial efforts, 7–8
Psychosocial factors, 110–124
  associated with presence of cancer or its
    prognosis, 111
  and immune system, 129
  and incidence and/or progression of cancer,
    125–126
  variables confounding results, 113
  variety of, 110–111
Psychosocial interventions, 203–204, 218
  clinical implications and recommendations,
    235–236
  life-extending, 730–742
  mediators, 736
  studies, 130
  and survival, 730–742
Psychosocial issues, 161–172
Psychosocial sequelae, 867–877
  in childhood cancer survivors, 926
Psychostimulants, 310, 444, 458, 461, 489,
  534, 537
Psychotherapeutic interventions, 120–121,
  440
Psychotherapy, 676, 694–700
  in anxiety disorders, 559
  applicability, 694
  in bereavement, 1028–1029
  in childhood cancer, 946–953
  definition, goals and methods, 695
  efficacy, 694
  framework, 695–699
  and pain, 461–462
  provision, 695
Psychotropic drugs, 260, 308, 617
Pubertal timing, 931
Puberty, 931

Publications, 12

Quality-adjusted life years (QALYs), 1112
Quality health care delivery, patient concerns,
  286
Quality of life (QOL), 10, 147, 155, 156, 157,
  1112, 1135–1146, 1148, 1149, 1151
  bone marrow transplantation (BMT), 294,
    415
  breast cancer, 395–396
  cancer of unknown primary (CUP),
    431–432
  chemotherapy, 285
  CNS tumors, 312
  colorectal cancer, 333
  definition, 1135–1137
  female first-degree relatives (FDRs), 395
  gynecologic cancer, 367–368
  lung cancer, 344–345
  measurement, 486, 1137–1138
  questionnaire reliability and validity,
    1138–1139
  and rehabilitation, 834
  research issues, 1139–1143
Quality of Life scale, 692
Quasi-prospective studies, 121–122

Radiotherapy, 19–20, 269–276
  acute side effects, 272–273
  adjustment to, 270
  anxiety in, 270, 554
  brain edema in, 273
  breast cancer, 388
  central nervous system, 501–502
  compliance with cancer treatment, 68
  delayed effects, 273–274
  endocrine effects in, 274
  fatigue, 273, 487–488
  nausea in, 272–273
  neuropsychiatric side effects of, 273
  nutritional effects in, 274
  preparation for treatment, 271
  principles, 269–270
  prostate cancer, 274
  psychiatric consultation, 272
  sexual dysfunction in, 274
  smoking cessation, 29–30
  sterility in, 274
  types, 20
Radium, 7
Randomized control trials (RCTs), 514
Rare familial cancers, genes in, 180
Reach-to-Recovery, 8
Rectal cancer. *See* Colorectal cancer
Recurrence
  and marital status, 103
  and social integration, 105
  and support functions, 106
Refractory symptoms in childhood cancer, 920
Regression and medical illness, 622–623
Rehabilitation, 828–836
  following surgery, 265
  head and neck cancer, 319–320
  interface with psycho-oncology, 833–834
  interventions, 830–832
  palliative, 829
  preventive, 829
  and quality of life, 834
  restorative, 829
  staff education, 834
  supportive, 829

Rehabilitation Act of 1973, 228
Relaxation techniques in pain, 463
Relaxation training, 559
Religion, 780–789
  and cancer prevalence, 782–784
  clinical implications, 787
  and coping with cancer, 784–787
  coping with dying and death, 785–786
  defining and measuring, 780
  and family coping, 786
  and general physical health, 781
  interpretive framework or worldview, 785
  interventions in support of intellectual
    aspects of faith, 804–806
  interventions to support emotional aspects
    of faith, 803
  and living with cancer, 786–787
  measuring in research, 798–800
  and mental health, 781–782
  participation in community, 785
  potential mechanisms of effect, 781
  prevalence of religious behaviors, 782
  private practices, 785
  research directions, 787
  self-assessment, 802–803
  See also Spiritual assessment
Religious interventions, 802
Renal carcinoma, 279
  diagnosis and management, 356
  epidemiology, 356
Reproductive counseling, 189–190
Research
  developments, 12–14
  efforts, 12
  ethical issues, 1091
  funding, 12
  informed consent, 1091
  model, 13
  quality of life (QOL), 1139–1143
  regulations governing, 1092–1093
  special dilemmas, 1093
Resource allocation, 1112–1122
  Africa, 1119–1120
  AIDS, 1120
  Australia, 1118–1119
  ethical principles, 1116–1117
  key elements, 1113
  levels of, 1114
  North America, 1118
  UK, 1119
Respiratory depression, 458
Restlessness, 919
Retinoblastoma, 180
Retroperitoneal lymph node dissection
  (RPLND), 232, 354
Risk. *See* Cancer risk
Risperidone, 473, 572
RNA, 16
Rotterdam Symptom Checklist (RSCL), 549,
  691, 1152

St. Christopher's Hospice, 10
Sarcomas, 402–405
  bone, 402–403
  psychological interventions, 404
  soft-tissue, 403–404
Schizoid personality disorder, 627
Schizophrenia, 116, 614–618
  and cancer risk factors, 615
  diagnostic considerations, 615–616
  epidemiology, 614–615

management, 616
psychopharmacology, 616–617
Schizophreniform symptoms, differential diagnosis, 615–616
Schizotypal personality disorder, 627
SCL-90-R, 683, 687
Screening, 161
adherence to, 200
alcoholism, 658
breast cancer, 198
children, 657–658
colorectal cancer, 164
criteria, 161
future directions, 169
genetic, 183
and health beliefs, 162–168
home care needs, 658
noncompliance, 164
ovarian cancer, 166
physiological symptoms, 658
prostate cancer, 349–350
psychosocial distress, 653–661
recommendations for specific cancers, 162
spiritual, 800
See also Tumor markers
Second malignant neoplasms (SMN), 413
Second malignant tumors (SMT), and smoking cessation, 30
Sedation, 489
Seizure disorders, 306–307
Seizures in childhood cancer, 919
Selective serotonin reuptake inhibitors (SSRIs), 140, 442–443
Selenium intake, 50
Self-blame, 869
Self-importance, 626–627
Self-Rating Symptom Scale, 679
Self-report screening measures, 655
Self-sacrifice, 625–626
Sense of vulnerability, 196
Separation anxiety, 621
Sepsis and anxiety disorders, 555
Serotonin. *See* 5-Hydroxytryptamine (5-HT, serotonin)
Serotonin-norephinephrine reuptake inhibitor (SNRI), 443
Serotonin receptor antagonists, 480
Serotonin specific reuptake inhibitors (SSRIs), 260, 261, 310, 460, 534, 535, 956, 957
Sertraline, 443, 535
Sexual function/dysfunction, 231–233, 328, 494–499
bladder cancer, 331, 355
breast cancer, 395–396
breast surgery, 233
colorectal cancer, 331
gynecologic cancer, 331, 362
management across timeline of cancer treatment, 496–498
men after cancer, 495
problems related to cancer, 494–498
radiotherapy, 274
rehabilitation, 495
research needs, 498
stoma surgery, 332
testis cancer, 233
Shame, 803–804
Short tandem repeat (STR) markers, 177
Short tandem repeat (STR) sequences, 182
Siblings of cancer patients, 985

Signal transduction, 16
Single gene traits, 187
Skin cancer, 58–66, 371–379
diagnosis, 376
etiology, 375
nonmelanoma (NMSC), 60, 62, 371, 377
prevention, 63, 375
prognosis, 376–378
psychological factors, 375–378
psychological interventions, 378
self-examination, 63
treatment, 376
warning signs, 374
See also Sun exposure, and specific types
Skin type and sun exposure interaction, 62
See also Sun exposure
Smoking cessation, 27–44
AHCPR guidelines, 32
behavioral interventions, 39
benefits to cancer patients, 29
combined patch and gum use, 37
current treatment recommendations, 32
dose effects and interactions using TN, 36
dose effects of nicotine gum and self-help intervention, 36
intervention format, 33–38
interventions in cancer patients, 39–40
mortality ratios, 28
mortality risk, 28
nicotine nasal spray (NNS), 37–38
nicotine replacement in general population, 35
nicotine replacement therapy (NRT), 34–35
nicotine replacement update, 35
patient-provider interaction intensity, duration and frequency, 33–34
in radiotherapy, 29–30
scope of the problem, 27
screening advice and providers, 32
and second malignant tumors (SMT), 30
self-help, 38–39
self-help, individual and group interventions, 33
self-quitting in the general population, 30–31
self-selection of NRT, 38
in surgical recovery, 29
transdermal nicotine (TN), 34–35
treatment content, 34
and treatment efficacy, 30–31
treatment interventions and components, 33
treatment recycling and long-term use of NRT, 36–37
Smoking quit programs, 851
Social activities and relationships with friends, 229, 230–231
Social environment, 99–109
and cancer, 99
limitations and future directions of research, 107–108
relation to cancer incidence and mortality among healthy persons, 100
relation to survival and recurrence among people with prior diagnosis of cancer, 101
review of the literature, 100–106
Social factors in adaptation, 211–222
Social Family Well-Being (SWB) scale, 1136

Social functioning, relationships with spouse, family, friends, and social activities, 229–231
Social integration
and incidence, 104
and mortality, 104
and network size, 104
and recurrence, 105
and survival, 104
Social Network Index (SNI), 102, 105
Social networks, 99
Social support
in adaptation, 213–214
interventions, 102
and mortality, 119
Social workers, training, 1061–1068
Societal views of cancer, 1
Socioeconomic conditions, 167
Socioeconomic status (SES), 78–90, 163, 167, 848
and cancer, 78–85
and health status, 78, 85
and incidence patterns, 79–82
methodologic issues, 85–86
and mortality patterns, 82–85
as risk factor, 84
Socioracial status, 848
Soft-tissue sarcomas, 403–404
Solitary site of disease, CUP, 429
Somatic cell genetics, 178–180
Somatization, 608
Somatization disorder, undifferentiated, 609–610
Somatoform disorders, 608–612
Spiritual assessment, 790–808
background issues, 790
early models, 791–792
future directions, 801–802
guidelines for evaluating models, 797–798
selected models, 792–798
7 × 7 model, 793–797
Spiritual beliefs, 780–789
Spiritual dimension in palliative home care, 1008–1009
Spiritual interventions, 802
Spiritual screening, 800
future directions, 801–802
Spiritual Well-Being Scale (SWBS), 799–800
Spirituality, defining and measuring, 780
Sporadic cancer, 183
Spouse of cancer patient, 984
Squamous cell carcinoma, 60–61
diagnosis, 372
etiology, 371–372
incidence, 371
mortality, 371
prevention, 372
prognosis, 373
treatment, 372
Staff stress, 1035–1048
current research, 1036
interventions, 1041–1044
Staff support groups, 1044–1046
Starvation, 468
State-Trait Anxiety Inventory, 551
State-Trait Anxiety scale, 683
Sterility in radiotherapy, 274
Steroid-induced anxiety, 556
Steroids, psychiatric side effects, 270
Stigmatization, 868
Stimulants, 958

Stomach cancer, 325
    initial symptoms, diagnosis and surgery, 325
    recovery after surgery and rehabilitation, 325
Stress, 111–114, 512–513
    anatomy, 1036–1041
    animal stress, 111–112
    chronic stress, 867–868
    human stress, 112–114
    and immune system, 129–130
    management, 735–736
    responses, 518
Stress-related HPA axis, hyperactivity and tumor growth, 138–139
Stressors, 513
    decisional, 1124–1125
    environmental, 1125–1126
    major categories, 1124
    in PTSD, 596–597
Substance abuse disorders, 576–586
    addiction, 579–580
    clinical management, 581–586
    conceptual problems, 578–579
    definition, 577
    drug-free recovery, 585
    history-taking, 583
    inpatient management, 584–585
    outpatient management, 585
    prevalence, 577
    spectrum of attitudes and behaviors, 581–582
Suicide, 533, 541–547
    aftermath, 545
    delirium in, 543
    demographics, 541–542
    depression in, 543
    fatigue in, 543
    ideation, 544–545
    impact on family and health care providers, 545
    incidence, 541
    intent, 1020
    loss of control and helplessness in, 543
    management principles, 546
    and pain, 452
    pain as risk factor for, 544
    patient evaluation, 546
    and preexisting psychopathology, 544
    prior history and family history, 544
    risk following surgery, 262
    risk management, 546
    and site of cancer, 542
    vulnerability variables, 542, 546
    See also Physician-assisted suicide
Sulpiride, 572
Sun exposure, 58–66
    beneficial effect, 62
    cancer risk related to, 60
    current research, 59–62
    and cutaneous melanoma, 61
    human behavior, 59–60
    and non-Hodgkin's lymphoma, 62
    psychological research, 63
    reaction and overreaction, 62–63
    and risk of nonmelanoma skin cancer, 60
    role in cancer etiology, 63–64
    and skin type interaction, 62
Sun protection factor number (SPF), 372
Sunscreen, 372

Support functions
    groups, 761–763
    and incidence, 105–106
    interventions, 106
    and mortality, 105
    and recurrence, 106
    and survival, 106
Supportive environment, 734
Supportive psychotherapy, 440, 445
Suppressors of emotion, 117–118
Surgery, 18–19, 257–268
    consent issues, 261
    early efforts, 6, 7
    and fatigue, 488
    historical milestones, 258
    postoperative delirium, 262
    preoperative panic, 261
    preventive, 258
    prophylactic, 258
    psychiatric syndromes in, 260–262
    psychological management, 259
    psychological preparation, 259–260
    psychological responses to impending, 257–259
    psychosocial issues related to site of, 262–265
    refusal, 261
    rehabilitation following, 265
    smoking cessation, 29
    types, 19
Survival
    adaptation, 223–254
    childhood cancer, 960
        cognitive sequelae, 927, 940–945
        coping style, 926
        family adaptation to, 924–925
        family environment, 926
        medical sequelae in, 925
        neuropsychological sequelae, 927
        physical sequelae in, 925
        post-traumatic symptoms, 925
        psychiatric sequelae, 924
        psychological sequelae, 924
        psychosexual sequelae, 930–939
        psychosocial sequelae, 923–924, 926
        PTSD, 923–929
    and marital status, 103
    and psychosocial interventions, 730–742
    and social integration, 104
    and support functions, 106
    survivor perspectives, 981
    underserved patients, 853–854
Susceptibility genes, 201
Suspiciousness, 627–628
Swallowing disorders, 832
Symbolic belief systems, 869
Symptomatology, 18
Symptom assessment and measurement
    clinical applications, 1149–1151
    instrumentation, 1151–1157
    principles, 1147–1149
    research applications, 1151
    in special populations, 1157–1158
Syndrome of inappropriate antidiuretic hormone (SIADH), 640, 646–647
Systematic desensitization (SD), 481, 559

Tamoxifen, 335, 391, 392
Tardive dyskinesia (TD), 309
Teleconferences, 761
Telephone bulletin board helplines, 763–764

Telephone counseling, 758–766
Telephone groups, 762–763
Temazepam, 439
Tennessee Self-Concept Scale, 679
Terminal care, 437–439
    childhood cancer, 960
    family issues, 447
    hope in, 803
    See also Death and dying
Testicular cancer
    diagnosis and medical work-up, 353–354
    epidemiology, 353
    management of psychosocial issues, 354–355
    medical management/treatment, 354
    and sexual dysfunction, 233
Theory of Reasoned Action (TRA), 168
Therapist Rating Form, 677
Thioridazine, 440, 532
Three Mile Island (TMI), 870–871
Thyroid carcinomas, 429
Thyroid hormone (thyroxine), 642
Thyroid-stimulating hormone (TSH), 642
Thyrotoxicosis, 642
Thyrotropin (TSH), 136, 137
Thyrotropin-releasing hormone (TRH), 136
Thyroxin-releasing hormone (TRH), 335
Ticarcillin, 634
TNM system, 18
Tobacco use
    and colorectal adenomas and carcinomas, 326
    and head and neck cancer, 318
    and lung cancer, 345
    See also Smoking cessation
Tobramycin, 635
Topical agents, 917
Total body irradiation (TBI), 232
Total Mood Disturbance score (TMD), 683
Total parenteral nutrition (TPN), 410
Training
    medical staff, 1074–1082
    nurses, 1069–1073
    psychiatrists, 1055–1060
    psychologists, 1055–1060
    social workers, 1061–1068
Tranquilizers, 260, 261
Transcutaneous electrical nerve stimulation (TENS), 832, 912
Transdermal fentanyl patch system, 457
Transdermal nicotine (TN), 34–35
Transitional cell carcinomas (TCC), 355
Trazodone, 444, 460, 535
Treatment advances, 7–8
Trial Outcome Index (TOI), 1137
Tricyclic antidepressants (TCAs), 260, 261, 310, 441, 442, 534, 536, 558, 605, 617, 916, 956, 957
Trifluoperazine, 532
Truth telling, 1085–1095
Tumor markers, 147–160
    cancer of unknown primary (CUP), 428
    defined, 147
    in determination of prognosis, 150, 155
    false negatives, 153
    false positives, 154
    monitoring for relapse and evaluation during course of metastatic disease, 155–157
    monitoring for relapse and evaluation of course of metastatic disease, 150–151

performance characteristics, 148
psychological consequences, 151–157
risk assessment, 151
screening of healthy individuals, 152–155
statistical biases, 148
true negatives, 153
true positives, 154
use in clinical practice, 149–151
utilities, 147
Tumor necrosis factor (TNF), 139, 140, 489
Tumor suppressor genes, 183, 184
Tumor suppressor proteins, 17
Type A behavior pattern, 96
Type C behavior pattern, 96

Ultraviolet radiation (UVR), 58–59, 62, 372
Underserved patients, 845–856
    barriers to adequate cancer detection,
        848–850
    definition, 845–846
    early identification, 853
    entry into treatment, 853
    health promotion in, 852
    historical perspective, 846–848

interventions targeting, 850
    palliative care, 854
    role of psycho-oncologist in, 852–854
    survivors, 853–854
    treatment adherence, 853
Uterine cancer, 366
    tamoxifen-related, 391
UVA radiation, 58, 59, 372
UVB radiation, 58–59, 62, 372
UVC radiation, 58

Vaginal cancer, 367
Venipuncture, 973
Venlafaxine, 443
Verbal rating scale (VRS), 1154
Vinblastine, 232, 356, 409, 445, 633
Vinca alkaloids, 633
Vincristine, 223, 304, 409, 414, 445, 633
Vindesine, 633
Vinorelbine, 633
Violence, 959–960
Visual analogue scale (VAS), 1154, 1155
Visual analogue scale-fatigue (VAS-F), 1155
Vitamin D, 58, 372

Vitamin D_3, 60, 62
Vocational functioning, 227–229
Voicemail bulletin board, 763–764
Vomiting. *See* Nausea and vomiting
Von Hippel-Lindau's disease, 181
Vulnerability model, 237
Vulvar cancer, 367

Wernicke-Korsakoff's syndrome, 590
Wilms' tumor, 181, 183, 881
Women's Intervention Nutrition Study
    (WINS), 54
World Health Organization Collaborating
    Center in Quality of Life
    Measurement, 10
World Health Organization (WHO), 1112
    Analgesic Ladder, 454

X chromosome, 177
X-rays, 19

Zidovudine (AZT), 422, 635